ROSSI'S PRINCIPLES OF TRANSFUSION MEDICINE

THIRD EDITION

Editors

TOBY L. SIMON, MD

Chief Medical Officer
Chief Operating Officer
TriCore Reference Laboratories
Clinical Professor of Pathology
University of New Mexico School of Medicine
Albuquerque, New Mexico

WALTER H. DZIK, MD

Associate Professor of Pathology
Harvard Medical School
Co-Director
Blood Transfusion Service
Massachusetts General Hospital
Boston, Massachusetts

EDWARD L. SNYDER, MD

Professor
Department of Laboratory Medicine
Yale University School of Medicine
Director, Blood Bank/Apheresis Unit
Yale–New Haven Hospital
New Haven, Connecticut

CHRISTOPHER P. STOWELL, MD, PHD

Assistant Professor of Pathology
Harvard Medical School
Co-Director
Blood Transfusion Service
Massachusetts General Hospital
Boston, Massachusetts

RONALD G. STRAUSS, MD

Professor, Pathology and Pediatrics
Departments of Pathology and Pediatrics
University of Iowa College of Medicine
Medical Director
DeGowin Blood Center
University of Iowa Hospitals and Clinics
Iowa City, Iowa

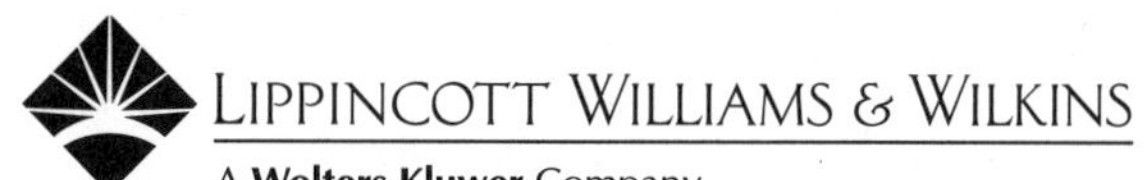

LIPPINCOTT WILLIAMS & WILKINS
A **Wolters Kluwer** Company
Philadelphia • Baltimore • New York • London
Buenos Aires • Hong Kong • Sydney • Tokyo

Acquisitions Editor: Ruth W. Weinberg
Developmental Editors: Tanya Lazar and Nicole Wagner
Production Manager: Toni Ann Scaramuzzo
Production Editor: Michael Mallard
Manufacturing Manager: Benjamin Rivera
Cover Designer: Christine Jenny
Compositor: Maryland Composition
Printer: Maple Press

530 Walnut Street
Philadelphia, PA 19106 USA
LWW.com

Printed in the USA

Library of Congress Cataloging-in-Publication Data

Rossi's principles of transfusion medicine / editors, Toby L. Simon . . . [et al.].—3rd ed.
p. ; cm.
Rev. ed. of: Principles of transfusion medicine / editors, Ennio C. Rossi . . . [et al.]. 2nd ed. c1996.
Includes bibliographical references and index.
ISBN 0-7817-3024-4
1. Blood—Transfusion. I. Title: Principles of transfusion medicine. II. Rossi, Ennio Claudio, 1931-III. Simon, Toby L.
[DNLM: 1. Blood Transfusion. 2. Blood Banks—organization & administration. 3. Blood Grouping and Crossmatching. WB 356 R835 2002]
RM171 .P75 2002
615′0.39—dc21

2001050582

10 9 8 7 6 5 4 3 2

CONTENTS

SECTION V: Special Topics

SECTION VI: Delivery of Blood Services

CONTRIBUTORS

Harvey J. Alter, MD Chief, Infectious Diseases Section, Associate Director for Research, Department of Transfusion Medicine, National Institutes of Health, Bethesda, Maryland; Clinical Professor, Department of Medicine, Georgetown University Medical School, Washington, D.C.

Ernest Beutler, MD Professor and Chairman, Department of Molecular and Experimental Medicine, The Scripps Research Institute, La Jolla, California

Celso Bianco, MD Executive Vice President, America's Blood Centers, Washington, D.C.

Morris A. Blajchman, MD, FRCP(C) Professor, Departments of Pathology and Medicine, McMaster University; Medical Director, Canadian Blood Services, Hamilton Centre, Hamilton, Ontario, Canada

José Orlando Bordin, MD, PhD Associate Professor, Department of Hematology and Transfusion Medicine, Escola Paulista de Medicina; Chief, Department of Hematology and Transfusion Medicine, Hospital São Paulo, São Paulo, Brazil

Arthur W. Bracey, MD Clinical Associate Professor of Pathology, Department of Pathology and Laboratory Medicine, University of Texas Medical School, Houston; Medical Director, Transfusion Service, St. Luke's Episcopal Hospital, Houston, Texas

Mark E. Brecher, MD Professor, Department of Pathology and Laboratory Medicine, University of North Carolina; Director, Transplantation and Transfusion Services, McLendon Clinical Laboratories, University of North Carolina Hospitals, Chapel Hill, North Carolina

Paul Brown, MD Senior Investigator, National Institutes of Health, Bethesda, Maryland

Silvana Z. Bucur, MD Assistant Professor, Winship Cancer Institute, Emory University, Atlanta, Georgia

Michael P. Busch, MD, PhD Professor, Department of Laboratory Medicine, University of California, San Francisco; Vice President, Department of Research and Scientific Affairs, Blood Centers of the Pacific and Blood Systems, Inc., San Francisco, California and Scotsdale, Arizona

Patricia M. Carey, MD Assistant Professor, Clinical Transfusion Medicine, University of Cincinnati Medical Center; Medical Director, Hoxworth Blood Center, Cincinnati, Ohio

Jeffrey L. Carson, MD Richard C. Reynolds Professor and Chief, Department of Medicine - General Internal Medicine, Robert Wood Johnson Medical School; Chief, Division of General Internal Medicine, Department of Medicine, Robert Wood Johnson University Hospital, New Brunswick, New Jersey

Li Chai, MD Blood Bank Fellow, Department of Laboratory Medicine, Yale University School of Medicine; Yale-New Haven Hospital, New Haven, Connecticut

Richard E. Champlin, MD Professor of Medicine and Chair, Blood and Marrow Transplantation, University of Texas MD Anderson Cancer Center, Houston, Texas

Robert D. Christensen, MD Professor and Chairman, Department of Pediatrics, University of South Florida College of Medicine; Physician-in-Chief, Department of Pediatrics, All Children's Hospital, St. Petersburg, Florida

Kendall P. Crookston, MD, PhD Assistant Professor of Medicine, Director, Transfusion Medicine and Coagulation, Department of Pathology, University of New Mexico School of Medicine and Tricore Reference Laboratories; Medical Director, United Blood Services of New Mexico, Albuquerque, New Mexico

Brian R. Curtis, MS, MT(ASCP)SBB Technical Director, Platelet and Neutrophil Immunology Lab, The Blood Center of Southeastern Wisconsin, Milwaukee, Wisconsin

David C. Dale, MD Professor, Department of Medicine, University of Washington, Seattle, Washington

Robertson D. Davenport, MD Associate Professor, Department of Pathology, University of Michigan; Medical Director, Blood Bank and Transfusion Service, University of Michigan Health Center, Ann Arbor, Michigan

Richard J. Davey, MD, FACS Chief Medical Officer, New York Blood Center, New York, New York

Kimberly A. Davis, MD Assistant Professor, Department of Surgery, Loyola University Stritch School of Medicine, Maywood, Illinois

Jules L. Dienstag, MD Associate Professor of Medicine, Harvard Medical School; Physician, Medical Services (Gastrointestinal Unit), Massachusetts General Hospital, Boston, Massachusetts

Thomas P. Duffy, MD Professor of Medicine, Department of Internal Medicine and Hematology, Yale University School of Medicine; Attending Physician, Department of Internal Medicine, Yale New Haven Hospital, New Haven, Connecticut

Walter H. Dzik, MD Associate Professor of Pathology, Harvard Medical School; Co-Director, Blood Transfusion Service, Massachusetts General Hospital, Boston, Massachusetts

Richard S. Eisenstaedt, MD Professor and Acting Chair, Department of Medicine, Temple University School of Medicine, Temple University Hospital, Philadelphia, Pennsylvania

Eberhard Fiebig, MD Assistant Professor, Department of Laboratory Medicine, University of California, San Francisco; Chief, Transfusion Service and Hematology Divisions, Clinical Laboratories, San Francisco General Hospital, San Francisco, California

James L. Gajewski, MD Associate Professor of Medicine, Blood and Marrow Transplantation; Medical Director, Managed Care and Strategic Planning, University of Texas MD Anderson Cancer Center, Bellaire, Texas

Richard L. Gamelli, MD, FACS The Robert J. Freeark Professor and Chair, Department of Surgery, Director, Burn and Shock Trauma Institute, Chief, Burn Center, Loyola University Medical Center, Maywood, Illinois

Ronald O. Gilcher, MD President/CEO and Medical Director, Oklahoma Blood Institute; Adjunct Professor of Pathology and Clinical Associate Professor of Medicine, Departments of Pathology and Medicine, The University of Oklahoma College of Medicine; Oklahoma City, Oklahoma

David W. Gjertson, PhD Associate Professor, Department of Biostatistics and Pathology, University of California Los Angeles, Los Angeles, California

Stuart L. Goldberg, MD Assistant Clinical Professor, Department of Medicine, University of Medicine and Dentistry of New Jersey, Newark, New Jersey; Section Head, Leukemia Service, Cancer Center, Blood and Marrow Transplant Program, Hackensack University Medical Center, Department of Hematology and Oncology, Hackensack, NJ

Lawrence T. Goodnough, MD Professor of Medicine, Pathology and Immunology, Department of Pathology, Washington University School of Medicine; Director, Transfusion Services, Donor/Apheresis Unit and Cryopreservation Laboratory, Barnes-Jewish Hospital, St. Louis, Missouri

Jerome L. Gottschall, MD Professor, Pathology Department, Medical College of Wisconsin; Vice President, Medical Services, The Blood Center of Southeastern Wisconsin, Inc., Milwaukee, Wisconsin

Marcia D. Haimowitz, MD Clinical Assistant Professor, Department of Pathology, University of Southern California Keck School of Medicine; Assistant Medical Director, American Red Cross Blood Services, Southern California Region, Los Angeles, California

Paul Clarence Hebert, MD, FRCPC, MHSC(EPID) Associate Professor, Medicine and Epidemiology, University of Ottawa; Director, Clinical Epidemiology Program, Ottawa Hospital Research Institute, Ottawa, Ontario

George R. Honig, MD, PhD Professor and Head, Department of Pediatrics, University of Illinois College of Medicine, Chicago, Illinois

P. Ann Hoppe, BA, MT (ASCP)SBB Hoppe Regulatory Consultants, Decatur, Georgia

Kai Hübel, MD Visiting Research Fellow, Department of Medicine, University of Washington, Seattle, Washington; Clinical Fellow, Department of Internal Medicine, University of Cologne, Cologne, Germany

Cindy Ippoliti, PharmD Clinical Hematology Coordinator, Department of Pharmacy/BMT, MD Anderson Cancer Center, Houston, Texas

Petr Jarolim, MD, PhD Assistant Professor, Department of Pathology, Harvard Medical School; Associate Pathologist, Department of Pathology, Brigham and Women's Hospital, Boston, Massachusetts

W. John Judd, FIBMS, MIBiol Professor of Immunohematology, Department of Pathology, University of Michigan, Ann Arbor, Michigan

Steven Kleinman, MD Clinical Professor, Department of Pathology, University of British Columbia, Vancouver, British Columbia Canada

Mark J. Koury, MD Professor of Medicine, Department of Medicine, Vanderbilt University; Staff Physician, Medical Service, VA Medical Center, Nashville, Tennessee

Diane S. Krause, MD, PhD Associate Professor, Laboratory Medicine, Yale University School of Medicine; Associate Director, Department of Transfusion Medicine, Yale-New Haven Hospital, New Haven, Connecticut

Margot S. Kruskall, MD Associate Professor of Pathology and Medicine, Harvard Medical School; Director, Division of Laboratory and Transfusion Medicine, Beth Israel Deaconess Medical Center, Boston, Massachusetts

Steven R. Lentz, MD, PhD Associate Professor, Department of Internal Medicine, The University of Iowa, Iowa City, Iowa

W. Conrad Liles, MD, PhD Associate Professor, Department of Medicine, University of Washington, Seattle, Washington

Jeanne V. Linden, MD, MPH Director, Blood and Tissue Resources, New York State Department of Health; Adjunct Associate Professor, Biomedical Sciences, School of Public Health, New York State Department of Health and State University of New York; Clinical Associate Professor, Pathology and Laboratory Medicine, Albany Medical College, Albany, New York

Naomi L.C. Luban, MD Professor, Department of Pediatrics and Pathology, Vice Chairman for Academic Affairs, The George Washington University School of Medicine; Chairman, Laboratory Medicine and Pathology; Director, Transfusion Medicine/Donor Center, Children's National Medical Center, Washington, D.C.

Jeanne M. Lusher, MD Distinguished Professor of Pediatrics, Marion I. Barnhart Hemostasis Research Professor, Wayne State University School of Medicine; Director, Hemostasis-Thrombosis Program; Co-Director, Division of Hematology-Oncology, Children's Hospital Michigan, Detroit, Michigan

Yan Ma, MBS, BS University of Texas, MD Anderson Cancer Center, Houston, Texas

James L. MacPherson, MS, MPh CEO, America's Blood Centers, Washington, D.C.

Edward M. Mansfield, JD Attorney, Belin, Lamson, McCormick, Zumbach and Flynn, Des Moines, Iowa

Janice McFarland, MD Consultant to Laboratories, Platelet and Neutrophil Immunology, The Blood Center of Southeastern Wisconsin, Inc., Milwaukee, Wisconsin

Bruce C. McLeod, MD Professor, Department of Medicine and Pathology, Rush Medical College; Director, Blood Center, Rush-Presbyterian-St. Luke's Medical Center, Chicago, Illinois

Jay E. Menitove, MD Executive Director and Medical Director, Community Blood Center of Greater Kansas City; Clinical Professor of Medicine, University of Missouri, Kansas City, Missouri; Kansas University School of Medicine, Kansas City, Kansas

Paul Mintz, MD Associate Chair and Professor of Pathology, Professor of Internal Medicine; Director, Clinical Laboratories and Blood Bank, University of Virginia Health System, Charlottesville, Virginia

Paul J. Mohacsi, MD, FESC Head, Heart Failure and Cardiac Transplantation, Department of Cardiology, Swiss Cardiovascular Center, University Hospital, Bern, Switzerland

Kenneth J. Moise, MD Upjohn Distinguished Professor of Obstetrics and Gynecology, Department of Obstetrics and Gynecology, University of North Carolina at Chapel Hill, Chapel Hill, North Carolina; Director, Division of Maternal-Fetal Medicine, University of North Carolina Hospitals, Chapel Hill, North Carolina

Scott Murphy, MD Chief Medical Officer, American Red Cross Blood Services-Penn Jersey Region; Adjunct Professor of Medicine, University of Pennsylvania, Philadelphia, Pennsylvania

Urs E. Nydegger, MD Titular Professor, Department of Surgery, University of Bern; Head, Research and Development, Clinica Cardiovascular Surgery, University Hospital, Bern, Switzerland

Alvaro A. Pineda, MD Professor, Department of Laboratory Medicine, Mayo Medical School; Consultant, Department of Laboratory Medicine and Pathology, Mayo Clinic, Rochester, Minnesota

Gregory J. Pomper, MD Assistant Professor, Laboratory Medicine, Yale University School of Medicine; Assistant Director, Transfusion Service, Laboratory Medicine, Yale-New Haven Hospital, New Haven, Connecticut

Thomas H. Price, MD Professor of Medicine, Department of Medicine, University of Washington; Medical Director, Puget Sound Blood Center, Seattle, Washington

Thomas J. Raife, MD Associate Medical Director, The Blood Center of Southeastern Wisconsin, Inc., Milwaukee, Wisconsin

Glenn Ramsey, MD Associate Professor, Department of Pathology, Northwestern University Medical School; Medical Director, Blood Bank, Northwestern Memorial Hospital, Chicago, Illinois

Henry M. Rinder, MD Associate Professor, Laboratory Medicine, Yale University School of Medicine; Director, Coagulation Laboratory, Laboratory Medicine, Yale-New Haven Hospital, New Haven, Connecticut

Stephan B. Rosenfeld, MD Fellow Associate, Department of Internal Medicine, The University of Iowa, Iowa City, Iowa

Ennio C. Rossi, MD Professor Emeritus, Department of Medicine, Northwestern University School of Medicine, Chicago, Illinois

Scott D. Rowley, MD, FACP Chief, Adult Allogenic Stem Cell Transplant Program, Department of Medicine, Hackensack University Medical Center, Hackensack, New Jersey

Ronald A. Sacher, MD, FRCPC Professor and Director, Hoxworth Blood Center, University of Cincinnati Medical Center, Cincinnati, Ohio

Bruce I. Sharon, MD Associate Professor of Clinical Pediatrics, Department of Pediatrics, University of Illinois College of Medicine; Attending Physician, Department of Pediatrics, University of Illinois Hospital, Chicago, Illinois

Ira A. Shulman, MD Professor and Vice Chair, Department of Pathology, and Director of Transfusion Medicine, Keck School of Medicine, University of Southern California; Associate Director of Laboratories, Department of Pathology, LAC/USC Medical Center, Los Angeles, California

Don L. Siegel, PhD, MD Associate Professor, Department of Pathology and Laboratory Medicine, University of Pennsylvania Medical Center; Director, Blood Bank Transfusion Medicine Section, Department of Pathology and Laboratory Medicine, University of Pennsylvania Medical Center, Philadelphia, Pennsylvania

Toby L. Simon, MD Chief Medical Officer and Chief Operating Officer, TriCore Reference Laboratories; Clinical Professor of Pathology, University of New Mexico, Albuquerque, New Mexico

Kenneth J. Smith, MD Professor of Medicine, Winship Cancer Institute, Emory University, Director, Hematology/Oncology, Emory University Hospital, Atlanta, Georgia

Edward L. Snyder, MD Professor, Department of Laboratory Medicine, Blood Bank, Yale University School of Medicine; Director, Blood Bank/Aphresis Unit, Yale-New Haven Hospital, New Haven, Connecticut

Martha C. Sola, MD Assistant Professor, Department of Pediatrics, University of Florida; Attending Neonatologist, Department of Pediatrics, Shands Children's Hospital, Gainesville, Florida

Susan M. Sorensen, MD Assistant Clinical Professor, Internal Medicine, Wright State University; Staff Physician, Internal Medicine, VA Medical Center, Dayton, Ohio

Bruce D. Spiess, MD Professor and Vice Chair, Department of Anesthesiology, Virginia Commonwealth University; Director, VCURES Shock Center; Director, Cardiothoracic Anesthesia, Medical College of Virginia, Richmond, Virginia

Patrice F. Spitalnik, MD Assistant Professor, Department of Pathology and Laboratory Medicine, University of Rochester Medical Center, Rochester, New York

Steven L. Spitalnik, MD Professor and Chair, Pathology and Laboratory Medicine, University of Rochester Medical Center, Rochester, New York

Gary Stack, MD, PhD Assistant Professor, Department of Laboratory Medicine, Yale University School of Medicine; Chief, Pathology and Laboratory Medicine Service, VA Connecticut Healthcare System, New Haven, Connecticut

Christopher P. Stowell, MD, PhD Assistant Professor, Department of Pathology, Harvard Medical School; Co-Director, Blood Transfusion Service, Massachusetts General Hospital, Boston, Massachusetts

Ronald G. Strauss, MD Professor, Pathology and Pediatrics, Departments of Pathology and Pediatrics, University of Iowa College of Medicine; Medical Director, DeGowin Blood Center, University of Iowa Hospitals and Clinics, Iowa City, Iowa

Aaron Tomer, MD Associate Professor of Medicine, Faculty of Health Sciences, Ben Gurion University of Negev; Director, Blood Bank and Transfusion Medicine, Soroka University Medical Center, Beer-Sheva, Israel

Pearl Toy, MD Professor, Department of Laboratory Medicine; Chief, Blood Bank, University of California San Francisco, San Francisco, California

C. Robert Valeri, MD Director, Naval Blood Research Laboratory, Boston University School of Medicine, Boston, Massachusetts

Eleftherios C. Vamvakas, MD, PhD Associate Professor, Department of Pathology, New York University; Director, Blood Bank and Transfusion Service, New York University Medical Center, New York, New York

Willem G. van Aken, MD, PhD Consultant and former Director, Products and Medical Affairs, Sanguin Blood Supply Foundation, Amsterdam, The Netherlands

Stephen J. Wagner Senior Scientist, Product Development Department, American Red Cross Holland Laboratory for the Biomedical Sciences, Rockville, Maryland

Theodore E. Warkentin, MD, FRCP(C), FACP Associate Professor, Department of Pathology and Molecular Medicine, McMaster University; Associate Head, Transfusion, Hamilton Regional Laboratory Medicine Program, Hamilton General Hospital, Hamilton Health Sciences, Hamilton, Ontario, Canada

Iain J. Webb, MD Millennium Pharmaceuticals, Cambridge, Massachusetts

Connie M. Westhoff, SBB, PhD Research Associate, Department of Pathology and Laboratory Medicine, University of Pennsylvania, Philadelphia, Pennsylvania

Thomas M. Williams, MD Associate Professor, Department of Pathology, University of New Mexico; Director, Department of Genetics and Cytometry, TriCore Reference Laboratories, Albuquerque, New Mexico

Edward C. C. Wong, MD Assistant Professor, Departments of Pediatrics and Pathology, The George Washington University School of Medicine; Director, Hematology/Associate Director, Transfusion Medicine, Department of Laboratory Medicine, Children's National Medical Center, Washington, D.C.

Robert D. Woodson, MD Professor, Department of Medicine, University of Wisconsin-Madison; Attending Physician, Department of Medicine, University of Wisconsin Hospitals and Clinics, Madison, Wisconsin

Thomas F. Zuck, MD, LLB Professor, Hoxworth Blood Center, University of Cincinnati Medical Center, Cincinnati, Ohio

PREFACE

Transfusion medicine as a multidisciplinary clinical specialty emerging from classic blood banking continues the dynamic and increasingly complex evolution that was noted in the first edition of Rossi's Principles of Transfusion Medicine. The goal of the first edition was to enhance the reader's understanding of this newly defined specialty through an approach aligned with other medical specialties, while preparing the newcomer and the experienced individual alike for the changes to come as transfusion medicine expanded as a discipline. This blending of transfusion sciences with clinical concerns continued in the second edition, which also added chapters reflecting the transition of blood services into a highly-regulated manufacturing environment based on a pharmaceutical model.

We believe the format of the first two editions has served our readers well, and we present this third edition based on the same organizational principles. In this new edition, we have addressed areas where the book could be further improved to meet the needs of a diverse group of professionals. We have slightly altered the format by dividing the material into six major sections: blood components and derivatives, clinical practice, apheresis, adverse sequelae, special topics, and delivery of blood services. Within these sections are sub-sections that are organized around the biology and clinical use of various blood components (red blood cells, platelets, white cells, and plasma); the transfusion needs of specific patient groups (medical, pediatric, obstetric, oncologic and surgical); and disease transmission and transfusion reactions. At the same time, we have made the clinical approach section more comprehensive and strengthened the more traditional blood banking material on red cell antigens and antibodies with new chapters. In recognition of the most recent changes in the evolution of the field, we have added new chapters in specialized therapeutic hemapheresis procedures, an overview of risk of transfusion-transmitted disease, prion transmission, and pathogen reduction. This creates a comprehensive resource for transfusion medicine and transfusion science while leaving the primarily technical material to other books.

To further improve the accessibility of information in the text and to help the reader find related material of interest more easily, we have consolidated chapters from the previous edition, enhanced the use of tables and figures and limited the references to the most comprehensive and important ones. This makes the book even more user-friendly.

Our most notable change from the prior editions is the addition of case studies, which consist of a description of a clinical situation and a discussion. The cases were chosen to illustrate different diagnostic or management problems, emphasize important points from the preceding chapter, and highlight the role of the transfusion medicine specialist in patient care. These cases are based on real patients. This serves to bring the technical and clinical issues to life and demonstrate the application of knowledge of transfusion medicine to real-life situations that may not be as clear-cut as the description in a text. This new feature establishes the book as a practical (hands-on) introduction to the field for trainees and provides a platform for teaching.

Editors and authors from the prior editions established the foundation on which we continue to build. New editors and authors have brought their insights and talents to bear on our most recent efforts. The editors thank the individual chapter authors who have provided an authoritative, up-dated presentation of the subject. The editors also express their appreciation to Ms. Ruth Weinberg and Ms. Tanya Lazar from Lippincott Williams & Wilkins for their continued support. The addition of Dr. Ennio Rossi's name to the title of the book recognizes his leadership in creating the book and sustaining it through its first two editions. It also emphasizes our belief that the book will remain an essential part of the ongoing evolution of transfusion medicine for many years to come.

Toby L. Simon, MD
Walter H. Dzik, MD
Edward L. Snyder, MD
Christopher P. Stowell, MD, PhD
Ronald G. Strauss, MD

ROSSI'S PRINCIPLES OF TRANSFUSION MEDICINE

THIRD EDITION

1

TRANSFUSION IN THE NEW MILLENNIUM

ENNIO C. ROSSI
TOBY L. SIMON

Prehistoric man left drawings of himself pierced by arrows (1). This means he was as aware of blood as he was of his own limbs. The flint implements he used as tools and weapons distinguished him from other creatures and contributed to the violence of his era. As he hunted food and fought enemies, he observed bleeding and the properties of blood. A cut, received or inflicted, yielded a vivid red color. If the cut was shallow, there was little blood. But if the cut was deep, a red torrent flowing from the stricken victim quickly led to death, with shed blood congealed and darkening in the sun. Fatal hemorrhage was commonplace. Nonetheless, the sight must have been fearful and possibly existential as life flowed red out of the body of an enemy or a wounded animal (2). It is no wonder, then, that at the dawn of recorded history, blood was already celebrated in religious rites and rituals as a life-giving force. The cultural expressions of primitive and ancient societies, though separated by time or space, can be strikingly similar. Whether these expressions emerged independently or were diffused about the world by unknown voyagers will probably always remain clouded in mystery (2). Nonetheless, there is a common thread in the ancient rituals that celebrate blood as a mystical vital principle. In Leviticus 17:11, "the life of the flesh is in the blood," and the Chinese Neiching (circa 1000 BC) claims the blood contains the soul (2). Pre-Columbian North American Indians bled their bodies "of its greatest power" as self-punishment (3), Egyptians took blood baths as a recuperative measure, and Romans drank the blood of fallen gladiators in an effort to cure epilepsy (4). The Romans also practiced a ceremony called taurobolium—a blood bath for spiritual restoration. A citizen seeking spiritual rebirth descended into a pit or fossa sanguinis. Above him on a platform, a priest sacrificed a bull, and the animal's blood cascaded down in a shower upon the beneficiary. Then, in a powerful visual image, the subject emerged up from the other end of the pit, covered with blood and reborn (1).

The legend of Medea and Aeson taken from Ovid's *Metamorphoses* and quoted in Bulfinch's *Mythology* (5) also ascribed rejuvenating powers to blood. Jason asked Medea to "take some years off his life and add them to those of his father Aeson." Medea, however, pursued an alternative course. She prepared a cauldron with the blood of a sacrificed black sheep. To this she added magic herbs, hoarfrost gathered by moonlight, the entrails of a wolf, and many other things "without a name." The boiling cauldron was stirred with a withered olive branch, which became green and full of leaves and young olives when it was withdrawn. Seeing that all was ready,

> Medea cut the throat of the old man and let out all his blood, and poured into his mouth and into his wound the juices of her cauldron. As soon as he had imbibed them, his hair and beard laid by their whiteness and assumed the blackness of youth; his paleness and emaciation were gone; his veins were full of blood, his limbs of vigour and robustness. Aeson is amazed at himself, and remembers that such as he now is, he was in his youthful days, forty years before.

This legend seems to echo in the apocryphal story of Pope Innocent VIII, who is said to have received the blood of three young boys in 1492 while on his deathbed. As the story goes, a physician attempted to save the pope's life by using blood drawn from three boys 10 years of age, all of whom died soon thereafter. Some nineteenth-century versions of this tale suggest

E.C. Rossi: Division of Internal Medicine, Northwestern University School of Medicine, Chicago, Illinois.

T.L. Simon: TriCore Reference Laboratories, Department of Pathology, University of New Mexico, School of Medicine, Albuquerque, New Mexico.

the blood was transfused. However, earlier renditions more plausibly suggest that the blood was intended for a potion to be taken by mouth. In any event, there is no evidence the pope actually received any blood in any form (6,7).

The folklore that flowed with blood was not accompanied by a great deal of accurate information. The ancient Greeks believed that blood formed in the heart and passed through the veins to the rest of the body, where it was consumed. Arteries were part of an independent system transporting air from the lungs. Although Erasistratos (circa 270 BC) had imagined the heart as a pump, his idea was ahead of its time. As long as veins and arteries were dead-end channels transporting blood and air, there was little need for a pump in the system. Although Galen (131–201 AD) finally proved that arteries contain blood, communication with the venous system was not suspected. Blood, formed in the liver, merely passed through the blood vessels and heart on its way to the periphery (1). These teachings remained in place for 1,400 years until they were swept away in 1628 by Harvey's discovery of the circulation.

The realization that blood moved in a circulating stream opened the way to experiments on vascular infusion. In 1642 George von Wahrendorff injected wine (8) and in 1656 Christopher Wren and Robert Boyle injected opium and other drugs (9) intravenously into dogs. The latter studies, performed at Oxford, were the inspiration for Richard Lower's experiments in animal transfusion.

THE FIRST ANIMAL TRANSFUSION

Richard Lower (1631–1691) was a student at Oxford when Christopher Wren and Robert Boyle began their experiments on infusion. In due course, Lower joined their scientific group and studied the intravenous injection of opiates, emetics, and other substances into living animals (10). In time, the transfusion of blood itself became the objective. The announcement of the first successful transfusion, performed by Richard Lower at Oxford in February 1665, was published on November 19, 1666, in the *Philosophical Transactions of the Royal Society* in a short notation entitled, "The Success of the Experiment of Transfusing the Blood of One Animal into Another" (11). The entire notation is as follows (11):

> This experiment, hitherto look'd upon to be of an almost insurmountable difficulty, hath been of late very successfully perform'd not only at Oxford, by the directions of that expert anatomist Dr. Lower, but also in London, by order of the R. Society, at their publick meeting in Gresham Colledge: the Description of the particulars whereof, and the Method of Operation is referred to the next opportunity.

The December 17, 1666, issue of the *Transactions* contained the full description as promised (12). It was taken from a letter (13) written by Lower to Robert Boyle on July 6, 1666, in which Lower described direct transfusion from the carotid artery of one dog to the jugular vein of another. After describing the insertion of quills into the blood vessels of the donor and recipient dogs, Lower wrote (13):

> When you have done this you may lay the dogs on their side and fasten them densely together as best you may to insure the connection of the two quills. Quickly tighten the noose around the neck of the receiving animal as in venasection, or at all events compress the vein on the opposite side of the neck with your finger, then take out the stopper and open the upper jugular quill so that while the foreign blood is flowing into the lower quill, the animal's own blood flows out from the upper into suitable receptacles—until at last the second animal, amid howls, faintings, and spasms[,] finally loses its life together with its vital fluid.
>
> When the tragedy is over, take both quills out of the jugular vein of the surviving animal, tie tightly with the former slipknots, and divide the vein. After the vessel has been divided, sew up the skin, slacken the cords binding the dog, and let it jump down from the table. It shakes itself a little, as though aroused from sleep, and runs away lively and strong, more active and vigorous perhaps, with the blood of its fellow than its own.

These studies inevitably led to the transfusion of animal blood to humans. In England, this occurred on November 23, 1667, when Lower and Edmund King transfused sheep blood into a man named Arthur Coga (14). Described by Samuel Pepys as "a little frantic," Coga was paid 20 shillings to accept this transfusion, with the expectation that it might have a beneficial "cooling" effect. One week later, Coga appeared before the society and claimed to be a new man, although Pepys concluded he was "cracked a little in the head" (13). However, this was not the first transfusion performed in a human. The credit for that accomplishment belongs to Jean Baptiste Denis (1635–1704), who had performed the first human transfusion several months earlier in Paris.

THE FIRST ANIMAL-TO-HUMAN TRANSFUSION

The founding of the Royal Society in London in 1662 was followed in 1666 by the establishment of the Academie des Sciences in Paris under the patronage of King Louis XIV. The new Academie reviewed the English reports on transfusion with great interest. Denis probably read of Lower's experiments in the *Journal des Savants* on January 31, 1667, and he began his own studies approximately one month later (15,16). The first human transfusion was then performed on June 15, 1667, when Denis administered the blood of a lamb to a 15-year-old boy (17) (Fig. 1.1).

Although discovery of the circulation had suggested the idea of transfusion, indications for the procedure remained uninformed. Transfusion was still thought to alter behavior and possibly achieve rejuvenation. The blood of young dogs made old dogs seem frisky; the blood of lions was proposed as a cure for cowardice; and 5 months later, Arthur Coga would receive a transfusion of sheep blood because of its presumed "cooling" effect. Denis used animal blood for transfusion because he thought it was "less full of impurities" (17):

> Sadness, Envy, Anger, Melancholy, Disquiet and generally all the Passions, are as so many causes which trouble the life of man, and corrupt the whole substance of the blood: Whereas the life of Brutes is much more regular, and less subject to all these miseries.

It is thus ironic that the symptoms of the first transfusion recipient may have been explained in part by profound anemia and that the single transfusion of lamb blood may have produced

(489) *Numb. 27.*

A LETTER

Concerning a new way of curing ſundry diſeaſes by Transfuſion of Blood, Written to Monſieur de MONTMOR, *Counſellor to the* French King, *and Maſter of* Requeſts.

By J: DENIS *Profeſſor of* Philoſophy, *and the* Mathematicks.

Munday July 22. 1667.

SIR,

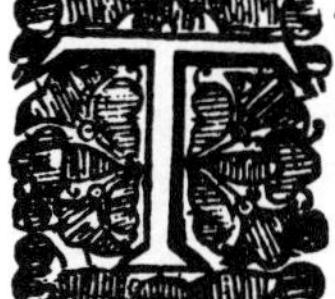

HE project of cauſing the Blood of a healthy animal to paſſe into the veins of one diſeaſed, having been conceived *a-bout ten years agoe*, in the illuſtrious Society of *Virtuoſi* which aſſembles at your houſe, and your goodneſs having received M. *Emmeriz*, & my ſelf, very favorably at ſuch times as we have preſum'd to entertain you either with diſcourſe concerning it, or the ſight of ſome not inconſiderable effects of it: You will not think it ſtrange that I now take the liberty of troubling you with this Letter, and deſign to inform you fully of what purſuances and ſucceſſes we have made in this Operation; wherein you are juſtly intitled to a greater ſhare than any other, conſidering that it was firſt ſpoken of in your *Academy*, & that the Publick is beholding to you for this as well as for many other diſcoveries, for the benefits & advantages it ſhall reap from the ſame. But that I may give you the reaſons of our procedure & con-

Ccc vince

FIGURE 1.1. The first human transfusion. (From Denis J. A letter concerning a new way of curing sundry diseases by transfusion of blood. *Philos Trans R Soc Lond* 1667;2:489.)

temporary amelioration owing to increased oxygen transport. Denis described the case as follows (17):

> On the 15 of this Moneth, we hapned upon a Youth aged between 15 and 16 years, who had for above two moneths bin tormented with a contumacious and violent fever, which obliged his Physitians to bleed him 20 times, in order to asswage the excessive heat.
>
> Before this disease, he was not observed to be of a lumpish dull spirit, his memory was happy enough, and he seem'd chearful and nimble enough in body; but since the violence of this fever, his wit seem'd wholly sunk, his memory perfectly lost, and his body so heavy and drowsie that he was not fit for anything. I beheld him fall asleep as he sate at dinner, as he was eating his Breakfast, and in all occurrences where men seem most unlikely to sleep. If he went to bed at nine of the clock in the Evening, he needed to be wakened several times before he could be got to rise by nine the next morning, and he pass'd the rest of the day in an incredible stupidity.
>
> I attributed all these changes to the great evacuations of blood, the Physitians had been oblig'd to make for saving his life.

Three ounces of the boy's blood were exchanged for 9 ounces of lamb arterial blood. Several hours later the boy arose, and "for the rest of the day, he spent it with much more liveliness than ordinary." Thus the first human transfusion, which was heterologous, was accomplished without any evident unfavorable effect.

This report stimulated a firestorm of controversy over priority of discovery (18,19). The letter by Denis was published in the *Philosophical Transactions of the Royal Society* on July 22, 1667, while the editor, Henry Oldenburg, was imprisoned in the Tower of London. Oldenburg, following some critical comments concerning the Anglo-Dutch War then in progress (1665–1667), had been arrested under a warrant issued June 20, 1667. After his release 2 months later, Oldenburg returned to his editorial post and found the letter published in his absence. He took offense at Denis's opening statement, which claimed that the French had conceived of transfusion "about ten years agoe, in the illustrious Society of Virtuosi . . . " (Fig. 1.1). This seemed to deny the English contributions to the field. Oldenburg cited these omissions in an issue of the *Transactions* published September 23, 1667, "for the Months of July, August, and September." By numbering this issue 27 and beginning pagination with 489, Oldenburg attempted to suppress the letter by Denis (18). However, as is evident, this did not ultimately succeed. Nonetheless, subsequent events created even greater difficulties for Jean Denis.

Although the first two subjects who underwent transfusion by Denis were not adversely affected, the third and fourth recipients died. The death of the third subject was easily attributable to other causes. However, the fourth case initiated a sequence of events that put an end to transfusion for 150 years.

Anthony du Mauroy was a 34-year-old man who suffered from intermittent bouts of maniacal behavior. On December 19, 1667, Denis and his assistant Paul Emmerez removed 10 ounces of the man's blood and replaced it with 5 or 6 ounces of blood from the femoral artery of a calf. Failing to note any apparent improvement, they repeated the transfusion 2 days later. After the second transfusion, du Mauroy experienced a classic transfusion reaction (20):

> His pulse rose presently, and soon after we observ'd a plentiful sweat over all his face. His pulse varied extremely at this instant, and he complain'd of great pains in his kidneys and that he was not well in his stomach.

Du Mauroy fell asleep at about 10 o'clock in the evening. He awoke the following morning and "made a great glass full of urine, of a colour as black, as if it had been mixed with the soot of chimneys" (20). Two months later, the patient again became maniacal, and his wife again sought transfusion therapy. Denis was reluctant but finally gave in to her urgings. However, the transfusion could not be accomplished, and du Mauroy died the next evening.

The physicians of Paris strongly disapproved of the experiments in transfusion. Three of them approached du Mauroy's widow and encouraged her to lodge a malpractice complaint against Denis. She instead went to Denis and attempted to extort money from him in return for her silence. Denis refused and filed a complaint before the Lieutenant in Criminal Causes. During the subsequent hearing, evidence was introduced to indicate that Madame du Mauroy had poisoned her husband with arsenic. In a judgment handed down at the Chatelet in Paris on

April 17, 1668, Denis was exonerated, and the woman was held for trial. The court also stipulated "that for the future no Transfusion should be made upon any Human Body but by the approbation of the Physicians of the Parisian Faculty" (21). At this point, transfusion research went into decline, and within 10 years it was prohibited in both France and England.

THE BEGINNINGS OF MODERN TRANSFUSION

After the edict that ended transfusion in the seventeenth century, the technique lay dormant for 150 years. Stimulated by earlier experiments by Leacock, transfusion was "resuscitated" and placed on a rational basis by James Blundell (1790–1877), a London obstetrician who had received his medical degree from the University of Edinburgh (22). Soon after graduation, Blundell accepted a post in physiology and midwifery at Guy's Hospital. It was there that he began the experiments on transfusion that led to its rebirth. The frequency of postpartum hemorrhage and death troubled Blundell. In 1818 he wrote (23):

> A few months ago I was requested to visit a woman who was sinking under uterine hemorrhage . . . . [H]er fate was decided, and notwithstanding every exertion of the medical attendants, she died in the course of two hours.
>
> Reflecting afterwards on this melancholy scene . . . [,] I could not forbear considering, that the patient might very probably have been saved by transfusion; and that . . . the vessels might have been replenished by means of the syringe with facility and prompitude.

This opening statement introduced Blundell's epoch-making study entitled, "Experiments on the Transfusion of Blood by the Syringe" (23) (Fig. 1.2). Blundell described in detail a series of animal experiments. He demonstrated that a syringe could be used effectively to perform transfusion, that the lethal effects of arterial exsanguination could be reversed by the transfusion of either venous or arterial blood, that the injection of 5 drams (20 cc) of air into the veins of a small dog was not fatal, but that transfusion across species ultimately was lethal to the recipient (23). Thus Blundell was the first to state clearly that only human blood should be used for human transfusion. The latter conclusion was confirmed in France by Dumas and Prevost, who demonstrated that the infusion of heterologous blood into an exsanguinated animal produced only temporary improvement and was followed by death within 6 days (24). These scientific studies provided the basis for Blundell's subsequent efforts in clinical transfusion.

EXPERIMENTS

ON THE

TRANSFUSION OF BLOOD

BY THE

SYRINGE.

By JAMES BLUNDELL, M.D.

LECTURER ON PHYSIOLOGY AT GUY'S HOSPITAL.

COMMUNICATED

By MR. CLINE.

Read Feb. 3, 1818.

FIGURE 1.2. The beginnings of modern transfusion. (From Blundell J. Experiments on the transfusion of blood by the syringe. *Med Chir Trans* 1818;9:56.)

The first well-documented transfusion with human blood took place on September 26, 1818 (25). The patient was an extremely emaciated man in his mid-thirties who had pyloric obstruction caused by carcinoma. He received 12 to 14 ounces of blood in the course of 30 or 40 minutes. Despite initial apparent improvement, the patient died 2 days later. Transfusion in the treatment of women with postpartum hemorrhage was more successful. In all, Blundell performed 10 transfusions of which five were successful. Three of the unsuccessful transfusions were performed on moribund patients; the fourth was performed on a patient with puerperal sepsis; and the fifth was performed on the aforementioned patient with terminal carcinoma. Four of the successful transfusions were given for postpartum hemorrhage, and the fifth was administered to a boy who bled after amputation (22). Blundell also devised various instruments for the performance of transfusion. They included an "impellor," which collected blood in a warmed cup and "impelled" the blood into the recipient via an attached syringe, and a "gravitator" (26) (Fig. 1.3), which received blood and delivered it by gravity through a long vertical cannula.

The writings of Blundell provided evidence against the use of animal blood in humans and established rational indications for transfusion. However, the gravitator (Fig. 1.3) graphically demonstrated the technical problems that remained to be solved. Blood from the donor, typically the patient's husband, flowed into a funnel-like device and down a flexible cannula into the patient's vein "with as little exposure as possible to air, cold and inanimate surface" (25). The amount of blood transfused was estimated from the amount spilled into the apparatus by the donor. In this clinical atmosphere, charged with apprehension and anxiety, the amount of blood issuing from a donor easily could be overstated. Clotting within the apparatus then ensured that only a portion of that blood actually reached the patient. Thus the amount of blood actually transfused may have been seriously overestimated. This may explain the apparent absence of transfusion reactions. Alternatively, reactions may have been unrecognized. Patients who underwent transfusion frequently were agonal. As Blundell (26) stated, "it seems right, as the operation now stands, to confine transfusion to the first class of cases only, namely, those in which there seems to be no hope for the patient, unless blood can be thrown into the veins." Under these circumstances, "symptoms" associated with an "unsuccessful" transfusion might be ascribed to the agonal state rather than the transfusion itself. For a time, the problem of

VOL. II.] LONDON, SATURDAY, JUNE 13. [1828-9.

OBSERVATIONS

ON

TRANSFUSION OF BLOOD.

BY DR. BLUNDELL.

*With a Description of his Gravitator.**

STATES of the body really requiring the infusion of blood into the veins are probably rare; yet we sometimes meet with cases in which the patient must die unless such operation can be performed; and still more frequently with cases which seem to require a supply of blood, in order to prevent the ill health which usually arises from large losses of the vital fluid, even when they do not prove fatal.

In the present state of our knowledge respecting the operation, although it has not been clearly shown to have proved fatal in any one instance, yet not to mention possible, though unknown risks, inflammation of the arm has certainly been produced by it on one or two occasions; and therefore it seems right, as the operation now stands, to confine transfusion to the first class of cases only, namely, those in which there seems to be no hope for the patient, unless blood can be thrown into the veins.

The object of the Gravitator is, to give help in this last extremity, by transmitting the blood in a regulated stream from one individual to another, with as little exposure as may be to air, cold, and inanimate surface; ordinary venesection being the only operation performed on the person who emits the blood; and the insertion of a small tube into the vein usually laid open in bleeding, being all the operation which it is necessary to execute on the person who receives it.

The following plate represents the whole apparatus connected for use and in action :—

* The instrument is manufactured by Messrs. Maw, 55, Aldermanbury.

Tab. 1.

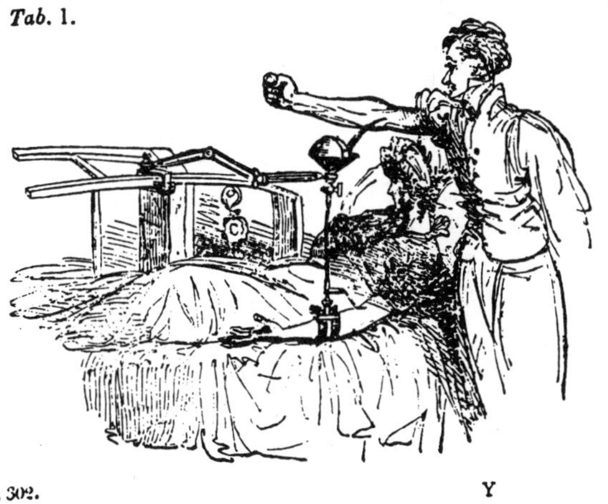

No. 302. Y

FIGURE 1.3. Blundell's gravitator. (From Blundell J. Observations on transfusions of blood. *Lancet* 1828;2:321.)

coagulation during transfusion was circumvented by the use of defibrinated blood. This undoubtedly increased the amount of blood actually transfused. However, there were numerous deaths. Interestingly, these deaths were attributed to intravascular coagulation when in actuality they were probably fatal hemolytic reactions caused by the infusion of incompatible blood (27).

Transfusion at the end of the nineteenth century, therefore, was neither safe nor efficient. The following description, written in 1884, illustrates this point (28):

> Students, with smiling faces, are rapidly leaving the theatre of one of our metropolitan hospitals. The most brilliant operator of the day has just performed immediate transfusion with the greatest success. By means of a very beautiful instrument, the most complex and ingenious that modern science has yet produced, a skilful surgeon has transfused half a pint, or perhaps a pint, of blood from a healthy individual to a fellow creature profoundly collapsed from the effects of severe haemorrhage. Some little difficulty was experienced prior to the operation, as one of the many stop-cocks of the transfusion apparatus was found to work stiffly; but this error was quickly rectified by a mechanic in attendance. Towards the close of the operation the blood-donor, a powerful and heavy young man, swooned. Two porters carried him on a stretcher into an adjoining room.

In the latter half of the nineteenth century, there were many attempts to render transfusion a more predictable and less arduous procedure. In 1869, Braxton-Hicks (29), using blood anticoagulated with phosphate solutions, performed a number of transfusions on women with obstetric bleeding. Many of the patients were in extremis, and ultimately all died. Unfortunately, a detailed description of terminal symptoms was not provided (29). Some investigators attempted to rejuvenate animal-to-human transfusion, and Hasse persisted in this approach despite disastrous results. Studies by Ponfick and by Landois finally put an end to this practice. Ponfick, in carefully controlled studies, confirmed the lethality of heterologous transfusion and identified the resulting hemoglobinuria along with its donor erythrocyte source. Landois documented the poor results of animal-to-human transfusion and demonstrated the lysis of sheep erythrocytes by human serum in vitro (8).

Frustration with blood as a transfusion product led to even more bizarre innovations. From 1873 to 1880, cow, goat, and even human milk was transfused as a blood substitute (30). The rationale derived from an earlier suggestion that the fat particles of milk could be converted into blood cells. Milk transfusion was particularly popular in the United States (30), where the practice of animal-to-human transfusion was recorded as late as 1890 (31). Fortunately, these astonishing practices were discontinued when saline solutions were introduced as "a life-saving measure" and "a substitute for the transfusion of blood" (32). A passage from an article written by Bull in 1884 (32) is particularly instructive:

> [T]he danger from loss of blood, even to two-thirds of its whole volume, lies in the disturbed relationship between the calibre of the vessels and the quantity of the blood contained therein, and not in the diminished number of red blood-corpuscles; and . . . This danger concerns the volume of the injected fluids also, it being a matter of indifference whether they be albuminous or containing blood corpuscles or not . . . .

Mercifully, volume replacement with saline solutions deflected attention from the unpredictable and still dangerous practice of blood transfusion. Accordingly, transfusions were abandoned until interest was rekindled by the scientific and technical advances of the early twentieth century.

THE TWENTIETH CENTURY

The twentieth century was ushered in by a truly monumental discovery. In 1900, Karl Landsteiner (1868–1943) observed that the sera of some persons agglutinated the red blood cells of others. This study, published in 1901 in the *Wiener Klinische Wochenschrift* (33) (Fig. 1.4), showed for the first time the cellular differences in individuals from the same species. In his article, Landsteiner (34) wrote:

> In a number of cases (Group A) the serum reacts on the corpuscles of another group (B), but not, however, on those of group A, while, again, the corpuscles of A will be influenced likewise by serum B.

Aus dem pathologisch-anatomischen Institute in Wien.

Ueber Agglutinationserscheinungen normalen menschlichen Blutes.

Von Dr. **Karl Landsteiner,** Assistenten am pathologisch-anatomischen Institute.

FIGURE 1.4. Landsteiner's description of blood groups. (From Landsteiner K. Ueber Agglutinationserscheinungen normalen menschlichen Blutes. *Wien Klin Wochenschr* 1901;14:1132.)

> The serum of the third group (C) agglutinates the corpuscles of A and B, while the corpuscles of C will not be influenced by the sera of A and B. The corpuscles are naturally apparently insensitive to the agglutinins which exist in the same serum.

With the identification of blood groups A, B, and C (subsequently renamed group O) by Landsteiner and of group AB by Decastello and Sturli (35), the stage was set for the performance of safe transfusion. For this work, Landsteiner somewhat belatedly received the Nobel Prize in 1930. But even that high recognition does not adequately express the true magnitude of Landsteiner's discovery. His work was like a burst of light in a darkened room. He gave us our first glimpse of immunohematology and transplantation biology and provided the tools for important discoveries in genetics, anthropology, and forensic medicine. Viewed from this perspective, the identification of human blood groups is one of only a few scientific discoveries of the twentieth century that changed all of our lives (34). Yet the translation of Landsteiner's discovery into transfusion practice took many years.

At the turn of the century, the effective transfer of blood from one person to another remained a formidable task. Clotting, still uncontrolled, quickly occluded transfusion devices and frustrated most efforts. In 1901 the methods used in transfusion were too primitive to demonstrate the importance of Landsteiner's discovery. Indeed, the study of in vitro red blood cell agglutination may have seemed rather remote from the technical problems that demanded attention. An intermediate step was needed before the importance of Landsteiner's breakthrough could be perceived and the appropriate changes could be incorporated into practice. This process was initiated by Alexis Carrel (1873–1944), another Nobel laureate, who developed a surgical procedure that allowed direct transfusion through an arteriovenous anastomosis.

Carrel (36) introduced the technique of end-to-end vascular anastomosis with triple-threaded suture material. This procedure brought the ends of vessels in close apposition and preserved luminal continuity, thus avoiding leakage or thrombosis. This technique paved the way for successful organ transplantation and brought Carrel the Nobel Prize in 1912. It was also adapted by Carrel (37) and others (38,39) to the performance of transfusion. Crile (38) introduced the use of a metal tube to facilitate placement of sutures, and Bernheim (39) used a two-piece cannula to unite the artery to the vein (Fig. 1.5). Because all of these procedures usually culminated in the sacrifice of the two vessels, they were not performed frequently. Direct transfusion was also fraught with danger. In a passage written two decades later, the procedure was recalled in the following manner (40):

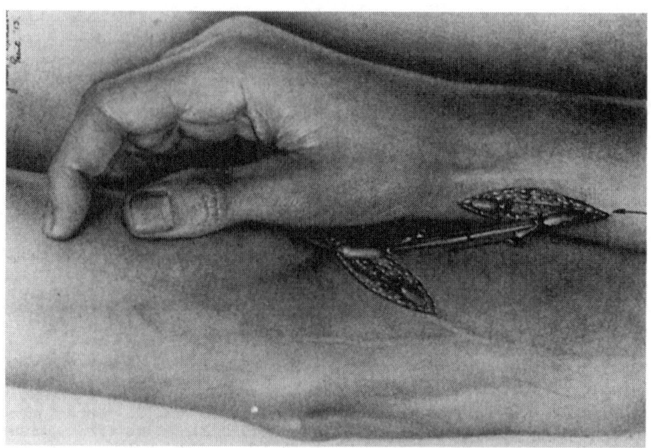

FIGURE 1.5. Direct transfusion by means of arteriovenous anastomosis through the two-pieced cannula of Bernheim. (From Bernheim BM. *Blood transfusion: hemorrhage and the anaemias.* Philadelphia: JB Lippincott, 1917.)

> [T]he direct artery to vein anastomosis was the best method available but was often very difficult or even unsuccessful. And, what was almost as bad, one never knew how much blood one had transfused at any moment or when to stop (unless the donor collapsed). (I remember one such collapse in which the donor almost died—and the surgeon needed to be revived.)

Despite these many difficulties, direct transfusion through an arteriovenous anastomosis for the first time efficiently transferred blood from one person to another. The process also disclosed fatal hemolytic reactions that were undeniably caused by transfusion (41) (Fig. 1.6). However, the relation of these fatal reactions to Landsteiner's discovery was not recognized until Reuben Ottenberg (1882–1959) demonstrated the importance of compatibility testing.

Ottenberg's interest in transfusion began in 1906 while he was an intern at German (now Lenox Hill) Hospital in New York. There Ottenberg learned of Landsteiner's discovery and in 1907 began pretransfusion compatibility testing (42). Ottenberg accepted an appointment at Mount Sinai Hospital the next year and continued his studies on transfusion. In 1913, Ottenberg published the report that conclusively demonstrated the impor-

A CASE OF FATAL HEMOLYSIS FOLLOWING DIRECT TRANSFUSION OF BLOOD BY ARTERIOVENOUS ANASTOMOSIS.*

WILLIAM PEPPER, M.D.
Instructor in Medicine, University of Pennsylvania.
AND
VERNER NISBET, M.D.
Assistant Instructor in Medicine, University of Pennsylvania; Assistant Director of the William Pepper Laboratory of Clinical Medicine.
PHILADELPHIA.

FIGURE 1.6. Report of a fatal transfusion reaction. (From Pepper W, Nisbet V. A case of fatal hemolysis following direct transfusion of blood by arteriovenous anastomosis. *JAMA* 1907;49:385.)

ACCIDENTS IN TRANSFUSION

THEIR PREVENTION BY PRELIMINARY BLOOD EXAMINATION: BASED ON AN EXPERIENCE OF ONE HUNDRED TWENTY-EIGHT TRANSFUSIONS *

REUBEN OTTENBERG, M.D.
AND
DAVID J. KALISKI, M.D.
NEW YORK

Accidents following transfusion have been sufficiently frequent to make many medical men hesitate to advise transfusion, except in desperate cases. It has been our opinion since we began making observations on this question in 1908 that such accidents could be prevented by careful preliminary tests, leading to the exclusion of agglutinative or hemolytic donors. Our observations on over 125 cases have confirmed this view and we believe that untoward symptoms can be prevented with absolute certainty.

FIGURE 1.7. Report of the importance of testing before transfusion. (From Ottenberg R, Kaliski DJ. Accidents in transfusion: their prevention by preliminary blood examination: based on an experience of 128 transfusions. *JAMA* 1913;61:2138.)

tance of preliminary blood testing for the prevention of transfusion "accidents" (43) (Fig. 1.7). This was not Ottenberg's only contribution. He observed the mendelian inheritance of blood groups (44), and he was the first to recognize the relative unimportance of donor antibodies and consequently the "universal" utility of type O blood donors (45).

Further advances in immunohematology were to occur in succeeding decades. The M, N, and P systems were described in the period between 1927 and 1947 (46). The Rh system was discovered in connection with an unusual transfusion reaction. In 1939, Levine and Stetson (47) described an immediate reaction in a group O woman who had received her husband's group O blood soon after delivery of a stillborn fetus with erythroblastosis. This sequence of events suggested that the infant had inherited a red blood cell agglutinogen from the father that was foreign to the mother. At about the same time, Landsteiner and Wiener (48) harvested a rhesus monkey red blood cell antibody from immunized guinea pigs and rabbits. This antibody agglutinated 85% of human red blood cell samples (Rh positive) and left 15% (Rh negative) unaffected. When the experimentally induced antibody was tested in parallel with the serum from Levine's patient, a similar positive and negative distribution was observed, and the Rh system had been discovered. Other red blood cell antigen systems were subsequently described, but when Rh immune globulin was introduced as a preventive measure for hemolytic disease of the newborn, it became one of the major public health advances of the century.

Despite the introduction of compatibility testing by Ottenberg, transfusion could not be performed frequently as long as arteriovenous anastomosis remained the procedure of choice. Using this method, Ottenberg needed 5 years (Fig. 1.7) to accumulate the 128 transfusions he reported in his study on pretransfusion testing (43). New techniques, such as Unger's two-syringe method introduced in 1915 (49) (Fig. 1.8), eventually put an end to transfusion by means of arteriovenous anastomosis. However, transfusions did not become commonplace until anticoagulants were developed and direct methods of transfusion were rendered obsolete.

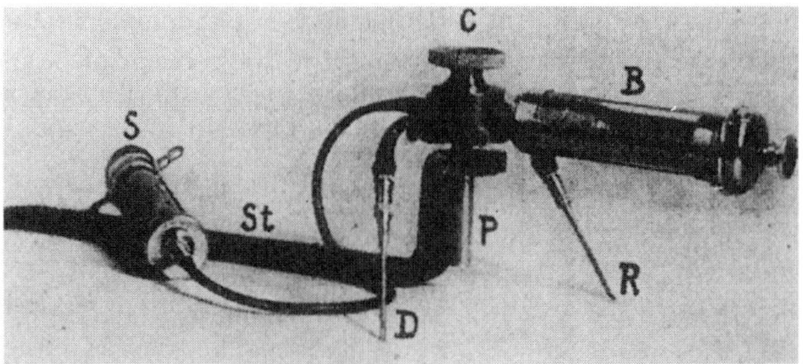

FIGURE 1.8. Apparatus for Unger's two-syringe, four-way stopcock method of indirect transfusion. (From Unger LJ. A new method of syringe transfusion. *JAMA* 1915;64:582.)

ANTICOAGULANTS, THE BLOOD BANK, AND COMPONENT THERAPY

The anticoagulant action of sodium citrate completely transformed the practice of transfusion. Early reports from Belgium (50) and Argentina (51) were followed by the work of Lewisohn (52) that established the optimal citrate concentration for anticoagulation. The work of Weil (53) then demonstrated the feasibility of refrigerated storage. Subsequently, Rous and Turner (54) developed the anticoagulant solution that was used during World War I (55). Despite its very large volume, this solution remained the anticoagulant of choice until World War II, when Loutit and Mollison (56) developed an acid-citrate-dextrose (ACD) solution. Used in a ratio of 70 ml ACD to 450 ml blood, ACD provided 3 to 4 weeks of preservation of a more concentrated red blood cell infusion. Thus, the two world wars were the stimuli for the development of citrate anticoagulants and the introduction of indirect transfusion (46). For the first time, the donation process could be separated, in time and place, from the actual transfusion. Blood drawn and set aside now awaited the emergence of systems of storage and distribution. Again, it was the provision of medical support during armed conflict that stimulated these developments.

A blood transfusion service, organized by the Republican Army during the Spanish Civil War (1936–1939), collected 9,000 L of blood in citrate-dextrose anticoagulant for the treatment of battle casualties (57). At about that same time, Fantus (58) began operation of the first hospital blood bank at Cook County Hospital in Chicago. His interest had been stimulated by Yudin's report (59) on the use of cadaveric blood in Russia. Apart from certain scruples attached to the use of cadaveric blood, Fantus reasoned that a transfusion service based on such a limited source of supply would be impractical. Accordingly, he established the principle of a "blood bank" from which blood could be withdrawn, provided it had previously been deposited. As Fantus (58) himself stated, "just as one cannot draw money from a bank unless one has deposited some, so the blood preservation department cannot supply blood unless as much comes in as goes out. The term 'blood bank' is not a mere metaphor. The development of anticoagulants and the concept of blood banks provided an infrastructure upon which a more elaborate blood services organization could be built. World War II was the catalyst for these further developments.

At the beginning of World War II, blood procurement programs were greatly expanded (46). In Great Britain an efficient system had been developed through the organization of regional centers. When the war started, these centers, already in place, were able to increase their level of operation. In the United States the use of plasma in the management of shock had led to the development of plasma collection facilities (60). The efficient long-term storage of plasma had been further facilitated by the process of lyophilization developed by Flosdorf and Mudd (61). In 1940, the United States organized a program for the collection of blood and the shipment of plasma to Europe. The American Red Cross, through its local chapters, participated in the project, which collected 13 million units by the end of the war (46).

The national program of the American Red Cross ceased at the end of the war. However, many of the local chapters continued to help recruit donors for local blood banks, and in 1948, the first regional Red Cross blood center was begun in Rochester, New York. By 1949–1950 in the United States, the blood procurement system included 1,500 hospital blood banks, 1,100 of which performed all blood bank functions. There were 46 non-hospital blood banks and 31 Red Cross regional blood centers. By 1962, these numbers had grown to 4,400 hospital blood banks, 123 non-hospital blood banks, and 55 American Red Cross regional blood centers, and the number of units collected had grown to between 5 and 6 million per year (62).

During this time, blood was collected through steel needles and rubber tubing into rubber-stoppered bottles. After washing and resterilization, the materials were reused. On occasion, "vacuum bottles" were used to speed up the collection. However, the high incidence of pyrogenic reactions soon led to the development of disposable plastic blood collection equipment.

In a classic article written in 1952, Walter and Murphy (63) described a closed, gravity technique for whole-blood preservation. They used a laminar flow phlebotomy needle, an interval donor tube, and a collapsible bag of polyvinyl resin designed so that the unit could be assembled and ready for use after sterilization with steam. The polyvinyl resin was chemically inert to biologic fluids and nonirritating to tissue. Soon thereafter, Gibson et al. (64) demonstrated that plastic systems were more flexible and allowed removal of plasma after sedimentation or centrifugation. In time, glass was replaced with plastic, and component therapy began to emerge.

Component and derivative therapy began during World War II when Edwin J. Cohn and his collaborators developed the cold ethanol method of plasma fractionation (65). As a result of their work, albumin, globulin, and fibrinogen became available for clinical use. As plastic equipment replaced glass, component separation became a more widespread practice, and the introduction of automated cell separators provided even greater capabilities in this area.

Clotting factor concentrates for the treatment of patients with hemophilia and other hemorrhagic disorders also were developed during the postwar era. Although antihemophilic globulin had been described in 1937 (66), unconcentrated plasma was the only therapeutic material until Pool discovered that factor VIII could be harvested in the cryoprecipitable fraction of blood (67). This resulted in the development of cryoprecipitate, which was introduced in 1965 for the management of hemophilia. Pool showed that cryoprecipitate could be made in a closed-bag system and urged its harvest from as many donations as possible. The development of cryoprecipitate and other concentrates was the dawn of a golden age in the care of patients with hemophilia. Self-infusion programs, made possible by technologic advances in plasma fractionation, allowed early therapy and greatly reduced disability and unemployment. This golden age came abruptly to an end with the appearance of the acquired immunodeficiency syndrome (AIDS) virus.

TRANSFUSION IN THE AGE OF TECHNOLOGY

In contrast to the past century's long ledger of lives lost because of the lack of blood, transfusion in the twentieth century has saved countless lives. In 1937, during those early halcyon days of transfusion, Ottenberg wrote (40):

> Today transfusion has become so safe and so easy to do that it is seldom omitted in any case in which it may be of benefit. Indeed the chief problem it presents is the finding of the large sums of money needed for the professional donors who now provide most of the blood.

It is ironic that Ottenberg's statement should refer to paid donors and foreshadow difficulties yet to come. However, experience to that point had not revealed the problem of viral disease transmission. More transfusions would have to be administered before that problem would be perceived.

After the introduction of anticoagulants, blood transfusions were given in progressively increasing numbers. At Mount Sinai Hospital in New York, the number of blood transfusions administered between 1923 and 1953 increased 20-fold (68,69) (Table 1.1). This increase was particularly notable after the establishment of blood banks. It was during this period that Beeson wrote

TABLE 1.1. INCREASE IN THE NUMBER OF BLOOD TRANSFUSIONS AT MOUNT SINAI HOSPITAL, NEW YORK, 1923–1953

Year	No. of Transfusions
1923	143
1932	477
1935	794
1938	Blood bank started
1941	2097
1952	2874
1953	3179

Adapted from Lewisohn R. Blood transfusion: 50 years ago and today. *Surg Gynecol Obstet* 1955;101:362.

JAUNDICE OCCURRING ONE TO FOUR MONTHS AFTER TRANSFUSION OF BLOOD OR PLASMA

REPORT OF SEVEN CASES

PAUL B. BEESON, M.D.

ATLANTA, GA.

The purpose of this communication is to report 7 cases of jaundice which occurred one to four months after transfusions of whole blood or plasma and to suggest that these illnesses were probably caused by the transfusions.

FIGURE 1.9. The first description of posttransfusion hepatitis. (From Beeson PB. Jaundice occurring one to four months after transfusion of blood or plasma. *JAMA* 1943;121:1332.)

his classic description of transfusion-transmitted hepatitis (70) (Fig. 1.9). He had been alerted to the problem by the outbreaks of jaundice that followed inoculation programs with human serum during World War II. Thus we entered a new era. Blood components not only saved lives but also transmitted disease. The discovery of the Australian antigen (71) and the subsequent definition of hepatitis A and B still left residual non-A and non-B disease (72), a gap that has been largely filled by the discovery of the hepatitis C virus (73). However, it was the outbreak of AIDS that galvanized public attention to blood transfusion.

The AIDS epidemic was first recognized in the United States, and the first case of AIDS associated with transfusion was observed in a 20-month-old infant (74). Subsequently the suspicion that AIDS could be transmitted by means of transfusion was confirmed (75). The human immunodeficiency virus (HIV) was identified (76), and an effective test to detect the HIV antibody was developed (76).

CONCERN FOR BLOOD SAFETY

Since 1943, transfusion therapy has been shadowed by the specter of disease transmission. In that year, Beeson described posttransfusion hepatitis and unveiled a problem that has grown with time. As transfusion increased, so did disease transmission. In 1962, the connection between paid donations and posttransfusion hepatitis was made (77). A decade later, the National Blood Policy mandated a voluntary donation system in the United States. And yet, blood utilization continued to increase.

Concern about posttransfusion hepatitis was not sufficient to decrease the number of transfusions. Although the use of whole blood declined as blood components became more popular, total blood use in the United States doubled between 1971 and 1980 (78) (Table 1.2). This pattern changed as the emergence of AIDS exposed all segments of society to a revealing light.

AIDS probably arose in Africa in the mid-1970s and spread quietly for several years before it was detected. By 1980 an estimated 100,000 persons were infected, and by 1981, when the first cases were reported, a worldwide pandemic lay just beneath

TABLE 1.2. TRANSFUSIONS IN THE UNITED STATES (IN MILLIONS OF UNITS)

Year	Whole Blood and Red Blood Cells	Platelets	Plasma	Total
1971	6.32	0.41	0.18	6.91
1979	9.47	2.22	1.29	12.98
1980	9.99	3.19	1.54	14.72
1982	11.47	4.18	1.95	17.60
1984	11.98	5.53	2.26	19.77
1986	12.16	6.30	2.18	20.64
1987	11.61	6.38	2.06	20.05
1989	12.06	7.26	2.16	21.48
1992	11.31	8.33	2.26	21.90
1994	11.11	7.87	2.62	21.60
1997	11.52	9.04	3.32	23.88
1999	12.39	9.05	3.32	24.76

Adapted from Surgenor DM, Schnitzer SS. The nation's blood resource: a summary report, National Institutes of Health (NIH) publication no. 85-2028, Bethesda, MD: US Department of Health and Human Services, Public Health Service, NIH, 1985; Surgenor DM, Wallace EL, Hao SHS, et al. Collection and transfusion of blood in the United States, 1982–1988. *N Engl J Med* 322:1646, 1990; Wallace EL, Surgenor DM, Hao HS, et al. Collection and transfusion of blood and blood components in the United States, 1989. *Transfusion* 33:139, 1993; Wallace EL, Churchill DN, Surgenor DM, et al. Collection and transfusion of blood and blood components in the United States, 1994. *Transfusion* 38:625, 1998; Comprehensive report on blood collection and transfusion in the United States in 1997 (NBDRC, 1999), Report on Blood Collection and Transfusion in the United States in 1999 (NBDRC, 2001).

the surface (79). The initial response of the public and officials seemed trifling and insufficient as the outbreak grew to proportions few had foreseen. Criticism was levied against the news media for initially ignoring the story, the government for delay in acknowledging the problem, gay civil rights groups for resistance to epidemiologic measures, research scientists for unseemly competition, blood services for delayed response in a time of crisis, and the U.S. Food and Drug Administration for inadequate regulatory activity. Historians with the perspective of time will determine whether there really were more villains than the virus itself (80).

Improved donor screening and increased donation testing have greatly decreased the risk of disease transmission and rendered the blood supply safer than it has ever been (80). Nonetheless, the realization that transfusion can transmit an almost invariably fatal disease had a chilling effect on the public. Two major changes in blood services have occurred in the aftermath of the AIDS epidemic. The Food and Drug Administration, using pharmaceutical manufacturing criteria not "tailored to . . . blood banks," has become more aggressive in regulatory actions against blood collection establishments (81). And, finally, blood use moderated for approximately 10 years. Through the 1980s and early 1990s, red blood cell and plasma transfusion peaked and began to stabilize (Table 1.2). Only platelet use, driven by the demands of cancer chemotherapy, continued to increase (82–84). Educational programs to encourage judicious use of blood have been initiated, and they have been favorably received by practicing physicians.

A GLIMPSE AT THE FUTURE

As the end of the century approached, relentless public pressure for a "zero risk" blood supply though not achieved in full began to result in dividends through continued scientific and technologic improvements. Enhanced sensitivity and better use of serologic testing, along with improved scrutiny of donors, resulted in major reductions in risk of transmitted disease by the mid-1990s (85). Discovery that pools of units subjected to nucleic acid testing almost closed the window for HIV and hepatitis C virus resulted in application of this testing for both whole blood and plasma donations in 1998–2000 time frame (86). This, combined with viral reduction and inactivation of final product, resulted in plasma derivatives that have not transmitted AIDS or hepatitis since 1994 (87). For whole blood and platelet products, risks have become low, and there is a solvent detergent fresh frozen plasma product.

On the horizon is pathogen inactivation of red blood cell and platelet products that potentially eliminates nearly all viral and bacterial risks. Red blood cell "substitutes"—substances that carry oxygen to tissues—remain in clinical trial. Finally "mad cow disease," which has generated concern that a new variant of Creutzfeldt-Jakob disease (vCJD) could be transmitted by transfusion, has led in some countries to universal leukoreduction of red blood cell and platelet products. Paradoxically, this is probably ineffective for CJD or its variant form but has stimulated a controversy in the United States over universal application to prevent other issues (88). Finally, focus on medical errors may lead to progress against a remaining nemesis—hemolytic transfusion reactions due to clinical error.

Although zero risk still has not been achieved and emerging infections remain a future potential threat, increased public and physician confidence in the safety of the blood supply combined with both increased aggressiveness of therapies and aging of the population has resulted in an increase in blood use as we enter the new millennium (89).

In 1965, before the AIDS era, Dr. Louis Diamond (46) wrote: "Few medical school curricula and rare residency training programs or postgraduate courses contain lectures on transfusion practices and the proper materials to use in specific situations. As a result, blood is often used wastefully, improperly, and dangerously." Recent events surely have emphasized the wisdom of these words written more than 30 years ago.

During the 1980s, innovative programs were developed to address educational needs, and *transfusion medicine* emerged as the term to describe these educational innovations. In Europe, the Committee on Blood Transfusion of the Council of Europe proposed the establishment of blood transfusion centers within teaching hospital complexes to serve as centers of excellence in transfusion medicine. In the United States, transfusion medicine academic awards granted by the National Heart, Lung, and Blood Institute provided a mechanism to introduce transfusion medicine curricula into undergraduate medical education. These initiatives, occurring independently on two continents, were mutually reinforcing and emphasize the importance of clinical training for the transfusion specialist and of transfusion education for the future medical practitioner. Thus there has been a transition from blood banking to transfusion medicine (90). This transition encourages the cooperation of clinical disciplines in studies of blood use. It also increases emphasis on alternatives to homologous blood, such as autologous transfusion and the use of growth factors and other products of genetic engineering.

Snyder has called for another major innovation: the development of transfusion immunobiology and transfusion oncology (91). This emphasizes the role of transfusion medicine specialists in bone marrow and peripheral blood stem cell transplantation, cord blood banking, ex vivo expansion, and progenitor cell graft engineering. Transfusion medicine specialists have always played a role in support of these patients. They now are asked to develop technologically complex processes that are central to more aggressive and effective therapy and conform to the highest standards of good manufacturing and laboratory practices. Similarly, an enhanced role for transfusion medicine specialists in support of surgery has emerged because of the choice of interventions such as acute normovolemic hemodilution, erythropoietin to reduce red blood cell transfusion needs, cell saving, and application of rational guidelines for perioperative transfusion.

The emergence of transfusion-transmitted disease has added a clinical dimension to the laboratory discipline that brought transfusion from Karl Landsteiner's laboratory to its present stage of development. Laboratory progress must continue to provide ever safer and more effective blood components and derivatives. But as hemotherapy becomes more complex, the specialty of transfusion medicine must develop pari passu to ensure that the "life-giving force" of blood is always used wisely and sparingly.

REFERENCES

1. Majno G. *The healing hand.* Cambridge, MA: Harvard University Press, 1975:330–332,402–403.
2. Garrison FH. *An introduction to the history of medicine.* Philadelphia: WB Saunders, 1928:17–74.
3. Ficarra BJ. *Essays on historical medicine.* New York: Froben Press, 1948: 96.
4. Zimmerman LM, Howell KM. History of blood transfusion. *Ann Med Hist* 1932;4:415–433.
5. Bulfinch T. *Mythology.* New York: Random House, 1855:111–112.
6. Brown HM. The beginnings of intravenous medication. *Ann Hist Med* 1917;1:177–197.
7. Lindeboom GA. The story of a blood transfusion to a pope. *J Hist Med* 1954;9:455–459.
8. Maluf NSR. History of blood transfusion. *J Hist Med* 1954;9:59–107.
9. Wren C. An account of the rise and attempts, of a way to conveigh liquors immediately into the mass of blood. *Philos Trans R Soc Lond* 1665;1:128–130.
10. Hollingsworth MW. Blood transfusion by Richard Lower in 1665. *Ann Hist Med* 1928;10:213–225.
11. Lower R. The success of the experiment of transfusing the blood of one animal into another. *Philos Trans R Soc Lond* 1666;1:352.
12. Lower R. The method observed in transfusing the blood out of one animal into another. *Philos Trans R Soc Lond* 1666;1:353–358.
13. Hoff EC, Hoff PM. The life and times of Richard Lower, physiologist and physician (1631–1691). *Bull Hist Med* 1936;4:517–535.
14. Lower R. An account of the experiment of transfusion practised upon a man in London. *Philos Trans R Soc Lond* 1667;2:557–559.
15. Brown H. Jean Denis and transfusion of blood, Paris, 1667–1668. *Isis* 1948;39:15–29.
16. Hoff HE, Guillemin R. The first experiments on transfusion in France. *J Hist Med* 1963;18:103–124.

17. Denis J. A letter concerning a new way of curing sundry diseases by transfusion of blood. *Philos Trans R Soc Lond* 1667;2:489–504.
18. Farr AD. The first human blood transfusion. *Med Hist* 1980;24: 143–162.
19. Walton MT. The first blood transfusion: French or English? *Med Hist* 1974;18:360–364.
20. Denis J. An extract of a letter: touching a late cure of an inveterate phrenisy by the transfusion of blood. *Philos Trans R Soc Lond* 1668; 3:617–623.
21. Denis J. An extract of a printed letter: touching the differences risen about the transfusion of blood. *Philos Trans R Soc Lond* 1668;3: 710–715.
22. Jones HW, Mackmull G. The influence of James Blundell on the development of blood transfusion. *Ann Hist Med* 1928;20:242–248.
23. Blundell J. Experiments on the transfusion of blood by the syringe. *Med Chir Trans* 1818;9:56–92.
24. Transfusion and infusion. *Lancet* 1828;2:324–326.
25. Blundell J. Some account of a case of obstinate vomiting in which an attempt was made to prolong life by the injection of blood into the veins. *Med Chir Trans* 1819;10:296–311.
26. Blundell J. Observations on transfusions of blood. *Lancet* 1828;2: 321–324.
27. Moss WL. A simple method for the indirect transfusion of blood. *Am J Med Sci* 1914;147:698–703.
28. Jennings CE. *Transfusion: its history, indications, and modes of application.* New York: CH Goodwin, 1884:101.
29. Braxton-Hicks J. Cases of transfusion with some remarks on a new method of performing the operation. *Guys Hosp Rep* 1869;14:1–14.
30. Oberman HA. Early history of blood substitutes: transfusion of milk. *Transfusion* 1969;9:74–77.
31. Schmidt PJ. Transfusion in America in the eighteenth and nineteenth centuries. *N Engl J Med* 1968;279:1319–1320.
32. Bull WT. On the intra-venous injection of saline solutions as a substitute for transfusion of blood. *Med Rec* 1884;25:6–8.
33. Landsteiner K. Ueber Agglutinationserscheinungen normalen menschlichen Blutes. *Wien Klin Wochenschr* 1901;14:1132–1134.
34. Dixon B. Of different bloods. *Science* 84 1984;5:65–67.
35. Decastello A, Sturli A. Ueber die Isoagglutinine im Serum gesunder und kranker Menschen. *Munch Med Wochenschr* 1902;49:1090–1095.
36. Carrel A. The transplantation of organs: a preliminary communication. *JAMA* 1905;45:1645–1646.
37. Walker LG Jr. Carrel's direct transfusion of a five day old infant. *Surg Gynecol Obstet* 1973;137:494–496.
38. Crile GW. The technique of direct transfusion of blood. *Ann Surg* 1907;46:329–332.
39. Bernheim BM. *Blood transfusion: hemorrhage and the anaemias.* Philadelphia: JB Lippincott, 1917:259.
40. Ottenberg R. Reminiscences of the history of blood transfusion. *J Mt Sinai Hosp* 1937;4:264–271.
41. Pepper W, Nisbet V. A case of fatal hemolysis following direct transfusion of blood by arteriovenous anastomosis. *JAMA* 1907;49:385–389.
42. Ottenberg R. Transfusion and arterial anastomosis. *Ann Surg* 1908; 47:486–505.
43. Ottenberg R, Kaliski DJ. Accidents in transfusion: their prevention by preliminary blood examination: based on an experience of 128 transfusions. *JAMA* 1913;61:2138–2140.
44. Epstein AA, Ottenberg R. A simple method of performing serum reactions. *Proc N Y Pathol Soc* 1908;8:117–123.
45. Ottenberg R. Studies in isoagglutination, I: transfusion and the question of intravascular agglutination. *J Exp Med* 1911;13:425–438.
46. Diamond LK. The story of our blood groups. In: Wintrobe MM, ed. *Blood, pure and eloquent.* New York: McGraw-Hill, 1980:658–717.
47. Levine P, Stetson RE. An unusual case of intragroup agglutination. *JAMA* 1939;113:126–127.
48. Landsteiner K, Wiener AS. An agglutinable factor in human blood recognized by immune sera for rhesus blood. *Proc Soc Exp Biol Med* 1940;43:233.
49. Unger LJ. A new method of syringe transfusion. *JAMA* 1915;64: 582–584.
50. Hustin A. Principe d'une nouvelle methode de transfusion. *J Med Bruxelles* 1914;12:436.
51. Agote L. Nuevo procediemento para la transfusion del sangre. *An Inst Mod Clin Med Buenos Aires* 1915;2:24–30.
52. Lewisohn R. A new and greatly simplified method of blood transfusion. *Med Rec* 1915;87:141–142.
53. Weil R. Sodium citrate in the transfusion of blood. *JAMA* 1915;64: 425–426.
54. Rous P, Turner JR. The preservation of living red blood cells in vitro. *J Exp Med* 1916;23:219–248.
55. Robertson OH. Transfusion with preserved red blood cells. *Br Med J* 1918;1:691–695.
56. Loutit JF, Mollison PL. Advantages of a disodium-citrate-glucose mixture as a blood preservative. *Br Med J* 1943;2:744–745.
57. Duran-Jorda F. The Barcelona blood transfusion service. *Lancet* 1939; 1:773–775.
58. Fantus B. The therapy of the Cook County Hospital. *JAMA* 1937; 109:128–131.
59. Yudin SS. Transfusion of cadaver blood. *JAMA* 1936;106:997–999.
60. Strumia MM, McGraw JJ. The development of plasma preparations for transfusions. *Ann Intern Med* 1941;15:80–87.
61. Flosdorf EW, Mudd S. Procedure and apparatus for preservation in "lyophile" form of serum and other biological substances. *J Immunol* 1935;29:389–425.
62. Diamond LK. History of blood banking in the United States. *JAMA* 1965;193:40–45.
63. Walter CW, Murphy WP Jr. A closed gravity technique for the preservation of whole blood in ACD solution utilizing plastic equipment. *Surg Gynecol Obstet* 1952;94:687–692.
64. Gibson JG II, Sack T, Buckley ES Jr. The preservation of whole ACD blood, collected, stored and transfused in plastic equipment. *Surg Gynecol Obstet* 1952;95:113–119.
65. Cohn EJ. The separation of blood into fractions of therapeutic value. *Ann Intern Med* 1947;26:341–352.
66. Patek AJ, Taylor FHL. Hemophilia, II: some properties of a substance obtained from normal human plasma effective in accelerating the coagulation of hemophilic blood. *J Clin Invest* 1937;16:113–124.
67. Pool JG, Shannon AE. Production of high-potency concentrates of antihemophilic globulin in a closed-bag system. *N Engl J Med* 1965; 273:1443–1447.
68. Lewisohn R. Blood transfusion: 50 years ago and today. *Surg Gynecol Obstet* 1955;101:362–368.
69. Rosenfeld RE. Early twentieth century origins of modern blood transfusion therapy. *Mt Sinai J Med* 1974;41:626–635.
70. Beeson PB. Jaundice occurring one to four months after transfusion of blood or plasma. *JAMA* 1943;121:1332–1334.
71. Blumberg BS, Alter HJ, Visnich S. A "new" antigen in leukemia sera. *JAMA* 1965;191:541–546.
72. Feinstone SM, Kapikian AZ, Purcell RH, et al. Transfusion-associated hepatitis not due to viral hepatitis type A or B. *N Engl J Med* 1975; 292:767–770.
73. Choo QL, Kuo G, Weiner AJ, et al. Isolation of a cDNA clone derived from a blood-borne non-A non-B viral hepatitis genome. *Science* 1989; 244:359–362.
74. Ammann JA, Cowan MJ, Wara DW, et al. Acquired immunodeficiency in an infant: possible transmission by means of blood products. *Lancet* 1983;1:956–958.
75. Curran JW, Lawrence DN, Jaffe H, et al. Acquired immunodeficiency syndrome (AIDS) associated with transfusions. *N Engl J Med* 1984; 310:69–75.
76. Sarngadharan MG, Popovic M, Bruch L, et al. Antibodies reactive with a human T-lymphotropic retrovirus (HTLV-III) in the serum of patients with AIDS. *Science* 1984;224:506–508.
77. Allen JG, Sayman WA. Serum hepatitis from transfusions of blood. *JAMA* 1962;180:1079–1085.
78. Surgenor DM, Schnitzer SS. The nation's blood resource: a summary report. National Institutes of Health (NIH) publication no. 85-2028. Bethesda, MD: US Department of Health and Human Services, Public Health Service, NIH, 1985.
79. Essex M. Origin of AIDS. In: DeVita VT, Hellman S, Rosenberg

SA, eds. *AIDS: etiology, diagnosis, treatment, and prevention,* 3rd ed. Philadelphia: JB Lippincott, 1992:3–11.
80. Starr D. *Blood: an epic history of medicine and commerce.* New York: Alfred A Knopf, 1998;147–357.
81. Solomon JM. The evolution of the current blood banking regulatory climate. *Transfusion* 1994;34:272–277.
82. Surgenor DM, Wallace EL, Hao SHS, et al. Collection and transfusion of blood in the United States, 1982–1988. *N Engl J Med* 1990;322: 1646–1651.
83. Wallace EL, Surgenor DM, Hao HS, et al. Collection and transfusion of blood and blood components in the United States, 1989. *Transfusion* 1993;33:139–144.
84. Wallace EL, Churchill DM, Surgenor GS, et al. Collection and transfusion of blood and blood components in the United States, 1994. *Transfusion* 1998;38:625–636.
85. Schreiber GB, Busch MP, Kleinman SH, et al. The risk of transfusion-transmitted viral infection. *N Engl J Med* 1996;334:1685–1690.
86. Busch MP, Kleinman SH. Report of the interorganizational task force on nucleic acid amplification testing of blood donors: nucleic acid amplification testing of blood donors for transfusion-transmitted infectious diseases. *Transfusion* 2000;40:143–159.
87. Tabor E. The epidemiology of virus transmission by plasma derivatives: clinical studies verifying the lack of transmission of hepatitis B and C viruses and HIV type 1. *Transfusion* 1999;39:1160–1168.
88. Goodnough LT. The case against universal WBC reduction (and for the practice of evidence-based medicine). *Transfusion* 2000;40: 1522–1527.
89. Sullivan M, National Blood Data Resource Center. Comprehensive Report on Blood Collection and Transfusion in the United States in 1997 (NBDRC, 1999). Report on Blood Collection and Transfusion in the United States in 1999 (NBDRC, 2001).
90. Klein HG. Transfusion medicine: the evolution of a new discipline. *JAMA* 1987;258:2108–2109.
91. Snyder E, Kuter D. Apoptosis in transfusion medicine: of death and dying—is that all there is? *Transfusion* 2000;40:135–137.

Rossi's Principles of Transfusion Medicine, Third Edition, edited by Toby L. Simon, Walter H. Dzik, Edward L. Snyder, Christopher P. Stowell, and Ronald G. Strauss. Lippincott Williams & Wilkins, Philadelphia © 2002.

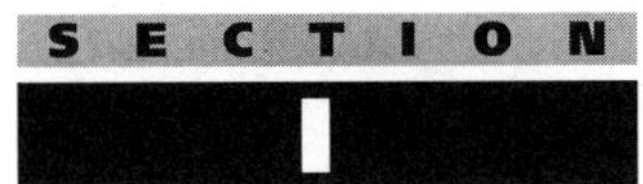

BLOOD COMPONENTS AND DERIVATIVES

PART I

Red Blood Cell

2

RED BLOOD CELL PRODUCTION AND KINETICS

MARK J. KOURY

Depending on the age and sex of a person, the red blood cells (erythrocytes) compose between one third and one half of the volume of blood. For any healthy person, however, the number of erythrocytes in the circulation is maintained in an extremely narrow range over long periods. Although erythrocytes play important roles in the transport of carbon dioxide and nitric oxide, their main function is to transport oxygen from the lungs to the other tissues of the body. This delivery of oxygen is finely controlled by the number of circulating erythrocytes, which is a function of the rate of old erythrocyte removal from the circulation and the rate of new erythrocyte production. Older, senescent erythrocytes are normally removed from the circulation at a rate of 1% per day. These older cells have developed altered surface membrane proteins that lead to their phagocytosis by macrophages. The 1% of circulating erythrocytes removed daily by this mechanism represent approximately 200 billion erythrocytes in a healthy adult.

Because the numbers of circulating erythrocytes are maintained in an extremely narrow range, the normal bone marrow produces almost exactly the same number of new erythrocytes each day as is lost through senescence. When much greater numbers of circulating erythrocytes are lost, such as with bleeding or hemolysis, the production of new erythrocytes increases rapidly to maintain the steady-state number of erythrocytes in a healthy person. This rapid expansion of erythrocyte production in response to bleeding or hemolysis is so well regulated that rebound polycythemia or overproduction of erythrocytes never occurs. This exquisitely controlled production of erythrocytes is mediated through a negative feedback mechanism that involves oxygen delivery to and utilization by the kidneys, the hormone erythropoietin (EPO) that is produced by specialized cells in the kidneys, and the erythroid progenitor cells in the bone marrow that respond to EPO. This chapter explores the production of erythrocytes and its regulation by this feedback mechanism under normal conditions and in various diseases.

ERYTHROPOIESIS

Erythropoiesis: A Component of Hematopoiesis

The production of erythrocytes is termed *erythropoiesis* and is one component of the more complex process of hematopoiesis. Hematopoiesis is the process by which a stem cell proliferates

M.J. Koury: Division of Hematology/Oncology, Vanderbilt University, Nashville, Tennessee.

and differentiates to form all the cell types in the blood and immune system (1). The end products of hematopoiesis include platelets, granulocytes, monocytes-macrophages, T lymphocytes, and B lymphocytes as well as erythrocytes. Thus normally regulated hematopoiesis is required for effective hemostasis, inflammation, immune response, and tissue oxygenation. Among these various functions, tissue oxygenation through erythropoiesis is the first required during embryonic development and the most tightly regulated in postnatal life. Erythropoiesis has two sequential phases during normal development—the primitive phase, during weeks 3 to 8 of human gestation, when nucleated erythrocytes are produced in "blood islands" of the yolk sac and the subsequent definitive phase in which enucleated erythrocytes are produced in the fetal liver and spleen and later in the bone marrow (2–4). In humans, the hemoglobin of the primitive erythrocytes contains embryonic ϵ- and ζ-globins, whereas the hemoglobin of the definitive erythrocytes contain adult α-globin and either fetal γ-globin from midgestation through the first few postnatal months or adult β-globin after the first few postnatal months. Results of embryologic studies suggest that primitive and definitive erythropoiesis arises from different stem cells in the early embryo (2,3,5,6). The primitive erythroid cells arise in the inner cell mass of the yolk sac blood islands whereas the definitive erythroid cells arise from the aortogonadomesonephros region of the mesoderm.

Current concepts of hematopoiesis are derived from studies involving mainly two species— mice and humans. These studies have included direct morphologic and immunologic analyses of cells in hematopoietic tissues, in vitro culture of hematopoietic progenitor cells and hematopoietic stromal cells, transplantation studies with hematopoietic cells, and genetic studies of mice with natural mutations, transgene expressions, or targeted gene knockouts. These studies have led to a hematopoietic model (Fig. 2.1) that applies to postnatal as well as prenatal hematopoiesis because turnover of both blood and immune cells requires new cell production throughout life (7). In this model, pluripotent hematopoietic stem cells (HSC), which have an incidence in bone marrow of one per 10^4 to 10^5 nucleated cells, have two functions—self-replication and production of progenitor cells committed to differentiation into all lymphoid and myeloid cell types. Hematopoietic stem cells appear to be immediate progeny of an even more primitive stem cell, the hemangioblast, which can give rise to both hematopoietic cells and vascular cells during embryonic development (8). If hemangioblasts persist into post-

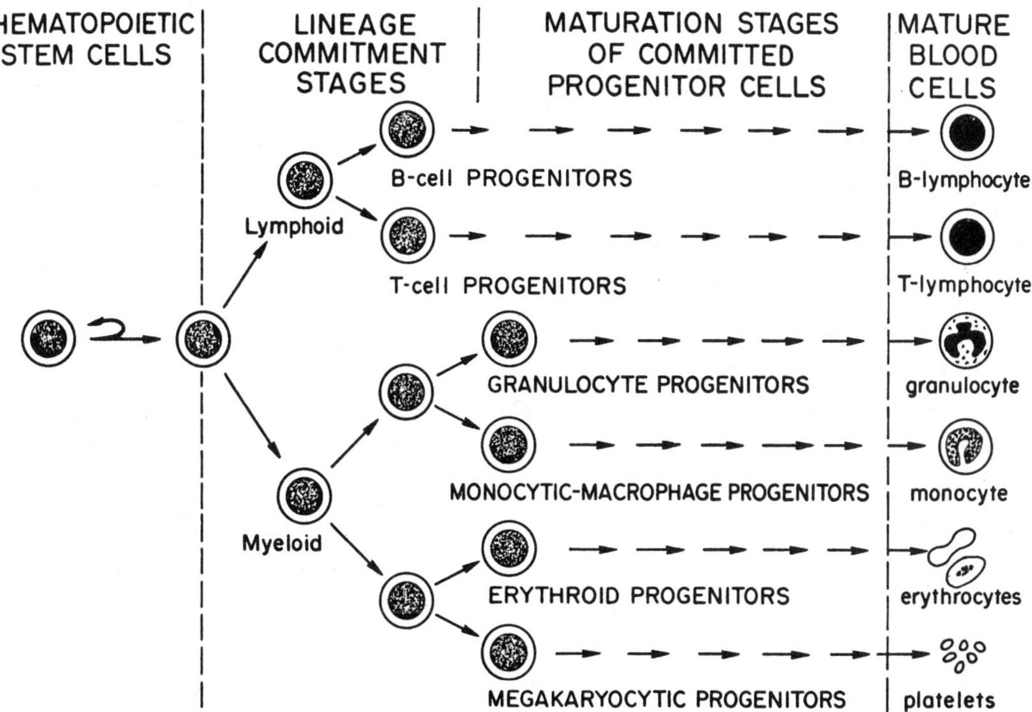

FIGURE 2.1. Hematopoietic stem cell differentiation. Pluripotent hematopoietic stem cels (HSC) can self-replicate (*curved arrow*) and give rise to progenitor cells committed to differentiation. Because of uncertainty about events leading to commitment and about self-replication of HSC around the time of commitment, a hypothetical cell has been placed at the border between the HSC and lineage commitment stages. Progeny of HSC become committed to differentiation along specific cell lineages. After lineage commitment, progenitor cells mature and acquire the characteristics of terminally differentiated cells in blood (e.g., erythroid cells produce hemoglobin and enucleate). During this maturation phase, lineage-specific hematopoietic growth factors act on progenitor cells. The stages of HSC differentiation are shown, but the proliferation that accompanies the differentiation is not. Proliferative potential decreases as cells progress through various stages toward mature blood cells. (From *News in Physiological Sciences* 1993;8:171, with permission.)

natal life, they may help maintain the numbers of HSC in addition to self-replication of HSC. However, the postnatal existence and function of hemangioblasts remain to be proved.

Differentiation of HSC requires a process called *commitment* in which the stem cell loses self-renewal capacity and its fate becomes limited to either further differentiation or death. Further differentiation involves cellular proliferation and additional commitment steps. Commitment at these early stages of differentiation restricts the hematopoietic progenitor cells to differentiation along either the lymphoid or the myeloid pathway and subsequently to the specific, single-cell lineages as shown in Figure 2.1.

Two possible mechanisms of hematopoietic cell commitment are a deterministic one and a stochastic one (1). Most experimental evidence indicates that commitment in hematopoietic cells is stochastic and not deterministic. In the deterministic mechanism, molecules from the cell's environment react with specific receptors on or in the cell and thereby lead to changes in specific gene structure or expression that in turn determine the commitment status of that cell. These environmental molecules can be either soluble growth factors or fixed ligands on other cells or extracellular matrix components in the hematopoietic microenvironment. In the stochastic mechanism, the fate of a hematopoietic cell is determined by the outcome of random intracellular events that change the structure or expression of specific genes (9,10). Two examples of such changes in hematopoietic cells are immunoglobulin gene rearrangement in B-lymphocyte progenitors and binding of specific transcription factors such as TAL-1 or GATA-1 to the promoters of erythroid-specific genes (11, 12). With the stochastic mechanism, environmental signals such as concentrations of a specific hematopoietic growth factor or the interactions with bone marrow stromal cells promote survival or death but do not affect commitment. Thus these environmental factors influence the size of hematopoietic cell populations that have had commitment decisions made by random intracellular events.

Stages of Erythropoiesis

The stages of erythropoiesis beginning at the HSC and extending through the mature erythrocyte are shown in Figure 2.2. Hematopoietic cell transplantation experiments with mice have demonstrated murine bone marrow cells that possess the properties of HSC (13–15). Through analyses of murine HSC and comparisons with human hematopoietic cell populations, a subset of hematopoietic cells that is highly enriched in human HSC can be identified with cellular markers (1,7). This human HSC-enriched population displays the CD34 and CD90 (Thy 1) antigens and has low uptake of rhodamine-123 and weak expression of HLA-DR antigens.

After commitment of HSC progeny to the erythroid lineage, the first stages of differentiation that can be recognized are called *burst-forming units–erythroid* (BFU-E) because they proliferate and differentiate in semisolid tissue culture medium to form large colonies or groups of colonies called *bursts of erythroblasts* (16). Human BFU-E need 2 to 3 weeks of culture to form bursts that contain as many as several thousand erythroblasts. The more immature BFU-E need the longest culture period and form the larger bursts. In some large bursts, megakaryocytes are present and represent the progeny of the erythroid-megakaryocytic progenitor. These very immature BFU-E demonstrate the close relation of the erythroid and megakaryocytic lines.

The next well-defined stage of erythroid development is the *colony-forming unit–erythroid* (CFU-E), which needs only 7 days in vitro to proliferate and differentiate into small colonies, usually composed of up to 64 erythroblasts (17). After the CFU-E stage is the proerythroblast stage, the last erythroid progenitor with a nonspecific morphologic appearance in the differentiation scheme shown in Figure 2.2. The proerythroblast gives rise to the successive stages of the basophilic, polychromatophilic, and orthochromatic erythroblasts that are recognized at light microscopic examination of stained marrow samples. The enucleation of erythroblasts in the orthochromatic stage gives rise to the reticulocytes. The reticulocyte stage lasts only a few days when the cells are very irregular in shape. The cells contain residual organelles, the "reticulum," that allow the cells to be recognized from the more mature erythrocytes.

The final stage of differentiation, the erythrocyte, is achieved after the reticulocytes rid themselves of their residual organelles and remodel their irregular shapes to become uniform biconcave disks. Although these stages of erythroid differentiation are defined physiologically and morphologically, they are part of a continuum that begins with HSC and ends with erythrocytes. Each progenitor cell loses proliferative potential as it differentiates along this continuum until it reaches the late erythroblast stages in which the cells do not divide. Thus between the BFU-E and the CFU-E stages are a series of intermediate stages called *mature burst-forming units,* which need more than 1 week but less than 2 weeks in culture to develop into colonies with sizes intermediate between those of typical erythroid bursts and colonies (18). Similarly, the reticulocyte population has early, intermediate, and late stages of development based on their relative RNA content, which steadily declines with maturation (19).

During the CFU-E stage through the early reticulocyte stages, many of the key proteins that compose the mature erythrocyte are either made or assembled (Fig. 2.2). At the CFU-E proerythroblast stages, both α- and β-spectrin are synthesized, but they are degraded in the cytoplasm rather than becoming associated with the cytoskeleton (20). Glycophorin A is present in the plasma membrane of these cells, but the band 3/anion transporter protein is not made until the basophilic erythroblast stage, and band 4.1 does not begin to accumulate until the polychromatophilic stage. Once the band 3/anion transporter protein is present in the membrane, α- and β-spectrin become membrane associated in the characteristic 1:1 ratio (20). Synthesis of hemoglobin begins as the erythroblasts are making the transition from the basophilic to the polychromatophilic stages. Production of these late proteins of erythroid differentiation, such as hemoglobin, the band 3/anion transporter, and band 4.1, can continue through enucleation and reticulocyte formation because the messenger RNA molecules encoding them and ribosomes and endoplasmic reticulum persist in the newly formed reticulocytes.

Requirements for Normal Erythroid Differentiation

A series of intracellular and extracellular events are needed for successful completion of the erythroid differentiation scheme

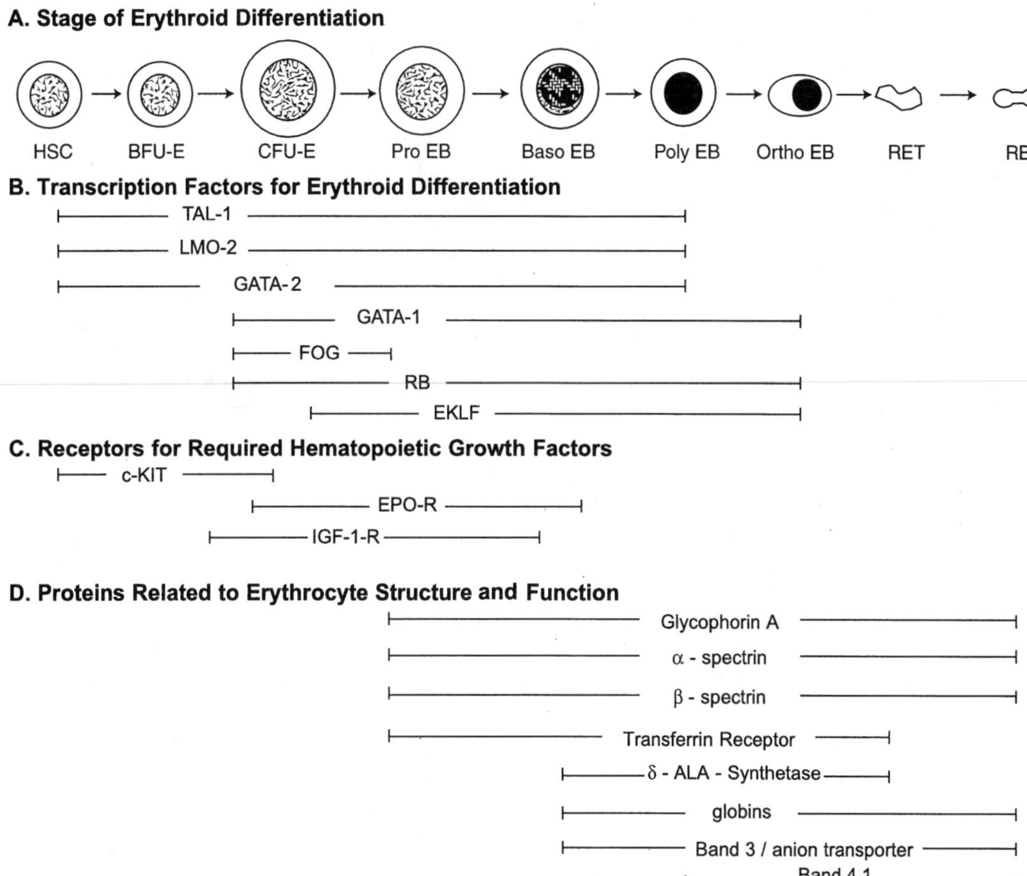

FIGURE 2.2. Cellular events in erythroid differentiation. **A:** The relative sizes and the known or presumed morphologic appearances of erythroid cells at various stages of differentiation—pluripotent hematopoietic stem cell (*HSC*); burst-forming unit–erythroid (*BFU-E*); colony-forming unit–erythroid (*CFU-E*); proerythroblasts (*Pro EB*); basophilic erythroblasts (*Baso EB*); polychromatophilic erythroblasts (*Poly EB*); orthochromatic erythroblasts (*Ortho EB*), reticulocytes (*RET*); erythrocytes (*RBC*). **B:** Erythroid transcription factors—basic helix-loop-helix factor (*TAL-1*); Lim-domain partner of TAL-1 (*LMO-2*); zinc finger factors that bind GATA sequences (*GATA-1, GATA-2*); GATA-1 partner, "friend of GATA" (*FOG*); retinoblastoma protein (*RB*); erythroid Krüppel-like factor (*EKLF*). **C:** Receptors for hematopoietic growth factors—stem cell factor receptor (*c-KIT*); erythropoietin receptor (*EPO-R*); insulin-like growth factor-1 receptor (*IGF-1-R*). **D:** Proteins related to erythrocyte structure and function. Periods of expression for erythroid-specific forms of proteins are shown. Transferrin receptors are present in all stages, but a period of large up-regulation is shown. For each transcription factor, growth factor receptor, and erythrocyte-related protein, the degree of expression can vary greatly during the period shown.

as shown in Figure 2.2. The intracellular events include the expression of (a) general hematopoietic and erythroid-specific transcription factors, (b) receptors for hematopoietic growth factors, and (c) erythroid-specific proteins such as hemoglobin and some membrane and membrane skeleton proteins. Extracellular requirements include (a) the adequate supply of required hematopoietic growth factors, (b) the presence of stromal cell and matrix support, and (c) a sufficient supply of nutrients required for progenitor cell proliferation and differentiation. In Figure 2.2, the transcription factors, growth factor receptors, and hematopoietic growth factors necessary for normal erythropoiesis are shown for the period of differentiation when they are known to be needed. The nutrients that play an important role in erythropoiesis—folate, vitamin B_{12}, and iron—are required at all stages of erythroid cell differentiation, but most importantly in the later stages. Deficiency of any of these three nutrients results in decreased erythrocyte production, and anemia will develop in a patient with a deficiency. These three nutrients and their roles in the erythropoiesis are discussed later.

ERYTHROPOIETIN

Regulation of Erythropoietin Production by Tissue Hypoxia

Although many intracellular and extracellular factors play important roles in the erythropoietic process, the one event that controls the rate of erythrocyte production under normal circumstances is the interaction of EPO with the EPO receptor (EPO-R) on the erythroid progenitor cells. Erythropoietin is a

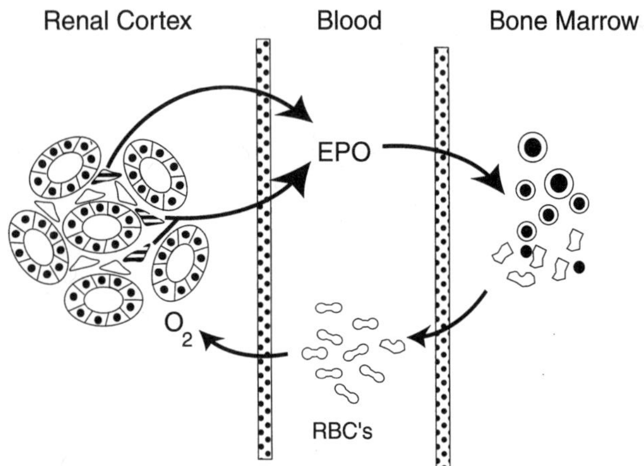

FIGURE 2.3. The oxygenation-erythropoietin (EPO) negative feedback mechanism. The number of circulating erythrocytes (*RBCs*) determines the amount of oxygen (*O_2*) delivered from the lungs to other tissues. In the renal cortex, a specific subset of interstitial cells (*hatched*) produce EPO when they perceive hypoxia. The EPO is immediately secreted into the blood and acts in the bone marrow to prevent the programmed death (apoptosis) of erythroid progenitor cells. Those erythroid progenitors that survive the EPO-dependent period of differentiation mature into reticulocytes (irregularly shaped anucleate cells in marrow and blood) and subsequently into erythrocytes. Increased numbers of erythrocytes resulting from increased plasma EPO levels deliver more oxygen to the kidneys and thereby lower the amount of EPO produced as renal hypoxia is relieved.

30.4-kd glycosylated protein, most of which is produced by the kidneys and a small amount of which is produced by the liver (21). The kidneys are a major component of the oxygenation-EPO negative feedback mechanism shown in Figure 2.3. The other components are the bone marrow, the blood erythrocytes, and EPO itself. The negative feedback characteristics of this mechanism account for the fine control of erythrocyte numbers that occur in each individual. The major determinant of oxygen delivery from the lungs to the peripheral tissues is the number of circulating erythrocytes. When erythrocyte numbers decrease, as occurs with bleeding or hemolysis, oxygen delivery decreases and the peripheral tissues become hypoxic. All tissues experience hypoxia, but the only ones that respond with EPO production are the kidneys and the liver. The same cells that sense hypoxia are the ones that produce EPO (22). The EPO-producing cells sense hypoxia by a mechanism involving a heme-containing protein (23) that in turn leads to induction by posttranslational mechanisms of a specific transcription factor, hypoxia-inducible factor-1 (HIF-1) (24,25). HIF-1 has two components, HIF-1α and HIF-1β, which form a complex that binds to a hypoxia-inducible transcription enhancer located at 120 bp 3′ to the human *EPO* gene polyadenylation signal (26–28) as shown in Figure 2.4B. HIF-1β is constitutively produced, and its intracellular levels are not influenced by hypoxia. HIF-1α also is constitutively produced, but under normoxic conditions, it is essentially undetectable because it is rapidly degraded along a ubiquitin-proteasome pathway (29) (Fig. 2.4A). However, when a cell experiences hypoxia, this rapid degradation ceases and intracellular HIF-1α levels promptly increase (Fig. 2.4B). This posttranslation regulation of HIF-1α levels in the cell is the key component in controlling the assembly of the factor complex that binds to the hypoxia-inducible enhancer and interacts with the promoter region and thereby regulates *EPO* gene transcription (Fig. 2.4B). Components of this complex other than HIF-1 include hepatocyte nuclear factor-4 (HNF-4) and the protein p300 (26–28). HIF-1α can be induced in other cell types that do not produce EPO and can bind to DNA sequences in other genes, including those involved in glucose metabolism and vascular biologic processes. Thus the specificity for EPO production in response to hypoxia is caused by factors other than HIF-1α within the EPO-producing cells. Once hypoxia reaches the threshold that triggers *EPO* transcription, the resultant EPO messenger RNA is translated into the EPO glycoprotein, which is immediately secreted (21). When an individual cell is triggered to produce EPO, it does so in an all-or-none manner (22,30). Thus EPO concentrations in the blood increase sharply within 2 hours after loss of blood, hemolysis, or a sudden decrease in atmospheric oxygen.

In the kidney, the cells that produce EPO are a subset of cortical interstitial cells adjacent to proximal tubules (31,32) and appear to be fibroblasts (33,34) (Fig. 2.3). In mild anemia, small foci of the EPO-producing cells are present in the inner cortex. In moderate anemia, they are present in larger areas within the inner half of the cortex. In severe anemia, they are present throughout the renal cortex (30). These progressive increases in the areas of EPO production in the kidney correspond to increasing areas of renal cortical hypoxia that are a function of oxygen supply from the blood and local oxygen utilization by rapidly metabolizing cells, such as the adjacent proximal tubular epithelium (30,35). Thus the rapid and sharp increase in EPO production after blood loss or hemolysis is not due to an increase in the rate of production by each EPO-producing cell but rather by the recruitment to active EPO production of increased numbers of cells with the potential to produce EPO (30). This increase in the number of cells actively producing EPO is exponential with a linear decrease in hematocrit. It results in a parallel exponential increase in blood plasma EPO levels. This exponential increase in blood EPO levels with a linear decrease in hematocrit is a characteristic of almost all studies except for those involving patients with renal disease (36).

Interaction of Erythropoietin and Erythroid Progenitor Cells

After being secreted, EPO is carried through the blood to the bone marrow, where it binds to a specific transmembrane glycoprotein receptor, the EPO-R (37). The mature, fully glycosylated EPO-R is displayed on the surface of erythroid progenitor cells beginning just before the CFU-E stage and extending through the basophilic erythroblast stage (38,39) (Fig. 2.2). The stages with the most EPO-Rs are the CFU-E and proerythroblasts, which have an average of approximately 1,000 surface receptors (38,39). The EPO-R is structurally homologous with the receptors for a large number of hematopoietic growth factors and cytokines that include granulocyte colony-stimulating factor, granulocyte-macrophage colony-stimulating factor, thrombo-

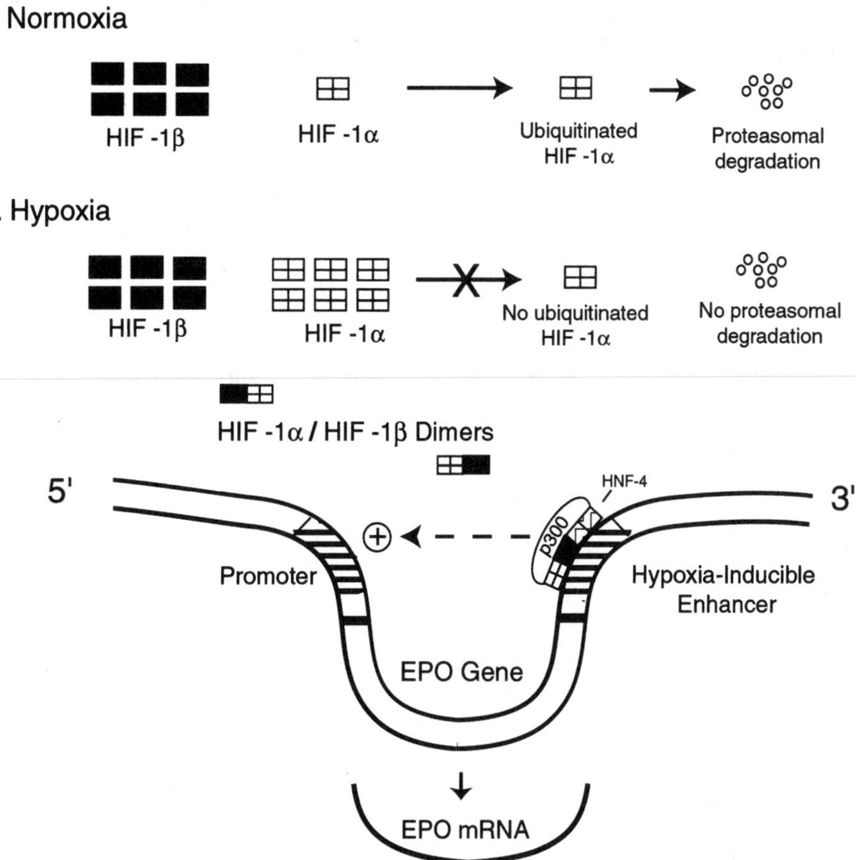

FIGURE 2.4. Induction of erythropoietin (EPO) gene transcription by hypoxia. **A:** In cells capable of producing EPO, the two components of hypoxia-inducible factor (HIF-1α and HIF-1β) are constitutively produced under normoxic conditions; HIF-1α are rapidly ubiquitinated and are degraded in proteasomes, whereas HIF-1β is stable and does not turn over rapidly. As a result, the heterodimers of HIF-1α and HIFβ are constitutively produced. Under normoxic conditions, HIF-1α and HIF-1β that bind to the hypoxia-inducible enhancer 120 bp 3′ to the *EPO* polyadenylation signal are not formed. Thus *EPO* and other genes containing hypoxia-inducible enhancer element are not transcriptionally active. **B:** When EPO-producing cells become hypoxic, HIF-1α is not ubiquitinated and its steady-state concentration increases in the cells. It forms heterodimers with HIF-1β that bind to specific sequences in the hypoxia-inducible enhancer 3′ to the *EPO* gene and to similar sequences in other hypoxia-inducible genes. The HIF-1α/HIF-1β heterodimer is part of a factor complex that includes hepatocyte nuclear factor-4 (HNF-4) and p300. This factor complex binds the 3′ hypoxia-inducible enhancer and increases *EPO* promoter activity with a resultant increase in *EPO* transcription and accumulation of EPO messenger RNA accumulation.

poietin, the interleukins, growth hormone, and prolactin (40). The binding of EPO to the EPO-R leads to three major changes, as follows: (a) dimerization of the EPO-R, (b) initiation of intracellular signaling by the EPO-R, and (c) endocytosis of the EPO/EPO-R complex, which is subsequently proteolyzed (27,38, 41–44). The homodimerization of EPO-R after EPO binding appears to trigger both signaling and endocytosis. This endocytosis and digestion of the EPO/EPO-R complex appears to be the normal mechanism for clearance of EPO from the blood (45).

The EPO receptors, like the other members of their hematopoietic growth factor–cytokine receptor family, have no intrinsic enzyme activity (40). However, like the other family members, EPO-Rs interact with several known signal transduction pathways that alter the phosphorylation state and the enzymatic activities of various intracellular proteins (27,38,41–44). The most studied pathway associated with the EPO-R involves the Janus tyrosine kinase-2 (JAK2) and the signal transduction and activator of transcription-5 (STAT5) proteins. With EPO binding to the EPO-R, JAK2 kinase associates with the cytoplasmic part of the EPO-R resulting in phosphorylation of multiple tyrosines in the cytoplasmic part of the EPO-R. STAT5 also becomes phosphorylated and translocates to the nucleus after EPO binding to the EPO-R. Although experiments with knockout mice confirm the important role of the JAK2/STAT5 pathway in EPO signal transduction, other pathways have been implicated as playing a role in EPO signal transduction. These include the RAS-raf-MAP kinase and the phosphoinositol-3 kinase/Akt kinase (protein kinase B) pathways that lead to specific protein phosphorylations as well as the SHP-1 and SHP-2 phosphatases that lead to specific dephosphorylations in signaling pathways. The exact roles of each of these pathways, including the JAK2/STAT5 pathway are not certain. Further studies are needed of both EPO-dependent cell lines and erythroid progenitor cells from hematopoietic tissues.

Effects of Erythropoietin on Erythroid Progenitor Cells

Three biologic effects on erythroid progenitor cells are possible: (a) stimulation of proliferation, (b) induction of terminal differentiation, and (c) promotion of survival (7,21). Stimulation of proliferation has for the most part been suggested by studies in continuous cell lines and one study with BFU-E (46,47). However, CFU-E, the normal erythroid progenitor that displays the most EPO-Rs, and continuous erythroid cell lines are both in an active proliferative state—most are in the DNA synthesis (S phase) of the cell cycle—and stimulation of proliferation is difficult to discern. Any direct effect of EPO on BFU-E is difficult to confirm because (a) a pure population of these progenitors is difficult to obtain and (b) EPO-Rs have not been found in BFU-E. Induction of terminal differentiation by EPO has been suggested from studies with continuous cell lines. However, cell lines only partially differentiate in response to EPO. Promotion of survival by EPO through the prevention of programmed cell death (apoptosis) has been found in several different systems, including CFU-E from various hematopoietic tissues (48–51), EPO-dependent cell lines (44,46), and knockout mice that are either *EPO* null (52) or *EPO-R* null (53). These studies with CFU-E and proerythroblasts from hematopoietic tissues and in situ examination of *EPO* null or *EPO-R* null mice have shown that the period of dependence on EPO for survival includes CFU-E, proerythroblasts, and basophilic erythroblasts. How EPO signaling results in the prevention of apoptosis is unknown. However, one key modulator of apoptosis in these EPO-dependent erythroid progenitor cells is the antiapoptotic member of the Bcl-2 family of proteins named Bcl-X_L (54,55). Bcl-X_L, which binds the proapoptotic protein Bax, is induced in erythroid progenitors by EPO and reaches extremely high levels in the orthochromatic erythroblasts and reticulocytes (55).

During the period of EPO dependence, individual erythroid cells in the same stage of differentiation from the same hematopoietic tissue display wide variation in degree of dependence on EPO for survival (56). Some of the erythroid cells need very low levels of EPO, such as those in the plasma of patients with chronic renal failure. Other erythroid cells need very high levels of EPO, such as those in patients with acute blood loss or hemolysis. Thus this broad spectrum of EPO requirements covers the more than 1,000-fold range of EPO concentrations in the blood under various physiologic and pathologic conditions. The mechanism responsible for this heterogeneity in EPO dependence is not known, but it does not appear to be due to differences in either the numbers of EPO-Rs or the EPO-binding affinities of EPO-Rs in the dependent progenitors (56).

A model that incorporates the wide range of plasma EPO levels and the wide heterogeneity in EPO dependence among the EPO-responsive cells of the hematopoietic tissues has been proposed to explain the regulation of erythrocyte production by EPO in various physiologic and pathologic conditions (57). In a representation of this model in Figure 2.5, the erythroid progenitor cells enter an EPO-dependent period of differentiation extending from the CFU-E through the early erythroblast stages and encompassing two cell divisions. In Figure 2.5, the proportion of total cells that survive in a generation is shown immediately under the population. The surviving cells in any population are represented by circles, each of which contains a large black dot representing an intact nucleus. The cells lost to apoptosis are shown by circles, each of which contains an *X*. For erythroid cell populations that are proliferating, the number of surviving cells in a generation results in twice that number for the total cells in the subsequent generation. Under normal conditions, the approximately 200 billion erythrocytes produced daily by a healthy adult are the progeny of a minority of all the erythroid progenitor cells that reach the CFU-E stage. Most cells reaching the CFU-E stage need more EPO than the low levels found in normal plasma to sustain them through the EPO-dependent period of differentiation. As a result, under normal conditions most of these cells undergo apoptosis (Fig. 2.5A). However, when anemia or decreased atmospheric oxygen is encountered, the resultant increases in plasma EPO allow the survival of many of EPO-dependent progenitors that would die by apoptosis under normal conditions (Fig. 2.5B). As a result of this enhanced survival, reticulocyte production increases within a few days after blood loss or suddenly decreased atmospheric oxygen. The increased reticulocytosis leads to increasing erythrocyte numbers until oxygen delivery recovers to normal and then plasma EPO levels decline toward normal. In pathologic states of decreased oxygen delivery, such as lung disease or cardiac diseases with right-to-left shunts, the persistently increased EPO levels allow greater than normal survival among the EPO-dependent cells at a sustained rate such that the total number of erythrocytes is maintained in the polycythemic range. On the other hand, when plasma EPO levels fall below normal because of decreased production in the kidneys as occurs in chronic renal disease, some of the erythroid progenitor cells that would survive the EPO-dependent period of differentiation under normal conditions do not survive (Fig. 2.5C).

In patients with renal disease, only the most EPO-sensitive progenitors escape apoptosis and give rise to reticulocytes. The result is anemia due to lower than normal rates of erythrocyte production. The treatment of patients with renal failure with exogenously administered EPO rescues the erythroid progenitor cells that need normal plasma levels of EPO. With this increased survival of erythroid progenitor cells, the rate of erythrocyte production in renal failure becomes closer to normal. Thus administration of EPO in the management of renal disease represents hormonal replacement therapy for an EPO deficiency state. The fourth scenario shown in Figure 2.5D is ineffective erythropoiesis, in which pathologic losses of erythroblasts to apoptosis in addition to the physiologic apoptosis related to EPO levels occurs during and after the period of EPO dependence. In ineffective erythropoiesis, the population of progenitor cells in the EPO-dependent period expand owing to increased EPO levels. The number of reticulocytes formed, however, is less than normal because of the increased rates of pathologic apoptosis in the EPO-dependent and post-EPO-dependent periods of differen-

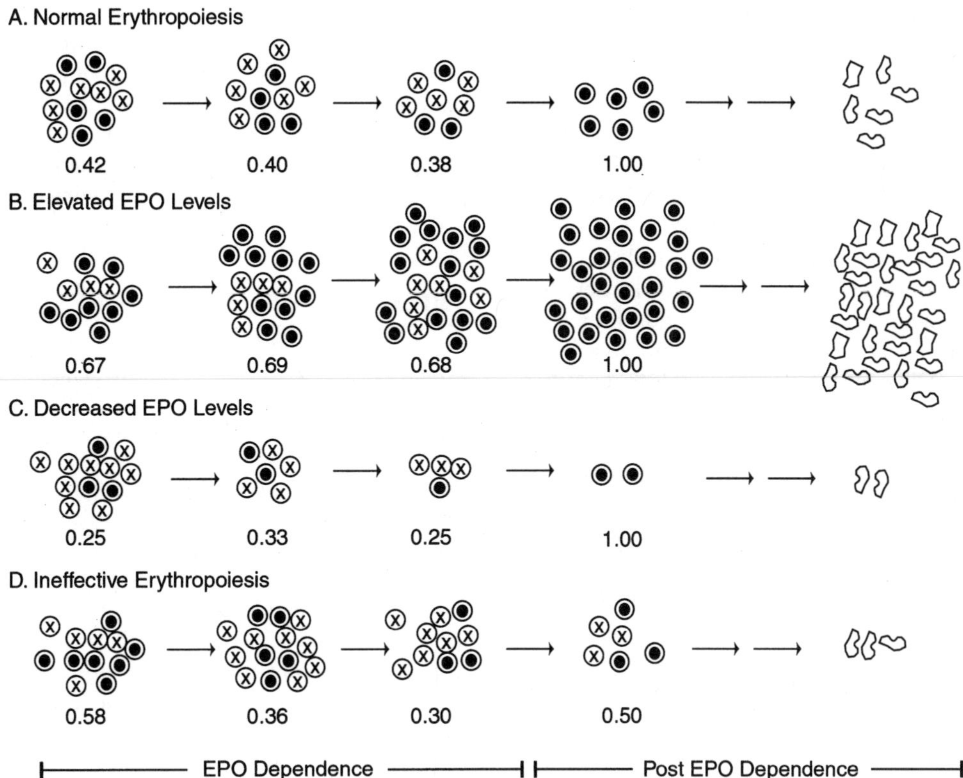

FIGURE 2.5. Model of erythropoiesis from CFU-E through reticulocyte stages based on (a) suppression of programmed cell death (apoptosis) by erythropoietin (EPO) and (b) heterogeneity in the degree of EPO dependence among the erythroid cells. Erythroid progenitors at the CFU-E stage of differentiation enter a period in which they depend on EPO for survival. This period lasts for more than one cell division and ends at the basophilic erythroblast stage. In this scheme, the EPO-dependent period encompasses three generations and two cell divisions. One cell division may occur after the EPO-dependent period (not shown). The surviving cells are shown as *circles* each of which contains a *large black dot* representing an intact nucleus. The proportion of the total cells that survive is shown below each generation. Cells succumbing to apoptosis are shown as *circles,* each of which contains an *X*. For erythroid cell populations that are proliferating, the number of surviving cells in a generation results in double that number for the total cells in the subsequent generation. **A:** Normal erythropoiesis with an average survival rate of 40% in each of the EPO-dependent generations. Normal EPO levels result in erythropoiesis with a daily production of 200 billion new erythrocytes, but only a minority of all potential cells survive the EPO-dependent period. **B:** Elevated EPO levels as found after acute blood loss or hemolysis with an average survival rate of 68% in each EPO-dependent generation. Daily erythrocyte production is increased five-fold above normal. **C:** Decreased EPO levels as found in renal failure with an average survival rate of 28% in each EPO-dependent generation. Daily erythrocyte production is one third of normal. **D:** Ineffective erythropoiesis with high EPO levels but increased rates of apoptosis due to a pathologic process such as folate or vitamin B_{12} deficiency. The high EPO levels expand the population in the EPO-dependent generations, but the increased rate of apoptosis due to folate or vitamin B_{12} deficiency results in relatively decreased survival rates. Daily erythrocyte production is one half of the normal rate. The apoptosis in the post EPO-dependent period is totally due to the pathologic process. In severe thalassemia (not shown), ineffective erythropoiesis is even more exaggerated in that almost all of the apoptosis occurs in the post-EPO-dependent period with enormously expanded EPO-dependent generations.

tiation. Common examples of ineffective erythropoiesis are megaloblastic anemia and thalassemia.

NUTRITIONAL REQUIREMENTS FOR ERYTHROPOIESIS

Although erythropoiesis is finely regulated by the oxygenation-EPO feedback mechanism shown in Figure 2.3, the erythropoietic process is frequently limited by an insufficient supply of three essential nutrients. These nutrients are folate, vitamin B_{12}, and iron. Although all proliferating cell populations need folate and vitamin B_{12}, the large numbers of erythrocytes that must be produced each day results in a large DNA synthesis requirement for erythropoiesis. Although iron also is needed by all proliferating cell populations, the erythroblasts need much more iron than any other cell type because they produce hemoglobin. When any of these three nutrients is not present in sufficient amounts for the differentiation of the erythroid cell population of the bone marrow, production of erythrocytes decreases, and anemia occurs. Through the hypoxia feedback mechanism, this anemia increases EPO production (36). Elevated levels of EPO can only partially compensate for the decreased erythropoiesis caused by the specific nutrient deficiency. Administration of the deficient nutrient, however, results in resolution of anemia in each of the deficiency states.

Folate deficiency results in decreased intracellular levels of all folate coenzymes in the erythroid progenitor cells. Deficiency of vitamin B_{12} results in trapping of folate in the methyltetrahydrofolate form, making it unavailable in the methylenetetrahydrofolate form required for thymidine synthesis or the formyltetrahydrofolate form required for purine synthesis (58). As a result, vitamin B_{12} deficiency, like folate deficiency, leads to decreased intracellular levels of the specific folate coenzymes needed for de novo synthesis of all of the deoxynucleotides used in DNA synthesis, except for deoxycytidine (59). The inability to synthesize DNA caused by an inadequate supply of thymidine and purines causes accumulation of erythroid progenitors in the S phase of the cell cycle, which appears to be rapidly followed by the induction of apoptosis (60,61). The stages of erythroid differentiation that appear to be most susceptible to this apoptosis are the end of the EPO-dependent stage and the beginning of the period of hemoglobin synthesis. EPO-induced expansion of the EPO-dependent population at the CFU-E and proerythroblast stages leads to the presence of even greater numbers of these progenitor cells that subsequently undergo apoptosis just as they are beginning to produce hemoglobin (62). The resultant clinical disease is megaloblastic anemia. The prominent feature of megaloblastic anemia is ineffective erythropoiesis (Fig. 2.5D) characterized by increased numbers of CFU-E with decreased numbers of reticulocytes and by enhanced death between these two stages as indicated by increases in iron turnover, serum bilirubin, and serum lactate dehydrogenase.

The mechanism of decreased erythropoiesis in iron deficiency is not as clear as it is in the case of folate or vitamin B_{12} deficiency. Although the life span of erythrocytes may be slightly shortened in patients with iron deficiency, the main cause of anemia is a decreased rate of erythrocyte production relative to the degree of anemia. Iron uptake by the erythroid progenitor cells is greatest just before hemoglobin synthesis (63), during the period of EPO dependence and coinciding with the greatest rate of cell proliferation during erythropoiesis. During iron deficiency anemia, the levels of EPO in the blood are elevated (36) and the number of CFU-E in the hematopoietic organs are increased while the numbers of erythroblasts in all stages are decreased compared with normal (64). These results suggest some ineffective erythropoiesis in the erythroblast stage of differentiation is present during iron deficiency. Indirect measurement of ineffective erythropoiesis by means of ferrokinetics or rates of bilirubin formation indicate some turnover of erythroblasts in iron deficiency anemia but not to the degree found in comparable anemia due to folate or vitamin B_{12} deficiency or thalassemia (65,66). When iron-deficient erythroid progenitor cells are compared with their normal, iron-replete counterparts, no effect on the proliferative state or distribution of cell cycle phases has been found (64,67). Although the rate of cell division may not play a role in iron deficiency anemia, retardation of maturation may play a role in that erythrocytes produced during iron deficiency have smaller volumes and lesser amounts of hemoglobin than normal. The increased levels of free intracellular protoporphyrin in iron deficiency indicate the limiting factor is the iron needed to form heme and subsequently hemoglobin. Thus in iron deficiency, several mechanisms contribute to the development of anemia, including ineffective erythropoiesis, retarded maturation of late-stage erythroblasts, and a shortened life span of circulating erythrocytes.

INFLUENCE OF PATHOLOGIC STATES ON ERYTHROPOIESIS

The erythropoietic process can be influenced by diseases that are intrinsic to the erythropoietic cells or that secondarily affect the erythropoietic cells. Among the intrinsic diseases are several that decrease the number of erythropoietic cells. These include myelodysplasia, myeloid leukemia, aplastic anemia, pure red cell aplasia, and Fanconi anemia. Increased apoptosis of hematopoietic cells or failure to differentiate, in the case of acute leukemia, are considered the mechanisms of population reduction in these diseases. On the other hand, polycythemia vera results in increased numbers of erythropoietic progenitor cells that have an increased sensitivity to EPO (68) and insulin-like growth factor-1 (69). This increased sensitivity to a trophic hematopoietic growth factor is presumed to be due to an enhanced intracellular signaling mechanism present in all myeloid cell lineages in polycythemia vera. Thus in patients with polycythemia vera, the erythroid progenitor cells in the EPO-dependent stages survive much better than do normal progenitors in the lower-than-normal EPO levels in polycythemia vera patients.

Diseases that can secondarily decrease erythropoiesis include those that directly displace the hematopoietic cells in the bone marrow, such as metastatic neoplasms, lymphoid neoplasms, and myelofibrosis. However, the most common cause of secondary inhibition of erythropoiesis is anemia of chronic disease. This anemia occurs in chronic infections, neoplasms, and inflammatory diseases and appears to be the result of direct and indirect effects of inflammatory cytokines on the erythropoietic cells (70, 71). Like iron deficiency, anemia of chronic disease has been shown to have multiple mechanisms that play a role in pathogenesis. These include increased sequestration of iron by macrophages, inflammatory cytokine-mediated decreases in both EPO production in the kidneys (relative to the degree of anemia), and suppression of erythroid cell growth by the inflammatory cytokines such as interferon-γ, tissue necrosis factor-α, and interleukin-1 (70,71). In addition to this inhibition of erythropoietic cell growth, some increased apoptosis of erythropoietic cells may result from the decrease in EPO level or the direct effects of the inflammatory cytokines. Although these forms of anemia may partially respond to exogenously administered EPO, resolution requires the effective treatment of the primary disease responsible for increased cytokine production.

SUMMARY

Erythropoiesis is a component of the larger process of hematopoiesis, in which a pluripotent HSC gives rise through proliferation and differentiation to all the mature cells of the blood and the immune system. Within the erythroid differentiation process, the rate of erythrocyte production is regulated by EPO. EPO acts by increasing the number of erythroid progenitors that can survive during a specific period when they are dependent on EPO for the prevention of apoptosis. Levels of EPO are controlled by oxygen delivery and utilization in the renal cortex, where hypoxia induces EPO production. This oxygen-EPO feedback mechanism results in finely controlled rates of erythrocyte production. This mechanism responds promptly to physiologic changes such as blood loss or changes in atmospheric oxygen. In pathologic conditions, it provides compensatory changes in the rates of erythrocyte production that partially correct the abnormal oxygen delivery to the peripheral tissues. Although the use of EPO in clinical medicine is now routine for patients with the anemia of renal disease, further research is needed to understand the molecular mechanisms involved in the production of EPO in response to hypoxia and the intracellular signaling by the EPO-R that leads to increased erythroid cell survival. Understanding of these EPO-related mechanisms will facilitate investigations into the effects of deficiencies of nutrients such as iron, folate, and vitamin B_{12}, which are needed for normal erythropoiesis. Knowledge about these EPO-related mechanisms will also help in studies of disorders caused by abnormal rates of erythrocyte production, such as polycythemia vera, myelodysplasia, and anemia of chronic disease.

REFERENCES

1. Bondurant MC, Koury MJ. Origin and development of blood cells. In: Lee GR, Foerster R, Lukens J, et al, eds. *Wintrobe's clinical hematology,* 10th ed. Baltimore: Williams & Wilkins, 1998;145–168.
2. Tavian M, Coulombel L, Luton D, et al. Aorta-associated CD34+ hematopoietic cells in the early human embryo. *Blood* 1996;87:67–72.
3. Dzierzak E, Medvinsky A. Mouse embryonic hematopoiesis. *Trends Genet* 1995;11:359–366.
4. Palis J, Segel GB. Developmental biology of erythropoiesis. *Blood Rev* 1998;12:106–114.
5. Zon LI. Developmental biology of hematopoiesis. *Blood* 1995;86: 2876–2891.
6. Ciau-Uitz A, Walmsley M, Patient R. Distinct origins of adult and embryonic blood in *Xenopus. Cell* 2000;102:787–796.
7. Koury MJ, Bauer C. Hematopoiesis and the red blood cell. In: Greger R, Windhorst U, eds. *Comprehensive human physiology.* Berlin: Springer-Verlag 1996;1679–1693.
8. Jaffredo T, Gautier R, Eichmann A, et al. Intraaortic hematopoietic cells are derived from endothelial cells during ontogeny. *Development* 1998;125:4575–4583.
9. Till JE, McCulloch EA, Siminovich L. A stochastic model of stem cell proliferation, based on the growth of spleen colony-forming cells. *Proc Natl Acad Sci U S A* 1964;51:29–36.
10. Ogawa M, Porter PN, Nakahata T. Renewal and commitment to differentiation of hemopoietic stem cells: an interpretive review. *Blood* 1983; 61:823–829.
11. Sieweke MH, Graf T. A transcription factor party during blood cell differentiation. *Curr Opin Genet Dev* 1998;8:545–551.
12. Orkin SH. Diversification of haematopoietic stem cells to specific lineages. *Nat Rev Genet* 2000;1:57–64.
13. Jordan CT, Lemischka IR. Clonal and systemic analysis of long-term hematopoiesis in the mouse. *Genes Dev* 1990;4:220–232.
14. Capel B, Hawley RG, Mintz B. Long- and short-lived murine hematopoietic stem cell clones individually identified with retroviral integration markers. *Blood* 1990;75:2267–2270.
15. Keller G, Snodgrass R. Life span of multipotential hematopoietic stem cells in vivo. *J Exp Med* 1990;171:1407–1418.
16. Axelrad AA, McLeod DL, Shreeve MM, et al. Properties of cells that produce erythrocytic colonies in vitro. In: Robinson WA, ed. *Proceedings of the Second International Workshop on Hematopoiesis in Culture.* DHEW publication no. NIH 74-205 1974;226–234.
17. Stephenson JR, Axelrad AA, McLeod DL, et al. Induction of colonies of hemoglobin-synthesizing cells by erythropoietin in vitro. *Proc Natl Acad Sci U S A* 1971;68:1542–1546.
18. Gregory CJ, Eaves AC. Three stages of erythropoietic progenitor cell differentiation distinguished by a number of physical and biologic properties. *Blood* 1978;51:527–537.
19. Brugnara C. Reticulocyte cellular indices: a new approach in the diagnosis of anemias and monitoring of erythropoietic function. *Crit Rev Clin Lab Sci* 2000;37:93–130.
20. Koury MJ, Bondurant MC, Rana SS. Changes in erythroid membrane proteins during erythropoietin-mediated terminal differentiation. *J Cell Physiol* 1987;133:438–448.
21. Koury MJ, Bondurant MC. The molecular mechanism of erythropoietin action. *Eur J Biochem* 1992;210:649–663.
22. Goldberg MA, Glass GA, Cunningham JM, et al. The regulated expression of erythropoietin by two human hepatoma cell lines. *Proc Natl Acad Sci U S A* 1987;84:7972–7976.
23. Goldberg MA, Dunning SP, Bunn HF. Regulation of the erythropoietin gene: evidence that the oxygen sensor is a heme protein. *Science* 1988;242:1412–1415.
24. Beck I, Weinmann R, Caro J. Characterization of hypoxia-responsive enhancer in the human erythropoietin gene shows presence of hypoxia-inducible 120-Kd nuclear DNA-binding protein in erythropoietin-producing and nonproducing cells. *Blood* 1993;82:704–711.
25. Wang GL, Semenza GL. Characterization of hypoxia-inducible factor 1 and regulation of DNA binding activity by hypoxia. *J Biol Chem* 1993;268:21513–21518.
26. Semenza GL. Regulation of erythropoietin production. *Hematol Oncol Clin North Am* 1994;8:863–884.
27. Lacombe C, Mayeux P. Biology of erythropoietin. *Haematologica* 1998; 83:724–732.
28. Ebert BL, Bunn HF. Regulation of the erythropoietin gene. *Blood* 1999;94:1864–1877.
29. Salceda S, Caro J. Hypoxia-inducible factor 1 alpha (HIF-1 alpha) protein is rapidly degraded by the ubiquitin-proteasome system under normoxic conditions: its stabilization by hypoxia depends on redox-induced changes. *J Biol Chem* 1997;272:22642–22647.
30. Koury ST, Koury MJ, Bondurant MC, et al. Quantitation of erythropoietin-producing cells in kidneys of mice by in situ hybridization: correlation with hematocrit, renal erythropoietin mRNA and serum erythropoietin concentration. *Blood* 1989;74:645–651.
31. Koury ST, Bondurant MC, Koury MJ. Localization of erythropoietin synthesizing cells in murine kidneys by in situ hybridization. *Blood* 1988;71:524–527.
32. Lacombe C, DaSilva JL, Bruneval P, et al. Peritubular cells are the site of erythropoietin synthesis in the murine hypoxic kidney. *J Clin Invest* 1988;81:620–623.
33. Bachmann S, LeHir M, Eckardt KU. Co-localization of erythropoietin mRNA and ecto-5′-nucleotidase immunoreactivity in peritubular cells of rat renal cortex indicates that fibroblasts produce erythropoietin. *J Histochem Cytochem* 1993;41:335–341.
34. Maxwell PH, Osmond MK, Pugh CW, et al. Identification of the renal erythropoietin-producing cells using transgenic mice. *Kidney Int* 1993; 44:1149–1162.
35. Bauer C. Physiologic determinants of erythropoietin production. *Semin Hematol* 1991;28[Suppl 3]:9–13.
36. Erslev AJ. Erythropoietin. *N Engl J Med* 1991;324:1339–1344.
37. D'Andrea AD, Lodish HF, Wong GG. Expression cloning of murine erythropoietin receptor. *Cell* 1989;57:277–285.
38. Sawyer ST, Penta K. Erythropoietin cell biology. *Hematol Oncol Clin North Am* 1994;8:895–911.
39. Youssoufian H, Longmore G, Neumann D, et al. Structure, function, and activation of the erythropoietin receptor. *Blood* 1993;81: 2223–2236.

40. Bazan JF. Haemopoietic receptors and helical cytokines. *Immunol Today* 1990;11:350–354.
41. Damen JE, Krystal G. Early events in erythropoietin-induced signaling. *Exp Hematol* 1996;24:1455–1459.
42. Klingmuller U. The role of phosphorylation in proliferation and maturation of erythroid progenitor cells. *Eur J Biochem* 1997;249:637–647.
43. Wojchowski DM, Gregory RC, Miller CP, et al. Signal transduction in the erythropoietin receptor system. *Exp Cell Res* 1999;253:143–156.
44. Sawyer ST, Jacobs-Helber SM. Unraveling distinct intracellular signals that promote survival and proliferation: study of erythropoietin, stem cell factor, and constitutive signaling in leukemic cells. *J Hematother Stem Cell Res* 2000;9:21–29.
45. Cazzola M, Guarnone R, Cerani P, et al. Red blood cell precursor mass as an independent determinant of serum erythropoietin level. *Blood* 1998;91:2139–2145.
46. Spivak JL, Pham T, Isaacs M, et al. Erythropoietin is both a mitogen and a survival factor. *Blood* 1991;77:1228–1233.
47. Dessypris EN, Krantz SB. Effect of pure erythropoietin on DNA synthesis by human marrow day 15 erythroid burst-forming units in short-term liquid culture. *Br J Haematol* 1984;56:295–306.
48. Koury MJ, Bondurant MC. Erythropoietin retards DNA breakdown and prevents programmed death in erythroid progenitor cells. *Science* 1990;248:378–381.
49. Boyer SH, Bishop TR, Rogers OC, et al. Roles of erythropoietin, insulin-like growth factor 1, and unidentified serum factors in promoting maturation of purified murine erythroid colony-forming units. *Blood* 1992;80:2503–2512.
50. Yu H, Bauer G, Lipke GK, et al. Apoptosis and hematopoiesis in murine fetal liver. *Blood* 1993;81:373–384.
51. Muta K, Krantz SB. Apoptosis of human erythroid colony-forming cells is decreased by stem cell factor and insulin-like growth factor-1 as well as erythropoietin. *J Cell Physiol* 1993;156:264–271.
52. Wu H, Liu X, Jaenisch R, et al. Generation of committed erythroid BFU-E and CFU-E progenitors does not require erythropoietin or the erythropoietin receptor. *Cell* 1995;83:59–67.
53. Lin CS, Lim SK, D'Agati V, et al. Differential effects of an erythropoietin receptor gene disruption on primative and definitive erythropoiesis. *Genes Dev* 1996;10:154–164.
54. Silva M, Grillot D, Benito A, et al. Erythropoietin can promote erythroid progenitor survival by repressing apoptosis through Bcl-XL and Bcl-2. *Blood* 1996;88:1576–1582.
55. Gregoli PA, Bondurant MC. The roles of Bcl-xL and apopain in the control of erythropoiesis by erythropoietin. *Blood* 1997;90:630–640.
56. Kelley LL, Koury MJ, Bondurant MC, et al. Survival or death of individual proerythroblasts resulting from differing erythropoietin sensitivities: a mechanism for controlled rates of erythrocyte production. *Blood* 1993;82:2340–2352.
57. Koury MJ, Bondurant MC. Control of erythrocyte production: the roles of programmed cell death (apoptosis) and erythropoietin. *Transfusion* 1990;30:673–674.
58. Herbert V, Zalusky R. Interrelations of vitamin B_{12} and folic acid metabolism: folic acid clearance studies. *J Clin Invest* 1962;41:1263–1276.
59. Shane B, Stokstad ELR. Vitamin B_{12}–folate interrelationships. *Annu Rev Nutr* 1985;5:115–141.
60. Koury MJ, Price JO, Hicks GG. Apoptosis in megaloblastic anemia occurs during DNA synthesis by a p53-independent, nucleoside-reversible mechanism. *Blood* 2000;96:3249–3255.
61. Koury MJ, Horne DW. Apoptosis mediates and thymidine prevents erythroblast destruction in folate deficiency anemia. *Proc Natl Acad Sci U S A* 1994;91:4067–4071.
62. Koury MJ, Horne DW, Brown ZA, et al. Apoptosis of late stage erythroblasts in megaloblastic anemia: association with DNA damage and macrocyte production. *Blood* 1997;89:4617–4623.
63. Sawyer ST, Krantz SB. Transferrin receptor number, synthesis, and endocytosis during erythropoietin-induced maturation of Friend virus-infected erythroid cells. *J Biol Chem* 1986;261:9187–9195.
64. Kimura H, Finch CA, Adamson JW. Hematopoiesis in the rat: quantitation of hematopoietic progenitors and the response to iron deficiency anemia. *J Cell Physiol* 1986;126:298–306.
65. Finch CA, Deubelbeiss K, Cook JD, et al. Ferrokinetics in man. *Medicine (Baltimore)* 1970;49:17–53.
66. Robinson SH. Increased formation of early-labeled bilirubin in rats with iron deficiency anemia: evidence for ineffective erythropoiesis. *Blood* 1969;33:909–917.
67. Wickramasinghe SN, Cooper EH, Chalmers DG. A study of erythropoiesis by combined morphologic, quantitative cytochemical and autoradiographic methods. *Blood* 1968;31:304–313.
68. Eaves CJ, Eaves AC. Erythropoietin (Ep) dose-response curves for three classes of erythroid progenitors in normal human marrow and in patients with polycythemia vera. *Blood* 1978;52:1196–1210.
69. Correa PN, Eskinazi D, Axelrad AA. Circulating erythroid progenitors in polycythemia vera are hypersensitive to insulin-like growth factor-1 in vitro: studies in an improved serum-free medium. *Blood* 1994;83:99–112.
70. Means RT, Jr. Pathogenesis of the anemia of chronic disease: a cytokine-mediated anemia. *Stem Cells* 1995;13:32–37.
71. Weiss G. Iron and anemia of chronic disease. *Kidney Int* 1999;55[Suppl 69]:S12–S17.

Rossi's Principles of Transfusion Medicine, Third Edition, edited by Toby L. Simon, Walter H. Dzik, Edward L. Snyder, Christopher P. Stowell, and Ronald G. Strauss. Lippincott Williams & Wilkins, Philadelphia © 2002.

3

HEMOGLOBIN SYNTHESIS, STRUCTURE, AND OXYGEN TRANSPORT

ROBERT D. WOODSON

Central to oxygen and carbon dioxide transport by blood is the respiratory pigment hemoglobin. Hemoglobin is a tetrameric protein. Each subunit is composed of globin, an unbranched chain of amino acid residues, and heme, a tetrapyrrole ring with a central iron atom.

HEMOGLOBIN BIOSYNTHESIS

Globin Synthesis

Synthesis of globin chains depends on transcription of precursor messenger RNA (mRNA) for globin from genomic DNA in the erythroid nucleus. This is followed by processing of the mRNA molecule to mature cytoplasmic mRNA and translation of the mature mRNA to produce globin molecules. A wealth of information about these various steps has been accumulated in recent years (1–3), and this complex process is only briefly described in this chapter.

Figure 3.1 shows the organization of the globin genes in humans. The genes for β, γ, δ, and ϵ globin (collectively called the *β-globin-like gene cluster* or the *non-α-globin gene cluster*) are located on chromosome 11. The genes for α and ζ globin (collectively called the *α-globin gene cluster*) are located on chromosome 16. Of great importance for regulation of globin (and other) gene transcription are a variety of specific, highly conserved DNA sequences a short distance upstream and downstream from each gene and, in some cases, within an intron of the gene. They are the promoters, enhancers, insulators, and silencers. These loci, called *cis*-acting elements, are binding sites for a number of *trans*-acting factors, which are nuclear protein products of remote genes. Each globin gene is flanked by such regulatory elements. For example, Figure 3.2 shows the *trans*-acting factors associated with the promoter for the β-globin gene. These factors bind to defined loci. Although there are similarities, each gene has its own specific set of regulatory sequences and accompanying mix of *trans*-acting factors (2).

Relatively far (5 to 25 kb) upstream from the β-globin gene cluster is the locus control region (LCR), a separate complex of important binding sites for *trans*-acting factors. The LCR comprises at least five separate domains, called *HS-1, HS-2,* and so on. Each contains a number of binding sites for various factors. The LCR, however, differs in several respects from regulatory sequences that flank each gene. First, its function is essential for transcription of all of the globin genes on this chromosome. Thus its deletion, whether naturally occurring, as in certain forms of thalassemia, or experimental, drastically reduces or totally silences all β-globin genes. Second, the LCR remains functional when its location is experimentally varied in relation to the gene cluster. Third, the LCR is required for significant expression of novel genes inserted into erythroid cells. Finally,

R.D. Woodson: Section of Hematology, Department of Medicine, University of Wisconsin–Madison, Madison, Wisconsin.

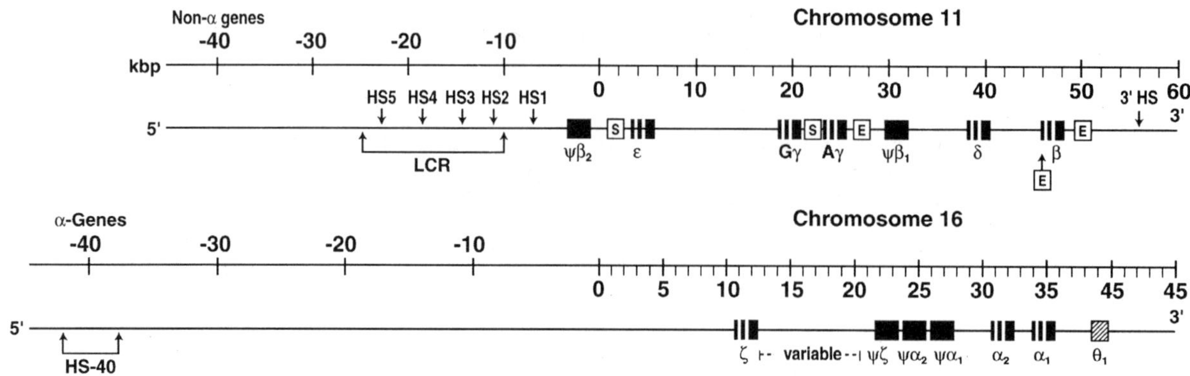

FIGURE 3.1. Map of human chromosomes. ζ- and α-globin genes are located on chromosome 16, whereas ϵ-, γ-, δ-, and β-globin genes are located on chromosome 11. Genes preceded by the letter ψ are functionless pseudogenes bearing structural homology to their namesakes. The θ_1 gene on chromosome 16 is transcribed but not translated. *Open areas* within each gene represent intervening sequences or introns. *Filled areas* represent exons. *E* and *S* symbolize the presence of enhancer and silencer sequences, as well as insulators, which are present at various points throughout the gene cluster. A promoter sequence (not shown) is located immediately upstream from each gene. Each normal hemoglobin type (Table 3.2) comprises one gene product from chromosome 16 and one from chromosome 11.

and most significantly, the LCR is essential for high-level expression, copy number dependent, of human β-globin genes in transgenic mice (4–6). A distant (40 kb) upstream regulatory complex on chromosome 11, called *HS-40,* serves a somewhat similar function for the α-globin gene cluster. Its deletion largely silences α-gene expression, and it is required for expression of *trans* genes; however, it differs from the β-globin LCR in a number of other respects.

A host of *trans*-acting factors bind to these nearby and distant regulatory domains. Of special note are GATA-1, friend of GATA (FOG) and erythroid Krüppel-like factor (EKLF). All are quite specific regulators of hematopoietic cell function with little or no expression or known function in nonhematopoietic tissues. It is clear from knockout experiments that each is indispensable for expression of globin, death from anemia during fetal life otherwise occurring (7–10). Some ubiquitous factors such as XH-2 also are essential for transcription. Other *trans*-acting factors, some essentially restricted to hematopoietic tissue (AP-1/NF-E2 and related family proteins, basic Krüppel-like factor (BKLF), possibly others (11–16)), and some ubiquitous, probably modulate globin transcriptional control, but none is currently known to be absolutely essential for globin gene expression (2,17).

It is now quite clear that this system of regulatory domains and various binding factors constitutes an elaborate control system for gene expression that accounts for both tissue-specific gene expression and the timing and level of expression. Exactly how these distant and nearby domains and related binding factors interact to activate and modulate gene transcription is the subject of intense study. A variety of physical models (DNA looping, DNA tracking through translocation, long-range DNA topology-related interactions) have been proposed to explain how the remote and nearby sequences collaborate to initiate (or de-repress) transcription, but none is able to account for all experimental data (11,18–20). In short, at this point in time, the interactions among these factors and their target sequences represent a three-dimensional jigsaw puzzle—capable of producing not one but multiple pictures–that is just beginning to take

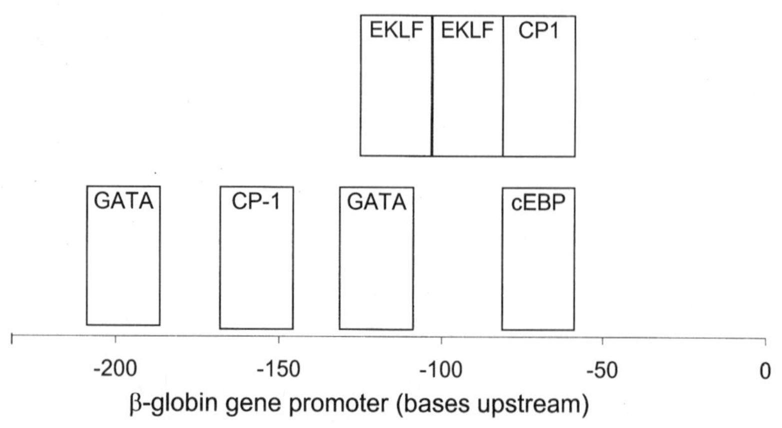

FIGURE 3.2. Diagram shows the β-globin gene promoter and implicated *trans*-acting factors and their binding sites. (Adapted from Stamatoyannopoulos G, Grosveld F. Hemoglobin switching. In: *The molecular basis of blood diseases.* Stamatoyannopoulos G, Majerus PW, Perlmutter RM, et al., eds. Philadelphia: WB Saunders, 2001:135–182, with permission.)

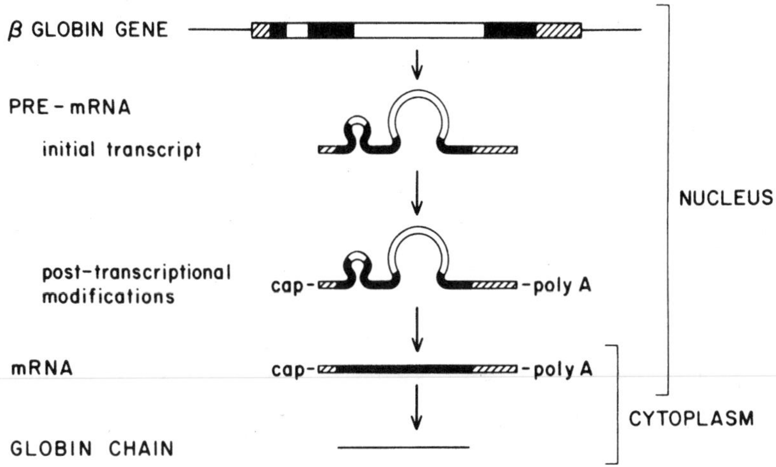

FIGURE 3.3. Overview of globin chain production. *Blackened areas* of the gene and mRNA transcripts contain the codes for the amino acid sequences of the protein. (From Bunn HF, Forget BG. *Hemoglobin: molecular, genetic and clinical aspects.* Philadelphia: WB Saunders, 1986:177, with permission.)

shape. A similarly complex control system is believed to regulate transcription of many other erythroid enzymes.

Once initiated, transcription of a globin (or other) gene entails the formation by RNA polymerase of a completely complementary RNA molecule, called *precursor mRNA,* in the nucleus (Fig. 3.3). This mRNA transcript contains many more triplets than the number of amino acids appearing in the final protein. It extends 41 to 57 bases upstream beyond the 5′ end of the portion of DNA that codes for the particular globin. It also extends 91 to 135 bases downstream (in the 3′ direction) beyond the structural portion and is fitted at the end with a tail of 100 or more adenylic acid residues, the poly(A) tail.

This precursor mRNA then undergoes a series of important modifications called *processing.* By a process called *capping,* its 5′ end is fitted with two or three specific nucleotides, which are linked and methylated in a specific manner. This cap and at least three well-conserved sequences of bases between the cap and the upstream end of the gene have important functions in later protein synthesis. The terminal poly(A) tail is shortened to 50 to 75 residues.

Analysis of the structural portion of the gene and its initial complementary RNA transcript shows that both are interrupted by two lengths of bases that do not code for the ultimate protein. These intervening sequences, or introns, are surrounded by specific nucleotide sequences. Spliceosomes recognize these sequences and excise the introns, splicing the exon transcripts to produce mature mRNA. Each of the now juxtaposed exons codes for functionally or structurally important domains of the protein product.

Mature mRNA is transported to the cytoplasm, where it attaches to a number of ribosomal subunits and serves as the template for synthesis of the globin molecule (Fig. 3.4). A large number of translation initiation factors are needed. Translation is initiated at a unique start codon, and each amino acid is added by a specific transfer RNA along the template in the 5′ to 3′ direction (i.e., beginning with the amino terminus) until a stop codon is encountered. At this point, the complete protein chain is released into the cytoplasm. The mRNA is reused for production of additional globin chains. Globin mRNA, in comparison

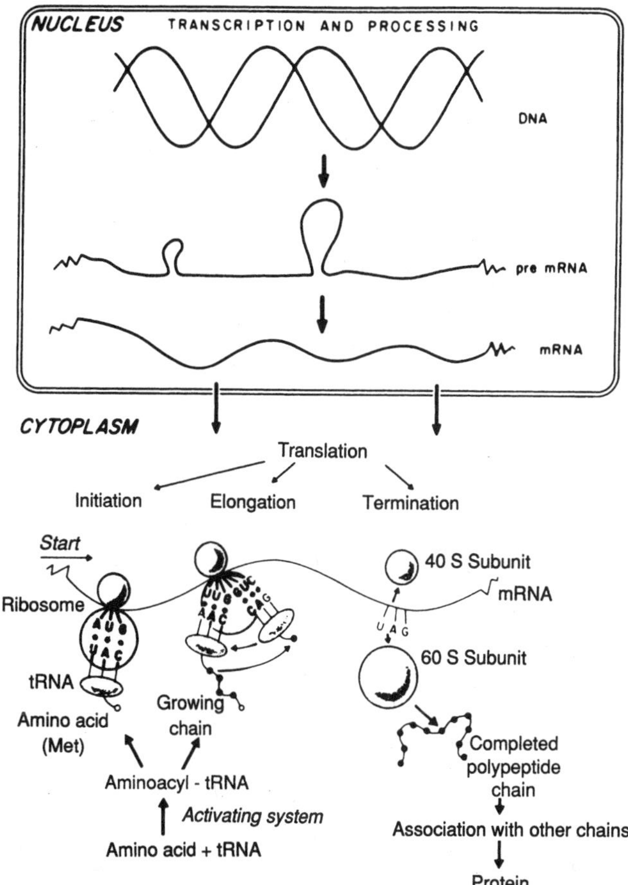

FIGURE 3.4. Schematic of messenger RNA (*mRNA*) translation. The two ribosomal subunits attach to mRNA and temporarily bind the specific transfer RNA (*tRNA*), which is complementary to the mRNA triplet. Once the amino acid carried by the tRNA is attached to the peptide chain, the tRNA is released, and another is bound. This process continues until the stop codon is encountered. (From Bunn HF, Forget BG. *Hemoglobin: molecular, genetic and clinical aspects.* Philadelphia: WB Saunders, 1986:170, with permission.)

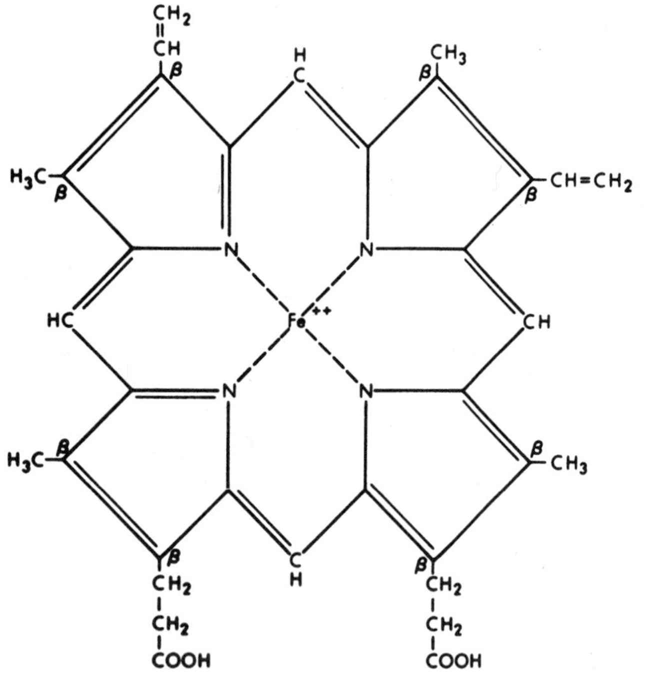

FIGURE 3.5. Structure of heme (Fe-protoporphyrin IX).

with mRNA elsewhere, is unusually stable, an essential feature that allows hemoglobin production to continue in reticulocytes for several days after nuclear extrusion (21).

In a genetic version of Parkinson's law, disorders of almost every step in this complex process have now been observed and have contributed immeasurably to our understanding of the overall process, with respect to both globin production specifically and molecular biology in general. It is possible to account precisely for the several hundred hemoglobin structural mutants (hemoglobinopathy) on the basis of base sequence abnormalities (single-base substitutions, deletions, insertions, missense mutations, frame shifts, crossovers) within an exon of the gene (3, 22–24). A similar situation exists with respect to thalassemia, which with minor exceptions is a disorder in which production of a globin chain is reduced or altogether absent. It is caused by genetic abnormalities that govern and illuminate every step in the process of globin production. Also numbering in the hundreds, these steps likewise comprise single base substitutions, missense mutations, frame shifts, and deletions that affect flanking regulatory domains, the LCR, HS-40, the genes themselves (introns, exons, an entire gene or cluster of genes), the poly(A) signal sequence, the cap site, mRNA processing, translation of mature RNA and *trans*-acting factors (3,23–25).

Heme Synthesis

Heme is a tetrapyrrole ring or porphyrin with a central iron atom linked to four nitrogen atoms (Fig. 3.5). Its capacity for reversibly binding oxygen or electrons is used in many settings, including hemoglobin, myoglobin, cytochromes (*b*, c_1, *c*, *a*, a_3, b_5, and P-450), peroxidases, catalase, and tryptophan pyrrolase. Heme absorbs light strongly. This accounts for the characteristic color of hemoglobin and myoglobin and their changes in color with oxygenation and oxidation.

Synthesis of heme begins with formation of δ-aminolevulinic acid (ALA) from succinylcoenzyme A and glycine by ALA synthase with pyridoxal 5′-phosphate as a cofactor (26) (Fig. 3.6). This reaction occurs on the inner mitochondrial membrane. The requirement for pyridoxal 5′-phosphate undoubtedly explains the response to pharmacologic doses of pyridoxine sometimes observed in patients with mutant ALA synthase enzymes causing the hereditary X-linked form of sideroblastic anemia (27). Two molecules of ALA combine in the cytoplasm to form porphobilinogen under the influence of ALA dehydratase. Four molecules of porphobilinogen then condense to form one molecule of uroporphyrinogen III. This is a two-step process, the enzyme porphobilinogen deaminase producing mainly the intermediate hydroxymethylbilane with subsequent conversion to uroporphyrinogen III by uroporphyrinogen III cosynthase. Uroporphyrinogen III is then converted to coproporphyrinogen III by uroporphyrinogen decarboxylase, which converts the four acetates to methyl residues. The remaining steps occur again in the mitochondrion. Coproporphyrinogen III is converted to protoporphyrin IX. This two-step process entails oxidative decarboxylation of propionate groups to vinyl residues by coproporphyrinogen III oxidase and oxidation by protoporphyrin oxidase of the four methylene bridges between the pyrrole groups. The last step is the insertion of iron by ferrochelatase (heme synthase).

Deficiencies and abnormalities of these enzymes underlie a variety of disorders (28). These are listed in Table 3.1. With minor qualifications, these explain all of the inherited forms of porphyria, the most common X-linked version of hereditary sideroblastic anemia and certain other hematologic disorders (29). The principal source of overproduction of porphyrin in most of these disorders is the liver, except in the case of congenital erythropoietic protoporphyria and protoporphyria, where it is bone marrow.

Much of the underlying molecular biologic process of heme synthesis was clarified in the 1990s (30). All of the genes have been cloned and mapped to their chromosomal loci (Table 3.1), and many of the mutations have been identified. Unlike the rate in liver and other tissues, the extremely high rate of heme synthesis in erythroid cells requires a different set of controls, and appearance of this pathway is temporally related to normoblast maturation and tightly linked to iron availability and globin synthesis. The first enzyme in red blood cell precursors, ALA synthase (ALAS2), unlike its ubiquitous relative in other tissues (ALAS1), arises from a gene on the X chromosome that is expressed only in erythroid cells (31). Its transcription appears to be triggered by erythropoietin binding to its receptor and to depend on the erythroid factors GATA-1, TATA basic protein (TBP), and very possibly EKLF. In contrast, its ALAS1 cousin is encoded by a housekeeping gene with different regulatory sequences on chromosome 3 that is expressed constitutively.

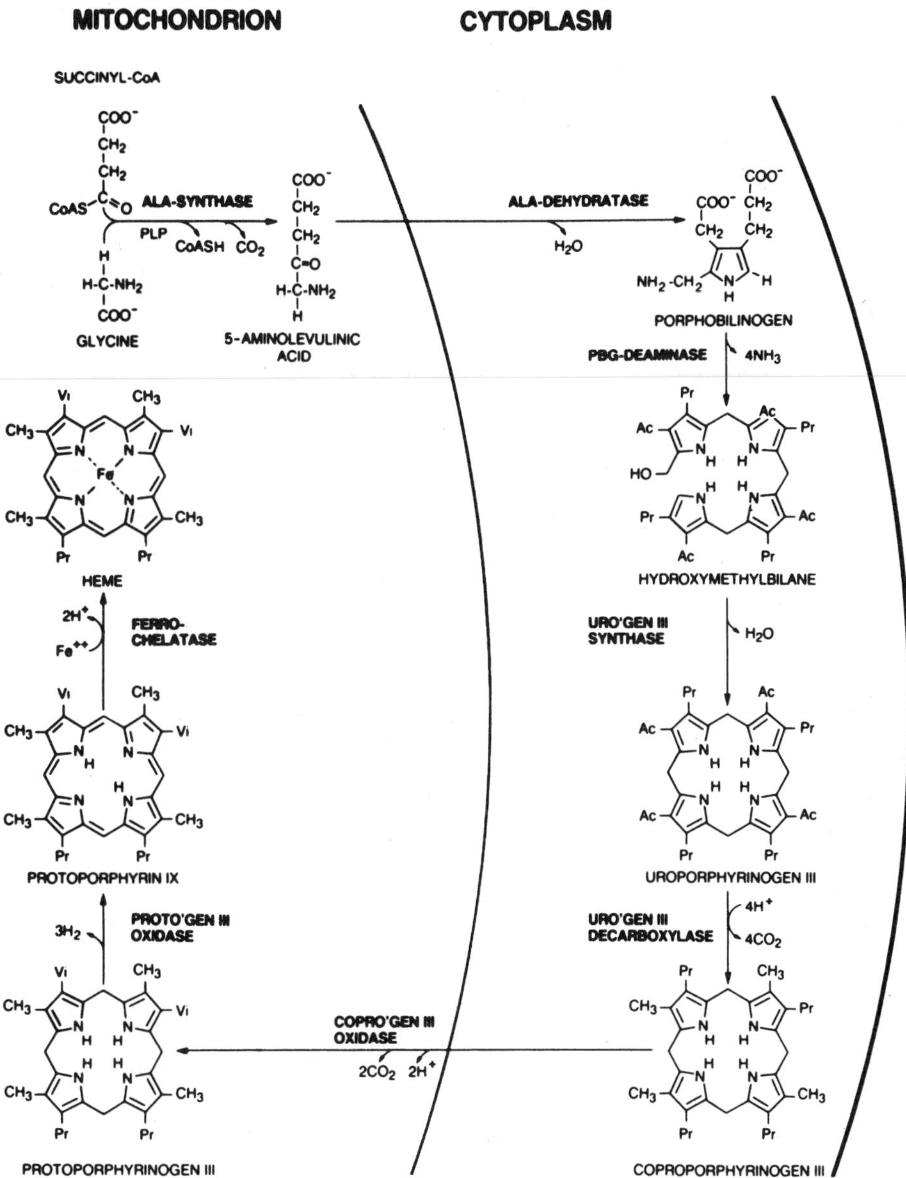

FIGURE 3.6. Pathway of heme synthesis. *PLP,* pyridoxal-5′-phosphate; *ALA,* δ-aminolevulinic acid; *PBG,* porphobilinogen; *URO'GEN,* uroporphyrinogen; *COPRO'GEN,* coproporphyrinogen; *PROTO'GEN,* protoporphyrinogen; *Ac,* acetate; *Pr,* propionate; *Vi,* vinyl. (From Bottomley SS, Muller-Eberhard U. Pathophysiology of heme synthesis. *Semin Hematol* 1988; 25:284, with permission.)

Synthesis of several other heme synthetic enzymes apparently is regulated in relation to ALAS2 synthesis, inasmuch as inhibition of ALAS2 production by an antisense strategy impairs synthesis of the enzymes as well as globin synthesis. The erythroid and ubiquitous versions of the second enzyme, ALA dehydratase, are products of the same gene and have identical exons, but an arrangement called *alternative splicing* equips them, respectively, with either erythroid or ubiquitous promoters. In a variation on the same theme, the erythroid and ubiquitous isoforms of the third enzyme, porphobilinogen deaminase, are constructed by means of alternative splicing from different combinations of exons from the same gene. Both ALA dehydratase and porphobilinogen deaminase possess putatively regulatory GATA-1 and NF-E2 domains, again indicating erythroid-specific control. Erythroid-specific regulatory domains also are present in the last three genes, coproporphyrinogen III oxidase, protoporphyrin oxidase, and ferrochelatase.

Although the enzyme steps in heme synthesis are the same in erythroid cells as in other cells, control of erythroid heme production differs from elsewhere in that it is tightly linked to iron availability and globin synthesis and is not directly inhibited by heme. First, translation of ALAS2 appears to be regulated by an iron-responsive element in its mRNA (Fig. 3.7). This is the binding site for an iron regulatory protein (IRP), such as

TABLE 3.1. ABNORMAL HEME BIOSYNTHETIC PATHWAY ENZYMES AND RELATED SYNDROMES

Enzyme Abnormality	Gene Locus	Clinical Disorder
ALA synthase (ALAS2)	Xp11.21	X-linked hereditary sideroblastic anemia
ALA dehydratase	9q34	ALA dehydratase deficiency porphyria; acquired deficiency caused by lead
Porphobilinogen deaminase	11q24.1-q24.2	Acute intermittent porphyria
Uroporphyrinogen III synthase	10q25.2-q26.3	Congenital erythropoietic porphyria
Uroporphyrinogen decarboxylase	1p34	Porphyria cutanea tarda (associated with liver disease, especially hepatitis C, and hereditary hemochromatosis), hepatoerythropoietic porphyria
Coproporphyrinogen oxidase	3q12	Coproporphyria; harderoporphyria; acquired deficiency caused by lead
Protoporphyrinogen oxidase	1q21-q23	Variegate porphyria
Ferrochelatase (heme synthase)	18q21.3	Erythropoietic protoporphyria; acquired deficiency due to lead inhibition

ALA, aminolevulinic acid.

IRP-1, which is known to regulate translation of mRNA for ferritin and transferrin receptors (26,32). Accordingly, the likely steps up-regulating ALAS2 production are increased ferritin, decreased IRP binding to ALAS2 mRNA, stabilization of the message, and increased translation. This serves to link heme synthesis and cellular iron availability. The final product, heme, when excessive, inhibits cellular iron uptake and may inhibit ALAS2 transport to mitochondria. Control also may exist at the next enzyme, porphobilinogen deaminase, which has low basal activity, increases severalfold with acceleration of erythropoiesis, and manifests product inhibition. Finally, it is noteworthy that heme and globin synthesis are tightly coordinated; that is, heme synthesis induces globin synthesis and does not proceed or proceeds at a reduced level when globin synthesis is blocked or diminished (26,30,31). Likewise, globin synthesis does not proceed if ALAS2 is nonfunctional. The final result is a multilayered con-

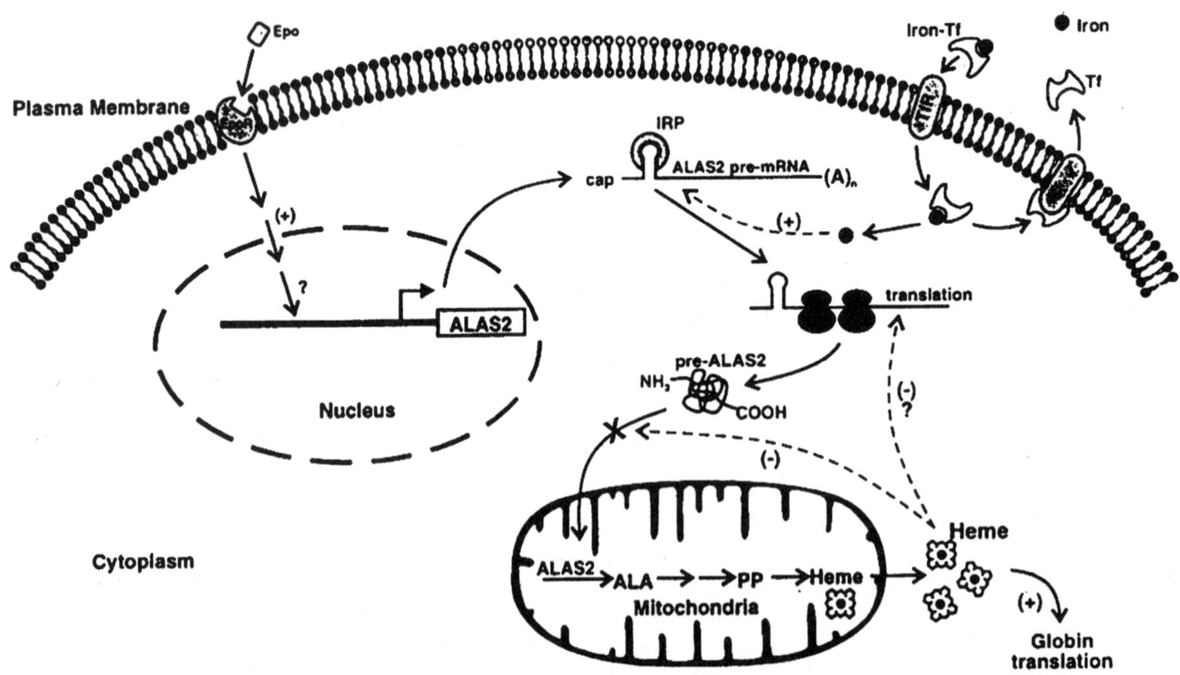

FIGURE 3.7. Overview of positive (+) and negative (−) control of heme synthesis in erythroid precursors. *ALAS2,* erythrocyte isoform of ALA-synthase; *Epo,* erythropoietin; *EpoR,* erythropoietin receptor; *Tf,* transferrin; *TfR,* transferrin receptor; *IRP,* iron regulatory protein; *PP,* protoporphyrin. (From Sadlon TJ, Dell'Oso T, Surinya KH, et al. Regulation of erythroid 5-aminolevulinate synthase expression during erythropoiesis. *Int J Biochem Cell Biol* 1999; 31:1153–1167, with permission.)

trol system that allows hemoglobin production at a high rate but avoids free heme or globin accumulation.

Tetramer Assembly

Final assembly of the hemoglobin molecule occurs in the cytoplasm. Binding of the heme ring to the globin monomer probably occurs during or just after globin transcription as the chain is adopting its secondary or tertiary configuration. Dimers comprising an α chain and a non-α chain (almost entirely αβ dimers after the first few months of life in healthy persons) then form spontaneously in the increasingly thick cytoplasm of the developing normoblast and reticulocyte.

Formation of dimers comprising an α and a non-α chain (rather than two like chains) is facilitated first by the difference in electrostatic charge at physiologic pH between α-globin chains (positive charge) and β-globin chains (negative charge) and, second, by the large number of specific contacts along the α-β interface. This charge-dependent association also explains why, in the case of heterozygosity for mutant hemoglobins, the ratio of hemoglobin A (HbA) to hemoglobin X is not normally 1:1 (33). Thus common β-chain mutants such as S, C, and E have a less negative net charge than do normal α chains. This places the mutant β chain at a relative disadvantage in dimer formation with the result that less of the mutant hemoglobin is produced. This phenomenon is further accentuated when the presence of α thalassemia, a common disorder, limits α-chain availability.

Assembly of tetramers from dimers also occurs spontaneously in the cytoplasm. Any unpaired globin chains, except when quite excessive (thalassemia), are removed by cellular proteases. Tetramer formation is strongly favored at the hemoglobin concentration that exists within the red blood cell, which eventually reaches 34 g/dl (~5 mmol/L), a value close to maximal solubility. When hemoglobin concentration is lower, as occurs in plasma during intravascular hemolysis, the tetramer dissociates into dimers. When two or more types of dimers are produced in a cell (e.g., $\alpha\beta^A$ and $\alpha\beta^S$), the resulting tetramers are commonly represented as combinations of like dimers ($\alpha_2{\beta^A}_2$ and $\alpha_2{\beta^S}_2$). This notation implies that each hemoglobin species forms its own tetramer. However, a mixture of dimer species leads to hybrid ($\alpha_2\beta^A\beta^S$) as well as nonhybrid tetramers within the erythrocyte. These tetramers dissociate into dimers under most conditions of hemoglobin analysis.

Hemoglobin Species in Humans

The normal human hemoglobins are shown in Table 3.2. The principal hemoglobin species produced in the normal adult is HbA, which has the structural formula $\alpha_2\beta_2$. HbF ($\alpha_2\gamma_2$) and HbA_2 ($\alpha_2\delta_2$) are present in small amounts. A succession of embryonic and fetal hemoglobins appears and disappears during intrauterine development (Fig. 3.8).

HbF is the principal hemoglobin after the first few weeks of gestation and is gradually replaced by HbA during late pregnancy and the first few months of extrauterine life. As discussed later, HbF under physiologic conditions binds oxygen more tightly than does HbA (i.e., the partial pressure of oxygen at which hemoglobin is 50% saturated with oxygen [P_{50}] of HbF is lower) and is therefore better suited for oxygen transport during intrauterine life. The molecular basis for this phenomenon of hemoglobin switching is under intensive investigation but not yet well understood (2). Insight into the beauty of the process is furnished by the fact that the order of genes in the β-globin gene cluster is the same as the order of appearance of the respective hemoglobins during fetal development. That this is not coincidence is suggested by the fact that experimentally varying the order of the globin genes changes their order of appearance in the embryo (34,35).

Hemoglobin undergoes progressive nonenzymatic glycation during the life span of the red blood cell. The most prevalent form is HbA_{Ic}, which is produced by glucose attachment to the N-terminus of the β chain by a ketoamine linkage. Because the quantity of HbA_{Ic} formed is determined by the glucose concentration, the level of HbA_{Ic}, given the lengthy erythrocyte life span, provides a useful overall measure of control in diabetes mellitus. Although HbA_{Ic} has detectably altered oxygen affinity, the amount present is too small to affect oxygen delivery significantly.

HEMOGLOBIN FUNCTION

Specific aspects of hemoglobin function relate directly to its role as an oxygen transporter. These are reversible oxygenation with cooperativity, the Bohr effect, the carbon dioxide effect, the chloride effect, the effect of 2,3-bisphosphoglycerate (2,3-BPG; formerly known as 2,3-diphosphoglycerate), effects associated with nitric oxide, and the temperature effect.

TABLE 3.2. NORMAL HUMAN HEMOGLOBINS

Name	Formula	Function
A	$\alpha_2\beta_2$	Predominant adult hemoglobin
A_2	$\alpha_2\delta_2$	Minor adult hemoglobin (<2.5%)
F	$\alpha_2\gamma_2$ ($\alpha_2{}^G\gamma_2$, $\alpha_2{}^A\gamma_2$)	Major hemoglobin in the fetus; replaced by hemoglobin A during late gestation and first months after birth; normally <1% in adult
Gower-1	$\zeta_2\epsilon_2$	Embryonic hemoglobins; replaced by hemoglobin F in early gestation
Gower-1	$\alpha_2\epsilon_2$	
Portland	$\zeta_2\gamma_2$	

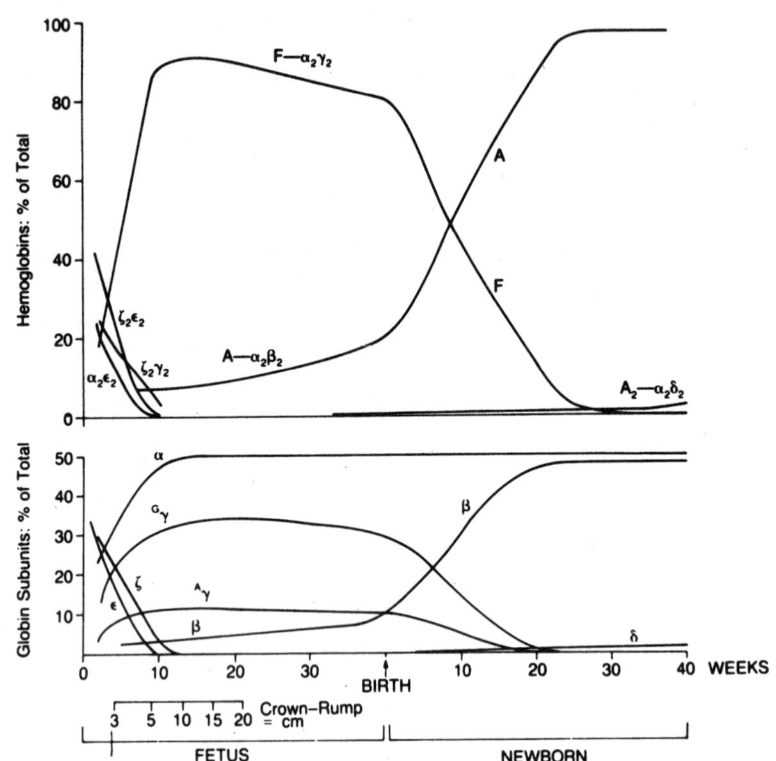

FIGURE 3.8. Ontogeny of globin chain production. (From Bunn HF, Forget BG. *Hemoglobin: molecular, genetic and clinical aspects.* Philadelphia: WB Saunders, 1986:68, with permission.)

Reversible Oxygen Binding

One molecule of hemoglobin (Hb) can bind four molecules of oxygen:

$$Hb + 4O_2 \rightleftharpoons Hb\,(O_2)_4 \qquad [3.1]$$

This translates to a theoretical maximal binding of 1.39 ml oxygen per gram of hemoglobin. Because of the small amounts of methemoglobin and carboxyhemoglobin normally present, and allowing for the small amount of dissolved oxygen, approximately 20 ml oxygen per deciliter is present in normal arterial blood when the hemoglobin concentration is 15 g/dl.

Figure 3.9 shows oxygen equilibrium curves (OEC) for myoglobin and hemoglobin under physiologic conditions. The curve for myoglobin is a hyperbola, whereas the hemoglobin curve is sigmoidal. This sigmoidicity is the result of cooperativity or heme-heme interaction, a phenomenon in which the oxygenation of one subunit of the hemoglobin tetramer alters the oxygen affinity of other subunits. Because myoglobin is monomeric, it cannot show heme-heme interaction. Cooperativity also depends on the presence of two different types of globin chains. A tetramer composed of four identical chains such as hemoglobin Bart (β_4) shows no cooperativity.

The degree of cooperativity can be quantitated when the data of Figure 3.8 are replotted as:

log (O_2 saturation/1 − O_2 saturation) (Fig. 3.10).

This yields a slope of 1.0 for myoglobin (no cooperativity) but a slope of 2.8 for hemoglobin. This latter value may be compared with the theoretical maximum of 4.0.

Evidence indicates that the oxygenation of hemoglobin begins in one of the α-heme subunits, which under physiologic conditions are thought to have higher affinity for oxygen. Binding of the first oxygen causes the oxygen affinity of other subunits to increase. Thus oxygenation of the second subunit occurs at a lower PO_2 than would be required without cooperativity. By

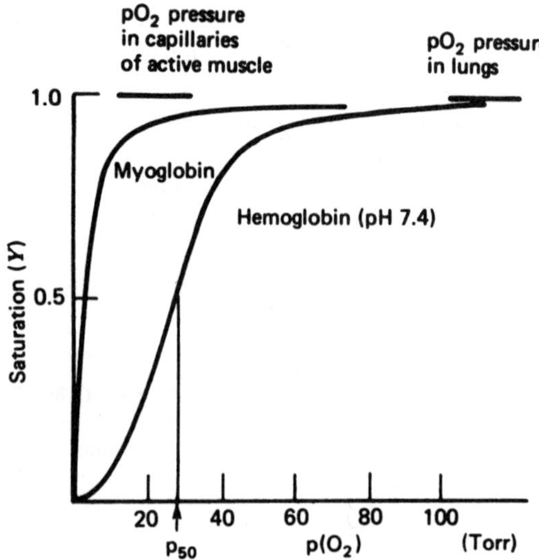

FIGURE 3.9. Oxygen equilibrium curves for myoglobin and hemoglobin under physiologic conditions. Myoglobin remains highly saturated as the blood PO_2 falls to low levels. (Modified from Schultz RM. Proteins, II: physiological proteins. In: Devlin TM, ed. *Textbook of biochemistry with clinical correlations,* 2nd ed. New York: John Wiley & Sons, 1986, with permission.)

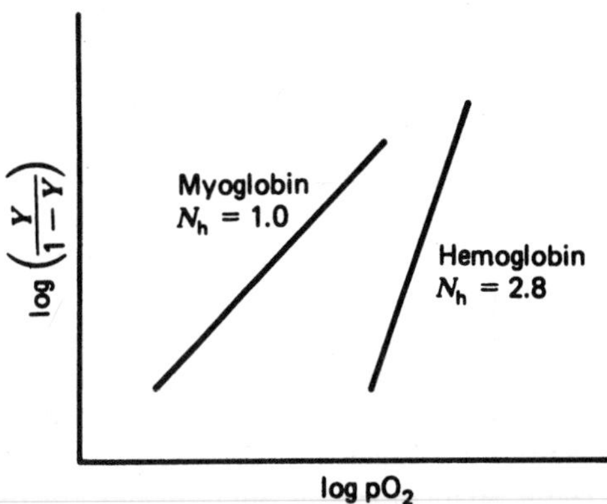

FIGURE 3.10. Hill plots for myoglobin and hemoglobin with log of the fractional hemoglobin oxygen saturation plotted against log PO_2. The slope, equal to the value *n* of the Hill equation, is a measure of the degree of cooperativity. (From Schultz RM. Proteins, II: physiological proteins. In: Devlin TM, ed. *Textbook of biochemistry with clinical correlations,* 2nd ed. New York: John Wiley & Sons, 1986, with permission.)

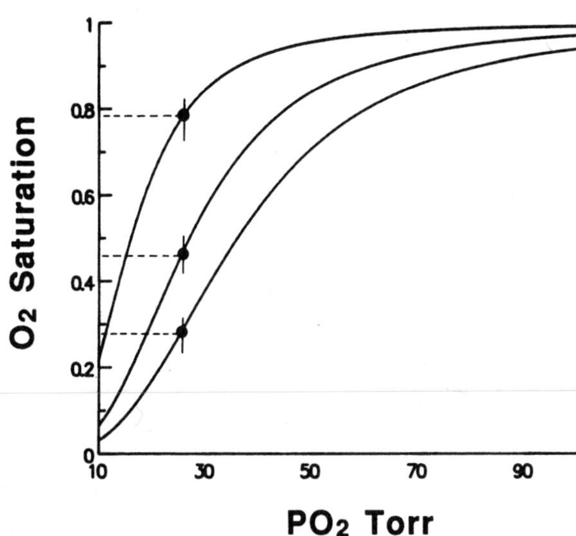

FIGURE 3.11. Blood oxygen equilibrium curves show effects of right and left shifts on oxygen release when alveolar PO_2 is normal. P_{50} values for the three curves are (*left to right*) 16 mm Hg (torr) (typical of stored blood with no 2,3-bisphopsphoglycerate [2,3-BPG]), 27 mm Hg (normal blood with a normal 2,3-BPG level), and 36 mm Hg (markedly right shifted).

the time the fourth subunit is oxygenated, its heme group binds oxygen approximately 300 times more tightly than does the first subunit. Conversely, *cooperativity* means that release of the first molecule of oxygen from hemoglobin facilitates release of subsequent molecules; that is, oxygen affinity decreases. It is almost as if the molecule has thoughtfully concluded that when some oxygen is bound, it should bind oxygen more tightly and that when oxygen is released, it should release its remaining oxygen molecules more liberally. A necessary consequence of this phenomenon is that in partially oxygenated hemoglobin, all molecules are not equally oxygenated; rather, most molecules tend toward being fully oxygenated or fully deoxygenated, with comparatively few intermediates present.

The shape of the hemoglobin OEC, a reflection of this cooperativity, has great biologic importance, because it allows nearly full saturation of hemoglobin at PO_2 values ordinarily present in the alveolus. Likewise, the steep down slope means that a large fraction of bound oxygen can be released as blood flows through tissue with a relatively modest decrease in PO_2. For example, 25% of oxygen is released when PO_2 falls from arterial levels to 40 mm Hg (torr) but nearly double this amount is released when PO_2 decreases from 40 to 20 mm Hg. Maintenance of relatively high microvascular blood PO_2 is necessary to provide the pressure head for oxygen diffusion from the red blood cell interior to cells distant from the microvasculature. The ideal shape and position of the hemoglobin OEC for maintaining nearly complete saturation of myoglobin at PO_2 values of 10 to 30 mm Hg are apparent from an inspection of Figure 3.9.

Figure 3.11 shows more quantitatively the effect of a given shift of the OEC to the right (P_{50}, 36 mm Hg) or left (16 mm Hg). When the curve is shifted to the right, more oxygen is released for any given decrease in pressure. At a microvessel PO_2 of 25 mm Hg, the normal adult curve for whole blood (Fig. 3.11, middle curve) releases 54% of its bound oxygen, whereas the right-shifted curve releases 72%. The curve to the left, typical of stored blood, releases only 22% of oxygen for the same decrease in PO_2. Stated another way, as blood passes through the microvasculature, the PO_2 also is higher at any point outside the vessel for a given volume of oxygen released when the curve is shifted to the right. Thus if conditions in an organ are such that 60% of the oxygen is released by the time the blood reaches a certain point in the microvasculature, the blood with the right-shifted curve is able to deliver oxygen to a cell 1.3 times farther from the capillary than is normal blood. The blood with the left-shifted curve is able to deliver oxygen to a distance only 0.61 times as great as the normal curve.

Figure 3.12 shows that a left-shifted OEC delivers more oxygen when alveolar PO_2 is markedly reduced, as at very high altitudes. Under these circumstances, 28% more oxygen is released in the microvasculature when PO_2 decreases from an arterial value of 35 to 15 mm Hg with the left-shifted curve (the vertical distance between A2 and V2) than with the right-shifted curve (the vertical distance between A1 and V1). This explains why the fetal OEC of almost all species lies to the left of the maternal (adult) curve and why animals native to high altitudes have a left-lying OEC. This benefit of a left-shifted curve has been confirmed experimentally by means of direct tests of altitude tolerance.

The OEC has been discussed so far under equilibrium conditions. Like all equilibria, the reversible reaction between hemoglobin and oxygen (Equation 3.1) implies a forward reaction with a rate constant (k' or "on" constant) and a backward reaction (k or "off" constant). The relative rates of these reactions determine the final concentrations of reactants and products. Because hemoglobin combines with four molecules of oxygen, there are a number of intermediate compounds and a family of forward and backward reaction rates. Factors that modify the OEC do so by altering the ratios between the on and off constants.

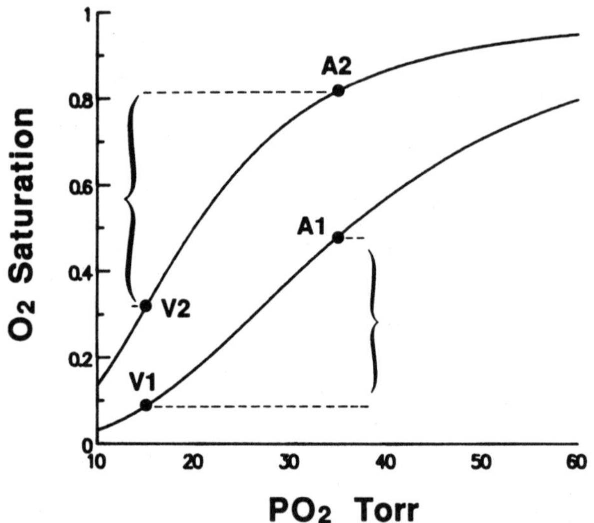

FIGURE 3.12. Blood oxygen equilibrium curves show the effects of rightward and leftward curve positions on oxygen release when alveolar PO_2 is appreciably reduced as at a high altitude. P_{50} values are 20 and 36 mm Hg (torr). More oxygen is released with the leftward curve at the selected loading and unloading PO_2 values.

Molecular Basis

One of the genuine triumphs of biologic research over the past several decades has been progressive clarification of the precise molecular basis of hemoglobin function (36–39). This entails explaining mechanistically how oxygenation of one heme group influences oxygen affinity of heme groups in distant subunits as well as explaining the interactions among ligands. Central to this understanding is the theory, originally advanced in 1965, that cooperative effects in an enzyme (or hemoglobin) arise from an equilibrium between two different physical structures that occurs as a result of ligand binding (40).

In brief, tetrameric hemoglobin has a molecular weight of 64,500 daltons. It is globular in shape with its diameters in the range of 5.0 to 6.5 nm (50 to 65 Å). Each globin chain exists for the most part as an α helix, which is folded on itself at several nonhelical inflection points (Fig. 3.13). The heme group is bound in an interior crevice of the folded globin chain (between the E and F helices) and is surrounded by mostly uncharged amino acid residues. This nonpolar environment serves to exclude water molecules, rendering the iron less susceptible to oxidation. The external portion of the molecule contains polar amino acids, which are necessary for its solubility. The iron atom is held at four of its six possible coordination positions to the four tetrapyrrole rings (Fig. 3.5). The fifth position is linked covalently to the N of a particular histidine (F8; residue 87 in α chains and 92 in β chains), which is termed the *proximal histidine* (Fig. 3.14). This portion of the molecule is very similar in all globin chains studied to date. In the deoxygenated (five-coordinated) state, the outermost electrons of iron are located in a higher orbital. The atomic diameter is such that the iron cannot quite fit in the plane of the ring between the four pyrrole nitrogens. As a result, it is forced slightly outside the plane of the ring (0.022 nm [0.22 Å] in α subunits, 0.019 nm [0.19 Å] in β_1 subunits, 0.044 nm [0.44 Å] in β_2 subunits) (Fig. 3.14) (37). This displaces the respective proximal histidines, causing tenting of the ring and strain within that subunit. When oxygenation occurs, the oxygen molecule binds to the iron on the side of the heme ring opposite from the proximal histidine, and the more distal of the two oxygen atoms forms a hydrogen bond with the imidazole nitrogen of the distal histidine (E7; residue 58 in α chains and 63 in β chains). With oxygen binding, the outer electrons of iron drop into a lower orbital, the diameter of the iron decreases, and the iron moves into the plane of the ring. This allows the proximal histidine to move toward the ring and reduces the strain triggering shifts in other parts of the subunit (Fig. 3.14). These shifts involve particularly the FG helical corner (of which histidine F8 is a part), which has a series of important contacts with the C corner of the β chain (β_2) of the opposite dimer (Fig. 3.13) (37). The C-terminal salt bridge is weakened. As oxygenation proceeds, like changes occur in the next subunit. As a result of these movements, a number of the 14 salt bridges in deoxyhemoglobin between subunits and within β subunits loosen or break. After two to three subunits are oxygenated, the entire tetramer, because of salt bond rupture (41), flips from a taut, constrained (lower oxygen affinity) state (T) to a relaxed (higher oxygen affinity) state (R):

$$Hb_T \overset{O_2}{\rightleftharpoons} Hb_R \qquad [3.2]$$

This relaxation sharply decreases oxygen affinity. This T → R transition is accompanied by a rotation of the two αβ dimers away from one another by 12 to 15 degrees and a lateral movement of one with respect to the other of 0.08 nm (0.8 Å). Thus the process of oxygenation and deoxygenation causes the heme molecule, like the lungs, to breathe. These intramolecular movements of the molecule were detected with x-ray crystallography by Dr. Max Perutz. He formulated these into a comprehensive model, an achievement for which he was awarded the Nobel Prize. A huge number of careful studies by a small army of scientists and by Perutz himself have since further interrogated various parts of the molecule by means of a variety of insightful physical and chemical techniques. Meanwhile the resolution of structure has been improved such that the location of every atom is known within 0.21 nm (2.1 Å). These studies have now established that the model originally proposed by Perutz, a few minor adjustments notwithstanding, was remarkably correct (37,39). Hemoglobin is thus the example par excellence of a complex functional protein for which there is a detailed, mechanistic understanding of the relation between structure and function.

Linked Functions of Hemoglobin

Oxygenation and deoxygenation of hemoglobin are not isolated events. Pari passu with the aforedescribed changes in oxygen-related intrasubunit and tetrameric movements are changes in the binding affinity of hemoglobin for its other ligands. These are hydrogen ions, carbon dioxide, chloride ions, 2,3-BPG, and nitric oxide. Likewise, when oxygen saturation is held constant,

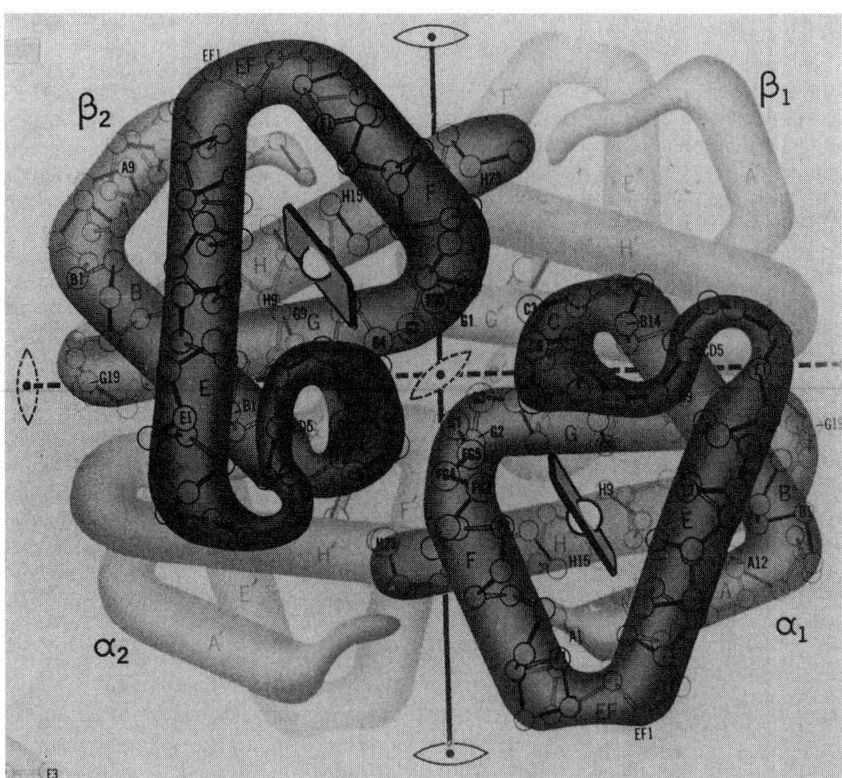

FIGURE 3.13. Interrelation of globin chains within the hemoglobin tetramer. The FG corner of the α_1 chain is in close contact with the C helix of the β_2 chain. Oxygenation of the α_1 chain weakens salt bridges and allows slippage between these chains. This raises the oxygen affinity of the neighboring β_2 chain and accounts for the cooperativity phenomenon (37). (From Dickerson RE, Geis I. *Hemoglobin: structure, function, evolution, and pathology.* Menlo Park, CA: Benjamin/Cummings, 1983. Illustrations by Irving Geis. Copyright by Howard Hughes Medical Institute, 2000, with permission.)

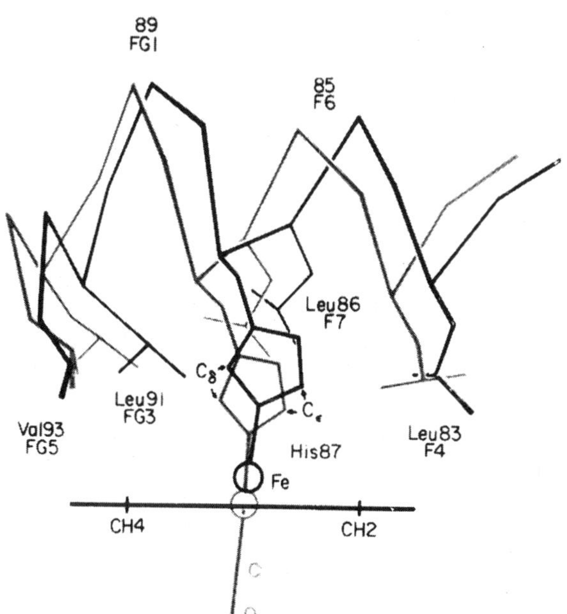

FIGURE 3.14. Schematic of conformational changes in the globin chain that are caused by oxygenation of the iron atom. *Heavy lines* show the configuration in the deoxygenated state. (From Baldwin J, Chothia C. Hemoglobin: the structural changes related to ligand binding and its allosteric mechanism. *J Mol Biol* 1979;129:192–220, with permission.)

a change in the amount of any other bound ligand evokes changes in the affinity of hemoglobin for the other ligands. The effects of various ligands, methemoglobin formation, and temperature on oxygen affinity are summarized in Table 3.3.

Bohr Effect

The alkaline Bohr effect describes the relation between hydrogen ions and oxygen affinity. An increase in hydrogen ions shifts the OEC to the right, and a decrease shifts it to the left. A corollary is that oxygenation of deoxyhemoglobin liberates hydrogen ions and that deoxygenation causes uptake of hydrogen ions. This effect, as originally described by Christian Bohr, is the change in oxygen affinity caused by a change in carbon dioxide concentration. As was subsequently shown, this effect with carbon diox-

TABLE 3.3. EFFECTS OF LIGANDS, OXIDATION, AND TEMPERATURE ON HEMOGLOBIN-OXYGEN AFFINITY

Increased Oxygen Affinity	Decreased Oxygen Affinity
Oxygen binding by deoxyhemoglobin	Oxygen release from oxyhemoglobin
H^+ (pH <6)	H^+ (pH >6)
Decrease in temperature	Increase in temperature
Carbon monoxide	2,3-bisphosphoglycerate
Methemoglobin Fe^{+3}	Chloride ion
	Nitric oxide?

ide comprises a major pH effect and a smaller pH-independent, carbon dioxide–specific effect on blood oxygen affinity. Consequently, physiologists often use the term *carbon dioxide Bohr effect* to denote the change in oxygen affinity caused by a change in PCO_2 (pH and carbon dioxide–specific effects combined) and the term *hydrogen ion Bohr effect* to denote the change in P_{50} caused by a change in pH at constant PCO_2 (pH effect per se). Chemists by convention use the term *Bohr effect,* or *alkaline Bohr effect,* to refer to the hydrogen ion Bohr effect. At low (subphysiologic) pH ($<$6.0), an increase or decrease in hydrogen ion concentration has the opposite effect on oxygen affinity, which is termed the *acid Bohr effect.*

When hydrogen ions are added to hemoglobin, amino acid residues throughout the molecule with pK values close to physiologic pH (principally the imidazole ring of histidine) are titrated. Because of the high concentration of hemoglobin present in blood, hemoglobin serves as a powerful buffer, a fact of considerable physiologic significance. Connected to this titration is a change in oxygen affinity, which can be simplistically formulated as Equation 3.3:

$$\text{HbO}_2\text{-imidazole (N, NH)} + H^+ \rightleftharpoons \text{Hb-imidazole (NH}^+\text{, NH)} + O_2 \qquad [3.3]$$

The Bohr effect occurs partly because protonation favors hydrogen bond formation at the C termini. This strengthens the T structure, shifting Equation 3.2 to the left. For example, when the imidazole of the β_{146} histidine is protonated, a salt bridge forms with β_{94} aspartate. This increases intramolecular constraints and favors the T state. A second effect of protonation is an increase in charge density of cationic groups lining the central cavity. This increases mutual repulsion and shifts the molecule toward the T structure (Equation 3.2). This portion of the alkaline Bohr effect requires the presence of chloride (see later), whereas that associated with hydrogen bonds is chloride independent (37). Under physiologic conditions, the relation between oxygen affinity and pH in whole blood is as follows:

$$\frac{\Delta \log P_{50}}{\Delta pH} = -0.40 \qquad [3.4]$$

Thus a decrease in pH of 0.10 increases the P_{50} of whole blood 2.5 to 3.0 mm Hg. This reciprocal relation between hydrogen ion and oxygen binding is one of the so-called linked functions of hemoglobin.

Carbon Dioxide Effect

Carbon dioxide affects hemoglobin oxygen affinity independently of its effect through pH. This is because carbon dioxide is in equilibrium with hemoglobin according to the carbamate reaction:

$$HbO_2\text{-}NH_2 + CO_2 \rightleftharpoons Hb\text{-}NH\text{-}CO_2^- + H^+ + O_2 \qquad [3.5]$$

This reaction takes place primarily at the N-terminal amino groups of β chains under physiologic conditions. An increase in carbon dioxide binding decreases the affinity of the molecule for oxygen, and oxygen uptake causes carbon dioxide binding to decrease. Accordingly, hemoglobin also participates directly, albeit modestly, in carbon dioxide transport. When oxygen saturation is 50%, and other factors are at physiologic levels and constant, a 40 mm Hg increase in PCO_2 increase whole-blood P_{50} about 0.8 mm Hg, a physiologically trivial change. This effect, however, is appreciably larger at a low oxygen saturation and a low 2,3-BPG concentration. The reciprocal relation between carbon dioxide and oxygen binding is a second linked function of hemoglobin.

Chloride Effect

In a manner somewhat analogous to pH and carbon dioxide, inorganic ions, mainly chloride, interact with certain positively charged sites on the hemoglobin molecule and alter oxygen affinity, as follows:

$$Hb\text{-}NH_{3+}Cl^- + O_2 \rightleftharpoons HbO_2\text{-}NH_2 + H^+ + Cl^- \qquad [3.6]$$

The chloride ion accounts for approximately one half of the Bohr effect; that is, in the absence of chloride, the Bohr effect is substantially reduced. The principal mechanism for the chloride effect is neutralization of positively charged residues within the central cavity. This is thought to increase the P_{50} by decreasing mutual repulsion. This allows the central cavity to decrease in size, which shifts the equilibrium toward the T structure (42–44). Thus hydrogen and chloride ions both decrease oxygen affinity, even though their charges are opposite. When the concentration of chloride ion decreases from 0.15 to 0.02 mol/L in a stripped (2,3-BPG-free) hemoglobin solution, P_{50} decreases from 16 to 10 mm Hg, and the Bohr effect decreases approximately 50%. The reciprocal relation between chloride and oxygen binding is a third linked function of hemoglobin.

2,3-Bisphosphoglycerate Effect

Red blood cells of most mammalian species contain 2,3-BPG, a highly charged molecule with approximately 3.5 negative charges at pH 7.2. This molecule, present in roughly equal molar concentrations with hemoglobin in humans, binds to specific molecular groups—β-terminal amino (NA1) valines, β_{143} (H21) histidine, and β_{82} (EF6) lysine—of deoxyhemoglobin (Fig. 3.15), constraining the tetramer internally and appreciably reducing its oxygen affinity:

$$Hb{\cdot}BPG + O_2 \rightleftharpoons HbO_2 + BPG \qquad [3.7]$$

Adenosine triphosphatase behaves in a similar manner toward hemoglobin but is less abundant than is 2,3-BPG under physiologic conditions. The quantitative effect of 2,3-BPG is such that a drop in its intracellular concentration from normal (~5 mmol/L) to 0 decreases the P_{50} from approximately 27 to 16 mm Hg (Fig. 3.11, center and left curves). When the level of 2,3-BPG increases to more than a 2,3-BPG to hemoglobin molar ratio of 1.0, there is no further effect on P_{50} attributable to specific hemoglobin–2,3-BPG binding. However, because 2,3-BPG is an acidic molecule, it lowers intraerythrocytic pH and thereby

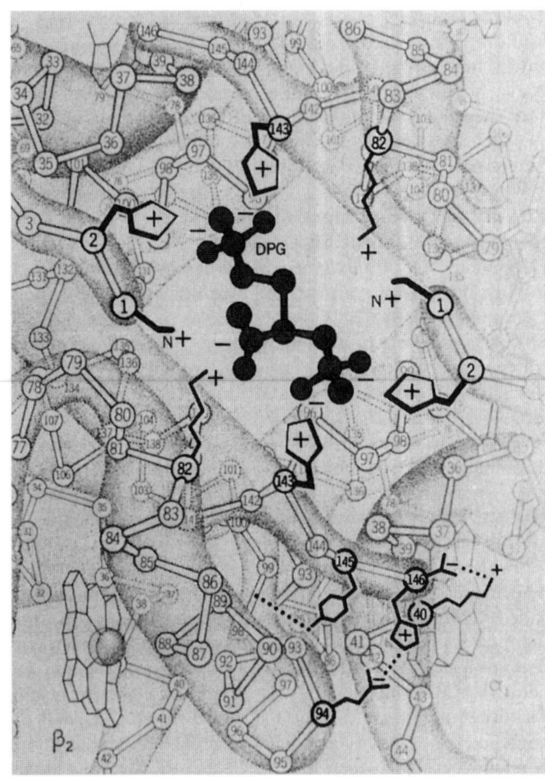

FIGURE 3.15. Binding site of 2,3-BPG (here labeled *DPG,* its former name) within the hemoglobin molecule. The polar attractions with certain residues constrain the molecule, shifting Equation 3.2 to the left. (From Dickerson RE, Geis I. *Hemoglobin: structure, function, evolution, and pathology.* Menlo Park, CA: Benjamin/Cummings, 1983. Illustrations by Irving Geis. Copyright by Howard Hughes Medical Institute, 2000, with permission.)

increases the P_{50} through the Bohr effect. Unlike the situation for HbA, 2,3-BPG does not interact significantly with HbF. This is mainly a result of replacement of the β_{143} histidine, a principal site of 2,3-BPG interaction, with serine. As a result, the oxygen affinity of fetal and neonatal cells increases significantly in comparison with that of adult cells. The reciprocal relation between binding of oxygen and 2,3-BPG (or certain other polyanions) is a fourth linked function of hemoglobin.

Nitric Oxide Effect

It is known that nitric oxide reacts with the Fe^{2+} of a deoxygenated subunit to generate Hb-Fe^{2+}-NO and with oxyhemoglobin to yield methemoglobin (Fe^{3+}-Hb) and nitrate:

$$\text{Hb-Fe}^{2+} + \text{NO} \rightleftharpoons \text{Hb-Fe}^{2+}\text{-NO} \quad [3.8]$$

$$\text{HbO}_2\text{-Fe}^{2+} + \text{NO} \rightleftharpoons \text{Hb-Fe}^{3+} + \text{NO}_3^{-} \quad [3.9]$$

Methemoglobin is well known to increase oxygen affinity of unaffected subunits (see later). Hemoglobin has also been classically regarded as the body's scavenging system for removal of nitric oxide. Stamler and Bonaventura and their colleagues have published a series of interesting studies concerning a possible third reaction of hemoglobin with nitric oxide (45–49). Nitric oxide binds to the β_{93} cysteine thiol group, a residue the biologic importance of which is suggested by the fact that it is invariant across mammals and birds, producing the adduct SNO-Hb. SNO binding affinity at β_{93} reportedly depends on oxygen saturation, SNO binding decreasing with deoxygenation and vice versa. That is, this reaction may also be oxygen linked. Only a small number of hemoglobin molecules actually contain the SNO adduct under physiologic conditions at any moment. It has been proposed that this linked reaction liberates SNO in the microvasculature as oxygen is released and that this nitric oxide modulates small-vessel tone and thus blood flow. This putative role, which depends on released nitric oxide reaching the endothelium in appropriate amounts, has been difficult to reconcile with the assumed role of hemoglobin as a major nitric oxide scavenger and with kinetic considerations. This paradox was addressed in data from Gow et al., suggesting that nitric oxide scavenging does not occur in vivo (45,46). Furthermore, the nitric oxide liberated as SNO is said to enjoy protection from rebinding by Fe^{2+} (Equation 3.8) and to facilitate diffusion through erythrocyte glutathione across the red blood cell to the endothelium. However, results have appeared that appear to be in conflict with some of the foregoing data (52–54). Studies in this area are methodologically difficult because of the small amounts of SNO-Hb present, the presence of alternative nitric oxide pathways (Equations 3.8, 3.9), the transfer of nitric oxide between Fe^{2+} and the β93cys, the reactions of nitric oxide with glutathione, and the fact that any Fe^{3+} produced by nitric oxide also influences oxygen affinity. Finally, the results of investigations attempting to clarify these questions through physiologic studies with recombinant and chemically modified hemoglobins having altered nitric oxide reactivity have yielded somewhat differing results (54–56) and are difficult to interpret because the hemoglobin is extracellular. Future clarification of this area will be germane not only to normal hemoglobin function and the physiologic mechanism of oxygen transport but also to development of blood substitutes in particular and the biologic role of nitric oxide in general.

Temperature Effect

An increase in temperature shifts the OEC to the right. The relation, other factors being constant and in the physiologic range, is given by the equation:

$$\frac{\Delta \log P_{50}}{\Delta T} = 0.023 \quad [3.10]$$

Thus an increase in temperature of 5°C increases P_{50} approximately 7 mm Hg.

Interactions

Although presented for simplicity as a series of individual interactions with hemoglobin, the foregoing factors are mutually interactive. For example, the magnitude of the Bohr effect (expressed as the number of hydrogen ions liberated per mole of hemoglobin oxygenated) is influenced by pH, PCO_2, anion and 2,3-BPG concentration, and temperature (57–60).

Effects of Carbon Monoxide and Hemoglobin Oxidation

Hemoglobin-oxygen affinity is affected greatly by the binding of carbon monoxide to heme iron (forming carboxyhemoglobin) and oxidation of the iron atom from Fe^{2+} to Fe^{3+} (forming methemoglobin). Both affect hemoglobin function by rendering the normal oxygen-binding site unavailable though this effect is greater than carbon monoxide. Both also shift the OEC of the remaining unaltered subunits to the left. Restated, carbon monoxide binding to, or oxidation of, one or two heme irons stabilizes the T structure, shifting Equation 3.3 to the left. These dual effects on hemoglobin (decreased total oxygen binding and increased affinity for the oxygen that is bound) explain the clinical severity of carbon monoxide poisoning and, to a lesser extent, methemoglobinemia.

Mutant Hemoglobins

Mutant hemoglobins are those that have one or more amino acid substitutions or deletions in some part of the molecule. Most of these mutations produce no alteration of function. If, however, the mutation occurs in a portion of the molecule affecting any of the intramolecular movements that underlie the relation shown in Equation 3.2, the hemoglobin display an OEC altered in position or shape. Examples with rightward and leftward OEC shifts and diminished cooperativity are well known. Similarly, mutations in sites at which hydrogen ions, 2,3-BPG, or other ligands attach cause functional consequences, such as a reduced Bohr effect or a decreased or absent 2,3-BPG effect. Other mutations lead to methemoglobin formation, susceptibility to heme loss with denaturation of the hemoglobin molecule, shortened red blood cell survival, and sickling.

It is somewhat daunting to realize that this elegant understanding of hemoglobin function—with details of intramolecular movement in hemoglobin crystals resolved at the subangstrom level, detailed functional study of hundreds of mutants, and recent ultrarapid ligand reaction experiments—is not yet complete despite several decades of research and thousands of insightful publications (39). Perhaps even more daunting is the realization that thousands of other functional proteins are ripe for equally detailed study of structure-function relations.

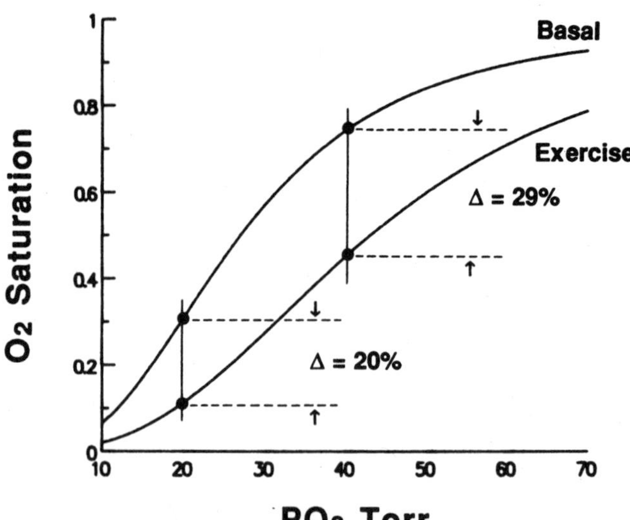

FIGURE 3.16. Effect of changes in pH, carbon dioxide, and temperature on oxygen release in blood from muscle at near maximal exercise in comparison with basal conditions. The estimated P_{50} of 43 mm Hg (torr) in muscle capillary blood is based on measurements of temperature, pH, and PCO_2 in deep femoral venous blood during exercise. At a PO_2 of 20 mm Hg, the percentage of oxygen released will increase 20% because of the curve shift. The effect is even greater at a PO_2 of 40 mm Hg (29%).

PHYSIOLOGIC AND PATHOPHYSIOLOGIC IMPLICATIONS OF SHIFTS IN THE OXYGEN EQUILIBRIUM CURVE

Ph, Carbon Dioxide, Temperature, and 2,3-Bisphosphoglycerate

The effects of the hydrogen ion, carbon dioxide, and temperature on blood oxygen affinity have obvious benefits to the organism when metabolism is increased (Table 3.3). First, the high concentration of hemoglobin present in the blood produces powerful buffering of hydrogen ions. Thus large amounts of acid, as in muscular exercise or other metabolic processes, are taken up by hemoglobin with relatively little change in red blood cell and plasma pH until excretion can occur. Second, the relation between oxygen affinity and hydrogen ions, carbon dioxide, and temperature means that more oxygen is released locally when tissues are metabolically active or hyperthermic. Thus during exercise, hydrogen ion and carbon dioxide concentrations and temperature in the muscle microvasculature increase, and the increases facilitate local oxygen release and diffusion to the tissues (Fig. 3.16). Conversely, the temperature of blood decreases after it leaves the muscle, and blood PCO_2 decreases and pH increases in the lungs. These effects increase the oxygen affinity of blood and allow efficient oxygen loading in the pulmonary capillaries.

An important factor affecting the position of the OEC in vivo is the concentration of erythrocyte 2,3-BPG. The level of 2,3-BPG often is increased in anemia and heart disease. This shifts the OEC to the right and improves oxygen release in these conditions in which oxygen availability is limited.

Some mutant hemoglobins are associated with a shift of the OEC to the left or to the right. This change in oxygen affinity usually leads, through the renal erythropoietin response, to erythrocytosis or anemia (22–24), which tends to compensate for the change in the OEC. Likewise the degree of rightward OEC shift in persons with sickle cell disease, in which the hemoglobin level varies inversely (61), helps to explain why persons with this disease tolerate the anemia per se relatively well, even when the anemia is severe.

The pH interacts with 2,3-BPG in determining the oxygen affinity of blood in the following way. A change in pH produces an immediate change in oxygen affinity (Bohr effect) and a delayed effect, through erythrocyte 2,3-BPG, that is opposite in direction (62,63). For example, a decrease in pH shifts the OEC to the right at once. During a period of many hours, the attendant rise in intraerythrocytic pH causes a decrease in 2,3-BPG concentration and restores the OEC to approximately its starting

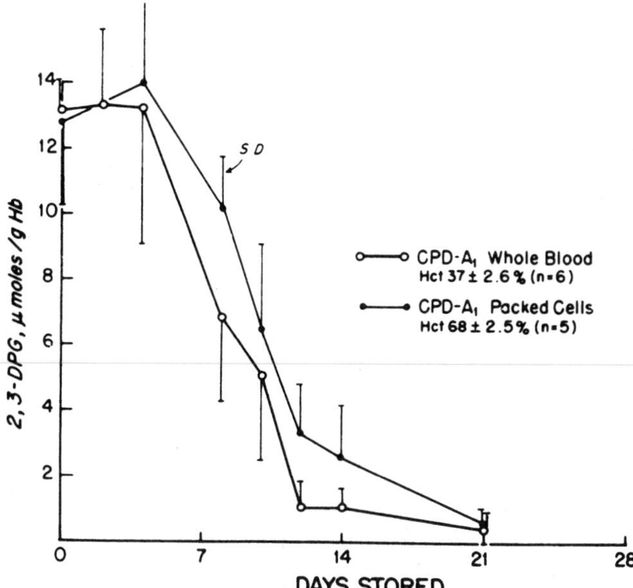

FIGURE 3.17. Effect on 2,3-bisphosphoglycerate (2,3-BPG) levels of storage time of whole blood and packed cells in citrate-phosphate-dextrose supplemented with 0.25 mmol/L adenine. (From Valeri CR, Valeri DA, Gray A, et al. Viability and function of red blood cell concentrates stored at 4C for 35 days in CPDA-1, CPDA-2, or CPDA-3. *Transfusion* 1982; 22:212, with permission.)

position. Alkalosis has the converse effect. Thus the sudden induction of respiratory or metabolic alkalosis or the abrupt correction of acidosis that has been present for some hours leaves the OEC appreciably left shifted for many hours until 2,3-BPG synthesis can occur. The decrease in oxygen availability caused by the OEC shift is compounded in the brain and heart by the direct vasoconstrictor effect of alkalosis and the likelihood of hypoxia (64).

Stored Blood

The OEC of stored blood is shifted appreciably to the left of normal (ultimate P_{50} of approximately 16 mm Hg versus the normal of 27 mm Hg; Fig. 3.11). This is because with all standard liquid storage methods, the level of 2,3-BPG in the red blood cells decreases to very low levels by about 10 days (Figs. 3.17, 3.18). Although the rate of decrease in 2,3-BPG level depends on a number of variables (rate of cooling to room temperature, actual room temperature, duration of room temperature holding as whole blood before preparation and refrigeration of the red blood cell concentrate in additive solution temperature during refrigeration, and especially solution pH), all currently licensed additive systems and storage conditions yield low levels of 2,3-BPG after 7 to 10 days (65,67,69). When such low-2,3-BPG blood is transfused, many hours are required for the 2,3-BPG and P_{50} of the transfused cells to increase to normal (70). When stored blood is transfused in limited quantities, this is probably of little concern. However, massive transfusion with

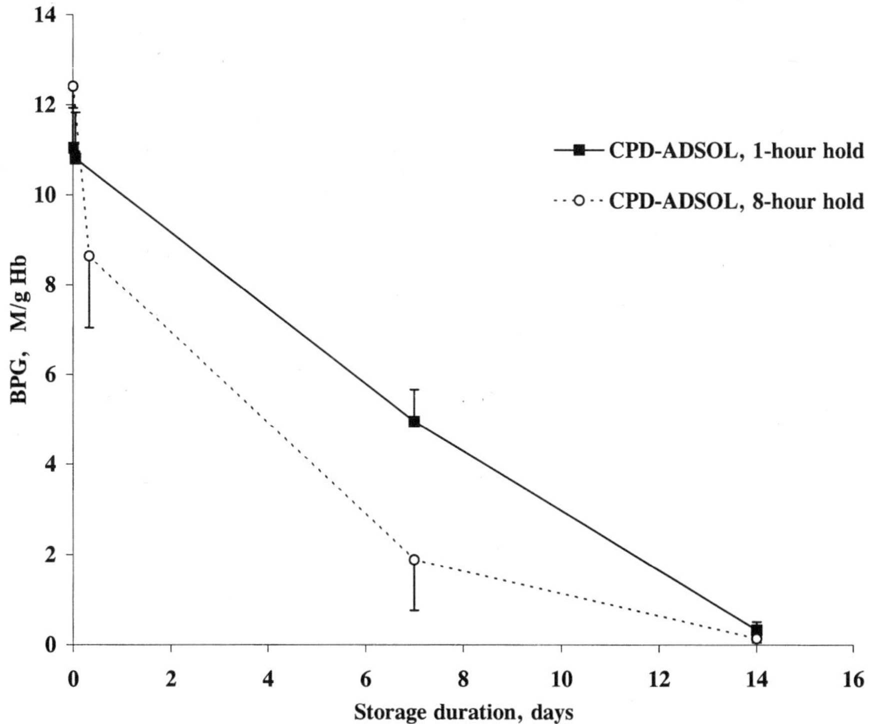

FIGURE 3.18. Effect on 2,3-bisphosphoglycerate (*BPG*) levels of storage time of packed cells collected in citrate-phosphate-dextrose (CPD) and then stored in an adenine-glucose-mannitol solution (Adsol). Similar results are observed after collection in CPD and an adenine-glucose-mannitol solution with differing solute concentrations (SAGM) (65,66). The rapid decline of 2,3-BPG level during the initial 8 hours of room temperature storage is evident (*circles, dashed line*). This early decrease continues when the room temperature holding period is prolonged further (66–68). (From Moroff G, Holme S, Keegan T, et al. Storage of ADSOL-preserved red cells at 2.5 and 5.5 degrees C: comparable retention of in vitro properties. *Vox Sang* 1990; 59:136–139, with permission.)

units of blood stored for more than 7 to 10 days produces a marked increase in oxygen affinity in vivo. The effect of this on the amount of oxygen that can be released as blood moves through the microvasculature is discussed earlier. Although acidosis, if present, would tend to counteract this result (through the Bohr effect), in vivo blood oxygen affinity nevertheless is considerably greater than it would be with 2,3-BPG-replete blood at any given pH. Whether this harms patients already compromised by considerable blood loss and underlying disease is unclear. Clinical data are sparse and difficult to interpret because of multiple confounding variables. Objective end points used to assess the adequacy of oxygenation in patients who undergo transfusion also are lacking. A number of studies, however, have been performed to examine the effect of increases in blood oxygen affinity in appropriate experimental models. Taken as a whole, these data allow the following conclusions. First, when blood flow is free to respond, an increase in oxygen affinity elicits a significant increase in cerebral and coronary flow, which sustains normal oxygenation (71). Thus a healthy subject probably has a sufficient physiologic reserve to deal with the limitation imposed by the leftward OEC shift. Conversely, when the blood flow response is blocked, an increase in oxygen affinity decreases oxygen consumption and greatly impairs the function of the heart and brain (72). Although there is no proof that these conclusions are directly applicable to the clinical setting, patients who need massive transfusions are precisely the ones who are least able to mount the blood flow responses needed to compensate for a left-shifted OEC. Coexistent coronary or cerebral vascular disease would further diminish the likelihood of an adequate cardiovascular response. Consequently, a reasonable case can be made for avoiding massive transfusion of blood with high oxygen affinity (low or absent 2,3-BPG) in seriously ill patients.

Novel Therapies

Clinical trials of novel methods of modifying the OEC are in progress. One promising approach is the drug 2-[4-[[3,5-dimethylanilino)carbonyl]methyl]phenoxyl]-2-methylproprionic acid (RSR13). This compound, a derivative of the antilipemic drug bezafibrate, crosses the red blood cell membrane and interacts with hemoglobin at a locus different from that of other ligands and shifts the OEC to the right (73). This drug has shown benefit in various animal models of ischemia (74–76), which affords further support for the concept that shifts of the OEC are clinically relevant. It is currently undergoing human trials both in the management of ischemic disorders (77) and as an adjunct to radiation therapy for malignant tumors (78, 79). It could also presumably be used in conjunction with stored blood transfusion to obviate the potential problems described earlier.

A second investigational approach is modification of erythrocytes by means of incorporation of inositol hexaphosphate, a naturally occurring hemoglobin ligand that regulates the OEC in some species. This compound has a powerful effect on the OEC of human hemoglobin. Refined methods for incorporating inositol hexaphosphate into erythrocytes now exist (80). This approach has the advantage that blood so treated, whether autologous or allogeneic, would presumably retain its rightward OEC shift during the erythrocyte lifespan (81). Clinical studies are in progress with various purified hemoglobins, both as blood substitutes and for other purposes. This topic is addressed in Chapter 13.

ACKNOWLEDGMENT

The author gratefully acknowledges sabbatical support from University Hospital, Linköping, Sweden, and from the University of Wisconsin–Madison, Madison, Wisconsin.

REFERENCES

1. Orkin SH: Transcription factors that regulate lineage decisions. In: Stamatoyannopoulos G, Majerus PW, Perlmutter RM, eds. *The molecular basis of blood diseases.* Philadelphia: WB Saunders, 2001:80–102.
2. Stamatoyannopoulos G, Grosveld F. Hemoglobin switching. In: Stamatoyannopoulos G, Majerus PW, Perlmutter RM, eds. *The molecular basis of blood diseases.* Philadelphia: WB Saunders, 2001:135–182.
3. Weatherall DJ. The thalassemias. In: Stamatoyannopoulos G, Majerus PW, Perlmutter RM, eds. *The molecular basis of blood diseases.* Philadelphia: WB Saunders, 2001:183–226.
4. Grosveld F, van Assendelft GB, Greaves DR, Kollias G. Position-independent, high-level expression of the human beta-globin gene in transgenic mice. *Cell* 1987;51: 975–985.
5. Grosveld F, de Boer E, Dillon N, et al. The dynamics of globin gene expression and position effects. *Novartis Foundation Symposium* 1998; 214:67–79.
6. Grosveld F. Activation by locus control regions? *Curr Opin Genet Dev* 1999;9:152–157.
7. Tsang AP, Fujiwara Y, Hom DB, et al. Failure of megakaryopoiesis and arrested erythropoiesis in mice lacking the GATA-1 transcriptional cofactor FOG. *Genes Dev* 1998;12:1176–1188.
8. Perkins AC, Sharpe AH, Orkin SH. Lethal beta-thalassaemia in mice lacking the erythroid CACCC-transcription factor EKLF. *Nature* 1995;375:318–322.
9. Nuez B, Michalovich D, Bygrave A, et al. Defective haematopoiesis in fetal liver resulting from inactivation of the EKLF gene. *Nature* 1995;375:316–318.
10. Pevny L, Simon MC, Robertson E, et al. Erythroid differentiation in chimaeric mice blocked by a targeted mutation in the gene for transcription factor GATA-1. *Nature* 1991;349:257–260.
11. Bagga R, Armstrong JA, Emerson BM. Role of chromatin structure and distal enhancers in tissue-specific transcriptional regulation in vitro. *Cold Spring Harbor Symposia on Quantitative Biology* 1998;63: 569–576.
12. Chae JH, Lee YH, Kim CG. Transcription factor CP2 is crucial in hemoglobin synthesis during erythroid terminal differentiation in vitro. *Biochem Biophys Res Comm* 1999;263:580–583.
13. Filipe A, Li Q, Deveaux S, et al. Regulation of embryonic/fetal globin genes by nuclear hormone receptors: a novel perspective on hemoglobin switching. *EMBO J* 1999;18:687–697.
14. Partington GA, Patient RK. Factor binding to the human gamma-globin gene distal CCAAT site: candidates for repression of the normal gene or activation of HPFH mutants. *Br J Haematol* 1998;102: 940–951.
15. Bean TL, Ney PA. Multiple regions of p45 NF-E2 are required for beta-globin gene expression in erythroid cells. *Nucleic Acids Res* 1997; 25:2509–2515.
16. Asano H, Li XS, Stamatoyannopoulos G. FKLF-2: a novel Kruppel-like transcriptional factor that activates globin and other erythroid lineage genes. *Blood* 2000;95:3578–3584.
17. Perkins A. Erythroid Kruppel like factor: from fishing expedition to gourmet meal. *Int J Biochem Cell Biol* 1999;31:1175–1192.
18. Dillon N, Sabbattini P. Functional gene expression domains: defining

the functional unit of eukaryotic gene regulation. *Bioessays* 2000;22: 657–665.

19. Muchardt C, Yaniv M. ATP-dependent chromatin remodelling: SWI/SNF and Co. are on the job. *J Mol Biol* 1999;293:187–198.
20. Engel JD, Tanimoto K. Looping, linking, and chromatin activity: new insights into beta-globin locus regulation. *Cell* 2000;100:499–502.
21. Russell JE, Morales J, Liebhaber SA. The role of mRNA stability in the control of globin gene expression. *Prog Nucleic Acid Res Mol Biol* 1997;57:249–287.
22. Bunn HF, Forget BG. *Hemoglobin: molecular, genetic and clinical aspects.* Philadelphia: WB Saunders, 1986:381–633.
23. Miller W, Hardison R, Chui HK, et al. Globin Gene Server. Available at: http://globin.cse.psu.edu.
24. Huisman THJ, Carver MFH, Efremov GD. *A syllabus of human hemoglobin variants.* Augusta, GA: The Sickle Cell Anemia Foundation, 1998.
25. Ho PJ, Thein SL. Gene regulation and deregulation: a beta globin perspective. *Blood Rev* 2000;14:78–93.
26. Ponka P. Tissue-specific regulation of iron metabolism and heme synthesis: distinct control mechanisms in erythroid cells. *Blood* 1997;89: 1–25.
27. Bottomley SS. Sideroblastic anemias. In: Lee GR, Foerster J, Lukens J, et al., eds. *Wintrobe's clinical hematology.* Baltimore: Williams & Wilkins, 1998:1022–1045.
28. Bottomley SS, Lee GR. Porphyria. In: Lee GR, Foerster J, Lukens J, et al., eds. *Wintrobe's clinical hematology.* Baltimore: Williams & Wilkins, 1998:1071–1108.
29. Sassa S. Hematologic aspects of the porphyrias. *Int J Hematol* 2000; 71:1–17.
30. Ponka P. Cell biology of heme. *Am J Med Sci* 1999;318:241–256.
31. Sadlon TJ, Dell'Oso T, Surinya KH, et al. Regulation of erythroid 5-aminolevulinate synthase expression during erythropoiesis. *Int J Biochem Cell Biol* 1999;31:1153–1167.
32. Rouault T, Klausner R. Regulation of iron metabolism in eukaryotes. *Curr Top Cell Regul* 1997;35:1–19.
33. Bunn HF. Subunit assembly of hemoglobin: an important determinant of hematologic phenotype. *Blood* 1987;69:1–6.
34. Li Q, Peterson KR, Stamatoyannopoulos G. Developmental control of epsilon- and gamma-globin genes. *Ann N Y Acad Sci* 1998;850: 10–17.
35. Dillon N, Trimborn T, Strouboulis J, et al. The effect of distance on long-range chromatin interactions. *Mol Cell* 1997;1:131–139.
36. Perutz MF. Stereochemistry of cooperative effects in haemoglobin. *Nature* 1970;228:726–385.
37. Perutz MF, Wilkinson AJ, Paoli M, et al. The stereochemical mechanism of the cooperative effects in hemoglobin revisited. *Annu Rev Biophys Biomol Struct* 1998;27:1–34.
38. Perutz MF. Mechanisms regulating the reactions of human hemoglobin with oxygen and carbon monoxide. *Annu Rev Physiol* 1990;52:1–25.
39. Eaton WA, Henry ER, Hofrichter J, et al. Is cooperative oxygen binding by hemoglobin really understood? *Nat Struct Biol* 1999;6:351–358.
40. Monod J, Wyman J, Changeux JP. On the nature of allosteric transitions: a plausible mode. *J Mol Biol* 1965;12:88–118.
41. Bettati S, Mozzarelli A, Perutz MF. Allosteric mechanism of haemoglobin: rupture of salt-bridges raises the oxygen affinity of the T-structure. *J Mol Biol* 1998;281:581–585.
42. Ueno H, Manning JM. The functional, oxygen-linked chloride binding sites of hemoglobin are contiguous within a channel in the central cavity. *J Protein Chem* 1992;11:177–185.
43. Perutz MF, Fermi G, Poyart C, et al. A novel allosteric mechanism in haemoglobin: structure of bovine deoxyhaemoglobin, absence of specific chloride-binding sites and origin of the chloride-linked Bohr effect in bovine and human haemoglobin. *J Mol Biol* 1993;233:536–545.
44. Perutz MF, Shih DT, Williamson D. The chloride effect in human haemoglobin: a new kind of allosteric mechanism. *J Mol Biol* 1994; 239:555–560.
45. Gow AJ, Stamler JS. Reactions between nitric oxide and haemoglobin under physiological conditions. *Nature* 1998;391:169–173.
46. Gow AJ, Luchsinger BP, Pawloski JR, et al. The oxyhemoglobin reaction of nitric oxide. *Proc Natl Acad Sci U S A* 1999;96:9027–9032.
47. Jia L, Bonaventura C, Bonaventura J, et al. S-nitrosohaemoglobin: a dynamic activity of blood involved in vascular control. *Nature* 1996; 380:221–226.
48. Stamler JS, Jia L, Eu JP, et al. Blood flow regulation by S-nitrosohemoglobin in the physiological oxygen gradient. *Science* 1997;276: 2034–2037.
49. Spencer NY, Zeng H, Patel RP, et al. Reaction of S-nitrosoglutathione with the heme group of deoxyhemoglobin. *J Biol Chem* 2000;275: 36562–36567.
50. Gross SS, Lane P. Physiological reactions of nitric oxide and hemoglobin: a radical rethink. *Proc Natl Acad Sci U S A* 1999;96:9967–9969.
51. McMahon TJ, Stamler JS. Concerted nitric oxide/oxygen delivery by hemoglobin. *Methods Enzymol* 1999;301:99–114.
52. Gladwin MT, Shelhamer JH, Schechter AN, et al. Role of circulating nitrite and S-nitrosohemoglobin in the regulation of regional blood flow in humans. *Proc Natl Acad Sci U S A* 2000;97:11482–11487.
53. Gladwin MT, Ognibene FP, Pannell LK, et al. Relative role of heme nitrosylation and beta-cysteine 93 nitrosation in the transport and metabolism of nitric oxide by hemoglobin in the human circulation. *Proc Natl Acad Sci U S A* 2000;97:9943–9948.
54. Doherty DH, Doyle MP, Curry SR, et al. Rate of reaction with nitric oxide determines the hypertensive effect of cell-free hemoglobin. *Nat Biotechnol* 1998;16:672–676.
55. Rohlfs RJ, Bruner E, Chiu A, et al. Arterial blood pressure responses to cell-free hemoglobin solutions and the reaction with nitric oxide. *J Biol Chem* 1998;273:12128–12134.
56. Winslow RM. Artificial blood: ancient dream, modern enigma. *Nat Biotechnol* 1998;16:621–622.
57. Hlastala MP, Woodson RD. Bohr effect data for blood gas calculations. *J Appl Physiol* 1983;55:1002–1007.
58. Hlastala MP, Woodson RD. Saturation dependency of the Bohr effect: interactions among H^+, CO_2, and DPG. *J Appl Physiol* 1975;38: 1126–1131.
59. Hlastala MP, Woodson RD, Wranne B. Influence of temperature on hemoglobin-ligand interaction in whole blood. *J Appl Physiol* 1977; 43:545–550.
60. Wranne B, Woodson RD, Detter JC. Bohr effect: interaction between H^+, CO_2, and 2,3-DPG in fresh and stored blood. *J Appl Physiol* 1972;32:749–754.
61. Serjeant G, Serjeant B, Stephens A, et al. Determinants of haemoglobin level in steady-state homozygous sickle cell disease. *Br J Haematol* 1996; 92:143–149.
62. Bellingham AJ, Detter JC, Lenfant C. Regulatory mechanisms of hemoglobin oxygen affinity in acidosis and alkalosis. *J Clin Invest* 1971; 50:700–706.
63. Hsia CC. Respiratory function of hemoglobin. *N Engl J Med* 1998; 338:239–247.
64. Beech JS, Williams SC, Iles RA, et al. Haemodynamic and metabolic effects in diabetic ketoacidosis in rats of treatment with sodium bicarbonate or a mixture of sodium bicarbonate and sodium carbonate. *Diabetologia* 1995;38:889–898.
65. Högman CF. Preparation and preservation of red cells. *Vox Sang* 1998; 74[Suppl 2]:177–187.
66. Solheim BG, Bergerud UE, Kjeldsen-Kragh J, et al. Improved blood preservation with 0.5CPD erythro-sol. Coagulation factor VIII activity and erythrocyte quality after delayed separation of blood. *Vox Sang* 1998;74:168–175.
67. Pietersz RN, de Korte D, Reesink HW, et al. Storage of whole blood for up to 24 hours at ambient temperature prior to component preparation. *Vox Sang* 1989;56:145–150.
68. Farrugia A, Douglas S, James J, et al. Red cell and platelet concentrates from blood collected into half-strength citrate anticoagulant: improved maintenance of red blood cell 2,3-diphosphoglycerate in half-citrate red cells. *Vox Sang* 1992;63:31–38.
69. Moroff G, Holme S, Keegan T, et al. Storage of ADSOL-preserved red cells at 2.5 and 5.5 degrees C: comparable retention of in vitro properties. *Vox Sang* 1990;59:136–139.
70. Heaton A, Keegan T, Holme S. In vivo regeneration of red cell 2,3-diphosphoglycerate following transfusion of DPG-depleted AS-1, AS-3 and CPDA-1 red cells. *Br J Haematol* 1989;71:131–136.

71. Woodson RD, Auerbach S. Effect of increased oxygen affinity and anemia on cardiac output and its distribution. *J Appl Physiol* 1982;53: 1299–1306.
72. Woodson RD, Fitzpatrick JHJ, Costello DJ, et al. Increased blood oxygen affinity decreases canine brain oxygen consumption. *J Lab Clin Med* 1982;100:411–424.
73. Abraham DJ, Wireko FC, Randad RS, et al. Allosteric modifiers of hemoglobin:2-[4-[[(3,5-disubstituted anilino)carbonyl]methyl]phenoxy]-2-methylpropionic acid derivatives that lower the oxygen affinity of hemoglobin in red cell suspensions, in whole blood, and in vivo in rats. *Biochemistry* 1992;31:9141–9149.
74. Weiss RG, Mejia MA, Kass DA, et al. Preservation of canine myocardial high-energy phosphates during low-flow ischemia with modification of hemoglobin-oxygen affinity. *J Clin Invest* 1999;103:739–746.
75. Kilgore KS, Shwartz CF, Gallagher MA, et al. RSR13, a synthetic allosteric modifier of hemoglobin, improves myocardial recovery following hypothermic cardiopulmonary bypass. *Circulation* 1999;100: II351–II356.
76. Watson JC, Doppenberg EM, Bullock MR, et al. Effects of the allosteric modification of hemoglobin on brain oxygen and infarct size in a feline model of stroke. *Stroke* 1997;28:1624–1630.
77. Wahr JA, Gerber M, Venitz J, et al. Allosteric modification of oxygen delivery by hemoglobin. *Anesth Analg* 2001;92:615–620.
78. Rowinsky EK. Novel radiation sensitizers targeting tissue hypoxia. *Oncology (Huntingt)* 1999;13:61–70.
79. Kleinberg L, Grossman SA, Piantadosi S, et al. Phase I trial to determine the safety, pharmacodynamics, and pharmacokinetics of RSR13, a novel radioenhancer, in newly diagnosed glioblastoma multiforme. *J Clin Oncol* 1999;17:2593–2603.
80. Bruggemann U, Roux EC, Hannig J, et al. Low-oxygen-affinity red cells produced in a large-volume, continuous-flow electroporation system. *Transfusion* 1995;35:478–486.
81. Teisseire B, Ropars C, Villereal MC, et al. Long-term physiological effects of enhanced O_2 release by inositol hexaphosphate-loaded erythrocytes. *Proc Natl Acad Sci U S A* 1987;84:6894–6898.

Rossi's Principles of Transfusion Medicine, Third Edition, edited by Toby L. Simon, Walter H. Dzik, Edward L. Snyder, Christopher P. Stowell, and Ronald G. Strauss. Lippincott Williams & Wilkins, Philadelphia © 2002.

4

RED BLOOD CELL METABOLISM

ERNEST BEUTLER

It lacks a nucleus and mitochondria, cannot divide, and lives for only 120 days. It cannot synthesize protein, use oxygen for the extraction of energy from its fuel, or synthesize nucleotides from simple precursors. Yet the human red blood cell is far from simple. It is admirably suited to its primary function—transporting oxygen to the tissues from the lungs and carrying carbon dioxide from the tissues to the lungs. These functions do not require the expenditure of energy. Nonetheless, maintaining the hemoglobin of the cell and maintaining the membrane that holds it in a functioning state does require active metabolism. A red blood cell that is unable to extract energy from glucose properly is unable to circulate. From the point of view of the transfusionist, such an erythrocyte is quite useless. It is essential, therefore, to understand the metabolism of the red blood cell to make possible the development of successful strategies for the long-term storage of red blood cells.

METABOLISM OF GLUCOSE

Under physiologic circumstances, the energy that the red blood cell requires is derived almost entirely through the breakdown of glucose to lactate or pyruvate. The sequence of reactions that perform the necessary chemical transformations is generally known as the glycolytic or the Embden-Meyerhof pathway (1, 2). This pathway is phylogenetically very old, and the sequence of reactions is the same in *Escherichia coli,* yeast, and humans. Except for the exaggerated production of 2,3-diphosphoglycerate (2,3-DPG) (also known as 2,3 bisphosphoglycerate) in the red blood cell, the pathway is the same in all tissues.

Main Glycolytic Pathway

The reactions of the glycolytic pathway are shown in Figure 4.1. Eleven enzymes are needed to break glucose down to lactate. In the sequential series of reactions that these enzymes catalyze, the six-carbon sugar glucose is phosphorylated, isomerized to fructose, phosphorylated again, and cleaved into three-carbon sugars. The three-carbon sugars are again phosphorylated. Eventually the carbohydrate-bound phosphate that has been gained is transferred to adenosine diphosphate (ADP), producing the high-energy compound, adenosine triphosphate (ATP). The ATP synthesized is used by ATPase for the pumping of ions against concentration gradients, for the phosphorylation of membrane proteins and lipids, and very importantly for the phosphorylation of additional glucose so that the ADP that has been formed from ATP can be rephosphorylated.

2,3-Diphosphoglycerate and the Rapoport-Luebering Shunt

The production of large quantities of 2,3-DPG (Fig. 4.2) is a unique feature of glycolysis in the red blood cell. This phosphorylated sugar acid is not found only in erythrocytes. Some 2,3-DPG is present in all cells, because it is needed for the functioning of the monophosphoglycerate mutase reaction. This reaction is on the main pathway of glycolysis. Red blood cells, however, contain vastly greater amounts of 2,3-DPG—a quantity approximately equimolar with the concentration of hemoglobin itself. It is the interaction of 2,3-DPG with hemoglobin that accounts

E. Beutler: Department of Molecular and Experimental Medicine, Scripps Research Institute, La Jolla, California.

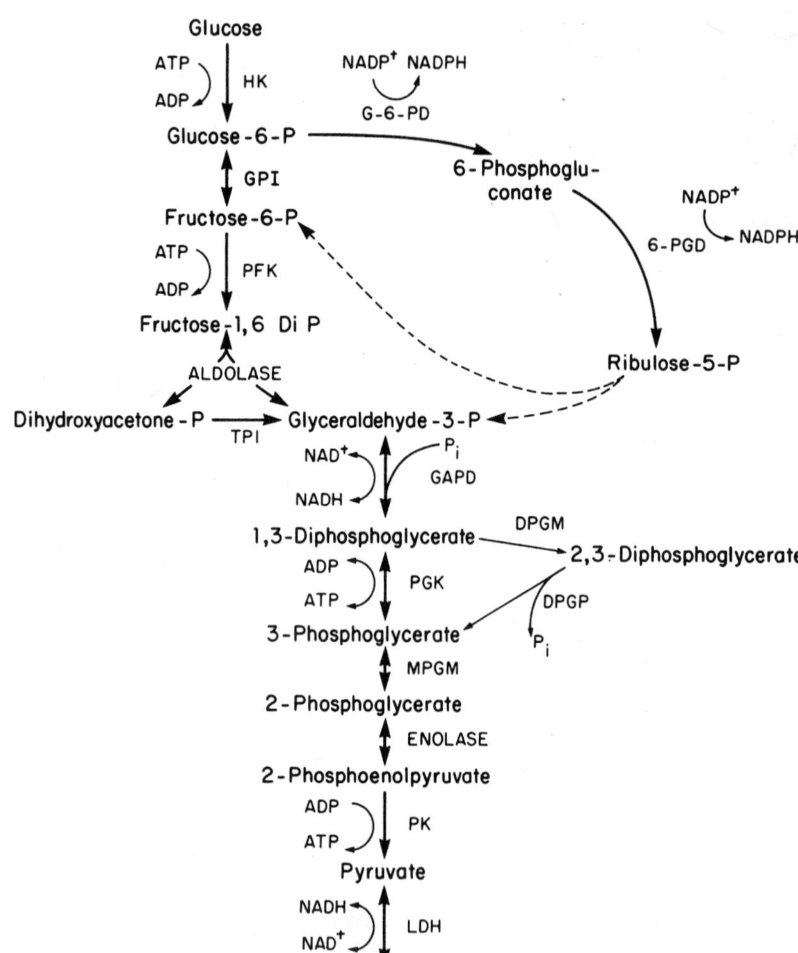

FIGURE 4.1. The glycolytic pathway and partial hexose monophosphate pathway of red blood cell metabolism. *ATP*, adenosine triphosphate; *ADP*, adenosine diphosphate; *HK*, hexokinase; *NADP+, nicotinamide adenine dinucleotide phosphate, oxidized form; NADPH,* nicotinamide adenine dinucleotide phosphate, reduced form; *6-PGD*, 6-phosphogluconate dehydrogenase; *P*, phosphate; *G-6-PD*, glucose-6-phosphate dehydrogenase; *PFK*, phosphofructokinase; *TPI*, triosephosphate isomerase; *NAD+*, nicotinamide adenine dinucleotide, oxidized form; *NADH*, nicotinamide adenine dinucleotide, reduced form; *GAPD*, glyceraldehyde-3-phosphate dehydrogenase; *PGK*, phosphoglycerate kinase; DPGM, diphosphoglycerate mutase. *DPGP*, diphosphoglycerate phosphatase; *MPGM*, monophosphoglycerate mutase; *PK*, pyruvate kinase; *LDH*, lactate dehydrogenase;

for its special role in the erythrocyte. Binding to the β subunits of deoxyhemoglobin, it serves to stabilize this low-affinity conformation. At a physiologic pH, solutions of pure hemoglobin become one-half saturated with oxygen at a partial oxygen pressure (PO_2) of only approximately 11 mm Hg (torr) (3). When equimolar concentrations of 2,3-DPG are present, however, one-half saturation requires a much higher PO_2, approximating 27 mm Hg.

Production of 2,3-DPG is the function of a special side pathway that branches from the main glycolytic pathway after the formation of 1,3-diphosphoglycerate (1,3-DPG) and returns to it with the formation of 3-phosphoglyceric acid (3-PGA). The pathway consists of the formation of 2,3-DPG from 1,3-DPG, and then the dephosphorylation of 1,3-DPG to 3-PGA. Both reactions are catalyzed by the same enzyme (4,5). The most probable mechanism of action of this phosphatase-mutase enzyme is based on the presumed capacity of the enzyme itself to undergo phosphorylation and to donate its phosphate to 3-PGA or, alternatively, to water. If the enzyme is phosphorylated by 1,3-DPG, it can transfer the phosphate it has received to the 3-position of 3-PGA. This makes it a mutase, forming 2,3-DPG while consuming 1,3-DPG. If, on the other hand, the 2-phosphate of 2,3-DPG is the phosphate donor and the enzyme-phosphate complex is hydrolyzed to free enzyme and phosphoric acid, the enzyme is acting as a phosphatase, forming 3-PGA and phosphate while consuming 2,3-DPG (6). This putative series of reactions is illustrated in Figure 4.3.

Hexose Monophosphate Pathway

Under normal, steady-state conditions, most glucose is metabolized by red blood cells by way of the main glycolytic pathway, but there is another metabolic pathway that can be important under some circumstances. This is the hexose monophosphate (HMP) shunt or pathway (7–9). Some of the glucose-6-phosphate (G-6-P) formed when glucose is phosphorylated in the hexokinase reaction may enter this pathway. Glucose-6-phosphate dehydrogenase (G-6-PD) catalyzes the oxidation of G-6-P to 6-phosphogluconolactone, reducing nicotinamide adenine dinucleotide phosphate (NADP) to NADPH. After hydrolysis of the lactone to 6-phosphogluconic acid by a specific lactonase (10,11), another oxidative step reduces additional NADP to NADPH, and releases carbon dioxide from the six-carbon compound, forming the five-carbon sugar ribose-1-phosphate. After

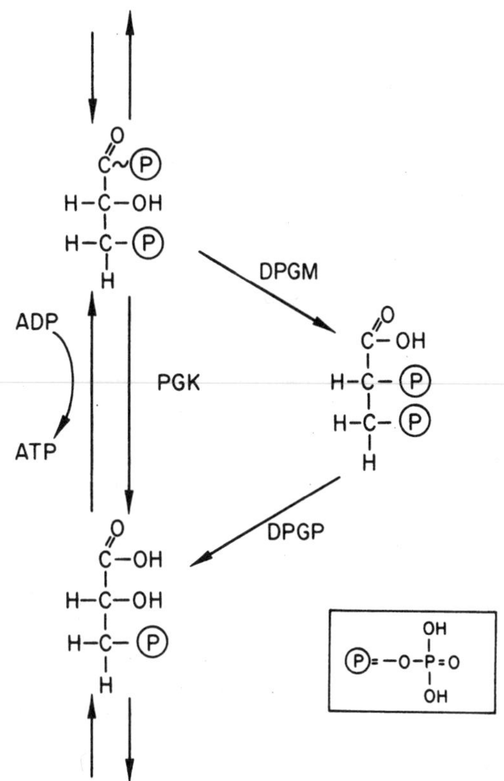

FIGURE 4.2. Rapoport-Luebering shunt pathway. The structure of 2,3-DPG is shown at the *left*. It is formed from 1,3-DPG (*top*) by DPGM. It is broken down to 3-phosphoglyceric acid (*bottom*) by DPGP. Abbreviations are as in Figure 4.1.

a series of rearrangements, two normal intermediates of the main glycolytic pathway, fructose-6-phosphate and glyceraldehyde-3-phosphate, are formed and rejoin the main metabolic stream.

The HMP pathway is important to the red blood cell primarily as a source of NADPH. It is this reduced nucleotide that maintains glutathione (12) and glutathione-protein disulfides (13) in the reduced form. Reduced glutathione also serves to detoxify electrophilic xenobiotics by forming thioether conjugates that are transported out of the red blood cell (14) and broken down elsewhere in the body. The pentose formed in the HMP pathway also plays an important role in the economy of

1) 1,3-DPG + [E] ⟶ 3-PGA + [E-P]

2) [E-P] + 3-PGA ⇄ 2,3-DPG + [E]

3) [E-P] + H_2O ⟶ [E] + P_i

FIGURE 4.3. Reactions between phosphoglycerates and a single multifunctional enzyme (*[E]*) and its phosphorylated form (*[E-P]*). These reactions convert 1,3-DPG to 2,3-DPG, the DPGM reaction, and 2,3-DPG to 3-phosphoglyceric acid, the DPGP reaction. The sum of reactions 1 and 2 results in conversion of 1,3-DPG to 2,3-DPG, the DPGM reaction. The reverse of reaction 2 plus reaction 3 results in conversion of 2,3-DPG to 3-PGA, the DPGP reaction.

the red blood cell by providing ribose-5-phosphate needed for phosphoribosyl pyrophosphate (PRPP), an essential substrate for the synthesis of adenine nucleotides (see later). Red blood cells from patients with a deficiency of G-6-PD, the most common hereditary enzyme deficiency among humans, do not maintain ATP levels in adenine-containing media as well as do cells without such a deficiency (15), probably because of inability to generate sufficient amounts of pentose phosphates.

ALTERNATIVE SUBSTRATES FOR RED BLOOD CELL METABOLISM

Glucose is the natural substrate for human red blood cell energy metabolism, but the capability of red blood cells to metabolize other substrates has been exploited in the design of experimental blood preservatives. Fructose (16,17) and mannose (18) are isomers of glucose that like glucose are phosphorylated at the 6-position by hexokinase and ATP. Fructose-6-phosphate is a normal intermediate in the glycolytic pathway (Fig. 4.1), and it is the direct product of fructose phosphorylation. The product of mannose phosphorylation, mannose-6-phosphate, is converted to fructose-6-phosphate by mannose phosphate isomerase (18). However, the activity of this enzyme is relatively low, and mannose is therefore more slowly used by red blood cells than are fructose and glucose. Galactose, another isomer of glucose, is also metabolized by red blood cells (19), but it is phosphorylated at the 1-position by galactokinase (20), an enzyme with very low activity in the erythrocyte. Such quantities of galactose-1-phosphate that are formed, however, are converted to glucose-1-phosphate and hence to the normal glycolytic intermediate G-6-P. The three-carbon sugar dihydroxyacetone is phosphorylated by red blood cell triokinase to form the normal glycolytic intermediate dihydroxyacetone phosphate (21). The rate of phosphorylation is comparable with that of glucose by hexokinase and is less sensitive to the inhibitory effect of hydrogen ions. It therefore has been found useful in the design of blood preservatives (see Chapter 5).

The presence in red blood cells of the enzyme nucleoside phosphorylase makes it possible for red blood cells to use nucleosides such as inosine (22–24):

$$\text{Inosine} + P_i \rightarrow \text{Ribose-1-P} + \text{Hypoxanthine}$$

In this reaction, phosphorylated carbohydrate is formed without the expenditure of ATP. Ribose-1-phosphate is readily converted to fructose-6-phosphate, a normal intermediate in the glycolytic pathway, by the HMP pathway (see earlier). Thus even ATP-depleted red blood cells are able to prime their metabolic pump when they are provided with nucleosides as fuel.

Erythrocytes are generally regarded as impermeable to phosphorylated metabolic intermediates, but phospho (enol) pyruvate (PEP) appears to be an exception to this rule (25). For this reason, storage media containing PEP have been studied, but the special conditions required for the penetration of this phosphate compound make it difficult or impossible to use PEP for the purpose of maintaining phosphorylated intermediates (26).

REGULATION OF ENERGY METABOLISM

Rate of Glucose Metabolism

In most tissues, metabolic regulation can be achieved, at least in part, by increasing or decreasing the rate of transcription of DNA or the translation of messenger RNA. Red blood cells do not have this option, lacking the capacity for protein synthesis. Instead, the rate of glucose metabolism is regulated by a series of elegant feedback mechanisms. These have been studied extensively and used as the basis for computer modeling of red blood cell metabolism (27–29). Yet our understanding of control of glucose metabolism by red blood cells is incomplete. It is, however, obvious that the rate of glucose metabolism by red blood cells is influenced by a great many factors other than the mere unrestrained activity of red blood cell enzymes. The activity of the first enzyme of the pathway, hexokinase, is the lowest of the entire series of reactions. Yet its unrestrained capacity to phosphorylate glucose and thus to admit substrate into the pathway is more than ten times the rate at which glucose is actually consumed by erythrocytes. The activity of this enzyme is markedly inhibited by glucose-6-phosphate, its product, and by 2,3-DPG (9,30–33). The level of these intermediates is influenced by the activators and inhibitors acting at other levels of glycolysis. Phosphofructokinase also is regulated by numerous effector molecules. For example, it is inhibited by ATP and by 2,3-DPG, so that its activity adjusts automatically to requirements for these vital compounds (34–36). Ammonia stimulates the enzyme (37), and both hexokinase and phosphofructokinase are readily inhibited by hydrogen ions. This is one of the principal reasons that the rate of glycolysis slows markedly during blood storage—the accumulation of lactic acid lowers the pH.

In addition to feedback regulation of glycolysis, it has been proposed that the cytoplasmic portion of membrane band 3 may exert a regulatory effect through reversible binding of glyceraldehyde phosphate dehydrogenase (38–40), but the evidence for such a mechanism is largely indirect.

Hexose Monophosphate Pathway

The activity of the HMP pathway is regulated largely by the availability of NADP and by the level of NADPH. Normally most of this nucleotide is in the reduced (NADPH) form, and the pathway operates very slowly. In the face of oxidative stress, NADPH, a potent inhibitor of G-6-PD, is oxidized to NADP. This process both disinhibits G-6-PD and provides rate-limiting substrate for the G-6-PD reaction. As a consequence, metabolism by way of the HMP pathway increases immediately to fill the need for additional production of NADPH.

2,3-Diphosphoglycerate

The steady state level of 2,3-DPG depends on the rate of its formation and degradation. Only two reactions, the diphosphoglycerate mutase (DPGM) and diphosphoglycerate phosphatase (DPGP) reactions, both catalyzed by the same enzyme, are involved. Many effectors determine whether the mutase or the phosphatase activity of the enzyme predominates (Fig. 4.4). The hydrogen ion concentration is one of the most important physiologic modulators. At low pH, phosphatase activity is stimulated and mutase activity is inhibited. Thus a high pH favors good 2,3-DPG maintenance during storage, whereas a low pH leads to rapid loss (see Chapter 6). Another effector that may be of particular importance is 2-phosphoglycolate. Shown to be present in red blood cells in trace quantities (41,42), this two-carbon compound can accelerate the phosphatase reaction more than 1,000-fold. Red blood cells also contain a specific phosphoglycolate phosphatase that rapidly hydrolyzes 2-phosphoglycolate, thereby serving to protect 2,3-DPG (43,44). However, the source of 2-phosphogycolate and the regulation of the amount present remain unknown (45–47). Modulation of red blood cell metabolism by pH and by inhibitors such as oxalate, alanine, and xanthone compounds (see Chapter 5), has been one of the principal means used to retard the decline of 2,3-DPG levels that occurs during liquid storage of red blood cells.

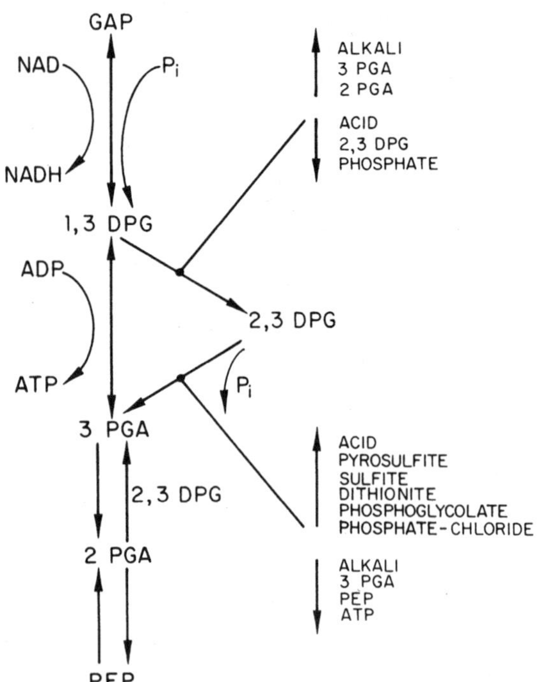

FIGURE 4.4. Regulation of the formation and breakdown of 2,3-DPG. The steady-state concentration of 2,3-DPG is governed by the rate of its formation from 1,3-DPG and by its breakdown to 3-phosphoglyceric acid. Both reactions are catalyzed by a multifunctional DPGM-DPGP enzyme modulated by a variety of substances. Abbreviations are as in Figure 4.1.

Adenosine Triphosphate

Regulation of ATP levels is complex, especially because this compound is synthesized from ADP in two different metabolic steps. ATP is used in a number of different metabolic pathways, particularly by kinases such as hexokinase, phosphofructokinase and protein kinase, and by ATPases such as Na^+-K^+-ATPase, Mg^{2+}-ATPase, and Ca^{2+}-ATPase. Moreover, ATP is in equilibrium with ADP and adenosine monophosphate (AMP) through the adenylate kinase reaction. As the level of ADP increases, some of it is converted to AMP. Adenosine monophosphate, in turn, is deaminated in the AMP deaminase reaction. This reaction seems to be particularly important in regulating the size of the adenine nucleotide pool in the erythrocyte. When the enzyme is absent, the level of ATP in red blood cells increases (48).

Guanine Nucleotides

Red blood cells contain and turn over guanine nucleotides (49–51) and guanosine triphosphatase (GTPase) (52), and GTP-binding activity is present (53,54). Guanosine triphosphatase inhibits transglutaminase (55), but the function of guanine nucleotides in red blood cells remains unknown.

SYNTHETIC PROCESSES

Although red blood cells have lost their protein-synthetic capabilities and to a large extent the ability to synthesize lipids, they are able to assemble some important molecules from simpler precursors. They retain the capacity to synthesize nucleotides through the "salvage pathway" and to synthesize glutathione from its precursor amino acids. Adenine is able to enter the erythrocyte through both saturable and unsaturable transport systems (56). Purine nucleotides are synthesized through the adenine phosphoribosyl transferase (APRT) reaction:

$$\text{Adenine} + \text{PRPP} \rightarrow \text{AMP} + \text{PP}$$

This reaction is critical in blood storage. The beneficial effect of addition of adenine to stored blood depends on it. Phosphoribosyl pyrophosphate (PRPP), one of the substrates for the formation of AMP in this reaction, is synthesized from pentose-phosphate formed in the HMP pathway. Guanine nucleotides form in an analogous reaction and are catalyzed by a different enzyme, hypoxanthine-guanine phosphoribosyl transferase. Red blood cells also actively synthesize a number of other small molecules, including reduced glutathione, nicotinamide adenine dinucleotide (NAD) (57), and *S*-adenosyl-L-methione (58).

MEMBRANE METABOLISM

The red blood cell membrane is the boundary between the plasma or other suspending medium and the hemoglobin-containing interior of the cell. It is composed of a phospholipid bilayer containing cholesterol molecules and membrane proteins (59). The phospholipids are asymmetrically disposed with a predominance of phosphatidyl choline and sphingomyelin in the outer leaflet and phosphatidylinositol, phosphatidylethanolamine, and phosphatidylserine in the inner leaflet. "Intrinsic" membrane proteins such as glycophorin and band 3 extend through the lipid membrane (59,60). Branches of carbohydrates anchored to membrane proteins protrude from the outer surface of the membrane. The inner surface of the membrane is lined by a network of "extrinsic" proteins, including spectrin and actin. The red blood cell membrane contains transport proteins such as the glucose transporter, the Ca^{2+}-ATPase, the Na^{+}-K^{+}-ATPase, the GSSG (oxidized glutathione) transport ATPases, and amino acid transporters.

Although the macromolecules of the membrane are produced by the red blood cell precursor in the bone marrow, at least some of the components of the membrane are metabolically quite active. For example, phosphatidylinositol undergoes active phosphorylation at two of the positions on the inositol ring (61). Membrane proteins are phosphorylated by protein kinases (62) and dephosphorylated by phosphatases (63). Cholesterol in the membrane exchanges readily with cholesterol in the plasma. It is presumed that these reactions influence the functional status of membrane components, although their importance is not yet fully understood. It has been proposed that interaction of membrane components, particularly band 3, may play a role in modulation of red blood cell glycolysis (38–40).

MOLECULAR BIOLOGY

Lacking DNA and RNA, red blood cells depend on the proteins synthesized early in their life. Therefore understanding of erythrocyte metabolism depends on appreciation of the kinetic properties of red blood cell enzymes. Our understanding of red blood cell metabolism therefore has not been much affected by the modern revolution in molecular biology. However, the genes that encode many of the red blood cell enzymes and membrane proteins have been cloned (64,65), and this has provided insights into protein structure that may aid in understanding their function and regulation.

SUMMARY

In the circulation, the erythrocyte metabolizes glucose in the glycolytic and hexose monophosphate pathways and uses the energy extracted to maintain hemoglobin in the reduced state so that it can bind and deliver oxygen and to provide ATP to maintain concentration gradients between the plasma and erythrocyte. The metabolic pathways involved have been studied extensively, and their characteristics are well known. Improvements in storing red blood cells can be based on understanding of red blood cell metabolism of glucose, and of other substrates, such as inosine and adenine, that can be added in the context of in vitro storage.

REFERENCES

1. Beutler E. *Hemolytic anemia in disorders of red cell metabolism.* New York: Plenum Publishing, 1978.
2. Beutler E. The red cell: a tiny dynamo. In: Wintrobe MM, ed. *Blood pure and eloquent.* New York: McGraw-Hill, 1980;141–168.
3. Paniker NV, Beutler E. Effect of normal metabolites on the oxygen-hemoglobin equilibrium. *Proc Soc Exp Biol Med* 1970;135:389–391.
4. Rosa R, Audit I, Rosa J. Evidence for three enzymatic activities in one electrophoretic band of 3-phosphoglycerate mutase from red cells. *Biochim Biophys Acta* 1975;57:1059–1063.

5. Chiba H, Ikura K, Narita H, et al. Regulation of 2, 3 bisphosphoglycerate metabolism in erythrocytes by a multifunctional enzyme. *Acta Biol Med Ger* 1977; 36:491–505.
6. Rose ZB. The enzymology of 2, 3-bisphosphoglycerate. *Adv Enzymol* 1980;51:211–253.
7. Beutler E. Abnormalities of the hexose monophosphate shunt. *Semin Hematol* 1971;8:311–347.
8. Horecker BL, Hiatt HH. Pathways of carbohydrate metabolism in normal and neoplastic cells. *N Engl J Med* 1958;258:177–184.
9. Dische Z. The pentose phosphate metabolism in red cells. In: Bishop C, Surgenor DM, eds. *The red blood cell.* New York: Academic Press, 1964:189–209.
10. Beutler E, Kuhl W. Limiting role of 6-phosphogluconolactonase in erythrocyte hexose monophosphate pathway metabolism. *J Lab Clin Med* 1985;106:573–577.
11. Bauer HP Srihari T, Jochims JC, et al. 6-Phosphogluconolactonase: purification, properties and activities in various tissues. *Eur J Biochem* 1983;133:163–168.
12. Chang JC, Van Der Hoeven LH, Haddox CH. Glutathione reductase in the red blood cells. *Ann Clin Lab Sci* 1978;8:23–29.
13. Srivastava SK, Beutler E. Glutathione metabolism of the erythrocyte: the enzymic cleavage of glutathione-haemoglobin preparations by glutathione reductase. *Biochem J* 1970;119:353–357.
14. Board PG. Transport of the S-2, 4 dinitrophenyl conjugate of glutathione from erythrocytes. *Br J Haematol* 1984;58:200–201.
15. Orlina AR, Josephson AM, McDonald BJ. The poststorage viability of glucose-6-phosphate dehydrogenase–deficient erythrocytes. *J Lab Clin Med* 1970;75:930–936.
16. Torrance JD. The role of fructose in restoration of organic phosphate compounds in outdated bank blood. *J Lab Clin Med* 1973;82: 489–499.
17. Moses SW, Bashan N. Fructose metabolism in the human red blood cell. *Isr J Med Sci* 1974;10:707–711.
18. Beutler E, Teeple L. Mannose metabolism in the human erythrocyte. *J Clin Invest* 1969;48:461–466.
19. Hjelm M, de Verdier CH. Über die Bestimmung des Galaktose-Verbrauchs in menschlichen Erythrozyten mit Galaktose-Oxydase. *Folia Haematol (Leipz)* 1965;83:347–349.
20. Blume KG, Beutler E. Galactokinase from human erythrocytes. *Methods Enzymol* 1975;42:47–53.
21. Beutler E, Guintto E. Dihydroxyacetone metabolism by human erythrocytes: demonstration of triokinase activity and its characterization. *Blood* 1973;41:559–568.
22. Zannis V, Doyle D, Martin DW. Purification and characterization of human erythrocyte purine nucleoside phosphorylase and its subunits. *J Biol Chem* 1978;253:504–510.
23. Kim BK, Cha S, Parks RE Jr. Purine nucleoside phosphorylase and human erythrocytes, II: Kinetic analysis and substrate-binding studies. *J Biol Chem* 1968;243:1771–1776.
24. Gabrio BW, Finch CA, Huennekens FM. Erythrocyte preservation: a topic in molecular biochemistry. *Blood* 1956;11:103–113.
25. Hamasaki N, Matsuyama H, Hirota-Chigita C. Characterization of phosphoenolpyruvate transport across the erythrocyte membrane: evidence for involvement of band 3 in the transport system. *Eur J Biochem* 1983;132:531–536.
26. Matsuyama H, Ericson Å, Högman CF, et al. Lack of success with a combination of alanine and phosphoenolpyruvate as an additive for liquid storage of red cells at 4°C. *Transfusion* 1990;30:339–343.
27. Heinrich R, Rapoport SM. The utility of mathematical models for the understanding of metabolic systems. *Biochem Soc Trans* 1983;11: 31–35.
28. Schuster R, Jacobasch G, Holzhötter HG. Mathematical modelling of metabolic pathways affected by an enzyme deficiency: energy and redox metabolism of glucose-6-phosphate—dehydrogenase–deficient erythrocytes. *Eur J Biochem* 1989;182:605–612.
29. Ni TC, Savageau MA. Application of biochemical systems theory to metabolism in human red blood cells: signal propagation and accuracy of representation. *J Biol Chem* 1996;271:7927–7941.
30. Rijksen G, Staal GEJ. Regulation of human erythrocyte hexokinase: the influence of glycolytic intermediates and inorganic phosphate. *Biochim Biophys Acta* 1977; 485:75–86.
31. Rose IA, Warms JVB, Kosow DP. Specificity for the glucose-6-p inhibition site of hexokinase. *Arch Biochem Biophys* 1974;164:729–735.
32. Beutler E. 2, 3-Diphosphoglycerate affects enzymes of glucose metabolism in red blood cells. *Nature* 1971; 232:20–21.
33. Brewer GJ. Erythrocyte metabolism and function: hexokinase inhibition by 2, 3- diphosphoglycerate and interaction with ATP and Mg2 +. *Biochim Biophys Acta* 1969;192:157–161.
34. Vora S. Isozymes of human phosphofructokinase: biochemical and genetic aspects. In: Rattazzi MC, Scandalios JG, Whitt GS, eds. *Isozymes: current topics in biological and medical research.* New York: Alan R. Liss, 1983:3–23.
35. Uyeda K, Furuya E, Luby LJ. The effect of natural and synthetic d-fructose 2, 6-bisphosphate on the regulatory kinetic properties of liver and muscle phosphofructokinases. *J Biol Chem* 1981;256:8394–8399.
36. Tarui S, Kono N, Uyeda K. Purification and properties of rabbit erythrocyte phosphofructokinase. *J Biol Chem* 1972;247:1138–1145.
37. Layzer RB, Rowland LP, Bank WJ. Physical and kinetic properties of human phosphofructokinase from skeletal muscle and erythrocytes. *J Biol Chem* 1969;244:3823–3831.
38. Moriyama R, Lombardo CR, Workman RF, et al. Regulation of linkages between the erythrocyte membrane and its skeleton by 2, 3-diphosphoglycerate. *J Biol Chem* 1993;268:10990–10996.
39. Low PS, Rathinavelu P, Harrison ML. Regulation of glycolysis via reversible enzyme binding to the membrane protein, band 3. *J Biol Chem* 1993;268:14627–14631.
40. Messana I, Ferroni L, Misiti F, et al. Blood bank conditions and RBCs: the progressive loss of metabolic modulation. *Transfusion* 2000;40: 353–360.
41. Vora S, Spear D. Demonstration and quantitation of phosphoglycolate in human red cells. *Clin Res* 1986;34:664A.
42. Rose ZB, Salon J. The identification of glycolate-2-P as a constituent of normal red blood cells. *Biochem Biophys Res Comm* 1979;87:869–875.
43. Badwey JA. Phosphoglycolate phosphatase in human erythrocytes. *J Biol Chem* 1977;252:2441–2443.
44. Beutler E, West C. An improved assay and some properties of phosphoglycolate phosphatase. *Anal Biochem* 1980;106:163–168.
45. Sasaki H, Fujii S, Yoshizaki Y, et al. Phosphoglycolate synthesis by human erythrocyte pyruvate kinase. *Acta Haematol* 1987;77:83–86.
46. Fujii S, Beutler E. Where does phosphoglycolate come from in red cells? *Acta Haematol* 1985;73:26–30.
47. Somoza R, Beutler E. Phosphoglycolate phosphatase and 2, 3-diphosphoglycerate in red cells of normal and anemic subjects. *Blood* 1983; 62:750–753.
48. Ogasawara N, Goto H, Yamada Y, et al. Deficiency of erythrocyte type isozyme of AMP deaminase in human. *Adv Exp Med Biol* 1986;195: 123–127.
49. Ericson A, Niklasson F, de Verdier CH. Metabolism of guanosine in human erythrocytes. *Vox Sang* 1985;48:72–83.
50. Sidi Y, Gelvan I, Brosh S, et al. Guanine nucleotide metabolism in red blood cells: the metabolic basis for GTP depletion in HGPRT and PNP deficiency. *Adv Exp Med Biol* 1990;253A:67–71.
51. Parks RE Jr, Brown PR, Kong CM. Incorporation of purine analogs into the nucleotide pools of human erythrocytes. In: Sperling O, De Vries A, Wyngaarden JB, eds. *Purine metabolism in man.* New York: Plenum Publishing, 1973;117–127.
52. Beutler E, Kuhl W. Guanosine triphosphatase activity in human erythrocyte membranes. *Biochim Biophys Acta* 1980;601:372–379.
53. Damonte G, Morelli A, Piu M, et al. "In situ" characterization of guanine nucleotide-binding properties of erythrocyte membranes. *Biochem Biophys Res Comm* 1989;159:41–47.
54. Carty DJ, Iyengar R. A 43 kDa form of the GTP-binding protein Gi3 in human erythrocytes. *FEBS Lett* 1990;262:101–103.
55. Bergamini CM, Signorini M, Poltronieri L. Inhibition of erythrocyte transglutaminase by GTP. *Biochim Biophys Acta* 1987;916:149–151.
56. Kraupp M, Marz R, Prager G, et al. Adenine and hypoxanthine trans-

port in human erythrocytes: distinct substrate effects on carrier mobility. *Biochim Biophys Acta* 1991;1070:157–162.
57. Micheli V, Simmonds HA. NAD synthesis by erythrocytes in phosphoribosylpyrophosphate synthetase (PRPPs) superactivity. *Adv Exp Med Biol* 1990;253A:1–8.
58. Oden KL, Clarke S. S-Adenosyl-L-methionine synthetase from human erythrocytes: role in the regulation of cellular S-adenosylmethionine levels. *Biochemistry* 1983;22:2978–2986.
59. Gallagher PG, Forget BG. The red cell membrane. In: Beutler E, Lichtman MA, Coller BS, et al., eds. *Williams hematology.* New York: McGraw-Hill, 2001:333–343.
60. Chasis JA, Shohet SB. Red blood cell biochemical anatomy and membrane properties. *Annu Rev Physiol* 1987;49:237–248.
61. Dale GL. Quantitation of adenosine-5′-triphosphate used for phosphoinositide metabolism in human erythrocytes. *Blood* 1985;66: 1133–1137.
62. Tuy FPD, Henry J, Rosenfield C, et al. Protein kinases in normal human blood cells. *Am J Hematol* 1983;15:105–115.
63. Usui H, Imazu M, Maeta K, et al. Three distinct forms of type 2A protein phosphatase in human erythrocyte cytosol. *J Biol Chem* 1988; 263:3752–3761.
64. Beutler E. The molecular biology of enzymes of erythrocyte metabolism. In: Stamatoyannopoulos G, Nienhuis AW, Majerus PW, et al., eds. *The molecular basis of blood diseases.* Philadelphia: WB Saunders, 1993:331–349.
65. Beutler E. Energy metabolism and maintenance of erythrocytes. In: Beutler E, Lichtman MA, Coller BS, et al., eds. *Williams hematology.* New York: McGraw-Hill, 2001:319–332.

Rossi's Principles of Transfusion Medicine, Third Edition, edited by Toby L. Simon, Walter H. Dzik, Edward L. Snyder, Christopher P. Stowell, and Ronald G. Strauss. Lippincott Williams & Wilkins, Philadelphia © 2002.

5

LIQUID PRESERVATION OF RED BLOOD CELLS

ERNEST BEUTLER

The storage of red blood cells at 4°C has traditionally been the mainstay of blood transfusion services. Even with the development of many other important blood products, providing red blood cells for transfusion is probably the single largest function of the average blood bank.

GENERAL PRINCIPLES

To be useful to the recipient, transfused red blood cells must survive in the circulation and must carry oxygen efficiently to the tissues. The *viability* of red blood cells is defined as their capability to circulate for 24 hours after reinfusion. The *function* of red blood cells is defined as their capability to deliver oxygen to tissues in a normal manner.

Studies performed on red blood cells stored in acid-citrate-dextrose (ACD) established that stored blood cells could be divided into two populations of cells—those that survive less than 24 hours and those that survive normally (1). The lesion sustained by red blood cells during storage apparently renders them either unfit for circulation, in which case the cells are destroyed, or completely repaired, in which case they circulate for their normal life span. Although such studies have not been conducted for all preservative solutions, the division of stored erythrocytes into viable and nonviable cells seems to be a generally valid formulation. The ability of red blood cells to deliver oxygen in an efficient manner is almost entirely a function of its 2,3-diphosphoglycerate (2,3-DPG; also known as 2,3-bisphosphoglycerate) level (2).

The ideal red blood cell preservative would be one that allowed the cells to be stored for an unlimited length of time without impairment of viability or function. This ideal has not been achieved, and it is unlikely that it ever will be in the context of liquid storage. At temperatures greater than 0°C, red blood cells metabolize actively, albeit at a greatly reduced rate. Thus the surrounding medium contains increasing amounts of metabolic products, gradually producing changes in the cells that impair its function or its viability.

HISTORY

Stored red blood cells were first transfused on the battlefields of France during World War I. O.H. Robertson, a young officer in the Canadian Expeditionary Force who later became a distin-

E. Beutler: Department of Molecular and Experimental Medicine, Scripps Research Institute, La Jolla, California.

guished scientist, collected blood in a large volume of sodium citrate and dextrose (3). At the end of the storage period, the red blood cells were allowed to sediment, the supernatant solution was discarded, and the red blood cells infused. Robertson's studies antedated the development of methods of measuring red blood cell survival, developed a few years later by Winifred Ashby (4). Thus the criterion of success was that at least in some cases, the wounded soldier survived.

Not much progress was made in preservation of red blood cells until World War II. Loutit and Mollison (5) added citric acid to a mixture of sodium citrate and dextrose because they were annoyed by the necessity of separately autoclaving glucose and citrate solutions to avoid the caramelization that occurs at neutral or alkaline pH. Thus, ACD solution was born. Loutit and Mollison measured the viability of the stored blood cells and determined that red blood cells from blood stored in ACD survived even better than red blood cells stored in unacidified citrate preservatives. Their well-designed preservative was to occupy center stage in blood preservation for more than a quarter of a century.

Finch et al. recognized that red blood cells that had lost their organic phosphate compounds, particularly adenosine triphosphate (ATP), during storage did not survive well (6). They therefore turned their attention toward better ATP maintenance. Initially adding adenosine to act as a substrate for ATP synthesis, they soon recognized that it was rapidly deaminated to inosine, and the latter compound became the focus of their studies (7). As pointed out in Chapter 4, metabolism of inosine by purine nucleoside phosphorylase results in the production of phosphorylated carbohydrate without consumption of ATP. But the addition of inosine to stored blood proved to be disappointing (8). Earlier promising results may have been due to the use of impure inosine preparations contaminated with adenine (9). Indeed, although inosine could provide energy to the red blood cell, it could not replenish the gradual loss of the adenine moiety from stored red blood cells. The deamination of adenine was irreversible. Only by supplying the cells with fresh adenine could the adenine nucleotide pool be replenished through the adenine phosphoribosyl transferase reaction (see Chapter 4). It was the addition by Nakao et al. (10) of adenine to blood that had been depleted of adenine nucleotides during storage that overcame this problem. Simon (11) soon showed that inclusion of adenine in blood preservatives also was highly effective in prolonging the shelf life of blood cells.

While these advances were being made, citrate-phosphate-dextrose (CPD) solution was designed by Gibson et al. (12) as an improvement over ACD, but the better survival of red blood cells in this solution was probably largely illusory (13). Only later, when the role of 2,3-DPG in red blood cell function was appreciated, did it become apparent that CPD had one advantage over ACD—the rate of 2,3-DPG loss was distinctly slower because of the higher pH of the preservative.

The discovery in 1967 by Chanutin and Curnish (14) and by Benesch and Benesch (15) that 2,3-DPG was an important modulator of the oxygen dissociation curve of hemoglobin quickly focused attention on this phosphate compound. Although it had been known that 2,3-DPG was depleted early in blood storage, the loss of this compound had not been regarded as important because 2,3-DPG was not associated with alterations of red blood cell survival.

Efforts to maintain 2,3-DPG at higher levels led to the development of a new generation of red blood cell preservatives, the additive solution. Removing plasma and platelets before storage of red blood cells not only was consistent with the growing trend toward administration of blood components but also allowed a degree of flexibility in the use of buffers that could not be achieved if the red blood cells were suspended in their own plasma. The first group of additive solutions were described by Wood and Beutler (16). These investigators subsequently designed a bicarbonate-based additive solution named bicarbonate-adenine-glucose-phosphate-mannitol (BAGPM) (17). The mannitol was needed to prevent excessive hemolysis of the plasma-deprived red blood cells (18,19). It was not until several years later when Högman et al. (20) introduced a simple additive solution saline-adenine-glucose (SAG) and subsequently SAG plus mannitol (SAGMAN) that such solutions were actually used clinically on a large scale. Because such solutions do not buffer the red blood cells, however, loss of 2,3-DPG remains a problem (21).

COMPOSITION OF PRESERVATIVE SOLUTIONS

The compositions of preservative solutions used for whole blood are summarized in Table 5.1. All of these solutions have certain components in common. Glucose serves as a source of metabolic energy. Adenine is supplied to allow the red blood cells to replenish the adenine nucleotide pool as adenine is deaminated to

TABLE 5.1. COMPOSITION OF SOME OF THE COMMON ACID CITRATE PRESERVATIVE SOLUTIONS

Solution	ACD-A	ACD-B	CPD	CPD-A1	CPD-A2	0.5 CPD
Citric acid ($C_6H_8O_7H_2O$)	8.0	4.8	3.27	3.27	3.27	1.64
Sodium citrate ($C_6H_5O_7Na_32H_2O$)	22.0	13.2	26.3	26.3	26.3	1.32
Dextrose	24.5	14.7	25.5	31.8	44.6	23.2
Sodium biphosphate ($NaH_2PO_4H_2O$)	—	—	2.22	2.22	2.22	3.26
Adenine	—	—		0.275	0.550	—
Ratio (ml anticoagulant:ml blood)	1.5:10	2.5:10	1.4:10	1.4:10	—	1.4:10

All concentrations are in g/L (48).
ACD, acid-citrate-dextrose formulas A and B; CPD, citrate-phosphate-dextrose; CPDA-1, CPDA-2, CPD-adenine; 0.5 CPD, half-strength CPD.

TABLE 5.2. CONCENTRATION (MMOL/L) OF COMPONENTS OF ADDITIVE SOLUTIONS

Component	BAGPM	SAG	SAGMAN	AS-1 (Adsol)	AS-3 (Nutricel)	PAGGS-M
Bicarbonate	115.7	0	0	0	0	0
Saline	0	150.0	150.0	154.0	70.15	72.0
Phosphate	1.0	0	0	0	23.00	10.5
Adenine	1.0	1.25	1.25	2.0	2.22	1.44
Guanosine	0	0	0	0	0	1.44
Glucose	55.0	45.00	45.0	111.0	55.51	52.2
Mannitol	27.5	0	30.0	41.2	0	54.9

BAGPM, bicarbonate-adenine-glucose-phosphate-mannitol; SAG, saline-adenine-glucose; SAGMAN, SAG plus mannitol; AS, additive solution; PAGGS-M, phosphate, adenine, guanosine, glucose, saline plus mannitol.

hypoxanthine during storage. These are the traditional preservatives, and they are being superseded for red blood cell storage by additive solutions. In modern blood banking practice, blood is collected into one of the solutions listed in Table 5.1, plasma and platelets are removed, and one of the solutions listed in Table 5.2 is added to the packed red blood cells.

In addition to solutions designed to preserve red blood cells that have been recently collected, rejuvenation solutions designed for use with red blood cells that have been stored for several weeks are occasionally used (22) sometimes before frozen storage (see Chapter 6). Such solutions are designed to restore depleted ATP and 2,3-DPG. Inosine is used as a substrate, because it can be metabolized in the absence of ATP (see Chapter 6). These solutions also contain pyruvate to make more of the oxidized form of nicotinamide adenine dinucleotide (NAD^+) available to facilitate metabolism through the glyceraldehyde phosphate dehydrogenase reaction (23,24). Rejuvenation solutions are not widely used, largely for economic reasons. Salvage of a portion of outdated blood can cost as much or more as recruiting and obtaining blood from a new donor.

USE OF ADDITIVE SOLUTIONS

There is no reason to believe that blood plasma is the ideal medium in which to preserve red blood cells at 4°C for several weeks. Its use for that purpose was simply a convenient outgrowth of the way that whole blood was collected and stored for many decades. Suspension of red blood cells in a solution specifically designed to preserve erythrocytes has two major advantages. First, valuable blood components are removed and processed immediately after collection. Second, the additive solution can be tailored to the specific metabolic needs of erythrocytes.

In the use of additive systems, blood is collected into a primary collection bag containing a standard anticoagulant, usually CPD. Satellite bags, one of which contains 100 ml of the additive solution, are attached in a closed system. After collection, the whole blood is centrifuged to produce the components—red blood cells, platelets, and plasma. The additive solution is added to and mixed with the red blood cells in the primary bag, and the red blood cells are stored until used. Figure 5.1 is a diagram of such a system.

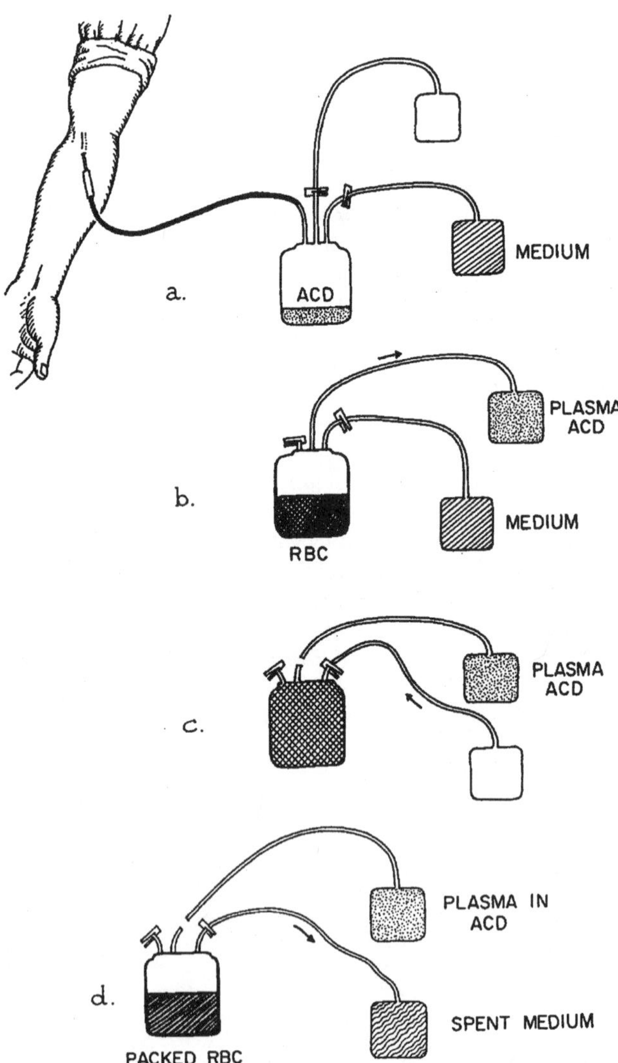

FIGURE 5.1. Schematic of the use of additive solutions. Blood is collected into a standard preservative (acid-citrate-dextrose when this figure was originally published, now more commonly citrate-phosphate-dextrose or citrate-phosphate-dextrose with adenine-1. (From Wood L, Beutler E. Storage of erythrocytes in artificial media. *Transfusion* 1971; 11:123–133, with permission.)

The components of the approved additive solutions are such that the entire suspension of red blood cells can be infused. The hematocrit of the suspension is low enough to allow relatively rapid transfusion of cells. To minimize the volume of infused fluid or of the potassium that invariably leaks from stored blood cells, some or most of the additive solution can be "pressed off" before infusion.

TEMPERATURE OF RED BLOOD CELL STORAGE

The temperature at which blood is stored is traditionally 4°C. Other storage temperatures have been studied (25,26). Lower temperatures somewhat improve maintenance of the biochemical integrity of stored blood, but also increase the risk of freezing. Higher temperatures are undesirable, because the rate of metabolism of stored red blood cells increases, resulting in a more rapid decrease in pH and consequent loss of 2,3-DPG and ATP.

CHANGES IN RED BLOOD CELLS DURING STORAGE

When red blood cells are stored at refrigerated temperatures, certain physical and biochemical changes occur. Although some of these changes are retarded or accelerated by changing the composition of the storage medium, they are not completely prevented. The alterations that occur during cold storage of erythrocytes are quite distinct from those that occur as red blood cells age in the circulation. Indeed, old red blood cells maintain viability during storage in a better manner than do young red blood cells (27).

Physical Changes

The volume of red blood cells undergoes little change during storage (28), but the shape of the cells changes from that of a discocyte to that of an echinocyte or spheroechinocyte (29,30). After prolonged storage, some of the membrane lipid is shed in the form of vesicles (30,31). Hemolysis of some of the cells occurs gradually during storage and proceeds much more rapidly in additive solutions than when the cells are stored in their own plasma. In additive solutions, mannitol has a pronounced effect in preventing hemolysis (18,19,28,32). Mannitol, or sorbitol in phosphate-adenine-guanosine-glucose-saline plus sorbitol (PAGGS-S) (33), is uniformly added to such solutions for this reason. Although the use of mannitol was originally proposed because it was thought that this agent served as an osmotically active substitute for plasma proteins, this is apparently not the mechanism of its action (28). Precisely how mannitol or sorbitol actually prevents hemolysis is not known.

In the case of red blood cells stored as whole blood or packed cells in media such as ACD or CPD in the usual polyvinyl chloride plastic blood bags, hemolysis occurs more gradually. However, if plastic films that do not contain leachable plasticizers are used, hemolysis is much more rapid and can be prevented by the addition of an emulsion of a plasticizer such as di-2-ethylhexylphthalate (34–36). Because phthalates may have toxic side effects (37–39), efforts have been made to introduce metabolizable substitutes such as butyl-*n*-trihexyl-citrate (40).

Osmotic fragility measurements have led to the erroneous conclusion that red blood cells become osmotically very fragile during storage (41). In reality, they accumulate lactate formed from glucose metabolized during storage. Because they are only rather slowly permeable to lactate, red blood cells become swollen and may burst when suspended in isotonic salt solution. Freshly drawn red blood cells equilibrated with lactate behave in an identical manner (42). If stored blood cells are equilibrated with an isotonic salt solution, their osmotic fragility is nearly normal, even after prolonged storage. There is, however, lipid loss during storage, indicating that the membrane area of some of the red blood cells has been compromised. Accordingly, a small tail of osmotically fragile cells has been detected in stored erythrocytes (43). During storage, red blood cells progressively lose deformability as demonstrated at ektacytometry (44).

Biochemical Changes

Red blood cells consume glucose during storage. The lactic and pyruvic acids that are products of glycolysis (see Chapter 4) accumulate, and as a consequence the pH of the stored blood cells gradually decreases. Hexokinase and phosphofructokinase are both quite pH sensitive, and as the pH decreases, the rate of glycolysis slows progressively. The fact that the metabolism of dihydroxyacetone and inosine are less pH sensitive than is that of glucose is one of the reasons that the addition of these substrates may be advantageous (see later).

As glycolysis slows, the ATP level of the red blood cells decreases, and the entire adenine nucleotide pool declines with it as AMP is deaminated to inosine monophosphate IMP by adenosine deaminase (45). The ammonium level of the blood increases. If adenine is included in the preservative mixture, there actually may be an increase in initial ATP level, and the subsequent rate of decrease in ATP level slows (46). Increasing the initial storage pH does not overcome this problem (47). In reality, an initially high pH of preservative is associated with a rapid decrease in ATP level. This occurs because hexokinase and phosphofructokinase are activated at high pH to the point that they consume more ATP in phosphorylating glucose than is produced in the later steps of glycolysis. The effects of adenine and pH on ATP and 2,3-DPG levels are illustrated in Figure 5.2.

Red blood cells lose potassium and gain sodium during the first 2 or 3 weeks of storage (48). This loss is essentially unrelated to the decrease in ATP level. It occurs because the Na^+-K^+-ATPase that normally pumps sodium out of the cell and replaces it with potassium has a very high temperature coefficient and scarcely functions at the temperature of cold storage (49). The degree of potassium depletion is even greater in the presence of ouabain (28), however, indicating that some active transport does take place, even at 4°C.

The level of 2,3-DPG decreases rapidly during storage, particularly if the pH of the preservative is very low. Thus a major portion of 2,3-DPG is already depleted after 1 week of storage in ACD (pH, 5.0), but in CPD (pH, 5.62), 2,3-DPG levels are maintained for approximately 1 week. After this, however, there

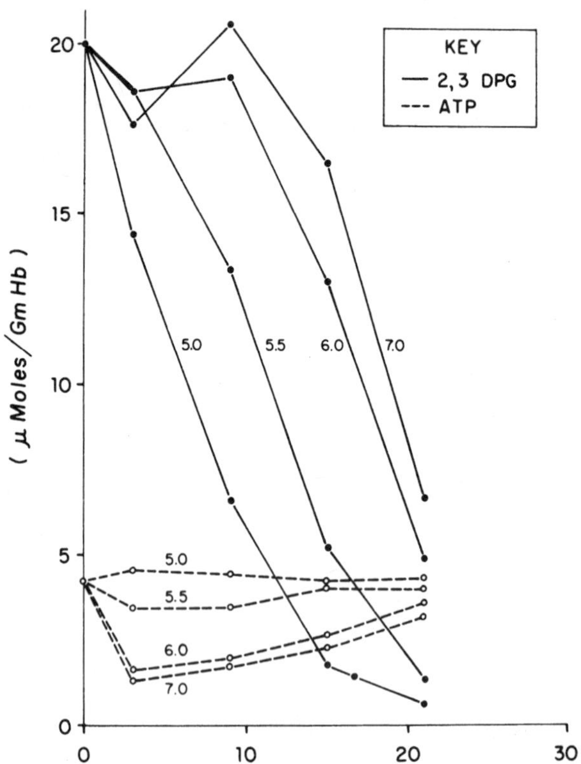

FIGURE 5.2. Levels of adenosine triphosphate (*ATP*) and 2,3-diphosphoglycerate (2,3-DPG) in blood collected in citric dextrose solutions containing 5 mM adenine. The numbers indicate the pH of the preservative solution into which the blood was drawn. (From Beutler E, Meul A, Wood LA. Depletion and regeneration of 2,3-diphosphoglyceric acid in stored red blood cells. *Transfusion* 1969;9:109–114, with permission.)

is a rapid decline in 2,3-DPG level even in CPD solution (Fig. 5.2). Although addition of adenine increases the level of ATP in stored red blood cells, the effect is to slightly hasten the decline of 2,3-DPG level (46,50). The activities of most red blood cell enzymes are well maintained during prolonged cold storage (51). Exceptions include phosphofructokinase, diphosphoglycerate mutase, diphosphoglycerate phosphatase, glyceraldehyde-3-phosphate dehydrogenase, and triosephosphate isomerase. Decreases in glutathione level are well maintained during blood storage.

Changes in membrane proteins found with sodium dodecyl sulfate polyacrylamide gel electrophoresis have been documented (52). The intensity of bands 1 + 2, 4.1, 4.2, 5, and 6 increases after 4 weeks of storage in CPD solution, and drug induced endocytosis decreases. However, these changes do not correlate with viability (53). Changes in the extractability of spectrin from red blood cell ghosts occur during storage (54), but this effect does not become prominent within normal storage periods (55). A defect in association between spectrin, protein 4.1, and actin has been demonstrated (56), and the number of IgG anti-band 3 binding sites increases (57), but no relation between these changes and viability is known. Although exposure of phosphatidyl serine seems to play an important role in red blood cell senescence in the circulation (58), it does not seem to play an important role in the storage lesion (59,60).

ADDITIVES

Phosphate

Phosphate ion has long been known to influence the levels of ATP and 2,3-DPG in stored red blood cells (61). It is a component of classic CPD solution (12) and of BAGPM, the original additive solution (62). This ion stimulates glycolysis, at least in part by relieving inhibition of hexokinase by glucose-6-phosphate (63). It also provides some buffering, but its stimulation of glycolysis counterbalances the buffering effect by increasing the production of lactic acid. Phosphate has been incorporated into a variety of recently devised additive solutions (64–66), sometimes along with citrate and ammonium ions (see later).

Inosine

Inosine is rapidly metabolized by red blood cells to form phosphorylated carbohydrate without the expenditure of ATP. Its addition to red blood cell preservatives greatly improves maintenance of 2,3-DPG levels (67). In the presence of adenine, inosine also aids in the maintenance of ATP (10,68,69). Despite these desirable properties, inosine has been used in practical blood banking only in rejuvenation solutions that are removed by means of washing before the salvaged red blood cells are stored again. It has not been possible to include inosine in blood preservatives because the product of its metabolism, hypoxanthine, is rapidly converted to uric acid in the body when inosine-containing preservatives are reinfused (70). Because many patients who receive blood transfusions have impaired liver function or may already have hyperuricemia because of hereditary or acquired factors, a blood product that increases plasma uric acid level cannot be considered safe.

Dihydroxyacetone

A simple and apparently nontoxic sugar, dihydroxyacetone (DHA) is phosphorylated to DHA-phosphate by the red blood cell enzyme triokinase (71). Triokinase is not as pH sensitive as hexokinase is, and the addition of DHA to blood storage media improves 2,3-DPG levels. Because it is much more slowly metabolized than inosine and because it requires the presence of ATP for its utilization, DHA is not useful as a rejuvenating solution (72). DHA is very stable in pure solution, but when combined with CPD or ACD, it seems to be less so, probably undergoing polymerization. Dihydroxyacetone is a promising additive that has never been used in commercially available preservatives.

Oxalate

Ascorbate seemed to greatly improve 2,3-DPG maintenance in stored red blood cells (73,74) and ascorbate phosphate had the same effect (75). The mechanism of the ascorbate effect remained unknown for many years, but eventually was clarified.

Pure ascorbate was found to have no effect at all on 2,3-DPG. Rather it was the oxalate universally contaminating commercial ascorbate preparations that was responsible for the better maintenance of 2,3-DPG (76). The effect of oxalate seems to be largely due to inhibition of pyruvate kinase, although it is possible that inhibition of lactate dehydrogenase with an effect on the ratio of NAD to the reduced form of NAD (NADH) also may play a role (77). Glyoxylate also has an effect on 2,3-DPG level (78), but this effect seems to be due to rapid conversion of glyoxylate in the lactate dehydrogenase reaction to oxalate (79).

Alanine

The addition of the amino acid alanine has a modest effect on 2,3-DPG level during storage (80). Attributed to a "glycolate shuttle" that seems to be kinetically unlikely to exist (81), the effect of alanine is most likely to be due to the well-known inhibitory effect of alanine on the pyruvate kinase reaction. Phenylalanine (82) and L-phenylalanyl-L-alanine (78) have a similar effect. These amino acids have not been used in any commercially available blood preservative.

Phospho(enol)pyruvate

Phospho(enol)pyruvate is a normal intermediate in red blood cell metabolism. It plays a role as a substrate for pyruvate kinase in the phosphorylation of ADP to ATP. Because it is in equilibrium with 2-phosphoglyceric acid and 3-phosphoglyceric acid, elevation of phospho(enol)pyruvate also causes elevation of 2,3-DPG levels. It had been assumed that the red blood cell is impermeable to this phosphorylated intermediate as it is to others, but it has been shown that under appropriate conditions, phospho(enol)pyruvate can enter the erythrocyte (83). The conditions required include incubation with sucrose at a low pH. There is serious question whether it will be possible to develop practical systems through which this compound can play an important role in blood preservation. Studies with a combination of alanine and phospho(enol)pyruvate have shown no advantage over control preservatives (84).

Xanthones

Xanthone derivatives were known to interact directly with hemoglobin to produce a right shift in the oxygen dissociation curve. Through serendipity it was discovered that they also exerted an effect on 2,3-DPG levels (85). These compounds are potent inhibitors of 2,3-DPG phosphatase, and it is likely that their 2,3-DPG-sparing effect is a consequence of the inhibition of this enzyme (86).

Ammonia

Ammonia has been considered an undesirable side product of blood storage, because the amino group of the adenine moiety of adenine nucleotides gives rise to this substance during storage. The storage of red blood cells in an ammonia-containing medium resulted in remarkably good preservation of 2,3-DPG levels and viability (87). Ammonium ions relieve phosphofructokinase from inhibition by ATP, allowing red blood cell ATP to increase to higher levels (88). Additive solutions containing ammonium and phosphate have been found to allow maintenance of superior viability for long storage periods. For example, although AS-1 solution provided average viability of only 72.6% after 8 weeks storage, an average of 87% of red blood cells stored in an ammonium and phosphate containing preservative (EAS-2) were viable at this time (89).

Citrate

Citrate has been used as a component of primary blood collection media such as ACD and CPD as a means for preventing coagulation of blood. However, it has long been known that as a result of the Donnan membrane equilibrium effect, citrate changes the pH gradient from inside to outside the cell, increasing the internal pH (90,91). It is presumably for this reason that the inclusion of citrate in additive media results in better preservation of 2,3-DPG (92–94).

EFFECT OF IRRADIATION

Irradiation of blood products has become commonplace to prevent graft-versus-host disease in the treatment of immunocompromised patients. Irradiation of red blood cells with up to 30 Gy 1 and up to 14 days after collection and stored in additive solution (AS-1) did not adversely affect viability (95,96).

STERILIZATION OF RED BLOOD CELL PREPARATIONS

Increasing public concern about the transmission of viral disease through blood transfusion has stimulated efforts to treat red blood cell preparations in such a way as to kill viruses, but not affect the viability of the red blood cells. This is a much more difficult task than is sterilization of plasma components, because the red blood cell membrane, like the membrane of viruses, is a lipid bilayer and is likely to be disrupted by any method used to disrupt the viral membrane. Methods under investigation include phototreatment after addition of methylene blue (97), a benzoporphyrin derivative (98,99), aluminum phthalocyanine sulfonates (100), merocyanine 540 (99), phthalocyanines (101–103), or psoralen derivatives (99). Because several of the infectious agents that can be transmitted by means of transfusion are harbored in leukocytes, removal of white blood cells may be useful in preventing transmission of such agents. Moreover, leukocyte reduction may decrease damage to red blood cells during storage (104).

IN VITRO AND IN VIVO EVALUATION OF THE VIABILITY OF RED BLOOD CELLS IN STORAGE MEDIA

In Vivo Studies of Viability

Red blood cells that do not survive for more than a few hours can, at best, provide only the most transient benefit. Stored blood cells that do not survive 24 hours are considered failures. It is generally required that more than 70% of stored red blood cells be viable at 24 hours if a preservative is to be considered satisfactory. It has been suggested (105) that nonviable cells actually are harmful to the recipient, producing reticuloendothelial blockade and increasing susceptibility to infection.

Evaluation of the viability of stored red blood cells can only be accomplished by actually labeling the stored blood cells and following their fate in the circulation. This is generally done using ^{51}Cr (see Chapter 61). Methods in which nonradioactive chromium is used to determine viability also have been described (106–108), but they require instrumentation that is not generally available.

To calculate the percentage of cells that survive, it is necessary to know precisely the dilution of the infused cells. This requires that the red blood cell mass be accurately measured. The most convenient way to perform this measurement is to back-extrapolate the early disappearance of the infused cells to the time that represents the midpoint of the infusion. Because complete mixing of the infused cells with the circulating red blood cells takes approximately 3 minutes (109), there is a short time during which valid sampling is impossible. Back-extrapolation is based on the assumption that the exponential rate constant of loss during this "blind" period is the same as that during the period when sampling is possible. More rapid early loss of the infused cells would result in a falsely high estimate of the red blood cell mass and consequently a spuriously high red blood cell viability estimate at 24 hours.

The theoretic problem just posed can be overcome by means of measuring red blood cell mass independently of the labeled stored red blood cells. Some investigators have attempted to accomplish this by measuring the plasma volume with radioiodinated albumin and estimating the red blood cell mass from the plasma volume (110). Because the "correction" for the difference between the total body and venous hematocrits is only an approximation, and the true value differs considerably from subject to subject (110), the red blood cell mass estimated also is only an approximation. However, results of some studies suggest that this approximation is reasonably accurate (111).

Fortunately, the development of the ^{99m}Tc method by Jones and Mollison (112) provides an accurate independent method for measurement of red blood cell mass. The distribution volume of freshly drawn ^{51}Cr-labeled and ^{99m}Tc-labeled cells is essentially identical, differing less than 1% (113). It has been claimed that unreliable results are obtained with this method (105), but this occurs only when the originally described technique is inappropriately modified. Using freshly drawn red blood cells labeled with ^{99m}Tc and stored blood cells labeled with ^{51}Cr, my colleagues and I have confirmed that there is a slight upward bias in red blood cell viability calculated from back-extrapolation of the ^{51}Cr activity of stored red blood cells after re-infusion (113) (Fig. 5.3). The absolute percentage of this bias is small (approximately 3%) and constant for cells with all degrees of impairment of viability. In a relative sense, of course, the error is much larger in poorly viable cells, but this is not of much practical importance. It would rarely matter whether the true viability were, for example, 18% or 21%. One factor in the study of red blood cell viability with ^{51}Cr has not been considered. After labeling of red blood cells with ^{51}Cr, the cells are washed in saline solution. It may be that this treatment has an effect on the viability of the stored blood cells. After prolonged storage in adenine-containing media, red blood cells contain a great deal of lactate. Because lactate leaves the cell only slowly, the cells swell rapidly when placed into an isotonic medium (42). In the circulation, such cells may swell sufficiently to be trapped by the spleen, but washed cells would have lost enough of their lactate so that much less swelling would occur.

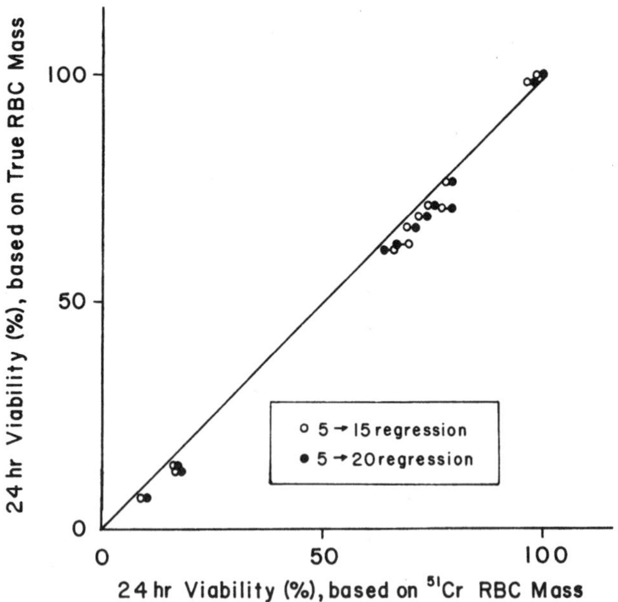

FIGURE 5.3. Relation between viability of stored red blood cells (RBCs) based on two methods of determining red blood cell mass. True red blood cell mass was estimated from fresh ^{99m}Tc-labeled erythrocytes. The ^{51}Cr red blood cell mass was determined by means of back-extrapolation from ^{51}Cr labeled stored red blood cells. *Solid dots,* results of back extrapolation between the 5th and the 20th minute after infusion of the cells. *Open circles,* results of back-extrapolation from the 5th to the 15th minute after infusion. (From West C. Measurement of the viability of stored red blood cells by the single-isotope technique using 51-Cr: analysis of validity. *Transfusion* 1984;24:100–104, with permission.)

In Vitro Studies of Viability

The documentation of in vivo viability—the standard for the evaluation of a preservative—is cumbersome and exposes volunteers to radioactivity. A great deal of attention therefore has been devoted to in vitro prediction of viability after storage.

Red blood cell ATP levels have a poorly deserved reputation as an indicator of viability. The facts are quite uniformly to the contrary and this has so frequently been pointed out (18,61, 114) that it is quite difficult to understand why so many investigators insist on depending on this measurement as a surrogate for viability. Perhaps it is because, unreliable as it is, there is no better substitute. In point of fact, there is a relation between viability and ATP level, but it manifests mostly at very low ATP

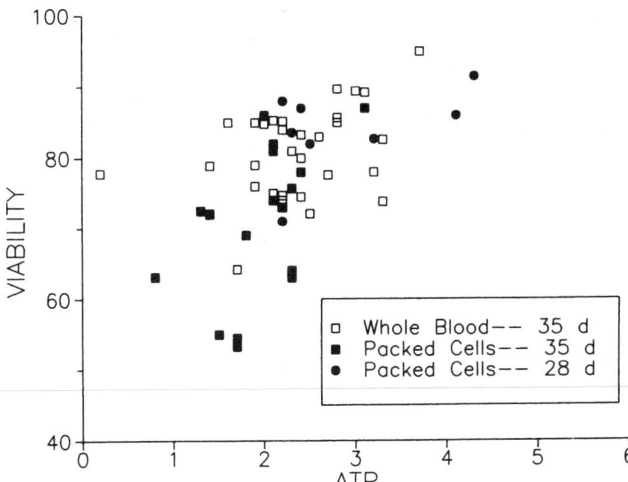

FIGURE 5.4. Relation between poststorage adenosine triphosphate (ATP) level and the viability of red blood cells stored for 28 or 35 days in citrate-phosphate-dextrose-adenine-1, either as concentrated (packed cells) or whole blood. (Data from Zuck TF, Bensinger TA, Peck CC, et al. The in vivo survival of red blood cells stored in modified CPD with adenine: report of a multi-institutional cooperative effort. *Transfusion* 1977;17:374–382, with permission.)

concentrations (Fig. 5.4). Red blood cells with very low ATP levels cannot survive in the circulation; they have no way to phosphorylate glucose, their natural energy source (see Chapter 4). The reverse is not true. Red blood cells with high ATP levels often are nonviable, especially after prolonged periods of storage. Moreover, the mean red blood cell ATP concentration in the stored blood cells provides no information about the distribution of ATP between cells. Suppose one makes the reasonable assumption that the critical level of ATP for red blood cell survival in the circulation is 10% of normal. It is quite conceivable that a preservative that maintains mean ATP level at 15% of normal might maintain the ATP level of all the cells at more than 10% of normal. To the extent that ATP is the limiting factor, all would survive. Another preservative that maintains a mean ATP level at 15% of normal might maintain the ATP level of 37% of the cells at 40% of normal, and the ATP level of many others might be vanishingly low. The latter 63% of the total number of cells would quickly perish.

Many other properties of stored red blood cells have been examined as predictors of viability, but none has been found at all satisfactory. Sometimes a logical error has been made in interpreting viability data. Red blood cell viability is a function of the length of storage. If it is examined at several different storage times, viability will be correlated with any other property that also is a function of the time of storage. Even the levels of clotting factors will correlate with the viability of the red blood cells (43), although one would not want to use one to predict the other. It is for this reason, for example, that the relation between red blood cell structure and viability, once proposed as a powerful means for predicting viability (115), is actually of relatively little value. The morphologic "scores" of stored red blood cells do not correlate well with viability at single storage periods. They do so only when data from several storage times are pooled. Similarly, the results of other attempts to develop means for predicting viability from in vitro data have been disappointing. These include measurements of the proportion of osmotically fragile cells (43), extractability of membrane spectrin (55), drug-induced endocytosis (53), deformability estimated by means of ektacytometry (44), complement binding (116), and measurement of total adenine nucleotides but not the "energy charge" of the cells (45). Each of these methods has some predictive value, but not enough to be useful.

Oxygen-delivering Function of Stored Red Blood Cells

In contrast to the great difficulty in assessing the capability of stored red blood cells to circulate after reinfusion, their ability to deliver oxygen is easily measured in vitro. This can be done by means of measuring the oxygen dissociation curve after correcting the greatly lowered pH of the stored blood cells or by measuring their content of 2,3-DPG. The latter measurement is simpler to perform for most laboratories and correlates so well with the oxygen dissociation curve (Fig. 5.5) that either measurement is probably sufficient (2).

The level of 2,3-DPG declines rapidly during blood storage, and red blood cells that have maintained their viability very well may have lost almost all of their 2,3-DPG. The oxygen dissociation of such cells is markedly shifted to the left. However, such cells rapidly regain their 2,3-DPG as they circulate in the recipient's blood stream. This was apparent from the early studies of Valtis and Kennedy (117), who first described the left shift of the oxygen dissociation curve. It was confirmed by means of direct isolation of transfused cells from the circulation of the recipient (46,118) (Fig. 5.6).

Over the long term, 2,3-DPG depletion is probably irrelevant, because the oxygen delivery properties of the red blood cells become normal after reinfusion. What about the short term? The importance of 2,3-DPG depletion in the acute situation, in which there is not yet reconstitution of this metabolite by

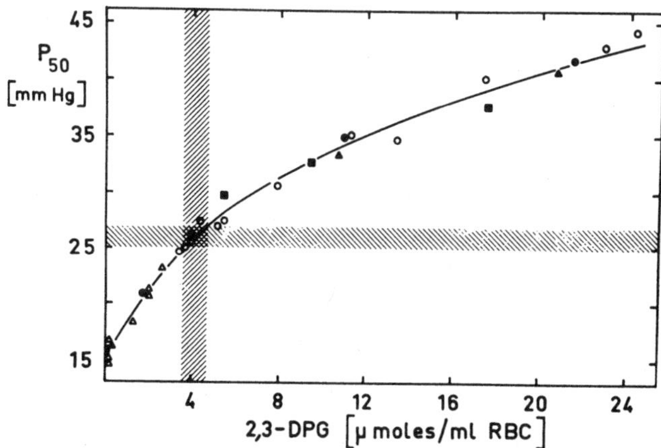

FIGURE 5.5. Relation between 2,3-diphosphoglycerate (2,3-DPG) level and P_{50}. (From Duhm J, Deuticke B, Gerlach E. Complete restoration of oxygen transport function and 2,3-diphosphoglycerate concentration in stored blood. *Transfusion* 1971;11:147–151, with permission.)

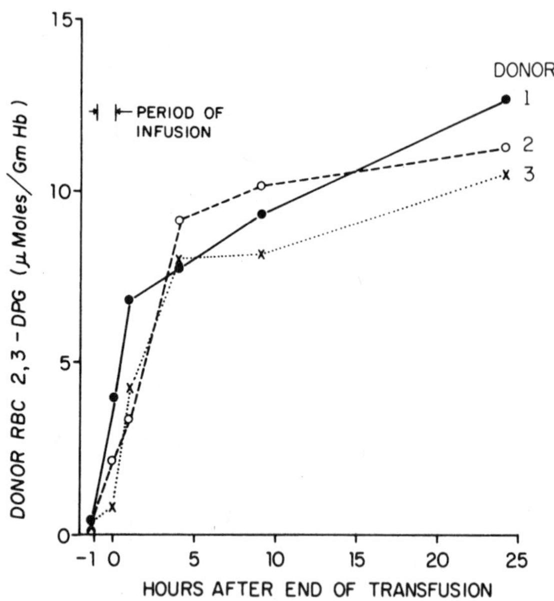

FIGURE 5.6. Regeneration of 2,3-diphosphoglycerate (2,3-DPG) in red blood cells transfused into three patients. The patients' own red blood cells were labeled with ^{51}Cr. The transfused red blood cells were recovered by means of differential agglutination, and correction for any agglutinable cells was made with the ^{51}Cr label. (From Beutler E, Wood L. The in vivo regeneration of red cell 2,3-diphosphoglyceric acid (DPG) after transfusion of stored blood. *J Lab Clin Med* 1969;74:300–304, with permission.)

the red blood cell, remains somewhat controversial (119–122; Hedian KA, Dawson RB. The effects of transfusing low-2,3 DPG blood into patients in differing physiological states, *unpublished data,* 1977). It is a difficult problem to approach experimentally, but a number of studies lean toward the conclusion that 2,3-DPG depletion may play a role. One of the more compelling arguments is the evolutionary one: Natural selection has eschewed hemoglobins with high oxygen affinities and has apparently favored the development of the 2,3-DPG (Rapoport-Luebering) shunt. It seems reasonable to suppose that transfusing cells that are as close as possible to normal ones is in the best interest of the recipient. Nonetheless, one should not underestimate the marvelous compensatory mechanisms that exist. The acidosis that results from tissue oxygen deprivation produces a profound right shift in the oxygen dissociation curve of hemoglobin. This may compensate in large measure for the 2,3-DPG loss that occurs during storage.

SUMMARY: FUTURE NEEDS AND FUTURE DEVELOPMENTS

Refrigerated red blood cell storage has advanced greatly since its introduction early in the twentieth century. The system that has gradually developed is quite satisfactory for current needs. Yet improved viability and longer storage life would be an advantage. Although blood stored for 42 days is considered satisfactory for transfusion because 70% of the cells are viable, the other side of the coin is that 30% are nonviable. Thus almost one and one-half times as much blood must be given to achieve the same increase in red blood cell mass. Fine-tuning of the content of additive solutions seems to be improving the viability of stored erythrocytes. The second challenge in improving blood preservation at refrigerated temperatures is the maintenance of 2,3-DPG levels. This may well be achieved with the implementation of what has been learned about red blood cell metabolism. In particular, solutions that maintain the pH of the blood-preservative mixture at sufficiently high levels achieve this aim. Future technologic advances may lead to the implementation of such improved additive solutions.

REFERENCES

1. Gabrio BW, Stevens AR, Finch CA. Erythrocyte preservation, III: the reversibility of the storage lesion. *J Clin Invest* 1954;33:252–256.
2. Duhm J, Deuticke B, Gerlach E. Complete restoration of oxygen transport function and 2,3-diphosphoglycerate concentration in stored blood. *Transfusion* 1971;11:147–151.
3. Robertson OH. Transfusion with preserved red blood cells. *Br Med J* 1918;1:691–695.
4. Ashby W. The determination of the length of life of transfused blood corpuscles in man. *J Exp Med* 1919;29:267–281.
5. Loutit JF, Mollison PL. Advantages of a disodium-citrate-glucose mixture as a blood preservative. *Br Med J* 1943;2:744–745.
6. Gabrio BW, Finch CA, Huennekens FM. Erythrocyte preservation: a topic in molecular biochemistry. *Blood* 1956;11:103–113.
7. Gabrio BW, Donohue DM, Huennekens FM, et al. Erythrocyte preservation, VII: acid-citrate-dextrose-inosine (ACDI) as a preservative for blood during storage at 4 degrees C. *J Clin Invest* 1956;35: 657–663.
8. Lange RD, Crosby WH, Donohue DM, et al. Effect of inosine on red cell preservation. *J Clin Invest* 1958;37:1485–1493.
9. Finch CA. Adenine-supplemented blood. *Vox Sang* 1985;48: 319–322.
10. Nakao K, Wada T, Kamiyama T, et al. A direct relationship between adenosine triphosphate level and in vivo viability of erythrocytes. *Nature* 1962;194:877–878.
11. Simon ER. Red cell preservation: further studies with adenine. *Blood* 1962;20:485–491.
12. Gibson JG, Rees SB, McManus TJ, et al. II. A citrate-phosphate-dextrose solution for the preservation of human blood. *Am J Clin Pathol* 1957;28:569–578.
13. Valeri CR, Szymanski IO, Zaroulis CG. 24–Hour survival of ACD- and CPD-stored red cells, 1: evaluation of nonwashed and washed stored red cells. *Vox Sang* 1972;22:289–308.
14. Chanutin A, Curnish RR. Effect of organic and inorganic phosphates on the oxygen equilibrium of human erythrocytes. *Arch Biochem Biophys* 1967;121:96–102.
15. Benesch R, Benesch RE. The effect of organic phosphates from the human erythrocyte on the allosteric properties of hemoglobin. *Biochem Biophys Res Comm* 1967;26:162–167.
16. Wood L, Beutler E. Storage of RBC in artificial media. *Clin Res* 1970; 18:134.
17. Beutler E, Wood LA. Preservation of red cell 2,3-DPG and viability in bicarbonate-containing medium: the effect of blood-bag permeability. *J Lab Clin Med* 1972;80:723–728.
18. Beutler E. Viability, function, rejuvenation of liquid-stored red cells. In: Chaplin H Jr, Jaffe ER, Lenfant C, et al., eds. *Preservation of red blood cells.* Washington, DC: National Academy of Sciences, 1973: 195–214.
19. Beutler E. Red cell suspensions. *N Engl J Med* 1979;300:984.
20. Högman CF, Hedlund K, Zetterstroem H. Clinical usefulness of red cells preserved in protein-poor mediums. *N Engl J Med* 1978;299: 1377–1382.

21. Matthes G, Strunk S, Siems W, et al. Posttransfusional changes of 2,3-diphosphoglycerate and nucleotides in CPD-SAGM-preserved erythrocytes. *Infusionsther Transfusionsmed* 1993;20:89–92.
22. Valeri CR, Pivacek LE, Cassidy GP, et al. The survival, function, hemolysis of human RBCs stored at 4 degrees C in additive solution (AS-1, AS-3, or AS-5) for 42 days and then biochemically modified, frozen, thawed, washed, stored at 4 degrees C in sodium chloride and glucose solution for 24 hours. *Transfusion* 2000;40:1341–1345.
23. Paniker NV, Beutler E. Pyruvate effect in maintenance of ATP and 2,3-DPG of stored blood. *J Lab Clin Med* 1971;78:472–482.
24. McManus TJ, Borgese TA. Effect of pyruvate on metabolism of inosine by erythrocytes. *Fed Proc* 1961;21:68.
25. Hughes-Jones NC. Storage of red cells at temperatures between +10°C and −20°C. *Br J Haematol* 1958;4:249–255.
26. Högman CF, Knutson F, Lööf H. Storage of whole blood before separation: the effect of temperature on red cell 2,3 DPG and the accumulation of lactate. *Transfusion* 1999;39:492–497.
27. Gabrio BW, Finch CA. Erythrocyte preservation, I: the relation of the storage lesion to in vivo erythrocyte senescence. *J Clin Invest* 1954; 33:242–246.
28. Beutler E, Kuhl W. Volume control of erythrocytes during storage: the role of mannitol. *Transfusion* 1988;28:353–357.
29. Högman CF, de Verdier CH, Ericson A, et al. Studies on the mechanism of human red cell loss of viability during storage at +4°C in vitro, I: cell shape and total adenylate concentration as determinant factors for posttransfusion survival. *Vox Sang* 1985;48:257–268.
30. Greenwalt TJ, Zehner Sostok C, Dumaswala UJ. Studies in red blood cell preservation, 2: comparison of vesicle formation, morphology, membrane lipids during storage in AS-1 and CPDA-1. *Vox Sang* 1990; 58:90–93.
31. Greenwalt TJ, McGuinness CG, Dumaswala UJ. Studies in red blood cell preservation, 4: plasma vesicle hemoglobin exceeds free hemoglobin. *Vox Sang* 1991;61:14–17.
32. Högman CF, Hedlund K, Sahlestrom Y. Red cell preservation in protein-poor media, III: protection against in vitro hemolysis. *Vox Sang* 1981;41:274–281.
33. Saint-Blancard J, Allary M, Fabre G, et al. Properties of red blood cell concentrates stored in PAGGS-sorbitol. *Ann Pharm Fr* 1995;53: 220–229.
34. Stern IJ, Carmen RA. Hemolysis in stored blood: stabilizing effect of phthalate plasticizer. *Proceedings of the 16th Congress of the International Society of Hematology.* 1980:151.
35. Gulliksson H, Karlman G, Segerlind A. et al. Preservation of red blood cells: content of microaggregates and Di-2-ethylhexylphthalate (DEHP) in red blood cells stored in saline-adenine-glucose-mannitol (SAGM) medium. *Vox Sang* 1986;50:16–20.
36. Carmen R. The selection of plastic materials for blood bags. *Transfus Med Rev* 1993;7:1–10.
37. Jaeger RJ, Rubin RJ. Migration of a phthalate ester plasticizer from polyvinyl chloride blood bags into stored human blood and its localization in human tissues. *N Engl J Med* 1972;287:1114–1118.
38. Barry YA, Labow RS, Keon WJ, et al. Cardiotoxic effects of the plasticizer metabolite mono (2-ethylhexyl) phthalate (MEHP) on human myocardium. *Blood* 1987;70:326a.
39. Rock G, Labow RS, Franklin C, et al. Hypotension and cardiac arrest in rats after infusion of mono(2-ethylhexyl) phthalate (MEHP), a contaminant of stored blood. *N Engl J Med* 1987;316:1218–1219.
40. Seidl S, Gosda W, Reppucci AJ. The in vitro and in vivo evaluation of whole blood and red cell concentrates drawn on CPDA-1 and stored in a non-DEHP plasticized PVC container. *Vox Sang* 1991; 61:8–13.
41. Danon D, Frei YF, Rimon A. et al. Simple rapid osmotic fragility test proposed as a routine in blood banks. *Transfusion* 1964;4:339–342.
42. Beutler E, Kuhl W, West C. The osmotic fragility of erythrocytes after prolonged liquid storage and after reinfusion. *Blood* 1982;59: 1141–1147.
43. Beutler E, West C. Storage of red cell concentrates in CPD-A2 for forty-two and forty–nine days. *J Lab Clin Med* 1983;102:53–62.
44. Card RT, Mohandas N, Mollison PL. Relationship of post-transfusion viability to deformability of stored red cells. *Br J Haematol* 1983; 53:237–240.
45. Högman CF, de Verdier CH, Ericson A. et al. Cell shape and total adenylate concentration as important factors for posttransfusion survival of erythrocytes. *Biomed Biochim Acta* 1983;42:327–331.
46. Beutler E, Meul A, Wood LA. Depletion and regeneration of 2,3-diphosphoglyceric acid in stored red blood cells. *Transfusion* 1969;9: 109–114.
47. Beutler E, Duron O. Effect of pH on preservation of red cell ATP. *Transfusion* 1965;5:17–24.
48. Mollison PL, Engelfriet CP, Contreras M. *Blood transfusion in clinical medicine.* Oxford, UK: Blackwell Scientific Publications, 1987.
49. Wood L, Beutler E. Temperature dependence of sodium-potassium activated erythrocyte adenosine triphosphatase. *J Lab Clin Med* 1967; 70:287–294.
50. Sugita Y, Simon ER. The mechanism of action of adenine in red cell preservation. *J Clin Invest* 1965;44:629–642.
51. Beutler E. *Red cell metabolism: a manual of biochemical methods.* New York: Grune & Stratton, 1984.
52. Messana I, Ferroni L, Misiti F, et al. Blood bank conditions and RBCs: the progressive loss of metabolic modulation. *Transfusion* 2000;40: 353–360.
53. Schrier SL, Sohmer PR, Moore GL, et al. Red blood cell membrane abnormalities during storage: correlation with in vivo survival. *Transfusion* 1982;22:261–265.
54. Lux SE, John KM, Ukena TE. Diminished spectrin extraction from ATP-depleted human erythrocytes evidence relating spectrin to changes in erythrocyte shape and deformability. *J Clin Invest* 1978; 61:815–826.
55. Beutler E, Villacorte D. Spectrin extractability in blood storage. *Transfusion* 1981;21:96–99.
56. Wolfe LC, Byrne AM, Lux SE. Molecular defect in the membrane skeleton of blood bank-stored red cells: abnormal spectrin-protein 4.1-actin complex formation. *J Clin Invest* 1986;78:1681–1686.
57. Ando K, Beppu M, Kikugawa K, et al. Increased susceptibility of stored erythrocytes to anti–band 3 IgG autoantibody binding. *Biochim Biophys Acta* 1993;1178:127–134.
58. Boas E, Forman L, Beutler E. Phosphatidyl serine exposure and red cell viability in red cell ageing and in hemolytic anemia. *Proc Natl Acad Sci U S A* 1998;85:3077–3071.
59. Geldwerth D, Kuypers FA, Butikofer P, et al. Transbilayer mobility and distribution of red cell phospholipids during storage. *J Clin Invest* 1993;92:308–314.
60. Boas FE, Forman L, Beutler E. Phosphatidylserine exposure and red cell viability in red cell ageing, storage, in hemolytic anemia. *Blood* 1997;90[Suppl 1]:272a.
61. Wood L, Beutler E. The viability of human blood stored in phosphate adenine media. *Transfusion* 1967;7:401–408.
62. Wood L, Beutler E. Storage of erythrocytes in artificial media. *Transfusion* 1971;11:123–133.
63. Gerber G, Kloppick E, Rapoport S. Über den Einfluss des Anorganischen Phosphats auf die Glykolyse: seine Unwirksamkeit auf die Hexokinase des Menschenerythrozyten. *Acta Biol Med Ger* 1967; 18: 305–312.
64. Hess JR, Lippert LE, Derse-Anthony CP, et al. The effects of phosphate, pH, AS volume on RBCs stored in saline-adenine-glucose-mannitol solutions. *Transfusion* 2000;40:1000–1006.
65. Hess JR, Rugg N, Knapp AD, et al. Successful storage of RBCs for 9 weeks in a new additive solution. *Transfusion* 2000;40:1007–1011.
66. Babcock JG, Lippert LE, Derse-Anthony CP, et al. A hypotonic storage solution did not prolong the viability of red blood cells. *Transfusion* 2000;40:994–999.
67. Chanutin A. Effect of storage of blood in ACD–adenine–inorganic phosphate plus nucleosides on metabolic intermediates of human red cells. *Transfusion* 1967;7:409–419.
68. Strumia MM, Strumia PV. The preservation of blood for transfusion, IX: the effect of increased pH and addition of inosine only or adenine and inosine on the red cell function. *J Lab Clin Med* 1972;79: 863–872.
69. de Verdier CH, Strauss D, Ericson A, et al. Purine metabolism of

erythrocytes preserved in adenine, adenine-inosine, adenine-guanosine supplemented media. *Transfusion* 1981;21:397–404.

70. Seidl S. Survival studies on the effect of the addition of adenine and different combinations of nucleosides in red cell preservation. *Bibl Haematol* 1971;38:190–195.
71. Beutler E, Guinto E. Dihydroxyacetone metabolism by human erythrocytes: demonstration of triokinase activity and its characterization. *Blood* 1973;41:559–568.
72. Beutler E, Guinto E. The metabolism of dihydroxyacetone by intact erythrocytes. *J Lab Clin Med* 1973;82:534–545.
73. Beutler E. The maintenance of red cell function during liquid storage. In: Schmidt PJ, ed. *Progress in transfusion and transplantation.* Chicago: American Association of Blood Banks, 1972:285–297.
74. Wood LA, Beutler E. The effect of ascorbate on the maintenance of 2,3-diphosphoglycerate (2,3-DPG) in stored red cells. *Br J Haematol* 1973;25:611–618.
75. Moore GL, Marks DH, Carmen RA, et al. Ascorbate-2-phosphate in red cell preservation: clinical trials and active components. *Transfusion* 1988;28:221–225.
76. Kandler R, Grode G, Symbol R, et al. Oxalate is the active component that produces increased 2,3-DPG in ascorbate stored red cells. *Transfusion* 1986;26:563.
77. Beutler E, Forman L, West C. Effect of oxalate and malonate on red cell metabolism. *Blood* 1987;70:1389–1393.
78. Vora S, West C, Beutler E. The effect of additives on red cell 2,3-DPG levels in CPDA preservatives. *Transfusion* 1989;29:226–229.
79. Warren WA. Catalysis of both oxidation and reduction of glyoxylate by pig heart lactate dehydrogenase isozyme 1. *J Biol Chem* 1970;245: 1675–1681.
80. Dawson RB, Ottinger WE, Chiu WM, et al. Control of red cell 2,3-DPG levels in vitro and a proposal for in vivo control in response to hypoxia and metabolic demand. *Prog Clin Biol Res* 1985;195: 349–365.
81. Fujii S, Beutler E. Glycolate kinase activity in human red cells. *Blood* 1985;65:480–483.
82. Vora S. Metabolic manipulation of key glycolytic enzymes: a novel proposal for the maintenance of red cell 2,3-DPG and ATP levels during storage. *Biomed Biochim Acta* 1987;46:285–289.
83. Hamasaki N, Ideguchi H, Ikehara Y. Regeneration of 2,3-bisphosphoglycerate and ATP in stored erythrocytes by phosphoenolpyruvate: a new preservative for blood storage. *Transfusion* 1981;21:391–396.
84. Matsuyama H, Ericson Å, Högman CF, et al. Lack of success with a combination of alanine and phosphoenolpyruvate as an additive for liquid storage of red cells at 4°C. *Transfusion* 1990;30:339–343.
85. Paterson RA, Dawson J, Hyde RM, et al. Xanthone additives for blood storage which maintains its potential for oxygen delivery, I: 2-hydroxyethoxy- and 2-ethoxy-6-(5-tetrazoyl) xanthones in citrate-phosphate-dextrose-adenine (CPDA-1) blood. *Transfusion* 1988;28: 34–37.
86. Beutler E, Forman L, West C, et al. The mechanism of improved maintenance of 2,3-diphosphoglycerate in stored blood by the xanthone compound BW A440C. *Biochem Pharmacol* 1988;37: 1057–1060.
87. Meryman HT, Hornblower MLS, Syring RL. Prolonged storage of red cells at 4 degrees C. *Transfusion* 1986;26:500–505.
88. Kay A, Beutler E. The effect of ammonium, phosphate, potassium, hypotonicity on stored red blood cells. *Transfusion* 1992;32:37–41.
89. Greenwalt TJ, Dumaswala UJ, Dhingra N, et al. Studies in red blood cell preservation, 7: in vivo and in vitro studies with a modified phosphate-ammonium additive solution. *Vox Sang* 1993;65:87–94.
90. Poyart CF, Bursaux E, Freminet A. Citrate and the Donnan equilibrium in human blood p507.4 or p507.2. *Biomedicine* 1973;19:52–55.
91. Minakami S, Tomoda A, Tsuda S. Effect of intracellular pH (pHi) change on red cell glycolysis. *Prog Clin Biol Res* 1975;1:149–166.
92. Lovric VA, Prince B, Bryant J. Packed red cell transfusions: improved survival, quality and storage. *Vox Sang* 1977;33:346–352.
93. Högman CF, Eriksson L, Gong J, et al. Half-strength citrate CPD combined with a new additive solution for improved storage of red blood cells suitable for clinical use. *Vox Sang* 1993;65:271–278.
94. Meryman HT, Hornblower M. Manipulating red cell intra- and extracellular pH by washing. *Vox Sang* 1991;60:99–104.
95. Mintz PD, Anderson G. Effect of gamma irradiation on the in vivo recovery of stored red blood cells. *Ann Clin Lab Sci* 1993;23:216–220.
96. Davey RJ, McCoy NC, Yu M, et al. The effect of prestorage irradiation on posttransfusion red cell survival. *Transfusion* 1992;32: 525–528.
97. Wagner SJ, Storry JR, Mallory DA, et al. Red cell alterations associated with virucidal methylene blue phototreatment. *Transfusion* 1993;33: 30–36.
98. North J, Neyndorff H, King D, et al. Viral inactivation in blood and red cell concentrates with benzoporphyrin derivative. *Blood Cells* 1992;8:129–140.
99. Friedman LI, Stromberg RR. Viral inactivation and reduction in cellular blood products. *Rev Fr Transfus Hemobiol* 1993;36:83–91.
100. Horowitz B, Rywkin S, Margolis-Nunno H, et al. Inactivation of viruses in red cell and platelet concentrates with aluminum phthalocyanine (AIPc) sulfonates. *Blood Cells* 1992;18:141–149.
101. Margolis-Nunno, H, Ben-Hur E, Gottlieb P, et al. Inactivation by phthalocyanine photosensitization of multiple forms of human immunodeficiency virus in red cell concentrates. *Transfusion* 1996;36: 743–750.
102. Ben-Hur E, Barshtein G, Chen S, et al. Photodynamic treatment of red blood cell concentrates for virus inactivation enhances red blood cell aggregation: protection with antioxidants. *Photochem Photobiol* 1997; 66:509–512.
103. Moor AC, Lagerberg JW, Tijssen K, et al. In vitro fluence rate effects in photodynamic reactions with AIPcS4 as sensitizer. *Photochem Photobiol* 1997;66:860–865.
104. Andreu G. Early leukocyte depletion of cellular blood components reduces red blood cell and platelet storage lesions. *Semin Hematol* 1991;28 Suppl.5:22–25.
105. Valeri CR, Pivacek LE, Palter M, et al. A clinical experience with Adsol preserved erythrocytes. *Surg Gynecol Obstet* 1988;166:33–46.
106. Drysdale HC, Emerson PM, Holmes A. An improved method for the measurement of red cell survival using non-radioactive chromium. *J Clin Pathol* 1979;32:655–659.
107. Glomski CA, Pillay KKS, MacDougall LG. Erythrocyte survival in children as studied by labeling with stable 50Cr. *Am J Dis Child* 1976; 130:1228–1230.
108. Heaton A, Pleban P, Keegan T, et al. Non-radioisotopic chromium-52 for the quantitative determination of red cell volume. Presented at the XX Congress of the International Society of Blood Transfusion, 1988:283A.
109. Mollison PL. Blood-group antibodies and red-cell destruction. *Br Med J* 1959;2:1123–1130.
110. Button LN, Gibson JG II, Walter CW. Simultaneous determination of the volume of red cells and plasma for survival studies of stored blood. *Transfusion* 1965;5:143–148.
111. Fairbanks VF. Measurement of blood volume and red cell mass: re-examination of 51Cr and 125I methods. *Blood Cells Mol Dis* 1996; 22:186C–186D.
112. Jones J, Mollison PL. A simple and efficient method of labeling red cells with 99m Tc for determination of red cell volume. *Br J Haematol* 1978;38:141–148.
113. Beutler E, West C. Measurement of the viability of stored red cells by the single-isotope technique using 51-Cr: analysis of validity. *Transfusion* 1984;24:100–104.
114. Dern RJ, Brewer GJ, Wiorkowski JJ. Studies on the preservation of human blood, II: the relationship of erythrocyte adenosine triphosphate levels and other in vitro measures to red cell storageability. *J Lab Clin Med* 1967;69:968–978.
115. Haradin AR, Weed RI, Reed CF. Changes in physical properties of stored erythrocytes: relationship to survival in vivo. *Transfusion* 1969; 9:229–237.
116. Szymanski IO, Odgren PR, Valeri CR. Relationship between the third component of human complement (C3) bound to stored preserved erythrocytes and their viability in vivo. *Vox Sang* 1985;49:34–41.
117. Valtis DJ, Kennedy AC. Defective gas-transport function of stored red blood cells. *Nippon Rinsho* 1954;1:119–124.

118. Valeri CR, Hirsch NM. Restoration in vivo of erythrocyte adenosine triphosphate, 2,3- diphosphoglycerate, potassium ion, sodium ion concentrations following the transfusion of acid-citrate-dextrose-stored human red blood cells. *J Lab Clin Med* 1969;73:722–733.
119. Harken AH. The surgical significance of the oxyhemoglobin dissociation curve. *Surg Gynecol Obstet* 1977;144:935–955.
120. Beutler E. What is the clinical importance of alterations of the hemoglobin oxygen affinity in preserved blood, especially as produced by variations of red cell 2,3 DPG content? *Vox Sang* 1978;34:113–115.
121. Spector JI, Zaroulis CG, Pivacek LW, et al. Physiologic effects of normal- or low-oxygen-affinity red cells in hypoxic baboons. *Am J Physiol* 1977;232:H79–H84.
122. Woodson RD, Wranne B, Detter JC. Effect of increased blood oxygen affinity on work performance of rats. *J Clin Invest* 1973;52: 2717–2724.

6

FROZEN PRESERVATION OF RED BLOOD CELLS

C. ROBERT VALERI

Three primary methods have been used to freeze human red blood cells over the past 50 years. One approach uses the extracellular cryoprotectant hydroxyethyl starch (HES) in a 14% solution, freezing in liquid nitrogen at −197°C, and frozen storage of the red blood cells at −150°C. This method does not require postthaw washing. Another approach uses 20% weight/volume (wt/vol) glycerol, with freezing in liquid nitrogen at −197°C and storage at −150° C, and requires postthaw washing to reduce the glycerol concentration to less than 1% wt/vol. The third approach uses 40% wt/vol glycerol with frozen storage at −80°C and postthaw washing to reduce the glycerol concentration to less than 1% wt/vol (1).

The first method would appear to be ideal because postthaw washing is not necessary, but there is still some question about the safety and therapeutic effectiveness of the red blood cells frozen by this method. Red blood cells frozen by the other two methods requiring postthaw washing have been shown to be safe and therapeutically effective. The method using 20% wt/vol glycerol is not widely used because transporting these frozen red blood cells is difficult: the use of liquid nitrogen, which is necessary to maintain a temperature below −130°C to prevent hemolysis, is both expensive and complex (1). Red blood cells frozen with 40% wt/vol glycerol at −80°C, on the other hand, tolerate wide temperature fluctuations without deterioration, thus making this method the most acceptable.

C.R. Valeri: Naval Blood Research Laboratory, Boston University School of Medicine, Boston, Massachusetts.

PRINCIPLES OF FREEZING NONREJUVENATED AND INDATED- AND OUTDATED-REJUVENATED RED BLOOD CELLS

Outdated red blood cells can be salvaged by treatment with a rejuvenation solution before glycerolization and freezing (2). The 50-ml volume of rejuvenation solution is made up of 100 mmol/L pyruvate, 100 mmol/L inosine, 100 mmol/L phosphate, and 5 mmol/L adenine, with an osmolality of 500 mOsmol/kg water and a pH of 7.2 (Rejuvesol; Cytosol Laboratories, Braintree, MA). The solution, which remains stable for 1 year at room temperature and for 2 years at 4°C, is added to the red blood cells in the primary collection bag under sterile conditions. The primary bag is then overwrapped in a double plastic bag, which prevents wetting during incubation and also acts as an insulator as the temperature of the red blood cell rejuvenation mixture increases during incubation. Incubation of outdated red blood cells in the Rejuvesol solution at 37°C for 60 minutes results in increases in the adenosine triphosphate (ATP) and 2,3-diphosphoglycerate (2,3-DPG; also known as 2,3-bisphosphoglycerate) levels to 150% of normal. Red blood cells treated with Rejuvesol after 4°C storage for 3 to 6 days in citrate-phosphate-dextrose (CPD) or in CPD supplemented with 0.25 mmol adenine (CPDA-1) anticoagulant exhibit increases in 2,3-DPG and ATP to 250% and 150% of normal, respectively (3). Red blood cells stored for 7 to 21 days in CPD, for 7 to 35 days in CPDA-1, or for 42 days in CPD/AS-1, CP2D/AS-3, or CPD/AS-5 and biochemically treated with Rejuvesol have 2,3-DPG and ATP levels that are normal or moderately increased (4).

In 1979, a new blood collection system was developed for the processing of red blood cells frozen with 40% wt/vol glycerol.

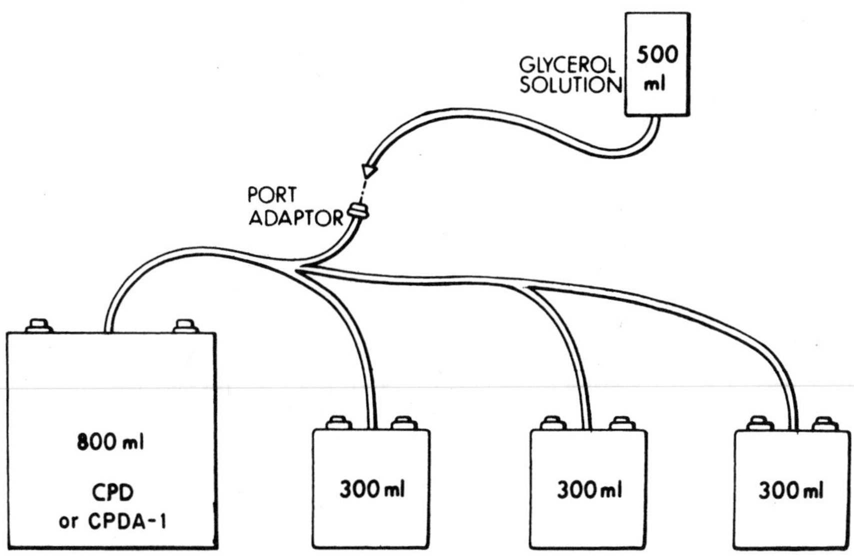

FIGURE 6.1. Diagram showing a modified PVC plastic quadruple-bag collection system with an 800-ml primary bag and three 300-ml transfer packs connected by plastic tubing integrally attached to an adapter port. A plastic tube connector with two stylets is used to add the glycerol solution into the 800-ml primary collection bag. (From Valeri CR. Cryobiology of the formed elements of human blood. In: Greenwalt TJ, ed. *Blood transfusion: methods in hematology.* Edinburgh: Churchill Livingstone, 1988;280, with permission.)

This system consisted of a 600-ml polyvinyl chloride (PVC) plastic collection bag attached to an empty 300-ml transfer pack with two ports, one port for addition of the rejuvenation solution and the other for the glycerol solution (5). Modification of the system in 1981 included replacing the 600-ml bag with an 800-ml primary collection bag and using three integrally attached transfer packs connected to the primary bag by plastic tubing attached to an adaptor port (6,7). Within this system blood is collected, components are prepared, the red blood cells are biochemically treated, glycerolized, and the supernatant glycerol is removed before freezing. The glycerolized red blood cells are frozen in the same 800-ml primary bag in which they are collected.

When red blood cells are not rejuvenated before freezing, the glycerol is added via a plastic tube with a male coupler at both ends, with one coupler inserted into the adaptor port and the other inserted into a glass bottle containing 500 ml of 6.2-mol/L glycerol solution (Fig. 6.1). The glycerol solution is delivered via an in-line 0.22-μm filter into the plastic bag containing the red blood cells, and a sterile connector device is used to connect the plastic tubing of the connector set to the tubing of the plastic bag.

When red blood cells are rejuvenated before freezing, a male coupler connecting the Y-type harness to the adapter port is used to add the rejuvenation solution to the 800-ml primary bag via the needle port; the other male coupler is used to add the glycerol solution (Fig. 6.2). In-line 0.22-μm filters and a sterile connector device are used to add the rejuvenation solution and the glycerol solution to the red blood cells in a manner similar to that used for nonrejuvenated red blood cells.

Red blood cells frozen with 40% wt/vol glycerol have been stored at −80°C for up to 37 years, with a mean in vitro freeze-thaw-wash recovery value of 75%, less than 1% hemolysis, and normal ATP, 2,3-DPG, and P_{50} levels, and 60% of normal red blood cell potassium levels (8). After 21 years of storage, red blood cell units frozen with 40% wt/vol glycerol have been thawed, washed, and stored in sodium chloride–glucose solution at 4°C for 3 days and have been shown to have a mean 24-hour posttransfusion survival value of 85% (9). These red blood cells can be transported on dry ice in polystyrene or polyurethane shipping containers and will tolerate wide fluctuations from the −80°C storage temperature without deterioration. Satisfactory results have been observed for red blood cells frozen with 40% wt/vol glycerol and stored at −40°C for 4 weeks or at −20°C for 2 weeks between periods of frozen storage at −80°C (10).

Irradiation of glycerol-frozen red blood cells with 2,500 or 4,000 cGy and postwash storage at 4°C in a sodium chloride–glucose solution for as long as 7 days does not adversely affect the freeze-thaw-wash recovery, percentage of hemolysis, or extracellular potassium or intracellular potassium levels. After postwash storage at 4°C for 3 days, in vitro measurements and in vivo survival values were similar for nonirradiated red blood cells and red blood cells treated with 2500 cGy (11). A new simplified method for washing red blood cells frozen with 40% wt/vol glycerol (7,8,9) (Fig. 6.3) employs the Haemonetics 115 (Haemonetics Corp., Braintree, MA) or the IBM-Cobe 2991-1 or 2991-2 (Cobe Laboratories, Cranbury, NJ). This method uses a 12% sodium chloride solution (Fenwal Laboratories, Deerfield, IL) and a solution containing 0.9% sodium chloride and 0.2% glucose, osmolality 290 mOsmol/kg water, pH 5.0, referred to as sodium chloride–glucose solution (Fenwal Laboratories). Red blood cells frozen with 40% wt/vol glycerol can be stored at 4°C in sodium chloride–glucose solution for at least 3 days after thawing and washing with satisfactory results (9–12).

If the supernatant glycerol is removed from the red blood cells before freezing in the 800-ml primary collection bag, then only 1.5 liters of postthaw wash solution is required instead of the customary 3.2 liters. This means that twice as many units can be stored in a −80°C mechanical freezer, the potential for

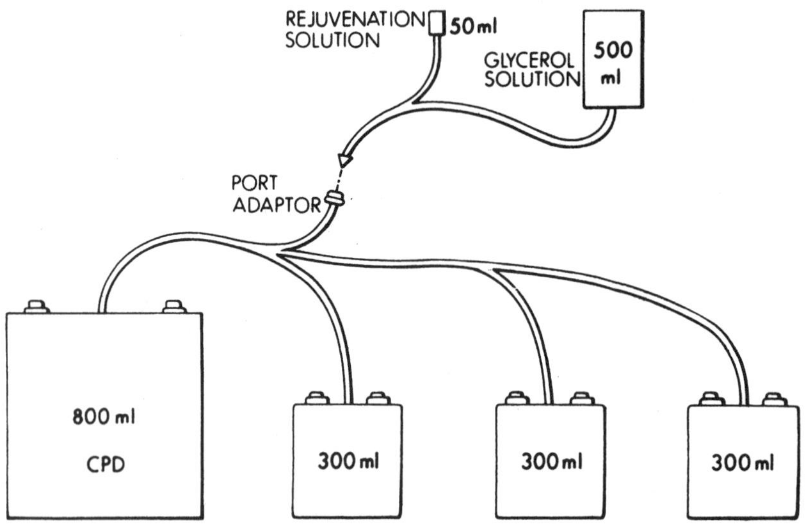

FIGURE 6.2. Diagram showing a modified PVC plastic quadruple-bag collection system with an 800-ml primary bag and three integrally attached 300-ml transfer packs connected by plastic tubing integrally attached to an adaptor port. A special harness is used to add the rejuvenation solution and the glycerol solution to the 800-ml primary collection bag. (From Valeri CR. Status report on rejuvenation and freezing of red blood cells. *Plasma Ther* 1981;2:164, with permission.)

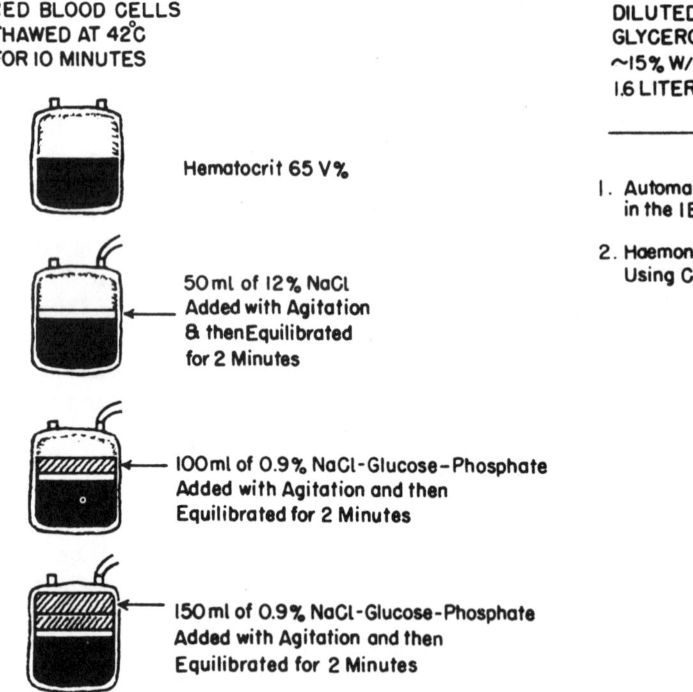

FIGURE 6.3. Diagram of thawing and washing of red blood cells frozen in the primary PVC plastic collection bag, including an outline of the three steps of dilution with 50 ml of 12% sodium chloride, 100 ml of 0.9% sodium chloride–0.2% glucose–40 mg/100 ml inorganic phosphorus or 0.9% sodium chloride–0.2% glucose, and 150 ml of 0.9% sodium chloride–0.2% glucose–40 mg/100 ml inorganic phosphorus or 0.9% sodium chloride–0.2% glucose. After dilution, the red blood cells were washed by automated serial centrifugation in the IBM-Cobe 2991-1 or 2991-2 blood processor or by continuous-flow centrifugation in the Haemonetics 115 blood processor. (From Valeri CR, Valeri DA, Anastasi J, et al. Freezing in the primary polyvinyl chloride plastic collection bag: a new system for preparing and freezing nonrejuvenated and rejuvenated red blood cells. *Transfusion* 1981;21:142, with permission.)

contamination is reduced, and breakage is less than 1% compared with 10% to 15% with special freezing bags (13,14). Moreover, the cost of freezing a unit of red blood cells is reduced by 20%. The ease with which O-positive and O-negative red blood cells that normally would be discarded can be salvaged by rejuvenation and cryopreservation makes this a very attractive approach for blood banks.

Food and Drug Administration (FDA) regulations now permit storage of red blood cells frozen with 40% wt/vol glycerol at −80°C for 10 years, but allow 4°C storage of the red blood cells after postthaw washing for only 24 hours. Notwithstanding these regulations, the Naval Blood Research Laboratory has observed satisfactory results when nonrejuvenated red blood cells were stored at 4°C for no more than 6 days after collection, frozen with 40% wt/vol glycerol, and stored at −80°C for as long as 21 years and, after thawing and washing, resuspended in a sodium chloride–glucose solution and stored at 4°C for 3 days. Before transfusion, the red blood cells are centrifuged, and the supernatant solution is removed into an attached transfer pack (15). The red blood cells exhibited a mean in vitro recovery value of 85%, a mean 24-hour posttransfusion survival of 85%, and normal or only slightly reduced oxygen transport function. When the washed red blood cells were stored sterilely at 4°C in the sodium chloride–glucose solution for 7 days, the mean 24-hour posttransfusion survival value was 75%, oxygen transport function was impaired, and hemolysis was excessive.

Outdated O-positive and O-negative rejuvenated red blood cells frozen with 40% wt/vol glycerol and stored for at least 10 years at −80°C, deglycerolized, and stored at 4°C in sodium chloride–glucose solution for 24 hours exhibited a mean in vitro recovery value of 85%, a mean 24-hour posttransfusion survival value of 75%, normal or only slightly impaired oxygen transport function, and minimal hemolysis (Figs. 6.4, 6.5). Indated-rejuvenated red blood cells treated in the same manner exhibited similar results, except that red blood cell 2,3-DPG levels were 200% to 250% of normal and ATP levels were 150% of normal (Figs. 6.4, 6.5). Bacterial contamination has not been observed in either the indated- or outdated-rejuvenated red blood cells after freezing, thawing, washing, and postwash storage for 1 week at 4°C.

QUALITY OF FROZEN RED BLOOD CELLS

Only limited data are available on the safety and therapeutic effectiveness of human red blood cells frozen with 14% HES and stored at −150°C in the gas phase of liquid nitrogen and transfused without postthaw washing.

Satisfactory results have been observed for human red blood cells frozen with 20% wt/vol glycerol and stored in liquid nitrogen at −150°C for at least 8 years, and after thawing and washing stored at 4°C for 24 hours before transfusion. Acceptable results also have been observed for red blood cells frozen with 40% wt/vol glycerol in either a special plastic bag or a PVC plastic 800-ml primary bag and stored at −80°C for 10 to 21 years (9).

Parameters used in the assessment of the quality of cryopreserved red blood cells include: red blood cell recovery after thawing and after washing, red blood cell in vivo survival measured by the 24-hour posttransfusion survival value, levels of 2,3-DPG

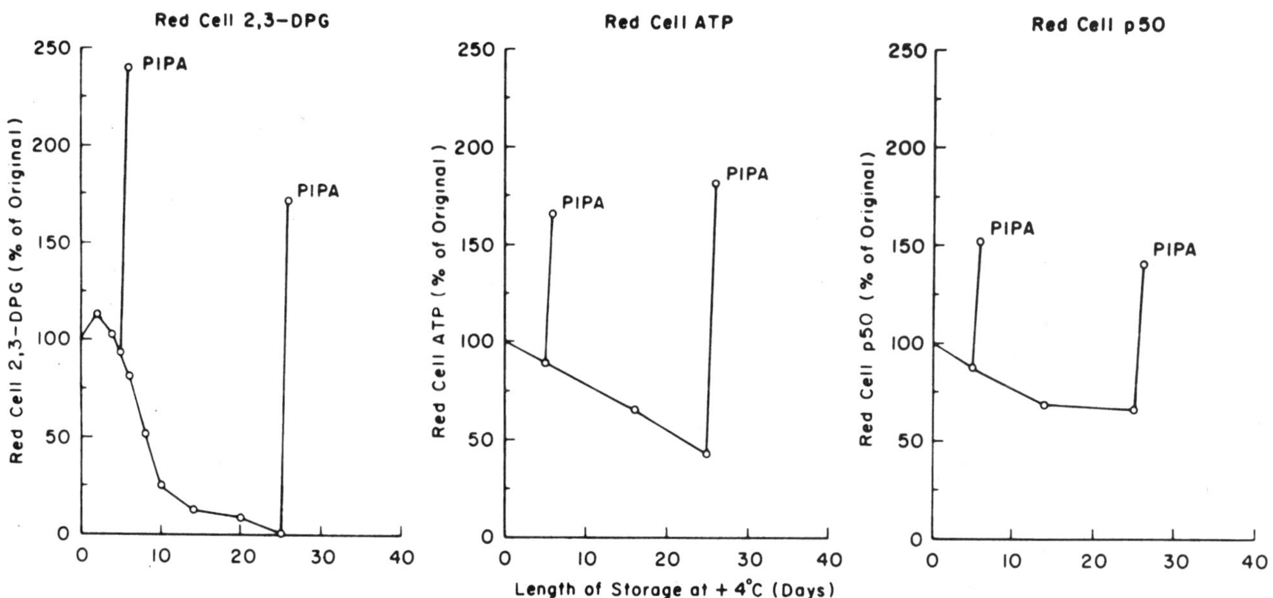

FIGURE 6.4. Red blood cell 2,3-DPG, ATP, and oxygen pressure at which hemoglobin is 50% saturated with oxygen (P_{50}) values for red blood cell concentrates with hematocrit values of 80 ± 5 V%, stored at 4°C in CPD for 6 to 8 days or for 25 days, biochemically treated with PIPA, frozen with 40% wt/vol glycerol in the original PVC collection bag at −80°C, thawed, and washed. (From Valeri CR. Use of rejuvenation solutions in red blood cell preservation. *Crit Rev Clin Lab Sci* 1982;17:332. CRC Press, Inc., Boca Raton, FL, with permission.)

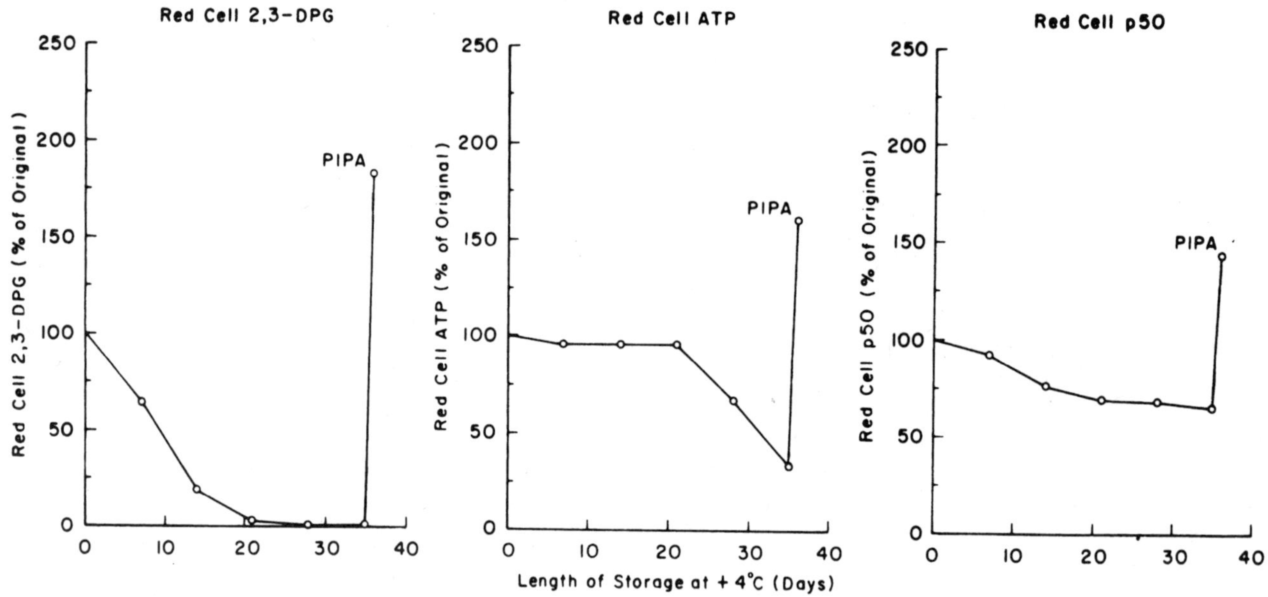

FIGURE 6.5. Red blood cell 2,3-DPG, ATP, and oxygen pressure at which hemoglobin is 50% saturated with oxygen (P_{50}) values for red blood cell concentrates with hematocrit values of 80 ± 5 V%, stored at 4°C in CPDA-1 for 35 days, biochemically treated with PIPA, frozen with 40% wt/vol glycerol in the original PVC collection bag at −80°C, thawed, and washed. (From Valeri CR. Use of rejuvenation solutions in red blood cell preservation. *Crit Rev Clin Lab Sci* 1982;17:332. CRC Press, Inc., Boca Raton, FL, with permission.)

and ATP, residual hemolysis, and sterility. Human red blood cells frozen with 20% wt/vol glycerol or 40% wt/vol glycerol have a mean freeze-thaw-wash recovery value of 85%. After post-wash storage at 4°C for 24 hours, these red blood cells exhibit a mean 24-hour posttransfusion survival value of 85%, normal oxygen transport function, minimal hemolysis, and no evidence of contamination.

APPLICATIONS FOR FROZEN RED BLOOD CELLS

Freezing of Red Blood Cells for Civilian Use

Civilian facilities are now involved in red blood cell cryopreservation in a limited manner. Autologous red blood cells are being frozen for anticipated surgical procedures and in anticipation of future red blood cell requirements. Rare and selected red blood cells are being frozen for allogeneic red blood cell transfusions, as are biochemically modified red blood cells with improved oxygen transport capability. In addition, allogeneic frozen red blood cells may be particularly useful in sensitized patients with immunoglobulin A deficiency.

Applications for cryopreserved red blood cells are listed in Table 6.1. It had been suggested that freezing and washing red blood cells prevents not only alloimmunization to platelet and leukocyte antigens but also transmission of posttransfusion hepatitis. The latter claim has not been borne out by studies in which posttransfusion hepatitis in chimpanzees and humans was observed after the transfusion of washed, previously frozen red blood cells (16,17). Freezing does not inactivate hepatitis B virus, hepatitis C virus, or human immunodeficiency virus, although postthaw washing does reduce the levels of these viruses. The reduction in the number of viable and nonviable white blood cells in the frozen red blood cell preparation reduces alloimmunization and transmission of leukocyte-associated viruses such as cytomegalovirus (and presumably human T cell lymphotropic viruses I and II) and might reduce the immunosuppressive effects of transfusion (1,18,19). Washing not only reduces the number of white blood cells in the unit but also the biologically active substances that may produce immunomodulation in recipients

TABLE 6.1. APPLICATIONS FOR FREEZE-PRESERVED RED BLOOD CELLS[a]

Rare and selected red blood cells lacking antigens that commonly sensitize patients
Autologous red blood cells
Preservation of universal donor (O-positive and O-negative) nonrejuvenated, indated-rejuvenated, and outdated-rejuvenated red blood cells
Indated-rejuvenated red blood cells with improved capacity to deliver oxygen for use in:
Hypothermic patients in hemorrhagic shock
Patients with fixed cerebral and/or coronary blood flow
Patients undergoing extracorporeal bypass and hypothermia
Red blood cells free of white blood cells, platelets, plasma proteins, and reduced amounts of microaggregates
Red blood cells free of citrate and vasoactive substances

[a]From Valeri CR, Valeri DA, Dennis RC, et al. Biochemical modification and freeze-preservation of red blood cells. *Crit Care Med* 1979;7:444.

(18,19). Washed, previously frozen red blood cells are not recommended for renal transplant recipients (20–25).

Freeze preservation may be used in blood banks to stockpile rare red blood cells and selected red blood cells to which patients commonly become sensitized. Another important benefit is the ability to quarantine frozen allogeneic universal donor–red blood cells for at least 6 months at −80°C, at which time the donor can be retested to avoid the potential for transfusion transmission of infectious diseases (26). Moreover, when combined with the rejuvenation procedure, cryopreservation also can be used to salvage outdated red blood cells that otherwise would be discarded. Blood banks also should stockpile nonrejuvenated and rejuvenated cryopreserved O-positive and O-negative red blood cells. O-positive and O-negative red blood cells of high quality can be used during low-donation periods and emergency situations to replenish inventory. Biochemically modified red blood cells with 2,3-DPG levels two to three times normal have enhanced oxygen transport function, which may benefit patients with fixed cerebral or coronary blood flow as well as those in hemorrhagic shock or subjected to hypothermia in the course of cardiopulmonary bypass surgery. The Department of Defense (DOD) now stockpiles nonrejuvenated and rejuvenated O-positive and O-negative frozen red blood cells for emergency situations (27).

Deployment of Frozen Blood Banks by the Department of Defense

The DOD has authorized the use of the 800-ml multiple-bag collection system with CPDA-1 as anticoagulant for all blood collections. Freezing red blood cells in the 800-ml primary bag is ideal for the military, because a greater number of units can be stored in each −80°C mechanical freezer, and the potential for contamination and incidence of breakage are reduced, as is the cost of freezing.

The DOD now deploys frozen blood banks to support combat casualties. At these frozen blood banks, O-positive and O-negative red blood cells frozen with 40% wt/vol glycerol in the 800-ml PVC plastic primary collection bag can be stored at −80°C for at least 21 years. Single-donor platelets frozen with 6% dimethyl sulfoxide in plasma can be stored at −80°C for up to 2 years, and AB fresh frozen plasma can be stored at −80°C for at least 7 years. About 60,000 units of frozen O-positive and O-negative red blood cells are now deployed by the DOD.

Cost of Frozen Storage

Frozen blood storage requires capital expenditures for freezers and cell washers in addition to the cost of supplies. The cost of supplies and labor for cryopreservation with 40% wt/vol glycerol is almost twice that for liquid preservation, but less than that for cryopreservation with 20% wt/vol glycerol and storage in liquid nitrogen. Although cost certainly is an important consideration, the benefits to the blood banking system are substantial. Red blood cells frozen with 40% wt/vol glycerol and stored at −80°C for as long as 21 years, deglycerolized, and stored at 4°C in sodium chloride–glucose solution for 24 hours have a mean 24-hour posttransfusion survival value of 85%, with normal or only slightly impaired oxygen transport function (9). These findings compare favorably with those for fresh red blood cells stored at 4°C for the commonly accepted period of 6 weeks (28). The additional costs to freeze an outdated unit or stockpile units during times when the community blood supply is adequate may not be excessive compared to the costs of collecting new units, particularly during low-donation periods.

RESEARCH TO EXPAND THE USE OF FROZEN RED BLOOD CELLS

One reason that red blood cell cryopreservation has been slow to gain acceptance has been the limitation on postwash storage to 24 hours. The two systems reported here for the deglycerolization of red blood cells, that is, the Haemonetics 115 blood processor and the IBM-Cobe 2991-1 or 2991-2 blood processor, are open systems (1). A sterile connector device and in-line 0.22-μm filters can be used to provide a functionally closed system during glycerolization and deglycerolization of red blood cells. Studies of artificial additive solutions in which to store deglycerolized red blood cells at 4°C for 3 weeks have been reported (29). FDA approval for the extension of the postthaw storage period at 4°C beyond the mandated 24 hours would stimulate a wider use of cryopreserved red blood cells by both civilian and military health care institutions.

The AS-3 additive solution (Nutricel) is an excellent medium in which to store liquid-preserved and washed previously frozen red blood cells at 4°C (18,19,30). Hemolysis is significantly reduced after storage of deglycerolized red blood cells in this medium (18,19).

The Naval Blood Research Laboratory has had satisfactory results with the Haemonetics Model 215, a functionally closed automated instrument for glycerolization and deglycerolization of human red blood cells. Previously frozen red blood cells processed in the Haemonetics 215 instrument and stored at 4°C in AS-3 solution for 15 days following deglycerolization were shown to be sterile and to have a mean 24-hour posttransfusion survival value of 77 ± 9% (SD) and 0.6 ± 0.2% hemolysis (18,19).

The Naval Blood Research Laboratory has submitted data to the FDA to extend the storage of red blood cells frozen with 40% wt/vol glycerol from 10 years to 22 years, and to store the red blood cells in AS-3 at 4°C for at least 15 days after deglycerolization in the functionally closed Haemonetics 215 system (18,19). The current limitation of 24 hours for postwash storage limits the use of frozen allogeneic universal donor–red blood cells as a primary source to balance the fluctuations in supply and demand and hampers efforts to provide rare, selected, and autologous red blood cells. FDA licensure of an automated and functionally closed system to glycerolize and deglycerolize human red blood cells and of an extension of the postwash storage period at 4°C to at least 15 days is anticipated and would be an important step in making previously frozen red blood cells available for emergency and inventory situations.

SUMMARY

Freezing human red blood cells with 40% wt/vol glycerol and storage at −80°C allows the stockpiling of universal-donor O-positive and O-negative red blood cells and rare and selected red blood cells for at least 10 years. In addition, frozen red blood cells can be quarantined for at least 6 months so that the donor can be retested for infectious disease markers.

Red blood cell biochemical modification can be used to salvage allogeneic O Rh-positive and O Rh-negative red blood cells and autologous and rare red blood cells prior to freezing. The recurring shortages experienced by most blood banks could be alleviated by maintaining a supply of frozen red blood cells with normal or improved oxygen transport function and acceptable 24-hour posttransfusion survival and lifespan values.

Previously frozen red blood cells are washed to remove the cryoprotectant, glycerol. Postthaw washing also reduces the number of white blood cells and biologically active substances that may produce immunomodulation in recipients.

FDA licensure of an automated and functionally closed system for glycerolization and deglycerolization of human red blood cells for storage at 4°C for at least 2 weeks will make previously frozen deglycerolized red blood cells available for emergency situations and for inventory control.

REFERENCES

1. Valeri CR. *Blood banking and the use of frozen blood products.* Boca Raton: Chemical Rubber Co., 1976.
2. Valeri CR, Zaroulis CG. Rejuvenation and freezing of outdated stored human red cells. *N Engl J Med* 1972;287:1307–1313.
3. Valeri CR. Use of rejuvenation solutions in red blood cell preservation. *Crit Rev Clin Lab Sci* 1982;17:299–374.
4. Valeri CR, Pivacek LE, Cassidy GP, et al. The survival, function, and hemolysis of human RBCs stored at 4°C in additive solution (AS-1, AS-3, or AS-5) for 42 days and then biochemically modified, frozen, thawed, washed, and stored at 4°C in sodium chloride and glucose solution for 24 hours. *Transfusion* 2000;40:1341–1345.
5. Valeri CR, Valeri DA, Dennis RC, et al. Biochemical modification and freeze-preservation of red blood cells. A new method. *Crit Care Med* 1979;7:438–447.
6. Valeri CR. Status report on rejuvenation and freezing of red blood cells. *Plasma Ther* 1981;2:155–170.
7. Valeri CR, Valeri DA, Anastasi J, et al. Freezing in the primary polyvinyl chloride plastic collection bag: a new system for preparing and freezing non-rejuvenated and rejuvenated red blood cells. *Transfusion* 1981;21:138–149.
8. Valeri CR, Ragno G, Pivacek LE, et al. An experiment with glycerol-frozen red blood cells stored at −80°C for up to 37 years. *Vox Sang* 2000;79:168–174.
9. Valeri CR, Pivacek LE, Gray AD, et al. The safety and therapeutic effectiveness of human red blood cells frozen with 40% to 45% (W/V) glycerol and stored at −80°C for as long as 21 years. *Transfusion* 1989;29:429–437.
10. Valeri CR, Pivacek LE, Cassidy GP, et al. In vitro and in vivo measurements of human RBC frozen with 40 percent W/V glycerol and subjected to different storage temperatures prior to deglycerolization and storage at 4°C for 3 days. *Transfusion* 2001;41(3):401–405.
11. Valeri CR, Pivacek LE, Cassidy GP, et al. In vitro and in vivo measurements of gamma irradiated frozen glycerolized red blood cells. *Transfusion* 2001;41(4):545–549.
12. Valeri CR. Cryobiology of the formed elements of human blood. In: Greenwalt TJ, ed. *Blood transfusion: methods in hematology.* Edinburgh: Churchill Livingstone, 1988;277–304.
13. Meryman HT, Hornblower M. A method for freezing and washing red blood cells using a high glycerol concentration. *Transfusion* 1972; 12:145–155.
14. Huggins CE. Frozen blood: principles of practical preservation. *Monogr Surg Sci* 1966;3:133–173.
15. Valeri CR, Pivacek LE, Cassidy GP, et al. Posttransfusion survival (24-hour) and hemolysis of previously frozen deglycerolized RBCs after storage at 4°C for up to 14 days in sodium chloride alone or sodium chloride supplemented with additive solutions. *Transfusion* 2000;40: 1337–1340.
16. Alter HJ, Tabor E, Meryman HT, et al. Transmission of hepatitis B virus infection by transfusion of frozen-deglycerolized red blood cells. *N Engl J Med* 1978;298:637–642.
17. Haugen RK. Hepatitis after the transfusion of frozen red cells and washed red cells. *N Engl J Med* 1979;301:393–395.
18. Valeri CR, Ragno G, Pivacek L, et al. In vivo survival of apheresed red cells, frozen with 40 percent W/V glycerol, deglycerolized with the Haemonetics Model 215, and stored at 4°C in AS-3 for up to 21 days. *Transfusion* 2001;41:928–932.
19. Valeri CR, Ragno G, Pivacek LE, et al. A multicenter study of in vitro and in vivo parameters of human red blood cells frozen with 40 percent W/V glycerol and stored after deglycerolization for 15 days at 4°C in AS-3: assessment of RBC processing in the Haemonetics Model 215. *Transfusion* 2001;41(7):933–939.
20. Dossetor JB, McKinnon KJ, Gault MH, et al. Cadaver kidney transplants. *Transplantation* 1967;5:844–853.
21. Morris PJ, Ting A, Stocker J. Leukocyte antigens in renal transplantation. I. The paradox of blood transfusion on renal transplantation. *Med J Aust* 1968;2:1088–1090.
22. Opelz G, Sengar DPS, Mickey MR, et al. Effect of blood transfusions on subsequent kidney transplants. *Transplant Proc* 1973;5:253–259.
23. Opelz G, Terasaki PI. Poor kidney transplant survival in recipients with frozen blood transfusions or no transfusions. *Lancet* 1974;2:696–698.
24. Opelz G, Terasaki PI. Prolongation effect of blood transfusions on kidney graft survival. *Transplantation* 1976;22:380–383.
25. Polesky HG, McCullough JJ, Yunis E, et al. The effects of transfusion of frozen-thawed deglycerolized red cells on renal graft survival. *Transplantation* 1977;24:449–452.
26. Petersen LR, Satten GA, Dodd R, et al. Duration of time from onset of human immunodeficiency virus type 1 infectiousness to development of detectable antibody. *Transfusion* 1994;34:283–289.
27. Valeri CR, Sims KL, Bates JF, et al. An integrated liquid-frozen blood banking system. *Vox Sang* 1983;45:25–39.
28. Valeri CR, Pivacek LE, Palter M, et al. A clinical experience with Adsol-preserved erythrocytes. *Surg Gynecol Obstet* 1988;166:33–46.
29. Moore GL, Hess JR, Ledford ME. In vivo viability studies of two additive solutions in the postthaw preservation of red cells held for 3 weeks at 4°C. *Transfusion* 1993;33:709–712.
30. Valeri CR, Pivacek LE, Cassidy GP, et al. 24-hour 51-Cr posttransfusion survival, 51-Cr lifespan, and hemolysis of red blood cells stored at 4°C for 56 days in AS-3. *Vox Sang* 2001;80(1):48–50.

Rossi's Principles of Transfusion Medicine, Third Edition, edited by Toby L. Simon, Walter H. Dzik, Edward L. Snyder, Christopher P. Stowell, and Ronald G. Strauss.
Lippincott Williams & Wilkins, Philadelphia © 2002.

7

RED BLOOD CELL IMMUNOLOGY AND COMPATIBILITY TESTING

W. JOHN JUDD

RED BLOOD CELL IMMUNOLOGY

Immune Response

Immune responses can be divided into two categories, humoral immunity and cell-mediated events. Humoral immunity is B-cell mediated and entails the generation of antibodies. Cell-mediated immunity is a reflection of the action of T cells, which regulate the immune response through the production of cytokines.

An individual's genetic constitution determines the characteristics of that person's cells and fluid-phase molecules; this is referred to as the "self" of the individual. All other ("nonself") molecules are considered foreign. During fetal development, and continuing through the neonatal period, B and T lymphocytes produce receptors that enable each lymphocyte to recognize a single specific antigen (1).

W.J. Judd: Professor of Immunohematology, Department of Pathology, University of Michigan, Ann Arbor, Michigan.

Antigen Receptors of T Cells and B Cells

The antigen receptors of both T and B cells consist of two polypeptide chains synthesized under the direction of two different chromosomal loci. The loci for B-cell receptors are on chromosome 14 and either on chromosome 2 or 22; the loci for T-cell receptors are on chromosome 7 and 14 (but not the same locus as for B-cell receptors). In the early stages of lymphocyte development, the genetic material at each of these loci undergoes a process of rearrangement that is unique to each cell (2).

Germline DNA at these loci contain numerous base-pair sequences, each capable of encoding different amino acid sequences. The gene rearrangement process entails selection of single base-pair sequences for each portion of the immunoglobulin molecule from the assortment (library) of base pairs available (Fig. 7.1), and also involves elimination of unused genetic material (3).

Each T-cell/B-cell receptor chain consists of a constant portion and a variable portion. Amino acid sequences of the variable portion determine the idiotypic specificity of the immunoglobulin molecule. For both receptors, one chain contains selections from three libraries (V, D, J), while the other chain contains

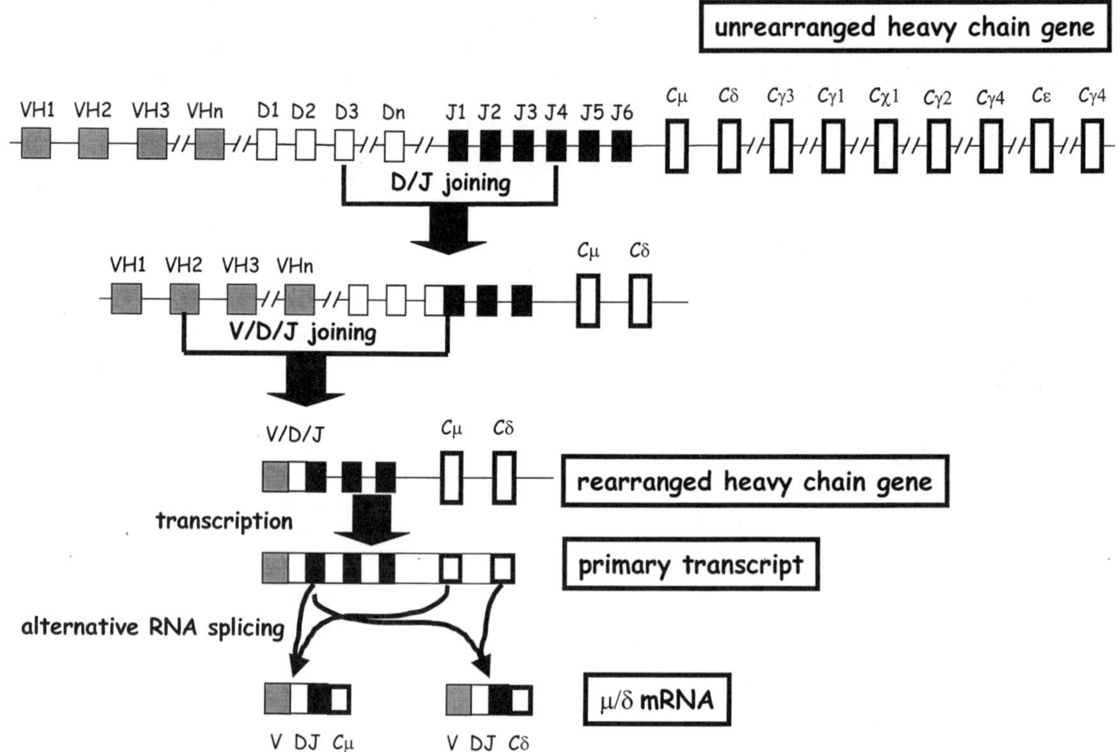

FIGURE 7.1. Diagram of the immunoglobulin heavy-chain locus on chromosome 14. In the unrearranged locus (top) V, D, and J libraries are on the left; sequences for the constant regions are on the right. Gene rearrangement occurs by selection of one D and one J exon to form a D/J unit. This is then joined by one V exon. The V/D/J unit is adjacent to the exons for μ- and δ-constant regions. Through alternative splicing, the primary transcript generates either μ or δ heavy chains with the same variable region configuration (idiotype). In later generations, clonal progeny can attach the V/D/J transcript to other sequences from the constant region (isotype switch).

selections from V and J libraries. Given that the heavy chain locus has as many as 400 exons in the V library, 20 in the J library, and six in the D library, the mathematically possible combinations for different protein configurations is astronomic. At the light chain loci there are some 300 possible selections in the V library, and four in the J library. Selection from each library is random, and further amino acid sequence variation is introduced by inaccurate splicing or when different exons are joined together. Consequently, 10^9 different receptor configurations can be generated (1).

Exposure to Foreign Protein Antigens

If foreign protein antigens enter the host, antigen-presenting cells (APCs) isolate the antigen and display the molecular configurations as epitopes on their cell surfaces. T and B lymphocytes with the appropriate receptor for the unique molecular configuration can then establish intimate contact with the APC. This contact initiates cellular events that generate clones of activated lymphocytes specific for the foreign antigen. Cytokines produced by APCs and by activated T cells cause B cells to evolve into immunoglobulin-secreting plasma cells. In turn, B cells capture antigen and present it back to T cells in a manner that causes the T cells to secrete cytokines that promote more focused antibody production.

Most plasma cells have a short but active life of antibody production. Some, however, become memory cells that retain intracellular changes resulting from exposure to APCs; these persist in the circulation long after their initial activation.

Primary Response

The first immunoglobulin class to appear in the blood stream is always immunoglobulin M (IgM); the lag phase (time between sensitizing event and appearance of antibody) can vary from days to months. Shortly after the appearance of IgM antibody, immunoglobulin G (IgG) antibody of the same specificity usually becomes detectable. The IgM component disappears over time, while the IgG component persists indefinitely. Cytokines from activated T cells are essential for this isotype switching and for generation of memory cells.

T Cell–Independent Response

It is of note that antibodies to carbohydrate antigens are invariably IgM. This is because B-cell APCs can interact directly with complex polysaccharides such as those that carry blood group A or B activity. Structures that have multiple identical repeat carbohydrate chains can initiate B-cell proliferation and antibody secretion without the action of T cells. In the absence of the immunomodulatory effects of T cells, isotype switching does not occur, and no memory cells develop (4).

Secondary (Anamnestic) Response

Within a few hours or days after subsequent exposure to T-dependent antigen, there is a sharp rise in the level of IgG antibody. Because there has been prior clonal expansion, the number of participating B cells will be high, resulting in production of significantly (e.g., 100-fold) more IgG than was produced in the primary response. Cytokines secreted by T cells promote more focused antibody production, resulting in a greater affinity of the antibody molecules for specific antigen.

Clonality

Only antigen-specific B cells proliferate and mature into antibody-secreting plasma cells. The number of progenitor B cells that are initially activated will determine the heterogeneity (clonality) of the immune response. The response will range from polyclonal (when many different B cells are activated simultaneously) to monoclonal (when the antibody-producing cells originate from a single ancestral B cell). Monoclonal antibodies for reagent use can also be produced in vitro using hybridoma technology (5).

Immunoglobulin Molecules

Figure 7.2 portrays the basic structure of an antibody molecule, which consists of four polypeptide chains: two identical light chains of 214 amino acids, and two identical heavy chains of 440 or more amino acids. Antigenic specificity is conferred by the 134 N-terminal amino acids of the light chains and the 144 N-terminal amino acids of the heavy chains; these are described as variable regions. The remaining portions of both chains are referred to as constant regions (6).

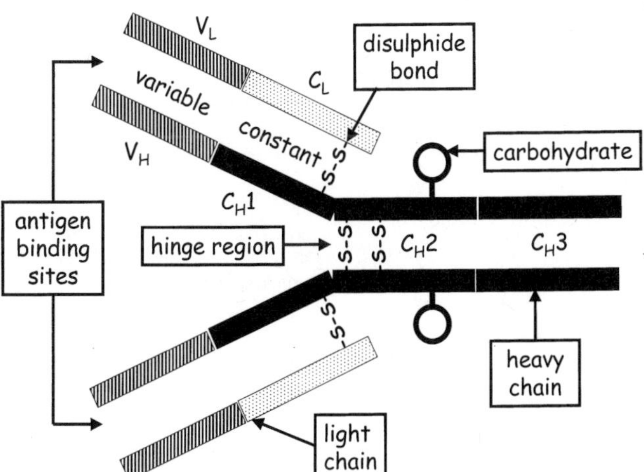

FIGURE 7.2. Basic structure of an immunoglobulin molecule.

Light Chains

The constant region of the light chains can have one of two different amino acid sequences, designated kappa (κ) and lambda (λ). κ chains are encoded by a locus on chromosome 2, λ chains by a locus on chromosome 22. A single cell will synthesize an immunoglobulin molecule containing either κ or λ chains, but never both.

Heavy Chains

The constant region of heavy chains can manifest one of five amino acid sequences, designated by the Greek letters α (alpha), δ (delta), ε (epsilon), γ (gamma), and μ (mu). These give rise to five types of immunoglobulin classes termed IgA, IgD, IgE, IgG, and IgM, respectively. The site on chromosome 14 that governs the manufacture of heavy chains contains DNA sequences for all five types of heavy chain.

Antibody Diversity

Serologic studies have revealed a number of antigenic markers on the heavy and light chains of immunoglobulin molecules. The results of such studies are strongly supported by molecular analysis of the immunoglobulin genes (3,6). Differences between these antigenic markers are illustrated in Fig. 7.3.

Isotypes

Isotypes result from structural changes to the constant region heavy and light chains. Genes encoding the various isotypes (IgA, IgD, IgE, IgG, IgM, κ, and λ) are all present in the human genome. Antibodies for isotype determination can be prepared by heterologous immunization (e.g., mouse immunization with human serum).

Allotypes

Allotypic distinctions between antibodies are the result of genetic polymorphisms, and each marker is not present in every individual. This genetic variation results from different alleles at structural loci. Antibodies to allotypic variants can be raised by same species (homologous, allogeneic) immunization, and are often found in the sera of women who have given birth to infants with different allotypic markers. These markers usually represent amino acid changes in the constant regions of antibody molecules.

Idiotypes

Idiotypic variation is the result of differences in amino acid sequence of the variable regions of either light or heavy chains. Antibodies to idiotypes may recognize sequences either within or outside the antigen-combining site, and can be prepared by either homologous or heterologous immunization.

Blood Group Antibodies

Blood group antibodies are immunoglobulins that react with antigens on the surface of red blood cells. They can either be acquired naturally or through immunization with foreign red blood cells (7). Most blood group antibodies are either IgG or

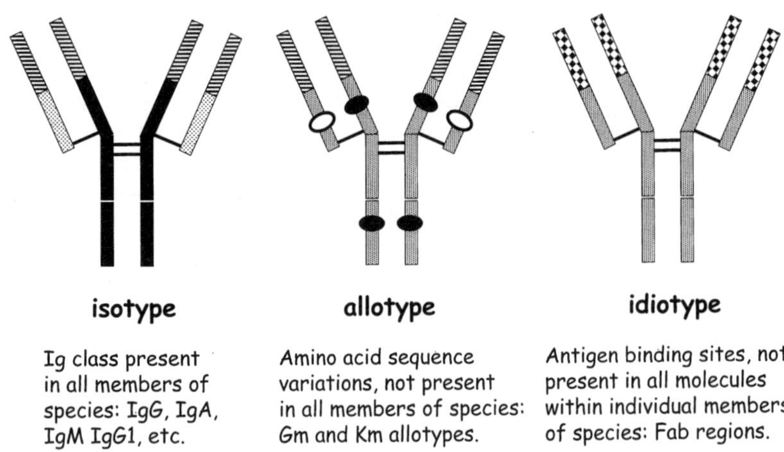

FIGURE 7.3. Diversity of antibody molecules.

IgM, occasionally they may be IgA. The IgD and IgE immunoglobulins have not been implicated as blood group antibodies (8) and will not be discussed further.

Physical Properties

The physical properties and serologic characteristics of the three immunoglobulin classes involved with blood group specificity are summarized in Table 7.1. IgM antibodies have ten available antigen binding sites, a wide spanning distance, and often fix complement to red blood cells. Antibodies to A and B antigens are predominantly IgM; they are found normally in persons whose red blood cells lack the corresponding antigen. They are stimulated by antigens present in the environment. Bacteria constituting normal intestinal flora carry blood group A- and B-like polysaccharides. As these flora establish themselves in the gut, they provide the immune stimulus for anti-A and anti-B (7). Anti-A and anti-B formed in this manner are often referred to as "natural" antibodies. They are also called "expected" antibodies, because in adults with a normal immune system these antibodies are almost always present when the corresponding antigens are absent on the red blood cells.

In contrast to anti-A and anti-B, most other blood group antibodies are IgG, which are immune in origin and do not appear in plasma/serum unless the host is exposed directly to foreign red blood cell antigens. The usual stimulating event is blood transfusion or pregnancy. IgG antibodies are smaller than IgM and have only two sites for antigen binding.

All antibodies to red blood cell antigens, other than naturally occurring anti-A and anti-B, are considered unexpected. They can either be alloantibodies, directed toward non–ABO-system antigens absent on the red blood cells of the antibody producer, or autoantibodies, directed toward self-antigens. The latter may cause autoimmune hemolytic anemia. Unexpected antibodies in donor plasma may destroy recipient red blood cells, while antibodies in the recipient may cause accelerated destruction of transfused red blood cells. In pregnant women, such antibodies may cross the placenta and cause hemolytic disease of the newborn (8).

Close to 300 different blood group alloantibodies have been described (9). Each antibody reacts with its specific antigen on the surface of red blood cells. The immunoglobulin class and clinical relevance of some of the antibodies encountered during compatibility testing are shown in Table 7.2.

TABLE 7.1. CHARACTERISTICS OF BLOOD GROUP–ACTIVE IMMUNOGLOBULINS

Immunoglobulin	IgM	IgG	IgA
H-chain isotype	μ	γ	α
Subclasses	1	4	2
L-chain types	$\kappa\lambda$	$\kappa\lambda$	$\kappa\lambda$
Sedimentation constant	19 S	7 S	11 S
Molecular weight	900–1000 kda	150 kda	180–500 kda
Electrophoretic mobility	between β and γ	γ	γ
Serum concentration (mg/dl)	85–205	1,000–1,500	200–350
Antigen binding sites	10 (5)	2	4
Fixes complement	Often	Some	No
Placental transfer	No	Yes	No
Direct agglutinin	Yes	Usually not	Usually not
Hemolytic in vitro	Often	No	No
Example	Anti-A, anti-B	Rh antibodies	Anti-Lu^a

TABLE 7.2. CHARACTERISTICS OF BLOOD GROUP ALLOANTIBODIES

Antibody	Agglutinating	Coating*	Ig Class†	C3-binding	Effect of Ficin	HDN‡	HTR	% Compatible	Comments
A	✓	✓	M, G	✓	↑	✓	✓	56	no dosage
A_1	✓	S	M	χ	↑	χ	R	64	in 2% A_2, 25% A_2B
At^a		✓	G	χ		χ	✓	R	in African-Americans
B	✓	✓	M, G	✓	↑	✓	✓	85	no dosage
Bg		✓	G	χ		χ	χ		to HLA**
C	S	✓	G, M	χ	↑	✓	✓	30	
c	S	✓	G, M	χ	↑	✓	✓	0	often with anti-E
Ch		✓	G	χ	↓	χ	χ	2	HTLA††; to C4d‡‡
C^w	S	✓	G, M	χ	↑	✓	✓	98	
Co^a		✓	G	χ		✓	✓	R	
Co^b		✓	G	R		✓	✓	91	
Cr^a		✓	G	χ		χ	✓	R	in African-Americans
Cs^a		✓	G	χ		χ	χ	2	HTLA
D	S	✓	G, M	χ	↑	✓	✓	15	no dosage
Di^a	S	✓	G	χ		✓	✓	>99	§§
Di^b		✓	G	χ		✓	✓	R	
Do^a		✓	G	✓	↑	χ	✓	33	
Do^b		✓	G	✓	↑	χ	✓	13	
E	S	✓	G, M	χ	↑	✓	✓	70	often with anti-c
e	S	✓	G, M	χ	↑	R	✓	3	auto in WAIHA¶¶
f(ce)	S	✓	G, M	χ	↑	✓	✓	36	compatible with c–
Fy^a	R	✓	G	R	↓	✓	✓	33	
Fy^b		✓	G	R	↓	✓	✓	20	
Ge	S	✓	G, M	✓	↓S	χ	✓	R	
H	✓	✓	M, G	✓	↑	✓	✓	R	in O_h bloods
Hy		✓	G	χ		χ	✓	R	in African-Amerians
I	✓	S	M, G	✓	↑	χ		R	in i adults
Jk^a	S	✓	G	✓	↑	✓	✓	25	
Jk^b	S	✓	G	✓	↑	✓	✓	25	
JMH		✓	G	χ	↓	χ	χ	R	HTLA
Js^a		✓	G	χ		✓	✓	>99	
Js^b		✓	G	χ		✓	✓	R	in African-Americans
K	S	✓	G, M	R		✓	✓	90	
k		✓	G	χ		✓	✓	R	
Kn^a		✓	G	χ	↓	χ	χ	2	HTLA
Kp^a		✓	G	χ		✓	✓	98	
Kp^b		✓	G	χ		✓	✓	R	
Lan		✓	G	S		✓	✓	R	
Le^a	✓		M	✓	↑	χ	R	78	
Le^{bL}	✓		M	✓	↑	χ	χ	28	true anti-Le^b
Le^{bH}	✓		M	✓	↑	χ	χ	48	in A_1 and A_1B
Lu^a	✓	S	G, A	R		R	χ	92	
Lu^b		✓	G, A	R		✓	✓	R	
M	✓	S	M, G	R	↓	R	R	22	
McC^a		✓	G	χ	↓	χ	χ	1.5	HTLA
N	✓	S	M, G	χ	↓	R	R	28	potent in N–U–
P_1	✓	S	M	S	↑	χ	R	21	no dosage
$P+P_1+P^k$	✓	✓	M, G	✓	↑	✓	✓	R	
Rg		✓	G	χ	↓	χ	χ	3	HTLA; to C4d
S	R	✓	G	S	↓	✓	✓	45	
s	R	✓	G	R	↓	✓	✓	11	
Sc1		✓	G	✓		χ	χ	R	
Sc2		✓	G	χ		✓	χ	99	
Sl^a		✓	G	χ	↓	χ	χ	2	HTLA
U		✓	G	χ		✓	✓	R	in African-Americans
V	S	✓	G	χ	↑	✓	✓	>99	
Vel	S	✓	M, G	✓	↑	χ	✓	R	
Wr^a	S	✓	M, G	χ		✓	✓	>99	
Xg^a		✓	G	χ	↓	χ	χ	23	
Yk^a		✓	G	χ	↓	χ	χ	8	HTLA
Yt^a		✓	G	χ	↓S	χ	S	R	
Yt^b		✓	G	χ		χ	χ	92	

* Coating antibodies detected primarily through the use of the indirect antiglobulin test (Table 2).
† Predominant immunoglobulin class shown first.
‡ HDN, reported to cause hemolytic disease of the newborn.
§ HTR, reported to cause hemolytic transfusion reactions.
S, some examples.
R, rare.
✓, yes.
χ, no.
** HLA, antibody to antigen present on white blood cells that is variably expressed on red blood cells.
†† HTLA, antibody, usually of high titer, to antigen of low–site density on red cells. Incorrectly called high-titer, low-avidity antibody.
‡‡ C4d, antibody to epitopes found on the fourth component of human complement (C4).
§§ Rare in Caucasians and African-Americans. Seen almost exclusively in individuals of Mongolian ancestry (South American Indians, Chippewa Indians, Chinese, Japanese).
¶¶ WAIHA, seen as an autoantibody in some cases of warm autoimmune hemolytic anemia.

Red Blood Cell Antigen-antibody Interactions

Red blood cells normally repel one another. The force of repulsion (ζ-potential) that exists at the red blood cell surface depends not only on the electronegative surface charge, but on the ionic cloud that normally surrounds it (10,11). The electronegative charge is imparted primarily by the carboxyl ($C00^-$) group of N-acetyl-neuraminic acid (12), a constituent of alkali-labile tetrasaccharides that are attached to MN and Ss sialoglycoproteins (glycophorins A and B, respectively) (9). At a minimum, there are 3.2×10^7 of these charged groups per red blood cell. The magnitude of this charge is modified by the formation of an ionic cloud of positively charged (+) sodium ions and negatively charged (−) chloride ions that align in alternating sequence extending from the red blood cell membrane surface (Fig. 7.4). The net effect of this ionic cloud is to decrease the electrostatic repulsion between red blood cells.

In considering the interaction of red blood cell antigens with blood group antibodies, three variables must be considered: the surface charge of the red blood cells, the dielectric constant of the medium (a relative measure of its charge dissipation), and the mutual attraction between antigen and antibody. The latter involves electrostatic (Coulombic) and hydrogen bonds and van der Waals interactions, which hold antigen and antibody together (10). Further, there must be structural complementarity between antigen and its binding site on antibody molecules (13).

There are two phases of red blood cell antigen-antibody interactions; these often occur simultaneously. The first phase is one of association, involving binding of antibody to antigens on the red blood cell membrane. The second phase involves the formation of an agglutination lattice of antibody-coated cells. For the latter to occur, antibody molecules must be able to span the distance between adjacent red blood cells.

Interaction between red blood cells and blood group antibodies can be observed either directly by examination of red blood cell and antibody mixtures for agglutination (or clumping) and/or hemolysis, or indirectly by use of the antiglobulin test. These two serologic techniques are summarized in Table 7.3.

Direct Agglutination

IgM-antibody molecules can span the distance that exists between red blood cells when suspended in saline and cause direct

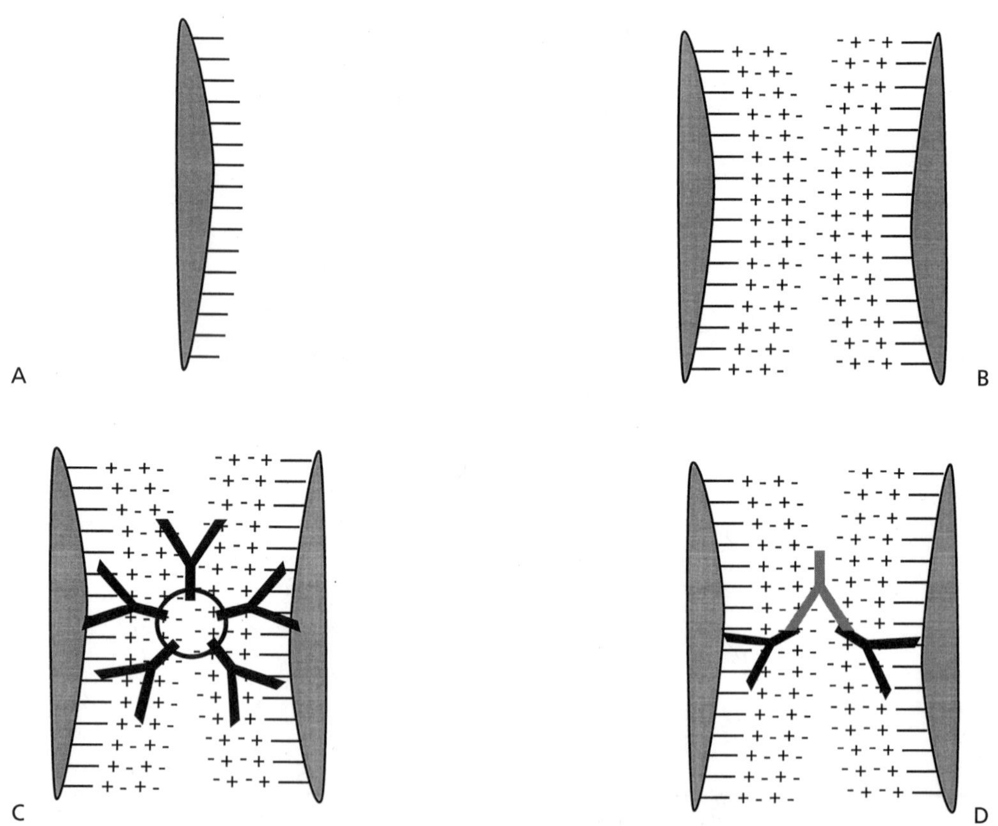

FIGURE 7.4. **A:** Red blood cells carry a strong negative electric charge, imparted primarily by the carboxyl (COO−) group of N-acetyl-neuraminic acid. **B:** When suspended in a saline medium, red blood cells are kept apart by virtue of their negative surface charge. The magnitude of this charge is modified by the formation of an ionic cloud of positively charged (+) sodium ions and negatively charged (−) chloride ions that align in alternating sequence extending from red blood cell membrane surface. The force of repulsion that exists between red blood cells in suspension is referred as the ζ-potential. **C:** In order for antibody molecules to cause agglutination of adjacent red blood cells, the antigen binding sites must be able to span the intercellular distance. Pentameric IgM antibody molecules can readily bridge the distance between adjacent red blood cells. **D:** IgG molecules *(black)* cannot readily affect direct agglutination. However, they are able to coat red blood cells. This antibody coating can be detected by a second IgG antibody (e.g., rabbit antihuman IgG), depicted here in gray.

TABLE 7.3. TWO TYPES OF RED BLOOD CELL SEROLOGIC TESTS

Direct Tests	Indirect Tests
mix serum and red cells	mix serum and red cells*
incubate (room temperature)†	incubate (37°C)
centrifuge	centrifuge
examine for agglutination and hemolysis	examine for agglutination and hemolysis†
	wash, to remove unbound globulins
	add antihuman globulin reagent
	centrifuge
	examine for agglutination‡

*An enhancement reagent, to promote antibody uptake, may be incorporated here.
†This step is optional.
‡Confirm negative tests with IgG coated red cells.

agglutination of those cells if they carry the corresponding antigen. This direct agglutination can be observed when red blood cells are mixed with IgM antibody, briefly incubated at room temperature, and centrifuged. Examination for hemagglutination may be performed either macroscopically or microscopically, but the latter is not encouraged because it leads to the detection of nonspecific reactivity. The strength of the observed reactions can be graded and numeric values assigned based on a scoring system in common use (14).

Hemolysis

IgM antibodies, in particular anti-A and anti-B, can also cause direct lysis of antigen-positive red blood cells, especially if tests are incubated at 37°C. This hemolysis results from the action of complement, a series of α and β globulins that act in sequence as enzymes (e.g., esterases) to form a complex (membrane attack complex) that causes holes to be formed in the red blood cell membrane through which the intracellular hemoglobin can escape (Fig. 7.5). For initiation of the complement cascade, the "tails" (Fc portions) of two pairs of immunoglobulin heavy chains must be in close proximity to each other on the red blood cell surface. Initiation of the complement cascade readily occurs when a single pentameric IgM antibody molecule is bound; for it to occur with IgG antibodies there must be closely adjacent heavy chain regions of two IgG molecules at the cell surface. Further, not all IgM antibodies bind complement to red blood cells, and complement binding does not always proceed to complete red blood cell lysis by membrane attack complex (intravascular hemolysis). Rather, activated C3b may be cleaved to C3d, which does not initiate the binding of C5; hence no membrane attack complex is formed. However, C3d remains bound to red blood cells and can be detected by the antiglobulin test (see below) (8,14).

Red blood cells coated with C3b are also removed by cells of the reticuloendothelial system (extravascular hemolysis). However, there are no receptors on macrophages for C3d. Thus, inactivators of C3b serve to limit the degree of both intravascular and extravascular hemolysis.

Antiglobulin Test

IgG antibodies do not readily cause direct agglutination of red blood cells, because intercellular distances are wider than the spanning distance of the antigen-binding sites of the IgG molecule. However, some IgG antibodies will cause direct agglutination if the red blood cell ζ-potential is reduced. This can be accomplished by treating the cells with proteolytic enzymes such as papain or ficin, which remove the proteins that carry the negatively charged neuraminic acid residues. Alternatively, ζ-potential can be decreased by raising the dielectric constant of the red blood cell–suspending medium by the addition of colloids such as bovine serum albumin (8).

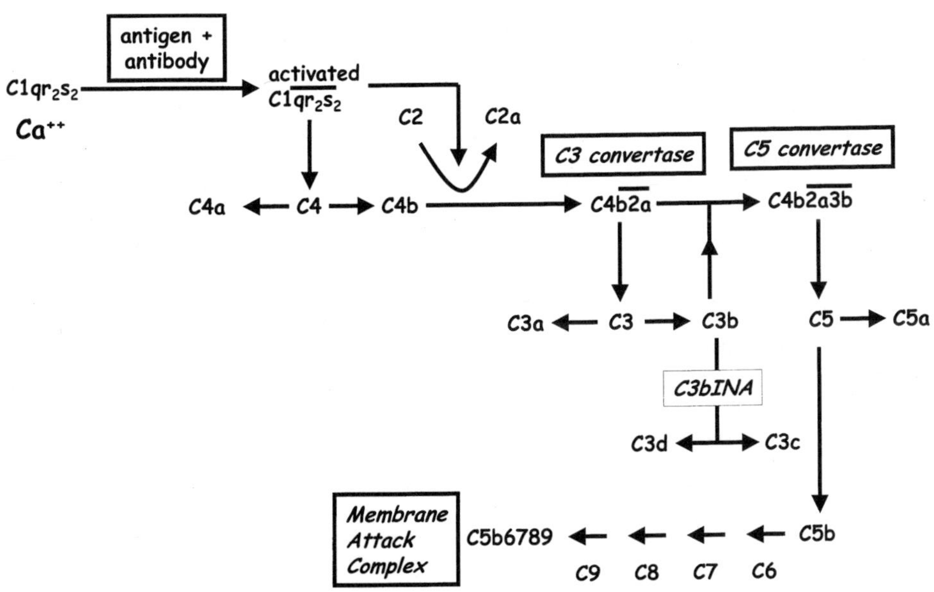

FIGURE 7.5. Classic pathway for complement activation.

IgG antibodies, as well as complement components bound to red blood cells by either IgM or IgG antibodies, are best detected by the antiglobulin test. This test, commonly called the Coombs test, entails the use of antibodies raised in animals (usually rabbit or sheep), or prepared by hybridoma technology (5), to detect human IgG and complement bound to red blood cells. The principles of this test are as follows:

1. Antibody molecules and complement components are globulins.
2. The injection of human globulins, either purified or in whole serum, into an animal stimulates the animal to produce antibodies against the foreign globulins. These antibodies are referred to as antihuman globulins. The antihuman globulins that are important for blood group serologic work are anti-IgG and anticomplement (anti-C3d).
3. Antihuman globulin (AHG) will react with human globulins, either bound to red blood cells or free in serum. Thus, red blood cells must be washed free of unbound globulins before testing with AHG. This is crucial to the avoidance of false-negative tests due to neutralization of AHG by unbound globulins.
4. Washed red blood cells coated with human globulin are agglutinated by AHG.

Antiglobulin tests can be performed either indirectly following in vitro incubation of red blood cells with serum, or directly to demonstrate that red blood cells are coated with globulins in vivo. The indirect antiglobulin test (IAT) is used to detect and identify unexpected antibodies in the serum of blood donors, prospective transfusion recipients, and prenatal patients. The direct antiglobulin test (DAT) is used to detect antibodies bound to red blood cells in vivo; such antibodies may be seen in patients with hemolysis due to autoantibodies or drugs, infants with hemolytic disease of the newborn, and patients manifesting an alloimmune response to a recent transfusion (14).

COMPATIBILITY TESTING

Pretransfusion compatibility testing comprises a series of policies and procedures, including laboratory tests, the goals of which are to provide blood for transfusion that will have the optimal clinical effect without causing undue harm to the recipient. These elements of pretransfusion testing can be placed into one of three categories: those related to donor unit testing and processing, those related to patient sample collection and testing, and those that serve as a final check between the donor unit and intended recipient (Table 7.4). Proper performance of each element will enable the right unit of blood to be transfused to the right patient (15).

TABLE 7.4. REQUIRED ELEMENTS OF PRETRANSFUSION TESTING*

Patient Sample Collection	
Identification	Positive identification of intended recipient and blood sample at time of collection (5.1.6.6)†
	Mechanism to identify phlebotomist (5.1.6.6.3)
Label	Two independent identifiers (e.g., first and last name, patient unique number) (5.1.6.6.1)
	Date of collection (5.1.6.6.1)
	Attached to tube before leaving side of intended recipient (5.1.6.6.2)
Timing	Within 3 days of red blood cell transfusion if patient transfused or pregnant within previous 3 months, or if history uncertain or unavailable (5.12.3.2)
Donor Unit Confirmatory Testing	
First-time donors or if electronic crossmatch used	From an attached segment, after the ABO and Rh label has been affixed (5.11.3.1; 5.11.3.2.2; 5.13.2.6)
	Anti-A and anti-B on units labeled group A or group B
	Anti-A,B on units labeled group O
	Direct tests with anti-D on units labeled Rh-negative
Repeat donors	A computer system (validated to prevent release of ABO–and Rh–mislabeled units) may be used (5.11.3.2)
Unexpected Antibodies	Confirmatory testing not required
Patient Sample Testing	
ABO	Red blood cells with anti-A and anti-B; serum or plasma with A1 and B red blood cells; concordance between red blood cell and serum results (5.12.1)
Rh	Test with anti-D; test for weak D not required (5.12.2)
Unexpected Antibodies	By a method that will demonstrate clinically significant antibodies; 37°C incubation preceding an antiglobulin test (alternative methods of documented equivalency acceptable); using reagent red cells that are not pooled (5.12.3)
	Confirm negative tests with IgG-coated red cells (or alternative method recommended by manufacturer) (5.12.3.4)
Donor/Patient Testing	
Crossmatch	Antiglobulin test (5.13.1); applies if clinically significant antibodies detected, currently or in past
	Serologic tests for ABO incompatibility if no clinically significant antibodies detected, currently or in past (5.13.1.1)
	Computer system validated on site to prevent release of ABO-incompatible blood may be used to detect to ABO incompatibility (5.13.2.1)

*Derived from AABB Standards.[11]
†Number refers to specific standard.

Donor Testing

Collection Facility

The initial ABO, Rh, and antibody detection tests on donor bloods, tests for infectious diseases, the interpretation of these tests, and correct labeling of donor units are functions normally carried out by a regional donor center. However, some hospital-based transfusion services continue to procure a portion of their blood needs from the population at large (allogeneic donors), and in recent years efforts have been made for patients awaiting elective surgical procedures to deposit their blood for later use (autologous donors). In addition, some patients request that they receive blood from relatives or friends (directed donations). Regardless of the type of donor, each unit of blood must be subjected to tests for ABO, Rh, and unexpected antibodies, as well as for markers of infectious disease. (See Chapter 66.)

The volume of testing that needs to be done at donor centers often necessitates use of automated equipment. Instrumentation currently in use is often based on microplate technology, and test results may be interpreted electronically. ABO grouping entails testing both donor red blood cells and serum/plasma. Red blood cells are tested with anti-A and anti-B; and the serum/plasma is tested with A_1 and B red blood cells. Although not required, anti-A,B and A_2 red blood cells may also be used, because results with these reagents serve to detect subgroups of A that may be nonreactive in direct tests with anti-A alone.

Rh typing is performed with anti-D. Because D is highly immunogenic (8), it is presumed that even weak expression of the antigen will evoke an immune response; consequently donor red blood cells that initially type as Rh-negative in direct agglutination tests are tested further for weak D (formerly D^u), usually by the IAT (Table 7.3). Only those units that are negative with anti-D by this method, or an equivalent procedure, can be labeled Rh-negative (16). All straightforward D-positive and weak D-positive bloods are considered Rh-positive.

Transfusing Facility

The ABO group of all units of whole blood or red blood cells, and the Rh group of those labeled Rh-negative, must be confirmed prior to transfusion (16). For first-time donors, this confirmatory testing must be done after the original ABO and Rh label has been affixed using a sample from a segment attached to the donor unit. Only tests with reagent antisera and donor red blood cells need be done; units labeled group O can be tested with anti-A,B alone (17). For D-typing of units labeled Rh-negative, only direct tests with anti-D are necessary; testing for weak expression of D is not required, nor is repeat testing for unexpected antibodies or for markers of infectious diseases (16). For repeat donors, the ABO/Rh may be confirmed by an electronic record check of previous donations, provided that tests for ABO compatibility are to be performed serologically. If blood is to be released using an electronic crossmatch process (see later), the ABO/Rh of the donor unit must be confirmed serologically by testing an attached segment.

Patient Testing

Sample Collection

The importance of the following measures cannot be overemphasized, because the major cause of fatal, hemolytic transfusion reactions is ABO-incompatible transfusion resulting from patient/sample misidentification.

1. Requisition. Forms requesting blood and blood components must contain the first and last names and a unique numeric identifier of the intended recipient, such as their hospital registration number (16). The name of the requesting physician, sex and date of birth of the patient, clinical diagnosis, and previous transfusion or pregnancy history are additional useful pieces of information.
2. Patient identity. The collection of a properly labeled blood sample for pretransfusion testing from the correct patient is critical to safe blood transfusion. The person collecting the sample must positively identify the patient (16). This is facilitated through use of a wristband, containing the patient's full name and unique hospital registration number that remains attached to the patient throughout the hospitalization. The information on the requisition form should be compared with that on the wristband; blood samples should not be collected if there is a discrepancy.

   In the absence of a wristband, the nursing staff should identify the patient; this should be documented on the requisition form. Nursing staff should be reminded to attach a wristband to the patient to validate patient identity at the time of transfusion. In an emergency, a temporary identification number should be used and cross-referenced with the patient's name and hospital identification number once they are known.
3. Labeling. Blood samples must be drawn into correctly labeled tubes. The tubes must be clearly labeled at the bedside with the patient's first and last names, the patient's unique hospital identification number, and the date of collection (11). The phlebotomist should initial the tube and sign or initial the requisition form so that there is a means of identifying the person who collected the sample. By filing the requisition form with the patient's medical records, a permanent record is made of the phlebotomist's name (14).
4. Confirmation of sample identity. Upon receipt of blood samples for pretransfusion testing, the information on the label must be compared with that on the requisition. A new sample must be obtained whenever there are discrepancies or if there is any doubt about the identity of the sample. It is unacceptable to correct an incorrectly labeled sample.
5. Type of sample. Either serum or plasma may be used for pretransfusion testing, but most workers use serum to avoid introducing small fibrin clots into serologic tests. Such clots may be mistaken for agglutination. Fibrin clots may also form when samples from heparinized patients are collected into nonanticoagulated tubes. These samples will clot properly following the addition of protamine sulfate (14).

   Some workers prefer to use serum rather than plasma for compatibility testing, to facilitate detection of antibodies that primarily coat red blood cells with the C3d component of complement. Bound C3d will not activate the lytic phase of the complement cascade but can be detected with AHG reagents containing anti-C3d.8, 18 EDTA, and citrate. Other commonly used anticoagulants chelate calcium ions that are essential for complement activation. However, as discussed later, the use of AHG reagents containing anti-C3d for compatibility testing is not mandatory (14).

6. Age of specimen. To ensure that the specimen used for compatibility testing is representative of a patient's current immune status, serologic studies must be performed using blood collected no more than 3 days in advance of the transfusion when the patient has been transfused or pregnant within the preceding 3 months, or when such information is uncertain or unavailable (16). From a practical standpoint, it is simpler to stipulate that all pretransfusion samples must be collected within 3 days before red blood cell transfusions, rather than ascertain whether or not each patient has been recently transfused or pregnant.
7. Storage. Blood samples used for compatibility testing, including donor red blood cells, must be kept at 1° to 6°C for at least 1 week after each transfusion (16). This ensures that appropriate samples are available for investigational purposes should adverse responses to transfusion occur.

ABO Typing

Both reagent antisera and red blood cells for ABO typing are available commercially. Anti-A and anti-B are monoclonal antibodies prepared by hybridoma technology. Reagent red blood cells are usually suspended in a preservative medium containing EDTA to prevent lysis of the red blood cells by complement-binding anti-A and anti-B (14). ABO grouping is performed using a direct agglutination technique (Table 7.3) (19). Red blood cells are tested with anti-A and anti-B, and the serum or plasma with known A_1 and B red blood cells. Use of anti-A,B and A_2 red blood cells is optional but generally considered unnecessary when ABO typing potential transfusion recipients (17).

The expected findings for each of the four common ABO phenotypes are shown in Table 7.5. When interpreting the results of ABO grouping tests, it is important to note the reciprocal relationship that exists between the absence of A and/or B antigens on red blood cells and the presence of the expected anti-A and/or anti-B in the serum. If there is conflict between cell and serum ABO tests, group O blood should be provided for transfusion until the discrepancy is resolved and reliable conclusions of the patient's ABO type can be made (14).

TABLE 7.5. THE EXPECTED REACTIONS OF THE FOUR COMMON ABO PHENOTYPES: RESULTS OF BLOOD-TYPING TESTS

Blood Type	Anti-A	Anti-B	A_1 Red Blood Cells	B Red Blood Cells
O	0*	0	4+*	4+
A	4+	0	0	4+
B	0	4+	4+	0
AB	4+	4+	0	0

*0 denotes no agglutination; 4+ denotes strong agglutination.

Rh Typing

Only tests for D are performed routinely on the red blood cells of prospective transfusion candidates. There are two different types of reagent anti-D available for Rh typing. High-protein reagents are prepared with human IgG anti-D diluted in bovine albumin and other substances that potentiate agglutination. Their final protein concentration may be greater than 20 g/dl. Such a high protein level is needed to potentiate IgG antibody reactivity so that positive and negative tests can be recognized almost instantaneously using a direct agglutination technique. In the United States, low-protein reagents (protein content >7 g/dl) are a blend of monoclonal IgM and monoclonal-polyclonal human IgG anti-D. With monoclonal-polyclonal anti-D blends, the IgM component causes direct agglutination of Rh-positive red blood cells and the IgG component permits detection of the weak expression of D by application of the antiglobulin test (14).

Only direct tests with anti-D are required on patient samples; the test for weak D (previously called D^u) is not necessary (16). To avoid incorrect designation of an Rh-negative recipient as Rh-positive because of autoantibodies or abnormal serum proteins, a control system appropriate to the anti-D reagent in use is required (14). For low protein anti-D, a concurrent negative test with anti-A and/or anti-B is considered an appropriate control system. Apparent AB Rh-positive samples should be retested concurrently with anti-D and an inert Rh control reagent (19).

Tests for Unexpected Antibodies

Methods for detecting unexpected antibodies in the serum or plasma of prospective transfusion recipients must be those that detect clinically significant antibodies (16). An IAT, after 37°C incubation of patient's serum or plasma with reagent red blood cells that are not pooled, is usually required. Table 7.2 lists many of the blood group alloantibodies that can be detected during pretransfusion testing and provides the approximate percentage of compatible units that are likely to be encountered in a predominantly white blood donor population, except as otherwise noted.

A number of options exist regarding the selection of methods for pretransfusion antibody detection (Tables 7.6, 7.7). Decisions relative to these options are within the purview of the blood bank medical director. They should be made based on the type of patient served, the causes and frequency of previous significant antibody-mediated transfusion reactions, the availability of resources, and with the realization that no one method will detect all clinically significant antibodies.

Tube Test Methods

A variety of red blood cell–suspending media or additives are used either to enhance antibody uptake or to potentiate the agglutination phase of antibody-antigen interactions (Table 7.7).

TABLE 7.6. ACCEPTABLE METHODS FOR PRETRANSFUSION ANTIBODY DETECTION

	Serum	Red Blood Cells	Incubation	AHG*
Saline	2–3 drops	1 drop, 3–5%	30–60′; 37°C	IgG/PS†
Albumin	2–3 drops	1 drop, 3–5%	15–30′; 37°C	IgG/PS
Low–ionic strength saline	2 drops‡	2 drops, 2%‡	10–15′; 37°C	IgG/PS
Gel	25 μL	50 μL, 0.8%	15′; 37°C	IgG
Polyethylene glycol	2 drops§	1 drop	15–30′; 37°C	IgG
Solid phase adherence	1 drop	¶	10–15′; 37°C	IgG
Low-ionic polycation	100 μL	1 drop, 1%	1′; RT	None

*AHG, antihuman globulin reagent.
†PS, polyspecific AHG.
‡Drop volumes should be equal.
§Plus-4 volumes of 20% polyethylene glycol.
¶Predetermined by reagent supplier.
RT, room temperature.

Low–ionic-strength saline (LISS) solution (20), normal saline, or red blood cell preservatives (modified Alsever's solution) are used as red blood cell–suspending media. Bovine serum albumin (22% or 30% weight/volume), LISS-additives, or polyethylene glycol (PEG) are commonly added directly to serum–red blood cell mixtures (19,21).

Antibody uptake (the first stage of an antigen-antibody interaction) is accelerated when red blood cells are suspended in LISS or PEG. The magnitude of the ionic cloud (Fig. 7.4) that forms around negatively charged red blood cells suspended in LISS (~0.03 mol) is lower than that surrounding red blood cells suspended in normal saline (0.15 mol NaCl). Not only does this cloud decrease intercellular distances by reducing the ζ-potential imparted by negatively charged carboxyl groups, but it hinders association between antibody and antigen; thus reducing the magnitude of the ionic cloud promotes antibody association (10). Weakening of ionic cloud also causes an increase in attraction between the negatively charged red blood cell membrane and positive charges on the antigen-binding sites of antibody molecules. In addition, PEG competes for and removes water molecules at the red blood cell surface. Similar to the ionic cloud of Na^+ and Cl^- ions that forms around red blood cells suspended in saline, these water molecules also sterically hinder antibody association. The net effect of these phenomena is that more antibody can be bound in a shorter period of time using LISS or PEG than by using saline. Consequently, incubation times can be reduced to 10 to 15 minutes for LISS, or 15 to 30 minutes for PEG, compared with 30 to 60 minutes for saline (22).

TABLE 7.7. OPTIONS IN PRETRANSFUSION TESTING

Option	Laboratories Performing[25]
ABO/Rh	
Recipient ABO red blood cell tests with anti-A,B	50.9%
Recipient ABO serum tests with group A_2 red blood cells	8.4%
Detection of weak D on recipient red blood cells	Unknown
Antibody Screen	
Immediate-spin test	65.7%
Room temperature incubation	6.9%
Polyspecific antihuman globulin, containing both anti-IgG and anti-C3d	31.4%
Pretransfusion direct antiglobulin test or autocontrol performed concurrently with screening tests for unexpected antibodies	55.4%
Microscopic examination of antiglobulin tests	52.8%
More than two reagent red blood cell samples for detection of unexpected antibodies	61%
37°C reading—for direct agglutination after 37°C incubation	86.7%

In contrast, albumin promotes the second stage of antigen-antibody interactions, namely the agglutination of antibody-coated red blood cells. It does so by increasing the dielectric constant of the suspending medium, thereby reducing the ζ-potential (force of repulsion) between red blood cells (11). Because of this effect, albumin can promote the direct agglutination of IgG-coated red blood cells (19). However, it should be noted that albumin is not used in the United States in a manner that promotes direct agglutination of antibody-coated red blood cells. Rather, the enhancing effect of albumin on red blood cell antigen interactions can be attributed to its formulation as a low-ionic solution.

In the low-ionic polycation technique, serum is incubated with red blood cells suspended in LISS to enhance antibody uptake (23). The second phase of the reaction is facilitated by aggregating red blood cells with the polycation, Polybrene. Aggregation is reversed with sodium citrate, but agglutinates formed by antigen-antibody interactions are not dispersed.

It is common practice to examine saline, albumin, and LISS tests for direct agglutination before subjecting them to the IAT. These examinations can be made immediately after mixing cells and serum together (immediate-spin tests) and again after incubation at 37°C. For antiglobulin testing, either anti-IgG or polyspecific AHG, containing anti-IgG and anti-C3, may be used

(14). However, use of polyspecific AHG leads to the detection of an inordinate number of unwanted positive tests (24), and its use in routine antibody detection tests is not recommended (17). Due to nonspecific aggregation and uptake of complement components that can occur in PEG tests, they should not be examined for direct agglutination and should not be tested with antiglobulin reagents containing anti-C3 (21).

Column Technologies

A gel test for detecting red blood cell antigen-antibody interactions was first described in 1990 by Lapierre et al. (25). Cards consisting of six microcolumns, each containing agarose gel suspended in anti-IgG, are commercially available. Atop each card is an incubation chamber in which reagent red blood cells and test plasma are dispensed. The cards are incubated at 37°C, then centrifuged. As the red blood cells pass through the gel, they are separated from the serum/plasma and come into contact with anti-IgG. If the red blood cells become coated with antibody during incubation, they will be agglutinated by anti-IgG. The agglutinated red blood cells become trapped in the gel; unagglutinated red blood cells pellet to the bottom of the microcolumn. A procedure for the gel test is depicted in Fig. 7.6.

The gel test has proven to be equivalent to standard tube technologies (LISS; PEG) for the detection of unexpected antibodies. In one study, the sensitivity and specificity of gel for potentially significant antibodies was 92% and 96%, respectively. This compares to 98% (sensitivity) and 90% (specificity) for a tube LISS procedure (26).

Column technologies offer several advantages over conventional test tube procedures:

1. Testing is simplified, as follows:
   a. Dispense measured volumes of test plasma/serum and red blood cells (in LISS) into gel card incubation chambers.
   b. Transfer cards to an incubator (15 minutes) and then to a centrifuge (10 minutes).
   c. Read and record results.
2. When compared to conventional tube tests, there is no centrifugation/reading for direct agglutination after incubation, no addition of antiglobulin reagent, and no need to validate negative tests utilizing IgG-coated red blood cells. Omission of these manipulations (especially the associated, repetitive transfer of test tubes between racks and centrifuges) provides significant "hands-on" time savings.
3. Batch testing increases time savings; a technologist can perform 36 to 48 antibody screens in about the same amount of time it takes to process 12 samples by conventional tube techniques (26).
4. Increased reproducibility of results is obtained through use of measured volumes of reactants, elimination of the washing process, and less subjective reading of tests.
5. Reactions are stable, facilitating validation of results by second technologist. With conventional tube methods, there is only one opportunity to read reactions; with the gel test, reactions can be read as many times as needed up to 48 hours after centrifugation.
6. Detection of cold agglutinins (anti-I/HI -M, -P_1, -Le) of no or doubtful clinical significance is reduced, with consequential reduction in the number of samples requiring antibody identification.
7. Procedure can be automated or semiautomated using liquid sample-handling devices, thereby further reducing "hands-on" time.

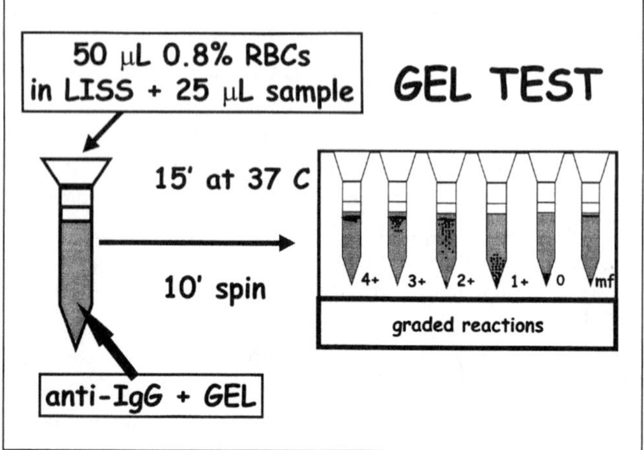

FIGURE 7.6. The gel test for detecting unexpected antibodies.

Solid-phase Adherence Methods

Two forms of solid-phase adherence assays are available for red blood cell serologic testing. For direct tests, antibody is fixed to wells of a microplate, and red blood cells are added (e.g., anti-A and anti-B for direct testing of donor-recipient ABO typing). Following centrifugation, red blood cells expressing the corresponding antigen will efface across the well; red blood cells lacking the antigen will pellet to the bottom of the well.

For indirect tests, (e.g., for detecting unexpected antibodies to red blood cell antigens) red blood cell membranes are affixed to microplate wells; test serum or plasma are added and the plates washed to remove unbound globulins. Indicator red blood cells, which are coated with anti-IgG, are then added and the plates centrifuged. The indicator red blood cells efface across the well in a positive test and pellet to the center of the well in a negative test (27). An overview of a solid-phase adherence assay for antibody detection is depicted in Fig. 7.7.

Quality Assurance for Antiglobulin Tests

All negative IATs must be validated using IgG-coated red blood cells (16). The agglutination of these red blood cells confirms that negative tests for unexpected antibodies are not due to either inadequate washing prior to the addition of antiglobulin reagent or to inactivation of the antiglobulin reagent by contamination with human serum. This testing is applicable to tube tests; for gel and solid-phase assays, the control system specified by the manufacturer should be used.

Reagent Red Blood Cells for Antibody Detection

The Food and Drug Administration (FDA) (28) currently mandates that sets of reagent red blood cell samples licensed for use

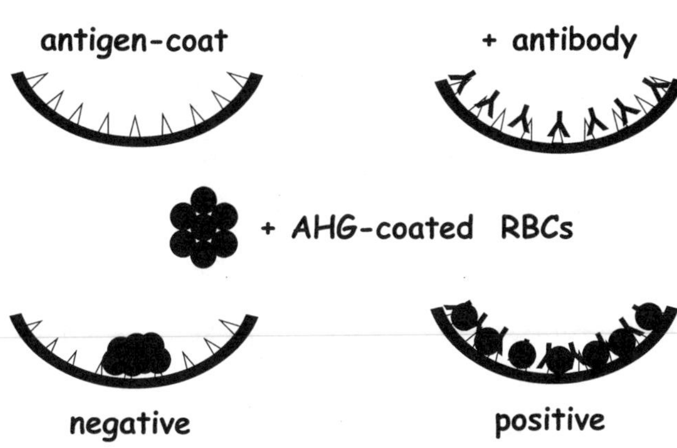

FIGURE 7.7. Solid-phase adherence assays.

in pretransfusion antibody detection tests carry C, c, D, E, e, Fy^a, Fy^b, Jk^a, Jk^b, K, k, Le^a, Le^b, P_1, M, N, S, and s antigens. Such red blood cells must not be pooled (16).

It is impossible to find a single donor with red blood cells that carry all of the above antigens, for adults rarely, if ever, have strong expression of both Le^a and Le^b on their red blood cells. Thus, reagent red blood cells for antibody detection are available commercially as sets of either two or three samples. The Rh phenotypes of red blood cells used in two-sample sets are R_1R_1 (D+C+c−E−e+) and R_2R_2 (D+C−c+E+e−). In three sample sets, an rr (D−C−c+ −E−e+) sample is provided, in addition to R_1R_1 and R_2R_2 red blood cells. Use of three red blood cell samples facilitates the inclusion of red blood cells from individuals homozygous for particular blood group genes. Such red blood cells tend to have a stronger expression of an antigen when compared to red blood cells from individuals heterozygous for the same gene; this phenomenon is known as dosage. It is easier to find double-dose expression of blood group antigens among three reagent red blood cell samples than among two samples; however, use of three samples increases the workload for antibody detection by 50% and rarely affords detection of significant alloantibodies that are not detected with two reagent red blood cell samples (29).

Further Options

Anti-IgG Versus Anti-IgG + C3

In addition to the selection of test methods and reagent red blood cells for detection of unexpected antibodies, there are other options in pretransfusion testing. Table 7.7 shows the approximate number of transfusion services still performing tests that some workers consider redundant, because such testing is neither mandatory nor required by accrediting agencies (30). Use of polyspecific AHG reagents, which contain anticomplement activity in addition to anti-IgG, may facilitate detection of some antibodies that coat red blood cells with complement components including, notably, anti-Jk^a and anti-Jk^b. Failure to detect such antibodies may lead to acute intravascular destruction of antigen-positive red blood cells (8). However, use of polyspecific AHG also facilitates detection of IgM complement-binding autoantibodies that are of no clinical significance (24). Many of these antibodies are autoantibodies directed toward the I antigen and are found naturally in virtually all normal adult human sera (8).

Room-temperature Incubation

The detection of some agglutinating alloantibodies, as well as the detection of IgM autoantibodies, is facilitated by the use of a room-temperature incubation phase. However, antibodies that do not react at body temperatures rarely, if ever, cause significant destruction of transfused incompatible red blood cells (8). Although room-temperature incubation of tests was commonly used as recently as the early 1980s, many laboratories have since abandoned the practice (30).

Microscopic Examination of Tests

Examination for agglutination may be macroscopic, performed using an illuminated concave mirror, or microscopic. The latter is rarely necessary in routine practice; indeed, such critical examination of serologic tests can result in incorrectly recording negative tests as positive (17,18).

Autocontrol

Some transfusion services routinely perform an autocontrol (AC) as part of pretransfusion testing. The AC consists of testing the serum against the patient's own red blood cells under the same conditions as those to which screening tests for unexpected antibodies are subjected. This test, or a DAT, is performed to detect globulins bound to the patient's red blood cells in vivo. Such in vivo coating of red blood cells occurs in patients with autoimmune hemolytic anemia or hemolytic disease of the newborn, and may also be seen following therapy with certain drugs or transfusion with incompatible blood (14). Moreover, a positive DAT may be the earliest manifestation of an alloimmune response to a previous, recent transfusion (31).

Inclusion of the DAT or AC as part of routine pretransfusion testing is no longer advocated; in the absence of detectable serum antibodies, the predictive value of a positive DAT is so low (0.29%) that routine testing is not cost effective (31). However, the DAT/AC is a good predictive test for immune-mediated hemolysis when performed on patients with clinical manifestations of hemolytic anemia (32).

Principles of Antibody Identification

When unexpected antibodies are present, as indicated by positive screening tests, they must be identified. At a minimum, this involves testing the patient's serum against a panel of fully phenotyped reagent red blood cell samples as well as the patient's own cells. A typical panel is shown in Table 7.8, which also includes the results of antibody identification tests with a serum containing a mixture of anti-M and anti-K. It should be noted that the tests performed in this example do include a reading for direct agglutination after room temperature incubation and

TABLE 7.8. RESULTS OF TESTS BETWEEN A PANEL OF REAGENT RED BLOOD CELLS AND A SERUM CONTAINING ANTI-M AND ANTI-K

	RH							MNS				P1	LE		KEL				JK		FY		XG		LISS			FICIN	
Panel	D	C	c	C^w	E	e	f	M	N	S	s	P_1	Le^a	Le^b	K	k	Kp^a	Js^a	Jk^a	Jk^b	Fy^a	Fy^b	Xg^a		RT	37	IgG	37	IAT
1 r′r	0	+	+	0	0	+	+	+	+	+	0	0	0	+	0	+	0	0	+	+	0	+	+	1	3+	1+	0	0	0
2 R1R1	+	+	0	0	0	+	0	0	+	+	+	+	+	0	0	+	0	0	+	+	+	+	+	2	0	0	0	0	0
3 R1R1	+	+	0	+	0	+	0	+	0	0	+	+	0	+	+	+	0	0	+	+	+	0	+	3	4+	3+	3+	0	3+
4 R2R2	+	0	+	0	+	0	0	0	+	0	+	+	0	+	0	+	0	0	0	+	+	+	+	4	0	0	0	0	0
5 r″r	0	0	+	0	+	+	+	+	0	+	0	+	0	+	0	+	0	0	+	+	0	+	+	5	4+	3+	3+	0	0
6 rrV	0	0	+	0	0	+	+	+	+	0	+	+	0	0	0	+	0	0	0	+	0	+	+	6	3+	1+	0	0	0
7 rr	0	0	+	0	0	+	+	0	+	0	+	+	0	+	+	0	0	0	0	+	+	0	0	7	0	0	4+	0	4+
8 rr	0	0	+	0	0	+	+	+	+	+	+	+	+	0	0	+	0	0	+	0	+	+	0	8	3+	1+	0	0	0
9 rr	0	0	+	0	0	+	+	+	0	+	0	+	0	+	0	+	0	0	+	0	0	+	+	9	4+	3+	3+	0	0
10 rr	0	0	+	0	0	+	+	+	+	+	+	0	+	0	+	+	0	0	+	+	+	0	+	10	3+	1+	3+	0	3+
11 Ror	+	0	+	0	0	+	+	+	+	0	0	+	0	+	0	+	0	+	+	+	0	0	0	11	3+	1+	0	0	0
PATIENT																								AC	0	0	0		

after incubation at 37°C. The results of tests with ficin-treated red blood cells are also displayed. This example will be used to illustrate a process by which the antibody specificities can be ascertained whenever there are reactive and nonreactive red blood cell samples. A typical approach follows.

1. The reactions of the AC are examined. Alloantibodies, by definition, should not react with the red blood cells of the antibody producer. When the AC is reactive, autoantibodies may be present or the AC may react, because alloantibodies have formed to recently transfused red blood cells that are still circulating in the recipient. In other cases, both auto- and alloantibodies may be present. Therapy with certain drugs, such as intravenous penicillin or a cephalosporin, can also cause the DAT/AC to be positive (14). The AC is negative in the case shown in Table 7.8, so autoantibodies likely are not present.
2. The graded reaction strengths are examined. If all positive tests are equally reactive, then only a single antibody may be present. If there are no negative tests with reagent red blood cells but the AC is nonreactive, the presence of antibody to a high-prevalence antigen should be considered. Variability in reaction strength may be an indication of dosage; that is, the antibody reacts stronger with red blood cells from homozygotes (double dose) than with red blood cells from heterozygotes (single dose). Except for antibodies to D, P_1, and Xg^a antigens, most blood group antibodies manifest dosage. There is variable expression of P_1 and Xg^a antigen on red blood cells from different donors, but this is unrelated to their zygosity. Given the varying degrees of reactivity of positive red blood cell samples in Table 7.8, more than one antibody appears to be present, and M+N− red blood cells react significantly stronger than M+N+ red blood cells.
3. A process of crossing out is undertaken. This process involves evaluating the antigens present on nonreactive red blood cells. Only reagent red blood cell samples 2 and 4 of Table 6.8 are nonreactive. Antibodies to any of the antigens (D, C, c, E, e, N, S, s, P_1, Le^a, Le^b, Jk^a, Jk^b, Fy^a, Fy^b, and Xg^a) present on these two cell samples can be eliminated from initial consideration This leaves only antibodies to M, K, C^w, f, Kp^a, and Js^a. However, C^w, Kp^a, and Js^a are low-prevalence antigens and are not likely to have been present on the reagent red blood cells used for antibody detection. Similarly f antigen will not be present on a two-sample screening set of R_1R_1 and R_2R_2 cells. Thus a provisional specificity of anti-M and anti-K can be assigned to this serum.
4. The test phase at which reactivity is observed is evaluated. Antibodies that are usually IgM (Table 7.2), such as anti-M, -N, -Le^a, and -P_1, react as direct agglutinins at room temperature. They do not react solely by the IAT, although there may be carry-over of direct agglutination that can be observed in antiglobulin tests. Similarly, those antibodies that are usually IgG (e.g., anti-Rh, -K, -Fy, -Jk, -S) react preferentially by the IAT. However, IgM antibodies of these specificities can be encountered, especially during the early stages of the immune response.

   If hemolysis of reagent red blood cells has been observed, a complement-binding antibody such as anti-Le^a or anti-Jk^a may be present. This complement-binding activity is often enhanced in tests with ficin-treated red blood cells, and in the absence of direct lysis of test red blood cells can best be observed through the use of polyspecific AHG.

   With the case under discussion, the anti-M appears to react best at room temperature and the anti-K reacts best by IAT. This is consistent with the anti-M being IgM, although many anti-M do have an IgG component (9), while the anti-K is most likely IgG (Table 7.2). The Rh antibody anti-f does not appear to be present because f-positive cell samples 1, 6, 8, and 11 are nonreactive by IAT.
5. The results of tests with enzyme-treated red blood cells, if performed, are evaluated. Knowledge of the anticipated behavior of certain antibodies with enzyme-treated red blood cells can be very helpful when identifying antibodies, especially when dealing with sera containing mixtures of alloantibodies. Antigens of the MNS, FY, and XG systems are cleaved by treatment of red blood cells with proteolytic enzymes such as papain or ficin. The high prevalence antigens Ch, En^a, JMH, In^b, Rg, Yt^a, and some Ge antigens are also cleaved by proteolytic enzymes (9). Negative or weak reactions are

observed when antibodies to these antigens are tested with ficin- or papain-treated red blood cells. In contrast, treatment of red blood cells with proteolytic enzymes enhances their reactivity with Rh antibodies, as well as complement-binding antibodies such as anti-Le^a, -P$_1$ and -Jk^a.

With the case under discussion, the double-dose M-positive red blood cell samples (3,5,9) react in LISS tests at 37°C and by IAT. These cells are nonreactive in ficin tests, which of course is expected for anti-M. In contrast, K antigen is not affected by ficin treatment, so there is no difference in the IAT reactions of ficin and LISS tests with cell samples 3, 7, and 10. Anti-f can now be completely eliminated from consideration because, if present, it should have reacted with all the K-negative ficin-treated cells from donors with *r (ce)* haplotype.

6. The data are reviewed to ensure that all other antibodies that must be excluded (by virtue of the FDA's requirements for reagent red blood cells) are not present in the serum. In this case, this was accomplished in Step 3. Although antibodies to C^w, Js^a and Kp^a *could* be present, this should not be of concern; they are no more likely to be present in this case than they are in patients with negative screening tests for unexpected antibodies.

   Some workers believe that exclusion tests should be done with double-dose red blood cells. Their rationale appears to be based on the notion that a patient who has made one alloantibody is likely to make another, more so than a nonalloimmunized patient is likely to make the first antibody following transfusion. To detect newly forming antibodies, they advocate the use of red blood cells from apparent homozygotes. However, there are no data to support this notion.

   Use of double-dose red blood cells for pretransfusion antibody detection is not required by either the FDA (28) or American Association of Blood Banks (AABB) (14,16). (See requirements for reagent red blood cells.) Reagent manufacturers do provide red blood cells with double-dose expression of Rh antigens, and some workers have established institutional policies regarding the required expression of other antigens on these cells. It would seem appropriate to use the same policies for exclusion purposes whenever practical; that is, ensure absence of anti-Jk^a with Jk(a+b−) cells if such apparent double-dose expression is required for antibody detection. It would not, however, be practical to exclude anti-E in a patient found to have anti-D using D-negative cells carrying double-dose expression of E, because this would require use of rare r″r″ cells.

7. The data are subjected to statistical analysis. Before final conclusions can be made regarding antibody specificity, there must be sufficient negative tests with red blood cells that lack the corresponding and sufficient positive tests with red blood cells that carry that antigen. To obtain a confidence level of >95% ($p = 0.05$), there should be at least three nonreactive antigen-negative red blood cell samples and at least three reactive antigen-positive red blood cells. This requirement has been met for both the anti-M and the anti-K of Table 7.8.

8. The patient's red blood cells lack the corresponding antigen. As discussed earlier, this is fundamental to the formation of alloantibodies following transfusion or pregnancy. The red blood cells from the patient of Table 7.8 should be tested with anti-M and anti-K. They should lack both M and K antigens. There are, however, exceptional cases of alloantibody formation when the corresponding antigen appears to be present on the autologous red blood cells. Most notably, this is seen with Rh-positive individuals of the partial-D phenotype who make antibody to the portions of D antigen that are absent from their red blood cells.

The above illustration represents but a basic approach to antibody identification. More complex cases involving autoantibodies, multiple alloantibodies, mixtures of both auto- and alloantibodies, and antibodies to high-prevalence antigens will require the resources of an immunohematology reference laboratory. The interested reader is referred elsewhere (14,19) for information regarding the investigation of complex antibody problems.

Donor-recipient Testing

Selection of Blood for Transfusion

ABO and Rh

Red blood cells and whole blood selected for transfusion must be compatible with the serum of the intended recipient. To avoid the hemolytic and often fatal consequences of an ABO mismatched transfusion, red blood cells carrying A and/or B antigens should not be transfused to a patient unless the patient's red blood cells also carry those antigens. Group O individuals should receive group O red blood cells, but group AB individuals can receive red blood cells of any ABO type. Rh-negative individuals, particularly females with child-bearing potential, should receive Rh-negative blood. Rh-positive individuals may receive blood of either Rh type (14).

Unexpected Antibodies

When the identified antibodies are known to cause accelerated destruction of transfused incompatible red blood cells, blood selected for transfusion should be shown to lack the corresponding antigen or antigens (14,16). This entails testing donor units with reagent antisera that are available commercially or prepared in-house from previously investigated samples. Examples of potentially significant antibodies include those directed toward antigens of the RH, JK, KELL and FY systems, and the S and s antigens of the MNS system, as well as most other antibodies active at 37°C and/or by the IAT (Table 7.2). When antibodies with specificities directed toward M, N, P$_1$, and LE antigens are present, particularly when the antibodies react best at or below room temperature, blood selected for transfusion need only be shown to be compatible by IAT following 37°C incubation; demonstrating that compatible units lack the relevant antigen(s) is not required (33,34). In instances when autoantibodies are present, least-incompatible units should be selected for transfusion once it has been established that the autoantibody is not masking a concomitant, clinically significant alloantibody (32).

Serologic Crossmatch

Before whole blood or red blood cells are administered, except in an emergency, a major crossmatch must be performed. This usually entails tests between donor red blood cells selected for transfusion and the prospective recipient's serum or plasma sample that was used for ABO, Rh, and antibody detection tests. The methods used should be capable of detecting ABO incompatibility and include the IAT. However, in the absence of unexpected antibodies (and absence of records of prior detection of such antibodies) in the intended recipient's serum, only testing to detect ABO incompatibility is required (16).

Antiglobulin Crossmatch

When clinically significant unexpected antibodies are present, or a patient's records indicate that such antibodies have been detected previously, blood selected for transfusion must be tested with the patient's serum or plasma by an IAT. Any of the methods described earlier for antibody detection can be used. An antiglobulin crossmatch can also be done routinely on patients with nonreactive screening tests for unexpected antibodies. This will detect ABO incompatibility and may detect unexpected antibodies that were missed in pretransfusion screening tests. Unexpected antibodies to low-incidence antigens and antibodies manifesting dosage may be detected in this manner, as may antibodies missed in screening tests due to technical error. However, the predictive value of a positive IAT crossmatch following nonreactive screening tests for unexpected antibodies is sufficiently low that many large hospital transfusion services do not perform the IAT crossmatch, except as required when unexpected antibodies are present or there are records of such antibodies (30).

Detection of ABO Incompatibility

Only a procedure for detecting ABO incompatibility is required when screening tests for unexpected antibodies are negative and there is no record of the patient having had such antibodies in the past. Detection of ABO incompatibility can be done serologically or, in certain situations, electronically through the use of computers. An immediate-spin crossmatch between the prospective recipient's serum or plasma and donor red blood cells suspended in EDTA-saline, to prevent false-negative tests due to prozone by complement-fixing high-titer anti-A and -B, is an acceptable serologic method for the detection of ABO incompatibility (35). Alternatively, the ABO groups of both the donor units and a blood sample from the intended recipient can be confirmed immediately before the units are released for transfusion (16).

Electronic Crossmatch

With the emergence of blood bank information systems, laboratories are beginning to use computer software to detect ABO incompatibility between the sample submitted for pretransfusion testing and the donor unit selected for transfusion (36). EXM replaces the immediate-spin test for detecting ABO incompatibility. Currently, an EXM is performed in over 50 North American facilities (30) and in other countries (Canada, Sweden, Australia, United Kingdom, Hong Kong) (37–42).

An EXM may be used instead of an immediate-spin crossmatch provided that:

1. The computer system has been validated on-site to ensure that only ABO-compatible red blood cell–containing products have been selected for transfusion.
2. No clinically significant antibodies are detected in the recipient's serum/plasma and there is no record of previous detection of such antibodies.
3. There are concordant results of at least two determinations of the recipient's ABO type on record, one of which is from a current sample.
4. The system contains the donor unit number, component name, ABO/Rh type, and the interpretation of confirmatory tests; and recipient information and ABO/Rh.
5. A method exists to verify the correct entry of data prior to release of blood or components.
6. The computer contains logic to alert the user to discrepancies between donor-unit labeling and confirmatory test interpretation, and to ABO incompatibilities between the recipient and the donor unit.
7. The donor unit blood type has been confirmed serologically using red blood cells from an attached segment.

These requirements are promulgated in AABB Standards (16), which should be consulted for the precise wording. While the FDA no longer requires facilities wishing to implement an EXM to submit a request for variance to 21 CFR 606.151 (compatibility testing). The EXM process must meet the requirements outlined in an FDA internal document (43). Table 7.9 summarizes the FDA requirements. Facilities implementing an EXM should expect their process to be evaluated during their next FDA inspection. Flow diagrams for EXM processes are depicted in Fig. 7.8 (44–46).

Advantages of the Electronic Crossmatch

The advantages of implementing an EXM are as follows:

1. Technologist time savings. This is the major advantage, and equates to approximately 2.5 minutes per unit crossmatched (36).
2. Reduced sample volume requirements. A 5- to 7-ml sample is more than adequate, and can be used for EXM for at least 30 days after collection provided other pretransfusion tests are performed soon after collection. The latter greatly facilitates same-day admission programs.
3. Reduced sample handling. Significant reduction in exposure to biohazardous materials results from elimination of the need to prepare donor red blood cell suspensions from attached segments and the need to use the patient's sample for the immediate-spin crossmatch.
4. No unwanted "false"-positive tests. Cold agglutinins, rouleaux, etc., are a frequent cause of a positive immediate-spin crossmatch following a negative antibody screen. These unwanted positive tests are avoided using an EXM.
5. Improved accuracy (no unwanted "false"-negative tests). Unlike the immediate-spin crossmatch, which is prone to yield false-negative tests between some 50% of group B sera and eclectic A_2B red blood cells (47,48), the EXM will detect such incompatibilities; it will provided the patient and donor ABO types are accurately entered into the computer and

TABLE 7.9. FDA'S EXPECTATIONS OF FACILITIES PERFORMING AN ELECTRONIC CROSSMATCH

Standard Operating Procedures

Standard operating procedures shall include:

1. Identification of the source(s) of the application software (name of software vendor or developer, the name and version of the software package). (Is the "computer" crossmatch function one designed by a commercial vendor or a modification or extended usage under the control of the blood bank or transfusion service?)
2. The location(s) where the system will be used.
3. Institution-specific, detailed instructions that address all facets of the procedure, including all circumstances for which the SOP will be used.

Software Requirements

The software requires (will not permit electronic release of blood products) unless there are:

1. Records of two determinations of the recipient's ABO group, one of which is from a current sample.
2. A record of a negative test for clinically significant antibodies from a current specimen and no record of previous detection of such antibodies.

Information

The software contains:

1. Donor unit information:
   a) Unit number.
   b) Component name.
   c) ABO and Rh type.
   d) The interpretation of the ABO confirmatory test (for units collected, processed and labeled by a separate facility).
2. ABO and Rh type of the recipient.
3. Detection of ABO incompatibility:
   a) The complete decision table is defined in the software; e.g., expected response for each possible combination of recipient/donor ABO combinations.
   b) Appropriate restrictions based on component type are defined in the software; e.g., most facilities will use decision tables to approve/reject release of a number of different red blood cell products (decision tables must be validated for each product code).
4. Logic to alert the user to:
   a) Missing required information.
   b) Donor unit labeling and confirmatory test interruption do not match.
   c) ABO incompatibilities between the recipient and the donor unit.
   d) Any other user-defined criteria.

Validation

1. The validation design must cover both "automated" software decision-making and decisions made "manually" by users following SOP.
2. The validation must be performed on-site using same hardware and software that will be employed in routine use.
3. Validation documentation includes:
   a) Testing strategies.
   b) Test acceptance and completion criteria.
   c) Copies of the documentation and testing results.
4. There is a method to review and validate entry of data before it can be used in the decision process. For manual entry this may be double entry of data or an affirmation response after reviewing on-screen display in addition to initial entry.
5. Validation testing must include:
   a) At least one case of each possible combination of decision variables.
   b) A reasonable number of cases where one or more required data elements are missing (the system should alert the user of the missing required element).
   c) A reasonable number of challenges for the selection of blood and/or components that do not meet specified criteria.
6. If the decision tables govern issues other than ABO (e.g., donor/recipient Rh match), they must be adequately tested in the validation protocol.

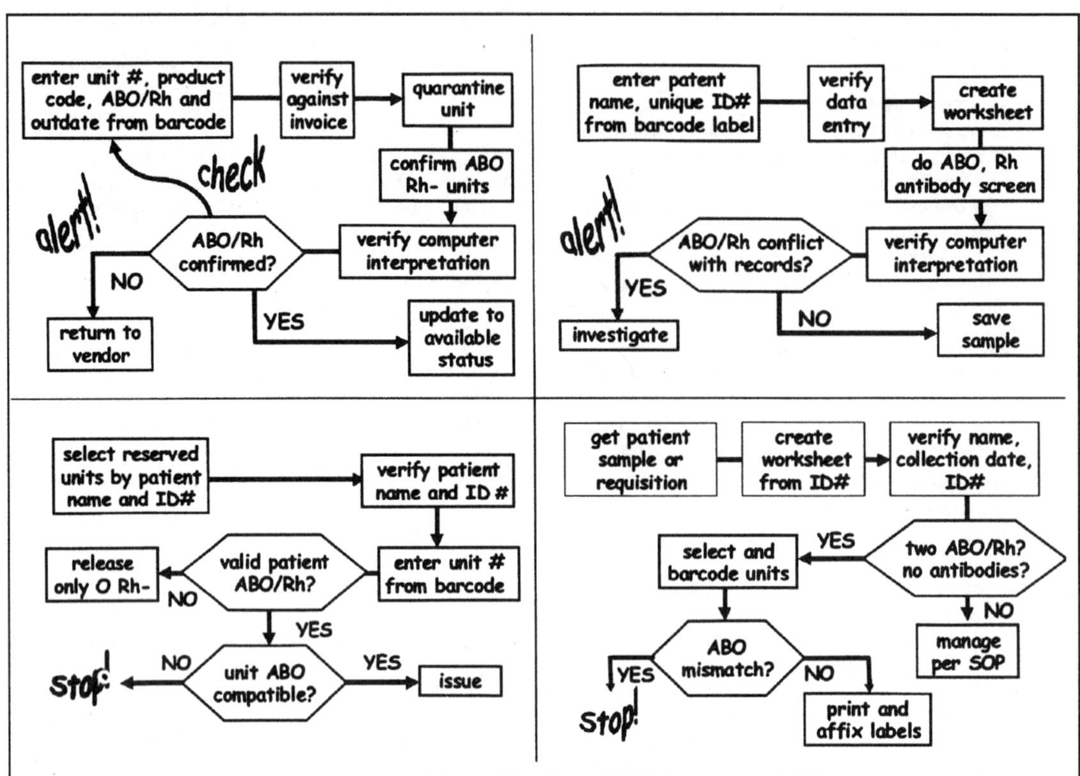

FIGURE 7.8. Flow diagrams for the electronic crossmatch. From the top left: process for donor unit entry and confirmatory ABO/Rh typing, process for initial patient ABO/Rh typing and detecting unexpected antibodies, electronic crossmatch process, dispense (release) process.

the EXM system has been properly designed, validated, and implemented. Moreover, unwanted negative tests associated with potent, prozoning anti-A and anti-B[35] are avoided.

6. Decreased turnaround time. This can lead to a decrease in the crossmatched to transfused ratio (C:T ratio).

Disadvantages of the EXM

The disadvantages of implementing an EXM are few. Barriers to implementation include availability of a laboratory information system with software for blood bank applications, the effort required to develop a system that conforms to AABB and FDA requirements, and the on-site validation process that must be undertaken to obtain FDA approval. EXM may cost more, but given current health care reimbursement practices and policies (managed care, diagnostic related groups), this may not be a real issue. One can, and should, bill for the second ABO and Rh compatibility tests, if required. A current procedural terminology (CPT) code of 909090 has been assigned to the EXM. This code can be used to track activity but does not generate a charge (49).

Release of Blood for Transfusion

Prior Records Check

As part of ongoing quality assurance and for compliance with the Standards for Blood Banks and Transfusion Services of the AABB (16), the results of current ABO, Rh, antibody detection, and compatibility tests must be checked against records of previous tests, if performed. This must be done before blood is released for transfusion, preferably at the time pretransfusion tests are completed. The specific records that must be checked are those for ABO and Rh typing performed within the previous 12 months, and any difficulties in typing, unexpected antibodies, severe adverse reactions to transfusion, and any special transfusion requirements. Any discrepancies between past and present ABO and Rh typing results must be thoroughly investigated; the most likely explanation is that the present sample is not from the same individual whose blood was tested previously. Further, even in the absence of detectable unexpected antibodies in the current sample, a record of such unexpected antibodies in previous samples must be taken into consideration when selecting and crossmatching blood for present and future transfusions.

Labeling

Before blood is released for transfusion the container shall have an affixed label or tie tag indicating the recipient's first and last names, unique identification number, the donor unit number, and the interpretation of compatibility tests, if performed (16). The unit must be inspected visually before release; if any abnormality in color or appearance is noted the unit should not be issued. A record should be made of this inspection. The expiration date must also be checked to avoid issuing an outdated unit (14).

Release Records

At the time blood and blood components are issued, there must be a final check of records maintained in the transfusion service (16). These records shall include:

1. The recipient's name and unique identification number; ABO type, and Rh type if required.
2. The donor unit number or pool identification number (for platelets), and the ABO and Rh type of the donor.
3. The interpretation of compatibility tests; if performed.
4. The date and time of issue.

Documentation that this process occurred can be facilitated by use of a log book, in which the name of the person performing the release check can be recorded (14).

Emergency Release

When a patient's ABO type is not known, only group O red blood cells can be issued (16). For female patients with child-bearing potential, these should also be Rh-negative. If the ABO and Rh type have been determined on a current sample, type-specific whole blood or ABO-compatible red blood cells may be issued. The container label or tie tag should indicate that compatibility testing was not completed at the time the unit was released. Testing should be completed expeditiously, and the records should contain a statement, signed by the requesting physician, indicating the need for transfusion before completion of compatibility testing.

Bedside Check

Before administering blood, the physician's written order should be reviewed to verify the request for transfusion (14). The transfusionist is responsible for this and for performing a final errors check. Verification of the following information must occur (16):

1. Recipient identification. The name and identification number on the patient's wristband must be identical to the name and number on the form attached to the unit.
2. Unit identification. The unit number on the blood container must match the unit number on the transfusion form.
3. ABO/Rh. The ABO and Rh type on the donor unit primary label must agree with that recorded on the transfusion form.
4. Expiration date. The expiration date of the unit should be checked and the unit verified as acceptable for transfusion.

CONCLUSION

Compatibility testing constitutes a quality assurance program designed to detect serologic incompatibility between donor unit and the intended recipient and to prevent both clerical and technical errors that may have serious, if not fatal, consequences. Assurance of quality requires proper performance of each individual task. There can be no substitute for proper patient identification, proper sample labeling, and proper performance of serologic tests.

REFERENCES

1. Alt F, Blackwell TK, Yancopoulos GD. Development of the primary antibody repertoire. *Science* 1987;248:1079–1087.
2. Kuby J. *Immunology,* 3rd ed. New York: WH Freeman & Company, 1997.
3. Parslow TC. Immunoglobulins and immunoglobulin genes. In: Stites DP, Terr AL, Parslow TC, eds. *Medical immunology,* 9th ed. Stamford, CT: Appleton & Lange, 1997;95–114.
4. Chestnut RW, Grey HM. Antigen presentation by B cells and its significance in T-B interactions. *Adv Immunol* 1986;39:51–64.
5. Kohler G, Milstein C. Derivation of specific antibody-producing tissue culture and tumor lines by cell fusion. *Eur J Immunol* 1976;6:511–519.
6. Silberstein LE. The antibody response to antigen. In: Nance S, ed. *Alloimmunity: 1993 and beyond.* Bethesda, MD: American Association of Blood Banks, 1993:25–47.
7. Race RR, Sanger R. *Blood groups in man,* 6th ed. Oxford: Blackwell Scientific Publications, 1965.
8. Mollison PL, Engelfriet CP, Contreras M. *Blood transfusion in clinical medicine,* 10th ed. Oxford: Blackwell Scientific Publications, 1997.
9. Reid ME, Lomas-Francis C. *The blood group antigen factsbook.* London: Academic Press, 1997.
10. Pollack W. Some physicochemical aspects of hemagglutination. *Ann N Y Acad Sci* 1965;127:892–900.
11. Pollack W, Hager HJ, Reckel R, et al. A study of the forces involved in the second stage of hemagglutination. *Transfusion* 1965;5:158–183.
12. Cook GMW, Heard DH, Seamen GVF. A sialomucopeptide liberated by trypsin from the human erythrocyte. *Nature (Lond)* 1960;188: 1011–1012.
13. Judd WJ. Antibody elution from red cells. In: Bell CA, ed. *Antigen-antibody reactions revisited.* Arlington, VA: American Association of Blood Banks, 1982:175–221.
14. Vengelan-Tyler V, ed. *Technical manual,* 13th ed. Bethesda, MD: American Association of Blood Banks, 1999.
15. Shulman IA. Controversies in red cell compatibility testing. In: Nance SJ, ed. *Immune destruction of red cells.* Arlington, VA: American Association of Blood Banks, 1989:171–199.
16. Menitove J, ed. *Standards for blood banks and transfusion services,* 20th ed. Bethesda, MD: American Association of Blood Banks, 2000.
17. Oberman HA, Judd WJ. Cost containment in transfusion medicine: a view from the United States. In: Cash JD, ed. *Progress in transfusion medicine,* vol 3. Edinburgh: Churchill Livingstone, 1988.
18. Issitt PD. *Applied blood group serology,* 4th ed. Durham, NC: Montgomery Scientific Publications, 1998.
19. Judd WJ. *Methods in immunohematology,* 2nd ed. Durham, NC: Montgomery Scientific Publications, 1994.
20. Löw B, Messeter L. Antiglobulin tests in low–ionic strength salt solution for rapid antibody screening and crossmatching. *Vox Sang* 1974; 26:53–61.
21. Nance S, Garratty G. A new technique to enhance antibody reactions using polyethylene glycol (abstract). *Transfusion* 1985;25:475.
22. Fitzsimmons JM, Morel PA. The effects of red blood cell suspending media on hemagglutination and the antiglobulin test. *Transfusion* 1979;19:81–85.
23. Lalezari P, Jiang AF. The manual Polybrene test: a simple and rapid procedure for detection of red cell antibodies. *Transfusion* 1980;20: 206–211.
24. Garratty G. The role of complement in blood group serology. *Crit Rev Clin Lab Sci* 1985;20:25–56.
25. Lapierre Y, Rigal D, Adam J, et al. The gel test: a new way to detect red cell antigen-antibody reactions. *Transfusion* 1990;30:109–113.

26. Judd WJ, Steiner EA, Knafl PC. The gel test: sensitivity and specificity for unexpected antibodies to blood group antigens. *Immunohematology* 1997;13:132–135.
27. Judd WJ. 'New' blood bank technologies. *Clin Lab Sci* 1998;11: 106–113.
28. Code of federal regulations (21-CFR), parts 606 and 660. Washington DC: US Government Printing Office, current edition.
29. Judd WJ. Testing for unexpected red cell antibodies—two or three reagent red cell samples. *Immunohematology* 1997;13:90–92.
30. Maffei LM, Johnson ST, Shulman IA, et al. Survey on pretransfusion testing. *Transfusion* 1998;38:343–349.
31. Judd WJ, Barnes BA, Steiner EA, et al. The evaluation of a positive direct antiglobulin test (autocontrol) revisited. *Transfusion* 1986;26: 220–224.
32. Judd WJ. Investigation and management of immune hemolysis—autoantibodies and drugs. In: Wallace ME, Levitt J, eds. *Current applications and interpretation of the direct antiglobulin test.* Arlington, VA: American Association of Blood Banks, 1988;47–103.
33. Cronin CA, Pohl BA, Miller WV. Crossmatch-compatible blood for patients with anti-P1. *Transfusion* 1978;18:728–730.
34. Issitt PD. Antibodies reactive at 30°Centigrade, room temperature and below: a technical workshop. In: Butch SH, ed. *Clinically significant and insignificant antibodies: a technical workshop.* Washington, DC: American Association of Blood Banks, 1979;13–28.
35. Judd WJ, Steiner EA, O'Donnell DB, et al. Discrepancies in ABO typing due to prozone: how safe is the immediate-spin crossmatch? *Transfusion* 1988;28:334–338.
36. Butch SH, Judd WJ, Steiner EA, et al. Electronic verification of donor-recipient compatibility: the computer crossmatch. *Transfusion* 1994; 34:105–109.
37. Sawfenberg J, Hogman CF, Cassemar B. Computerized delivery control: a useful and safe complement to the type and screen compatibility testing. *Vox Sang* 1997;72:162–168.
38. Cox C, Enno A, Deveridge S, et al. Remote electronic release blood system. *Transfusion* 1997;37:960–964.
39. Chan A, Chan JC, Wong LY, et al. From maximum surgical blood ordering schedule to unlimited computer crossmatching: evolution of blood transfusion for surgical patients at a tertiary hospital in Hong Kong. *Transfus Med* 1996;6:121–124.
40. British Committee for Standardization in Haematology, Blood Transfusion Task Force. Guidelines for pre-transfusion compatibility procedures in blood transfusion laboratories. *Transfus Med* 1996;6:273–283.
41. Georgsen J, Jensen F, Jeppesen S, et al. Transfusion service of the county of Funen. Organizational and economic aspects of restructuring. *Ugeskr Laeger* 1997;159:1758–1762.
42. Barratt PG, Russel PG, Rowell JA. Eighteen months experience with a computer crossmatch minus the computer. *Transfusion* 1993; 33[Suppl]:74(abst).
43. Center for Biologics Evaluation and Research. Computer Crossmatch Reviewer's Checklist. Rockville, MD: US Food and Drug Administration, 1997.
44. Butch SH, Judd WJ. Requirements for the computer crossmatch [Letter]. *Transfusion* 1994;34:187.
45. Judd WJ. Requirements for the electronic crossmatch. *Vox Sang* 1998; 74[Suppl 2]:409–417.
46. Judd WJ. The electronic crossmatch: an alternative method the immediate-spin crossmatch to detect ABO incompatibility. *Advance* 1998; 10(15):16–23.
47. Steane EA, Steane SM, Montgomery SR, et al. A proposal for compatibility testing incorporating the manual hexadimethrine bromide (Polybrene) test. *Transfusion* 1985;25:176–178.
48. Berry-Dortch S, Woodside C, Boral LI. Limitations of the immediate spin crossmatch when used for detecting ABO incompatibility. *Transfusion* 1985;25:540–544.
49. Physician's current procedural terminology: CPT '98. Chicago: American Medical Association; 1998.

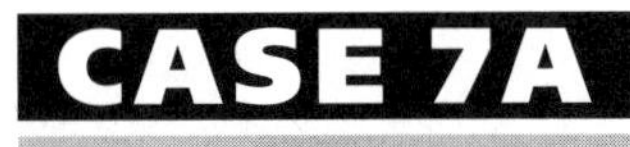

KNOWING WHEN TO ASK FOR HELP

An Immunohematologic Laboratory Problem

CASE HISTORY

Gladys G. is a spry 60-year-old lady with a chronic myelodysplastic syndrome who comes to our outpatient department for red blood cell transfusion. On physical exam there is no splenomegaly. Her medications include only an antihypertensive agent and a mild antidepressant. She is group B, Rh-negative with prior nonreactive antibody screening tests. She had two uncomplicated pregnancies decades earlier. She has received fewer than six transfusions in her life and was last transfused 2 months ago. Today, however, her antibody screen shows 3+ reactivity with all three screening cells at the antiglobulin phase of testing.

LABORATORY FINDINGS

An initial panel showed 3+ reactivity with all panel cells at the antiglobulin phase. The autocontrol included in that panel was nonreactive.

Interpretation

Failure of the patient's plasma to react with her own cells under the same conditions under which it reacts 3+ with all other cells of a large panel is most consistent with one or more alloantibodies. The very uniform strength of reactivity in the panel suggests the likelihood of a single alloantibody directed against a high-frequency antigen. Antibodies to high-frequency antigens can be very problematic for the patient and for the transfusion service. In this case, we told the patient that more work needed to be done and rescheduled her outpatient transfusion for a few days hence.

LABORATORY FINDINGS

A direct Coombs test reacted microscopically using polyvalent antisera and using anti-IgG antisera, and was nonreactive using anticomplement antisera. Treatment of the patient's cells with a glycine-acid mixture rendered the microscopic Coombs test negative.

Interpretation

The microscopic direct antiglobulin test suggests the presence of a weak autoantibody. Some laboratories would pay little attention to reactions detectable only with the aid of a microscope. Indeed, many question the utility of keeping a microscope in the serology laboratory.

LABORATORY FINDINGS

An extended phenotype of the patient's red blood cells was done to determine if she lacked a high-frequency antigen. Her cells initially typed C-weak; E-weak; c 4+; e 4+; and D-negative. Using monoclonal Rh typing sera, however, her results were: C-negative; E-negative; c 4+; e 4+; D-negative. Additional typing results were: Kell-weak; Cellano 4+; Fy^a 3+; Fy^b 3+; Jk^a 3+; Jk^b 3+; S-weak; s 4+; M 3+; N 2+; P_1 4+; Di^b 2+; Ge: 2 2+; Cr 2+.

Interpretation

The initial typings for C and E were weakly positive using reagents that require the antiglobulin phase of testing. When repeated with monoclonal reagents, the results were nonreactive. Monoclonal reagents have the advantage that they are IgM direct agglutinins and can be used for typing without the requirement for an antiglobulin phase of testing. The weak reactivity with nonmonoclonal reagents and nonreactivity with monoclonal reagents is consistent with the weak direct antiglobulin test observed earlier. The other phenotype results showed weak reactivity with Kell and S. However, the patient had been transfused 2 months earlier with two units of red blood cells. Investigation showed that one of these was Kell-positive and one was S-positive. The other phenotype results are not ambiguous. We note that patient was not lacking the high-incidence antigens Cellano, Di^b, Ge:2, and Cr.

LABORATORY FINDINGS

Even though the direct antiglobulin test was only microscopically positive, an acid eluate was performed. The eluate reacted 3+ with all target cells. The plasma was adsorbed against the patient's papain-treated cells. Four serial autoadsorptions were done using fresh autologous cells each time. The residual plasma (adsorbed plasma) was found to react 3+ with all target cells.

Interpretation

The strongly reactive eluate is consistent with an autoantibody. Another possibility is that the microscopic direct antiglobulin test has resulted from the coating of previously transfused cells with the new high-frequency alloantibody. In this case the eluate would react as the plasma does. The plasma antibody failed to be depleted by autoadsorptions. This finding is typical of an alloantibody to a high-frequency antibody.

LABORATORY FINDINGS

The patient's plasma was tested against a selected panel of target cells, each of which lacked a particular high-frequency antigen. Her plasma reacted 3+ at the antiglobulin phase of testing with cells lacking Cellano, Js[b], Co[a], Kp[b], Chido, Vel, Yt[a], Rg, and Yk[a].

TABLE 7A.1. DIFFERENTIAL EXPRESSION OF SOME BLOOD GROUP ANTIGENS

Reduced by Ficin	Reduced by DTT	Reduced by EGA[a]	Reduced on Cord Cells
Fy[a], Fy[b]	Kell	Kell	I
M, N, S, s	Cr	Er[a]	Sd[a]
Ch/Rg	Kn	Bg	Ch/Rg
In	In		Lewis
JMH	JMH		P_1
Ge2, Ge4	Sc		Lu[a], Lu[b]
Yt[a]	Yt[a]		Yt[a]
	LW		Vel
			Dombrock
			Kn
			AnWj

[a]EGA is an EDTA and glycine-acid mixture (Gamma Biologicals, Houston, TX).

Interpretation

Failure to react with a selected cell that lacks a common antigen would have provided strong evidence that the alloantibody was directed against that antigen. Unfortunately, all cells were reactive to equal strength, so the antibody must be directed against some other high-incidence antigen.

LABORATORY FINDINGS

The patient's plasma reacted 3+ against all cells in a panel of ficin-treated cells and 3+ with a different panel of cells treated with dithiothreitol. Her plasma also reacted 3+ against a cord blood cell. Her plasma was adsorbed with a suspension of human platelet concentrate and the adsorbed plasma reacted 3+ with all target cells. A review of her peripheral blood smear showed no elliptocytes, acanthocytes, or stomatocytes.

Interpretation

Target cells can be chemically modified in order to selectively remove expression of particular antigens. The effect of different chemical treatments are shown in Table 7A.1 below. Nonreactivity of the plasma with treated cells provides evidence that the patient's antibody is directed against one of the antigens destroyed by that chemical. In this case, her plasma reacted with all treated cells. Human cord blood cells also fail to strongly express some antigens (Table 7A.1). Because her plasma reacted with cord blood cells, we felt her antibody could not have been directed to a high-frequency antigen absent on cord blood cells. Patients lacking some high-frequency antigens can show characteristic abnormalities on peripheral blood smear; for example, Gerbich-negative individuals have elliptocytes, but our patient demonstrated no abnormally shaped red blood cells.

LABORATORY FINDINGS

Twofold serial dilutions of the patient's plasma were tested against a randomly selected untreated ABO-compatible target cell. The undiluted serum reacted 3+ and the serum reacted macroscopically at a dilution of 1 to 2,048.

Interpretation

This patient has a high-titer alloantibody to an undefined high-frequency antigen. This is a serious problem for transfusion support.

At this juncture, her elective transfusion was further postponed. The patient is of mixed European ancestry. She was not the product of a consanguineous marriage. She has no living relatives. Options at this point include additional testing by another laboratory with access to different reagent antisera or cells or the infusion of a small aliquot of radiolabeled cells to determine if the alloantibody is clinically significant. Fortunately, the patient was able to tolerate her anemia. Erythropoietin therapy was considered but deemed unlikely to benefit her because her native erythropoietin synthesis was expected to be normal, and because her anemia was secondary to decreased bone marrow production due to myelodysplasia. It was now 2 weeks after the initial positive antibody screen. New samples were sent to the National Reference Laboratory of the American Red Cross.

NATIONAL REFERENCE LABORATORY FINDINGS

The National Reference Laboratory confirmed many of the findings of the hospital laboratory. The reference laboratory also found that the antiglobulin test was microscopically positive with polyvalent, anti-IgG, and anti-C3b,-C3d antisera. The eluate was panreactive as before. The plasma reacted to a dilution greater than 1 to 512 with a random target cell. The undiluted plasma was tested against an extensive panel of selected rare blood cells. Each cell lacked a different high-incidence antigen including: Kp[b], Kn[a], Vel, I, U, Rg, Cellano, Yt[a], hr[B], McC[a], Js[b], Co[a], Lu[b], Hy, JMH, Di[b], Lu(a−b−), At[a], Jr[a], Cr[a], Lan, Tj[a], Jk3, Er(a), Au[a], Jo[a], Wr[b], H, Wj, In[b], Yk[a], Ch[a], Cs[a], Sc:

− 1, and Ge: − 2 − 3. The patient's plasma reacted 3 + with all cells tested, except 2 + with a Yt(a)-negative cell; and 1 + with a rare blood cell that was Lu(a − b −). The plasma was adsorbed with an R_1/R_1, R_2/R_2 and r/r cell. These adsorptions removed the high-incidence alloantibody and the residual adsorbed plasma showed no additional reactivity. The laboratory concluded that the high-frequency antibody could not be identified and that transfusion was not recommended.

Interpretation

It is unusual for the National Reference Laboratory to be unable to identify a high-incidence antibody. The work at the national laboratory confirmed and extended the information about this patient. In addition, adsorptions with normal cells suggested that all the reactivity was confined to the single high-frequency alloantibody with no additional antibodies demonstrable. While this latter news was reassuring, we still did not have a practical strategy for her transfusion support.

We discussed the findings in detail with the patient. Although her hematocrit was in the 20 to 25 range and although she had lost much of her exercise tolerance, she agreed to one final attempt to identify her antibody before proceeding with a blind test of infusion of radiolabeled incompatible cells. We wondered whether or not she may have made an antibody to an, as yet, undiscovered red blood cell antigen, and our attention shifted from a serologic investigation to a molecular investigation. We contacted the International Blood Grouping Reference Laboratory at Bristol, UK. Dr. David Anstee, Director of the Laboratory, agreed to investigate the case, commenting that the laboratory would perform serologic investigation before looking for a molecular polymorphism.

INTERNATIONAL REFERENCE LABORATORY FINDINGS

The laboratory in England received a sample drawn 1 month after the original positive antibody screen at the hospital. On initial testing, the laboratory found a moderately strong direct antiglobulin test reacting with anti-IgG reagent. The eluate (autoantibody) showed enhanced reactivity with papain-treated cells. Using chloroquine diphosphonate, they treated the patient's cells to render them nonreactive in the antiglobulin phase of testing. Using these treated cells and rare antisera, they were able to test the patient for the presence of high-frequency antigens and found the patient to be Yt(a − b +). The laboratory performed three serial autoadsorptions of the patient's plasma onto her own cells. The residual autoadsorbed plasma reacted strongly with routine target cells but failed to react with six different examples of Yt(a −) cells. These compatible cells ruled out the presence of anti-C, anti-D, anti-E, anti-S, and anti-K_1. The laboratory concluded that the patient had a strong anti-Yt^a in the presence of an autoantibody.

SUMMARY

Reactivity with all target cells usually means either an autoantibody or an alloantibody to a high-frequency antigen. This patient had both conditions simultaneously, and that led to great difficulty resolving her problem. The hospital laboratory and National Reference Laboratory were initially led away from the correct trail by the very weak nature of the direct Coombs test (microscopic reactivity only) and the initial nonreactive autocontrol. As a result, the hospital laboratory focused the case on the high-frequency alloantibody and tested rare target cells with undiluted and unadsorbed plasma. Although enzyme treatment (ficin, papain) of target cells greatly reduces expression of the Yt^a antigen, the unadsorbed plasma contained the autoantibody whose reactivity was enhanced against enzyme-treated cells (as is typical with autoantibodies). Time passed between the initial samples and the samples sent to England. During that time, the direct antiglobulin test reacted more strongly, and the international reference laboratory began their investigation by acknowledging the existence of both kinds of antibodies. Using this starting point, the international reference laboratory used rare antisera and cells plus expert investigation to arrive at the correct solution. The case illustrates not only the importance of considering all findings (including the microscopically reactive direct antiglobulin test), but also the value of repeating the investigation of a difficult case after the passage of a few weeks.

Yt^a, also called Cartwright (YT1 or 011.001), is a high-frequency member of the YT blood group system. Yt^a is a ubiquitous antigen found in 99.8% of all populations (1). The antigen resides on the red blood cell surface protein acetylcholinesterase (AChE). AChE (and thus Yt^a) are linked to the red blood cell via the phosphoinositol glycan anchor. AChE levels are reduced in patients with paroxysmal nocturnal hemoglobinuria and in some patients with myelodysplasia associated with chromosome 7 abnormalities. Interestingly, our patient has myelodysplasia but a normal karyotype. Although not considered a potently hemolytic antibody, some examples of anti-Yt^a have been implicated in delayed hemolytic reactions, and injection of ^{51}Cr-labeled Yt^a red blood cells demonstrated greatly reduced posttransfusion survival ($T_{1/2}$ = 96 hours) (2). Our patient required four additional units of red blood cells. On subsequent testing during the next several months, her autoantibody disappeared and the anti-Yt^a remained very strong. We transfused her with Yt^a-negative units without problem.

Case contributed by Walter H. Dzik, M.D., Massachusetts General Hospital, Boston, MA

REFERENCES

1. Reid ME, Lomas-Francis C. *The blood group antigen factsbook.* New York: Academic Press, 1997.
2. Davey RJ, Simpkins SS. 51Chromium survival of Yt(a +) red cells as a determinant of the in vivo significance of anti-Yta. *Transfusion* 1981; 21:702–705.

8

HUMAN CARBOHYDRATE BLOOD GROUP SYSTEMS

PATRICE F. SPITALNIK AND STEVEN L. SPITALNIK

Many important human blood group antigens are glycoconjugates. These are grouped together in this chapter because there are similarities in their biosynthesis, in the human immune response to these antigens, and in the outcome in vivo after transfusion of incompatible blood.

The antigens in the ABH, Lewis, P, and I blood group systems are synthesized by interrelated pathways. These oligosaccharide antigens may exist free in solution. In addition, they may be covalently attached to lipids (i.e., ceramides) to form glycosphingolipids, or to polypeptides to form mucins, integral membrane glycoproteins, or soluble glycoproteins. Specific glycosyltransferase enzymes catalyze formation of the relevant glycosidic linkages (i.e., the bonds between monosaccharides). Some glycosyltransferases, found in all individuals, form framework structures. The genes encoding other glycosyltransferases are allelically inherited and the resulting enzymes specify the synthesis of variable structures. Because of their variable inheritance and expression, the latter may form immunologically recognized blood group antigens. The absence of particular blood group antigens in certain individuals may result in specific antibody production after stimulation by the foreign antigen. As described below, antigens in the ABH, Lewis, P, and I blood group systems are synthesized on common precursor framework molecules. Competition between genetically inherited blood group–specific glycosyltransferases results in a rich mixture of antigenic molecules. In addition, a single oligosaccharide may encode several different blood group antigens.

The immune response to carbohydrate antigens, particularly when presented as repetitive epitopes, is typically thymus independent (1). The repetitive, multivalent antigens can thus directly stimulate B cells to synthesize antibodies without the aid of helper T cells. Thymus-independent immune responses classically produce IgM antibodies, and most antibodies to carbohydrate blood group antigens are of the IgM class. Individuals lacking a particular carbohydrate blood group antigen on their red blood cells often have "naturally occurring" IgM antibodies to that antigen in their serum, even if they were not previously exposed to human blood products. Most evidence suggests that these antibodies did not arise spontaneously without prior antigenic stimulation, but rather that cross-reacting antigens present in the environment, such as on gut bacteria, stimulate specific IgM production (2). In contrast, high-titered IgG antibodies to carbohydrate antigens can be found in certain individuals. The IgG antibodies may be induced by a thymus-dependent form of these oligosaccharides, perhaps as individual epitopes on glycoproteins, in which T-cell help leads to an isotype switch from IgM to IgG. However, a complete understanding of this phenomenon is not yet available.

Because antibodies to carbohydrate blood group antigens are predominantly IgM, these decavalent molecules directly agglutinate antigen-positive human red blood cells without the aid of an antiglobulin reagent. Agglutination by these antibodies in vitro is typically greater at temperatures $<37°C$. Because most IgM molecules directly fix complement, these antibodies can cause immediate intravascular hemolysis after transfusion of incompatible, antigen-positive red blood cells. In unusual cases, carbohydrate-specific IgG antibodies can coat red blood cells in vivo, leading to extravascular hemolysis after incompatible transfusion. In addition, the latter may cross the placenta resulting in hemolytic disease of the newborn (3,4).

P.F. Spitalnik and S.L. Spitalnik: Department of Pathology and Laboratory Medicine, University of Rochester Medical Center, Rochester, New York.

ABH, SECRETOR, AND LEWIS SYSTEMS

ABH Antigens: Introduction

The ABO blood group system is the most important one with respect to blood transfusion and renal transplantation. Karl Landsteiner was the first to discover human alloantigens by using a conceptually simple experiment (Table 8.1). The red blood cells of each individual were found either to lack or to have one or both of two antigens, A and B. In addition, the serum of each subject contained "naturally occurring" directly agglutinating antibodies that recognized the antigens absent from their own red blood cells. The modern explanation of this experiment is that cross-reacting carbohydrate structures on environmental agents stimulate thymus-independent production of IgM anti-A and/or anti-B antibodies in individuals not tolerant to these antigens. The IgM antibodies then directly agglutinate the corresponding antigen-positive red blood cells.

Although the ABH antigens (the H antigen is the relevant carbohydrate structure present on group O red blood cells) are typically described as "blood group antigens" because of their presence on red blood cells, they are also found on other tissues, and are more appropriately termed "histo–blood group antigens" (5). In blood they are both membrane bound (e.g., on platelets [6]) and soluble, as blood group–active glycosphingolipids contained in plasma lipoprotein particles. They also are membrane antigens on such diverse cells as vascular endothelial cells and intestinal, cervical, urothelial, and mammary epithelial cells. Soluble forms are found in various secretions and excretions, such as saliva, milk, urine, meconium, and feces. Their expression in some tissues is developmentally regulated (7). Despite their wide distribution, genetic inheritance, developmental regulation, and importance in transfusion and transplantation, their normal physiologic function, if any, remains a mystery.

ABH Antigens: Biochemistry

To appreciate the structure and antigenicity of ABH antigens, and their relationship to other blood group systems, it is necessary to understand the underlying biochemistry. Early studies indicated that anti-A, anti-B, and anti-H specifically recognize epitopes composed of the terminal trisaccharides or disaccharides

TABLE 8.1. ABO BLOOD GROUP ANTIGENS AND ANTIBODIES

	Red Blood Cell Antigens		Serum Antibodies	
Blood Group	**A**	**B**	**Anti-A**	**Anti-B**
A	+	−	−	+
B	−	+	+	−
AB	+	+	−	−
O	−	−	+	+

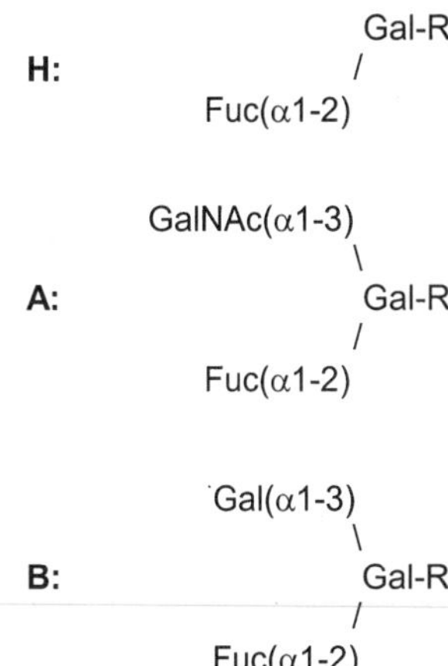

FIGURE 8.1. Carbohydrate structures of the A, B, and H antigens. The monosaccharides are abbreviated as follows: D-galactose is Gal; N-acetyl-D-galactosamine is GalNAc; and L-fucose is Fuc.

illustrated in Fig. 1. From these results it was possible to conclude that the A, B, and H antigens are not directly encoded by the corresponding genes; rather the genes encode glycosyltransferases, commonly called the A, B, and H transferases, or equivalently, the A, B, and H enzymes. The H enzyme is a fucosyltransferase that specifically adds fucose in an α1-2 linkage to a terminal galactose. The A and B enzymes then add N-acetylgalactosamine or galactose, respectively, in an α1-3 linkage to the same terminal galactose. Nonetheless, the substrate for the A and B enzymes is the H antigen sequence; these enzymes do not transfer the relevant sugar to galactose in the absence of (α1-2)-linked fucose. Similarly, the H enzyme does not function if this galactose is substituted with a different sugar. Thus, the biosynthetic pathway is as follows:

$$\text{Gal-R} \xrightarrow{1} \text{H} \xrightarrow{2} \text{A or B}$$

where reaction 1 is catalyzed by the H enzyme and reaction 2 by the A or B enzyme.

The finding that the *A* and *B* genes encode glycosyltransferases explains some classic results from analysis of family pedigrees. In particular, the *A* and *B* genes are inherited in a strict mendelian fashion and are dominant compared to *O*, but *A* and *B* are codominant with each other. That is, an individual with the genotype *AO* (or *BO)* is phenotypically A (or B), an individual of genotype *AB* is phenotypically AB, and an individual of genotype *OO* is phenotypically O. Because both the A and B enzymes use the H antigen as substrate, even the presence of only approximately 50% of these enzyme proteins in an *AO* (or *BO)* heterozygote is sufficient to convert the red blood cells to the corresponding A (or B) phenotype. Similarly, if both the A and B enzymes are present, they each convert approximately 50% of the available H-antigen substrate, yielding red blood cells expressing both the A and B antigens.

Much of the molecular biology of the ABH system has been elucidated recently. The allelic *A* and *B* genes are located on chromosome 9 (8,9) (Table 8.2). They encode membrane-

TABLE 8.2. CHROMOSOMAL ASSIGNMENT OF CLONED GENES IN THE ABH, SE, LE, I, AND P BLOOD GROUP SYSTEMS

Gene	Gene Product	Location	Reference
H (FUT1)	(α1-2)fucosyltransferase (Fuc-TI)	19q13.3	54
Se (FUT2)	(α1-2)fucosyltransferase (Fuc-TII)	19q13.3	54
Sec1	Pseudogene (nonfunctional; homolog of *FUT1* and *FUT2*)	19q13.3	50, 52
Le (FUT3)	(α1-3/4)fucosyltransferase (Fuc-TIII)	19p13.3	54, 81
A	(α1-3)N-acetylgalactosaminyl transferase	9q34.1-q34.2	8, 11
B	(α1-3)galactosyltransferase	9q34.1-q34.2	8, 11
I	(β1-6)N-acetylglucosaminyl transferase	9q21	104
Pk	(α1-4)galactosyltransferase	22q13.2	114
Pl	(α1-4)galactosyltransferase	22q12.3-q13.1	115, 116

The *A* and *B* genes are allelic. The *H, Se,* and *Sec1* genes are encoded at distinct, but closely linked, loci and are not alleles of each other. Although the *H, Se, Sec1, Le, A, B, Pk,* and *I* cDNA sequences and some genomic sequences have been determined, neither the *Pl* gene nor its cDNA have yet been cloned.

-bound glycosyltransferases containing 354 amino acids (Fig. 8.2). Interestingly, these two enzymes exhibit a great degree of homology and differ at only four amino acid residues (10,11). Their substrate specificity is primarily determined by two adjacent residues near the C-terminus of the protein, amino acids 266 and 268 (12,13) (Fig. 8.2). The availability of molecular genetic techniques has allowed the identification of not only the original (wild type) *A* and *B* genes (herein denoted A^{1-1} and B^{1-1}), but also several fully functional variants of each (i.e., A^{1-2}, A^{1-3}, A^{1-4}, B^{1-2}, and B^{1-3}) (Figs. 8.3, 8.4). These variants contain silent nucleotide polymorphisms that do not affect the function of these enzymes (11,14–18). A common allele corresponding to blood group O, O^1, is highly homologous to the *A* and *B* alleles, but contains a single nucleotide deletion near the N-terminus of the protein. This leads to a shift in reading frame and a prematurely terminated translation product that lacks enzymatic activity (Fig. 8.2) (11). Many other *O* alleles have been identified that do not encode functional glycosyltransferases (Fig. 8.2) (15,16,19–26). For example, the O^2 allele has a missense mutation that abolishes enzymatic activity (19,20,24).

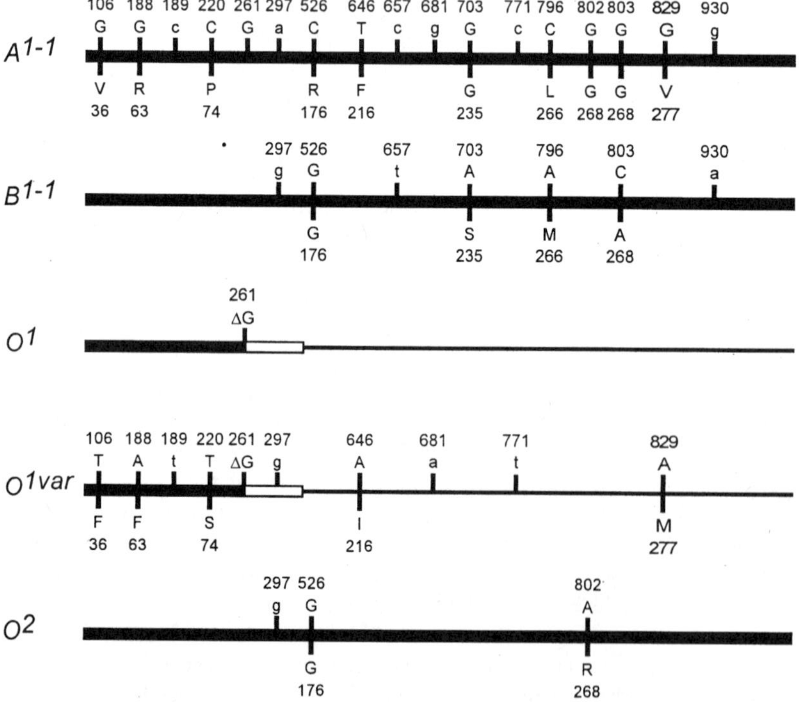

FIGURE 8.2. Nucleotide and amino acid sequences of the cDNA's derived from the *A, B,* and *O* genes. The A^{1-1} and B^{1-1} glycosyltransferases are 354 amino acid, Type II, membrane glycoproteins. All sequences in this figure are compared to the A^{1-1} sequence. Above each bar is the relevant nucleotide sequence; upper case letters denote a mutation leading to a change in amino acid sequence, lower case letters denote a silent mutation. Below each bar is the corresponding amino acid sequence using the single letter code. The open portions of the bar indicate that a frameshift mutation resulted in translation of a significant length of amino acid sequence that differs from the A^{1-1}sequence. The thin portion of the bar indicates that these sequences are not translated due to a frameshift mutation leading to a premature stop codon. The term "ins" indicates that there is a one nucleotide insertion. There is no generally agreed upon nomenclature for naming variant alleles of the *A, B,* or *O* genes; the system chosen here is based on the literature, but is otherwise arbitrary (Figs. 8.3, 8.4).

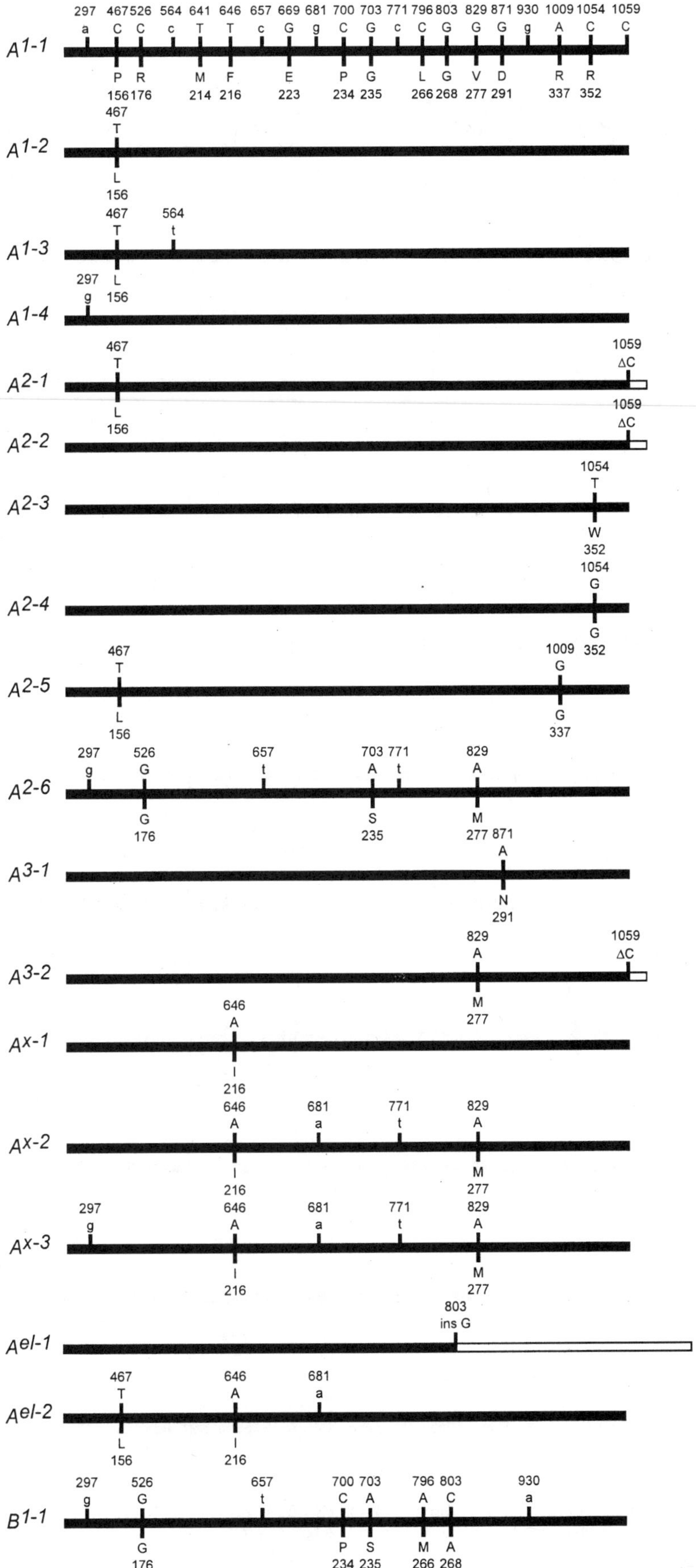

FIGURE 8.3. Weak subgroups of A: cDNA sequences. As in Figure 8.2, all sequences in this figure are compared with the A^{1-1} sequence. The B^{1-1} sequence is provided for comparison.

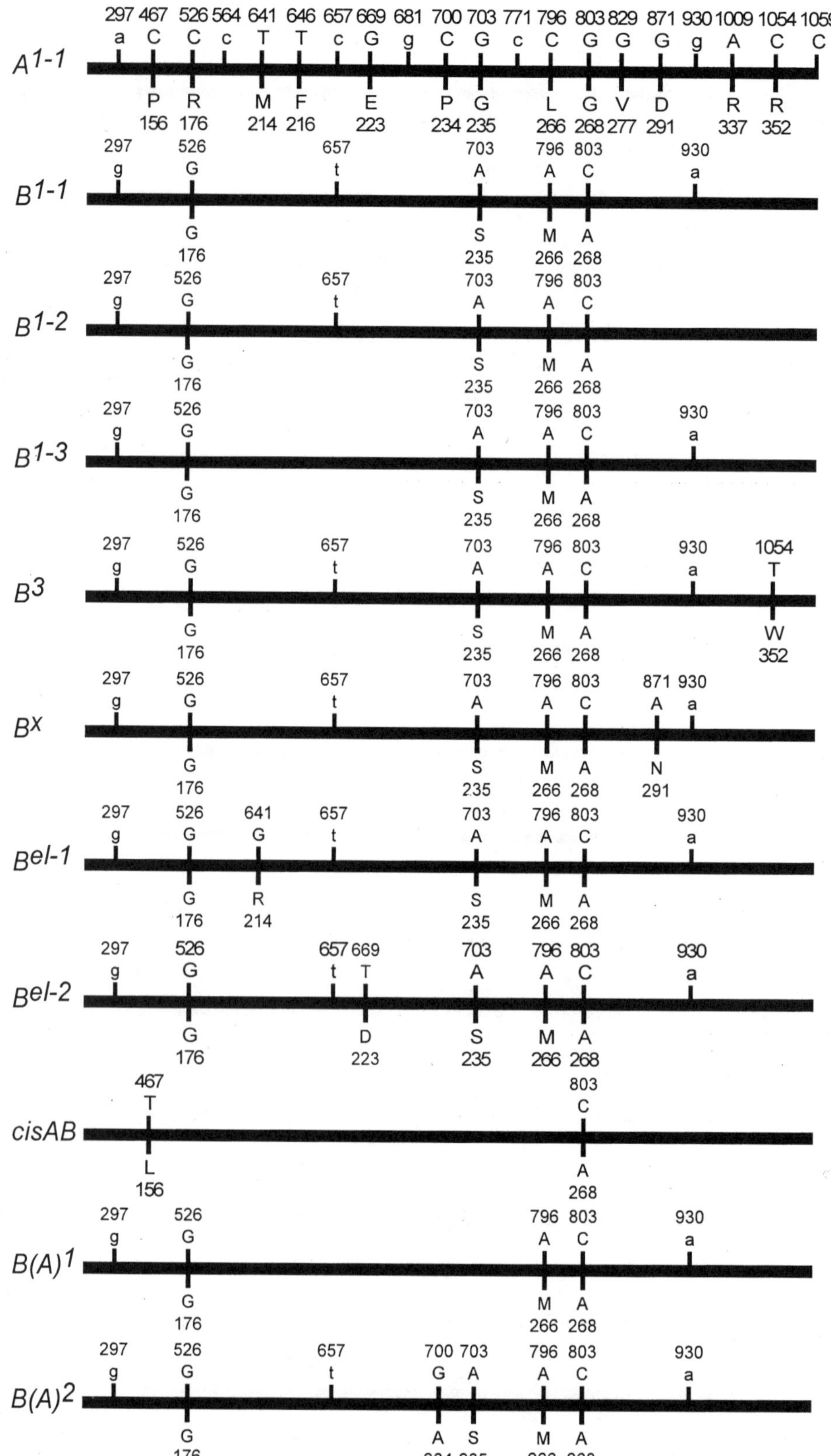

FIGURE 8.4. Weak subgroups of B and the B(A) and cis AB phenotypes: cDNA sequences. As in Figure 8.2, all sequences in this figure are compared with the $A^{1\text{-}1}$ sequence.

These findings using molecular biology not only confirm and extend the results obtained from carbohydrate biochemistry and enzymology, but they also suggest new ways of blood typing (26–28).

Antigenic Variants in the ABH System

Some relatively common variations in the ABH system relate to the "strength" of the A antigen on group A red blood cells. Several subgroups of A that have weak expression of the A antigen have been identified. The red blood cells of most group A individuals (e.g., 80% of whites) type as A_1 due to their inheritance of one of the A_1 alleles. Most of the remaining group A individuals have weaker expression of this antigen and are denoted A_2. Other rarer subgroups of A (e.g., A_3, A_x, A_m, A_{el}) have progressively weaker A-antigen expression. Interestingly, many individuals with weak A expression produce an antibody, anti-A_1, which does not agglutinate their own red blood cells but does agglutinate A_1 red blood cells. This phenomenon is explained by quantitative and qualitative differences in antigen expression. For example, the number of A antigen sites per red blood cell varies from approximately 800,000 sites for A_1 cells to 250,000 sites for A_2 cells to 700 sites for A_m cells (29). The finding that A_2 individuals can synthesize A_1-specific antibodies suggests that there are also qualitative differences. Recent biochemical investigations demonstrate that A antigens on A_1 red blood cells differ from those on cells of the various subgroups of A (30,31). In addition, the molecular biologic approach has identified mutations in the cDNA and genomic DNA sequences of the A alleles of individuals with red blood cells expressing weak A activity (Fig. 8.3) (16,17,32–38). For example, the A transferase in A_2 individuals that is encoded by the $A^{2\text{-}1}$ allele has a 156 P → L missense mutation and a frame shift mutation near the 3′-end of the coding sequence (34). In addition, some A_3 individuals have an allele, $A^{3\text{-}1}$, containing a 291 D → R mutation in the coding sequence (33). These findings are summarized in Fig. 8.3. In some cases, transfection studies have been employed to prove that these mutations result in weakened or variant enzyme activity of the encoded glycosyltransferases (34). Interestingly, when evaluating the coding sequence alone, there is not always a one-to-one correspondence between genotype and phenotype. As an example, even within a given family the red blood cells of individuals inheriting the $A^{2\text{-}2}$ allele can have either the A_2 or A_3 phenotype (38). In another family, the red blood cells of individuals inheriting the $A^{2\text{-}1}$ allele were typed as either A_2 or A_x (35). A complete understanding of these results is not yet available, but it may be important to investigate the regulation of expression of these genes in greater detail, particularly by focusing on the promoter and enhancer regulatory regions (39–42). Finally, the identification of individuals with weak subgroups of A has allowed the successful transplantation of "incompatible" A_2 renal allografts into group O recipients (43).

By analogy with the subgroups of A, "weak" subgroups of B have also been described (e.g., B_3, B_x, B_{el}). For example, the gene encoding the B^3 allele responsible for the B_3 subgroup has an additional 352 R → W mutation in the coding sequence that is not found in the wild-type $B^{1\text{-}1}$ allele (Fig. 8.4) (33).

The B(A) and cis AB phenotypes are interesting and unusual variations in the ABH system. In each case, one chromosome in the affected individual apparently encodes for a gene (or genes) that leads to the synthesis of both the A and B antigens. In the B(A) phenotype, the red blood cells predominantly have B antigens with small amounts of A antigens (32). In the cis AB phenotype, the red blood cells have equivalent amounts of A and B antigens (44). Molecular studies demonstrated that the coding sequence of one B(A) transferase, $B(A)^1$, is virtually identical to the wild-type $B^{1\text{-}1}$ allele, except that it lacks the 235 G → S mutation (32). Thus, at three of the relevant amino acid positions the $B(A)^1$ allele is identical to $B^{1\text{-}1}$ and at one position it is identical to $A^{1\text{-}1}$; this then allows the resulting glycosyltransferase to create small amounts of A antigen in addition to large amounts of B antigen (32). In contrast, the sequence of the $B(A)^2$ allele is identical to $B^{1\text{-}1}$ except for the addition of a 700 P → A mutation (Fig. 8.4) (45). In the two cases of cis AB that have been studied, the *cisAB* allele has mutations resulting in two amino acid substitutions (Fig. 8.4) (46). The 156 P → L mutation is identical to that found in the weak A allele, $A^{2\text{-}1}$; the 268 G → A mutation is a change that is important for conferring B-transferase activity to the resulting enzyme (12,13). Thus, these changes result in an enzyme that functions as an AB-transferase chimera. Evidence for an alternative model, in which crossing over results in one chromosome that contains *both* an intact *A* gene and a separate, intact *B* gene, is not yet available.

Secretion of ABH Antigens

The ABH antigens are found not only on red blood cells but also in secretions, particularly saliva and plasma. The ability to secrete ABH antigens is genetically inherited: approximately 80% of whites are secretors and 20% are nonsecretors. This trait is inherited as a single locus gene in simple mendelian fashion. The secretor gene *(Se)* is dominant; nonsecretor *(se)* is recessive. The terminal carbohydrate sequences of the ABH antigens in saliva and plasma are identical to those on red blood cells. However, the backbone or framework carbohydrate structures are different. ABH antigens on glycosphingolipids and glycoproteins synthesized by red blood cell precursors are primarily coupled to framework Type 2 chains (i.e., Gal[β1-4]GlcNAc-R); the same antigens on plasma glycosphingolipids and salivary mucins are coupled to Type 1 chains (i.e., Gal[β1-3]GlcNAc-R) (Table 8.3). Because ABH blood group–active glycosphingolipids on plasma lipoproteins are also passively transferred onto red blood cells, red blood cells of secretors have ABH antigens not only on Type 2 precursor chains but also on small numbers of Type 1 chains. In contrast, red blood cells of nonsecretors have ABH antigens only on Type 2 chains.

Initially, it was thought that the *H* gene was a structural gene coding for the H enzyme and the secretor locus encoded a regulatory gene that permitted expression of the *H* gene in the relevant tissues. This hypothesis suggested that a single H enzyme transferred fucose in an α1-2 linkage to the terminal galactose residue on either Type 1 or Type 2 chains. In this model, the H enzyme is always expressed in red blood cell precursors, but its expression in "secretory" tissues (e.g., salivary epithelium)

TABLE 8.3. BIOCHEMICAL STRUCTURES OF ABH ANTIGENS

Blood Group	Secretions (Type 1 Chain)	Red Blood Cells (Type 2 Chain)
H	Fuc(α1-2) ⟩ Gal(β1-3)GlcNAc-R	Fuc(α1-2) ⟩ Gal(β1-4)GlcNAc-R
A	GalNAc(α1-3), Fuc(α1-2) ⟩ Gal(β1-3)GlcNAc-R	GalNAc(α1-3), Fuc(α1-2) ⟩ Gal(β1-4) GlcNAc-R
B	Gal(α1-3), Fuc(α1-2) ⟩ Gal(β1-3)GlcNAc-R	Gal(α1-3), Fuc(α1-2) ⟩ Gal(β1-4) GlcNAc-R

is controlled by the *Se* gene. However, this model did not explain all the available data, and multiple biochemical, immunologic, and genetic studies supported an alternative model (47,48). The latter postulated two different H transferases: one adding fucose to Type 1 chains (an H Type 1 enzyme) and one acting on Type 2 chains (an H Type 2 enzyme). In this model, the H Type 1 enzyme is the structural protein encoded by the secretor gene *(Se)* and is only expressed in secretory tissues.

Se and *H* Genes

Recent cloning of genes and cDNAs encoding multiple mammalian fucosyltransferases (for review, see [49]) show that *Se* is the *FUT2* gene and that the product of the *Se* gene, the H Type 1 enzyme, is the Se (or Fuc-TII) enzyme (50,51). At least one copy of the *Se* gene is found in approximately 80% of individuals and leads to ABH-antigen expression in secretions. Indeed, *FUT2* mRNA expression is found in both normal epithelial cells (50) and cell lines derived from carcinomas (52), but not in cell lines derived from hematopoietic neoplasms (52). By contrast, the traditional *H* locus encodes the H Type 2 enzyme; the latter is equivalent to the H (or Fuc-TI) fucosyltransferase (53). This gene, *(H* or *FUT1),* is active in virtually all individuals (for exceptions, see below) and leads to ABH antigen expression on red blood cells and other tissues. The *FUT1* (or *H*) and *FUT2* (or *Se*) genes are closely linked on chromosome 19 (Table 8.2) (54). In addition, a third gene in this region, *Sec1,* has been cloned (50). *Sec1* is a pseudogene of *FUT2* (50) and, although it is actively transcribed in human cell lines (52), but perhaps not in normal human tissues (50), it has no intrinsic enzymatic activity. These genes are arranged on chromosome 19 in the following 5′ to 3′ sequence: *Sec1* → *FUT2* → *FUT1*. In addition, the high homology of these three genes and the proximity of many *Alu* sequences make this region a hot spot for mutation and genetic recombination (52) (see below).

Se (Fuc-TII) Glycosyltransferase

The Se enzyme is a Type II membrane glycoprotein containing 332 amino acids, a short cytosolic domain, and a large lumenal domain (Fig. 8.5) (51). There are three potential N-glycosylation sites in the lumenal domain at N177, N271, and N297. As such, its overall structure is similar to that of other mammalian glycosyltransferases, including the A and B enzymes. By analyzing the sequences of many eukaryotic and prokaryotic (α1-2)fucosyltransferases, three highly conserved sequence motifs were identified (49). Motifs I, II, and III encompass amino acid residues 184 to 204, 226 to 239, and 278 to 288, respectively; Motif I may be responsible for binding the nucleotide sugar substrate, GDP-fucose, required for the catalytic action of this enzyme.

Following cloning of *Se* (50,51), multiple functional and nonfunctional variants of this gene have been described. For example, many individuals have a normally functioning variant, Se^1, which contains a silent mutation: 357 c → t (Fig. 8.6) (55–58). In other individuals, normally functioning genes are found that contain only missense mutations (e.g., Se^2, Se^3, Se^4) or combinations of silent and missense mutations (e.g., Se^6 and Se^7) (58). In addition, the Se^w mutant encodes a functional, but significantly less active, enzyme (56,59,60). This allele contains a missense mutation that leads to partial expression of the secretor phenotype; individuals with this allele can have red blood cells with the unusual Le(a+b+) Lewis blood group phenotype (see below). Interestingly, none of the mutations found in functional Se variants occur in any of the three highly conserved (α1-2)fucosyltransferase motifs (Figs. 8.5, 8.6).

In contrast, at least ten nonenzymatically active variants of the Se gene have been described (Fig. 8.7). Most of these are caused by nonsense (i.e., se^1, se^2, se^3, se^4, se^5, se^8) or small deletion (i.e., se^9) mutations that yield premature stop codons resulting in the expression of truncated, nonfunctional enzyme proteins (51,55,57,58,61–63). However, the se^7 allele contains one missense mutation at amino acid 101 that presumably encodes a full-length nonfunctional enzyme; nonetheless the effect of this

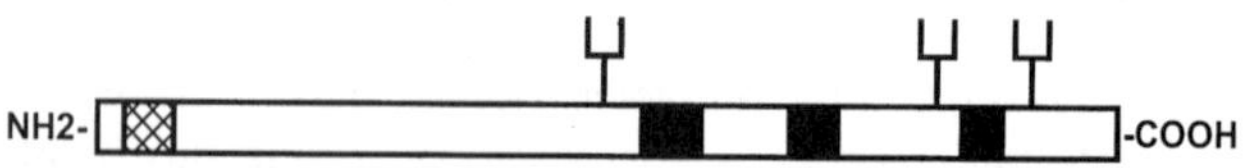

FIGURE 8.5. Structure of the Se (Fuc-TII) glycoprotein. The amino acids are numbered from the second initiation codon, as described (51); by this convention the *Se* gene encodes a protein containing 332 amino acids. The hatched region represents the transmembrane domain comprising amino acids 4 to 17. The filled regions represent the three fucosyltransferase motifs, I (amino acids 184 to 204), II (amino acids 226 to 239), and III (amino acids 278 to 288), respectively. The locations of the three potential N-glycosylation sites at N177, N271, and N297 are indicated by the "goalposts."

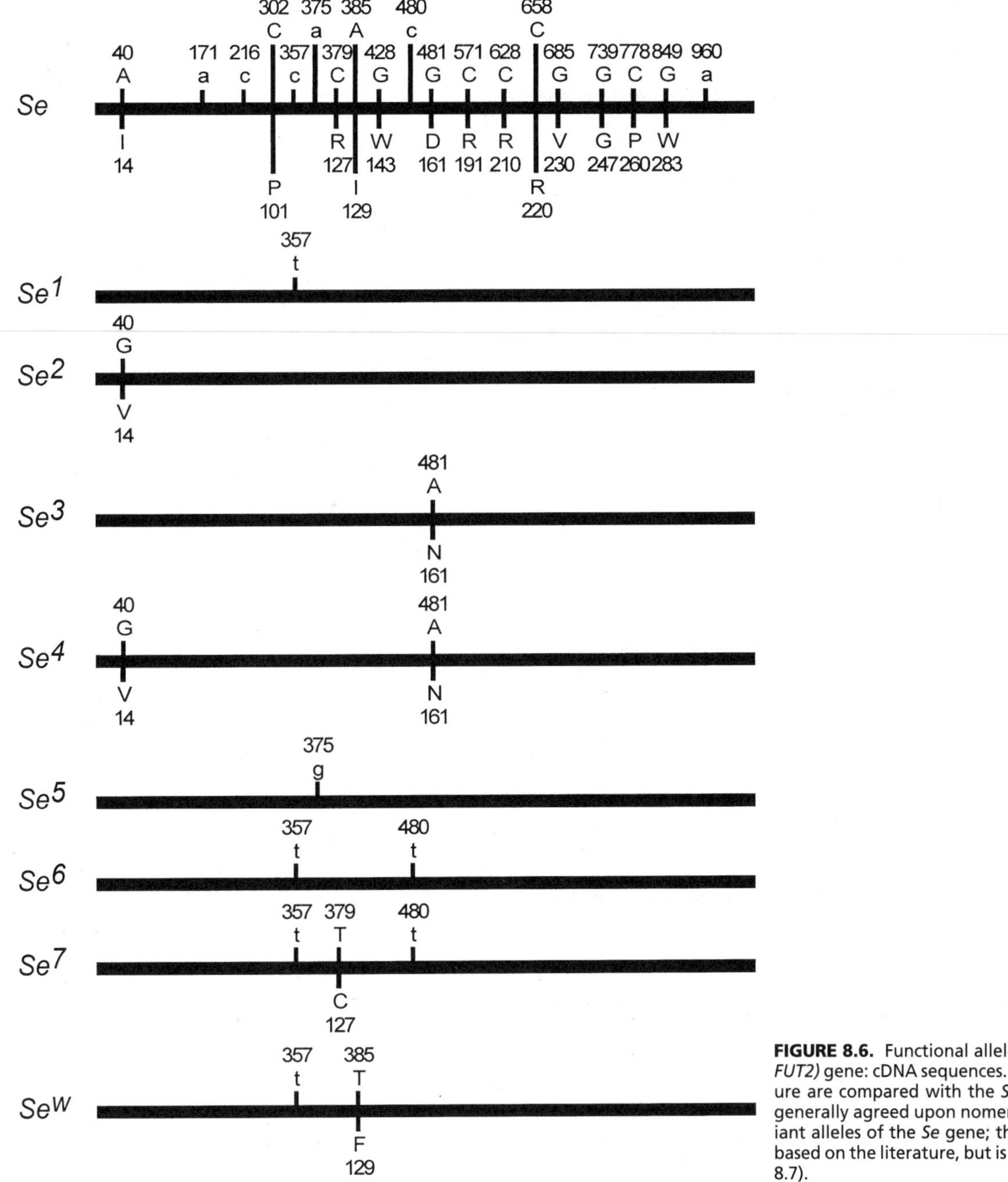

FIGURE 8.6. Functional alleles of the *Secretor (Se or FUT2)* gene: cDNA sequences. All sequences in this figure are compared with the *Se* sequence. There is no generally agreed upon nomenclature for naming variant alleles of the *Se* gene; the system chosen here is based on the literature, but is otherwise arbitrary (Fig. 8.7).

mutation on enzyme function was not directly tested with recombinant protein (64). Similarly, the se^{10} allele contains a three-bp deletion resulting in the deletion of a single amino acid, V230; although the encoded protein is presumably nonfunctional, this has not yet been verified by transfection studies (65, 66). Interestingly, the mutation in the se^{10} allele occurs in the highly conserved (α1-2)fucosyltransferase Motif II (Figs. 8.5, 8.7). One nonfunctional allele, se^{6}, is the result of a fusion gene between *FUT2 (i.e., Se)* and the adjacent upstream *Sec1* pseudogene (57,61). Although the recombinant se^{6} protein has low, but measurable, enzymatic activity using model substrates in vitro, it does not produce H antigen when expressed in transfected cells; the reasons for this lack of enzymatic function in red blood cells or transfected cells remain to be clarified. Finally, the complete deletion of the entire *FUT2* gene is seen in individuals with the classic Bombay phenotype (see below); this allele is denoted as se^{del} (67,68). This large deletion is mediated by the presence of *Alu* sequences (69), which are abundant in this region of the chromosome (52).

Given the abundance of sequencing data now available, it is

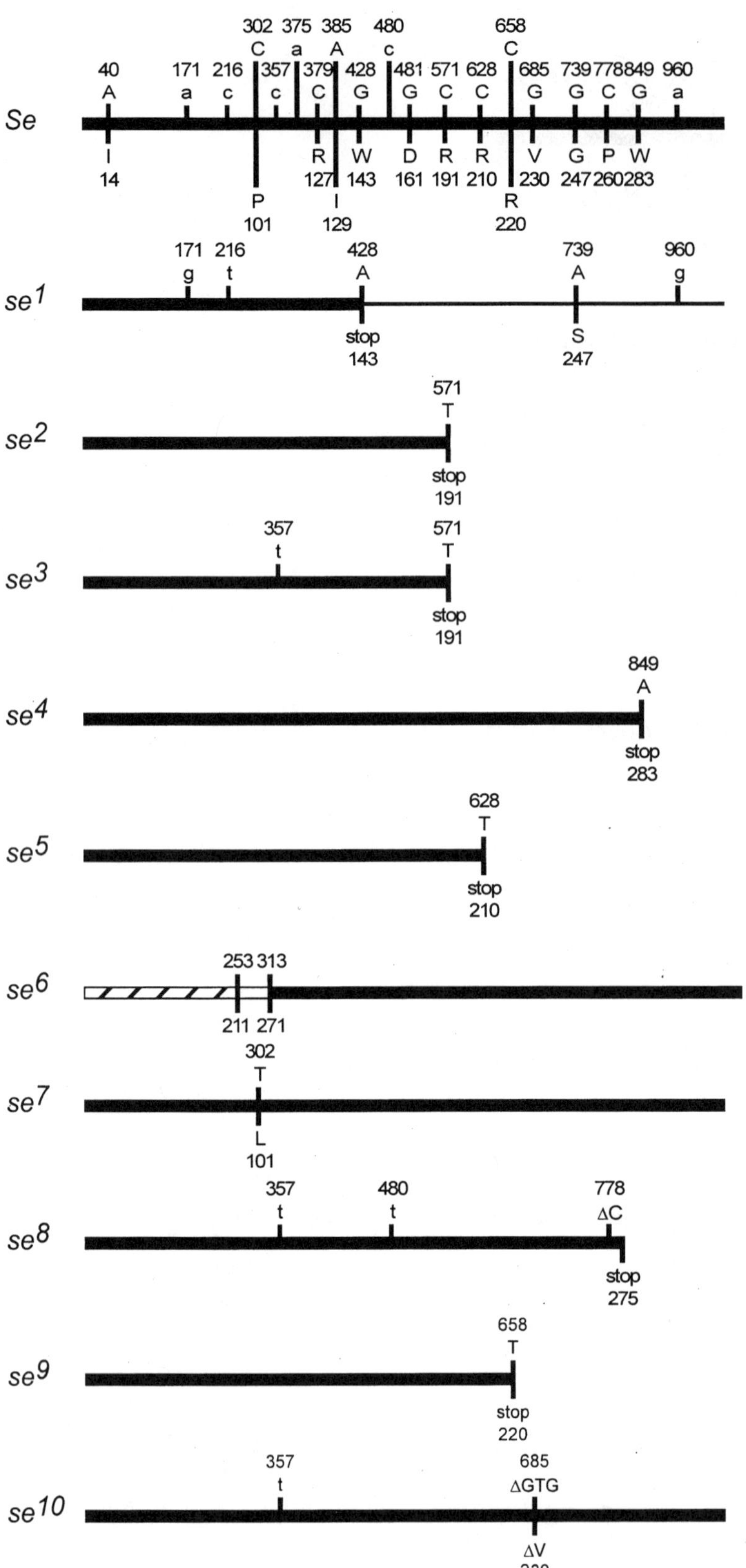

FIGURE 8.7. Nonfunctional alleles of the *Se* gene: cDNA sequences. All sequences in this figure are compared with *Se*. The hatched portion of the bar in *se*[6] represents sequences derived from the homologous pseudogene *Sec1*. The open portion of the bar in *se*[6] represents a length of sequence in which *Sec1* and *Se* are identical; the fusion between these two genes occurred in this region (57). The thin portion of the bar in *se*[1] represents untranslated cDNA sequence as a result of a missense mutation encoding a premature stop codon.

possible to speculate on the temporal sequence during which the various mutations in the Se gene developed. One possible sequence is provided below:

$$
\begin{array}{ccccccc}
 & & se^{10} & & & & \\
 & & \uparrow & & & & \\
Se & \rightarrow & Se^{1} & \rightarrow & Se^{6} & \rightarrow & Se^{7} \\
 & & \downarrow & & \downarrow & & \\
 & & Se^{w} & & se^{8} & &
\end{array}
$$

Interestingly, this model supports the "out of Africa" hypothesis for the evolution of human populations. To this end, the *Se* and Se^1 genes are commonly found in black, white, and Asian populations. In contrast, se^{10} and Se^w have been found only in Asian populations (56,59,60,65). In addition, Se^6 has been found in black and white, but not Asian, populations (58). Finally, se^8 and Se^7 have been found only in black and white populations, respectively (58).

H (Fuc-TI) Glycosyltransferase

The H enzyme contains 365 amino acids and is highly homologous to Se (51). In particular, it also contains the three highly conserved (α1-2)fucosyltransferase sequence motifs: Motifs I, II, and III comprise amino acids 214 to 224, 256 to 269, and 308 to 318, respectively (49). Based on the premise that the *H* gene codes for the H Type 2 glycosyltransferase (FUT1), then the allelic *h* gene codes for a nonfunctional enzyme. Because of the cloning and sequencing of the *H* gene (53), various groups have investigated the molecular nature of the defective *h* alleles (67,70–75). More than 20 different *h* alleles have been identified to date, variously containing missense, nonsense, and frameshift mutations (Table 8.4). It is noteworthy that virtually every family examined in these studies had a different mutation leading to inactivation of Fuc-TI activity. In addition, several missense mutations occurred in the (α1-2)fucosyltransferase motifs; for example, the amino acid substitution 220 R → C occurs in Motif I, 259 V → E and 262 S → K occur in Motif II, and 315 A → V occurs in Motif III. The mutation at position 220 is particularly interesting in that the arginine at this position in the putative nucleotide sugar-binding domain is absolutely conserved in all (α1-2)- and (α1-6)fucosyltransferases throughout evolution from bacteria to mammals (76). Although, the 327 N → T mutation does not occur in an (α1-

TABLE 8.4. *h* ALLELES: WEAK OR INACTIVE ALLELES OF *FUT1*

Nucleotide Change	Amino Acid Change	Enzymatic Activity	Reference
	Missense Mutations		
349 C → T	117 H → Y	Weak	67
442 G → T	148 D → Y	Weak	71, 72
460 T → C	154 Y → H	Weak	71, 72, 74
460 T → C	154 Y → H	Weak or absent	71, 74
1042 G → A	348 E → K		
461 A → G	154 Y → C	None	73
491 T → A	164 L → H	None	70
513 G → C	171 W → C	None	73
658 C → T	220 R → C	None	72
721 T → C	241 Y → H	Weak	71
725 T → G	242 L → R	None	67, 68, 69
776 T → A	259 V → E	None	73
785 G → A	262 S → K	None	75
786 C → A			
944 C → T	315 A → V	None	73
980 A → C	327 N → T	None	72
1042 G → A	348 E → K	Weak	71, 74
1047 G → C	349 W → C	None	73
	Nonsense Mutations		
547 ΔAG	182 R → frameshift	None	72
695 G → A	232 W → stop	None	71
826 C → T	276 S → stop	None	70
880 ΔTT	294 F → frameshift	None	72
948 C → G	316 Y → stop	None	70
969 ΔCT	323 V → frameshift	None	73
990 ΔG	330 L → frameshift	Weak	71

The table summarizes results published in peer-reviewed papers; several additional mutations have been reported in abstract form.
The activity of each *h* allele was determined by transfection and expression of the recombinant protein and/or inferred on the basis of serological studies of the red blood cells of the propositus.
The *h* allele containing the 327 N → T amino acid mutation also contains an amino acid mutation at position 12 (A → V). However, because the latter is a conservative change in the putative transmembrane domain, it probably is not involved in the function of this enzyme. One *h* allele has been identified in which there are no mutations in the coding sequence; the lack of enzymatic activity is presumably due to a mutation(s) in a regulatory sequence (73).

2)fucosyltransferase motif, it does destroy a potential N-glycosylation site, suggesting that this posttranslational modification is important in the activity of this enzyme. In addition to the variants described above, one individual had a completely normal coding sequence but an absence of enzyme activity (73), suggesting a defect in transcriptional regulation rather than in protein structure. This latter result also shows that caution is required when molecular approaches for blood typing based on genotype are used, rather than classic methods, which directly determine blood group phenotype.

H-Deficient Phenotypes and Genotypes

Based on the information described above, it should be clear that there are multiple molecular mechanisms by which an individual could express low amounts of H antigens on their red blood cells and/or in their secretions.

The most common example of an H-deficient individual is a "classic nonsecretor," that is, an individual with the general genotype *Hh sese* or *HH sese* (Table 8.5). This individual has normal amounts of H Type 2 antigens on red blood cells but does not express H Type 1 antigens in secretions. In this case, the individual would carry two *se* alleles, which could theoretically be combinations of any of the following: se^{1}, se^{2}, se^{3}, se^{4}, se^{5}, se^{6}, se^{7}, se^{8}, se^{9}, se^{10}, or se^{del}.

"Classic weak secretors" are those individuals who are either homozygous or heterozygous for wild-type *H* and are either Se^{w}-Se^{w} or $Se^{w}se$ at the secretor locus. Se^{w} is a weak secretor allele (see above) that can synthesize small amounts of H Type 1 antigens and allows expression of the unusual Le(a+b+) phenotype (see below).

The most striking example of an H-deficient phenotype is the "classic Bombay phenotype," often denoted O_h (77). These individuals were originally identified in Bombay, India, their red blood cells type as group O, and they are nonsecretors of ABH antigens. In addition, they do not express any H antigens on their red blood cells and their sera contain high-titered, hemolytic anti-H antibodies that lyse red blood cells of individuals of any ABO group, except those from another individual with a similar type of global deficiency of H antigens. Individuals with the classic Bombay phenotype are homozygous for an *h* allele with the amino acid substitution 242 L → R; they are also homozygous for a deletion of the entire *FUT2* gene, that is, the se^{del} allele of *Se* (67–69). In this way, they are incapable of synthesizing either H Type 1 or H Type 2 structures. Although some of these individuals do express active A and/or B enzymes, the A (or B) antigen is not detected because the appropriate substrate for these enzymes (H Type 1 or H Type 2 chains) is not synthesized (Fig. 8.8). Nonetheless, the functional *A* (or *B*) genes can be transmitted to the next generation, yielding the apparently paradoxical pedigree O × O → A (or B).

On rare occasions, individuals are identified with ABH-deficient red blood cells but with ABH antigens in their secretions; this is often referred to as the "para-Bombay phenotype" (70–72,74,78). However, the literature can be confusing on this point, and this broad phenotypic description can encompass individuals with functional *Se* alleles and nonfunctional *H* alleles, or with weakly functioning *H* alleles and nonfunctional *Se* alleles (Table 8.5). Thus, individuals with the "red blood cell H-deficient, secretor," "red blood cell H-deficient, weak se-

TABLE 8.5. PHENOTYPES AND GENOTYPES INVOLVING *FUT1* AND *FUT2*

Phenotype	RBC ABH Antigen Level	Salivary ABH Antigen Level	*H (FUT1)* Gene	*Se (FUT2)* Gene
Classical secretor	Normal	Normal	*HH* or *Hh*	*SeSe* or *Sese*
Classical nonsecretor	Normal	Absent	*HH* or *Hh*	*sese*
Classical weak secretor	Normal	Weak	*HH* or *Hh*	$Se^{w}Se^{w}$ or $Se^{w}se$
Classical Reunion phenotype	Weak	Absent	*hh*: 117 H → Y	$se^{l}se^{l}$
RBC weak H, nonsecretor	Weak	Absent	*hh*: e.g., 241 Y → H	*sese*
RBC weak H, weak secretor	Weak	Weak	*hh*: e.g., 241 Y → H	$Se^{w}Se^{w}$ or $Se^{w}se$
RBC weak H, secretor	Weak	Normal	*hh*: e.g., 241 Y → H	*SeSe or Sese*
Classic Bombay phenotype	Absent	Absent	*hh*: 242 L → R	$se^{del}se^{del}$
Other "Bombay" phenotype	Absent	Absent	*hh*	*sese*
RBC H-deficient, weak secretor	Absent	Weak	*hh*	$Se^{w}Se^{w}$ or $Se^{w}se$
RBC H-deficient, secretor	Absent	Normal	*hh*	*SeSe* or *Sese*

Where the type of *Se*, *se*, or *h* allele is not specified, various alleles described in Table 8.4 and Figures 8.6 and 8.7 could theoretically be used. Most, if not all, of the phenotypes in this table have been described in the literature using serologic and/or genetic methods. The "RBC H-deficient, weak secretor" and the "RBC H-deficient, secretor" phenotypes are often described as para-Bombay phenotypes; however, on occasion, the "RBC weak H, non-secretor" phenotype can also be described as a "para-Bombay" phenotype, which can lead to confusion.

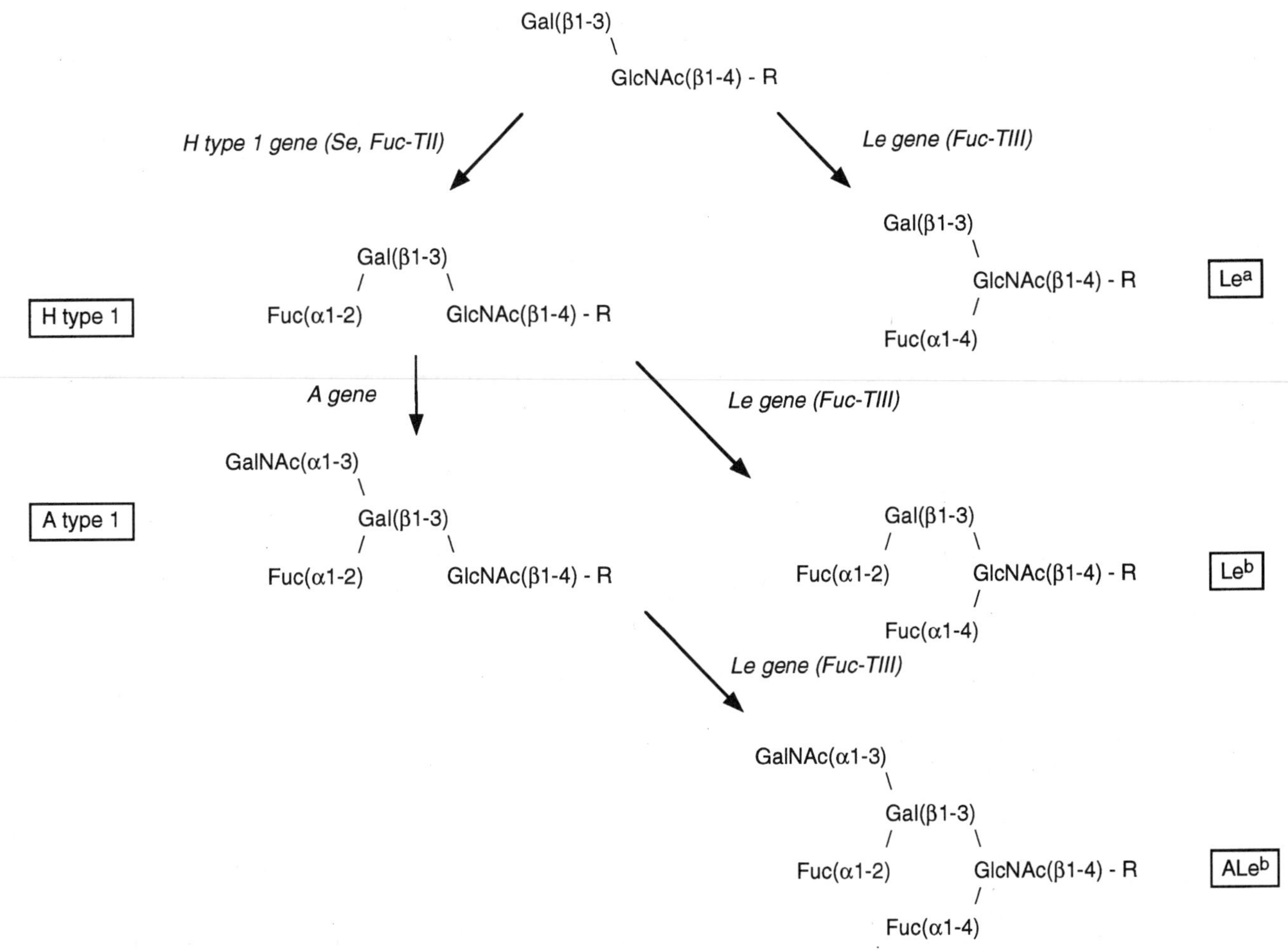

FIGURE 8.8. Biosynthesis of blood group antigens with Type 1 chains. The genes encoding the relevant glycosyltransferases are denoted in italics and the reactions catalyzed are indicated by arrows. The names of the blood group antigens are in boxes next to the relevant structures. The abbreviations for the monosaccharides are as described in Figures 8.1 and 8.9.

cretor," and "red blood cell weak H, nonsecretor" phenotypes could all be described as having the para-Bombay phenotype. Therefore, confusion can be avoided by using more specific terms that describe the types of alleles an individual has at the *Se* and *H* loci (Table 8.5).

Lewis System

The two Lewis blood group antigens Le^a (Lewis a) and Le^b (Lewis b) were discovered in the 1940s (79). Virtually all individuals fall into one of three different Lewis types: Le(a+b−), Le(a-b+), and Le(a−b−) (Table 8.6). These molecules are not intrinsic red blood cell antigens; they are synthesized in another tissue (probably the intestinal epithelium), circulate in plasma attached to lipoproteins, and then passively transfer onto red blood cells (80). Biochemically these are carbohydrate antigens on glycosphingolipids (Fig. 8.9). They are structurally similar to the Type 1 ABH antigens found on plasma glycosphingolipids, which can also transfer onto red blood cells.

The Lewis gene *(Le)* resides on chromosome 19 (54,81) and

TABLE 8.6. THE LEWIS BLOOD GROUP SYSTEM

	Red Blood Cell Antigens		Secretor Status	Serum Antibodies	
Blood Group	**Le^a**	**Le^b**		**Anti-Le^a**	**Anti-Le^b**
Le(a+b−)	+	−	Nonsecretor	−	Very rarely
Le(a−b+)	−	+	Secretor	Very rarely	−
Le(a−b−)	−	−	Secretor or nonsecretor	Occasionally	Occasionally

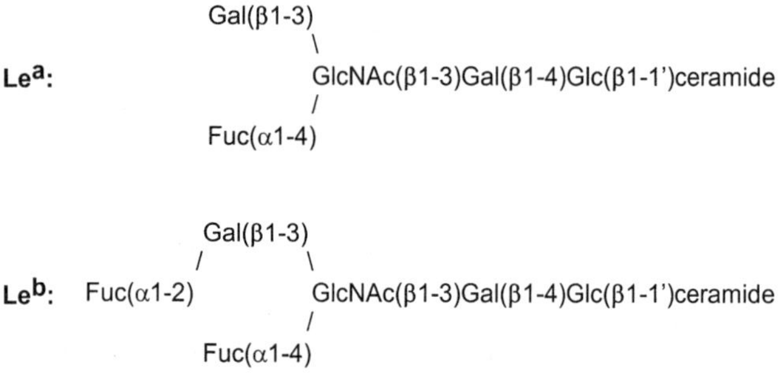

```
            Gal(β1-3)
                    \
Leª:                 GlcNAc(β1-3)Gal(β1-4)Glc(β1-1')ceramide
                    /
            Fuc(α1-4)


            Gal(β1-3)
           /        \
Leᵇ: Fuc(α1-2)       GlcNAc(β1-3)Gal(β1-4)Glc(β1-1')ceramide
                    /
            Fuc(α1-4)
```

FIGURE 8.9. Biochemical structures of the Lewis-active glycosphingolipid antigens. The monosaccharides are abbreviated as follows: D-glucose is Glc and N-acetyl-D-glucosamine is GlcNAc. Ceramide is abbreviated as cer. Other abbreviations are as in Figure 8.1.

is distantly linked to the *H* and *Se* loci (Table 8.2). The gene encodes an (α1-4)fucosyltransferase, denoted Fuc-TIII, and thus behaves in a dominant fashion. A human cDNA derived from the *Le* gene (equivalently, the *FUT3* gene) was cloned and encodes a 361 amino acid Type II membrane-bound glycoprotein (82). Interestingly, in addition to adding fucose in an α1-4 linkage to the GlcNAc residue on a Type 1 chain, it can also add fucose in an α1-3 linkage to the GlcNAc on a Type 2 chain. Although the latter reaction is relatively inefficient, it forms the Lewis x antigen, Le^x. Thus, Fuc-TIII is a very unusual glycosyltransferase in that it can transfer a monosaccharide to two very different substrates using different glycosidic linkages; therefore, it is technically an (α1-3/4)fucosyltransferase (82). The sequence near its NH2-terminus is important for determining its acceptor specificity (83–87). Thus, mutating the sequence of Fuc-TIII at residues 111 and 112 to that which is found in the (α1-3)fucosyltransferase Fuc-TVI (i.e., from WD in Fuc-TIII to RE in Fuc-TVI), significantly improves its ability to use Type 2 chains as substrates (83). By sequence analysis, Fuc-TIII is a member of a family of (α1-3)fucosyltransferases that is conserved from bacteria to mammals (49,76). As such, there are two highly conserved sequence motifs: Motif I comprising amino acids 152–171 and Motif II comprising amino acids 239–272. Fuc-TIII also contains two potential N-glycosylation sites; the site at N154 is in sequence Motif I.

The transfer of fucose to a Type 1 chain by Fuc-TIII results in formation of the Le^a antigen; the addition of (α1-4)-linked fucose to the H Type 1 structure leads to formation of Le^b. Thus, the latter is formed by the cooperation of two glycosyltransferases encoded by two genes, one from the Lewis system (*Le* on chromosome 19) and one from the ABH system (*Se* at a different locus on chromosome 19). The biosynthetic pathways connecting the ABH, Secretor, and Lewis systems (encoded by genes at three distinct loci on chromosomes 9 and 19) are shown in Figure 8.8. Interestingly, cooperation of the *Le, Se,* and *A (*or *B)* genes leads to the formation of a minor antigen, ALe^b (or BLe^b), recognized by both anti-A (or anti-B) and anti-Le^b antibodies. Because the Se enzyme (i.e., Fuc-TII) converts virtually all Type 1 chains into H Type 1, whether or not Fuc-TIII is present, Lewis-positive secretors have virtually no Le^a antigen and their red blood cells type as Le(a − b +). By contrast, Lewis-positive nonsecretors have Le(a + b −) red blood cells. This is summarized in Table 8.6.

Individuals whose red blood cells type as Le(a + b +) are very unusual among whites but are relatively common in Asian populations. In these individuals the *Le* gene is normal but the Se (Fuc-TII) enzyme is partially defective due to a variant allele *(Se^w)* containing the 129 I → F mutation (56,59,60) (Fig. 8.6). Because the Se^w enzyme has partial activity, some Type 1 chains are converted to H Type 1, which are then converted to Le^b by the normal Lewis enzyme, Fuc-TIII (Fig. 8.8). In addition, some Type 1 chains avoid α1-2 fucosylation by the partially defective Se^w enzyme and are converted into Le^a by the normal Lewis Fuc-TIII enzyme (Fig. 8.8). Thus, the red blood cells of these individuals contain both the Le^a and Le^b antigens and type as Le(a + b +).

The presence of defective Le alleles is relatively common, and approximately 5% of whites and 25% of blacks type as Le(a − b −). To date, at least ten different defective *Le* alleles *(le^1 to le^{10})* have been identified (Fig. 8.10) (88–95). Based both on family studies and expression of transfected chimeric cDNAs in vitro, the mutations at amino acids 68 (94), 170 (89,90,92), 223 (96), 270 (96), and 356 (89–91) severely inhibit or abolish enzyme activity. One of these mutations occurs in (α1-3)fucosyltransferase Motif I and one in Motif II. Interestingly, the mutation at amino acid 20, which is in the transmembrane domain, affects Golgi localization of this enzyme and its activity with glycosphingolipid and glycoprotein substrates, thus yielding a paradoxical "nongenuine" Lewis-negative phenotype (89–92). That is, although red blood cells of individuals homozygous for *le^3* lack Lewis-active glycosphingolipids and type as Le(a − b −), their salivary mucins do contain Lewis antigens (91,97).

Although hemolytic transfusion reactions and hemolytic disease of the newborn are rarely caused by antibodies to the Lewis blood group antigens, this blood group system may be important in renal transplantation (98), coronary heart disease (99,100), gastrointestinal cancer (101), and infection by *Helicobacter pylori* (102,103).

II BLOOD GROUP SYSTEM

The Ii antigens are oligosaccharides that form the Type 2 chain precursors for the ABH antigens (Fig. 8.11). The best available evidence indicates that the difference between the I and i antigens relates to branching of the oligosaccharide chain; anti-i antibodies recognize an unbranched oligosaccharide chain, and anti-I antibodies recognize a similar chain that is also branched. Fetal and cord red blood cells contain mostly i antigen with small amounts of I; adult red blood cells demonstrate the opposite pattern. This suggests that the glycosyltransferase necessary for synthesis of the branched structure, a (β1-6)N-acetylglucosaminyltransferase, is developmentally regulated. The availability of the cloned cDNA encoding both this enzyme (104) and the "i-extension" enzyme (105) (Table 8.2) has allowed this hypothesis to be tested. Rare adults have red blood cells that type as i; presumably their red blood cell precursors lack the branching glycosyltransferase. Antibodies specific for the Ii antigens are

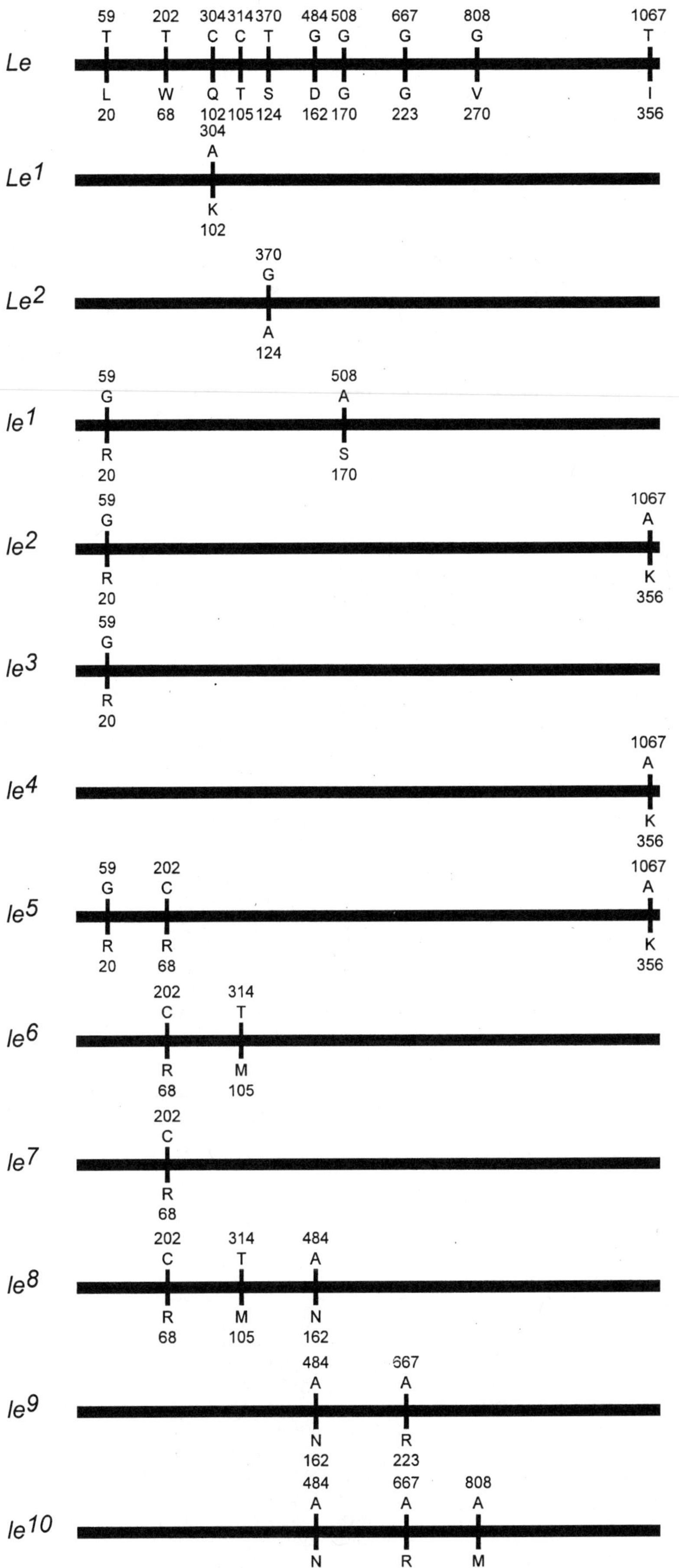

FIGURE 8.10. Functional and nonfunctional alleles of the *Lewis (Le)* gene: cDNA sequences. All sequences are compared with the *Le* sequence. There is no generally agreed upon nomenclature for naming variant alleles of the *Le* gene; the system chosen here is based on the literature, but is otherwise arbitrary.

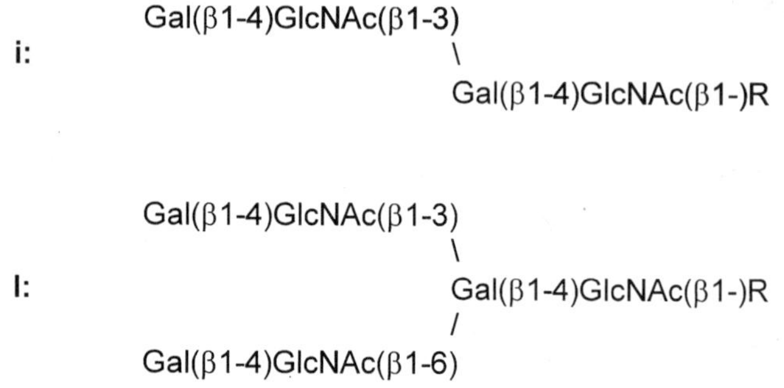

```
          Gal(β1-4)GlcNAc(β1-3)
i:                            \
                               Gal(β1-4)GlcNAc(β1-)R

          Gal(β1-4)GlcNAc(β1-3)
                              \
I:                             Gal(β1-4)GlcNAc(β1-)R
                              /
          Gal(β1-4)GlcNAc(β1-6)
```

FIGURE 8.11. Biochemical structures of the Ii blood group antigens. The monosaccharide abbreviations are as described in Figures 8.1 and 8.9.

clinically relevant in the setting of cold-type autoimmune hemolytic anemia. The sera of these patients typically contain high titers of a monoclonal antibody, usually with anti-I specificity. In patients demonstrating hemolysis in vivo, the antibodies bind to red blood cells at or near 37°C in vitro and have the ability to fix complement. Surprisingly, almost all normal individuals have low titers of anti-I; these autoantibodies agglutinate red blood cells only at room temperature or below and do not cause accelerated red blood cell destruction in vivo. Patients with particular infectious diseases such as infectious mononucleosis and mycoplasma pneumonia often develop cold agglutinins, typically with anti-i and anti-I specificity, respectively (106). In unusual cases, this may result in immune-mediated hemolytic anemia. At present, there is not a complete understanding of the mechanisms underlying the differences between cold agglutinins that cause hemolysis in vivo and those that do not (107–109).

P BLOOD GROUP SYSTEM

The P blood group system consists of at least three well-defined glycosphingolipid antigens (P^k, P, and P_1) and associated structures such as LKE, Globo-H, and Globo-A (Table 8.7) (110). These carbohydrate chains are related structurally and biosynthetically (111). Each has a common precursor, Gal(β1-4)Glc-ceramide (also called lactosylceramide). The P^k antigen is the biosynthetic precursor of the P antigen and both P^k and P_1 share a common disaccharide structure, Gal(α1-4)Gal(β1-4)-R, at the nonreducing end of the glycosphingolipid. These antigenic structures are not found on red blood cell–membrane glycoproteins (112). The glycosyltransferase that converts lactosylceramide to the P^k antigen is denoted as P^k synthase, that which converts P^k to P is denoted as P synthase, and that which converts paragloboside to P_1 is denoted as P_1 synthase (Tables 8.7, 8.8 and Fig. 8.12). The human P^k synthase has recently been cloned (113,114). In contrast, the gene encoding the P_1 synthase has been localized to chromosome 22 but has not yet been cloned (Table 8.2) (115,116).

Five different red blood cell phenotypes have been described in which various combinations of these three antigens are expressed (Table 8.8). The P_1 and P_2 phenotypes are common and account for almost the entire population. The serum of some P_2 individuals contains anti-P_1 antibodies. These antibodies are usually low-titered IgM cold agglutinins and are rarely of clinical significance; however, rare acute hemolytic transfusion reactions have been described (117). In contrast, the unusual individuals with the P_1^k, P_2^k, and p phenotypes have naturally occurring high-titered IgM antibodies with specificity either for the P antigen (i.e., anti-P) or for all the antigens in the P blood group system (i.e., anti-P_1PP^k or, equivalently, anti-Tj^a). These antibodies are clinically relevant in that they can cause severe hemolytic transfusion reactions. An unusual syndrome of recurrent spontaneous abortions has also been associated with these antibodies (118), presumably due to the presence of P^k- and P-active glycosphingolipids on trophoblastic tissue (119). In addition, the syndrome of paroxysmal cold hemoglobinuria, originally associated with syphilis, is caused by Donath-Landsteiner antibodies. The latter are complement-fixing IgG antibodies with anti-P specificity that cause immune-mediated hemolysis in vivo (120).

The P blood group antigens are present on multiple cell types in addition to red blood cells and have various functions. For example, the P antigen is the receptor for parvovirus B19 on erythropoietic precursors (121,122). This virus causes both transient aplastic crises in patients with underlying hemolysis and anemia in immunocompromised patients (123). In addition, the P^k antigen, also denoted as CD77, is the receptor on endothelial

TABLE 8.7. STRUCTURES OF P BLOOD GROUP AND RELATED GLYCOSPHINGOLIPID ANTIGENS

Lactosylceramide	Galβ1-4Glcβ1-1′cer
P^k	Galα1-4Galβ1-4Glcβ1-1′cer
P	GalNAcβ1-3Galα1-4Galβ1-4Glcβ1-1′cer
Gal-globoside	Galβ1-3GalNAcβ1-3Galα1-4Galβ1-4Glcβ1-1′cer
LKE	NeuAcα2-3Galβ1-3GalNAcβ1-3Galα1-4Galβ1-4Glcβ1-1′cer
Globo-H	Fucα1-2Galβ1-3GalNAcβ1-3Galα1-4Galβ1-4Glcβ1-1′cer
Globo-A	GalNAcα1-3[Fucα1-2]Galβ1-3GalNAcβ1-3Galα1-4Galβ1-4Glcβ1-1′cer
Lacto-N-neotriaosylceramide	GlcNAcβ1-3Galβ1-4Glcβ1-1′cer
Lacto-N-neotetraosylceramide	Galβ1-4GlcNAcβ1-3Galβ1-4Glcβ1-1′cer
P_1	Galα1-4Galβ1-4GlcNAcβ1-3Galβ1-4Glcβ1-1′cer
H Type 2	Fucα1-2Galβ1-4GlcNAcβ1-3Galβ1-4Glcβ1-1′cer
A Type 2	GalNAcα1-3[Fucα1-2]Galβ1-4GlcNAcβ1-3Galβ1-4Glcβ1-1′cer

TABLE 8.8. RED BLOOD CELL PHENOTYPES IN THE P BLOOD GROUP SYSTEM

Phenotype	Frequency	Red Blood Cell Antigens	Enzymes Present	Serum Antibodies
P_1	75%	P_1, P, P^k	P_1, P, P^k synthases	None
P_2	25%	P, P^k	P, P^k synthases	Anti-P_1
P_1^k	Rare	P_1, P^k	P_1, P^k synthases	Anti-P
P_2^k	Rare	P^k	P^k synthase	Anti-P_1, anti-P
p	Rare	None	None	Anti-P_1PP^k (anti-Tj^a)

cells for *Escherichia coli* verotoxins, which are important in the pathogenesis of the hemolytic uremic syndrome (124). The LKE antigen also functions as a receptor for uropathogenic *E. coli* (125). Finally, the P^k antigen appears to be important in signal transduction following binding of α-interferon and also in apoptosis (126,127).

SUMMARY

The carbohydrate blood group antigens that are most relevant for the practice of transfusion medicine are found in the ABH, Secretor, Lewis, Ii, and P human blood group systems. These may be more appropriately regarded as "histo–blood group antigens" in that their expression is not restricted to red blood cells. The oligosaccharide structures in these systems are related to each other biochemically and immunologically. Great progress has been made in understanding the enzymatic pathways involved in synthesizing these antigens and in the molecular biology of the genes encoding these glycosyltransferases. Although the normal biologic functions of these structures are not yet fully understood, many of them are important as receptors for human pathogens.

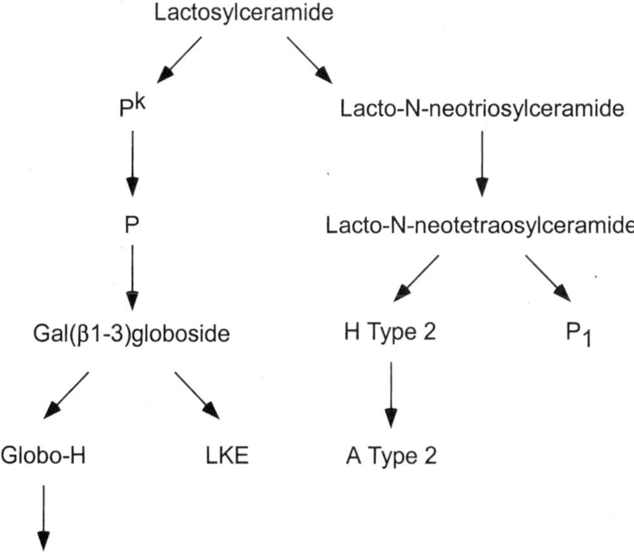

FIGURE 8.12. Biosynthetic pathway of P blood group system antigens and related structures. The biochemical structures of these glycosphingolipids are shown in Table 8.7.

REFERENCES

1. Mond JJ, Lees A, Snapper CM. T cell-independent antigens type 2. *Ann Rev Immunol* 1995;13:655–692.
2. Springer GF, Horton RE. Blood group isoantibody stimulation in man by feeding blood group–active bacteria. *J Clin Invest* 1969;48: 1280–1291.
3. Waldron P, de Alarcon P. ABO hemolytic disease of the newborn: a unique constellation of findings in siblings and review of protective mechanisms in the fetal-maternal system. *Am J Perinatol* 1999;16: 391–398.
4. McDonnell M, Hannam S, Devane SP. Hydrops fetalis due to ABO incompatibility. *Arch Dis Child Fetal Neonatal Ed* 1998;78: F220–221.
5. Clausen H, Hakomori SI. ABH and related histo-blood group antigens: immunochemical differences in carrier isotypes and their distribution. *Vox Sang* 1989;56:1–20.
6. Curtis BR, Edwards JT, Hessner MJ, et al. Blood group A and B antigens are strongly expressed on platelets of some individuals. *Blood* 2000;96:1574–1581.
7. Ravn V, Dabelsteen E. Tissue distribution of histo-blood group antigens. *APMIS* 2000;108:1–28.
8. Ferguson-Smith MA, Aitken DA, Turleua C, et al. Localization of the human ABO, Np-1: AK-1 linkage group by regional assignment of AK-1 to 9q34. *Hum Genet* 1976;34:35–43.
9. Yamamoto F. Molecular genetics of the ABO histo-blood group system. *Vox Sang* 1995;69:1–7.
10. Yamamoto FI, Marken J, Tsuji T, et al. Cloning and characterization of DNA complementary to human UDP-GalNAc:Fucα1-2Galα1-3GalNAc transferase (histo-blood group A transferase) mRNA. *J Biol Chem* 1990;265:1146–1151.
11. Yamamoto FI, Clausen H, White T, et al. Molecular genetic basis of the histo-blood group ABO system. *Nature* 1990;345:229–233.
12. Yamamoto FI, McNeill PD. Amino acid residue at codon 268 determines both activity and nucleotide-sugar donor substrate specificity of human histo-blood group A and B transferases. *J Biol Chem* 1996; 271:10515–10520.
13. Yamamoto FI, Hakomori SI. Sugar-nucleotide donor specificity of histo-blood group A and B transferases is based on amino acid substitutions. *J Biol Chem* 1990;265:19257–19262.
14. Watanabe G, Umetsu K, Yuasa I, et al. Amplified product length polymorphism (APLP): a novel strategy for genotyping the ABO blood group. *Hum Genet* 1997;99:34–37.
15. Ogasawara K, Bannai M, Saitou N, et al. Extensive polymorphism of ABO blood group gene: three major lineages of the alleles for the common ABO phenotypes. *Hum Genet* 1996;97:777–783.
16. Ogasawara K, Yabe R, Uchikawa M, et al. Different alleles cause an imbalance in A2 and A2B phenotypes of the ABO blood group. *Vox Sang* 1998;74:242–247.

17. Ogasawara K, Yabe R, Uchikawa M, et al. Molecular genetic analysis of variant phenotypes of the ABO blood group system. *Blood* 1996; 88:2732–2737.
18. Stroncek DF, Konz R, Clay ME, et al. Determination of ABO glycosyltransferase genotypes by use of polymerase chain reaction and restriction enzymes. *Transfusion* 1995;35:231–240.
19. Grunnet N, Steffensen R, Bennett EP, et al. Evaluation of histo-blood group ABO genotyping in a Danish population: frequency of a novel O allele defined as O_2. *Vox Sang* 1994;67:210–215.
20. Yamamoto F, McNeill PD, Yamamoto M, et al. Molecular genetic analysis of the ABO blood group system: 4. Another type of O allele. *Vox Sang* 1993;64:175–178.
21. Olsson ML, Santos SE, Guerreiro JF, et al. Heterogeneity of the O alleles at the blood group ABO locus in Amerindians. *Vox Sang* 1998; 74:46–50.
22. Olsson ML, Guerreiro JF, Zago MA, et al. Molecular analysis of the O alleles at the blood group ABO locus in populations of different ethnic origin reveals novel crossing-over events and point mutations. *Biochem Biophys Res Commun* 1997;234:779–782.
23. Olsson ML, Chester MA. Frequent occurrence of a variant O_1 gene at the blood group ABO locus. *Vox Sang* 1996;70:26–30.
24. Olsson ML, Chester MA. Evidence for a new type of O allele at the ABO locus, due to a combination of the A_2 nucleotide deletion and the A_{el} nucleotide insertion. *Vox Sang* 1996;71:113–117.
25. Yip SP. Single-tube multiplex PCR-SSCP analysis distinguishes 7 common ABO alleles and readily identifies new alleles. *Blood* 2000; 95:1487–1492.
26. Gassner C, Schmarda A, Nussbaumer W, et al. ABO glycosyltransferase genotyping by polymerase chain reaction using sequence-specific primers. *Blood* 1996;88:1852–1856.
27. Rozman P, Dovc T, Gassner C. Differentiation of autologous ABO, RHD, RHCE, KEL, JK, and FY blood group genotypes by analysis of peripheral blood samples of patients who have recently received multiple transfusions. *Transfusion* 2000;40:936–942.
28. Tsai LC, Kao LG, Chang JG, et al. Rapid identification of the ABO genotypes by their single-stand conformation polymorphism. *Electrophoresis* 2000;21:537–540.
29. Cartron JP. Etude quantitative et thermodynamique des phenotypes erythrocytaines "A faible." *Rev Fr Transfus Immunohematol* 1976;19: 35–54.
30. Clausen H, Levery SB, Nudelman E, et al. Further characterization of Type 2 and Type 3 chain blood group A glycosphingolipids from human erythrocyte membranes. *Biochemistry* 1986;25:7075–7085.
31. Hakomori S. Antigen structure and genetic basis of histo-blood groups A, B and O: their changes associated with human cancer. *Biochim Biophys Acta* 1999;1473:247–266.
32. Yamamoto F, McNeill PD, Yamamoto M, et al. Molecular genetic analysis of the ABO blood group system: 3. A_x and $B_{(A)}$ alleles. *Vox Sang* 1993;64:171–174.
33. Yamamoto FI, McNeill PD, Yamamoto M, et al. Molecular genetic analysis of the ABO blood group system: 1. Weak subgroups: A^3 and B^3 alleles. *Vox Sang* 1993;64:116–119.
34. Yamamoto RI, McNeill PD, Hakomori SI. Human histo-blood group A^2 transferase coded by A^2 allele, one of the A subtypes, is characterized by a single base deletion in the coding sequence, which results in an additional domain at the carboxyl terminal. *Biochem Biophys Res Commun* 1992;187:366–374.
35. Olsson ML, Chester MA. Heterogeneity of the blood group Ax allele: genetic recombination of common alleles can result in the Ax phenotype. *Transfus Med* 1998;8:231–238.
36. Olsson ML, Thuresson B, Chester MA. An A_{el} allele-specific nucleotide insertion at the blood group ABO locus and its detection using a sequence-specific polymerase chain reaction. *Biochem Biophys Res Commun* 1995;216:642–647.
37. Olsson ML, Chester MA. Polymorphisms at the *ABO* locus in subgroup A individuals. *Transfusion* 1996;36:309–313.
38. Barjas-Castro ML, Carvalho MH, Locatelli MF, et al. Molecular heterogeneity of the A3 subgroup. *Clin Lab Haematol* 2000;22:73–78.
39. Irshaid NM, Chester MA, Olsson ML. Allele-related variation in minisatellite repeats involved in the transcription of the blood group ABO gene. *Transfus Med* 1999;9:219–226.
40. Iwamoto S, Withers DA, Handa K, et al. Deletion of A-antigen in a human cancer cell line is associated with reduced promoter activity of CBF/NF-Y binding region, and possibly with enhanced DNA methylation of A transferase promoter. *Glycoconj J* 1999;16:659–666.
41. Kominato Y, Hata Y, Takizawa H, et al. Expression of human histo-blood group ABO genes is dependent upon DNA methylation of the promoter region. *J Biol Chem* 1999;274:37240–37250.
42. Yu LC, Chang CY, Twu YC, et al. Human histo-blood group ABO glycosyltransferase genes: different enhancer structures with different transcriptional activities. *Biochem Biophys Res Commun* 2000;273: 459–466.
43. Nelson PW, Landreneau MD, Luger AM, et al. Ten-year experience in transplantation of A2 kidneys into B and O recipients. *Transplantation* 1998;65:256–260.
44. Bennett M, Levene C, Greenwell P. An Israeli family with six cisAB members: serologic and enzymatic studies. *Transfusion* 1998;38: 441–448.
45. Yu LC, Lee HL, Chan YS, et al. The molecular basis for the B(A) allele: an amino acid alteration in the human histoblood group B α-(1,3)-galactosyltransferase increases its intrinsic α-(1,3)-N-acetylgalactosaminyltransferase activity. *Biochem Biophys Res Commun* 1999; 262:487–493.
46. Yamamoto F, McNeill PD, Kominato Y, et al. Molecular genetic analysis of the ABO blood group system: 2. cis-AB alleles. *Vox Sang* 1993;64:120–123.
47. Oriol R, Le Pendu J, Mollicone R. Genetics of ABO, H, Lewis, X, and related antigens. *Vox Sang* 1986;51:161–171.
48. Sarnesto A, Kohlin T, Hindsgaul O, et al. Purification of the secretor-type β-galactoside α 1-2-fucosyltransferase from human serum. *J Biol Chem* 1992;267:2737–2744.
49. Oriol R, Mollicone R, Cailleau A, et al. Divergent evolution of fucosyltransferase genes from vertebrates, invertebrates, and bacteria. *Glycobiology* 1999;9:323–334.
50. Rouquier S, Lowe JB, Kelly RJ, et al. Molecular cloning of a human genomic region containing the H blood group α(1,2)fucosyltransferase gene and two H locus–related DNA restriction fragments. *J Biol Chem* 1995;270:4632–4639.
51. Kelly RJ, Rouquier S, Giorgi D, et al. Sequence and expression of a candidate for the human Secretor blood group α(1,2)fucosyltransferase gene (FUT2). *J Biol Chem* 1995;270:4640–4649.
52. Koda Y, Soejima M, Wang B, et al. Structure and expression of the gene encoding secretor-type galactoside 2-α-L-fucosyltransferase (FUT2). *Eur J Biochem* 1997;246:750–755.
53. Larsen RD, Ernst LK, Nair RP, et al. Molecular cloning, sequence, and expression of a human GDP-L-fucose:β-D-galactoside 2-α-L-fucosyltransferase cDNA that can form the H blood group antigen. *Proc Natl Acad Sci U S A* 1990;87:6674–6678.
54. Reguigne-Arnould I, Faure S, Chery M, et al. Physical mapping of 49 microsatellite markers on chromosome 19 and correlation with the genetic linkage map. *Genomics* 1996;32:458–461.
55. Yu LC, Broadberry RE, Yang YH, et al. Heterogeneity of the human Secretor α(1,2) fucosyltransferase gene among Lewis (a+b+) non-secretors. *Biochem Biophys Res Commun* 1996;222:390–394.
56. Yu LC, Yang YH, Broadberry RE, et al. Correlation of a missense mutation in the human Secretor α1,2-fucosyltransferase gene with the Lewis (a+b+) phenotype: a potential molecular basis for the weak Secretor allele (Se^w). *Biochem J* 1995;312:329–332.
57. Koda Y, Soejima M, Liu Y, et al. Molecular basis for secretor type α(1,2)-fucosyltransferase gene deficiency in a Japanese population: a fusion gene generated by unequal crossover responsible for the enzyme deficiency. *Am J Hum Genet* 1996;59:343–350.
58. Liu Y, Koda Y, Soejima M, et al. Extensive polymorphism of the FUT2 gene in an African (Xhosa) population of South Africa. *Hum Genet* 1998;103:204–210.
59. Henry S, Mollicone R, Fernandez P, et al. Molecular basis for erythrocyte Le(a+b+) and salivary partial-secretor phenotypes: expression of a FUT2 secretor allele with an A → T mutation at nucleotide 385

correlates with reduced α(1,2)fucosyltransferase activity. *Glycoconj J* 1996;13:985–993.
60. Henry S, Mollicone R, Fernandez P, et al. Homozygous expression of a missense mutation at nucleotide 385 in the FUT2 gene associates with the Le(a + b +) partial-secretor phenotype in an Indonesian family. *Biochem Biophys Res Commun* 1996;219:675–678.
61. Liu YH, Koda Y, Soejima M, et al. The fusion gene at the ABO-secretor locus (FUT2): absence in Chinese populations. *J Hum Genet* 1999;44:181–184.
62. Peng CT, Tsai CH, Lin TP, et al. Molecular characterization of secretor type α(1, 2)-fucosyltransferase gene deficiency in the Philippine population. *Ann Hematol* 1999;78:463–467.
63. Henry S, Mollicone R, Lowe JB, et al. A second nonsecretor allele of the blood group α(1,2)fucosyltransferase gene (FUT2). *Vox Sang* 1996;70:21–25.
64. Chang JG, Yang TY, Liu TC, et al. Molecular analysis of secretor type α(1,2)-fucosyltransferase gene mutations in the Chinese and Thai populations. *Transfusion* 1999;39:1013–1017.
65. Yu LC, Lee HL, Chu CC, et al. A newly identified nonsecretor allele of the human histo-blood group α(1,2)fucosyltransferase gene (FUT2). *Vox Sang* 1999;76:115–119.
66. Svensson L, Petersson A, Henry SM. Secretor genotyping for A385T, G428A, C571T, C628T, 685delTGG, G849A, and other mutations from a single PCR. *Transfusion* 2000;40:856–860.
67. Fernandez-Mateos P, Cailleau A, Henry S, et al. Point mutations and deletion responsible for the Bombay H null and the Reunion H weak blood groups. *Vox Sang* 1998;75:37–46.
68. Koda Y, Soejima M, Johnson PH, et al. Missense mutation of FUT1 and deletion of FUT2 are responsible for Indian Bombay phenotype of ABO blood group system. *Biochem Biophys Res Commun* 1997; 238:21–25.
69. Koda Y, Soejima M, Johnson PH, et al. An Alu-mediated large deletion of the FUT2 gene in individuals with the ABO-Bombay phenotype. *Hum Genet* 2000;106:80–85.
70. Kelly RJ, Ernst LK, Larsen RD, et al. Molecular basis for H blood group deficiency in Bombay (Oh) and para-Bombay individuals. *Proc Natl Acad Sci U S A* 1994;91:5843–5847.
71. Kaneko M, Nishihara S, Shinya N, et al. Wide variety of point mutations in the H gene of Bombay and para-Bombay individuals that inactivate H enzyme. *Blood* 1997;90:839–849.
72. Yu LC, Yang YH, Broadberry RE, et al. Heterogeneity of the human H blood group α(1,2)fucosyltransferase gene among para-Bombay individuals. *Vox Sang* 1997;72:36–40.
73. Wagner FF, Flegel WA. Polymorphism of the h allele and the population frequency of sporadic nonfunctional alleles. *Transfusion* 1997; 37:284–290.
74. Wang B, Koda Y, Soejima M, et al. Two missense mutations of H type α(1,2)fucosyltransferase gene (FUT1) responsible for para-Bombay phenotype. *Vox Sang* 1997;72:31–35.
75. Wagner T, Vadon M, Staudacher E, et al. A new h allele detected in Europe has a missense mutation in α(1,2)-fucosyltransferase motif II. *Transfusion* 2001;41:31–38.
76. Breton C, Oriol R, Imberty A. Conserved structural features in eukaryotic and prokaryotic fucosyltransferases. *Glycobiology* 1998;8:87–94.
77. Bhatia HM, Sathe MS. Incidence of "Bombay" (Oh) phenotype and weaker variants of A and B antigen in Bombay (India). *Vox Sang* 1974;27:524–532.
78. Le Pendu J, Clamagirand-Mulet C, Cartron JP, et al. H-deficient blood groups of Reunion Island. III. α-2-L-fucosyltransferase activity in sera of homozygous and heterozygous individuals. *Am J Hum Genet* 1983;35:497–507.
79. Henry S, Oriol R, Samuelsson B. Lewis histo-blood group system and associated phenotypes. *Vox Sang* 1995;69:166–182.
80. Marcus DM, Cass LE. Glycosphingolipids with Lewis blood group activity: uptake by human erythrocytes. *Science* 1969;164:553–555.
81. Reguigne-Arnould I, Couillin P, Mollicone R, et al. Relative positions of two clusters of human α-L-fucosyltransferases in 19q (FUT1-FUT2) and 19p (FUT6-FUT3-FUT5) within the microsatellite genetic map of chromosome 19. *Cytogenet Cell Genet* 1995;71:158–162.
82. Kukowska-Latallo JF, Larsen RD, Nair RP, et al. A cloned human cDNA determines expression of a mouse stage-specific embryonic antigen and the Lewis blood group α(1,3/1,4)fucosyltransferase. *Genes Dev* 1990;4:1288–1303.
83. Dupuy F, Petit JM, Mollicone R, et al. A single amino acid in the hypervariable stem domain of vertebrate α1,3/1,4-fucosyltransferases determines the type 1/type 2 transfer. Characterization of acceptor substrate specificity of the lewis enzyme by site-directed mutagenesis. *J Biol Chem* 1999;274:12257–12262.
84. de Vries T, Srnka CA, Palcic MM, et al. Acceptor specificity of different length constructs of human recombinant α 1,3/4-fucosyltransferases. Replacement of the stem region and the transmembrane domain of fucosyltransferase V by protein A results in an enzyme with GDP-fucose hydrolyzing activity. *J Biol Chem* 1995;270:8712–8722.
85. Legault DJ, Kelly RJ, Natsuka Y, et al. Human α(1,3/1,4)-fucosyltransferases discriminate between different oligosaccharide acceptor substrates through a discrete peptide fragment. *J Biol Chem* 1995; 270:20987–20996.
86. Nguyen AT, Holmes EH, Whitaker JM, et al. Human α1,3/4-fucosyltransferases. I. Identification of amino acids involved in acceptor substrate binding by site-directed mutagenesis. *J Biol Chem* 1998; 273:25244–25249.
87. Xu Z, Vo L, Macher BA. Structure-function analysis of human α1,3-fucosyltransferase. Amino acids involved in acceptor substrate specificity. *J Biol Chem* 1996;271:8818–8823.
88. Pang H, Liu Y, Koda Y, et al. Five novel missense mutations of the Lewis gene (FUT3) in African (Xhosa) and Caucasian populations in South Africa. *Hum Genet* 1998;102:675–680.
89. Nishihara S, Yazawa S, Iwasaki H, et al. α (1,3/1,4)fucosyltransferase (FucT-III) gene is inactivated by a single amino acid substitution in Lewis histo-blood type negative individuals. *Biochem Biophys Res Commun* 1993;196:624–631.
90. Nishihara S, Narimatsu H, Iwasaki H, et al. Molecular genetic analysis of the human Lewis histo-blood group system. *J Biol Chem* 1994; 269:29271–29278.
91. Mollicone R, Reguigne I, Kelly RJ, et al. Molecular basis for Lewis α(1,3/1,4)-fucosyltransferase gene deficiency (FUT3) found in Lewis-negative Indonesian pedigrees. *J Biol Chem* 1994;269:20987–20994.
92. Koda Y, Kimura H, Mekada E. Analysis of Lewis fucosyltransferase genes from the human gastric mucosa of Lewis-positive and -negative individuals. *Blood* 1993;82:2915–2919.
93. Elmgren A, Borjeson C, Svensson L, et al. DNA sequencing and screening for point mutations in the human Lewis (FUT3) gene enables molecular genotyping of the human Lewis blood group system. *Vox Sang* 1996;70:97–103.
94. Elmgren A, Mollicone R, Costache M, et al. Significance of individual point mutations, T202C and C314T, in the human Lewis (FUT3) gene for expression of Lewis antigens by the human α(1,3/1,4)-fucosyltransferase, Fuc-TIII. *J Biol Chem* 1997;269:21994–21998.
95. Elmgren A, Rydberg L, Larson G. Genotypic heterogeneity among Lewis negative individuals. *Biochem Biophys Res Commun* 1993;196: 515–520.
96. Pang H, Koda Y, Soejima M, et al. Significance of each of three missense mutations, G484A, G667A, and G808A, present in an inactive allele of the human Lewis gene (FUT3) for α(1,3/1,4)fucosyltransferase inactivation. *Glycoconj J* 1998;15:961–967.
97. Nishihara S, Hiraga T, Ikehara Y, et al. Molecular behavior of mutant Lewis enzymes in vivo. *Glycobiology* 1999;9:373–382.
98. Spitalnik S, Pfaff W, Cowles J, et al. Humoral immunity to Lewis blood group antigens correlates with renal transplant rejection. *Transplantation* 1984;37:265–268.
99. Salomaa V, Pankow J, Heiss G, et al. Genetic background of Lewis negative blood group phenotype and its association with atherosclerotic disease in the NHLBI family heart study. *J Intern Med* 2000; 247:689–698.
100. Ellison RC, Zhang Y, Myers RH, et al. Lewis blood group phenotype as an independent risk factor for coronary heart disease (the NHLBI Family Heart Study). *Am J Cardiol* 1999;83:345–348.
101. Weston BW, Hiller KM, Mayben JP, et al. Expression of human α(1, 3)fucosyltransferase antisense sequences inhibits selectin-mediated ad-

hesion and liver metastasis of colon carcinoma cells. *Cancer Res* 1999; 59:2127–2135.

102. Boren T, Falk P, Roth KA, et al. Attachment of *Helicobacter pylori* to human gastric epithelium mediated by blood group antigens. *Science* 1993;262:1892–1895.
103. Clyne M, Drumm B. Absence of effect of Lewis A and Lewis B expression on adherence of *Helicobacter pylori* to human gastric cells. *Gastroenterology* 1997;113:72–80.
104. Bierhuizen MFA, Mattei MG, Fukuda M. Expression of the developmental I antigen by a cloned human cDNA encoding a member of a β-1,6-N-acetylglucosaminyltransferase gene family. *Genes Dev* 1993;7:468–478.
105. Sasaki K, Kurata-Miura K, Ujita M, et al. Expression cloning of cDNA encoding a human β-1,3-N-acetylglucosaminyltransferase that is essential for poly-N-acetyllactosamine synthesis. *Proc Natl Acad Sci U S A* 1997;94:14294–14299.
106. Feizi T, Loveless RW. Carbohydrate recognition by *Mycoplasma pneumoniae* and pathologic consequences. *Am J Respir Crit Care Med* 1996; 154[Suppl]:133–136.
107. Jefferies LC, Carchidi CM, Silberstein LE. Naturally occurring anti-i/I cold agglutinins may be encoded by different VH3 genes as well as the VH4.21 gene segment. *J Clin Invest* 1993;92:2821–2833.
108. Silberstein LE. B-cell origin of cold agglutinins. *Adv Exp Med Biol* 1994;347:193–205.
109. Havouis S, Dumas G, Ave P, et al. A murine transgenic model of human cold agglutinin disease. *Haematologica* 1999;84:67–69.
110. Spitalnik PF, Spitalnik SL. The P blood group system: Biochemical, serological, and clinical aspects. *Transfus Med Rev* 1995;9:110–122.
111. Bailly P, Piller F, Gillard B, et al. Biosynthesis of the blood group P^k and P_1 antigens by human kidney microsomes. *Carbohydr Res* 1992;228:277–287.
112. Yang Z, Bergstrom J, Karlsson KA. Glycoproteins with Gal α 4Gal are absent from human erythrocyte membranes, indicating that glycolipids are the sole carriers of blood group P activities. *J Biol Chem* 1994;269:14620–14624.
113. Kojima Y, Fukumoto S, Furukawa K, et al. Molecular cloning of globotriaosylceramide/CD77 synthase, a glycosyltransferase that initiates the synthesis of globo series glycosphingolipids. *J Biol Chem* 2000; 275:15152–15156.
114. Steffensen R, Carlier K, Wiels J, et al. Cloning and expression of the histo-blood group Pk UDP-galactose: Galβ-4G1cβ1-cer α1, 4-galactosyltransferase. Molecular genetic basis of the p phenotype. *J Biol Chem* 2000;275:16723–16729.
115. Tippett P, Kaplan JC. Report of the Committee on the Genetic Constitution of Chromosomes 20, 21, and 22. *Cytogenet Cell Genet* 1985; 40:268–295.
116. Julier C, Lathrop GM, Reghis A, et al. A linkage and physical map of chromosome 22, and some applications to gene mapping. *Am J Hum Genet* 1988;42:297–308.
117. Arndt PA, Garratty G, Marfoe RA, et al. An acute hemolytic transfusion reaction caused by an anti-Pi that reacted at 37 degrees C. *Transfusion* 1998;38:373–377.
118. Iseki S, Masaki S, Levine P. A remarkable family with the rare human isoantibody anti-Tj^a in four siblings; anti-Tj^a and habitual abortion. *Nature* 1954;173:1193–1194.
119. Hansson G, Wazniowska K, Rock JA, et al. The glycosphingolipid composition of the placenta of a blood group P fetus delivered by a blood group P_1^k woman and analysis of the anti-globoside antibodies found in maternal serum. *Arch Biochem Biophys* 1988;260:168–176.
120. Schwarting GA, Kundu SK, Marcus DM. Reaction of antibodies that cause paroxysmal cold hemoglobinuria (PCH) with globoside and Forssman glycosphingolipids. *Blood* 1979;53:186–192.
121. Brown KE, Anderson SM, Young NS. Erythrocyte P antigen: cellular receptor for B19 parvovirus. *Science* 1993;262:114–117.
122. Brown KE, Hibbs JR, Gallinella G, et al. Resistance to parvovirus B19 infection due to lack of virus receptor (erythrocyte P antigen). *New Engl J Med* 1994;330:1192–1196.
123. Brown KE, Young NS. Human parvovirus B19 infections in infants and children. *Adv Pediatr Infect Dis* 1997;13:101–126.
124. Lingwood CA. Glycolipid receptors for verotoxin and *Helicobacter pylori:* role in pathology. *Biochim Biophys Acta* 1999;1455:375–386.
125. Stroud MR, Stapleton AE, Levery SB. The P histo-blood group-related glycosphingolipid sialosyl galactosyl globoside as a preferred binding receptor for uropathogenic *Escherichia coli:* isolation and structural characterization from human kidney. *Biochemistry* 1998; 37:17420–17428.
126. Maloney MD, Binnington-Boyd B, Lingwood CA. Globotriaosyl ceramide modulates interferon-α-induced growth inhibition and CD19 expression in Burkitt's lymphoma cells. *Glycoconj J* 1999;16;821–828.
127. Taga S, Carlier K, Mishal Z, et al. Intracellular signaling events in CD77-mediated apoptosis of Burkitt's lymphoma cells. *Blood* 1997; 90:2757–2767.

Rossi's Principles of Transfusion Medicine, Third Edition, edited by Toby L. Simon, Walter H. Dzik, Edward L. Snyder, Christopher P. Stowell, and Ronald G. Strauss. Lippincott Williams & Wilkins, Philadelphia © 2002.

CASE 8A

A FRENCH CANADIAN WITH A RARE BLOOD TYPE

CASE HISTORY

Mrs. Roulx is a 69-year-old woman referred to our hospital because of a history of progressive shortness of breath upon exertion and the detection of a lung mass by chest radiograph. She was in good health until just a few weeks ago, when she developed pain on deep breathing and shortness of breath when walking quickly.

Her physical exam showed no cyanosis or clubbing of the fingers or toes and no unusual findings on percussion or auscultation of the lungs. She had a systolic murmur at the base of the heart. There was no abnormal lymphadenopathy. The patient is of French Canadian ancestry and lives in Maine. She is married and has no children. She has never smoked cigarettes and had never been transfused.

Her initial chest radiograph and computed tomography (CT) scan at this hospital showed a prominent mass located within the pulmonary artery. A pulmonary arteriogram showed that the mass had nearly occluded blood flow in the left main branch of the pulmonary artery, had extended into the main pulmonary artery, and was growing into the first portion of the right pulmonary artery. No wonder she became short of breath upon exertion! She underwent pulmonary function testing which demonstrated that she could tolerate a complete left pneumonectomy, if required. She was scheduled for elective thoracotomy and resection of the mass. Four units of red blood cells were requested for the operating room.

Her pretransfusion testing showed her to be group O, Rh-negative. Her antibody screen was markedly reactive with all three screening cells at all phases of testing. The direct antiglobulin test was negative. Upon further questioning, the patient said that she had an unusual blood type but could not recall what it was. Because she appeared to be a group O individual with an antibody that was strongly reactive against all targets at immediate spin, 37°C and the antiglobulin phase, the Bombay blood group was considered. Her cells were completely nonreactive with Ulex europeus, a lectin known to react with Type 2 H-structures. This finding provides very strong evidence that she has group O_h (Bombay) blood. Bombay individuals make a potent anti-H which reacts with all non-Bombay cells. To rule out the presence of additional alloantibodies, her plasma was adsorbed onto three separate group O cells: R1/R1, R2/R2, and r/r. These cells adsorbed the anti-H and the residual plasma was nonreactive when tested against antibody screening cells, thereby ruling out any likely additional alloantibodies. Her phenotype was found to be C-negative, E-negative, D-negative, c-positive, e-positive, K1-negative, Fy(a−b+), Jk(a+b+), S+, s+, M+, N+, and Le(a+b−).

The surgical team and the patient were notified of the findings and the surgery was postponed until an adequate supply of Bombay-type blood could be obtained. We contacted the American rare-donor registry. Bombay blood is quite rare and Rh-negative Bombay blood even rarer! Nevertheless, the registry was able to identify four units of O_h Rh-negative blood and two units of O_h Rh-positive blood which were sent to the hospital as frozen glycerolized units. Because of the urgency of her surgery, her difficulty breathing, and her low preoperative hematocrit (30%), we felt she was not a candidate for preoperative autologous blood donation. She had no siblings who might be O_h donors for her.

DISCUSSION

Group O_h (Bombay) blood is perhaps the most famous of the rare blood groups. It was recognized in 1952 when a woman with a group-AB parent was found to be apparently group O. Bombay patients with anti-H are ABO incompatible with all non-Bombay individuals. Group O_h individuals are homozygous for a gene mutation in the H-enzyme, a fucosyltransferase that is necessary for making the ABH antigens (Fig. 8A.1). A simplified view of the Bombay blood group follows. There are two fucosyltransferases that create H structures. One enzyme (H enzyme) preferentially attaches a fucose to Type 2 chains. The other fucosyltransferase (Se enzyme) preferentially uses Type 1 chains as its substrate. Most complete Bombay individuals have a mutation that disrupts not only the *H* gene but also the adjacent Se gene. For this reason, complete Bombay individuals fail to express ABH substances in their secretions and type as Le(a+b−) if they possess the Le gene. Some Bombay individuals lack only the transferase that uses Type 2 chains as substrate (H enzyme), but still express the fucosyltransferase that use Type 1 chains as substrate (Se enzyme). These individuals—called para-Bombays—continue to make Type 1–ABH substances and can therefore type as Le(a−b+) and express limited amounts of Type-1 A or B substance on the surface of their red blood cells. Thus, they often weakly express group A or B. Para-Bombay individuals may or may not develop anti-H.

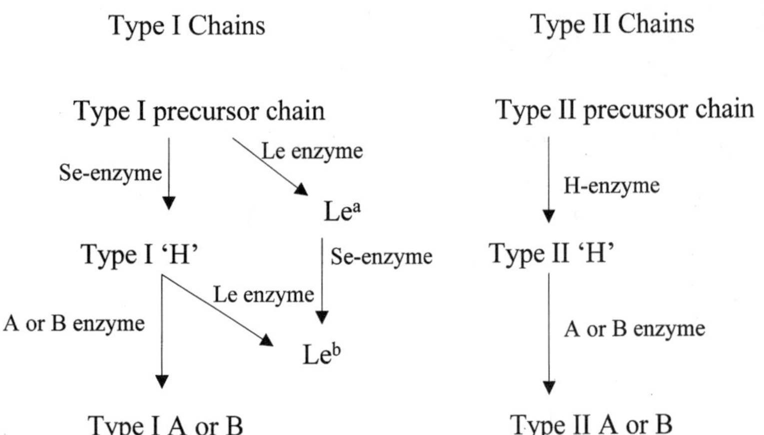

FIGURE 8A.1. Simplified view of ABH synthesis. The H-enzyme is absent in O_h individuals.

The *H* gene is found on chromosome 19. Several different single nucleotide point mutations account for the recognized defects in the *H* gene of Bombay individuals (1,2). This rare blood group was originally identified in an individual of Asian Indian descent who lived in Bombay, India. The genetic lesion is not limited to people from the subcontinent, however. Indeed, it is felt that the original founder mutation originated in Europe, probably in France. French explorers who rounded the Cape of Good Hope during the seventeenth-century expeditions probably brought the gene with them. Indeed, the French established a settlement on Reunion Island off the southeast coast of Africa (near Madagascar). This island has one of the highest rates of the Bombay blood group in the world. From Reunion Island, it was just a short sail for the intrepid explorers to reach India and the city of Bombay. From France, explorers also carried the rare gene with them to the New World. Our patient's known French-Canadian name and ancestry may be a link to that original genetic migration.

CODA

Mrs. Roulx underwent a complex and difficult operation to have the tumor removed. She was placed on cardiopulmonary bypass, her heart was fibrillated, and her entire left lung was removed. In addition, her main pulmonary artery and the left main pulmonary artery were removed. A frozen cadaver aortic allograft was used to connect the outflow tract of her right ventricle to the right pulmonary artery. Following this, her heart was restored to normal rhythm and she was taken off cardiopulmonary bypass. Multiple surgical drains were placed and her chest cavity was closed. Despite the complex surgery and with the aid of intraoperative blood recovery, she required only the four Rh-negative units of deglycerolized red blood cells. At the close of surgery, a collective sigh of relief was heard in both the operating room and the blood bank. The pathology confirmed that the mass was a malignant fibrous histiocytoma and the tumor was noted to extend along the vascular intima. The patient recovered from the tumor resection without complication and was discharged from the hospital to home.

Case contributed by Walter H. Dzik, M.D., Massachusetts General Hospital, Boston, MA

REFERENCES

1. Kaneko M, Nishihara S, Shinya N, et al. Wide variety of point mutations in the H gene of Bombay and para-Bombay individuals that inactivate H enzyme. *Blood* 1997;90:839–849.
2. Wagner T, Vadon M, Staudacher E, et al. A new h allele detected in Europe has a missense mutation α (1,2)-fucosyltransferase motif II. *Transfusion* 2001;41:31–38.

9

RH AND LW BLOOD GROUP SYSTEMS

CONSTANCE M. WESTHOFF AND DON L. SIEGEL

Although it is now clear that the Rh and LW antigens are carried on entirely different proteins, they are incorporated together in this chapter based on a historic serologic connection (and confusion), and more recently on evidence that they are physically associated within the red blood cell (RBC) membrane.

RH BLOOD GROUP SYSTEM

History and Nomenclature

The Rh system is second only to the ABO system in importance in transfusion medicine because Rh antigens, especially D, are highly immunogenic and cause hemolytic disease of the newborn (HDN) and transfusion reactions. HDN was first described by a French midwife in 1609 in a set of twins, one of which was hydropic and stillborn, while the other was jaundiced and died of kernicterus (1). That a wide range of observed clinical scenarios involving RBC hemolysis were related—from severely hydropic stillborn fetuses to infants with mild or significant levels of jaundice and kernicterus—was not realized until 1932 (2). However, the cause of RBC hemolysis remained elusive until 1939, when a case was described of a woman who delivered a stillborn fetus and also suffered a severe hemolytic reaction when transfused with blood from her husband. Levine and Stetson correctly surmised that the mother had been immunized by a fetal RBC antigen inherited from the father and suggested that the cause of the erythroblastosis fetalis was maternal antibody in the fetal circulation (3). They did not give the target blood group antigen a name. Meanwhile Landsteiner and Wiener, in an effort to discover new blood groups, injected rabbits and guinea pigs with rhesus monkey RBCs. The antiserum they obtained agglutinated not only rhesus monkey RBCs, but also the RBCs of 85% of whites, who they called "Rh positive"; the remaining 15% were termed "Rh negative" (4). The "anti-Rhesus" serum seemed to be reacting similarly to the maternal antibody in serologic testing, hence the blood group system responsible for HDN came to be known as "Rh." It is now clear that the anti-Rhesus serum was detecting the LW antigen (subsequently named for Landsteiner and Wiener), which is present in greater amounts on D-positive than on D-negative RBCs (5). Years of debate followed concerning whether the human antibodies and the anti-Rhesus antibodies were detecting the same antigen and extended long after serologic profiles suggested they were reacting with different structures. Landsteiner and Wiener never accepted the LW terminology, because doing so would imply that they had not discovered the cause of HDN (6).

It was soon obvious that Rh was not a simple, single antigen system. In 1941, Fisher named the C and c antigens (A and B had been used for ABO), and used the next letters of the alphabet, D and E, to define antigens recognized by additional antibodies. In 1945, the e antigen was identified (4).

It is important for transfusion medicine specialists to appreciate that the often confusing nomenclature used to describe Rh antigens results from the difference in opinion that existed concerning the number of genes that were involved in their expression. The Fisher-Race nomenclature suggested that three closely linked genes, C/c, E/e, and D were responsible, while the Wiener nomenclature (Rh-Hr) was based on his belief that a single gene encoded one "agglutinogen" that carried several blood group

C.M. Westhoff and D.L. Siegel: Blood Bank/Transfusion Medicine Section, Department of Pathology and Laboratory Medicine, University of Pennsylvania Medical Center, Philadelphia, Pennsylvania.

TABLE 9.1. NOMENCLATURE AND INCIDENCE FOR Rh HAPLOTYPES

Haplotype Based on Antigens Present (Fisher/Race)	Shorthand for Haplotype (Modified Wiener)	Incidence (%)		
		Whites	Blacks	Asians
DCe	R_1	42	17	70
DcE	R_2	14	11	21
Dce	R_0	4	44	3
DCE	R_z	<0.01	<0.01	1
ce	r	37	26	3
Ce	r′	2	2	2
cE	r″	1	<0.01	<0.01
CE	r^y	<0.01	<0.01	<0.01

factors. Even though neither theory was correct (there are two genes—*RHD* and *RHCE*—correctly proposed by Tippett) (7), for written communication the Fisher-Race designation (CDE) for haplotypes is preferred, and for spoken communication a modified version of Wiener's nomenclature is preferred (Table 9.1). The "R" indicates that D is present and use of a lowercase "r" (or "little r") indicates that it is not. The C or c and E or e Rh antigens carried with D are represented by subscripts: 1 for Ce (R_1), 2 for cE (R_2), 0 for ce (R_0), and Z for CE (R_z). The CcEe antigens present without D (r) are represented by superscript symbols: "prime" for Ce (r′), "double-prime" for cE (r″), and "y" for CE (r^y). The "R" versus "r" terminology allows one to convey the common Rh antigens present on one chromosomal haplotype in a single term (a phenotype).

The major Rh antigens are D, C, c, E, and e, but the Rh blood group system is one of the most complex because of the number of additional antigens (approximately 45) that have been reported (Table 9.2). These additional antigens include compound antigens in *cis* [e.g., f (ce), Ce, CE], high- and low-incidence antigens arising from partial-D hybrid proteins (e.g., D^w, Go^a, Evans), and antigens arising from various point mutations in the RhCE protein (e.g., C^w, C^x, VS). Table 9.2 also includes the numeric designations for Rh antigens that Rosenfield introduced in 1962 in anticipation of the computer era (8). With a few exceptions (Rh17, Rh29, Rh32, Rh33), the numeric designations are not widely used in the clinical laboratory.

Genes and Their Expressed Proteins

Two genes designated *RHD* and *RHCE* encode the Rh proteins (9). They are 97% identical, each has ten exons, and are the result of a gene duplication on chromosome 1p34–36 (10). Rh-

TABLE 9.2. ROSENFIELD NUMERICAL TERMINOLOGY FOR Rh ANTIGENS

Numeric	Symbol	Numeric	Symbol	Numeric	Symbol
Rh1	D	Rh27	cE	Rh48	JAL
Rh2	C	Rh28	hr^H	Rh49	STEM
Rh3	E	Rh29	"total"	Rh50	FPTT
Rh4	c	Rh30	Go^a	Rh51	MAR
Rh5	e	Rh31	hr^B	Rh52	BARC
Rh6	ce or f	Rh32	Rh32**		
Rh7	Ce	Rh33	Rh33***		
Rh8	C^W	Rh34	Hr^B		
Rh9	C^X	Rh35	Rh35****		
Rh10	V	Rh36	Be^a		
Rh11	E^W	Rh37	Evans		
Rh12	G	Rh39	Rh39		
Rh17	Hr_0*	Rh40	Tar		
Rh18	Hr	Rh41	Rh41		
Rh19	hr^S	Rh42	Rh42		
Rh20	VS	Rh43	Crawford		
Rh21	C^G	Rh44	Nou		
Rh22	CE	Rh45	Riv		
Rh23	D^W	Rh46	Sec		
Rh26	c-like	Rh47	Dav		

Note: Rh13 through 16, 24 and 25 are obsolete.
*High frequency antigen. The antibody is made by D−/D− and similar phenotypes.
**Low incidence antigen expressed by $\bar{\bar{R}}^N$ and DBT phenotypes.
***Original described on R_0Har phenotype but also found on $\bar{\bar{R}}^N$, D^{VIa}(C)−, R_0^{JoH}, R_1^{Lisa}.
****Low frequency antigen on D(C)(E) cell.

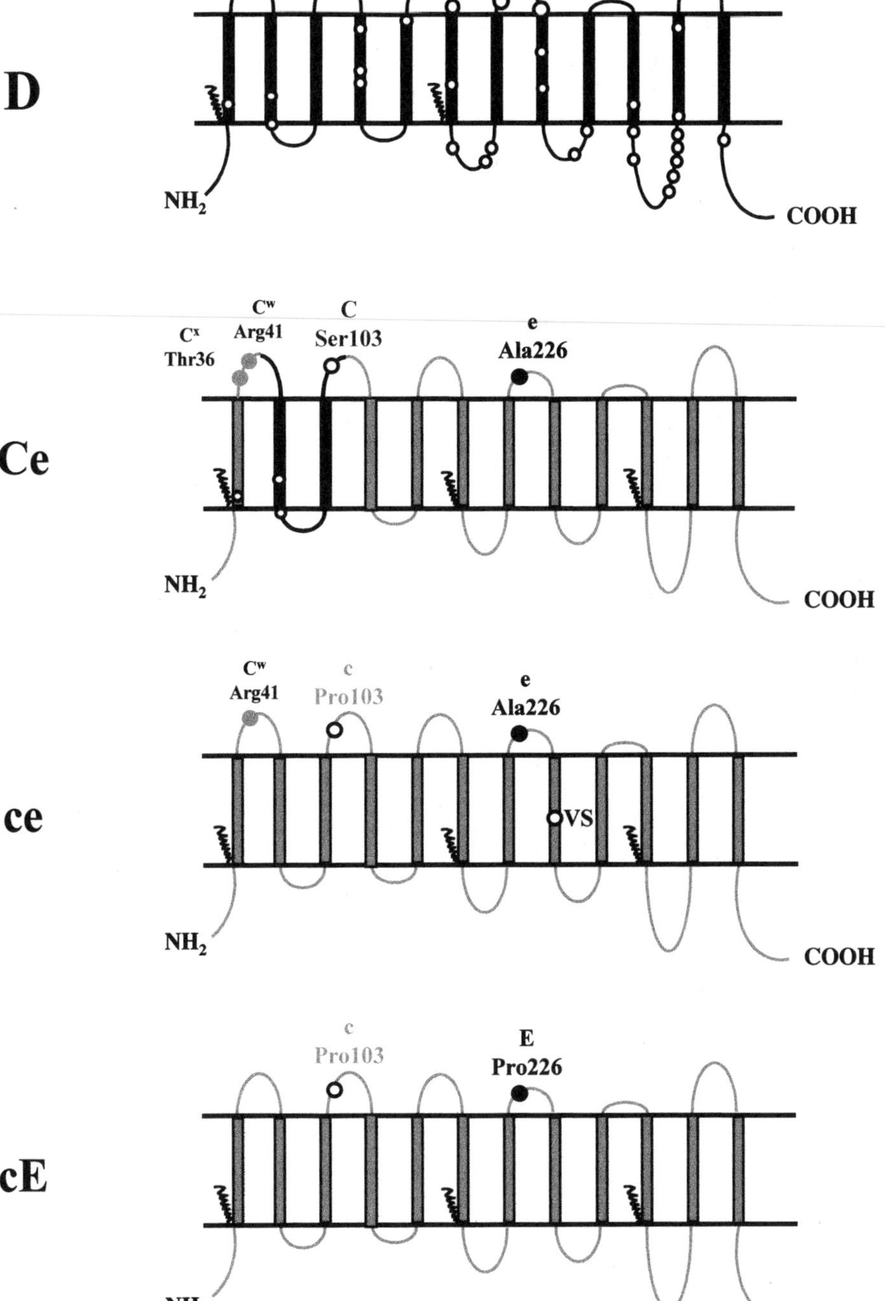

FIGURE 9.1. Predicted membrane topology of D and the major CE proteins. The amino and carboxy termini are cytoplasmic and the proteins are predicted to transverse the membrane 12 times. The location of the amino acid residues that differ between D and CE are represented by open circles, only nine of which are predicted to be extracellular. The C/c (Ser103Pro) located on the second extracellular loop and the e/E (Ala226Pro) polymorphism on the fourth extracellular loop are shown. The shared exon 2 between D and Ce, responsible for expression of the G antigen, is shown in black. Amino acid changes responsible for C^X and C^W are located on the first extracellular loop of Ce and Ce or ce, respectively, and the VS antigen, common in blacks, is located in the eighth transmembrane domain of ce. The zigzag line represents covalent linkage to fatty acid in the lipid bilayer.

positive individuals have both genes, while most Rh-negative individuals have only the *RHCE* gene (see below).

RhD and RhCE are 417-amino acid, nonglycosylated proteins. One protein carries the D antigen, and the other carries various combinations of the CE antigens (ce, cE, Ce, or CE). RhD differs from RhCE by 32 to 35 amino acids, depending on which form of RhCE is present (Fig. 9.1) (11–14). This degree of difference may explain why D is the most immunogenic of all the blood group proteins, because most other blood group antigen polymorphisms result from single amino acid changes in the respective protein. The Rh proteins migrate in sodium dodecyl sulphate-polyacrylamide (SDS-PAGE) gels with an approximate M_r of 30 to 32 kd and hence are often referred to as the Rh30 proteins. They are predicted to span the membrane twelve times and are covalently linked to fatty acids (palmitate) in the lipid bilayer (Fig. 9.1) (15).

Molecular Basis for Antigen Expression

D Antigen

"Rh-positive" and "Rh-negative" refer to the presence or absence of the D antigen, respectively. The Rh-negative phenotype occurs in 15% to 17% of whites, but is not as common in other ethnic populations (4). The absence of D in people of European descent was caused by a complete deletion of the *RHD* gene (16) and probably occurred on a Dce (R_o) haplotype because the allele most often carried with the deletion is *ce*. In contrast, inactive or silent *RHD* rather than a complete gene deletion causes D-negative phenotypes in Asians or Africans. D-negative phenotypes in Asians occur with a frequency of <1% (4), and most carry mutant *RHD* genes associated with *Ce*, indicating that they probably originated on a DCe (R_1) haplotype. Only 3% to 7% of South African blacks are D-negative, but 66% have *RHD* genes that contain a 37-bp internal duplication, which results in a premature stop codon. The 37-bp insert *RHD*-pseudogene was also found in 24% of D-negative African-Americans. Additionally, 15% of D-negative phenotypes in Africans result from a hybrid *RHD-CE-D*[s] gene characterized by expression of VS, weak C and e, and no D antigen. In total, only 18% of D-negative Africans and 54% of D-negative African-Americans completely lack *RHD* (17). This is important when designing polymerase chain reaction (PCR) -based methods to predict the D status of the fetus and the possibility of HDN. The population being tested and the different molecular events responsible for D-negative phenotypes must be considered. Even among D-negative whites, rare cases of an *RHD* gene that is not expressed because of a premature stop codon, a 4-bp insertion at the intron 3/exon 4 junction, or a gross deletion of *RHD* exons 2 to 9 have been reported (18). All were associated with the infrequent CCee (r′r′) haplotype.

Weak D

An estimated 0.2% to 1% of whites (and a greater number of blacks) have reduced expression of the D antigen (5), which is characterized serologically as failure of such RBCs to agglutinate directly with anti-D typing reagents and requiring the use of the indirect antiglobulin test for detection. The molecular basis of weak-D expression is heterogeneous and has been associated with the presence of various point mutations in *RHD*. The mutations cause amino acid changes predicted to be intracellular or in the transmembrane regions of RhD rather than on the outer surface of the RBC (Fig. 9.2) (19). This suggests that these mutations affect the efficiency of insertion, and therefore the quantity, of protein in the membrane, but do not affect the expression of D epitopes. This explains why individuals with a weak-D phenotype can safely receive D-positive blood and do not make anti-D.

It is important that donor center typing procedures detect and label weak-D RBCs as D-positive, because they can stimulate D-negative recipients. However, weak-D typing is not required for transfusion recipients, who would then receive D-negative units without untoward effects.

A very weak form of D (D_{el}), detected by absorption and elution of anti-D, has a high incidence in Hong Kong Chinese and Japanese and results from a deletion of exon 9 of *RHD* (18).

Partial D

The D antigen has long been described as a "mosaic" based on the observation that some Rh-positive individuals make alloanti-D when exposed to normal D antigen. It was hypothesized that the RBCs of these individuals lack some part of D and that they can produce antibodies to the missing portion. Molecular analysis has shown that this is correct, but what was not predicted is that the missing portions of *RHD* are replaced by corresponding portions of *RHCE* in the great majority of cases (Fig. 9.3) (18,20). The novel sequences of amino acids and the conformational changes that result from segments of RhD joined to segments of RhCE can generate new antigens (e.g., Go^a, Evans, D^w, BARC, FPTT, Rh32) (Fig. 9.3 and Table 9.2). The replacements are due to gene conversion, the hallmark being that the donor gene is unchanged. Some replacements involve single exons (e.g., D^{IIIb}, D^{IIIc}) or multiple exons (e.g., D^{IVb}, D^{VI},

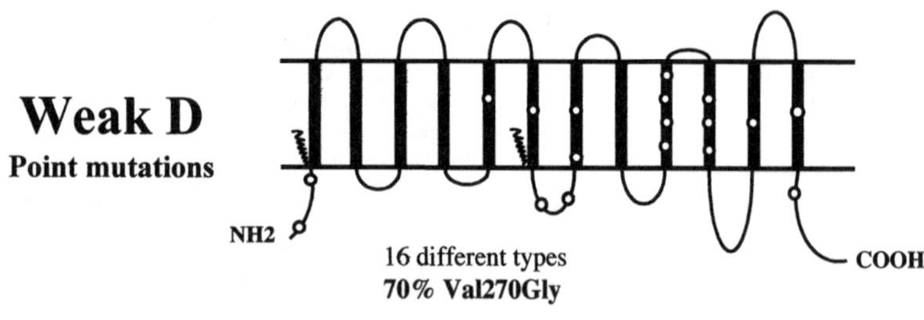

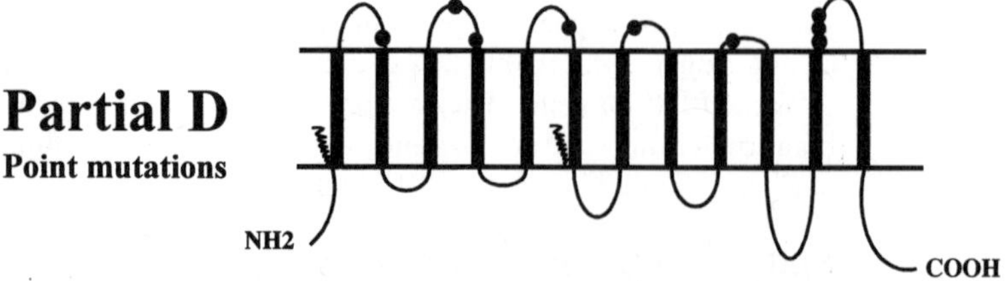

FIGURE 9.2. Predicted location of point mutations that cause weak D compared to those that cause partial-D phenotypes. Weak D carry mutations in *RHD* that primarily cause amino acid changes predicted to be intracellular or in the less conserved transmembrane regions of D (*upper panel*). Some partial D's carry mutations in *RHD* predicted to be located on extracellular loops of D (*lower panel*). These individuals can recognize conventional D as foreign.

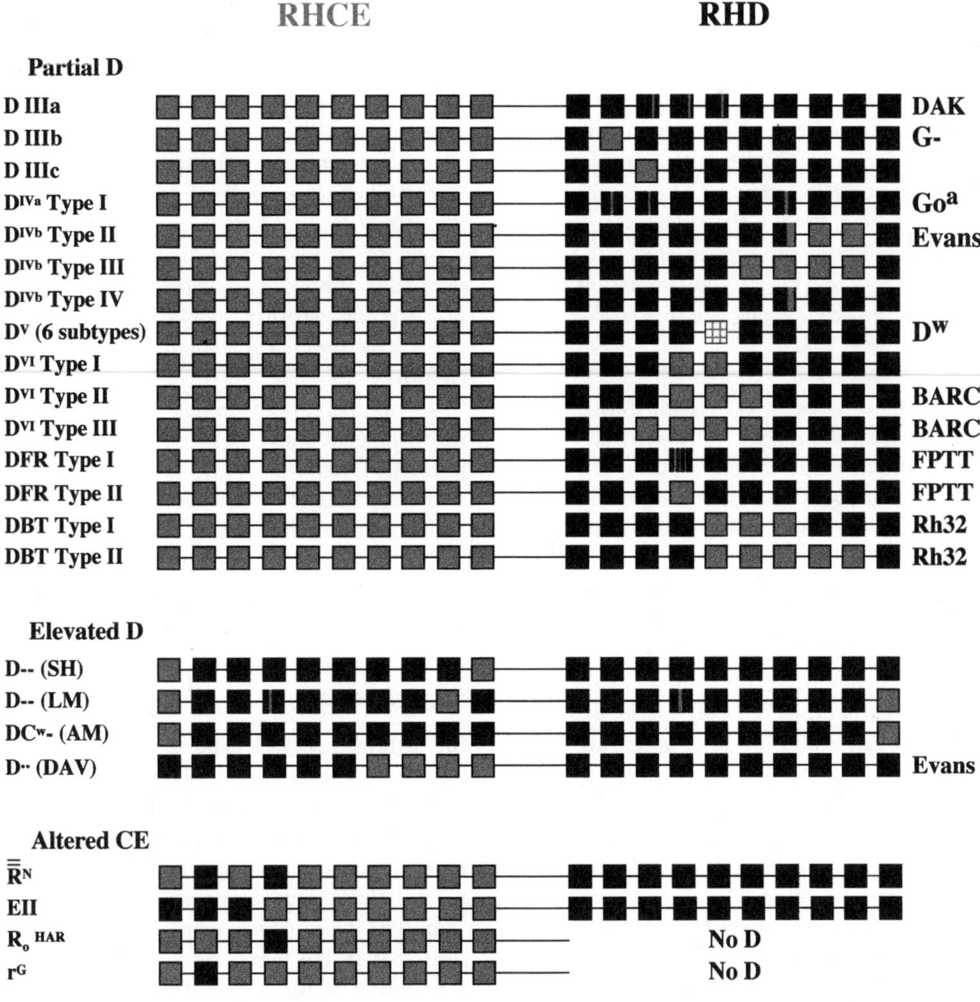

FIGURE 9.3. Gene conversion events between *RHCE* and *RHD* produce chimeric Rh proteins. Gray (RHCE) and black boxes (RHD) represent the 10 exons that encode Rh polypeptides. Gene conversion events involve amino acids (*vertical bars*) or whole exons (*filled boxes*). Replacement of portions of *RHD* by *RHCE* (*upper panel*) causes many of the partial-D phenotypes, some of which are shown here. Replacement of portions of *RHCE* by *RHD* cause elevated D phenotypes with concurrent loss of expression of CE antigens (*middle panel*) or altered CE expression (*lower panel*).

DBT), while others involve short stretches of amino acids (e.g., D^{IVb} Type IV, DFR Type I) (Fig. 9.3). Some also result from only single amino acid changes (e.g., DMH, DFW, D^{II}) (Fig.9.2). In contrast to the single amino acid changes that cause weak D (above), which are predicted to be cytoplasmic or transmembrane in location, those that cause partial-D phenotypes are predicted to be located on the extracellular loops of the protein (Fig 9.2). The extracellular location of the changes explains why these individuals recognize conventional D as foreign. From a clinical standpoint, individuals with partial-D antigens ideally should receive D-negative blood, but in practice most will type as D-positive (especially if a weak-D test is performed) and will only be recognized after they have made anti-D following a transfusion with D-positive cells.

Elevated D

Several phenotypes, including D− −, Dc−, and DC^{w}−, have an enhanced expression of D antigen and no, weak, or variant CE antigens, respectively (5). These phenotypes are analogous to the partial D rearrangements described above, only they involve the opposite situation, that is, replacement of portions of *RHCE* by *RHD* (Fig. 9.3). The additional *RHD* sequences in *RHCE* along with a normal *RHD* may explain the enhanced D and account for the reduced or missing CE antigens. Although these represent altered *RHCE* genes (see below), they are included here because of their elevated D phenotype. Individuals with such altered CE phenotypes can make anti-Rh17 when immunized.

C/c and E/e Antigens

The four major forms of the *RHCE* gene encode four different proteins: RhCe, -ce, -cE and -CE (Fig. 9.1) (11). C versus c differ by four amino acids: Cys16Trp encoded by exon 1, and Ile60Leu, Ser68Asn, and Ser103Pro encoded by exon 2 (Fig. 9.1, *open circles*). Of those four amino acids, only the residue at

103 is predicted to be extracellular and is located on the second loop of CE. Interestingly, all the amino acids encoded by exon 2 of *RHCe* are identical to those encoded by exon 2 of *RHD* (Fig. 9.1, *black*). This suggests that *RHCe* arose from the transfer of exon 2 from an *RHD* into an *RHce* gene. The sharing of exon 2-encoded amino acids by *D* and *Ce* alleles accounts for the expression of the G antigen on RBCs that are D or C positive. E and e differ by one amino acid, Pro226Ala, predicted to reside on the fourth extracellular loop of the protein (Fig. 9.1, *solid circle*). The E antigen arose from a single point mutation that occurred in exon 5 of a *RHce* gene, giving rise to *RHcE*.

Altered CE

C^W and C^X are low-incidence antigens that result from single amino acid changes (Gln41Arg and Ala36Thr, respectively) predicted to be located on the first extracellular loop of CE (Fig. 9.1, *gray circles*) (21). These antigens are more common in Finns (4%), and are most often present on Ce. C^w is also associated with the deletion phenotype DC^w-.

V and VS antigens, which are expressed on RBCs of more than 30% of blacks, result from a Leu245Val substitution located in the predicted eighth transmembrane segment of ce (Fig. 9.1) (22). The V−VS+ phenotype results from a Gly336Cys change on the 245Val background (23). Many blacks that are V+ and VS+ have weakened expression of e, indicating that Leu245Val probably causes a local conformation change on the fourth extracellular loop where the e-specific amino acid resides.

Most individuals have e-positive RBCs, but the e antigen has been considered to be second in complexity to D because variant expression has frequently been observed (24). The e antigen is altered in several phenotypes that are known to carry hybrids of *RHCE* that contain portions of *RHD* (R^N, R_0^{Har}, r^G, r'^s or e^s, e^u) (Fig. 9.3) (20). Extensive discussion is beyond the scope of this chapter, but several deserve mention because they are not uncommon in certain ethnic groups. When encountered in a donor center or by a transfusion service, they often appear as discrepant typing results when compared to previous records. R^N RBCs are found in people of African origin, result from the inheritance of an altered *RHCe* (Fig. 9.3), and carry weak expression of C and e. These RBCs were often typed as e-negative with polyclonal reagents but are e-positive with some monoclonal anti-e (25). D^{HAR} (R_o^{Har}) are found in individuals of German ancestry, carry weak or altered e, but are more notable for their D typing. They have been found more frequently since implementation of monoclonal anti-D reagent blends for routine typing, and present as having been classified as D-negative (including weak-D–negative) with polyclonal anti-D, but type as D-positive with monoclonal anti-D reagents (even without a weak-D test) (26). These individuals have only one D-specific exon (exon 4) and would be better served to be treated as D-negative for transfusion and should receive Rh immune globulin prophylaxis when indicated.

Altered expression of e also results from loss of the codon for Arg229 (18). Altered e has also been shown to be associated with the presence of a 16Cys residue in ce and to occur frequently on the R_0 haplotype, which is common in blacks (27).

E variants are not common and included EI, EII, and EIII, which result from a point mutation (EI) or gene conversion replacement of RhcE amino acids with RhD residues (EII and EIII) with concurrent loss of some E epitope expression. Category EIV RBCs, which have an amino acid substitution in an intracellular domain, do not lack E epitopes but have reduced E expression (28).

Variants of c are infrequent. The very rare RH:-26 results from a Gly96Ser transmembrane amino acid change which abolishes Rh 26 and weakens c expression (29). The lack of c antigen variants in humans compared to the other Rh antigens, and the preservation of expression of c on the RBCs of nonhuman primates suggests that the two proline residues involved form a stable structure that is resistant to perturbations and changes in ce (30).

In summary, point mutations and genetic exchange, mainly involving gene conversion events between *RHD* and *RHCE,* are primarily responsible for the large number of Rh antigens. Additional complexity results because many of the Rh epitopes are highly conformational and single amino acid changes in one part of the protein, including changes within the transmembrane regions, can affect the expression of cell-surface–exposed antigen epitopes.

Rh_{null} Phenotype

Rh_{null} individuals lack expression of all Rh antigens. They suffer from a compensated hemolytic anemia, have variable degrees of spherocytosis, stomatocytosis, and increased RBC osmotic fragility (31). The phenotype is rare and occurs on two different genetic backgrounds: the "regulator" type, caused by a gene at an unlinked locus (previously referred to as X^0r), and the "amorph" type, which maps to the RH locus (6). It is now clear that in the more common, regulator type of Rh_{null}, the suppression of Rh is caused by a lack of, or a mutant, RhAG (Rh50) protein (32). RhAG (Rh-associated glycoprotein) is a 409-amino acid glycosylated protein that coprecipitates with the Rh30 proteins (D and CE) and is often called Rh50 to reflect its apparent molecular weight (33). RhAG shares 37% amino acid identity with the Rh30 proteins and has the same predicted membrane topology. RhAG is not polymorphic, does not carry Rh antigens, but is important for targeting the Rh proteins to the membrane during erythroid development. RhAG has one N-glycan chain that carries ABO and Ii specificities (34). It is encoded by a single gene, *RHAG,* located at chromosome 6p11-21.1 (33).

The amorph type of Rh_{null} results from mutations in *RHCE* on a D-negative background (35). Amorph-type RBCs express no Rh protein and have reduced amounts (~20%) of RhAG.

Rh-membrane Complex

Additional complexity in Rh protein structure arises because they exist in the RBC membrane as a complex with several other proteins. Rh and RhAG are associated in the membrane, possibly as a tetramer consisting of two molecules of each as a core complex (36). That several other proteins interact with the Rh-core complex come from observations on Rh_{null} cells (18,20). These RBCs have reduced expression of CD47, an integrin-associated protein (IAP) that has wide tissue distribution, binds β_3 integrins, and is required for integrin-regulated Ca^{2+} entry into endothelial cells. Its function on the RBCs is unknown; however a role in RBC senescence has recently been suggested (37). Rh_{null} cells also have reduced glycophorin B (GPB), a sialoglycoprotein that carries S or s and U antigens. GPB appears to aid RhAG trafficking to the membrane, because the RhAG protein in GPB-deficient cells has increased glycosylation. Null cells lack LW, a glycoprotein of unknown function that belongs to the family of intercellular adhesion molecules (ICAM-4, see below). Recently, it was shown that band 3 (the anion exchanger) enhanced the expression of the Rh antigens in transfected cells, suggesting that band 3 may also be associated with the Rh–core complex as well (38). The complex may also be associated with the membrane skeleton, but the molecules to which it may connect are not known.

Rh Function

Clues to the function of Rh proteins come from analysis of their predicted membrane-spanning structure, which suggests a role as putative transporters (39). In particular, amino acid sequence analysis links them to the family of ammonium (NH_4^+) transporters present in bacteria, fungi, and plants (40). A relationship to the ammonium transporters from yeast has recently been verified (41), and direct evidence for transport of amonium ions has recently been shown (62). Functional studies have been hampered by difficulties in obtaining high levels of heterologous expression of the Rh-erythroid proteins. Recently, two nonerythroid Rh homologs were revealed in expressed sequence tag (EST) database searches and were found to be expressed in kidney, testis, and brain (RhCG) and in kidney and liver (RhBG) (42,43). These nonerythroid Rh family members share 56% amino acid identity with each other and 30% to 51% with erythroid Rh and RhAG, and have the same predicted 12-transmembrane spanning structure. The discovery that homologs of the erythrocyte Rh proteins are present in the kidney and liver supports their possible function in transport and homeostasis and expands the Rh family of proteins beyond the RBC. Additionally, Rh-related proteins are also present in the worm *(C. elegans),* the fruit fly *(Drosophila),* the sponge *(Geodia),* the slime mold *(Dictyostelium),* and the frog *(Xenopus)* (18). The evolutionary conservation of Rh proteins suggests that they perform an important function in many different organisms.

Immune Response to Rh

Medical Aspects

Human RBCs can express more than 400 different blood group antigens. Typing patient and donor cells for every known antigen with the intention of providing perfectly matched blood would be a practical and fiscal impossibility. Fortunately, such extensive testing is not required for a number of reasons, the most important of which is that exposure to the majority of foreign RBC antigens through transfusion does not lead to the production of clinically-significant alloantibodies. The D antigen is one notable exception. As many as 80% of D-negative patients exposed to D-positive RBCs may develop high-titer, high-affinity, anti-D IgG antibodies that may persist for the rest of their lives even if they are never exposed to the antigen again. The resulting antibodies can cause hemolytic transfusion reactions (HTRs) and can cross the placenta causing HDN when present in an D-negative pregnant individual carrying a D-positive fetus. Therefore, because of its extraordinary immunogenicity and clinical significance, the D antigen is the only blood group antigen for which it is routine to prophylactically match blood prior to transfusion. Although antibodies to C, c, E, and e can cause HTRs and HDN, they are much less immunogenic than D (~1% rate of sensitization) and the use of RBCs lacking one or more of those antigens are indicated only after sensitization has occurred.

In practice, D-positive patients can be transfused with either D-positive or D-negative RBCs—the absence of D will cause no harm—but it is deemed prudent to reserve the rarer units of D-negative blood (~15% of donor units) for D-negative individuals who must receive them. In cases of trauma and/or massive transfusion in which the patient's D-status is unknown, efforts are made to provide D-negative blood until the appropriate testing can be completed. When D-negative blood is in short supply, it may be necessary to transfuse D-negative patients with D-positive units. In such scenarios, D-negative units are reserved for women of child-bearing age and for patients whose serum contains anti-D from a previous sensitization.

Unlike a number of other blood group antigens which are expressed by all transfused blood cells including platelets, the D antigen is present only on RBCs. Theoretically, the selection of platelet units for transfusion should be independent of the D-status of the donor. However, a transfusion of pooled platelet concentrates may introduce as much as 5 milliliters of donor RBCs, which may be sufficient to alloimmunize a D-negative patient. Therefore, the standard of care is to avoid transfusing D-negative patients, particularly women of child-bearing age, with platelet units derived from D-positive donors. If such units are unavailable and platelet transfusion must be undertaken, the administration of Rh(D) immune globulin (RhIg) can be considered. A standard 300-μg dose of RhIg, which may inhibit the immunizing potential of up to 15 milliliters of D-positive RBCs, would therefore neutralize the effects of D-positive cells from several mismatched platelet transfusions. With respect to the transfusion of plasma products, the D status of the donor is not an issue because they do not contain cellular or soluble material capable of inducing anti-D immune responses.

Serologic Aspects

The immune response to Rh, like that to other peptide antigens, is typically thymus-dependent, requiring T-cell help. Upon exposure to a foreign Rh antigen, an IgM response may develop, but this is quickly followed by the production of IgG antibodies. Consequently, nearly all examples of Rh antibodies are IgG molecules (mostly IgG_1 and IgG_3), which bind optimally to RBCs at 37°C and require the addition of an antiglobulin reagent to produce hemagglutination. Although IgG_1 and IgG_3 subclasses classically initiate complement activation, the vast majority of anti-Rh–containing sera do not do so. The usual explanation for this cites the relatively low copy number of Rh antigens per

RBC, which results in Rh molecules situated too far apart on the RBC surface to permit the simultaneous binding of C1q by multiple anti-Rh IgG. Therefore, hemolysis from the transfusion of Rh-incompatible RBCs is generally extravascular due to phagocytosis of IgG-coated erythrocytes by cells of the reticuloendothelial system.

After anti-D, the Rh antibodies most commonly found in the sera of alloimmunized individuals are anti-E > anti-c > anti-e > anti-C. In approximately 50% of cases of warm-type autoimmune hemolytic anemia (WAIHA), autoantibodies are believed to be directed to Rh antigens by virtue of their "panreactivity" with all RBC phenotypes except Rh_{null} cells. However, direct binding of autoantibodies to putative epitopes common to D and C/E polypeptides or to other components of the Rh-membrane complex (Rh50, CD47, etc.) has yet to be demonstrated in WAIHA. The difficulties in approaching this problem are largely technical in nature and relate to both the inability to produce workable quantities of pure patient autoantibody in vitro (i.e., clone the autoantibody-producing B lymphocytes) and the inability to purify Rh proteins in a way that retains their native conformationally-dependent epitopes.

Molecular Aspects

The characterization of Rh antibodies on a molecular level, particularly that of anti-D, has been the focus of much study not only because of their clinical significance, but because of the need to develop suitable in vitro methods for their production. Ironically, due to better transfusion practice and the use of RhIg, alloimmunization of antigen-negative individuals is significantly less common (as are sera donors willing to be purposely hyperimmunized), so that supplies of Rh antibodies for use as typing reagents and for the preparation of RhIg are dwindling. To better understand the molecular make-up of Rh antibodies, investigations have focused on analyzing their variable regions in order to determine whether there are commonly shared genetic and/or structural features among anti-Rh antibodies made by different individuals.

Early work using rabbit antisera specific for different human heavy chain–variable region gene products suggested a restriction in the use of certain heavy chain gene families by the anti-D contained in polyclonal sera from several dozen anti-D donors (44). Subsequent studies with rodent antiidiotypic antibodies demonstrated cross-reactive idiotypes among polyclonal anti-D preparations (45,46) and among different examples of human monoclonal anti-C, -c, -D, -E, -e, and -G produced by transformed B cells (47). A more direct approach using nucleotide sequencing to examine immunoglobulin gene diversity examined a cohort of four IgM and ten IgG monoclonal anti-D variable regions (48). A restricted use of the human heavy chain variable region genes V_H3-33 and V_H4-34 was found with a shift in repertoire usage toward V_H3-33 for anti-D that had isotype switched to the more clinically relevant IgG. The restriction of anti-D heavy chains to the use of these and other highly related V_H genes has been confirmed and extended through the analysis of many additional examples of anti-D produced through both tissue culture and recombinant means (49,50). More recently, the use of molecular approaches such as site-directed mutagenesis (51) and complementarity-determining region (CDR) sequence randomization (52) has demonstrated the genetic relatedness among anti-D molecules directed against different D epitopes as well as among antibodies with anti-D and anti-E specificity. These studies have suggested that a process termed "epitope migration" (49) may play a role in the molding of the anti-Rh immune repertoire (53).

Although the precise significance of immunoglobulin germline gene restriction by anti-Rh antibodies is not fully understood, it may have practical significance for the preparation of anti-D for both therapeutic and diagnostic use. For example, the V_H genes used to encode anti-D are among the most cationic of the human germline V_H genes (54) and may account for the relatively high pI of polyclonal anti-D–containing antisera originally noted over 40 years ago (55). Although the cationic nature of the antibodies may be important for binding to D, it has also been suggested that a constitutive net-positive charge may be necessary to permeate the highly negative RBC ζ-potential, thus permitting antibody to contact antigen (56). Secondly, while IgM anti-D monoclonal antibodies are well-suited for antigen typing as they may serve as direct agglutinins, the fact that they are most often encoded by V_H4-34 (the germline gene to which cold agglutinins are also restricted) (57), may explain why many IgM monoclonal anti-D typing reagents falsely agglutinate D-negative cells when used at cooler-than-recommended temperatures. This phenomenon may also explain the body of literature claiming that the D antigen was present on numerous non-erythroid cells. Using IgM anti-D, these investigators may have been detecting the I blood group antigen.

LW BLOOD GROUP SYSTEM

History and Nomenclature

The LW antigens are the "true" Rhesus antigens shared by humans and the rhesus monkey. As discussed earlier, the confusion occurred because LW antigens are more abundant on D-positive than on D-negative RBCs. When the situation was clarified, the term "Rh" remained associated with the human antigen, so the real Rhesus antigen was renamed LW in honor of Landsteiner and Wiener (6). The confusion can be understood today in the transfusion service when a weak example of anti-LW^a often appears initially to be anti-D. The LW system has undergone additional terminology revisions. The historic terminology of LW_1, LW_2, LW_3, LW_4, and LW_0 to describe phenotypes was based on both the LW and the D status of the RBCs but is now obsolete (6). The phenotypes are LW(a+b−), LW(a−b+), LW(a+b+), and the rare LW(a−b−), and the antigens are designated LW^a and LW^b and LW^{ab}.

Genes and Their Expressed Proteins

LW is encoded by a single gene located on chromosome 19. The 42-kd LW glycoprotein is a member of the family of ICAMs and has been renamed ICAM-4. LW passes through the RBC membrane once, and the N-terminal extracellular region is organized into two immunoglobulin superfamily (IgSF) domains (58).

Molecular Basis for Antigen Expression

LW^a is the common antigen while LW^b has an incidence of less than 1% in most Europeans (5). The LW^a/LW^b polymorphism is due to a single amino acid substitution, Gln70Arg, on the LW glycoprotein (59). An increased frequency of the uncommon LW^b antigen in Latvians and Lithuanians (6%), Estonians (4%), Finns (3%), and Poles (2%) suggests that the LW^b mutation originated in the people of the Baltic region. The LW^{ab} antigen was originally defined by an alloantibody made by the only known (genetically-verified) LW(a−b−) person, who lacks expression of all LW antigens (6). The *LW* gene in this rare LW(a−b−) individual has a 10-bp deletion and a premature stop codon in the first exon (60). Rh_{null} RBCs also lack LW antigens but do not have defective *LW* genes. Rh proteins appear to be required for LW to traffic to the membrane, and association with the D antigen is preferred.

LW antigens require divalent cations (e.g., Mg^{2+}) for expression and have intramolecular disulfide bonds that are sensitive to dithiothreitol (DTT) treatment (6). This is helpful to differentiate anti-LW from anti-D, because the D-antigen is resistant to DTT. Also helpful in identifying anti-LW is that LW antigens are expressed equally well on D-positive and D-negative cord blood RBCs (5).

Transient loss of RBC LW antigens has been described in pregnancy and patients with diseases, particularly Hodgkin's disease, lymphoma, leukemia, sarcoma, and other forms of malignancy. Transient loss of LW antigens is associated with the production of autoanti-LW that can appear to be alloantibody (5).

LW Function

LW glycoprotein, ICAM-4, is a ligand for the β_2 integrins LFA-1, Mac-1, CD11/CD18 (58). Its function on mature RBCs, if any, is not clear, but LW might contribute to adhesive interactions involved in the formation of erythroblastic islands and attachment to stroma cells and extracellular matrix (ECM) (61).

SUMMARY

The molecular basis for the Rh antigens has now been elucidated. A gene deletion or silent *RHD* gene explains the absence of the D antigen in Rh-negative individuals. The large number of amino acid differences between the RhD and RhCE proteins explains why exposure in an individual lacking D often results in a vigorous immune response characterized by a very heterogeneous population of antibodies. The proximity of *RHD* and *RHCE,* duplicated genes on the same chromosome, has resulted in numerous exchanges by gene conversion between them. This has generated new polymorphisms and explains the many antigens observed in this blood group system. Molecular analysis has also revealed that Rh antigen expression is affected not only by changes in extracellular amino acids, but is also significantly affected by intracellular changes, highlighting the conformational nature of these blood group antigens and complicating attempts to map the epitopes to specific amino acid residues. Anti-Rh antibodies show restriction in their use of particular variable region germline genes. Antibodies to serologically distinct epitopes may be genetically related, and epitope migration may be an important process that helps shape the composition of the anti-Rh immune repertoire. Questions remain concerning the function of the Rh proteins. The discovery that Rh protein homologs also exist in the liver and kidney indicates that the Rh blood group antigens belong to a larger, conserved family of proteins and will contribute to the elucidation of their function. Similarly, the function of LW on the mature RBC is not clear but may play a role in erythroid migration and development.

REFERENCES

1. Bowman JM. RhD hemolytic disease of the newborn. *N Engl J Med* 1998;339:1775–1777.
2. Diamond LK, Blackfan KD, Baty JM. Erythroblastosis fetalis and its association with universal edema of the fetus, icterus gravis neonatorum and anemia of the newborn. *J Pediatr* 1932;1:269–309.
3. Levine P, Burnham L, Katzin WM, et al. The role of isoimmunization in the pathogenesis of erythroblastosis fetalis. *Am J Obstet Gynecol* 1941; 42:925–937.
4. Race RR, Sanger R. *Blood groups in man,* 6th ed. Oxford, England: Blackwell Science, 1975.
5. Daniels G. *Human blood groups,* ed. Oxford: Blackwell Science, 1995.
6. Issitt PD, Anstee DJ. *Applied blood group serology,* 4th ed. Durham, NC: Montgomery Scientific Publications, 1998.
7. Tippett P. A speculative model for the Rh blood groups. *Ann Hum Genet* 1986;50:241–247.
8. Rosenfeld RE, Allen FH, Swisher SN, et al. A review of Rh serology and presentation of a new terminology. *Transfusion* 1962;2:287–312.
9. Colin Y, Cherif-Zahar B, Le Van Kim C, et al. Genetic basis of the RhD-positive and RhD-negative blood group polymorphism as determined by Southern analysis. *Blood* 1991;78:2747–2752.
10. Cherif-Zahar B, Mattei MG, Le Van Kim C, et al. Localization of the human Rh blood group gene structure to chromosome 1p34.3–1p36.1 region by in situ hybridization. *Hum Genet* 1991;86:398–400.
11. Mouro I, Colin Y, Cherif-Zahar B, et al. Molecular genetic basis of the human Rhesus blood group system. *Nat Genet* 1993;5:62–65.
12. Cherif-Zahar B, Bloy C, Le Van Kim C, et al. Molecular cloning and protein structure of a human blood group Rh polypeptide. *Proc Natl Acad Sci U S A* 1990;87:6243–6247.
13. Arce MA, Thompson ES, Wagner S, et al. Molecular cloning of RhD cDNA derived from a gene present in RhD-positive, but not RhD-negative individuals. *Blood* 1993;82:651–655.
14. Simsek S, de Jong CAM, Cuijpers HTM, et al. Sequence analysis of cDNA derived from reticulocyte mRNAs coding for Rh polypeptides and demonstration of E/e and C/c polymorphism. *Vox Sang* 1994;67: 203–209.
15. Cartron J-P, Agre P. Rh blood group antigens: protein and gene structure. *Semin Hematol* 1993;30:193–208.
16. Wagner FF, Flegel WA. RHD gene deletion occurred in the Rhesus box. *Blood* 2000;95:3662–3668.
17. Singleton BK, Green CA, Avent ND, et al. The presence of an RHD pseudogene containing a 37 base pair duplication and a nonsense mutation in Africans with the Rh D-negative blood group phenotype. *Blood* 2000;95:12–18.
18. Huang CH, Liu PZ, Chen JG. Molecular biology and genetics of the Rh blood group system. *Semin Hematol* 2000;37:150–165.
19. Wagner FF, Gassner C, Muller TH, et al. Molecular basis of weak D phenotypes. *Blood* 1999;93:385–393.
20. Avent ND, Reid ME. The Rh blood group system: a review. *Blood* 2000;95:375–387.
21. Mouro I, Colin Y, Sistonen P, et al. Molecular basis of the RhC^W (Rh8) and RhC^X (Rh9) blood group specificities. *Blood* 1995;86:1196–1201.
22. Faas BHW, Beckers EAM, Wildoer P, et al. Molecular background of VS and weak C expression in blacks. *Transfusion* 1997;37:38–44.

23. Daniels G, Faas BHW, Green CA, et al. The VS and V blood group polymorphisms in Africans: a serological and molecular analysis. *Transfusion* 1998;38:951–958.
24. Issitt PD. An invited review: the Rh antigen e, its variants, and some closely related serological observations. *Immunohematology* 1991;7: 29–36.
25. Rouillac C, Gane P, Cartron J, et al. Molecular basis of the altered antigenic expression of RhD in weak D (D^u) and RhC/e in R^N phenotypes. *Blood* 1996;87:4853–4861.
26. Beckers Ea, Faas BHW, von dem Borne AE, et al. The R_oHar Rh:33 phenotype results from substitution of exon 5 of the RHCE gene by the corresponding exon of the RHD gene. *Br J Haematol* 1996;92: 751–757.
27. Westhoff CM, Silberstein LE, Wylie DE, et al. 16Cys encoded by the RHce gene is associated with altered expression of the e antigen and is frequent in the R_o haplotype. *Br J Haematol* 2001;113:666–671.
28. Noizat-Pirenne F, Mouro I, Gane P, et al. Heterogeneity of blood group RhE variants revealed by serological analysis and molecular alteration of the RHCE gene and transcript. *Br J Haematol* 1998;103: 429–436.
29. Faas BHW, Ligthart PC, Lomas-Francis C, et al. Involvement of Gly96 in the formation of the Rh26 epitope. *Transfusion* 1997;37: 1123–1130.
30. Westhoff CM, Silberstein LE, Wylie DE. Evidence supporting the requirement for two proline residues for expression of c. *Transfusion* 2000;40:321–324.
31. Ballas S, Clark MR, Mohandas N, et al. Red cell membranes and cation deficiency in Rhnull syndrome. *Blood* 1984;63:1046–1055.
32. Cherif-Zahar B, Raynal V, Gane P, et al. Candidate gene acting as a suppressor of the RH locus in most cases of Rh-deficiency. *Nat Genet* 1996;12:168–173.
33. Ridgwell K, Spurr NK, Laguda B, et al. Isolation of cDNA clones for a 50 kDa glycoprotein of the human erythrocyte membrane associated with Rh (Rhesus) blood-group antigen expression. *Biochem J* 1992; 287:223–228.
34. Moore S, Green C. The identification of specific Rhesus polypeptide blood group ABH-active glycoprotein complexes in the human red cell membrane. *Biochem J* 1987;244:735–741.
35. Huang CH, Chen Y, Reid ME, et al. Rhnull disease: the amorph type results from a novel double mutation in RhCe gene on D-negative background. *Blood* 1998;92:664–671.
36. Ridgwell K, Eyers SAC, Mawby WJ, et al. Studies on the glycoprotein associated with Rh (Rhesus) blood group antigen expression in the human red blood cell membrane. *J Biol Chem* 1994;269:6410–6416.
37. Oldenborg P-A, Zheleznyak A, Fang Y-F, et al. Role of CD47 as a marker of self on red blood cells. *Science* 2000;288:2051–2053.
38. Beckmann R, Smythe JS, Anstee DJ, et al. Functional cell surface expression of band 3, the human red blood cell anion exchange protein (AE1) in K562 erythroleukemia cells: band 3 enhances the cell surface reactivity of Rh antigens. *Blood* 1998;92:4428–4438.
39. Henderson PJF. The 12-transmembrane helix transporters. *Curr Opin Cell Biol* 1993;5:708–721.
40. Marini A-M, Urrestarazu A, Beauwens R, et al. The Rh (Rhesus) blood group polypeptides are related to NH_4^+ transporters. *Trends Biochem Sci* 1997;22:460–461.
41. Marini AM, Matassi G, Raynal V, et al. The human Rhesus-associated RhAG protein and a kidney homologue promote ammonium transport in yeast. *Nat Genet* 2000;26:341–344.
42. Liu Z, Chen Y, Mo R, et al. Characterization of human RhCG and mouse Rhcg as novel nonerythroid Rh glycoprotein homologues predominantly expressed in kidney and testis. *J Biol Chem* 2000;275: 25641–25651.
43. Liu Z, Peng J, Mo R, et al. Rh type B glycoprotein is a new member of the Rh superfamily and a putative ammonia transporter in mammals. *J Biol Chem* 2001;276:1424–1433.
44. Natvig JB, Forre O, Michaelsen TE. Restriction of human immune antibodies to heavy-chain variable subgroups. *Scand J Immunol* 1976; 5:667–675.
45. Natvig JB, Kunkel HG, Rosenfield RE, et al. Idiotypic specificities of anti-Rh antibodies. *J Immunol* 1976;116:1536–1538.
46. Forre O, Natvig JB, Michaelsen TE. Cross-idiotypic reactions among anti-Rh(D) antibodies. *Scand J Immunol* 1977;6:997–1003.
47. Thompson KM, Sutherland J, Barden G, et al. Human monoclonal antibodies against blood group antigens preferentially express a V_H4-21 variable region gene-associated epitope. *Scand J Immunol* 1991;34: 509–518.
48. Bye JM, Carter C, Cui Y, et al. Germline variable region gene segment derivation of human monoclonal anti-Rh(D) antibodies. *J Clin Invest* 1992;90:2481–2490.
49. Chang TY, Siegel DL. Genetic and immunological properties of phage-displayed human anti-Rh(D) antibodies: Implications for Rh(D) epitope topology. *Blood* 1998;91:3066–3078.
50. Siegel D. Research and clinical applications of antibody phage display in transfusion medicine. *Transfus Med Rev* 2001;15:35–52.
51. Siegel DL, Chang TY. Epitope migration: Anti-Rh(D) antibodies as a model for human immunogenicity. *Blood* 1998;92:671a.
52. Hughes-Jones NC, Bye JM, Gorick BD, et al. Synthesis of Rh Fv phage-antibodies using VH and VL germline genes. *Br J Haematol* 1999;105:811–816.
53. Chang T. Towards a quantitative model of immunogenicity: counting pathways in sequence space. *J Theor Biol* 2000;206:255–278.
54. Boucher G, Broly H, Lemieux R. Restricted use of cationic germline V_H gene segments in human Rh(D) red cell antibodies. *Blood* 1997; 89:3277–3286.
55. Abelson N, Rawson A. Studies of blood group antibodies. II. Fractionation of Rh antibodies by anion-cation cellulose exchange chromatography. *J Immunol* 1959;83:49–56.
56. Mollison PL, Engelfreit CP, Contreras M. *Blood transfusion in clinical medicine,* 10th ed. Oxford: Blackwell Science, 1997.
57. Siegel DL, Silberstein LE. Structural analyses of red cell autoantibodies. In Garratty G, ed: *Immunobiology of transfusion medicine.* New York: Dekker, 1994;387–399.
58. Bailly P, Tontti E, Hermand P, et al. The red cell LW blood group protein is an intercellular adhesion molecule which binds to CD11/ CD18 leukocyte integrins. *J Immunol* 1995;25:3316–3320.
59. Hermand P, Gane P, Mattei MG, et al. Molecular basis and expression of the LWa/LWb blood group polymorphism. *Blood* 1995;86: 1590–1594.
60. Hermand P, Le Pennec PY, Rouger P, et al. Characterization of the gene encoding the human LW blood group protein in LW+ and LW− phenotypes. *Blood* 1996;87:2962–2967.
61. Bony V, Gane P, Bailly P, et al. Time-course expression of polypeptides carrying blood group antigens during human erythroid differentiation. *Br J Haematol* 1999;107:263–274.
62. Westhoff CM, Ferrari-Jacobic M, Fuskett JK. Functional expression of Rh-glycoprotein (RhAG) in xeropus oocytes. *Transfusion* 2001;41: 15A.

Rossi's Principles of Transfusion Medicine, Third Edition, edited by Toby L. Simon, Walter H. Dzik, Edward L. Snyder, Christopher P. Stowell, and Ronald G. Strauss. Lippincott Williams & Wilkins, Philadelphia © 2002.

CASE 9A

WHO'S MY DADDY?

CASE HISTORY

A 28-year-old gravida-5, para-4 woman from a small town in Morocco came to the United States for management of her pregnancy after having lost one infant to hemolytic disease of the newborn. Upon arrival at the high-risk obstetrics clinic, she was at approximately 14 weeks of gestation by dates. According to the patient, her first child was Rh(D)-positive, and the second was Rh(D)-negative. The third infant, who was Rh(D)-positive, was extremely anemic and jaundiced at birth, while the fourth infant was stillborn with hydrops fetalis. The patient denied any history of transfusion and had never sustained surgery or trauma. She also had never received Rh immune globulin. A specimen sent to the blood bank showed the woman to be group O, rr (C−, c+, D−, E−, e+), with a positive antibody screen. The antibody identification panel was consistent with anti-D plus anti-C and the titres were 1:16 and 1:8, respectively, at antiglobulin phase. A specimen from the husband was also sent, and he was found to be group A, and a probable R_2r (C−, c+, D+, E+, e+).

The obstetrician reviewed the results and called a transfusion medicine physician, somewhat confused about the finding of an anti-C in the mother but the absence of the C antigen in the father (according to the patient) of all of her children. To this alert obstetrician, the serologic findings raised the possibility of nonpaternity in a couple who, from all appearances, were strictly observant of the cultural and religious mores of their society. The transfusion medicine physician reviewed the serologic testing on the patient and her husband and suggested to the obstetrician that the patient had anti-G and possibly anti-D. The obstetrician then wanted to know if Rh immune globulin would be helpful.

DISCUSSION

The G antigen is found on all red blood cells which are either D(+) or C(+), with only very rare exceptions. The *RHCe* gene probably arose from the transfer of exon 2 of the *RHD* gene into an *RHce* allele, hence the shared amino acid sequence on Ce and D proteins which express the G antigen (Fig. 9.1). Anti-G will therefore bind to red blood cells bearing either the D or the C antigen because both also carry the G antigen. As a result, it is impossible to distinguish between anti-G (with or without anti-D or anti-C) and anti-D plus anti-C using routine antibody identification panels. There is a very rare phenotype which expresses G but not D or C (r^Gr) and which can be used to differentiate anti-G from the others, but such cells are not available for routine serologic testing. In addition, some r^G express a "C-like" antigen which reacts with some anti-C. The reactions of anti-G, anti-C, and anti-D with representative panel cells are shown in Table 9A.1.

Because very few laboratories have access to such rare cells, the more commonly used approach to distinguish between anti-G and anti-D plus anti-C is to use a series of adsorption/elution steps (1) which are shown in Table 9A.2. The alloantibodies in question are first adsorbed onto a cell which is D(+) but C(−), for example, R_0R_0. Anti-D or anti-G would bind to this cell, but anti-C would not and would be left in the supernatant. The bound alloantibodies are then eluted off and the eluate is adsorbed against cells which are D(−) C(+), for example, r′r′. Anti-D obviously would not be adsorbed by these cells, although anti-G would be. The eluate from these adsorbing cells is then tested against R_0R_0 and r′r′ cells. Anti-D and anti-C will have been winnowed out leaving only anti-G.

Although the identification of an anti-G would help to re-

TABLE 9A.1. REACTIONS OF RH ALLOANTIBODIES WITH SELECTED CELLS

		Alloantibodies			
Cell	Antigens Present	Anti-C	Anti-D	Anti-C + Anti-D	Anti-G
R_1R_1	C D G e	+	+	+	+
r′r′	C − G e	+	−	+	+
R_0R_0	c D G e	−	+	+	+
r^Gr	c − G e	−	−	−	+
rr	c − − e	−	−	−	−

TABLE 9A.2. ADSORPTION ELUTION PROCEDURES TO DISTINGUISH AMONG Rh ALLOANTIBODIES

		Plasma Containing:			
Adsorbing Cells (Antigens)	**Fraction**	**Anti-D Anti-C**	**Anti-D Anti-C Anti-G**	**Anti-D Anti-G**	**Anti-C Anti-G**
R_0R_0 (c D G e)	Supernatant	Anti-C	Anti-C	—	Anti-C
	Eluate	Anti-D	Anti-D Anti-G	Anti-D Anti-G	Anti-G
r′r′ (C − G e)	Supernatant	Anti-D	Anti-D	Anti-D	—
	Eluate	—	Anti-G	Anti-G	Anti-G

solve the paternity issue in this case, it is much more important to establish whether or not the patient has anti-D for the purposes of both prognosis and management. Hemolytic disease of the newborn is much more severe with anti-D than with anti-C, while anti-G is rarely found in high titre and is unlikely to cause serious disease. Hence the prognosis is quite different for a patient with anti-D plus anti-C or anti-G, and one with anti-C plus anti-G. It is also important to make these distinctions in order to decide whether or not to offer Rh immune globulin prophylaxis. Although anti-G is usually accompanied by anti-D, several examples of sensitized D(−) pregnant women with anti-G plus anti-C have been described (2,3). Such women should receive Rh immune globulin because it will prevent D alloimmunization and its consequences.

In this case, the husband is clearly heterozygous for D (one child was reported to be Rh(D)-negative), hence the desirability to establish the red blood cell phenotype for the fetus early in pregnancy. The finding that the fetus expresses the target antigen commits the patient and her obstetrician to close monitoring of the pregnancy including invasive procedures, such as percutaneous umbilical blood sampling and amniocentesis, which carry low but real risks to the fetus. There have been several reports in recent years of the use of amplification techniques to detect fetal DNA in the maternal circulation and determine whether or not the fetus carries the RHD gene (4). Although not yet generally available, such techniques offer a minimally invasive assessment of the red blood cell genotype of the fetus and its risk of hemolytic disease of the newborn.

CODA

The patient's plasma was adsorbed and eluted as described and found to contain anti-D and anti-G, but not anti-C, consistent with exposure to the R_2 haplotype inherited by several of the children from her husband. The finding of anti-D also correlated with the clinical picture of severe hemolytic disease of the newborn. Because the patient had already been alloimmunized to D, Rh immune globulin offered no benefit and was not recommended.

Maternal alloantibody titres were performed biweekly over the ensuing 6 weeks but did not change, and ultrasound examinations were unremarkable. At almost 20 weeks of gestation, percutaneous umbilical blood sampling was performed. The fetal red blood cells were found to be group A and RhD(−) (rr). The patient returned to Morocco and was delivered of a healthy girl at 38 weeks of gestation.

Case contributed by Christopher P. Stowell, M.D., Ph.D., Massachusetts General Hospital, Boston, MA.

REFERENCES

1. Issit PD. *Applied blood group serology,* 4th ed. Miami: Montgomery Scientific Publications, 1998:350–352.
2. Shirey RS, Mirabella DC, Lumadue JA, et al. Differentiation of anti-D, -C, and -G: clinical relevance in alloimmunized pregnancies. *Transfusion* 1997;37:493–496.
3. Palfi M, Gunnarsson C. The frequency of anti-C + anti-G in the absence of anti-D in alloimmunized pregnancies. *Transfus Med* 2001;11: 207–210.
4. Lo YM, Hjelm NM, Fidlar C, et al. Prenatal diagnosis of fetal RhD status by molecular analysis of maternal plasma. *N Engl J Med* 1998; 339:1734–1738.

10

OTHER PROTEIN BLOOD GROUP ANTIGENS

PETR JAROLIM

Antigens of only five of the 25 currently known blood group systems are formed by carbohydrates. Antigens of the remaining 20 blood group systems are carried by proteins. Two of these twenty systems, the most important, Rh (ISBT 004), and the closely associated LW (ISBT 016) blood group systems, were discussed in detail in the previous chapter. The remaining 18 systems are summarized in Table 10.1.

Many of the proteins carrying blood group antigens are functionally important, however, antibodies in only a few blood group systems represent a problem for the transfusion service. We discuss here in greater detail only those antigens that elicit formation of clinically significant antibodies and briefly comment on the other blood group systems. Further details may be found in review articles (1–4) and comprehensive textbooks (5–7).

P. Jarolim: Department of Pathology, Brigham and Women's Hospital, Harvard Medical School, Boston, Massachusetts, and Institute of Hematology and Blood Transfusion, Prague, Czech Republic.

KELL AND KX BLOOD GROUP SYSTEMS (ISBT 006 AND 019)

Structure, Function, and Interaction of the Kell and XK Proteins

Antigens of the Kell blood group system are carried by a 93-kd red blood cell membrane glycoprotein (8). The glycoprotein contains a short cytoplasmic N-terminal portion, a single membrane-spanning α-helical segment, and a large, 665 amino acid extracellular C-terminal portion held in a globular conformation by multiple disulfide bonds (Fig. 10.1). Kell antigens are inactivated by reducing agents such as dithiothreitol, suggesting that disulfide bonds are important in maintaining its antigenic conformation (9). Proteolytic cleavage with chymotrypsin or trypsin also destroys Kell antigens.

The Kell protein is a member of the neprilysin (M13) family of zinc metalloproteases. This family currently consists of Kell, neutral endopeptidase 24.11, two different endothelin-converting enzymes, the product of the PEX gene, and XCE (10,11). Members of the M13 subfamily of membrane zinc endopepti-

TABLE 10.1. OVERVIEW OF THE PROTEIN BLOOD GROUP SYSTEMS OTHER THAN Rh AND LW

ISBT Number	System Name	ISBT Symbol	Red Blood Cell Component Membrane	Number of Antigens	Examples of Antigens
002	MNS	MNS	Glycophorins A and B	40	M, N, S, s, U
005	Lutheran	LU	Lutheran glycoprotein	18	Lu^a, Lu^b
006	Kell	KEL	Kell protein	22	K, k, Js^a, Js^b, Kp^a, Kp^b
008	Duffy	FY	Chemokine receptor	6	Fy^a, Fy^b
009	Kidd	JK	Urea transporter	3	Jk^a, Jk^b
010	Diego	DI	Anion exchanger	20	Di^a, Di^b, Wr^a, Wr^b
011	Cartwright	YT	Acetylcholinesterase	2	Yt^a, Yt^b
012	Xg	XG	Xg glycoprotein	1	Xg^a
013	Scianna	SC	Scianna protein	3	Sc^a, Sc^b
014	Dombrock	DO	Dombrock glycoprotein	5	Do^a, Do^b
015	Colton	CO	Aquaporin	3	Co^a, Co^b
017	Chido/Rodgers	CH/RG	Complement component C4	9	Ch1, Ch2, Ch3, Rg^1, Rg^2
019	Kx	XK	XK protein	1	Kx
020	Gerbich	GE	Glycophorins C and D	7	Ge2, Ge3, Ge4
021	Cromer	CROM	Decay accelerating factor (DAF, CD55)	10	Cr^a
022	Knops	KN	Complement receptor 1 (CR1, CD35)	5	Kn^a
023	Indian	IN	CD44	2	In^a, In^b
024	OK	OK	CD147	1	Ok^a
025	RAPH	RAPH	Unknown	1	MER2

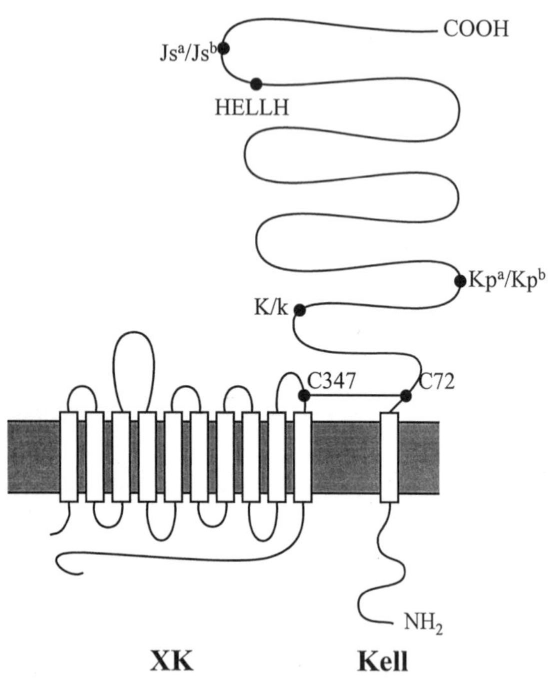

FIGURE 10.1. Schematic representation of the Kell/XK complex in the red blood cell membrane. The XK protein is a membrane protein with ten α-helical transmembrane segments, while Kell has only one transmembrane domain, most of which is exposed on the ectoplasmic side. Due to multiple disulfide bonds, the ectoplasmic portion of Kell is a globular structure; however, it is represented here schematically so that the positions of the main alleles can be shown. A disulfide bond between Cys72 of Kell and Cys347 of XK connects the two proteins. The position of the pentameric sequence HELLH is shown. Sequences HEXXH are involved in zinc binding and catalytic activity of zinc endopeptidases. The K/k polymorphism at amino acid 193 changes the consensus sequence for N-glycosylation at Asn191, which is not glycosylated in K. This difference in glycosylation may be important for the marked antigenicity of K. Positions of two additional sets of antithetical antigens Kp^a/Kp^b and Js^a/Js^b at amino acids 281 and 597 are indicated.

dases have widely different roles, including processing of opioid peptides, Met- and Leu-enkephalin, oxytocin, bradykinin, angiotensin, endothelins, and parathyroid hormone. Kell protein has been shown to preferentially activate endothelin-3 (12) however, the in vivo physiologic role of Kell protein is probably complex, because K_0(null) persons are healthy.

The Kell protein interacts in the membrane with the 37-kd protein XK, which plays an important role in the expression of Kell system antigens. In contrast to the Kell protein, XK spans the membrane ten times and both of its N- and C-termini are located intracellularly (Fig. 10.1). The function of XK is not known. Structurally, XK resembles the glutamate transporters but it has very little amino acid sequence homology with this group of transport proteins. The Kell and XK proteins are covalently associated in the membrane by a disulfide link between cysteine 72 of Kell and cysteine 347 of XK (13–15) (Fig. 10.1). The gene encoding the Kx antigen is located on the short arm of the X chromosome near the loci for X-linked chronic granulomatous disease (CGD) and Duchenne of Becker muscular dystrophy (DMD, BMD).

Kell in Transfusion Medicine

The Kell blood group system is the second most important protein blood group system in transfusion medicine after Rh, because the antibodies can cause hemolytic transfusion reactions and hemolytic disease of the newborn (HDN). The most important antigens in this system are KEL1, or K, and the antithetical KEL2, or k. K and k are codominant autosomal alleles; approximately 9% of whites and 2% of blacks are K-positive (i.e., KK or Kk); the remainder are K-negative (i.e., kk). Antigens of the Kell blood group system are highly immunogenic and, excluding ABO, K is second only to RhD in its potential to elicit production of alloantibodies.

Anti-K antibodies are commonly found. Fortunately, because

more than 90% of donor units are K-negative, it is easy to obtain blood for transfusion into individuals with anti-K antibodies. In contrast, although anti-k is relatively rare, it is also of clinical significance, and only 1 in 500 random-donor units is antigen negative. The other two sets of well-defined antithetical antigens are Kp^a/Kp^b and Js^a/Js^b (Fig. 10.1).

Mothers with anti-K antibodies are relatively rare, but since the introduction of Rh prophylaxis, anti-K accounts for nearly 10% of cases of severe HDN. In contrast to RhD, anti-K titers are not good predictors of fetal anemia. In addition, affected Kell alloimmunized babies have lower reticulocyte counts and amniotic fluid bilirubin concentrations than anti-RhD–sensitized babies. Anti-K has been hypothesized to suppress erythropoiesis at the progenitor cell level. It is important to determine if a fetus is at risk when the mother has anti-K. The prospective father should be typed and if he carries the K antigen, genotyping from amniocentesis can be performed using molecular techniques.

Kell Variants

There are two rare but clinically interesting variants in the Kell blood group system. Rare individuals have red blood cells that completely lack the common Kell antigens. Interestingly, although these cells exhibit the null phenotype (K_0), they are morphologically normal and survive normally in vivo. In contrast, individuals lacking the Kx antigen exhibit depressed levels of the Kell protein (8,9). This phenotype, known as the McLeod syndrome, is associated with acanthocytic red blood cells and a mild chronic hemolytic anemia. The frequently reported neuromuscular symptoms in subjects with McLeod phenotype may be caused by lack of Kx expression. At the same time, association of the McLeod phenotype with other rare syndromes, most frequently with CGD and DMD or BMD, is caused by large gene deletions encompassing *XK* together with adjacent genes *CYBB* that encodes a large subunit of cytochrome b_{558} and is associated with X-linked CGD, and *DMD* that encodes dystrophin (16, 17).

DUFFY BLOOD GROUP SYSTEM (ISBT 008)

Structure and Function of the Duffy Protein

The Duffy gene encodes a glycoprotein of 336 amino acids with a molecular weight of 36 kd. The Duffy glycoprotein has seven transmembrane α-helical domains. The N-terminus is ectoplasmic and the C-terminus intracellular (Fig. 10.2). Duffy protein functions as a chemokine receptor and is frequently called the Duffy antigen receptor for chemokines (DARC) (18,19). Duffy binds both CXC chemokines, such as interleukin-8 (IL-8) and melanocyte growth-stimulating activity (MGSA), as well as CC chemokines, such as regulated on activation, normal T-cell expressed and secreted (RANTES) and macrophage chemoattractant protein (MCP-1) (18). It is currently not known why a red blood cell with its limited metabolism and response to chemokine binding would carry a significant number of chemokine receptors at its surface. One possible explanation is that the chemokine receptor acts as a scavenger for locally released chemokines. However, individuals who do not express the Duffy protein either on erythrocytes or in all tissues are phenotypically normal, suggesting that the Duffy protein is dispensable.

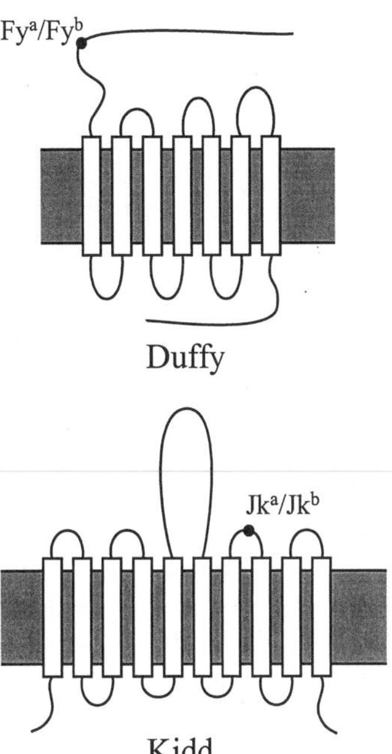

FIGURE 10.2. Schematic depiction of proteins carrying the Duffy and Kidd blood group antigens. The Duffy antigen receptor for chemokines (DARC) consists of seven transmembrane segments. The N-terminus is located extracellularly, functions as both the chemokine and *P. vivax* attachment site, and carries the Fy^a/Fy^b polymorphism. Kidd protein has ten transmembrane segments, both N- and C-termini are intracellular and the amino acid determining the Jk^a/Jk^b polymorphism is located in the fourth ectoplasmic loop.

Duffy also functions as a receptor for the human malarial parasite *Plasmodium vivax,* which infects only erythrocytes of Duffy-positive individuals (20). The binding site for *P. vivax* is located in the N-terminal ectoplasmic domain of Duffy. *P. vivax* merozoites invade primarily reticulocytes, although reticulocytes and mature erythrocytes do not substantially differ in Duffy expression. This suggests that an additional receptor has to play a role in erythrocyte invasion.

Duffy in Transfusion Medicine

The two main alleles of the Duffy blood group system are the antithetical codominant antigens Fy^a and Fy^b, whose genetic determinant is a Gly/Asp polymorphism in position 44 (Fig.10.2) (21). These two alleles occur with similar frequencies in whites, Fy^a being somewhat more common. The Fy(a − b −) phenotype is extremely rare among whites, but approximately two-thirds of African-Americans and more than 90% of native West Africans are Fy(a − b −). This is most likely caused by the genetic adaptation for resistance to *P. vivax* malaria. However, it is not clear why this genetic advantage would lead almost to fixation of the Fy(a − b −) phenotype in the indigenous population of West Africa, because *P. vivax,* in contrast to the other malarial parasites, causes a relatively mild form of malaria (18).

A longstanding and well-known conundrum of immunohematology has been that transfused Fy(a − b −) people of African ancestry never develop anti-Fy^b antibodies. This problem was solved by the recent characterization of the mutation causing the Fy(a − b −) phenotype in native West Africans. The underlying mutation is a T → C substitution in the GATA site of the promoter region (22). This substitution prevents binding of the erythroid transcription factor GATA-1 and abolishes transcription of the gene in the erythroid cells while leaving the transcription of the *FY* gene in other tissues unaffected. Because the mutation occurred in the *FY*B* allele, the Fy^b antigen remains expressed in certain endothelial, epithelial, and brain cells and, consequently, the transfusion recipient does not form antibodies against Fy^b.

Anti-Fy^a antibodies are found relatively frequently, comprising 6% to 10% of the clinically significant antibodies identified by immunohematology laboratories. For reasons not quite understood, Fy^b is a relatively poor immunogen and, consequently, anti-Fy^b antibodies are considerably less common. Both immediate and delayed transfusion reactions due to Fy^a incompatibility have been described, ranging from mild to severe hemolysis. HDN is usually mild; only a few cases of severe HDN have been reported. In contrast, anti-Fy^b is associated only rarely with cases of mild HDN and is usually found in delayed transfusion reactions, although on rare occasions it has caused severe acute hemolysis.

KIDD BLOOD GROUP SYSTEM (ISBT 009)

The two main antigens of the Kidd blood group system, Jk^a and Jk^b, are found with almost identical frequencies in the white population. Jk^a is a better immunogen and anti-Jk^a is found more frequently than anti-Jk^b. Anti-Jk^a may cause severe immediate or delayed hemolytic transfusion reactions and, occasionally, HDN. It is one of the most dangerous immune antibodies because of its tendency to fall to undetectable levels between transfusions and its relatively low affinity for Jk^a-positive red blood cells. For these reasons, it accounts for a large proportion of delayed hemolytic transfusion reactions. Anti-Jk^b may also cause immediate or delayed hemolytic transfusion reactions, albeit less severe than those caused by anti-Jk^a. Several cases of mild HDN caused by anti-Jk^b have been reported.

The finding that cells of the Jk(a − b −) phenotype are resistant to lysis by 2-mol urea led to the discovery of the function of the protein carrying the Kidd antigens. Based on this finding and on in vitro expression of the cloned Kidd cDNA (23–25), it is now known that the protein is a urea transporter, although the importance of urea transport for erythrocytes is not completely understood. Its presence or absence may not be critical for red blood cell structure and function, because carriers of the Jk(a − b −) phenotype have red blood cells indistinguishable from those of controls.

Kidd is an integral protein with ten transmembrane domains and both N- and C-termini located intracellularly (Fig.10.2). Out of the five ectoplasmic loops, the longest, third loop is N-glycosylated, and the relatively short fourth loop carries an Asp280Asn polymorphism corresponding to the Jk^a/Jk^b antigens (26). Kidd protein is expressed not only on the red blood cell surface but also on neutrophils and in the kidney.

MNS BLOOD GROUP SYSTEM (ISBT 002)

Structure and Function of Glycophorins A and B

Antigens of the MNS blood group system are carried by glycophorin A (GPA) and glycophorin B (GPB). Both molecules are present in a very high copy number in the plasma membrane; 0.5 to 1.0 × 10^6 copies of GPA and 1 to 3 × 10^5 molecules of GPB. GPA and GPB are encoded by homologous genes at chromosome 4q28-q31 that undoubtedly arose by gene duplication. Both glycoproteins are integral membrane proteins with a single transmembrane α-helical segment and with the N-termini located extracellularly (Fig. 10.3). GPA was the first protein whose primary structure was determined by amino acid sequencing (27).

GPA carries the M and N antigens. The antigenic difference is due to substitutions in positions 1 and 5. Serine in position 1 and glycine in position 5 correspond to the M antigen, while the N allele has leucine and glutamic acid in these positions (Fig. 10.3 and Table 10.2). An important requirement for recognition of these antigens by human antibodies is that serines in positions 2 and 4 and threonine in position 3 are O-glycosylated.

GPB is homologous with GPA. Although the genes are >95% identical, *GYPB* encodes a shorter protein because a point mutation at the 5′ splicing site of the third intron prevents incorporation of exon 3 into the translated mRNA. Because *GYPB* arose by duplication of the *N* allele of *GYPA, GYPA*N,* and the first 26 amino acids of GPB are therefore identical to those of GPA with N specificity, GPB expresses an N-like antigen designated as 'N' (Table 10.2 and Fig. 10.3). The S and s alleles of GPB differ at amino acid position 29. The S allele contains methionine and the s allele, threonine. GPB also carries the U antigen whose epitope is adjacent to the point where GPB enters into the lipid bilayer (Fig. 10.3).

As is frequently the case with genes arising by duplication and located next to each other, unequal crossing over or gene conversion may easily occur. Consequently, numerous hybrid molecules containing portions of GPA and GPB have been described. This phenomenon is partly responsible for the 45 currently known antigens of the MNS blood group system, particularly for many of the Miltenberger (Mi) variants.

GPA associates in the red blood cell membrane with the band 3 protein. Interestingly, the epitope of the Wr^b antigen from the Diego blood group system (see below) is formed by both GPA and band 3. This clearly demonstrates the intimate association of GPA and band 3 in the plasma membrane (28) (Fig. 10.3).

MNS in Transfusion Medicine

The most commonly encountered antibodies are directed against the M, N, S, and s antigens. Anti-M is often found in the sera of persons who have not been exposed to the human red blood cells. Anti-M antibodies are mostly IgM, however they fre-

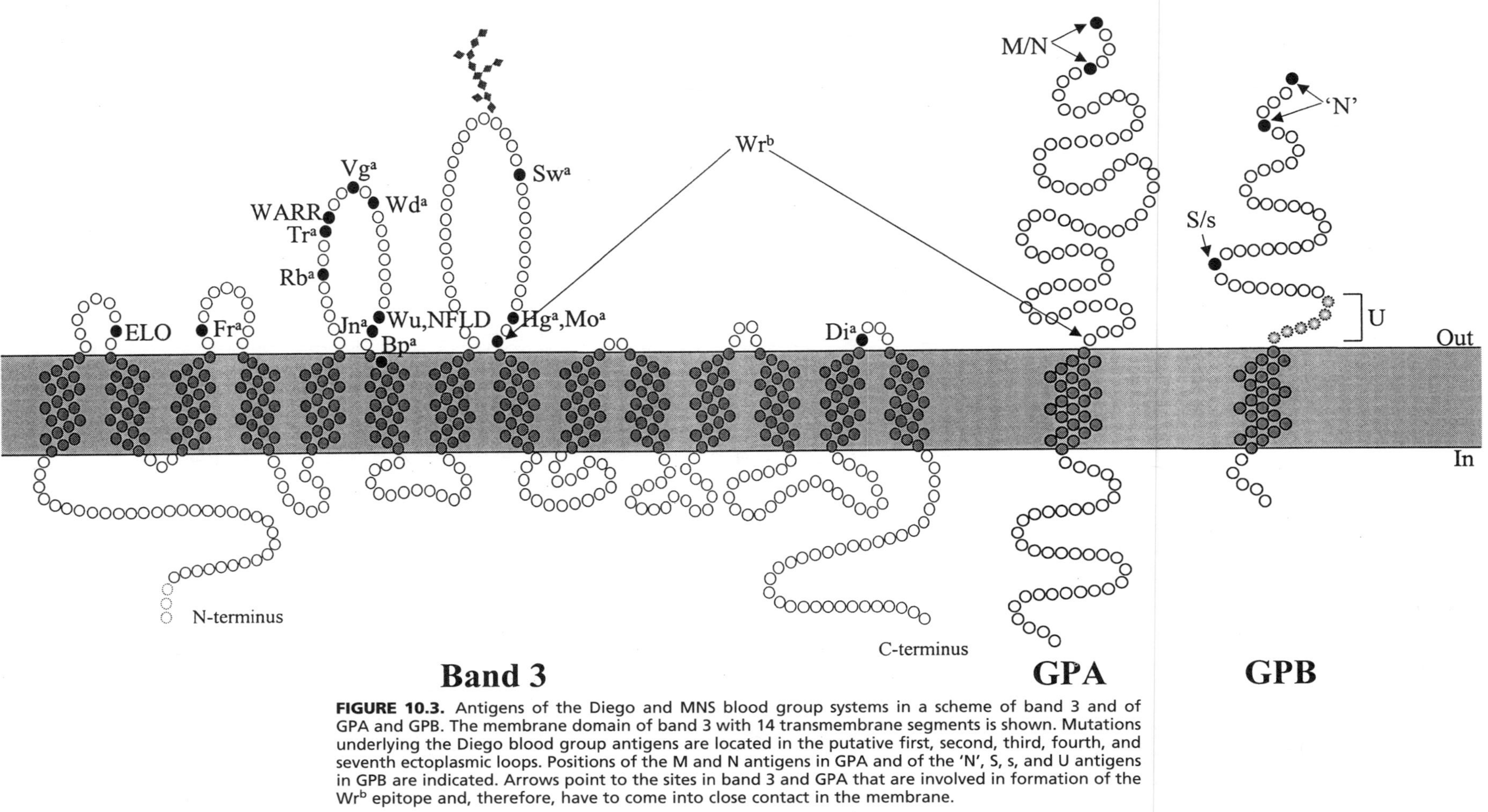

FIGURE 10.3. Antigens of the Diego and MNS blood group systems in a scheme of band 3 and of GPA and GPB. The membrane domain of band 3 with 14 transmembrane segments is shown. Mutations underlying the Diego blood group antigens are located in the putative first, second, third, fourth, and seventh ectoplasmic loops. Positions of the M and N antigens in GPA and of the 'N', S, s, and U antigens in GPB are indicated. Arrows point to the sites in band 3 and GPA that are involved in formation of the Wr^b epitope and, therefore, have to come into close contact in the membrane.

TABLE 10.2. N-TERMINAL SEQUENCES OF THE M AND N ALLELES OF GLYCOPHORIN A (GPA) AND OF THE S AND s ALLELES OF GLYCOPHORIN B (GPB)

Antigen	Amino Acid Sequence (1 ↓ 5 ↓ … 26 ↓ 29 ↓)
M (GPA)	**SSTTG**VAMHTSTSSSVTKSYISSQTNDTHKRDTYAATPRA..
N (GPA)	**LSTTE** VAMHTSTSSSVTKSYISSQTNDTHKRDTYAATPRA..
S (GPB)	**LSTTE** VAMHTSTSSSVTKSYISSQTNGE**M**GQLVHRFTVPA..
S (GPB)	**LSTTE** VAMHTSTSSSVTKSYISSQTNGE**T**GQLVHRFTVPA..
	<- - -> M/N; 'N' … ↑ S/s

Differences between M and N reside in amino acids 1 and 5. First 26 amino acids of GPB are identical to GPA, and GPB, therefore expresses an N-like antigen 'N'. The differences between the S and s antigens correspond to a M/T polymorphism in position 29 of GPB.
S, Ser; L, Leu; G, Gly; E, Glu; M, Met; T, Thr.

quently contain an IgG component and, occasionally, are exclusively IgG. Anti-M is rarely clinically significant; hemolytic anti-M are usually IgG and reactive at 37°C. Anti-N is rare, most likely due to the immune tolerance induced by the 'N' antigen on GPB. Strong and potentially clinically significant antibodies have been observed in persons of the rare phenotype M+N−S−s−U− who do not express GPB (hence 'N'). In contrast to anti-M and anti-N, antibodies to S, s, and U usually occur after exposure to allogeneic red blood cells. All are capable of causing hemolytic transfusion reactions and HDN. The most important antibodies of the MNS system are compared in Table 10.3.

DIEGO BLOOD GROUP SYSTEM (ISBT 010)

Antigens of the Diego blood group system are carried by erythrocyte band 3 protein (anion exchanger 1), the most abundant integral protein of the red blood cell membrane together with GPA (see above). Band 3 is also one of the most important proteins for the structure and function of the membrane, because it maintains red blood cell integrity by linking the red blood cell membrane to the underlying spectrin-based membrane skeleton. It also mediates exchange of chloride and bicarbonate anions across the plasma membrane, thereby increasing severalfold the carrying capacity of blood for carbon dioxide.

TABLE 10.3. COMPARISON OF THE MOST FREQUENTLY ENCOUNTERED ANTIBODIES IN THE MNS SYSTEM

Anti-M and -N	Anti-S, -s, and -U
Naturally occurring	Exposure is required
Cold IgM	Warm IgG
Dosage	Minimal dosage
Clinically insignificant	Clinically significant

Band 3 consists of a cytoplasmic and a membrane domain. The membrane domain contains 14 transmembrane helices connected by ecto- and endoplasmic loops (29,30) (Fig. 10.3). The fourth loop of band 3 is N-glycosylated and the attached carbohydrate chain carries over half of the red blood cell ABO blood group epitopes (31). Several disorders of red blood cell structure and function have been associated with mutations in the band 3 gene, including Southeast Asian ovalocytosis (32), autosomal dominant spherocytosis (33–35), and distal renal tubular acidosis (36).

Despite being the most abundant protein of the red blood cell membrane, band 3 until recently has not been known to carry any red blood cell antigens with the exception of the ABO antigens residing on the attached carbohydrate chains. It was only in 1992 that Spring et al. reported that the Memphis II variant of erythroid band 3 protein carries the Di^a blood group antigen (37). Di^a was originally described in South American Indians by Layrisse et al. in 1955 (38). The antithetical antigen Di^b was reported by Thompson et al. in 1967 (39). Di^a and Di^b represent codominantly expressed gene products. Di^a is a low-incidence blood group antigen in whites who carry the antithetical high-incidence antigen Di^b. Prevalence of Di^a is as high as 8% in certain areas of Southeast Asia and reaches up to 40% in some groups of South American Indians (38). Interestingly, Di^a was used as one of the markers for studying migration of people from Southeast Asia across the Bering Strait and southward through the American continent. Cloning and sequencing of band 3 gene identified the substitution 854 Pro→Leu in the last ectoplasmic loop of band 3 as the molecular basis of the Di^a antigen. Di^b corresponds to the wild type band 3 with proline in position 854 (40).

Subsequently, the low-incidence blood group antigen Wr^a was mapped to the fourth ectoplasmic loop (28). The antithetical Wr^b antigen is seen only when both GPA and band 3 protein are expressed in the erythrocyte membrane, which helped to characterize the site of interaction between band 3 and GPA (Fig. 10.3). During the last several years, numerous additional low-incidence antigens have been associated with single point mutations on band 3 and included in the Diego system (41, 42). Positions of the mutated amino acids in the band 3 molecule are shown in Fig. 10.3, which also indicates the regions of band 3 and GPA that interact in the membrane and are involved in formation of the Wr^b antigen.

Some antigens of the Diego blood group system have been localized to the regions of band 3 protein that have been implicated in the adhesion of abnormal red blood cells, such as sickle cells or malaria-infected erythrocytes, to vascular endothelium (43,44). Erythrocytes from carriers of low-incidence blood group antigens in ectoplasmic loops of band 3 may serve as a model for evaluation of the sequence requirements for adhesion. Interestingly, the so-called *senescent,* or *aging,* red blood cell antigen may also be located in the ectoplasmic loops of band 3.

GERBICH BLOOD GROUP SYSTEM (ISBT 020)

Similarly to the MNS system, antigens of the Gerbich system are located on glycophorins C (GPC) and D (GPC). The glycophorin terminology is the only common feature of these two classes of glycophorins. There is otherwise no homology between the Gerbich and MNS genes. Unlike GPA and GPB, GPC and GPD are the products of a single gene and, unlike *GYPA* and *GYPB,* this gene is expressed in multiple tissues. The considerably less abundant and smaller GPD is produced from a shorter transcript than GPC. Although present in much smaller copy numbers than GPA and GPB, GPC plays an important role in the structural integrity of the red blood cell membrane. In the Leach phenotype, in which neither GPC nor CPD is expressed, red blood cells are elliptic and prone to hemolysis (45,46). Antibodies in the Gerbich system are rare and, in the vast majority of cases, clinically insignificant.

COLTON BLOOD GROUP SYSTEM (ISBT 015)

Antibodies against the two antigens of the Colton blood group system, Co^a and Co^b, are rare and have only rarely been associated with mild transfusion reactions and mild HDN. The antigens are carried by aquaporin-1 (47), a member of a large family of water channels (48). It is present in the membrane as a tetramer. Expression of aquaporin-1 in Xenopus oocytes is associated with dramatic swelling and lysis of the cell (49). At the same time, the Co(a − b −) phenotype is associated with only slightly abnormal red blood cells and with normal kidney function despite aquaporin-1's role as the major water channel of human kidney (50,51).

LUTHERAN BLOOD GROUP SYSTEM (ISBT 005)

The Lutheran blood group system contains multiple antigens; however, clinically significant antibodies are rarely encountered. The most important antigens are Lu^a and Lu^b. The frequency of Lu^a is less than 10% in most populations, while Lu^b is a high frequency antigen with an average prevalence of 99.8% in all populations. Lutheran antigens are poorly developed at birth and, not surprisingly, anti-Lu^a has been associated only rarely with mild cases of HDN. It does not cause transfusion reactions. Lu^b is somewhat more immunogenic and anti-Lu^b have caused mild or moderate transfusion reactions and mild HDN. Of historic note, Lu and Se (Chapter 8) were the first two loci for which an autosomal linkage in humans was demonstrated.

Lutheran antigens reside on B-CAM/LU (Fig. 10.4), a pair of spliceosomes (protein products arising from the same gene due to alternative splicing of hnRNA) that belong to the immunoglobulin superfamily (52). Basal cell adhesion molecule (B-CAM) is involved in adhesion of the basal surface of epithelial cells to the basement membrane. B-CAM/LU has recently been shown to function as a receptor for laminin (53). Expression of B-CAM/LU is increased on red blood cells from patients with sickle cell disease (53) and on a number of malignant epithelial tumors, which also lose the polarity of B-CAM/LU expression found in normal tissues (52).

The null phenotype, Lu(a − b −), is rare but quite interesting. It may result from three different patterns of inheritance. A recessive pattern of inheritance is associated with an exceedingly

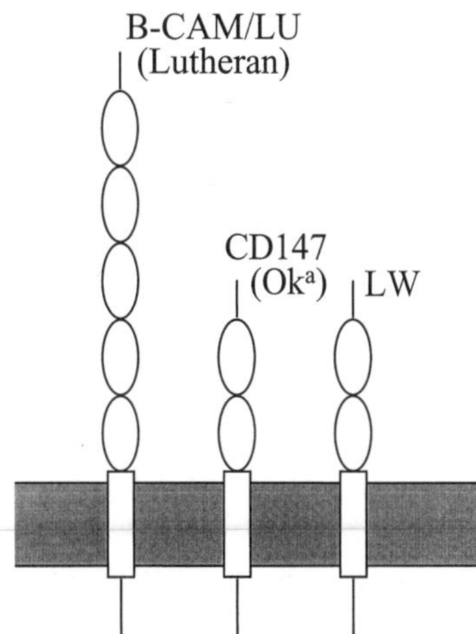

FIGURE 10.4. Members of the immunoglobulin superfamily carrying blood group antigens. B-CAM/LU contains five immunoglobulin domains and carries antigens of the Lutheran blood group system. CD147, or neurothelin, contains two Ig domains and carries the Ok^a antigen. CD147 is similar to the LW protein, which was discussed in chapter 9.

rare null allele. In the most common dominant type of inheritance, the expression of *Lu* can be suppressed by a single copy of the suppressor gene *In(Lu)* (54). In addition to reducing the expression of Lutheran antigens to levels undetectable by standard serologic techniques, *In(Lu)* also decreases the expression of antigens P_1, i, In^a and In^b (see below), and AnWj, a receptor for *Haemophilus influenzae.* The third cause of the Lu(a − b −) phenotype is the presence of an X-linked recessive suppressor gene *XS2* (55).

INDIAN BLOOD GROUP SYSTEM (ISBT 023)

The two antigens of this system, In^a and In^b, reside on CD44, an adhesion molecule expressed in leukocytes, fibroblasts, epithelial cells, and other tissues. CD44 is an important lymphocyte marker, which functions as a hyaluronan receptor (56) and a lymphocyte homing receptor (Fig. 10.4). Transfection of nonadherent cell lines with CD44 cDNA confers an adherent phenotype (57). Similarly to the Lutheran antigens, expression of In^a and In^b is suppressed by *In(Lu).*

XG BLOOD GROUP SYSTEM (ISBT 012)

The only antigen of the Xg system, Xg^a, is carried by a glycoprotein of 180 amino acids (58). Designation of this blood group system reflects that the *PBDX* gene (59), which encodes Xg, is located on the X chromosome. Xg is 48% homologous to CD99, an adhesion molecule. Anti-Xg^a antibodies are clinically insignificant.

SCIANNA BLOOD GROUP SYSTEM (ISBT 013)

The molecular basis of the Scianna blood group system (60) has not been elucidated. The Scianna locus on chromosome 1 encodes a glycoprotein but the corresponding gene has not been cloned. Mild HDN and mild posttransfusion hemolysis due to anti-Sc-2 and anti-Sc-3 antibodies have been reported.

CHIDO/RODGERS BLOOD GROUP SYSTEM (ISBT 017)

Antigens of the Chido/Rodgers blood group system are the only protein antigens that are not produced by red blood cells but instead adhere to the red blood cell surface (Lewis antigens are glycolipids). They are carried by the complement component C4. Although antibodies against the nine known antigens of the system are generally benign, a severe anaphylactic reaction following a transfusion of platelets to a patient with anti-Ch3 was described (61).

KNOPS BLOOD GROUP SYSTEM (ISBT 022)

Antigens are located on the C3b/C4b complement receptor (CR1, CD35) (Fig. 4). CR1 is a large 190- to 280-kd molecule. It contains 30 complement control protein domains (CCPD) of about 60 amino acids. Seven CCPDs form a long homologous repeat (LHR) of about 450 amino acids. Various forms of CR1 contain up to 6 LHRs. Erythrocyte CR1 binds immune complexes and carries them to the liver and spleen for removal. Expression of CR1 on erythrocytes varies widely from 20 to 1,500 molecules and is decreased in hemolytic anemias, acquired immunodeficiency syndrome (AIDS), and systemic lupus erythematosus and other autoimmune disorders. *Plasmodium falciparum*–infected erythrocytes deficient in CR1 have greatly reduced rosetting capacity, indicating an essential role for CR1 in rosette formation and raising the possibility that CR1 polymorphisms in Africans that influence the interaction between erythrocytes and parasite-encoded protein PfEMP1 may protect against severe malaria. CR1 could therefore be a potential target for future therapeutic interventions to treat severe malaria (62, 63).

BLOOD GROUP ANTIGENS ON PHOSPHATIDYLINOSITOL-LINKED PROTEINS—CARTWRIGHT (ISBT 011), DOMBROCK (ISBT 014), CROMER (ISBT 021)

The common denominator of these antigens is the linkage of the carrier protein to the glycosylated phosphatidylinositol (GPI) anchor (Fig. 10.5). The Cartwright (Yt) blood group system consists of two antigens, Yt[a] and Yt[b], which are located on red blood cell acetylcholinesterase. Most examples of anti-Yt[a] are benign.

The five antigens of the Dombrock system are located on a recently characterized glycoprotein (64). Homology studies suggest that the Dombrock molecule is a member of the adenosine 5′-diphosphate (ADP)-ribosyltransferase ectoenzyme gene family. Dombrock expression is developmentally regulated during erythroid differentiation and occurs at highest levels in the fetal liver. Do[a] and Do[b] antigens differ in a single amino acid substitution within the RGD motif of the molecule (64).

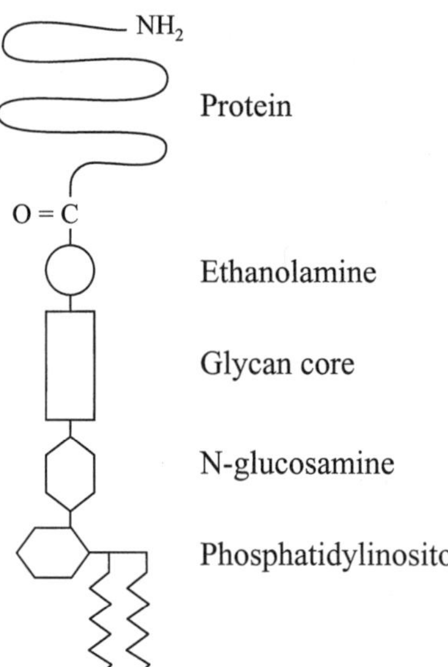

FIGURE 10.5. Schematic representation of a GPI-anchored protein. The membrane anchor is provided by phosphatidylinositol. The inositol moiety binds to a glycan core via a molecule of N-glucosamine. The glycan core is attached via ethanolamine to the C-terminus of the protein.

The Cromer blood group system contains ten antigens located on decay accelerating factor (DAF, CD55), a complement regulatory protein. Although DAF is the first complement regulatory protein identified, it plays only a minor role in complement-mediated lysis, the more important being the membrane inhibitor of reactive lysis (MIRL, CD59) molecule. This was clearly demonstrated in the case of the null phenotype, Inab, which is associated with lack of DAF expression on all circulating cells but not with increased hemolysis.

Antibodies in these three blood group systems have been associated with only occasional mild transfusion reactions or HDN. Expression of all GPI-linked antigens is, not surprisingly, decreased in paroxysmal nocturnal hemoglobinuria, a disorder caused by defects in the X-linked *PIG-A* (phosphatidylinositol glycan class A) gene, which participates in an early step of GPI anchor synthesis.

OK AND RAPH BLOOD GROUP SYSTEM (ISBT 024 AND 025)

Each of these two newly defined blood group systems contains only one antigen. Ok[a] is a high-incidence antigen; rare Ok(a−) individuals have so far been reported only in Japan. It is carried on an N-glycosylated protein with an apparent molecular weight of 35 to 69 kd, which is expressed in multiple tissues. The Ok[a] glycoprotein is a member of the immunoglobulin superfamily. Similarly to LW, its extracellular domain contains two immunoglobulin domains.

MER2 is the only antigen of the RAPH system. All anti-

MER2 antibodies so far reported have been found in patients on hemodialysis. The molecular basis of the antigen is not known.

SUMMARY

The century-long history of modern transfusion medicine and immunohematology practice led to the characterization of an enormous number of blood group antigens with often confusing terminology. These antigens have been arranged into a complex framework of blood group systems, collections, and low- and high-frequency antigens. Fortunately, advances in biochemical and molecular biology techniques in the last two decades led to a detailed structural characterization of most proteins carrying blood group antigens and to a better understanding of the relation between gene variations, amino acid polymorphisms, protein structure, and immunogenicity of individual antigens. Better understanding of the molecular biology, biochemistry, and immunogenicity of proteins carrying blood group antigens will undoubtedly contribute to accurate compatibility testing and to safe transfusion of red blood cells.

REFERENCES

1. Daniels G. Functional aspects of red cell antigens. *Blood Rev* 1999;13:14–35.
2. Cartron JP, Bailly P, Levankim C, et al. Insights into the structure and function of membrane polypeptides carrying blood group antigens. *Vox Sang* 1998;74[Suppl 2]:29–64.
3. Reid ME, Oyen R, Marsh WL. Summary of the clinical significance of blood group alloantibodies. *Semin Hematol* 2000;37:197–216.
4. Reid ME, Rios M, Yazdanbakhsh K. Applications of molecular biology techniques to transfusion medicine. *Semin Hematol* 2000;37:166–176.
5. Reid M, Lomas-Francis C. *The blood group antigen factsbook.* San Diego: Academic Press, 1997;12.
6. Daniels G. *Human blood groups,* 1st ed. London: Blackwell Science, 1995.
7. Issitt PD, Anstee DJ. *Applied blood group serology,* 4th ed. Durham, NC: Montgomery Scientific Publications, 1998.
8. Lee S, Russo D, Redman CM. The Kell blood group system: Kell and XK membrane proteins. *Semin Hematol* 2000;37:113–121.
9. Lee S, Russo D, Redman C. Functional and structural aspects of the Kell blood group system. *Transfus Med Rev* 2000;14:93–103.
10. Valdenaire O, Richards JG, Faull RLM, et al. XCE, a new member of the endothelin-converting enzyme and neutral endopeptidase family, is preferentially expressed in the CNS. *Brain Res Mol Brain Res* 1999;64:211–221.
11. Turner AJ, Tanzawa K. Mammalian membrane metallopeptidases: NEP, ECE, KELL, and PEX. *FASEB J* 1997;11:355–364.
12. Lee S, Lin M, Mele A, et al. Proteolytic processing of big endothelin-3 by the kell blood group protein. *Blood* 1999;94:1440–1450.
13. Khamlichi S, Bailly P, Blanchard D, et al. Purification and partial characterization of the erythrocyte Kx protein deficient in McLeod patients. *Eur J Biochem* 1995;228:931–934.
14. Russo D, Lee S, Redman C. Intracellular assembly of Kell and XK blood group proteins. *Biochim Biophys Acta* 1999;1461:10–18.
15. Russo D, Redman C, Lee S. Association of XK and Kell blood group proteins. *J Biol Chem* 1998;273:13950–13956.
16. Francke V, Ochs HD, De Martinville B, et al. Minor Xp21 chromosome deletion in a male associated with expression of Duchenne muscular dystrophy, chronic granulomatous disease, retinitis pigmentosa and McLeod's syndrome. *Am J Hum Genet* 1985;37:250.
17. Swash M, Schwartz MS, Carter ND, et al. Benign X-linked myopathy with acanthocytes (McLeod syndrome): its relationship to X-linked muscular dystrophy. *Brain* 1983;106:717.
18. Pogo AO, Chaudhuri A. The Duffy protein: a malarial and chemokine receptor. *Semin Hematol* 2000;37:122–129.
19. Horuk R, Martin A, Hesselgesser J, et al. The Duffy antigen receptor for chemokines: structural analysis and expression in the brain. *J Leukoc Biol* 1996;59:29–38.
20. Chaudhuri A, Polyakova J, Zbrzezna V, et al. Cloning of glycoprotein D cDNA, which encodes the major subunit of the Duffy blood group system and the receptor for the *Plasmodium vivax* malaria parasite. *Proc Natl Acad Sci U S A* 1993;90:10793–10797.
21. Tournamille C, Kim CLV, Gane P, et al. Molecular basis and PCR-DNA typing of the Fy^a/Fy^b blood group polymorphism. *Hum Genet* 1995;95:407–410.
22. Tournamille C, Colin Y, Cartron JP, et al. Disruption of a GATA motif in the Duffy gene promoter abolishes erythroid gene expression in Duffy negative individuals. *Nat Genet* 1995;10:224–228.
23. Olives B, Neau P, Bailly P, et al. Cloning and functional expression of a urea transporter from human bone marrow cells. *J Biol Chem* 1994;269:31649–31652.
24. Olives B, Martial S, Mattei MG, et al. Molecular characterization of a new urea transporter in the human kidney [Letter]. *FEB S Letters* 1996;386:156–160.
25. Olives B, Mattei MG, Huet M, et al. Kidd blood group and urea transport function of human erythrocytes are carried by the same protein. *J Biol Chem* 1995;270:15607–15610.
26. Olives B, Merriman M, Bailly P, et al. The molecular basis of the Kidd blood group polymorphism and its lack of association with type 1 diabetes susceptibility. *Hum Mol Genet* 1997;6:1017–1020.
27. Tomita M, Marchesi VT. Amino-acid sequence and oligosaccharide attachment sites of human erythrocyte glycophorin. *Proc Natl Acad Sci U S A* 1975;72:2964–2968.
28. Bruce LJ, Ring SM, Anstee DJ, et al. Changes in the blood group Wright antigens are associated with a mutation at amino acid 658 in human erythrocyte band 3: a site of interaction between band 3 and glycophorin A under certain conditions. *Blood* 1995;85:541–547.
29. Lux SE, John KM, Kopito RR, et al. Cloning and characterization of band 3, the human erythrocyte anion-exchange protein (AE1). *Proc Natl Acad Sci U S A* 1989;86:9089–9093.
30. Tanner MJA, Martin PG, High S. The complete amino acid sequence of the human erythrocyte membrane anion-transport protein deduced from the cDNA. *Biochem J* 1988;256:703–712.
31. Fukuda M, Fukuda MN. Changes in red cell surface glycoproteins and carbohydrate structures during the development and differentiation of human erythroid cells. *J Supramol Struct* 1981;17:324.
32. Jarolim P, Palek J, Amato D, et al. Deletion in erythrocyte band 3 gene in malaria-resistant Southeast Asian ovalocytosis. *Proc Natl Acad Sci U S A* 1991;88:11022–11026.
33. Jarolim P, Rubin HL, Liu S-C, et al. Duplication of 10 nucleotides in the erythroid band 3 (AE1) gene in a kindred with hereditary spherocytosis and band 3 protein deficiency (band 3^{PRAGUE}). *J Clin Invest* 1994;93:121–130.
34. Jarolim P, Rubin HL, Brabec V, et al. Mutations of conserved arginines in the membrane domain of erythroid band 3 lead to a decrease in membrane-associated band 3 and to the phenotype of hereditary spherocytosis. *Blood* 1995;85:634–640.
35. Jarolim P, Murray JL, Rubin HL, et al. Characterization of 13 novel band 3 gene defects in hereditary spherocytosis with band 3 deficiency. *Blood* 1996;88:4366–4374.
36. Jarolim P, Shayakul C, Prabakaran D, et al. Autosomal dominant distal renal tubular acidosis is associated in three families with heterozygosity for the R589H mutation in the AE1 (band 3) Cl-/HCO3- exchanger. *J Biol Chem* 1998;273:6380–6388.
37. Spring FA, Bruce LJ, Anstee DJ, et al. A red cell band 3 variant with altered stilbene disulphonate binding is associated with the Diego (Di^a) blood group antigen. *Biochem J* 1992;288:713–716.
38. Layrisse M, Arends T, Dominguez-Sisco R. Nuevo grupo sanguineo encontrado en descencientes de Indios. *Acta Med Venez* 1955;3:132.
39. Thompson PR, Childers DM, Hatcher DE. Anti-Di^b. First and second examples. *Vox Sang* 1967;13:314.

40. Bruce LJ, Anstee DJ, Spring FA, et al. Band 3 Memphis variant II. Altered stilbene disulfonate binding and the Diego (Di^a) blood group antigen are associated with the human erythrocyte band 3 mutation $Pro^{854}\rightarrow Leu$ *J Biol Chem* 1994;269:16155–16158.
41. Jarolim P, Murray J, Rubin H, et al. Blood group antigens Rb^a, Tr^a and Wd^a are located in the third edoplasmic loop of erythrocyte band 3 protein. *Transfusion* 1997;37:605–615.
42. Jarolim P, Murray JL, Rubin HL, et al. A Thr552->Ile substitution in erythroid band 3 gives rise to the Warrior blood group antigen. *Transfusion* 1997;37:398–405.
43. Crandall I, Collins WE, Gysin J, et al. Synthetic peptides based on motifs present in human band 3 protein inhibit cytoadherence/sequestration of the malaria parasite *Plasmodium falciparum. Proc Natl Acad Sci U S A* 1993;90:4703–4707.
44. Thevenin BJM, Crandall I, Ballas SK, et al. Band 3 peptides block the adherence of sickle cells to endothelial cells in vitro. *Blood* 1997; 4172–4179.
45. Daniels GL, Shaw MA, Judson PA, et al. A family demonstrating inheritance of the Leach phenotype: a Gerbich negative phenotype associated with elliptocytosis. *Vox Sang* 1986;50:117–121.
46. Anstee DJ, Parsons SF, Ridgwell K, et al. Two individuals with elliptocytic red cells apparently lack three minor erythrocyte membrane sialoglycoproteins. *Biochem J* 1984;218:615–619.
47. Smith BL, Preston GM, Spring FA, et al. Human red cell aquaporin CHIP. I. Molecular characterization of ABH and Colton blood group antigens. *J Clin Invest* 1994;94:1043–1049.
48. Preston GM, Agre P. Isolation of the cDNA for erythrocyte integral membrane protein of 28 kilodaltons: member of an ancient channel family. *Proc Natl Acad Sci U S A* 1991;88:11110–11114.
49. Preston GM, Carroll TP, Guggino WB, et al. Appearance of water channels in xenopus oocytes expressing red cell CHIP28 protein. *Science* 1992;256:385–387.
50. Preston GM, Smith BL, Zeidel ML, et al. Mutations in aquaporin-1 in phenotypically normal humans without function CHIP water channels. *Nature* 1994;265:1585–1587.
51. Mathai JC, Mori S, Smith BL, et al. Functional analysis of aquaporin-1 deficient red cells—the Colton-null phenotype. *J Biol Chem* 1996; 271:1309–1313.
52. Campbell IG, Foulkes WD, Senger G, et al. Molecular cloning of the B-CAM cell surface glycoprotein of epithelial cancers: a novel member of the immunoglobulin superfamily. *Cancer Res* 1994;54:5761–5765.
53. Udani M, Zen Q, Cottman M, et al. Basal cell adhesion molecule Lutheran protein—the receptor critical for sickle cell adhesion to laminin. *J Clin Invest* 1998;101:2550–2558.
54. Taliano V, Guevin RM, Tippett P. The genetics of a dominant inhibitor of the Lutheran antigens. *Vox Sang* 1973;24:42–47.
55. Norman PC, Tippett P, Beal RW. An Lu(a − b −) phenotype caused by an X-linked recessive gene. *Vox Sang* 1986;51:49–52.
56. Aruffo A, Stamenkovic I, Melnick M, et al. CD44 is the principal cell surface receptor for hyaluronate. *Cell* 1990;61:1303–1313.
57. St John T, Meyer J, Idzerda R, et al. Expression of CD44 confers a new adhesive phenotype on transfected cells. *Cell* 1990;60:45–52.
58. Ellis NA, Tippett P, Petty A, et al. PBDX is the XG blood group gene. *Nat Genet* 1994;8:285–290.
59. Ellis NA, Ye TZ, Patton S, et al. Cloning of PBDX, an MIC2-related gene that spans the pseudoautosomal boundary on chromosome Xp. *Nat Genet* 1994;6:394–400.
60. Lewis M, Kaita H, Chown B. Scianna blood group system. *Vox Sang* 1974;27:261–264.
61. Westhoff CM, Sipherd BD, Wylie DE, et al. Severe anaphylactic reactions following transfusions of platelets to a patient with anti-Ch. *Transfusion* 1992;32:576–579.
62. Rowe JA, Moulds JM, Newbold CI, et al. *P. falciparum* rosetting mediated by a parasite-variant erythrocyte membrane protein and complement-receptor 1. *Nature* 1997;388:292–295.
63. Rowe JA, Rogerson SJ, Raza A, et al. Mapping of the region of complement receptor (CR) 1 required for *Plasmodium falciparum* rosetting and demonstration of the importance of CR1 in rosetting in field isolates. *J Immunol* 2000;165:6341–6346.
64. Gubin AN, Njoroge JM, Wojda U, et al. Identification of the Dombrock blood group glycoprotein as a polymorphic member of the ADP-ribosyltransferase gene family. *Blood* 2000;96:2621–2627.

Rossi's Principles of Transfusion Medicine, Third Edition, edited by Toby L. Simon, Walter H. Dzik, Edward L. Snyder, Christopher P. Stowell, and Ronald G. Strauss. Lippincott Williams & Wilkins, Philadelphia © 2002.

CASE 10A

THE AWFUL ALLOS: TREATING A PATIENT WITH MULTIPLE ALLOANTIBODIES

CASE HISTORY

A 74-year-old woman was seen by her primary care physician with a 1-week history of melena and a hematocrit that had decreased to 28.8% from a baseline level of approximately 35%. The international normalized ratio was 6.2 on warfarin sodium (Coumadin) which the patient had been taking since the placement of prosthetic mitral and aortic valves 15 years ago. The patient had been admitted several times over the past 5 years for gastrointestinal bleeding caused by erosive gastropathy and diverticulosis, although it had not always been possible to find a well-defined source of each bleeding episode. The patient had undergone frequent transfusions during the previous admissions. Other medical problems included class II congestive heart failure secondary to hypertensive and rheumatic heart disease, cardiac dysrhythmia controlled with a dual-chamber pacemaker and a calcium channel blocker, and insulin-dependent diabetes mellitus.

The patient was admitted to the hospital with a blood pressure of 100/60 mm Hg and a heart rate of 90 beats/min. The electrocardiogram showed normal sinus rhythm and nonspecific ST-T wave changes but no signs of acute ischemia. Warfarin was discontinued, and parenteral vitamin K was administered (5 mg subcutaneously). The patient also received four units of fresh frozen plasma. However, the hematocrit continued to decrease and reached 23.9%. At this point, the ST-T wave changes became more pronounced. Depression was noted despite judicious volume replacement. Volume replacement was complicated by the underlying congestive heart failure.

On admission, a blood sample was sent for typing and crossmatching. The patient was well known to the blood bank staff, who had identified multiple alloantibodies over the past several years, including anti-C, anti-e, anti-S, and anti-Jk^a. At this point, however, only the anti-C and anti-e were evident, even when a variety of techniques were used to detect the anti-S and anti-Jk^a antibodies (e.g., polyethylene glycol, gel test, ficin-treated cells). The patient's red blood cells were group O, probable R_2R_2 and lacked the S, Jk^a, Kell, and Fy^b antigens.

The patient's physician was aware of the serologic problems because they had delayed transfusions and provoked cries of anguish from the blood bank in the past. He consulted with a transfusion medicine physician to discuss both immediate and long-term management of the patient's transfusion needs. The immediate concerns were the need for red blood cell transfusion and the ability to obtain compatible units rapidly. The long-term issues for this patient included preparation for subsequent gastrointestinal bleeding, and quite possibly repeat valvuloplasty.

DISCUSSION

The care of patients with multiple antibodies is always a trial for the transfusion service, even for elective transfusions, as in the treatment of patients with sickle cell disease or β thalassemia major. But the presence of multiple antibodies poses even greater challenges in the treatment of bleeding patients, in which the options are further constrained by time. The first objective is to stop the bleeding. In this case, the rate of blood loss appeared to be too great to wait safely for 12 to 24 hours until vitamin K reversed the effects of warfarin, so fresh frozen plasma was given.

The second objective in the treatment of a bleeding patient with multiple alloantibodies is to delay red blood cell transfusion for as long as it takes for the blood bank to locate suitable units. This requires careful assessment of the patient for evidence of ongoing blood loss and signs or symptoms of anemia. Because the signs and symptoms of anemia are difficult to differentiate from those of hypovolemia, it is extremely important to maintain intravascular volume with crystalloid solutions. Many of the untoward effects of blood loss can be averted or mitigated with volume replacement. When this patient was admitted, she appeared to be tolerating the blood loss reasonably well. However, over the course of the first day, the decreasing hematocrit and signs of cardiac ischemia forced the physician's hand, and he decided to perform a transfusion.

Finding compatible units for this patient was more easily said than done. All four of her red blood cell alloantibodies are clinically significant and cause hemolytic transfusion reactions. The blood bank needed to find units that lacked C, e, S, and Jk^a. Because fewer than one unit in 1,000 would lack all four antigens (Table 10A.1), it is unlikely that the average transfusion service, or for that matter any but the larger donor centers, would have several such units in the liquid inventory. If the donor center were to keep an inventory of frozen, phenotyped red

TABLE 10A.1. FREQUENCY OF DONOR RED CELLS NEGATIVE FOR ANTIGEN TARGETS FOR CLINICALLY SIGNIFICANT ALLOANTIBODIES

Blood Group System	% Donor Units Negative for Antigen		
	Antigen	European	African
Rh	C	20[a]	64[a]
	c	23[a]	4[a]
	E	68[a]	77[a]
	e	3[a]	2[a]
Kell	K	91	98
	k	0.2	Rare
Glycophorin A/B	M	22	30
	N	28	26
	S	45	69
	s	11	3
Duffy	Fy^a	34	88[b]
	Fy^b	17	77[b]
Kidd	Jk^a	23	9
	Jk^b	9	57

[a]Based on antigen frequencies in D(+) donor units.
[b]Approximately 68% of African Americans are Fy(a−, b−).

blood cells, it might be able to locate a few suitable units. When the local supply of suitable units is inadequate, transfusion services and donor centers have recourse to the American Rare Donor Program, which maintains a national listing of rare and uncommon units. The American Rare Donor Program, which can be contacted by telephone or e-mail (1), can locate special units of blood throughout the United States and provide contact information. Arrangements for shipping and billing these units can be made directly with the facility providing them or through the National Blood Exchange (NBE), a service of the American Association of Blood Banks (AABB). The NBE acts as a national clearinghouse to facilitate the movement of blood from areas with temporary excess inventory to areas where it is needed.

If units lacking all four antigens are not available, what are the alternatives? It may be necessary to disregard some of the alloantibodies. Not all red blood cell alloantibodies cause hemolytic transfusion reactions. Room temperature–reactive anti-M, anti-Le^a and anti-P_1, for example, usually can be ignored. In this instance, unfortunately, all four alloantibodies were clinically significant. However, because only anti-C and anti-e were detectable, a reasonable alternative might have been to transfuse R_2R_2 cells. If these units were S positive or Jk^a positive, they would certainly elicit an anamnestic response resulting in a delayed serologic or hemolytic transfusion reaction. Anti-Jk^a antibodies are notorious for their role in delayed hemolytic transfusion reactions. Because anti-Jk^a antibodies also can cause intravascular hemolysis, it is probably unwise to disregard them. Therefore the best option if units lacking all four antigens cannot be found would be to screen R_2R_2 cells for the Jk^a antigen and remain vigilant for signs of a delayed serologic or hemolytic reaction due to anti-S antibodies. Although this is certainly not the safest course of action, these risks must be weighed against the hazards of severe anemia in an elderly woman with already compromised cardiac function and hints of ischemia.

In his conversation with the clinician, the transfusion medicine physician outlined the difficulties posed by the patient's alloantibodies, the likelihood of finding compatible units, the time that might be required to obtain them, and the risks of transfusing incompatible units. Because these risks had to be assessed in the context of the patient's other medical problems, the gastroenterologist and the cardiologist contributed to the discussion as well.

CASE HISTORY, CONTINUED

The transfusion medicine physician's predictions were too pessimistic. In fact, four units lacking the C, e, S and Jk^a antigens were found in the inventories of frozen blood of the hospital blood bank and the local blood donor center. An additional six frozen units were located through the American Rare Donor Program and shipped over the next several days.

The patient underwent several enteroscopic procedures, although no focal bleeding sites were identified. Bleeding stopped with reversal of anticoagulation but not before the patient received all ten units of red blood cells, which finally stabilized the hematocrit at 28% to 30%. The patient underwent slow reanticoagulation and was brought to an international normalized ratio of 3.5 to 5.0 with no evidence of bleeding. Doppler ultrasonographic evidence of increasing mitral and aortic valve insufficiency led to the possibility that either or both of the prosthetic valves would have to be replaced within the next several years.

DISCUSSION, CONTINUED

Although the blood bank had been fortunate in locating ten units with a rare phenotype within a few days, the serology gods may not smile so benignly in the future. A plan was needed for providing red blood cell transfusion support for this patient in the likely event that she should bleed again or need cardiac surgery. As part of planning for follow-up care of this patient after discharge, the transfusion medicine physician reviewed the options with the clinicians. One option in this kind of situation is for the donor center or hospital blood bank to designate their own donors with suitable phenotypes and put those units into frozen storage when they arrive in the bank. Such donors could even be specifically recruited. The other possible option is to collect and freeze autologous units from the patient. In this instance, the patient tended to have mild anemia (hematocrit, ~35%) even without bleeding and may not have been able to donate many units successfully. The transfusion medicine physician therefore proposed starting administration of erythropoietin, which has been used successfully to augment presurgical autologous blood donation (2).

CODA

In this case, the hospital blood bank had discovered that two of its own donors had a suitable red blood cell phenotype and designated their donations for frozen storage. The patient began erythropoietin therapy and was able to give approximately one unit every month while maintaining a hematocrit of 38% to 40%. An inventory of ten frozen units was accumulated, which should provide reasonable transfusion support in the event of renewed gastrointestinal bleeding or valve replacement. In addition, the elevated hematocrit also provided the patient with a more substantial margin of safety for the time she was receiving erythropoietin.

Case contributed by Christopher P. Stowell, M.D., Ph.D., Massachusetts General Hospital, Boston, MA.

REFERENCES

1. American Rare Donor Program, Musser Blood Center, 700 Spring Garden St, Philadelphia, PA, 19123. Phone: 215-451-4900; Fax: 215-451-2538; e-mail: ardp@usa.redcross.org.
2. Price TH, Goodnough LT, Vogler WR, et al. Improving the efficacy of preoperative autologous blood donation in patients with low hematocrits: a randomized, double-blind, controlled trial of recombinant human erythropoietin. *Am J Med* 1996;101:22S–27S.

11

ERYTHROCYTOSIS AND THERAPEUTIC PHLEBOTOMY

RICHARD S. EISENSTAEDT

Erythrocytosis may occur in a variety of conditions ranging from ectopic cytokine production to neoplastic hematopoietic clonal proliferation, or it may develop as a physiologic adaptation to inadequate tissue oxygen delivery. This chapter reviews the relation between erythrocytosis and blood viscosity and outlines an approach to classifying and determining the cause of erythrocytosis. The indications and risks of phlebotomy in the management of erythrocytosis and other disorders are discussed. The potential for a significant increase in the numbers of patients undergoing therapeutic phlebotomy for hereditary hemochromatosis is reviewed. The disposition of blood obtained by means of therapeutic phlebotomy also is considered.

BLOOD VISCOSITY

Viscosity, the flow-determining property of fluids, is defined as the relation between the horizontal force applied to a contact area moving across a liquid surface and the velocity gradient of the contact area with increasing distance or depth from the plane of application of the force. The force applied per unit area also is called *shear stress,* and the velocity gradient is the *shear rate* (1). Viscosity, thus considered the ratio of shear stress to shear rate, is calculated in units of poise (dyne-seconds per square centimeter). The viscosity of water at 20°C is approximately 1 centipoise. Blood, a suspension of cells within plasma, is a nonhomogeneous fluid described as non-newtonian in that the ratio of shear stress to shear rate is not constant (as is the case for a newtonian, homogeneous fluid such as water). Blood varies with changes in factors known to affect red blood cell agglutination, such as vessel luminal diameter, flow rate, and fibrinogen concentration. The viscosity of blood increases as shear rate decreases in areas of reduced blood flow that favor cell clumping.

Although large molecules such as fibrinogen and macroglobulins produce a plasma viscosity approximately 1.2 to 1.3 times that of water, red blood cell volume, or hematocrit, is the main contributor to whole-blood viscosity. The changes in viscosity that occur with changes in hematocrit less than 40% to 45% have been considered insignificant, a supposition apparently corroborated when viscosity is measured in vitro in capillary viscometers. However, such devices measure viscosity at high shear rates that may bear little resemblance to areas of the circulation with a low flow rate. Thus these instruments can underestimate important contributions to the rheologic properties of blood (2). Indeed, the hemodynamic benefits ascribed to perioperative hemodilution may relate to diminished viscosity as the hematocrit decreases from apparently normal values. Increases in hematocrit greater than 50% unequivocally increase viscosity and resistance to blood flow. Reduction of the hematocrit by means of phlebotomy in patients with erythrocytosis therefore decreases blood viscosity and improves blood flow.

Although decreasing blood viscosity by means of phlebotomy predictably improves blood flow, the ultimate circulatory goal is tissue oxygenation. The relation between erythrocytosis, viscosity, and blood flow on one hand and oxygen delivery to tissue

R.S. Eisenstaedt: Department of Medicine, Temple University School of Medicine and Temple University Hospital, Philadelphia, Pennsylvania.

TABLE 11.1. CLASSIFICATION OF ERYTHROCYTOSIS BY MECHANISM

Myeloproliferative disease
- Polycythemia rubra vera
- Pure erythrocytosis

Secondary erythrocytosis
- Physiologically appropriate
  - Hypoxia
    - High altitude
    - Cyanotic heart disease
    - Hypoxic lung disease
  - Increased hemoglobin-oxygen affinity
    - Hemoglobinopathy
    - Disordered 2,3-diphosphoglycerate metabolism
    - Carbon monoxide intoxication
- Physiologically inappropriate
  - Hypernephroma and other tumors
  - Benign renal disease
  - Disordered erythropoietin regulation
  - Relative erythrocytosis: plasma volume contraction

on the other may be complicated. Removal of red blood cells decreases viscosity but simultaneously decreases blood oxygen content. This may produce an overall negative effect on oxygen delivery. The effects of phlebotomy on cardiac output, vasoregulatory mechanisms, peripheral vascular resistance, pulmonary gas exchange, and oxygen-hemoglobin dissociation may be more difficult to predict and certainly are influenced by additional factors such as the presence or absence of peripheral vascular disease, myocardial dysfunction, chronic pulmonary insufficiency, and in some instances, the cause of the underlying erythrocytosis.

CLASSIFICATION OF ERYTHROCYTOSIS

Diseases characterized by erythrocytosis can be classified into two categories. (Table 11.1). In myeloproliferative disorders such as polycythemia rubra vera, neoplastic proliferation of marrow stem cells is independent of the growth factors and inhibitors that normally regulate hematopoiesis. Secondary erythrocytosis is erythropoietin mediated and may be a physiologically appropriate compensation for faulty oxygen delivery to peripheral tissue or from inappropriate excess erythropoietin in the absence of a relevant physiologic stimulus. Phlebotomy decisions flow from this conceptual scheme. In circumstances in which there is no physiologic basis for the erythrocytosis, phlebotomy is clearly indicated to reduce viscosity and decrease thromboembolic risk. Phlebotomy thus is indicated in polycythemia vera and in the secondary erythrocytosis caused by ectopic erythropoietin secretion. Phlebotomy also may be indicated in the compensatory erythrocytosis caused by hypoxia and abnormal tissue delivery of oxygen, but these decisions are much more complicated, weighing the advantage of lowering blood viscosity against the risk of reducing the oxygen-carrying capacity of blood.

Erythrocytosis also can be classified by erythropoietin response (Table 11.2). The excessive red blood cell proliferation in the myeloproliferative disease polycythemia vera is independent of erythropoietin and suppresses endogenous renal erythropoietin secretion to low or undetectable levels (3). Secondary erythrocytosis in response to tissue hypoxia is mediated by erythropoietin, and measured erythropoietin levels are in the "normal" range but, in theory, too high when matched with the elevated red blood cell count. The highest measured levels are present in ectopic erythropoietin secretion. Classification of erythrocytosis by erythropoietin level may be useful in outlining a diagnostic algorithm.

POLYCYTHEMIA RUBRA VERA

Polycythemia vera was probably recognized by Hippocrates and has been associated with pathologic thrombosis for more than two centuries (4). Polycythemia vera may be discovered when an elevated hemoglobin level is noted on a routine screening blood count. Patients may have nonspecific symptoms such as headache, tinnitus, weakness, and dizziness or may report pruritus that is worse after a warm shower (5) or burning pain in the hands and feet, called *erythromelalgia* (6). Classic physical findings include facial plethora and hepatosplenomegaly, which may reflect extramedullary erythropoiesis. Characteristic laboratory features include elevation in hematocrit with increased red

TABLE 11.2. CLASSIFICATION OF ERYTHROCYTOSIS: BY ERYTHROPOIETIN LEVEL

Low	Normal	Elevated
Polycythemia rubra vera	Hypoxia	Ectopic erythropoietin secretion
Pure erythrocytosis	Pulmonary insufficiency	Tumor
	Congenital cyanotic heart disease	Hypernephroma
	High altitude	Hepatocellular carcinoma
	Increased hemoglobin oxygen binding	Other renal disease
	Hemoglobinopathy	Renovascular disease
	Disordered 2,3-diphosphoglycerate metabolism	Polycystic renal disease
	Carbon monoxide intoxication	Aftermath of transplantation
	Relative erythrocytosis, plasma volume contraction	

blood cell mass, thrombocytosis, and leukocytosis, occasionally with basophilia. The bone marrow is hypercellular with increased collagen and reticulin fibrosis. Studies involving patients with a cytogenetic marker or women with polycythemia vera who were heterozygotes for glucose-6-phosphate dehydrogenase isoenzymes have shown a clonal neoplastic expansion of hematopoietic stem cells. Erythropoietin levels are low. Red blood cell precursors in patients with polycythemia vera that are grown in vitro do not require exogenous erythropoietin to proliferate (7) and overexpress Bcl-x, an apoptosis-inhibiting oncoprotein (8). These features of in vitro cell growth shed insight on the biologic mechanisms of the disease and offer diagnostic clues. The diagnosis is made when the characteristic clinical features are found and when disorders associated with physiologically appropriate or inappropriate secondary erythrocytosis are excluded.

Patients with polycythemia vera have two possible predispositions to intravascular thrombosis. Hyperviscosity per se can slow blood flow and directly facilitate thrombosis. A second risk arises from abnormal platelet function. Megakaryocytes in patients with polycythemia vera also evolve from a defective stem cell clone that may produce excessive numbers of platelets as well as platelets that, individually, possess subtle intrinsic defects. These quantitative and qualitative defects can cause measurable abnormalities of platelet function and, ironically, have been clinically linked to both an increased likelihood of bleeding and to a predisposition to hypercoagulable events (9). The incidence of thrombotic complications is clearly increased in comparison with that among patients with comparable erythrocytosis unrelated to myeloproliferative disease (10).

Typically found in the elderly, polycythemia vera is a relatively indolent disease with a mean survival period of a decade or more. Morbidity and mortality are caused by progressive marrow fibrosis, evolution to acute leukemia, especially among patients with previous alkylator agent or phosphorus 32 therapy, or from excess thromboembolic events related to erythrocytosis and hyperviscosity, abnormal platelet function, or both (11). Therapeutic phlebotomy is the mainstay of therapy; it reduces red blood cell mass and prolongs survival.

Debate continues to focus on how aggressively phlebotomy should be performed and on what constitutes a safe hematocrit. Epidemiologists have identified "high normal" hematocrit as a risk factor in cerebral infarction (12). In the Framingham population study, the incidence of cerebral infarction doubled among men with hemoglobin levels greater than 15 g/dl, although some of that risk was explained by dependent factors such as hypertension and smoking (13). Thomas et al. (14) found improved cerebral blood flow and reduced viscosity among patients with neurologic disorders whose mean hematocrit decreased from 49% to 42% after phlebotomy. Such data, along with the recognition that vascular occlusive episodes in patients with polycythemia vera strongly correlate with hematocrit (15), have led investigators in both Great Britain and the United States to recommend that phlebotomy be used to maintain the hematocrit at 45% or less (11,16).

Despite such treatment, patients with polycythemia vera continue to have thromboembolic disease and excessive mortality, especially during the first 3 years after diagnosis. Because reductions in thromboembolic mortality with phosphorus 32 or chlorambucil therapy are offset by an excessive death rate from leukemia (11) and because aspirin, at least in high doses, and dipyridamole are ineffective (17), efforts are focused on identification of agents that are myelosuppressive but not leukemogenic. Hydroxyurea plus phlebotomy seems superior to phlebotomy alone in the treatment of patients with additional risks for thromboembolic disease, such as very high platelet count, previous thromboembolism, or age older than 70 years. The advantage of hydroxyurea was most evident in the first several years of therapy and eventually was offset by an increased risk of leukemia compared with the risk of phlebotomy alone (18). The earlier polycythemia vera aspirin trial that showed a higher risk of bleeding and no therapeutic benefit was conducted with a higher dose of aspirin than has proved beneficial in decreasing mortality among patients with coronary artery or cerebrovascular disease. A trial has examined the role of low-dose aspirin in the treatment of patients with polycythemia vera (19). Newer therapy options, including interferon to control red blood cell mass (20) or anagrelide to decrease platelet count (21), are being evaluated.

TABLE 11.3. INCREASED RISK OF THROMBOSIS ASSOCIATED WITH POLYCYTHEMIA RUBRA VERA

Age >70 y
Recent diagnosis
More intense phlebotomy requirements
Hematologic features
Hemoglobin >15 g/dl
Platelet count >1,500 × 10^9/L
Previous thromboembolic event
Hypertension
Hyperlipidemia
Tobacco use

Phlebotomy of 1 U (500 ml) of blood may be performed once or twice a week to treat patients with polycythemia vera until the target hematocrit is reached. Patients typically develop iron deficiency and, possibly, thrombocytosis as phlebotomy treatments proceed. Iron deficiency eventually decreases phlebotomy requirements but may have deleterious effects on nonhematopoietic tissue (22). Some investigators have suggested that the microcytic hypochromic red blood cells and thrombocytosis associated with iron deficiency may increase blood viscosity and thrombotic risk (23).

The risk of thrombosis among patients with polycythemia vera treated with phlebotomy alone is greatest in the first few years after diagnosis. It increases among older patients, patients with previous thrombotic events, those with higher platelet counts, and, curiously, among patients with increased phlebotomy rates (Table 11.3) (17). Whether increased phlebotomy rates designate patients with more accelerated hematopoiesis in whom high thrombotic risk might be assumed or whether there are secondary responses to increased phlebotomy that independently add to hypercoagulability is unknown.

PURE ERYTHROCYTOSIS

Familial erythrocytosis (24) or erythremia occurs among persons whose red blood cell precursors mimic the defect of polycythemia vera but whose nonerythroid precursors seem uninvolved, leading clinically to pure erythrocytosis. An autosomal dominant form may be caused by enhanced precursor cell sensitivity to erythropoietin (25) associated with a mutation in the erythropoietin receptor gene (26). An alternative mechanism remains to be elicited to explain erythrocytosis in other kindreds (27). The risk of hyperviscosity and thrombosis warrants phlebotomy as used in polycythemia vera.

SECONDARY ERYTHROCYTOSIS: ERYTHROPOIETIN MEDIATED

Physiologically Appropriate

Erythrocytosis also can occur among patients with excess erythropoietin secretion arising from impaired oxygen release to peripheral tissue. This situation can occur in persons with chronic severe hypoxia and hemoglobin-oxygen desaturation, such as those living at high altitude, those inspiring air with low oxygen tension, those with chronic pulmonary insufficiency, or those with congenital cyanotic heart disease. A second setting is normal oxygen saturation but abnormal oxygen-hemoglobin dissociation, so that adequately oxygenated hemoglobin does not deliver oxygen efficiently to peripheral tissues. In this situation, the renal tissue relying on oxygen delivery to regulate erythropoietin secretion senses the same lack of oxygen delivery as in anemia or hypoxia and responds analogously by secreting erythropoietin and stimulating erythropoiesis. Such oxygen-avid hemoglobins are present in persons with certain inherited hemoglobin mutations or in patients, often heavy cigarette smokers, with carbon monoxide exposure and elevated carboxyhemoglobin levels (28). Decisions about phlebotomy in the treatment of patients with physiologic explanations for erythrocytosis are more complicated than those in the care of patients with polycythemia vera.

High Altitude

There is little information about the course of erythrocytosis in persons residing at high altitudes or the physiologic effect of phlebotomy on those with long-term exposure. Mountaineers experience decreased exercise tolerance and reduced alertness that may improve after phlebotomy, but data are too scant to promote use of this therapy for mountain sickness (29).

Chronic Pulmonary Insufficiency

Most patients with erythrocytosis from respiratory insufficiency have obvious hypoxia and a baseline reduction in oxygen saturation. The predisposing desaturation sometimes can be demonstrated only during sleep (30). The secondary erythrocytosis that occurs in patients with respiratory insufficiency and sustained hypoxia, initially an adaptive mechanism to increase oxygen content and oxygen delivery, at some point may prove maladaptive as hyperviscosity retards tissue oxygenation and contributes to pulmonary artery hypertension, right ventricular dilation, and right-sided heart failure (31). Investigators have shown that phlebotomy in the treatment of patients with chronic obstructive pulmonary disease and erythrocytosis may improve right ventricular function (32) and increase exercise tolerance (33,34). Mean pulmonary arterial pressure and pulmonary vascular resistance decrease (35). Phlebotomy may be useful to these patients to complement chronic oxygen treatment and other pharmacologic interventions aimed at optimizing cardiopulmonary function. Phlebotomy is most useful in the care of patients with overt cor pulmonale and a hematocrit greater than 70%. The target postphlebotomy hematocrit for these patients should be conservative, approximately 55%. Removal of smaller volumes, approximately 250 ml per phlebotomy, with careful monitoring seems prudent to avoid an intravascular volume flux that can be acutely deleterious (36,37).

Cyanotic Congenital Heart Disease

The initially appropriate increase in hematocrit in patients with cyanotic heart disease can become exaggerated and adversely affect tissue oxygenation and cardiac output. Thrombotic complications, hemorrhagic diathesis, and central nervous system symptoms are reported in such patients with a hematocrit greater than 70%. If the congenital defect is not surgically correctable and the erythropoietic response is excessive, phlebotomy may be beneficial. Rosenthal et al. decreased hematocrit from 73% to 62% with isovolemic albumin replacement and observed improved stroke volume, systemic blood flow, and oxygen transport (38). Oldershaw and Sutton (39) found improved exercise performance that persisted for 2 weeks after phlebotomy. Phlebotomy generally is not needed in the care of patients with a hematocrit less than 60%. Phlebotomy performed on a patient with a markedly higher hematocrit should be done euvolemically to maintain cardiac output (40). Iron replacement is recommended for children (41), and avoiding iron deficiency in adults with congenital cyanotic heart disease may decrease the risk of stroke (42).

Hemoglobinopathy

There are more than 30 known hemoglobin mutations, generally occurring at strategic portions of the molecule involved in oxygen binding, that increase oxygen avidity (43). The normal hemoglobin tetramer exists in equilibrium between the so-called relaxed state of fully oxygenated quaternary protein conformation and the tense fully deoxygenated state. All of these mutations either stabilize the oxygenated state or destabilize the deoxygenated state, resulting in decreased tissue oxygen delivery and secondary polycythemia. Some of these mutations occur at sites that reduce hemoglobin affinity for 2,3-diphosphoglycerate (2, 3-DPG; also known as 2,3-bisphosphoglycerate). Although some of these abnormal hemoglobins may migrate with a normal electrophoretic pattern, all are revealed with measurement of altered P_{50}, the oxygen pressure at which hemoglobin is 50% saturated with oxygen.

Patients with congenital methemoglobinemia, usually from a deficiency of cytochrome 5b reductase, have ferric hemes of methemoglobin that are unable to bind oxygen and ferrous hemes with increased oxygen affinity. A familial deficiency of 2,3-DPG is a rare cause of increased oxygen affinity (44). The molecular mechanism of other inherited causes of polycythemia remains elusive (45).

Thrombotic complications have been reported anecdotally in the care of some patients with oxygen-avid hemoglobinopathy (46,47). Other patients have had symptoms similar to those of polycythemia vera. However, a large number may have asymptomatic mutations found during evaluation of incidentally detected benign erythrocytosis (48,49). Whether oxygen-avid hemoglobinopathy and the resulting erythrocytosis place patients sufficiently at risk to justify phlebotomy is unknown. Phlebotomy effects in a small number of these patients have been studied. Although reasonably well tolerated, effects on exercise performance were inconsistent (50–52). Increased hemoglobin-oxygen avidity also can occur after carbon monoxide intoxication through carboxyhemoglobin formation. This mechanism has been implicated in erythrocytosis found in cigarette smokers (28).

Physiologically Inappropriate

Hypernephroma or, less commonly, neoplasms in other organs such as the liver, cerebellum, or uterus can secrete ectopic erythropoietin and cause erythrocytosis (53). The blood abnormality may be the initial manifestation of the underlying tumor and lead to early diagnosis and tumor resection that not only corrects the erythrocytosis but also may lead to long tumor-free survival.

Renovascular disease or other renal lesions that compress blood flow to renal tissue sites where erythropoietin is secreted in response to oxygen delivery can lead to erythrocytosis. A variety of benign renal lesions, from polycystic kidney disease to glomerulonephritis, have been associated with excessive erythropoietin and erythrocytosis. As many as 20% of recipients of renal transplants experience erythrocytosis, often in the first year after transplantation while the graft seems to be functioning well. Although phlebotomy may be the most direct therapy to prevent associated thromboembolic complications, enalapril also decreases erythropoietin secretion and corrects erythrocytosis (54). Angiotensin II receptor antagonists also are effective (55). Theophylline decreases posttransplantation erythrocytosis but is less predictably effective and more potentially toxic than are either angiotensin-converting enzyme inhibitors or angiotensin II receptor antagonists (56). Patients with congenital defects in erythropoietin regulation may secrete excessive hormone independently of normal oxygen delivery (57).

RELATIVE ERYTHROCYTOSIS

Relative erythrocytosis, also called *pseudopolycythemia, spurious, stress,* or *benign polycythemia,* or *Gaisbock syndrome,* occurs in persons whose total red blood cell mass is at the upper limit of normal or mildly elevated and who may or may not also have contracted plasma volume. That this syndrome is neither benign nor spurious is supported by studies suggesting chronic symptoms and increased thromboembolic mortality similar to those of polycythemia vera (58,59).

Although the effects of phlebotomy on viscosity and cerebral blood flow are similar to those of polycythemia vera (60), the need for phlebotomy is uncertain. This procedure may not be warranted when a patient has asymptomatic, mild erythrocytosis, especially if the patient does not have other thrombotic risk factors such as smoking or hypertension (61). Moreover, patients with contracted plasma volumes may not tolerate a phlebotomy volume of 500 ml.

EVALUATION OF ERYTHROCYTOSIS

A carefully obtained history and physical examination often point to the cause of erythrocytosis, especially for patients with severe pulmonary or cyanotic heart disease or those with fully expressed polycythemia vera. Patients who are young and entirely healthy are likely to have a hemoglobinopathy, but more ominous causes, such as hypernephroma, have to be excluded. Patients who smoke cigarettes may have relative erythrocytosis, carbon monoxide intoxication, or both (Fig. 11.1).

The laboratory evaluation of all patients with erythrocytosis should include a complete blood cell count, pulse oximetry or arterial blood gas measurement to asses PO_2, urinalysis, and abdominal ultrasonography to assess for hepatosplenomegaly that may be difficult to detect during the physical examination and to rule out hypernephroma or other structural renal disease (Table 11.4). The cause may be evident with these initial studies.

Some experts include bone marrow aspiration and measurement of erythropoietin levels in the initial evaluation, but these studies may be superfluous and are rarely definitive in ascertaining the cause. The bone marrow is apt to mimic the peripheral blood and is highly suggestive in the evaluation of patients with a complete blood cell count that is highly suggestive, that is, leukocytosis, basophilia, and thrombocytosis. The results are less convincing in the evaluation of a patient with early polycythemia vera who have less dramatic elevation of other cell lines. The bone marrow also shows increased reticulin and collagen fibrosis that is not evident in the peripheral blood smear and may be studied in specialized laboratories to assess characteristics of cell culture growth and oncogene expression that could also support a diagnosis of polycythemia vera.

The erythropoietin level, if markedly elevated, strongly points to an ectopic source of secretion. Most of these causes are revealed at abdominal ultrasonography that shows a renal tumor (or more rarely a liver neoplasm) or asymmetry in kidney size consistent with renovascular disease. Abnormal results of urinalysis and an elevated creatinine level suggest another underlying renal disease. In the absence of overt renal disease or a liver neoplasm, all of which are usually seen at ultrasonography, the elevated erythropoietin level can lead to other diagnostic studies in pursuit of ectopic production, including imaging of the central nervous system. A low erythropoietin level is characteristic of polycythemia vera or pure erythrocytosis but in itself is unlikely to establish those etiologic factors without corroborating clinical features. Furthermore, patients with polycythemia vera

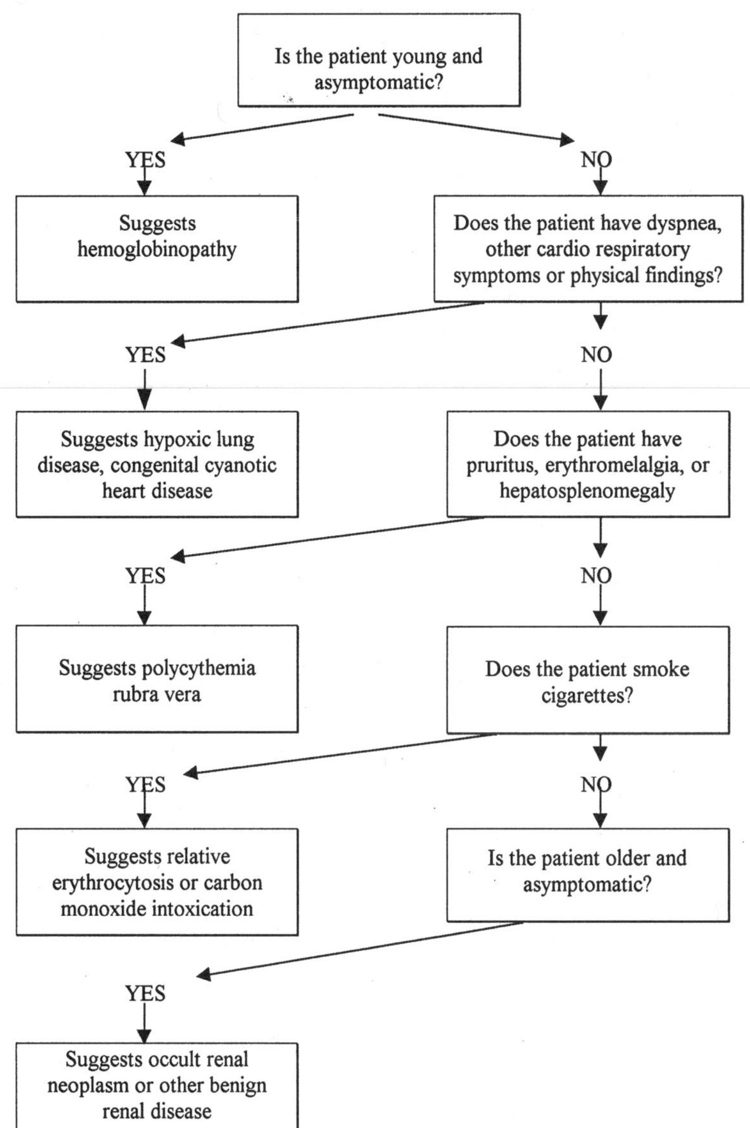

FIGURE 11.1. Approach to the management of erythrocytosis—history, physical examination.

TABLE 11.4. LABORATORY EVALUATION FOR ERYTHROCYTOSIS

Initial laboratory evaluation
Complete blood cell count
Pulse oximetry or arterial blood gas measurement
Urinalysis
Abdominal ultrasonography
Optional additional laboratory studies
Bone marrow aspiration
Erythropoietin levels
Determination of P_{50}
Red blood cell mass and plasma volume

may have erythropoietin levels that fluctuate between low and normal (62).

Measurement of the P_{50} establishes impaired oxygen delivery as the mechanism of erythrocytosis. Hemoglobinopathy is the likely cause in young patients and those without symptoms. Carbon monoxide intoxication should be suspected in heavy cigarette smokers.

Older algorithms recommended measuring red blood cell mass and plasma volume with radionuclear techniques as the first step in differentiating true erythrocytosis from relative erythrocytosis caused by contracted plasma volume. Those studies may be useful in the care of patients with modest erythrocytosis, but one can assume that hemoglobin levels greater than 18 g/dl are invariably a reflection of a true increase in red blood cell mass. The laboratory investigation of erythrocytosis is outlined in Figure 11.2.

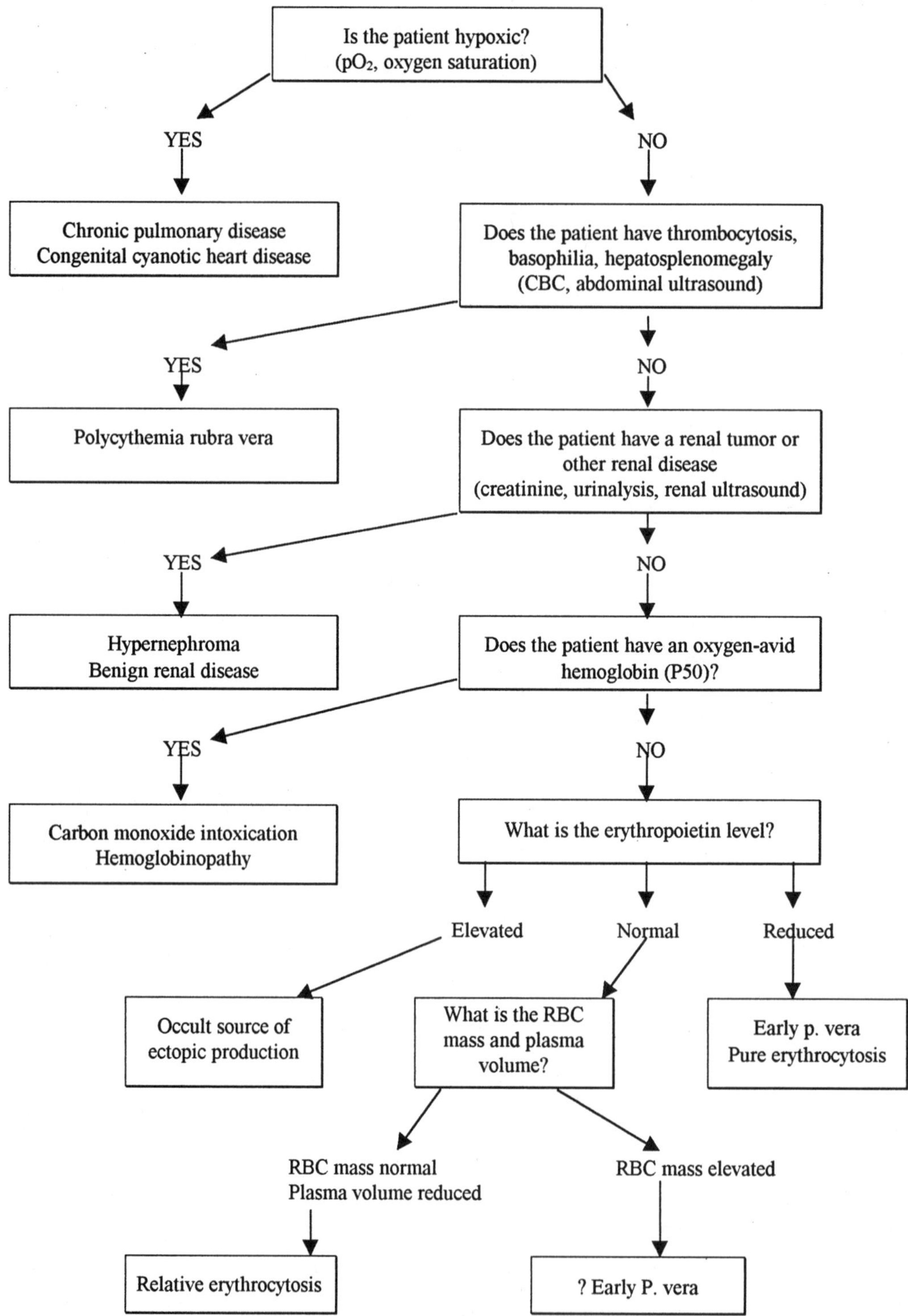

FIGURE 11.2. Approach to the management of erythrocytosis—laboratory studies.

TABLE 11.5. INDICATIONS FOR THERAPEUTIC PHLEBOTOMY

Disease	Guidelines	Comments
Polycythemia vera	Maintain hematocrit <45%	Myelosuppressive chemotherapy may also be needed with increased thrombotic risk (Table 11.3). Therapy for iron deficiency debatable
Pure erythrocytosis	See Polycythemia vera	
Hypoxic lung disease	For patients with hematocrit >70%; cor pulmonale	Reduced-volume (250 ml or less) phlebotomy Euvolemic technique Benefits with hematocrit >60% but <70% less clear
Cyanotic heart disease	For patients with hematocrit >70%	See Hypoxic lung disease Iron replacement may decrease stroke risk.
Oxygen-avid hemoglobinopathy	Unknown	—
Ectopic erythropoietin secretion	Short-term therapy before surgical correction Hematocrit <45%	—
Relative erythrocytosis	See polycythemia vera (??)	Especially indicated for patients with additional thromboembolic risk factors Reduced volume for those with contracted plasma volume
Hemochromatosis	Weekly until ferritin <300 μg/dl	With caution in patients with overt cardiomyopathy (see hypoxic lung disease, first two comments) Will not reduce mortality or decrease hepatoma risk in patients who already have cirrhosis

PHLEBOTOMY DECISIONS

The benefit of phlebotomy is most apparent when erythrocytosis has evolved independently of physiologic need, that is, the red blood cell expansion of myeloproliferative disease or ectopic erythropoietin secretion. Under those circumstances, phlebotomy reduces the thromboembolic risk of erythrocytosis, with no cost attached to the sacrificed oxygen content, which was not needed in the first place. Phlebotomy decisions are more complex when erythrocytosis evolves in response to a pathophysiologic deficit, such as hypoxia or impaired oxygen delivery.

The relative safety of therapeutic phlebotomy is to some extent borne out by the low morbidity among 10 million volunteers who donate blood yearly in the United States. Vasovagal reactions, local discomfort, and hematoma at the venesection site occasionally occur. Age and the lack of underlying medical problems, however, differentiate volunteer donors from patients undergoing therapeutic phlebotomy, who may need additional precautions. Serious complications and death have been reported (37). Elderly patients, those who are unusually thin, and those with active cardiopulmonary problems may not tolerate a 500-ml phlebotomy. Such patients initially should be treated with removal of 250 ml or less. In some cases, it may be advisable to administer a simultaneous infusion of crystalloid or colloid solution. For patients with hypoxia or other appropriate stimuli for secondary erythrocytosis, the benefits and risks of hematocrit reduction should be carefully weighed (Table 11.5).

PHLEBOTOMY THERAPY FOR IRON OVERLOAD

Dramatic advances in identifying the genetics of hereditary hemochromatosis have underscored the frequency of this disorder. The hemochromatosis gene, *HFE,* is located near the major histocompatibility complex on the short arm of chromosome 6, and two missense mutations have been identified (63). With approximately one in 250 white persons homozygous for this disorder, hereditary hemochromatosis is likely the most common inherited disease in the United States (64). The molecular pathogenesis of the disorder is not yet identified, but individuals with the genetic defect do not curtail intestinal iron absorption when body iron stores are normal or increased. With iron excretion fixed to a small amount of daily gastrointestinal loss plus additional menstrual blood loss for women, the continued excessive iron absorption eventually leads to iron overload and multiple-organ injury, including cardiomyopathy, cirrhosis with a high risk of hepatocellular cancer, diabetes mellitus, arthritis, and pituitary-linked endocrinopathy.

Phlebotomy to reduce iron stores is extremely effective in preventing morbidity and mortality from cardiac and liver disease. Unfortunately, once cirrhosis is diagnosed, phlebotomy therapy is not effective in preventing the complications of liver failure or in decreasing the risk of liver cancer (65). Similarly, phlebotomy treatment is much less effective once overt heart failure has developed.

Early signs of iron overload in patients with hereditary hemochromatosis can be diagnosed through inexpensive blood screening tests. A high transferrin saturation or elevated ferritin level indicates that a patient is at risk (66). The diagnosis usually is made when a patient with vague symptoms is found to have abnormal results of liver function tests. The disorder also is discovered in the evaluation of unexplained heart failure or cirrhosis. At present, all relatives of patients found to have hemochromatosis are screened. Arguably, relatives of patients who die of heart disease or liver disease of unknown causation and otherwise healthy persons who have abnormal transaminase levels on routine screening chemistry tests also should be screened. The frequency of the disorder, the ease and expense of screening, and the availability of phlebotomy therapy that can prevent morbidity but that is ineffective once advanced organ injury is present all suggest that more routine primary care screening should be instituted. Such widespread screening is likely to identify many cases of early disease and dramatically increases the numbers of patients undergoing therapeutic phlebotomy.

Iron overload also seems important in the pathogenesis of porphyria cutanea tarda, a disorder characterized by liver disease and cutaneous eruptions caused by a decrease in uroporphyrinogen decarboxylase. The hemochromatosis gene is found more commonly in these patients (67), and phlebotomy is indicated. A syndrome of iron overload in African patients that otherwise closely resembles hereditary hemochromatosis is not related to the *HFE* gene mutation and not linked to the histocompatibility complex (68). An uncommon form of hemochromatosis, termed *juvenile hemochromatosis,* occurs among much younger patients, is associated with more extensive end-organ damage, and has been linked to a mutation on the long arm of chromosome 1 not heretofore known to be involved in iron metabolism. These patients and all patients with hereditary hemochromatosis need phlebotomy therapy until the serum ferritin level is less than 300 μg/dl (69).

Signs of iron overload also can be found among patients with liver disease and chronic hepatitis. Results of early studies suggested that phlebotomy therapy might improve the response to interferon therapy among patients with chronic hepatitis C infection. More recent randomized, clinical trials, however, have shown no advantage to reduction of iron stores in enhancing the efficacy of antiviral therapy (70). The role of phlebotomy therapy in treating patients with alcoholic hepatitis and increased iron stores is unknown.

DISPOSITION OF BLOOD FROM THERAPEUTIC PHLEBOTOMY

The safety of the blood supply in the United States is based on a two-tier process. In the first tier, a detailed interview is conducted to identify known illness or behavioral risks that increase the likelihood that those persons harbor a transfusion-transmitted disease. The interview, brief examination, and hemoglobin measurement also focus on the personal health of the potential donor to assure the safety of phlebotomy. Persons with behavioral risks or known problems that increase the likelihood that they harbor a transfusion-transmitted disease are disqualified from donating blood. In the second tier, all apparently healthy persons undergo phlebotomy, but before the donated blood is transfused, a detailed battery of serologic tests is performed to exclude asymptomatic infection.

Inherent in achieving the initial goal of the healthiest possible donor pool is the principle of altruism as the prime motivation for blood donation and the avoidance of financial incentives that might influence the honesty of response to interview questions and perhaps increase the prevalence of transmissible diseases in that cohort. Many experts have argued that reliance on an all-volunteer donor population motivated by altruism is the single most important factor ensuring the safety of the blood supply. Indeed, an inevitable lag exists with each newly recognized transfusion-transmitted pathogen from recognition of the complication to establishment of tests to eliminate risky donors.

The U.S. Food and Drug Administration (FDA) has explicitly defined blood withdrawn to promote the health of the donor as different from the broader volunteer pool. Although the FDA in theory allows such blood to be used in transfusion, it requires that the unit be labeled to indicate the disease that necessitated phlebotomy. Recently FDA has allowed an exception for blood drawn from donors with hemochromatosis providing that the collecting facility does not charge patients/donors for therapeutic phlebotomy and submits a request for variance (71). The Standards of the American Association of Blood Banks permit the use of therapeutic phlebotomy units from patients/donors with hemochromatosis as specified by FDA.

If patients with hereditary hemochromatosis must pay for phlebotomy, were it for purely therapeutic purposes, but could have the procedure performed free of charge, were the blood to be used for subsequent transfusion, the financial difference could be seen as analogous to a paid blood donation. In reality, the situation entails avoiding payment for a therapeutic procedure rather than actually receiving payment for the donation. Whether the distinction is ethically meaningful is debatable. Similar debate has centered on other non-financial rewards for donation, such as time off from work, gifts, or other free screening tests.

It does not appear that patients with hereditary hemochromatosis are an inherently riskier donor population (72). There are, however, no data or even a theoretical basis for assuming that patients with hereditary hemochromatosis in early stage, identified before pathologic iron overload has led to organ injury, are at increased risk of harboring transfusion-transmitted diseases.

In 1999, the American Medical Association (AMA) recommended that blood drawn therapeutically from patients with hereditary hemochromatosis continue to be labeled as such. The AMA continues to require the consent of the physician ordering the transfusion and, presumably, the consent of the patient undergoing transfusion. The AMA recommended that such policy continue until therapeutic phlebotomy is universally available at no charge to patients independently of the future use of the phlebotomized blood. The AMA also recommended that physicians be encouraged to "explain to their patients that HH has a genetic basis, that the disease is not transmissible via blood transfusions, and that the blood from persons with HH is not necessarily unsuitable for direct transfusion" (73). The clear impact of this recommendation is to maintain the status quo.

Two evolving factors may modify the status quo independently of the cautious language of the AMA policy. First, the blood supply, although of unparalleled safety, has become endangered in its limited quantity, as more and more stringent safety regulations eliminate potential donors. The demographics of our aging population suggest that transfusion demand continues to increase. Options to increase the donor pool without compromising safety are already sought with fervor. Second, the potential number of healthy patients with early stages of excess iron overload from hereditary hemochromatosis will increase enormously if primary care physicians adopt the practice of routine screening of all patients. These two issues may promote change in the current attitudes toward the use of therapeutic phlebotomy and, at a minimum, provide impetus for research to rigorously assess the safety of such blood in transfusion.

SUMMARY

A wide array of conditions lead to erythrocytosis. Recognizing the cause of erythrocytosis is crucial in formulating treatment decisions to ensure that the risks of phlebotomy are small and readily offset by benefits in reducing blood viscosity and avoiding thromboembolic complications. Phlebotomy therapy is crucial in the treatment of patients with hereditary hemochromatosis. The frequency of this disorder and the ease of screening suggest that the number of patients undergoing phlebotomy for early stages of iron overload will increase dramatically.

REFERENCES

1. Berne RM, Levy MN. *Cardiovascular physiology,* 5th ed. St Louis: Mosby, 1986:105–124.
2. Replogle RL, Meiselman HJ, Merrill EW. Clinical implications of blood rheology studies. *Circulation* 1967;36:148–160.
3. Messinezy M, Westwood NB, Woodcock SP, et al. Low serum erythropoietin: a strong diagnostic criterion of primary polycythemia even at normal hemoglobin levels. *Clin Lab Haematol* 1995;17:217–220.
4. Wasserman LR. Polycythemia vera study group: a historical perspective. *Semin Hematol* 1986;23:183–187.
5. Steinman HK, Kobza-Black A, Lotti TM et al. Polycythaemia rubra vera and water induced pruritus: blood histamine levels and cutaneous fibrinolytic activity before and after water challenge. *Br J Dermatol* 1987;116:329–333.
6. Michiels JJ. Erythromelalgia and vascular complications in polycythemia vera. *Semin Thromb Hemost* 1997;23:441–445.
7. Partanens A, Juvonen E, Ikkala E, et al. Spontaneous erythroid colony formation in the differential diagnosis of erythrocytosis. *Eur J Haematol* 1989;42:327–329.
8. Silva M, Richard C, Benito A, et al. Expression of Bcl-x in erythroid precursors from patients with polycythemia vera. *N Engl J Med* 1998; 338:564–571.
9. Schafer AI. Bleeding and thrombosis in the myeloproliferative disorders. *Blood* 1984;64:1–12.
10. Schwarcz TH, Hogan LA, Endean ED, et al. Thromboembolic complications of polycythemia: polycythemia vera versus smokers' polycythemia. *J Vasc Surg* 1993;17:518–523.
11. Berk PD, Goldberg JD, Silverstein MW, et al. Increased incidence of acute leukemia in polycythemia vera associated with chlorambucil therapy. *N Engl J Med* 1981;304:441–447.
12. Toghi H, Yananouchi H, Murakaml M, et al. Importance of the hematocrit as a risk factor in cerebral infarction. *Stroke* 1978;9:369–374.
13. Kannel VS, Gordan T, Wolf PA, et al. Hemoglobin and the risk of cerebral infarction: the Framingham study. *Stroke* 1972;3:409–420.
14. Thomas DJ, duBoulay GH, Marshall J, et al. Effect of haemotocrit on cerebral blood flow in man. *Lancet* 1977;2:941–943.
15. Pearson JC, Weatherley-Mein G. Vascular occlusive episode and venous haemotocrit in primary proliferative polycythaemia. *Lancet* 1978; 2:1219–1222.
16. Thomas DJ, duBoulay GH, Marshall J, et al. Cerebral blood flow in polycythemia. *Lancet* 1977;2:161–163.
17. Berk PD, Goldberg JD, Donovan PB, et al. Therapeutic recommendations in polycythemia vera based on polycythemia vera study group protocols. *Semin Hematol* 1986;23:132–143.
18. Fruchtman SM, Mack K, Kaplan ME, et al. From efficacy to safety: a Polycythemia Vera Study Group report on hydroxyurea in patients with polycythemia vera. *Semin Hematol* 1997;34:17–23.
19. Landolfi R, Marchioli R. European Collaboration on Low-dose Aspirin in Polycythemia Vera (ECLAP): a randomized trial. *Semin Thromb Hemost* 1997:23:473–478.
20. Silver RT. A new treatment for polycythemia vera: recombinant interferon alfa. *Blood* 1990;76:664–665.
21. Silverstein MN. Anagrelide, a therapy for thrombocythemic states: experience in 577 patients. *Am J Med* 1992;92:69–76.
22. Birgegard G, Carlsson M, Sandhagen B, et al. Does iron deficiency in treated polycythemia vera affect whole blood viscosity? *Acta Med Scand* 1984;16:165–169.
23. Rector WG Jr, Fortuin NJ, Conley CL. Non-hematologic effects of chronic iron deficiency. *Medicine (Baltimore)* 1982;61:382–389.
24. Greenberg BR, Golde DW. Erythropoiesis in familial erythrocytosis. *N Engl J Med* 1977;296:1080–1084.
25. Juvonen E, Ikkala E, Fyhrquist F, et al. Autosomal dominant erythrocytosis caused by increased sensitivity to erythropoietin. *Blood* 1991; 78:3066–1069.
26. de la Chapelle A, Sistonen P, Lehvaslaiho H, et al. Familial erythrocytosis genetically linked to erythropoietin receptor gene. *Lancet* 1993; 341:82–84.
27. Emanuel PD, Eaves CJ, Broudy VC, et al. Familial and congenital polycythemia in three unrelated families. *Blood* 1992;79:3019–3030.
28. Smith JR, Landaw SA. Smoker's polycythemia. *N Engl J Med* 1978; 298:6–10.
29. Sarnquist FH, Schoene RB, Hackett PH, et al. Hemodilution of polycythemia in mountaineers: effects on exercise and mental function. *Aviat Space Environ Med* 1986;54:313–317.
30. Messinezy M, Aubry S, O'Connell G, et al. Oxygen desaturation in apparent and relative polycythaemia. *Br Med J* 1991;302:216–217.
31. Harrison BDW, Stokes TC. Secondary polycythaemia: its causes, effects and treatment. *Br J Dis Chest* 1982;76:313–339.
32. Erickson AD, Golden WA, Claunch BC, et al. Acute effects of phlebotomy on right ventricular size and performance in polycythemic patients with COPD. *Am J Cardiol* 1983;52:163–166.
33. Wedzicha JA, Cotter FE, Rudd RM, et al. Erythropheresis compared with placebo aphaeresis in patients with polycythaemia secondary to hypoxic lung disease. *Eur J Respir Dis* 1984;65:579–585.
34. Chetty KG, Brown SE, Light RW. Improved exercise tolerance of the polycythemic lung patient following phlebotomy. *Am J Med* 74:1983; 415–420.
35. Wiedemann HP, Matthay RA. Cor pulmonale in chronic obstructive pulmonary disease: circulatory pathophysiology and management. *Clin Chest Med* 1990;11:523.
36. Fishman AP. Pulmonary hypertension and cor pulmonale. In: Fishman AP, ed. *Pulmonary diseases and disorders.* New York: McGraw-Hill, 1988:999–1048.
37. Kiraly JF, Feldmann JE, Wheby MS. Hazards of phlebotomy in polycythemia patients with cardiovascular disease. *JAMA* 1976;236: 2080–2081.
38. Rosenthal A, Nathan DG, Marty AT, et al. Acute hemodynamic effects of red cell volume reduction in polycythemia of cyanotic congenital heart disease. *Circulation* 1970;42:297–307.
39. Oldershaw PJ, Sutton SJ. Haemodynamic effects of haemotocrit reduction in patients with polycythaemia secondary to cyanotic congenital heart disease. *Br Heart J* 1980;44:584–587.
40. Territo MC, Rosove MH. Cyanotic congenital heart disease: hematological management. *J Am Coll Cardiol* 1991;18:320–322.
41. Liberthson RR. Congenital heart disease in the child adolescent and adult patient. In: Johnson RA, Haber E, Austen WG, eds. *The practice of cardiology.* Boston: Little, Brown, 1980:755–896.
42. Ammash N, Warnes CA. Cerebrovascular events in adult patients with cyanotic congenital heart disease. *J Am Coll Cardiol* 1996;28:768–772.
43. Jandl JH. *Blood: textbook of hematology.* Boston: Little, Brown, 1987: 392–394.
44. Lemarchandel V, Joulin V, Valentin C, et al. Compound heterozygosity in a complete erythrocyte bisphosphoglycerate mutase deficiency. *Blood* 1992;80:2643–2649.
45. Sergeyeva A, Gordeuk VR, Tokarev YN, et al. Congenital polycythemia in Chuvashia. *Blood* 1997;89:2148–2154.
46. White JM, Szui L, Gillies IDS, et al. Familial polycythaemia caused by

a new haemoglobin variant: Hg Heathrow, B 103 (65) phenylalanine leucine. *Br Med J* 1973;3:665–667.
47. Gau GT, Fairbanks VF, Maldonado JE, et al. Cardiac dysfunction in a patient with hemoglobin Malmo treated with repeated transfusions. *Clin Res* 1974;22:276A(abst).
48. Bunn HF, Forget BG. *Hemoglobin: molecular, genetic and clinical aspects.* Philadelphia: WB Saunders, 1980.
49. Stephen AD. Annotation: polycythemia and high affinity hemoglobins. *Br J Haematol* 1977;36:153–159.
50. Poyart C, Bursaux E, Teisseire B, et al. Hemoglobin Creteil: oxygen transport by erythrocytes. *Ann Intern Med* 1978;88:758–763.
51. Charache S, Schuff S, Winslow R, et al. Variability of the homeostatic response to altered p50. *Blood* 1978;52:1156–1162.
52. Winslow RM, Butler WM, Kork JA, et al. The effect of bloodletting on exercise performance in a subject with high-affinity hemoglobin variant. *Blood* 1983;62:1159–1164.
53. Balcerzak SP, Bromberg PA. Secondary polycythemia. *Semin Hematol* 1975;12:353–382.
54. Conlon PJ, Farrell J, Donohoe J, et al. The beneficial effect of enalapril on erythrocytosis after renal transplantation. *Transplantation* 1993;56: 217–219.
55. Julian BA, Brantley RR Jr, Barker CV, et al. Losartan, an angiotensin II type 1 receptor antagonist, lowers hematocrit in post transplant erythrocytosis. *J Am Soc Nephrol* 1998;9:1104–1108.
56. Ok E, Akcicek F, Toz H, et al. Comparison of the effects of enalapril and theophylline on polycythemia after renal transplantation. *Transplantation* 1995;59:1623–1626.
57. Kulkarni V, Ritchey K, Howard D, et al. Heterogeneity of erythropoietin-dependent erythrocytosis: case report on a child and synopsis of primary erythrocytosis syndromes. *Br J Haematol* 1985;60:751–758.
58. Burge PS, Johnson WS, Prankerd TAJ. Morbidity and mortality in pseudopolycythemia. *Lancet* 1975;1:1266–1269.
59. Weinreb NJ, Shih CF. Spurious polycythemia. *Semin Hematol* 1975; 12:397–407.
60. Humphrey PRD, duBoulay GH, Marshall J, et al. Cerebral blood flow and viscosity in relative polycythaemia. *Lancet* 1979;2:873–877.
61. Lederle FA. Relative erythrocytosis: an approach to the patient. *J Gen Intern Med* 1987;2:128–130.
62. Birgegard G, Wide L. Serum erythropoietin in the diagnosis of polycythaemia and after phlebotomy treatment. *Br J Haematol* 1992;81: 603–606.
63. Powell LW, Subramaniam VN, Thomas R. Hemochromatosis in the new millennium. *J Hepatol* 2000;1[Suppl]:48–62.
64. Edwards CQ, Griffin LM, Goldgar D, et al. Prevalence of hemochromatosis among 11,065 presumably healthy blood donors. *N Engl J Med* 1988;318:1355–1362.
65. Niederau C, Fischer R, Sonnenberg A, et al. Survival and causes of death in cirrhotic and noncirrhotic patients with primary hemochromatosis. *N Engl J Med* 1985;313:1256–1262.
66. Edwards CQ, Kushner JP. Screening for hemochromatosis. *N Engl J Med* 1993;328:1616–1620.
67. Roberts AG, Whatly SD, Morgan RR, et al. Increased frequency of the hemochromatosis Cys282Tyr mutation in sporadic porphyria cutanea tarda. *Lancet* 1997;349:321–323.
68. Gordeuk V, Mukibi J, Hasstedt SJ, et al. Iron overload in Africa: interaction between a gene and dietary iron content. *N Engl J Med* 1992;326:95–100.
69. Roetto A, Totaro A, Cazzola M, et al. Juvenile hemochromatosis locus maps to chromosome 1q. *Am J Hum Genet* 1999;64:1388–1393.
70. Fontana RJ, Israel J, LeClair P, et al. Iron reduction before and during interferon therapy of chronic hepatitis C: results of a multicenter, randomized, controlled trial. *Hepatology* 2000;31:730–736.
71. Variances for blood collection from individuals with hereditary hemochromatosis. Guidance for Industry, August, 2001. Center for Biologies Evaluation and Research, Food and Drug Administration.
72. Sanchez AM, Schreiber GB, Bethel J, et al. Prevalence, donation practices, and risk assessment of blood donors with hemochromatosis. JAMA 2001;286:1475–1481.
73. Tan L, Khan MK, Hawk JC III. Use of blood therapeutically drawn from hemochromatosis patients. *Transfusion* 1999;30:1018–1026.

12

ANEMIA AND RED BLOOD CELL TRANSFUSION

JEFFREY L. CARSON
PAUL HÉBERT

Red blood cell transfusion is an extremely common medical intervention. In the United States, 11.5 million units were donated in 1997 (1,2). Approximately 2.5 million donations are issued annually in England and Wales. Typically, between 60% and 70% of all red blood cell units are transfused in the surgical setting. Other common uses are in the treatment of patients in intensive care units, those with cancer, and patients with blood loss from medical conditions such as gastrointestinal bleeding (1).

In this chapter we review the current knowledge about red blood cell transfusion and the risk posed by anemia. We begin by describing the physiologic adaptations to blood loss and anemia. We review oxygen transport, adaptive mechanisms in anemia, and microcirculatory effects of anemia. We then review the clinical outcomes of anemia and red blood cell transfusion. In that discussion, we present data from studies with animal and with human subjects that form the basis of our understanding of the consequences of anemia. We then summarize observational studies and clinical trials that examined the effect of red blood cell transfusion on mortality, morbidity, and functional recovery. We then review the guidelines on transfusion practices. The first three sections are based on systematic reviews of the literature. In the fourth section, we describe our approach to decision making in red blood cell transfusion. Our recommendations are based on evidence, when available. However, the section represents our views on this controversial subject.

J.L. Carson: Division of General Internal Medicine, Department of Medicine, University of Medicine and Dentistry of New Jersey, Robert Wood Johnson Medical School, New Brunswick, New Jersey.

P. Hébert: University of Ottawa Centre for Transfusion Medicine Research, Clinical Epidemiology Unit, University of Ottawa, Ontario, Canada.

PHYSIOLOGIC ADAPTATIONS TO BLOOD LOSS AND ANEMIA

Overview of Oxygen Transport

Hemoglobin is a complex molecule that consists of four globin moieties, each incorporating an iron-containing heme ring where oxygen is bound according to its partial pressure (PO_2). The oxygen-binding affinity of hemoglobin is graphically represented by a sinusoidal relation between hemoglobin oxygen saturation and PO_2. This relation, referred to as the *oxyhemoglobin dissociation curve,* enables both efficient loading in the lungs at high PO_2 and efficient unloading in the tissues at low PO_2 (Fig. 12.1). However, the affinity of hemoglobin for oxygen (the degree to which oxygen molecules saturate the hemoglobin binding sites at a given PO_2) may be altered by various disease states and may play a significant adaptive role in the response to anemia. The amount of oxygen delivered, either to the whole body or to specific organs, is the product of blood flow and arterial oxygen content. For the whole body, oxygen delivery (DO_2) is the product of total blood flow or cardiac output (CO) and arterial oxygen content (CaO_2), represented by the equation:

$$DO_2 = CO \times CaO_2 \qquad [1]$$

When ambient air is breathed under normal conditions, the

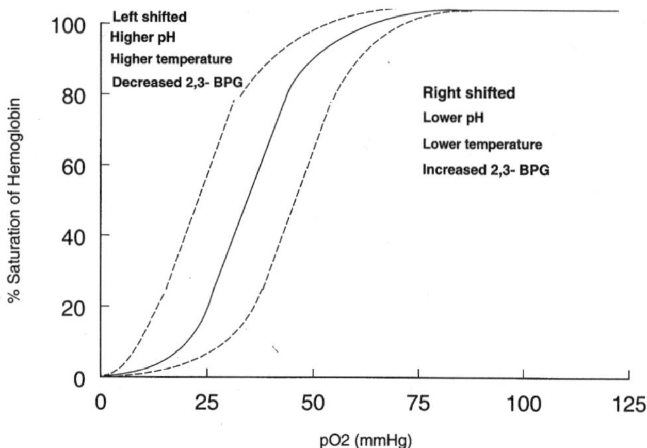

FIGURE 12.1. Oxyhemoglobin dissociation curve. The *solid line* represents oxygen-binding affinity to the hemoglobin molecule at standard temperature (37°C) and pH (7.4). The *dashed lines* represent hypothetical shifts in the curve. A rightward shift may be related to increased levels of 2,3-bisphosphoglycerate (2,3-BPG) or decreased temperature or pH. A shift to the left results from decreased level of 2,3-BPG or increased temperature or pH.

oxygen present in arterial blood is bound to hemoglobin. When fully saturated, 1 g of hemoglobin binds 1.39 ml of oxygen. In addition, a small amount also is dissolved in plasma water. The negligible amount of dissolved oxygen is directly proportional to the partial pressure and may be calculated by multiplying PO_2 by a constant ($k = 0.00301$ ml/ml per millimeter mercury), called the *solubility coefficient.* Thus under most circumstances, arterial oxygen content can be approximated from the portion bound to hemoglobin with the following equation:

$$CaO_2\ (\text{ml/L}) = \%\ \text{Sat} \times 1.39\ (\text{ml/g}) \times [\text{Hb}]\ (\text{g/dl}) \quad [2]$$

If we substitute CaO_2 from equation 2 into equation 1, then

$$DO_2 = CO \times (\%\text{Sat} \times 1.39 \times [\text{Hb}]) \quad [3]$$

Where CO is cardiac output in liters per minute, %Sat is hemoglobin oxygen saturation in percent, and [Hb] is hemoglobin concentration in grams per deciliter.

Tissue hypoxia and anoxia eventually occur if oxygen delivery decreases to a level at which it is no longer adequate to meet the metabolic demands of the tissues. From Equations 1 and 3, it is apparent that tissue hypoxia can be caused by decreased oxygen delivery due to decreases in either hemoglobin concentration (anemic hypoxia), cardiac output (stagnant hypoxia), or hemoglobin saturation (hypoxic hypoxia). Each of the determinants of DO_2 has substantial physiologic reserves thereby enabling the human body to adapt to significant increases in oxygen requirements or decreases in one of the determinants of DO_2 as a result of various diseases.

In health, the amount of oxygen delivered to the whole body exceeds resting oxygen requirements twofold to fourfold. For example, if we assume a hemoglobin level of 15 g/dl, a hemoglobin oxygen saturation of 99% and a cardiac output of 5 L/min, oxygen delivery is 1,032 ml/min. At rest, the amount of oxygen required or consumed by the whole body ranges from 200 to 300 ml/min. A decrease in hemoglobin concentration to 10 g/dl would result in an oxygen delivery of 688 ml/min. Despite this 33% decrease in oxygen delivery, there remains a twofold excess of oxygen delivered compared with oxygen consumed. However, a further decrease in hemoglobin concentration to 5 g/dl with all other parameters, including cardiac output, remaining constant decreases oxygen delivery to a critical level of 342 ml/min. Under stable experimental conditions, this dramatic decrease in oxygen delivery still exceeds oxygen consumption. However, at the critical level or threshold of oxygen—DO_2(crit)—oxygen delivery equals oxygen consumption. Further decreases in hemoglobin concentration result in inadequate oxygen delivery to tissues. There is, therefore, a biphasic relation between oxygen delivery and consumption (Fig. 12.2). One phase is an oxygen delivery–independent portion of the relation above a threshold value—DO_2(crit)—at which oxygen consumption is independent of oxygen delivery. The other is a delivery or supply-dependent portion, in which oxygen delivery is linearly related to oxygen consumption. The latter portion of this relation below DO_2(crit) indicates the presence of tissue hypoxia. Both laboratory and clinical studies have attempted to determine DO_2(crit). In the most rigorous clinical study (3), the investigators found a threshold value of 4 ml/min per kilogram. In other clinical and laboratory studies, investigators found values in the range of 6 to 10 ml/min per kilogram (3,4). The DO_2(crit), or the anaerobic threshold, is not a single, fixed value but varies substantially depending on factors such as basal metabolic rate, the specific organ or tissue, some disease states, and perhaps such complex factors as patient age or genetic composition. In the previous example, cardiac output did not increase as would otherwise be expected in anemia.

Once it is oxygenated, blood is distributed to all organs and tissues through the arterial tree into the microcirculation. Organ blood flow is controlled by arterial tone in medium-sized vessels and is primarily responsive to changes in autonomic stimulation

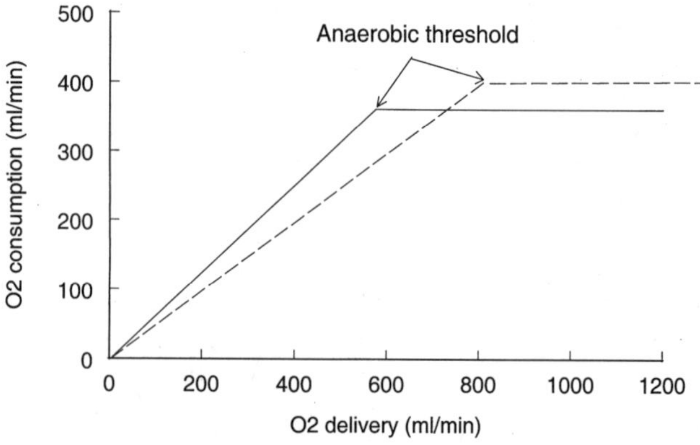

FIGURE 12.2. Relation between oxygen consumption and oxygen delivery. The *solid line* shows the biphasic relation between consumption and delivery. The *dashed line* illustrates the postulated changes in the relation with diseases such as sepsis and acute respiratory distress syndrome. The anaerobic threshold is shifted to the right, suggesting that patients need increased levels of delivery to avoid ongoing ischemic damage to vital organs.

and the release of locally generated vasodilating substances. Within organ systems, red blood cells are carried into the microcirculation, where oxygen is released to the tissues through a thin-walled capillary network. Once released, oxygen diffuses through the interstitial space, finally finding its way into the cell and its mitochondria to be used in cellular respiration. Each of these physiologic mechanisms can be altered in disease, as described later. Additional adaptive changes in the microcirculation enhance oxygen delivery in anemia (5).

Adaptive Mechanisms in Anemia

In anemia, oxygen-carrying capacity decreases, but tissue oxygenation is preserved at hemoglobin levels well below 10 g/dl (Table 12.1). After the development of anemia, adaptive changes include a shift in the oxyhemoglobin dissociation curve, hemodynamic alterations, and microcirculatory alterations. The shift to the right of the oxyhemoglobin dissociation curve in anemia is primarily the result of increased synthesis of 2,3-bisphosphoglycerate (2,3-BPG; also known as 2,3-diphosphoglycerate) in red blood cells (6–8). This rightward shift enables more oxygen to be released to the tissues at a given PO_2, offsetting the effect of reduced oxygen-carrying capacity of the blood. In vitro studies have shown rightward shifts in the oxyhemoglobin dissociation curve with decreases in temperature and pH (9). Although clinically important shifts have been documented in a number of studies, hemoglobin oxygen saturation generally is measured in arterial specimens processed at standard temperature and pH. Therefore current measurement techniques do not reflect oxygen-binding affinity or unloading conditions in the patient's microcirculatory environment, which may be affected by temperature, pH, and a number of disease processes. The shift in the oxyhemoglobin dissociation curve caused by decreases in pH (increase in hydrogen ion concentration) is the Bohr effect (9, 10). Because changes in pH rapidly affect the ability of hemoglobin to bind oxygen, this mechanism has been postulated to be an important early adaptive response to anemia (11). However, the equations describing the physical process indicate that a very large change in pH is needed to modify the partial pressure of oxygen at which hemoglobin is 50% saturated with oxygen (P_{50}) by a clinically important amount (~10 mm Hg). As a result, the Bohr effect is unlikely to have significant clinical consequences (9,10).

TABLE 12.1. PHYSIOLOGIC CHANGES ASSOCIATED WITH ANEMIA

Oxyhemoglobin dissociation curve

Anemia shifts the oxyhemoglobin curve to the right because of increased levels of 2,3-diphosphoglycerate.

Anemia causes clinically significant rightward shifts in the oxyhemoglobin curve because of the Bohr effect.

The shift in the oxyhemoglobin curve has been clearly established in many forms of anemia (excluding hemoglobinopathy).

The shift in the oxyhemoglobin curve has been clearly established in a number of human diseases.

Cardiac output

Cardiac output increases with increasing degrees of normovolemic anemia.

Increased cardiac output in normovolemic anemia is a result of increased stroke volume.

The contribution of increased heart rate to the increase in cardiac output after normovolemic anemia is variable.

Other hemodynamic alteration

Changes in blood viscosity result in many of the hemodynamic changes in normovolemic anemia.

Normovolemic anemia is accompanied by increased sympathetic activity.

Normovolemic anemia causes increased myocardial contractility.

Normovolemic anemia causes a decrease in systemic vascular resistance.

Normovolemic anemia results in a redistribution of cardiac output toward the heart and brain and away from the splanchnic circulation.

Maximal global oxygen delivery occurs at hemoglobin values of 10 to 11 g/dl.

Global oxygen delivery declines above and below hemoglobin values of 10 to 16 g/dl.

Coronary and cerebral blood flow

Coronary blood flow increases during anemia.

Cerebral blood flow increases during anemia.

Coronary artery disease in the presence of moderate degrees of anemia (hemoglobin values less than 9 g/dl) results in impaired left ventrical contractility or ischemia.

Moderate anemia does not aggravate cerebral ischemia in patients with cerebrovascular disease.

Several hemodynamic alterations occur after the development of anemia. The most important determinant of cardiovascular response is the patient's volume status, or more specifically left ventricular preload. The combined effect of hypovolemia and anemia often occurs as a result of blood loss. Acute anemia thus can cause tissue hypoxia or anoxia through both diminished cardiac output resulting in stagnant hypoxia and decreased oxygen-carrying capacity (anemic hypoxia) (12). The body primarily attempts to preserve oxygen delivery to vital organs by compensatory increases in myocardial contractility and heart rate as well as increased arterial and venous vascular tone mediated through increased sympathetic discharge. In addition, a variety of mechanisms redistribute organ blood flow. The adrenergic system plays an important role in altering blood flow to and within specific organs. The renin-angiotensin-aldosterone system is stimulated to retain both water and sodium. Losses ranging from 5% to 15% in blood volume result in variable increases in resting heart rate and diastolic blood pressure. Orthostatic hypotension often is a sensitive indicator of relatively small losses in blood volume not sufficient to cause a marked decrease in blood pressure. Larger losses result in progressive increases in heart rate and decreases in arterial blood pressure accompanied by evidence of organ hypoperfusion. The increased sympathetic tone diverts an ever decreasing global blood flow (cardiac output) away from the splanchnic, skeletal, and cutaneous circulation toward the coronary and cerebral circulation. Once vital organ systems such as the kidneys, the central nervous system, and the heart are affected, the patient is considered in hypovolemic shock. Although the American College of Surgeons Committee on Trauma (13) has categorized the cardiovascular and systemic response to acute blood loss according to degree of blood loss, many of these responses are modified by the rapidity of blood loss and patient characteristics, such as age, coexisting illnesses, preexisting volume status, hemoglobin value, and the use of

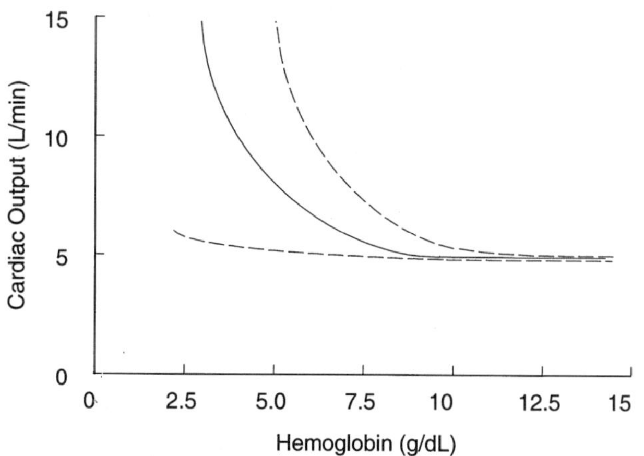

FIGURE 12.3. The theoretic effect of hemoglobin concentration on cardiac output. The series of *curves* illustrate how cardiac output increases as hemoglobin concentration decreases. The *solid curve* is meant to describe the increase in a healthy adult. The *dashed line on the top* shows how the cardiac output response can be accentuated in a young athlete while the *lower dashed line* might correspond to someone with poor cardiovascular function.

medications having cardiac (β-blockers) or peripheral vascular effects (antihypertensives).

The compensatory changes in cardiac output most thoroughly studied are the cardiovascular consequence of normovolemic anemia. When intravascular volume is stable or high after the development of anemia (as opposed to hypovolemic anemia and shock), increases in cardiac output have been consistently reported. Indeed, an inverse relation between hemoglobin level (or hematocrit) and cardiac output has been clearly established in well-controlled laboratory studies (11,14–17) (Fig. 12.3). Similar clinical observations have been made in the perioperative setting (18) and for chronic anemia (14). Unfortunately, the strength of inferences from clinical studies is limited by confounding factors arising from major coexisting illnesses such as cardiac disease, a lack of appropriate control patients, and significant weaknesses in study design. Researchers have attempted to determine the level of anemia at which cardiac output begins to rise. Reported thresholds for this phenomenon identified in primary clinical and laboratory studies have ranged from 7 to 12 g/dl of hemoglobin (14). Two major mechanisms are thought to be principally responsible for the physiologic processes underlying increased cardiac output during normovolemic anemia: (a) reduced blood viscosity and (b) increased sympathetic stimulation of the cardiovascular effectors (19). Blood viscosity affects both preload and afterload, two major determinants of cardiac output (19–21), whereas sympathetic stimulation primarily increases the two other determinants, heart rate and contractility. Unlike the situation for hypovolemic anemia, in this setting the effects of blood viscosity appear to predominate (20,21).

There are complex interactions between blood flow, blood viscosity, and cardiac output. In vessels, blood flow alters whole-blood viscosity, and blood viscosity modulates cardiac output. Under experimental conditions in a rigid hollow cylinder, blood flow is directly related to the fourth power of the diameter and to driving pressure. It is inversely related to the length of the vessel and to blood viscosity (Poiseuille-Hagen law) (5,19). Also, blood viscosity increases as flow decreases because of increasing aggregation of red blood cells. Thus viscosity is highest in postcapillary venules, where flow is the lowest, and viscosity is lowest in the aorta, where flow is highest. In postcapillary venules, there is a disproportionate decrease in blood viscosity as anemia worsens, consequently augmenting venous return at a given venous pressure. If cardiac function is normal, the increase in venous return or left ventricular preload is the most important determinant of increased cardiac output during normovolemic anemia. The conclusion is based on experiments in which viscosity was maintained during anemia by means of high-viscosity colloidal solutions. In such studies, the cardiovascular effects of hemodilution were attenuated (20) compared with similar levels of hemodilution accompanied by reduced whole-blood viscosity. Decreased left ventricular afterload, another cardiac consequence of decreased blood viscosity, also may be an important mechanism for the increase in cardiac output as anemia worsens (20).

Sympathetic stimulation can result in increased cardiac output through enhanced myocardial contractility (22) and increased venomotor tone (16,23). The effects of anemia on left ventricular contractility in isolation have not been clearly determined, given the complex changes in preload, afterload, and heart rate. Only one before-and-after hemodilution study was performed with load-independent measures to document increased left ventricular contractility (22). Chapler and Cain (16) summarized several well-controlled animal studies indicating that venomotor tone increases and that it results from stimulation of the aortic chemoreceptors. If sympathetic stimulation is significant in the specific clinical setting, contractility is increased from stimulation of the β-adrenergic receptors (19,24).

The inverse relation between cardiac output and hemoglobin level has led investigators to attempt to determine the hemoglobin level that maximizes oxygen transport. Richardson and Guyton (25) evaluated the effects of hematocrit on cardiac performance in a canine model. They established that optimal oxygen transport occurred between hematocrits of 40% and 60%. Others determined maximum oxygen delivery to be in the lower end of the range, at a hematocrit of 40% to 45% (13 to 15 g/dl) (26,27). However, in one of the most widely quoted studies addressing this topic (28), investigators found peak oxygen transport to occur at a hematocrit of 30% (hemoglobin concentration, 10 g/dl). Unfortunately, global indices of optimal oxygen delivery mask any differences in blood flow between specific organs (29,30). In addition, attempting to identify a single optimal hemoglobin concentration that maximizes oxygen delivery neglects the large number of factors interfering with adaptive mechanisms when dealing with anyone other than healthy, young patients with anemia.

Will the transfusion of allogeneic red blood cells reverse any adaptive response to acute or chronic normovolemic anemia? It is expected that if oxygen-carrying capacity is not impaired in the red blood cell storage process and that hematocrit is restored after a transfusion, the cardiovascular consequences will be reversed, if there has been no irreversible ischemic organ damage. However, the storage process alters the properties of red blood cells, and the alteration may impair flow and oxygen release from hemoglobin (7) in the microcirculation.

Microcirculatory Effects of Anemia and Red Blood Cell Transfusion

At the level of the microcirculation, three putative adaptive mechanisms may increase the amount of oxygen supplied to tissues by capillary networks. In a model of the microcirculation proposed by Krogh (31), oxygen supply to the tissues may be enhanced through recruitment of previously closed capillaries, increased capillary flow, and increased oxygen extraction from existing capillaries. The degree of anemia, the specific tissue bed, and a variety of disease processes all may affect microcirculatory blood flow and oxygen supply (5,32). As the degree of hemodilution becomes more pronounced and hematocrit decreases, blood viscosity decreases disproportionately in capillary networks. This occurs because the hematocrit is highest in the capillary network and therefore results in a larger decrease in viscosity. This effect results in progressive increases in flow velocities of red blood cells through capillaries and proportionate decreases in the time red blood cells spend in capillaries (transit time) (33). With moderate degrees of anemia, the increased red blood cell flow velocities may increase the amount of oxygen delivered to tissues (5). However, during profound anemia, the transit times may be so brief as to interfere with the diffusion of oxygen to cells (34). Indeed, increases in flow velocity may be one of the important reasons for the onset of anaerobic metabolism. Whereas the effect of hemoglobin levels (hematocrit) on systemic oxygen transport in the central circulation have been well studied, it remains unclear how an increased hematocrit influences oxygen delivery in the microcirculation (35). Until recently, few interpretable results were published in this area because of difficulty in obtaining in situ measurements of blood viscosity, microcirculatory flow, oxygen delivery, and cellular respiration (36). One group (33) suggested that microcirculatory stasis and impaired oxygen delivery to the tissues may be directly related to changes in hematocrit. They theorized that normovolemic hemodilution improves microcirculatory flow and oxygen delivery. Other authors have suggested that hematocrit has limited effects on microcirculatory flow (37).

Banked red blood cells have properties that differ from those of their in vivo counterparts; many are related to the duration of storage. Characteristically, older units of red blood cells have lower levels of 2,3-BPG. The result is a leftward shift in the oxyhemoglobin dissociation curve, which can impede delivery of oxygen to the tissues (11). In addition, storage of red blood cells may decrease the deformability of the red blood cell membrane (38). As a consequence, stored red blood cells may impede flow in the microcirculation (39) and may have limited ability to release oxygen to tissues. However, these storage lesions are reversible within 24 to 48 hours (40).

There are reports (41) suggesting that disease processes such as sepsis impair red blood cell deformability. In conjunction with significant systemic microcirculatory dysfunction, the decrease in red blood cell deformability may dramatically affect tissue oxygen delivery in sepsis and septic shock (41). This body of evidence suggests that red blood cell transfusions increase systemic oxygen delivery but may have adverse effects on microcirculatory flow.

Interaction between Pathophysiologic Processes and Anemia

A number of disease processes affecting either the entire body or specific organs potentially limit adaptive responses and make patients more vulnerable to the effects of anemia. Specifically, heart, lung, and cerebrovascular diseases have been proposed to increase the risk of adverse consequences of anemia. Age, severity of illness, and therapeutic interventions also may affect adaptive mechanisms.

The heart, specifically the left ventricle, may be particularly prone to adverse consequences of anemia. This is because the myocardium consumes 60% to 75% (extraction ratio) of all oxygen delivered by the coronary circulation (26,29,42). Such a high extraction ratio is unique to the coronary circulation. As a result, oxygen delivery to the myocardium can increase substantially only with an increase in blood flow (43). Moreover, most left ventricular perfusion is restricted to the diastolic period, and any shortening of its duration (e.g., tachycardia) constrains blood flow. Laboratory studies have been performed to investigate the effects of normovolemic anemia on the coronary circulation (27,42,44). There appear to be minimal consequences of anemia with hemoglobin levels in the range of 7 g/dl if the coronary circulation is normal (17,22,45). However, myocardial dysfunction and ischemia either occur earlier or are greater in anemic animal models with moderate to high-grade coronary stenosis compared with controls with normal hemoglobin values (45).

Data from studies with human subjects are inconsistent. Several clinical studies with patients with coronary artery disease undergoing normovolemic hemodilution have not shown any increase in cardiac complications or silent ischemia during electrocardiographic monitoring (46). In addition, a retrospective analysis involving 224 patients undergoing coronary artery bypass graft surgery did not show a significant association between hemoglobin level and coronary sinus lactate level (an indicator of myocardial ischemia) (47). In two recent cohort studies, moderate anemia was poorly tolerated by perioperative (48) and critically ill patients (49) with cardiovascular disease. The results confirmed observations made in the laboratory. Anemia also can result in considerable increases in morbidity and mortality among patients with other cardiac diseases, including heart failure and valvular heart disease, presumably because of the greater burden of the adaptive increase in cardiac output.

During normovolemic anemia, cerebral blood flow increases as hemoglobin values decrease. Investigators have observed increases ranging from 50% to 500% of baseline value in laboratory studies (50) and in one study with human subjects (51). Cerebral blood flow increases because of overall increases in cardiac output, which is preferentially diverted to the cerebral circulation. As oxygen delivery begins to decrease, cerebral tissues are able to increase the amount of oxygen extracted from blood. A number of factors, including degree of hemodilution, type of fluid used for volume expansion, volume status (preload), and extent of cerebrovascular disease, are capable of potentially modifying global or regional cerebral blood flow during anemia (52). The increase in global cerebral blood flow combined with the potential for improved flow characteristics across areas of vascular stenosis (improved rheologic properties of blood because of decreased viscosity) prompted a number of laboratory and clinical (52–55) studies to investigate hemodilution as therapy for acute ischemic stroke (53–55).

The results of laboratory studies suggest that moderate degrees of anemia alone should rarely result in or worsen cerebral ischemia. None of the randomized, clinical trials showed hemodilution as therapy for acute ischemic stroke produced significant overall improvement in clinical outcome. Because of the variety of variables that affect clinical outcome, the negative findings may not fully rule out the possibility that hemodilution may offer therapeutic benefit. Thus the currently available evidence indicates that cerebrovascular disease does not appear to predispose patients to serious morbidity from anemia.

Changes in oxygen delivery to the brain during normovolemic anemia (either increases or decreases in blood flow) do not uniformly affect various cerebral pathologic conditions. For example, patients with high intracranial pressure from traumatic brain injury may be adversely affected by increased cerebral blood flow. However, after subarachnoid hemorrhage, mild degrees of normovolemic or hypervolemic anemia may improve overall oxygen delivery, possibly by overcoming the effects of cerebral vasospasm and thereby improving cerebral blood flow through decreased viscosity (56). However, the effects of moderate to severe anemia in subarachnoid hemorrhage have not been assessed in laboratory or clinical studies.

One of the major consequences of redistributing some of the available cardiac output toward the coronary and cerebral circulation during normovolemic anemia is shunting of flow away from other organs, including the kidneys and intestines. Critically ill patients may be adversely affected by this redistribution (57), which could result in increased intestinal ischemia, bacterial translocation, and multiple-system organ failure (58). Critical illness also can tax many of the body's adaptive responses. Specifically, cardiac performance may be impaired (59) or may already be at maximal capacity in response to increased metabolic demands. Pathologic processes affecting the microcirculation, particularly prevalent among critically ill patients, also may affect the patient's response to anemia and transfusions.

CLINICAL OUTCOMES OF ANEMIA AND RED BLOOD CELL TRANSFUSION

Every medical decision must weigh risk versus benefit. The decision to administer red blood cells must consider the risks of blood transfusion (see Chapters 48 through 60), the risk of anemia, and the level of anemia at which blood transfusion prevents the associated adverse outcomes. In this section, we review data from studies with animal and human subjects on the risk of anemia. We then review the evidence used to evaluate the efficacy of allogeneic blood transfusion in reducing risk.

Risk of Anemia

Data on Animals

Results of studies suggest that healthy animals can tolerate hemoglobin levels between 3 and 5 g/dl after normovolemic hemodilution. Electrocardiographic changes consistent with ischemia occur at hemoglobin levels less than 5 g/dl, whereas lactate production, depressed ventricular function, and death have occurred at hemoglobin levels of 3 g/dl or less. Some animals survive with hemoglobin levels as low as 1 to 2 g/dl (60). However, results of studies with animals suggest a decreased ability to tolerate anemia in the presence of cardiac disease. In dogs with experimentally induced coronary stenosis varying from 50% to 80%, ST-segment changes or locally depressed cardiac function occurred at hemoglobin levels in the range of 7 to 10 g/dl (61, 62).

Data on Humans

Studies with patients who decline blood transfusion for religious reasons provide critical insight into the effect of anemia on humans. The largest study was performed with 1,958 adult surgical patients who refused transfusion for religious reasons (48). The mortality was greatest among patients with the lowest preoperative hemoglobin levels. Among patients with underlying cardiovascular disease, the risk of death was markedly greater among patients with a hemoglobin level of 10 g/dl or less. Among patients without underlying cardiovascular disease, the difference in mortality at hemoglobin levels greater than and less than 10 g/dl was not as great (Fig. 12.4). These results, as well as data on animals and physiologic data, suggest that anemia is not tolerated as well in the presence of cardiovascular disease.

In a series of studies, the effect of anemia was evaluated among healthy volunteers who underwent isovolemic reduction of hemoglobin level to 5 g/dl. Transient and asymptomatic electrocardiographic changes were found in 5 of 87 volunteers included in two studies (63,64). These changes occurred when the hemoglobin level was between 5 and 7 g/dl and in patients with faster heart rates (64). Changes in critical oxygen delivery were not measured. Subtle but reversible changes in cognition were identified in 9 volunteers younger than 35 years at a hemoglobin level between 5 and 7 g/dl (65). Self-rated fatigue was found in 8 volunteers when the hemoglobin level decreased to 7 g/dl. Fatigue increased as hemoglobin level decreased to 5 g/dl (66). The results of these studies suggest that important clinical effects can be measured in young, healthy humans with hemoglobin levels between 5 and 7 g/dl. It is uncertain how these results apply to older patients with comorbid factors who are also under stress from surgery or acute illness. However, it is possible that the changes measured in these young healthy volunteers would occur at higher hemoglobin levels in older patients.

Efficacy of Transfusion

Observational Studies

Seven observational studies have been performed to investigate the importance of anemia or transfusion practices in various settings. The characteristics of six of these studies are summarized in Table 12.2. Four large cohort studies concerned intensive care (67), coronary artery bypass surgery (68), hip fracture (69), and myocardial infarction (89). Each of these studies came to a different conclusion. In the first study, investigators evaluated 4,470 critically ill patients admitted to six tertiary level intensive care units in Canada (67). The need for transfusion

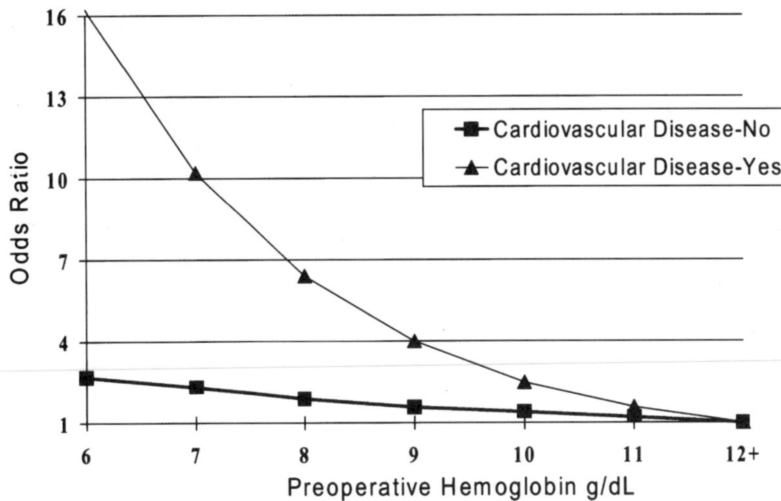

FIGURE 12.4. Association between preoperative hemoglobin level and mortality among patients with and without cardiovascular disease (48). In a population of patients who declined blood transfusion, the risk of death was higher among patients with cardiovascular disease (*top line*) than among patients without cardiovascular disease (*bottom line*) for each preoperative hemoglobin level.

was associated with a worse outcome. The outcomes were better for intensive care unit patients who had undergone transfusion, especially those with cardiovascular disease. In the second study, 2,202 patients undergoing coronary artery bypass graft surgery were divided into three groups corresponding to hematocrit on admission to the intensive care unit, as follows: high, >34%; medium, 25% to 33%; and low, <24% (68). Patients in the high-hematocrit group were more than twice as likely to have myocardial infarction than were those in the low-hematocrit group. In the third study, the subjects were 8,787 consecutively enrolled patients with hip fracture who underwent surgical repair. The 30-day and 90-day mortality was not increased or

TABLE 12.2. SUMMARY OF NONRANDOMIZED STUDIES

Study	Clinical Setting	Subjects	Transfusion Trigger
Nelson et al., 1997 (71)	Vascular surgery (N = 27)	Patients at high-risk who had undergone elective infrainguinal bypass vascular procedures Anemic group: n = 13 Nonanemic group: n = 14	MI occurred in 14% of patients with Hct >28% compared with 77% with Hct <28% No deaths in either group
Hébert et al., 1997 (67)	Critical care (N = 4,470)	Critically ill patients admitted to ICU Survivors n = 3,469 Nonsurvivors n = 1,001	Survivors had higher Hgb levels than of nonsurvivors
Paone and Silverman, 1997 (70)	Cardiac surgery (N = 100)	Patients undergoing isolated CABG Transfusion group: n = 13 No transfusion group: n = 87 Allogeneic RBC were transfused during bypass for low SvO_2 (<55%) and transfused postoperatively for a Hct <20% or at any Hct if deemed clinically warranted	No difference in clinical outcomes Length of ICU stay longer for transfusion patients: 2.6 ± 0.3 d vs 1.6 ± 0.1 d
Carson et al., 1998 (69)	Orthopedic surgery (N = 8,787)	Hip fracture patients 60 years or older who underwent surgical repair Transfusion group: n = 3,699 No transfusion group: n = 5,088	No difference in 30- or 90-d mortality.
Spiess et al., 1998 (68)	Cardiac surgery (N = 2,202)	CABG High ICU Hct ≥34% group n = 410 Medium ICU Hct group 25% to 33%, n = 1,544 Low ICU Hct ≤24% group n = 248; mean age ± (sD), 64.3 ± 10.2	MI highest in high Hct group (8.3%), compared to medium Hct groups (5.5%) and low Hct (3.6%)
Wu et al., 2001 (89)	Myocardial infarction (N = 78,794)	Myocardial infarction patients 65 years or older	Transfusion associated with reduction in 30 day mortality in group with admission HCT 5.0% to 33.0%

MI, myocardial infarction; Hct, hematocrit; ICU, intensive care unit; Hgb, hemoglobin; CABG, coronary artery bypass grafting; RBC, red blood cells.

decreased by perioperative transfusion (69). Three smaller studies were performed to evaluate the relation between anemia and adverse outcome among surgical patients (70–72). More ischemic events occurred among anemic patients in all three of these studies. The validity of these studies is uncertain because the decision to perform transfusion often correlates with the illness burden of the patient. It is possible that comorbidity was not adequately adjusted for in these studies. Only randomized clinical trials can overcome this limitation.

Clinical Trials

Ten randomized, clinical trials contrasted the effects of different transfusion thresholds (Table 12.3) (73–82). The clinical settings varied, although each trial randomized patients to transfusion on the basis of a restrictive or a liberal strategy. Restrictive triggers (specified hemoglobin concentrations that had to be attained) ranged from 7 to 9 g/dl.

Two trials specified a hematocrit of 25% or 30%. The liberal transfusion strategies specified the following triggers: 100% of normal red blood cell volume, two units of blood (immediately in one trial, postoperatively in another) irrespective of clinical state, and transfusion sufficient to maintain hemoglobin level at or above 10 g/dl in three trials and above 9 g/dl in another. Two trials specified the liberal triggers as transfusion to maintain hematocrit at 32% and 40% or greater. There is overlap between the liberal and restrictive transfusion groups in these trials. One trial (involving patients in intensive care), contributed 47% of the patients and 82% of the recorded deaths. There were a total of 1,780 trial participants.

Of the ten trials, only three included more than 100 patients, and only one of these evaluated a transfusion strategy that included assessment for symptoms. In one of these trials, 428 patients undergoing first-time, elective coronary artery bypass surgery were randomized to arms with transfusion triggers of 9 g/dl versus 8 g/dl (81). The differences between perioperative hemoglobin levels was small, and the mean reduction in hemoglobin level during the admission was equal between the groups. The event rates were very low, and there were no differences in any outcome. The second trial included 127 patients undergoing knee arthroplasty. Patients were randomized to receive autologous blood transfusion immediately after the operation (first unit in recovery room and second unit on return to the ward) versus autologous blood only if the hemoglobin level decreased to less than 9 g/dl (82). The mean postoperative hemoglobin level was approximately 0.7 g/dl different, although only 25% of the restrictive group received a transfusion. There were no differences in outcome. In a third trial (pilot study), 84 patients with hip fracture undergoing surgical repair were randomized to a 10 g/dl threshold or to transfusion for symptoms (transfusion was allowed if hemoglobin level was less than 8 g/dl) (79). The mean prerandomization hemoglobin level was 9.1 g/dl. The lowest mean hemoglobin level after randomization in the group with symptoms was 8.8 g/dl, and the highest mean hemoglobin level in the threshold group was 11.1 g/dl. There were no differences in outcome (including functional recovery, mortality, and morbidity), although 60 days after the operation, 5 patients in the symptomatic group had died, as had 2 patients in the 10 g/dl group. In all of these trials (and the other five trials in Table 12.3), the numbers of patients were much too small to evaluate the effect of lower transfusion triggers on clinically important outcomes such as mortality, morbidity, and functional status.

The Transfusion Requirement in Critical Care (TRICC) trial (80,83) is the only adequately powered study to evaluate clinically important outcome. In the main study, the investigators randomized 838 volume-resuscitated intensive care unit patients to a restrictive strategy in which patients received allogeneic red blood cell transfusions at hemoglobin levels of 7 g/dl (and were maintained between 7 to 9 g/dl) or to a liberal strategy of receiving red blood cells at 10 g/dl (and were maintained between 10 and 12 g/dl). Average hemoglobin levels (8.5 versus 10.7 g/dl) and red blood cell units transfused (2.6 versus 5.6 units) were significantly lower in the restrictive as opposed to the liberal group. The 30-day mortality was slightly lower in the restrictive transfusion group (18.7% versus 23.3%), although the finding was not statistically significant ($P = .11$).

A metaanalysis combined data from five or more trials for six outcomes: probability of red blood cell transfusion, volume of red blood cells transfused, hematocrit, cardiac events, mortality at 30 days, and overall length of hospital stay (84). The pooled data indicated that on average, a restrictive transfusion trigger reduced the probability of red blood cell transfusion by a proportional 42% (an average saving of 0.93 units of red blood cells per transfused patient) and resulted in a hematocrit 5.6% lower on average than in patients who received more liberal transfusions. The effect on length of hospital stay and the rate of cardiac events were not increased significantly by the use of restrictive transfusion triggers. Restrictive transfusion triggers were not associated with an increase in mortality (Fig. 12.5). The TRICC trial involving patients in intensive care units contributed 83% of the information on mortality data in the metaanalysis.

Functional recovery is another potentially important benefit of higher hematocrit. Only one small pilot study evaluated the effect of red blood cell transfusion on the functional ability of patients with anemia (79). The number of subjects was too small for detection of clinically important differences. Most of the other published data relating anemia to function were generated from clinical trials performed to evaluate the use of recombinant human erythropoietin in end-stage renal failure and patients undergoing cancer chemotherapy. These limited data suggest that increasing the hemoglobin level of patients with marked anemia (hemoglobin, <10 g/dl) may increase exercise tolerance (85). The studies with negative findings (86) evaluated the effect of increasing hemoglobin level beyond the 10-g/dl threshold. A review of the use of erythropoietin in the care of patients with cancer-related anemia (86) concluded that patients receiving erythropoietin had increased levels of energy and function.

TRANSFUSION GUIDELINES

Guidelines have been issued by organizations with the intent of aiding clinical decisions. The administration of red blood cells is based on the balance of benefits, risks, and costs. Physicians making transfusion decisions are faced with massive amounts of sometimes conflicting information. Since 1985, concerns about

TABLE 12.3. RESULTS OF RANDOMIZED, CONTROLLED TRIALS

Study	Setting	Subjects: Eligibility and Comparability	Transfusion Strategy	Blood Usage in Units/pt [mean (sD)]	Proportion Transfused [% (n)]	Hb (g/dl)/ Hct (%) [mean (sD)]	30-Day Mortality [% (n)]	Length of Hospital Stay in Days [mean (sD)]
Topley et al., 1956 (73)	Trauma (N = 22)	>1 L blood loss; considered to be at no clinical risk in raising the blood volume ≥100% of normal, or allowing it to reach 30% below normal	*Liberal:* to achieve RBC volume ≥100% of normal	11.3 (6.9)	100 (10)	Lowest Hb 15.6 (2.0)	—	—
			Restrictive: maintain RBC volume 70–80% of normal	4.8 (6.7)	67 (8)	Lowest Hb 11.3 (0.7)	—	—
Blair et al., 1986 (74)	Gastrointestinal bleeding (N = 50)	Acute severe upper gastrointestinal hemorrhage	*Liberal:* patients received at least 2 units of PRBC immediately on admission to hospital	4.6 (1.5)	100 (24)	Admission Hct 28 (5.9) Discharge Hct 37 (7.8)	8.3 (2)	—
			Restrictive: patients were not given PRBC during the first 24 h unless Hb <8.0 g/dl or shock persisted after initial resuscitation with colloid	2.6 (3.1)	19.2 (5)	Admission Hct 29 (8.2) Discharge Hct 37 (7.1)	0 (0)	—
Fortune et al., 1987 (75)	Trauma, acute hemorrhage (N = 25)	Patients who had sustained class III or class IV hemorrhage and had clinical signs of shock	*Liberal:* Hct was brought up to 40% slowly over a period of several hours by the infusion of PRBC	—	—	Average Hct for 3-d period 38.4 (2.1)	—	—
			Restrictive: Hct was kept close to 30% by the administration of PRBC	—	—	Average Hct for 3-d period 29.7 (1.9)	—	—
Johnson et al., 1992 (76)	Cardiac surgery (N = 38)	Patients undergoing elective coronary revascularization and able to donate at least three units of PRBC preoperatively	*Liberal:* patients received blood transfusion to achieve a Hct of 32% as long as autologous blood was available	2.05 (0.93)	100 (18)	Hct 4 hr postop, 31.3	—	7.6 (1.9)
			Restrictive: patients received transfusions only if the Hct fell below 25%	1.0 (0.86)	75 (15)	Hct 4 hr postop, 28.7	—	7.9 (4.3)
Hébert et al., 1995 (77)	Critical care (N = 69)	Critically ill patients admitted to 1 of 5 tertiary level intensive care units with normovolemia after initial treatment who had Hb concentrations <9.0 g/dl within 72 h	*Liberal:* patients were given PRBC if Hb was 10.0–10.5 g/dl or less; Hb concentration maintained at 10.0–12.0 g/dl	Mean units per patient, 4.8 Total units 174	—	Admission Hb 9.3 (13) Average daily Hb 10.9	25 (9)	Median (IQR) 31 (13–64)
			Restrictive: patients were given PRBC only if Hb was 7.0–7.5 g/dl Hb concentration maintained at 7.0–9.0 g/dl	Mean units per patient 2.5 Total units 82	—	Admission Hb 9.7 (14) Average daily Hb 9.0	24 (8)	Median (IQR) 38 (25–62)

(continued)

TABLE 12.3. (Continued)

Study	Setting	Subjects: Eligibility and Comparability	Transfusion Strategy	Blood Usage in Units/pt [mean (sD)]	Proportion Transfused [% (n)]	Hb (g/dl)/ Hct (%) [mean (sD)]	30-Day Mortality [% (n)]	Length of Hospital Stay in Days [mean (sD)]
Bush et al., 1997 (78)	Vascular surgery (N = 99)	Patients undergoing elective aortic and infrainguinal arterial reconstruction	*Liberal:* transfusion with PRBC to maintain Hb >10.0 g/dl	Total units 3.7 (3.5) Intraop 2.4 (2.5)	88 (43)	Hb during 48 h postop period 11.0 (1.2)	8% (4)	11 (9)
			Restrictive: Transfusion only if Hb level fell below 9.0 g/dl	Total units 2.8 (3.1) Intraop 1.5 (1.7)	80 (40)	Hb during 48 h postop period 9.8 (1.3)	8 (4)	10 (6)
Carson et al., 1998 (79)	Orthopedic surgery (N = 84)	Hip fracture patients undergoing surgical repair who had postoperative Hb levels less than 10.0 g/dl	*Liberal:* patients received 1 unit of PRBC at random assignment and then as needed to maintain Hb >10.0 g/dl	Total median 2 (1–2)	98.8 (83)	Lowest Hb 9.4 (1.0)	2.4 (1)	6.3 (3.4)
			Restrictive: transfusion delayed until symptoms or consequences of anemia developed or Hb value <8.0 g/dl in the absence of symptoms	Total median 0 (0–2)	45.2 (38)	Lowest Hb 8.8 (1.2)	2.4 (1)	6.4 (3.4)
Hébert et al., 1999 (80)	Critical care (N = 838)	Critically ill patients admitted to 1 of 22 tertiary level and 3 community intensive care units with normovolemia after initial treatment who had Hb concentrations <9.0 g/dl within 72 h	*Liberal:* PRBC transfused to maintain Hb concentration at 10.0–12.0 g/dl	Total 5.6 (5.3)	100 (420)	Mean daily Hb 10.7 (0.7)	23.3 (98)	35.5 (19.4)
			Restrictive: transfused given to maintain Hb concentration between 7.0 and 9.0 g/dl	Total 2.6 (4.1)	77 (280)	Mean daily Hb 8.5 (0.7)	18.7 (78)	34.8 (19.5)
Bracey et al., 1999 (81)	Cardiac surgery (N = 428)	Patients undergoing first-time elective coronary revascularisation	*Liberal:* received RBC transfusions on the instructions of individual physicians, who considered the clinical assessment of the patient and the institutional guidelines, which propose a Hb level <9.0 g/dl as the postoperative threshold for RBC transfusion	Postop 1.4 (1.8)	Postop 48 (104)	Mean net reduction in Hb (admission to discharge) 4.2 (1.9)	2.7 (6)	7.9 (4.9)

(continued)

TABLE 12.3. (Continued)

Study	Setting	Subjects: Eligibility and Comparability	Transfusion Strategy	Blood Usage in Units/pt [mean (sD)]	Proportion Transfused [% (n)]	Hb (g/dl)/ Hct (%) [mean (sD)]	30-Day Mortality [% (n)]	Length of Hospital Stay in Days [mean (sD)]
Bracey et al., 1999 (81) cont'd			*Restrictive:* received RBC transfusion in the postoperative period for a Hb level <8.0 g/dl, unless the patient experienced blood loss >750 ml since the last transfusion, hypovolemia with hemodynamic instability and excessive acute blood loss, acute respiratory failure or inadequate cardiac output and oxygenation, or hemodynamic instability requiring vasopressors	Postop 0.9 (1.5) Total 2.0 (2.2)	Postop 35 (74) Total 60 (127)	Mean net reduction in Hb (admission to discharge) 4.2 (1.7)	1.4 (3)	7.5 (2.9)
Lotke et al., 1999 (82)	Orthopedic surgery (N = 127)	Patients undergoing primary total knee arthroplasty who were able to donate 2 units of autologous blood preoperatively	*Liberal:* received autologous blood immediately after operation, first unit beginning in the recovery room and second unit on return to the ward		Postop 100 (65)	Mean Postop Hb Day 1 (11.4) Day 3 (10.7)	—	—
			Restrictive: received all autologous blood if Hb level had fallen below 9.0 g/dl	—	Postop 26 (16)	Mean Postop Hb Day 1 (10.6) Day 3 (10.0)	—	—

Hb, hemglobin; Hct, hematocrit; RBC, red blood cell; PRBC, packed RBCs; IQR, interquartile range.

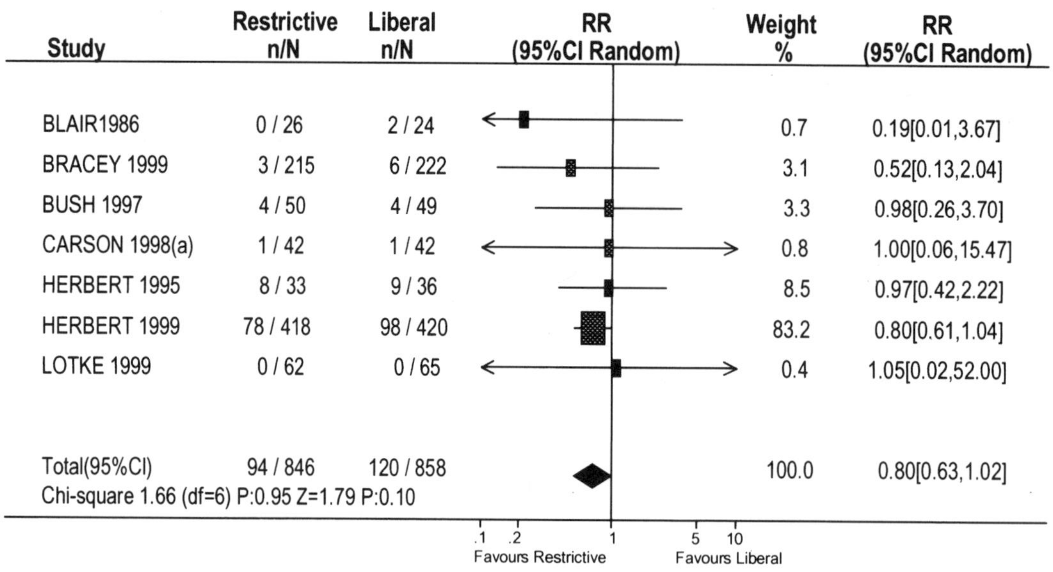

FIGURE 12.5. Effect of restrictive transfusion triggers on 30-day all-cause mortality. Summary of data from randomized, clinical trials comparing effect of restrictive versus liberal transfusion strategies on mortality (expressed as relative risk).

the transmission of human immunodeficiency virus and other viruses through blood products have significantly modified both real and perceived risks and benefits. Many agencies responded by issuing clinical practice guidelines advocating a more restrictive approach to the use of allogeneic red blood cells and other components.

Seventeen clinical practice guidelines on blood transfusion have been published (84). Thirteen guidelines address the use of allogeneic red blood cells. All guidelines were formulated by expert panels without a description of the specific consensus process. Only one organization reported the use of a computerized literature search strategy and graded both the evidence and the strength of each of the recommendations (87). None of the organizations cited or discussed the results of the few randomized, controlled, clinical trials published at least 6 months before the appearance of the guideline.

Recommendations varied among the guidelines. Only one set of guidelines recommended a transfusion trigger; six advocated a range of transfusion thresholds based on clinical judgment, one recommended using clinical judgment only, and five did not comment on either clinical judgment or a transfusion trigger. Because of the paucity of clinical trials, the guidelines relied heavily on expert opinion, which sometimes (particularly more recently) valued the risks of virus transmission through blood products above all other consequences of the transfusion decision.

The guidelines developed by the American Society of Anesthesiology are by far the most rigorously developed and methodologically sound (87). As with several other guidelines, the American Society of Anesthesiology task force advised against a transfusion trigger, although it did suggest a hemoglobin range to guide clinicians. This task force recommended that the decision to perform transfusion should be based on a patient's risk of complications of inadequate oxygenation, as well as all other important physiologic and surgical factors. Since 1995, the College of American Pathologists is the only major medical organization that has updated its guidelines.

DECISION MAKING IN RED BLOOD CELL TRANSFUSION

Approach to Evaluating a Bleeding Patient

In the care of a bleeding patient, the physician must first determine the degree of blood loss and rate of bleeding. Initial assessment of hemodynamic status must be made. Vital signs (supine, sitting, and standing) are immediately assessed. The history interview and physical examination are performed quickly. The focus is on possible causes of bleeding and important comorbid conditions, such as cardiovascular disease. An emergency complete blood cell count, type and cross-match, prothrombin time (PT), and partial thromboplastin time are obtained. From these data, the source and rate of bleeding are estimated, and a decision can be made about red blood cell transfusion and correction of coagulopathy. For patients with gastrointestinal bleeding, consultations may be requested from the gastroenterology and possibly surgery departments. In the care of patients with postoperative bleeding, exploratory surgery should be considered.

In patients with active bleeding, hemodynamic status and need for emergency intervention must be determined. Crystalloid is administered to maintain intravascular volume. Red blood cell transfusions are administered rapidly to maintain adequate oxygen-carrying capacity. Clinical judgment is needed to estimate how much more bleeding may occur, how much lower the hemoglobin level will decrease, and then to perform expectant transfusion. Vital signs are examined for a decrease in blood pressure and for tachycardia. The patient is asked about symptoms that can result from anemia, including cardiac ischemia (chest pain), congestive heart failure (dyspnea, paroxysmal nocturnal dyspnea, edema), fatigue, dizziness, weakness, and orthostatic hypotension unresponsive to intravenous fluids. The hemoglobin level is measured at regular intervals.

It is important to determine the presence of coronary artery disease because results of studies with animal and with human subjects suggest that patients with coronary artery disease are less tolerant of anemia. Review of the medical history for angina, myocardial infarction, and coronary artery bypass surgery is essential. The electrocardiogram is examined for evidence of old myocardial infarction or ischemic changes. The chest radiograph is examined for cardiomegaly and other changes consistent with congestive heart failure. Patients with a history of peripheral or cerebral vascular disease are more likely also to have asymptomatic coronary artery disease.

In the care of patients with moderate to severe blood loss that has abated, there is more time for complete assessment of the source of bleeding, development of a course of management, and thorough evaluation of the patient. After bleeding has stopped and equilibration has occurred, hemoglobin level stabilizes and the nadir hemoglobin level can be determined.

Surgical Patient

Patients undergoing major surgical intervention often experience hemodynamic instability and frequently need blood products as a consequence of considerable blood loss. One of the goals of resuscitation is to maintain oxygen delivery well beyond the anaerobic threshold. Hemoglobin concentration should be maintained above a value that maintains adequate DO_2 and minimizes exposure to allogeneic red blood cell transfusion. However, optimal intraoperative thresholds have not been established. Current methods of monitoring effective circulatory blood volume and utilization of oxygen at the tissue level have limitations. Therefore maintenance of adequate hemoglobin level has been recommended (87). Frequent measurement can assist the anesthesiologist in administering red blood cell transfusion one unit at a time when blood loss is predictable. Blood loss exceeding 20% of blood volume in a short time may necessitate transfusion of multiple units of red blood cells as well as administration of plasma and platelets. Reliable intraoperative measurements can be easily performed at the point of care with hemoglobin measurements obtained with standard blood gas analyzers. However, the accuracy of this value is influenced by the amount of intravenous fluid administered by the anesthesiologist and the fact that the time period is too short for equilibration to occur. Therefore, expert clinical judgment is required.

Standard anesthetic practice mandates intraoperative monitoring of cardiac function with measurement of continuous electrocardiographic and noninvasive or invasive blood pressure monitoring. Both monitoring techniques are essential but are insensitive to significant blood loss. This can delay recognition until late in the process. Monitoring of respiratory function usually includes continuous oxygen saturations and measurement of end tidal carbon dioxide. A patient can have profound anemia without appreciable changes in either measurement. More sophisticated and invasive monitoring of cardiac function includes measurement of right- and left-sided ventricular filling pressure by means of central venous pressure and pulmonary artery catheters. Both techniques provide estimates of the effective circulating blood volume and are frequently used in high risk surgery and in intensive care units. Repeated measurement of central pressure and fluid challenges provide much more reliable assessment of effective circulating blood volume than does an isolated single measurement. Continuous monitoring of cardiac output with either pulmonary arterial catheters or esophageal Doppler techniques can be performed in many centers. Most of these techniques are reliable and are used frequently intraoperatively and during critical illness (88). However, current monitoring techniques have a number of major limitations in guiding transfusion requirements. Careful clinical observation in conjunction with the physiologic data provide many of the necessary tools in the diagnosis and detection of clinically important anemia. The more difficult task is knowing how best to administer red blood cells, intravenous solutions such as colloids and crystalloids, and vasoactive drugs.

There are few data on whether invasive monitoring and different treatment strategies cause more good than harm. Most experienced anesthesiologists and critical care physicians have developed an approach to management of blood loss and hemodynamic instability. There is still enormous practice variation in selecting specific therapies. Randomized clinical trials are needed to assist in clinical decision making.

Chronic Anemia

In chronic anemia, there is time for compensation to develop and for careful observation of the patient. Anemia is associated with an increase in blood flow resulting from decreased viscosity, greater release of oxygen caused by higher levels of 2,3-BPG, and an increase in cardiac output. There is time to determine whether these physiologic events are clinically important in the individual patient and carefully determine whether the patient has symptoms. Besides cardiac symptoms (angina, dyspnea), anemia can lead to nonspecific symptoms, such as fatigue, weakness, dizziness, reduced exercise tolerance, and impaired performance of activities of daily living. There also may be time to implement alternative treatments to correct anemia depending on the cause. Iron, vitamin B_{12}, and folate can be replaced. Erythropoietin can be administered. Patients vary in ability to tolerate low hemoglobin levels.

Transfusion Threshold

The optimal threshold for transfusion is uncertain in most clinical situations. The only adequately powered randomized clinical trial showed it is safe to withhold blood until the hemoglobin level falls to less than 7 g/dl. The study was performed with intensive care unit patients and should guide therapy in this setting. However, these patients are unique in that they are extremely ill, monitored very closely, and usually bedridden. It is uncertain whether the results may be applied to other clinical situations, such as care of surgical patients. No other adequately powered studies have been performed in other clinical settings.

Outcomes such as functional recovery have not been evaluated. Transfusion thresholds have not been adequately examined in the care of patients with underlying cardiac disease.

In the absence of evidence, it is necessary to rely on clinical judgment. Our opinion is that for patients who have no symptoms and do not have cardiovascular disease, a transfusion trigger of 7 g/dl should be used. For patients with cardiovascular disease, we suggest using a higher transfusion threshold such as 10 g/dl. Patients with symptoms of anemia should be transfused as needed. No set of guidelines applies to every patient. In the end, careful clinical assessment with thoughtful consideration of risks and benefits should guide the transfusion decision.

Dose and Administration

Packed red blood cells should be transfused through a standard filter. For acute blood loss, the rate of administration is guided by the rate of bleeding and hemodynamic compromise. In the treatment of rapidly bleeding patients, blood can be given at the rate of blood loss. In the care of patients with chronic anemia, enough blood is given to control symptoms. In the average adult patient, 1 unit of blood increases the hemoglobin level approximately 1 g/dl and hematocrit approximately 3%. Ordinarily, 1 unit of blood is given over 1 to 2 hours. For patients at risk of fluid overload, blood should be administered at a rate of 1 ml/kg per hour. It also may be prudent to administer a loop diuretic (furosemide) before the transfusion. After transfusion of each unit of blood, measurement of hemoglobin level is repeated, and the patient reassessed.

FUTURE

During the next decade, advances and risks may dramatically alter transfusion practice. Research is underway to develop safe red blood cell products. Further clinical trials should be performed to better describe the clinical effect of different transfusion strategies. It is likely that within the next one or two decades a cost-effective oxygen carrier will be developed that will reduce the use of allogeneic red blood cells.

SUMMARY

Red blood cell transfusion is an extremely common treatment throughout the world. Blood is administered to improve oxygen delivery. Patients compensate for anemia by increasing cardiac output and through redistribution of blood flow to the cardiac and cerebral circulation. Particular attention must be paid to maintaining adequate oxygen delivery to the heart. Results of the one adequately powered clinical trial, performed with intensive care unit patients, suggest a hemoglobin level of 7 g/dl is a safe threshold for red blood cell transfusion. For patients with cardiovascular disease, a higher transfusion threshold is advised. Blood transfusion usually should be administered one unit at a time, and the patient and hemoglobin level reassessed. Transfusion decisions should consider whether anemia is acute or chronic, the rate of bleeding, the presence of underlying medical problems, hemodynamic status, and the presence of symptoms.

REFERENCES

1. Goodnough LT, Brecher ME, Kanter MH, et al. Transfusion medicine, I: blood transfusion. *N Engl J Med* 1999;340:438–447.
2. Wallace EL, Churchill WH, Surgenor DM, et al. Collection and transfusion of blood and blood components in the United States, 1994. *Transfusion* 1998;38:625–636.
3. Ronco JJ, Fenwick JC, Tweeddale MG, et al. Identification of the critical oxygen delivery for anaerobic metabolism in critically ill septic and nonseptic humans. *JAMA* 1993;270:1724–1730.
4. Nelson DP, King CE, Dodd SL, et al. Systemic and intestinal limits of O_2 extraction in the dog. *J Appl Physiol* 1987;63:387–394.
5. Tuman KJ. Tissue oxygen delivery: the physiology of anemia. *Anesthesiol Clin North America* 1990;8:451–469.
6. Rodman T, Close HP, Purcell MK. The oxyhemoglobin dissociation curve in anemia. *Ann Intern Med* 1960;52:295–309.
7. Kennedy AC, Valtis DJ. The oxygen dissociation curve in anemia of various types. *J Clin Invest* 1954;33:1372–1381.
8. Brecher ME, Zylstra-Halling VW, Pineda AA. Rejuvenation of erythrocytes preserved with AS-1 and AS-3. *Am J Clin Pathol* 1991;96: 767–769.
9. Wyman J. Hemoglobin function. In: Bunn HF, Forget BG, eds. *Hemoglobin: molecular, genetic and clinical aspects.* Philadelphia: WB Saunders, 1986:37–60.
10. Bohr C, Hasselbalch KA, Krogh A. Ueber einen in biologischer beziehung wichtigen Einfluss, den die Kohlensaurespannung des Blutes auf dessen Sauerstoff Binding uebt. *Scand Arch Physiol* 1904;16:402–412.
11. Welch HG, Meehan KR, Goodnough LT. Prudent strategies for elective red blood cell transfusion. *Ann Intern Med* 1992;116:393–402.
12. Finch CA, Lenfant C. Oxygen transport in man. *N Engl J Med* 1972; 286:407–415.
13. Alexander RH, Ali J, Aprahamian C, et al. *Advanced trauma life support: program for physicians,* 5th ed. Chicago: American College of Surgeons, 1993.
14. Brannon ES, Merrill AJ, Warren VJ, et al. The cardiac output in patients with chronic anemia as measured by the technique of right atrial catheterization. *J Clin Invest* 1945;24:332–336.
15. Duke M, Abelmann WH. The hemodynamic response to chronic anemia. *Circulation* 1969;39:503–515.
16. Chapler CK, Cain SM. The physiologic reserve in oxygen carrying capacity: studies in experimental hemodilution. *Can J Physiol Pharmacol* 1985;64:7–12.
17. Crystal GJ, Salem MR. Myocardial oxygen consumption and segmental shortening during selective coronary hemodilution in dogs. Anesth Analg 1988;67:500–508.
18. Laks H, Pilon RN, Klovekorn WP, et al. Acute hemodilution: its effect on hemodynamics and oxygen transport in anesthetized man. *Ann Surg* 1974;180:103–109.
19. Spahn DR, Leone BJ, Reves JG, et al. Cardiovascular and coronary physiology of acute isovolemic hemodilution: a review of nonoxygen-carrying and oxygen-carrying solutions. *Anesth Analg* 1994;78: 1000–1021.
20. Murray JF, Escobar E, Rapaport E. Effects of blood viscosity on hemodynamic responses in acute normovolemic anemia. *Am J Physiol* 1969; 216:638–642.
21. Fowler NO, Holmes JC. Blood viscosity and cardiac output in acute experimental anemia. *J Appl Physiol* 1975;39:453–456.
22. Habler OP, Kleen MS, Podtschaske AH, et al. The effect of acute normovolemic hemodilution (ANH) on myocardial contractilty in anesthetized dogs. *Anesth Analg* 1996;83:451–458.
23. Chapler CK, Stainsby WN, Lillie MA. Peripheral vascular responses during acute anemia. *Can J Physiol Pharmacol* 1981;59:102–107.
24. Glick G, Plauth WH Jr, Braunwald E. Role of autonomic nervous system in the circulatory response to acutely induced anemia in unanesthetized dogs. *J Clin Invest* 1964;43:2112–2124.

25. Richardson TQ, Guyton AC. Effects of polycythemia and anemia on cardiac output and other circulatory factors. *Am J Physiol* 1959;197: 1167–1170.
26. Fan FC, Chen RYZ, Schuessler GB, et al. Effects of hematocrit variations on regional hemodynamics and oxygen transport in the dog. *Am J Physiol* 1980;238:H545–H552.
27. Jan KM, Heldman J, Chien S. Coronary hemodynamics and oxygen utilization after hematocrit variations in hemorrhage. *Am J Physiol* 1980;239:H326–H332.
28. Messmer K, Lewis DH, Sunder-Plassmann L, et al. Acute normovolemic hemodilution. *Eur Surg Res* 1972;4:55–70.
29. Murray JF, Rapaport E. Coronary blood flow and myocardial metabolism in acute experimental anaemia. *Cardiovasc Res* 1972;6:360–367.
30. Kiel JW, Shepherd AP. Optimal hematocrit for canine gastric oxygenation. *Am J Physiol* 1989;256:H472–H477.
31. Krogh A. The number and distribution of capillaries in muscles with calculations of the oxygen pressure head necessary for supplying the tissue. *J Physiol* 1919;52:409–415.
32. Kuo L, Pittman RN. Effect of hemodilution on oxygen transport in arteriolar networks of hamster striated muscle. *Am J Physiol* 1988;254: H331–H339.
33. Mirhashemi S, Ertefai S, Messmer K. Medol analysis of the enhancement of tissue oxygenation by hemodilution due to increased microvascular flow velocity. *Microvasc Res* 1987;34:290–301.
34. Gutierrez G. The rate of oxygen release and its effect on capillary O_2 tension: a mathematical analysis. *Respir Physiol* 1986;63:79–96.
35. Messmer KFW. Acceptable hematocrit levels in surgical patients. *World J Surg* 1987;11:41–46.
36. Ellis CG, Ellsworth ML, Pittman RN. Determination of red cell oxygenation in vivo by dual video densitometric image analysis. *Am J Physiol* 1990;258:H1216–H1223.
37. Sarelius IH. Microcirculation in striated muscle after acute reduction in systemic hematocrit. *Respir Physiol* 1989;78:7–17.
38. LaCelle PL. Alteration of deformability of the erythrocyte membrane in stored blood. *Transfusion* 1969;9:238–245.
39. Simchon S, Jan KM, Chien S. Influence of reduced red cell deformability on regional blood flow. *Am J Physiol* 1987;253:H898–H903.
40. Valeri CR, Hirsch NM. Restoration in vivo of erythrocyte adenosine triphosphate, 2,3-diphosphoglycerate, potassium ion, and sodium ion concentrations following the transfusion of acid-citrate-dextrose–stored human red blood cells. *J Lab Clin Med* 1969;73:722–733.
41. Hurd TC, Dasmahapatra KS, Rush BF, et al. Red blood cell deformability in human and experimental sepsis. *Arch Surg* 1988;123: 217–220.
42. Brazier J, Cooper N, Maloney JV Jr, et al. The adequacy of myocardial oxygen delivery in acute normovolemic anemia. *Surgery* 1974;75: 508–516.
43. Jan KM, Chien S. Effect of hematocrit variations on coronary hemodynamics and oxygen utilization. *Am J Physiol* 1977;233:H106–H113.
44. Most AS, Ruocco NA, Gewirtz H. Effect of a reduction in blood viscosity on maximal myocardial oxygen delivery distal to a moderate coronary stenosis. *Circulation* 1986;74:1085–1092.
45. Spahn DR, Smith LR, Veronee CD, et al. Acute isovolemic hemodilution and blood transfusion: effects on regional function and metabolism in myocardium with compromised coronary blood flow. *J Thorac Cardiovasc Surg* 1993;105:694–704.
46. Spahn DR, Schmid ER, Seifert B, et al. Hemodilution tolerance in patients with coronary artery disease who are receiving chronic β-adrenergic blocker therapy. *Anesth Analg* 1996;82:687–694.
47. Doak GJ, Hall RI. Does hemoglobin concentration affect perioperative myocardial lactate flux in patients undergoing coronary artery bypass surgery? *Anesth Analg* 1995;80:910–916.
48. Carson JL, Duff A, Poses RM, et al. Effect of anaemia and cardiovascular disease on surgical mortality and morbidity. *Lancet* 1996;348: 1055–1060.
49. Lam HTC, Schweitzer SO, Petz L, et al. Effectiveness of a prospective physician self-audit transfusion-monitoring system. *Transfusion* 1997; 37:577–584.
50. Korosue K, Heros RC. Mechanism of cerebral blood flow augmentation by hemodilution in rabbits. *Stroke* 1992;23:1487–1493.
51. Tu YK, Liu HM. Effects of isovolemic hemodilution on hemodynamics, cerebral perfusion, and cerebral vascular reactivity. *Stroke* 1996; 27:441–445.
52. Wood JH, Simeone FA, Kron RE, et al. Experimental hypervolemic hemodilution: physiological correlations of cortical blood flow, cardiac output, and intracranial pressure with fresh blood viscosity and plasma volume. *Neurosurgery* 1984;14:709–723.
53. Scandinavian Stroke Study Group. Multicenter trial of hemodilution in acute ischemic stroke: results of subgroup analyses. *Stroke* 1988;19: 464–471.
54. The Hemodilution in Stroke Study Group. Hypervolemic hemodilution treatment of acute stroke: results of a randomized multicenter trial using pentastarch. *Stroke* 1989;20:317–323.
55. Strand T. Evaluation of long-term outcome and safety after hemodilution therapy in acute ischemic stroke. *Stroke* 1992;23:657–662.
56. Awad IA, Carter LP, Spetzler RF, et al. Clinical vasospasm after subarachnoid hemorrhage: response to hypervolemic hemodilution and arterial hypertension. *Stroke* 1987;18:365–372.
57. Nelson DP, Samsel RW, Wood LDH, et al. Pathological supply dependence of systemic and intestinal O_2 uptake during endotoxemia. *J Appl Physiol* 1988;64:2410–2419.
58. Gutierrez G, Lund N, Bryan-Brown CW. Cellular oxygen utilization during multiple organ failure. *Crit Care Clin* 1989;5:271–287.
59. Parrillo JE, Parker MM, Natanson C, et al. Septic shock in humans: advances in the understanding of pathogenesis, cardiovascular dysfunction, and therapy. *Ann Intern Med* 1990;113:227–242.
60. Wilkerson DK, Rosen AL, Sehgal LR, et al. Limits of cardiac compensation in anemic baboons. *Surgery* 1988;103:665–670.
61. Anderson HT, Kessinger JM, McFarland WJ Jr, et al. Response of the hypertrophied heart to acute anemia and coronary stenosis. *Surgery* 1978;84:8–15.
62. Hagl S, Heimisch W, Meisner H, et al. The effect of hemodilution on regional myocardial function in the presence of coronary stenosis. *Basic Res Cardiol* 1977;72:344–364.
63. Weiskopf RB, Viele MK, Feiner J, et al. Human cardiovascular and metabolic response to acute, severe isovolemic anemia. *JAMA* 1998; 279:217–221.
64. Leung JM, Weiskopf RB, Feiner J, et al. Electrocardiographic ST-segment changes during acute, severe isovolemic hemodilution in humans. *Anesthesiology* 2000;93:1004–1010.
65. Weiskopf RB, Kramer JH, Viele M, et al. Acute severe isovolemic anemia impairs cognitive function and memory in humans. *Anesthesiology* 2000;92:1646–1652.
66. Toy P, Feiner J, Viele MK, et al. Fatigue during acute isovolemic anemia in healthy, resting humans. *Transfusion* 2000;40:457–460.
67. Hébert PC, Wells G, Tweeddale M, et al. Does transfusion practice affect mortality in critically ill patients? Transfusion Requirements in Critical Care (TRICC) Investigators and the Canadian Critical Care Trials Group. *Am J Respir Crit Care Med* 1997;155:1618–1623.
68. Spiess BD, Ley C, Body SC, et al. Hematocrit value on intensive care unit entry influences the frequency of Q-wave myocardial infarction after coronary artery bypass grafting. The Institutions of the Multicenter Study of Perioperative Ischemia (McSPI) Research Group. *J Thorac Cardiovasc Surg* 1998;116:460–467.
69. Carson JL, Duff A, Berlin JA, et al. Perioperative blood transfusion and postoperative mortality. *JAMA* 1998;279:199–205.
70. Paone G, Silverman NA. The paradox of on-bypass transfusion thresholds in blood conservation. *Circulation* 1997;96[Suppl 9]:II-205–II-208.
71. Nelson AH, Fleisher LA, Rosenbaum SH. Relationship between postoperative anemia and cardiac morbidity in high-risk vascular patients in the intensive care unit. *Crit Care Med* 1993;21:860–866.
72. Hogue CW, Goodnough LT, Monk TG. Perioperative myocardial ischemic episodes are related to hematocrit level in patients undergoing radical prostatectomy. *Transfusion* 1998;38:924–931.
73. Topley E, Fischer MR. The illness of trauma. *Br J Clin Pract* 1956; 1:770–776.
74. Blair SD, Janvrin SB, McCollum CN, et al. Effect of early blood transfusion on gastrointestinal haemorrhage. *Br J Surg* 1986;73:783–785.
75. Fortune JB, Feustel PJ, Saifi J, et al. Influence of hematocrit on cardio-

pulmonary function after acute hemorrhage. *J Trauma* 1987;27: 243–249.
76. Johnson RG, Thurer RL, Kruskall MS, et al. Comparison of two transfusion strategies after elective operations for myocardial revascularization. *J Thorac Cardiovasc Surg* 1992;104:307–314.
77. Hébert PC, Wells G, Marshall J, et al. Transfusion requirements in critical care: a pilot study. Canadian Critical Care Trials Group [published erratum appears in *JAMA* 1995;274:944]. *JAMA* 1995;273: 1439–1444.
78. Bush RL, Pevec WC, Holcroft JW. A prospective, randomized trial limiting perioperative red blood cell transfusions in vascular patients. *Am J Surg* 1997;174:143–148.
79. Carson JL, Terrin ML, Barton FB, et al. A pilot randomized trial comparing symptomatic vs. hemoglobin-level–driven red blood cell transfusions following hip fracture. *Transfusion* 1998;38:522–529.
80. Hébert PC, Wells G, Blajchman MA, et al. A multicenter, randomized, controlled clinical trial of transfusion requirements in critical care. Transfusion Requirements in Critical Care Investigators, Canadian Critical Care Trials Group. *N Engl J Med* 1999;340:409–417.
81. Bracey AW, Radovancevic R, Riggs SA, et al. Lowering the hemoglobin threshold for transfusion in coronary artery bypass procedures: effect on patient outcome. *Transfusion* 1999;39:1070–1077.
82. Lotke PA, Barth P, Garino JP, et al. Predonated autologous blood transfusions after total knee arthroplasty: immediate versus delayed administration. *J Arthroplasty* 1999;14:647–650.
83. Hébert PC, Wells G, Marshall J, et al. Transfusion requirements in critical care: a pilot study. Canadian Critical Care Trials Group *JAMA* 1995;273:1439–1444.
84. Carson JL, Hill S, Carless P, et al. Transfusion triggers: a systematic review of the literature. *Transfusion Med Rev* 2002 *(in press).*
85. Clyne N, Jogestrand T. Effect of erythropoietin treatment on physical exercise capacity and on renal function in predialytic uremic patients. *Nephron* 1992;60:390–396.
86. Cella D, Bron D. The effect of epoetin alfa on quality of life in anemic cancer patients. *Cancer Pract* 1999;7:177–182.
87. Practice guidelines for blood component therapy: a report by the American Society of Anesthesiologists Task Force on Blood Component Therapy. *Anesthesiology* 1996;84:732–747.
88. Marik PE. Pulmonary artery catheterization and esophageal Doppler monitoring in the ICU. *Chest* 1999;116:1085–1091.
89. Wu WC, Rathove SS, Wang Y, et al. Blood transfusion in elderly patients with acute myocardial infarction. *N Engl J Med* 2001;345: 1230–1236.

Rossi's Principles of Transfusion Medicine, Third Edition, edited by Toby L. Simon, Walter H. Dzik, Edward L. Snyder, Christopher P. Stowell, and Ronald G. Strauss. Lippincott Williams & Wilkins, Philadelphia © 2002.

13

RED BLOOD CELL SUBSTITUTES

CHRISTOPHER P. STOWELL

Concerns about the adequacy of the blood supply and transfusion-transmitted infectious diseases in the 1980s stimulated interest in the development of blood substitutes, materials that could be used to deliver oxygen to tissues in place of donated red blood cells (RBCs). However, as the safety of the blood supply reached unparalleled levels in the 1990s, the advantages of a synthetic or semisynthetic RBC substitute seemed to become less compelling. Ironically, as we enter the new century, we are again faced with impending blood shortages as the donor pool contracts and an aging population strains medical resources. In addition, we have new concerns about the possibility that recently recognized infectious agents, such as prions, might be transmissible by means of transfusion. As a result, interest in the development of RBC substitutes remains high, largely because of the clinical potential but to some extent because of the insight into oxygen delivery and its regulation that has been gained through study of these materials.

The search for a substitute for the RBC has led to the investigation of three different classes of oxygen carriers—perfluorocarbons (PFCs), modified hemoglobin, and liposome-encapsulated hemoglobin. The development of the last remains in the preclinical stage, but several PFC- and hemoglobin-based substitutes have advanced to the level of phase III trials and may be available for clinical use within a few years. This chapter focuses on PFC- and hemoglobin-based RBC substitutes. In addition to the literature cited, the reader is referred to several recent reviews and monographs on this subject (1–7).

The desirable characteristics of an RBC substitute are listed in Table 13.1. Absence of infectious risk and abundance are key attributes. An RBC substitute also must be able to transport high concentrations of oxygen, and preferably of carbon dioxide, and to load and unload these gases in the appropriate milieu. The substitute also must have a suitable intravascular half-life. Most of the materials currently under study have a half-life of 1 day or less, which is adequate for perioperative use or in the setting of acute blood loss. As plasma half-life increases, so do the possible clinical applications.

The initial working assumption guiding the development of RBC substitutes was that it would be desirable to produce a material approximately isoncotic and isosmotic with blood that had a low viscosity. The theory was that reduction in systemic vascular resistance would improve hemodynamics. This systemic effect may not be predictive of the hemodynamics at the microcirculatory level, however (8). Reduction in blood viscosity, when not compensated for by increased flow velocity, reduces shear stress on vascular endothelial cells, which respond by curtailing the output of various relaxing factors, such as endothelin and prostacyclin (9–11). As a result, local vasoconstriction may decrease regional blood flow despite favorable systemic hemodynamics.

In addition to being efficacious, RBC substitutes also must be safe. Given the current safety of the donor blood supply, the side-effect profile of the candidate substitute must be exemplary. The ideal RBC substitute must be free of infectious risk and be minimally immunogenic. Perfluorocarbons carry no infectious or immunologic risk. Although hemoglobin is a weak immunogen, the same may not be true of neoantigens formed by means of chemical alteration of hemoglobin or expression of xenoantigens by bovine hemoglobin. Among the practical considerations for a candidate RBC substitute are its ease of use, stability, and cost. The ideal substitute would require no preparation and could be used off the shelf. Because there are no compatibility issues, a substitute could be stocked much as other intravenous fluids at the point of care, for example in an ambulance, in which case stability under a wide variety of storage conditions would be advantageous.

C.P. Stowell: Blood Transfusion Service, Massachusetts General Hospital, Boston, Massachusetts.

TABLE 13.1. DESIRABLE CHARACTERISTICS FOR RED BLOOD CELL SUBSTITUTES

Characteristic	Requirement
Efficacy	High capacity for oxygen and carbon dioxide
	Physiologic gas exchange
	Suitable intravascular half-life
	Approximately isoncotic and isosmotic
	Favorable rheologic properties
Safety	Minimal infectious risk
	Minimal immunogenicity (e.g., neoantigens, xenoantigens)
	Lack of toxicity
	Limited extraneous physiologic effects
Logistics	Stability under a wide range of conditions
	Immediate availability
	Abundance
	Low cost

HEMOGLOBIN-BASED RED BLOOD CELL SUBSTITUTES

Background

Hemoglobin is an obvious candidate for an RBC substitute and has a number of desirable attributes (Table 13.2). The first is its ability to carry high concentrations of oxygen and carbon dioxide and, at least potentially, to load and unload these gases in response to the appropriate physiologic cues, such as hypoxemia and acidemia. Hemoglobin solutions can be prepared to be approximately isoncotic and isosmotic with plasma and to have low viscosity, which is not clearly beneficial. The absence of the RBC membrane eliminates the complications caused by the presence of blood group antigens. The purification procedures remove other cell components that could produce undesirable effects, and a variety of processes are used to eliminate or inactivate infectious agents. In purified form, hemoglobin solutions are stable and can be stored for a much longer time than can units of RBCs and under more permissive conditions (e.g., room temperature).

TABLE 13.2. POTENTIAL ADVANTAGES AND DISADVANTAGES OF UNMODIFIED HEMOGLOBIN

Advantages	Disadvantages
High capacity for oxygen and carbon dioxide	Rapid clearance
Functions at physiologic PO_2	Renal toxicity
Low viscosity (?)	Vasoactivity
High oncotic pressure	Increased oxygen affinity
Absence of red blood cell antigens	Autoxidation
Prolonged shelf life	Immunogenicity (modified or nonhuman)
Purification and viral inactivation possible	Potentiation of sepsis (?)

Potential Problems with Unmodified Hemoglobin

Hemoglobin is a highly active molecule and in its unmodified state can produce a number of deleterious effects (Table 13.2). For this reason, all of the hemoglobin-based oxygen carriers (HBOCs) being studied make use of hemoglobin preparations that have been chemically modified in an effort to eliminate or mitigate some of these potential toxicities.

The first problem with free hemoglobin in plasma is that it dissociates into $\alpha\beta$ dimers and is rapidly cleared by means of glomerular filtration. The hemoglobin leaves the bloodstream too rapidly to be clinically useful and is toxic to the renal tubular cells (12). Various modifications have been made to all hemoglobin-based substitutes under study that have had the effect of increasing the plasma half-life and eliminating nephrotoxicity. Three types of modifications have been used to achieve these ends—intramolecular stabilization of the hemoglobin tetramer, intermolecular cross-linking (polymerization of the tetramer), and surface conjugation of hemoglobin with other macromolecules (Fig. 13.1).

Baxter Healthcare prepared stabilized hemoglobin tetramer by using the bifunctional reagent bis-(3,5-dibromosalicyl) fumarate (diaspirin) to cross-link the α chains, a technique initially developed by the U.S. Army (Table 13.3) (13–15). Somatogen used recombinant technology to produce a single di-α chain, which when associated with two β chains resulted in a cross-

Cross Linked Hemoglobin

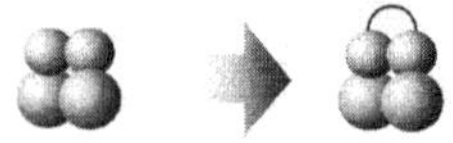

Polymerized Hemoglobin

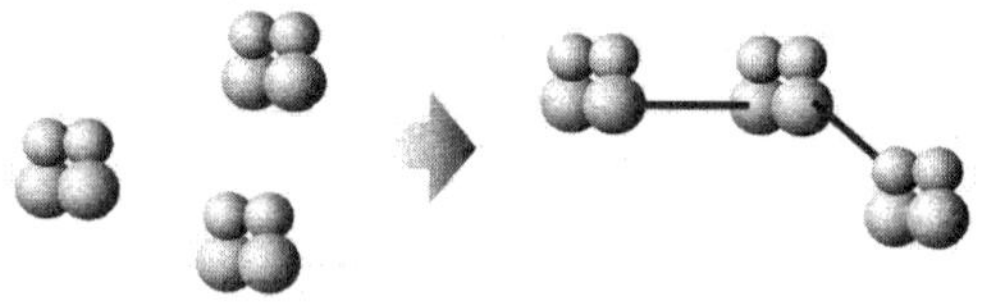

Conjugated Hemoglobin

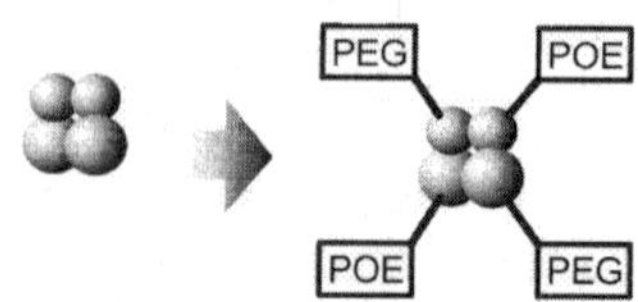

FIGURE 13.1. Three techniques to prevent rapid clearance of cell-free hemoglobin—intramolecular cross-linking, intermolecular cross-linking (polymerization), and surface modification by means of conjugation with macromolecules. (From Stowell CP, Levin J, Spiess BD, et al. Progress in the development of RBC substitutes. *Transfusion* 2001;41: 287–299, with permission.)

TABLE 13.3. MODIFICATIONS TO PREVENT RAPID CLEARANCE AND NEPHROTIXICITY OF HEMOGLOBIN

Class	Technique	Company/Product	Product
Intramolecular cross-linking	Di-aspirin	Baxter/HemAssist	Hb tetramers (64 kd)
	Recombinant di-α chain	Somatogen/Optro	Hb tetramers (64 kd)
Intermolecular cross-linking	Gluteraldehyde	Northfield/PolyHeme	Hb oligomers (150 kd)
	Gluteraldehyde	Biopure/Hemopure	Hb oligomers (240 kd)
	o-Raffinose	Hemosol/HemoLink	Hb oligomers (156 kd)
Surface conjugation	PEG	Enzon/PEG Hemoglobin	Hb tetramers (117 kd)
	POE	Ajinomoto/Apex/PHP	Hb tetramers (97 kd)

PEG, polyethylene glycol; Hb, hemoglobin; POE, polyoxyethylene.

linked tetramer (16). The reagents gluteraldehyde and open-chain *o*-raffinose were used to form a combination of intramolecular and intermolecular cross-links, producing a distribution of oligomers of the hemoglobin tetramer that compose the products PolyHeme (17), Hemopure (18), and Hemolink (19). Conjugation of macromolecules such as polyethylene glycol (PEG) or polyxyethylene to the hemoglobin tetramer markedly increases its molecular weight, molecular radius, and colloid oncotic pressure (20), thereby reducing its renal clearance and perhaps its immunogenicity (21). Both PEG-hemoglobin (22,23) and pyridoxylated hemoglobin polyxyethylene (24) make use of this approach.

A second concern with the hemoglobin molecule is its vasoactivity. The hypertensive effects of cell-free hemoglobin have been observed in animals (25,26) and humans (27) and are attributed in part to nitric oxide scavenging by heme iron and the resulting vasoconstriction (28). In an intact red blood cell, some nitric oxide is present in a membrane-associated compartment as *S*-nitrosothiol adducts, which can dissociate to release nitric oxide and perhaps function to regulate vascular tone (29). Other factors that play a role in the vasoactivity of hemoglobin are its effects on endothelin-mediated and adrenergic receptor-mediated regulation of vascular tone (30,31) and the influence of reduced viscosity (10). Delivery of oxygen by the substitute also may exert local vasoconstrictive effects by triggering an oxygen-sensitive autoregulatory response (32,33). The degree of vasoactivity varies among the different HBOCs and is generally more prominent in preparations with a large proportion of hemoglobin tetramer and low viscosity (8). The hypertensive effect has been exploited by Baxter (15,34) and by Apex/Ajinomoto (35) in trials in which the HBOC was given to patients with septic and hemorrhagic shock, states in which nitric oxide levels usually are elevated.

Another characteristic of hemoglobin in solution is the loss of 2,3-bisphosphoglycerate (2,3-BPG; formerly known as 2,3-diphosphoglycerate) which has the effect of decreasing the P_{50} (the partial pressure of oxygen at which hemoglobin is 50% saturated). The theoretic concern is that oxygen unloading from 2,3-BPG–depleted hemoglobin may be impaired, as is thought to be the case with banked blood (36). Several techniques have been used to increase P_{50} (Fig. 13.2). The diaspirin linkage modification used in HemAssist also has the effect of shifting the oxyhemoglobin dissociation curve to the right (37), as does the ββ cross-linking into the 2,3-BPG pocket of Hemolink (38). Pyridoxylation has been used in PolyHeme (39) and pyridoxylated hemoglobin polyxyethylene (24) to achieve the same effect. Bovine hemoglobin, which is used in Hemopure and PEG-hemoglobin, is not regulated by 2,3-BPG but rather has a similar allosteric response to chloride. Hence, at physiologic chloride concentrations, the oxyhemoglobin dissociation curve of bovine hemoglobin resembles that of human hemoglobin with bound 2,3-BPG. The recombinant hemoglobin used in Somatogen's Optro is based on a naturally occurring human hemoglobin variant with a high P_{50} (Hemoglobin Presbyterian). Although the initial assumption was that a low P_{50} was an undesirable characteristic for an HBOC, it may be counterbalanced by several mitigating factors. Among them is blunting of the autoregulatory response by the more parsimonious release of oxygen (40). In addition, by retaining oxygen in the face of a greater degree of hypoxemia, the modified hemoglobin may produce a steeper oxygen gradient. Because oxygen delivery beyond the vascular space depends on diffusion, the steeper oxygen gradient may drive oxygen more deeply into the tissue (41).

Hemoglobin in solution autooxidizes to methemoglobin, which does not carry oxygen, then to irreversibly altered metabolites, including free radicals (42), which can have deleterious effects on tissues exposed to them. Methemoglobin formation has been measured in all of the HBOCs studied to date and found to be less than 15% in all with little tendency to accumulate during storage (43).

The possibility that an HBOC might be immunogenic is low but is being assessed in various clinical trials (44). Human hemoglobin is a poor immunogen, but chemically modified human hemoglobin, or bovine hemoglobin, which has 90% sequence homology with the human form, could conceivably be more highly immunogenic. Surface modification with macromolecules such as PEG and polyoxyethylene may shield hemoglobin from the immune system and reduce the frequency or magnitude of the response (21).

A theoretic concern with HBOCs is the potentiation of bacterial sepsis. This concern has emerged from a number of studies of animal models of bacterial sepsis in which the presence of an HBOC increased mortality (45). The mechanism of action is not known. The HBOC may enhance bacterial growth or impede clearance of opsonized bacteria by the reticuloendothelial system (RES). There also is evidence that hemoglobin binds to endotoxins and enhances their effects (46,47).

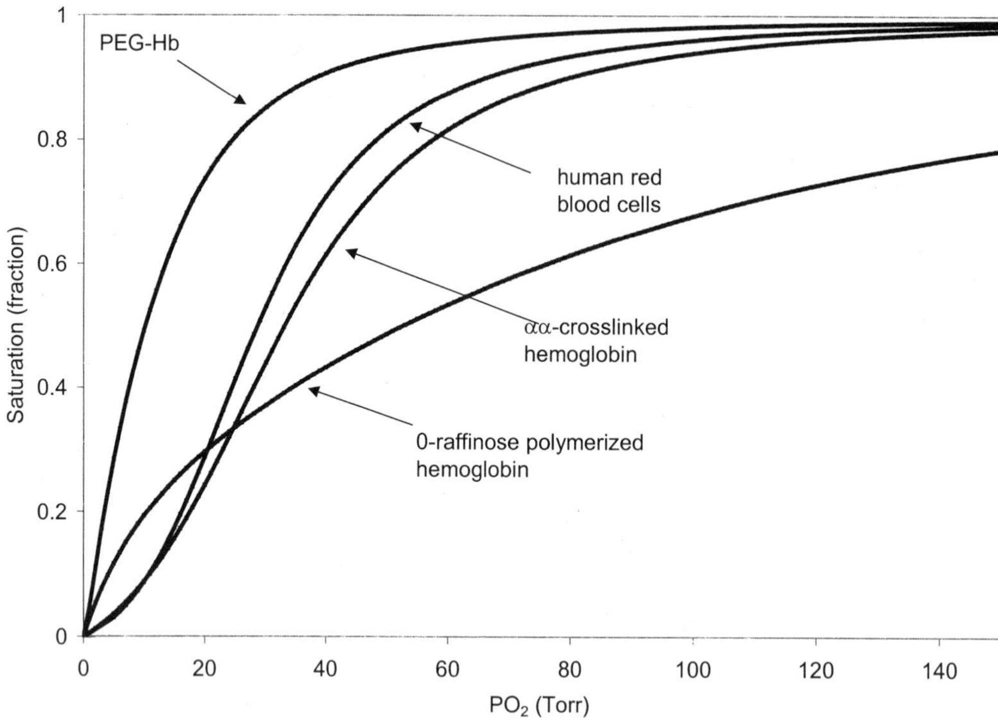

FIGURE 13.2. Oxyhemoglobin dissociation curves (fractional saturation versus PO_2) for red blood cells and the main classes of hemoglobin-based oxygen carriers—intramolecular cross-linked (data for U. S. Army diaspirin linked αα hemoglobin) (37); intermolecular cross-linked (data for *o*-raffinose polymerized human hemoglobin) (38); and surface modified human hemoglobin (data for polyethylene glycol-conjugated hemoglobin). (From Stowell CP, Levin J, Spiess BD, et al. Progress in the development of RBC substitutes. *Transfusion* 2001;41:287–299, with permission.)

Hemoglobin Sources

The HBOCs under development have been based on hemoglobin from three sources—human from outdated units of donor RBCs, bovine from designated herds of beef cattle, and recombinant technology. Several attributes of these sources are compared in Table 13.4. The most striking difference between sources is availability. The outdate rate for donor RBC units is less than 10% (48) and is likely to shrink as increasing demands for blood are superimposed on a contracting donor base (49). The supply of bovine hemoglobin, on the other hand, is almost unlimited. Most recombinant proteins in clinical use are active in microgram to milligram quantities. Because the equivalent of a two-unit transfusion would require approximately 100 g of hemoglobin, the production of source hemoglobin would have to occur on an almost unprecedented scale for a recombinant protein (50). Even if adequate scale-up can be achieved, the costs may substantially exceed those incurred in obtaining bovine or human hemoglobin. The differences in P_{50} and the risk of immunogenicity of hemoglobins from different sources have been discussed and remain, so far, theoretic considerations. The risk of infection associated with any of these source products is likely to be similar to that of plasma derivatives subject to robust viral inactivation techniques. As with any product based on pooled human blood or plasma, there is theoretic concern that a new, uncharacterized human pathogen could be present. It also is conceivable that a bovine pathogen or commensal organism could become pathogenic in humans. There is concern that prion-mediated diseases can be transmitted by transfusion (see Chapter 54) (51,52). To date, there is no evidence of transfusion transmission among humans. There has been a preliminary report of possible transfusion transmission of bovine spongiform encephalopathy in a sheep model system (53), although the study is still in progress. In any of these possible situations, the infectious agent would also have to survive the rigorous pathogen inactivation processes in place for all HBOCs. One company

TABLE 13.4. COMPARISON OF HEMOGLOBIN SOURCES

Property	Human	Bovine	Recombinant (Human)
Quantity	Limited[a]	Abundant	Moderate
P_{50}[b]	↓	↔	↔
Immunogenicity[c]	Very low	Low	Very low
Infection risk	Very low	Very low	Very low
	? New pathogen	? Bovine pathogens	

[a] Outdated red blood cells.
[b] Unmodified hemoglobin.
[c] May depend on modification procedures.
↓, decreased; ↔, unchanged.

TABLE 13.5. MODIFIED HEMOGLOBIN-BASED RED BLOOD CELL SUBSTITUTES

Product (Manufacturer)	Hemoglobin Source	Trial Level	Application
PolyHeme (Northfield)	Human	Phase III	Trauma, surgery
Hemolink (Hemosol)	Human	Phase II	Cardiopulmonary bypass—ANH; orthopedic surgery—acute blood loss, dialysis
		Phase III	Cardiac surgery
HemAssist (Baxter)	Human	Phase II	Septic shock, hemodialysis, hemorrhagic shock, cardiopulmonary bypass
		Phase III (all trials terminated)	Acute blood loss—surgery, trauma Stroke
PHP (Ajinomoto/Apex)	Human	Phase III	Nitric oxide–induced shock
PEG Hemoglobin (Enzon)	Bovine	Phase Ib	Radiosensitizer solid tumors
Hemopure (Biopure)	Bovine	Preclinical	Erythropoiesis
		Phase I	Radiosensitizer, glioblastoma
		Phase II	Sickle cell crisis, oncology, Surgery—orthopedic, urologic, vascular, cardiac, trauma
		Phase III[a]	Surgery—cardiac, orthopedic
Oxyglobin (Biopure)	Bovine	Approved	Veterinary—anemia, acute blood loss
Optro (Somatogen Baxter)	Recombinant	Phase I	Erythropoiesis—ESRD, refractory anemia
		Phase II (all trials terminated)	ANH, acute blood loss, surgery

Information current to April 2001.
[a]Approved in South Africa.
ANH, acute normovolemic hemodilution; ESRD, end-stage renal disease.

(Biopure) has developed a process that produces substantial reduction of the scrapie prion agent (43).

Human Hemoglobin-based Oxygen Carriers

Seven HBOCs, four of them based on human hemoglobin, have been studied in clinical trials. Three of the four human hemoglobin-based HBOC (and one of the bovine hemoglobin-based HBOCs) have reached the phase III level. The clinical trial information is summarized in Table 13.5 and as follows.

PolyHeme

PolyHeme consists of glutaraldehyde-polymerized human hemoglobin that has been pyridoxylated and extensively purified to remove residual hemoglobin tetramers (17). Some characteristics of this product are listed in Table 13.6. It is being developed by Northfield Laboratories (Evanston, IL) as an alternative to RBCs in surgery and trauma (54–56). Trauma patients who received PolyHeme needed fewer transfusions of banked blood (54).

Hemolink

Hemosol has prepared this product by means of polymerization with open-chain *o*-raffinose followed by a reduction step (19). Chemical modification is followed by extensive purification and virus-inactivation procedures. Some characteristics of this product are listed in Table 13.6. It has been studied in phase II clinical trials in dialysis and as an oxygen-carrying replacement fluid in acute normovolemic hemodilution (ANH). It is in phase III trials in Canada, the United States, and Europe.

Hemassist

Baxter Healthcare (Deerfield, IL) prepared a stabilized hemoglobin tetramer using the diaspirin linkage technique followed by purification and heat inactivation (13). The product is stored frozen. In 1998, the company halted phase III clinical trials of use of this product in trauma, surgery, and acute ischemic stroke and discontinued development citing safety concerns (57). In both the stroke trial (58) and the trauma trial (59), administration of HemAssist was a significant predictor of worse outcome.

Pyridoxal Hemoglobin Polyoxyethylene

Pyridoxal hemoglobin polyxyethylene is prepared by Apex Bioscience (Research Triangle Park, NC) by means of pyridoxylation of human hemoglobin followed by conjugation with polyxyethylene (24). This preparation has a hypertensive effect and is being studied in the care of patients with septic or hemorrhagic shock.

Bovine Hemoglobin-based Oxygen Carriers

Hemopure

The Biopure Corporation (Cambridge, MA) uses glutaraldehyde to polymerize bovine hemoglobin followed by extensive purification and viral inactivation steps to produce a substitute with less than 3 % hemoglobin tetramers. Some characteristics of this product are listed in Table 13.6. This product has been studied

TABLE 13.6. CHARACTERISTICS OF HEMOGLOBIN-BASED OXYGEN CARRIERS IN PHASE III CLINICAL TRIALS

Characteristic	PolyHeme	Hemopure	Hemolink
Hemoglobin source	Human	Bovine	Human
Modification	Glutaraldehyde pyridoxal-5-phosphate	Glutaraldehyde borohydride	*o*-Raffinose dimethylamineborane
Molecular weight (kd)	150	240	156
Percentage tetramer (64 kd)	<1	<3	35
P_{50} (mm Hg)	28–30	38	39 ± 12
Percentage methemoglobin	<3	<3	<15
Grams of hemoglobin per unit	50	30	25
Hemoglobin concentration (g/dl)	10	13	10
Vol/unit (ml)	500	250	250
Colloid oncotic pressure (mm Hg)	20–25	17	24
Change in mean arterial pressure	↔	↑ 15%	↑ 14%
Plasma half-life (h)	24	20	18
Shelf life	1 y (4–10°C)	3 y (RT)	60 d (RT)

↔, no change; ↑, increased; RT, room temperature.

principally for perioperative use as a bridge to delay the need for banked RBCs until the patient's condition has been stabilized and blood loss curtailed (60–62). Enrollment has been completed in several phase III trials in noncardiac surgery in the United States and abroad. The Biopure Corporation was the first to obtain licensure for a blood substitute product. In 1997, a veterinary formulation of its HBOC Oxyglobin was licensed by the U.S. Food and Drug Administration for use in animals. In April 2001, Biopure announced that Hemopure had been approved for clinical use in South Africa. Hemopure has also been studied in a phase II trial in the management of sickle cell crisis, in which it improved exercise tolerance (63).

Hemopure has been infused on a compassionate use basis into a patient with warm autoimmune hemolytic anemia refractory to treatment that necessitated RBC transfusion support (64). This patient received 11 units of Hemopure over several days. This treatment improved hemodynamics and relieved ischemic symptoms until therapy eventually produced remission of hemolysis.

Polyethylene Glycol Hemoglobin

Polyethylene glycol hemoglobin is being developed by Enzon (Piscataway, NJ) for use as a sensitizer for radiation therapy for solid tumors (65). Although adequate oxygenation of tumor tissue is required for optimal effectiveness of radiation therapy, the anomalous vasculature of many tumors impedes the flow of erythrocytes. Polyethylene glycol hemoglobin, which is much smaller, can navigate through the vessels of the tumor more readily than can RBCs, deliver oxygen, and enhance the effect of radiation. Polyethylene glycol hemoglobin is prepared by means of conjugating PEG to bovine hemoglobin tetramer followed by purification. Polyethylene glycol hemoglobin has a much larger molecular radius than does native hemoglobin. It has a slightly longer plasma half-life (48 hours) than do the other HBOCs and is hyperoncotic compared with the others.

Recombinant Human Hemoglobin

Somatogen (Boulder, CO) has developed a product called Optro that is based on recombinant human hemoglobin cross-linked by a di-αα chain to produce a stabilized, hemoglobin tetramer (16). Optro was in phase I (66) and II clinical trials when Baxter Healthcare, the parent company, discontinued development when it closed down trials with HemAssist.

PERFLUOROCARBON-BASED RED BLOOD CELL SUBSTITUTES

Background

Perfluorocarbons are a class of compounds consisting of a linear or cyclic carbon backbone highly substituted with fluorine (Fig. 13.3). They were initially developed as chemically inert materials for the handling of unstable radioisotopes and have gone on to fame as nonstick coatings for cookware and fabrics. Most of the PFCs are liquid at room temperature and are highly soluble for respiratory gases including oxygen, nitrogen, and carbon dioxide. The amount of gas that can be dissolved into a PFC is directly proportional to its ambient partial pressure (Fig. 13.4). Theoretically, at a high enough PO_2, a PFC could contain the same amount of oxygen as blood. Perfluorocarbons are not miscible in water, however, and must be prepared as emulsions for any biologic applications, with the exception of liquid ventilation (see later). The need to prepare PFCs as emulsions decreases the oxygen-carrying capacity. As shown in Figure 13.4, PFCs have a much lower capacity for oxygen than does blood at physiologic PO_2. Therefore patients need supplemental oxygen when a PFC emulsion is used.

Perfluorocarbon emulsions are cleared by the RES (as are HBOCs) but eventually are exhaled. The half-life in the RES of some of the first PFCs studied was quite long. The two PFCs under development recently have a half-life in the RES on the order of a few days. The effect on the RES of ingestion of large amounts of PFCs or emulsifying agents remains to be determined. The clearance rate of PFC emulsions from the circulation

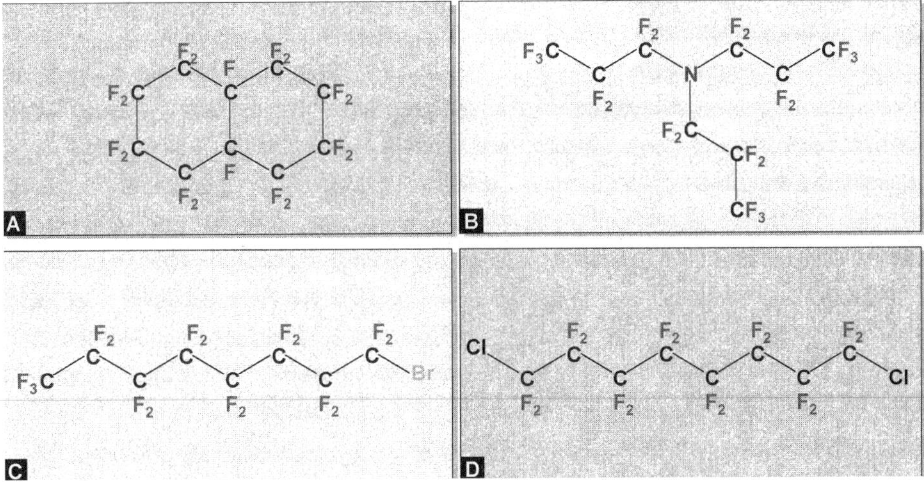

FIGURE 13.3. Perfluorocarbons studied in clinical trials. Perfluorodecalin **(A)** and perfluorotripropylamine **(B)** are components of Fluosol-DA. Perfluorooctylbromide (perflubron) **(C)** is a component of Oxygent, Imavist, and Liquivent. α,ω-dichloroperfluorooctane **(D)** is a component of Oxyfluor. (From Stowell CP, Levin J, Spiess BD, et al. Progress in the development of RBC substitutes. *Transfusion* 2001;41:287–299, with permission.)

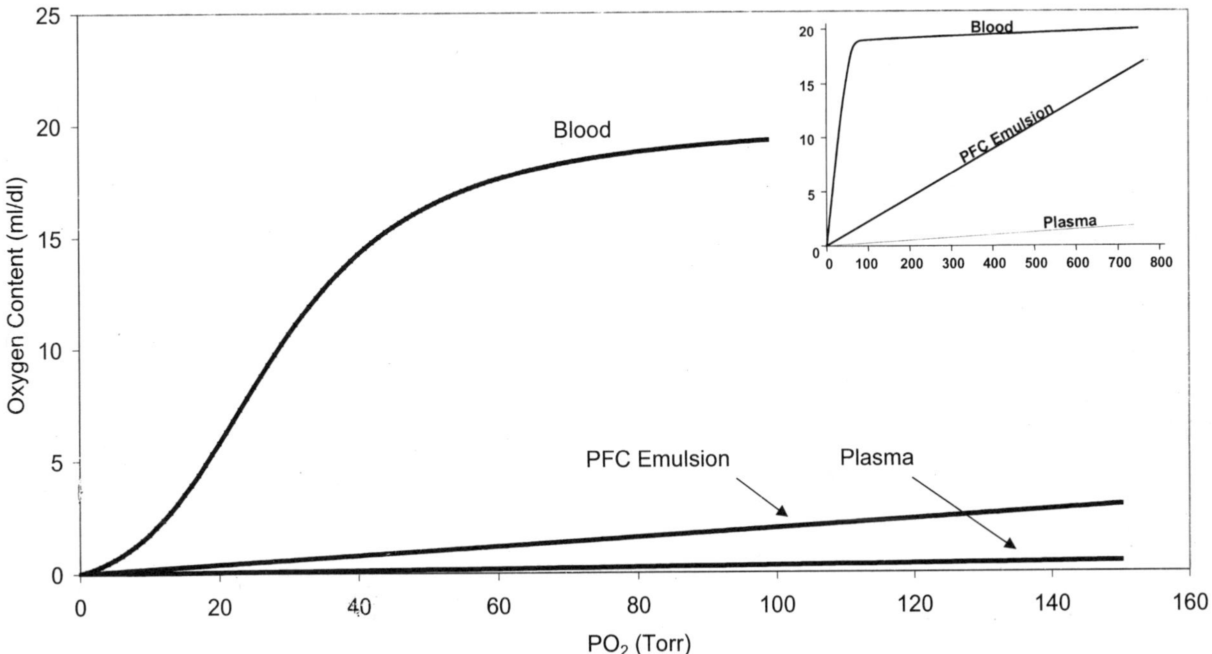

FIGURE 13.4. Oxygen-carrying capacity of whole blood, a perfluorocarbon emulsion (Oxygent) (70), and plasma, as a function of PO_2. The data for whole blood and plasma are from healthy humans at a hemoglobin concentration 15 g/dl (71). *Inset,* the same at higher PO_2. (Modified from Stowell CP, Levin J, Spiess BD, et al. Progress in the development of RBC substitutes. *Transfusion* 2001;41:287–299, with permission.)

TABLE 13.7. POTENTIAL ADVANTAGES AND DISADVANTAGES OF PERFLUOROCARBON RED BLOOD CELL SUBSTITUTES

Advantages	Disadvantages
Control of composition	Requirement for emulsification and stabilization
Possibility of specific modification	Heterogeneous particle size
Large-scale production	Variable (long) reticuloendothelial clearance
Low production costs	High FiO_2 required
Prolonged shelf life	Low oxygen capacity at physiologic PO_2
Minimal infectious risk	Rapid plasma clearance
Minimal immunogenicity	
Low viscosity (?)	

increases as the particle size of the emulsion decreases. Reproducible and predictable preparation of emulsions with the appropriate distribution of particle sizes is one of the technical challenges that the developers of these materials have faced. The plasma half-life of the PFC emulsions under study is approximately 12 to 24 hours, which compares favorably with the half-life of HBOCs.

Additional potential advantages and disadvantages of the PFCs are summarized in Table 13.7. Given the synthetic origin, it is possible to prepare a PFC itself in large quantities and to alter its structure to affect its characteristics. Because they are chemically inert, PFCs are not subject to degradation and are unlikely to be immunogenic. The PFC emulsions are not as stable and depending on the emulsifying agent may be immunogenic. The synthetic origin and biologic inertness entirely remove the risk of transmission of infectious disease.

Fluosol-DA

The first blood substitute tested in clinical trials was Fluosol-DA (Table 13.8), a PFC emulsion prepared by the Green Cross Corporation (Osaka, Japan) and managed in the United States by Alpha Therapeutics (Los Angeles, CA). This product consisted of two PFCs (Fig. 13.3), a surfactant, and an emulsion stabilizer. In a phase II trial of the treatment of patients with acute hemorrhage, Fluosol-DA was not efficacious (67). The lack of efficacy has been attributed to the low oxygen-carrying capacity of the product, the small amounts infused, and the extremely acute condition of the patients in the trial. Although further investigation of Fluosol-DA as a RBC substitute was halted, this product eventually was licensed for use in percutaneous transluminal coronary angioplasty. It is used in this procedure to perfuse and oxygenate capillary beds distal to the balloon (68,69). Fluosol-DA was removed from the market 5 years after being licensed because of the requirement for product preparation immediately before use, the instability of the emulsion, and improvements in catheter technology that eliminated the need. The experience with Fluosol-DA did provide proof of concept and indicated where improvements were needed. This experience was capitalized on for the development of a second generation of PFCs represented by perflubron and Oxyfluor.

Perflubron

Alliance Pharmaceutical Corporation (San Diego, CA) has conducted trials of a substitute based on a new PFC, perfluorooctylbromide (perflubron; Fig. 13.3), which is emulsified with egg yolk phospholipid (lecithin) (70). Perflubron emulsion, named Oxygent, has a much higher capacity for oxygen than did Fluosol-DA. In safety trials perflubron has been shown to be well tolerated. The principal adverse effects are mild, reversible thrombocytopenia (72) and transient flulike symptoms attributed to the release of cytokines and arachidonic acid metabolites from the cells of the RES as they ingest PFC emulsion particles (73). Oxygent has been studied as a sensitizing agent for radiation therapy for solid tumors (74), but the primary application is as an extender in ANH in general and cardiac surgery (75, 76). Phase III clinical trials are in progress (Table 13.8).

Alliance has pursued other applications for perflubron. Because perflubron has one bromine substituent, it is radiopaque

TABLE 13.8. PERFLUOROCARBON RED BLOOD CELL SUBSTITUTES STUDIED

Product (Manufacturer)	Perfluorocarbon	Trial Level	Application
Fluosol-DA (Green Cross/Alpha)	Perfluorodecalin	Phase II (discontinued)	Acute blood loss
	Perfluoropropylamine	Approved (withdrawn)	PTCA
Oxygent (Alliance)	Perflubron	Phase II	CABG-ANH
			Orthopedic surgery—acute blood loss
		Phase III	Cardiac surgery
			Surgery—ANH
Imagent GI	Perflubron	Approved	GI imaging
Imavist (Alliance)	Perflubron	Phase III	Cardiac ultrasonography
Liquivent (Alliance)	Perflubron (neat)	Phase Ib/II	Liquid ventilation—IRDS
		Phase II/III	Liquid ventilation—pediatric and adult ARDS
Oxyfluor (HemaGen/PFC)	Perfluorodichlorooctane	Phase II (discontinued)	Surgery, neuroprotectant, bypass

Information current to 4/01.
PCTA, percutaneous transluminal coronary angioplasty; CABG, coronary artery bypass graft; ANH, acute normovolemic hemodilution; GI, gastrointestinal; IRDS, infant respiratory distress syndrome; ARDS, adult respiratory distress syndrome.

and has been studied as a contrast agent for several imaging applications. One formulation, Imagent GI, has been licensed for use in gastrointestinal radiography (77). Another formulation, Imavist, is in phase III clinical trials for use in cardiac ultrasonography because of its propensity to form stable microbubbles that are highly echogenic (78).

One particularly novel application that Alliance is studying is partial liquid ventilation in which oxygenated perflubron (neat) is instilled into the lungs of patients with respiratory distress syndrome. The PFC was intended not only to deliver oxygen but also to act as a surfactant to improve gas diffusion. Early results in the treatment of infants with acute respiratory distress syndrome (79) were promising. Enrollment has been completed for a phase III trial of the treatment of adult patients with acute respiratory distress syndrome or acute lung injury syndrome.

Oxyfluor

HemaGen/PFC (Waltham, MA) produced a PFC emulsion based on perfluorodichlorooctane (Fig. 13.3) stabilized with lecithin and safflower oil (triglycerides). Oxyfluor could be stored for 1 year at room temperature (72). In safety trials in the treatment of humans, it elicited side effects similar to those of Oxygent. Oxyfluor was studied for use as an RBC substitute in surgery. The principal application pursued by HemaGen was as a scavenger of the microbubbles that form in blood exposed to the oxygenation systems of cardiopulmonary bypass circuits (80, 81). These microbubbles are thought to be responsible for occlusion of the microvasculature of the brain, which produces some of the characteristic neuropsychiatric symptoms that occur among patients who have undergone cardiopulmonary bypass (82,83). In model systems, Oxyfluor protected animals from central nervous system damage when air was introduced into the carotid artery (84). However, further development of this product has been halted.

POTENTIAL IMPACT OF RED BLOOD CELL SUBSTITUTES

The extent to which any RBC substitute will affect blood banking and transfusion medicine will depend on a number of factors, which are listed in Table 13.9. Because of their unique characteristics, many of these RBC substitutes may find roles not currently fulfilled by donated RBCs. Table 13.10 lists possible uses for these oxygen-carrying materials. Products licensed for uses other than RBC transfusion equivalents or extenders in ANH will have little effect on blood banking. Plasma half-life, a key consideration for products licensed as RBC substitutes, will determine the range of possible applications. The half-life of the products in development is suitable for trauma management or surgery. Modest increases in plasma half-life to even a few days would be adequate for most in-hospital applications for the care of patients with reasonable erythropoiesis.

TABLE 13.9. FACTORS INFLUENCING USE OF BLOOD SUBSTITUTES

Indication
Half-life
Safety
Abundance
Cost
Competing technology
Safety and availability of donor red blood cells

TABLE 13.10. APPLICATIONS FOR RED BLOOD CELL SUBSTITUTES

Acute blood loss—trauma, surgery
Acute blood loss—Jehovah's Witnesses, multiple red blood cell alloantibodies, rare blood type, endemic infection in donor blood supply
Extender in acute normovolemic hemodilution
Septic shock
Antiischemic-sickle cell crisis, PTCA, MI, cardiopulmonary bypass, vasoocclusive stroke
Ex vivo organ, tissue preservation
Neuroprotectant—cardiopulmonary bypass
Sensitizer for chemotherapy and radiation therapy
Imaging
Partial liquid ventilation—ARDS, near drowning, smoke inhalation, infection
Erythropoiesis

PTCA, percutaneous transluminal coronary angioplasty; MI, myocardial infarction; ARDS, adult respiratory distress syndrome.

As the safety of the conventional blood supply increases (48), tolerance of adverse effects of RBC substitutes will diminish. However, patient perceptions that the conventional blood supply carries high risk of infection or their fears of unknown but catastrophic complications of allogeneic blood transfusion may fuel demand for the substitutes just as they support continued interest in expensive autologous transfusion practices (85). Another significant driver for the use of RBC substitutes may be the adequacy of the conventional blood supply. If the margin between blood donations and transfusions continues to decrease (49), RBC substitutes may be needed to fill the gap, particularly at times of the year when shortages are common. Paradoxically, the availability of substitutes based on discarded donor RBCs may be limited by dwindling donations unless an alternative source can be found. Abundance of the source material for the substitute may therefore also affect the degree to which it supplants conventional donor RBCs. Cost of the substitute will also play a role in its acceptance and may determine whether the product would be used routinely or in a more restricted manner, perhaps limiting its use to specific patient populations or periods of blood shortages. Finally, new alternatives to the substitutes studied to date may prove superior. Several of these potentially competing technologies are listed in Table 13.11.

Once one of these preparations is licensed for use as a substitute, hospitals will have to make a series of decisions about how to handle it. The first decision will be whether to add the substitute to the formulary at all. If the hospital decides to stock a

TABLE 13.11. ALTERNATIVES TO TRANSFUSION OF DONOR RED BLOOD CELLS IN DEVELOPMENT

In vitro red blood cell culture
Persistent oxygen bubbles (86)
Protein (hemoglobin) "bubbles" (87)
Intravenous allosteric modifiers
Hemoglobin from transgenic swine (88)

product, a decision will have to be made about what, if any, restrictions should be put on distribution and who should monitor its use. These decisions may be made by the transfusion committee, the pharmacy and formulary committee, or a committee with oversight for new technology. Another consideration will be which department in the hospital will have the responsibility for stocking, issuing, and tracking these products. Given the permissive storage conditions, universal compatibility, and lack of a need for preparation, these products may be handled by the transfusion service or the pharmacy just as plasma derivatives are in many hospitals. If substitutes supplant a large proportion of donor RBC transfusions, there may be a shift of labor from the transfusion service to the pharmacy.

Depending on the breadth of applications and the abundance of RBC substitutes, donor centers may see a diminished need for whole blood collections and put more emphasis on collection of plasma and platelets by means of apheresis. However, the need for donor RBCs as source material for the preparation of HBOCs based on human hemoglobin may open up a new opportunity to donor centers in the collection of source hemoglobin. It is conceivable that an entirely new classification of donor with somewhat less restrictive qualification criteria might be established to fulfill the manufacturing needs for HBOCs.

SUMMARY

In the 100 years since Landsteiner's discovery of the ABO blood group system made transfusion clinically feasible, we have come to the verge of having a synthetic oxygen-carrying product available to take the place of donated RBCs, at least in some circumstances. Although the various preparations studied have in common the ability to transport oxygen, they are quite distinct from one another and certainly very different from RBCs. If these products are to be used to best advantage, transfusion medicine specialists will need to be familiar with the capabilities and liabilities of the substitutes that find their way into the clinical arena. The development of these RBC substitutes has shed considerable light on the mechanisms of oxygen delivery and regulation and forced us to reconsider some long-held assumptions. To adequately fulfill the role of consultant, the transfusion medicine specialist will need an even greater understanding of the physiologic mechanisms of RBC transfusion and oxygen delivery.

REFERENCES

1. Winslow RM, Vandegriff KD, Intaglietta M, eds. *Blood substitutes: physiological basis of efficacy.* Boston: Birkhäuser, 1995.
2. Winslow RM, Vandegriff KD, Intaglietta M, eds. *Blood substitutes: new challenges.* Boston: Birkhäuser, 1996.
3. Winslow RM, Vandegriff KD, Intaglietta M, eds. *Advances in blood substitutes: industrial opportunities and medical challenges.* Boston: Birkhäuser, 1997.
4. Chang TMS. *Blood substitutes: principles, methods, products and clinical trials.* Vol 1. Basel: Karger Landes, 1997.
5. Rudolph AS, Rabinovici R, Feuerstein GZ, eds. *Red blood cell substitutes. basic principles and clinical applications.* New York; Marcel Dekker, 1998.
6. Winslow RM. New transfusion strategies: red cell substitutes. *Annu Rev Med* 1999;50:337–353.
7. Stowell CP, Levin J, Spiess BD, et al. Progress in the development of RBC substitutes. *Transfusion* 2001;41:287–299.
8. Winslow RM, Gonzales A, Gonzales M, et al. Vascular resistance and the efficacy of red cell substitutes in a rat hemorrhage model. *J Appl Physiol* 1998;85:993–1003.
9. Intaglietta M, Johnson PC, Winslow RM. Microvascular and tissue oxygen distribution. *Cardiovasc Res* 1996;32:632–643.
10. Karmaker N, Dhar P. Effect of steady shear stress on fluid filtration through the rabbit arterial wall in the presence of macromolecules. *Clin Exp Pharmacol Physiol* 1996;23:299–304.
11. Garcia-Sepulcre ME, Carnicer F, Mauri M, et al. Increased plasma endothelin in liver cirrhosis and response to plasma volume expansion (letter). *Am J Gastroenterol* 1996;91:2452–2453.
12. Lieberthal W. Renal effects of hemoglobin-based blood substitutes. In: Rudolph AS, Rabinivici R, Feuerstein GZ, eds. *Red blood cell substitutes: basic principles and clinical applications.* New York: Marcel Dekker, 1998:189–217.
13. Chatterjee R, Welty EV, Walder TY, et al. Isolation and characterization of a new hemoglobin derivative cross-linked between the α chains (lysine 99α1-99α2). *J Biol Chem* 1986;26:9929–9937.
14. Przybelski R, Kisicki J, Dailey E, et al. Diaspirin cross-linked hemoglobin (DCLHb): phase I clinical safety assessment in normal healthy volunteers. *Crit Care Med* 1994;22:A231(abst).
15. Swan SK, Halstenson CE, Collins AJ, et al. Pharmacologic profile of diaspirin cross-linked hemoglobin in hemodialysis patients. *Am J Kidney Dis* 1995;26:918–923.
16. Looker D, Abbott-Brown D, Cozart P, et al. A human recombinant hemoglobin designed for use as a blood substitute. *Nature* 1992;356: 258–260.
17. Sehgal SA, Gould LR, Rowen AL, et al. Polymerized pyridoxylated hemoglobin: a red cell substitute with normal O_2 capacity. *Surgery* 1984;95:433–438.
18. Hughes GS, Antal EJ, Locker PK, et al. Physiology and pharmacokinetics of a novel hemoglobin-based oxygen carrier in humans. *Crit Care Med* 1996;24:756–764.
19. Adamson JG, Bonaventura BJ, Song SE, et al. Production, characterization, and clinical evaluation of Hemolink, an oxidized raffinose cross-linked hemoglobin–based blood substitute. In: Rudolph AS, Rabinovici R, Feuerstein GZ, eds. *Red blood cell substitutes.* New York: Marcel Dekker, 1998:335–351.
20. Vandegriff KD, McCarthy M, Rohlfs RH, et al. Colloid osmotic properties of modified hemoglobins: chemically cross-linked versus polyethylene glycol surface-conjugated. *Biophys Chem* 1999;69:23–30.
21. Chang TMS, Lister C, Nishiya T, et al. Immunological effects of hemoglobin, encapsulated hemoglobin, polyhemoglobin and conjugated hemoglobin using different immunization schedules. *Biomater Artif Cells Blood Substit Immobil Biotechnol* 1992;20:611–618.
22. Conover CD, Malatesta P, Lejeune L, et al. The effects of hemodilution with polyethylene glycol bovine hemoglobin (PEG-Hb) in a conscious porcine model. *J Invest Med* 1996;44:238–246.
23. Nho K, Linberg R, Johnson M, et al. PEG-hemoglobin: an efficient oxygen delivery system in the rat exchange transfusion and hypovolemic shock models. *Biomater Artif Cells Blood Substit Immobil Biotechnol* 1994;22:795–803.
24. Iwashita Y, Yabuki A, Yamaji K, et al. A new resuscitation fluid stabilized hemoglobin preparation and characteristics. *Biomater Artif Cells Artif Organs* 1988;16:271–280.
25. Hess JR, Macdonald VW, Brinkley WW. Systemic and pulmonary

hypertension after resuscitation with cell-free hemoglobin. *J Appl Physiol* 1993;74:1769–1778.
26. Keipert PE, Gonzales A, Gomez CL, et al. Acute changes in systemic blood pressure and urine output of conscious rats following exchange transfusion with diaspirin-crosslinked hemoglobin solution. *Transfusion* 1993;33:701–708.
27. Przybelski RJ, Dailey EK, Birnbaum ML. The pressor effect of hemoglobin: good or bad? In: Winslow RM, Vandegriff KD, Intaglietta M, eds. *Advances in blood substitutes: industrial opportunities and medical challenges.* Boston: Birkhäuser, 1997:71–85.
28. Rioux F, Drapeau G, Marceau F. Recombinant human hemoglobin (rHb1. 1) selectively inhibits vasorelaxation elicited by nitric oxide donors in rabbit isolated aortic rings. *J Cardiovasc Pharmacol* 1995;25: 587–594.
29. Pawloski JR, Hess DT, Stamler JS. Export by red blood cells of nitric acid bioactivity. *Nature* 2001;409:622–626.
30. Schultz SC, Grady B, Cole F, et al. A role for endothelin and nitric oxide in the pressor response to diaspirin cross-linked hemoglobin. *J Lab Clin Med* 1993;122:301–308.
31. Gulati A, Singh S, Rebello S, et al. Effect of diaspirin cross-linked and stroma-reduced hemoglobin on mean arterial pressure and endothelin-1 concentration in rats. *Life Sci* 1995;56:1433–1442.
32. Gulati A, Sharma AC, Burhop KE. Effect of stroma-free hemoglobin and diaspirin cross-linked hemoglobin on the regional circulation and systemic hemodynamics. *Life Sci* 1994;55:827–837.
33. Ulatowski JA, Nishikawa T, Matheson-Urbaitis B, et al. Regional blood flow alterations after bovine fumaryl ββ-crosslinked hemoglobin transfusion and nitric oxide synthase inhibition. *Crit Care Med* 1996;24: 558–565.
34. Reah G, Bodenham AR, Mallick A, et al. Initial evaluation of diaspirin cross-linked hemoglobin (DCLHb) as a vasopressor in critically ill patients. *Crit Care Med* 1997;25:1480–1488.
35. Yabuki A, Matsushita S, Malchesky PS, et al. In vitro evaluation of a pyridoxalated hemoglobin polyoxyethylene conjugate in reversing cell sickling. *ASAIO Trans* 1998;34:773–777.
36. Marik PE, Sibbald WJ. Effect of stored-blood transfusion on oxygen delivery in patients with sepsis. *JAMA* 1993;269:3024–3029.
37. Vandegriff KD, Medina F, Marini MA, et al. Equilibrium oxygen binding to human hemoglobin cross-linked between the α chains by bis(3,5-dibromosalicyl) fumarate. *J Biol Chem* 1989;64:17824–17833.
38. Rohlfs RJ, Bruner E, Chiu A, et al. Arterial blood pressure responses to cell-free hemoglobin solutions and the reaction with nitric oxide. *J Biol Chem* 1998;273:12128–12134.
39. Sehgal LR, Rosen AL, Noud G, et al. Large volume preparation of pyridoxylated hemoglobin with high P_{50}. *J Surg Res* 1981;30:14–20.
40. Winslow RM, Vandegriff KD. Hemoglobin oxygen affinity and the design of red cell substitutes. In: Winslow RM, Vandegriff KD, Intaglietta M, eds. *Advances in blood substitutes: industrial opportunities and medical challenges.* Boston: Birkhäuser, 1997:167–188.
41. Intaglietta M. Microcirculatory basis for the design of artificial blood. *Microcirculation* 1999;6:247–258.
42. Vandegriff KD. Stability and toxicity of hemoglobin solutions. In: Winslow RM, Vandegriff KD, Intaglietta M, eds. *Blood substitutes: physiological basis of efficacy.* Boston: Birkhäuser, 1995:105–131.
43. Light WR, Jacobs EE, Rentko VT, et al. Use of HBOC-201 as an oxygen therapeutic in the preclinical and clinical settings. In: Rudolph AS, Rabinovici R, Feuerstein GZ, eds. *Red blood cell substitutes.* New York: Marcel Dekker, 1998:421–436.
44. Patel MJ, Webb EJ, Shelbourn TE, et al. Absence of immunogenicity of diaspirin cross-linked hemoglobin in humans. *Blood* 1998;91: 710–716.
45. Griffiths E, Cortes A, Gilbert N, et al. Haemoglobin-based blood substitutes and sepsis. *Lancet* 1995;345:158–160.
46. Kaca W, Roth RI, Levin J. Hemoglobin, a newly recognized lipopolysaccharide (LPS)–binding protein that enhances LPS biological activity. *J Biol Chem* 1994;269:25078–25084.
47. Su D, Roth RI, Yoshida M, et al. Hemoglobin increases mortality from bacterial endotoxin. *Infect Immunol* 1997;65:1258–1266.
48. Goodnough LT, Brecher ME, Kanter MH, et al. Transfusion medicine, I: blood transfusion. *N Engl J Med* 1999;340:438–447.
49. Sullivan MT, Wallace EL, Umana WO. Trends in the collection and transfusion of blood in the United States, 1987–1997. *Transfusion* 2000;332:719–724.
50. Kobayaski K, Nakamura N, Sumi A, et al. The development of recombinant human serum albumin. *Ther Apheresis* 1998;2:257–262.
51. Murphy MF. New variant Creutzfeldt-Jakob disease (nvCJD): the risk of transmission by blood transfusion and the potential benefit of leukocyte-reduction of blood components. *Transfus Med Rev* 1999;13: 75–83.
52. Brown P, Rohwer PG, Dunstan BC, et al. The distribution of infectivity in blood components and plasma derivatives in experimental models of transmissible spongiform encephalopathies. *Transfusion* 1998;38: 810–816.
53. Houston F, Foster JD, Chong A, et al. Transmission of BSE by blood transfusion in sheep. *Lancet* 2000;356:999–1000.
54. Gould SA, Moore EE, Hoyt DB, et al. The first randomized trial of human polymerized hemoglobin as a blood substitute in acute trauma and emergent surgery. *J Am Coll Surg* 1998;187:113–120.
55. Gould SA, Moore EE, Moore FA, et al. Clinical utility of human polymerized hemoglobin as a blood substitute following acute trauma and urgent surgery. *J Trauma* 1997;43:325–332.
56. Moore EE, Gould SA, Hoyt DB, et al. Clinical utility of human polymerized hemoglobin as a blood substitute following trauma and emergent surgery. *Shock* 1997;7[Suppl 1]:145.
57. Burton TM. Baxter suspends trial of blood substitute. *Wall Street Journal* 1998;Jun3.
58. Saxena R, Wijnhoud AD, Carton H, et al. Controlled safety study of a hemoglobin-based oxygen carrier, DCLHb, in acute ischemic stroke. *Stroke* 1999;30:993–996.
59. Sloan EP, Koenigsberg M, Gens D, et al. Diaspirin cross-linked hemoglobin (DCHLb) in the treatment of severe traumatic hemorrhagic shock: a randomized controlled efficacy trial. *JAMA* 1999;282: 1857–1864.
60. Hughes GS, Francom SF, Antal EJ, et al. Effects of a novel hemoglobin-based oxygen carrier on percent oxygen saturation as determined with arterial blood gas analysis and pulse oximetry. *Ann Emerg Med* 1996; 27:164–169.
61. LaMuraglia GM, O'Hara PJ, Baker WH, et al. The reduction of allogeneic transfusion requirement in aortic surgery with hemoglobin-based solution. *J Vasc Surg* 2000;31:299–308.
62. Kasper SM, Walter M, Grune F, et al. Effects of a hemoglobin-based oxygen carrier (HBOC-201) on hemodynamics and oxygen transport in patients undergoing preoperative hemodilution for elective abdominal aortic surgery. *Anesth Analg* 1996;83:921–927.
63. Hughes GS, Yancey EP, Albrecht R, et al. Hemoglobin-based oxygen carrier preserves submaximal exercise capacity in humans. *Clin Pharmacol Ther* 1995;58:434–443.
64. Mullon J, Giacoppe G, Clagett C, et al. Transfusions of polymerized bovine hemoglobin in a patient with severe autoimmune hemolytic anemia. *N Engl J Med* 2000;342:1638–1643.
65. Robinson MF, Dupuis NP, Kusumoto T, et al. Increased tumor oxygenation and radiation sensitivity in two rat tumors by a hemoglobin-based, oxygen-carrying preparation. *Artif Cells Blood Substit Immobil Biotechnol* 1995;23:431–438.
66. Murray JA, Ledlow A, Launspach J, et al. The effects of recombinant human hemoglobin on esophageal motor functions in humans. *Gastroenterology* 1995;109:1241–1248.
67. Gould SA, Rosen A, Sehgal L et al. Fluosol-DA as a red cell substitute in acute anemia. *N Engl J Med* 1986;314:1653–1656.
68. Kerins DM. Role of perfluorocarbon Fluosol-DA in coronary angioplasty. *Am J Med Sci* 1994;307:218–221.
69. Williams G, Kent S. Specific identification of hemoglobin and myoglobin in renal tubular casts by the fluorescent antibody technic on fixed embedded tissues. *Am J Clin Pathol* 1981;75:726–730.
70. Flaim SF. Perflubron-based emulsion: efficacy as temporary oxygen carrier. In: Winslow R, Vandegriff K, Intaglietta M, eds. *Advances in blood substitutes: industrial opportunities and medical challenges.* Boston: Birkhäuser, 1997:91–132.
71. Winslow RM, Swenberg ML, Berger RL, et al. Oxygen equilibrium

curve of normal human blood and its evaluation by Adair's equation. *J Biol Chem* 1977;252:2331–2337.
72. Kaufman RJ. Clinical development of perfluorocarbon-based emulsions as red cell substitutes. In: Winslow RM, Vandegriff KD, Intaglietta M, eds. *Blood substitutes: physiological basis of efficacy.* Boston: Birkhäuser, 1995:53–75.
73. Keipert PE, Otto S, Flaim SF, et al. Influence of perflubron emulsion particle size on blood half-life and febrile response in rats. *Artif Cells Blood Substit Immobil Biotechnol* 1994;22:1169–1174.
74. Rockwell S, Kelley M, Irvin CG, et al. Preclinical evaluation of Oxygent (TM) as an adjunct to radiotherapy. *Biomater Artif Cells Immobil Biotechnol* 1992;20:883–893.
75. Wahr JA, Trouwborst A, Spence RK, et al. A pilot study of the effects of perflubron emulsion, AF0104, on mixed venous oxygen tension in anesthetized surgical patients. *Anesth Analg* 1996;82:103–107.
76. Stern SA, Dronen SC, McGoron AJ. Effect of supplemental perfluorocarbon administration on hypotensive resuscitation of severe uncontrolled hemorrhage. *Am J Emerg Med* 1995;13:269–275.
77. Rubin DL, Muller HH, Nino-Murcia M, et al. Intraluminal contrast enhancement and MR visualization of the bowel wall: efficacy of PFOB. *Radiology* 1991;22:371–380.
78. Andre M, Nelson T, Mattrey R. Physical and acoustical properties of perfluorooctyl-bromide, an ultrasound contrast agent. *Invest Radiol* 1990;25:983–987.
79. Leach CL, Greenspan JS, Rubenstein DS, et al. Partial liquid ventilation with perflubron in premature infants with severe respiratory distress syndrome. *N Engl J Med* 1996;335:761–767.
80. Blauth CI, Arnold JV, Schulenberg WE, et al. Cerebral microembolism during cardiopulmonary bypass: retinal microvascular studies in vivo with fluorescein angiography. *J Thorac Cardiovasc Surg* 1988;95:668–676.
81. Blauth CI, Smith P, Newman S, et al. Retinal microembolism and neuropsychological deficit following clinical cardiopulmonary bypass: comparison of a membrane and a bubble oxygenator—a preliminary communication. *Eur J Cardiothorac Surg* 1989;3:135–138.
82. Shaw PJ, Bates D, Cartlidge EF, et al. Neurologic and neuropsychological morbidity following major surgery: comparison of coronary artery bypass and peripheral vascular surgery. *Stroke* 1987;18:700–707.
83. Roach GW, Kanchugar M, Mangano CM, et al. Adverse cerebral outcomes after coronary artery bypass surgery. *N Engl J Med* 1996;335:1857–1863.
84. Cochran RP, Kunzelman KS, Vocelka CR, et al. Perfluorocarbon emulsion in the cardiopulmonary bypass prime reduces neurologic injury. *Ann Thorac Surg* 1997;63:1326–1332.
85. Lee SJ, Liljas B, Churchill WH, et al. Perceptions and preferences of autologous blood donors. *Transfusion* 1998;38:757–763.
86. Burkard ME, Van Liew HD. Oxygen transport to tissue by persistent bubbles: theory and simulations. *J Appl Physiol* 1994;77:2874–2878.
87. Sakai H, Hamada K, Takeoka S, et al. Physical properties of hemoglobin vesicles as red cell substitutes. *Biotechnol Prog* 1996;12:119–125.
88. O'Donnell JK, Martin MJ, Logan JS, et al. Production of human hemoglobin in transgenic swine: an approach to a blood substitute. *Cancer Detect Prev* 1993;17:307–312.

Rossi's Principles of Transfusion Medicine, Third Edition, edited by Toby L. Simon, Walter H. Dzik, Edward L. Snyder, Christopher P. Stowell, and Ronald G. Strauss. Lippincott Williams & Wilkins, Philadelphia © 2002.

PART II
Platelets

14

MEGAKARYOCYTOPOIESIS, KINETICS, AND PLATELET RADIOLABELING

AARON TOMER

Human blood platelets circulate at a concentration of 250 × 10^9/L (range, 150 to 400 × 10^9/L) with a lifespan of 9 to 10 days. Megakaryocytes give rise to circulating platelets through a process of progenitor cell proliferation, endoreduplication, differentiation, and release of cytoplasmic fragments as circulating platelets. To maintain the platelet count within that narrow range, the production of platelets is regulated by alterations in megakaryocytopoiesis to compensate for changes in platelet demand. Megakaryocytopoiesis is primarily controlled by thrombopoietin, which induces the expansion of early progenitors as well as the proliferation, endoreduplication, and differentiation of megakaryocytes. Thrombopoietin avidly binds to the c-Mpl receptors on platelets and megakaryocytes. Accordingly, circulating levels of unbound thrombopoietin induce concentration-dependent proliferation and maturation of megakaryocyte progenitors. Circulating platelets compete for the binding of thrombopoietin and produce negative feedback regulation of megakaryocytopoiesis by diminishing the concentrations of unbound thrombopoietin available for stimulation of megakaryocytes. On the other hand, a decrease in platelet turnover rate results in an increase in the concentration of unbound thrombopoietin followed by augmentation of the stimulus for megakaryocytopoiesis. Thrombocytopenia may result from impaired production, increased destruction, or altered sequestration into liver and spleen. Peripheral platelet levels of 5,000 to 10,000/μl may avert spontaneous bleeding. However, in the presence of conditions that increase bleeding tendency, such as sepsis, acute leukemia, or altered hemostasis, a higher concentration, up to 100,000 platelets/μl, may be required to maintain normal hemostasis. Thrombocytopenia secondary to impaired production or blood loss may be restored by means of allogeneic platelet transfusion, which usually results in successful restoration of hemostasis. Thrombopoietin therapy may be useful in the future in supporting platelet production in chronic thrombocytopenic states. In this chapter, the quantitative alterations in marrow megakaryocytopoiesis and platelet kinetics in health and disease are reviewed.

A. Tomer: Faculty of Health Sciences, Ben Gurion University of the Negev, Blood Bank and Transfusion Medicine, Soroka Medical Center, Beer-Sheva, Israel.

DEVELOPMENT AND MATURATION OF MEGAKARYOCYTES

Normal Megakaryocytopoiesis

Megakaryocytes give rise to circulating platelets (thrombocytes) through a process of proliferation, endoreduplication, differen-

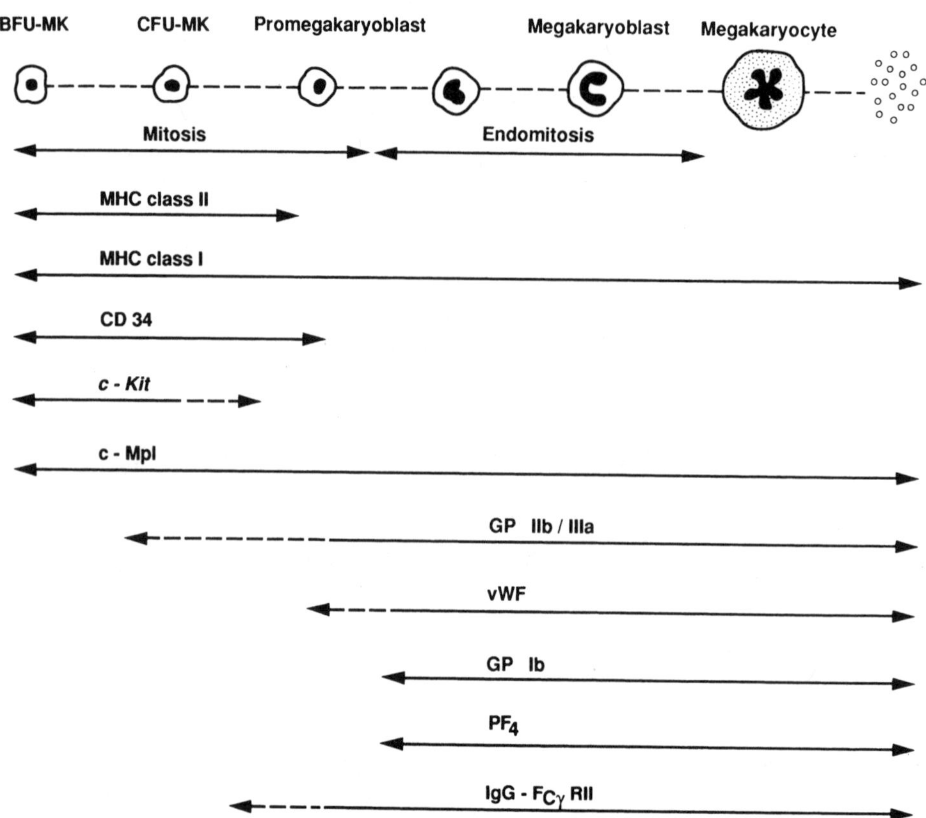

FIGURE 14.1. Differentiation markers of the megakaryocytic lineage. *BFU-MK,* megakaryocytic burst-forming units; *CFU-MK,* megakaryocytic colony-forming units; *MHC,* histocompatibility complex; *CD,* cluster designation; *c-Kit,*cellular *Kit* gene encodes for the receptor to stem cell factor; *c-Mpl,* cellular *mpl* gene encodes for the receptor to thrombopoietin.

tiation, and release of cytoplasmic fragments as circulating platelets. This process involves the commitment, proliferation, and differentiation of hematopoietic progenitor cells in the megakaryocytic lineage as well as acquisition of the cytoplasmic functional and structural characteristics necessary for platelet action (1–5).

The cellular anatomic features and differentiation of the platelet-megakaryocyte system are shown in Figure 14.1. According to this schema, megakaryocytes arise from multipotent stem cells capable of differentiating into erythrocytic, granulocytic, monocytic, and megakaryocytic series. The pluripotent stem cell becomes progressively restricted to a unilineage megakaryocytic stem cell. This cell develops into diploid megakaryocytes (megakaryoblasts) that at some point lose their capability for cell division but retain their capability for DNA replication (endoreduplication). The cytoplasm increases in mass and forms the organelles and biochemical apparatus characteristic of functional platelets. Mature megakaryocytes are large, granular, and polyploid cells. Their size may reach 48 μm, and their ploidy ranges from 8 to 128N with modal ploidy of 16N (6–11).

Cells giving rise to megakaryocytes, erythrocytes, and granulocytes were originally designated as spleen colony-forming units (CFU-S) (12). In the original experiments, mice receiving lethal marrow irradiation and subsequent injection of normal bone marrow cells had macroscopic colonies on the splenic surface after 7 to 10 days. These colonies were composed of hematopoietic cells of megakaryocytic, granulocytic, macrophagic, and erythroid lineage. Studies with genetic markers showed that each cell of an individual spleen colony arose from a single cell capable of both self-renewal and differentiation (13,14).

Evidence in humans for the existence of multipotent stem cells has been provided through studies of pathologic states. Philadelphia chromosomal translocation in chronic myelogenous leukemia has been found in megakaryocytes, red blood cells, and granulocytes, suggesting the occurrence of a mutation in a stem cell common for these lineages (15). In addition, studies of patients heterozygous at the locus for glucose-6-phosphate dehydrogenase (G-6-PD) have shown that the skin fibroblasts of patients with chronic myeloproliferative disorders have equal proportions of G-6-PD isoenzymes A and B, whereas the platelets, red blood cells, and granulocytes contain either one or the other isoenzyme type but not both (16–19). The existence of a pluripotent stem cell giving rise to the megakaryocytic lineage has been confirmed in healthy persons by means of bone marrow transplantation and in vitro studies, including cultures of single human bone marrow stem cells (20,21).

Regulation of Megakaryocytopoiesis

Megakaryocytes respond to changes in requirements for peripheral blood platelets. In experiments, mechanisms that regulate megakaryocytopoiesis operate at the levels of proliferation, differentiation, and platelet release (22–30). The hematopoietic growth factor specific for the growth and development of megakaryocyte lineage is variously referred to as *thrombopoietin* (analogous to erythropoietin for the erythroid lineage), *megakaryocyte growth and development factor* (MGDF), or c-Mpl ligand (31–35). After 30 years of searching for the factor regulating megakaryocytopoietic activities, four different groups in 1994 reported simultaneously its isolation, cloning, molecular, and physiologic characterization (31–35). The complementary DNA for human and murine thrombopoietin belongs to the cytokine family of genes encoding for a glycoprotein homologous with erythropoietin that binds with its receptor (c-Mpl) on megakaryocytes and selectively initiates proliferation, maturation, and cytoplasmic delivery of platelets into the circulation. This remarkable coincidence of discovery stems from the report in 1990 by Souyri et al. (36) of a cellular gene (c-*Mpl*) homologous with genes encoding for a family of hematopoietic growth factor receptors. Moreover, the addition of c-Mpl antisense oligodeoxynucleotides in excess selectively abolishes megakaryocyte colony formation (37). Subsequent cloning of the c-Mpl receptor from engineered blood cell lines provided the essential tool for isolating and cloning thrombopoietin, the c-Mpl ligand. The ligand was purified from thrombocytopenic plasma, sequenced, cloned, and characterized (31–35). One group successfully isolated and characterized thrombopoietin from a transfected cell clone that produced the growth factor (32,33). The identical molecule has been isolated and cloned by all four groups of investigators. Thrombopoietin is now produced as a recombinant protein for both investigation of physiologic regulation in experimental animals and clinical trials. Both the megakaryocyte colony-stimulating activity and platelet-elevating activity in thrombocytopenic plasma are neutralized by the addition of c-Mpl receptor in excess (34).

Thrombopoietin is a heavily glycosylated protein composed of 332 amino acids that share homology in the amino terminal region (21% sequence identity) with erythropoietin. The gene for thrombopoietin is located in chromosome 3 (bands 26 to 28). Interestingly, abnormalities in chromosome 3 (inversion or deletion) are found in megakaryocytic leukemia and other myeloproliferative disorders associated with thrombocytosis (38, 39). Thrombopoietin-specific messenger RNA is found in the liver, kidney, and marrow stroma (31,32,35). Megakaryocytopoiesis is regulated by plasma levels of unbound thrombopoietin. The plasma levels of thrombopoietin in normal state (95 $\pm$ 6 pg/L) increase several orders of magnitude in patients with thrombocytopenia secondary to marrow suppression and decrease after platelet transfusions or recovery of hematopoiesis (35,40).

Thrombopoietin avidly binds to the c-Mpl receptors on platelets ($\sim$200 receptors per platelet). Because plasma thrombopoietin level is not primarily dependent on gene transcriptional regulation (41), it is conceivable that negative feedback regulation is produced by the circulating concentration of platelets through binding of thrombopoietin and shedding of soluble c-Mpl-receptor in plasma. Thus circulating levels of unbound thrombopoietin induce concentration-dependent receptor-mediated proliferation and differentiation of early megakaryocyte progenitors, thereby modulating platelet production rate.

Several pleiotropic hematopoietic growth factors have been shown to exert stimulatory activity on megakaryocytes both in vivo and in vitro, including interleukin-3 (IL-3) (multi-CSF), IL-6, IL-11, granulocyte-macrophage colony-stimulating factor (GM-CSF), and leukemia inhibitory factor (9,43–49). A schematic of the regulation of megakaryocytopoiesis appears in Figure 14.2. Interleukin-1 may stimulate megakaryocytes indirectly (43,50), and erythropoietin has exhibited colony-stimulating activity in animal studies (51,52). The stem cell factor (also called

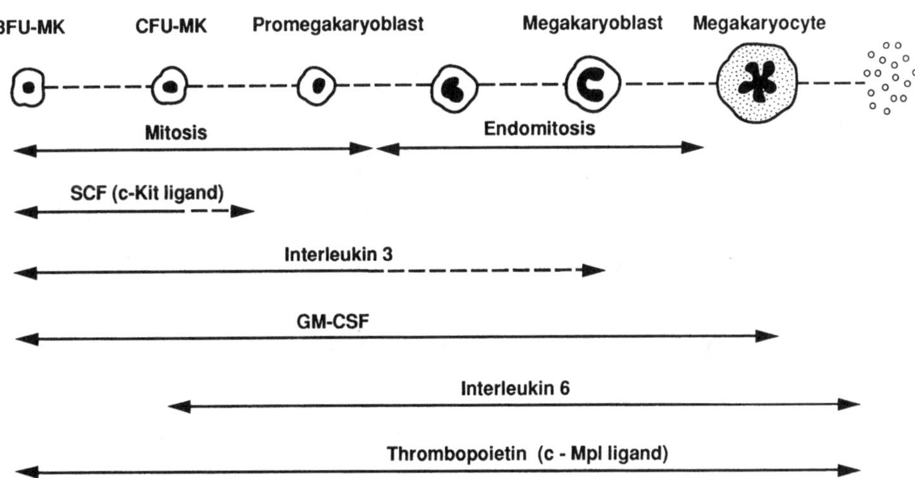

FIGURE 14.2. Schematic outline of the regulation of megakaryocytopoiesis. *BFU-MK,* megakaryocytic burst-forming units; *CFU-MK,* megakaryocytic colony-forming units; *SCF,* stem cell factor; *GM-CSF,* granulocyte macrophage colony-stimulating factor.

mast cell growth factor, steel factor, and *c*-kit *ligand*) has been shown to promote megakaryocytic burst-forming units with IL-3 and megakaryocytic colony-forming units in synergy with both IL-3 and GM-CSF (53). Granulocyte-macrophage colony-stimulating factor may induce megakaryocytic maturation in vivo, as shown in humans (48) and nonhuman primates (49), although there is no corresponding increase in circulating platelet count (54). The direct stimulatory effect of GM-CSF on megakaryocytes is evident in cultures of megakaryocytes purified directly from bone marrow aspirates from humans (10). Interleukin-6 primarily affects megakaryocyte maturation (42,50), although the combination of IL-6 and IL-3 promotes megakaryocyte proliferation (43). The administration of IL-6 to primates markedly increases platelet count and the size and ploidy of megakaryocytes (45). Interleukin-11 and leukemia inhibitory factor also affect both the size and the ploidy of megakaryocytes (44,46). In addition, combined effects have been found for IL-6 and IL-3 (43), IL-3 and GM-CSF (43,47,50), and IL-3 and IL-11 (46). Thus different stages of megakaryocytes can be modulated by dose and by additive or synergistic effects among growth factors. There is also evidence of negative control of megakaryocytopoiesis. One of the relatively well-characterized inhibitory factors is transforming growth factor β derived from platelets (55). In addition, megakaryocytes appear to be capable of synthesizing and secreting hematopoietic growth factors, including IL-1, IL-6, and GM-CSF (42,56).

In vivo administration of recombinant human GM-CSF (rHuGM-CSF) to rhesus monkeys resulted in a prompt increase in megakaryocyte ploidy and average volume (Fig. 14.3B) (54). Treatment with IL-6 resulted in a similar response (45). However, unlike administration of IL-6, administration of rHuGM-CSF was not associated with a notable increase in platelet count (54). In baboons, administration of recombinant human thrombopoietin or polyethylene glycol (PEG) derivative, referred to as *PEG–recombinant human megakaryocyte growth and development factor* (PEG-rHuMDGF), produced a log-linear increase in marrow megakaryocyte mass (cell number multiplied by volume) up to 6.5 fold associated with a marked increase in cell ploidy (Fig. 14.3C). There was a concordant increase in platelet count up to fivefold; peak value was reached after 2 to 4 weeks of subcutaneous injections (Fig. 14.4). Because megakaryocyte volume and ploidy attained predictable maximum values simultaneously, megakaryocyte ploidy is an accurate measure of the Mpl-ligand stimulation of megakaryocytopoiesis (57–60).

Compared with other megakaryocyte-stimulating growth factors, thrombopoietin increases platelet production to previously unattainable levels. The two recombinant Mpl ligands, recombinant human thrombopoietin and PEG-rHuMDGF, are the most potent growth factors for inducing megakaryocytopoiesis (31–34,57–60). It was assumed that the lineage-specific recombinant thrombopoietin had negligible toxicity, similar to that for the other two late-acting hematopoietic growth factors, erythropoietin and granulocyte colony-stimulating factor. Thrombopoietin was expected to have had many uses in the care of patients with platelet transfusion–dependent thrombocytopenia or other thrombocytopenic disorders responsive to exogenously stimulated platelet production (61–64). However, the development of cross-reacting neutralizing antibody to endogenous thrombopoietin in healthy volunteers, as well as in patients, after several subcutaneous injections of PEG-rHu-MGDF led to withdrawal of the drug from study and termination of clinical trials.

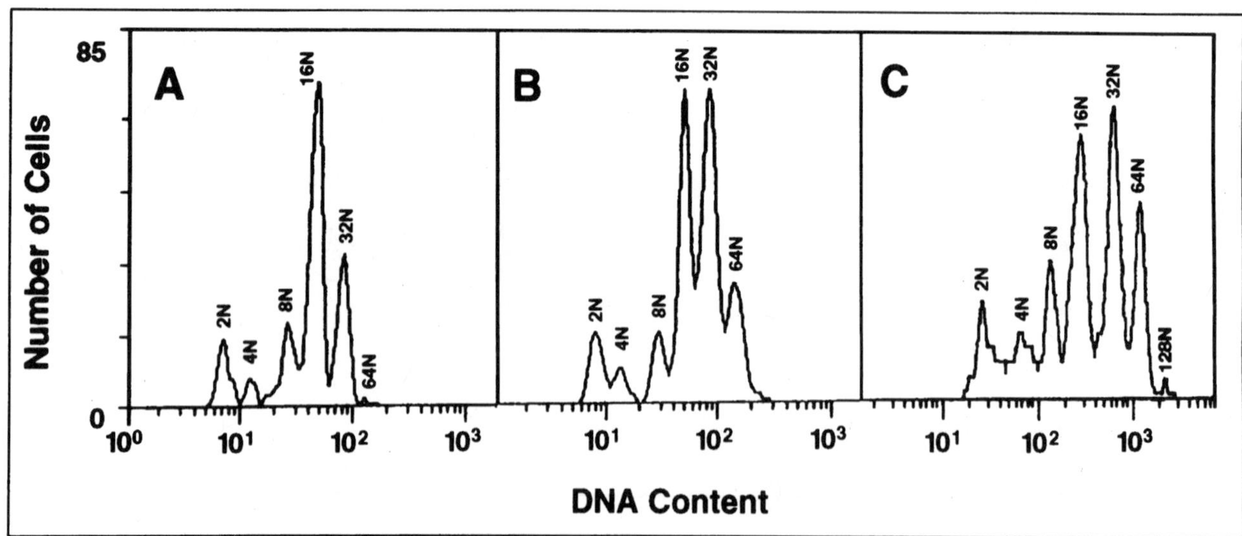

FIGURE 14.3. Effect of in vivo administration of megakaryocyte-stimulating factors on megakaryocyte ploidy in nonhuman primates. **A:** Rhesus monkeys or baboons before treatment. **B:** After treatment with recombinant human granulocyte-macrophage colony-stimulating factor for 8 days, rhesus monkey have a markedly right shift. A similar response was observed with interleukin 6. **C:** Baboon after treatment with recombinant human megakaryocyte growth and development factor for 7 days. The right shift is more prominent than that in **B.** Megakaryocyte ploidy correlates with cell size.

greater than those of controls. In contrast, serum IL-6 levels of patients with primary thrombocytosis were not significantly different from those of healthy controls (115).

The results obtained in studies with human subjects suggest that in humans, megakaryocytes respond to altered platelet demand in a manner similar to that in experimental animals. These changes are primarily mediated by thrombopoietin, which may have considerable application in thrombocytopenic states secondary to impaired platelet production.

PLATELET KINETICS

Platelet Production and Destruction

Platelet Production

The overall rate of platelet production in healthy humans ranges from 35,000 to 44,000 platelets/µl per day (76,116–119). These estimates of platelet production have been measured indirectly by means of determining the turnover of circulating platelets (platelet count divided by the platelet survival time and corrected for recovery) under steady-state conditions. This estimation assumes that platelet removal is equivalent to platelet production when the platelet count is constant. Thus platelet turnover has been used as a measure of the delivery of viable platelets into the general circulation. As expected, megakaryocytic mass generally correlates directly with platelet turnover in healthy persons. However, intramedullary destruction of platelets can occur or abnormalities of megakaryocytopoiesis can result in impaired delivery of the cytoplasmic mass to circulating viable platelets. This discrepancy detected between megakaryocytic mass and platelet turnover is called *ineffective thrombocytopoiesis.*

The reliability of platelet turnover estimates depends on the accuracy with which each of the three variables used in calculating platelet turnover can be determined—mean platelet life span, recovery of platelets in the circulation, and blood platelet count. This summation error may be considerable, as occurs among patients with ITP (117).

Distribution of Platelets

In humans, approximately two thirds of platelets are in the general circulation. The other platelets are reversibly sequestered, primarily in the spleen. The distribution between the general and the splenic pool of platelets can be determined by means of measuring the proportion of radiolabeled platelets remaining in the general circulation after infusion. The size of the splenic pool has been estimated to be approximately 30% of whole-body platelet mass (76,116,119–121). In persons without a spleen, nearly 100% of infused platelets are recovered. In patients with splenomegaly, as much as 90% of total-body platelet mass can be sequestered in the spleen (121). Platelet accumulation in the spleen reached 90% of the maximum activity within approximately 12.5 minutes after reinjection of labeled platelets (116,120). Although the role of the spleen in the regulation of platelet count is controversial, the splenic pool appears to be reversible. For example, intravenous infusion of epinephrine, which reduces blood flow in the spleen and causes the organ to empty passively into the circulation, normally causes platelet level to increase 30% to 50% but does not affect platelet concentration in persons without a spleen (121). Hepatic pooling of labeled platelets is also significant initially, reaching a maximum of approximately 16% of the whole-body radioactivity 6 to 8 minutes after reinjection of labeled platelets. However, the activity reaches a steady state approximately 45 minutes after reinfusion of the platelets. At equilibrium, hepatic radioactivity is approximately 10% of total-body radioactivity (116,120).

Platelet Survival

The finite platelet life span in healthy persons is 9.5 ± 0.6 days (76). Platelet disappearance is generally linear over the first week, primarily reflecting platelet senescence (122). However, in patients with consumptive thrombocytopenia, the platelet life span is shorter and the disappearance pattern becomes exponential, primarily reflecting random platelet removal (123,124).

Platelet survival time has been shown to shorten progressively as the platelet count decreases to less than 100,000/µl (118, 125). Therefore, a shortened platelet survival time in patients with thrombocytopenia may not necessarily indicate a pathologic destructive process. Hanson and Slichter (118) proposed a model for platelet removal that predicted shortening of platelet survival time in relation to the level of thrombocytopenia. The analysis indicated that 82% of platelet turnover in healthy persons is caused by senescence, and approximately 18% is due to a fixed requirement of platelets removed randomly to support vascular integrity. Thus in severe thrombocytopenia, the proportion of the fixed daily requirement of platelets removed randomly increases relative to total platelet turnover (>60%) with consequent shortening of platelet life span (126).

At present, platelet survival studies are usually performed (a) to evaluate patients with thrombocytopenia to discriminate between disorders of decreased production and increased platelet destruction (destructive or consumptive thrombocytopenia), (b) to determine the rate and site of platelet consumption associated with thrombotic disease or to evaluate the efficacy of antiplatelet drugs that interfere with platelet-thrombogenic surface interaction, or (c) to assess platelet viability in platelet concentrates after storage.

Sites of Platelet Destruction

When platelets disappear from the circulation, they are taken up by the mononuclear phagocytic system (120,125,127,128). The accumulation of platelet radioactivity in the spleen and liver has been quantified, and it is evident that these organs are major sites of removal of the labeled platelets. After injection of ^{111}In-labeled platelets, radioactivity in the liver increased significantly and linearly with time from a level of 9.6% at equilibrium to 28.7% of total-body radioactivity (116,120). Mean splenic radioactivity also increased significantly from 31.1% to 35.6% during the clearance of labeled platelets. After labeled platelets are removed from circulation (approximately 10 days after administration), 30.3% of whole-body platelet radioactivity is neither in the liver nor in the spleen. Platelets not removed by these two organs are presumably removed by the mononuclear phagocytic cells of the bone marrow. In nonhuman primates, it has been found by means of quantification of organ radioactivity that approximately 15% of labeled platelets are destroyed in the bone marrow (129).

Methods for Measuring Platelet Survival Times

A number of methods have been used to measure platelet life span (130). The most commonly used procedure in humans is measurement of the disappearance time of platelets labeled isotopically in vitro. Theoretically, a labeled cohort of cells would provide the most accurate survival data. In human beings, [^{75}Se]selenomethionine has been proposed as a platelet cohort label (131,132). This γ-emitting analogue of the amino acid methionine is incorporated directly into a component of megakaryocytic proteins, including thrombosthenin (133). In studies with rats, this method has provided a reproducible but imperfect cohort survival curve (133). This complex method, however, has not been practical for studies with human subjects.

Because cohort survival studies generally are not feasible, labeling of a random platelet population (autologous or homologous) has been widely used for platelet survival measurements in humans. To be suitable for random platelet labeling in vitro, the ideal radiolabel should have the following characteristics: (a) be platelet specific, (b) be efficiently incorporated, (c) be retained intracellularly without considerable reutilization, (d) have a half-life long enough to allow measurement of the entire life span of the labeled cell but short enough to eliminate unnecessary irradiation, (e) not affect the viability or function of the labeled cell, and (f) emit γ irradiation with sufficient energy for external imaging. Unfortunately, not one of the commercially available radiolabels is platelet specific. Therefore, in vitro labeling must be performed on isolated platelet preparations. These manipulations involved in the separation of platelets from other blood cells and plasma proteins have potential adverse effects on the test platelets (collection injury) (116,134–136). Currently most platelet survival studies are performed with either ^{51}Cr-chloride or ^{111}In-oxine.

Radiolabels

Chromium 51

Chromium 51 was first introduced as a tracer for platelet labeling by Robertson et al. (137). The platelet uptake of ^{51}Cr is rapid; as much as 50% of the binding occurs in 30 minutes (138) at 37°C. The extent of ^{51}Cr elution from labeled platelets or reutilization of the isotope in vivo is controversial (117,139). Until recently, platelet labeling with ^{51}Cr has been the standard method for measurement of platelet survival (140). The radionuclide, however, suffers from several disadvantages, including a relatively long half-life (28 days), low incorporation rate into platelets (low labeling efficiency, 10% on the average), and γ-photon emission not well suited for external imaging. Therefore body localization by external detection is inefficient, and accurate data cannot be obtained unless large quantities of radioactivity are used (130). This requirement demands that a large volume of blood (200 to 500 ml) be obtained to provide sufficient numbers of platelets (139). For these reasons, ^{51}Cr now has largely been replaced by ^{111}In-oxine.

Indium-111-Oxine

Indium 111 oxine as a platelet label was introduced by Thakur et al. in 1976 (141,142) and is now firmly established as the preferred isotope (120,143,144). Indium 111 forms a stable lipophilic chelate with oxine (8-hydroxyquinoline), which is readily incorporated into platelets (and other cells) by means of passive processes (128). Indium 111 has a half-life of 2.8 days, which is long enough for platelet survival measurements and γ-photon emissions suitable for external detection. Labeling with ^{111}In-oxine has not been shown to affect platelet function (120, 130,141,143,144), and no significant portion of the ^{111}In taken up is subsequently lost from platelets (141,144). Indium 111 oxine is incorporated efficiently into platelets, and the labeling efficiency in normal preparations reaches the levels of 80% to 95% (116,117,140,145). Consequently, ^{111}In-oxine is commonly used for platelet kinetic studies, especially in thrombocytopenia (117,126,134). The major limitation of the labeling technique with ^{111}In-oxine is lack of specificity for platelets and high avidity for plasma proteins, particularly transferrin (128, 142). Therefore high labeling efficiency necessitates not only that platelets are isolated by differential centrifugation but also that plasma proteins be eliminated. This procedure results in a loss (that may be preferential) of as many as 40% of platelets (146) and manipulation of platelets in the absence of protein that can cause collection injury (144). Although the agents ^{111}In-mercaptopyridine-*N*-oxide (^{111}In-Merc) and ^{111}In-tropolone have been shown to allow relatively efficient cell labeling in plasma (147–149), there are insufficient data to recommend these agents over oxine (150).

In healthy subjects, mean platelet survival times estimated with ^{111}In and ^{51}Cr are similar (117,122). However, in thrombocytopenia, ^{111}In appears to be a superior label. The survival of ^{111}In-labeled autologous platelets is significantly longer than that of either homologous or autologous platelets labeled with ^{51}Cr (117,120,139,150–152). In addition, ^{111}In allows accurate estimation of the size of the splenic pool by means of quantitative imaging (117,120,151).

Procedures for Labeling Platelets

The recommended method for the use of ^{51}Cr as a platelet radiolabel was published by the International Committee for Standardization in Hematology (ISCH) in 1977 (140). A consensus regarding a standard method appeared only in 1986 when the Ad Hoc Committee of the Symposium on Radiolabeling of Stored Platelet Concentrates proposed the use of a standard procedure to facilitate comparison of results from different laboratories (150). This protocol was recommended for platelet survival studies performed on healthy persons with fresh platelets or for studies with stored platelet concentrates. The ISCH-recommended method for study of platelet survival with ^{111}In was published in 1988 (153). The recommended method for calculation of platelet life span is the γ-function model for nonlinear estimation (150,153).

Platelet Labeling in Thrombocytopenia

Whereas several different ^{111}In labeling methods appear to be adequate for patients with normal or moderately reduced platelet counts, direct application of these methods to patients with platelet counts less than 50,000 /μl is less suitable. The ISCH protocol recommends increasing the volume of blood required for the study of patients with platelet counts of 20,000/μl to 30,000/μl from 43 ml to 200 ml and indicates that lower platelet counts may be too low for study. Heyns et al. (117,134) studied autologous platelet labeling in evaluation of patients with moderate to severe thrombocytopenia. Although the results obtained were satisfactory, it appeared that harvesting efficiency depended on the initial platelet count (mean harvest of 55% ± 21% compared with 87% ± 74% in normal conditions), and the labeling efficiency was markedly reduced to 48% ± 24% compared with the normal value of 80% ± 3%. The reduced labeling efficiency was attributed to decreased platelet concentration in the labeled platelet preparation with an increase in contaminating plasma.

In studies performed with a modified method for patients with severe thrombocytopenia (platelet counts reduced to 10,000/μl), high uptake of ^{111}In-oxine (91% ± 2.1%) by autologous platelets has been achieved (126). The high labeling efficiency allowed a decrease in the blood volume required for survival studies and the elimination of the pelleting and resuspension step after incubation with the radioisotope. This method decreased the risk of collecting injury. Recovery of the labeled platelets in circulation at equilibrium was normal, and the survival time in patients with near-normal platelet counts also was normal.

When platelet life span measurements have been prospectively studied in patients with moderate to severe thrombocytopenia (10,000/μl to 150,000/μl) (126), the results in patients with megakaryocytic hypoplasia have been predicted with the platelet count. However, platelet life span in patients with ITP has been much shorter than the predicted value (Fig. 14.6). Thus measurement of platelet survival time in patients with thrombocytopenia is useful to discriminate between patients with megakaryocytic hypoplasia and patients with thrombocytopenia caused by increased platelet destruction.

In patients with thrombocytopenia with equivocal clinical presentations, measurement of platelet survival together with assays for antiplatelet glycoprotein autoantibodies (124,126, 154–156) and flow cytometric analysis of marrow megakaryocytes (11) may be useful in characterizing pathogenetic mechanisms of thrombocytopenia.

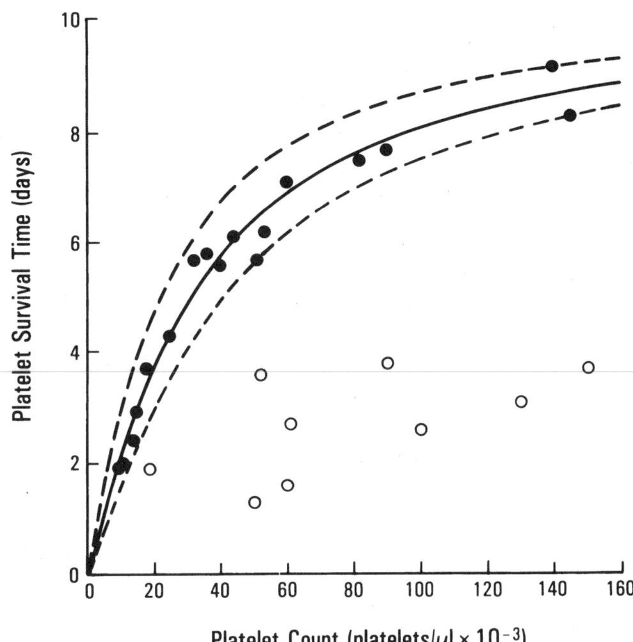

FIGURE 14.6. Relation between the survival time of ^{111}In-oxine-labeled autologous platelets and the circulating platelet count. *Closed circles* indicate patients with megakaryocytic hypoplasia. *Open circles* represent patients with idiopathic thrombocytic purpura. *Solid line* represents the best fit to data obtained with the first patient group. Platelet survival therefore could be predicted on the basis of the platelet count in these patients. All data points contained within the *interrupted lines* were consistent with a value of random platelet turnover that ranged from 15.1% to 28.0% of overall platelet turnover.

Platelet Transfusion Therapy

Platelet survival time shortens progressively as the platelet count decreases to less than 100,000/μl (118,125,126). Therefore shortened platelet survival in patients with thrombocytopenia may not necessarily indicate a pathologic destructive process (126). In a state of thrombocytopenia, the fixed daily requirement of platelets needed to maintain hemostasis constitutes a greater proportion (>60%) (126) of the overall platelet turnover and can be predicted with a mathematical model (118,126). Thus it is predicted that transfusion of sufficient platelets to increase the circulating count, for example from 10,000 to 20,000/μl to 75,000 to 100,000/μl, should result in prolonged platelet survival from 2 to 3 days to 8 to 9 days. The required frequency of platelet transfusion consequently would be significantly decreased.

In preliminary reports (61), administration of PEG-rHuMDGF to platelet donors resulted in a twofold to threefold increase in platelet count. This strategy may be useful in the care of patients with thrombocytopenia as an alternative to platelet transfusion (61–64). In these studies, the posttransfusion increment of platelets was proportionally higher in recipients of high-dose platelet concentrates than in those recipients receiving a low dose. In addition, it appears that less frequent transfusion of larger doses of platelets confers more effective platelet hemostatic function. Therefore transfusion of high-yield ($>8 \times 10^{11}$) platelet concentrates may provide hemostatic protection more effectively than is achieved with conventional platelet concentrates (2 to 4×10^{11}). This approach may result in decreasing the frequency of transfusion approximately one half (e.g., from every other day to every 4 days) without increasing the total number of platelets infused, largely because of the increasing platelet life span at higher counts.

This conclusion was corroborated by a recent analysis of the platelet dose-response relation in patients with nonrefractory disease (157). By means of a decision analysis model, it was estimated that a 38% reduction in mean platelet dose, within the commonly prescribed dose range, would result in the average patient's requiring approximately 60% more transfusions. Thus efforts to decrease costs by using lower-dose platelet transfusions are predicted to result in a disproportionate increase in the number of transfusions per patient, with a corresponding increase in overall hospital transfusion costs. In thrombocytopenia secondary to increased platelet destruction, however, platelet transfusions are less effective because of the high platelet turnover rate, which exceeds the normal rate several times (117,126,134). Because a high transfusion rate may result in refractoriness owing to alloimmunization, platelet transfusion in the treatment of these patients should be used cautiously and perhaps be reserved for life-threatening bleeding or preparation for an invasive procedure or childbirth. Administration of high-dose human γ-globulin before transfusion may reduce platelet removal rate as well.

SUMMARY

Abnormal circulating platelet counts result from quantitative alterations in megakaryocytopoiesis and platelet kinetics. Megakaryocytopoiesis involves the commitment, proliferation, and differentiation of the megakaryocytic cell lineage together with cytoplasmic acquisition of functional and structural properties of platelets. Megakaryocytes respond to increased demand for peripheral blood platelets by modifying the progenitor cell compartment, cellular replication, endoreduplication, cytoplasmic differentiation, and platelet shedding. Flow cytometry of aspirated marrow is a powerful technique for quantitative characterization of megakaryocytic number, size, ploidy, and cytoplasmic differentiation. The regulation of megakaryocytopoiesis is mediated through several hematopoietic growth factors, primarily thrombopoietin. Stimulated megakaryocytopoiesis typically manifests as an increase in megakaryocytic number, size, and ploidy and a shortened cytoplasmic maturation time.

Platelet production can be measured indirectly by means of determining platelet turnover (circulating concentration divided by platelet survival time corrected for splenic pooling). In general, platelet turnover correlates directly with the megakaryocytic cytoplasmic mass. A discrepancy between the available megakaryocytic cytoplasmic substrate and platelet turnover reflects ineffective thrombocytopoiesis. Autologous platelet survival time can be reliably measured, even for patients with thrombocytopenia, by means of ^{111}In-oxine labeling. In normal conditions, platelets survive approximately 9 to 10 days in the circulation, and approximately one third of the blood platelets are pooled within the splenic circulation. To discriminate between disorders of platelet production and platelet destruction, platelet kinetic measurements in patients with low platelet counts are interpreted by means of relating the measured survival time to the circulating concentration. Platelet transfusion is an effective method to restore platelet hemostasis in thrombocytopenia of decreased production. With the development of new nonneutralizing forms of thrombopoietin, administration of recombinant thrombopoietic growth factor may one day be useful as an alternative to platelet transfusion in the treatment of patients with thrombocytopenia.

REFERENCES

1. Burstein SA, Harker LA. Control of platelet production. *Clin Haematol* 1983;12:3–22.
2. Gewirtz AM. Human megakaryocytopoiesis. *Semin Hematol* 1986; 23:27–42.
3. Vainchenker W, Kieffer N. Human megakaryocytopoiesis: in vitro regulation and characterization of megakaryocytic precursor cells by differentiation markers. *Blood Rev* 1988;2:102–107.
4. Breton-Gorius J, Vainchenker W. Expression of platelet proteins during the in vitro and in vivo differentiation of megakaryocytes and morphological aspects of their maturation. *Semin Hematol* 1986;23: 43–67.
5. Schick BP, Schick PK. Megakaryocyte biochemistry. *Semin Hematol* 1986;23:68–87.
6. Levine RF. Isolation and characterization of normal human megakaryocytes. *Br J Haematol* 1980;45:487–497.
7. Levine RF, Hazzard KC, Lamberg JD. The significance of megakaryocyte size. *Blood* 1982;60:1122–1127.
8. Mazur EM, Lindquist DL, de Alarcon PA, et al. Evaluation of bone marrow megakaryocyte ploidy distributions in persons with normal and abnormal platelet counts. *J Lab Clin Med* 1988;111:194–202.
9. Tomer A, Harker LA, Burstein SA. Purification of human megakaryocytes by fluorescence-activated cell sorting. *Blood* 1987;70: 1735–1742.
10. Tomer A, Harker LA, Burstein SA. Flow cytometric analysis of normal human megakaryocytes. *Blood* 1988;71:1244–1252.
11. Tomer A, Friese P, Conklin R, et al. Flow cytometric analysis of megakaryocytes from patients with abnormal platelet counts. *Blood* 1989;74:594–601.
12. Till JE, McCulloch EA. A direct measurement of the radiation sensitivity of normal mouse bone marrow cells. *Radiat Res* 1989;14: 213–222.
13. Becker AJ, McCulloch EA, Till JE. Cytological demonstration of the clonal nature spleen colonies derived from transplanted mouse marrow cells. *Nature* 1993;197:452–455.
14. McCullouch EA, Till JE. A direct measurement of the radiation sensitivity of normal mouse bone marrow cells. *Radiat Res* 1961;14:213.
15. Whang J, Frei E III, Tjio JH. The distribution of the Philadelphia chromosome in patients with chronic myelogenous leukemia. *Blood* 1963;22:664–673.
16. Adamson JW, Fialkow PJ. Polycythemia vera: stem cell and probable clinical origin of the disease. *N Engl J Med* 1976;245:913–916.
17. Fialkow PJ, Jacobson RJ, Papayannopoulos T. Chronic myelocytic leukemia: clonal origin in a stem cell common to the granulocyte, erythrocyte, platelet and monocyte/macrophage. *Am J Med* 1977;63: 125–130.
18. Jacobson RJ, Salo A, Fialkow PJ. Agnogenic myeloid metaplasia: a clonal proliferation of hematopoietic stem cells with secondary myelofibrosis. *Blood* 1978;51:189–194.
19. Fialkow PJ, Faguet SB, Jacobson RJ. Evidence that essential thrombocythemia is a clonal disorder with origin in a multipotent stem cell. *Blood* 1981;58:916–919.
20. Fauser AA, Messner HA. Identification of megakaryocytes, macrophages and eosinophils in colonies of human bone marrow containing neutrophilic granulocytes and erthroblasts. *Blood* 1979;53: 1023–1027.
21. Huang S, Terstappen LW. Formation of haematopoietic microenvironment and haematopoietic stem cells from single human bone marrow stem cells. *Nature* 1992;360:745–749.
22. Metcalf D, MacDonald HR, Odartchenko N, et al. Growth of mouse megakaryocyte colonies in vitro. *Proc Natl Acad Sci U S A* 1975;72: 1744–1748.
23. Jackson CW, Brown KL, Somerville BC, et al. Two-color flow cytometric measurement of DNA distributions of rat megakaryocytes in unfixed, unfractionated marrow cell suspensions. *Blood* 1984;63:768.
24. Williams N, McDonald TP, Rabellino EM. Maturation and regulation of megakaryocytopoiesis. *Blood Cells* 1979;5:43–55.
25. Corash L, Chen HY, Levin J, et al. Regulation of thrombopoiesis:

effects of the degree of thrombocytopenia on megakaryocyte ploidy and platelet volume. *Blood* 1987;70:177–185.
26. Ebbe S, Stohlman F Jr, Overcash J, et al. Megakaryocyte size in thrombocytopenic and normal rats. *Blood* 1968;32:383–392.
27. Greenberg SM, Kuter DJ, Rosenberg RD. In vitro stimulation of megakaryocyte maturation by megakaryocyte stimulatory factor. *J Biol Chem* 1987;262:3269–3277.
28. Odell TT, Murphy JR, Jackson CW. Stimulation of megakaryocytes by acute thrombocytopenia in rats. *Blood* 1976;48:765–775.
29. Rolovic Z, Baldini M, Dameshek W. Megakaryocytopoiesis in experimentally induced immune thrombocytopenia. *Blood* 1970;35:173.
30. Burstein SA, Adamson JW, Erb SK, et al. Megakaryocytopoiesis in the mouse: response to varying platelet demand. *J Cell Physiol* 1981; 109:333.
31. deSauvage FJ, Hass PE, Spencer SD, et al. Stimulation of megakaryocytopoiesis and thrombopoiesis by the c-Mpl ligand. *Nature* 1994; 369:533.
32. Lok S, Kaushansky K, Holly RD, et al. Cloning and expression of murine thrombopoietin cDNA and stimulation of platelet production in vivo. *Nature* 1994;369:565.
33. Kaushansky K, Lok S, Holly RD, et al. Promotion of megakaryocyte progenitor expansion and differentiation by the c-Mpl ligand thrombopoietin. *Nature* 1994;369:568.
34. Wendling F, Maraskovsky E, Debili N, et al. c-Mpl ligand is a humoral regulator of megakaryocytopoiesis. *Nature* 1994;369:571.
35. Bartley TD, Bogenberger J, Hunt P, et al. Identification and cloning of a megakaryocyte growth and development factor that is a ligand for the cytokine receptor Mpl. *Cell* 1994;77:1117–1124.
36. Souyri M, Vigon I, Penciolelli JF, et al. A putative truncated cytokine receptor gene transduced by the myeloproliferative leukemia virus immortalizes hematopoietic progenitors. *Cell* 1990;63:1137–1147.
37. Methia N, Louache F, Vainchenker W, et al. Oligodeoxynucleotides antisense to the proto-oncogene c-mpl specifically inhibit in vitro megakaryocytopoiesis. *Blood* 1993;82:1395–1401.
38. Pinto MR, King MA, Goss GD, et al. Acute megakaryoblastic leukaemia with 3q inversion and elevated thrombopoietin (TSF): an autocrine role for TSF? *Br J Haematol* 1985;61:687–694.
39. Yamamoto K, Nagata K, Tzurukubo Y, et al. A novel translocation t(3; 22)(q21;q11) involving 3q21 in myelodysplastic syndrome–derived overt leukemia with thrombocytosis. *Leuk Res* 2000;24:453–457.
40. Nichol JL, Hokonm MM, Hornkohl A. et al, Megakaryocyte growth and development factor: analyses of in vitro effects on human megakaryocytopoiesis and endogenous serum levels during chemotherapy-induced thrombocytopenia. *J Clin Invest* 1995;95:2973–2978.
41. Stoffel R, Wiestner A, Skoda RC. Thrombopoietin in thrombocytopenic mice: evidence against regulation at the mRNA level and for a direct regulatory role of platelets. *Blood* 1996: 87:567–572.
42. Navarro S, Debili N, LeCouedic JP, et al. Interleukin-6 and its receptor are expressed by human megakaryocytes: in vitro effects on proliferation and endoreplication. *Blood* 1991;77:32.
43. Bruno E, Cooper RJ, Briddell RA, et al. Further examination of the effects of recombinant cytokines on the prolifcration of human megakaryocyte progenitor cells. *Blood* 1991;77:23–39.
44. Metcalf D, Nicola NA. Leukemia inhibitory factor can potentiate murine megakaryocyte production in vitro. *Blood* 1991;77:21–50.
45. Stahl CP, Zucker-Franklin D, Evatt BL, et al. Effects of human interleukin-6 on megakaryocyte development and thrombocytopoiesis in primates. *Blood* 1991;78:1467–1475.
46. Bruno E, Briddell RA, Cooper RJ, et al. Effects of recombinant interleukin-11 on human megakaryocyte progenitor cells. *Exp Hematol* 1991;19:378.
47. Robinson BE, McCrath HE, Quesenberry PJ. Recombinant murine granulocyte macrophage colony-stimulating factor has megakaryocyte colony stimulating activity and augments megakaryocyte colony stimulation by interleukin 3. *J Clin Invest* 1987;79:1648–1652.
48. Aglietta M, Monzeglio C, Sanavio F, et al. In vivo effect of human granulocyte-macrophage colony-stimulating factor on megakaryocytopoiesis. *Blood* 1991;77:1191–1194.
49. Stahl CP, Winton EF, Monroe MC, et al. Recombinant human granulocyte-macrophage colony-stimulating factor promotes megakaryocyte maturation in nonhuman primates. *Exp Hematol* 1991;19:810.
50. Hoffman R. Regulation of megakaryocytopoiesis. *Blood* 1989;74: 1196.
51. Vainchenker W, Bouguet J, Guichard J, et al. Megakaryocyte colony formation from human bone marrow precursors. *Blood* 1979;54: 940–945.
52. Dessypris EN, Gleaton JH, Armstrong OL. Effect of human recombinant erythropoietin on human marrow megakaryocyte colony formation in vitro. *Br J Haematol* 1987;65:265–269.
53. Briddell RA, Bruno E, Cooper RJ, et al. Effect of c-kit ligand in vitro human megakaryocytopoiesis. *Blood* 1991;78:2854–2859.
54. Tomer A, Stahl CP, McClure HM, et al. Effects of recombinant human granulocyte-macrophage colony-stimulating factor on platelet survival and activation using a nonhuman primate model. *Exp Hematol* 1993;21:1577–1582.
55. Solberg LA, Tucker RF, Grant MN, et al. Transforming growth factor–β inhibits colony formation from human megakaryocytic, erythroid and multipotent stem cells. In: Najman A, Guigen M, eds. *The inhibitors of hematopoiesis.* London: John Libbey Eurotext, 1987: 111–121.
56. Fuse A, Kakuda H, Shima Y, et al. Interleukin 6, a possible autocrine growth and differentiation factor for the human megakaryocytic cell line, CMK. *Br J Haematol* 1991;77:32–36.
57. Tomer A, Harker LA. Measurements of in vivo megakaryocytopoiesis: studies in nonhuman primates and patients. *Stem Cells* 1996;14[Suppl 1]:18–30.
58. Harker LA, Marzec UM, Kelly AB, et al. Prevention of thrombocytopenia and neutropenia in a non-human model of marrow suppressive chemotherapy by combining pegylated recombinant human megakaryocyte growth and development factor and recombinant human granulocyte colony stimulating factor. *Blood* 1997;89:155–165.
59. Harker LA, Hunt P, Kelly AB, et al. Regulation of platelet production and function by megakaryocyte growth and development factor in nonhuman primates. *Blood* 1996;87:1833–1844.
60. Harker LA, Marzec UM, Hunt P, et al. Dose-response effect of pegylated human megakaryocyte growth and development factor on platelet production and function in nonhuman primates. *Blood* 1996;88: 511–521.
61. Kuter DJ. Future directions with platelet growth factors. *Semin Hematol.* 2000;37[2 suppl 4]:41–49.
62. Vadhan-Raj S. Clinical experience with recombinant TPO in chemotherapy-induced thrombocytopenia. *Semin Hematol* 2000;37[2 suppl 4]:28–34.
63. Linker C. Thrombopoietin in the treatment of acute myeloid leukemia and in transplantation. *Semin Hematol* 2000;37[2 suppl 4]: 35–40.
64. Demetri GD. Pharmacologic options in patients with thrombocytopenia. *Semin Hematol* 2000;37[2 Suppl 4]:11–18.
65. Williams N, Levine RF. Annotation: the origin, development and regulation of megakarycytes. *Br J Haematol* 1982;52:173–180.
66. Feinendegen LE, Odartchenko N, Cottier N. Kinetics of megakaryocyte proliferation. *Proc Soc Exp Biol Med* 1962;111:177–182.
67. Breton-Gorius J, Reyes R. Ultrastructure of human bone marrow cell maturation. *Int Rev Cytol* 1976;46:251–314.
68. Ebbe S, Stohlman F Jr. Megakaryocytopoiesis in the rat. *Blood* 1965; 26:20–35.
69. Ebbe S. Experimental and clinical megakaryocytopoiesis. *Clin Haematol* 1979;8:371–394.
70. Lichtman MA, Chamberlain JK, Simon W, et al. Parasinusoidal location of megakaryocytes in marrow: a determinant of platelet release. *Am J Hematol* 1978;4:303–312.
71. Wright JJ. The histogenesis of the blood platelets. *J Morphol* 1910; 21:203.
72. Theiry JP, Bessis M. Mecanisme de la plaquettogenese: etude in vivo par la microcinematographie. Rev Hematol 1956;11:162.
73. Behnke O. An electron microscopic study of the rat megakaryocyte, II: some aspects of platelet release and microtubules. *J Ultrastruct Res* 1969;26:111.

74. Tavassoli M, Aoki M. Migration of entire megakaryocytes through the marrow blood barrier. *Br J Haematol* 1981;48:35–39.
75. Tomer A, Scharf RE, McMillan R, et al. Bernard-Soulier syndrome: quantitative characterization of megakaryocytes and platelets by flow cytometric and platelet kinetic measurements. *Eur J Haematol* 1994; 52:193–200.
76. Harker LA, Finch CA. Thrombokinetics in man. *J Clin Invest* 1969; 48:963–974.
77. Tomer A, Harker LA. Quantitative cytometric measurement of normal human megakaryocytes. *J Exp Clin Hematol* 1989;31:37.
78. Tomer A. Effects of anagrelide on megakaryocyte proliferation and maturation in essential thrombocythemia. *Blood* 2002;99: 1602–1609.
79. Lichtman MA, Brennan JK. Megakaryocyte structure, maturation and ecology. In: Colman RW, Hirsh J, Marder VJ, et al., eds. *Hemostasis and thrombosis. basic principles and clinical practice.* Philadelphia: JB Lippincott, 1987:395–417.
80. Rabellino EM, Nachman RL, Williams N, et al. Human megakaryocytes, 1: characterization of the membrane and cytoplasmic components of isolated marrow megakaryocytes. *J Exp Med* 1979;149:1273.
81. Mazur EM, Hoffman R, Chasis J, et al. Immunofluorescent identification of human megakaryocyte colonies using an antiplatelet glycoprotein antiserum. *Blood* 1981;57:277–286.
82. Vinci G, Tabilio A, Deschamps JF, et al. Immunological study of in vitro maturation of human megakaryocytes. *Br J Haematol* 1984;56: 589–605.
83. Asch AS, Barnwell J, Silverstein RL, et al. Isolation of the thrombospondin membrane receptor. *J Clin Invest* 1987;79:1054–1061.
84. Cramer EM, Debili N, Martin JF. Uncoordinated expression of fibrinogen compared with thrombospondin and von Willebrand factor in maturing human megakaryocytes. *Blood* 1989;73:1123–1129.
85. Cramer EM, Vainchenker W, Vinci G, et al. Gray platelet syndrome: immunoelectron microscopy localization of fibrinogen and von Willebrand factor in platelets and megakaryocytes. *Blood* 1985;66: 1309–1316.
86. Rabellino EM, Goodwin L, Bussel JB, et al. Studies of human marrow megakaryocytes. In: Evatt R, Levine RF, Williams N, eds. *Megakaryocyte biology and precursors: in vitro cloning and cellular properties.* New York: Elsevier, 1981.
87. Nakeff A. Megakaryocytic cells. *Bibl Haematol* 1984;48:131.
88. Berkow RL, Straneva JE, Bruno ED, et al. Isolation of human megakaryocytes by density centrifugation and counterflow centrifugal elutriation. *J Lab Clin Med* 1984;103:811.
89. Nakeff A, Valeriote F, Gray JW, et al. Application of flow cytometry and cell sorting to megakaryocytopoiesis. *Blood* 1979;53:732.
90. Worthington RE, Nakeff A, Micko S. Flow cytometric analysis of megakaryocyte differentiation. *Cytometry* 1984;5:501–508.
91. Parks DR, Herzenberg LA. Fluorescence-activated cell sorting: theory, experimental optimization, and applications in lymphoid cell biology. *Methods Enzymol* 1984;108:197.
92. Tomer A, Vergara CM, Harker LA. Human megakaryocyte differentiation: multiparameter correlative analysis using three-color flow cytometry. *Blood* 1993;82[Suppl 1]:260.
93. Tomer A. Flow cytometry as a universal tool in megakaryocyte research. NHLBI Workshop, Washington, DC, August 1994.
94. Levin J. Thrombopoiesis. In: Colman RW, Hirsh J, Marder VJ, et al., eds. *Hemostasis and thrombosis: basic principles and clinical practice.* Philadelphia: JB Lippincott, 1987:418–430.
95. Odell TT Jr, Jackson CW. Polyploidy and maturation of rat megakaryocytes *Blood* 1968;32:102–110.
96. Paulus JM. DNA metabolism and development of organelles in guinea pig megakaryocytes: a combined ultrastructural, autoradiographic and cytophotometric study. *Blood* 1970;35:298–311.
97. DeLeval M. Etude cytochimique quantitative des acides desoxyribonucleiques au cours de la maturation megacaryocytaire. *Nouv Rev Fr Hematol* 1968;8:392–394.
98. Kinet-Denoel, C, Bassleer R, Andrien JM, et al. Ploidy histograms in ITP. In: Paulus JM, ed. *Platelet kinetics: radioisotopic, cytological, mathematical and clinical aspects.* Amsterdam: North Holland, 1971: 280–284.
99. Penington DG, Weste SM. Ploidy histograms in ITP. In: Paulus JM, ed. *Platelet kinetics: radioisotopic, cytological, mathematical and clinical aspects.* Amsterdam: North Holland, 1971:284–286.
100. Ishibashi T, Ruggeri ZM, Harker LA, et al. Separation of human megakaryocytes by state of differentiation on continuous gradients of Percoll: size and ploidy analysis of cells identified by monoclonal antibody to glycoprotein IIb/IIIa *Blood* 1986;67:1286.
101. Queisser U, Queisser W, Spiertz B. Polyploidization of megakaryocytes in normal humans, in patients with idiopathic thrombocytopenia and with pernicious anaemia. *Br J Haematol* 1971;20:489.
102. Lagerlof B. Cytophotometric study of megakaryocyte ploidy in polycythemia vera and chronic granulocyte leukemia. *Acta Cytol* 1972; 16:240.
103. Harker LA. Kinetics of thrombopoiesis. *J Clin Invest* 1968;47: 458–465.
104. Pizzolato P. Sternal marrow megakaryocytes in health and disease. *Am J Clin Pathol* 1948;18:891.
105. Tragnor JE, Ingram M. A membrane filler technique for enumerative megakaryocytes. *J Lab Clin Med* 1965;66:705.
106. Harker LA. Megakaryocyte quantitation. *J Clin Invest* 1968;47:452.
107. Cullen WC, McDonald TP. Comparison of stereologic techniques for the quantification of megakaryocyte size and number. *Exp Hematol* 1986;14:782.
108. Shapiro HM. *Practical flow cytometry,* 2nd ed. New York: Alan R. Liss, 1988.
109. Odell TT Jr, Jackson CW, Friday TJ, et al. Effects of thrombocytopenia on megakaryocytopoiesis. *Br J Haematol* 1969;17:91–101.
110. Odell TT, Jackson CW, Reiter RS. Depression of megakaryocyte-platelet system in rats by transfusion of platelets. *Acta Haematol* 1967; 38:34–42.
111. Sullivan LW, Adams W II, Liu YK. Induction of thrombocytopenia by thrombopheresis in man: patterns of recovery in normal subjects during ethanol ingestion and abstinence. *Blood* 1977;49:197–207.
112. Adams WH, Liu YK, Sullivan LW. Humoral regulation of thrombopoiesis in man. *J Lab Clin Med* 1978;91:941–947.
113. Burstein SA, Adamson JW, Thorning DJ, et al. Characteristics of murine megakaryocytopoiesis in vitro. *Blood* 1979;54:169.
114. Bessman JD. The relation of megakaryocyte ploidy to platelet volume. *Am J Hematol* 1984;16:161–170.
115. Hollen CW, Henthorn J, Koziol JA, et al. Elevated serum interleukin-6 levels in patients with reactive thrombocytosis. *Br J Haematol* 1991; 79:286–290.
116. Wessels P, Heyns AD, Pieter H, et al. An improved method for the quantification of the in vivo kinetics of a representative population of 111-In-labelled human platelets. *Eur J Nucl Med* 1985;10:522.
117. Heyns AD, Badenhorst PH, Lotter MG, et al. Platelet turnover and kinetics in immune thrombocytopenic purpura: results with autologous 111-In-labeled platelets and homologous 51-CR-labeled platelets differ. *Blood* 1986;67:8692.
118. Hanson SR, Slichter SJ. Platelet kinetics in patients with bone marrow hypoplasia: evidence for a fixed platelet requirement. *Blood* 1985;66: 1105–1109.
119. Paulus JM, Aster RH. Platelet kinetics: production, distribution, lifespan, and fate of platelets. In: Williams N, Beutler E, Erslev O, et al., eds. *Hematology.* New York: McGraw-Hill, 1983:1185.
120. Heyns AD, Lotter MG, Badenhorst PN, et al. Kinetics, distribution and sites of destruction of indium-111-labelled human platelets. *Br J Haematol* 1980;44:269–280.
121. Aster RH. Pooling of platelets in the spleen: role in the pathogenesis of "hypersplenic" thrombocytopenia. *J Clin Invest* 1966;45:645–657.
122. Peters AM, Lavender JP. Platelet kinetics with indium-111 platelets: comparison with chromium-51 platelets. *Semin Thromb Hemost* 1983; 9:100.
123. Harker LA. The kinetics of platelet production and destruction in man. *Clin Haematol* 1977;6:671–693.
124. Tomer A, Schreiber AD, McMillan R, et al. Menstrual cyclic thrombocytopenia. *Br J Haematol* 1989;71:519–524.
125. Davey MG. The survival and destruction of human platelets. *Bibl Haematol* 1966;22:1–136.
126. Tomer A, Hanson SR, Harker LA. Autologous platelet kinetics in patients with severe thrombocytopenia: discrimination between disor-

ders of production and destruction. *J Lab Clin Med* 1991;118: 546–554.
127. Aster RH. Studies of the fate of platelets in rats and man. *Blood* 1969; 34:117–128.
128. Scheffel U, Tsan MF, Mitchell G, et al. Human platelets labeled with In-111-8-hydroxyquinoline: kinetics, distribution and estimates of radiation dose. *J Nucl Med* 1982;23:149.
129. Heyns AD, Lotter MG, Kotze HF, et al. Quantification of in vivo distribution of platelets labeled with indium-111-oxine. *J Nucl Med* 1982;23:943–945.
130. Shulman NR, Jordan JV Jr. Platelet kinetics. In: Colman RW, Hirsh J, Marder VJ, et al., eds. *Hemostasis and thrombosis: basic principles and clinical practice.* Philadelphia: JB Lippincott, 1987:431–451.
131. Ardaillou N, Najean Y, Eberlin A. Study of platelet kinetics using 75-Se-selenomethionine. In: Paulus JM, ed. *Platelet kinetics.* Amsterdam: North Holland, 1971:131–142.
132. Brodsky, I, Ross EM, Petkov G, et al. Platelet and fibrinogen kinetics with 75-Se-selenomethionine in patients with myeloproliferative disorders. *Br J Haematol* 1972;22:179.
133. Dassin E, Najean, Y. The use of 75-Se-methionine as a tracer of thrombocytopoiesis. In vivo incorporation of the tracer into platelet proteins: a biochemical study. *Acta Haematol* 1979;61:61.
134. Heyns AD, Badenhorst PN, Wessels P, et al. Indium-111-labelled human platelets: a method for use in severe thrombocytopenia. *Thromb Haemost* 1984;52:226–229.
135. Kelton JG. Platelet survival studies: an overview of the factors affecting the efficiency and reliability of platelet radiolabeling. *Transfusion* 1986;26:19–22.
136. Slichter SJ. Post-storage platelet viability in thrombocytopenic recipients is reliably measured by radiochromium-labeled platelet recovery and survival measurements in normal volunteers. *Transfusion* 1986; 26:8–12.
137. Robertson JS, Milne WL, Cohn SH. Labeling and tracing of rat blood platelets with chromium-51. In: *Proceedings of the Second International Radioisotopic Congress,* July 19–22, 1954. London: Butterworth, 1954:205–209.
138. Tsukada T, Steiner M, Baldini M. Mechanism and kinetics of chromate transport in human platelets. *Am J Physiol* 1971;221: 1697–1705.
139. Heaton WAL. Indium-111 (^{111}In) and chromium–51 (^{51}Cr) labeling of platelets: are they comparable? *Transfusion* 1986;26:16–19.
140. International Committee for Standardization in Hematology. Panel for Standardization in Hematology: recommended methods of radioisotope platelet survival studies. *Blood* 1977;50:1137–1144.
141. Thakur ML, Welch MJ, Joist JH. Indium-111-labeled platelets: studies on preparation and evaluation of in vitro and in vivo function. *Thromb Res* 1976;9:345–357.
142. Thakur ML. Radioisotopic labeling of platelets: an historical perspective. *Semin Thromb Hemost* 1983;9:79.
143. Hawker RJ, Hawker LM, Wilkinson AR. (111-In) labeled human platelets: optimal methods. *Clin Sci (Colch)* 1980;58:243–248.
144. Joist JH, Baker RK, Thakur ML, et al. Indium-111-labeled human platelets: uptake and loss of label and in vitro function of labeled platelets. *J Lab Clin Med* 1978;92:829–836.
145. Vigneron N, Dassin E, Najean Y. Double radioactive labeling for the simultaneous study of autologous and homologous human platelets' life span. *Nouv Presse Med* 1980;9:1835–1837.
146. Corash L, Shafer B, Perlow M. Heterogenicity of human whole blood platelet subpopulation, II: use of subhuman primate model to analyze the relationship between density and platelet age. *Blood* 1978;52: 726–734.
147. Thakur ML, McKenney SL, Park CH. Simplified and efficient labeling of human platelets in plasma using indium-111-2-mercaptopyridine-N-oxide: preparation and evaluation. *J Nucl Med* 1985;26: 510–517.
148. Thakur M.L, McKenney SM. Indium 111-mercaptopyridine N-oxide-labeled human leukocytes and platelets: mechanism of labeling and intracellular location of 111-indium and mercaptopyridine N-oxide. *J Lab Clin Med* 1986;107:141–147.
149. Dewanjee megakaryocyte, Wahner HW, Dunn WL, et al. Comparison of three platelet markers for measurement of platelet survival time in healthy volunteers. *Mayo Clin Proc* 1986;61:327–336.
150. Snyder EL, Moroff G, Simon TS, et al. Recommended methods for conducting radiolabeled platelet survival studies. *Transfusion* 1986; 26:37.
151. Heyns AP, Lotter MG, Badenhorst PN. Methodology of platelet imaging. In: Harker LA, Zimmerman TS, eds. *Methods in hematology: measurements of platelet function.* New York: Churchill Livingstone, 1983:216–234.
152. Schmidt KG, Rasmussen JW. Kinetics and distribution in vivo of 111-In-labelled autologous platelets in idiopathic thrombocytopenic purpura. *Scand J Haematol* 1985;34:47.
153. International Committee for Standardization in Hematology. Panel on diagnostic applications of radionuclides, recommended method for indium-111 platelet survival studies. *J Nucl Med* 1988;29:564.
154. McMillan R, Tani P, Millard F, et al. Platelet-associated and plasma anti-glycoprotein autoantibodies in chronic ITP. *Blood* 1987;70: 1040–1045.
155. Tomer A, Hanson SR, McMillan R, et al. Mechanisms of thrombocytopenia in man. *Thromb Haemost* 1989;62:1574.
156. Tomer A, Kasey S. Autoimmune thrombocytopenia: determination of circulating autoantibodies to platelet specific receptors using flow cytometry. *Blood* 1998;92[Suppl 1]:3369.
157. Ackerman SJ, Klumpp TR, Guzman GI, et al. Economic consequences of alterations in platelet transfusion dose: analysis of a prospective, randomized, double-blind trial. *Transfusion* 2000;40: 1457–1462.

Rossi's Principles of Transfusion Medicine, Third Edition, edited by Toby L. Simon, Walter H. Dzik, Edward L. Snyder, Christopher P. Stowell, and Ronald G. Strauss. Lippincott Williams & Wilkins, Philadelphia © 2002.

15

PLATELET KINETICS AND HEMOSTASIS

HENRY M. RINDER

Platelets in the blood are essential for normal hemostasis, and thrombocytopenia is associated with an increased risk of both spontaneous and traumatic bleeding. Platelet transfusions are therefore a critical part of the support of thrombocytopenic patients with malignancies and critically ill medical patients with either thrombocytopenia or platelet dysfunction. The use of platelet transfusions has increased dramatically during the past 30 years, more than doubling during the 1980s in the United States alone (1). This increase is primarily caused by patients receiving prophylactic platelet transfusions for thrombocytopenia. Therefore, it is important to understand the kinetics of platelet turnover and the hemostatic function of both native and transfused platelets in order to appreciate the indications for and clinical efficacy of platelet transfusions. This chapter will detail the current understanding of the normal physiology of platelet turnover and platelet function, as well as provide a brief discussion of platelet kinetics and hemostasis associated with platelet transfusion.

PLATELET KINETICS

Platelet Production

Platelets in the circulation are anucleate cells between 2 and 4 μm in diameter with a volume between 6 and 11 fl. Platelets are derived from the megakaryocyte cytoplasm after a maturation time of about 4 days. The processes of megakaryocyte proliferation, endoreduplication, differentiation, and release of the cytoplasmic megakaryocyte fragments into the circulation as true platelets are described in detail in the preceding chapter. When platelets are released into the circulation, they survive for 7 to 10 days. The normal platelet count ranges from 150,000 to 450,000/μl. In isotopic studies of platelet survival after transfusion, it has been reasonably estimated that platelet removal over time is approximately equivalent to platelet production when the platelet count is at a steady state. Therefore, platelet turnover, measured as the survival of radioactively labeled platelets (2) has been used as a surrogate measure of platelet production, that is, the delivery of viable platelets into the circulation. Using these isotopic methods, the rate of platelet production in normal humans is estimated to range from 35,000 to 44,000 platelets/μl per day (3). Platelet survival, and by extension platelet production, has also been estimated by nonisotopic methods, which include monitoring of platelet enzyme activities over time after administration of either aspirin (cyclooxygenase) or phenelzine (monoamine oxidase) (4,5). Newer methods, such as thiazole orange labeling of platelets, now allow for direct quantitation of the release of young "reticulated" platelets into the circulation from megakaryocytes (Fig. 15.1).

Reticulated platelets (RP) are identified by their detectable RNA content (6). Because platelets are anucleate, their RNA content is maximal at the time of release from the megakaryocyte into the blood, and this RNA level declines over time as the platelet ages in the circulation. Measurement of RP in animal studies has directly confirmed that RP are those platelets which have been most recently released from the megakaryocyte into the peripheral circulation (7,8). In humans, the percentage of circulating RP correlates with thrombopoietic activity (9). Analogous to red blood cell reticulocytes, the RP percentage increases in the setting of a normal hyperproductive marrow response to destructive thrombocytopenia; by contrast, the percentage of young platelets in the blood falls in association with thrombocytopenia caused by megakaryocyte hypoproliferation due to chemotherapy or intrinsic marrow aplasia (10). Unpublished

H.M. Rinder: Laboratory Medicine, Yale University School of Medicine and Yale–New Haven Hospital, New Haven, Connecticut.

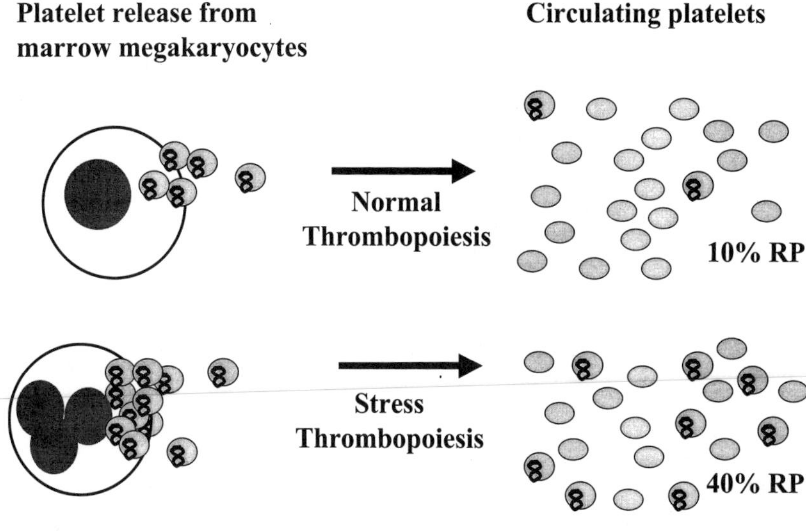

FIGURE 15.1. Release of reticulated platelets (RP) into peripheral blood. Megakaryocytes normally undergo cytoplasmic fragmentation, thereby releasing platelets into the periphery. Because platelets are anucleate and cannot transcribe additional RNA, their RNA content is maximal at the time of release into peripheral blood, and this RNA content is significantly higher than levels seen in older circulating platelets. Detection of that percentage of newly released "reticulated" platelets in peripheral blood provides a direct measure of thrombopoietic function. Stress thrombopoiesis results in increased megakaryocyte ploidy and overall mass, resulting in larger numbers of platelets released into the circulation and a corresponding increase in the percentage of RP in blood.

studies in our laboratory have demonstrated that the average number of RP which are estimated to be released into the circulation per day agrees well with estimates of platelet production by radioactive labeling. We found that the absolute reticulated platelet count in healthy volunteers with normal platelet counts was 24,000 platelets/μl on average (ranging from 15,000 to 48,000 platelets/μl/day). In animal studies, RP appear to be identifiable as such for approximately 18 hours; similar RP data in humans would therefore suggest that platelet production averages 32,000 platelets/μl/day, similar to the indirect estimates of platelet production by isotopic labeling studies. Differences among laboratories in the techniques for detecting RP (11) have led to different reference ranges (12) and difficulty in applying a "standard" test. Recently, we have developed an RNAse-based RP analysis, which corrects for platelet size (13), thereby setting a protocol-defined standardized RP% measurement amenable to interlaboratory use (14). In addition, this standard method now allows for the determination of an RP maturation index, analogous to the immature red blood cell reticulocyte fraction, which further refines the sensitivity of the RP assay to early increases in platelet production, such as following chemotherapy-induced thrombocytopenia.

Platelet Distribution

Platelets are distributed in humans in the general blood circulation and in the spleen. Transfusion studies have shown that approximately 25% to 35% of the total platelet mass is present in the splenic pool at any one time (15) and correspondingly, asplenic patients show 100% of infused platelets to be present in their circulation. Although there is some evidence that hepatic pooling of platelets can occur in normal humans, liver sequestration of platelets occurs to a much lesser extent than splenic pooling (16). In addition, those platelets which are initially sequestered in the liver are released into the blood much more rapidly than those platelets which enter the splenic pool directly after transfusion. It is currently controversial whether splenic pooling alters platelet survival. Splenectomy has been shown in some studies to cause prolongation of platelet lifespan (17), while other studies found no change in platelet survival after splenectomy (18). However, data from an animal model demonstrated a significant (>40%) increase in platelet lifespan postsplenectomy (19). Similar to leukocytes, the splenic pool of platelets in humans can be released into the general circulation with stress, as demonstrated by studies using intravenous epinephrine to mobilize platelets from the spleen into the blood. Splenic pooling of platelets becomes clinically important in patients with splenomegaly. Massive splenomegaly may result in sequestration of as much as 90% of the total platelet population within the enlarged spleen (20). In patients with more moderate splenomegaly, such as seen in patients with cirrhosis and portal hypertension, mild thrombocytopenia results from splenic sequestration, and platelet counts in the range of 60,000 to 100,000/μl are common.

Platelet Destruction

Platelet survival has been modeled in different ways, but most schema generally depict two main mechanisms by which platelets are lost from the circulation (21). In healthy individuals with normal platelet counts, the vast majority, 83% on average, of platelets are lost through senescence, that is, normal platelet aging. The factors which appear to naturally cause senescent platelets to be removed have been postulated to include irreversible changes in membrane glycoproteins, increased platelet-associated immunoglobulin (with subsequent clearance of those high-immunoglobulin–expressing platelets by splenic macrophages), increased exposure of the negatively-charged procoagulant lipid, phosphatidylserine, on the external platelet membrane, and decreased levels of surface sialic acid (22). As opposed to those platelets lost from the circulation through normal aging, the remainder of the platelets, approximately 17%, are estimated to be lost on a daily basis through maintenance of hemostasis (23), the preservation of the structural integrity of the vascular endothelium. Taking into account the splenic pool, this amount of hemostatic loss represents about 7,000 platelets/μl/day for daily hemostatic turnover. Interestingly, this loss of platelets for hemostatic integrity appears to be a fixed absolute number; thus, when marrow hypoplasia results in thrombocytopenia, the daily proportion of platelets removed by hemostatic consumption rises dramatically, approaching 80% to 85%, similar to levels normally removed by senescence.

In diseases characterized by increased hemostatic consumption of platelets, initial increases in platelet turnover may not be detectable because of the early compensatory megakaryocyte response maintaining platelet counts at a steady state. Under these circumstances, RP measurements have been valuable for detecting changes in platelet turnover and for predicting thrombotic risk. In patients recovering from allogeneic hematopoietic stem cell transplantation, a sudden increase in the RP% was associated with subsequent development of graft-versus-host disease (24). In asymptomatic pregnant women at risk for development of preeclampsia, an increase in the RP% from the first to second trimester was retrospectively associated with those women who subsequently went on to develop signs and symptoms of preeclampsia (25), despite normal platelet counts and the absence of proteinuria and hypertension at the time of sampling in the second trimester. The potential for the RP% to predict disease complications associated with increased platelet turnover is further illustrated in a study of thromboembolism associated with thrombocytosis (26). Asymptomatic patients with thrombocytosis at a steady state (platelet counts unchanging) were shown to be at increased risk for subsequent thrombotic events (mostly arterial) if they demonstrated an elevated RP% or absolute RP count; the relative risk associated with these laboratory findings was higher than the risk associated with a high platelet count alone. Furthermore, the RP% was shown to decrease with successful aspirin therapy in patients with thrombocytosis treated for thromboembolic complications, similar to data using isotopic survival that demonstrated decreased platelet turnover in aspirin-treated patients with thrombocytosis (27).

Platelet Turnover with Thrombocytopenia

Platelet transfusions are frequently given to thrombocytopenic patients receiving chemotherapy, either for bleeding or for prophylaxis of bleeding when the platelet count is less than 20,000/μl. Thrombocytopenic patients receiving platelet transfusions can be monitored for adequate platelet recovery by determining the increase in platelet count within 60 minutes of platelet transfusion. The need for repeated platelet transfusion, especially when platelet survival is decreased by inherent clinical factors, can be assessed by obtaining serial platelet counts over the days following a platelet transfusion (28). Clinical factors which may further decrease platelet survival in thrombocytopenic patients via increased hemostatic consumption include fever, bacterial or viral infection, shock (29) (especially secondary to sepsis), vascular disease, thrombosis, disseminated intravascular coagulation, and drugs (Table 15.1) (30). Alloimmunization to platelets, which commonly occurs in patients receiving chronic platelet transfusions, is another cause of decreased platelet recovery and survival following platelet transfusion (discussed in the following chapters). In adult patients who are relatively stable (lacking the consumptive factors noted above) despite chemotherapy-induced thrombocytopenia, a single unit of random-donor platelet concentrate will raise the platelet count by 5,000 to 10,000 platelets/μl. A more formal approach is to estimate the expected corrected count increment (CCI) after transfusion based on the patient's body surface area (BSA), change in platelet count, and the number of platelets transfused, as follows (31):

TABLE 15.1. DRUGS COMMONLY ASSOCIATED WITH THROMBOCYTOPENIA

Enhanced Peripheral Platelet Destruction
Amphotericin B
Anticonvulsants
Antihypertensives
Gold salts
Heparin
Procainamide
Psychotropics
Quinidine/quinine
Sulfonamides
Suppression of Megakaryopoiesis
Anticonvulsants
Chemotherapy agents
Estrogens
Ethanol
Thiazide diuretics

$$\text{CCI} = \text{BSA} \times \frac{(\text{post-tx plt.ct—pre-tx ptt.ct})}{(\text{Number of platelets transfused} \times 10^{-11})}$$

The marrow's capacity for rapidly increasing platelet production is perhaps best illustrated by patients with immune thrombocytopenic purpura (ITP). In ITP, antibodies to platelet membrane epitopes (32) bind to platelets, and these antibody-coated platelets adhere to splenic macrophage Fc receptors, removing the platelets from the circulation (33). Platelet survival in ITP can be so severely decreased that the platelet lifespan is measured in hours rather than days. When platelet destruction occurs to this severe extent, the marrow is able to increase the megakaryocyte mass by nearly ten-fold (34); yet, this increase may be insufficient to maintain a normal platelet count. Patients with ITP demonstrate increased numbers of megakaryocytes on bone marrow examination and an increased percentage of RP in the peripheral blood, further confirming the compensatory marrow production response to destructive thrombocytopenia. As patients' platelet counts recover with successful therapy (steroids, intravenous immune globulin, anti-D therapy) (35), the RP% has been observed to fall just prior to the start of the platelet count recovery; the RP% then continues to fall as the platelet count increases back to normal or supranormal levels. These data indicate that restoration of a normal platelet lifespan rapidly down-regulates the brisk release of RP.

Patients with ITP appear to have relatively normal hemostasis despite extremely low platelet counts (36), and most patients, especially children, do not have significant blood loss despite very low platelet counts. Platelet transfusion is not generally recommended in patients with ITP, because the survival of those transfused platelets is too short to impact on their overall course (thrombocytopenia will recur rapidly) and, as noted below, the hemostatic function of young platelets in ITP appears to be well-preserved. Transfused platelets do not have a survival advantage over native platelets in ITP, most likely because the autoantigens in ITP are common to all platelets, unlike the platelet polymorphisms which can result in neonatal alloimmune thrombocytopenia or posttransfusion purpura (Chapter 16). However, when life-threatening bleeding, especially cerebral hemorrhage, occurs in patients with ITP, platelet transfusion can be effective, and there appear to be no significant adverse effects of platelet transfusions in these patients (37). Platelet transfusions can yield transient but nonetheless impressive platelet count increments in even patients with severe ITP without generally aggravating the course of the disease.

One reason for the lack of significant bleeding in ITP is that the function of the circulating platelets is preserved or even increased because of the higher proportion of robust, young platelets in the blood, especially when compared with the function of older circulating platelets. In studies of human platelets after recovery from thrombocytopenia, cohorts of younger platelets had greater aggregation and adherence responses to agonists when compared with older platelet subsets (38), as if younger platelets had higher procoagulant potential. In an animal model, RP had a lesser threshold for α-granule release to agonist compared with older circulating platelets (39). We directly examined human RP in comparison with older circulating platelets in normal patients and in patients with ITP. We found that, compared with controls, all platelets in patients with ITP were primed to undergo α-granule release (both RP and older non-RP) (40). In both controls and patients, RP did not have a lower threshold for α-granule release; instead, RP always demonstrated increased α-granule content, approximately twice as much as older circulating platelets, suggesting that RP may contribute more granule content to the hemostatic microenvironment. These factors may explain why patients with ITP tend to have less bleeding than chemotherapy patients with similar levels of thrombocytopenia.

PLATELET HEMOSTASIS

The platelet serves as the cellular-based engine of hemostasis. Platelet membrane receptors mediate primary hemostasis, allowing platelets to bind directly to endothelium and to subendothelial sites of damage. Platelet adhesion triggers transmembrane signaling, thereby inducing activation and expression of procoagulant platelet function. These procoagulant mechanisms are mediated through translocation of adhesive and signaling receptors to the membrane surface, receptor conformational change to promote adhesion, release of agonistic granule contents, and exposure of internal membrane phospholipids. The procoagulant surface of the platelet then serves as a platform for assembly of the coagulation cascade and the ultimate formation of thrombin which (a) feeds back on both platelets and the clotting cascade to amplify the procoagulant response, and (b) produces fibrin to provide a platelet matrix for secondary, long-acting hemostasis. The platelet also assists in clot consolidation and terminal protection from fibrinolysis by respectively contributing factor XIII and platelet factor 4 to the clot milieu (Table 15.2).

TABLE 15.2. PROTHROMBOTIC ASPECTS OF PLATELET FUNCTION

Membrane Components
Thromboxane A_2 formation (cyclooxygenase-dependent)
Phosphatidylserine expression (translocation from the internal membrane surface)
Platelet Microparticles
Receptor:Ligand Interactions Promoting Adhesion or Activation
GP Ib/V/IX:von Willebrand factor (vWF)
GP IIb/IIIa:fibrinogen and GP IIb/IIIa:vWF
GP Ia/IIa:collagen
GP Ib:thrombin
GP VI:collagen
PAR-1:thrombin
α2-Adrenergic receptor:epinephrine
ADP receptor:ADP
Secreted Proteins/Agonists from α Granules and Dense Granules
Ligands (fibrinogen, fibronectin, thrombospondin, vitronectin, vWF)
Enzymes (α2-antiplasmin, factors V, VIII, and XI)
Anti-heparin (platelet factor 4)
ADP, serotonin
Secreted Cytosolic Factor XIII

Platelet Interaction with Blood Vessels

The normal endothelial cell lining of the vasculature strives to maintain a nonthrombogenic surface by secretion of factors which block soluble coagulation activity, including heparan sulfates, production of thrombomodulin, and synthesis of tissue plasminogen activator. Antiplatelet factors are similarly part of the anticoagulant activity which is intrinsic to the healthy endothelial cell lining, and these include (a) net negative surface charge, which repels similarly charged platelets, (b) constitutive release of nitric oxide and prostacyclin which inhibit platelet aggregation, and (c) constitutive surface expression of an adenosine 5′-diphosphatase (ADPase) which inactivates platelet-released ADP (41,42), limiting activation of nearby platelets.

The platelet–vessel wall interaction is best illustrated at the high flow velocities of the arterial circulation. The interaction between the vasculature and flowing blood, as shown in Figure 15.2, creates parallel planes of blood moving at different velocities; the blood closest to the vessel wall moves more slowly than the blood at the center of the vessel (43). These different velocities create shear stress, which is greatest at the blood vessel wall and least at the center of the vessel. Shear rate, therefore, changes inversely with the vessel diameter, with levels estimated to vary between 500 sec^{-1} in larger arteries to 5,000 sec^{-1} in the smallest arterioles. Shear rates at the surface of atherosclerotic plaques

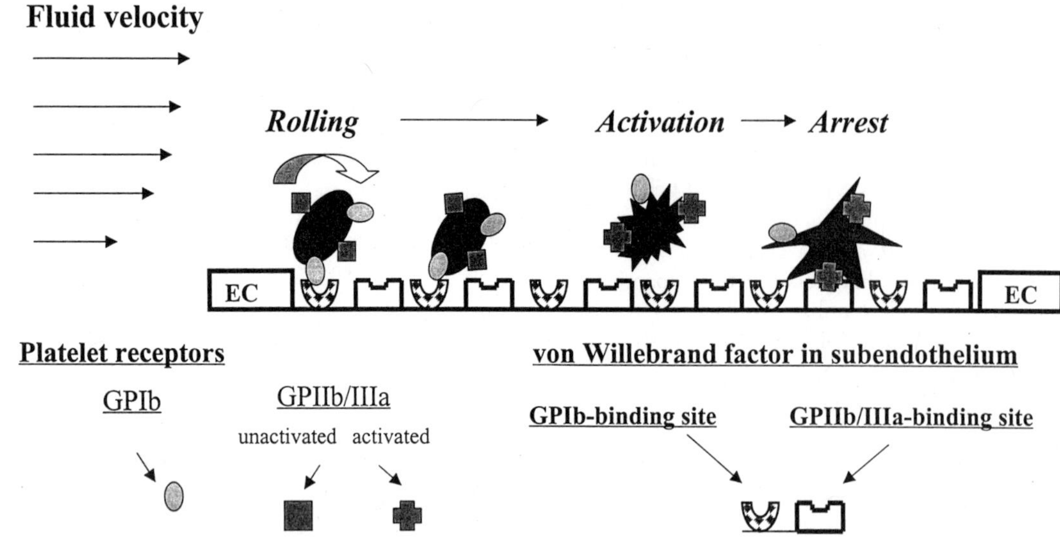

FIGURE 15.2. Adhesive mechanisms resulting in platelet adherence to subendothelial von Willebrand factor (vWF) in flowing blood. Endothelial injury exposes subendothelial collagen, which binds vWF and presents vWF attachment sites to platelets streaming along the vessel wall. GP Ib rapidly attaches to its binding site on vWF, but this adhesion is relatively weak and short lived, resulting in platelet rolling in close proximity to the subendothelium. The vWF-GP Ib interaction causes transmembrane signaling, activating the platelet, and transforming the GP IIb/IIIa receptor into a conformation, which avidly binds the RGD domain on vWF. This secondary adhesion is essentially irreversible, resulting in anchoring of the platelet to the exposed subendothelium, and allowing subsequent propagation of a platelet-fibrin clot.

with modest (50%) stenosis reach 3,000 to 10,000 sec^{-1}, and even greater shear can be seen in clinically significant stenoses. The high-velocity arterial blood flow opposes the tendency to form clot by (a) limiting the time available for localized procoagulant reactions to occur and (b) disrupting cells and proteins which are not tightly adherent to the vessel wall. However, once the vessel wall is damaged and bleeding occurs, platelets rapidly and decisively respond to the loss of endothelial integrity via their adherent mechanisms and simultaneously resist the tendency to be swept downstream.

One of the forces enhancing platelet adhesion to the vessel wall in the arterial circulation is radial dispersion, the tendency of larger cells (erythrocytes and leukocytes) to stream in the center of the vessel where shear is lowest; this phenomenon effectively pushes the smaller platelets out of the central flow and toward the vessel wall, optimally positioning platelets to respond to hemostatic challenges. This size-dependent flow may also explain the seemingly paradoxical ability of red blood cell transfusions to slow or stop bleeding simply by correcting severe anemia (44). This effect also underscores the importance of platelets in arterial hemostasis; reductions in platelet number or function may be associated with catastrophic arterial hemorrhage. By contrast, the lesser shear forces experienced in the venous circulation (20 to 200 sec^{-1}) permit more random cell movement and greater time for localized coagulation reactions to occur, making the minimal requirements for platelet number and function correspondingly less stringent than those found in the arterial circulation.

Given the velocity of blood flow at an arterial bleeding site, platelets must activate and adhere to the injured vessel nearly instantaneously. Two molecules present in the subendothelium are critical for this process: von Willebrand factor (vWF) (45) and collagen. Control of bleeding in vessels under the highest shear stresses is absolutely dependent on adequate amounts and normal function of vWF (46). A large molecule synthesized in endothelial cells and megakaryocytes, vWF polymerizes in the blood to form a range of large multimers. The largest multimeric forms of vWF, which are immobilized by adherence to exposed subendothelial collagen, bind to the glycoprotein Ib (GP Ib) receptor (47) on the platelet surface in response to high shear stress (Fig. 15.2). The binding of vWF to GP Ib is an extremely rapid but low-affinity event, which markedly slows the platelets but does not firmly adhere them to the subendothelial surface. With platelets no longer streaming by but, instead, tumbling over the subendothelium, the high shear stress in tandem with transmembrane signaling produced by the GP Ib-vWF interaction (48) results in loss of the normal platelet discoid shape (shape change) and conformational change in another critical platelet receptor, glycoprotein IIb/IIIa (GP IIb/IIIa). The conformationally activated GP IIb/IIIa can now undergo binding either to fibrinogen or to the larger vWF multimers at a locus on the vWF molecule which is distinct from the GP Ib binding epitope; this secondary adhesion of GP IIb/IIIα-vWF is a higher affinity interaction than the GP Ib-vWF bond and serves to adhere the platelet firmly to the subendothelium.

At more moderate shear, vWF-GP Ib adhesion is supplemented by a second binding mechanism produced by subendothelial collagen, which is itself an adhesive moiety capable of arresting the platelet via binding to the platelet receptor GP Ia/IIa (Table 15.2) (49). Thus, subendothelial vWF and collagen act cooperatively to initiate platelet adhesion, with the former predominating at higher shear rates. Collagen is unique as a platelet receptor in that it can act to both anchor platelets at one locus via binding to platelet GP Ia/IIa and simultaneously activate platelets at a second collagen locus by binding to platelet GP VI (50). The congenital absence of any of the critical platelet adhesion receptors, GP IIb/IIIa, GP Ib (52), GP VI (52), or GP Ia/IIa (53), results in a significant hemostatic defect, correctable only by platelet transfusion (see congenital platelet disorders, later in this chapter). Similarly, decreases in the concentration of vWF, especially the larger multimeric forms, or abnormal vWF function can predispose to bleeding (54). Once a layer of platelets is adherent to the subendothelial site of bleeding, vWF bound to GP Ib on the uppermost adherent platelets, which are exposed to flowing blood, serves to recruit additional platelets from the vascular flow into the growing platelet plug.

Platelet Activation

Platelets which become adherent to this platelet plug undergo a series of interdependent processes which are collectively referred to as "activation." Platelet activation has five major sequelae: (a) local release of adhesive ligands essential to stabilizing the platelet-platelet matrix, (b) continued recruitment of additional platelets from flowing blood, (c) vasoconstriction of smaller arteries to slow bleeding, (d) localization and acceleration of platelet-associated fibrin formation in the plug and, finally, (e) clot protection from fibrinolysis.

The basis of the platelet plug is a platelet-ligand-platelet matrix with both fibrinogen and vWF serving as bridging ligands. Both fibrinogen and vWF are stored within α granules inside the resting platelet. The α granules are translocated to the platelet external membrane with platelet activation, thereby releasing both fibrinogen and vWF to now bind to a GP IIb/IIIa receptor on each of two platelets, linking the platelets. Platelet GP IIb/IIIa undergoes a calcium-dependent conformational change during platelet activation which allows it to bind to loci containing the amino acid sequence arginine-glycine-aspartate (RGD) on either fibrinogen or vWF. Each fibrinogen molecule has two RGD sites on its polar ends and the larger vWF multimers have several RGD sites, all of which are capable of binding to conformationally altered GP IIb/IIIa and creating the platelet-ligand-platelet matrix (55). GP IIb/IIIa is the most abundant glycoprotein on the platelet surface, with approximately 50,000 copies on the *resting* platelet; additional GP IIb/IIIa receptors within the cytosol are mobilized to the surface after activation, further increasing the surface density of this critical ligand. The importance of these platelet adhesive mechanisms is underscored by the successful development of potent antiplatelet drugs which target these particular binding ligands and receptors (Table 15.3).

Platelets are continuously recruited from the blood and then cemented into the platelet plug by the actions of local agonists (collagen, epinephrine, and thrombin) and by release of additional agonists from adherent platelets into the local microenvironment. Both collagen (as noted above) and thrombin interact with specific platelet receptors to strongly activate platelets; although epinephrine by itself is not a powerful platelet agonist, stimulation of the α-adrenergic receptor on platelets primes them for synergistic activation to other agonists, even relatively weak ones like ADP. One activating compound released directly from activated platelets is thromboxane A_2, which is formed in the platelet cytosol after cyclooxygenase cleavage of arachidonic acid and then released into the clot milieu (56). Thromboxane A_2 is both a platelet agonist and a vasoconstrictor, and it is rapidly degraded to its inert by-product, thromboxane B_2. Cyclooxygenase activity is *irreversibly* inhibited by aspirin, thereby blocking thromboxane A_2 formation for the lifetime of that platelet, unlike other nonsteroidal antiinflammatory drugs (e.g., indomethacin) which *reversibly* inhibit cyclooxygenase activity for 24 to 48 hours after discontinuation of the drug.

TABLE 15.3. DRUGS WHICH INHIBIT PLATELET FUNCTION

ADP receptor blockers—clopidogrel/ticlopidine
Antibiotics (penicillins, cephalosporins, nitrofurantoin)
Anti-GP IIb/IIIa or anti-RGD compounds (abciximab, eptifibatide [Integrilin])
Aspirin
Heparin (both unfractionated and low-molecular-weight)
Hetastarch
Nitroglycerin
Nitroprusside
Nonsteroidal antiinflammatory drugs (NSAIDs, COX-1/2 nonselective)

Other platelet agonists are liberated into the clot microenvironment by fusion of platelet dense and α granules with the platelet external membrane, producing extrusion of granule contents (Table 15.2). α Granules contain adhesive proteins (fibrinogen, fibronectin, vWF, and thrombospondin), which contribute to platelet aggregation upon release into the extracellular milieu. α-Granule translocation to the platelet membrane also results in external expression of P-selectin, which contributes directly to platelet-heterotypic cell adhesion (57). Adherence of activated platelets via P-selectin to neutrophils and monocytes in the blood has been demonstrated to be a marker for platelet activation in several clinical circumstances, including cardiopulmonary bypass (58), thrombotic thrombocytopenic purpura (59), and unstable coronary syndromes (60). This P-selectin–mediated adhesive interaction may serve to target heterotypic cell populations to areas of inflammation or thrombosis (61), upregulate procoagulant (tissue factor) (62) and/or inflammatory (TNFα) activity (63), as well as promote transcellular metabolic cooperation (64).

Platelet-dense granules contain serotonin which, like thromboxane A_2, is both a platelet agonist and a vasoconstrictor (65). Another dense granule constituent, ADP, acts purely as a platelet agonist without vasoactive properties (Table 15.2). The importance of thromboxane A_2- and serotonin-induced vasoconstriction is not entirely clear; however, vasoconstriction, by decreasing the vessel diameter, may increase shear stress and thereby facilitate additional recruitment of platelets to the injured site. The importance of dense granule release to the maintenance of hemostasis is manifested by the severe hemorrhage noted in patients with congenital dense-granule deficiencies (e.g., Hermansky-Pudlak syndrome and storage pool disease). Platelet activation therefore serves to amplify platelet adhesion and optimize the platelet surface for fibrin-generating procoagulant activity by interaction of platelets with the soluble coagulation cascade.

Platelet Interaction with Soluble Coagulation Factors

Tissue injury and low levels of circulating activated clotting factors physiologically initiate the clotting cascade, which is then propagated by clotting enzyme complexes that function most effectively on a phospholipid membrane surface, predominantly supplied by platelets. Tissue factor expressed after EC injury binds to circulating VIIa, and the VIIa-TF complex subsequently binds to its zymogen substrates, IX and X, on the activated platelet membrane to form the extrinsic "tenase" complex (66). Activated platelets undergo a redistribution of membrane phospholipids, increasing the external membrane expression of the negatively charged, procoagulant phosphatidylserine (PS) moiety. PS on the platelet surface can be detected either by calcium-dependent binding to annexin V or procoagulant assays, the latter because PS on the activated platelet surface enhances both the tenase and prothrombinase reactions. Activated platelets also provide specific receptors for factors Xa, IXa, and Va (67); factor V is also secreted from the α granule of the activated platelet, and platelet-derived V appears to contribute to the overall function of factor V derived from the plasma pool (68). These platelet-bound coagulation factors are spatially oriented in the platelet plasma membrane such that they interact closely with PS; this physical association not only accelerates procoagulant enzymatic reactions, it simultaneously protects the activated factors on the platelet surface from circulating inhibitors, culminating in accelerated thrombin generation (69).

Physiologic clotting can therefore be modeled as follows: TF-VIIa converts X to Xa and IX to IXa, both of which are bound to platelet receptors. The intrinsic tenase complex on the platelet membrane is formed initially by TF-induced IXa formation; IXa binds to its cofactor, VIIIa, and its zymogen substrate X to amplify production of Xa on the platelet surface (Fig. 15.3). The platelet Xa receptor is closely associated with platelet-bound Va; together with free Ca^{2+} and platelet membrane PS, these factors bind prothrombin (II) to form the prothrombinase complex (70), thereby generating thrombin, albeit in relatively small amounts (Fig. 15.3). This initially formed thrombin feeds back to activate VIII to VIIIa (which binds to platelet-bound IXa), V to Va (which binds to its platelet receptor), and XI to XIa. Once these initial amounts of thrombin activate more platelets and generate appreciable quantities of XIa (71) and cofactors Va and VIIIa on the platelet surface (72), activation of the more kinetically favorable intrinsic pathway occurs to amplify the clotting cascade, thereby increasing the rate of Xa and thrombin generation exponentially (73).

This rapid thrombin generation cleaves fibrinogen to fibrin monomers, which rapidly combine to form a fibrin matrix integrated with adherent platelets. Factor XIIIa, a transamidase produced by the action of thrombin on either plasma or platelet-released XIII, converts the soluble fibrin clot into an insoluble fibrin polymer and effectively incorporates α2-antiplasmin into the clot to inhibit plasmin-mediated dissolution (74). Finally,

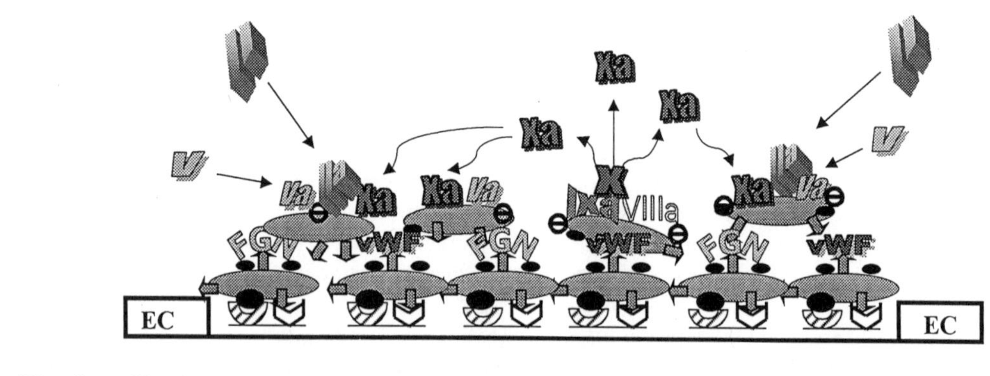

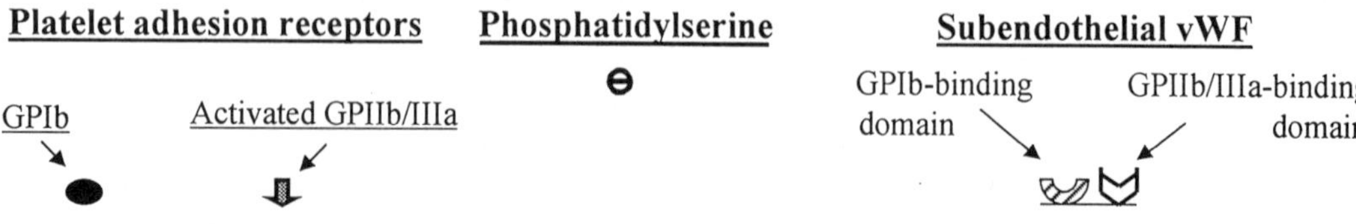

FIGURE 15.3. Activated platelet interaction with the soluble coagulation cascade. Platelets which are adherent to a thrombus via vWF and fibrinogen become activated and express the procoagulant phospholipid moiety phosphatidylserine (PS) on the external surface of the platelet membrane. Circulating activated factor IXa binds to its specific receptor on the platelet surface and to its cofactor, VIIIa, as well as its zymogen substrate, unactivated X. In combination with calcium and PS, this intrinsic tenase complex amplifies production of Xa on the platelet surface, and both Xa and Va (either plasma- or platelet-derived) bind to their closely associated platelet surface receptors, thereby forming the prothrombinase complex when their zymogen substrate, II, is subsequently bound, again in combination with calcium and PS. Thrombin generation in this manner feeds back on itself to further activate platelets and the intrinsic clotting pathways.

the platelet plug undergoes clot retraction, which additionally protects the platelet-fibrin matrices from lysis by plasmin (75). These antilytic mechanisms, largely linked to platelet activation, may explain the relative resistance of platelet-rich clots to thrombolysis.

Acquired Qualitative Platelet Defects

Normal platelet function, the ability of platelets to adhere to damaged vessels and to recruit additional platelets into the clot, is critical for primary hemostasis, especially when patients are hemostatically challenged by trauma or surgery. Aspirin irreversibly acetylates cyclooxygenase and thereby blocks normal arachidonic acid metabolism. All exposed platelets are irreversibly affected and will not respond to arachidonic acid for their lifetimes even if aspirin is discontinued. Nonsteroidal antiinflammatory drugs (e.g., indomethacin) *reversibly* inhibit cyclooxygenase; platelet function is restored within 24 to 48 hours after discontinuation of the drug. Yet surgical bleeding in the setting of concomitant aspirin or nonsteroidal antiinflammatory drug therapy is usually mild (76), and aspirin is often continued through surgery in patients who are at risk for stroke or myocardial infarction. However, excessive bleeding due to aspirin-induced platelet dysfunction may require treatment. Desmopressin acetate (DDAVP; [1-deamino, 8-D-arginine] vasopressin) has been shown to shorten the bleeding time and reduce bleeding in patients with aspirin-induced platelet dysfunction (77); transfusion of platelets is appropriate when DDAVP by itself does not restore hemostasis. In most cases, platelet transfusion consisting of four to six random donor units or a single apheresis unit will restore primary hemostasis in aspirin-treated patients. Platelet dysfunction and bleeding caused by other drugs (Table 15.3) can be similarly treated by discontinuation of the drug, administration of DDAVP, and if necessary, platelet transfusion (78).

Uremic bleeding is caused by proteins which accumulate in renal failure and which effectively poison platelet adhesive function (79). Control of renal failure with dialysis and maintenance of the hematocrit will usually preserve platelet function, but bleeding with acute renal failure is a common inpatient problem. Acute treatment of uremic platelet dysfunction includes DDAVP, which has been shown to shorten the bleeding time significantly, or cryoprecipitate (80). Platelet transfusions may also be useful in life-threatening bleeding with acute renal failure, but this effect is short lived because the transfused platelets rapidly acquire the uremic defect. Long-term estrogen therapy has also been shown to be efficacious in patients with renal failure who are prone to hemorrhage.

Congenital Platelet Dysfunction

Inherited qualitative platelet defects include abnormalities of platelet receptors, platelet procoagulant activity, and granules. Two relatively rare, but well-characterized, platelet receptor disorders are Bernard-Soulier syndrome (BSS) (81) and Glanzmann thrombasthenia (GT) (82). BSS is caused by decreased surface expression of platelet GP Ib (the primary vWF receptor) and more rarely by normal antigenic expression of GP Ib but diminished GP Ib function, a mutation that blocks vWF binding to platelets. BSS is characterized by mild thrombocytopenia, an increased bleeding time, large platelets, and a mild-to-moderate bleeding disorder. The diagnosis is usually made in children but occasionally may not be manifest until adulthood. Laboratory testing for BSS shows an absent platelet aggregation response to ristocetin despite having adequate plasma vWF antigenic levels and a normal ristocetin cofactor activity in plasma. GT is characterized by an increased bleeding time and abnormally low levels of platelet GP IIb/IIIa expression (the receptor for both vWF and fibrinogen) or more rarely, normal expression but absent GP IIb/IIIa function. Patients commonly seek treatment for bleeding in childhood. Platelet aggregation testing in GT shows absent or diminished response to all agonists (ADP, epinephrine, collagen, arachidonic acid) except ristocetin, which agglutinates platelets primarily through GP Ib interaction. Platelet transfusions are effective for bleeding symptoms in both BSS and GT. However, because of the high risk of alloimmunization with frequent platelet transfusions (83) this therapy is usually reserved for life-threatening bleeding, and most patients are successfully managed with conservative therapy.

Inherited platelet granule disorders are defined by the type of granule which is absent or defective (84). Storage pool disease is characterized by a relative decrease or absence of dense granules, resulting in symptoms of moderate-to-severe mucosal bleeding. Defective release of dense granule constituents impairs the ability of platelets themselves to recruit and activate other platelets in the microenvironment. The laboratory diagnosis of storage pool disease is characterized by diminished or absent secondary wave aggregation to weak platelet agonists such as ADP (85). Hermansky-Pudlak syndrome is one form of dense-granule deficiency, which is accompanied by oculocutaneous albinism and mild thrombocytopenia. Patients with Hermansky-Pudlak syndrome demonstrate excessive bleeding with trauma or surgery and occasionally have spontaneous bleeding. Chediak-Higashi disease is a general granule disorder characterized by mild bleeding, partial albinism, and recurrent pyogenic infections. Gray platelet syndrome is characterized by platelets which lack the normal staining on the peripheral smear; electron microscopy has confirmed the absence of α granules and/or their contents (86). Patients with gray platelet syndrome have a mild bleeding history, and aggregation testing exhibits diminished responses to epinephrine, ADP, and collagen. Patients with platelet granule disorders are successfully treated by avoidance of aspirin and other antiplatelet drugs (Table 15.3), hormonal control of menses, and when bleeding occurs, with platelet transfusions.

Patients with bleeding due to Scott syndrome (87) have normal platelet aggregation and secretion (88), but their platelets are unable to translocate anionic phospholipids from the internal to the external platelet membrane with platelet activation (89). Examination of this platelet lesion has further demonstrated impairment in the ability to generate platelet microparticles in response to agonist, as well as a decrease in the number and function of inducible factor Va receptors on the platelet surface. Thus, platelets in Scott syndrome do not provide a membrane surface that optimally provides sites for assembly of the intrinsic tenase and prothrombinase complexes (90). Like other rare disorders of platelet procoagulant function (Factor V Quebec, a platelet defect in which most proteins of the α granules are probably degraded) (91,92), platelet transfusion is effective for clinically significant bleeding symptoms.

Platelet Survival and Function After Transfusion

Preparation and storage of platelets for subsequent transfusion results in a lesion characterized by partial platelet activation and some loss of metabolic function. Functionally, the platelets' ability to aggregate to agonists declines, and platelet-matrix adhesion capabilities are similarly compromised as measured by in vitro assays (93–95), described in more detail in Chapter 17. The longer platelets are stored, the shorter their subsequent survival in animal models (96), but in humans, the clinical status of the transfusion recipient may significantly influence the initial recovery and subsequent survival of transfused platelets (97). However, despite these factors and the platelet storage lesion, a significant proportion of transfused platelets will appear in the circulation and restore hemostasis in patients bleeding from thrombocytopenia or platelet dysfunction. In a study of patients with chemotherapy-induced thrombocytopenia, platelet transfusion resulted in an immediate increase in whole blood platelet aggregation and ATP release, and this effect persisted for several hours, suggesting that transfused platelets do not require acclimation in order to regain function posttransfusion. In human studies, modeling of platelet survival has suggested that stored platelets can survive after transfusion for an average of 6 days (98), and these findings have been confirmed by in vivo studies in humans (99,100). Thus, a major challenge in transfusion therapy, rather than simply providing functional platelets for transfusion, has been to find ways to preserve stored platelets for longer periods without compromising function or increasing the risk of bacterial contamination.

SUMMARY

Platelet survival in the circulation is dependent on the complex interplay of megakaryocyte production and release, platelet distribution within the spleen, and the clearance of platelets by senescence and hemostatic mechanisms. The pathologic processes that impose abnormal clearance may be detected by the enumeration of young RP in the circulation. Our understanding of the numerous and redundant hemostatic mechanisms residing within platelets has led to an improved ability to treat platelet dysfunction and bleeding and, conversely, to better strategies for blocking pathologic platelet-dependent thromboses. The investigation of platelet kinetics and hemostasis will ideally result in stored platelets for transfusion with preserved ability to maintain physiologic molecular interactions and provide maximum hemostatic benefit to the transfusion recipient.

REFERENCES

1. Surgenor DM, Wallace EL, Hao SHS, et al. Collection and transfusion of blood in the United States, 1982–1988. *N Engl J Med* 1990; 322:1646–1652.
2. Holme S, Heaton A, Roodt J. Concurrent label method with ^{111}In and ^{51}Cr allows accurate evaluation of platelet viability of stored platelet concentrates. *Brit J Haematol* 1993;84:717–723.
3. Harker LA, Finch CA. Thrombokinetics in man. *J Clin Invest* 1969; 48:963–974.
4. Catalano PM, Smith JB, Murphy S. Platelet recovery from aspirin inhibition in vivo: differing patterns under various assay conditions. *Blood* 1981;57:99–105.
5. Chamberlain KG, Tong M, Chiu E. The relationship of human platelet density to platelet age: platelet population labeling by monoamine oxidase inhibition. *Blood* 1989;73:1218–1225.
6. Kienast J, Schmitz G. Flow cytometric analysis of thiazole orange uptake by platelets: a diagnostic aid in the evaluation of thrombocytopenic disorders. *Blood* 1990;75:116–121.
7. Ault KA, Knowles C. In vivo biotinylation demonstrates that reticulated platelets are the youngest platelets in circulation. *Exp Hematol* 1995;23:996–1001.
8. Dale GL, Friese P, Hynes LA. Demonstration that thiazole orange–positive platelets in the dog are less than 24 hours old. *Blood* 1995;85:1822–1825.
9. Ault KA, Rinder HM, Mitchell JG, et al. The significance of platelets with increased RNA content (reticulated platelets): a measure of the rate of thrombopoiesis? *Am J Clin Pathol* 1992;98:637–646.
10. Rinder HM, Munz U, Ault KA, et al. Utility of reticulated platelets in the evaluation of thrombopoietic disorders. *Arch Pathol Lab Med* 1993;117:606–610.
11. Richards EM, Baglin TP. Quantitation of reticulated platelets: methodologic and clinical application. *Br J Haematol* 1995;91:445–451.
12. Bonan JL, Rinder HM, Smith BR. Determination of the percentage of thiazole orange (TO)-positive "reticulated" platelets using autologous erythrocyte TO fluorescence as an internal standard. *Cytometry* 1993; 14:790–794.
13. Saxon BR, Mody M, Blanchette VS, et al. Reticulated platelet counts in the assessment of thrombocytopenic disorders. *Acta Paediatr* 1998; 424[Suppl]:65–70.
14. Rinder HM, Smith BR, Ault KA. Stress thrombocytes are detectable in blood and predict imminent recovery from chemotherapy-induced thrombocytopenia. *Blood* 2000;96[Suppl]:260a.
15. Aster RH. Pooling of platelets in the spleen: role in the pathogenesis of "hypersplenic" thrombocytopenia. *J Clin Invest* 1966;45:645–657.
16. Heyns ADP, Lotter MG, Badenhorst PN. Kinetics, distribution, and sites of destruction of ^{111}In-labeled human platelets. *Brit J Haematol* 1980;44:269–280.
17. Hill-Zobek RL, McCandless B, Kang SA. Organ distribution and fate of human platelets: studies of asplenic and splenomegalic individuals. *Am J Hematol* 1986;23:231–238.
18. Kutti J, Safai-Kutti S. In vitro labeling of platelets: an experimental study on healthy asplenic subjects using two different incubation media. *Br J Haematol* 1975;31:57–64.
19. Dale GL, Wolf RF, Hynes LA. Quantitation of platelet lifespan in splenectomized dogs. *Exp Hematol* 1996;24:518–523.
20. Heyns ADP, Badenhorst PN, Lotter MG. Platelet turnover and kinetics in immune thrombocytopenic purpura: results with autologous ^{111}In-labeled platelets and homologous ^{51}Cr-labeled platelets. *Blood* 1986;67:86–92.
21. Hersh JK, Hom EG, Brecher ME. Mathematical modeling of platelet survival with implications for optimal transfusion practice in the chronically platelet transfusion–dependent patient. *Transfusion* 1998; 38:637–644.
22. Kotze HF, van Wyk V, Badenhorst PN. Influence of platelet membrane sialic acid and platelet-associated IgG on aging and sequestration of blood platelets in baboons. *Thromb Haemost* 1993;70: 676–680.
23. Hanson SR, Slichter SJ. Platelet kinetics with bone marrow hypoplasia: evidence for fixed platelet requirement. *Blood* 1985;66: 1105–1109.
24. Romp KG, Peters WP, Hoffman M. Reticulated platelet counts in patients undergoing autologous bone marrow transplantation: an aid in assessing marrow recovery. *Am J Hematol* 1994;46:319–324.
25. Rinder HM, Bonan JL, Anandan S, et al. Noninvasive measurement

of platelet kinetics in normal and hypertensive pregnancies. *Am J Obstet Gynecol* 1994;170:117–122.
26. Rinder HM, Schuster JE, Rinder CS, et al. Correlation of thrombosis with increased platelet turnover in thrombocytosis. *Blood* 1998;91: 1288–1294.
27. Van Genderen PJ, Lucas IS, van Strik R, et al. Platelet consumption in thrombocythemia complicated by erythromelalgia: reversal by aspirin. *Thromb Haemost* 1995;73:210–219.
28. Currie LM, Lichtiger B, Livesey SA, et al. Enhanced circulatory parameters of human platelets cryopreserved with second messenger effectors: an in vivo study of 16 volunteer platelet donors. *Brit J Haematol* 1999;105:826–831.
29. Isarangkura P, Tuchinda S. The behavior of transfused platelets in dengue hemorrhagic fever. *Southeast Asian J Trop Med Public Health* 1993;24:222–224.
30. Hussein MA, Fletcher R, Long TJ, et al. Transfusing platelets 2 h after the completion of amphotericin-B decreases its detrimental effect on transfused platelet recovery and survival. *Transfus Med* 1998;8: 43–47.
31. Herman J. Platelet transfusion therapy. In: Mintz PD, ed. *Transfusion therapy: clinical principles and practice.* American Association of Blood Banks, 1999:65–79.
32. Kuwana M, Kaburaki J, Ikeda Y. Autoreactive T cells to platelet GPIIb-IIIa in immune thrombocytopenic purpura. Role in production of anti-platelet autoantibody. *J Clin Invest* 1998;102:1393–1402.
33. Wright JF, Blanchette VS, Wang H, et al. Characterization of platelet-reactive antibodies in children with varicella-associated acute immune thrombocytopenic purpura (ITP). *Br J Haematol* 1996;95:145–152.
34. Adams WH, Liu YK, Sullivan LW. Humoral regulation of thrombopoiesis in man. *J Lab Clin Med* 1978;91:941–947.
35. Scaradavou A, Bussel JB. Clinical experience with anti-D in the treatment of idiopathic thrombocytopenic purpura. *Semin Hematol* 1998; 35:52–57.
36. Gewirtz AM. Human megakaryocytopoiesis. *Semin Hematol* 1986; 23:27–42.
37. Chandramouli NB, Rodgers GM. Prolonged immunoglobulin and platelet infusion for treatment of immune thrombocytopenia. *Am J Hematol* 2000;65:85–86.
38. Hirsh J, Glynn MF, Mustard JF. The effect of platelet age on platelet adherence to collagen. *J Clin Invest* 1968;47:466–473.
39. Peng J, Friese P, Heilmann E. Aged platelets have an impaired response to thrombin as quantitated by P-selectin expression. *Blood* 1994;83:161–166.
40. Rinder HM, Tracey JB, Recht M, et al. Differences in platelet α-granule release between normals and immune thrombocytopenic patients and between young and old platelets. *Thromb Haemost* 1998; 80:457–462.
41. Marcus AJ, Safier SV, Hajjar KA, et al. Inhibition of platelet function by an aspirin-insensitive endothelial cell ADPase: thromboregulation by endothelial cells. *J Clin Invest* 1991;88:1690.
42. Marcus AJ, Broekman MJ, Drosopuolos JH, et al. The endothelial cell ecto-ADPase responsible for inhibition of platelet function is CD39. *J Clin Invest* 1997;99:1351–1360.
43. Ruggeri ZM. Mechanisms initiating platelet thrombus formation. *Thromb Haemostas* 1997;78:611–616.
44. Livio M, Gotti E, Marchesi D, et al. Uraemic bleeding: role of anaemia and beneficial effect of red cell transfusions. *Lancet* 1982;2: 1013–1015.
45. Ikeda Y, Handa M, Kawano K. The role of von Willebrand factor and fibrinogen in platelet aggregation under varying shear stress. *J Clin Invest* 1991;87:1234.
46. Ruggeri ZM. von Willebrand Factor. *J Clin Invest* 1997;99:559–564.
47. Ruggeri ZM, Dent JA, Saldivar E. Contribution of distinct adhesive interactions to platelet aggregation in flowing blood. *Blood* 1999;94: 172–178.
48. Kroll MH, Harris TS, Moake HL, et al. von Willebrand factor binding to platelet gpIb initiates signals for platelet activation. *J Clin Invest* 1991;88:1568–1573.
49. Saelman EUM, Niewenhuis HK, Hese KM, et al. Platelet adhesion to collagen types I through VIII under conditions of stasis and flow is mediated by GPIa/IIa. *Blood* 1994;83:1244–1250.
50. Kehrel B, Wierwille S, Clemetson KJ, et al. Glycoprotein VI is a major collagen receptor for platelet activation: it recognizes the platelet-activating quaternary structure of collagen, whereas CD36, glycoprotein IIb/IIIa, and von Willebrand factor do not. *Blood* 1998;91: 491–499.
51. Dunlop LC, Andrews RK, Lopez JA, et al. Congenital disorders of platelet function. In: Loscalzo J, Shafer A, eds. *Thrombosis and hemorrhage.* Baltimore: Williams & Wilkins, 1998:685–689.
52. Moroi M, Jung SM, Okuma M, et al. A patients with platelets deficient in glycoprotein VI that lack both collagen-induced aggregation and adhesion. *J Clin Invest* 1989;84:1440–1445.
53. Nieuwenhuis HK, Akkerman JWN, Houdijk WPM, et al. Human blood platelets showing no response to collagen fail to express surface glycoprotein Ia. *Nature* 1985;318:4770–4772.
54. Nichols WC, Coone KA, Ginsburg D, et al. von Willebrand disease. In: Loscalzo J, Shafer A, eds. *Thrombosis and hemorrhage.* Baltimore: Williams & Wilkins, 1998:729–756.
55. Lefkovits J, Plow EF, Topol EJ. Platelet glycoprotein IIb/IIIa receptors in cardiovascular medicine. *N Engl J Med* 1995;332:1553–1559.
56. Zucker MB, Nachmias VT. Platelet activation. *Arteriosclerosis* 1985; 5:2–18.
57. Hamburger SA, McEver RP. GMP-140 mediates adhesion of stimulated platelets to neutrophils. *Blood* 1990;75:550–558.
58. Rinder CS, Bonan JL, Rinder HM, et al. Cardiopulmonary bypass induces leukocyte-platelet adhesion. *Blood* 1992;79:1201–1205.
59. Smith BR, Rinder HM. Interactions of platelets and endothelial cells with erythrocytes and leukocytes in thrombotic thrombocytopenic purpura. *Semin Hematol* 1997;34:90–97.
60. Ott I, Neumann FJ, Gawaz M, et al. Increased neutrophil-platelet adhesion in patients with unstable angina. *Circulation* 1996;94: 1239–1246.
61. Lefer A, Campbell B, Scalia T. Synergism between platelets and neutrophils in provoking cardiac dysfunction after ischemia and reperfusion. *Circulation* 1998;98:1322–1328.
62. Osterud B. Tissue factor expression by monocytes: regulation and pathophysiological roles. *Blood Coagul Fibrinolysis* 1998;9[Suppl 1]: 9–14.
63. Koike J, Nagata K, Kudo S, et al. Density-dependent induction of TNFα release from human monocytes by immobilized P-selectin. *FEB S Letters* 2000;477:84–88.
64. Marcus AJ. Thrombosis and inflammation as multicellular processes: pathophysiologic significance of transcellular metabolism. *Blood* 1990; 76:1903–1907.
65. Anderson GM, Hall LM, Yang JX, et al. Platelet dense granule release reaction monitored by HPLC-fluorometric determination of endogenous serotonin. *Anal Biochem* 1992;206:64.
66. Rapaport SI. Regulation of the tissue factor pathway. In: Ruggeri ZM, Fulcher CA, Ware J, eds. *Progress in vascular biology, hemostasis, and thrombosis.* New York: New York Academy of Sciences, 1991: 51.
67. Scandura JM, Walsh PN. Factor X bound to the surface of activated human platelets is preferentially activated by platelet-bound factor IXa. *Biochemistry* 1996;35:8890–8901.
68. Camire RM, Pollak ES, Kaushansky K, et al. Secretable human platelet–derived factor V originates from the plasma pool. *Blood* 1998; 92:3035–3041.
69. Swords NA, Mann KG. The assembly of the prothrombinase complex on adherent platelets. *Arterioscler Thromb* 1993;13:1602–1612.
70. Larson PJ, Camire RM, Wong D, et al. Structure/function analyses of recombinant variants of human factor Xa: factor Xa incorporation into prothrombinase on the thrombin-activated platelet surface is not mimicked by synthetic phospholipid vesicles. *Biochemistry* 1998;37: 5029–5038.
71. Gailani D, Broze GJ Jr. Factor XI activation in a revised model of blood coagulation. *Science* 1991;253:909.
72. Mann KG, Bovill EG, Krishnaswamy S. Surface-dependent reactions in the propagation phase of blood coagulation. In: Ruggeri ZM,

Fulcher CA, Ware J, eds. *Progress in vascular biology, hemostasis, and thrombosis.* New York: New York Academy of Sciences, 1991:63.
73. Ofosu FA, Longbin L, Freedman J. Control mechanisms in thrombin generation. *Semin Thromb Hemost* 1996;22:303–308.
74. Muszbek L, Pogar J, Boda Z. Platelet factor XIII becomes active without the release of activation peptide during platelet activation. *Thromb Haemost* 1993;69:282–285.
75. Braaten JV, Jerome WG, Hantgan RR. Uncoupling fibrin from integrin receptors hastens fibrinolysis at the platelet-fibrin interface. *Blood* 1994;83:982–993.
76. Schafer AI. Effects of nonsteroidal anti-inflammatory therapy on platelets. *Am J Med* 1999;106:25s–36s.
77. Flordal PA, Sahlin S. Use of desmopressin to prevent bleeding complications in patients treated with aspirin. *Brit J Surg* 1993;80:723–724.
78. George JN, Shattil SJ. The clinical importance of acquired abnormalities of platelet function. *N Engl J Med* 1991;324:327.
79. Escolar G, Cases A, Bastida E. Uremic platelets have a functional defect affecting the interaction of von Willebrand factor with glycoprotein IIb-IIIa. *Blood* 1990;76:1336.
80. Remuzzi G. Bleeding in renal failure. *Lancet* 1988;1:1205–1208.
81. Nurden AT, Caen JP. Specific roles for platelet surface glycoproteins in platelet function. *Nature* 1975;255:720–722.
82. Degos L, Dautigny A, Brouet JC, et al. A molecular defect in thrombasthenic platelets. *J Clin Invest* 1975;56:236–245.
83. Kunicki TJ, Bull B, Furihata K, et al. The immunogenicity of platelet membrane glycoproteins. *Transfus Med Rev* 1987;1:21–33.
84. Weiss HJ, Witte LD, Kaplan KL. Heterogeneity in storage pool deficiency: studies on granule-bound substances in 18 patients including variants deficient in α granules, platelet factor 4, β thromboglobulin, and platelet derived growth factor. *Blood* 1979;54:1296–1319.
85. White JG, Gerrard JM. Ultrastructural features of abnormal blood platelets. *Am J Pathol* 1976;83:590–632.
86. White JG. Ultrastructural studies of the gray platelet syndrome. *Am Assoc Pathol* 1979;95:445–453.
87. Weiss HJ, Lages B. Platelet prothrombinase activity and intracellular calcium responses in patients with storage pool deficiency, glycoprotein IIb-IIIa deficiency, or impaired platelet coagulant activity—a comparison with Scott syndrome. *Blood* 1997;89:1599–1611.
88. Weiss HJ. Scott syndrome: a disorder of platelet coagulant activity. *Semin Hematol* 1994;31:312–319.
89. Sims PJ, Wiedmer T, Esmon CT, et al. Assembly of the platelet prothrombinase complex is linked to vesiculation of the platelet plasma membrane. Studies in Scott syndrome: an isolated defect in platelet procoagulant activity. *J Biol Chem* 1989;264:17049–17057.
90. Rosing J, Bevers EM, Comfurius P. Impaired factor X and prothrombin activation associated with decreased phospholipid exposure in platelets from an individual with a bleeding disorder. *Blood* 1985;65:1557–1561.
91. Tracy PB, Giles AR, Mann KG. Factor V Quebec: a bleeding diathesis associated with a qualitative platelet factor V deficiency. *J Clin Invest* 1984;74:1221–1228.
92. Janeway CM, Rivard GE, Tracy PB, et al. Factor V Quebec revisited. *Blood* 1996;87:3571–3578.
93. Seghatchian J, Krailadsiri P. The platelet storage lesion. *Transfus Med Rev* 1997;11:130–144.
94. Rosenfeld BA, Herfel B, Faraday N, et al. Effects of storage time on quantitative and qualitative platelet function after transfusion. *Anesthesiology* 1995;83:1167–1172.
95. Boomgaard MN, Gouwerok CWN, Homburg CHE, et al. Platelet adhesion capacity to subendothelial matrix and collagen in a flow model during storage of platelet concentrates for 7 days. *Thromb Haemost* 1994;72:611–616.
96. Rothwell SW, Maglasnag P, Krishnamurti C. Survival of fresh human platelets in a rabbit model as traced by flow cytometry. *Transfusion* 1998;38:550–556.
97. Norol F, Kuentz M, Cordonnier C, et al. Influence of clinical status on the efficiency of stored platelet transfusion. *Brit J Haematol* 1994;86:125–129.
98. Saeki Y, Tada K, Sano T, et al. Platelet kinetics after transfusion. *Biopharm Drug Dispos* 1996;17:71–79.
99. Holme S, Heaton A. In vitro platelet aging at 22°C is reduced compared to in vivo aging at 37°C. *Brit J Haematol* 1995;91:212–218.
100. Holme S, Heaton WA, Whitley P. Platelet storage lesions in second-generation containers: correlation with in vivo behavior for up to 14 days. *Vox Sang* 1990;59:12–18.

16

PLATELET IMMUNOLOGY AND ALLOIMMUNIZATION

BRIAN R. CURTIS
JEROME L. GOTTSCHALL
JANICE G. MCFARLAND

Platelets express a variety of immunogenic markers on the cell surface. Some of these antigens are shared with other cell types as in the case of human leukocyte antigens (HLAs), which are shared with virtually all nucleated cells in the body; whereas others are observed to be essentially platelet specific. This chapter will review the antigens expressed on the platelet, the various patterns of alloimmunization to these antigens, and their impact on platelet transfusion responses. Strategies to treat and prevent alloimmunization will also be summarized.

ANTIGENS ON THE PLATELET SURFACE

Antigens Shared with Other Tissues

HLA Antigens

Class I HLA antigens are the principal antigens shared by platelets and lymphocytes. Indeed, platelets are the major source of Class I HLA antigens in whole blood.

Although platelets ultimately derive from nucleated precursors (the megakaryocytes) and hence might be anticipated to acquire their HLA antigens through mechanisms in common with other nucleated cells, consensus as to the source of Class I HLA structures in circulating, mature platelets has developed only recently. Early studies (1,2) demonstrated that, in vitro, platelets do absorb and express soluble HLA antigens after incubation in plasma. Other studies showing that Class I HLA molecules can apparently be eluted from platelets by incubation in low pH chloroquine or citrate solutions (3,4) suggested that these antigens were not firmly embedded in the membrane and were likely absorbed from the surrounding plasma. These studies suggested that HLA absorbed from plasma contributed significantly to the total Class I HLA present on platelets. However, only small amounts of HLA were absorbed by platelets in these studies, and it is now recognized that low-pH treatment of platelets does not "strip" the Class I HLA heavy chain from the cell membrane of platelets. Rather, acid treatment of platelets actually disrupts the trimolecular complex of Class I HLA heavy chain, peptide, and β2-microglobulin, destroying antigenic epitopes and preventing the binding of specific HLA antibodies (5, 6).

More recent evidence indicates that most Class I HLA molecules on platelets are integral membrane proteins persisting from the megakaryocyte stage of development. Phorbol ester stimulation of platelets results in phosphorylation of their HLA molecules, which is consistent with these molecules being an integral part of the platelet membrane (7). mRNA from platelets is capable of producing small amounts of Class I HLA (8). Peptides presented by HLA-A2 molecules on human platelets have been isolated and sequenced, and most of these peptides are com-

B.R. Curtis, J.L. Gottschall, and J.G. McFarland: The Blood Center of Southeastern Wisconsin, Inc., Milwaukee, Wisconsin.

monly expressed by HLA-A2 on nucleated cells (6). One ubiquitously expressed peptide is derived from the megakaryocyte-platelet–specific GP IX glycoprotein. Detectable Class I HLA surface molecules that were removed by treatment with pH 3.0 citrate could be restored only after addition of exogenous β2-microglobulin and peptide ligand, indicating that platelets themselves are not able to load HLA molecules with endogenous peptides, but that this occurs during HLA protein synthesis at the megakaryocyte stage (6). The vast majority of Class I HLA molecules on platelets are intrinsic transmembrane proteins synthesized and acquired at the megakaryocyte stage before platelets become cytoplasmic fragments (5–9).

Another controversy centers around the number of Class I HLA molecules expressed on the platelet surface. Estimates vary from approximately 15,000 to 120,000 (10,11). Using a direct assay with a ^{125}I-labeled monoclonal antibody specific for the Fc portion of human immunoglobulin G (IgG), the number of anti-HLA Ig molecules binding to specific HLA antigens at saturation ranged from 870 to 11,000 per platelet per antigen, depending on the antigen (10). The same number of Class I HLA antigens on platelets were found in a study of density-fractionated platelets (12). A competitive binding assay to quantitate platelet-associated HLA found a much higher number of molecules per platelet (up to 120,000) (11). A mean of 81,587 molecules per platelet was found in 12 healthy individuals.

Several studies attempting to quantitate HLA on platelets demonstrated variable expression of specific antigens in different individuals (10,13,14). The covariation of the quantity of Bw4/6 antigens with specific private HLA-B antigens and the variability of B44 expression have been repeatedly demonstrated (10, 14). Platelets from the same individual also seem to differ in HLA antigen expression in that lower-density platelet cohorts were found to have 42% more HLA-A2 molecules than high-density cohorts (12). More recently, variability in A2, B35, and B62 antigen expression on platelets was measured among different individuals. Here again the levels of specific antigens varied three- to five-fold among individuals and also on the platelets of the same individual (13).

Only Class I HLA molecules appear to be present on the platelet membrane, and of the Class I loci, only the A and B antigens are significantly represented (15). An exception is detection of Class II structures on platelets of a patient with acute autoimmune thrombocytopenia (16). Although Class II antigens have been detected on megakaryoblasts from patients with myeloproliferative diseases and in colony-forming unit–megakaryoblast colonies in cultures of normal bone marrow, this was the first report of Class II antigen expression on circulating platelets. The implications of this finding in the pathogenesis of autoimmunity are intriguing.

ABH Blood Group Antigens

Second only to HLA, the ABH blood group system is an important non–platelet-specific antigen system on platelets. Similar to HLA antigens, the amount of ABH substance on platelets varies not only from person to person but also among platelets in the same person. The variable distribution of group A substance has been demonstrated on platelets using flow cytometry (17). This distribution of ABH could explain why, in some platelet transfusions, there is a rapid destruction of a subset of ABO-incompatible cells followed by near-normal survival of the remaining cells (18). Greater recovery was seen for group B platelets than for group A platelets, attributable perhaps to the lower levels of B antigens on donor platelets (19) and the lower levels of B-specific isoagglutinins in recipient plasma (18).

The number of A antigens per platelet estimated using an IgG murine monoclonal antibody specific for A substance and immunofluorescence flow cytometry showed a wide range (2, 100 to 16,000 molecules/platelet) and was donor dependent (19). Individuals of the subgroup A_2 have no detectable A antigens on their platelets (19–21) (Fig. 16.1), and A_2 platelets can be substituted successfully for group O, even for transfusion to refractory group O patients with high-titer anti-A,B (20). The number of B sites on platelets are considered to be about one-half the numbers reported for A. For many years it was thought that most ABH antigens on platelets (like HLA antigens) were absorbed from the plasma. Group O platelets incubated in group A or group B plasma could be shown to acquire soluble A or B substance detectable with anti-A or anti-B typing reagents in agglutination tests (22). In one study (23), about 6,000 molecules of A substance were acquired by group O platelets in 24 hours. Alternatively, incubation of group A platelets in group O plasma resulted in loss of approximately 50% of group A sites. Studies by the same researchers, using a monoclonal probe specific for Type II H chains, demonstrated that this membrane-intrinsic form of H substance is present on platelets and detectable in varying quantities according to the ABO type of the platelet donor (greatest in group O platelets, less in groups B, A_1, and A_1B, and least in O_h [Bombay]) (23). More recent studies show that a great majority of blood group A, B, and H antigens on platelets are expressed on many of the integral platelet membrane glycoproteins (GP) including, GP IIb, GP IIIa, GP IV, GP V, PECAM-1 (platelet-endothelial cell adhesion molecule-1), GP Ib/IX, and GP Ia/IIa (19,21,24–26) with GP Ia/IIa expressing the most ABH substance per molecule of GP, and GP IIb and PECAM-1 expressing the majority of ABH per platelet (19,21). Although it is likely that a small, but significant, amount of ABH on platelets is acquired by absorption of glycolipids expressing these antigens from the surrounding plasma, the majority, like HLA, is intrinsically derived at the megakaryocyte stage.

One report from Japan described a group O patient who failed to respond to 2 of 12 ABO-incompatible HLA-matched platelet transfusions (24). Further evaluation determined that the platelets in the two unsuccessful transfusions were from donors who expressed unusually high amounts of group B substance on their platelets, up to 20 times that found on group B, HLA-matched platelets that were successfully transfused in this patient. In studies of 313 healthy Japanese blood donors, they found that approximately 7% had platelets that carried significantly more A or B antigen than the mean level of these antigens on platelets determined for the entire group. This phenotype, designated "high expresser," was found to be inherited as a dominant trait and was unrelated to secretor phenotype, but did correlate with elevated serum glycosyltransferase activity (24). Recently, these findings were confirmed in studies of 200

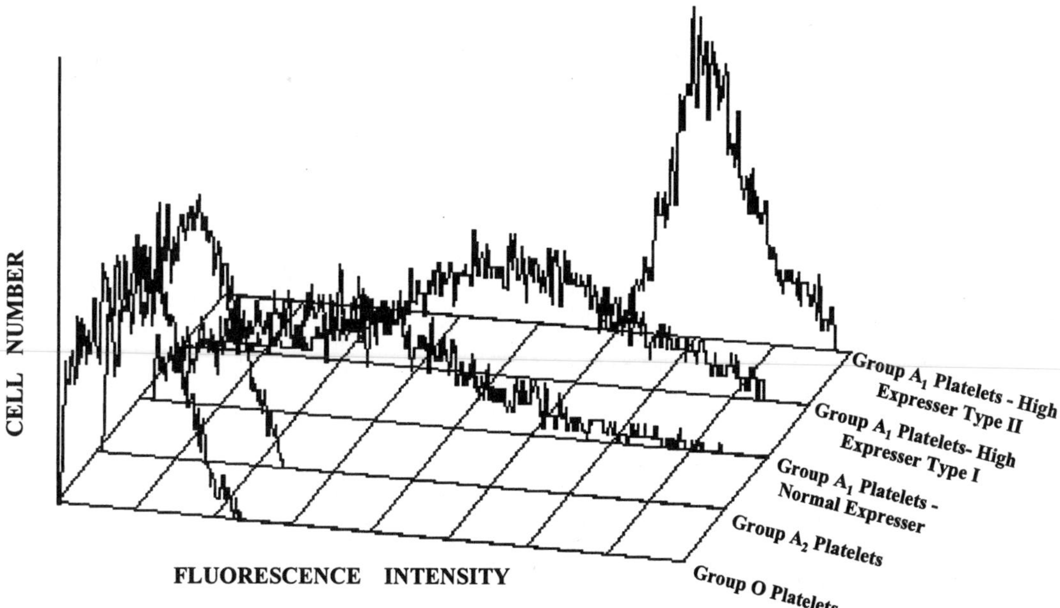

FIGURE 16.1. Fluorescence histograms of platelets after incubation with a fluorescent-labeled monoclonal antibody specific for the blood group A antigen and immunofluorescence detection by flow cytometry. Group A2 platelets are not distinguishable from group O platelets—no A antigens detected. Normal group A1 platelets (*middle histogram*) show great variation in A antigen expression—broad histogram. Platelets from a Type I high expresser, like the normal expresser, give a broad histogram, but have overall higher levels (*histogram shifted to the right*) of A antigen. Type II high expressers have much higher levels and show a more homogeneous (*narrow histogram at top*) expression of A antigens per platelet.

white blood donors that further defined two subgroups of high expressers of platelet A_1 antigens, termed Type I and Type II (19). Type I high expressers had elevated platelet A_1 antigen levels (about three times the normal expression), elevated serum A^1-glycosyltransferase activity, and a heterogeneous distribution of A_1 antigens on individual platelets (Fig. 16.1). Type II high expressers were characterized as having platelet A_1 antigen levels that averaged seven times the normal expression, higher A^1-transferase activity than even Type I individuals, a homogeneous distribution of platelet A_1 antigens (Fig.16.1), and the majority of the antigens were found to be expressed on platelet GP IIb and PECAM (19). This marked interdonor variability in A and B substance expression on platelets may offer an explanation for the nonuniform refractory response some patients develop to ABO-incompatible platelet transfusions (see below). The high-expression phenomenon might explain some cases of neonatal alloimmune thrombocytopenia (NAIT), because two unresolved cases of suspected NAIT, in which the fathers were both Type II high expressers of platelet A antigens, were recently evaluated (19).

Other Antigens

Other red blood cell antigens have been sought on the platelet surface. Ii, Lewis, and P antigens were demonstrated by using flow cytometry (25), but Rh, Duffy, Kidd, Kell, and Lutheran-b were not detected by a two-stage radioimmunometric assay (27).

Platelet GP IV, or CD36, is expressed on various human cells including, platelets, macrophages, capillary endothelium, erythroblasts, and adipocytes (28,29). Some apparently normal individuals lack CD36 on their platelets (Type II deficiency) or platelets and monocytes (Type I deficiency) (30). CD36 deficiency is common in Asians (3% to 11%) (31) and Africans (3% to 6%) (32), but is extremely rare in white populations (0.1%) (32). It is interesting that the most common gene mutations responsible for CD36 deficiency in Asians and Africans are different—$C \rightarrow T_{478}$ point mutation in exon 4 (Asians [29,30]) and $T \rightarrow G_{1264}$ stop mutation in exon 10 (Africans [33]). The higher frequency of CD36 deficiency in the former groups is thought to be related to their living in regions of the world endemic for malaria. CD36 is a known receptor for red blood cells infected with *Plasmodium falciparum,* thus it is believed that CD36 deficiency may afford partial resistance to malarial infection. One recent report suggests CD36 deficiency may actually be a risk factor for more severe forms of malarial infection (33). Type I CD36–deficient people can become immunized from transfusion or pregnancy and make isoantibodies against CD36 that have been implicated in cases of NAIT, posttransfusion purpura (PTP), and multiple platelet transfusion refractoriness (31,34,35).

CD109 is a 175-kd glycoprotein found on activated T cells, cultured endothelial cells, several tumor cell lines, and platelets (36). The sequence and function of this protein are yet to be determined. Recently, two new alloantigens, Gov^a and Gov^b, were found on platelet CD109 (36), and unlike most platelet-

TABLE 16.1. HUMAN PLATELET ALLOANTIGENS[a]

Alloantigen System	Other Names	Allelic Forms	Phenotypic Frequency	Glycoprotein[b] Location/ Amino Acid Change
HPA-1	$P1^A$, Zw	HPA-1a ($P1^{A1}$) HPA-1b ($P1^{A2}$)	72% a/a 26% a/b 2% b/b	GP IIIa[b] Leu ↔ Pro_{33}
HPA-2	Ko, Sib	HPA-2a (Ko^b) HPA-2b (Ko^a)	85% a/a 14% a/b 1% b/b	GP Ib/Thr ↔ Met_{145}
HPA-3	Bak, Lek	HPA-3a (Bak^a) HPA-3b (Bak^b)	37% a/a 48% a/b 15% b/b	GP IIb/Ile ↔ Ser_{843}
HPA-4	Pen, Yuk	HPA-4a (Pen^a) HPA-4b (Pen^b)	>99.9% a/a <0.1% a/b <0.1% b/b	GP IIIa/Arg ↔ Gln_{143}
HPA-5	Br, Hc, Zav	HPA-5a (Br^b) HPA-5b (Br^a)	80% a/a 19% a/b 1% b/b	GP Ia/Glu ↔ Lys_{505}
HPA-6w	Ca, Tu	HPA-6wb (Ca^a)	<1% b/b	GP IIIa/Arg ↔ Gln_{489}
HPA-7w	Mo	HPA-7wb (Mo^b)	<1% b/b	GP IIIa/Pro ↔ Ala_{407}
HPA-8w	Sr^a	HPA-8wb (Sr^a)	<0.1% b/b	GP IIIa/Arg ↔ Cys_{636}
HPA-9w	Max^a	HPA-9wb (Max^a)	<1% b/b	GP IIb/Val: Met_{837}
HPA-10w	La^a	HPA-10wb (La^a)	1%	GP IIIa/Arg: Gln_{62}
HPA-11w	Gro^a	HPA-11wb(Gro^a)	<0.5% b/b	GP IIIa/Arg: His_{633}
HPA-12w	Iy^a	HPA-12wb (Iy^a)	1% b/b	GP Ib_β/Gly: Glu_{15}
HPA-13w	Sit^a	HPA-13wb (Sit^a)	<1% b/b	GP Ia/Met: Thr_{799}
HPA-?[b]	Oe^a	ND[c]	1%	GP IIIa/De1 Lys_{611}
HPA-?	Va^a	ND	<1%	GP IIIa/ND
HPA-?	Pe^a	ND	<1%	GP Ib_α/ND
HPA-?	Gov	Gova/a Gova/b Govb/b	26% 55% 19%	CD109/ND

[a]Phenotypic frequencies for the antigen systems shown are for the white population only. Significant differences in gene frequencies may be found in African and Asian populations.
[b]?, Antigen number not yet assigned.
GP, glycoprotein; ND, Not determined.

specific alloantigens, both alleles are highly expressed: 81% (Gov^a) and 74% (Gov^b) in whites (Table 16.1). The number of Gov antigens expressed on platelets is small (<2,000 molecules/platelet) and the antigens are labile in storage, making detection of Gov antibodies difficult using currently available serologic assays. These properties of Gov would suggest that alloimmunization to these antigens may be underreported. Using optimal assay conditions, antibodies to Gov^a or Gov^b (37) were detected in 14 of 605 (2.3%) serum samples collected from patients with NAIT, PTP, and platelet transfusion refractoriness. These data suggest that Gov may be as immunogenic as the HPA-5 (Br) antigen system, which is second only to the highly immunogenic HPA-1a (Pl^{A1}) platelet antigen system.

Platelet-specific Antigens

Antibodies recognizing platelet-specific antigens have been discovered in three clinical situations including mothers who give birth to infants with NAIT, patients who develop dramatic thrombocytopenia after blood transfusion (PTP), and patients who have received multiple transfusions. To date, 21 platelet-specific alloantigens have been described, including localization to platelet surface GP structures, quantification of their density on the platelet surface, and determination of DNA polymorphisms in genes encoding for them (Table 16.1) (38). Several others have been described serologically, but genetic polymorphisms underlying these have not yet been determined (38). Many of the recognized platelet alloantigens have been implicated in cases of NAIT and PTP (Chapter 27). Some also have been determined to be relevant in platelet transfusion responses.

ALLOIMMUNIZATION TO PLATELET ANTIGENS

Immunization to HLA Antigens

Pregnancy and blood transfusion account for the development of HLA alloimmunization. There are no naturally occurring anti-HLA antibodies described. The natural history of HLA alloimmunization in patients receiving platelet transfusions was studied in 1978 (39). Sixty-three patients who required transfusions of random-donor platelets were followed. By actuarial analysis, 60% of those not positive for lymphocytotoxic antibodies at the beginning of the study were projected to develop lymphocytotoxic (LCT) antibodies as early as 10 days after primary exposure or 4 days after secondary exposure in patients who had been transfused or pregnant in the past. The number of transfusions was not related to the likelihood of immunization, an observation that was confirmed in a later study (40).

Patients alloimmunized at the beginning of the study had the poorest responses to transfusion of random platelets; those who did not develop LCT antibodies had the best; and those whose LCT antibodies developed during the period of observation had an intermediate response to platelet transfusion (39). A more recent study followed 50 patients who received multiple transfusions for various hematologic and oncologic conditions (41). Four (8%) were immunized to HLA at the start, and a further nine (18%) developed anti-HLA reactivity after the transfusion period was completed.

The risk of HLA alloimmunization is related to the underlying disease. Patients undergoing induction chemotherapy for acute myelogenous leukemia (AML) were more likely to become alloimmunized to HLA antigens than were patients being treated for acute lymphoblastic leukemia (ALL) (42). Although both groups of patients received similar intensive chemotherapy and required roughly the same level of transfusion support, HLA antibodies developed in 44% of the patients with AML in the study, whereas they did so in only 18% of the patients with ALL ($P = .00002$). The authors postulated that the difference may be attributable to either an additional immunosuppressive effect of the high-dose corticosteroids given in ALL or to a decreased immune responsiveness in patients with ALL caused by their underlying disease (42). Others have corroborated this finding and noted, moreover, that alloimmunization seems to occur sooner in patients with AML than in those with ALL (43).

There is some disagreement in the literature regarding the importance of a dose-response relationship between platelet transfusions from different donors and the risk of alloimmunization. One study failed to note such a relationship in a group of patients with AML receiving induction therapy. However, only 1 of the 106 patients included in the study received fewer than ten platelet donor exposures (40). Although there did not seem to be an overall trend linking the rate of alloimmunization (as measured by reactivity in a standard lymphocytotoxicity [LCT] test) and the number of donor exposures, it was of interest that only 2 of 9 patients receiving fewer than 20 donor exposures became alloimmunized, whereas 27 of 65 (41%) of those receiving more than 20 donor exposures were alloimmunized. Patients receiving more than 60 donor exposures had a lower rate of forming HLA antibodies. Although the findings are compatible with a lack of a dose-response relationship between platelet dose and alloimmunization rate, it is equally plausible that alloimmunization in this setting (induction therapy of acute leukemia) occurs on a very steep dose-response curve and that a better correlation might have been evident had patients received single-donor platelets instead of pools of random-donor platelet concentrates. Indeed, animal data (44) and human transfusion trials (45) suggest that when dealing with fewer donor exposures (i.e., fewer than 20), there is a dose-response relationship between the number of exposures and the rate of alloimmunization. There does seem to be general agreement that primary alloimmunization to HLA antigens is unlikely to occur before 3 to 4 weeks after the first transfusion in patients receiving multiple transfusions. HLA antibodies that are detected sooner than this most likely represent secondary immune response in patients with remote histories of transfusion or pregnancy. Although one might anticipate that prior pregnancy in women may increase their risk of developing LCT antibodies during transfusion therapy, there is conflicting data in transfusion trials (40,43,46). In a study of patients with AML and ALL, only 12% of women with prior pregnancies who received untreated blood products developed LCT antibodies compared with 38% of those not previously pregnant or transfused (43). In the Trial to Reduce Alloimmunization to Platelets (TRAP) study, 62% of previously pregnant women with AML receiving nontreated blood products (control product) developed LCT antibodies. These women also developed LCT antibodies sooner and at higher rates than women who had never been pregnant or men. However, only 33% of women with prior pregnancies who received leukocyte-reduced platelets developed LCT antibodies (46).

Despite the established correlation between broadly reactive HLA antibodies and refractoriness to platelet transfusions (47, 48), LCT antibodies are frequently a transient complication. Studies document that 17% to 67% of patients demonstrating these antibodies eventually lose them (42,43,49–52) (Table 16.2). The loss of LCT antibodies may be related to discontinuance of the antigenic exposure after bone marrow recovery or to switching of platelet transfusion support to HLA-matched homologous or frozen autologous platelets; but it can occur despite continued exposure to random-donor platelet transfusions (42,49,50,53). One interesting report (51) found that two-thirds of patients with decreasing anti-HLA reactivity despite continued exposure had developed antiidiotypic (anti-id) antibodies that reacted with the V region of anti-HLA IgG. In 36% of these, the serum actually inhibited binding of the patient's own prior anti-HLA to appropriate lymphocyte targets. A history of pregnancy did not affect the ability to produce these anti-id antibodies. In contrast, those patients with persistently detectable anti-HLA did not develop anti-id reactivity.

HLA antibodies that are detected before the onset of transfusion therapy (i.e., because of remote transfusion or pregnancy) tend to persist throughout the current period of transfusion therapy, whereas those antibodies that develop *de novo* during a transfusion support episode are more likely to be transient and to decrease in strength or disappear altogether, despite continued exposure to allogeneic blood and platelets (49) (Table 16.2).

The major immunizing source of HLA in transfused platelets is the donor leukocytes. In vitro experiments showed that highly purified HLA-A2+ platelets could not induce allocytotoxicity in HLA-A2–negative peripheral blood mononuclear cells (PBMCs)—not even in the presence of helper HLA-A2 PBMCs (6). Studies in animals and humans show that when platelets devoid of lymphocytes are transfused, primary immunization to HLA is very much delayed or does not occur at all (46,54–56), whereas unmodified platelet concentrates are associated with a rate of HLA immunization ranging from 25% to 93% (39,42, 43,46,49,50,53,55–56) (Table 16.2). These observations implicate the contaminating leukocytes in both platelet and red blood cell transfusions as the source of primary immunization. In addition, animal studies suggest that cell-free plasma supernatants from platelet concentrates stored without prior leukodepletion

TABLE 16.2. PLATELET ALLOIMMUNIZATION IN MULTITRANSFUSED PATIENTS[a]

Ref.	(Yr)	N pts	Anti-HLA[b]	Anti-PSA[c]	Loss/Decrease in Antibody
48	1992	50	13/50 (26%)	4/50 (8%)	
94	1989	22	10/22 (45%)		
56	1987	154	55/154 (36%)	5/154 (3%)	30/55 (54%)
50	1989	49	20/49 (41%)	11/49 (22%)	12/20 (59%)
59	1993	106	37/106 (35%)	45/106 (42%)	29/45 (64%)
57	1993	134	95/134 (71%)		43/95 (38%)
53	1997	131	59/131 (45%)	11/131 (8%)	

[a] Frequency of anti-HLA antibody and anti-platelet–specific antibody formation in studies of patients with hematologic and oncologic diagnoses requiring repeated platelet transfusion. The final column contains frequencies of antibody loss or decline in these studies.
[b] Anti-HLA antibodies determined by lymphocytotoxicity testing.
[c] Anti-platelet–specific antibodies determined by a variety of methods.

contain immunizing fragments thought to have been derived from white blood cells (57), and these fragments are not significantly removed by leukoreduction filters (58).

Immunization to Platelet-specific Antigens

The importance of platelet-specific antigen systems in the clinical syndromes NAIT and PTP is undisputed and is described in Chapter 27. Their relevance to platelet transfusion practice is controversial.

One kind of evidence implicating platelet-specific antigens in the destruction of transfused platelets is that not all transfusions of HLA-matched platelet concentrates in patients refractory to random-donor platelets are successful (54). The failure of platelet transfusions, despite HLA matching, indicates that other antigens, perhaps platelet specific, are involved. The other kind of evidence involves the demonstration of platelet-reactive antibodies in the absence of LCT activity. The conclusion drawn is that these "platelet-specific" reactions are caused by antibodies directed at platelet-specific antigens (53,54,59).

Although there are a few well-documented cases of transfusion failures attributable to platelet-specific antibodies (60–62), most "platelet-specific reactivity" in transfusion refractory recipients does not seem to influence transfusion responses (41,47, 52). In 2 of the 50 patients in one study, possible platelet-specific alloantibodies with ill-defined specificities developed, and a further two had what were thought to be platelet-directed autoantibodies. In none of these four patients was the platelet reactivity clearly correlated with poor transfusion responses (41). Many of the best-documented platelet-specific antibodies detected in patients who receive transfusions are directed against platelet antigens, the phenotypic frequency of which is less than 30% in the blood donor population (60,63). Therefore, it is difficult to attribute refractory responses in random-donor and/or HLA-matched platelet transfusions to these antibodies. Alloimmunization to high-frequency platelet-specific antigens would be expected to present a major challenge in finding compatible platelets to support a patient requiring multiple platelet transfusions. Fortunately these cases are extremely rare (63,64). However, recently there have been several reports of platelet transfusion refractoriness caused by antibodies to GP IV (CD36) in patients who are GP IV deficient (31,65,66). These patients are difficult to support because virtually all platelet products available for transfusion would be incompatible (GP IV-positive). In a single report, GP IV-negative platelets were obtained by large-scale screening of donor populations with a higher frequency of GP IV deficiency (African), and transfusion of those platelets resulted in good platelet increments for the patients (65).

One interesting report suggests that in 42% of a cohort of 106 patients who received multiple transfusions, platelet-specific antibody developed, as detected by chloroquine-treated platelets in a platelet antibody screening test. Western blotting on these sera identified a number of bands to which IgG in the sera reacted, most commonly with molecular weights of 80 to 83 kd. In three of the sera the reactivity was not detected against thrombin-treated platelets, indicating that the antibodies might be directed against platelet glycoprotein V. No correlation with platelet transfusion responses was reported, and more than half of these "platelet-specific" antibodies were transient and not detected in follow-up testing (67).

A number of investigators have described what seem to be autoantibodies to platelet-specific proteins developing in patients who receive multiple transfusions. However, few if any of these have been linked to refractoriness to platelet transfusions, and therefore their significance is unclear (41).

Immunization to Blood Group Antigens

Several studies have documented the effect of ABO incompatibility on platelet transfusion therapy. One study found that in 91 alloimmunized thrombocytopenic patients receiving 389 transfusions, 24-hour transfused platelet recovery was reduced by 23% in ABO-incompatible donor-recipient pairs (donor group A, B, or AB; recipient group O, B, or A) (68). The impact of ABO incompatibility on transfused platelet recovery was confirmed in a second study from the same institution (69). Moreover, the effect of ABO incompatibility, apparent 1 hour after transfusion, was not augmented at 24 hours. In the latter study, a subset of group O patients refractory to all group A HLA-matched platelets was identified (5 of 23). In these patients, ABO incompatibility was a significant clinical problem, whereas in the remainder of the patients, it was statistically significant but not clinically relevant to their response to HLA-matched platelets.

In the aggregate, patients receiving multiple platelet transfusions have been thought to demonstrate a statistically significant but clinically unimportant decrease in platelet recovery after transfusion of ABO-incompatible platelets (especially group A). In a subset, however, as many as 20% of group O patients could develop severe refractoriness to group A platelets (20,24,70). Failure to respond to HLA-matched platelet transfusions in the absence of nonimmune clinical factors should prompt the clinician to examine the ABO types of the recipient and of the donors to determine whether ABO incompatibility might be responsible for the unexpected poor responses.

The importance of ABO blood groups in platelet transfusion therapy has been reexamined by Heal's group. Forty patients with hematologic diseases receiving platelet transfusions were randomized to receive either ABO-identical or ABO-unmatched platelets (71). The responses in the group of patients receiving ABO-unmatched transfusions (i.e., when either the recipient would be expected to have isoagglutinins to the ABH antigens on the transfused platelets, or the donor had such antibodies directed at the recipient's blood type) were significantly worse than those observed in patients receiving ABO-identical platelet transfusions. Analyzing the first 25 transfusions in each group, a significantly better response was seen in the ABO-identical arm (mean corrected count increment [CCI] 6,600 versus 5,200; $P < .01$). This effect was most important in the first ten transfusion episodes and tended to predict subsequent alloimmunization and refractoriness to platelet transfusions (71). This finding seemed to be in conflict with earlier reports in which a minor, clinically insignificant impact of ABO mismatching was observed. The newer data were then reanalyzed using the earlier definitions of ABO "compatibility" (the patient lacks isoagglutinins to recipient ABO antigens) and "incompatibility" (the patient has isoagglutinins reactive with donor ABO antigens). In the reanalysis, no benefits of ABO compatibility were detected (72), suggesting that there is a significant negative impact of both major and minor ABO incompatibility in platelet transfusions. An increased frequency of refractoriness in patients receiving ABO-unmatched platelet transfusions was also observed in a study of 26 patients (69% versus 58%; $P = .001$) (73).

The mechanism for platelet destruction in platelet ABO-incompatible transfusions (the recipient has isoagglutinins against donor ABH) is not difficult to ascertain. Presumably, IgM and IgG anti-A or anti-B in the recipient interact with A and B substances on the transfused platelets, resulting in their premature exit from the circulation. Explanations offered for the biphasic survival curves of ABO-incompatible platelets include (a) the elution of a portion of group A substance from the platelet surface, (b) the nonhomogeneous distribution of group A substance with resultant rapid destruction of heavily coated platelets, and (c) secondary injury to a subset of transfused platelets caused by the reaction between anti-A isoagglutinins and A red blood cells contaminating the platelet concentrate (18,19).

The suboptimal response of the plasma-incompatible transfusions (the donor has isoagglutinins against recipient ABH) is more difficult to explain. One report postulates that immune complexes involving soluble recipient ABH substance and donor anti-A or -B antibodies form. These immune complexes secondarily interact with the transfused platelets via the FcγRIIα receptor, or the complement receptors cC1q-R and gC1q-R, and mediate their destruction (74). Some experimental evidence supports this theory, in that anti-A has been detected in an immune complex fraction of group A recipient plasma after transfusion with group O platelets, and that these immune complexes bind to IgG FcγRIIα and the cC1q-R and gC1q-R receptors on group O platelets (74). Indeed, in at least one study, plasma-incompatible platelet transfusions were even less effective than platelet-incompatible transfusions (71).

Immune complexes involving other plasma proteins such as C2, C4, albumin, and fibrinogen likewise have been implicated in refractory responses to platelet transfusion (74,75). Although one independent report seems to lend support to this conjecture (76), further observations are required before accepting this as a bona fide cause of poor platelet transfusion responses.

TRANSFUSION REFRACTORINESS

Alloimmunization is an immunologic state referring to the immune system's response to foreign antigen(s), most often involving the production of antibodies directed at the antigen(s). The refractory state describes a clinical condition in which a patient does not achieve the anticipated platelet count increment from a platelet transfusion.

The detection of alloimmunization is straightforward using standard laboratory techniques to detect antibodies in the patient's serum reactive with HLA or platelet-specific antigens. In contrast, the definition of the refractory state is less precise (77, 78). A standard dose of platelets (six units of pooled random-donor platelet concentrates or one apheresis platelet) generally increases the platelet count by about 5,000 to 7,000 platelets/μl per each random concentrate in a 70-kg man. This would result in a postplatelet increment of about 30,000 to 40,000 platelets/μl 1 hour after platelet transfusion (78). The TRAP study defines the refractory state as a CCI (normalizing transfusion responses for patient blood volume estimated using body surface area [BSA] and platelet dose) of <5,000 after two sequential ABO-compatible platelet transfusions (46). Another measure of platelet transfusion response is the percent platelet recovery (PPR). Similar to the CCI, the PPR uses platelet dose and patient blood volume; the latter is estimated using the patient's body weight in kilograms rather than BSA. Studies in normal autologous platelet donors show an average 1-hour PPR of approximately 66% (48).

Recently, the PPR and CCI have been criticized as measures of posttransfusion platelet response, because both calculations yield information about the likelihood of an individual's platelet recovery only (79). Therefore, a small dose of platelets given to a large patient might result in an acceptable PPR or CCI but a poor absolute platelet count increment. A modification of these formulas using a regression analysis of posttransfusion platelet increments was suggested, because such an analysis combines the effect of platelet dose, filtration, and patient size. It was further suggested that CCI and PPR not be used to define platelet refractoriness because these measures are biased in favor of platelet preparation techniques that provide fewer platelets. Regardless of which method is used, the actual platelet increment in patients who are highly refractory due to alloimmunization is extremely small to negligible.

It is important to recognize that refractoriness does not necessarily imply alloimmunization. Indeed, the major cause of refractoriness to platelet transfusion is not alloimmunization, but rather nonimmune factors that result in shortened platelet survival and/or markedly decreased platelet recoveries in patients who receive transfusions. Multiple linear regression analysis has been used to demonstrate a number of factors related to clinical refractoriness, including HLA alloimmunization as well as splenomegaly, amphotericin B therapy, disseminated intravascular coagulation, or a recent allogeneic bone marrow transplant (80). Other studies have also demonstrated factors such as sepsis, fever, and drugs that have a negative impact on platelet response (81, 82). It is important to realize that individual patients may have significantly different responses to the nonimmune causes of refractoriness, with some patients experiencing minimal impact while others have markedly impaired response to platelet transfusions.

Some patients, particularly those with multiple clinical complications (sepsis, fever), appear to respond poorly to platelets that are approaching the end of the recommended storage interval (5 days). Such patients may experience an improvement in their platelet response after receiving "fresh platelets"—platelets that are within 48 hours of collection (78).

TREATMENT OF THE ALLOIMMUNIZED PATIENT

The refractory state in which patients fail to benefit from random-donor platelet transfusions develops in between 13% and 100% of patients receiving multiple transfusions (43,46,83,84). The refractoriness, if related to HLA immunization, can be transient or persistent. Several approaches can be considered to provide such patients with adequate platelet support including provision of HLA-matched platelets, platelets selected by crossmatch tests, and maneuvers to reduce alloimmunization.

Platelet Selection

HLA-selected Platelet Transfusions

A standard approach to supporting a patient refractory to random-donor platelet transfusions is to supply HLA-matched single-donor platelet concentrates (85). Because the primary cause of immune refractoriness to platelet transfusion is alloimmunization to Class I HLA antigens, it follows that avoidance of incompatible HLA specificities should result in a more successful platelet transfusion response. In practice, up to 90% of refractory patients benefit from an HLA-matched product. This was first demonstrated in a study that showed patients refractory to random-donor platelets could be successfully supported by HLA-matched family member platelet transfusions (86).

Certain "private" HLA antigens can be segregated into so-called *cross-reactive groups (CREGs),* defined by antisera that react with several different, but structurally related, HLA specificities. It was proposed that selection of platelet donors with antigens in the same CREGs as the antigens in the patient might result in a relative inability of the patient's immune system to recognize these cross-reactive antigens as different. This would greatly increase the number of potentially successful platelet donors in a given pool (85). The success of selectively mismatched platelet transfusions based on this system has been confirmed by others (87,88).

TABLE 16.3. CLASSIFICATION OF DONOR/RECIPIENT PAIRS ON THE BASIS OF HLA MATCH

A	All four antigens in donor identical to those in recipient
BIU	Only three antigens detected in donor; all present and identical in recipient
BIX	Three donor antigens identical to recipient; fourth antigen cross-reactive with recipient
B2U	Only two antigens detected in donor; both present and identical in recipient
B2UX	Only three antigens detected in donor; two identical in recipient, third cross-reactive
B2X	Two donor antigens identical to recipient; third and fourth antigens cross-reactive with recipient
C	One antigen of donor not present in recipient and non–cross-reactive with recipient
D	Two antigens of donor not present in recipient and non–cross-reactive with recipient

Cross-reactive associations were used to create HLA-match grades (Table 16.3). When refractory patients were supported with platelet transfusions selected using these match grades, platelet count increments were nearly as successful on average as those of transfusions from donors who were HLA identical to the patient (89).

The effect of LCT reactivity on the results of single HLA antigen–mismatched platelet transfusions to alloimmunized patients has been studied with good responses in patients with 73% of the one antigen–mismatched platelet transfusions being successful when the panel reactive antibody (PRA) in the LCT test was less than 60% (90). Even when the PRA was greater than 60%, 58% of all such transfusions were successful. Based on these data, some experts suggest extending donor searches for alloimmunized patients to include single-antigen mismatches, particularly if the PRA is less than 60% reactive (90).

The HLA antibodies formed in refractory patients who receive multiple transfusions are typically broadly reactive when tested against panels of randomly chosen lymphocytes. In the past, this was thought to represent the accumulation of many different HLA antibodies. Subsequent studies revealed that broad HLA reactivity often represents one or few antibodies directed against "public" determinants shared by HLA antigens in the same CREG (91). Indeed, these shared public determinants are the basis for the cross-reactivity and are different from the private determinants, which account for the highly polymorphic HLA system.

In another study, 18 alloimmunized thrombocytopenic patients who received multiple transfusions were evaluated for HLA reactivity (92). Sera from these patients reacted with 53% to 100% of cells on lymphocyte panels. Eleven of these 18 patients had antibodies against public antigens alone—three had antibodies with only private specificities and two had both kinds of reactivity. The reactivity in the serum of the remaining two patients could not be identified. Comparing HLA types of both patients and platelet donors, these investigators were able to predict positive or negative LCT cross-matches in nearly 80% using cross-reactive associations. The correlation might have been even higher had they used an antiglobulin enhancement to the standard LCT test. In another study, the majority of patients in a cohort of multiply transfused dialysis patients had preformed CREG-reactive antibodies. Indeed, 90% of the HLA reactivity in this group could be attributed to reactivity to public epitopes (91).

Recently, the use of HLA-typed platelets has been extended by using the patient's HLA antibody specificity as the basis for selecting a platelet product. A and B match-grade platelets are frequently unavailable for some patients, and cross-matching of platelet transfusions has limitations. Using antibody specificity prediction (ASP) (93), platelet products from donors who lacked HLA antigens to which the patient had raised an antibody were selected. These platelet products were often frank mismatches for some or all of the Class I antigens. For comparison, platelets were selected by standard HLA-matching criteria and by platelet cross-matching using a solid phase red cell adherence (SPRCA) assay. PPR was determined in 1,621 platelet transfusions in 114 patients. HLA-matched, cross-matched, and ASP-selected platelet transfusions were found to have similar platelet recoveries, while randomly selected control platelets had significantly lower PPR. Interestingly, for 29 alloimmunized, typed patients, the mean number of potential donors found in a file of 7,247 donors was only six when grade-A HLA matches were required and 39 when BU matches were added. However, 1,426 potential donors (20% of total) were identified by the ASP method. It was recommended that careful HLA-antibody–specificity identification could greatly enhance the number of potential donors by identifying nonmatched products that lack these HLA antigens. Other investigators using a computerized analysis of the LCT assay for private and public HLA Class I epitopes in platelet recipients confirmed that there is a value in carefully identifying HLA antibody specificities, allowing selection of many more donors by simply avoiding the HLA antigens against which the antibodies are directed (94).

In a small number of patients who fail to respond to HLA-matched platelets and for whom no other explanation can be found for refractoriness, it is important to evaluate for platelet-specific alloantibodies. Approximately 7% of multiple platelet–transfused patients develop platelet-specific antibodies (46, 95). Many of these patients are also alloimmunized against HLA. One recent report described six patients who were highly alloimmunized to HLA but also had human platelet alloantibodies to HPA-1b or HPA-5b (96). These patients were successfully supported with a pool of HLA-matched platelets that were typed for the HPA antigens.

Platelet Cross-matching

Although the use of HLA-matched and selectively mismatched donors provides support for the majority of patients refractory to random-donor platelet transfusions, as many as 20% to 25% of refractory patients fail to respond adequately to HLA-matched platelets. In the absence of nonimmunologic clinical factors that can decrease platelet transfusion recovery and survival, these failures might be explained by ABO incompatibility, platelet-specific antibodies, and undetected HLA incompatibility (97).

Platelet compatibility testing has been attempted using a wide variety of platelet and leukocyte antibody detection methods. A cross-matching method that has gained wide acceptance is the commercially available SPRCA assay. The test is rapid and sensitive, particularly for the detection of anti-HLA antibodies, and is therefore suitable for routine platelet cross-matching (98,99).

The degree to which a patient is alloimmunized has an impact on the success of platelet transfusions selected by compatibility assays. Using random-donor platelet concentrates from whole blood units and a radiolabeled antiglobulin technique one study found that 70% of transfusions selected by the test were successful in supporting moderately alloimmunized patients (100). In contrast, others found that only 41% of transfusions selected by either a microenzyme-linked immunosorbent assay (micro-ELISA) or a SPRCA test were successful in a highly alloimmunized group of leukemia patients (101). Moreover, only 15% to 24% of random platelet concentrate segments tested were negative, indicating that very large numbers of random-donor platelet concentrates had to be screened to provide only a limited number of "compatible" transfusions to the refractory patients. In the latter study, the most compatible platelet products selected by cross-matching were less successful in supporting the refractory patients than HLA-matched platelets (mean CCI with "cross-matched compatible" platelets, 4,300 to 9,500; compare with a mean CCI of 17,100 with HLA-matched platelets).

A SPRCA method for all patients refractory to platelet transfusions has been used without determining whether it was on an immunologic or nonimmunologic basis (102). A significant improvement in the mean CCI was found when cross-matched compatible platelets were used versus randomly selected platelets with a mean increase of 8,000 ± 6,100. It was suggested that routine cross-matching for patients refractory to randomly selected platelets will lead to transfusion response improvement in about one-half of the patients, even when the patients are not preselected for having alloimmunization.

Another multicenter study compared available cross-matching techniques with HLA selection for support of refractory patients (103). This study used three different platelet antibody tests depending on the site; ELISA, the indirect immunofluorescence test for platelets, and a radioimmunoassay. At least one set of two single-donor platelet components was transfused to each patient. One unit was selected by HLA matching and the other by cross-matching. The results of the two donor selection methods were compared. Although the difference was not statistically significant, HLA-selected transfusions were slightly more successful than the cross-match–selected transfusions when 1-hour posttransfusion recoveries were compared. However, after 24 hours the HLA-selected transfusions were significantly more successful. This was even more apparent when only A and BU matches were considered. The authors concluded that when HLA-typed donors are available, A or BU matches were preferable to random products selected by any of the cross-matched methods used in their study. The quality of the HLA match is paramount to the transfusion success rate as shown in a study in which HLA matching did not apparently improve the success rate of cross-match–selected platelets (104). Here the HLA-selected platelets were seldom of A or BU match grade with the recipients.

Flow cytometry has been used as a cross-matching technique and has met with variable success (105). Its effectiveness was demonstrated when compared to both a monoclonal antibody-specific immobilization of platelet antigen (MAIPA) tests and the LCT assay (106). Sensitivities and efficiencies of 70% and 88.6% were noted for the flow cytometric assay. It was also noted that the flow cytometric assay was able to detect some positive results with antigens known to have variable expression on platelets such as the HLA B-44, B-45 antigens.

Experience using both LCT and SPRCA assays for analyzing antibodies to HLA and platelet antigens has been reported (107). With LCT, they found that if the PRA was <70%, adequate transfusion responses were seen in approximately 80% of transfusions that were selected simply by HLA criteria (avoidance of HLA antigens to which patients have an antibody and CREGs). However, when the PRA was >70%, only about 25% of patients did well. When analyzing the results using cross-matching, patients with PRAs <80% did well with cross-match–selected platelets; but when the PRA was 80% to 100%, there were a high number of failures with the cross-match–compatible products. It was suggested that at high levels of alloimmunization, cross-matching misses significant antibodies.

Finally, a recent report comparing a MAIPA assay to the LCT test showed the MAIPA to be more sensitive in detecting HLA antibodies, and that MAIPA-positive, LCT test–negative HLA antibodies are clinically relevant and affect posttransfusion platelet count increment (108).

Overcoming Established Alloimmunization

A number of strategies have attempted to reverse established alloimmunity to HLA antigens, but these have met with only limited success to date. Previously attempted methods include (a) methods to temporarily block the immune-mediated destruction of platelets, (b) suppression of the immune response to decrease the production of relevant antibodies, and (c) provision of alternative (nonplatelet) hemostatic compounds.

Intravenous IgG

A number of studies investigated the utility of high-dose intravenous immune globulin (IVIG) to increase the platelet count in association with transfusion in refractory patients. The results of these studies have been highly variable (109,110,111). Initial uncontrolled trials were done on very small numbers of patients using random-donor platelet transfusions. Studies using somewhat larger numbers of patients have been inconclusive. One study treated 11 refractory patients with 0.4 g/kg per day for 5 days with no benefit in the 1-hour posttransfusion recoveries (109). Another study found a modest beneficial effect of IVIG in a randomized placebo-controlled trial with 12 alloimmunized thrombocytopenic patients (110). The same donor platelets were used before and after treatment with IVIG. The posttreatment 1-hour CCIs in the IVIG group (seven patients) were significantly greater than in the five patients receiving placebo treatment, 8,413 versus 1,050, respectively. However, by 24 hours after the transfusion, there was no residual benefit of IVIG. The authors concluded that the use of IVIG could not replace HLA-matched platelet transfusions in supporting alloimmunized refractory patients.

Using very–high-dose (6 g/kg) IVIG, other investigators could reverse the refractory response in some patients who failed to respond to HLA-selected LCT-compatible platelet transfusions (111). Prior to treatment with IVIG, the patients had been refractory to HLA-matched platelet products. Following therapy, 13 of 19 patients responded with improvement in 1-hour posttransfusion platelet count increment using HLA-matched platelets. Those patients with PRAs <85% responded better than those who were highly alloimmunized.

Other Strategies

Other strategies evaluated to overcome the platelet refractory state include use of vinblastine-loaded platelet transfusions (112), treatment with cyclosporin A (113), immunoabsorption using staphylococcal protein A columns, and plasmapheresis (114,115). Each strategy has had some limited success. A novel approach has recently been developed involving transfusion with acid treated random-donor platelets. Treatment of platelets with citric acid modifies Class I antigens on the platelet surface making them less recognizable to the immune system (5,6). A small number of patients have been treated with such products but with very limited success, and studies are still ongoing (116).

The role of platelet growth factors in the treatment of patients who have undergone highly myeloablative therapy is not totally defined. There may be a subgroup of such refractory patients who may benefit from treatment with platelet growth factors by having a more rapid return of their platelet count to more normal levels. Currently, only one product, recombinant HUIL-11 (NEUMEGA Genetics Institute, Cambridge, MD) is licensed in the United States for the prevention of severe thrombocytopenia and the reduction of the need for platelet transfusion following myelosuppressive, but not myeloablative, chemotherapy in patients with nonmyeloid malignancies (117,118).

A number of potential platelet substitutes are currently in investigative stages. These include lyophilized platelets, infusible platelet membranes, thromboerythrocytes, and thrombospheres. Whether these will have clinical relevancy remains for future investigation (119,120,121).

It has been shown in a small number of patients who are refractory to platelet transfusions and anemic, that treating the anemia with red blood cell transfusions can shorten the bleeding time and impact bleeding episodes. In a patient who was refractory to platelet transfusions and had epistaxis for two weeks, the bleeding could not be controlled with platelets and standard therapy. The patient was then transfused, with hemoglobin rising from 8 gm/dl to a >12 g/dl and kept at this level. The epistaxis gradually improved over the next 4 days and no further bleeding was noted (122).

Prevention of Alloimmunity

Although alloimmunization to HLA antigens appears to be transient in some patients, for most, once the alloimmune refractory state is established, it is very difficult to reverse. Therapy for the refractory state is expensive and frequently requires more transfusions than for patients who are not refractory (123). Therefore, attention has turned to prevention of alloimmunization as a more practical way to assure continued successful platelet support.

Several strategies have been employed in attempts to prevent alloimmunization to platelet products. Donor antigenic exposure can be limited by providing single-donor platelet transfusions. Although this method showed some promise in early studies, it is no longer a standard means of preventing alloimmunization (124). A second promising method is treatment of blood products with ultraviolet B (UVB) irradiation (125). UVB irradiation prevents the interaction of dendritic cells contained in the transfusion product with recipient T lymphocytes, which is probably the major route of primary HLA alloimmunization to platelet transfusions. Additional studies have provided evidence that the inability of donor and recipient immune cells to interact following UVB irradiation may indicate a state of immunologic tolerance to a blood transfusion. Preliminary studies with UVB-treated platelets in thrombocytopenic patients with cancer demonstrated a reduced rate of formation of HLA antibodies. A definitive study to be discussed below, the TRAP study found that UVB irradiation could reduce the incidence of alloimmunization and platelet refractoriness (46). Despite its being shown to work in this regard, at the present time UVB irradiation is not used, because it is more cumbersome and not any more effective for preventing alloimmunization than a third approach, leukocyte reduction. A large number of studies have evaluated leukocyte reduction as means to prevent alloimmunization, and these are discussed below.

A primary immune response against Class I HLA antigens requires that they be presented in the context of Class II HLA molecules. Therefore, significant work has centered on removing the Class II HLA-bearing cells, the leukocytes, from the donor blood products as a means of preventing alloimmunization. Both the Food and Drug Administration (FDA) and the American Association of Blood Banks define a leukocyte-reduced blood product as one that contains fewer than 5×10^6 leukocytes. Removal of leukocytes is most often accomplished by passing the blood products through so-called third-generation leukocyte reduction filters. These filters remove the leukocytes by a combination of adhesion and pore size and are capable of producing a three- to four-log reduction in contaminating leukocytes that results in products that easily meet the FDA's requirement for leukocyte-reduced blood products. Although such filters can be used at the bedside, the preferred methodology is prestorage leukocyte reduction in the laboratory. The latter allows leukocyte-reduced blood products to be manufactured under Good Manufacturing Practices with well-defined quality control. Leukocyte reduction of platelet products can also be accomplished using apheresis technology by which the equivalent of six units of random-donor platelets can be obtained from a single donor, and the product is leukoreduced as it is collected.

The majority of trials to date support the use of leukocyte reduction to reduce alloimmunization to blood products. Eighteen clinical trials, both randomized controlled and nonrandomized, using leukocyte-reduced red blood cells and platelets to prevent alloimmunization, have been reviewed (126). Fourteen of the trials showed positive results using leukocyte-reduced blood to prevent HLA alloimmunization and platelet refractoriness, while three of the trials showed no benefit. In addition, a recent meta-analysis of eight randomized control trials demonstrated a clear, protective effect of white blood cell reduction in the prevention of HLA alloimmunization and platelet refractoriness (127).

The most definitive clinical trial demonstrating the importance of leukocyte reduction in the prevention of alloimmunization and refractoriness to platelet transfusion was the TRAP study (46). This trial had four groups for comparison: (a) patients receiving pooled platelet concentrates (control), (b) patients receiving leukocyte reduced (filtered), pooled platelet concentrates, (c) patients receiving UVB-irradiated pooled platelet concentrates, and (d) patients receiving filtered platelets obtained by apheresis from single donors.

All patients received leukocyte-reduced red blood cell products. Evidence of alloimmunization by LCT developed in 45% of the control group compared with 17% to 21% in the treated groups ($P \leq 0.0001$ for each treated group as compared with controls). There were no differences among the treated groups in rates of alloimmunization. Thirteen percent of patients in the control group became refractory compared to 3% to 5% in the treated groups ($P \leq 0.03$ for each treated group as compared to the control). Again, individual treatments did not differ.

The following other important findings were noted in the TRAP study: (a) Clinical outcomes were similar in all four groups of the study with no significant difference in the incidence of deaths due to hemorrhage. (b) The incidence of refractoriness to platelet transfusions was low in the control group relative to previous reported studies. (c) Patients who had never been pregnant had a lower risk of developing refractoriness than those who had. (d) Only about 8% of the patients in the study developed platelet-specific antibodies. The treatment groups had no impact on this type of immunization. (e) The presence of platelet-specific antibodies did not correlate with refractoriness. (f) A small percentage of patients in all groups were refractory to platelet transfusions yet did not have LCT antibodies. Most likely, these patients had either clinical factors or drug-related causes of refractoriness.

From the studies cited above, it is clear that both leukocyte reduction and UVB irradiation are capable of reducing the incidence of alloimmunization and platelet refractoriness. At the present time, leukocyte reduction of blood products is the most practical means of reducing the incidence of alloimmune platelet refractoriness and should be recommended for all patients at risk.

The identification and characterization of platelet antigens and increased understanding of immunologic responses to these markers have been crucial in developing optimal platelet transfusion practices. Our understanding of the causes and mechanisms of both the immunologic and nonimmunologic aspects of the refractory response allows for improved strategies in the care of the potentially refractory patient. Figure 16.2 represents an approach to managing platelet transfusions that encompasses both prevention of and platelet selection for refractoriness to platelet transfusions.

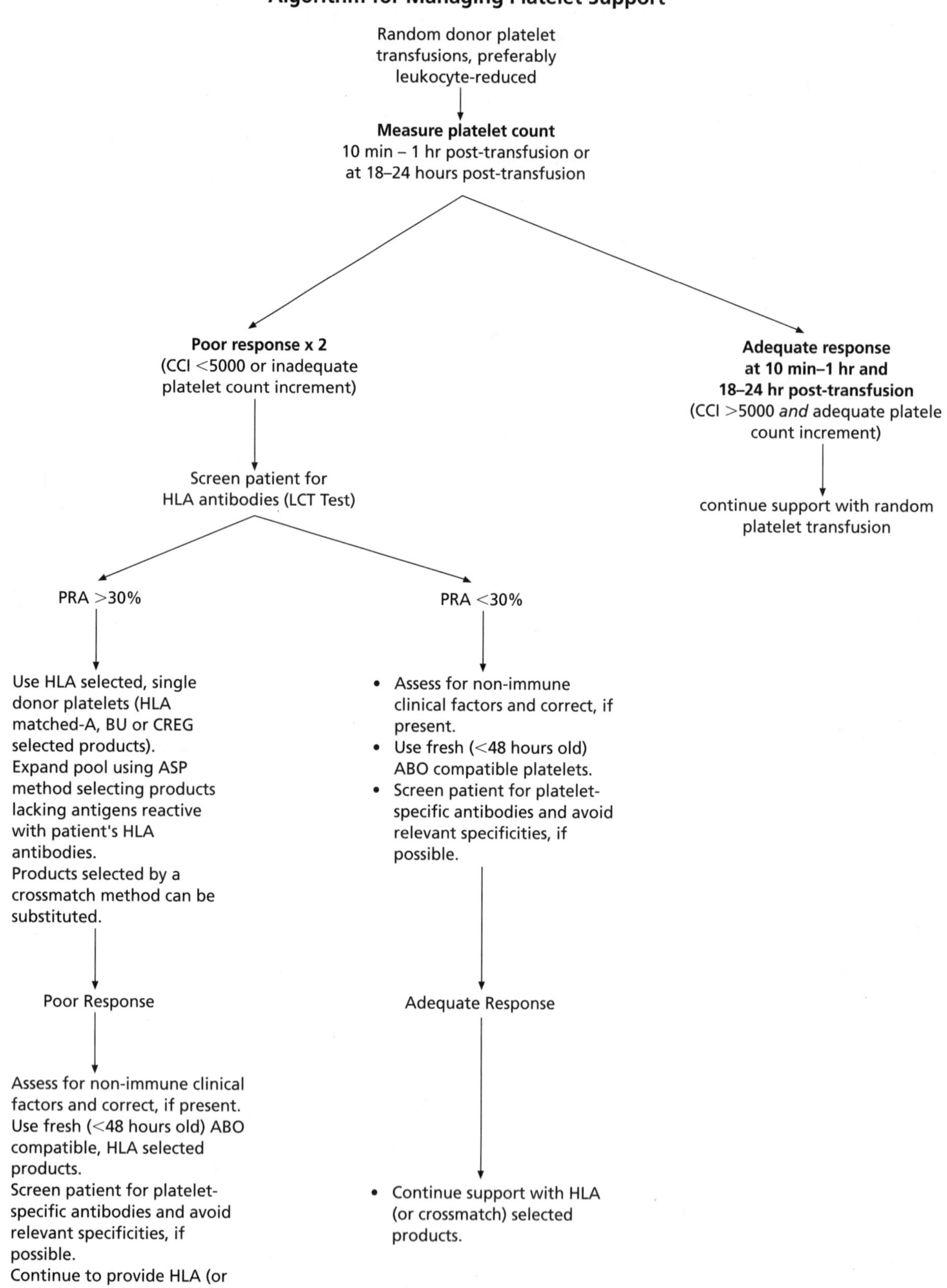

FIGURE 16.2. Algorithm for managing platelet support.

SUMMARY

Platelets express a variety of immunogenic markers on the cell surface. Some of these antigens are shared with other cell types as in the case of HLA antigens, which are shared with virtually all nucleated cells in the body. Other antigens are observed to be essentially platelet specific. This chapter has reviewed the antigens expressed on the platelet, the various patterns of alloimmunization to these antigens, and the impact on platelet transfusion responses. Strategies to treat and prevent alloimmunization were also summarized. The role of HLA and platelet immunogenic markers in modern transplantation cannot be overemphasized. The need for increased numbers of transplants to treat an ever-growing patient population in need of such therapies will require that even greater strides be made regarding our ability to understand and manipulate these complex antigen systems.

REFERENCES

1. Lalezari P, Driscoll AM. Ability of thrombocytes to acquire HLA specificity from plasma. *Blood* 1982;59:167–170.
2. Santoso S, Mueller-Eckhardt G, Keifel V, et al. HLA antigens on platelet membranes in vitro and in vivo studies. *Vox Sang* 1986;51: 327–333.
3. Kao KJ. Selective elution of HLA antigens and B2 microglobulin from human platelets by chloroquine diphosphate. *Transfusion* 1988; 28:14–17.
4. Sugawara S, Abo T, Kumagai K. A simple method to eliminate the antigenicity of surface Class I MHC molecules from the membrane of viable cells by acid treatment at pH 3. *J Immunol Methods* 1987; 10083–10090.
5. Neumuller J, Tohidast-Akrad M, Fisher M, et al. Influence of chloroquine or acid treatment of human platelets on the antigenicity of HLA and the "thrombocyte-specific" glycoproteins Ia/IIa, IIb, and IIb/IIIa. *Vox Sang* 1993;65:223–231.
6. Gouttefangeas C, Diehl M, Keilholz W, et al. Thrombocyte HLA molecules retain nonrenewable endogenous peptides of megakaryocyte lineage and do not stimulate direct allocytotoxicity in vitro. *Blood* 2000;95:3168–3175.
7. Feuerstein N, Mono DS, Cooper HL. Phorbolester effect in platelets, lymphocytes, and leukemic cells (HL-60) is associated with enhanced phosphorylation of Class I HLA antigens. *Biochem Biophys Res Commun* 1985;126:206–213.
8. Santoso S, Kalb R, Kiefel V, et al. The presence of messenger RNA for HLA Class I in human platelets and its capability for protein biosynthesis. *Br J Haematol* 1993;84:451–456.
9. Novotny VMJ, Doxiadis IIN, Brand A. The reduction of HLA class I expression on platelets: a potential approach in the management of HLA-alloimmunized refractory patients. *Transfus Med Rev* 1999;13: 95–105.
10. Janson M, McFarland J, Aster RH. Quantitative determination of platelet surface alloantigens using a monoclonal probe. *Hum Immunol* 1986;15:251–262.
11. Kao KJ, Cook DJ, Scornik JC. Quantitative analysis of platelet surface HLA by W6/32 anti-HLA monoclonal antibody. *Blood* 1986;68: 627–632.
12. Pereira J, Cretney C, Aster RH. Variation of Class I HLA antigen expression among platelet density cohorts: a possible index of platelet age? *Blood* 1988;71:516–519.
13. Kao KJ, Scornik JC, McQueen CF. Evaluation of individual specificities of class I HLA on platelets by a newly developed monoclonal antibody. *Hum Immunol* 1990;27:285–297.
14. Szatkowski NS, Aster RH. HLA antigens of platelets. IV. Influence of "private" HLA-B locus specificities on the expression of Bw4 and Bw6 on human platelets. *Tissue Antigens* 1980;15:361–368.
15. Mueller-Eckhardt G, Hauck M, Kayser W, et al. HLA-C on platelets. *Tissue Antigens* 1980;16:91–94.
16. Boshkov LK, Kelton JG, Halloran PF. HLA-DR expression by platelets in acute idiopathic thrombocytopenic purpura. *Br J Haematol* 1992;81:552–557.
17. Dunstan RA, Simpson MB. Heterogenous distribution of antigens on human platelets demonstrated by fluorescence flow cytometry. *Br J Haematol* 1985;61:603–609.
18. Aster RH. Effect of anticoagulant and ABO incompatibility on recovery of transfused human platelets. *Blood* 1965;26:732–743.
19. Curtis BR, Edwards JT, Hessner MJ, et al. Blood group A and B antigens are strongly expressed on platelets of some individuals. *Blood* 2000;96:1574–1581.
20. Skogen B, Rossebo Hansen B, Husebekk A, et al. Minimal expression of blood group A antigen on thrombocytes from A_2 individuals. *Transfusion* 1988;28:456–459.
21. Santoso S, Kiefel V, Mueller-Eckhardt C. Blood group A and B determinants are expressed on platelet glycoproteins IIa, IIIa, and Ib. *Thromb Haemost* 1991;65:196–201.
22. Kelton JG, Hamid C, Aker S, et al. The amount of blood group A substance on platelets is proportional to the amount in the plasma. *Blood* 1982;59:980–985.
23. Dunstan RA, Simpson MB, Knowles RW, et al. The origin of ABH antigens on human platelets. *Blood* 1985;65:615–619.
24. Ogasawara K, Ueki J, Takenaka M, et al. Study on the expression of ABH antigens on platelets. *Blood* 1993;82:993–999.
25. Mollicone R, Caillard T, Le Pendu J, et al. Expression of ABH and X (Lex) antigens on platelets and lymphocytes. *Blood* 1988;71: 1113–1119.
26. Stockelberg D, Hou M, Rydberg L, et al. Evidence for an expression of blood group A antigen on platelet glycoproteins IV and V. *Transfus Med* 1996;6:243–248.
27. Dunstan RH, Simpson MB, Rosse WF. Erythrocyte antigens on human platelets: absence of Rh, Duffy, Kell, Kidd, and Lutheran antigens. *Transfusion* 1984;24:243–246.
28. Greenwalt DE, Lipsky RH, Ockenhouse CF, et al. Membrane glycoprotein CD36: a review of its roles in adherence, signal transduction, and transfusion medicine. *Blood* 1992;80:1105–1115.
29. Yanai H, Chiba H, Morimoto M, et al. Human CD36 deficiency is associated with elevation in low-density lipoprotein-cholesterol. *Am J Med Genet* 2000;93:299–304.
30. Yanai H, Chiba H, Fujiwara H, et al. Phenotype-genotype correlation in CD36 deficiency Types I and II. *Thromb Haemost* 2000;84: 436–441.
31. Ikeda H, Mitani T, Ohnuma M, et al. A new platelet specific antigen Nak[a], involved in the refractoriness of HLA matched platelet transfusion. *Vox Sang* 1989;57:312–317.
32. Curtis BR, Aster RH. Incidence of the Nak[a]-negative platelet phenotype in African Americans is similar to that of Asians. *Transfusion* 1996;36:331–334.
33. Aitman TJ, Cooper LD, Norsworthy JP, et al. Malaria susceptibility and CD36 mutation. *Nature* 2000;405:1015–1016.
34. Bierling P, Godeau P, Fromont P, et al. Posttransfusion purpura-like syndrome associated with CD36 (Nak[a]) isoimmunization. *Transfusion* 1995;35:777–782.
35. Kankirawatana S, Kupatawintu P, Juji T, et al. Neonatal alloimmune thrombocytopenia due to anti-Nak[a]. *Transfusion* 2001;41:375–377.
36. Smith JW, Hayward CP, Horsewood P, et al. Characterization and localization of the Gova/b alloantigens to the glycosylphosphatidylinositol-anchored protein CDw109 on human platelets. *Blood* 1995; 86;2807–2814.
37. Berry JE, Murphy GA, Smith GA, et al. Detection of Gov system antibodies by MAIPA reveals an immunogenicity similar to HPA-5 alloantigens. *Br J Haematol* 2000;110:735–742.
38. Santoso S, Kiefel V. Human platelet-specific alloantigens: update. *Vox Sang* 1998;74[Suppl 2]:249–253.
39. Howard JE, Perkins HA. The natural history of alloimmunization to platelets. *Transfusion* 1978;18:496–503.
40. Dutcher JP, Schiffer CA, Aisner J, et al. Alloimmunization following platelet transfusion: the absence of a dose-response relationship. *Blood* 1981;57:395–398.

41. Godeau B, Fromont P, Seror T, et al. Platelet alloimmunization after multiple transfusions: a prospective study of 50 patients. *Br J Haematol* 1992;81:395–400.
42. Lee EJ, Schiffer CA. Serial measurement of lymphocytotoxic antibody and response to nonmatched platelet transfusions in alloimmunized patients. *Blood* 1987;70:1727–1729.
43. Pamphilon DH, Farrell DH, Donaldson C, et al. Development of lymphocytotoxic and platelet reactive antibodies: a prospective study in patients with acute leukaemia. *Vox Sang* 1989;57:177–181.
44. Slichter S, O'Donnell M, Weiden P, et al. Canine platelet alloimmunization: the role of donor selection. *Br J Haematol* 1986;63:713–727.
45. Gmur J, von Felten A, Osterwaider B, et al. Delayed alloimmunization using random single donor platelet transfusions: a prospective study in thrombocytopenic patients with acute leukemia. *Blood* 1983;62:473–479.
46. The Trial to Reduce Alloimmunization to Platelets Study Group. Leukocyte reduction and ultraviolet B irradiation of platelets to prevent alloimmunization and refractoriness to platelet transfusions. *N Engl J Med* 1997;337:1861–1869.
47. Novotny VMJ. Prevention and management of platelet transfusion refractoriness. *Vox Sang* 1999;76:1–13.
48. Delaflor-Weiss E, Mintz PD. The evaluation and management of platelet refractoriness and alloimmunization. *Tranfus Med Rev* 2000;14:180–196.
49. Murphy MF, Metcalf P, Ord J, et al. Disappearance of HLA and platelet-specific antibodies in acute leukaemia patients alloimmunized by multiple transfusions. *Br J Haematol* 1987;67:255–260.
50. Dutcher JP, Schiffer CA, Aisner J, et al. Long term followup of patients with leukemia receiving platelet transfusions: identification of a large group of patients who do not become alloimmunized. *Blood* 1981;58:1007–1011.
51. Atlas E, Freedman J, Blanchette V, et al. Downregulation of the anti-HLA alloimmune response by variable region reactive (anti-idiotypic) antibodies in leukemic patients transfused with platelet concentrates. *Blood* 1993;81:538–542.
52. Hogge DE, Dutcher JP, Aisner J, et al. Lymphocytotoxic antibody is a predictor of response to random donor platelet transfusion. *Am J Hematol* 1983;14:363–369.
53. McGrath K, Wolf M, Bishop J, et al. Transient platelet and HLA antibody formation in multitransfused patients with malignancy. *Br J Haematol* 1988;68:345–350.
54. Brand A, Claas FHJ, Voogt PJ, et al. Alloimmunization after leukocyte-depleted multiple random donor platelet transfusions. *Vox Sang* 1988;54:160–166.
55. Murphy MF, Metcalfe P, Thomas H, et al. Use of leucocyte poor blood components and HLA matched platelet donors to prevent HLA alloimmunization. *Br J Haematol* 1986;62:529–534.
56. Eernisse JG, Brand A. Prevention of platelet refractoriness due to HLA antibodies by administration of leukocyte poor blood components. *Exp Hematol* 1987;9:77–83.
57. Bordin J, Bardossy L, Blajchman M. Experimental animal model of refractoriness to donor platelets: the effect of plasma removal and the extent of white cell reduction on allogeneic alloimmunization. *Transfusion* 1993;33:798–801.
58. Ramos RR, Curtis BR, Duffy BF, et al. Low retention of WBC fragments by polyester fiber leukocyte reduction platelet filters. *Transfusion* 1994;34:31–34.
59. Kickler TS. Platelet-compatibility testing: an update. *Lab Management* 1987;1:33–39.
60. Taaning E, Jacobsen N, Morling N. Graft derived anti-HPA2b production after allogeneic bone-marrow transplantation. *Br J Haematol* 1994;86:651–653.
61. Murata M, Furihata K, Ishida F, et al. Genetic and structural characterization of an amino acid dimorphism in glycoprotein Ib-alfa involved in platelet transfusion refractoriness. *Blood* 1992;79:3086–3090.
62. Saji H, Maruya E, Fujii H, et al. New platelet antigen Siba involved in platelet transfusion refractoriness in a Japanese man. *Vox Sang* 1989;56:283–287.
63. Taaning E, Simonsen AC, Hjelms E, et al. Platelet alloimmunization after transfusion. *Vox Sang* 1997;72:238–241.
64. Lagenscheidt F, Kiefel V, Santoso S, et al. Platelet transfusion refractoriness associated with two rare platelet-specific alloantibodies (anti-Bak^{a} and anti-Pl^{A2}) and multiple HLA antibodies. *Transfusion* 1988;28:597–600.
65. Curtis BR, Donnelly SF, Mintz PD, et al. Platelet transfusion refractoriness in an African American patient due to anti-Nak^{a}. *Transfusion* 1997;37[Suppl 384]:96(abst).
66. Lee K, Godeau P, Fromont P. CD36 deficiency is frequent and can cause platelet immunization in Africans. *Transfusion* 1999;39:873–879.
67. Meenaghan M, Judson P, Yousaf K, et al. Antibodies to platelet glycoprotein V in polytransfused patients with hematological disease. *Vox Sang* 1993;64:167–170.
68. Duquesnoy RJ, Anderson AJ, Tomasulo PA, et al. ABO compatibility and platelet transfusions of alloimmunized thrombocytopenic patients. *Blood* 1979;54:595–599.
69. McElligott MC, McFarland JG, Anderson AJ, et al. ABO incompatibility in HLA-matched platelet transfusions. *Blood* 1984;67[Suppl 1]:823a(abst).
70. Brand A, Sintnicolaas K, Claas FHJ, et al. ABH antibodies causing platelet transfusion refractoriness. *Transfusion* 1986;26:463–466.
71. Heal J, Rowe J, McMican A, et al. The role of ABO matching in platelet transfusion. *Eur J Haematol* 1993;50:110–117.
72. Heal J, Rowe J, Blumberg N. ABO and platelet transfusion revisited. *Ann Hematol* 1993;66:309–314.
73. Carr R, Hutton J, Jenkins J, et al. Transfusion of ABO mismatched platelets leads to early platelet refractoriness. *Br J Haematol* 1990;75:408–413.
74. Heal JM, Masel D, Blumberg N. Interaction of platelet Fc and complement receptors with circulating immune complexes involving the ABO system. *Vox Sang* 1996;71:205–211.
75. Heal J, Cowles J, Masel D, et al. Antibodies to plasma proteins: an association with platelet transfusion refractoriness. *Br J Haematol* 1992;80:83–90.
76. Ohto H, Yasuda H, Abe R, et al. Platelet transfusion refractoriness associated with plasma proteins. *Br J Haematol* 1992;80:680–681.
77. Benson K. Criteria for diagnosing refractoriness to platelet transfusions. In: Kickler TS, Herman JH, eds. *Current issues in platelet transfusion therapy and platelet alloimmunity.* Bethesda: American Association of Blood Banks, 1999.
78. Slichter SJ. Algorithm for managing the platelet refractory patient. *J Clin Apheresis* 1997;12:4–9.
79. Davis KB, Slichter SJ, Corash L. Corrected count increment and percent platelet recovery as measures of posttransfusion platelet response: problems and a solution. *Transfusion* 1999;39:586–592.
80. Bishop J, McGrath K, Wolf M, et al. Clinical factors influencing the efficacy of pooled platelet transfusions. *Blood* 1988;71:383–387.
81. Alcorta I, Pereira A, Ordinas A. Clinical and laboratory factors associated with platelet transfusion refractoriness: a case-control study. *Br J Haematol* 1996;93:220–224.
82. McFarland JG, Anderson AF, Slichter SJ. Factors influencing the transfusion response to HLA-selected apheresis donor platelets in patients refractory to random platelet concentrates. *Br J Haematol* 1989;73:380–386.
83. Hogge DE, McDonnell M, Jacobson C, et al. Platelet refractoriness and alloimmunization in pediatric oncology and bone marrow transplant patients. *Transfusion* 1995;35:645–652.
84. Schiffer CA, Dutcher JP, Aisner J, et al. A randomized trial of leukocyte depleted platelet transfusion to modify alloimmunization in patients with leukemia. *Blood* 1983;62:815–820.
85. Duquesnoy RJ. Donor selection in platelet transfusions therapy of alloimmunized thrombocytopenic patients. In: Greenwalt TJ, Jamieson GA, eds. *The blood platelet in transfusion therapy,* New York: Alan R. Liss, 1978:229–243.
86. Yankee RA, Grumet FC, Rogentine GN. Platelet transfusion therapy: the selection of compatible platelet donors for refractory patients by lymphocyte HL-A typing. *New Engl J Med* 1969;281:1208–1212.
87. Jorgensen DW, McFarland JG, Hillman RS, et al. Platelet apheresis program II: computer selection of HLA compatible donors. *Transfusion* 1984;24:292–298.

88. Engelfriet CP, Reesink HW. Management of alloimmunized, refractory patients in need of platelet transfusions. *Vox Sang* 1997;73: 191–198.
89. Duquesnoy RJ, Filip DJ, Rodey GE, et al. Successful transfusion of platelets "mismatched" for HLA antigens to alloimmunized thrombocytopenic patients. *Am J Hematol* 1977;2:219–226.
90. Hussein MA, Lee EJ, Fletcher R, et al. The effect of lymphocytotoxic antibody reactivity on the results of single antigen mismatched platelet transfusions to alloimmunized patients. *Blood* 1996;87:3959–3962.
91. Oldfather J, Mora A, Phelan D, et al. The occurrence of crossreactive "public" antibodies in the sera of highly sensitized dialysis patients. *Transplant Proc* 1983;15:1212–1215.
92. MacPherson BR, Hammond PB, Maniscalco CA. Alloimmunization to public HLA antigens in multi-transfused platelet recipients. *Ann Clin Lab Sci* 1986;16:38–44.
93. Petz LD, Garratty G, Calhoun L, et al. Selecting donors of platelets for refractory patients on the basis of HLA antibody specificity. *Transfusion* 2000;40:1446–1456.
94. Zimmermann R, Wittmann G, Zingsem J, et al. Antibodies to private and public HLA Class I epitopes in platelet recipients. *Transfusion* 1999;39:772–780.
95. Kickler T, Kennedy SD, Braine HG. Alloimmunization to platelet-specific antigens on glycoproteins IIb-IIIa and Ib/IX in multiply transfused thrombocytopenic patients. *Transfusion* 1990;30:622.
96. Kekomäki S, Volin L, Koistinen P, et al. Successful treatment of platelet transfusion refractoriness: the use of platelet transfusions matched for both human leucocyte antigens (HLA) and human platelet alloantigens (HPA) in alloimmunized patients with leukaemia. *Eur J Haematol* 1998;60:112–118.
97. Kickler T. Pretransfusion testing for platelet transfusions [Editorial]. *Transfusion* 2000;40:1425–1426.
98. Shibata Y, Juji T, Nishizawa Y, et al. Detection of platelet antibodies by a newly developed mixed agglutination with platelets. *Vox Sang* 1981;41:25–31.
99. Rachel JM, Sinor LT, Tawfik OW, et al. A solid-phase red cell adherence test for platelet cross-matching. *Med Sci Lab* 1985;41:194–195.
100. Friedman J, Hooi C, Garvey MB. Prospective platelet crossmatching for selection of compatible random donors. *Br J Haematol* 1984;56: 9–18.
101. O'Connell BA, Schiffer CA. Donor selection for alloimmunized patients by platelet crossmatching of random-donor platelet concentrates. *Transfusion* 1990;30:314–317.
102. Gelb AB, Leavitt AD. Crossmatch-compatible platelets improve corrected count increments in patients who are refractory to randomly selected platelets. *Transfusion* 1997;37:624–630.
103. Moroff G, Garratty G, Hai JM, et al. Selection of platelets for refractory patients by HLA matching and prospective crossmatching. *Transfusion* 1992;32:633–640.
104. Friedberg R, Donnelly S, Mintz P. Independent roles for platelet crossmatching and HLA in the selection of platelets for alloimmunized patients. *Transfusion* 1994;34:215–220.
105. Sintnicolaas K, Löwenberg B. A flow cytometric platelet immunofluorescence crossmatch for predicting successful HLA matched platelet transfusions. *Br J Haematol* 1996;92:1005–1010.
106. Köhler M, Dittmann J, Legler TJ, et al. Flow cytometric detection of platelet-reactive antibodies and application in platelet crossmatching. *Transfusion* 1996;36:250–255.
107. Murphy S, Varma M. Selecting platelets for transfusion of the alloimmunized patient: a review. *Immunohematology* 1998;14:117–123.
108. Kurtz M, Khöbl P, Kalhs P, et al. Platelet-reactive HLA antibodies associated with low posttransfusion platelet increments: a comparison between the monoclonal antibody-specific immobilization of platelet antigens and the lymphocytotoxicity test. *Transfusion* 2001;41: 771–774.
109. Schiffer CA, Hogge DE, Aisner J, et al. High dose intravenous γglobulin in alloimmunized platelet transfusion recipients. *Blood* 1984; 64:937–940.
110. Kickler T, Braine HG, Piantadosi S, et al. A randomized, placebo controlled trial of intravenous γglobulin in alloimmunized thrombocytopenic patients. *Blood* 1990;75:313–316.
111. Ziegler ZR, Shadduck RK, Rosenfeld CS, et al. Intravenous γ globulin decreases platelet associated IgG and improves transfusion responses in platelet refractory states. *Am J Hematol* 1991;38:15–23.
112. Wong P, Hiruma K, Endoh N, et al. Vinblastine-loaded platelet transfusion in an alloimmunized patient. *Br J Haematol*1987;65:380–381.
113. Tilly H, Azagury M, Bastit D, et al. Cyclosporin for treatment of life-threatening alloimmunization. *Am J Hematol* 1990;34:75–76.
114. Christie D, Howe R, Lennon S, et al. Treatment of refractoriness to platelet transfusion by protein A column therapy. *Transfusion* 1993; 33:234–242.
115. Rock G. The application of protein A immunoadsorption to remove platelet alloantibodies. *Transfusion* 1993;33:192–194.
116. Novotny VMJ, Doxiadis LIN, Brand A. The reduction of HLA Class I expression on platelets: a potential approach in the management of HLA-alloimmunized refractory patients. *Transfus Med Rev* 1999;13: 95–105.
117. Kuter DJ, Cebon J, Harker LA, et al. Platelet growth factors: potential impact on transfusion medicine. *Transfusion* 1999;39:321–332.
118. Fanucchi M, Glaspy J, Crawford J, et al. Effects of polyethylene glycol-conjugated recombinant human megakaryocyte growth and development factor on platelet counts after chemotherapy for lung cancer. *New Engl J Med* 1997;336:404–409.
119. Chao FC, Kim BK, Houranieh AM, et al. Infusible platelet membrane microvesicles: a potential transfusion substitute for platelets. *Transfusion* 1996;36:536–542.
120. Vostal JG, Reid TJ, Mondoro TH. Summary of a workshop on in vivo efficacy of transfused platelet components and platelet substitutes. *Transfusion* 2000;40:742–750.
121. Sarkodee-Adoo CB, Heyman MR. Alternative management strategies in alloimmunized thrombocytopenic patients. In: Kickler TS, Herman JH, eds. *Current issues in platelet transfusion therapy and platelet alloimmunity.* Bethesda: American Association of Blood Banks, 1999: 135–159.
122. Ho C-H. The hemostatic effect of adequate red cell transfusion in patients with anemia and thrombocytopenia. *Transfusion* 1996; 36[Suppl]:290(abst).
123. Lill M, Snider C, Calhoun L, et al. Analysis of utilization and cost of platelet transfusions in refractory hematology/oncology patients. *Transfusion* 1997;37[Suppl]:26s (abst).
124. Gmur J, von Felten A, Osterwaider B, et al. Delayed alloimmunization using random single donor platelet transfusions: a prospective study in thrombocytopenic patients with acute leukemia. *Blood* 1983;62: 473–479.
125. Pamphilon DH. The rationale and use of platelet concentrates irradiated with ultraviolet-B light. *Transfus Med Rev* 1999;13:323–333.
126. Kao KJ. A critical analysis of clinical trials to prevent platelet alloimmunization. In: Kickler TS, Herman JH, eds. *Current issues in platelet transfusion therapy and platelet alloimmunity.* Bethesda: American Association of Blood Banks, 1998:103–133.
127. Vamvakas E. Meta-analysis of randomized controlled trials of the efficacy of white blood cell reduction in preventing HLA-alloimmunization and refractoriness to random-donor platelet transfusions. *Transfus Med Rev* 1998;12:258–270.

Rossi's Principles of Transfusion Medicine, Third Edition, edited by Toby L. Simon, Walter H. Dzik, Edward L. Snyder, Christopher P. Stowell, and Ronald G. Strauss. Lippincott Williams & Wilkins, Philadelphia

CASE 16A

IF AT FIRST YOU DON'T SUCCEED, SOMETIMES YOU SHOULD NOT TRY AGAIN

CASE HISTORY

A 77-year-old female was transferred from a suburban hospital with a 3-week history of chest tightness. Four days prior to transfer she was admitted to hospital with increasing shortness of breath. She was found to be in new congestive heart failure with newly developed mitral valve regurgitation. Her hematocrit was 28%, and she was transfused with two units of red blood cells without incident and transferred to our hospital for cardiac surgery. She was treated with diuretics and placed on subcutaneous heparin therapy.

She had a history of anemia, polymyalgia rheumatica, and temporal arteritis confirmed by biopsy 2 years before admission.

On examination she was able to lie flat in bed without acute shortness of breath. Her blood pressure was 128/60 mm Hg, pulse 89 beats/min and regular, and respiratory rate 18 breaths/min. A 3/6 holosystolic murmur was heard at the cardiac apex. There was no jugular venous distention and no leg edema. A transesophageal echocardiographic study of the heart documented a flail mitral valve leaflet due to a ruptured chordae tendinae. There was no left atrial thrombosis. She was anticoagulated with systemic heparin and underwent a coronary catheterization. Her medications were changed to include diuretics, a β-blocker, and an angiotensin-converting enzyme inhibitor.

On day 5, she underwent cardiac surgery for placement of a mechanical mitral valve. She received one unit of red blood cells and no other blood components. Immediately postoperatively, she was noted to have moderate thrombocytopenia (39,000/μl). The heparin was discontinued. On the first full postoperative day, her platelet count was found to be 6,000/μl. A heparin-PF4 antibody assay was ordered, six units of pooled platelet concentrates transfused, and a hematology consult requested. The hematologist noted the absence of schistocytes or platelet clumping on the peripheral blood smear and considered the thrombocytopenia due to a cephalosporin antibiotic, which was discontinued. The patient received two subsequent transfusions of apheresis platelets over the next 12 hours without a rise in platelet count.

During the second of these transfusions at 11:00 PM, her heart rate increased to 150 beats/min and she experienced "uncontrollable shaking, decreased oxygen saturation, and diaphoresis." The platelet transfusion was stopped and a transfusion reaction investigation was begun. The blood bank reported no immediate serologic incompatibility, and another dose of platelets was administered at 4:00 AM without a reaction. The next morning the platelet count was 5,000/μl. The heparin antibody test was negative. The hematology consultant recommended additional platelet transfusions. During the next infusion, the patient again developed shaking chills, temperature of 102°F, and tachycardia followed by a brief period of complete heart block and control of systole by an indwelling temporary pacemaker. That evening the clinical service requested high-dose intravenous immune globulin plus additional platelet transfusions using premedication with diphenhydramine, hydrocortisone (Solu-Cortef), furosemide, acetaminophen, and albuterol.

Because all requests for intravenous immune globulin are screened by a physician from the blood transfusion service, the patient was next seen by a transfusion medicine physician who considered the diagnosis of posttransfusion purpura (PTP). A test for antiplatelet antibodies was sent, and the patient was treated with high-dose intravenous immune globulin without additional platelet transfusions. The platelet serology test demonstrated an anti-HPA-1a antibody as shown from the worksheet below (Table 16A.1).

DISCUSSION

This patient had PTP which was not initially recognized. The sudden onset of intense thrombocytopenia about 10 days following a transfusion (in this case the transfusion given at the suburban hospital) is often the only clue to the diagnosis. Although heparin therapy is the most common cause of drug-induced thrombocytopenia, heparin usually does not induce such a profound depression of the platelet count. Nevertheless, PTP can be confused with heparin-induced thrombocytopenia (1). In contrast, platelet counts were found to be <10,000/μl in over 80% of PTP cases. The clinicians considered heparin-induced thrombocytopenia and ordered a diagnostic test, but then chose to administer platelet transfusions—a strategy which would not be recommended for patients with heparin-induced thrombocytopenia. The clinicians attributed the poor success to pooled platelets and asked for platelets from a single donor. Not surprisingly, these proved to be no more effective. Laboratory evaluation showed that the patient also had a moderate human lym-

TABLE 16A.1. PLATELET ANTIBODY WORKSHEET*

Test Well	Negative Control	Patient Result	Interpretation
GpIIb-IIIa HPA-1a/1a HPA-3a/3a HPA-4a	0.064	0.774	Positive
GpIIb-IIIa HPA-1b/1b HPA-3b/3b HPA-4a	0.071	0.084	Negative
GpIa-IIa HPA-5b/5b	0.074	0.093	Negative
GpIa-IIa HPA-5a/5a	0.074	0.097	Negative
GpIb-IX	0.035	0.034	Negative
GpIV	0.060	0.054	Negative
HLA Class I†	0.052	0.219	Positive
Positive control	–	0.574	Should be 2× highest negative control

* Numbers in table are the optical density of reactivity in EIA testing (Pak Plus assay, GTI Corp, Brookfield, WI).
† HLA panel reactive antibody by lymphocytotoxicity found to be 39%.

phocyte antigen (HLA) antibody sensitization which may have contributed to platelet refractoriness. The patient survived the attempts to "correct" her thrombocytopenia by repeated transfusion of incompatible products, but she experienced repeated serious transfusion reactions—one of which was life-threatening.

The case also demonstrates delayed recognition of the true diagnosis by the transfusion service. The transfusion reaction investigation represented a missed opportunity for the transfusion medicine physician to make the correct diagnosis. Rather than doing a full evaluation of the patient's case, the investigation focused on eliminating the possibility of a hemolytic transfusion reaction even though hemolysis is not a common consequence of platelet transfusions. The reaction workup was undoubtedly reviewed by the pathology resident and staff but without full knowledge of the patient's circumstances. It was only when intravenous immune globulin was requested that the transfusion medicine physician was brought more thoroughly into the case.

PTP is an unusual but dramatic complication of transfusion. The reaction occurs in rare individuals who lack the common platelet antigen, HPA-1a (also known as PL^{A1}). For unknown reasons, the disorder is much more common in females (95% of cases). When exposed to transfusion, the individual mounts an immune response against the HPA-1a antigen. Interestingly, the processing and immune response to HPA-1a appears restricted to individuals who carry the HLA-DRw52 antigen. This latter situation may possibly be due the ability of HLA-DRw52 allele to bind the relevant oligopeptide that carries the HPA-1a epitope.

PTP displays the paradoxical feature that the patient's immune response rapidly destroys the patient's own (HPA-1a negative) platelets, thereby inducing thrombocytopenia. A report from Taaning et al. helped to clarify this observation (2). They found that during the initial immune response in PTP, the susceptible blood recipient mounts an immunoglobulin M (IgM) response that is initially broadly reactive with the platelet glycoprotein IIb-IIIa structure. This indiscriminate IgM reacts with both the transfused platelets and the patient's own platelets. Thus, in the initial days of intense thrombocytopenia, the serology of the patient may be similar to that found among patients with autoimmune thrombocytopenia (ITP). Over the next several days to weeks, the patient's immune response "matures" and the resulting immunoglobulin G (IgG) antibody demonstrates reactivity with HPA-1a.

Like patients with ITP, those with PTP respond to high-dose intravenous immune globulin. The mechanism of response is unclear and can occur within hours of administration of immune globulin. Other treatments include steroids and plasmapheresis. Platelets are often given (as in this case) but are of little, if any, known value. Because the patient has antibodies against platelets, an increase in the platelet count does not generally occur, and reactions to infusion of large numbers of incompatible platelets can be dramatic. The true incidence of PTP is not known. Although generally regarded as a rare disorder, it was a leading cause of reported adverse events in the United Kingdom's Serious Hazards of Transfusion national reporting scheme (3).

Case contributed by Walter H. Dzik, M.D., Massachusetts General Hospital, Boston, MA.

REFERENCES

1. Lubenow N, Eichler P, Albrecht D, et al. Very low platelet counts in post-transfusion purpura falsely diagnosed as heparin-induced thrombocytopenia: report of four cases and review of literature. *Thromb Res* 2000; 100:115–125.
2. Taaning E, Finn T. Pan-reactive platelet antibodies in post-transfusion purpura. *Vox Sang*1999;76:120–123.
3. Williamson L, Cohen H, Love E, et al. The Serious Hazards of Transfusion (SHOT) initiative: the UK approach to hemovigilance. *Vox Sang* 2000;78[Suppl]:291–296.

17

PREPARATION AND STORAGE OF PLATELET CONCENTRATES

SCOTT MURPHY

PLATELET PREPARATIONS FOR TRANSFUSION

Platelets are transfused as platelet concentrates (PCs) prepared from routine donations of whole blood or by apheresis (AP-PC) using citrate as the anticoagulant. At present, the storage medium is primarily autologous plasma, although in many centers, particularly in Europe, some of the plasma is being replaced by synthetic media. There are two methods for preparing whole blood–derived PCs, the platelet-rich plasma (PRP) method and the buffy-coat (BC) method. The principles of storage are probably similar for all types of PC, but most of the basic knowledge has been derived from the study of storage of whole blood–derived PCs prepared by the PRP method.

Much attention is now being given to the number of contaminating leukocytes in PC as well as the appropriate platelet content. Problems related to contaminating leukocytes will be discussed in Chapter 21. PCs can be filtered during infusion at the bedside, but it may be preferable to perform leukoreduction at the time of preparation of the PC. In the United States, an AP-PC or a pool of PRP-PC is considered leukoreduced if it contains less than 5×10^6 leukocytes, while the standard in Europe is 1×10^6.

S. Murphy: Department of Medicine, University of Pennsylvania; American Red Cross Blood Services—Penn Jersey Region, Philadelphia, Pennsylvania.

PREPARATION OF WHOLE BLOOD–DERIVED PLATELET CONCENTRATES (PCS)

Platelet-rich Plasma Method

Platelets were first transfused in the 1950s and 1960s, a time when blood processing and storage were performed at refrigerated temperatures (1° to 6°C). Whole blood units (450 to 500 ml) were anticoagulated with acid-citrate-dextrose. PRP could be prepared by subjecting the blood to slow centrifugation, which sedimented the red blood cells and BC, leaving most of the platelets in 200 to 250 ml of supernatant plasma. However, when attempts were made to concentrate the platelets by high-speed centrifugation, the platelets invariably clumped irreversibly as they were resuspended from the pellet that formed at the bottom of the container.

In the mid-1960s, it was found that platelets from acid-citrate-dextrose PRP could be smoothly resuspended if the PRP was brought to room temperature before high-speed centrifugation and if the platelet pellet was allowed to rest undisturbed for 30 minutes at room temperature before resuspension (1) (Fig. 17.1). This principle has remained the standard of practice for 25 years. It allows preparation of PCs from blood anticoagulated with newer anticoagulants such as citrate-phosphate-dextrose (CPD) or CPD-adenine, although the "rest period" must be extended to 1 hour with those anticoagulants. Optimal speeds and durations of centrifugation have been determined empirically. In current practice, whole blood and PRP are kept at room

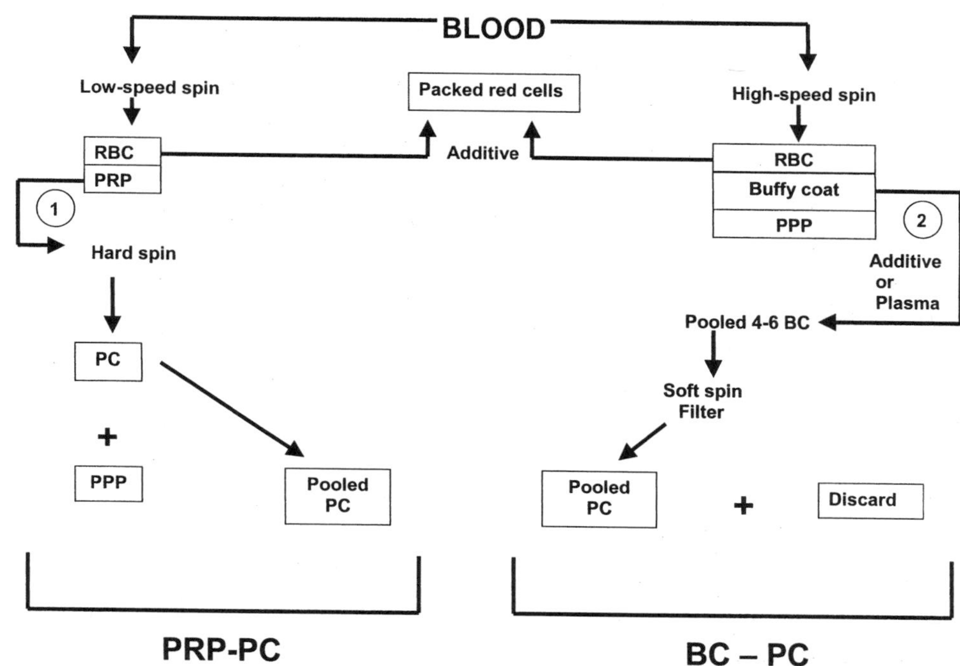

FIGURE 17.1. Two ways to prepare a pool of platelet concentrates (PCs) from units of whole blood. Pathway 1 is the platelet-rich plasma (PRP) method, the only method used in North America. Pathway 2 outlines the buffy-coat (BC) method, which is widely used in Europe. Both methods are described in the text. RBC, red blood cells; PPP, platelet-poor plasma.

temperature before and during processing until the platelets have been separated (2). In the United States, regulations require that this process be completed within 8 hours. In several European centers, very good results have been obtained holding the whole blood for up to 24 hours at ambient temperature before component preparation (3).

A unit of PRP-PC represents the platelets derived from one whole blood unit. An average unit of PRP-PC should contain 0.8 to 0.9 $\times$ 10^{11} platelets, but the range around the average is high, 0.4 to 1.8 $\times$ 10^{11} (4,5). One unit is adequate only for the transfusion of a small child who weighs less than 30 pounds. To transfuse adults, four to eight units are pooled to provide a therapeutic dose. Because of the wide range around the mean, it has been suggested that one must pool five units to be certain that the pool will contain at least 3 $\times$ 10^{11} platelets (5). Because each unit contains 0.1 to 0.5 $\times$ 10^9 leukocytes, predominantly lymphocytes, such pools contain 0.4 to 4.0 $\times$ 10^9 leukocytes, three orders of magnitude higher than a leukoreduced transfusion. There is a system which inserts a leukocyte-reduction filter between the primary blood bag and the bag that accepts the PRP (6,7). Thus, the PRP is leukoreduced at the time of its preparation. This system was introduced in early 1998 for the preparation of all PRP-PC in Canada and is gaining acceptance in the United States.

Buffy-coat Method

The PRP method for production of PCs may be traumatic for the platelets. The high-speed centrifugation against the wall of the plastic container and the 60-minute rest period during which the platelets form a compact mass may activate or injure the cells. During this process, there is evidence for thromboxane production (8), release of β-thromboglobulin (9), and expression on the platelet surface of the granular marker, P-selectin or CD-62 (10), all of which suggest platelet activation.

In a different approach to the preparation of PCs, the BC method, the initial centrifugation of whole blood is performed at a high speed so that the plasma, BC, and red blood cells can be collected in three separate containers (11) (Fig. 17.1). During centrifugation, the platelets at the top of the bag fall to the BC and, remarkably, the platelets at the bottom of the bag rise to the BC. Therefore, platelet yields in the BC are excellent. One can pool four to six BCs, add twice their volume of plasma or a synthetic storage medium, centrifuge the pool at low speed to remove red blood cells and leukocytes, and push the supernatant through a leukoreduction filter to produce a therapeutic, leukoreduced dose of platelets for an adult.

The PRP and BC methods have their advantages and disadvantages (12). Each produces platelets of acceptable quality, and platelet yields from a unit of blood are equivalent. In the BC method, 20 to 25 ml of red blood cells are lost with the BC so that they are not transfused to the recipients of the red blood cells. However, an extra 70 to 80 ml of plasma is collected.

Apheresis PC

One can obtain a therapeutic dose of platelets for one to three adults by apheresis of donors over 1 to 2 hours using a variety of devices (13–16). The details of this technology are presented in Chapter 45. The number of platelets obtained during the procedure varies with the platelet concentration in the blood of the donor, the volume of blood processed, and the efficiency of the device. In many centers, more than 95% of collections contain 3×10^{11} platelets and some contain more than 10×10^{11} platelets. Depending on their platelet content, these products must be distributed to one to three containers for storage, which will be discussed subsequently. The original intent of apheresis was to obtain a therapeutic dose for a single patient. However, many centers now divide these products to treat two or three patients. The separation technology of the various apheresis devices lends itself to the production of leukoreduced products during collection. Progressive improvements of those most recently available (13,14) has allowed the production of products with less than 1×10^6 leukocytes close to 100% of the time.

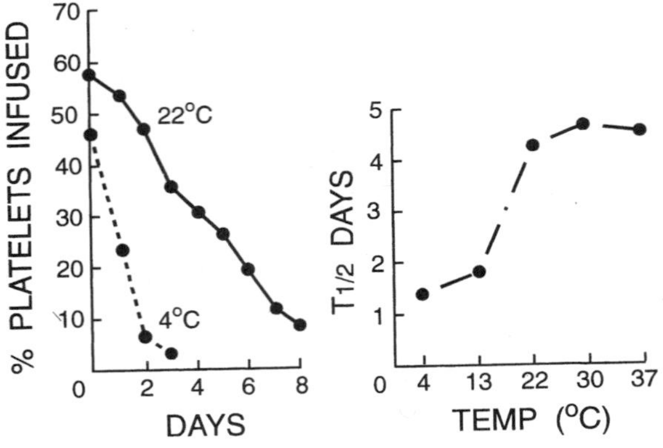

FIGURE 17.2. Autologous reinfusion studies in healthy volunteers of radiolabeled (chromium 51) platelets stored as PRP for 18 hours at various temperatures. The *graph* on the *left* shows the survival of platelets stored at 22°C is nearly equivalent to that of fresh platelets, whereas the survival of platelets stored at 4°C is very short. The initial recovery of 50% to 60% of the platelets infused results from physiologic pooling in the spleen (26) rather than from platelet injury. The half-life of fresh platelets is 3 to 5 days. The *graph* on the *right* shows that the half-life is normal after storage at 22°C but is reduced after storage at lower temperatures. (Data are redrawn from Murphy S, Gardner FH. Platelet preservation. Effect of storage temperature on maintenance of platelet viability-deleterious effect of refrigerated storage. *N Engl J Med* 1969; 280:1094–1098; and Murphy S. Platelet transfusion. *Prog Hemost Thromb* 1976;3:289–310, with permission.)

LIQUID STORAGE OF SINGLE WHOLE BLOOD–DERIVED PCS (PRP METHOD) IN PLASMA

Both whole blood–derived and AP-PC may be stored for 5 days using the same principles: (a) The temperature must be 20° to 24°C, (b) the storage container must be constructed of a plastic material that allows adequate diffusion of oxygen through its walls to meet the cells' metabolic needs, and (c) the PC must be agitated during storage.

Temperature of Storage

From the beginnings of platelet transfusion therapy, it was recognized that clinical efficacy correlated with a measurable, sustained rise in the platelet concentration in the blood of thrombocytopenic recipients (17). Therefore, research into the storage of PCs has always stressed the development of methods that allow the stored platelets to circulate normally after infusion. The ultimate test has been the result of transfusion in thrombocytopenic patients. However, such studies are too cumbersome and imprecise for developmental work because of the many clinical variables, such as infection and alloimmunization, that affect the results of platelet transfusion in these patients. Therefore, investigators have relied on autologous reinfusion studies in healthy volunteers in which the platelets are radiolabeled after storage and reinfused into the original donors. The data are generally reduced to two numbers: the percent recovery, reflecting the percentage of infused platelets that are present in the circulation 1 to 3 hours after infusion, and some measurement of subsequent survival, either mean cell life or half-life ($t^{1/2}$). Chromium 51 and indium-111 have been used for this purpose (18). Concurrent labeling of experimental and control platelets with two labels allows more precise conclusions to be drawn (19). As will be discussed subsequently, some in vitro tests have shown good correlation with in vivo results (20, 21).

In the 1950s and 1960s, PCs were stored in the cold. It was recognized that these stored platelets survived only briefly in the circulation after infusion. In the late 1960s, it was found that survival was normal, even after several days of storage, if storage was carried out at room temperature (20° to 24°C) rather than in the cold (22) (Fig. 17.2). Survival was equally compromised with storage at 13°C, and subsequent work indicated lesser but definite shortening of survival even after 24-hour storage at 18°C (23). In fact, the damage caused by cold temperature is a function of both the temperature and the time of exposure. Measurable damage occurs at 16°C for 16 hours, 12°C for 10 hours, and 4°C for 6 hours (24). Storage at temperatures warmer than 20° to 24°C seems to be inferior (22,24), although this has not been studied intensively.

Platelets lose their discoid shape and become spherical when they are damaged by cold (22,25). At the ultrastructural level, this change correlates with an irreversible loss of the circumferential band of microtubules that maintains the cell's discoid shape (25). There is a strong correlation between this morphologic change and shortening of survival in vivo (20–22).

Metabolic Patterns During PC Storage at 20° to 24°C

Figures 17.3 and 17.4 outline the major features of platelet energy metabolism, with emphasis on changes during storage in plasma at 20° to 24°C of whole blood–derived PCs prepared by the PRP method. For fresh PCs, the glycogen content is 0.05 mmol/L/10^{11} platelets (27). In 50 ml of PC containing 10^{11} platelets, this represents a concentration of 1 mmol/L in glucose equivalents. On the other hand, the initial glucose concentration is approximately 25 mmol/L, five times the physiologic concentration, because of the glucose added to the primary anticoagulant. Glycogen cannot be synthesized from glucose by platelets

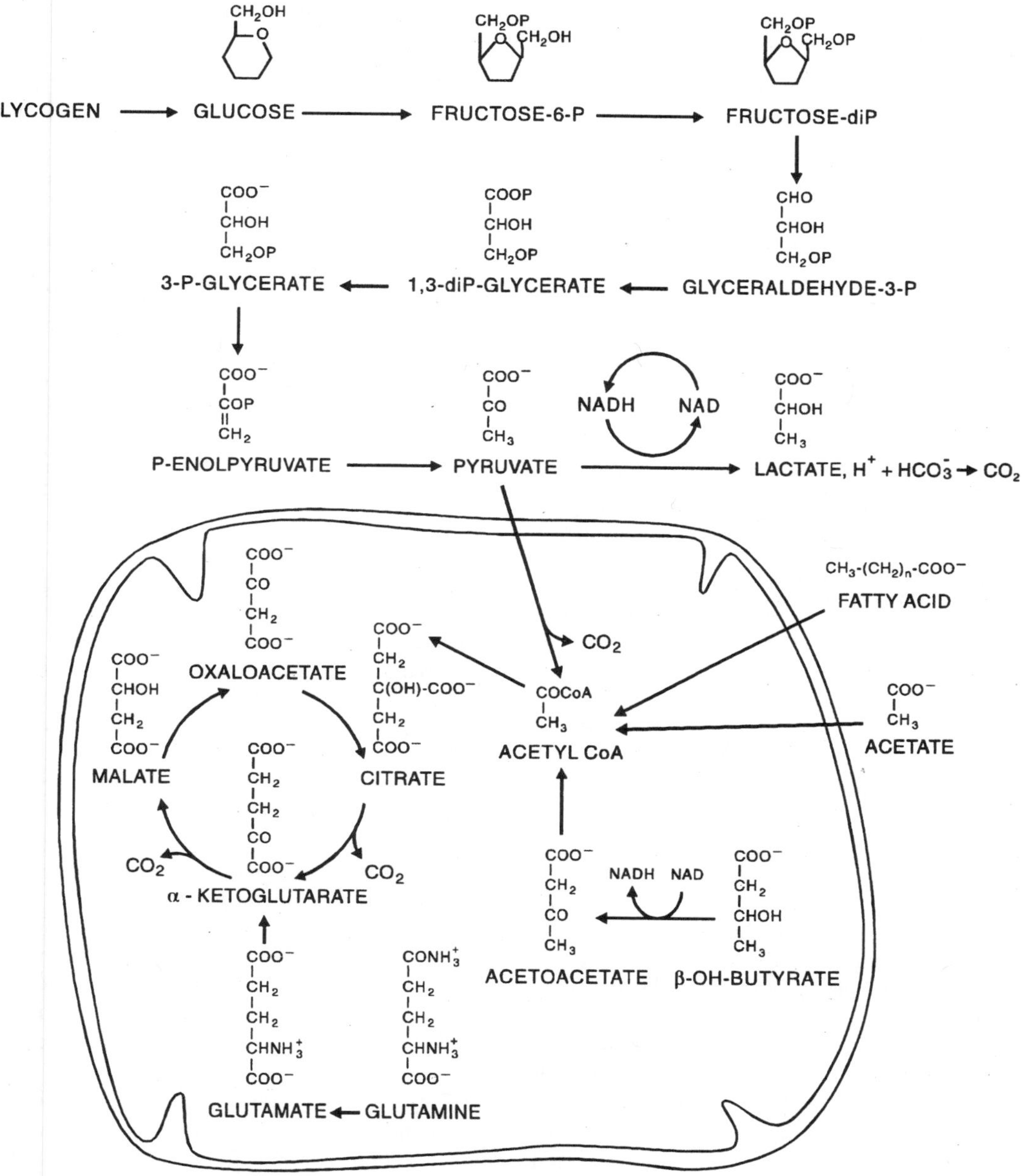

FIGURE 17.3. Metabolic pathways available to platelets. The oval with indentations represents the mitochondrial compartment. Most of these pathways are described in the text in the sections entitled, Metabolic Patterns During PC Storage at 20° to 24°C and Synthetic Storage Media. The circular pathway in the *upper left* portion of the mitochondrial compartment represents the TCA cycle. The pathway from β-OH-butyrate to acetyl CoA has been shown to be active in platelets (34). (Redrawn with modifications from Murphy S. The oxidation of exogenously added organic anions by platelets facilitates maintenance of pH during storage for transfusion at 22°C. *Blood* 1995;85:1929–1935, with permission.)

in vitro, and 80% of platelet glycogen is degraded during the first 24 hours of storage (27). During storage, glucose is converted to lactate essentially quantitatively, so that the lactate concentration rises by approximately 2.5 mmol/L/day (28).

Fortunately, oxygen can enter the PC through the walls of the plastic container. The rates of production of lactate and consumption of oxygen are approximately the same, 1.0 to 1.5 mmol/day/10^{12} platelets. Because the production of one lactate molecule fuels the regeneration of one adenosine triphosphate (ATP) molecule, and the consumption of one oxygen molecule fuels the regeneration of six ATP molecules, the cell derives 15% of its ATP regeneration through glycolysis and 85% through oxygen consumption through the tricarboxylic acid (TCA) cycle (28). Therefore, when completely deprived of oxygen, the cell will increase its rate of lactate production six- to seven-fold to compensate for the absence of ATP regeneration from oxidative

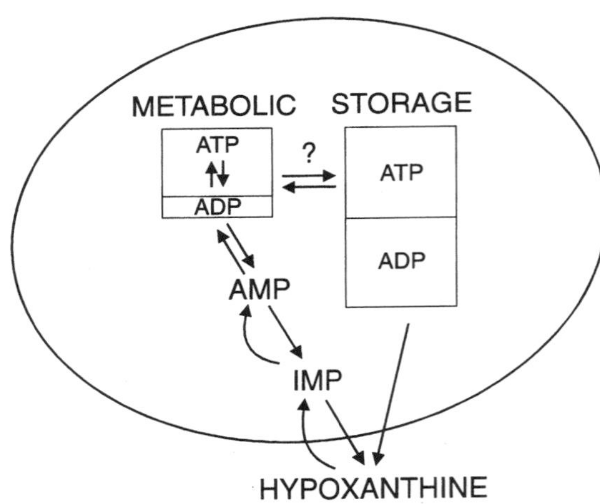

FIGURE 17.4. Adenine nucleotide metabolism during PC storage. The *oval* represents the cell wall. The metabolic and storage pools are drawn to scale. During storage, nucleotides from each pool are continuously degraded, with each pool contributing equally to the accumulation of hypoxanthine. Approximately 25% of hypoxanthine formed is reincorporated into adenine nucleotides through the hypoxanthine phosphoribosyl-transferase reaction. We do not know whether nucleotides are exchanged between two pools. (Redrawn from Ebenbrandt CM, Murphy. Adenine and guanine nucleotide metabolism during platelet storage at 22°C. *Blood* 1990;9:1884–1892, with permission.)

metabolism (27,28). This is the Pasteur effect, a response common to many cells.

Because almost all glucose metabolized is converted to lactate, even in the presence of adequate oxygen, the enzyme responsible for the conversion of pyruvate to acetylcoenzyme A (acetyl-CoA), pyruvate dehydrogenase, must be in an inactive state in platelets. The major substrate for oxidative metabolism of platelets during storage of PC in plasma appears to be free fatty acids, which are oxidized continuously to carbon dioxide with replenishment from triglycerides (29). Ammonia accumulates to a dramatic degree during storage of the PC, reaching 0.5 mmol/L after 7 days (30,31). This ammonia is derived from deamination of glutamine to glutamate by the mitochondrial enzyme glutaminase (31). It is not known whether this ammonia has a deleterious effect on platelets during storage. The glutamate formed is a potential fuel for oxidative metabolism, but little is used (31).

Oxidative metabolism generates a volatile acid, carbon dioxide, which can leave the PC by passing through the plastic walls of the storage container. Glycolysis of glucose yields lactate and a hydrogen ion that must be buffered if the pH is to remain stable. During storage of PC in plasma, the principal buffer is bicarbonate. For each mole of lactate produced, 0.8 mol of bicarbonate is converted to water and carbon dioxide. As long as bicarbonate is present, the pH will remain relatively stable at greater than 6.8. However, if lactate concentration rises to greater than 28 mmol/L, bicarbonate stores will be exhausted, and the pH will fall precipitously (28). Unless there is a stimulus to production of lactic acid, this generally does not happen until they've been stored for 7 to 10 days. A pH fall to less than 6.2 is associated with loss of platelet viability (32). As will be discussed subsequently, it is the accelerated production of lactic acid because of hypoxic conditions that accounts for inferior storage in first-generation containers.

Glycolytic and oxidative metabolism by platelets during storage of PCs allows regeneration of the ATP that breaks down to adenosine diphosphate (ADP) and adenosine monophosphate (AMP) as the cells' ongoing energy needs are being met. The stoichiometric production of lactate from glucose certainly seems wasteful in this regard, in that it yields only two ATP molecules per molecule of glucose metabolized, whereas the decarboxylation of pyruvate would yield three ATP molecules, and the subsequent oxidation of a molecule of acetyl-CoA would yield another 12 ATP molecules. In addition, as mentioned above, the continuous production of lactic acid eventually leads to a pH fall during storage of the PC, a problem that nature, of course, did not envision. Despite this ongoing metabolism, platelet adenine nucleotide levels fall during storage to approximately 75% and 50% of initial levels after 3 and 7 days of storage, respectively (30). The decline in platelet adenine nucleotides is matched quantitatively by a rise in their metabolic end product, hypoxanthine, in supernatant plasma (30). Platelet ADP and ATP are present in two pools, a metabolic pool, which meets the cell's ongoing metabolic needs, and a storage pool located in intracellular granules, which are released when the cell is stimulated. Each of the two pools contributes approximately equally to the decline in ADP and ATP during storage (Fig. 17.4) (30).

Hypoxanthine can be salvaged by hypoxanthine-guanine phosphoribosyltransferase to form inosine monophosphate, which can then be converted to AMP by a complex series of reactions in which adenylosuccinate synthetase converts inosine monophosphate and aspartate to adenylosuccinate which, in turn, is converted to AMP and fumarate by adenylosuccinate lyase. During storage of PCs, approximately 25% of the hypoxanthine formed is reincorporated back into adenine nucleotides by this salvage pathway (30). It is not known why this process cannot proceed more rapidly to allow better maintenance of adenine nucleotides. Enzymatic activities, concentration of the substrate, ribose 1-phosphate, or supply of necessary ATP may be deficient. Adenine is more readily incorporated into AMP than is hypoxanthine and, when adenine is present because of supplementation of the primary anticoagulant, this reaction is quite active. In one study, the presence of adenine allowed better maintenance of ATP during storage of PCs (30). However, to date there are no studies to show that inclusion of adenine improves the quality of platelets after storage of PCs in plasma (33).

Storage in First-generation Containers

The initial studies that showed the superiority of storage at 20° to 24°C were carried out with PRP. When, in the early 1970s, attempts were made to store PCs, the results were satisfactory but there were problems. First of all, it was shown that the containers had to be agitated to obtain satisfactory results after infusion in vivo (35). Second, among the polyvinyl chloride (PVC) plastic containers in use at the time, some were clearly better than others. For example, Fenwal's PL-146 was superior to its PL-130 (35), and Cutter's CL-3000 was superior to its CL-2399 (36). The differences seemed to be attributable to the presence of a secondary plasticizer, tetrahydrofurfuryl oleate, in PL-130 and CL-2399 (36). However, even with adequate agitation and the optimal available containers, some PCs had dramatic falls in pH to well less than 6.0 (35). Subsequent studies showed that, as the pH falls from 6.8 to 6.0, platelets swell and undergo a disc-to-sphere transformation (37). In the 6.2 to 6.8 range, these changes are reversible. However, when the pH falls to less than 6.2, the platelets become irreversibly swollen and eventually agglutinate together or lyse (35). When labeled and reinfused, these platelets do not circulate (32,35).

An understanding of the origins of pH change began with the serendipitous observation that a decline in pH did not occur in experimental containers constructed of plastic that had an increased permeability to oxygen and carbon dioxide (38). Plastics do not have pores through which gases pass, but the gases are soluble in the plastic and pass through to the other side when the plastic is saturated. Plastics vary in the ease with which gases penetrate. In retrospect, this major problem with first-generation containers can be explained by reference to Figure 17.3. The pH will remain stable during storage of PCs as long as the production of lactic acid does not exceed the capacity of plasma bicarbonate to buffer it, and the walls of the container are sufficiently permeable to allow the escape of the carbon dioxide produced by this buffering and by the oxidation of TCA-cycle substrates. First-generation containers were relatively impermeable to oxygen. PCs with high platelet counts were relatively hypoxic, so that there was inadequate generation of ATP from the TCA cycle. To compensate, according to the Pasteur effect, the rate of glycolysis and the production of lactate and hydrogen ion increased to the point that bicarbonate was exhausted, and the pH fell (28). Thus, a first-generation container is one with walls that permit insufficient oxygen to enter to meet the oxidative demands of the platelets within.

Storage in Second-generation Containers

A second-generation container for storage of PRP-PCs may be defined as one with plastic walls that have sufficient permeability to oxygen to meet the oxygen demand of the cells within. In practice, a container meets this qualification if there is a measurable oxygen tension (>40 mm Hg) throughout storage in PCs with the highest platelet counts encountered in practice (39) and if the rate of rise of the lactate concentration does not exceed 2 to 3 mmol/L/day. If the rate is faster than this and PO_2 is very low, it is likely that the cells are hypoxic and have accelerated glycolysis as a result of the Pasteur effect. With adequate oxygenation, there is enough bicarbonate to buffer the lactate produced at the baseline rate to maintain a stable pH for approximately 1 week.

Second generation has to be viewed as a relative term. Figure 17.5 contrasts the measured oxygen permeabilities of a series of second-generation containers with the platelet contents encoun-

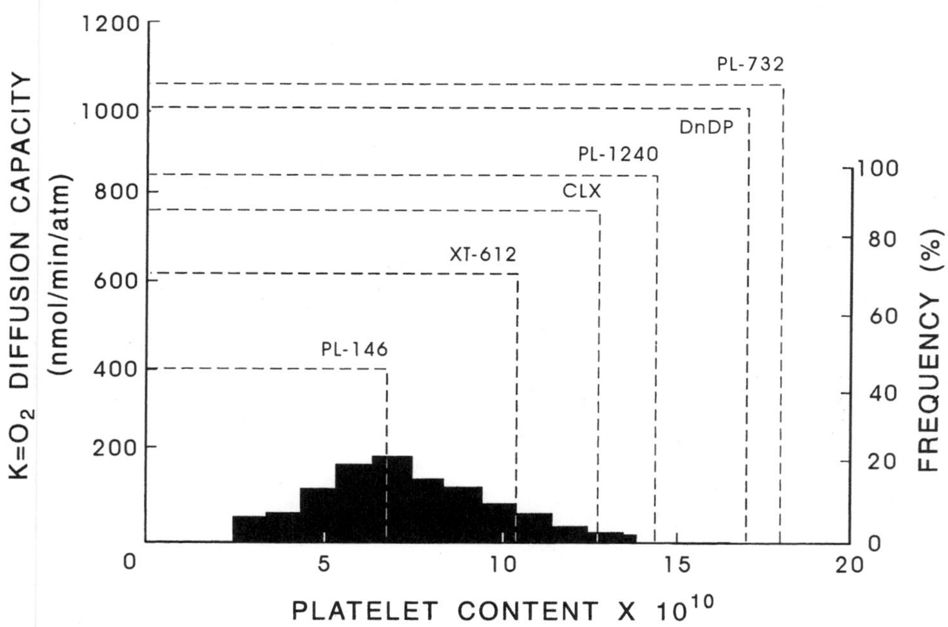

FIGURE 17.5. First- and second-generation containers for storage of PRP-PC. The capacity of a container to transport oxygen, *K*, can be measured (28) and compared with the distribution of platelet contents seen commonly in practice. For each container, the *vertical interrupted line* indicates that platelet content above which the PC will be hypoxic. The *vertical axis* on the *right* indicates the frequency of the PC with adequate oxygen supply. References for plastic types: PL-146 (39), XT-612 (40), CLX (41), PL-1240 (42), DnDP (43), and PL-732 (39). (Redrawn with modifications from Heaton WAL, Holme S. Storage of platelet concentrates. In: Rock G, Seghatchian MJ, eds. *Quality assurance in transfusion medicine.* Boca Raton, FL: CRC Press, 1992:122–139, with permission.)

tered commonly in practice. Furthermore, it indicates, for each container, the content of platelets above which the PC will be hypoxic and at risk for a fall in pH. Some containers are unsatisfactory, some are barely satisfactory, and some are more than satisfactory. However, even the most permeable container would revert to being a first-generation container if the platelet content were substantially increased over that seen commonly in current practice, for example greater than 20×10^{10}.

Changes in bag design that allow increased oxygen permeability generally will be associated with increased permeability to carbon dioxide. It might be expected that an accelerated exit of carbon dioxide would play a major role in preventing a pH fall. Actually, at the carbon dioxide tensions seen in practice, 10 to 100 mm Hg, the carbon dioxide concentration plays only a modulating role in this regard (28,32). On the other hand, early in storage when the lactate concentration is less than 10 mmol/L, a low carbon dioxide pressure (10 to 20 mm Hg) will allow the pH to be greater than 7.6. Such a high pH may also damage platelets during storage (39).

Even under optimal circumstances, there appears to be a platelet storage lesion. Autologous reinfusion studies of radiolabeled platelets stored for 5 to 7 days in second-generation containers have indicated a decline in the initial recovery of approximately 25%, with a modest shortening of survival time (39,40, 41,42). When pools of platelet units stored for this period have been infused into thrombocytopenic patients, increments in platelet counts at 1 hour after infusion have ranged from 50% to 80% of what would be expected for fresh platelets (39,41, 43,44,45). The prolonged bleeding times of thrombocytopenic patients, in general, have been shortened appropriately relative to the increment in platelet count achieved (39,41), at least at 24 hours after infusion. In three studies of PCs stored for 3 to 5 days (39,46,47), the bleeding times of some patients were not as short 1 to 3 hours after infusion as they were 4 to 24 hours after infusion. It is suggested, but far from established, that the function of stored platelets is impaired immediately after infusion, with normalization after several hours in the circulation.

Increased gas permeability in second-generation containers has been achieved by a variety of means, including the use of non-PVC plastic (39), different quantities and types of plasticizers (41–43), and thinner versions of traditional PVC (40). There is no evidence showing significant differences among the containers, particularly if in vivo studies are used as the major criteria, as long as the platelets receive adequate oxygenation.

Agitation During Storage

The role of agitation during PC storage is partially understood (48). For unknown reasons, when agitation is interrupted, oxygen consumption decreases and production of lactic acid increases. Agitation interruption does not interfere with the availability of oxygen. When the platelet concentration is high, lactate production can be so rapid that pH can fall to deleterious levels if agitation is interrupted for 2 to 3 days (Fig. 17.6). However, even at the highest platelet concentrations, agitation can be interrupted for 24 hours without platelet damage (48).

There have been clear differences when various forms of agitation were compared (39,42,49). In early studies (38) using a Ferris-wheel type of apparatus, the pH rose to the range of 7.6 to 7.8 in PCs with low platelet counts because of a rapid carbon dioxide escape from the container early in storage, as described above in the section on carbon dioxide loss. This was associated

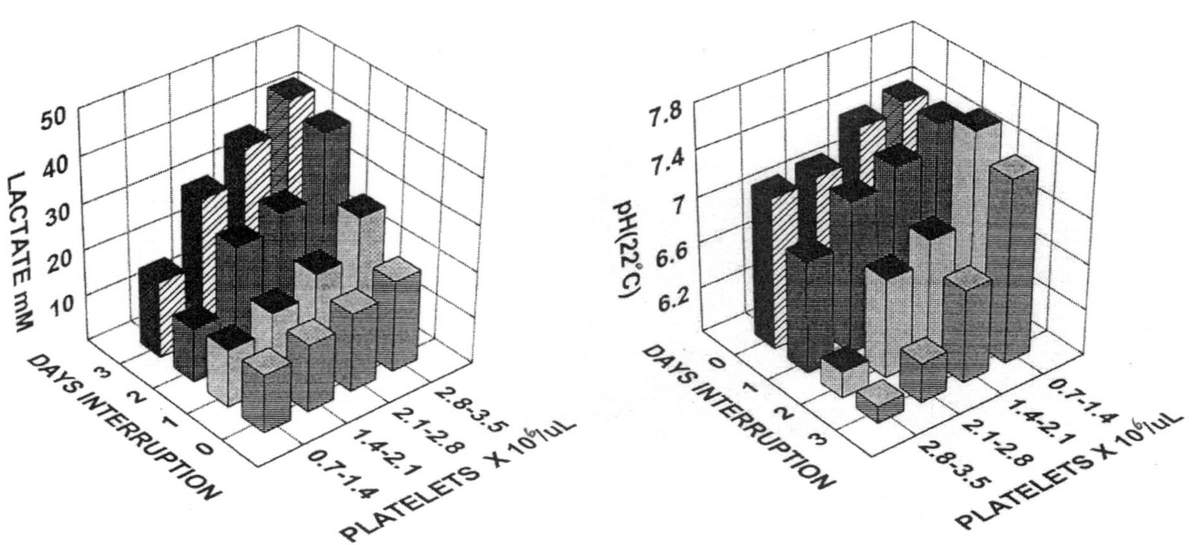

FIGURE 17.6. Effect of interruption of agitation for 1, 2, and 3 days on lactate concentration *(left)* and pH *(right)* on the fifth day of storage (48) of 50 ml PC. The results are also expressed relative to the PC platelet concentration. The combination of high platelet concentration and 2- to 3-day interruption of agitation results in acceleration of lactate production such that pH can reach levels of 6.2 or lower on the fifth day of storage. (Figure derived from data in Hunter S, Nixon J, Murphy S. The effect of interruption of agitation on platelet quality during storage for transfusion. *Transfusion* 2001;41:809–814, with permission.)

with marked morphologic abnormalities and a loss of viability after reinfusion in vivo. An identical lesion was observed when an elliptical, "end-over-end" form of agitation was used (39, 42). In the studies with the Ferris-wheel type of apparatus, storage with a 10% external carbon dioxide atmosphere prevented the pH rise and the morphologic changes and allowed maintenance of in vivo viability, indicating that the carbon dioxide escape and pH rise were critical components in causing the damage. However, even with the carbon dioxide atmosphere, results with a platform horizontal agitator were significantly better than with the Ferris-wheel type of apparatus (49), suggesting that the form of agitation was critical for obtaining optimal results even when the rise in pH was prevented. A reasonable hypothesis is that a rise in pH occurs early in storage in second-generation containers, sensitizing platelets to damage that is more marked with certain forms of agitation than with others. This damage slows metabolism, thereby reducing lactic acid and carbon dioxide production, leading to a further pH rise and a vicious cycle. In most studies, platform agitation and the Helmer tumbler "face-over-face" agitator (39) have produced satisfactory results, whereas elliptical and Ferris-wheel forms of agitation have not.

In addition, keeping PC volume above a certain minimum, 35 ml (50), is important. Results with 30 ml have been unsatisfactory (39).

SYNTHETIC STORAGE MEDIA

Ongoing research is directed toward developing synthetic storage media to replace some or all of the plasma that has been traditionally used. As a minimal goal, this would free this plasma for fractionation. In addition, platelet quality after storage might be enhanced. As mentioned previously, the use of a synthetic medium is ideally suited to the BC method of PC preparation, because four to six BCs can be pooled before storage and diluted in twice the pool volume of synthetic medium before the slow centrifugation, which removes contaminating erythrocytes and leukocytes (Figure 17.1). These platelets have had superior quality relative to PCs prepared by the PRP method after prolonged storage by both in vivo (51) and in vitro (52) criteria. Table 17.1 lists the ingredients of three synthetic media which have been used successfully for the storage of pooled BC-PC and AP-PC using one-third volume of plasma and two-thirds volume of medium. Notably absent from the media are glucose and bicarbonate, both of which introduce significant manufacturing problems (55). Fortunately, the one-third volume of plasma provides approximately 7.5 mmol/L glucose, which is sufficient for at least 7 days of storage.

Present in all synthetic media has been sodium acetate in concentrations in excess of 25 mmol/L. Perhaps 15 mmol/L would suffice for 7 days of storage (55). The inclusion of acetate in the medium is crucial because it acts as a substrate for oxidative metabolism (Fig. 17.3) and provides a buffering action by using a hydrogen ion for each molecule oxidized (34,55). In effect, acetate plays the role played by bicarbonate during storage in plasma. The requirements may be more stringent when the percentage of synthetic medium by volume is greater than 80% (55). Supplemental phosphate and citrate may be helpful, and there is debate about the necessity for supplemental glucose (55). The roles of potassium, magnesium, and gluconate present in Plasma Lyte A are still to be defined.

TABLE 17.1. SOME SYNTHETIC STORAGE MEDIA FOR PLATELETS

	PlasmaLyte A[b]	PAS-2[c]	PAS-3[d]
NaCl	90.0[a]	115.5	77.0
KCl	5.0	—	—
$MgCl_2$	3.0	—	—
Na_3 citrate	—	10.0	12.3
Na phosphate	—	—	28.0
Na acetate	27.0	30.0	42.0
Na gluconate	23.0	—	—

[a]Concentrations given in mmol/L
[b]Bertolini F, Rebulla P, Riccardi. Evaluation of platelet concentrates prepared from buffy coats and stored in a glucose-free crystalloid medium. *Transfusion* 1989;29:605–609.
[c]Gulliksson H, Eriksson L, Hogman CF, et al. Buffy-coat–derived platelet concentrates prepared from half-strength citrate CPD and CPD whole-blood units. *Vox Sang* 1995;68:152–159.
[d]Corash L, Behrman B, Rheinschmidt M, et al. Post-transfusion viability and tolerability of photochemically treated platelet concentrates (PC). *Blood* 1997;90:267a.

20° TO 24°C STORAGE LESION

Some authors have been unable to show any practical difference between fresh and stored platelets (56,57) but, as mentioned above, most find that in vivo recovery and subsequent platelet survival are reduced after 5 days of storage by at least 25% in both autologous reinfusion and patient studies. This loss of viability has been associated with morphologic, biochemical, and functional changes.

Atypical morphologic forms identified by phase and electron microscopy are observed after storage (58). These consist of crescent forms, discs resembling elm or dogwood leaves, elongated tubular forms, ring forms, and empty swollen cells. More objective techniques have shown that platelets undergo a disc-to-sphere transformation during storage. In addition, the mean platelet volume decreases by about 10%. Finally, we have observed a varying, although usually small, number of platelet fragments, platelet ghosts, and swollen (ballooned) platelets that create a tail of light platelets in the density distribution of stored platelets. These may be the platelets that are nonviable after infusion (37).

Many investigators have likened the platelet storage lesion to a form of activation (59,60). With activation, platelets undergo a disc-to-sphere transformation and secrete the contents of their granules. Platelet granules are of two types, the more numerous α granules, which contain platelet-specific proteins such as platelet factor 4 and β-thromboglobulin, and the dense granules, which contain ADP, ATP, and serotonin (Fig. 17.4). The decrease in dense-granule ADP and ATP during storage already has been described in the section on metabolic patterns during storage. In addition, several studies (60) have observed a continuous disappearance from platelets and appearance in plasma of β thromboglobulin during storage. Taken together, these results strongly suggest that both α and dense granules decrease during storage, even under optimal circumstances. In addition, during physiologic activation, the glycoprotein (GP) P-selectin or CD62, which is a component of the α-granule membrane of the resting platelet, becomes expressed on the surface of the cell, and membranous microparticles are released into the supernatant. Similar events occur during PC storage (59–61). Inhibitors of platelet activation reduce the extent of these changes, suggesting that their use might improve the quality of stored platelets (62).

After recovery from activation, platelets are less responsive to stimulation with agonists. Similarly, stored platelets have decreased reactivity to single aggregating agents such as ADP, epinephrine, and collagen when they are assessed in the platelet aggregometer (8). Platelet aggregation in response to physiologic agonists is mediated by the exposure of receptors for fibrinogen that reside on the GP IIb-IIIa complex. Calcium-dependent binding of fibrinogen to receptors on adjacent platelets mediates the attachment of these platelets to each other. Stored platelets have a normal content of GP IIb-IIIa. However, after stimulation with ADP or epinephrine, stored platelets bind significantly less fibrinogen than fresh platelets, suggesting that the function of the receptor is defective (63). It is not clear whether these observations have relevance for the function of stored platelets after infusion. The response of stored platelets to pairs of aggregating agents is much less impaired than that to single agents (8). Because platelet function in vivo undoubtedly occurs in response to several stimuli simultaneously, failure of response to a single agent in vitro may be of little importance. Furthermore, the responsiveness to single aggregating agents improves in the circulation after infusion (64).

More recently, some investigators have suggested that the platelet storage lesion may be a form of apoptosis (65). Most discussions of apoptosis have involved nucleated cells, but it is clear that apoptosis can occur in nonnucleated cells as well.

Some, but not all, in vitro abnormalities correlate with loss of in vivo viability (20). In particular, decreased response to hypotonic shock (49) and the extent of disc-to-sphere transformation (39, 49) predict decreased viability in vivo. However, aggregation abnormalities and the release of granule contents have not correlated with in vivo viability (42). Therefore, developmental work assessing new storage techniques should attempt to show that in vitro measurements that correlate with in vivo viability are well maintained. In addition, the retention of the disc shape, which predicts good in vivo viability, can be assessed noninvasively by examining the PC macroscopically for the so-called *swirling* or *shimmering* phenomenon (48,66). Blood bank and clinical personnel are urged to check PCs for this phenomenon prior to transfusion.

STORAGE OF APHERESIS-PCS

The same basic principles apply to the storage of AP-PC as to single PRP-PC (67). However, the situation is complicated by the great variation in volume and platelet content of the collections depending on the platelet count of the donor, the volume of the donor's blood processed, and the efficiency of the apheresis device. The collected platelet content may range from 2×10^{11} to 12×10^{11}. Individual collection containers have a 1-liter capacity so that the surface area for gas exchange is enhanced, perhaps 2.5-fold, relative to those used for PRP-PC. However, complexity is added because gas transport varies directly with the volume of the collection in the container. Furthermore, the plastics of the various manufacturers vary in their gas transport capacity so that there is variability in the maximum platelet content which a container can tolerate without risking hypoxia and pH fall (67). This range extends from 3.5×10^{11} to 5×10^{11} (67). Each manufacturer identifies this value for the customer. Thus, one needs to know the platelet content of each collection. A collection may be small enough to be stored in one container, but large collections may require two or even three containers.

Hematology analyzers vary by as much as 20% in the platelet count that they will record for a given sample (67). There is a danger that the manufacturer's analyzer may yield higher results than the blood center's. Thus, unexpected examples of pH fall may be observed (67).

COMPLICATIONS OF PLATELET TRANSFUSION RELATED TO PREPARATION AND STORAGE OF PCS

Some of the complications of platelet transfusion are related to the techniques used for preparation and storage. In some instances, modifications of and additions to these techniques can reduce the incidence and severity of these complications.

Bacterial Contamination

For many years (68), there has been concern that storage of PCs at 20° to 24°C will allow proliferation of the bacteria that occasionally may contaminate blood at the time of collection (see Chapter 55). Contamination may occur by skin organisms at the time of venipuncture or through asymptomatic bacteremia in the donor. There have been studies suggesting that bacterial contamination that might not be clinically significant after 3 days of storage might become so if bacterial multiplication continues for 7 days. Therefore, although the viability of platelets after storage of PCs for 5 and 7 days is similar (45), storage of PCs at 20° to 24°C is currently limited to 5 days. It is hoped that methods of viral inactivation (which also inhibit bacterial proliferation in PCs) (69) and methods for screening PCs for the presence of bacteria before infusion (70) will allow us to deal with this problem.

Benefits of Leukoreduction

There is evidence that leukoreduction can reduce the incidence of alloimmunization to HLA class I antigens and the transmission of cytomegalovirus (Chapter 21). Furthermore, as many as 20% of patients receiving platelet transfusion have febrile reactions. Leukocyte reduction at the time of infusion of red blood cells has reduced the incidence of these reactions, but this has not been true for platelets (71,72). It has been shown that contaminating leukocytes produce a variety of cytokines such as interleukin-1b, interleukin-6, interleukin-8, and tumor necrosis factor during PC storage (Chapter 58), and many reactions have been linked to these bioreactive substances in the plasma supernatants of PCs. These observations provide a strong argument for the routine removal of leukocytes from PCs during or soon after preparation.

FROZEN STORAGE OF PLATELETS

The most widely studied method for frozen storage employs controlled rate freezing (1°C per minute), 5% dimethyl sulfoxide (DMSO) as a cryoprotective agent, rapid thawing, graded reduction of the DMSO concentration, and washing prior to infusion. In vivo viability is approximately 40% to 50% relative to fresh platelets (73), but enhanced in vivo function has been claimed (74). Most find that this technology is more complex and expensive and less effective than liquid storage at 20° to 24°C (75). However, these preparations can be effective clinically and may be used for autologous transfusion of selected patients, particularly those who are highly alloimmunized. Platelets may be obtained before myelosuppressive therapy, frozen, and then administered during subsequent periods of thrombocytopenia (76). Newer approaches using second-messenger effectors may allow the use of lower concentrations of DMSO, which would in turn allow the direct infusion of platelets after thawing (77).

SUMMARY

Platelet storage technology has advanced to a remarkable degree since the very early days of 4°C–platelet storage. The ability to store platelets for longer than the currently Food and Drug Administration–approved limit of 5 days is restricted only by concerns over the growth of bacterial pathogens in the units of platelets. Storage of platelets for 7 days or more with maintenance of their metabolic and functional status is within the grasp of our technology. Concern over the presence of other pathogens in the blood supply, however, has led to the development of pathogen inactivation methodologies. Interestingly, pathogen inactivation may actually permit long-term platelet storage due to the elimination of concerns over bacterial growth. Advances in frozen storage technology are needed before platelets can be cryopreserved as successfully as red blood cells. Advances in surgical techniques for transplantation and treatment of trauma, as well as advances in oncologic therapy for patients with cancer, all require increased availability of platelets. This need for increasing numbers of platelets will doubtless provide the stimulus for further advances in platelet storage technology during the next decade.

REFERENCES

1. Mourad N. A simple method for obtaining platelet concentrates free of aggregates. *Transfusion* 1968;8:48.
2. Holme S, Moroff G, Whitley P, et al. Properties of platelet concentrates prepared after extended whole blood holding time. *Transfusion* 1989; 29:689–692.
3. Pietersz RNI, de Korte D, Reesink HW, et al. Storage of whole blood for up to 24 hours at ambient temperatures prior to component preparation. *Vox Sang* 1989;56:145–150.
4. Kelly DL, Fegan RL, Ng AT, et al. High-yield platelet concentrates attainable by continuous quality improvement reduce platelet transfusion cost and donor exposure. *Transfusion* 1997;37:482–486.
5. Hoeltge GA, Shah A, Miller JP. An optimized strategy for choosing the number of platelet concentrates to pool. *Arch Pathol Lab Med* 1999; 123:928–930.
6. Devine DV, Bradley AJ, Maurer E, et al. Effects of prestorage white cell reduction on platelet aggregate formation and the activation state of platelets and plasma enzyme systems. *Transfusion* 1999;39:724–734.
7. Sweeney JD, Kouttab NM, Penn CL, et al. A comparison of prestorage WBC-reduced whole-blood–derived platelets and bedside-filtered whole-blood–derived platelets in autologous progenitor cell transplant. *Transfusion* 2000;40:794–800.
8. DiMinnio G, Silver MJ, Murphy S. Stored human platelets retain full aggregation potential in response to pairs of aggregating agents. *Blood* 1982;59:563–568.
9. Rinder HM, Snyder EL. Activation of platelet concentrate during preparation and storage. *Blood Cells* 1992;18:4445–4456.
10. George JN, Pickett EB, Heinz R. Platelet membrane glycoprotein changes during the preparation and storage of platelet concentrates. *Transfusion* 1988;28:123–126.
11. Murphy S, Heaton WA, Rebulla P. Platelet production in the old world and the new. *Transfusion* 1996;36:751–754.
12. Heaton WAL, Rebulla P, Pappalettera M, et al. A comparative analysis of different methods for routine blood component preparation. *Transfus Med Rev* 1997;11:116–129.
13. Elfath D, Tahhan H, Mintz P, et al. Quality and clinical response to transfusion of prestorage white cell-reduced apheresis platelets prepared by use of an in-line white cell-reduction system. *Transfusion* 1999;39: 960–966.
14. Yockey C, Murphy S, Eggers L, et al. Evaluation of the Amicus separator in the collection of apheresis platelets. *Transfusion* 1998;38: 848–854.
15. Holme S, Andres M, Goermar N, et al. Improved removal of white cells with minimal platelet loss by filtration of apheresis platelets during collection. *Transfusion* 1999;39:75–82.
16. Zeiler T, Zingsem J, Moog R, et al. Periodic alternating interface positioning to lower WBC contamination of apheresis platelet concentrates: a multicenter evaluation. *Transfusion* 2000;40:687–692.
17. Hirsch EO, Gardner FH. The transfusion of human blood platelets. With a note on the transfusion of granulocytes. *J Lab Clin Med* 1952; 39:556–569.
18. Snyder EL, Moroff G, Simon T. Symposium on radiolabeling of stored platelet concentrates. *Transfusion* 1986;26:1–42.
19. Holme S, Heaton A, Roodt J. Concurrent labeling method with ^{111}IN and ^{51}Cr allows accurate evaluation of platelet viability of stored platelet concentrates. *Br J Haematol* 1993;84:717–723.
20. Murphy S, Rebulla P, Bertolini F, et al. In vitro assessment of the quality of stored platelet concentrates. *Transfus Med Rev* 1994;8:29–36.
21. Holme S, Moroff G, Murphy S. A multi-laboratory evaluation of in vitro platelet assays: the tests for extent of shape change and response to hypotonic shock. *Transfusion* 1998;38:31–40.
22. Murphy S, Gardner FH. Platelet preservation. Effect of storage temperature on maintenance of platelet viability–deleterious effect of refrigerated storage. *N Engl J Med* 1969;280:1094–1098.
23. Gottschall JL, Rzad L, Aster RH. Studies of the minimum temperature at which human platelets can be stored with full maintenance of viability. *Transfusion* 1986;26:460–462.
24. Holme S, Sawyer S, Heaton A, et al. Studies on platelets exposed to or stored at temperatures below 20°C or above 24°C. *Transfusion* 1997; 37:5–11.
25. White JG, Krivit W. Ultrastructural basis for shape changes induced in platelets by chilling. *Blood* 1967;30:625–635.

26. Aster RH, Jandl JH. Platelet sequestration in man. I. Methods. *J Clin Invest* 1964;43:843–855.
27. Murphy S, Gardner FH. Platelet storage at 22°C: metabolic, morphologic, and functional studies. *J Clin Invest* 1971;50:370–377.
28. Kilkson H, Holmes S, Murphy S. Platelet metabolism during storage of platelet concentrates at 22°C. *Blood* 1984;64:406–414.
29. Cesar J, DiMinnio G, Alam I, et al. Plasma free fatty acid metabolism during storage of platelet concentrates for transfusion. *Transfusion* 1987;27:434–437.
30. Edenbrandt CM, Murphy S. Adenine and guanine nucleotide metabolism during platelet storage at 22°C. *Blood* 1990;9:1884–1892.
31. Murphy S, Munoz S, Parry-Billings M, et al. Amino acid metabolism during platelet storage for transfusion. *Br J Haematol* 1992;81: 585–590.
32. Murphy S. Platelet storage for transfusion. *Semin Hematol* 1985;22: 165–177.
33. Simon TL, Nelson EJ, Murphy S. Extension of platelet concentrate storage to 7 days in second-generation bags. *Transfusion* 1987;27:6–9.
34. Murphy S. The oxidation of exogenously added organic anions by platelets facilitates maintenance of pH during their storage for transfusion at 22°C. *Blood* 1995;85:1929–1935.
35. Murphy S, Sayer SN, Gardner FH. Storage of platelet concentrates at 22°C. *Blood* 1970;35:549–557.
36. Lindberg JE, Slichter SJ, Murphy S, et al. In vitro function and in vivo viability of stored platelet concentrates. Effect of a secondary plasticizer component of PVC storage bags. *Transfusion* 1983;23:294–299.
37. Holme S, Murphy S. Platelet storage at 22°C for transfusion: interrrelationship of platelet density and size, medium pH, and viability after in vivo infusion. *J Lab Clin Med* 1983;101:161–174.
38. Murphy S, Gardner FH. Platelet storage at 22°C: role of gas transport across plastic containers in maintenance of viability. *Blood* 1975;46: 209–218.
39. Murphy S, Kahn RA, Holme S, et al. Improved storage of platelets for transfusion in a new container. *Blood* 1982;60:194–200.
40. Holme S, Heaton A, Momoda G. Evaluation of a new, oxygen-permeable, polyvinylchloride container. *Transfusion* 1989;29:159–164.
41. Simon TL, Nelson EJ, Carmen R, et al. Extension of platelet concentrate storage. *Transfusion* 1983;23:207–212.
42. Snyder EL, Pope C, Ferri PM, et al. The effect of mode of agitation and type of plastic bag on storage characteristics and in vivo kinetics of platelet concentrates. *Transfusion* 1986;26:125–130.
43. Shimizu T, Kouketsu K, Morishima Y, et al. A new polyvinylchloride blood bag plasticized with less-leachable phthalate ester analogue, di-n-decyl phthalate, for storage of platelets. *Transfusion* 1989;29:292–297.
44. Schiffer CA, Lee EJ, Ness PM, et al. Clinical evaluation of platelet concentrates stored for one to five days. *Blood* 1986;67:1591–1594.
45. Hogge DE, Thompson BW, Schiffer CA. Platelet storage for 7 days in second-generation blood bags. *Transfusion* 1986;26:131–135.
46. Slichter SJ, Harker LA. Preparation and storage of platelet concentrates. II. Storage variables influencing platelet viability and function. *Br J Haematol* 1976;34:403.
47. Filip DJ, Aster RH. Relative hemostatic effectiveness of human platelets stored at 40 and 22°C. *J Lab Clin Med* 1978;91:618–624.
48. Hunter S, Nixon J, Murphy S. The effect of interruption of agitation on platelet quality during storage for transfusion. *Transfusion* 2001; 41:809–814.
49. Holme S, Vaidja K, Murphy S. Platelet storage at 22°C: effect of type of agitation on morphology, viability, and function in vitro. *Blood* 1978;52:425–435.
50. Holme S, Heaton WA, Moroff G. Evaluation of platelet concentrates stored for 5 days with reduced plasma volume. *Transfusion* 1994;34: 39–43.
51. Bertolini F, Rebulla P, Riccardi. Evaluation of platelet concentrates prepared from buffy coats and stored in a glucose-free crystalloid medium. *Transfusion* 1989;29:605–609.
52. Bertolini F, Rebulla P, Porretti L, et al. Platelet quality after 15-day storage of platelet concentrates prepared from buffy coats and stored in a glucose-free crystalloid medium. *Transfusion* 1992;32:9–16.
53. Gulliksson H, Eriksson L, Hogman CF, et al. Buffy-coat–derived platelet concentrates prepared from half-strength citrate CPD and CPD whole-blood units. *Vox Sang* 1995;68:152–159.
54. Corash L, Behrman B, Rheinschmidt M, et al. Post-transfusion viability and tolerability of photochemically treated platelet concentrates (PC). *Blood* 1997;90:267a.
55. Murphy S. The efficacy of synthetic media in the storage of human platelets for transfusion. *Transfus Med Rev* 1999;13:153–163.
56. Shanwell A, Larsson S, Aschan J, et al. A randomized trial comparing the use of fresh and stored platelets in the treatment of bone marrow transplant recipients. *Eur J Haematol* 1992;49:77–81.
57. Leach MF, AuBuchon JP. Effect of storage time on clinical efficacy of single-donor platelet units. *Transfusion* 1993;33:661–664.
58. Fratantoni JC, Sturdivant B, Poindexter BJ. Aberrant morphology of platelets stored in five-day containers. *Thromb Res* 1984;33:607–615.
59. Metcalfe P, Williamson LM, Reutlingsperger CPM, et al. Activation during preparation of therapeutic platelets affects deterioration during storage: a comparative flow cytometric study of different production methods. *Br J Haematol* 1997;98:86–95.
60. Rinder HM, Snyder EL, Bonan JL, et al. Activation in stored platelet concentrates: correlates between membrane expression of P-selectin, glycoprotein IIb/IIIa, and thromboglobulin release. *Transfusion* 1993; 33:25–29.
61. Bode AP, Orton SM, Frye MJ, et al. Vesiculation of platelets during in vitro aging. *Blood* 1991;77:887–895.
62. Holme S, Bode A, Heaton WAL, et al. Improved maintenance of platelet in vivo viability during storage when using a synthetic medium with inhibitors. *J Lab Clin Med* 1992;119:144–150.
63. DiMinnio G, Capitanio AM, Thiagarajan P, et al. Exposure of fibrinogen receptors on fresh and stored platelets by ADP and epinephrine as single agents and as a pair. *Blood* 1983;61:1054–1059.
64. Owens M, Holme S, Heaton A, et al. Post-transfusion recovery of function of 5-day stored platelet concentrates. *Br J Haematol* 1992;80: 539–544.
65. Li J, Xia Y, Bertino AM, et al. The mechanism of apoptosis in human platelets during storage. *Transfusion* 2000;40:1320–1329.
66. Bertolini F. The absence of swirling in platelet concentrates is highly predictive of poor posttransfusion platelet count increments and increased risk of a transfusion reaction. *Transfusion* 2000;40:121–122.
67. Murphy S. Platelet function, kinetics, and metabolism: impact on quality assessment, storage, and clinical use. In: McLeod BC. *Apheresis principles and practice.* Bethesda: American Association of Blood Banks, 1997:123.
68. Klein HG, Dodd RY, Ness PM, et al. Current status of microbial contamination of blood components: summary of a conference. *Transfusion* 1997;37:95–101.
69. Lin L, Cook DN, Wiesehahn GP, et al. Photochemical inactivation of viruses and bacteria in platelet concentrates by use of a novel psoralen and long-wavelength ultraviolet light. *Transfusion* 1997;37:423–435.
70. Mitchell KM, Brecher ME. Approaches to the detection of bacterial contamination in cellular blood products. *Transfus Med Rev* 1999;13: 132–144.
71. Mangano MM, Chambers LA, Kruskall MS. Limited efficacy of leukopoor platelets for prevention of febrile transfusion reactions. *Am J Clin Pathol* 1991;95:733–738.
72. Goodnough LT, Riddell IVJ, Lazarus H, et al. Prevalence of platelet transfusion reactions before and after implementation of leukocyte-depleted platelet concentrates by filtration. *Vox Sang* 1993;65: 103–107.
73. Murphy S, Sayar SN, Abdou NL, et al. Platelet preservation by freezing. Use of dimethylsulfoxide as cryoprotective agent. *Transfusion* 1974;14: 139–144.
74. Barnard MR, MacGregor H, Ragno G, et al. Fresh, liquid-preserved, cryopreserved platelets: adhesive surface receptors and membrane procoagulant activity. *Transfusion* 1999;39:880–888.
75. Towell BL, Levine SP, Knight WA III, et al. A comparison of frozen and fresh platelet concentrates in the support of thrombocytopenic patients. *Transfusion* 1986;26:525–530.

76. Schiffer CA, Aisner J, Wiernik PH. Frozen autologous platelet transfusion for patients with leukemia. *N Engl J Med* 1978;299:7–12.
77. Pedrazzoli P, Nors P, Perotti C, et al. Transfusion of platelet concentrates cryopreserved with ThromboSol plus low-dose dimethylsulphoxide in patients with severe thrombocytopenia: a pilot study. *Br J Haematol* 2000;108:653–659.
78. Murphy S. Platelet transfusion. *Prog Hemost Thromb* 1976;3:289–310.
79. Ebenbrandt CM, Murphy. Adenine and guanine nucleotide metabolism during platelet storage at 22°C. *Blood* 1990;9:1884–1892.
80. Heaton WAL, Holme S. Storage of platelet concentrates. In: Rock G, Seghatchian MJ, eds. *Quality assurance in transfusion medicine.* Boca Raton, FL: CRC Press, 1992:122–139.

18

PLATELET TRANSFUSION AND ALTERNATIVES

GREGORY J. POMPER
LI CHAI
EDWARD L. SNYDER

THROMBOCYTOPENIA AND PLATELET DYSFUNCTION

Platelet transfusions are the primary therapy for thrombocytopenia of various causes. Thrombocytopenia is generally separated into three etiologic categories when formulating a differential diagnosis: disorders of platelet production (decreased production or dysfunction), platelet sequestration, and platelet destruction. Effective platelet transfusion therapy depends on a correct diagnosis of a patient's thrombocytopenia in order to select an appropriate platelet preparation. Numerous platelet products and laboratory manipulations of platelet products are available to treat the many different diseases amenable to platelet transfusions.

Disorders of Platelet Production

Decreased Platelet Production

The number of circulating platelets is determined by production in the bone marrow in conjunction with levels of endogenous thrombopoietin and other regulatory cytokines. Thrombocyto-

G.J. Pomper, L. Chai and E.L. Snyder: Blood Bank/Apheresis Service, Yale–New Haven Hospital, and Department of Laboratory Medicine, Yale University School of Medicine, New Haven, Connecticut.

penia ensues when toxic or pathologic insults damage megakaryocytes and interrupt the constant (steady state) production of platelets (approximately 40,000 platelets per µl per day).

Chemotherapeutic agents cause thrombocytopenia in cancer patients, and specific prophylactic platelet transfusion "triggers" or minimum levels have been studied to avoid hemorrhagic complications (see Platelet Dose, Prophylactic Transfusion Dose). Other toxins that can affect platelet production include ethanol, benzene, radiation, hydrochlorothiazide, and ganciclovir.

Numerous pathologic processes can cause decreased platelet production. Any space-occupying lesion that invades an excessive amount of marrow space can suppress normal hematopoiesis. Examples of neoplastic conditions that can involve the bone marrow include primary or secondary leukemias, myelodysplastic syndromes, or metastatic carcinomas. Nonneoplastic conditions, such as tuberculosis, can also infiltrate the bone marrow and suppress platelet production. Some diseases may suppress platelet production by means other than mass effect. Viral infections (e.g., acquired immune deficiency syndrome, measles, mumps), aplastic anemia, Fanconi anemia, nutritional deficiencies (vitamin B_{12} and folate), and hereditary thrombocytopenia can cause clinical complications of thrombocytopenia.

Thrombocytopenia due to decreased platelet production is treated with transfusion of either a unit of single-donor apheresis platelets (SDP), or with a pool of random-donor platelets (RDP). The size of the pool varies among institutions but is generally between four and eight units. For children, dosage of 0.1 unit of RDP/kg body weight (or 5 ml/kg body weight) can be used. For patients needing frequent transfusions, prestorage leukoreduced RDP or process leukoreduced SDP are recommended.

Platelet Dysfunction

Platelet dysfunction is caused by both congenital and acquired defects. Dysfunctional platelets are often present in normal amounts, but their function is abnormal. Patients typically have a normal (or slightly low) platelet count but a prolonged bleeding time. Disorders of platelet function usually appear clinically as mucocutaneous hemorrhage (such as menorrhagia), mucosal hemorrhage (epistaxis, gingival bleeding, and /or gastrointestinal bleeding), or easy bruising. Petechial hemorrhage results from thrombocytopenia or platelet dysfunction and small unsealed endothelial lesions. This is distinct from the clinical hemorrhage secondary to coagulation factor defects, characterized by hemarthrosis and larger soft tissue hematomas. Some dysfunctional platelet disorders also lead to more overt clinical hemorrhage requiring platelet transfusion.

Congenital Platelet Disorders

Congenital platelet disorders are caused by a pathophysiologic deficiency or defect that is necessary for normal platelet adhesion, aggregation, and procoagulant activity. Platelet transfusions are generally reserved for active clinical hemorrhage in order to avoid cumulative blood product exposures and to minimize the risk of platelet alloimmunization. Multiple platelet transfusions increase the risk of human lymphocyte antigen (HLA) alloimmunization (see Immune-mediated Refractoriness), febrile transfusion reactions, and cytomegalovirus (CMV) infection. Leukocyte reduction of platelet transfusions is recommended in this population to reduce the risks from multiple transfusions. In addition to the risk of HLA alloimmunization, multiply transfused patients with congenital platelet antigen deficiencies, such as those patients lacking the glycoprotein (GP) GPIIb/IIIa (Glanzmann thrombasthenia), are also at risk for developing platelet-specific antibodies (1). Immune-mediated alloimmunization can result in poor posttransfusion platelet increments, platelet refractoriness, and ineffective clinical hemostasis.

The first line of therapy for most congenital platelet disorders is pharmacotherapy. Desmopressin (DDAVP), antifibrinolytics, estrogens, recombinant FVIIa, and topical agents such as fibrin glue and gel foam have been used to control bleeding. Alternative approaches to therapy for congenital platelet disorders include avoidance of any medication with antiplatelet activity (i.e., nonsteroidal antiinflammatory drugs [NSAIDs]). In addition, the use of erythropoietin and nutritional supplements, such as iron and folate, to help the patient compensate for chronic blood loss may be recommended. Lastly, allogeneic bone marrow transplantation has been reported to have been successful in two patients with severe Glanzmann thrombasthenia (2).

Platelet Membrane Defects. Bernard-Soulier syndrome (BSS) and platelet-type von Willebrand disease (vWD) are two examples of disorders with impaired platelet adhesion (3,4). BSS is usually inherited as an autosomal recessive condition, although spontaneous mutations and autosomal dominant forms have been reported. BSS is characterized by thrombocytopenia, giant platelets, and an abnormal GPIb-IX-V complex, the platelet von Willebrand factor (vWF) receptor. Because vWF acts as glue between the subendothelium and the platelet, this defect leads to a failure of platelet adhesion. There is considerable variability in symptoms among patients, which ranges from epistaxis (70%) to retinal hemorrhage (2%). Laboratory features include thrombocytopenia, varying from 20,000/µl to near-normal counts, giant platelets, prolonged bleeding time, a failure of platelet aggregation in response to ristocetin or botrocetin (agents that require vWF-GPIb interactions), and normal or enhanced platelet aggregation in response to other agonists such as collagen, ADP, and epinephrine.

Platelet-type vWD (or pseudo-vWD) causes mild-to-moderate bleeding symptoms and has an autosomal dominant pattern of inheritance. The defect in this disease is a qualitative abnormality in GPIb, which causes an enhanced interaction between an abnormal platelet GPIb/IX receptor and normal plasma vWF. The increased GPIb/vWF binding results in a depletion of the plasma high–molecular weight von Willebrand multimers and shortened platelet survival. Laboratory findings in patients with pseudo-vWD include a prolonged bleeding time, thrombocytopenia, and enhanced platelet aggregation in response to low concentrations of ristocetin or botrocetin (5). However, similar abnormal platelet aggregation is seen in type 2b vWD, and only special assays can help to differentiate the platelet GPIb defect in platelet-type vWD from the vWF defect in type 2b vWD. In addition, due to the enhanced binding between GPIb and vWF in these diseases, administration of DDAVP or cryoprecipitate may exacerbate a patient's thrombocytopenia and/or cause spontaneous platelet aggregation. Pharmacotherapy, cryoprecipitate, and platelet transfusion therapy must be given with extreme caution in these patients. However, these therapies have been used successfully, usually preceded by preclinical test dosing with laboratory monitoring, in specific patients who do not demonstrate in vitro platelet hyperaggregation.

Glanzmann thrombasthenia is an autosomal recessive platelet disorder characterized by a failure of platelet aggregation in response to most physiologic agonists and impaired or absent clot retraction. Glanzmann thrombasthenia is due to either a qualitative or quantitative abnormality of platelet GPIIb/GPIIIa, which is the receptor for fibrinogen and other adhesive molecules (6). Patients usually have mild, intermittent mucocutaneous hemorrhage. There is a notable lack of correlation between the laboratory and clinical findings in this disorder. Platelet transfusions should be reserved for life-threatening hemorrhage, because these patients rapidly become refractory due to formation of antibodies to the GP IIb/IIIa receptor.

Platelet Granule Defects. The platelet granule defects can be subclassified to three groups based on the affected granules: (a) α-storage pool deficiency–gray platelet syndrome (also associated with Hermansky-Pudlak syndrome); (b) δ storage pool deficiency–dense granule substance deficiency, including ADP, ATP, serotonin, phosphate, and calcium; and (c) $\alpha\delta$ storage pool deficiency. Most patients have a mild-to-moderate bleeding tendency. Abnormal platelet aggregation is useful in differentiating these platelet disorders from other diagnoses. In δ-storage and $\alpha\delta$-storage pool deficiencies, typical findings are abnormal second-wave responses to platelet stimulation with adenosine phosphate and epinephrine. In α-storage pool deficiency, platelet aggregation abnormalities are variably reported with most abnormal aggregation observed in response to collagen and thrombin stimulation (7).

If a patient with one of these disorders suffers from serious bleeding, treatment would involve use of RDPs or SDPs. However, for less serious bleeding, DDAVP could be used.

Other congenital defects of platelet function include defects of collagen receptors (GPIa/IIa, GPIV, and GPVI), defects of platelet receptors (thromboxane A_2 receptor, adenosine diphosphate [ADP] receptor, epinephrine receptor, and platelet-activating factor receptor), and defects of platelet activation (cyclooxygenase deficiency, thromboxane synthase deficiency, and arachidonic acid release abnormalities).

Acquired Platelet Disorders

Medications. Many clinical conditions and therapeutic interventions can negatively affect platelet function. Medication is the most common cause of platelet dysfunction, and prostaglandin inhibitors, such as aspirin (acetylsalicylic acid), are the class of medications most often implicated. Aspirin inhibits thromboxane A_2 synthesis by irreversibly inactivating (acetylating) cyclooxygenase, the enzyme that converts arachidonic acid to the prostaglandin endoperoxides G2 and H2 (8). Thus, in vitro platelet aggregation responses to collagen, ADP, epinephrine, and arachidonic acid are reduced (9). Other NSAIDs, such as indomethacin, ibuprofen, and sulfinpyrazone, cause platelet dysfunction through a reversible inhibition platelet cyclooxygenase (10). Antibiotics such as penicillin and carbenicillin also inhibit platelet aggregation (11). Ticlopidine, abciximab, tirofiban, and eptifibatide, used as antithrombotic agents, are GPIIb/IIIa antagonists that inhibit platelet aggregation by blockage of the GP IIb/IIIa biding sites (12). The antiplatelet agent, dipyridamole, inhibits phosphodiesterase to increase platelet cyclic adenosine monophosphate (cAMP) accumulation, which potentiates the platelet deaggregating effects of prostacyclin.

The use of platelet transfusions for patients taking one of these medications can be problematic. For patients with acute bleeding, necessary platelet transfusions should be given at the dosage level normally used at the institution. Ideally one should wait for the aspirin or NSAID effect to reverse before giving a platelet transfusion. However, in a patient without a defect in any other aspect of hemostasis, that is, normal coagulation factors and no vascular problems (congenital or acquired), the prolongation of the bleeding time caused by these medications is minimal. Thus, platelets would not be needed prophylactically. If, however, a therapeutic platelet transfusion is needed for a patient taking one of these drugs, it should be given and the patient followed clinically.

Uremia. Uremia results in defects of platelet adhesion, aggregation, and procoagulant activity. In a uremic patient, clinical factors, such as anemia, anticoagulation therapy, and thrombocytopenia, may markedly compound the severity of even small hemorrhages. The cause of uremic bleeding is multifactorial; however, it has been shown that urea does not directly cause platelet dysfunction (13). Dialysis decreases the potential for bleeding in uremic patients possibly by the removal of guanidinosuccinic acid, a dialyzable substance that accumulates in uremia. Guanidinosuccinic acid inhibits platelet aggregation (14), and more recently it has been shown that the accumulation of guanidinosuccinic acid leads to excess nitric oxide production, which has negative effects on both platelet aggregation and vascular integrity (15).

Platelet transfusions in uremia are generally reserved for severe bleeding, because once transfused, the allogeneic platelets will also become dysfunctional. In addition, a hematocrit between 25% to 30%, achieved by the administration of red blood cell transfusions or erythropoietin, can reduce clinical bleeding in uremic patients (16,17). It has been postulated that a higher hematocrit redistributes platelets toward the intravascular periphery, thereby enhancing exposure of the platelet to the endothelial surface. In addition to the hematocrit, some medications have been used to improve hemostasis in uremic patients. DDAVP stimulates release of vWF from endothelial cells and enhances platelet aggregation and adhesion. Cryoprecipitate contains significant vWF and can also aid hemostasis in uremic patients through enhanced platelet aggregation and adhesion. Conjugated estrogen has been reported to be a very beneficial therapy for uremic bleeding (18). The mechanism of action is unclear, but it has been postulated to occur through estrogen binding to endothelial surface receptors, causing enhanced platelet binding and possibly through estrogen-mediated inhibition of nitric oxide production. Estrogens may be of particular benefit to women with uremia who suffer from menstrual hemorrhage. Treatment with rFVIIa has also been reported to decrease severe uremic bleeding in a small cohort of patients (19). However, more clinical trials are needed to establish the safety of rFVIIa in patients suffering from thrombocytopenia.

Cardiopulmonary Bypass. Cardiopulmonary bypass results in thrombocytopenia (consumptive and dilutional), platelet dysfunction, and hyperfibrinolysis. Platelet dysfunction, due to platelet damage and activation, is caused by contact with artificial surfaces during circulation of the platelets through the bypass machine. Similar platelet defects and profound hemorrhage are also encountered in the neonatal setting during extracorporeal membrane oxygenation (ECMO). After cardiopulmonary bypass, the hemorrhagic diathesis may be multifactorial and can continue for several hours to several days. The stresses imposed on the platelet during extracorporeal circulation deplete the platelet of ADP and ATP, causing reduced platelet aggregation and procoagulant activity. Acquired forms of storage pool deficiency have also been reported (20,21). Platelet dysfunction secondary to extracorporeal platelet damage is usually treated empirically with platelet transfusions and is based upon observed clinical bleeding and institutional protocols. Generally the goal is to maintain a platelet count of greater than 50,000/μl after bypass, with the caveat that the platelet count may rapidly increase over the 1 to 2 hours postbypass if there are no other significant complications.

Hematologic Disorders and Malignancies. Complicated platelet function defects have been noted in the myeloproliferative disorders: polycythemia vera, essential thrombocythemia, chronic myelogenous leukemia (CML), and myelofibrosis with myeloid metaplasia. Multiple intrinsic platelet defects have been described, and both bleeding and thrombosis are associated complications with a high incidence of morbidity and mortality. Approximately 17% of patients with myeloproliferative disorders have a prolonged bleeding time, and bleeding can occur in patients with a normal bleeding time (22,23). Acute leukemia is also associated with multiple platelet function defects, possibly due to abnormal megakaryocytopoiesis derived from leukemic stem cells or from megakaryocyte damage induced by the cytotoxic chemotherapy agents. In addition, dysproteinemia has been associated with platelet dysfunction due to the monoclonal protein interfering with platelet adhesion through interactions between immunoglobulins and platelet surfaces (24,25). Acquired vWD may occur with autoimmune or clonal hematologic diseases, such as multiple myeloma, low-grade non-Hodgkin lymphoma, chronic lymphocytic leukemia, and waldenström macroglobulinemia (26).

A patient with one of these disorders who is bleeding may benefit from platelet transfusions, as necessary, for platelet counts below 50,000/μl. When a paraprotein causes a thrombocytopathy, such as in waldenström macroglobulinemia, consideration should be given to a course of plasmapheresis to lower intravascular levels of the implicated protein and improve platelet function. For patients with vWD, depending on the type, treatment would be either with DDAVP, cryoprecipitate, or factor concentrates such as Humate-P.

Platelet Sequestration

Splenic blood flow occurs at a slow rate that facilitates interactions between the macrophage and pathogens and/or complement. Approximately one-third of the circulating platelet pool is normally sequestered in the spleen, but sequestration increases in conditions that upset the homeostatic balance of platelet removal. Hypersplenism of any etiology causes an increased sequestration of platelets in the splenic parenchyma. Patients with portal venous hypertension, due to liver cirrhosis or other etiology, develop congestive splenomegaly. Additionally, many diseases, such as CML, hairy cell leukemia, or infectious mononucleosis, may cause hypersplenism. Significant hypersplenism leads to pooling of platelets within the tortuous splenic sinusoids and retention of platelets through reversible adherence to macrophages during intrasplenic transit. As much as 90% of the total platelet mass becomes sequestered in the enlarged spleen. Fortunately, pure hypersplenism rarely causes such severe thrombocytopenia as to require platelet transfusion therapy; however, hypersplenism can worsen thrombocytopenia due to other etiologies. When hypersplenism exacerbates pathologic thrombocytopenia caused by another mechanism (such as decreased production associated with myelofibrosis or another myelophthisic process), patients sometimes become refractory to platelet transfusions even in the absence of a specific HLA or other immune-mediated platelet antibody. Nonimmune-mediated refractoriness to platelet transfusions is a difficult therapeutic problem.

In these cases, for a bleeding patient, transfusion of platelet concentrates is indicated. However, posttransfusion increments may be low in these patients. If cross-matched platelets or HLA-matched platelets do not provide a sustained rise in platelet count, the likelihood of maintaining a patient's platelet count at a high level is remote. In such cases in which a patient is either bleeding or preparing to undergo an invasive procedure, a continuous platelet infusion drip may be a useful therapeutic maneuver. One such protocol calls for three units of RDP given over 4 hours through an electromechanical intravenous pump. The patient's platelet count should be monitored periodically to assess response. It should be noted that for patients with nonimmune platelet refractoriness, cross-matched or HLA-matched platelets offer no advantage over random-donor platelets, either RDP or SDP.

In addition to the spleen, platelets may also be sequestered in giant, cavernous hemangiomas (Kasabach-Merritt syndrome). Although platelet sequestration in a large hemangioma causes thrombocytopenia, platelet destruction as a component of a localized disseminated intravascular coagulation (DIC) within the hemangioma has also been postulated to occur based on fibrinogen assays and laboratory evidence of a consumptive coagulopathy (27).

Platelet Destruction

Thrombocytopenia due to platelet destruction is often due to an immune-mediated platelet destruction. Conditions that cause immune-mediated platelet destruction include drug-induced thrombocytopenia (i.e., heparin, quinine, gold salts, abciximab), platelet autoantibody as in idiopathic thrombocytopenic purpura (ITP), and platelet alloantibody as in HLA alloimmunization or neonatal alloimmune thrombocytopenia (NAIT).

Immune-mediated Destruction

Immune-mediated thrombocytopenias are similar to immune-mediated red blood cell hemolytic anemias in their general pathobiology. Antibodies, reactive against antigens expressed on the patient's platelets, result in premature destruction of those cells in the patient's reticuloendothelial system. Both autoimmune antibodies and alloimmune antibodies have been found to cause thrombocytopenia, and there are clear associations between many autoimmune diseases and thrombocytopenia. Evans syndrome, the association of chronic ITP and autoimmune hemolytic anemia, is an example of the close association of platelet and red blood cell destruction via antibody-mediated immune mechanisms. In contrast, paroxysmal nocturnal hemoglobinuria is an example of platelet and red blood cell destruction via complement-mediated immune mechanisms (see Chapter 26).

Nonimmune-mediated Destruction

Nonimmune-mediated platelet destruction is also a cause of thrombocytopenia in many patients, including those with DIC and most forms of thrombotic thrombocytopenic purpura (TTP). Bacterial or other microbial infection, trauma, invasive surgery, burns, and obstetric conditions are associated with both thrombocytopenia and DIC.

TTP classically occurs as a pentad of clinical findings: fever, thrombocytopenia, microangiopathic hemolytic anemia, neurologic abnormalities, and renal involvement. However, the definition of TTP has evolved since its original description in 1925, and only a dyad of symptoms is usually needed to make the diagnosis in the appropriate clinical setting. TTP can be primary (idiopathic or hereditary), or secondary to a number of causes including pregnancy, verotoxins *(Escherichia coli* or *Shigella dysenteriae),* metastatic carcinoma, chemotherapeutic agents (mitomycin C, cisplatin, cyclophosphamide, gemcitabine), other medications (cyclosporine, tacrolimus, sirolimus, quinine, ticlopidine, clopidogrel, interferon alpha, and others), total body irradiation, and hematopoietic transplantation (28–33). The mechanical destruction of platelets may be exacerbated by a decreased production (bone marrow suppression) of platelets in the setting of postchemotherapy or bone marrow transplant–induced TTP.

The primary treatment for TTP is plasma exchange. Plasma exchange therapy is thought to ameliorate platelet aggregation by removing both high–molecular weight vWF multimers and an inhibitor to a metalloprotease necessary for degradation of the multimers, while replenishing fresh metalloprotease. Glucocorticoids are also sometimes used in combination with plasma exchange. The efficacy of antiplatelet medications, such as NSAIDs, immunosuppressive agents, and intravenous immune globulin (IVIG) have not been clearly demonstrated. There is controversy regarding the use of platelet transfusions in patients with TTP. Platelet transfusions have been reported to exacerbate microthrombosis leading to severe complications (32), whereas, others have reported improvement in thrombocytopenia without complication (31). Because of the reports of rapid clinical deterioration after platelet transfusions, they should be avoided in patients with TTP unless absolutely necessary to curb life-threatening hemorrhage. If platelets are needed, they should be given slowly and with close clinical monitoring for signs of ischemic complications.

The etiologies of other recognized forms of nonimmune thrombocytopenia are related to endothelial injury, vascular damage, and/or platelet activation. Pregnancy, preeclampsia, indwelling catheters, burns, adult respiratory distress syndrome (ARDS), renal vein thrombosis, cardiac valve lesions, intravascular prosthetics, and fever have been associated with consumptive thrombocytopenia. Data are accumulating that correlate cytokine production and inflammation with consumptive thrombocytopenia (34).

In consumptive thrombocytopenias, platelets should be transfused as necessary to treat a bleeding patient. It is often difficult to raise the patient's platelet count above a certain level, over 50,000 to 75,000/μl, despite multiple infusions of large numbers of pooled platelets. This is because in patients with these conditions, once transfused, platelets are consumed by the disease process and do not survive well. Thus, it may be necessary to resort to a continuous platelet infusion to provide sufficient platelets to affected individuals. As mentioned above, we suggest infusing three units of RDP every 4 hours. With an infusion, although the patient is getting around-the-clock platelet support, the peripheral platelet count may still not rise. In such patients the platelet count should be monitored periodically to assess individual responses to different therapeutic interventions. Additional platelet doses may be needed during infusion therapy for a recurrence or an exacerbation of clinical hemorrhage.

PLATELET DOSE

Product Dose

The Food and Drug Administration (FDA) and American Association of Blood Banks (AABB) require that 75% of RDP contain at least 5.5×10^{10} platelets and 75% of apheresis platelet products contain at least 3.0×10^{11} platelets (35). In practice, most blood centers produce random-donor units with a count exceeding 7×10^{10} platelets and apheresis units exceeding 3.5×10^{11} platelets. A six-unit pool of RDP concentrates or equivalent SDP is expected to raise the platelet count in a 70-kg adult by 30,000 to 60,000/μl. These platelet increment targets can be used clinically to detect platelet refractoriness, which occurs in 30% to 70% of multiply transfused patients (36). Platelet refractoriness often is revealed when appropriate platelet increments are not achieved following repeated platelet transfusions.

Prophylactic Transfusion Dose

The prophylactic threshold for platelet transfusions to prevent bleeding in uncomplicated patients with failure of platelet production, either due to malignancy or disease-related treatments, is a platelet count of 10,000/μl (37,38). The "trigger" for platelet transfusion in these situations is controversial, but a 5,000/μl threshold platelet count has been suggested. The major hemorrhagic events that occurred in several patients with leukemia who did not receive prophylactic transfusions when the platelet count was between 6,000 and 10,000/μl, however, suggests caution (39). In addition, the precision of low platelet count determinations is technically difficult (40). Currently there is a growing consensus to use a 10,000/μl count as a basis for daily prophylactic platelet transfusions. In patients with additional risk factors (such as sepsis), other hemostatic abnormalities, or in neonates, a higher trigger for prophylactic platelet transfusion (20,000 to 50,000/μl) should be used. Although there is no consensus on the threshold for invasive procedures (i.e., liver biopsy) most clinicians accept a 50,000/μl trigger level for prophylactic transfusions (41). When patients with low platelet counts are taken to surgery, the recommended approach is to administer platelets as the incision is being made so they are not consumed before they are needed for surgical hemostasis. In situations when platelet counts are marginal, supplemental stored platelets should be available, but not used, unless the platelet count drops significantly or severe bleeding ensues.

Therapeutic Transfusion Dose

Transfusion approaches have been modeled based on a consideration of the hemostatic requirement. A fixed platelet requirement for hemostasis is estimated to be 7,500/μl/day (42). Two platelet transfusion strategies, "low dose" and "high dose", have been debated (43). Platelet survival decreases with worsening thrombocytopenia and, therefore, platelet loss in patients with higher platelet counts is most likely due to platelet senescence. For example, in patients with a platelet count of 20,000/μl, the average platelet survival time is 1 to 2 days, while in those with normal platelet counts, platelet survival time is 5 to 7 days. Mathematic models suggest that increasing the platelet dose per transfusion would prolong the in vivo platelet survival time and thus decrease the platelet transfusion frequency, but at a cost of more total platelet transfusions and donor exposures (Fig.18.1). The model predicted that more frequent transfusions of smaller doses, using two RDPs instead of the usual six RDPs, could maintain a patient's platelet count above 10,000/μl for 100 thrombocytopenic days, with a 22% reduction in total number of platelet transfusions and donor exposures (44).

In a recent randomized clinical trial of patients receiving prophylactic platelet transfusions, three different apheresis platelet doses were compared: standard, high, and very high (means of 4.6×10^{11}, 6.5×10^{11}, and 8.9×10^{11}, respectively) (45). The high and very high dose cohorts had higher platelet increments and longer intervals between transfusions, when compared with the standard platelet dose (corroborating the mathematic model). However, there were no data regarding the total number of platelet transfusions or donor exposures among the three patients groups. Furthermore, in all cohorts the half-disappearance of the platelets (i.e., slope) was not significantly differ-

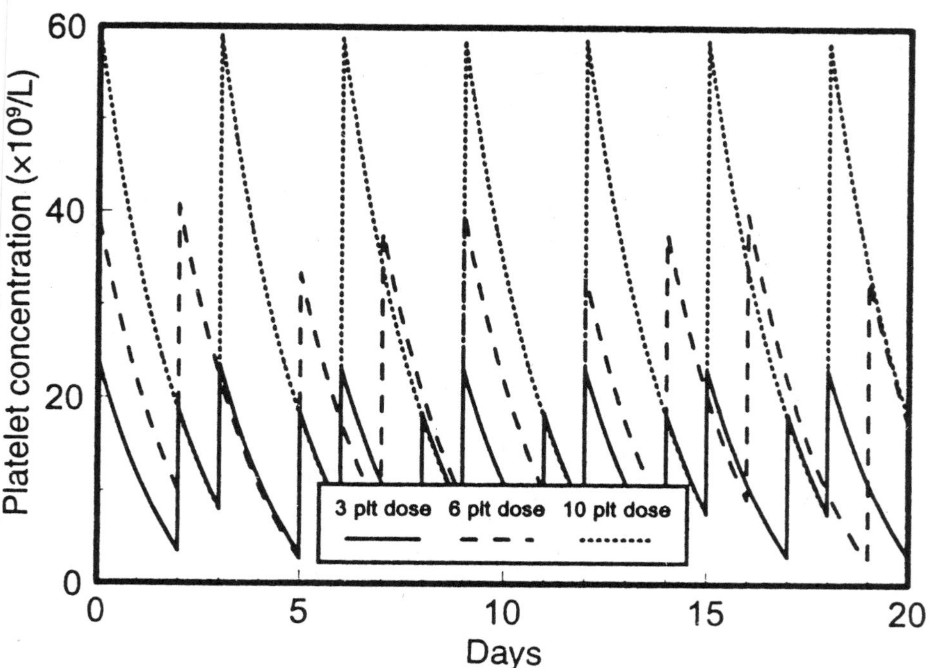

FIGURE 18.1. Mathematic model comparing platelet concentration with platelet transfusions of pool sizes of 3, 6, or 10 concentrates. A larger pool size was associated with a decreased frequency of transfusion but an increased use of platelet concentrates. (Reproduced from Hersh JK, Hom EG, Brecher ME. Mathematical modeling of platelet survival with implications for optimal transfusion practice in the chronically platelet transfusion–dependent patient. *Transfusion* 1998;38:637–644, with permission.)

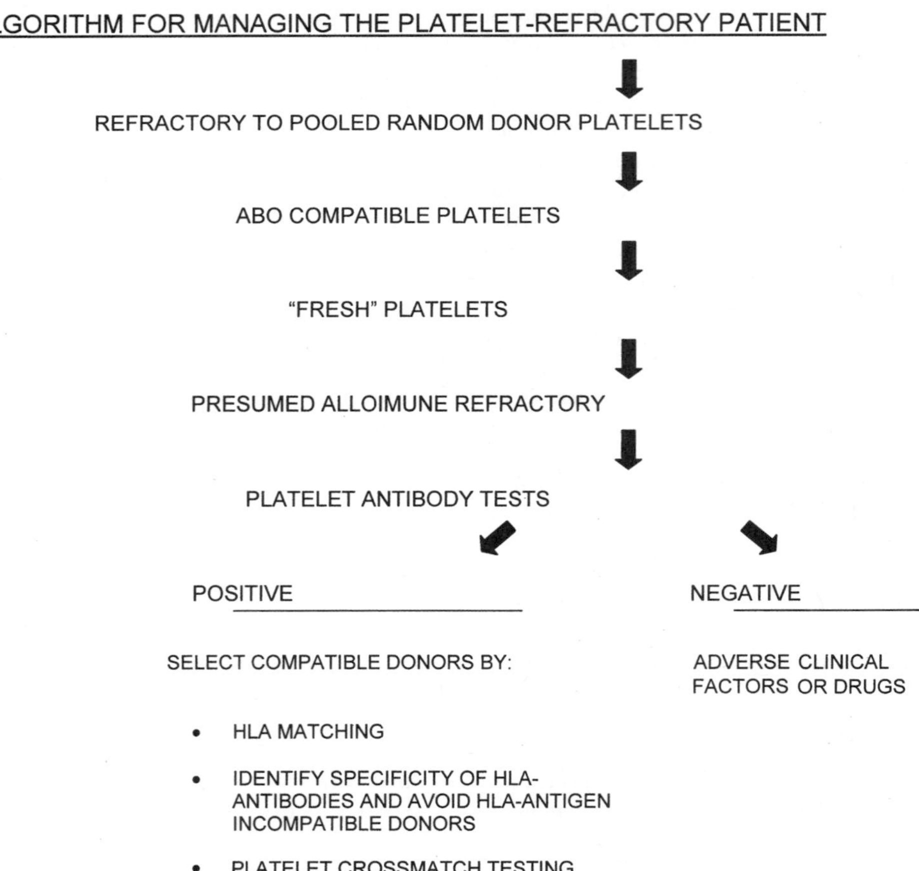

FIGURE 18.2. Platelet refractory algorithm. The sequence of steps to guide the evaluation and platelet product selection for the platelet refractory patient. (Reproduced from Slichter SJ. Algorithm for managing the platelet refractory patient. *J Clin Apheresis* 1997;12:4–9, with permission.)

ent over a 5-day posttransfusion period, indicating that in vivo platelet survival did not normalize at higher platelet counts. This suggested that larger doses of platelets may not improve in vivo platelet survival and that the rate of platelet clearance was constant for both high and low platelet counts. Therefore, in patients requiring platelet transfusions for active bleeding, we recommend giving a standard dose of platelets according to the institution's guidelines, followed by close monitoring of the posttransfusion platelet count. If the patient does not manifest a rise in platelet count after several infusions of RDP, the next step would be use of cross-matched or HLA-matched platelets. If this fails, a continuous platelet infusion might be indicated in addition to other measures aimed at treating the primary illness (Fig 18.2).

PLATELET PRODUCTS

There is a variety of platelet products available for transfusion (Table 18.1). The selection of a particular product for transfusion is based on several parameters including: the patient's diagnosis, patient's immune system status, transfusion and reaction history, urgency of transfusion (clinical hemorrhage), response to previous platelet transfusions, and current platelet count. Furthermore, the intention of a platelet transfusion is to protect against and/or treat clinically significant hemorrhage. However, research comparing the efficacy of different platelet products and alternatives is limited by the lack of availability of any simple test of platelet function that reliably predicts in vivo, clinical hemostasis. Because severe bleeding due to thrombocytopenia is a rare event, very large clinical trials are needed to adequately evaluate the efficacy of platelet products and substitutes (46).

Fresh Platelets

There are some conflicting data on whether fresh platelets (less than 2 days old) provide improved hemostasis compared to older products (3 to 5 days old) (47–49). Data have shown that older platelets have more markers of activation and shortened survival (50). Platelet products can accumulate cytokines or other substances (i.e., RANTES [regulated on activation, normal T cell expressed and secreted]) during storage that may be detrimental to the transfusion recipient. Additionally, the risk of bacterial contamination of the platelet product (stored at room temperature) increases with storage time (51–53). However, platelet

TABLE 18.1. RECOMMENDED PLATELET PRODUCT SELECTION AND LABORATORY TESTING BASED ON THE CLINICAL CONDITION

Clinical Condition	Recommended Testing	Platelet Product
Trauma patients	1. Serial platelet count 2. Serial coagulation testing (PT, PTT, fibrinogen)	RDP pool or SDP
Disseminated intravascular coagulopathy	1. Serial platelet count 2. Serial coagulation testing (PT, PTT, fibrinogen)	RDP pool or SDP
Oncology Patients		
Nonrefractory	1. Pretransfusion platelet count 2. 1 hour–posttransfusion platelet count	RDP pool or SDP —prestorage leukocyte reduced —irradiated
Refractory[a]	1. Pretransfusion platelet count 2. 1-hour–posttransfusion platelet count 3a. Platelet crossmatch or 3b. HLA match 4. Platelet-specific antibody testing (anti-PLA-1, anti-PLA-2, etc.) 5. Antiheparin-associated antibody (if patient on heparin) or consider other drug-associated etiology	1. SDP —prestorage leukocyte reduced or leukocyte reduced by apheresis —irradiated —cross-matched or HLA matched 2. RDP pool or continuous infusion if cross-matched or HLA-matched unavailable —prestorage leukocyte reduced —irradiated
Pediatric Patients	1. Platelet count 2. 1 hour–posttransfusion platelet count	SDP (5 ml/kg) preferred to limit exposure, but RDP (0.1 unit/kg or 5 ml/kg) may be used —volume reduced as needed —prestorage leukocyte reduced —irradiated if the recipient is less than 4 months of age
Neonatal alloimmune thrombocytopenia	1. Platelet count 2. 1 hour–posttransfusion platelet count 3. Platelet-specific antibody testing (anti-PLA-1, anti-PLA-2, etc.) on mother and patient 4. Platelet antigen typing (PLA-1, PLA-2, etc.) on patient and parents 5. Platelet crossmatch between maternal serum and paternal platelets	1. SDP preferred to limit exposure, but RDP may be used (unrelated allogeneic platelets are more readily available, with completed viral testing, and possibly safer) —volume reduced as needed —prestorage leukocyte reduced —irradiated 2. Maternal SDP (maternal platelets are always antigen-negative and compatible, best choice if patient unresponsive to unrelated, allogeneic platelets) —volume reduced —prestorage leukocyte reduced —irradiated —washed 3. Antigen-negative (PLA-1) unrelated allogeneic SDP (if available and maternal platelet collection not possible) —volume reduced as needed —prestorage leukocyte reduced —irradiated
Posttransfusion purpura	1. Platelet-specific antibody testing (anti-PLA-1, anti-PLA-2, etc.) 2. Platelet antigen typing (PLA-1, PLA-2, etc.) on patient	1. IVIG or therapeutic plasma exchange 2. Platelet transfusion reserved only for severe hemorrhage[b]
Thrombotic thrombocytopenic purpura	1. Platelet count 2. Complete blood count 3. LDH 4. Bilirubin 5. BUN and creatinine 6. Peripheral smear 7. Direct antiglobulin test 8. Coagulation testing	1. Therapeutic plasma exchange 2. Glucocorticoids 3. Platelet transfusion reserved only for severe hemorrhage[b]
Idiopathic thrombocytopenic purpura	1. Platelet-specific antibody testing 2. Bone marrow biopsy 3. Antiheparin-associated antibody (if patient on heparin) or consider other drug-associated etiology	1. Glucocorticoids 2. Splenectomy 3. Immunosuppressive therapy 4. IVIG or RhIG

(*continued*)

TABLE 18.1. (Continued)

Clinical Condition	Recommended Testing	Platelet Product
		5. Platelet transfusion may be of benefit to control bleeding, but patient responses are variable
Drug induced thrombocytopenia	1. Heparin-(or other drug)-associated platelet antibody testing 2. Platelet-specific antibody testing	1. Avoid heparin 2. Platelet transfusions reserved only for severe hemorrhage[b]
IgA deficiency or severe allergic/anaphylactic reaction	1. IgA antibody testing 2. IgG (anti-IgA) antibody testing	RDP pool or SDP —washed
TA-GVHD prevention	See chapter 59 for list of patients at risk for TA-GVHD 1. Immune-suppressed patients 2. Products donated from related family members 3. Pediatric patients less than 4 months of age	RDP pool or SDP —irradiated

[a]Patients other than oncology patients may develop refractoriness. The recommended laboratory testing and platelet selections are not limited to oncology patients and can be used for any refractory patient.
[b]Platelet transfusions should be given with caution. Thrombotic complications after platelet transfusion have been reported with this disease.
PT, prothrombin time; PTT, partial thromboplastin time; RDP, random-donor platelets; SDP, single-donor platelets; HLA, human lymphocyte antigen; PLA, platelet-specific antigen; IVIG, intravenous immune globulin; LDH, lactic dehydrogenase; BUN, blood urea nitrogen; RhIG, Rhesus immune globulin; IgA, immunoglobulin A; IgG, immunoglobulin G; TA-GVHD, transfision-associated graft-vesus-host disease.

products collected using good manufacturing practices and transfused within the standard 5-day storage time provide needed clinical hemostasis for thrombocytopenic patients. Under most clinical circumstances, platelet storage time should not a determining factor in the transfusion trigger. In addition, the initiation of nucleic acid testing (NAT) of blood products prevents blood centers from providing fresh platelets (less than 48 hours old) due to the time required for completion of all testing.

Random-donor Platelet Pools Versus Single-donor (Apheresis) Platelets

Several studies have been undertaken to compare the benefits of single-donor platelets (SDPs, collected from one donor by apheresis) over random-donor platelet pools (RDPs, collected by combining the removed platelet fractions of four to eight different whole blood donations) (54–57). The most notable advantage of SDPs over RDPs is the decreased number of blood exposures, resulting in a decreased risk of transfusion transmitted diseases for SDPs, although the risk is very small currently. SDPs express less P-selectin and more GPIb than RDPs, and these in vitro changes may translate into some in vivo advantages, because P-selectin has been associated with decreased platelet survival and GPIb is integral to platelet adhesion. However, prospective clinical studies, such as the Trial to Reduce Alloimmunization to Platelets (TRAP) study, did not show any advantage of SDPs compared to RDPs (58). Additionally, SDPs may be "process leukoreduced" at the time of apheresis collection, as compared to RDPs which require filtration, optimally performed prior to storage. Leukoreduction is possible for both products, but there may be some advantage to "process leukoreduction" because this method eliminates any mixing of leukocytes and platelets. By preventing leukocyte contamination of platelets during apheresis, degranulation of neutrophils and leukocyte enzyme activation, is minimized. Minimizing adverse leukocyte interactions with platelet glycoproteins may prevent unwanted platelet activation.

The potential disadvantages of SDPs compared with RDPs are cost and availability. SDPs cost more than RDPs per unit; however, four to six units of RDPs are often pooled and transfused as a single dose. When comparing the cost of a platelet transfusion per dose, the differential between SDPs and pooled RDPs is small. The cost of SDPs, however, can be decreased by using "split" SDPs from those units that contain a higher platelet yield (57), whereas the cost of RDPs can also be reduced by decreasing the number of RDPs pooled in the final product. As prices for platelet products vary among regions, the cost effectiveness of SDPs compared to RDPs also depends on local market pressures. Availability also has a role in the selection of SDPs or RDPs. There does not appear to be any advantage of SDPs over RDPs when considering platelet increment after transfusion, and it seems more likely that a random pool of platelets may contain a small dose of HLA-compatible product in the event that HLA-matched SDPs are unavailable for the alloimmunized patient. The advantages and disadvantages of these two commonly available platelet preparations, SDPs and RDPs, should be considered when selecting a product for transfusion, and concerns such as availability, patient population, and cost effectiveness need to be balanced. At present the products are comparable in safety and efficacy.

Continuous Platelet Infusion

A continuous platelet infusion is an alternative transfusion approach that can be employed in the platelet-refractory patient. A continuous infusion of platelets uses the "low dose" theory of therapeutic platelet transfusion (see above, Platelet Dose) to provide a continuous intravenous infusion of platelets. This approach can be used as a temporary measure in cases when refractory patients need platelets in emergent situations. The platelets may be administered as a pool of three RDPs transfused over 4 hours, or as a "split" (one-half) of an SDP administered over a similar interval. The clinical response to continuous platelet infusions is variable among patients and has not been well studied in prospective randomized trials. However, this approach provides a significantly high (18 RDPs or 3 SDP apheresis products per day), constant, and titratable dose of platelets for the patient, while providing a predictable impact on the blood bank inventory. Conversely, massive boluses of 20 pooled units have been reported to be effective in achieving hemostasis in an animal model of platelet refractoriness (59). Continuous platelet transfusions should be used only when a significant platelet increment cannot be obtained with any available platelet product as a single dose and/or continuous life-threatening hemorrhage exists.

ABO Blood Group Compatibility

A significant body of evidence supports the beneficial effect of transfusing ABO-identical platelets (60,61). The A and B oligosaccharide antigens are integral components of the platelet membrane, and soluble A and B antigens can be adsorbed onto the platelet surface. Depending on the individual, the expression of A and B antigens on platelets varies significantly (62). Furthermore, anti-A and anti-B present in the donor supernatant platelet-poor plasma is reactive against a recipient's red blood cells. Numerous case reports have documented significant hemolysis when out-of-group plasma in platelet products has been transfused, and this phenomenon is particularly relevant in pediatric patients who have a smaller blood volume and less ability to neutralize passive ABO antibodies (63,64).

ABO-mediated platelet destruction is one form of immune-mediated platelet destruction, and data support the findings of an improved platelet increment when ABO-identical (not simply compatible) platelets are transfused (60,65). However, supply problems preclude ABO-identical platelet transfusions as a policy for all patients. Most transfusion services attempt to issue ABO-identical platelets when possible given the general platelet demand of their service and the current status of their platelet supply. In most adult patients the risks of thrombocytopenia exceed the disadvantages of non–ABO-identical platelet products and these out-of-group products remain an acceptable option.

Rh Blood Group Compatibility

Rh blood group antigens are not expressed on platelets (66). Small amounts of red blood cells may contaminate both RDPs (less than 0.5 ml of red blood cells) and SDPs (less than 5 ml of red blood cells) (67). When platelets from Rh-positive donors are transfused into Rh-negative patients, there is a possibility that anti-D antibody formation will occur. One study reported an incidence of Rh alloimmunization to be 14% after an Rh-positive platelet transfusion in patients without hematologic diseases (68). Rh-negative patients with hematologic diseases rarely form anti-D antibodies after transfusion with platelets from Rh-positive donors, presumably due to immune suppression after receiving chemotherapy (68,69). A dose of 100 IU of Rh immune globulin has been protective when Rh-positive SDPs have been administered to Rh-negative patients (70). Alternatively, in collaboration with the blood bank physician, an appropriate dose of Rh immune globulin can be determined based on an estimate of the red blood cell contamination in the platelet product. Administration of Rh immune globulin prophylaxis should be considered when Rh-incompatible platelet products need to be administered to a female child or a woman who may subsequently become pregnant, especially in nonimmunosuppressed patients. Some Rh immune globulin preparations can only be administered intramuscularly, and hematoma formation may occur if given to thrombocytopenic patients. Therefore, the use of Rh immune globulin formulations that can be administered intravenously is preferable in such patients.

PLATELET TRANSFUSION FOR REFRACTORY PATIENTS

Definitions and Diagnosis

Patients who are refractory to platelet transfusions fall into two general categories: nonimmune mediated and immune mediated (Fig.18.2). The usual clinical pictures of nonimmune-mediated refractoriness include sepsis, fever, splenomegaly and sequestration (see above), ongoing hemorrhage, massive transfusion, hemodilution, DIC, burns, or a combination of these findings. Multiply transfused patients or multiparous women may develop immune-mediated platelet refractoriness resulting from alloimmunization (see Chapter 16). Additionally, patients with complex platelet refractoriness may have components of both nonimmune- and immune-mediated etiologies leading to severe, life-threatening thrombocytopenia.

A commonly used clinical criterion for defining platelet refractoriness is the failure to achieve an expected increment in the platelet count after two consecutive transfusions (71). To estimate the expected platelet increment from a transfusion, the platelet count should be sampled between 10 minutes and 1 hour after completion of the transfusion (72). Repeatedly low platelet counts determined at 24-hour intervals (i.e., standard morning blood counts) do not provide the needed information to assist in determining refractoriness, even when the patient has been transfused once daily. A platelet count taken 1 hour after completion of the transfusion provides in vivo platelet survival characteristics that help to distinguish nonimmune-mediated from immune-mediated refractoriness (73).

The two commonly used equations to help determine platelet refractoriness are the 1-hour posttransfusion corrected count increment (CCI) and the 1-hour posttransfusion percent platelet recovery (PPR) (74). The CCI and PPR are more often used to compare platelet increments when conducting research, but these formulas can be very useful clinically as well. The formulas are as follows:

$$\text{CCI} = \frac{[\text{post-tx plt.ct. } (/\mu\text{l}) - \text{pre-tx plt.ct. } (/\mu\text{l})] \times \text{BSA } (\text{m}^2)}{(\text{number of platelets transfused}) \times 10^{-11}}$$

The number of platelets transfused is taken from a platelet count of the unit(s) or an estimate based on experience. However, one can assume minimum doses of 5.5×10^{10} platelets per random donor concentrate (multiplied by the number of concentrates in the RDP pool) and 3.0×10^{11} platelets per SDP apheresis product. The CCI estimates the number of surviving donor platelets following transfusion. A CCI >7500 (per μl/m^2) from a sample drawn 10 minutes to 1 hour after transfusion, is considered appropriate for the platelet increment and indicates that refractoriness is unlikely (36,73).

$$\text{PPR} = \frac{(\text{platelet increment per } \mu\text{l}) \times (\text{weight in kg}) \times (\text{total blood volume in ml}) \times (100\%)}{(\text{platelet count of transfused product per } \mu\text{l}) \times (\text{volume of product in ml})}$$

One can expect a 66% platelet recovery in a patient with an intact spleen, and 100% platelet recovery in asplenic patients. Thrombocytopenic patients will often yield a 50% recovery, and as the recovery decreases below 50%, refractoriness becomes more likely.

Nonimmune-mediated Refractoriness

Severely ill patients may demonstrate a resistance to platelet transfusions that have no well-defined etiology, except possible splenomegaly. Clinical conditions associated with a refractory state include DIC, amphotericin B therapy, bone marrow transplantation (and graft-versus-host disease), γ-irradiation therapy, fever, sepsis, ARDS, hemorrhagic states, pregnancy, and venoocclusive disease (75). Some of these conditions may also contribute to and initiate a workup of immune-mediated refractoriness; however, negative immunologic results are often seen.

Immune-mediated Refractoriness

Alloimmunized Patients

Alloimmunization to platelet transfusions results from previous exposure to donor HLA antigens that are not expressed on recipient platelets (see Chapter 16). A history of multiple transfusions in either gender, or in multiparous women, are two common predisposing clinical situations in which previous donor antigen exposure can occur. The stimulated antibody response, after one or more exposures, leads to early clearance of the platelets by an immune-mediated reaction. Platelets express HLA class I (A and B) antigens and platelet specific antigens, but do not express HLA class II (DR, DP, or DQ antigens). Most clinical antiplatelet antibodies are actually formed against HLA antigens (45%) and fewer patients (8%) develop antibodies against platelet-specific glycoproteins. Alloimmunization against HLA antigens is usually due to exposure to contaminating leukocytes in transfused blood products, whereas platelet-specific glycoprotein alloimmunization occurs through exposure to allogeneic platelets, and not leukocytes. However, antigen exposure and subsequent alloimmunization requires the presence of functional antigen-presenting cells (APCs) plus antigen to engender an immune response (76). The leukocyte contamination in blood products provides an adequate milieu (HLA class I and II antigens plus APCs) to stimulate alloimmunization, and leukocyte reduction or UVB irradiation will substantially reduce (by 10% to 15%), but not entirely prevent, an alloimmune response. Reduction in alloimmunization is possibly due to the weaker antigen stimulus of UV-irradiated platelets in the former product and the reduced or dysfunctional APCs in the latter product. In the absence of functional donor APCs or a significant number of leukocytes, multiple platelet transfusions occasionally result in alloimmunization presumably due to functional recipient APCs (58). Alloimmune platelet transfusion reactions are sometimes accompanied by fever, chills, tachycardia, and other hallmarks of reactive humoral immunity. Accordingly, when incompatible platelets are administered, the posttransfusion platelet increment can be markedly diminished or even lower than the pretransfusion count.

Platelet Cross-matching and HLA Matching

Transfusion strategies for the alloimmunized patient are aimed at providing HLA antigen–negative platelets that are most compatible with the patient. Several platelet antibody tests reliably detect almost any HLA or platelet glycoprotein antibody reactivity. Some blood banks use platelet cross-match techniques, whereas others use HLA antibody–targeted approaches. The successful identification of a platelet product, using either approach, provides improved transfusion increments in about 60% of cases. Platelet cross-match techniques provide the advantages of screening for both HLA and platelet glycoprotein antibodies, in addition to a cost advantage and possibly a more rapid product procurement, but are limited by the supply of collected apheresis products available for testing. HLA-matching approaches permit the screening of a broader range of HLA-typed platelet donors but will not identify the 5% to 10% of patients with antiplatelet glycoprotein antibodies (71). Also, HLA-matched platelet donors may not be available for donation, and if available, the minimum procurement time is at least 48 hours. Using either the cross-match or HLA-matching techniques, at least 1 day (and usually more) is required to obtain a product. Furthermore, even under optimal conditions, the number of available products is often limited to one or two SDPs because the product is donor specific. A limited number of products can be collected from the same matched donor, although the FDA allows exceptions if physician examinations are done and the donor is dedicated to a single recipient. These sophisticated techniques are available only when a workup has already been completed.

Figure 18.2 summarizes a recommended approach to management of the platelet-refractory patient.

Neonatal Alloimmune Thrombocytopenia

NAIT is caused by antiplatelet antibodies in the mother that cross the placenta and react with incompatible fetal platelets. Newborns with NAIT may respond to allogeneic platelet transfusions, but maternal platelets are the preferred source, if plateletpheresis of the mother is safe for both the donor and the recipient of the product. Plateletpheresis of the mother is contraindicated if the mother is recovering from lacerations or other postpartum trauma that might introduce contamination into the platelet product. Nevertheless, maternal platelets will be compatible with the neonate and, if used, the platelets should be washed to remove residual antibody and irradiated to prevent transfusion-associated graft-versus-host disease. Therapy for NAIT often includes concomitant glucocorticoid therapy; IVIG may also be used.

Autoimmunized Patients

Idiopathic Thrombocytopenic Purpura

Patients with ITP, Evans syndrome, or other autoimmune conditions responsible for autoimmune thrombocytopenia will also more rapidly clear allogeneic platelet transfusions (see Chapter 27). However, these conditions do not pose an absolute contraindication to the option of platelet transfusion, and therapeutic transfusions can be successfully administered if life-threatening bleeding has occurred. If standard treatment doses of platelets do not survive, strategies considering ABO-identical blood group, larger dose, small frequent dosing, shorter storage time, HLA matching, and timing of transfusion to coincide with medical procedures or events should be employed. A continuous platelet infusion that is initiated prior to a procedure and maintained throughout the procedure can provide some coverage for the severely refractory patient with severe bleeding. In this fashion, potential transfusion reactions may be identified and treated prior to the procedure.

There are many alternative approaches to platelet transfusion for patients with autoimmune antibodies to platelets. Patient with ITP may respond to steroid therapy, splenectomy, splenic irradiation, azathioprine, vincristine, colchicine, cyclophosphamide, danazol, IVIG, Rh immune globulin, plasma exchange, or combination therapy. The blood bank director should work with the patient's primary physician to decide the best course of therapy for each patient.

Posttransfusion Purpura

Posttransfusion purpura (PTP) is an autoimmune phenomenon caused by an alloimmune antibody and usually occurs 1 week after blood transfusion in patients who lack a platelet-specific antigen, most often PLA-1. PTP is caused by antiplatelet antibodies that autoreact with the patient's antigen-negative platelets through passive transfer of antigen at the time of transfusion. Allogeneic platelet transfusions for PTP can result in significant transfusion reactions and are usually ineffective because the platelets are rapidly cleared. Therapy for PTP consists of glucocorticoids plus plasma exchange or IVIG. Interestingly, once a patient has recovered from PTP and the thrombocytopenia has resolved, PTP may not recur with additional blood transfusions.

ALTERNATIVES TO PLATELET TRANSFUSION

The use of platelet transfusions has steadily increased. In addition, the short storage time for platelets (5 days maximum) creates a need for continuous replenishment of the platelet supply, and low platelet inventories often occur over holidays, long weekends, and after inclement weather when platelet donations decrease. Chronic platelet shortages and limited platelet storage time have prompted the development of new agents (cytokines, antifibrinolytic agents, synthetic platelet substitutes) with potential to stimulate platelet production and reduce the need for platelet transfusion.

Cytokines

Cytokines, such as recombinant human thrombopoietin (rhTPO); human recombinant interleukin-6 (IL-6), interleukin-3 (IL-3), and interleukin-11 (IL-11); and amifostine, a cytoprotective agent, have been tested in thrombocytopenic patients for their role in the stimulation of platelet production (46,77). The TPO gene is located on chromosome 3q, and the TPO protein is composed of 332 amino acids with two domains. An erythropoietin-like domain, located on the N-terminus, has 163 amino acids and is responsible for the biologic activity of TPO. The second domain is a long carbohydrate chain on the C-terminus and functions as a stabilizer. TPO stimulates platelet production by inducing the proliferation of marrow progenitor cells and maturation of megakaryocytes. Limited clinical trials have been conducted in thrombocytopenic oncology patients and the results showed that, although platelet counts increased, treatment with TPO did not decrease the numbers of platelet transfusions (78). Larger clinical trials are needed to establish the therapeutic role of TPO in clinical practice. Additionally, one in vitro study of the platelet storage lesion reported that adding TPO to apheresis platelet products did not demonstrate any effect at 1 and 5 days of storage on markers such as pH, platelet count, LDH, and osmotic recovery, among others (79). In another clinical trial, a truncated form of TPO in which polyethylene glycol (PEG) replaced the second chain, was used to achieve a long half-life (80–82). Pegylated recombinant human megakaryocyte growth and development factor (PEG-rHuMGDF) was tested in a clinical trial on healthy donors to increase the donor's circulating platelet count and thereby increase the platelet apheresis yield. The trial was complicated by the development of an antibody, found in several of the healthy donors, that cross-reacted with endogenous TPO and resulted in severe thrombocytopenia secondary to iatrogenic ITP (83). This led to the termination of the clinical trial. A full-length TPO form is now being evaluated.

Other cytokines that have been studied for beneficial effect in thrombocytopenic patients include IL-11, IL-3, and IL-6, but only IL-11 has demonstrated promise. The IL-11 gene is located on chromosome 19q, and its protein has 199 amino acids. Limited clinical trials in oncology patients have shown that when administered at a dose of 50μg/kg/day, IL-11 reduces the number of platelet transfusions; however, these observations need to be verified in larger prospective randomized trials (84–86). Both IL-3 and IL-6 were used in clinical trials and have failed to show improvement of thrombocytopenia.

Antifibrinolytics

Several additional pharmacotherapeutic agents have been associated with reduced transfusion requirements and may be of benefit to the platelet-refractory and/or hemorrhaging patient. Antifibrinolytic agents such as tranexamic acid and ϵ-aminocaproic acid have been shown to reduce the platelet transfusion requirement in patients with leukemia (87,88). These agents are synthetic lysine analogs that bind to plasminogen and cause a conformational change in the plasminogen protein that prevents fibrin lysis. The use of antifibrinolytic therapy should be reserved for patients with severe, ongoing hemorrhage that is unresponsive to multiple platelet transfusions, and when other medical and surgical interventions have failed to achieve hemostasis.

Platelet Substitutes

A number of platelet substitutes are under development. One product, also known as lyophilized platelets or freeze-dried fixed platelets, is manufactured using platelet pools in a multistep, bovine serum albumin (BSA)-phosphate buffer wash, paraformaldehyde fixation process, followed by freezing and lyophilization. Phase I and II studies of toxicity, in vivo survival and function, immunogenicity and side effects are currently being evaluated (89,90).

An infusible platelet membrane (IPM) is made from older platelets that are lysed by freeze-thaw methods, pasteurized, sonicated (for uniformity of particle size), and then lyophilized. IPM is composed of membrane phospholipids, along with GPIb, but not GPIIb-IIIa. Studies in thrombocytopenic rabbits have demonstrated that IPM can reduce bleeding time. Clinical trials suggest the product has hemostatic effectiveness in humans; however, it remains under development (90,91).

Other potential platelet substitutes include (a) modified autologous erythrocytes with covalently bound fibrinogen or peptide sequences (92), which aggregate platelets (93); (b) fibrinogen-coated albumin microcapsules (also known as Synthocytes), which facilitate platelet adhesion to endothelial cell matrix (94); and (c) polyamide microcapsules, which are composed of synthetic bilayer membrane and modify platelet activation, adhesion, and platelet membrane vesicles (95).

TRANSFUSION ADMINISTRATION MODALITIES

Numerous specialized techniques are available through the blood bank to assist in a patient's transfusion requirements. Manipulations of platelet products, such as transfer to syringe storage, volume reduction, washing, and freezing, usually result in direct puncture of the blood bag prior to transfusion, opening the system. Once a platelet storage system has been opened, the product must either be infused within 4 hours to minimize the potential for bacterial growth or discarded. Therefore, coordination of the release and timely transfusion of specialized products is essential to hospital patient safety. In addition to a shortened expiration of specialized products, added manipulations of platelet products are time consuming and, subsequently, of limited utility when in urgent situations.

Recent advances in pathogen inactivation have used special processing of platelet products after collection to treat the product and inactivate any contaminating viral or bacterial constituents (96). Pathogen inactivation methods may help to extend the current 4-hour expiration of open-system blood products, but the technology is still under development and validation is needed.

Pumps, Syringes, and Blood Warmers

Platelets can be safely administered through standard hospital pumps without any significant detriment to the product. Platelet infusion using a mechanical pump enables a more controlled rate of platelet administration (97,98).

Syringes provide a convenient storage media in neonatal transfusion medicine. Platelet transfusions for premature infants and neonates are often subjected to filtration, centrifugation, and irradiation prior to issue in a syringe. In vitro data have shown no significant platelet storage lesion when held in gas-impermeable polypropylene syringes for up to 6 hours, although the product should be infused within 4 hours to avoid potential bacterial growth (99,100.)

Volume Reduction and Washing

Platelets can be volume reduced for the volume-sensitive patient. Volume reduction is usually performed concurrently with pharmacologic volume reduction of the patient's intravenous medications as part of an overall fluid restriction plan. Moreover, platelets can be washed, to remove the plasma, and resuspended in normal saline to avoid plasma exposures in patients with a history of severe allergic transfusion reactions to plasma proteins, such as can occur with immunoglobulin A (IgA) deficiency. Volume reduction and/or washing of platelets by the blood bank requires from one to several hours to perform, and the time restriction of these techniques limits their availability in emergent situations. Additionally, volume reduction of the product can result in some loss of platelets during processing and, therefore, a lower platelet dose for the patient.

SUMMARY

Platelet transfusion therapy can be of substantial benefit for patients with thrombocytopenia or platelet dysfunction, and there are numerous platelet products and alternatives available for transfusion. Additionally, significant advancements in the safety, purity, and efficacy of platelet preparations have been achieved. These remarkable advancements in platelet preparations provide clinicians with the ability to transfuse platelets without the risk of serious complications, and an increasing number of patients are receiving the benefits of platelet transfusion therapy. Unfortunately, due to the limitations of platelet storage time and platelet refractoriness in some patients, the availability of platelet products for all patients remains a challenge. Platelet substitutes and pharmacologic alternatives provide some additional avenues of therapy, and advancements in platelet donation and collection have also improved the quality and quantity of platelet preparations available for patients. Coordinated research efforts that combine knowledge of platelet function, storage, and transfusion are necessary to meet the increasing demand for this valuable product.

REFERENCES

1. Coller BS FD. Hereditary qualitative platelet disorders. In: Beutler ELM, Coller BS, Kipps TJ, eds. *Williams hematology.* New York: McGraw-Hill, 1995:1364–1385.
2. Bellucci S, Damaj G, Boval B, et al. Bone marrow transplantation in severe Glanzmann's thrombasthenia with antiplatelet alloimmunization. *Bone Marrow Transplant* 2000;25:327–330.
3. George JN. Platelets. *Lancet* 2000;355:1531–1539.
4. Mhawech P, Saleem A. Inherited giant platelet disorders. Classification and literature review. *Am J Clin Pathol* 2000;113:176–190.
5. Gralnick HR, Williams SB, Shafer BC, et al. Factor VIII/von Willebrand factor binding to von Willebrand's disease platelets. *Blood* 1982; 60:328–332.
6. French DL, Seligsohn U. Platelet glycoprotein IIb/IIIa receptors and Glanzmann's thrombasthenia. *Arterioscler Thromb Vasc Biol* 2000;20: 607–610.
7. Berrebi A, Klepfish A, Varon D, et al. Gray platelet syndrome in the elderly. *Am J Hematol* 1988;28:270–272.
8. Roth GJ, Calverley DC. Aspirin, platelets, and thrombosis: theory and practice. *Blood* 1994;83:885–898.
9. O'Brien JR. Effect of salicylates on human platelets. *Lancet* 1968;1: 1431.
10. McQueen EG, Facoory B, Faed JM. Non-steroidal anti-inflammatory drugs and platelet function. *N Z Med J* 1986;99:358–360.
11. Fass RJ, Copelan EA, Brandt JT, et al. Platelet-mediated bleeding caused by broad-spectrum penicillins. *J Infect Dis* 1987;155: 1242–1248.
12. McTavish D, Faulds D, Goa KL. Ticlopidine. An updated review of its pharmacology and therapeutic use in platelet-dependent disorders. *Drugs* 1990;40:238–259.
13. Shattil SJ, Bennett JS. Acquired qualitative platelet disorders due to diseases, drugs, and foods. In: Beutler ELM, Coller BS, Kipps TJ, eds. *Williams hematology.* New York: McGraw-Hill, 1995: 1386–1400.
14. Rabiner SF. Uremic bleeding. *Prog Hemost Thromb* 1972;1:233–250.
15. Noris M, Remuzzi G. Uremic bleeding: closing the circle after 30 years of controversies? *Blood* 1999;94:2569–2574.
16. Vigano G, Benigni A, Mendogni D, et al. Recombinant human erythropoietin to correct uremic bleeding. *Am J Kidney Dis* 1991;18: 44–49.
17. Akizawa T, Kinugasa E, Kitaoka T, et al. Effects of recombinant human erythropoietin and correction of anemia on platelet function in hemodialysis patients. *Nephron* 1991;58:400–406.
18. Heunisch C, Resnick DJ, Vitello JM, et al. Conjugated estrogens for the management of gastrointestinal bleeding secondary to uremia of acute renal failure. *Pharmacotherapy* 1998;18:210–217.
19. Revesz T, Arets B, Bierings M, et al. Recombinant factor VIIa in severe uremic bleeding. *Thromb Haemost* 1998;80:353.
20. Khuri SF, Wolfe JA, Josa M, et al. Hematologic changes during and after cardiopulmonary bypass and their relationship to the bleeding time and nonsurgical blood loss. *J Thorac Cardiovasc Surg* 1992;104: 94–107.
21. Abrams CS, Ellison N, Budzynski AZ, et al. Direct detection of activated platelets and platelet-derived microparticles in humans. *Blood* 1990;75:128–138.
22. Schafer AI. Essential thrombocythemia. *Prog Hemost Thromb* 1991; 10:69–96.
23. Kessler CM, Klein HG, Havlik RJ. Uncontrolled thrombocytosis in chronic myeloproliferative disorders. *Br J Haematol* 1982;50: 157–167.
24. McGrath KM, Stuart JJ, Richards F II. Correlation between serum IgG, platelet membrane IgG, and platelet function in hypergammaglobulinaemic states. *Br J Haematol* 1979;42:585–591.
25. Kasturi J, Saraya AK. Platelet functions in dysproteinaemia. *Acta Haematol* 1978;59:104–113.
26. Rinder MR, Richard RE, Rinder HM. Acquired von Willebrand's disease: a concise review. *Am J Hematol* 1997;54:139–145.
27. George J, El-Harke, M. Thrombocytopenia due to enhanced platelet destruction by nonimmunologic mechanisms. In: Beutler ELM, Coller BS, Kipps TJ, eds. *Williams hematology.* New York: McGraw-Hill, 1995:1290–1315.
28. Lacotte L, Thierry A, Delwail V, et al. Thrombotic thrombocytopenic purpura during interferon α treatment for chronic myelogenous leukemia. *Acta Haematol* 2000;102:160–162.
29. Bennett CL, Connors JM, Carwile JM, et al. Thrombotic thrombocytopenic purpura associated with clopidogrel. *N Engl J Med* 2000;342: 1773–1777.
30. Chen DK, Kim JS, Sutton DM. Thrombotic thrombocytopenic purpura associated with ticlopidine use: a report of 3 cases and review of the literature. *Arch Intern Med* 1999;159:311–314.
31. George JN. How I treat patients with thrombotic thrombocytopenic purpura–hemolytic uremic syndrome. *Blood* 2000;96:1223–1229.
32. Harkness DR, Byrnes JJ, Lian EC, et al. Hazard of platelet transfusion in thrombotic thrombocytopenic purpura. *JAMA* 1981;246: 1931–1933.
33. van der Plas RM, Schiphorst ME, Huizinga EG, et al. von Willebrand factor proteolysis is deficient in classic, but not in bone marrow transplantation–associated, thrombotic thrombocytopenic purpura. *Blood* 1999;93:3798–3802.
34. Takala A, Lahdevirta J, Jansson SE, et al. Systemic inflammation in hemorrhagic fever with renal syndrome correlates with hypotension and thrombocytopenia but not with renal injury. *J Infect Dis* 2000; 181:1964–1970.
35. Menitove JE. *Standards for blood banks and transfusion services.* Bethesda: American Association of Blood Banks, 2000.
36. Gelinas JP, Stoddart LV, Snyder EL. Thrombocytopenia and critical care medicine. *J Intensive Care Med* 2001;16:1–21.
37. Rebulla P, Finazzi G, Marangoni F, et al. The threshold for prophylactic platelet transfusions in adults with acute myeloid leukemia. *N Engl J Med* 1997;337:1870–1875.
38. Wandt H, Frank M, Ehninger G, et al. Safety and cost effectiveness of a 10 × 10(9)/L trigger for prophylactic platelet transfusions compared with the traditional 20 × 10^9/L trigger: a prospective comparative trial in 105 patients with acute myeloid leukemia. *Blood* 1998; 91:3601–3606.
39. Murphy WG. Prophylactic platelet transfusion in acute leukaemia. *Lancet* 1992;339:120–121.
40. Schiffer CA. Management of patients refractory of platelet transfusion. *Leukemia* 2001;15:683–685.
41. Stehling L, Luban NL, Anderson KC, et al. Guidelines for blood utilization review. *Transfusion* 1994;34:438–448.
42. Hanson SR, Slichter SJ. Platelet kinetics in patients with bone marrow hypoplasia: evidence for a fixed platelet requirement. *Blood* 1985;66: 1105–1109.
43. Harker LA, Roskos L, Cheung E. Effective and efficient platelet transfusion strategies that maintain hemostatic protection. *Transfusion* 1998;38:619–621.
44. Hersh JK, Hom EG, Brecher ME. Mathematical modeling of platelet survival with implications for optimal transfusion practice in the chronically platelet transfusion–dependent patient. *Transfusion* 1998; 38:637–644.
45. Norol F, Bierling P, Roudot-Thoraval F, et al. Platelet transfusion: a dose-response study. *Blood* 1998;92:1448–1453.
46. Vostal JG, Reid TJ, Mondoro TH. Summary of a workshop on in vivo efficacy of transfused platelet components and platelet substitutes. *Transfusion* 2000;40:742–750.
47. Shanwell A, Larsson S, Aschan J, et al. A randomized trial comparing the use of fresh and stored platelets in the treatment of bone marrow transplant recipients. *Eur J Haematol* 1992;49:77–81.
48. Holme S. Storage and quality assessment of platelets. *Vox Sang* 1998; 74:207–216.
49. Wasser MN, Houbiers JG, D'Amaro J, et al. The effect of fresh versus stored blood on post-operative bleeding after coronary bypass surgery: a prospective randomized study. *Br J Haematol* 1989;72:81–84.
50. Rinder HM, Murphy M, Mitchell JG, et al. Progressive platelet activation with storage: evidence for shortened survival of activated platelets after transfusion. *Transfusion* 1991;31:409–414.
51. Braine HG, Kickler TS, Charache P, et al. Bacterial sepsis secondary

to platelet transfusion: an adverse effect of extended storage at room temperature. *Transfusion* 1986;26:391–393.

52. Goldman M, Blajchman MA. Blood product–associated bacterial sepsis. *Transfus Med Rev* 1991;5:73–83.
53. Heal JM, Singal S, Sardisco E, et al. Bacterial proliferation in platelet concentrates. *Transfusion* 1986;26:388–390.
54. Sloand EM, Yu M, Klein HG. Comparison of random-donor platelet concentrates prepared from whole blood units and platelets prepared from single-donor apheresis collections. *Transfusion* 1996;36: 955–959.
55. Strindberg J, Berlin G. Transfusion of platelet concentrates—clinical evaluation of two preparations. *Eur J Haematol* 1996;57:307–311.
56. Chambers LA, Herman JH. Considerations in the selection of a platelet component: apheresis versus whole blood-derived. *Transfus Med Rev* 1999;13:311–322.
57. Goodnough LT, Kuter D, McCullough J, et al. Apheresis platelets: emerging issues related to donor platelet count, apheresis platelet yield, and platelet transfusion dose. *J Clin Apheresis* 1998;13: 114–119.
58. The Trial to Reduce Alloimmunization to Platelets Study Group. Leukocyte reduction and ultraviolet B irradiation of platelets to prevent alloimmunization and refractoriness to platelet transfusions. *N Engl J Med* 1997;337:1861–1869.
59. Nagasawa T, Kim BK, Baldini MG. Temporary suppression of circulating antiplatelet alloantibodies by the massive infusion of fresh, stored, or lyophilized platelets. *Transfusion* 1978;18:429–435.
60. Blumberg N, Heal JM, Kirkley SA, et al. Leukodepleted–ABO-identical blood components in the treatment of hematologic malignancies: a cost analysis. *Am J Hematol* 1995;48:108–115.
61. Blumberg N, Hicks GL, Risher WH. Association of ABO-mismatched platelet transfusions with morbidity and mortality in cardiac surgery. *Transfusion* 2001;41:790–793.
62. Curtis BR, Edwards JT, Hessner MJ, et al. Blood group A and B antigens are strongly expressed on platelets of some individuals. *Blood* 2000;96:1574–1581.
63. Larsson LG, Welsh VJ, Ladd DJ. Acute intravascular hemolysis secondary to out-of-group platelet transfusion. *Transfusion* 2000;40: 902–906.
64. McManigal S, Sims KL. Intravascular hemolysis secondary to ABO incompatible platelet products. An underrecognized transfusion reaction. *Am J Clin Pathol* 1999;111:202–206.
65. Heal JM, Rowe JM, McMican A, et al. The role of ABO matching in platelet transfusion. *Eur J Haematol* 1993;50:110–117.
66. Dunstan RA, Simpson MB, Rosse WF. Erythrocyte antigens on human platelets. Absence of Rh, Duffy, Kell, Kidd, and Lutheran antigens. *Transfusion* 1984;24:243–246.
67. Vengelen-Tyler V. *Technical manual. Blood transfusion practice.* Bethesda: American Association of Blood Banks, 1999; 451–482.
68. Atoyebi W, Mundy N, Croxton T, et al. Is it necessary to administer anti-D to prevent RhD immunization after the transfusion of RhD-positive platelet concentrates? *Br J Haematol* 2000;111:980–983.
69. Lichtiger B, Surgeon J, Rhorer S. Rh-incompatible platelet transfusion therapy in cancer patients. A study of 30 cases. *Vox Sang* 1983;45: 139–143.
70. Zeiler T, Wittmann G, Zingsem J, et al. A dose of 100 IU intravenous anti-D γ-globulin is effective for the prevention of RhD immunisation after RhD-incompatible single donor platelet transfusion. *Vox Sang* 1994;66:243.
71. Slichter SJ. Algorithm for managing the platelet refractory patient. *J Clin Apheresis* 1997;12:4–9.
72. O'Connell B, Lee EJ, Schiffer CA. The value of 10-minute posttransfusion platelet counts. *Transfusion* 1988;28:66–67.
73. Daly PA, Schiffer CA, Aisner J, et al. Platelet transfusion therapy. One-hour posttransfusion increments are valuable in predicting the need for HLA-matched preparations. *JAMA* 1980;243:435–438.
74. Vengelen-Tyler V. *Technical manual. Platelet and granulocyte antigens and antibodies.* Bethesda: American Association of Blood Banks, 1999; 339–356.
75. Bishop JF, McGrath K, Wolf MM, et al. Clinical factors influencing the efficacy of pooled platelet transfusions. *Blood* 1988;71:383–387.
76. Delaflor-Weiss E, Mintz PD. The evaluation and management of platelet refractoriness and alloimmunization. *Transfus Med Rev* 2000; 14:180–196.
77. Lee DH, Blajchman MA. Novel platelet products and substitutes. *Transfus Med Rev* 1998;12:175–187.
78. Gerotziafas G, Samama MM. Alternatives to platelet transfusion. In: Seghatchian J, Snyder EL, Krailadsiri P, eds. *Platelet therapy: current status and future trends.* New York: Elsevier Science, 2000:363–381.
79. Snyder E, Perrotta P, Rinder H, et al. Effect of recombinant human megakaryocyte growth and development factor coupled with polyethylene glycol on the platelet storage lesion. *Transfusion* 1999;39: 258–264.
80. Brereton ML, Adams JA, Briggs M, et al. The in vitro effect of pegylated recombinant human megakaryocyte growth and development factor (PEG-rHuMGDF) on megakaryopoiesis in patients with aplastic anaemia. *Br J Haematol* 1999;104:119–126.
81. Somlo G, Sniecinski I, ter Veer A, et al. Recombinant human thrombopoietin in combination with granulocyte colony–stimulating factor enhances mobilization of peripheral blood progenitor cells, increases peripheral blood platelet concentration, and accelerates hematopoietic recovery following high-dose chemotherapy. *Blood* 1999;93: 2798–2806.
82. Miller YM, Klein HG. Growth factors and their impact on transfusion medicine. *Vox Sang* 1996;71:196–204.
83. Kuter DJ, Cebon J, Harker LA, et al. Platelet growth factors: potential impact on transfusion medicine. *Transfusion* 1999;39:321–332.
84. Gordon MS, McCaskill-Stevens WJ, Battiato LA, et al. A phase I trial of recombinant human interleukin-11 (neumega rhIL-11 growth factor) in women with breast cancer receiving chemotherapy. *Blood* 1996;87:3615–3624.
85. Isaacs C, Robert NJ, Bailey FA, et al. Randomized placebo-controlled study of recombinant human interleukin-11 to prevent chemotherapy-induced thrombocytopenia in patients with breast cancer receiving dose-intensive cyclophosphamide and doxorubicin. *J Clin Oncol* 1997;15:3368–3377.
86. Vredenburgh JJ, Hussein A, Fisher D, et al. A randomized trial of recombinant human interleukin-11 following autologous bone marrow transplantation with peripheral blood progenitor cell support in patients with breast cancer. *Biol Blood Marrow Transplant* 1998;4: 134–141.
87. Avvisati G, ten Cate JW, Buller HR, et al. Tranexamic acid for control of haemorrhage in acute promyelocytic leukaemia. *Lancet* 1989;2: 122–124.
88. Shpilberg O, Blumenthal R, Sofer O, et al. A controlled trial of tranexamic acid therapy for the reduction of bleeding during treatment of acute myeloid leukemia. *Leuk Lymphoma* 1995;19:141–144.
89. Bode AP, Read MS. Lyophilized platelets for transfusion. In: Seghatchian J, Snyder EL, Krailadsiri P, eds. *Platelet therapy: current status and future trends.* Elsevier Science, 2000:131–168.
90. Snyder EL, Pisciotto PT. Platelet storage and metabolism. In: Anderson C, Ness P, eds. *Scientific basis of transfusion medicine.* Philadelphia: WB Saunders, 2000:217–218.
91. Galan AM, Bozzo J, Hernandez MR, et al. Infusible platelet membranes improve hemostasis in thrombocytopenic blood: experimental studies under flow conditions. *Transfusion* 2000;40:1074–1080.
92. Coller BS, Springer KT, Beer JH, et al. Thromboerythrocytes. In vitro studies of a potential autologous, semi-artificial alternative to platelet transfusions. *J Clin Invest* 1992;89:546–555.
93. Agam G, Livne AA. Erythrocytes with covalently bound fibrinogen as a cellular replacement for the treatment of thrombocytopenia. *Eur J Clin Invest* 1992;22:105–112.
94. Levi M, Friederich PW, Middleton S, et al. Fibrinogen-coated albumin microcapsules reduce bleeding in severely thrombocytopenic rabbits. *Nat Med* 1999;5:107–111.
95. Kono K, Ito Y, Kimura S, et al. Platelet adhesion on to polyamide microcapsules coated with lipid bilayer membrane. *Biomaterials* 1989; 10:455–461.
96. Lin L, Cook DN, Wiesehahn GP, et al. Photochemical inactivation

of viruses and bacteria in platelet concentrates by use of a novel psoralen and long-wavelength ultraviolet light. *Transfusion* 1997;37:423–435.
97. Norville R, Hinds P, Wilimas J, et al. The effects of infusion methods on platelet count, morphology, and corrected count increment in children with cancer: in vitro and in vivo studies. *Oncol Nurs Forum* 1994;21:1669–1673.
98. Snyder EL, Rinder HM, Napychank P. In vitro and in vivo evaluation of platelet transfusions administered through an electromechanical infusion pump. *Am J Clin Pathol* 1990;94:77–80.
99. Pisciotto PT, Snyder EL, Snyder JA, et al. In vitro characteristics of white cell-reduced single-unit platelet concentrates stored in syringes. *Transfusion* 1994;34:407–411.
100. Pisciotto PT, Snyder EL, Napychank PA, et al. In vitro characteristics of volume-reduced platelet concentrate stored in syringes. *Transfusion* 1991;31:404–408.

Rossi's Principles of Transfusion Medicine, Third Edition, edited by Toby L. Simon, Walter H. Dzik, Edward L. Snyder, Christopher P. Stowell, and Ronald G. Strauss. Lippincott Williams & Wilkins, Philadelphia © 2002.

CASE 18A

INTERCONNECTED CASCADES

CASE HISTORY

JK is a 58-year-old female with myelodysplasia and mild splenomegaly who comes to the outpatient department for transfusion. She has progressive pancytopenia with a hematocrit of 27%, white blood cell count of 1500/μl, and platelet count of 22,000/μl. Because of her thrombocytopenia, her oncologist requested a transfusion with irradiated, leukoreduced, apheresis platelets.

The platelets were administered via an electronic pump from 10:00 to 10:45 AM. At the completion of the transfusion, JK complained of pain in her legs and buttocks. She also had a spell of shivering that lasted a few minutes with no other symptoms. Her temperature was unchanged from before the transfusion and was 98.9°F. Her blood pressure was 160/78 mm Hg, which was not substantially different from before the transfusion. Her pulse had increased from 75 beats/min before the transfusion to 95 beats/min at the end. On examination there were no hives or other lesions found on the skin of the thighs or buttocks. Her legs and back were not tender to touch and during the examination she had another bout of shivering lasting less than 5 minutes. She was given acetaminophen, and a posttransfusion sample was sent for a complete blood count (CBC) and to the blood bank for evaluation of a suspected unusual transfusion reaction.

In the laboratory the clerical check was correct. The patient is group A with a nonreactive antibody screen. The posttransfusion serum sample had no visible evidence of hemolysis, and the direct antiglobulin test was negative using polyvalent antiglobulin reagent. The CBC drawn posttransfusion showed that the platelet count had risen to 40,000/μl. The hematocrit was unchanged. The donor was a regular, male group O donor. The unit appeared normal. A specimen of the donor unit was sent for bacterial culture. The laboratory reported back to the nurses' station that there was no evidence of hemolysis. The patient was observed. One hour after the transfusion, she still complained of upper leg and back pain but noted that the pain was fading. She had stopped shivering and temperature was now 101°F. She had passed urine that was clear and was negative for hemoglobin by dipstick analysis. During the next hour she felt much better and was discharged to home with her husband. The transfusion medicine physician on duty called her that evening at home. She felt "back to normal."

DISCUSSION

The following day the case was reviewed. First, the indication for the platelet transfusion was reviewed. The patient had chronic thrombocytopenia. The value of prophylactic platelet transfusions in outpatients with chronic thrombocytopenia has never been assessed in clinical trials. Bacterial culture of the donor product was negative. Because the patient developed a reasonable increment from the transfusion, acute destruction of the transfused platelets seemed unlikely. Indeed, the patient had a recent human lymphocyte antigen (HLA) antibody screen which was negative.

The platelets were administered over 45 minutes. Although the volume of a unit of apheresis platelets is equal to or greater than that of most units of packed red blood cells, it is surprising to find that in nearly all hospitals platelets are administered very quickly (15 minutes to 1 hour), while red blood cells are often administered over up to 4 hours. There is no specific rationale for this practice.

It was noted that the patient's initial temperature was not elevated, but that it rose 1°F after the transfusion. This is, in fact, a typical fever response to a pyrogenic stimulus. Immediately after the stimulus, patients will shiver. At that moment, the systemic temperature will not be elevated. Pyrogenic stimuli to the brain result in a resetting of the body's thermoregulatory center that causes shivering, an increased metabolic rate, heat-seeking behavior (patients want to get under the covers), and the deliberate turning off of cooling mechanisms, all of which combine to result in a raised body temperature. It is important to appreciate this time lag, because forms submitted to the laboratory with posttransfusion vital signs often include only the record of signs taken at the time of the transfusion reaction and before the patient has had a chance to mount a fever.

Because of the combination of chills, fever, and back pain, an ABO reaction was considered. The patient is group A and the donor unit was group O. The passive infusion of plasma ABO antibodies from the donor unit, which are incompatible with the recipient red blood cells, can cause significant ABO reactions, although these generally occur in recipients with small blood volumes, such as children (1). In retrospect it was noted that the patient weighed only 100 pounds. The donor unit was retrieved and ABO titers were done. The donor's anti-A and ani-B titers were found to be very high (>1:512).

When group O donors have high-titer ABO antibodies, the transfusion of single-donor (apheresis) platelets to non–group O recipients is more dangerous than pooled platelet concentrates, because the chance of pooling platelets from four to six donors, all of whom have such high-titer antibodies, is so unlikely. One should be particularly careful regarding the use of out-of-group apheresis platelets for children.

The posttransfusion clear serum, negative DAT, and the negative urine sample documented that the patient did not actually have hemolysis as a result of the transfusion. A small amount of hemolysis resulting in depression of the free haptoglobin without production of free intravascular hemoglobin was possible, but a haptoglobin was not measured. A trained technologist can observe a pink tinge to the posttransfusion serum specimen when the concentration of free hemoglobin is only 50 to 100 mg%. This corresponds to the lysis of 5 to 10 ml of blood in an adult. Thus, the visual inspection of the posttransfusion sample is a sensitive test for hemolysis and should be part of the evaluation of all transfusion reactions. Significant hemolysis due to passive transfer of ABO antibodies by apheresis platelet transfusions has been previously reported (1). In our case, we believe that the passively transferred anti-A bound to antigen sites on vascular endothelial cells and tissues.

Fever and chills are the most common first symptoms in major hemolytic reactions (2). Fever is also a hallmark of nonhemolytic reactions as well as incompatible platelet reactions. All three of these events share a common underlying mechanism—namely that antigen-antibody complexes are fully capable of triggering recipient macrophages to release cytokines that can result in the fever response (3). In our case, donor anti-A may have reacted with recipient soluble-A substance in the plasma and on recipient A antigens on platelets.

The pain of ABO reactions has been noted for centuries and remains unexplained. This pain is said to occur in anephric individuals who experience transfusion reactions and occurs (as in our patient) in the absence of overt hemolysis. Thus, back pain is *not* due to "pain in the kidneys as they filter free hemoglobin." Moreover, patients who are infused with immunologically compatible but lysed units and who pass large quantities of free hemoglobin in the urine do so painlessly. Because pain results from tissue swelling, activation of complement and/or bradykinin is much more likely to be the underlying cause of pain during ABO reactions. Anaphylatoxins such as C3a and C5a may cause local vasodilation and tissue swelling. Bradykinin is known to cause a local pain response through both tissue swelling and direct activation of pain receptors. ABO reactions are considered to activate the high–molecular-weight kininogen cascade leading to bradykinin formation. Why the back and upper legs? Although there is no answer yet, it is entirely possible that these parts of the body simply represent areas with large muscle beds susceptible to tissue swelling in response to complement and kinin activation.

The pathophysiology of ABO reactions remains an opportunity for continued research (4,5). We know that in major hemolytic reactions, at least three cascade systems participate: the coagulation system (disseminated intravascular coagulation [DIC] often accompanies severe hemolysis), the complement system, and the kinin system. In addition, recent in vitro experiments demonstrate that intravascular antigen-antibody complexes result in a cytokine response that causes the hallmark response of fever following transfusion (Fig. 18A.1).

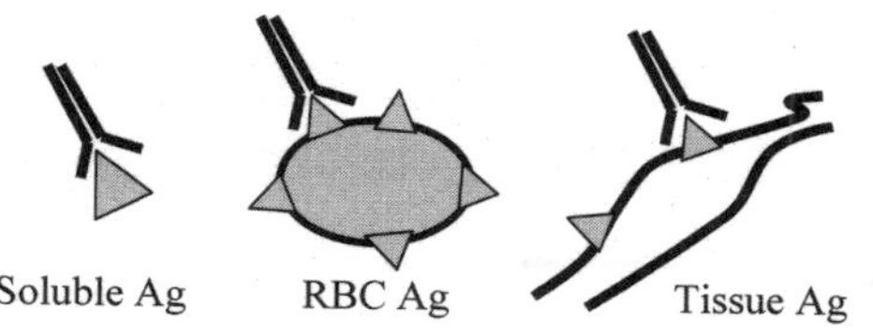

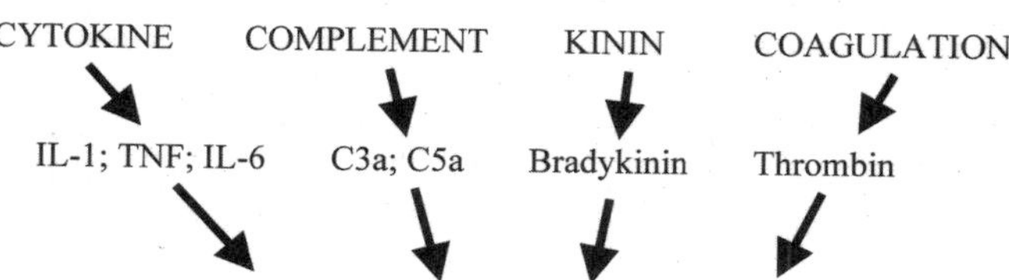

FIGURE 18A.1. Overview of the pathophysiology of ABO-mediated transfusion reactions. The sudden and explosive formation of immune complexes on soluble antigens, erythrocyte antigens, and tissue antigens triggers four interconnected cascade systems, leading to the production a variety of inflammatory mediators. These in turn lead to clinical symptoms that vary in individual patients.

Case contributed by Walter H. Dzik, M.D., Massachusetts General Hospital, Boston, MA.

REFERENCES

1. Pierce RN, Reich LM, Mayer K. Hemolysis following platelet transfusions from ABO-incompatible donors. *Transfusion* 1985;25:60–62.
2. Pineda AA, Brzica SM, Taswell HF. Hemolytic transfusion reaction: recent experience in a large blood bank. *Mayo Clin Proc* 1978;53: 378–390.
3. Dzik WH. Is the febrile response to transfusion due to donor or recipient cytokine? *Transfusion* 1992;32:594.
4. Goldfinger D. Acute hemolytic transfusion reactions—a fresh look at pathophysiology and considerations regarding therapy. *Transfusion* 1977;17:85–98.
5. Davenport R, Burdick M, Moore SA, et al. Cytokine production in IgG-mediated red cell incompatibility. *Transfusion* 1993;33:19–24.

PART III
White Blood Cell

19

NEUTROPHIL PRODUCTION AND KINETICS: NEUTROPENIA AND NEUTROPHILIA

THOMAS H. PRICE

The neutrophil, as the body's primary defense against bacterial infection, is especially equipped to locate, engulf, and destroy invading microorganisms. The system of neutrophil production in the bone marrow and distribution in the blood and tissues serves both to maintain a baseline cell concentration and, under situations of infection or inflammation, to effect the rapid delivery of large numbers of cells to areas of infection or inflammation.

BONE MARROW PRODUCTION

The pluripotent stem cell is capable of giving rise to any type of hematopoietic cell. With differentiation, a fraction of these cells become committed to the neutrophil line. Development beyond this committed progenitor stage proceeds sequentially in the marrow from the myeloblast, the earliest recognizable neutrophil precursor, to the mature segmented neutrophil. The mature cells are released into the circulation—a process that during the basal state takes approximately 10 to 12 days. There are two important features to bone marrow neutrophil production—cell proliferation and cell maturation. Proliferation is necessary to convert the small stem/progenitor cell population into a mass of mature cells large enough to adequately combat an actual or potential infectious challenge. Isotopic studies have shown that cell division is limited to the myeloblast, promyelocyte, and myelocyte compartments (1). Most cells probably undergo four or five divisions between the myeloblast and myelocyte stage, each division taking approximately 1 day (2). Cell maturation is required to ensure that the neutrophil will be able to function as a highly developed phagocyte. Maturation occurs continuously from the myeloblast to the mature neutrophil. An essential feature of this process is the ordered development of the four characteristic types of cytoplasmic granules of the neutrophil. Primary granules containing myeloperoxidase and serine proteases appear during the promyelocyte stage, secondary granules containing lactoferrin and collagenase and tertiary granules containing gelatinase at the myelocyte stage, and secretory vesicles at the stage of the mature cell. Studies have shown that this cytokine-driven chronology is based on the transcriptional regulation of sequentially expressed genes (3). Additional

T.H. Price: Puget Sound Blood Center, Seattle, Washington.

changes during maturation include increased adherence ability, increased deformability, increased responsiveness to chemoattractants, and development of the characteristic segmented nucleus of the neutrophil. Postmitotic neutrophil development in the marrow is a "first in, first out" phenomenon; that is, the cells exit the postmitotic compartment in the same order in which they enter it. Under normal circumstances, the transit time for the postmitotic pool is approximately 7 days (4), a value that can be shortened 2 to 3 days under stress. Normal baseline neutrophil production, based on the transit time and the size of the postmitotic compartment, has been calculated to be approximately 0.85×10^9 cells/kg per day (4).

One of the important requirements of the neutrophil defense system is that it be able to deliver a large number of neutrophils to a site of infection or inflammation quickly. To this end, approximately two thirds of the marrow postmitotic pool, which consists of the most mature cells, can be shifted rapidly from the marrow into the circulation. This pool of cells, which comprises segmented neutrophils and band forms, is known as the *marrow storage pool* or the *marrow reserve.* These cells are mobilized in situations of stress or increased tissue neutrophil demand (5). Mobilization also occurs as a response to stimuli such as corticosteroids, endotoxin, or granulocyte colony-stimulating factor (G-CSF) (6–8). Blood neutrophil counts typically increase dramatically within a few hours after stimulation with these agents, a pattern also observed in clinical situations associated with release of the marrow reserves. The extent of the shift in the storage pool depends on the intensity of the stimulus and is reflected in the magnitude of neutrophilia and the degree to which immature forms are present in the blood. The more intense the stimulus (e.g., the more severe the infection), the higher is the neutrophil count and the higher is the fraction of immature cells. The ability to mobilize additional neutrophils is an important aspect of host defense, and a decreased marrow reserve, as in patients with malnutrition or those previously treated with chemotherapy, compromises the ability of the patient to deal with bacterial infection.

BLOOD KINETICS

Most of the information about the kinetics of neutrophils in the blood has been derived from studies with radioisotopically labeled autologous cells. These studies have shown that neutrophils leave the circulation by means of first-order kinetics. The implication is that loss is random rather than caused by senescence. This finding is consistent with the fact that these cells function normally after they leave the bloodstream. The half-disappearance time from the blood is normally 6 to 8 hours (4, 9). Blood neutrophils are distributed between two freely exchangeable pools of approximately equal size—the circulating pool and the marginal pool (10). Cells in the circulating pool are those readily sampled by means of drawing blood. The anatomic nature of the marginal pool has not been settled. The cells in the marginal pool conventionally have been considered loosely adherent to the vascular endothelium of the small venules. This notion has arisen from direct observation of the microcirculation of animals. Investigators have seen neutrophils slowly rolling along the endothelial surfaces outside the main axial stream of the blood flow (11,12). They also have observed that cells in the marginal and circulating pools are freely exchangeable and rapidly achieve equilibrium (10). However, other information suggests that the marginal pool is not diffusely distributed throughout the vasculature but is largely localized to the liver, the spleen, or the pulmonary vasculature (13–19). In the pulmonary circulation, most sequestered or marginated neutrophils are in the capillary bed. In contrast, in the systemic circulation, they are in the precapillary and postcapillary microvasculature (19).

MIGRATION INTO TISSUES

The process of migrating from the blood to a site of inflammation is complex (18,19). The neutrophil first becomes loosely adherent to the vascular endothelium. It then becomes more firmly fixed to the endothelium and migrates between adjacent endothelial cells to the extravascular tissues. These events are governed by adhesion molecules on the surface of both the neutrophil and the endothelium (20). Three families of adhesive molecules have been described—selectins, integrins, and members of the immunoglobulin superfamily. Numerous studies have shown that the selectins (E, L, and P selectin) mediate the initial adherence of neutrophils to the vessel wall, which manifests as "rolling" under conditions of flow (18–23). Firmer attachment to the endothelial cell is mediated by the interaction of the β_2 integrin CD11/18 on the surface of the neutrophil with the intercellular adhesion molecule 1 on endothelial cells (18–20). Transendothelial migration involves two additional IgG superfamily molecules, CD31 and junctional adhesion molecule (18). The importance of these adhesion molecules for neutrophil emigration from the blood has been demonstrated by the effects of antibodies to these proteins (24,25) and by identification of patients who lack these molecules or their ligands (26–29). Patients with leukocyte adhesion deficiency types I and II are deficient in the β_2 integrin and in a selectin ligand, respectively, on the neutrophil surface. Both disorders are characterized by severe neutrophil dysfunction, neutrophilia, an inability to deliver neutrophils to sites of infection, and recurrent bacterial infection.

The nature and mechanisms of neutrophil margination and emigration appear to be different in the pulmonary than in the systemic vasculature. Neutrophil sequestration and migration in the lungs occur principally in the capillary bed rather than in the postcapillary venules (19). The degree of neutrophil sequestration in the pulmonary capillary bed may be related more to cell size and deformability than to the influence of adhesion proteins (30–32). The role of the adhesion proteins in neutrophil emigration to the alveolar space appears to depend on the particular inflammatory stimulus. For example, evidence has indicated that emigration after infection with gram-positive organisms is selectin and integrin independent, whereas emigration after infection with gram-negative organisms requires the involvement of these adhesion proteins (31,33).

Little is known about neutrophil kinetics once the cell leaves the vasculature. The cell probably survives only 1 to 2 days, after which it undergoes phagocytosis by macrophages. The neutrophil does not return to the blood.

Studies have shown that neutrophil survival in both the blood and the tissues depends on the rate of cellular apoptosis, the regulation of which is poorly understood. Proinflammatory stimuli such as G-CSF inhibit apoptosis; the result is prolongation of cell survival both in vitro and in vivo (34,35). Proapoptotic factors, which dampen the inflammatory response, have been identified in certain tissue inflammatory sites. Regulation of neutrophil apoptosis thus appears to be an important determinant of the intensity of the inflammatory process (36).

REGULATION OF NEUTROPHIL PRODUCTION

At least four cytokines appear to be important in the regulation of neutrophil production, survival, and function—G-CSF, granulocyte-macrophage colony-stimulating factor (GM-CSF), interleukin-3, and stem cell factor (1). Interleukin-3 and stem cell factor act early in hematopoieses. Granulocyte-macrophage colony-stimulating factor stimulates production of neutrophils, monocytes, and eosinophils, whereas G-CSF affects production of neutrophils only. Both G-CSF and GM-CSF stimulate the function of mature neutrophils. Although the exact roles of these and other factors in neutrophil production are incompletely understood, it is clear that G-CSF plays a pivotal role. Knockout mice for either G-CSF or the G-CSF receptor have severe neutropenia (37,38), as do animals treated with antibody to G-CSF (39). In vivo administration of G-CSF causes a dramatic increase in neutrophil production with marked neutrophilia (35,40). There is a presumed negative feedback system in which inflammatory stimuli or a paucity of mature neutrophils provides either a direct or an indirect stimulus to monocytes, T cells, endothelial cells, or fibroblasts, all of which are capable of elaborating cytokines such as G-CSF. Whether these factors are generated in the immediate microenvironment of the target progenitor cells or the developing myeloid cells and thus act over a short range or whether the target cells are primarily influenced by blood levels of these substances is not clear.

RESPONSE TO INFECTION

An essential function of the bone marrow is to increase the delivery of neutrophils to the tissues in the face of infection or the need for an inflammatory response. The kinetic features of such a reaction are shown in Figure 19.1. The first phase is characterized by a rapid shift of bands and segmented neutrophils from the marrow maturational pool into the blood. The sudden influx of neutrophils into the blood results in neutrophilia and is typically associated with an increase in the degree of margination of the blood neutrophils. At the same time, cell

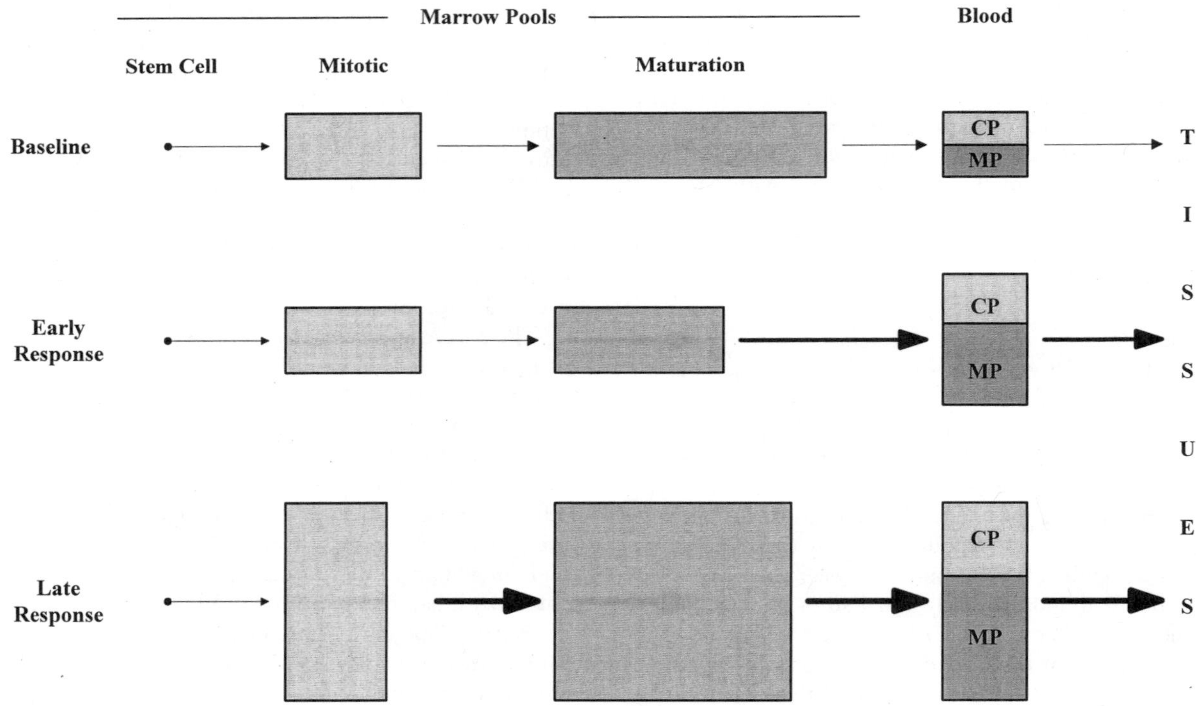

FIGURE 19.1. Marrow response to inflammation and infection. Pool size is represented by *height* of the box. Time spent in the early pool is represented by the *width* of box. The rate of cell flow between compartments is represented by the *size of arrows.* Early response is characterized by a shift of the marrow storage pool into the circulation and increased margination of blood neutrophils. A late response is characterized by proliferation of the mitotic pool and reduced transit time through the marrow pools. *CP,* circulatory pool; *MP,* marginal pool.

production in the mitotic pool expands owing to an increased rate of division of promyelocytes and myelocytes. It then takes 2 to 4 days for the leading edge of this wave of proliferation to proceed through the maturational pool and reach the blood. The result is a steadily increased supply of neutrophils that can be delivered to the tissues. When the infection clears or the inflammatory process runs its course, marrow proliferative activity returns to baseline over a few days.

BLOOD NEUTROPHIL COUNT

Although blood is merely the vehicle for transporting neutrophils from the bone marrow to the extravascular tissues, the blood neutrophil count remains the physician's most convenient measure of the status of the neutrophil defense system. Abnormalities of the neutrophil count are caused by alterations in the rate of effective marrow production, shifts from the marrow reserve into the circulation, or changes in the distribution or survival of blood neutrophils.

NEUTROPENIA

Classification

Neutropenia, defined as a blood neutrophil count less than 1.5 $\times$ 10^9/L, is important not only as an indicator of underlying abnormality but also because of its association, if severe (<0.5 $\times$ 10^9/L), with an increased incidence of bacterial or fungal infection. Neutropenia occurs in a variety of infectious, inflammatory, nutritional, malignant, and hematologic diseases and as a consequence of many chemotherapeutic agents. In most of these disorders, neutropenia is accompanied by marked degrees of anemia or thrombocytopenia. The following discussion focuses on selective neutropenia—conditions in which neutropenia is the dominant hematologic abnormality (Table 19.1).

By far the most common cause of isolated neutropenia is drug related. Cytotoxic drugs used to manage malignant disease or for immunosuppression regularly cause neutropenia and if given in large enough doses do so in all patients. Neutropenia also can result from an idiosyncratic reaction to a drug that in most patients does not cause neutropenia. In severe cases, the onset is sudden, and patients have a high fever, malaise, and perhaps evidence of localized infection. Blood neutrophils are few or absent; bone marrow examination reveals depletion of mature neutrophils and, in severe cases, absence of all myeloid cells. Many drugs have been reported responsible for these reactions (41), and probably any drug can be. These idiosyncratic drug reactions are thought to occur by one of two mechanisms. The first is dose-related toxicity to the developing myeloid cells in the marrow. Prototype drugs for this type of reaction include antithyroid drugs and phenothiazines. The second is an immunologic reaction, the patient having developed an antibody to the drug or a drug metabolite. The two mechanisms cannot be differentiated on the basis of the original clinical manifestations. However, if the patient is later rechallenged with the offending drug (not recommended), the syndrome rapidly recurs if the mechanism is immunologic. If the mechanism is toxic, the syndrome recurs only after enough drug has been administered to reproduce the effect.

TABLE 19.1. SELECTIVE NEUTROPENIA

Cause	Disorder
Drug effect	Cytotoxic
	Idiosyncratic
Decreased marrow production	
Congenital	Reticular dysgenesis
	Kostmann syndrome
	Schwachman-diamond syndrome
	Chediak-Higashi syndrome
	Myelokathexis
	Type 1b glycogen storage disease
	Cyclic neutropenia
Chronic idiopathic neutropenia	Various congenital and acquired disorders
Acquired	Nutritional deficiencies
	Pure white blood cell aplasia
	Neonates of hypertensive mothers
Increased utilization or turnover	
Alloimmune	Isoimmune neonatal neutropenia
Autoimmune	Idiopathic
	Systemic lupus erythematosis
	Rheumatoid arthritis
	Sjögren syndrome
Increased margination	Infection, inflammation
	Splenomegaly

Congenital neutropenia is a diverse collection of syndromes characterized by decreased neutrophil production in the bone marrow (41). Reticular dysgenesis is a neonatal disorder characterized by thymic aplasia and lack of lymphoid or myeloid development (42). Patients are prone to serious bacterial and viral infection, and death occurs in early infancy. Kostmann syndrome is an autosomal recessive disorder that manifests as severe neutropenia in the neonatal period (43). Examination of the marrow reveals a paucity of cells beyond the promyelocyte stage, and patients have repeated episodes of infection. Before G-CSF treatment became available, most patients did not survive to adulthood. Schwachman-Diamond syndrome is an autosomal recessive disorder characterized by short stature, pancreatic exocrine deficiency, and moderate neutropenia (44). Patients with Chediak-Higashi syndrome have cutaneous and ocular hypopigmentation, the presence of large abnormal granules in all granule-containing cells, frequent pyogenic infections, and the occurrence of a late lymphoma-like accelerated phase. Neutropenia usually is mild, and the neutrophils are dysfunctional (45). Myelokathexis is a disorder in which severe neutropenia is accompanied by hypersegmentation and degenerative changes in the neutrophils. The marrow neutrophil compartment is hypercellular. The underlying pathologic process appears to be accelerated neutrophil apoptosis with defective expression of the antiapoptotic *bcl*-x protooncogene (46). Severe neutropenia and neutrophil dysfunction frequently accompany type 1b glycogen storage disease, for unclear mechanistic reasons (47). Cyclic neutropenia is an autosomal dominant or sporadically occurring disorder characterized by regular oscillations of leukocytes, platelets, and reticulocytes with predictable severe neutropenia that occurs every 21 days (48). Studies have shown that both Kostmann syndrome and cyclic neutropenia appear to be attributable to mutations in the neutrophil elastase gene (49), the likely mechanism being alteration of the rate of neutrophil apoptosis.

Chronic idiopathic neutropenia may be congenital or acquired and is characterized by absence of other hematologic findings, splenomegaly, or chromosomal abnormalities (50). The bone marrow appears normal except for reduced mature neutrophils in certain patients. Clinical problems with infection tend to be more severe in patients with the lowest neutrophil counts and the fewest neutrophil precursors in the marrow. Susceptibility to infection is best judged, however, by the patient's previous experience, however, because some patients with very low counts have little clinical difficulty. Progression to malignant growth or more serious hematologic disease is unusual.

Isolated neutropenia can occur with deficiencies of folic acid, vitamin B_{12}, or copper, although these disorders are more often accompanied by other hematologic abnormalities. Pure white blood cell aplasia is a rare disorder characterized by absence of myeloid cells in the marrow. It is attributed to autoimmune suppression of neutrophil production (51). Moderate neutropenia is frequent in neonates born to hypertensive mothers (52). It is apparently attributable to transient suppression of neutrophil production and may persist for as long as 1 month.

Immune neutropenia and some types of neutropenia associated with splenomegaly are probably kinetically attributable to increased neutrophil turnover. Alloimmune neutropenia is a well-described but uncommon disorder caused by the transplacental transfer of maternal antibody to neonatal neutrophil antigens—the neutrophil equivalent of hemolytic disease of the newborn. The clinical course usually is benign. The disorder is transient and resolves after maternal antibody is metabolized. Autoimmune neutropenia is a poorly characterized syndrome, usually defined by the ability to detect an antibody directed toward a neutrophil antigen. In most cases, the clinical features are similar to those of chronic idiopathic neutropenia (53). Neutropenia is an occasional feature of immune-mediated diseases such as systemic lupus erythematosus, rheumatoid arthritis, and Sjögren syndrome (54,55).

Increased margination can occur in patients with splenomegaly or inflammation (15,56–58), and mild neutropenia may result. Whether the increased margination that occurs with inflammation is a generalized phenomenon or occurs only in the small vessels in the area of inflammation is not known.

Mild to moderate neutropenia can occur in association with a variety of bacterial, viral, parasitic, or rickettsial infections. The mechanisms are poorly understood but probably involve a combination of marrow suppression, increased adherence to endothelial cells, increased utilization, and splenic sequestration. In the face of overwhelming sepsis, neutropenia may be severe, reflecting increased utilization and exhaustion of the marrow reserves.

Management of Neutropenia

The principal complication of moderate to severe neutropenia is increased risk of infection. Patients with neutropenia and a fever should be carefully evaluated to identify infection and should be treated initially with broad-spectrum antibiotic therapy. Once an offending organism is identified, the antibiotic regimen can be adjusted accordingly. The use of prophylactic antibiotics is associated with complications such as the emergence of resistant organisms, gastrointestinal disorders, and allergic reactions. Nevertheless, use of these agents is common in the care of many patients with chronic neutropenia and frequent infections. Antibiotic therapy is not justified for patients who do not have difficulty with infection, even if neutropenia is severe.

With the availability of G-CSF over the last decade, it has been possible to increase neutrophil production in many patients with neutropenia to the point that the blood neutrophil count increases and problems with infection are greatly reduced or eliminated. A series of randomized trials first showed that G-CSF therapy was efficacious in shortening the duration of neutropenia and in reducing fever and infection in patients with neutropenia due to intensive chemotherapy or hematopoietic stem cell transplantation (59–61). In these studies, G-CSF, usually 5 to 10 μg/kg a day, was generally initiated approximately 24 hours after the completion of cytotoxic therapy.

Granulocyte colony-stimulating factor is useful in the management of severe chronic neutropenia. The largest body of information is available for patients with severe congenital neutropenia (Kostmann syndrome), cyclic neutropenia, and idiopathic neutropenia. Dale et al. (62) reported on a randomized, controlled trial of daily G-CSF treatment of 123 patients with recurrent infections and severe chronic neutropenia (absolute neutrophil count $<0.5 \times 10^9$/L). Patients were randomized to G-CSF treatment or 4 months of observation. Those in the observation arm were subsequently treated with G-CSF. Ninety-three percent of patients responded. With therapy, the mean blood neutrophil count was 1.5×10^9/L. Marrow examination revealed an increased proportion of mature neutrophils. The incidence and duration of infectious episodes decreased 50%, and the duration of antibiotic use decreased 70%. Subsequent studies have shown that these effects are sustained with long-term G-CSF therapy. Granulocyte colony-stimulating factor also has been shown effective in the management of neutropenia in neonates of hypertensive mothers (63) and patients with myelokathexis (64), Felty syndrome (65), autoimmune neutropenia (66), and glycogen storage disease type 1b (67). It is not effective in the care of patients with reticular dysgenesis, presumably because myeloid progenitors are not present in sufficient numbers (68). Myelodysplasia and acute leukemia have been observed to occur in approximately 9% of patients with Kostmann syndrome who are treated with G-CSF . This phenomenon, which is associated with additional acquired clonal abnormalities, has not been observed in patients with other disorders who are treated with G-CSF.

Patients with febrile neutropenia may benefit from G-CSF therapy. In a randomized, controlled study, investigators compared G-CSF–antibiotic therapy with antibiotic treatment alone and found that patients receiving G-CSF had shorter duration of neutropenia and fever and less likelihood of prolonged hospitalization (69). The greatest benefit appeared to be for patients with documented infection and severe neutropenia ($<0.1 \times 10^9$/L).

Case reports and results of small series suggest that patients with neutropenia secondary to idiosyncratic drug reactions may benefit from G-CSF therapy (70,71). In general, there seems to be less benefit if neutrophil precursors are absent from the marrow, but examples exist in which rapid return of the neutrophil count occurs even under these circumstances.

NEUTROPHILIA

Neutrophilia is generally defined as a blood neutrophil count in excess of 7.5×10^9/L and can be either acute or chronic (Table 19.2). Unlike the case with neutropenia, an elevated level of mature blood neutrophils usually has no clinical implications in itself; rather, it serves to alert the clinician to underlying events.

A shift of cells from the marginal pool to the circulating pool, resulting in neutrophilia, can occur as an effect of epinephrine, in situations of acute stress, or with vigorous exercise. The effect is rapid, usually within minutes, and is short lived, the neutrophil count rapidly returning to baseline when the stimulus is removed. Because the source of additional cells in the circulatory pool is the marginal pool, the neutrophil count usually is no more than double, and immature neutrophils are not present.

Acute neutrophilia can occur with mobilization of the marrow neutrophil reserves, most commonly as a result of infection or inflammation. The extent of the storage pool shift under these conditions depends on the intensity of the stimulus and is reflected in the magnitude of the neutrophilia and in the degree to which immature forms are present in the blood. The more intense the stimulus (e.g., the more severe the infection), the higher is the neutrophil count and the greater is the fraction of immature cells.

Chronic neutrophilia most commonly represents the normal reaction of the marrow to infection or inflammation. The marrow proliferative pool expands and increases marrow neutrophil production as much as severalfold over baseline. Chronic neutrophilia also is a feature of the myeloproliferative diseases, in which marrow neutrophil production is autonomous (72). These disorders usually can be differentiated from the more common benign reactive neutrophilia by the presence of additional features such as erythrocytosis, thrombocytosis, eosinophilia, basophilia, a more pronounced shift to the left, splenomegaly, a low leukocyte alkaline phosphatase level (in chronic myelocytic leukemia), chromosomal abnormalities, or the presence of the BCR gene rearrangement.

Chronic neutrophilia can be attributable to reduced migration of neutrophils from the blood to the tissues. This mechanism is responsible for the mild to moderate neutrophilia that occurs with long-term glucocorticoid therapy (73,74). It also is the principal cause of the marked neutrophilia that occurs in patients with leukocyte adhesion (CD11/18) deficiency.

Patients with reactive leukocytosis occasionally come to medical attention with a leukocyte profile indistinguishable from that of leukemia—so-called leukemoid reactions. Usually there is marked leukocytosis ($>50 \times 10^9$ cells/L) with immature forms. The confusion is with the myeloproliferative syndromes (most commonly chronic myelocytic leukemia), although acute leukemia may be simulated. The absence of the characteristics of the myeloproliferative disorders (e.g., basophilia, chromosomal

TABLE 19.2. MECHANISMS AND CAUSES OF NEUTROPHILIA

Mechanism	Causes of Acute Neutrophilia	Causes of Chronic Neutrophilia
Decreased margination	Stress Hypoxia Intoxication Exercise Epinephrine	
Mobilization from marrow	Infection Inflammation Stress Hypoxia Intoxication Prolonged exercise G-CSF Glucocorticoids	
Prolonged survival	Glucocorticoids G-CSF	Myeloproliferative disorders Glucocorticoids Leukocyte adhesion Deficiency
Increased marrow proliferation	Rebound from neutropenia	Infection Inflammation Myeloproliferative disorders

G-CSF, granulocyte colony-stimulating factor.

markers) often is helpful in the differential diagnosis. However, the diagnosis of a leukemoid reaction can be considered certain only if the leukocyte profile returns to normal when the underlying infectious or inflammatory disorder resolves.

REFERENCES

1. Babior BM, Golde DW. Production, distribution, and fate of neutrophils. In: Beutler E, Lichtman MA, Coller BS, et al., eds. *Williams hematology,* 6th ed. New York: McGraw-Hill, 2001:753–759.
2. Warner HR, Athens JW. An analysis of granulocyte kinetics in blood and bone marrow. *Ann New York Acad Sci* 1964;113:523–536.
3. Berliner N. Molecular biology of neutrophil differentiation. *Curr Opin Hematol* 1998;5:49–53.
4. Dancey JT, Deubelbeiss KA, Harker LA, et al. Neutrophil kinetics in man. *J Clin Invest* 1976;58:705–715.
5. Craddock CG Jr, Perry S, Lawrence JS. The dynamics of leukopoiesis and leukocytosis, as studied by leukopheresis and isotopic techniques. *J Clin Invest* 1956;35:285–296.
6. Craddock CG Jr, Perry S, Ventzke LE, et al. Evaluation of marrow granulocytic reserves in normal and disease states. *Blood* 1960;15: 840–855.
7. Vogel JM, Kimball HR, Wolff SM, et al. Etiocholanolone in the evaluation of marrow reserves in patients receiving cytotoxic agents. *Ann Intern Med* 1967;67:1226–1238.
8. Chatta GS, Price TH, Allen RC, et al. Effects of in vivo recombinant methionyl human granulocyte colony-stimulating factor on the neutrophil response and peripheral blood colony-forming cells in healthy young and elderly adult volunteers. *Blood* 1994;84:2923–2929.
9. Athens JW, Haab OP, Raab SO, et al. Leukokinetic studies, IV: the total blood, circulating and marginal granulocyte pools and the granulocyte turnover rate in normal subjects. *J Clin Invest* 1961;40:989–995.
10. Athens JW, Haab OP, Raab SO, et al. Leukokinetic studies, III: the distribution of granulocytes in the blood of normal subjects. *J Clin Invest* 1961;40:159–164.
11. Atherton A, Born GVR. Quantitative investigations of the adhesiveness of circulating polymorphonuclear leucocytes to blood vessel walls. *J Physiol (Lond)* 1972;222:447–474.
12. Mayrovitz HN, Wiedman MP, Tuma RF. Factors influencing leukocyte adherence in microvessels. *Thromb Haemost* 1977;38:823–830.
13. Ambrus CM, Ambrus JL, Johnson GC, et al. Role of lungs in regulation of the white blood cell level. *Am J Physiol* 1954;178:33–44.
14. Martin BA, Wright JL, Thommasen H, et al. Effect of pulmonary blood flow on the exchange between the circulating and marginating pool of polymorphonuclear leukocytes in dog lungs. *J Clin Invest* 1982; 69:1277–1285.
15. Rohrer C, Arni U, Deubelbeiss KA. Influence of the spleen on the distribution of blood neutrophils: quantitative studies in the rat. *Scand J Haematol* 1983;30:103–109.
16. Peters AM, Saverymuttu SH, Bell RN, et al. Quantification of the distribution of the marginating granulocyte pool in man. *Scand J Haematol* 1985;34:111–120.
17. Hogg JC. Neutrophil kinetics and lung injury. *Physiol Rev* 1987;67: 1249–1295.
18. Witko-Sarsat V, Rieu P, Descamps-Latscha B, et al. Neutrophils: molecules, functions and pathophysiological aspects. *Lab Invest* 2000;80: 617–653.
19. Wagner JG, Roth RA. Neutrophil migration mechanisms, with an emphasis on the pulmonary vasculature. *Pharmacol Rev* 2000;52: 349–374.
20. Carlos TM, Harlan JM. Leukocyte-endothelial adhesion molecules. *Blood* 1994;84:2068–2101.
21. Mayadas TN, Johnson RC, Rayburn H, et al. Leukocyte rolling and extravasation are severly compromised in P selectin–deficient mice. *Cell* 1993;74:541–554.
22. Doré, M, Korthuis RJ, Granger DN, et al. P-selectin mediates spontaneous leukocyte rolling in vivo. *Blood* 1993;82:1308–1316.
23. Ley K, Gaehtgens P, Fennie C, et al. Lectin-like cell adhesion molecular 1 mediates leukocyte rolling in mesenteric venules in vivo. *Blood* 1991; 77:2553–2555.
24. Harlan JM, Killen PD, Senecal FM, et al. The role of neutrophil membrane glycoprotein GP-150 in neutrophil adherence to endothelium in vitro. *Blood* 1985;66:167–178.
25. Price TH, Beatty PG, Corpuz SR. In vivo inhibition of neutrophil function in the rabbit using monoclonal antibody to CD18. *J Immunol* 1987;139:4174–4177.
26. Anderson DC, Springer TA. Leukocyte adhesion deficiency: an inherited defect in the Lac-1, LFA-1, and p150,95 glycoproteins. *Annu Rev Med* 1987;38:175–194.
27. Bowen TJ, Ochs HD, Altman LC, et al. Severe recurrent bacterial infections associated with defective adherence and chemotaxis in two patients with neutrophils deficient in a cell-associated glycoprotein. *J Pediatr* 1982;101:932–940.
28. Etzioni A, Frydman M, Pollack S, et al. Brief report: recurrent severe infections caused by a novel leukocyte adhesion deficiency. *N Engl J Med* 1992;327:1789–1792.
29. Price TH, Ochs HD, Gershoni-Baruch R, et al. In vivo neutrophil and lymphocyte function studies in a patient with leukocyte adhesion deficiency type II. *Blood* 1994;84:1635–1639.
30. Downey GP, Doherty DE, Schwab B, et al. Retention of leukocytes in capillaries: role of cell size and deformability. *J Appl Physiol* 1990; 69:1767–1778.
31. Doyle NA, Bhagwan SD, Meek BB, et al. Neutrophil margination, sequestration, and emigration in the lungs of L-selectin–deficient mice. *J Clin Invest* 1997;99:526–533.
32. Mizgerd JP, Kubo H, Kutkoski GJ, et al. Neutrophil emigration in the skin, lungs, and peritoneum: different requirements for CD11/ CD18 revealed by CD18-deficient mice. *J Exp Med* 1997;186: 1357–1364.
33. Mizgerd JP, Horwitz BH, Quillen HC, et al. Effects of CD18 deficiency on the emigration of murine neutrophils during pneumonia. *J Immunol* 1999;163:995–999.
34. Cohen DM, Bhalla SC, Anaissie EJ, et al. Effects of in vitro and in vivo cytokine treatment, leucapheresis and irradiation on the function of human neutrophils: implications for white blood cell transfusion therapy. *Clin Lab Haematol* 1997;19:39–47.
35. Price TH, Chatta GS, Dale DC. Effect of recombinant granulocyte colony-stimulating factor on neutrophil kinetics in normal young and elderly humans. *Blood* 1996;88:335–340.
36. Whyte M, Renshaw S, Lawson R, et al. Apoptosis and the regulation of neutrophil lifespan. *Biochem Soc Trans* 1999;27:802–807.
37. Lieschke GJ, Grail D, Hodgson G, et al. Mice lacking granulocyte colony-stimulating factor have chronic neutropenia, granulocyte and macrophage progenitor cell deficiency, and impaired neutrophil mobilization. *Blood* 1994;84:1737–1746.
38. Liu F, Wu HY, Wesselshmidt R, et al. Impaired production and increased apoptosis of neutrophils in granulocyte colony-stimulating factor receptor–deficient mice. *Immunity* 1996;5:491–501.
39. Hammond WP, Csiba E, Canin A, et al. Chronic neutropenia: a new canine model induced by human granulocyte colony-stimulating factor. *J Clin Invest* 1991;87:704–710.
40. Anderlini P, Przepiorka D, Champlin R, et al. Biologic and clinical effects of granulocyte colony-stimulating factor in normal individuals. *Blood* 1996;88:2819–2825.
41. Dale DC. Neutropenia and neutrophilia. In: Beutler E, Lichtman MA, Coller BS, et al., eds. *Williams hematology,* 6th ed. New York: McGraw-Hill, 2001:823–834.
42. Roper M, Parmley RT, Crist WM, et al. Severe congenital leukopenia (reticular dysgenesis): immunologic and morphologic characterizations of leukocytes. *Am J Dis Child* 1985;139:832–835.
43. Kostmann R. Infantile genetic agranulocytosis: a review with presentation of ten new cases. *Acta Paediatr Scand* 1975;64:362–368.
44. Aggett PJ, Cavanagh NP, Matthew DJ, et al. Shwachman's syndrome: a review of 21 cases. *Arch Dis Child* 1980;55:331–347.
45. Blume RS, Wolff SM. The Chediak-Higashi syndrome: studies in four patients and a review of the literature. *Medicine (Baltimore)* 1972;51: 247–280.
46. Aprikyan AA, Liles WC, Park JR, et al. Myelokathexis, a congenital

disorder of severe neutropenia characterized by accelerated apoptosis and defective expression of bcl-x in neutrophil precursors. *Blood* 2000; 95:320–327.

47. Calderwood S, Kilpatrick L, Douglas SD, et al. Recombinant human granulocyte colony-stimulating factor therapy for patients with neutropenia and/or neutrophil dysfunction secondary to glycogen storage disease type 1b. *Blood* 2001;97:376–382.
48. Dale DC, Hammond WP. Cyclic neutropenia: a clinical review. *Blood Rev* 1988;2:178–185.
49. Dale DC, Person RE, Bolyard AA, et al. Mutations in the gene encoding neutrophil elastase in congenital and cyclic neutropenia. *Blood* 2000;96:2317–2322.
50. Dale DC, Guerry D, Wewerka JR, et al. Chronic neutropenia. *Medicine (Baltimore)* 1979;58:128–144.
51. Marinone G, Roncoli B, Marinone MG. Pure white cell aplasia. *Semin Hematol* 1991;28:298–302.
52. Koenig JM, Christensen RD. Incidence, neutrophil kinetics, and natural history of neonatal neutropenia associated with maternal hypertension. *N Engl J Med* 1989;321:557–562.
53. Shastri KA, Logue GL. Autoimmune neutropenia. *Blood* 1993;81: 1984–1995.
54. Starkebaum G, Price TH, Lee MY, et al. Autoimmune neutropenia in systemic lupus erythematosus. *Arthritis Rheum* 1978;21:504–512.
55. Starkebaum G, Martin PJ, Singer JW, et al. Chronic lymphocytosis with neutropenia: evidence for a novel, abnormal T-cell population associated with antibody-mediated neutrophil destruction. *Clin Immunol Immunopathol* 1983;27:110–123.
56. Boggs DR, Athens JW, Cartwright GE, et al. "Masked" granulocytosis. *Proc Soc Exp Biol Med* 1965;118:753–755.
57. Uchida T, Kariyone S. Intravascular granulocyte kinetics and spleen size in patients with neutropenia and chronic splenomegaly. *J Lab Clin Med* 1973;82:9–19.
58. Brubaker LH, Johnson CA. Correlation of splenomegaly and abnormal neutrophil pooling (margination). *J Lab Clin Med* 1978;92:508–515.
59. Crawford J, Ozer H, Stoller R, et al. Reduction by granulocyte colony-stimulating factor of fever and neutropenia induced by chemotherapy in patients with small-cell lung cancer. *N Engl J Med* 1991;325: 164–170.
60. Gabrilove JL, Jakubowski A, Scher H, et al. Effect of granulocyte colony-stimulating factor on neutropenia and associated morbidity due to chemotherapy for transitional-cell carcinoma of the urothelium. *N Engl J Med* 1988;318:1414–1422.
61. American Society of Clinical Oncology. American Society of Clinical Oncology recommendations for the use of hematopoietic colony-stimulating factors: evidence-based, clinical practice guidelines. *J Clin Oncol* 1994;12:2471–2508.
62. Dale DC, Bonilla MA, Davis MW, et al. A randomized controlled phase III trial of recombinant human granulocyte colony-stimulating factor (filgrastim) for treatment of severe chronic neutropenia. *Blood* 1993;81:2496–2502.
63. Kocherlakota P, La Gamma EF. Preliminary report: rhG-CSF may reduce the incidence of neonatal sepsis in prolonged preeclampsia-associated neutropenia. *Pediatrics* 1998;102:1107–1111.
64. Weston B, Axtell RA, Todd RF III, et al. Clinical and biologic effects of granulocyte colony stimulating factor in the treatment of myelokathexis. *J Pediatr* 1991;118:229–234.
65. Wandt H, Seifert M, Falge C, et al. Long-term correction of neutropenia in Felty's syndrome with granulocyte colony-stimulating factor. *Ann Hematol* 1993;66:265–266.
66. Imoto S, Hashimoto M, Miyamoto M, et al. Response to granulocyte colony-stimulating factor in an autoimmune neutropenic adult. *Acta Haematol* 1999;101:153–156.
67. Bujan W, Ferster A, Azzi N, et al. Use of recombinant human granulocyte colony stimulating factor in reticular dysgenesis. *Br J Haematol* 1992;81:128–130.
68. Freedman MH, Bonilla MA, Fier C, et al. Myelodysplasia syndrome and acute myeloid leukemia in patients with congenital neutropenia receiving G-CSF therapy. *Blood* 2000;96:429–436.
69. Maher DW, Lieschke GJ, Green M, et al. Filgrastim in patients with chemotherapy-induced febrile neutropenia: a double-blind, placebo-controlled trial. *Ann Intern Med* 1994;121:492–501.
70. Tajiri J, Noguchi S, Okamura S, et al. Granulocyte colony-stimulating factor treatment of antithyroid drug-induced granulocytopenia. *Arch Intern Med* 1993;153:509–514.
71. Willfort A, Lorber C, Kapiotis S, et al. Treatment of drug-induced agranulocytosis with recombinant granulocyte colony-stimulating factor (rh G-CSF). *Ann Hematol* 1993;66:241–244.
72. Athens JW, Haab OP, Raab SO, et al. Leukokinetic studies. XI. Blood granulocyte kinetics in polycythemia vera, infection, and myelofibrosis. *J Clin Invest* 1965;40:778–788.
73. Bishop CR, Athens JW, Boggs DR, et al. Leukokinetic studies: a non-steady-state kinetic evaluation of the mechanism of cortisone-induced granulocytosis. *J Clin Invest* 1968;47:249–260.
74. Dale DC, Fauci AS, Wolff SM. Alternate-day prednisone: leukocyte kinetics and susceptibility to infections. *N Engl J Med* 1974;291: 1154–1158.

Rossi's Principles of Transfusion Medicine, Third Edition, edited by Toby L. Simon, Walter H. Dzik, Edward L. Snyder, Christopher P. Stowell, and Ronald G. Strauss. Lippincott Williams & Wilkins, Philadelphia © 2002.

20

NEUTROPHIL COLLECTION AND TRANSFUSION

RONALD G. STRAUSS

Life-threatening infections with bacteria, yeast, and fungus continue to be a consequence of severe neutropenia ($<0.5 \times 10^9$/L blood neutrophils) and disorders of neutrophil dysfunction. The most frequent situation is neutropenic fever and infection with yeast or fungus following either intense chemotherapy for hematologic malignant disease or preparative therapy for hematopoietic progenitor cell transplantation. Neutropenic infections cause considerable morbidity, occasionally are fatal, and add considerable cost to the treatment of these patients.

Previous attempts to prevent infection in severely neutropenic patients by transfusing neutrophil concentrates—commonly called prophylactic granulocyte transfusion (GTX)—achieved only questionable success. Although rates of certain infections were significantly reduced with prophylactic GTX, many adverse effects such as the occurrence of pulmonary infiltrates and cytomegalovirus infection were reported, and GTX was expensive. Similarly, use of therapeutic GTX to resolve existing infections has not gained broad acceptance, despite many reports documenting benefit (1). This lack of enthusiasm for GTX can be explained by the continuing development of effective antimicrobial drugs to prevent and manage infection, by the availability of recombinant hematopoietic growth factors and peripheral blood hematopoietic progenitor cell (PBHPC) transfusions to hasten patient recovery from myelotoxic therapy and shorten the period of risk of neutropenic infection, and by the lack of familiarity of some oncology and transplant physicians with the markedly improved neutrophil concentrates available for transfusion.

Historically, neutrophil concentrates collected for transfusion from unstimulated donors or those stimulated only with glucocorticoids contained woefully inadequate numbers of neutrophils. Currently, very large numbers of neutrophils can be collected from healthy donors by means of granulocyte-colony stimulating factor (G-CSF) plus glucocorticoid marrow stimulation followed by large-volume leukapheresis (2). This chapter discusses the current technology of neutrophil collection and provides a critical assessment of the potential for use of therapeutic and prophylactic GTX.

R.G. Strauss: Departments of Pathology and Pediatrics, University of Iowa College of Medicine, UI Degowin Blood Center, University of Iowa Hospitals and Clinics, Iowa City, Iowa.

COLLECTION OF NEUTROPHILS FOR TRANSFUSION

Donor Marrow Stimulation

A limitation of GTX has been the inability to transfuse satisfactory numbers of adequately functioning neutrophils. To ensure an adequate GTX dose, neutrophil concentrates must be collected from stimulated donors by means of leukapheresis with an erythrocyte-sedimenting agent (3). The bloodstream of an average-sized adult contains 2 to 4×10^{10} neutrophils. Under steady-state conditions, approximately 6×10^{10} neutrophils are produced daily by the marrow. With the stress of a severe bacterial infection, the marrow of a healthy adult produces between 10^{11} and 10^{12} neutrophils daily. Granulocyte concentrates collected from healthy donors whose marrow has not been stimulated with glucocorticoids or G-CSF contains between 0.2 and 0.8×10^{10} neutrophils, approximately 1% of the normal output of healthy marrow stressed by infection. Because donor neutrophils are collected with approximately 50% efficiency with modern centrifugation blood separators, it is unlikely that leukapheresis technology per se can be improved sufficiently to markedly increase neutrophil yields (even if improved to 100% collection efficiency, the neutrophil yield would only double). Hence donor marrow stimulation is mandatory to achieve even the hope of a reasonable neutrophil dose for each GTX.

Donor marrow stimulation with properly timed administration of glucocorticoids (4 hours before leukapheresis) produces granulocyte concentrates containing, at best, approximately 2×10^{10} neutrophils (4). Stimulation with G-CSF alone or in combination with glucocorticoids produces higher neutrophil yields but varies depending on the G-CSF dose and schedule of administration. Granulocyte concentrates with yields of 4 to 8×10^{10} neutrophils are achieved regularly. After transfusion, blood neutrophil counts in recipients often increase to more than 2×10^9/L, transfused neutrophils persisting in the bloodstream for more than 24 hours after GTX (5–7). For optimal donor stimulation, G-CSF is given subcutaneously at a dose of 300 to 600 μg. The glucocorticoid given orally is dexamethasone (8 to 12 mg) or prednisone (60 mg) usually approximately 12 hours before leukapheresis is begun. Although they experience minor pain in muscle, bone, or the head that is readily relieved with acetaminophen or ibuprofen, most donors given G-CSF have no long-term effects, and it is unusual that they refuse to donate again (7).

Although they are known to alter neutrophil function, G-CSF and glucocorticoids have relatively minor effects at the doses administered to donors for neutrophil collection (8). The functional properties of neutrophils collected from donors stimulated with G-CSF do not deviate greatly from those of normal neutrophils and cause no unusual reactions in recipients when transfused. After transfusion, neutrophils from G-CSF–stimulated donors have long intravascular survival times (5,9). The long survival time can be explained by multiple factors, including the shift of young neutrophils from the storage compartment of donor marrow into the bloodstream for collection, an alteration in expression of several membrane proteins on donor neutrophils associated with neutrophil adherence to vascular endothelium and egress from the circulation into the tissues, and possibly by specific antiapoptotic effects of G-CSF on neutrophils (8). Although it has been suggested that G-CSF–mobilized neutrophils may exhibit decreased migration into tissue sites because of their prolonged intravascular circulation, studies with transfused neutrophils indicate that they migrate satisfactorily into areas of inflammation and infection (7,9).

The ability to collect and store neutrophils may differ when donors are stimulated only once during a course of GTX therapy compared with when they are stimulated repeatedly on a daily basis for GTX. Neutrophils collected after several days of G-CSF stimulation are qualitatively different than neutrophils collected after a single dose of G-CSF (8). They are younger, exhibit increased metabolic activity and different surface markers, may possess enhanced antifungal properties, and may not have the same separation characteristics during centrifugation leukapheresis. Because the functional properties and possibly the efficacy and toxicity of neutrophils may differ when collected under conditions of single versus repeated G-CSF and glucocorticoid stimulation, additional studies are needed to define optimal donor stimulation and GTX therapy. Similarly, the presumed greater efficacy of granulocytes collected from donors stimulated with G-CSF and a glucocorticoid compared with granulocytes collected from donors stimulated only with glucocorticoids or with patients not given GTX at all but treated directly with recombinant growth factors and antibiotics has not been established with randomized, clinical trials.

Hydroxyethyl Starch

Use of an erythrocyte-sedimenting agent, such as hydroxyethyl starch or dextran, during centrifugation leukapheresis is mandatory. Although in the United States hydroxyethyl starch almost always has been used, the optimal type of hydroxyethyl starch for neutrophil collection is controversial. In an uncontrolled multicenter trial, pentastarch appeared to be an efficacious and safe erythrocyte-sedimenting agent for use during centrifugation leukapheresis (4). Its efficacy seemed established because neutrophil concentrates, prepared by means of a variety of centrifugation leukapheresis techniques with pentastarch in four cytapheresis centers, were found to contain quantities of neutrophils comparable with concentrates prepared previously with hetastarch at participating centers. Most granulocyte concentrates contained at least 2×10^{10} neutrophils, if collected with a continuous flow device (8 L of donor blood processed) from donors properly stimulated with glucocorticoids (4).

In 1995, the efficacy of pentastarch for neutrophil collection was challenged. In two studies (10,11), the effects of pentastarch and hetastarch on donor erythrocyte sedimentation rates were compared, and pentastarch exerted lesser effects than did hetastarch. Pentastarch consequently was predicted with a granulocyte collection efficiency equation to be less effective than hetastarch in enhancing neutrophil yields. This prediction was supported later in a controlled clinical trial (12) in which steroid-stimulated donors underwent paired neutrophil collections, separated by 2 weeks to 7 months, during which they received 500 ml of either 10% pentastarch or 6% hetastarch during centrifugation leukapheresis (7 L donor blood processed at a 1:13 starch to donor blood ratio). In 92% of the donors, hetastarch procedures were more efficient. The neutrophil yield was $2.3 \pm 0.7 \times 10^{10}$ with hetastarch versus $1.4 \pm 0.076 \times 10^{10}$ with pentastarch (12).

It is unclear why pentastarch performed so poorly in the later studies (10–12) compared with its performance in the initial multicenter trial (4). The pentastarch solutions used in all studies (4,10–12) appeared to have similar biochemical properties, but whether they were identical cannot be established because information about the C2/C6 hydroxyethylation ratio—a property that can influence erythrocyte sedimentation rates independently of molecular weight and overall degree of hydroxyethylation (13)—was not given in any report. Thus the possibility cannot be excluded that pentastarch solutions with different properties were studied by the different groups despite having identical molecular weights and overall degrees of hydroxyethylation. As another factor, the efficacy of different hydroxyethyl starch solutions may differ depending on the type of cell separator technology used for centrifugation leukapheresis.

Until the issue is resolved, it is prudent for each center preparing neutrophil concentrates to perform continuing quality assessment of its own leukapheresis program. The average neutrophil yield obtained by means of processing 10 L of donor blood after glucocorticoid stimulation alone and use of pentastarch at a 1: 13 starch to donor blood ratio should be between 1.5 and 2.5 $\times 10^{10}$. After G-CSF stimulation with or without a glucocorticoid, the neutrophil yield should be between 4 and 8 $\times 10^{10}$. If this is achieved, it seems reasonable to continue using pentastarch, particularly if donors experience repeated leukapheresis at short intervals. Pentastarch is more rapidly eliminated from the bloodstream than is hetastarch and avoids the problem with repeated leukapheresis in which hetastarch blood levels accumulate and increase in a stairstep manner. Pentastarch exerts lesser effects on coagulation than does hetastarch (14). If neutrophil yields are not satisfactory with pentastarch, leukapheresis methods should be reviewed and pentastarch possibly replaced by hetastarch.

NEUTROPHIL TRANSFUSION IN CLINICAL MEDICINE

Historical Overview of Therapeutic Granulocyte Transfusion

Thirty-four reports (15) of GTX from unstimulated donors or donors stimulated only with glucocorticoids and used to treat patients with infection and severe neutropenia ($<0.5 \times 10^9$/L blood neutrophils) are summarized here. Patients were entered into Table 20.1 according to the index infection that prompted GTX. Each patient was counted only once (e.g., patients with bacterial septicemia were listed only in the septicemia section, even if they had another infection such as pneumonia; those with pneumonia without septicemia were listed only under pneumonia). As an exception, all patients with invasive fungal and yeast infections (e.g., sepsis, pneumonia, sinusitis) were grouped into one category. All patients given GTX for a designated type of infection were entered under the treated heading of Table 20.1. Of all patients in the treated column, those for whom the actual course and mortality could be determined were entered again in the evaluable column. Treatment of the evaluable patients with GTX was deemed successful if so stated by the authors of the articles.

Several of the 34 reports described uncontrolled studies involving small numbers of patients with a diversity of underlying diseases, types of infections, antimicrobial therapies, and GTX management strategies (variable dose and quality of neutrophils), as well as varying definitions of success. To obtain more definitive information regarding efficacy, seven controlled studies (16–22) of therapeutic GTX from unstimulated donors or from donors stimulated only with glucocorticoids were analyzed in more detail (Table 20.2). In these studies, the response to treatment with antibiotics plus GTX (transfusion group) of patients with infection and neutropenia was compared with that of comparable patients given only antibiotics and evaluated concurrently (control group). Three of the studies showed a significant benefit overall for therapeutic GTX (16–18). In two additional studies (19,20), overall success of GTX was not demonstrated, but certain subgroups of patients were found to benefit considerably (amounting to partial success for GTX therapy). For example, in the first controlled study of GTX reported, many patients received an inadequate dose of neutrophils by current standards, and overall success was not demonstrated (20). However, when the transfusion group of 39 patients was subdivided, all of the patients survived if they received at least four GTXs, as did 80% of those receiving three GTXs. The survival rate was only 30% among the control subjects. In the other study in which partial success was found (19), no advantage to GTX was found when all of the patients were analyzed. However, when the subgroup of patients with persistent marrow failure was analyzed separately, after exclusion of those with marrow recovery during infection, 75% of those receiving GTX responded favorably compared with only 20% of the control subjects. Thus some measure of success of GTX was evident in five of the seven controlled studies—three overall (16–18) and two partial (19, 20). However, these results were counterbalanced by those of four studies that were negative in some respect—two overall (21,22) and two partial (19,20).

An explanation of these seemingly inconsistent results is evident on critical analysis of the adequacy of GTX support (Table 20.3). Patients in the three successful controlled trials received relatively high doses of neutrophils from donors selected to be leukocyte compatible (16–18). In contrast, the two controlled studies with negative results provided inadequate neutrophils

TABLE 20.1. INFECTIONS IN PATIENTS WITH NEUTROPENIA FROM 34 HISTORICAL REPORTS GIVEN TRANSFUSIONS OF GRANULOCYTES COLLECTED FROM UNSTIMULATED DONORS OR THOSE STIMULATED ONLY WITH GLUCOCORTICOIDS

Type of Infection	Treated	Evaluable	Success Rate
Bacterial septicemia	298	206	127/206 (62)
Sepsis organism unspecified	132	39	18/39 (46)
Pneumonia	120	11	7/11 (64)
Localized infection	143	47	39/47 (83)
Cause of fever unknown	184	85	64/85 (75)
Invasive fungus and yeast	83	77	28/77 (36)

Values in parentheses are percentages.
Reports from Strauss RG. Granulocyte transfusion therapy. In: Mintz PD, ed. *Transfusion therapy: clinical principles and practice*. Bethesda, MD: American Association of Blood Banks, 1999;81–96.

TABLE 20.2. RESULTS OF SEVEN HISTORICAL CONTROLLED STUDIES EVALUATING TREATMENT OF PATIENTS WITH NEUTROPENIA BY MEANS OF THERAPEUTIC TRANSFUSION OF GRANULOCYTES COLLECTED FROM UNSTIMULATED DONORS OR THOSE STIMULATED ONLY WITH GLUCOCORTICOIDS

		Transfusion Group		Control Group	
Investigators	**Success**	**N**	**Survival Rate (%)**	**N**	**Survival Rate (%)**
Higby et al. (16)	Yes	17	76	19	26
Vogler and Winton (17)	Yes	17	59	13	15
Herzig et al. (18)	Yes	13	75	14	36
Alavi et al. (19)	Partial	12	82	19	62
Graw et al. (20)	Partial	39	46	37	30
Winston et al. (21)	No	48	63	47	72
Fortuny et al. (22)	No	17	78	22	80

(21, 22). The dose of neutrophils transfused (0.4 to 0.5 $\times$ 10^{10}) was extremely low—approximately one-tenth the dose currently transfused (5 to 8 $\times$ 10^{10}). It is not surprising that GTX was unsuccessful when administered inadequately. Investigators in one of the two studies with negative results (21) made no provisions for the possibility of leukocyte alloimmunization and selected donors without attempting to improve leukocyte compatibility. Finally, control subjects responded so well to antibiotics alone in both of the studies with negative results (21,22) that it was impossible to demonstrate a statistically significant additional advantage to GTX.

The preceding qualitative analysis is imprecise because it combines data from studies that although controlled are not truly comparable. That is, they were not uniform in terms of patient clinical status, selection of control subjects, GTX dose, and leukocyte compatibility, for example. In 1996, data from the seven controlled GTX trials (16–22) were analyzed quantitatively by means of formal metaanalysis (23). Many of the impressions of the preceding qualitative analysis were confirmed, specifically that the dose of neutrophils transfused and the survival rates among control subjects were primarily responsible for the differing success rates of the reported controlled trials. When the survival rate among control subjects was low, subjects who underwent transfusion were found to benefit from adequate doses of neutrophils. On the basis of the results of the metaanalysis, the authors (23) concluded that patients with severe neutropenia and an infection known to carry a high mortality should be considered for GTX in an adequate dose.

Bacterial sepsis was the most common infection for which GTX was prescribed in the 34 historical studies (Table 20.1) in which therapeutic GTX from unstimulated donors or those stimulated only with glucocorticoids were used. Patients with neutropenic and bacterial sepsis responded to antibiotics alone if they experienced marrow recovery during the early days of infection. Most patients with newly diagnosed hematologic malignant disease currently undergo successful induction chemo-

TABLE 20.3. DESIGN OF SEVEN HISTORICAL CONTROLLED STUDIES EVALUATING TREATMENT OF PATIENTS WITH NEUTROPENIA BY MEANS OF THERAPEUTIC TRANSFUSION OF GRANULOCYTES COLLECTED FROM UNSTIMULATED DONORS OR THOSE STIMULATED ONLY WITH GLUCOCORTICOIDS

		Characteristics of Granulocytes Transfused				
Investigators	**Randomized**	**Collection Method**	**Dose $\times$ 10^{10}**	**Schedule**	**HLA[a]**	**WBC[a]**
Higby et al. (16)	Yes	Filtration	2.2	Daily	No	Yes
Vogler and Winton (17)	Yes	Centrifugation	2.7	Daily	Yes	Yes
Herzig et al. (18)	Yes	Filtration	1.7	Daily	No	Yes
		Centrifugation	0.4	Daily	No	Yes
Alavi et al. (19)	Yes	Filtration	5.9	Daily	No	No
Graw et al. (20)	No	Filtration	2.0	Daily	No	Yes
		Centrifugation	0.6	Daily	No	Yes
Winston et al. (21)	Yes	Centrifugation	0.5	Daily	No	No
Fortuny et al. (22)	No	Centrifugation	0.4	Daily	No	Yes

[a]Donors compatible with recipient by HLA typing (A and B loci matched, at least in part) or by leukocyte (WBC) cross-matching.

therapy and fit into this category of having relatively brief severe neutropenia without need for GTX. In contrast, patients with more prolonged severe neutropenia due to continuing marrow failure may benefit from GTX added to antibiotic therapy. Examples are patients with relatively high-risk leukemia (e.g., elderly patients or those with a relapse of leukemia and undergoing investigational chemotherapy) and recipients of hematopoietic progenitor cell grafts, particularly when progenitor cells are lymphocyte depleted or obtained from mismatched donors. For these patients, yeast and fungal infections pose serious problems.

Occasional case reports, experimental studies with animals, and experience with chronic granulomatous disease (24) support the success of GTX as treatment of some patients with yeast and fungal infections. In contrast, a large clinical study comparing GTX treatment of patients with infection after bone marrow transplantation (n = 50) with treatment without GTX (n = 37) showed no benefit of GTX (25). This retrospective study was not designed to provide definitive answers. Patients were not randomly assigned to the GTX or no transfusion groups; clinical heterogeneity was not balanced because neither the characteristics of patients nor infections being treated were distributed evenly between groups; and the dose of neutrophils transfused was known for only 15% of the GTX given and likely was quite low because suboptimal neutrophil collection techniques were used (25). Thus the efficacy of GTX therapy for yeast and fungal infections in patients with neutropenia has not been firmly established in historical reports and awaits future studies of modern GTX.

Historical Overview of Prophylactic Granulocyte Transfusion

Historical reports of 12 controlled trials (Table 20.4) indicate that prophylactic GTX from unstimulated donors or those stimulated only with glucocorticoids was of questionable value (26–37), and accordingly, this technique is not used in clinical practice. Overall benefits seemed few, whereas risks and expenses were substantial. Some measure of success was found in 7 of the 12 historical studies, generally in studies in which relatively high doses of neutrophils were transfused daily with some attempt at increasing donor-recipient leukocyte compatibility (26–32). Although the other 5 studies did not show benefit of prophylactic GTX (Table 20.4), in none of these studies with negative results was there daily transfusion of large numbers of neutrophils obtained from matched leukocyte donors (33–37). Thus in a situation somewhat analogous to that of the negative results of historical trials of therapeutic GTX, the failure of historical prophylactic GTX may be explained by inadequate neutrophil transfusions.

In 1997, data from 8 of the 12 historical controlled trials of prophylactic GTX were analyzed quantitatively by means of formal metaanalysis (38). The findings of the metaanalysis confirmed that variability in the dose of neutrophils transfused, inconsistent attempts to provide leukocyte-compatible GTX, and the varying duration of severe neutropenia in different patient groups were primarily responsible for the differing success rates in the reported controlled trials. It was recommended that high doses of compatible neutrophils be transfused in future trials (38).

Assessment of Modern Granulocyte Transfusion

A modern GTX is defined as a transfusion in which neutrophils were obtained from donors stimulated with G-CSF with or without glucocorticoids and collected by means of centrifugation leukapheresis with an erythrocyte-sedimenting agent during the processing of relatively large volumes of donor blood. Specifically, the requirements of an ideal neutrophil collection should include (a) at least 300 μg G-CSF given subcutaneously plus 8 mg dexamethasone given orally to the donor approximately 12 hours before leukapheresis is begun, (b) pentastarch or hetastarch

TABLE 20.4. TWELVE HISTORICAL CONTROLLED STUDIES OF TREATMENT OF PATIENTS WITH NEUTROPENIA BY MEANS OF PROPHYLACTIC TRANSFUSION OF GRANULOCYTES COLLECTED FROM UNSTIMULATED DONORS OR THOSE STIMULATED ONLY WITH GLUCOCORTICOIDS

Investigators	Success	Dose × 10^{10}	Schedule	HLA[a]	WBC[a]
Mannoni et al. (26)	Yes	2.1	Daily	No	Yes
Gomez-Villagran et al. (27)	Yes	1.2	Daily	No	Yes
Clift et al. (28)	Yes	1.5–2.2	Daily	Yes	Yes
Strauss et al. (29)	Partial	0.7	Daily	No	No
Hester et al. (30)	Partial	1.6	Daily	Yes	No
Buckner et al. (31)	Partial	Not reported	Daily	Yes	No
Curtis et al. (32)	Partial	0.07	Not reported	Yes	No
Schiffer et al. (33)	No	1.2	Alternate days	No	No
Sutton et al. (34)	No	0.9	Daily	No	No
Ford et al. (35)	No	1.5	Alternate days	No	No
Cooper et al. (36)	No	2.6	Twice a week	Yes	Yes
Winston et al. (37)	No	1.2	Daily	No	No

[a]Donors compatible with recipient by HLA typing (A and B loci matched, at least in part) or by leukocyte (WBC) cross-matching.

TABLE 20.5. THERAPEUTIC GRANULOCYTE TRANSFUSION WITH POLYMORPHONUCLEAR LEUKOCYTES COLLECTED FROM GRANULOCYTE COLONY-STIMULATING FACTOR–STIMULATED DONORS IN THE CARE OF ONCOLOGY AND TRANSPLANTATION PATIENTS WITH NEUTROPENIA

Author	PMNs × 10^{10} per Granulocyte Transfusion	Stimulation	Leukapheresis	Outcome
Hester et al. (39)	4.1	G-CSF 5 μg/kg	Pentastarch 7 L processed	60% (9 of 15) success with fungus (11 patients) and yeast (4 patients)
Clarke et al. (40)	5.3[a]	G-CSF 5–10 μg/kg	Dextran 10 L processed	One patient with fungus recovered
Catalano et al. (41)	1.9	G-CSF 300 μg/dose	Not described	One patient with fungus recovered
Ozsahin et al. (42)	3.1	G-CSF 5 μg/dose	Hetastarch 5–7L processed	One patient with fungus recovered
Bielorai et al. (43)	7.0[a]	G-CSF 5 μg/dose	Not described	One patient with fungus recovered
Grigg et al. (44)	5.9[a]	G-CSF 10 μg/kg	Dextran 10 L processed	100% (3 of 3) success with bacterial infection 0% (0 of 5) success with progressive fungus 67% (2 of 3) success with stable fungus
Peters et al. (45)	3.5[a]	G-CSF 5 μg/kg *or* Prednisolone	Hetastarch 6.4 L processed	82% (14 of 17) success with bacterial infection 54% (7 of 13) success with fungal infection
Price et al. (7)	8.2	G-CSF 600 μg/kg *plus* Dexamethasone 8 mg	Hetastarch 10 L processed	100% (4 of 4) success with bacterial infection 0% (0 of 8) success with invasive fungus 57% (4 of 7) success with yeast infection

[a]Assumptions made as PMN dose expressed × 10^{10} unclear in these reports. Dose calculated that would be given to a 70-kg recipient for Clark et al., Bielorai et al., and Peters et al. PMN dose calculated with values for range of leukocytes collected, percentage of collected cells being myeloid and volume of units collected (Grigg et al.).
PMNs, polymorphonuclear leukocytes; G-CSF, granulocyte colony-stimulating factor.

infused throughout the leukapheresis procedure at a ratio of 1 part starch to 12 to 14 parts donor blood, and (c) processing of 8 to 10 L of donor blood. The goal should be to transfuse 6 to 8 × 10^{10} neutrophils per GTX with a lower limit of 4 × 10^{10}.

At present, no results of randomized trials of therapeutic GTX collected after G-CSF donor stimulation have been reported to establish the efficacy or potential toxicity of modern GTX. However, several reports of uncontrolled studies (7, 39–45) contain varying findings (Table 20.5).

Hester et al. (39) administered transfusions to 15 patients with hematologic malignant disease and infection. Neutrophils were collected from donors stimulated only with G-CSF and selected without regard for leukocyte compatibility. Although GTX was successful for some patients, it was not possible to differentiate responses of fungal and yeast infections.

Clark et al. (40) and Catalano et al. (41) described patients with fungal infection and aplastic anemia who underwent progenitor cell transplantation and responded favorably to strikingly different doses of neutrophils. Ozsahin et al. (42) and Bielorai et al. (43) described patients with chronic granulomatous disease and fungal infection who responded favorably to GTX during the transplantation period. It is impossible in these complicated cases to firmly ascribe the good outcome to the GTX.

Grigg et al. (44) administered transfusions to 11 patients. Eight patients had hematologic malignant disease and progressive infection. Five of the eight underwent progenitor cell transplantation and three received chemotherapy. Three additional patients who were undergoing progenitor cell transplantation had stable fungal infections. Neutrophils were collected from donors stimulated only with G-CSF and selected without regard for leukocyte compatibility. Management of bacterial and stable fungal infections was successful, but that of progressive fungal infection with organ dysfunction was not.

Peters et al. (45) administered transfusions to 30 patients with hematologic disorders, 18 of whom underwent progenitor cell transplantation. Neutrophils were collected from donors stimulated with either G-CSF or prednisolone and selected without regard for leukocyte compatibility. The exact neutrophil dose transfused is uncertain because values from 0.9 × 10^{10} to 14.4 × 10^{10} can be calculated from data reported. It was impossible to differentiate the success of GTX with G-CSF–stimulated donors from that of GTX with prednisolone-stimulated donors. However, the outcome of bacterial infections appeared to be superior to that of fungal infection.

Price et al. (7) administered transfusions to 19 patients with hematologic malignant disease, 16 of whom had received progenitor cell transplants and three who were preparing for transplantation. Neutrophils were collected from donors stimulated with both G-CSF and dexamethasone. Although donors were selected without regard for leukocyte compatibility, recipients were documented not to have evidence of leukocyte alloimmunization at entrance into the study. Bacterial infection responded well and yeast infection modestly. Despite very high neutrophil doses, the results for management of invasive fungal infection were dismal (7).

No firm conclusions can be drawn from these somewhat anecdotal reports of modern therapeutic GTX for the following

TABLE 20.6. STUDIES OF PROPHYLACTIC GRANULOCYTE TRANSFUSION WITH POLYMORPHONUCLEAR LEUKOCYTES COLLECTED FROM GRANULOCYTE COLONY-STIMULATING FACTOR–STIMULATED DONORS IN THE CARE OF RECIPIENTS OF HEMATOPOIETIC PROGENITOR CELL TRANSPLANTS

Author	PMNs × 10^{10}	Stimulation	Leukapheresis	Outcome
Bensinger et al. (46)	4.2	G-CSF 3.5–6 μg/kg	Variable	Not reported
Adkins et al. (45)	4.1 (day 1) 5.1 (day 3) 6.1 (day 5)	G-CSF 5 μg/kg for 5 days after transplantation	Hetastarch 7 L processed days 1, 3, 5	60% (6 of 10) afebrile 40% (4 of 10) with fever; 3 culture positive
Adkins et al. (47)	5.6 (day 2) 7.0 (day 4) 8.5 (day 6) 9.9 (day 8)	G-CSF 10 μg/kg	Hetastarch 7 L processed days 2, 4, 6, 8	Reduction of fever and antibiotics if no leukocyte antibodies

PMNs, polymorphonuclear leukocytes; G-CSF, granulocyte colony-stimulating factor.

reasons: (a) no concurrent control subjects were included (i.e., no one was given either no GTX or GTX from donors stimulated only with glucocorticoids, (b) the number of patients was quite small, and (c) neutrophil collection methods were variable and a broad range of neutrophil doses were transfused. These preliminary findings showed that bacterial infections appeared to respond well to modern GTX. Relatively mild fungal and yeast infections responded only modestly well, whereas serious fungal infections with tissue damage resisted even the large doses of neutrophils transfused with modern GTX (7,44,45). Thus the precise role of modern therapeutic GTX from donors stimulated with G-CSF plus glucocorticoids awaits definition in randomized, clinical trials.

Similarly, the role of modern prophylactic GTX has not been established in definitive clinical trials. However, two factors suggest possible success. First, because of the rapid recovery from myeloablation hastened by PBHPC transfusions and treatment of patients with recombinant growth factors, the period of severe neutropenia may be as short as 1 week. Second, this relatively brief period of severe neutropenia may be eliminated by means of transfusion of large doses of neutrophils collected from donors stimulated with G-CSF plus glucocorticoids—cells often able to increase recipient neutrophil blood counts for more than 24 hours. A few studies have begun to explore this possibility (Table 20.6).

Bensinger et al. (46) treated seven recipients of allogeneic marrow by means of transfusion of neutrophils collected from HLA-identical or syngeneic marrow donors. Because donors experienced leukapheresis on consecutive days, collection techniques were quite variable in terms of quantity of hydroxyethyl starch infused and liters of donor blood processed, and the number of neutrophils collected varied from 0.3 to 14.4 × 10^{10}. Recipients received an average of 7.6 GTXs while awaiting marrow recovery and were given 5 μg/kg G-CSF daily to maintain a mean blood neutrophil count of 0.95 × 10^9/L measured 24 hours after transfusion. The goals of this study were to evaluate the feasibility and safety of collecting and transfusing neutrophils from G-CSF–stimulated donors. Patient outcomes were not reported.

Adkins et al. (7) treated ten recipients of allogeneic marrow by means of transfusion of neutrophils collected from HLA-matched sibling marrow donors. Leukapheresis was performed on the first, third, and fifth days after transplantation, and neutrophils were infused. Recipients were given 7.5 μg/kg G-CSF every 12 hours until the blood neutrophil count was 1.5 × 10^9/L. Recipient blood neutrophils were maintained at more than 0.5 × 10^9/L throughout the 5 days of posttransplantation GTX. In comparison, a historical group of control recipients treated with G-CSF and no GTX had mean blood neutrophil counts less than 0.5 × 10^9/L after transplantation. Prophylactic GTX seemed promising in this setting and perhaps would have been even more effective (higher recipient blood neutrophil count and fewer infections) if given daily.

Adkins et al. (47) treated 23 recipients of autologous PBHPCs by means of transfusion of neutrophils collected from first-degree relative donors. Leukapheresis was performed 2, 4, 6, and 8 days after transplantation, and neutrophils were infused. Recipients were given 5 μg/kg G-CSF daily until the blood neutrophil count was 1.5 × 10^9/L or more. Recipients were studied for the effects of lymphocytotoxic antibodies (leukocyte alloimmunization) on the effectiveness of GTX. The 15 recipients who did not have lymphocytotoxic antibodies during the 10-day study period had a mean of 4.1 febrile days and needed 7.3 days of antibiotic therapy. Values for the eight recipients with lymphocytotoxic antibodies were less desirable—6.3 febrile days and 10.5 days of antibiotics. Rates of documented infection were not reported. As in the earlier study (45), GTX given every other day did not completely eliminate febrile neutropenia, and daily GTX might have maintained higher recipient blood neutrophil counts and, consequently, reduced days of fever and antibiotics (47).

No firm conclusions can be drawn from these reports of prophylactic GTX because no control subjects who did not undergo transfusion were included; few patients were studied; and most patients were given GTX every other day rather than daily, possibly providing a less than optimal dose of neutrophils. In a preliminary report of a controlled but not randomized, trial (48), 16 patients undergoing PBHPC transplantation who received prophylactic GTX 3 and 6 days after transplantation had fewer days of fever (P = .05) and antibiotics (P = .007) than did 42 concurrent control patients not given GTX. Modern prophylactic GTX appears promising, but the efficacy, adverse effects, and economic analysis await definition in randomized, clinical trials.

SUMMARY AND RECOMMENDATIONS

The use of G-CSF with glucocorticoids to stimulate neutrophil donors has brought GTX therapy into a new era. It is now possible to collect relatively large numbers of neutrophils by means of modern leukapheresis techniques. This factor, along with the historical success of GTX in the management of bacterial infection even when neutrophils were given in low doses, suggests that both therapeutic and prophylactic GTX be reassessed.

To determine whether a need exists for therapeutic GTX, physicians should survey the outcome of neutropenic infections at their own institutions. If these infections respond promptly to antibiotics alone and the survival rate approaches 100%, therapeutic GTX is unnecessary and should not be used, because possible benefits are small and likely would not outweigh the risk and expense. In contrast, if patients with infection and neutropenia (fewer than 0.5×10^9 neutrophils/L) do not respond quickly and completely to antibiotics alone, the addition of therapeutic GTX should be considered along with other modifications of therapy, such as selection of different antibiotics, closer monitoring of antibiotic blood levels, intravenous γ-globulin therapy, and treatment with recombinant myeloid growth factors.

Prophylactic GTX is most likely to be useful in the setting of hematopoietic progenitor cell transplantation or rescue after myeloablation. Both autologous and allogeneic bone marrow transplantation is being supplanted by PBHPC transfusion and transplantation. This technique is used increasingly because it is convenient and economical and leads to relatively rapid engraftment. Recovery to a blood neutrophil count of at least 0.5×10^9/L occurs within 7 to 14 days after PBHPC transfusion. In the future, donors of PBHPCs may be stimulated with recombinant cytokines other than G-CSF alone, such as stem cell factor or interleukin-7, and the period of severe neutropenia may be shortened even more by means of transfusion of these cells. Thus complete elimination of severe neutropenia with a strategy of transplanting PBHPCs followed by prophylactic GTX is a distinct possibility that deserves careful study.

Once the decision has been made to provide either therapeutic or prophylactic GTX, neutrophils must be collected and transfused with optimal techniques. Recommendations include the following:

1. Collect neutrophils from allogeneic donors with a goal to transfuse 6 to 8×10^{10} neutrophils per GTX with a lower limit of 4×10^{10}. The need to select donors of modern (high neutrophil dose) GTX who are leukocyte compatible with recipients has not been established despite the historical importance of doing so when lower doses of neutrophils were transfused. In studies of modern GTX, Price et al. (7) found no apparent adverse effects of several leukocyte antibodies (granulocyte agglutinating, granulocyte immunofluorescent, lymphocytotoxic, and lymphocyte immunofluorescent) that became detectable in the recipient's blood during GTX therapy. Adkins et al. (48), however, found the presence of lymphocytotoxic antibodies to be a poor prognostic factor in general, even though actual donor-recipient incompatibility for individual GTX was rare. Until more data are available, it seems prudent to select donors who are leukocyte compatible (e.g., by means of HLA matching or leukocyte cross-matching) whenever feasible but not to delay or deny GTX therapy if selecting donors by these methods is not readily accomplished.
2. Stimulate donor neutrophilia by giving 300 to 600 μg G-CSF subcutaneously plus glucocorticoid orally 12 hours before beginning leukapheresis. A regimen reported to produce high neutrophil yields with well-tolerated adverse effects on the donor is 450 μg G-CSF subcutaneously plus 8 mg dexamethasone orally 12 hours before leukapheresis (49).
3. Process 10 L of donor blood using a continuous-flow, centrifugation blood separator with citrated hydroxyethyl starch (hetastarch or pentastarch) solution infused throughout the entire collection at a starch to donor blood ratio of 1:13.
4. Perform the GTX as soon as possible to minimize storage damage. Historical data suggest deterioration of neutrophil function begins within a few hours of storage. Until the efficacy of stored neutrophils from G-CSF–stimulated leukapheresis donors is documented, it seems wise to perform the transfusion promptly, certainly within 6 hours or so of collection. This timing may require agreement by the patient's physician to perform infectious disease testing on the donor before actual neutrophil collection (e.g., at the time G-CSF is administered before leukapheresis).
5. Give GTX daily as prophylactic GTX in an attempt to prevent infection during the period of severe neutropenia or as therapeutic GTX to resolve a documented infection—either as evidenced by clearing of tissue lesions, negative cultures, or resolution of fever or until marrow function recovers to produce adequate numbers of endogenous neutrophils. Determining marrow recovery may be difficult. Neutrophils collected from G-CSF and glucocorticoid-stimulated donors and transfused at doses of 4 to 8×10^{10} neutrophils may elevate the recipient's blood neutrophil count to more than 1×10^9/L for more than 24 hours. Accurate differentiation of transfused neutrophils from those produced endogenously is challenging, and marrow recovery must be based on a sustained increase in blood neutrophil count after GTX is discontinued.

REFERENCES

1. Strauss RG. Therapeutic granulocyte transfusions in 1993. *Blood* 1993; 81:1675–1678.
2. Strauss RG. Granulocyte transfusions. In: McLeod BC, Price TH, Drew MJ, eds. *Apheresis: principles and practice.* Bethesda, MD: American Association of Blood Banks, 1997:195–209.
3. Strauss RG, Rohert PA, Randels MJ, et al. Granulocyte collection. *J Clin Apheresis* 1991;6:241–245.
4. Strauss RG, Hester JP, Vogler WR, et al. A multi-center trial to document the efficacy and safety of a rapidly excreted analogue of hydroxyethyl starch for leukapheresis: with a note on steroid stimulation. *Transfusion* 1986;26:258–262.
5. Adkins D, Spitzer G, Johnston M, et al. Transfusions of granulocyte-colony-stimulating factor-mobilized granulocyte components to alloge-

neic transplant recipients: analysis of kinetics and factors determining posttransfusion neutrophil and platelet counts. *Transfusion* 1997;37: 737–748.

6. Liles WC, Huang JE, Llewellyn C, et al. A comparative trial of granulocyte colony-stimulating factor and dexamethasone, separately and in combination, for the mobilization of neutrophils in the peripheral blood of normal volunteers. *Transfusion* 1997;37:182–188.
7. Price TH, Bowden RA, Boeckh M, et al. Phase I/II trial of neutrophil transfusions from donors stimulated with G-CSF and dexamethasone for treatment of patients with infections in hematopoietic stem cell transplantation. *Blood* 2000;95:3302–3309.
8. Price TH, Chatta GS, Dale DC. Effect of recombinant granulocyte colony-stimulating factor on neutrophil kinetics in normal young and elderly humans. *Blood* 1996;88:335–340.
9. Adkins D, Goodgold H, Hendershott L, et al. Indium-labeled white blood cells apheresed from donors receiving G-CSF localize to sites of inflammation when infused into allogeneic bone marrow transplant recipients. *Bone Marrow Transplant* 1997;19:809–814.
10. Lee JH, Cullis H, Leitman SF, et al. Efficacy of pentastarch in granulocyte collection by centrifugal leukapheresis. *J Clin Apheresis* 1995;10: 198–202.
11. Lee JH, Klein HG. The effect of donor red cell sedimentation rate on efficiency of granulocyte collection by centrifugal leukapheresis. *Transfusion* 1995;35:384–388.
12. Lee JH, Leitman SF, Klein HG. A controlled comparison of the efficacy of hetastarch and pentastarch in granulocyte collections by centrifugal leukapheresis. *Blood* 1995;86:4662–4666.
13. Treib J, Haass A, Pindur G, et al. HES 200/0. 5 is not HES 200/ 0.5: influence of the C2/C6 hydroxyethylation ratio of hemorheology, coagulation and elimination kinetics. *Thromb Haemost* 1995;74: 1462–1466.
14. Strauss RG. Volume replacement and coagulation: a comparative review. *J Cardiothorac Anesth* 1988;2[Suppl 1]:24–32.
15. Strauss RG. Granulocyte transfusion therapy. In: Mintz PD, ed. *Transfusion therapy: clinical principles and practice.* Bethesda, MD: American Association of Blood Banks, 1999;81–96.
16. Higby DJ, Yates YW, Henderson ES, et al. Filtration leukapheresis for granulocytic transfusion therapy. *N Engl J Med* 1975;292:761–766.
17. Vogler WR, Winton EF. A controlled study of the efficacy of granulocyte transfusions in patients with neutropenia. *Am J Med* 1977;63: 548–555.
18. Herzig RH, Herzig GP, Graw RG Jr, et al. Successful granulocyte transfusion therapy for gram-negative septicemia. *N Engl J Med* 1977; 396:701–705.
19. Alavi JB, Root RK, Djerassi I, et al. A randomized clinical trial of granulocyte transfusions for infection in acute leukemia. *N Engl J Med* 1977;296:706–711.
20. Graw RG Jr, Herzig G, Perry S, et al. Normal granulocyte transfusion therapy. *N Engl J Med* 1972;287:367–376.
21. Winston DJ, Ho WG, Gale RP. Therapeutic granulocyte transfusions for documented infections: a controlled trial in 95 infectious granulocytopenic episodes. *Ann Intern Med* 1982;97:509–515.
22. Fortuny IE, Bloomfield CD, Hadlock DC, et al. Granulocyte transfusion: a controlled study in patients with acute non-lymphocytic leukemia. *Transfusion* 1975;15:548–558.
23. Vamvakas EC, Pineda AA. Meta-analysis of clinical studies of efficacy of granulocyte transfusions in the treatment of bacterial sepsis. *J Clin Apheresis* 1996;11:1–9.
24. Yomtovian R, Abramson J, Quie P, et al. Granulocyte transfusion therapy in chronic granulomatous disease: report of a patient and review of the literature. *Transfusion* 1981;21:739–744.
25. Bhatia S, McCullough JJ, Perry EH, et al. Granulocyte transfusions: efficacy in fungal infections in neutropenic patients following bone marrow transplantation. *Transfusion* 1994;34:226–231.
26. Mannoni P, Rodet M, Vernant JP, et al. Efficiency of prophylactic granulocyte transfusions in preventing infections in acute leukemia. *Rev Fr Transfus Immunohaematol* 1979;22:503–518.
27. Gomez-Villagran JL, Torres-Gomez A, Gomez-Garcia P, et al. A controlled trial of prophylactic granulocyte transfusions during induction chemotherapy for acute nonlymphoblastic leukemia. *Cancer* 1984;54: 734–738.
28. Clift RA, Sanders JE, Thomas ED, et al. Granulocyte transfusions for the prevention of infection in patients receiving bone-marrow transplants. *N Engl J Med* 1978;298:1052–1056.
29. Strauss RG, Connett JE, Gale RP, et al. A controlled trial of prophylactic granulocyte transfusions during initial induction chemotherapy for acute myelogenous leukemia. *N Engl J Med* 1981;305:597–603.
30. Hester JP, McCredie KB, Freireich EJ. Advances in supportive care: blood component transfusions. In: *Care of the child with cancer.* Atlanta: American Cancer Society, 1979:93–97.
31. Buckner CD, Clift RA, Thomas ED, et al. Early infections complications in allogenic marrow transplant recipients with acute leukemia: effects of prophylactic measures. *Infection* 1983;11:243–247.
32. Curtis JE, Hasselback R, Bergsagel DE. Leukocyte transfusions for the prophylaxis and treatment of infections associated with granulocytopenia. *Can Med Assoc J* 1977;117:341–345.
33. Schiffer CA, Aisner J, Daly PA, et al. Alloimmunization following prophylactic granulocyte transfusion. *Blood* 1979;54:766–770.
34. Sutton DMC, Shumak KH, Baker MA. Prophylactic granulocyte transfusions in acute leukemia. *Plasma Ther Transfus Technol* 1982;3:45–52.
35. Ford JM, Cullen MH, Roberts MM, et al. Prophylactic granulocyte transfusions: results of a randomized controlled trial in patients with acute myelogenous leukemia. *Transfusion* 1982;22:311–315.
36. Cooper MR, Heise E, Richards F, et al. A prospective study of histocompatible leukocyte and platelet transfusions during chemotherapeutic induction of acute myeloblastic leukemia. In: Goldman JM, Lowenthal RM, eds. *Leukocytes: separation, collection and transfusion.* San Diego: Academic Press, 1981:436–439.
37. Winston DJ, Ho WG, Young LS, et al. Prophylactic granulocyte transfusions during human bone marrow transplantation. *Am J Med* 1982; 68:893–900.
38. Vamvakas EC, Pineda AA. Determinants of the efficacy of prophylactic granulocyte transfusions: a meta-analysis. *J Clin Apheresis* 1997;12: 74–81.
39. Hester JP, Dignani MC, Anaisse EJ, et al. Collection and transfusion of granulocyte concentrates from donors primed with granulocyte stimulating factor and response of myelosuppressed patients with established infection. *J Clin Apheresis* 1995;10:188–193.
40. Clarke K, Szer J, Shelton M, et al. Multiple granulocyte transfusions facilitating successful unrelated bone marrow transplantation in a patient with very severe aplastic anemia complicated by suspected fungal infection. *Bone Marrow Transplant* 1995;16:723–726.
41. Catalano L, Fontant R, Scarpato N, et al. Combined treatment with amphotericin-B and granulocyte transfusion from G-CSF–stimulated donors in an aplastic patient with invasive aspergillosis undergoing bone marrow transplantation. *Haematologica* 1997;82:71–72.
42. Ozsahin H, von Planta M, Muller I, et al. Successful treatment of invasive aspergillosis in chronic granulomatous disease by invasive aspergillosis in chronic granulomatous disease by bone marrow transplantation, granulocyte colony-stimulating factor–mobilized granulocytes, and liposomal amphotericin-B. *Blood* 1998; 92:2719–2724.
43. Bielorai B, Toren A, Wolach B, et al. Successful treatment of invasive aspergillosis in chronic granulomatous disease by granulocyte transfusions followed by peripheral blood stem cell transplantation. *Bone Marrow Transplant* 2000; 26:1025–1028.
44. Grigg A, Vecchi L, Bardy P, et al. G-CSF stimulated donor granulocyte collections for prophylaxis and therapy of neutropenic sepsis. *Aust N Z J Med* 1996;26:813–818.
45. Peters C, Minkov M, Matthes-Martin S, et al. Leucocyte transfusions from rhG-CSF or prednisolone stimulated donors for treatment of severe infections in immunocompromised neutropenic patients. *Br J Haematol* 1999;106:689–696.
46. Bensinger WI, Price TH, Dale DC, et al. The effects of daily recombinant human granulocyte colony stimulating factor administration on normal granulocyte donors undergoing leukapheresis. *Blood* 1993;81: 1883–1888.

47. Adkins DR, Goodnough LT, Shenoy S, et al. Effect of leukocyte compatibility on neutrophil increment after transfusion of granulocyte colony-stimulating factor-mobilized prophylactic granulocyte transfusions and on clinical outcomes after stem cell transplantation. *Blood* 2000; 95:3605–3612.
48. Adkins D, Goodnough LT, Moellering J, et al. Reduction in antibiotic utilization and in febrile days by transfusion of G-CSF mobilized prophylactic granulocyte components: a randomized study. *Blood* 1999; 94:590a(abst).
49. Liles WC, Rodger E, Dale DC. Combined administration of G-CSF and dexamethasone for the mobilization of granulocytes in normal donors: optimization of dosing. *Transfusion* 2000;40:642–644.

Rossi's Principles of Transfusion Medicine, Third Edition, edited by Toby L. Simon, Walter H. Dzik, Edward L. Snyder, Christopher P. Stowell, and Ronald G. Strauss. Lippincott Williams & Wilkins, Philadelphia © 2002.

CASE 20A

IS GRANULOCYTE COLONY-STIMULATING FACTOR LEUKEMOGENIC?

CASE HISTORY

Tommy, a 9-year-old boy from Canada, was on spring break in Florida when he experienced a sore throat and fever. At an oceanside hospital emergency department, his throat was found to be erythematous with modest amounts of whitish exudate and a few small punched-out ulcers on the tonsillar pillars. Results of a complete blood cell count were hemoglobin, 9.4 g/dl; platelets, 43,000/ml, and leukocytes 28,000/ml, of which 78% were blasts, some of which contained Auer rods.

Hospital Evaluation

Tommy was admitted to the hospital, and antibiotic therapy was begun. Other than the pharyngitis, the physical examination was remarkable only for modest cervical lymphadenopathy and splenomegaly palpable 4 cm below the left costal margin. Blood cultures revealed streptococcal sepsis, which responded quickly to the antibiotics.

The medical history was significant for the presence of severe congenital neutropenia. Two weeks after a normal birth, Tommy had pneumonia and was found to have a blood neutrophil count of 100/μl. He responded well to antibiotics, but severe neutropenia (<200/μl) persisted, and Tommy was hospitalized for five episodes of bacterial infection during the first 6 months of life. Tommy's blood hemoglobin values were slightly low, ascribed to the recurrent infections, and platelet counts were normal. A bone marrow examination revealed normal maturation of erythrocyte and megakaryocyte lineages, but myeloid precursors showed a maturation arrest; that is, only myeloblasts and promyelocytes were seen. Results of cytogenetic studies were normal.

Because of the severe neutropenia and recurrent infections, when Tommy was 8 months of age, therapy with granulocyte colony-stimulating factor (G-CSF) was begun at a dosage of 10 μg/kg a day subcutaneously. Tommy responded nicely, and the G-CSF dose was adjusted over the years to maintain a blood neutrophil count between 1,000 and 2,000/μl. With the exception of occasional childhood "virus" infections, Tommy was in good health until the present illness.

Further Evaluation and Course

As soon as the streptococcal sepsis was under control, Tommy returned to Canada and was admitted to the hematology-oncology service at a local children's hospital. The diagnosis of acute myelocytic leukemia was made, and special studies of his myeloblasts revealed complete loss of chromosome 7, a mutation in the gene for the G-CSF receptor that resulted in a truncated C-terminal cytoplasmic region of the receptor and the ELA-2 mutation of the elastase gene.

Tommy was treated with combination chemotherapy and achieved complete remission. Both the monosomy chromosome 7 and the G-CSF receptor mutation disappeared. The ELA-2 elastase mutation persisted. After 8 weeks of remission, Tommy underwent successful bone marrow transplantation to control both severe congenital neutropenia and acquired myeloid leukemia.

DISCUSSION

Tommy had severe congenital neutropenia, often called Kostmann syndrome. It is an autosomal recessive disorder characterized by the onset of profound neutropenia (blood neutrophil count <200/μl) during infancy and a maturation arrest of marrow myeloid precursors at the myeloblast-promyelocyte stage of differentiation. Approximately 10% of these patients acquire a myelodysplasia-leukemia syndrome whether or not they receive G-CSF treatment. As the myelodysplasia-leukemia syndrome develops, patients acquire cytogenetic abnormalities—typically partial or complete loss of chromosome 7 and mutations of the G-CSF receptor gene that result in truncation of the carboxy-terminal region that renders cells hypersensitive to G-CSF. These mutations of the G-CSF receptor transduce signals that increase resistance to apoptosis and prolong cell survival.

Mutations of the G-CSF receptor in patients with severe congenital neutropenia are believed to be only one of numerous factors leading to the development of leukemia. That is, the G-CSF receptor mutation prolongs cell survival for a sufficient period to allow additional oncogenic events, which together induce leukemic transformation. The need for several factors is supported by the observation that some patients with severe congenital neutropenia acquire the G-CSF receptor mutation but do not have leukemia.

Tommy's case is relevant to decisions regarding administration of G-CSF to healthy persons donating neutrophils-granulocytes for transfusion or hematopoietic progenitor cells for transplantation because it provides evidence that G-CSF therapy is not directly leukemogenic. In severe congenital neutropenia, the predisposition to myelodysplasia-leukemia is ascribed to an inherent characteristic of the disorder because some patients have leukemia despite never being treated with G-CSF. The acquired mutation of the G-CSF receptor gene that appears in patients with severe congenital neutropenia, many of whom eventually have myelodysplasia-leukemia, is not confined to myeloblasts—cells that are obvious targets for G-CSF—but also has been found in lymphoblasts. Patients with cyclic neutropenia, who like patients with severe congenital neutropenia are treated with G-CSF, do not have myelodysplasia-leukemia at an increased rate, despite the presence in both disorders of ELA-2 mutations of the elastase gene. Importantly, the elastase gene mutation, when present in severe congenital neutropenia or in cyclic neutropenia, has been found in all affected family members, indicating germ-line rather than somatic mutation.

Although the long-term effects of G-CSF administered to healthy donors will only be known after comprehensive studies conducted over long periods, evidence to date suggests no serious hematopoietic complications of giving G-CSF to healthy persons. Most donors receiving G-CSF for 1 to 5 days experience a variety of musculoskeletal aches and pains and transient abnormalities of many laboratory values. With rare exceptions, these adverse effects have little clinical significance and are alleviated by analgesics. Follow-up studies performed 1 year after initial G-CSF administration (five daily doses at 2 to 10 μg/kg a day) revealed normal hematologic values after a repeated course of G-CSF.

Case contributed by Ronald G. Strauss, M.D., University of Iowa Hospitals, Iowa City, IA.

REFERENCES

1. Freedman MH, Bonnilla MA, Fier C, et al. Myelodysplasia syndrome and acute myeloid leukemia in patients with congenital neutropenia receiving G-CSF therapy. *Blood* 2000;15:429–436.
2. Hunter MG, Avalos BR. Granulocyte colony-stimulating factor receptor mutations in severe congenital neutropenia transforming to acute myelogenous leukemia confer resistance to apoptosis and enhance cell survival. *Blood* 2000;95:2132–2137.
3. Germeshausen M, Ballmaier M, Schulze H, et al. Granulocyte colony-stimulating factor receptor mutations in a patient with acute lymphoblastic leukemia secondary to severe congenital neutropenia. *Blood* 2001; 97:829–830.
4. Stroncek DF, Clay ME, Herr G, et al. Blood counts in healthy donors 1 year after the collection of granulocyte-colony-stimulating factor-mobilized progenitor cells and the results of a second mobilization and collection. *Transfusion* 1997;37:304–308.

21

LEUKOREDUCED BLOOD COMPONENTS: LABORATORY AND CLINICAL ASPECTS

WALTER H. DZIK

Recipient exposure to residual donor leukocytes present in cellular blood components has been linked to the wide range of transfusion complications. Some complications result directly from exposure to donor leukocytes, and leukoreduction or inactivation is a highly effective prevention strategy. For other complications, the association with donor leukocytes is less certain, and considerably more research is needed before specific transfusion practice can be established. The development of technology to reduce the residual leukocyte content of cellular components has sparked active investigation into the potential benefits of leukoreduced blood components. This chapter reviews both the laboratory and clinical aspects of leukocyte reduction. The reader is also referred to several recent reviews of this topic (1–3).

LABORATORY ASPECTS

Fresh cellular blood components contain considerable quantities of residual donor leukocytes (Table 21.1). However, during refrigerated storage of red blood cell concentrates, a substantial proportion of donor leukocytes undergo cellular degeneration and apoptosis, and surface antigens on residual cells change. Thus refrigerated storage itself may help prevent complications of use of donor leukocytes to a degree not completely appreciated. In the 1980s washed or frozen-deglycerolized red blood cell concentrates were used to prevent complications resulting from use of donor leukocytes. During the 1990s, several technologies were introduced to remove or inactivate residual donor leukocytes in blood components. High-performance leukocyte reduction filters are used for either red blood cell or platelet concentrates. Apheresis platelets can be leukoreduced at the time of collection without the use of filters. Chemical pathogen reduction systems designed specifically for red blood cell concentrates or platelet concentrates are undergoing clinical trials. These chemicals inactivate residual donor leukocytes. The potential of these diverse technologies to affect known complications of recipient exposure to donor leukocytes is shown in Table 21.2.

Technologies for Leukocyte Reduction

Centrifugation

Removal of the buffy coat from whole blood during initial component preparation is widely practiced in Europe and Japan. In one technique, called the *top and bottom method,* whole blood is subjected to centrifugation at relatively high gravity force to compress both platelets and leukocytes into the buffy coat (Fig. 21.1). Preparation of the buffy coat component is sensitive to minor changes in centrifugation and separation conditions. Machines have been developed to render the process more reproducible. Buffy coat–reduced red blood cell concentrates contain approximately 70% to 80% fewer leukocytes than do unmodified red blood cell concentrates. This advantage is offset to some degree by the loss of platelets and red blood cells that occurs

W.H. Dzik: Blood Transfusion Service, Massachusetts General Hospital, Department of Pathology, Harvard Medical School, Boston, Massachusetts.

TABLE 21.1. APPROXIMATE RESIDUAL NUMBER OF LEUKOCYTES IN CELLULAR BLOOD COMPONENTS

Component	No. of Leukocytes
Fresh whole blood	10^9
Red blood cell concentrate	10^8–10^9
Buffy coat–depleted red blood cells	10^8
Washed red blood cell concentrate	10^7
Frozen deglycerolized red blood cells	10^6–10^7
Whole blood platelet concentrate	10^7–10^8
Apheresis platelets	10^6–10^8
Leukoreduced red blood cell concentrate	$<5 \times 10^6$
Leukoreduced whole blood platelets	$<0.83 \times 10^5$
Leukoreduced apheresis platelets	$<5 \times 10^6$
Fresh frozen plasma	$<10^4$

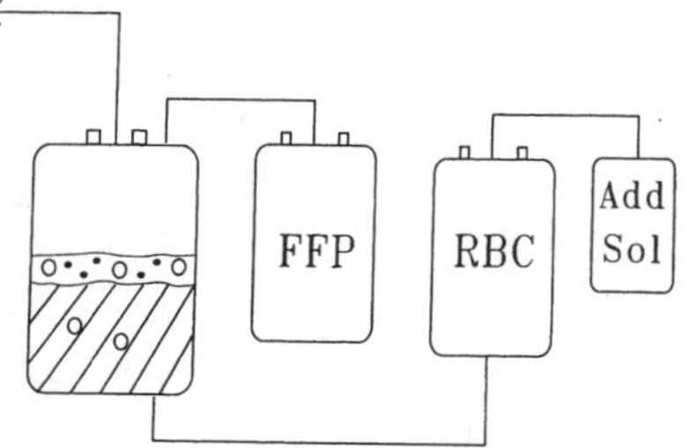

FIGURE 21.1. Preparation of buffy coat–depleted blood components from whole blood by means of the top and bottom method. The primary bag (*left*) has undergone centrifugation at a high-gravity force. The buffy coat–containing leukocytes and platelets are between the plasma (*open area*) and red blood cells (*hatched area*). The supernatant plasma is expressed out the top of the primary bag into a satellite bag while the red blood cells are expressed out the bottom into another satellite bag. The buffy coat–containing donor white blood cells and platelets are then pooled with other buffy coats, and the pool is subjected to centrifugation at a lower gravity force than used previously. After this centrifugation, the pooled platelet-rich plasma is expressed out the top of the pooling bag, and the residual cellular elements are discarded. *FFP,* fresh-frozen plasma; *RBC,* red blood cells; *Add Sol,* additive solution.

during the procedure. Buffy coat depletion is sufficient to prevent many febrile nonhemolytic (FNH) reactions to blood but is not considered sufficient to prevent human leukocyte antigen (HLA) alloimmunization.

Filtration

Filtration has emerged as the most commonly used method of leukoreduction. Because of rapid product development and enhancement in this area, the results of clinical studies may lead to underestimation of the potential clinical efficacy of current filters. Early leukocyte reduction achieved only 90% to 99% (1 to 2 $\log_{10}$) leukocyte reduction. Current high-performance leukocyte removal filters can reduce the residual white blood cell (WBC) content at least 3 logs. As a result, the proportion of filtered units with less than 10^6 residual leukocytes has steadily increased.

Mechanisms of Filtration

High-performance filters have been specifically designed to remove leukocytes (4). The plastic housing that contains the filtration medium is designed so that blood encounters a large surface area of medium; the volume of blood retained by the filter (hold-up volume) is minimal; and the medium fits tightly enough within the housing so that blood entering the device cannot bypass the filtration medium. Depletion of leukocytes results primarily from barrier retention in which the pore size of the filter medium is large enough to allow passage of red blood cells and platelets but small enough to impede passage of leukocytes. To achieve the small pore sizes required, manufacturers have

TABLE 21.2. POTENTIAL USE OF TECHNOLOGIES DESIGNED TO REDUCE THE RISK OF COMPLICATIONS ATTRIBUTED TO RESIDUAL DONOR LEUKOCYTES

Use	Leukoreduced Blood	γ Irradiation	Ultraviolet-B Irradiation	Chemical Inactivation
Reduce rate of HLA antibody formation	Yes	No	Yes	Uncertain
Reduce risk of transmission of leukotropic viruses	Yes	No	No	Yes
Reduce risk of FNH reactions due to donor cytokine	Yes, if prestorage	Unproven	Probable	Probable
Reduce risk of FNH reactions due to reaction against donor cells	Yes	No	No	Uncertain
Reduce risk of TA-GVHD	Unproven	Yes	Animal studies only	Animal studies only

FNH, febrile nonhemolytic; TA-GVHD, transfusion-associated graft-versus-host disease.

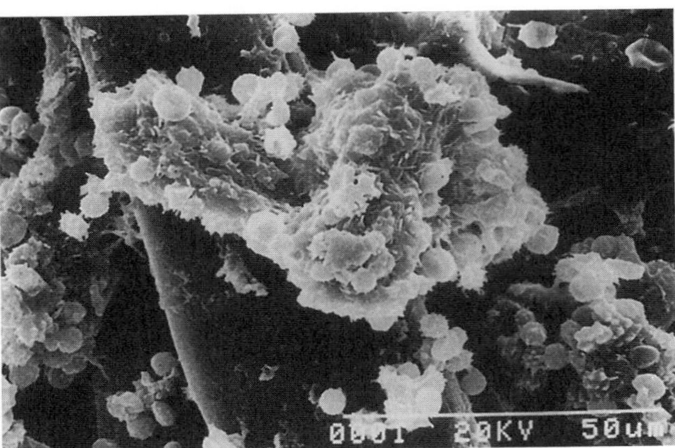

FIGURE 21.2. Electron photomicrograph shows fibers in the coarse filter (upstream layer) of a leukocyte removal filter designed for red blood cell concentrates. A microaggregate is present in the *center* of the figure. The diameter of the pore and the caliber of the fibers relative to individual cells are evident. (From Nishimura T, Kuroda T, Mizoguchi Y, et al. Advanced methods for leucocyte removal by blood filtration. In: Brozovic B, ed. *The role of leucocyte depletion in blood transfusion practice.* Oxford, UK: Blackwell Scientific, 1989:37.)

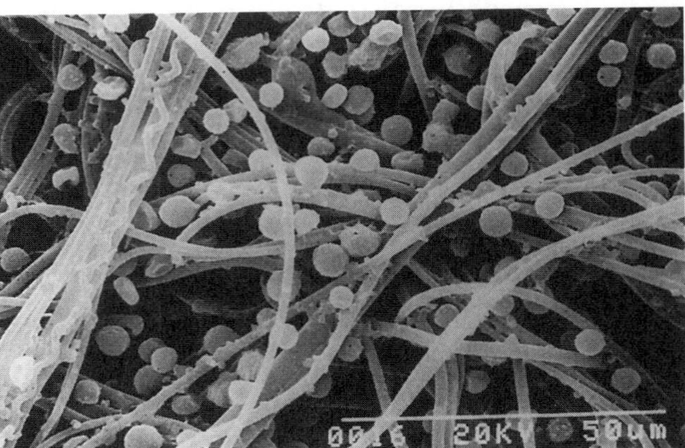

FIGURE 21.3. Electron micrograph shows fibers from the fine filter (downstream layer) of a leukocyte removal filter designed for red blood cells. The caliber of the fibers relative to that of individual cells is evident. (From Nishimura T, Kuroda T, Mizoguchi Y, et al. Advanced methods for leucocyte removal by blood filtration. In: Brozovic B, ed. *The role of leucocyte depletion in blood transfusion practice.* Oxford, UK: Blackwell Scientific, 1989:37.)

used three different fabrication strategies. In one method, polyester is melted and extruded through fine nozzles into a turbulent gas stream at high velocity. In the process, akin to the formation of cotton candy, the polyester is stretched and cooled to form fine threads of microfibers. These fibers are matted together (like teased hair) and compressed to a controlled fiber density. A variation of this technique is used in products made by Pall Corporation, Asahi Medical Company, and Fresenius AG. A second method is wet fiber formation with a method akin to paper making. Fibrous ingredients are put into water suspension and deposited onto a fine mesh screen. As the water is removed, the fibers settle into a soft mat, which is heated and dried to stabilize the structure into a fibrous sheet. This process is used by Hemasure Corporation. A third approach (used by Terumo Corporation) produces foamlike structures of porous polycarbonate with an open-cell geometric configuration containing interconnecting voids that necessitate a circuitous path of flow. On cross-section, this medium resembles Swiss cheese.

Polyester fiber filters consist of a series of layers of fiber material. At the upstream end of the filter, the fiber diameter and effective pore size are large (Fig. 21.2). As blood passes through the layers of medium, the fiber diameter becomes smaller, and the pore size decreases to approximately 4 μm (Fig. 21.3). Red blood cells, which are more deformable than leukocyte nuclei, can traverse these small pores. Differences in the viscoelastic properties of red blood cells and leukocytes are particularly pronounced at low temperatures. Because synthetic materials are naturally hydrophobic, they do not become "wet" easily in aqueous solutions. As a result, surface tension would prevent blood from flowing through very fine pore spaces under gravity. To overcome this obstacle, manufacturers have modified the surface of the filter medium fibers to increase their "wetability."

Factors Affecting Filter Performance

Because of the complex physical and biologic forces involved in leukocyte retention by the filter medium, it is not surprising that a variety of factors has been shown to affect the degree of leukoreduction obtained (Table 21.3). A primary factor is the capacity of the filter itself. The input load of WBCs to be filtered has a direct relation to the postfiltration WBC content. The temperature of filtration has a dominant effect on the performance of leukofiltration of red blood cell concentrates. Nearly all studies have found that the efficiency of filtration improves when the procedure is conducted at refrigerated temperatures. For example, Beaujean et al. (5) studied red blood cell concentrates suspended in saline-adenine-glucose plus mannitol (SAGMAN) that were stored for 2 to 10 days. The stored units were paired, pooled, and split. One member of each pair was filtered (R500; Asahi Medical, Tokyo, Japan) either at 4°C or 37°C. The mean postfiltration WBC content was 11×10^6 for units filtered at 4°C but 114×10^6 for units filtered at 37°C. Sirchia et al. (6) extended these results by showing that when red blood cell concentrates were filtered under conditions that mimicked bedside leukofiltration, the units warmed from refrigerated temperature to room temperature within 90 minutes. As the units warmed, filtration became less efficient such that most units filtered under bedside conditions over 3 to 4 hours did not meet minimum standards as leukoreduced red blood cell

TABLE 21.3. FACTORS AFFECTING FILTER PERFORMANCE

Capacity of the filter
Input number of leukocytes
Temperature (viscoelasticity)
Flow rate, pressure, priming, rinsing
Presence of hemoglobin S
Number and function of platelets
Holding time between blood collection and filtration
Plasma content of cell suspension media

concentrates. Improved performance of filtration at refrigerated temperatures has been observed by other investigators (7,8). The dominant effect of temperature on the performance of early filters designed for use with red blood cell concentrates may have had a subtle effect on the results of the cytomegalovirus (CMV) prevention trial conducted by Bowden et al. (9), which was conducted before the temperature effect was realized.

The cellular composition of the blood also affects retention of leukocytes. Blood from donors with sickle cell trait often does not become leukoreduced when filtered. Results of preliminary studies suggest that approximately 50% of units from donors with hemoglobin AS clog the filter and do not flow. Of the remaining 50%, approximately half of these flow normally but do not undergo adequate leukoreduction (10–12). The exact mechanism by which blood from sickle trait donors fails to undergo leukoreduction is unknown, but results of preliminary investigation suggest that sickle trait red blood cells are far more adhesive to the filter medium. As the filter medium is progressively coated with erythrocytes, there is less effective medium area for leukocyte trapping. The increased adhesion of sickle trait red blood cells to the medium may result from interaction of plasma proteins with elevated concentrations of integrin receptors expressed on sickle trait red blood cells.

Other factors that affect the performance of filtration include the protein content of the cell suspension. For example, as little as 5 to 10 ml of plasma added to red blood cell concentrates suspended in SAGMAN additive solution improved the leukocyte removal efficiency of an RC50 filter (Pall Corporation) tenfold (13). This observation suggests that adhesive proteins present in plasma contribute to leukocyte retention. The speed of filtration also has been shown to affect leukoreduction. If temperature is held constant, faster flow rates result in decreased performance (6). This is presumed to result from high shear rates and decreased contact time with the medium.

Low-Leukocyte Apheresis Devices

Manufacturers of apheresis devices have modified the machinery to collect platelets with low levels of residual donor leukocytes. The collections require no further filtration to meet standards as leukoreduced platelet concentrates. In the United States, two devices—the Gambro/COBE Spectra LRS and the Baxter Amicus—are approved for collection of leukoreduced platelet concentrates without filtration. These devices achieve a high degree of separation between the donor platelets and the donor leukocytes as a result of several design principles. Flow path geometry, counter-flow centrifugation, elutriation, and fluid particle bed separation all are used to separate platelets from leukocytes on the basis of differences in cell mass. Despite advanced design, apheresis systems can fail to collect platelet concentrates that meet standards as leukocyte is reduced. Failed collections may result from sudden changes in the donor bleed rate, paused collections that disturb centrifugal separation, or characteristics of the donor blood that interfere with optical sensors on the devices. As in the case of filtration-based systems, some form of process control is required to document that the collected products are leukoreduced.

Process Control of Leukoreduced Components

To achieve the expected clinical benefits of providing leukoreduced blood, facilities need to control the process by which such products are prepared. Process control of leukoreduction seeks to establish with a specified statistical confidence that a specified proportion of units conform to the standards for leukoreduction. Selecting an appropriate degree of confidence and conformance may depend on the expected use of the technology. For example, a greater degree of process control might be applied by facilities that use leukoreduction technology as the sole means to prevent transmission of CMV. In contrast, because FNH reactions are not serious events and because prevention of HLA alloimmunization has not been shown to result in improved clinical outcomes, a lower degree of process control may be appropriate if leukoreduction is to be used to achieve these two goals. Process control of leukoreduction also should document that the prepared products retain an adequate amount of the therapeutic blood cells intended for transfusion. Guidelines for statistical process control of leukoreduced blood have been published (14). New draft guidelines have been issued by the U.S. Food and Drug Administration (FDA) (15).

Methods of Counting Low-Leukocyte Residuals

The concentration of WBCs in a 300 ml leukoreduced blood component with 10^6 WBCs per unit is only 3.3 WBCs/μl. Because traditional automated cell counters are not accurate at leukocyte concentrations less than 100 WBCs/μl, special techniques are required to accurately count residual WBCs in leukoreduced components. The challenges of counting such low levels of leukocytes have been reviewed (16). All methods depend on counting the cells present in a large volume of blood. Sampling errors and the precision of different methods affect the confidence of the measured result. Several different methods have been published, including cytospin methods, Nageotte chamber counting, flow cytometric counting, volumetric cytometry, and counting based on the polymerase chain reaction (PCR). Leukocytes can be stained with either a crystal violet nuclear stain (Turks solution), fluorescent dye (propidium iodide), or other vital stains (e.g., Plaxan solution). Nageotte chamber counting with crystal violet stain is the most commonly used technique, requires only a light microscope, and has been used for both platelet and red blood cell concentrates. The Nageotte counting chamber has a 50 μl bed volume. The sample to be counted is mixed with a red blood cell or platelet lysing agent and a nuclear stain, allowed to settle undisturbed in the counting chamber, and then examined under 200× magnification. The Nageotte counting method has been shown in multicenter evaluations to be accurate to approximately 1 WBC/μl (17). Because of its simplicity, low cost, and low limit of detection, it is adequate for routine quality control programs. With concentration of a larger volume of blood sample before staining, the lower limit of accurate detection by means of Nageotte counting can be reduced by as much as 100-fold (18).

Flow cytometry can be used to achieve a lower limit of accurate detection (approximately 0.1 WBC/μl) because a larger volume of sample can be processed. The method requires an expensive instrument and relies on a fluorescent dye that is taken up by leukocyte DNA and emits light when struck by the cytometer laser. With adjustment of the conditions of data acquisition of the cytometer, signals from fluorescent residual leukocytes can be discriminated from those of residual red blood cells or platelets. Techniques are available for counting WBCs in red blood cell and platelet concentrates (16). Within the range detectable by means of Nageotte counting, the two methods show good correlation.

Because different transfusion complications have been associated with different leukocyte subsets, there has been investigation into the proportion of leukocyte subpopulations that remain after different techniques of leukoreduction. Although some investigators have found slight differences in the relative proportion of different leukocyte subsets, there is no evidence that these differences translate into differences in clinical outcome. The next several years are likely to see improved methods for chemically fixing cells so that samples can be transported to central sites for testing. The development of standardized concentrations of cells and cooperative proficiency testing programs are underway, especially in the United Kingdom.

Prestorage, Poststorage, or Bedside Leukoreduction

Leukocyte reduction by means of filtration can be performed at three different points in time—before storage, after storage before issue from the blood bank, and at the bedside. Bedside filtration was the first approach to leukocyte reduction and has been shown in clinical studies to be highly effective for the prevention of febrile reactions to red blood cell concentrates. Although bedside filtration is probably effective for prevention of CMV transmission, one study concluded that it was not effective for prevention of HLA alloimmunization (19). Bedside filtration has several disadvantages compared with laboratory filtration. These include reduced performance and poor quality control. In addition, there is evidence that febrile reactions to platelet concentrates may be more effectively prevented if leukocytes are removed before storage. Moreover, for some recipients taking angiotensin-converting enzyme (ACE) inhibitors, bedside filtration has been associated with hypotensive transfusion reactions. The principal advantage of leukoreduction at the bedside is that filters are used only for selected patients, and thus the cost of filtration is restricted.

Poststorage leukocyte reduction is filtration of components before issue from the blood bank. This approach allows development of an inventory of leukoreduced blood. Poststorage filtration is easy to standardize, can be incorporated into the laboratory procedure in a manner similar to that for other manipulations of blood components, and is easily adapted into a program of process control. For platelet concentrates, poststorage leukoreduction has the disadvantage that cytokines can accumulate during storage and are not removed by filtration. For red blood cell concentrates, there is no known disadvantage to poststorage leukoreduction.

Prestorage leukocyte reduction during or soon after component preparation is becoming the preferred method of leukoreduction and is ideally suited to process control. Opinions differ as to the definition of prestorage leukoreduction, but the FDA has suggested that 72 hours be used as the time from collection to filtration. For platelet concentrates, numerous investigators have documented that inflammatory cytokines including interleukin-1 (IL-1), tumor necrosis factor (TNF), and IL-6 can accumulate during storage in some units. The extent of cytokine accumulation correlates with the leukocyte content of the unit and the duration of room temperature storage. For some transfusion recipients, the passively transferred cytokines result in FNH reactions (see later). Prestorage leukoreduction of platelet concentrates prevents accumulation of these cytokines. There is speculation that prestorage leukoreduction would have additional advantages by preventing transfusion of leukocyte fragments that would otherwise develop during storage. Results of laboratory studies and preclinical animal studies have suggested that leukocyte breakdown may contribute to HLA alloimmunization (20), release of intracellular viruses (21), and immunosuppression (22). However, none of these effects has been documented in clinical trials. Results of a large, randomized, controlled study conducted in Europe with patients undergoing cardiac surgery showed no advantage of prestorage leukoreduced red blood cell concentrate over poststorage leukoreduced red blood cell concentrate for the prevention of postoperative infection, multiple organ failure, or death (23). Nevertheless, prestorage leukoreduction is evolving as the standard method.

CLINICAL INDICATIONS FOR LEUKOREDUCTION

The clinical indications for the use of leukocyte-reduced blood components continue to evolve. New higher-performance filters, the perception of clinical benefit, and the increasing use of prestorage leukoreduction have resulted in greater use of leukoreduced components. There has been considerable debate concerning whether all cellular blood components should undergo leukoreduction. Evidence-based clinical indications for the use of leukoreduced blood have been proposed (1) and are listed in Table 21.4. In October 2000, the University Health Consortium concluded that the available evidence was insufficient to recommend universal leukoreduction. In contrast, the U.S. Blood Safety and Availability Committee recommended in January 2001 that universal leukoreduction be implemented as "soon as is feasible." A recent large randomized prospective clinical trial was unable to demonstrate clinical benefit from conversion from selective leukoreduction to universal leukoreduction (82).

Reduction in Febrile Nonhemolytic Transfusion Reactions

Reduction in the rate of recurrent FNH reactions to red blood cell concentrates was among the earliest applications of leukocyte reduction. Washed red blood cells, frozen deglycerolized red blood cells, and red blood cells filtered through microaggregate blood filters all were effective at preventing FNH reactions. This success was based in large part on the fact that FNH reactions may be prevented with blood containing fewer than 5×10^8 WBCs per transfusion. This value represents 100-fold more leukocytes than a widely used benchmark for prevention of HLA

TABLE 21.4. CLINICAL INDICATIONS FOR LEUKOREDUCED BLOOD COMPONENTS

Established indications
Reduce frequency of recurrent febrile nonhemolytic transfusion reactions to red blood cells
Reduce rate of alloimmunization to leukocyte antigens for patients with hematologic malignant disease
Reduce risk of transmission of cytomegalovirus among persons at risk of infection by transfusion
Indications under investigation[a]
Prevention of bleeding due to platelet refractoriness
Prevention of postoperative bacterial infection
Prevention of immune modulation leading to tumor recurrence
Prevention of bacterial overgrowth of *Yersinia enterocolitica* in stored red blood cells
Contraindications[b]
Prevention of transfusion-associated graft-versus-host disease
Prevention of transfusion-related acute lung injury due to passive infusion of leukocyte antibody
Prevention of the red blood cell or platelet storage lesion
Prevention of viral reactivation among patients with human immunodeficiency virus infection

[a]Inadequate evidence to suggest benefit from leukoreduction.
[b]Evidence demonstrates no benefit of leukoreduction.

alloimmunization or CMV transmission—$<5 \times 10^6$ per transfusion.

Mechanisms of Febrile Nonhemolytic Reactions

At least three mechanisms may account for the development of FNH reactions (Fig. 21.4) (see Chapter 58). The final pathway for all three mechanisms is the elaboration of inflammatory cytokines such as IL-1 or TNF. These cytokines react with cell surface receptors in the hypothalamus and stimulate prostaglandin and leukotriene-mediated pathways that reset the thermoregulatory center of the brain.

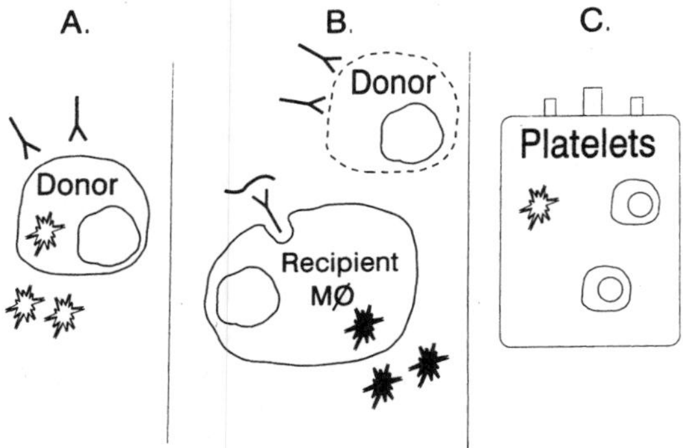

FIGURE 21.4. Three mechanisms for the development of febrile nonhemolytic reactions. **A:** Donor cells react with recipient antileukocyte antibody and cause a release of interleukin of donor origin. **B:** Donor cells react with recipient antibody and form antigen-antibody complexes that react with recipient monocytes to result in the release of recipient interleukin. **C:** Residual donor leukocytes present in platelet concentrates during storage release interleukin passively transfused to the recipient.

One mechanism of FNH reactions involves recipient antibodies reacting with donor leukocytes and stimulating the release of endogenous pyrogens (cytokines) from the donor cells. This mechanism is consistent with the prevention of FNH reactions by leukoreduction of donor blood and with the results of studies by Perkins et al. (24) and Brubaker (25) that documented the high prevalence of antilymphocyte or antigranulocyte antibodies in the sera of patients who experienced FNH reactions. The mechanism does not explain all FNH reactions, however. Patients with antibodies to platelet-specific antigens have febrile reactions when they receive transfusions of leukocyte-reduced platelet concentrates.

A second proposed mechanism for FNH reactions suggests that inflammatory cytokines are released by recipient cells in response to antigen-antibody complexes formed when incompatible donor cells are transfused into patients with reacting antibodies (26). This mechanism is consistent with the role of recipient antibodies, with the ease of preventing FNH reactions to red blood cell concentrates, and with the difficulty of preventing these reactions among alloimmunized patients receiving platelet concentrates. This mechanism also accounts for the fever and chills accompanying hemolytic transfusion reactions.

A third mechanism of FNH reactions is based on the passive transfer of inflammatory cytokines that accumulate in platelet concentrates during storage. Several investigators have found detectable levels of IL-1, TNF, and IL-6 in platelet concentrates after several days of storage (27). These substances do not accumulate in platelet concentrates that have undergone prestorage leukocyte reduction or in platelet concentrates prepared from buffy coats. Of note, the accumulation of IL-1 and TNF in platelet concentrates does not occur if platelet concentrates are stored at refrigerated temperatures (28). This may explain why IL-1 does not accumulate in red blood cell concentrates and may account for the relative ease of preventing FNH reactions to red blood cell concentrates.

Clinical evidence that FNH reactions to platelet concentrates result from passive transfer of cytokines was presented by Heddle et al. (29). They prepared pools of whole-blood platelet concentrates using 4- to 5-day-old concentrates. Before transfusion, the pooled platelet concentrates were subjected to centrifugation and the plasma supernatant was transferred to a sterile bag. The platelet pellet was then resuspended in fresh frozen plasma. The supernatant from the pool and the resuspended platelets were then transfused in random order with 2-hour intervals between transfusions. Among 64 paired transfusions, patients reacted to plasma alone in 20 instances, to resuspended cells alone in 6 instances, to both members of the pair in 8 instances, and to neither product in 30 instances. The severity of the reactions to the plasma supernatant correlated with the level of IL-1β and IL-6 present in the plasma. Although 34 transfusion pairs were associated with reactions, it is important to note that only 7 (20%) actually involved a temperature increase more than 1°C. However, the patients were given premedication with acetaminophen, which may have obscured the clinical signs and symptoms. The passive transfer of cytokines accumulated during storage of platelet concentrate may explain FNH reactions that occur in the absence of detectable antileukocyte or antiplatelet antibodies or the absence of a history of previous transfusions or

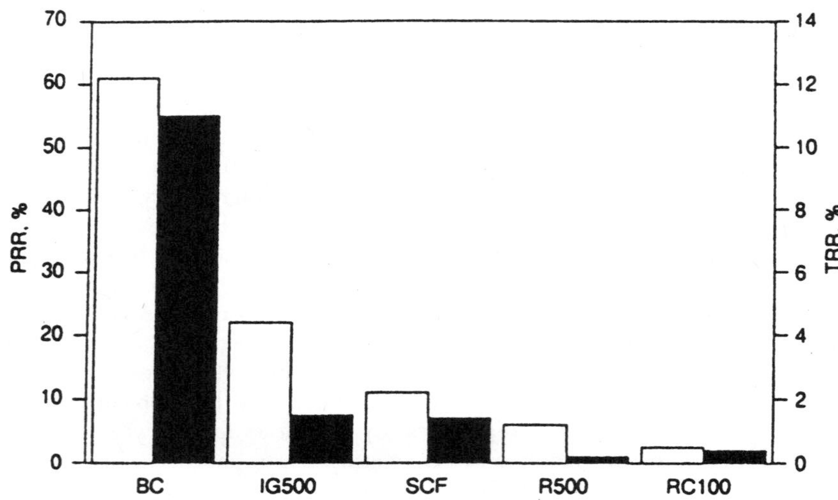

FIGURE 21.5. The incidence of febrile nonhemolytic reactions among 82 patients with thalassemia undergoing long-term transfusion therapy. The patient reaction rate (*PRR*) is shown in the *white bars* and the transfusion reaction rate in the *black bars.* Reaction rates from *left to right* parallel the use of improved filters over time. *BC,* Buffy coat removal only; *IG500,* Terumo filter; *SCF,* spin-cool filter (microaggregate filter); *R500,* Asahi filter; *RC100,* Pall filter. (From Sirchia G, Rebulla P, Parravicini A. Leukocyte depletion of red cells. In: Lane TA, Myllyla G, eds. *Leukocyte-depleted blood products: current studies in hematology and blood transfusion.* Basel: Karger, 1994: 60.)

pregnancies. It is also consistent with the observation that the incidence of FNH reactions to platelet concentrates increases with increasing duration of storage (30,31).

Clinical Studies of Leukoreduction and Febrile Nonhemolytic Reactions

Clinical experience has documented that modern leukoreduction filters effectively reduce but do not eliminate FNH reactions to red blood cell concentrates. Patients with thalassemia major have a lifelong transfusion requirement, are not otherwise immunosuppressed, and do not have the confounding clinical circumstances present among patients receiving oncologic chemotherapy. For such selected patients, leukoreduction filters have been particularly effective (Fig. 21.5).

In contrast to the experience with red blood cell concentrates, leukoreduction has proved less successful for the prevention of FNH reactions to platelet concentrates. Consistent with the role of passively transferred cytokines as mediators of reactions to platelet concentrates, Mangano et al. (32), Goodnough et al. (33), and Mintz (34) found that bedside leukoreduction of platelet concentrates did not substantially reduce the rate of FNH reactions. In contrast, prestorage leukoreduction of platelet concentrates is expected to result in a greater reduction in the rate of FNH reactions (35). However, in the Trial to Reduce Alloimmunization to Platelets (TRAP), there was no difference in the rate of reported transfusion reactions among patients randomly assigned to support with leukoreduced apheresis platelets (prestorage leukoreduction), leukoreduced pooled platelets (poststorage leukoreduction), or nonleukoreduced pooled platelets (36).

Reduction in HLA Alloimmunization

Leukocyte reduction is commonly used in an attempt to prevent alloimmunization to donor HLA antigens. Prevention of alloimmunization is of clear clinical value for patients awaiting renal transplantation and those with aplastic anemia awaiting bone marrow transplantation (BMT) (37). In addition, much attention has been given to the prevention of alloimmunization among patients undergoing chemotherapy. In 33 studies involving more than 3,000 patients, the median reported incidence of HLA alloimmunization when unmodified components were used was 39% (range, 20% to 71%). The use of leukoreduced components is expected to reduce the incidence of HLA alloimmunization and subsequent platelet refractoriness. Reduced refractoriness is expected to decrease morbidity or mortality caused by bleeding, but this has not yet been documented in any clinical trials.

The threshold level of leukocytes needed to provoke primary HLA alloimmunization is generally regarded to be 1 to 5 $\times$ 10^6 per transfusion. Fisher et al. (38) administered transfusions of small doses of platelet concentrate to two groups of 12 patients undergoing dialysis on three occasions at 14-day intervals. Five of 12 patients given a mean of 15 $\times$ 10^6 WBCs per transfusion made HLA antibodies, and none of 12 given fewer than 5 $\times$ 10^6 WBCs per transfusion made HLA antibodies. Although this study had numerous serious design flaws, results of a subsequent study by van Marwijk-Kooy et al. (39) also suggested that 5 $\times$ 10^6 represented a threshold dose for alloimmunization. In a prospective trial, patients with leukemia received filtered buffy coat–depleted red blood cell concentrates and were then randomized to receive either centrifuged platelet concentrates (mean WBC content, 35 $\times$ 10^6) or filtered platelet concentrates (mean WBC content 5 $\times$ 10^6). Clinical refractoriness occurred in 46% of those given centrifuged platelet concentrates but in only 11% of those given filtered platelet concentrates. Although significant individual variation is likely, 5 $\times$ 10^6 WBCs per transfusion was adopted during the 1990s as the standard for leukoreduced blood components. However, the threshold level was set at 1 $\times$ 10^6 WBCs per transfusion in Europe. In 2001 the FDA proposed a similar threshold level for the United States (15).

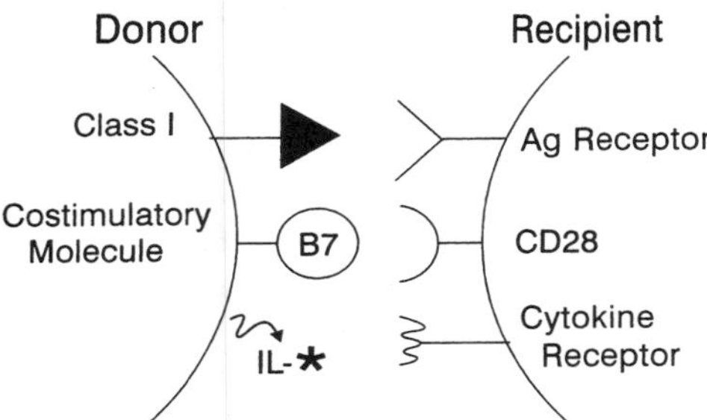

FIGURE 21.6. Direct HLA alloimmunization to class I antigen. The recipient cell directly recognizes foreign class I provided that a second costimulatory molecule also is expressed and provided that the appropriate cytokine is locally present. *Ag,* antigen.

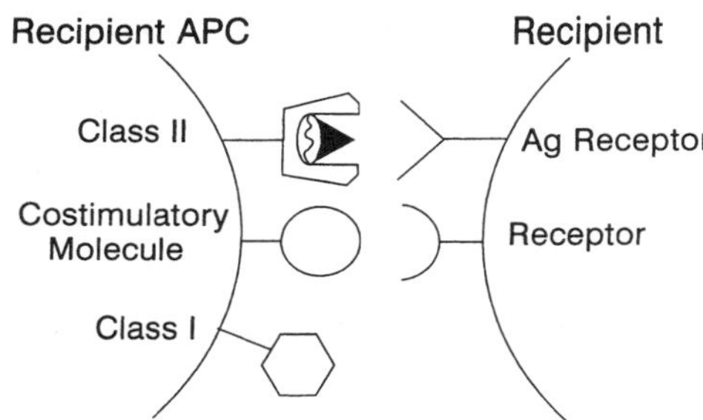

FIGURE 21.8. Indirect HLA alloimmunization to class I antigen. Recipient antigen presenting cells (*APC*) have digested donor cells or cell fragments and deposited a fragment of donor class I antigen in the peptide-binding groove of the recipient class II molecule.

Mechanism by Which Leukoreduction Decreases the Rate of HLA Alloimmunization

Decades of research provide unequivocal evidence that passenger leukocytes, which express donor HLA antigens, are a prime cause of recipient sensitization to HLA alloantigens. Experiments by Claas et al. (40) with a rodent transfusion model showed that residual donor leukocytes provoked major histocompatibility complex (MHC) alloimmunization and that leukoreduction could decrease the incidence of primary sensitization to MHC antigens. These investigators further documented that even very low numbers of donor leukocytes in previously sensitized animals induced secondary immunization, suggesting that leukoreduction would be less effective in the previously sensitized patient. The importance of donor leukocytes was confirmed in experiments by Kao (41) and Blajchman et al. (20), who also provided evidence for the possible role of antigens on microparticles in plasma (42).

Alloimmunization can occur by means of both direct and indirect immune recognition. Direct allorecognition is the process by which recipient immune cells respond directly to donor HLA antigens without the processing of donor antigens by recipient antigen-presenting cells (APCs) (Figs. 21.6, 21.7). The mixed lymphocyte reaction is an in vitro example of direct T-cell recognition. Direct allosensitization requires at least three fundamental elements—binding of the antigen to the antigen receptor, binding of costimulatory molecules mediating cell-cell contact, and local elaboration of cytokines and appropriate cytokine receptors. Recipients may recognize intact class I structures on the surface of donor leukocytes (Fig 21.6). An alternative explantation is that class II–positive donor cells may carry, within the peptide-binding groove, oligopeptides that represent the cell's own HLA class I antigen (Fig 21.7). In either case, depletion of donor class II–positive cells would reduce the chance of direct HLA immunization to class I antigens. The failure of the recipient to recognize donor class I antigens on platelets may reflect the fact that platelets lack critical costimulatory molecules required for direct allostimulation.

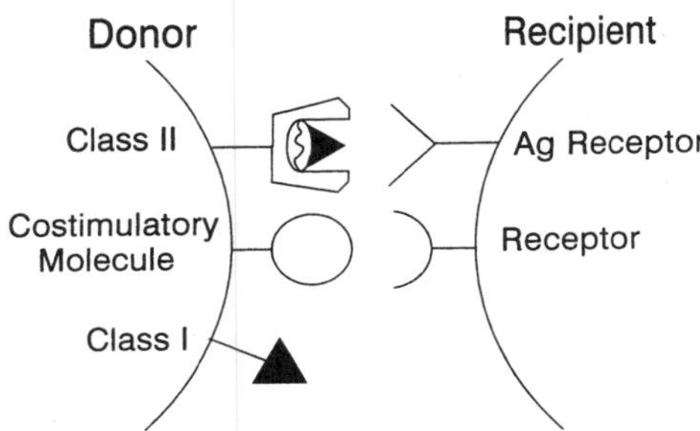

FIGURE 21.7. Direct HLA alloimmunization to class I antigen. The donor cell carries a fragment of its class I molecule within the peptide-binding groove of its own class II molecule. This model, suggested by the author of this chapter, provides one hypothesis to explain the frequency with which transfusion of unmodified cellular components results in antibodies to HLA class I. *Ag,* antigen; *IL,* interleukin.

Indirect allorecognition is the process by which recipient APCs first engulf donor cells and then process donor antigen for redisplay to the recipient immune system. Donor cells, cell fragments, or soluble donor antigens are engulfed and degraded within lysozymes of the recipient APCs. Small peptide fragments corresponding to the alloantigenic region of donor HLA are then deposited in the peptide-binding groove of class II structures on recipient APCs (Fig. 21.8). Recipient T and B cells then interact with recipient APCs in an MHC-restricted manner and respond to the donor peptide antigens displayed by the APCs. Indirect immune recognition is unlikely to account for the initial response in an in vitro mixed leukocyte reaction. However, the indirect pathway may be particularly relevant for secondary immune responses observed in vivo after transfusion. In addition, the indirect pathway may account for experimental evidence in favor of alloimmunization by donor cell microparticles.

Antibodies to Public versus Private HLA Antigens

Broad platelet alloimmunization can be measured by the percentage of a random lymphocyte panel to which the patient's serum will react—a percentage referred to as *percent reactive antibody* (PRA). Patients with a PRA greater than 60% to 80% do not achieve good posttransfusion increments with unselected platelet concentrate transfusions. Patients with a PRA greater than 95% are difficult to support with platelet transfusion. Although it is commonly thought that such patients have formed a large number of antibodies directed against different HLA antigens, study of patient sera suggests that these patients have formed antibodies directed against one or two HLA antigens that are highly prevalent. These common HLA antigens are called *public antigens.* For example, Duquesnoy et al. (43) analyzed sera from 132 highly immunized patients awaiting renal transplantation who had received numerous transfusions. Among those with 90% to 100% PRA, reactions could be accounted for by one or two antibody specificities in most (80%) of the patients. Only 10% of patients had more than three antibody specificities in their sera. The importance of public specificities in HLA alloimmunization among patients with hematologic disorders was reported by MacPherson et al. (44), who found public antibodies in 15 of 18 patients with a high PRA. This phenomenon explains why transfusion strategies that rely on limiting the number of donors (e.g., apheresis platelet concentrates) do not protect against broad HLA alloimmunization. Immunization to public antigens also emphasizes the importance of limiting the incidence of leukoreduction failures to prevent HLA alloimmunization.

Clinical Trials of the Prevention of HLA Alloimmunization by Leukocyte Reduction

A large number of clinical trials have investigated the usefulness of leukoreduction in the prevention of HLA alloimmunization and refractoriness. These studies have been reviewed by Heddle (45) and by Vamvakas (46). As of 2001, reports of 11 randomized, controlled clinical trials had been published (Table 21.5). Typically, in these trials patients with hematologic malignant disease were randomized to receive either filtered or unfiltered blood components. Filters have ranged from early devices that achieved only 1 to 1.5 log reduction in residual leukocytes to more recent filters that are capable of at least 3-log reduction. Some investigators measured the residual WBC content after filtration, whereas others assumed that patients in the filtration arm received components that had been adequately leukoreduced. Some investigators used in-laboratory leukocyte reduction, whereas others used bedside leukocyte filtration. Patients were followed with periodic measurement of HLA antibodies. The details of HLA antibody detection and the criteria for labeling a patient as alloimmunized varied among different clinical trials. Once a patient met the study criteria for alloimmunization, some trials censored the patient from further analysis in the study, whereas others continued to collect data on the patient. Because of these differences in study design and execution, strict comparison of the current randomized trials must be cautious. With these limitations, metaanalysis has identified a reduction in alloimmunization with leukoreduction for patients with hematologic malignant disease (45,46). There is insufficient evidence to demonstrate a beneficial effect of leukoreduction for the prevention of HLA alloimmunization among less immunosuppressed transfusion recipients.

The TRAP was the largest randomized trial to test the effect of leukoreduction for prevention of HLA alloimmunization (36). Five hundred thirty patients undergoing initial therapy for acute leukemia were randomized to one of four arms—pooled whole blood platelets (control), leukoreduced pooled whole blood platelets, leukoreduced apheresis platelets, and ultraviolet B–irradiated pooled platelets. All red blood cell products were leukoreduced. Patients were evaluated for 8 weeks. Blood products were leukoreduced in the laboratory under process control. Overall, 3% of transfusions were not of the assigned group. Alloimmunization was defined as cytotoxicity against one or

TABLE 21.5. PROSPECTIVE, CONTROLLED CLINICAL TRIALS OF LEUKOREDUCTION TO DECREASE HLA ALLOIMMUNIZATION

		Method of Leukoreduction		All Patients		Previously Immunized	
Author	Diagnosis	RBCs	PLTs	Control	Leukoreduced	Control	Leukoreduced
Elghouzzi	Solid tumor	Cellselect	None	26/93 (0.28)	10/67 (0.15)	27/73 (0.32)	10/52 (0.19)
Schiffer	AML	Deglyced	Pooled	13/31 (0.42)	5/25 (0.20)	9/19 (0.47)	1/10 (0.10)
Andreu	Heme malignancy	IG 500	IG 500	11/35 (0.31)	4/34 (0.12)	4/14 (0.28)	2/13 (0.15)
Sniecinski	AML, ALL, AA	IG 500	IG 500	10/20 (0.50)	3/20 (0.15)	6/12 (0.50)	2/10 (0.20)
Rebulla	AML, ALL	Cellselect	IG 500	5/15 (0.33)	4/16 (0.25)	2/5 (0.40)	2/4 (0.50)
van Marwjik	AML, ALL	Cellselect	Cellselect	11/26 (0.42)	2/27 (0.07)	2/6 (0.33)	1/5 (0.20)
Oksanen	AML, ALL BMT	Cellselect	IG 500	3/15 (0.20)	2/16 (0.12)	1/3 (0.33)	1/4 (0.25)
Handa	Heme malignancy	R500	PL10N	9/23 (0.39)	4/49 (0.08)	4/6 (0.66)	1/20 (0.05)
Lane	AML, CLL, CML	Filtration	Filtration	7/20 (0.35)	3/26 (0.11)	4/10 (0.40)	3/9 (0.33)
Williamson	Heme malignancy	Filtration	Filtration	21/56 (0.37)	15/67 (0.22)	—	—
Sintnicolaas	AML	Filtration	Filtration	—	—	9/21 (0.43)	11/25 (0.44)
TRAP	AML	Filtration	Filtration	59/131 (0.45)	25/137 (0.18)	30/48 (0.62)	17/53 (0.33)

Numbers in table are the proportion (%) demonstrating HLA antibodies.
RBCs, red blood cells; PLTs, platelets; AML, acute myelogenous leukemia; ALL, acute lymphocytic leukemia; AA, aplastic anemia; BMT, bone marrow transplantation; CLL, chronic lymphocytic leukemia; CML, chronic myelogenous leukemia.
Data derived from Heddle NM. The efficacy of leukoreduction to improve platelet transfusion response: a critical appraisal of clinical studies. *Tranfus Med Rev* 1994;8:15–28 and Vamvakas E. Meta-analysis of randomized controlled trials of the efficiency of white cell reduction in preventing HLA-alloimmunization and refractoriness to random-donor platelet transfusions. *Transfus Med Rev* 1998;12:258–270.

more wells of a 30- to 60-cell target HLA antibody panel. Seventy-five percent of patients had received transfusions (mostly nonleukoreduced) during the 2 weeks before enrollment and randomization. The results showed that platelet refractoriness was infrequent (10%) and was similar for all four treatment arms. Lymphocytotoxic antibodies developed in 45% of patients supported with nonleukoreduced pooled platelets compared with 21% in the ultraviolet B group, 18% in the group receiving leukoreduced pooled platelets, and 17% in the group receiving leukoreduced apheresis platelets. All three treatment groups had significantly lower rates of alloimmunization than did controls. The three treatment groups, however, had similar results; that is, no advantage of prestorage leukoreduced apheresis platelets over poststorage leukoreduced pooled platelets. It is also noteworthy that alloimmunization was defined as reactivity against a single target cell and so should not be confused with broad alloimmunization. Finally, the study was limited to 8 weeks; long-term rates of alloimmunization were not determined.

Will Leukocyte Reduction Prevent Secondary Alloimmunization?

Because a secondary or anamnestic immune response requires a far smaller antigenic challenge than does a primary response, the secondary antibody recall to MHC antigens is difficult to prevent with leukoreduced blood components (40). Most clinical studies of HLA alloimmunization have included patients with previous exposure to transfusion or pregnancy. Therefore, the issue of secondary alloimmunization seldom has been independently addressed. However, subgroup analysis of studies listed in Table 21.5 showed a higher rate of sensitization among pregnant patients or those who previously have received transfusions. The issue of secondary alloimmunization was directly addressed in the study by Sintnicolaas et al. (47). Female patients (n = 75) with hematologic malignant disease and a history of previous pregnancy were randomized to receive platelet concentrate support with either unmodified or leukoreduced apheresis platelet concentrates. Among the evaluable patients, HLA alloimmunization developed in 43% (9 of 21) of the standard platelet concentrate group and in 44% (11 of 25) of the filtration group. Refractoriness occurred in 41% (14 of 34) of women in the standard platelet concentrate group and in 29% (8 of 28) of the filtration group ($P = .52$). The time to development of refractoriness was similar in the two groups. The authors concluded that leukoreduction to fewer than 5×10^6 WBCs per transfusion did not prevent alloimmunization and refractoriness among previously sensitized recipients.

In the TRAP, however, analysis of patients who had been previously pregnant showed some benefit, albeit decreased, from the use of leukoreduced blood. In that study, 62% of patients with a history of pregnancy had HLA alloantibodies after transfusion of routine components; 33% did so after transfusion of leukoreduced components (36). Thus it appears that patients with hematologic malignant disease and a history of exposure to foreign HLA antigens from previous transfusion or pregnancy derive diminished benefit from the use of leukoreduced components. This benefit may not extend to patients with diagnoses other than hematologic malignant disease.

Will Prevention of Alloimmunization Decrease Bleeding Complications Caused by Platelet Refractoriness?

Although the clinical trials conducted to date provide meaningful information on the prevention of HLA alloimmunization by means of leukocyte reduction, measurement of alloimmunization is a poor proxy for prevention of bleeding caused by immune-mediated refractoriness and is no proxy for bleeding due to nonimmune causes (45). In addition, because bleeding is not limited to refractory patients, prevention of refractoriness will not prevent all bleeding complications. Finally, because serious bleeding complications are infrequent even when unmodified (nonleukoreduced) blood components are used, the potential gain resulting from the prevention of alloimmunization is small. These three factors make the clinical importance of leukocyte filtration technology difficult to assess. For example, in one study, 486 patients undergoing BMT were prospectively randomized to receive support with either filtered or unfiltered blood components to analyze the effect of filtration on transmission of CMV (9). Even among BMT patients who were at high risk of fatal bleeding complications, there was no difference in overall early mortality between the two treatment arms. Thus leukocyte filtration was not likely to have substantially affected the rate of fatal bleeding episodes. Similarly, the large TRAP was unable to demonstrate that the use of leukoreduced blood conferred any advantage to prevent bleeding due to HLA refractoriness. Moreover, survival rates, remission rates, and blood component support all were unaffected by leukoreduction. Because of the low incidence of bleeding due to platelet refractoriness, prevention of HLA alloimmunization by means of leukoreduction may not be cost-effective. For example, if one assumes that 2% of patients have serious bleeding with standard blood component support (45), that 75% of these events are caused by refractory states (only one-half of which are attributable to HLA antibodies), and that filtration can reduce the incidence of HLA alloimmunization 50% (45), then only 1 in 265 patients derives benefit. At $30 per filter and 33 transfusions per patient (36) ($1,000 per patient course), the cost to prevent a single episode of bleeding (not necessarily even associated with morbidity) would be more than $250,000. Thus leukoreduction has been shown to decrease the rate of HLA alloimmunization, but the effect on patient outcome has not been adequately assessed.

Reduced Risk of Transmission of Cytomegalovirus and Other Leukotropic Viruses

The human leukotropic viruses—CMV, Epstein-Barr virus, and human T-cell lymphotropic virus (HTLV-I/II)—reside within the leukocytes of infected individuals. These viruses are found in such a low copy number outside of cells that plasma from infected donors does not transmit infection. Unlike human immunodeficiency virus (HIV), these three viruses are not present in platelets. Thus substantial leukocyte reduction of blood components would be expected to prevent transmission of CMV, Epstein-Barr virus, and HTLV through blood transfusion. Epstein-Barr virus and HTLV viruses are rarely clinically important

TABLE 21.6. CLINICAL TRIALS OF CYTOMEGALOVIRUS PREVENTION BY LEUKOREDUCTION

			Method of Leukoreduction		No. of CMV Seroconversions	
Author	Design	Diagnosis	RBCs	PLTs	Unmodified	Leukoreduced
Murphy	Retrospective	Leukemia	Bedside filter	Centrifuge	2/9 (22)	0/11 (0)
Graan-Hentzen	Retrospective	Mixed	Bedside filter	Centrifuge	10/86 (12)	0/59 (0)
Eisenfield	Retrospective	Newborn	Bedside filter	—	—	0/48 (0)
Gilbert	Prospective randomized	Newborn	Bedside filter	—	9/42 (21)	0/30 (0)
Verdonck	Prospective	Auto/allo BMT	Filter	—	—	0/29 (0)
De Witte	Prospective	Allo BMT	Filter	Centrifuge	—	0/28 (0)
Bowden	Prospective randomized	Auto/allo BMT	Bedside filter	Centrifuge	7/30 (23)	0/35 (0)
Bowden	Prospective randomized	Auto/allo BMT	Bedside filter	Bedside filter	3/246 (1)	5/241 (2)

Values in parentheses are percentages.
RBCs, red blood cells; PLTs, platelets; CMV, cytomegalovirus; BMT, bone marrow transplantation.
Data derived from Bowden RA, Slichter SJ, Sayers M, et al. A comparison of filtered leukocyte-reduced and cytomegalovirus (CMV) seronegative blood products for the prevention of transfusion-associated CMV infection after marrow transplant. @TFN:*Blood* 1995;86:3599–3603 and Hillyer CD, Emmens RK, Zago-Novaretti M, et al. Methods for the reduction of transfusion-transmitted cytomegalovirus infection: filtration versus the use of seronegative donor units. *Transfusion* 1994;34:929–934.

transfusion-transmitted pathogens. In contrast, CMV is an important pathogen for immunosuppressed recipients and has been the subject of several clinical trials of leukoreduced blood components (9,48) (Table 21.6). In evaluating such trials, it is important to recognize that many patients, even if immunosuppressed, do not acquire primary CMV infection from unmodified blood transfusions. This may be attributed to the fact that among healthy blood donors only a small minority of leukocytes (estimated at less than 0.2%) carry CMV. Sensitive PCR techniques are needed to demonstrate the CMV genome in the blood of seropositive healthy donors. In one study, the PCR signal was removed when blood was leukoreduced by means of filtration (49). In the clinical trials described later, a distinction is drawn between CMV infection defined by laboratory evidence of viral infection and CMV disease defined by symptomatic infection.

Collection of blood from donors with negative test results for antibodies to CMV has been a traditional method to decrease the risk of transfusion-transmitted CMV. Although the use of CMV-seronegative blood has been shown to be an effective prevention strategy, the widely used term *CMV-negative* is an unfortunate one because it can be misinterpreted to mean the absence of CMV virus. Studies have documented that as many as 55% of CMV-seronegative donations have detectable CMV virus when tested by means of PCR (50). Thus the term *CMV reduced risk* is better than either *CMV negative* or *CMV safe.*

Transfusion-transmitted Cytomegalovirus among Low-birth-weight Neonates

Term neonates of normal birth weight with normal immunity do not acquire serious CMV disease as a result of exposure to blood components. However, low-birth-weight premature neonates, who frequently need small-volume blood transfusions, are at risk of CMV disease (see Chapter 52). Consequently, all low-birth-weight infants are appropriate candidates for strategies to prevent CMV transmission by means of transfusion. Because these infants are at times given fresh blood, protection against CMV resulting from leukocyte apoptosis during refrigerated storage is diminished. Early studies showed that the use of frozen deglycerolized red blood cell concentrates decreased the rate of transmission of CMV among at-risk neonates (51,52). As high-performance leukocyte removal filters replaced freezing technology, studies were performed to document the effectiveness of leukocyte depletion to prevent CMV transmission to at-risk neonates. Gilbert et al. (53) conducted a prospective, randomized, blinded trial in which 515 newborns were randomized to receive transfusion support with either unmodified red blood cell concentrates or red blood cell concentrates filtered through an IG500 (Terumo Corporation) filter capable of 1- to 1.5-log leukocyte removal. In the control arm, 29 infants weighed less than 1,500 g, and CMV infection developed in 9 (33%). In the filtration arm, among 24 neonates weighing less than 1,500 g who were CMV seronegative and received CMV-seropositive filtered blood, none acquired CMV infection. In another study, Eisenfield et al. (54) used less advanced filtration technology and documented prevention of CMV transmission to at-risk neonates. Because current filters are considerably more effective at leukocyte reduction than were those used in the studies, it is likely that filtration technology is completely adequate to prevent CMV transmission to at-risk neonates. The presence of a passively transferred antibody must be considered in interpretation of the results of CMV serologic testing after transfusion.

Transfusion-transmitted Cytomegalovirus after Bone Marrow Transplantation

Patients undergoing allogeneic BMT are at great risk of CMV infection and disease because of the intense immunosuppression needed for marrow engraftment and the persistent defects in cellular and humoral immunity resulting from the chimeric immune system present after transplantation. In this setting, uncontrolled CMV infection can represent a devastating illness with a high mortality. As a result, CMV-seronegative recipients of CMV-seronegative bone marrow should be protected from transfusion-transmitted CMV. When either the donor or the recipient is seropositive for CMV, the role of transfusion-transmitted CMV becomes much less important. In these latter cases, there is little evidence that the use of CMV-reduced risk blood components has any substantial clinical benefit.

For CMV-seronegative donor-recipient pairs, the traditional approach has been to use seronegative donor blood. Early reports documented that leukocyte filtration was an alternative approach to prevent transfusion-transmitted CMV infection among patients undergoing allogeneic BMT (2). The results of these studies were consistent with those of studies conducted with neonates. They showed that prevention of CMV transmission with use of platelet concentrates does not require extensive leukocyte reduction. Bowden et al. (9) conducted a large, randomized, prospective trial with CMV-negative patients who received transplants of CMV-negative bone marrow. The investigators compared support with CMV-seronegative blood with support with filtered blood from untested donors. They randomized 502 CMV-seronegative patients undergoing autologous or allogeneic BMT. Among 252 patients receiving CMV-seronegative blood components, two had CMV infection; none had CMV disease. Among 250 patients receiving filtered CMV-untested components, three CMV infections (three with CMV disease) were observed. Two additional CMV infections in the seronegative group and three in the filtration group occurred within 21 days of entrance to the study and were considered the result of transfusions before enrollment. The survival rate was equal in the two study arms.

Several features of the study by Bowden et al. (9) affect interpretation of the results. First, the filters used were not as effective as current devices. Second, filtration was conducted at the bedside under conditions now known to decrease filter performance. Third, patients could receive up to six units of blood to which they were not assigned (protocol violations) and still have the outcome included in the results. Although most observers interpreted this study to show no significant difference between the two strategies of CMV prevention, the results sparked controversy over the relative merits of the two methods. Subsequent advances in the performance of leukoreduction, application of laboratory process control, and recognition that many CMV-seronegative donors have positive results of PCR tests suggest that leukoreduction has become a standard method for preparation of CMV reduced-risk blood.

Transfusion-transmitted Cytomegalovirus among Recipients of Solid Organ Transplants

Although the morbidity and mortality associated with CMV among recipients of solid-organ transplants are not as severe as they are among recipients of allogeneic BMT, CMV still represents a serious infectious complication of solid-organ transplantation. In addition, CMV infection can promote rejection of the allograft. Because the graft is the most common site of post-transplantation CMV infection, the distinction between rejection and CMV infection can be difficult. Glomerulopathy, vanishing bile duct syndrome, accelerated atherosclerosis, and obliterative bronchiolitis may be the renal, hepatic, cardiac, and lung allograft expressions of CMV infection. The dominant factors controlling the development of CMV infection after transplantation are the serologic status of the organ donor and recipient and the degree of immunosuppression of the recipient (55–57). There is no evidence that patients who are CMV seropositive benefit from use of seronegative or leukoreduced blood components. Although infection with a second strain of CMV transmitted by blood transfusion is theoretically possible, there are no published reports of second-strain infections attributable to blood transfusion. Patients who are CMV seronegative and who receive organs from CMV-seropositive donors are at the greatest risk of postoperative CMV disease and acquire the infection from the allograft. Thus prevention of transfusion-transmitted CMV is currently an appropriate consideration only for CMV-seronegative recipients of allografts from CMV-seronegative donors.

No results of prospective, randomized trials document that leukoreduction prevents transfusion-transmitted CMV infection among seronegative recipients of seronegative solid organs. Experience with neonates, patients with hematologic malignant disease, and patients undergoing BMT, however, suggests it is highly likely that CMV-seronegative and leukoreduced blood are equivalent means to prevent transfusion-transmitted CMV infection. Liver transplantation often requires massive transfusion support, but the attack rate for transfusion-transmitted CMV in liver transplantation is very low. It is not practical to restrict these patients to seronegative or leukocyte-reduced blood components. For example, the deliberate use of CMV-untested, nonleukoreduced blood in the care of CMV-seronegative patients receiving CMV-seronegative liver allografts resulted in only a 10% incidence of CMV disease and no deaths attributed to CMV infection (2).

INVESTIGATIVE APPLICATIONS OF LEUKOREDUCTION

Viral Reactivation

Results of preclinical studies suggested that recipient exposure to allogeneic donor leukocytes might promote activation of latent recipient viruses. Research has focused on CMV and HIV. As early as 1972, Lang (58) suggested that allogeneic transfusion might induce reactivation of latent CMV infection in the recipient. However, results of animal studies have been conflicting; there has been evidence both for and against viral reactivation by donor leukocytes (59,60). More recently, Soderberg-Naucler et al. (61) used prolonged in vitro culture in the presence of cytokines to elicit reactivation of CMV with allogeneic human leukocytes.

For HIV infection, results of initial preclinical work also suggested a role of viral reactivation by donor leukocytes. Busch et al. (62) cocultured peripheral blood lymphocytes from a person with latent HIV-1 infection with normal uninfected allogeneic cells. When the infected cells were cultured in the presence of allogeneic erythrocytes, platelets, or plasma, there was no evidence of viral activation. However, when the cells were cocultured with allogeneic leukocytes, there was an increase in the concentration of HIV antigen (p24) in the culture supernatant. Release of HIV antigen occurred after several days and depended on the dose of allogeneic cells in coculture. The released virus infected previously uninfected cells in the culture.

Because of these preclinical findings, reactivation of CMV and HIV by donor leukocytes was specifically addressed in a large, multicenter, randomized clinical trial- the Viral Activation by Transfusion Study (63). The study was conducted to evaluate the ability of leukoreduced blood to prevent either HIV or CMV activation among a cohort of patients with HIV infection undergoing therapy for the infection. The study showed no beneficial effect of leukoreduction for prevention of early death, viral activation, or time to first infection-related complication. Among the subgroup of patients at greatest risk of HIV-related complications, the investigators found a statistically significant detrimental effect associated with leukoreduction.

Bacterial Overgrowth

It is unlikely that prestorage removal of leukocytes would have any measurable effect on the incidence of bacterial overgrowth in blood components. The mechanisms by which leukocyte reduction filters may deplete blood components of low levels of contaminating bacteria have been reviewed (64). Because bacterial overgrowth is infrequent, a clinical study would require an enormous number of observations. In the absence of a clinical trial, investigation of the potential role of prestorage filtration has entailed deliberate inoculation experiments. Units of blood are "spiked" with varying concentrations of bacteria and split into pairs, one of which is filtered. The paired units are stored and checked periodically for bacterial overgrowth. Many variables affect the results of such experiments. These include the strain of bacteria, the presence of bacterial plasmids, blood component characteristics, the filter selected, the inoculation dose, the holding time and temperature between inoculation and filtration, the method of assaying for bacterial overgrowth, the type of isolator used to culture bacteria, and the statistical power of the study (64). Because of these numerous variables, caution must be used when interpreting the results of in vitro experiments.

For red blood cell concentrates, Buchholz et al. (65) studied two serotypes of *Yersinia enterocolitica* at doses of inoculum ranging from 0.3 to 132 colony-forming units (CFU)/ml. In all cases, the investigators found a dramatic decline (approximately 100-fold) in the concentration of bacteria from the time of original inoculation to the time before filtration (7 hours at room temperature), attributable to the natural antibacterial properties of blood. During 42-day refrigerated storage, serotype O:3 grew in nearly all unfiltered units. Filtered units showed no growth if the concentration of bacteria just before filtration was 0 to 2 CFU/ml. However, *Yersinia* organisms grew during storage in filtered units if the concentration just before filtration was 2.0 to 3.7 CFU/ml. This study showed (within the constraints of the experimental model) that holding time significantly reduced bacterial concentration and that prestorage filtration of red blood cell concentrates prevented bacterial overgrowth with *Y. enterocolitica* in units containing low concentrations of bacteria (<2 CFU/ml) before filtration. Filtration did not sterilize units when the prefiltration concentration was more than 3 CFU/ml. Results of inoculation studies by other investigators were consistent with these results (2). Inoculation studies of coagulase-negative *Staphylococcus* and a variety of other organisms did not show a consistent beneficial effect of filtration on bacterial overgrowth.

For platelet concentrates, results of most inoculation experiments have suggested that prestorage leukocyte reduction by means of filtration would have little effect on subsequent bacterial overgrowth during storage (2). For example, Wenz et al. (66) examined a number of bacterial isolates including strains of *Staphylococcus epidermidis* and found similar growth patterns in filtered or unfiltered platelet concentrates during 5 days of storage. However, Buchholz et al. (67), using only 1 CFU/ml as an inoculating dose, found that in 6 of 24 cases bacterial proliferation during storage was less in filtered units than in unfiltered units. It is expected that chemical pathogen reduction systems will prove far more effective than leukoreduction for reducing the risk of bacterial overgrowth in stored blood components.

Transfusion-related Acute Lung Injury

Transfusion-related acute lung injury (TRALI) is an acute, immune-mediated transfusion reaction characterized by dyspnea, hypoxia, pulmonary edema, low pulmonary capillary wedge pressure, and alveolar infiltrates on chest radiographs. Three different mechanisms may contribute to the development of TRALI. First, results of serologic investigations suggest that TRALI occurs when donor plasma contains antibodies reactive against the recipient's HLA type or against recipient non-HLA leukocyte antigens (2). Second, TRALI may result when recipient antileukocyte antibodies react with residual donor leukocytes. However, an FNH reaction is more common in this setting. Why some patients with antileukocyte antibodies would experience TRALI in contrast to an FNH reaction is unresolved, but it may depend on the degree to which granulocytes rather than lymphocytes are involved (68). A third mechanism proposes a two-hit model involving lipid agents in donor blood which prime recipient neutrophils in the presence of specific cytokine activation (69). Currently, TRALI is best documented to result from the passive transfer of antibodies directed against recipient leukocyte antigens. Thus leukocyte reduction is not expected to play an important role in the prevention of TRALI.

Transfusion-associated Graft versus Host Disease

Transfusion-associated graft-versus-host disease (TA-GVHD) results from the unchecked clonal expansion of allogeneic donor leukocytes (see Chapter 59). Patients who experience TA-GVHD either do not eliminate donor leukocytes because of severe immunosuppression or do not recognize donor cells as foreign because of HLA similarity between the donor and recipient. The threshold number of donor leukocytes required to provoke human TA-GVHD cannot be determined and likely varies among different donor-recipient pairs. Because TA-GVHD depends on recipient exposure to viable allogeneic donor leukocytes, it might be anticipated that sufficient leukocyte reduction would prevent TA-GVHD. However, there are no conclusive clinical data to support this notion, and TA-GVHD has been reported among isolated patients who received transfusion of leukoreduced blood components (70). Therefore, γ-irradiation remains the only acceptable current means to prevent TA-GVHD. Nevertheless, two lines of information suggest the risk of TA-GVHD may be related to the residual leukocyte content of blood components. In an in vitro study in which the mixed lymphocyte reaction was used to model GVHD, a logarithmic decline in the number of cells available to respond resulted in a decline in lymphocyte reactivity similar to that after irradiation (71). Of greater in vivo relevance, the number of instances in which blood is transfused from a donor who is HLA homozygous for a haplotype shared by the recipient far exceeds the observed incidence of TA-GVHD. This finding, coupled with the observation that TA-GVHD is more common after transfusion of fresh blood components containing large numbers of leukocytes, suggests that under normal transfusion circumstances the decline in donor cell viability that occurs during routine blood storage may provide some degree of protection against TA-GVHD.

Storage Lesions of Red Blood Cells and Platelets

Several laboratories have investigated whether prestorage leukocyte reduction would improve the storage properties of red blood cell concentrates. Initially it was considered likely that leukocyte degeneration during storage would result in release of enzymes that would damage red blood cells. Lysosomal contents such as elastase, acid hydrolase, histamine, and serotonin were shown to accumulate during blood storage, and prestorage leukocyte reduction was shown to prevent this accumulation (2). Although free leukocyte elastase is able to induce hemolysis of red blood cells in the absence of plasma, the elevated levels of elastase measured during blood storage were measurements of elastase antigen, which is largely bound to and inactivated by natural plasma inhibitors. Thus no direct proof of red blood cell damage by free elastase released from leukocytes during storage was ever demonstrated. Nevertheless, paired storage studies have shown that red blood cell concentrates containing leukocytes undergo slightly more hemolysis during storage than do leukoreduced red blood cell concentrates (Table 21.7). However, the quantity of hemolysis attributed to the leukocytes is very small. Because leukoreduction results in loss of as much as 10% to 15% of the original red blood cell mass, any slight decrease in hemolysis during maximal storage of leukoreduced red blood cell concentrates is more than outweighed by the loss of red blood cells that occurs as a result of leukoreduction.

Several investigators have studied the effect of prestorage leukocyte reduction on the posttransfusion survival of chromium 51–labeled red blood cells (2,72) (Table 21.7). With one exception, there was no significant difference in the posttransfusion survival of red blood cells stored either with or without leukocytes. An additional study documented that the beneficial effect of plasticizer on red blood cell storage was greater than the effect of leukoreduction (73). Together these studies provide evidence that prestorage leukocyte reduction does not substantially improve the quality of stored red blood cells.

The effect of prestorage leukoreduction on the development of the platelet storage lesion also has been systematically investigated (2). Studies have shown no consistent significant difference among leukoreduced or unmodified platelet concentrates in levels of lactate dehydrogenase, β-thromboglobulin, response to hypotonic shock, aggregation to thrombin or other agonists, platelet adhesion capacity in flowing blood, platelet nucleotide content, expression of activation antigens, partial oxygen pressure, pH, partial carbon dioxide pressure, glucose consumption, or lactate production. Autologous posttransfusion survival of radiolabeled platelets was the same for both unmodified platelet concentrates and platelet concentrates leukoreduced before storage.

TABLE 21.7. RESULTS OF PAIRED STUDIES EXAMINING THE EFFECT OF PRESTORAGE LEUKOREDUCTION ON STORAGE OF RED BLOOD CELLS

	Percentage Hemolysis at End of Storage			24-hour ^{51}Cr Survival (mean ± SD)		
Author	No. of Pairs	WBC-reduced	Unmodified	No. of Pairs	WBC-reduced	Unmodified
Davey	6	0.41 ± 0.68	1.15 + 1.54	Lab A, 9	81.9 ± 6.4	79.9 ± 4.2
				Lab B, 8	78.1 ± 6.8	77.8 ± 5.7
Taylor	6	0.93	1.94	6	78	76.5
Brecher	10	0.34	0.83	6	82.3	82.3
Smith	10	0.12 ± 0.05	0.29 ± 0.15	10	81.6 ± 5	79.7 ± 5
Heaton	5	0.10 ± 0.06	0.40 ± 0.10	5	77 ± 9	74 ± 3
Kagen	10	0.17 ± 0.07	0.35 ± 0.07	10	88.9 ± 5.5	82.1 ± 3.8
Heaton	20	0.12 ± 0.04	0.29 ± 0.13	—	83 ± 4	79 ± 8
Stewart	5	0.10 ± 0.04	0.30 ± 0.20	—	NT	NT
Angue	24	0.27 ± 0.12	0.50 ± 0.18	—	NT	NT

WBC, white blood cell; NT, no test.
Data derived from Dzik WH. Leukoreduced blood components: laboratory and clinical aspects. In: Rossi EC, Simon TL, Moss GS, et al., eds. *Principles of transfusion medicine,* 2nd ed. Baltimore: Williams & Wilkins, 1996:353–374.

Transfusion-related Immunomodulation

Allogeneic transfusions have been associated with a variety of immune phenomena, including tolerance to subsequent solid-organ transplantation, increased susceptibility to viral or bacterial infection, and diminished immune surveillance against tumors (74) (see Chapter 60). This effect has not been unequivocally linked to transfusion, and a large body of research has investigated a number of possible mechanisms. Early hypotheses included patient selection bias, clonal deletion of primed cells by immunosuppressive drugs, the development of antiidiotype antibodies, and the development of suppressor T cells. Subsequent proposals have included central thymic tolerance, effects of microchimerism, persistence of donor veto cells, shifting of T-cell cytokine expression, inhibition of natural killer cell activity, and infusion of soluble HLA proteins or soluble mediators of apoptosis (74).

Several lines of evidence have suggested that recipient exposure to donor WBCs can result in improved survival of subsequent renal transplants. For example, the original studies of Opelz and Terasaki (75) showed that the use of frozen-deglycerolized (and thus leukoreduced) blood did not protect against rejection of renal transplants as well as did other red blood cell preparations. Okazaki et al. (76) subsequently found that the beneficial effect of pretransplantation transfusion could be obtained by means of transfusion of the buffy coat alone. In 1993, a prospective, double-blind, randomized trial showed that patients given postoperative transfusions of nonleukoreduced fresh red blood cell concentrates had better renal allograft survival than did patients given frozen-deglycerolized red blood cell concentrates (77). In this study, 90 patients were first treated with two fresh red blood cell concentrates before renal transplantation and then were randomized to receive three postoperative transfusions of either deglycerolized blood or three transfusions of fresh red blood cell concentrates packaged in a similar container. Those receiving fresh red blood cell concentrates had a 94% graft survival rate at 3 years compared with only 73% for patients receiving deglycerolized red blood cell concentrates ($P = .01$).

Recipient exposure to allogeneic leukocytes has been proposed to account for increased susceptibility to bacterial infections among persons receiving transfusions. Numerous studies with human subjects have shown that postoperative infection is more common among patients who undergo transfusion than among patients who do not. However, such studies are flawed in that these two groups do not have comparable infectious risk. Thus the observations do not shed light on the role of donor leukocytes or the value of leukoreduction. Unlike these studies, seven randomized, controlled trials have been performed to examine postoperative infection rates among recipients of leukoreduced or nonleukoreduced blood (Table 21.8). These studies have provided conflicting results; some show benefit of leukoreduction and others do not (74).

Recipient exposure to donor leukocytes has been said to account for an increased rate of relapse after resection of colorectal carcinoma. Preclinical studies with rodents have shown that the deliberate inoculation of tumor cells produces more pulmonary metastasis or tumor growth if it is followed by transfusion of blood that contains allogeneic leukocytes rather than transfusion of syngeneic or leukoreduced blood (74). Although several clinical studies have shown that patients who undergo transfusion have a higher relapse rate than do patients who do not undergo transfusion, such studies cannot be used to draw conclusions about the effect of leukoreduction. In three randomized, controlled, clinical trials with human subjects, investigators directly compared outcomes among patients receiving either leukoreduced or buffy coat–depleted blood. These studies did not show a beneficial effect of leukoreduction (74). In a 2001 randomized trial, investigators found no beneficial effect of leukoreduction on 5-year cancer recurrence rates among patients with colorectal carcinoma (78). In light of current evidence, leukoreduction cannot be considered indicated for the prevention of a purported immunodulatory effect of transfusion.

ADVERSE EFFECTS OF LEUKOREDUCTION

Little evidence suggests a serious clinical disadvantage of leukoreduction. The technology is expensive—estimated at more than $1 billion every 2 years for the United States alone. Concern has been raised that this cost will divert resources from other initiatives of greater consequence to safe transfusion practice (1). In addition to the cost, three disadvantages have been observed. First, filtration results in a substantial loss of the therapeutic blood element intended for transfusion. This problem may be

TABLE 21.8. RANDOMIZED CONTROLLED TRIALS OF LEUKOREDUCTION AND POSTOPERATIVE INFECTION

Author	Surgery	Single/Mulicenter N	LR Arm	Control Arm	95% CI of Relative Risk
Jensen	Colorectal	S 197	LR Whole blood	Whole blood	1.62–3.3
Heiss	Colorectal	S 120	Buffy coat	Autologous	1.05–7.24
Busch	Colorectal	M 470	Buffy coat	Autologous	0.59–1.34
Houbiers	Colorectal	M 697	LR RBCs	Buffy	0.64–1.19
Jensen	Colorectal	S 589	LR RBCs	Buffy	2.16–5.20
van de Watering	Cardiac	S 909	LR RBCs	Buffy	1.00–1.99
Tartter	Gastrointestinal	S 221	LR RBCs	RBCs	0.89–3.85

LR, leukoreduction; CI, confidence interval; S, single center; M, more than one center; RBCs, red blood cells.
Data derived from Vamvakas EC, Blajchman MA. *Immunomodulatory effects of blood transfusion.* Bethesda, MD: American Association of Blood Banks, 1999.

particularly important if filtration is combined with other manipulations, such as preparation of red blood cell concentrates by the buffy coat removal technique or preparation of washed platelet concentrates. Second, bedside leukoreduction has been associated with hypotensive reactions, especially among recipients treated with ACE inhibitors (79). These reactions are considered to occur when short-lived vasoactive proteins such as bradykinin are generated during filtration. For example, Takahashi et al. (79) found that some filters were associated with the production of bradykinin during filtration of platelet concentrates. Bradykinin level increased from 37 pg/ml to 6,794 pg/ml as a result of filtration. If an ACE inhibitor was added to the plasma, the level increased to 36,000 pg/ml because the ACE inhibitor also inhibits the kininases responsible for the breakdown of bradykinin. Thus patients taking ACE inhibitors and patients with inherited deficiencies of kininases are more susceptible to the hypotensive effects of administered bradykinin. Mair and Leparc reported numerous cases, including one death among patients undergoing cardiac surgery (79). Third, reports of allergic reactions characterized by acute conjunctivitis, pain at the site of blood infusion (80), or the sudden onset of back pain and hypertension (81) have been observed in some patients undergoing transfusion of leukoreduced blood. Although these events appear to occur in a very small proportion of patients who undergo transfusion, the studies highlight that even low-frequency adverse consequences attributed to leukofiltration will affect growing numbers of patients as the technology becomes more widely used.

SUMMARY

The use of leukocyte-reduced cellular blood components has expanded dramatically in the last decade. The development of high-performance blood filters and low-leukocyte apheresis devices have made leukocyte-reduced components available to all transfusion facilities. The technology represents an important advance in the purity of blood components. Several European nations and Canada have adopted universal leukoreduction of the blood supply. However, leukocyte reduction represents the largest incremental increase in the cost of producing blood components in history. Although billions of dollars in health care resources will be needed to implement universal leukoreduction in the developed world, clinical trials have shown benefit for only three selected indications—prevention of recurrent febrile reactions, reduction in HLA alloimmunization, and reduction of the risk of CMV transmission.

REFERENCES

1. Dzik S, Aubuchon J, Jeffries L, et al. Leukocyte reduction of blood components: public policy and new technology. *Transfus Med Rev* 2000;14: 34–52.
2. Dzik WH. Leukoreduced blood components: laboratory and clinical aspects. In: Rossi EC, Simon TL, Moss GS, et al., eds. *Principles of transfusion medicine,* 2nd ed. Baltimore: Williams & Wilkins, 1996: 353–374.
3. Vamvakas EC, Blajchman MA. Universal white-cell reduction: the case for and against. *Transfusion* 2001;41:691–712.
4. Dzik S. Leukoreduction blood filters: filter design and mechanisms of leukocyte removal. *Transfus Med Rev* 1993;7:65–77.
5. Beaujean F, Segier JM, le Forestier C, et al. Leukocyte depletion of red cell concentrates by filtration: influence of blood product temperature. *Vox Sang* 1992;62:242–243.
6. Sirchia G, Rebulla P, Sabbioneda L, et al. Optimal conditions for white cell reduction in red cells by filtration at the patient's bedside. *Transfusion* 1996;36:322–327.
7. Van der meer PF, Pietersz RN, Nelis JT, et al. Six filters for the removal of white cells from red cell concentrates, evaluated at 4 degrees C and/or at room temperature. *Transfusion* 1999;39:265–270.
8. Smith JD, Leitman SF. Filtration of RBC units: effect of storage time and temperature on filter performance. *Transfusion* 2000;40:521–526.
9. Bowden RA, Slichter SJ, Sayers M, et al. A comparison of filtered leukocyte-reduced and cytomegalovirus (CMV) seronegative blood products for the prevention of transfusion-associated CMV infection after marrow transplant. *Blood* 1995;86:3599–3603.
10. Gorlin JB, Adams CL, Stefan MM, et al. Variable leukoreduction on units from donors with sickle cell trait: a time-temperature, donor reproducibility study. *Transfusion* 2000;40[Suppl]:55S(abst).
11. Harbin K, Prihoda L, Thomas A. Residual WBCs in leukocyte-reduction filtered hemoglobin S positive RBCs. *Transfusion* 2000;40[Suppl]: 55S(abst).
12. Williamson LM, Beard M, Seghatchian J, et al. Leukocyte depletion of whole blood and red cells from donors with hemoglobin sickle trait. *Transfusion* 1999;39[Suppl]:108S(abst).
13. Ledent E, Berlin G. Does plasma influence the efficiency of leukocyte filtration? *Vox Sang* 1994;67[Suppl 2]:20(abst).
14. Dumont L, Dzik WH, Rebulla P. Practical guidelines for process control and validation of leukoreduced components. *Transfusion* 1996;36: 11–20.
15. US Department of Health and Human Services. Food and Drug Administration, Center for Biologics Evaluation and Research. Guidance for industry: pre-storage leukocyte reduction of whole blood and blood components intended for transfusion. Draft, January 2001.
16. Dzik S. Principles of counting low numbers of leukocytes in leukoreduced blood components. *Transfus Med Rev* 1997;11:44–55.
17. Dzik S, Moroff G, Dumont L. A multicenter study evaluating three methods for counting residual WBCs in WBC-reduced blood components: Nageotte hemocytometry, flow cytometry, and microfluorimetry. *Transfusion* 2000;40:513–520.
18. Szuflad P, Dzik WH. A general method for concentrating blood samples in preparation for counting very low numbers of white cells. *Transfusion* 1997;37:277–283.
19. Williamson LM, Wimperis JZ, Williamson P, et al. Bedside filtration of blood products in the prevention of HLA alloimmunization: a prospective randomized trial. *Blood* 1994;83:3028–3035.
20. Blajchman MA, Bardossy L, Carmen RA, et al. An animal model of allogeneic donor platelet refractoriness: the effect of the time of leukoreduction. *Blood* 1992;79:1371–1375.
21. James DJ, Sikotra S, Sivakumaran M, et al. The presence of free infectious cytomegalovirus (CMV) in the plasma of donated CMV-seropositive blood and platelets. *Transfus Med* 1997;7:123–126.
22. Bordin JO, Bardossy L, Blajchman MA. Growth enhancement of established tumors by allogeneic blood transfusions in experimental animals and its amelioration by leukoreduction: the importance of timing of the leukoreduction. *Blood* 1994;84:344–348.
23. Van der Watering, LMG, Hermans J, Houbiers JGA, et al. Beneficial effects of leukocyte depletion of transfused blood on postoperative complications in patients undergoing cardiac surgery: a randomized clinical trial. *Circulation* 1998;97:562–568.
24. Perkins HA, Payne R, Ferguson J, et al. Nonhemolytic febrile transfusion reactions: quantitative effects of blood components with emphasis on isoantigenic incompatibility of leukocytes. *Vox Sang* 1966;11: 578–600.
25. Brubaker DB. Clinical significance of white cell antibodies in febrile nonhemolytic transfusion reactions. *Transfusion* 1990;30:733–737.
26. Dzik WH. Is the febrile response to transfusion due to donor or recipient cytokine [letter]? *Transfusion* 1992;32:594.
27. Davenport RD, Snyder EL, eds. *Cytokines in transfusion medicine: a*

primer. Bethesda, MD: American Association of Blood Banks, 1997: 1–219.

28. Heddle N, Tan M, Klama L, et al. Factors affecting cytokine production in platelet concentrates. *Transfusion* 1994;34(suppl 1):67S(abst).
29. Heddle NM, Klama L, Singer J, et al. The role of the plasma from platelet concentrates in transfusion reactions. *N Engl J Med* 1994;331: 625–628.
30. Heddle NM, Klama LN, Griffith L, et al. A prospective study to identify the risk factors associated with acute reactions to platelet and red cell transfusions. *Transfusion* 1993;33:794–797.
31. Muylle L, Wouters E, DeBock R, et al. Reactions to platelet transfusion: the effect of the storage time of the concentrate. *Transfns Med* 1992; 2:289–293.
32. Mangano MM, Chambers LA, Kruskall MS. Limited efficacy of leukopoor platelets for prevention of febrile transfusion reactions. *Am J Clin Pathol* 1991;95:733–738.
33. Goodnough LT, Riddell JIV, Lazarus H, et al. Prevalence of platelet transfusion reactions before and after implementation of leukocyte-depleted platelet concentrates by filtration. *Vox Sang* 1993;65: 103–107.
34. Mintz PD. Febrile reactions to platelet transfusions. *Am J Clin Pathol* 1991;95:609–611.
35. Anderson NA, Gray S, Copplestone JA, et al. A prospective randomized study of three types of platelet concentrates in patients with haematological malignancy: corrected platelet count increments and frequency of non-haemolytic febrile transfusion reactions. *Transfus Med* 1996;6: 33–39.
36. Trial to Reduce Alloimmunization to Platelets Study Group. Leukocyte reduction and ultraviolet B irradiation of platelets to prevent alloimmunization and refractoriness to platelet transfusions. *N Engl J Med* 1997; 337:1861–1869.
37. Killick SB, Win N, Marsh JC, et al. Pilot study of HLA alloimmunization after transfusion with pre-storage leucodepleted blood products in aplastic anaemia. *Br J Haematol* 1997;97:677–684.
38. Fisher M, Chapman JR, Ting A, et al. Alloimmunization to HLA antigens following transfusion with leukocyte-poor and purified platelet suspensions. *Vox Sang* 1985;49:331–335.
39. van Marwijk-Kooy M, van Prooijen HC, Moes M. Use of leukocyte-depleted platelet concentrates for the prevention of refractoriness and primary HLA alloimmunization: a prospective, randomized trial. *Blood* 1991;77:201–205.
40. Claas FHJ, Smeenk RJJ, Schmidt R, et al. Alloimmunisation against the MHC antigens after platelet transfusions is due to contaminating leucocytes in the platelet suspension. *Exp Hematol* 1981;9:84–89.
41. Kao KJ. Effects of leukocyte depletion and UVB irradiation on alloantigenicity of major histocompatibility complex antigens in platelet concentrates: a comparative study. *Blood* 1992;80:2931–2937.
42. Bordin JO, Bardossy L, Blajchman MA. Experimental animal model of refractoriness to donor platelets: the effect of plasma removal and the extent of white cell reduction on allogeneic alloimmunization. *Transfusion* 1993;33:798–801.
43. Duquesnoy RJ, White LT, Fierst JW, et al. Multiscreen serum analysis of highly sensitized renal dialysis patients for antibodies toward public and private class I HLA determinants. *Transplantation* 1990;50: 427–437.
44. MacPherson BR, Hammond PB, Maniscalco CA. Alloimmunization to public HLA antigens in multitransfused platelet recipients. *Ann Clin Lab Sci* 1986;16:38–44.
45. Heddle NM. The efficacy of leukoreduction to improve platelet transfusion response: a critical appraisal of clinical studies. *Transfus Med Rev* 1994;8:15–28.
46. Vamvakas E. Meta-analysis of randomized controlled trials of the efficiency of white cell reduction in preventing HLA-alloimmunization and refractoriness to random-donor platelet transfusions. *Transfus Med Rev* 1998;12:258–270.
47. Sintnicolaas K, van Marwijk-Kooy M, van Prooijen HC, et al. Leukocyte depletion of random single donor platelet transfusions does not prevent secondary HLA alloimmunization and refractoriness: a randomized prospective study. *Vox Sang* 1994;67[Suppl 2]:101(abst).
48. Hillyer CD, Emmens RK, Zago-Novaretti M, et al. Methods for the reduction of transfusion-transmitted cytomegalovirus infection: filtration versus the use of seronegative donor units. *Transfusion* 1994;34: 929–934.
49. Smith KL, Cobain T, Dunstan RA. Removal of cytomegalovirus DNA from donor blood by filtration. *Br J Haematol* 1993;83:640–642.
50. Larsson S, Soderberg-Naucler C, Wang FZ, et al. Cytomegalovirus DNA can be detected in peripheral blood mononuclear cells from all seropositive and most seronegative healthy blood donors over time. *Transfusion* 1998;38:271–278.
51. Brady MT, Milam JD, Anderson DC, et al. Use of deglycerolized red blood cells to prevent posttransfusion infection with cytomegalovirus in neonates. *J Infect Dis* 1984;150:334–339.
52. Taylor BJ, Jacobs RF, Baker RL, et al. Frozen deglycerolized blood prevents transfusion-acquired cytomegalovirus infections in neonates. *Pediatr Infect Dis J* 1986;5:188–191.
53. Gilbert G, Hayes K, Hudson IL, et al. Prevention of transfusion-acquired cytomegalovirus infection in infants by blood filtration to remove leucocytes. *Lancet* 1989;i:1228–1231.
54. Eisenfield L, Silver H, McLaughlin J, et al. Prevention of transfusion-associated cytomegalovirus infection in neonatal patients by the removal of white cells from blood. *Transfusion* 1992;32:205–209.
55. Wiesner RH, Marin E, Porayko MK, et al. Advances in the diagnosis, treatment, and prevention of cytomegalovirus infections after liver transplantation. *Gastroenterol Clin North Am* 1993;22:351–366.
56. Farrugia E, Schwab TR. Management and prevention of cytomegalovirus infection after renal transplantation. *Mayo Clin Proc* 1992;67: 879–890.
57. Gorensek MJ, Stewart RW, Keys TF, et al. A multivariate analysis of the risk of cytomegalovirus infection in heart transplant recipients. *J Infect Dis* 1988;157:515–522.
58. Lang DJ. Cytomegalovirus infections in organ transplantation and posttransfusion: an hypothesis. *Arch Gesamte Virusforsch* 1972;37: 365–377.
59. Cheung KS, Lang DJ. Transmission and activation of cytomegalovirus with blood transfusion: a mouse model. *J Infect Dis* 1977;135: 841–845.
60. Bruggerman CA. Reactivation of latent CMV in the rat. *Transplant Proc* 1991;23[Suppl 3]:22–24.
61. Soderberg-Naucler C, Fish KN, Nelson JA. Reactivation of latent human cytomegalovirus by allogeneic stimulation of blood cells from healthy donors. *Cell* 1997;91:119–126.
62. Busch MP, Lee TH, Heitman J. Allogenic leukocytes but not therapeutic blood elements induce reactivation and dissemination of latent human immunodeficiency virus type 1 infection: implications for transfusion support of infected patients. *Blood* 1992;80:2128–2135.
63. Collier AC, Kalish LA, Busch MP, et al. Leukocyte-reduced red blood cell transfusions in patients with anemia and human immunodeficiency virus infection: the viral activation transfusion study—a randomized controlled trial. *JAMA* 2001;285:1592–1601.
64. Dzik WH. Removal of bacteria by leukocyte filtration. *Immunol Comm* 1995;24:95–115.
65. Buchholz DH, AuBouchon JP, Snyder EL, et al. Removal of *Yersinia enterocolitica* from AS-1 red cells. *Transfusion* 1992;32:667–672.
66. Wenz B, Ciavarella D, Freundlich L. Effect of prestorage white cell reduction on bacterial growth in platelet concentrates. *Transfusion* 1993;33:520–523.
67. Buchholz DH, AuBuchon JP, Snyder EL, et al. Effects of white cell reduction on the resistance of blood components to bacterial multiplication. *Transfusion* 1994;34:852–857.
68. Seeger W, Schneider U, Kreusler B, et al. Reproduction of transfusion-related acute lung injury in ex vivo lung model. *Blood* 1990;76: 1438–1444.
69. Silliman CC, Paterson AJ, Dickey WO, et al. The association of biologically active lipids with the development of transfusion-related acute lung injury: a retrospective study. *Transfusion* 1997;37:719–726.
70. Akahoshi M, Takanashi M, Masuda M, et al. A case of transfusion-associated graft-versus-host disease not prevented by white cell–reduction filters. *Transfusion* 1992;32:169–172.
71. Dzik WH, Jones KS. The effects of gamma irradiation versus white

cell reduction on the mixed lymphocyte reaction. *Transfusion* 1993;33:493–496.
72. Heaton WAL, Holme S, Smith K, et al. Effects of 3-5 log10 prestorage leucocyte depletion on red cell storage and metabolism. *Br J Haematol* 1994;87:363–368.
73. Davey RJ, Heaton WA, Sweat LT, et al. Characteristics of white cell–reduced red cells stored in tri-(2-ethylhexyl)trimellitate plastic. *Transfusion* 1994;34:895–898.
74. Vamvakas EC, Blajchman MA. *Immunomodulatory effects of blood transfusion.* Bethesda, MD: American Association of Blood Banks, 1999.
75. Opelz G, Terasaki PI. Improvement of kidney-graft survival with increased numbers of blood transfusions. *N Engl J Med* 1978;299:799–803.
76. Okazaki H, Takahashi M, Miura K, et al. Effect of buffycoat transfusions in living related and cadaveric renal transplantation. *Transplant Proc* 1985;17:1034–1036.
77. Lang P, Bierling P, Buisson C, et al. Influence of posttransplantation blood transfusion on kidney allograft survival: a one-center, double-blind, prospective, randomized study comparing cryopreserved and fresh red blood cell concentrates. *Transplant Proc* 1993;25:616–618.
78. van de Watering LMG, Brand A, Houbiers JGA, et al. Perioperative blood transfusions, with or without allogeneic leucocytes, relate to survival, not to cancer recurrence. *Br J Surg* 2001;88:267–272.
79. Klein HG, Dzik S, Slichter SJ, et al. Leukocyte-reduced blood components: current status. American Society of Hematology, 1998:154–177.
80. Podlosky LR, Boshkov LK. Infusion site pain related to bedside leukoreduction filters [letter]. *Transfusion* 1995;35:362.
81. Haley NR, Sledge LS, Gibble J, et al. An unusual transfusion reaction pattern to leukocyte reduced red cells. *Transfusion* 2000;40[Suppl]:40S(abst).
82. Dzik S, Anderson JK, O'Neill M, et al. A prospective randomized clinical trial of universal leukoreduction (abst.). *Transfusion* 2001;41:15.

Rossi's Principles of Transfusion Medicine, Third Edition, edited by Toby L. Simon, Walter H. Dzik, Edward L. Snyder, Christopher P. Stowell, and Ronald G. Strauss. Lippincott Williams & Wilkins, Philadelphia © 2002.

PART IV
Plasma

22

PLASMA COMPOSITION AND COAGULATION MECHANISM

KENNETH J. SMITH
SILVANA Z. BUCUR

The first portion of this chapter describes the composition of plasma and its protein components important for plasma transfusion therapy. The functions of the coagulation and fibrinolytic systems and the plasma content of these proteins are then discussed.

K.J. Smith and S.Z. Bucur: Winship Cancer Institute, Emory University, Atlanta, Georgia.

PLASMA COMPOSITION

Plasma, the aqueous part of blood, is composed of electrolytes and solutes, including protein, lipid, and carbohydrate macromolecules. It is the medium through which nutrients, hormones, waste products, and pharmaceuticals are transported through the body. In vivo, the fluidity of plasma is maintained through complex interactions between its coagulant and anticoagulant proteins. Plasma is collected with the addition of a variety of anticoagulants, including sodium citrate, heparin, and ethylenediaminetetraacetic acid (EDTA), to maintain its fluidity in vitro. The plasma constituents important for transfusion medicine are

TABLE 22.1. CLASSIFICATION OF PLASMA PROTEINS

I. Albumin family
  a. Albumin
  b. α-Fetoprotein
  c. Vitamin D–binding protein

II. Serine protease superfamily
  a. Coagulation proteins (prothrombin, proteins C, Z, factors VII, IX, X, XI, XII)
  b. Fibrinolytic proteins (plasminogen, prekallikrein)
  c. Complement proteins (C1r, C1s, C2, factors B, D, and I)
  d. Other (haptoglobin)

III. Immunoglobulin superfamily
  a. Immunoglobulins (IgG, IgA, IgM, IgD, IgE)
  b. β_2-microglobulin

IV. Serpin superfamily
  a. Serine protease inhibitors (ATIII, C1-inhibitor, heparin cofactor II, α_1-antitrypsin, protein C inhibitor, α_2-antiplasmin)
  b. Other (angiotensin, thyroxine-binding globulin)

V. α_2-Macroglobulin family
  a. Protease inhibitors (α_2-macroglobulin)
  b. Complement proteins (C3,C4,C5)

VI. Cystatin superfamily
  a. Thiolprotease inhibitors (HMW and LMW kininogens)
  b. Other (histidine-rich glycoprotein)

VII. Pentraxin superfamily (C-reactive protein, serum amyloid protein)

VIII. Ceruloplasmin superfamily (ceruloplasmin, factors V, VIII)

Proteins are grouped by structural homology. Superfamilies of proteins show those with divergent functions related by sequence homology and common ancestor genes. Families of proteins have homologous sequences and similar functions.
Adapted from Haupt H. Chemistry and clinical significance of human plasma proteins. *Behring Inst Mitt* 1990;86:1–66, with permission.

albumin, proteins with immune system functions, and coagulation proteins (Table 22.1).

Plasma Proteins

Proteins are present at concentrations ranging from 65 to 88 g/L in serum, compared with a plasma content of 6.6 g/L for chloride and 3.3 g/L for sodium. Plasma proteins usually are greater than 50 kd in molecular weight, and their anionic charge keeps them from being filtered through the glomerular membrane (1). The concentrations of many plasma proteins change dramatically in response to injury and inflammatory processes and are subject to variations in the nutritional state of the individual. Alterations in plasma protein levels also are caused by protein wasting diseases, including glomerulopathy and intestinal diseases.

Although human plasma contains more than 700 identified proteins, only a small number are available for clinical use as purified preparations (2). Through large-scale application of Cohn fractionation, several partially purified plasma derivatives have become available for clinical use, most notably albumin, immunoglobulin, and coagulation factor concentrates. Use of these substances has reduced the use of plasma for replacement therapy.

Albumin is the most abundant protein in plasma with a concentration of 35 to 50 g/L. The major physiologic roles of albumin are maintaining oncotic pressure and functioning as a transport protein. Immunoglobulins and complement system components have important roles in host defense. The most abundant immunoglobulin is IgG at a concentration of approximately 6 to 16 g/L. Among the complement components, C3 predominates at a concentration of 1.2 g/L. The coagulation and fibrinolytic proteins discussed herein are responsible for maintaining normal hemostasis. Fibrinogen is the most abundant coagulation protein with a concentration of 2.8 g/L of plasma collected in sodium citrate.

Plasma Processing

Human plasma can be collected directly by means of single-donor plasmapheresis or from whole-blood collections separated into units of packed red blood cells and plasma. Between 180 and 300 ml of plasma can be obtained after the processing of one unit of whole blood depending on the volume and red blood cell content of the unit collected. Plasmapheresis from single donors yields 500 to 800 ml of plasma depending on the donor's weight. Once plasma is collected, it can be stored frozen at −18°C or lower generally within 6 hours of collection as fresh frozen plasma (FFP) according to the specifications of the collecting system (3). When FFP is thawed at 4°C, a portion of the fibrinogen, factor VIII, von Willebrand factor, and fibronectin remains insoluble at the interface of liquid and frozen plasma. Centrifugation can be used to concentrate the insoluble cryoprecipitate after thawing. The supernatant plasma is termed *plasma, cryoprecipitate reduced* and usually is stored after refreezing. Fresh frozen plasma; plasma, cryoprecipitate reduced; and cryoprecipitate are the major plasma products in clinical use. Other plasma products include those separated from red blood cells under conditions other than those specified for FFP. These products are called *liquid plasma* if they are to be used for intravenous infusion, but they often are stored frozen or at room temperature as recovered plasma destined for manufacturing plasma derivatives. When plasma is to be used for components in replacement therapy of hemostatic defects, only plasma products collected and stored under conditions known to preserve labile coagulation factors are used in transfusion (FFP; plasma, cryoprecipitate reduced; or cryoprecipitate). Depending on storage conditions, other plasma products are used in the manufacturing of coagulation factor concentrates or less labile plasma derivatives, including albumin and immune globulin preparations.

The infectious potential of plasma resides primarily in the transmission of lipid-encapsulated viruses, including human immunodeficiency virus 1 and 2, hepatitis B virus, hepatitis C virus, and human T-lymphotropic virus I and II. Inactivation of lipid envelope viruses in plasma with a mixture of solvent [tri(n-butyl)phosphate (TNBP)] and a nonionic detergent (Triton X-100) has been recently approved by the U.S. Food and Drug Administration to limit the risk of transfusion-transmitted disease (4). Nonenveloped viruses, such as hepatitis A virus and Parvovirus B19, are not inactivated by the solvent-detergent method. This process involves pooling plasma from thousands of donors before solvent-detergent treatment. Thus solvent-detergent plasma may contain viruses not affected by this method of inactivation, although it is speculated that the presence of antiviral antibodies in pooled plasma may block transmission or attenuate any resulting infection. Prions are not known to be inactivated by the solvent-detergent method and remain a source of concern, although human-human transmission of prions through blood transfusion has not been documented (5).

Albumin

Albumin is the most abundant plasma protein. It is synthesized in the liver and has a high density of negative charges. Its 17 disulfide bridges allow the 67-kd albumin molecule to be tightly packed. Albumin contains one reduced cysteine residue and has no postsynthetic modifications (glycosylation) (6). In a normal adult, the half-life of albumin in plasma is 20 days, and the total body content of albumin is 300 to 350 g. Turnover is 4% to 5% of total albumin per day (7). Although 60% to 65% of albumin is present in extravascular fluid, albumin in the intravascular compartment is responsible for approximately 70% to 80% of plasma oncotic pressure and is the main protein contributor to maintenance of blood volume. Albumin not only binds and transports endogenous substances, including bilirubin, hormones, and nutrients such as amino acids, fatty acids, and minerals but also can bind exogenous substances with therapeutic or toxic effects. The thiol group on the surface of the albumin molecule enables it to function as a radical scavenger and is a site of binding for some of its ligands (8).

Albumin is extracted from plasma through Cohn fractionation as fraction V. Commercially available albumin preparations are pasteurized for viral inactivation. Available preparations contain either 5% or 25% albumin in buffered diluent. Plasma protein fraction contains 83% albumin and 17% globulins in a 5% protein solution.

Plasma albumin concentration is low in conditions that affect protein synthesis, metabolism, and distribution or produce intestinal or renal loss of protein. Impaired albumin synthesis occurs in liver disease and in malnutrition. Loss of albumin occurs in nephrotic syndrome, in protein-losing enteropathy, and after extensive burns. Although total body stores do not change, hypervolemia due to fluid administration decreases serum albumin concentration.

Hypoalbuminemia due to an underlying inflammatory condition improves as the underlying condition is controlled. However, there are clinical situations, including the practice of large volume paracentesis in the care of patients with portal hypertension and ascites, in which albumin repletion is necessary (9). During this procedure, albumin infusion prevents hypotension and renal dysfunction. It preserves sodium balance and may improve mortality rates. In nephrotic syndrome, the glomerular loss of albumin results in decreased plasma oncotic pressure and interstitial edema. Some studies have shown that patients with nephrotic syndrome refractory to conventional therapy may respond to infusions of 25% albumin with loop diuretics (10). The prophylactic use of albumin to maintain plasma oncotic pressure around the time of oocyte retrieval in women undergoing assisted reproductive manipulation may prevent or reduce the severity of ovarian hyperstimulation syndrome among women taking gonadotropins to induce ovulation (11). Albumin also is used as replacement fluid in therapeutic plasmapheresis.

Immunoglobulins and Complement Proteins

Immunoglobulins are synthesized by plasma cells and make up one third of the plasma protein content. Immunoglobulins are glycoproteins with molecular weights varying between 150 kd for IgG to more than 1,000 kd for IgM molecules. Immunoglobulins are composed of two heavy (H) and two light (L) peptide chains, each with variable and constant regions. Enzymatic digestion of IgG by papain produces a complement-activating, crystallizable Fc fragment and two antigen-binding domains (Fab). The antigen-binding domains contain light chain and heavy chain moieties. Seventy-five percent of plasma immunoglobulins have the IgG isotype, and IgG is the only isotype that is able to cross the placenta.

Polyvalent immune globulin preparations are made from pooled plasma and are primarily IgG with only trace amounts of other isotypes. Intravenous immune globulin (IVIG) preparations are made to minimize aggregates that bind complement in recipients and cause reactions during infusion.

Hyperimmune or high-titer, disease-specific immune globulin preparations are obtained from actively immunized healthy persons and are used to prevent postexposure viral illnesses, including hepatitis B, varicella-zoster, cytomegalovirus infection, and rabies (12–16). Passive immunity with IVIG is thought to be beneficial to patients with Parvovirus B19–associated pure red blood cell aplasia (17). Antibodies to tetanus toxoid can be used to provide passive protection to patients at risk of wound tetanus. Antibodies to the Rh blood group are used to block maternal immunization to fetal Rh-positive red blood cells (18).

Immune globulin preparations from source plasma or recovered plasma are used in clinical practice to decrease the incidence and severity of infections in patients with decreased humoral immunity. In patients with primary immunodeficiency syndromes, the use of prophylactic maintenance immune globulins have decreased morbidity and mortality by decreasing the incidence and severity of infectious episodes (19). In patients with secondary immunodeficiency due to lymphoid malignant disease (20,21) or human immunodeficiency virus infection (22, 23) and patients who have undergone bone marrow or solid organ transplantation (24,25), prophylactic administration of immune globulin preparations has some clinical benefit, but the cost of this treatment is prohibitive for routine use in these indications.

An important use of IVIG concentrates is in the management of immune cytopenia to produce macrophage Fc receptor blockade. Reduced clearance of antibody-coated red blood cells occurs in patients given 2 g/kg IVIG. Part of the prompt increase in platelet count is thought to be due to blockade of clearance of platelets by macrophage Fc receptors in idiopathic thrombocytopenic purpura (ITP) (26). In autoimmune disorders such as ITP and posttransfusion purpura, administration of high-dose immune globulin may have benefit through numerous mechanisms in addition to effects on macrophage Fc receptors (27). Intravenous immune globulin can modulate B-lymphocyte function, inhibit antibody production, and block interaction between autoantibodies and cellular antigens.

Administration of IVIG has been effective in inflammatory conditions such as Kawasaki disease (28) and in autoimmune disorders such as chronic demyelinating polyradiculoneuropathy and Guillain-Barré syndrome (29,30). There are anecdotal reports of clinical response in the management of antiphospholipid antibody syndrome (31), inflammatory myopathy (32,33), and acquired factor VIII inhibitors (34).

C1 Esterase Inhibitor

The complement system for inactivating and clearing pathogens is composed of more than 20 proteins that can be activated through either the classical immune complex or the alternative pathway involving properdin. Complement activation is initiated by the formation of immune complexes in the classical pathway and the subsequent conversion of zymogen C5 into the active C5b generating a cell membrane bound attack complex and release of C5a.

Of all the complement proteins, C3 predominates in plasma at a concentration of 1.3 g/L. Both inherited and acquired deficiencies of various complement proteins have been described. They have clinical manifestations ranging from recurrent infections as with C3 deficiency, to life-threatening angioedema associated with C1 inhibitor deficiency. The C1 inhibitor is a member of the serpin (serine protease inhibitor) family that binds and irreversibly inactivates C1 in the classical pathway of complement activation. C1 interacts with coagulation factors XIa and XIIa, plasmin, and kallikrein in vitro, but the physiologic significance of this potential regulatory function is not clear (35–37). Angioedema is a clinical manifestation of C1-inhibitor deficiency. This is a congenital or acquired disorder. The acquired disorder occurs in some patients with low-grade lymphoma with autoantibodies to C1 inhibitor or chronic complement activation and resulting consumption of C1 inhibitor. Both the inherited and acquired forms have been managed with plasma infusion or purified C1 inhibitor concentrate.

α_1-Antitrypsin

α_1-Antitrypsin is another member of the serpin family with inhibitory activity against a variety of serine proteases. Neutrophil elastase is the most important protease target. Uninhibited neutrophil elastase is present in the setting of quantitative or qualitative α_1-antitrypsin deficiency and causes pulmonary emphysema and cirrhosis of the liver. Concentrates of α_1-antitrypsin have been used for replacement therapy (38). Replacement of α_1-antitrypsin with solvent-detergent plasma may not be as effective as use of FFP. In vitro data have indicated that the solvent-detergent process decreases plasma α_1-antitrypsin activity (39).

Coagulation Factor Concentrates

Hereditary deficiencies of certain coagulation proteins are associated with increased risk of thrombosis (deficiencies of antithrombin III, protein C, and protein S), whereas other deficiencies increase the risk of bleeding, as in factor VIII deficiency or von Willebrand disease. Plasma can be used for replacement therapy in the care of patients with hereditary or acquired deficiencies of these proteins, but concentrates prepared from pooled plasma donations and treated to inactivate transfusion-transmitted viruses usually are the preferred product for transfusion. Use of concentrates of coagulation factors, when available, avoids the risk of volume overload when large amounts of plasma must be transfused to achieve hemostatically effective levels in recipients.

Cohn fractionation procedures have allowed the separation of plasma into several of its components. The result is better-targeted therapy, in which a recipient who needs immune globulin or albumin replacement can be treated with an appropriate component. Plasma-derived and recombinant coagulation factor products have become available for deficiencies of factors VII, VIII, IX, and XI, further limiting the use of plasma in the management of coagulation defects. Plasma remains useful for replacement therapy when there are deficiencies of multiple coagulation factors, as in disseminated intravascular coagulation (DIC) (40) or liver disease (41) or when plasma is used to reverse the warfarin effect (42). Plasma also is used for replacement therapy when commercial concentrates are not available for management of hereditary isolated coagulation factor deficiencies. Commercial concentrates of fibrinogen for replacement therapy were removed from the market because of high rates of transmission hepatitis before viral inactivation procedures became available. Cryoprecipitate and FFP are used for fibrinogen replacement. Fibrinogen concentrates are prepared from either allogeneic or autologous plasma (cryoprecipitate) and used in conjunction with bovine thrombin to enhance local surgical hemostasis with fibrin glue. A commercial preparation of vapor heat–treated human fibrinogen, human thrombin, and a bovine fibrinolytic inhibitor (Tisseal) has been approved as an adjunct to conventional hemostatic measures in various surgical procedures. The fibrin seal aids wound closure in plastic surgical, cardiovascular, and neurosurgical procedures in which synthetic materials or tissue grafts must be watertight after suturing (43–45).

COAGULATION MECHANISM

Plasma hemostatic proteins interact with a network of cellular and tissue responses to injury and inflammation. Cytokines from blood cells, tissue macrophages, and stromal cells affect the interaction of vascular tissue with platelets, the coagulation system, and complement pathways. Vascular tissue itself responds to changes in the local milieu after generation of thrombin and other proteases in the coagulation cascade, attraction of neutrophils and monocytes, and the appearance of platelet-derived growth factor after clotting is initiated. This chapter discusses coagulation factors and fibrinolytic system components in plasma. The functions of the vessel wall and platelets in hemostasis are presented in Chapter 15.

Electron microscopic examination of injured blood vessels has shown that platelets accumulate in seconds in areas where subendothelial connective tissue is exposed to blood (46). Two distinct processes are involved in formation of a platelet plug. Adhesion of platelets to subendothelial connective tissue involves a relatively small number of platelets with binding of von Willebrand factor and glycoprotein IIb/IIIa (integrin $\alpha IIb\beta 3$) to subendothelial collagen. Manyfold more platelets are involved in formation of platelet-platelet contact at the site of injury in a reaction that involves activation of integrin $\alpha IIb\beta 3$ receptors for fibrinogen and thrombospondin binding. Within minutes, platelets adherent to subendothelial connective tissue or in contact with other platelets have released their intracellular stores of adenosine diphosphate (ADP) and secretary proteins, including von Willebrand factor and thrombospondin, to recruit other platelets in the aggregation response. Arachidonic acid within the platelet membrane is converted to thromboxane A^2 by cyclooxygenase in activated platelets. Blockade of these pathways with competitive inhibitors of integrin, ligands, or monoclonal antibodies to integrins, aspirin for cyclooxygenase-1 inhibition, and clopidogrel for inhibition of the platelet response to ADP has been found to be useful clinically in maintaining vessel patency after angioplasty or in acute coronary syndromes (47–49).

Thrombin is essential for formation of a stable fibrin-platelet thrombus (50). Once the platelet plug is formed, fibrin strands are present in the loose aggregate approximately 5 minutes after injury, and platelet plug consolidation proceeds through further deposition of fibrin and contraction of the platelet cytoskeleton. Two receptors for thrombin that allow thrombin to recruit additional platelets after coagulation reactions have been initiated have been found on platelets (51). Deficiencies of coagulation factors lead to poor platelet plug formation. Although platelet plug formation occurs normally in factor VIII–deficient dogs with cuticle injury, electron microscopic examination of the platelet plug shows much less evidence of platelet activation within the platelet plug, and platelets are less dense within the clot than in animals with a normal level of factor VII. Factor VII–deficient dogs have less impairment of platelet plug consolidation. This finding suggests that the extrinsic pathway defects lead to more thrombin generation than in factor VIII deficient dogs. Fibrinolysis occurs over days, paralleling the appearance of leukocytes and fibroblasts in the fibrin clot. Mice with inactivated prothrombin genes or with inactivation of the thrombin receptor (PAR-1) do not survive in utero and have abnormal vessel development. This finding suggests a role of the cellular response to thrombin in vessel formation after wounding (52).

COAGULATION PATHWAYS

In vitro studies of coagulation reactions are performed with phospholipid vesicles containing negatively charged phospholipid (phosphatidylserine) to replace the function of membrane surfaces in vivo. Complexes of coagulation factor proteases and cofactors are thought to form in vivo on the surface of stimulated platelets or endothelial cells in which negatively charged phospholipid is accessible on the outer cell membrane. Assembly of complexes of coagulation factors and cofactors on the surface of platelets or phospholipid vesicles accelerates coagulation reactions and can protect the proteases from their plasma inhibitors (53). Kinetic measurements have shown that the catalytic efficiency of factor X activation by factor IXa, for example, is increased by a factor of approximately 10,000 to 100,000 in the presence of factor VIIIa and phospholipid vesicles.

Complexes of fibrinolytic system enzymes also direct physiologic clot lysis. The increased binding of tissue plasminogen activator to plasminogen on a fibrin surface is an example of assembly of protease and substrate in a complex that can form without phospholipid or calcium ion. The result is increased efficiency of the enzymatic reaction for plasminogen activation. Plasminogen activator inhibitor-1 (PAI-1) has less affinity for plasmin on the surface of a fibrin clot than it does in plasma. Plasmin formed on the surface of a fibrin clot is less likely to be neutralized by α_2-antiplasmin (54).

Intrinsic and Extrinsic Coagulation

Coagulation enzymes and cofactors often are grouped as components of the intrinsic and extrinsic coagulation systems, triggered by the contact activation system (factor XII dependent) and tissue factor– and activated factor VII–dependent systems, respectively. Factor XII and other components of the intrinsic system (prekallikrein and high-molecular-weight kininogen) are not essential for clot formation in vivo because patients with congenital deficiencies of these coagulation factors do not have clinical bleeding despite prolonged partial thromboplastin time (PTT) in vitro. Other pathways for factor XI activation must function in vivo. Factor XIa, once formed, activates factor IX at two cleavage sites.

Factor X may be activated by the complex containing factor IXa, phospholipid vesicles, calcium ions, and factor VIIIa or by the complex of factor VIIa and tissue factor. In the final common pathway, factor Xa converts prothrombin to thrombin in the presence of factor Va, calcium ions, and phospholipid vesicles. Both intrinsic and extrinsic pathways are needed for normal hemostasis because patients with hemophilia A or B bleed even though the extrinsic pathway is intact. Patients with factor VII deficiency bleed even with an intact extrinsic pathway.

Thrombin generated early in the response to injury through the extrinsic pathway may activate factor XI, but the importance of this reaction in vivo is not known. This reaction has been shown to occur in vitro but requires dextran sulfate or a negatively charged surface, such as that of silicates (55). This reaction is inhibited by the presence of fibrinogen and by formation of factor XI–high-molecular-weight kininogen complexes, as occurs in plasma (56). Activation of factor XI by thrombin in vivo would allow the intrinsic system to amplify an initial clotting stimulus generated by the factor VIIa–tissue factor pathway, which would involve functions of both pathways in normal hemostasis.

The concept of separate intrinsic and extrinsic pathways remains useful despite a number of crossover pathways linking the intrinsic and extrinsic pathways. The crossover pathways include activation of factor IX by the tissue factor–VIIa complex and activation of factor VII by activated factor IX. Clinical coagulation tests can be used to detect isolated defects in the intrinsic system with a normal prothrombin time (PT) and abnormal PTT or isolated factor VII deficiency when PT is prolonged and PTT is normal. Heparin, vitamin K deficiency, liver disease, and congenital deficiencies of coagulation factors in the final common pathway prolong results of both screening tests.

Contact Activation System

Patients with deficiencies of proteins in the contact activation system (factor XII, prekallikrein, and high-molecular-weight kininogen) do not need transfusion for support in surgery or trauma. Activation of the contact activation system with sepsis or consumption coagulopathy (DIC) may contribute to coagulopathy, and generation of kinins in vivo after transfusion of plasma derivatives can cause hypotensive reactions (57) after activation of the contact activation system.

Factor XII Activation

The interaction of plasma factor XII and a surface with a high density of negative charges generates small amounts of activated factor XII (factor XIIa). Surface-bound factor XIIa activates fluid-phase prekallikrein, which cleaves surface-bound factor XIIa to amplify the initial response. High-molecular-weight kininogen binds to surfaces with a high density of negative charges in association with factor XII. The rate of activation of factor XI by factor XIIa is greatly accelerated in vitro by the presence of high-molecular-weight kininogen. In addition to its role as a binding protein, high-molecular-weight kininogen is a substrate for kallikrein, which cleaves bradykinin from high-molecular-weight kininogen. Kinins cause smooth muscle contraction and vascular permeability in vitro. Infusion of Hageman factor fragments in vivo can cause hypotension, presumably resulting from activation of prekallikrein and subsequent release of kinins from high-molecular-weight kininogen (57). Complement activation and proteolysis of high-molecular-weight kininogen have been described as occurring when plasma passes through leukocyte-reduction filters, but the amount of bradykinin generated may not be sufficient to explain reactions (58). Patients taking angiotensin-converting enzyme inhibitors for control of hypertension have a prolonged response to kinins generated during contact of blood with membranes. This occurs during use of apheresis devices and leukocyte-reduction filters and has been attributed to medication effect in blocking degradation of kinins (59).

There is probably little activation of factor XI by factor XIIa in physiologic hemostasis. Activated factor XII does appear late in cardiac bypass operations, for example, but lags well behind factor Xa detected by generation of prothrombin fragments and thrombin detected by appearance of thrombin–antithrombin III complexes (60,61).

Prekallikrein Activation

The generation of kallikrein from prekallikrein is probably caused by the action of factor XIIa. Kallikrein activates plasminogen to plasmin in vitro, generates kinin from high-molecular-weight kininogen, and activates factor XII. The physiologic importance of plasminogen activation through kallikrein is doubtful, because the principal physiologic plasminogen activator is tissue plasminogen activator. Patients with prekallikrein deficiency have been reported to have thrombotic events, but it is difficult to know whether these events exceed the expected incidence (62).

Factor XI

Patients with factor XI deficiency have a bleeding disorder of variable severity in which the bleeding manifestations may be difficult to predict from the activity level in vitro. Heterozygotes with factor XI deficiency may have a mild bleeding disorder, although this is infrequent in carriers of hemophilia A or B. Clinical bleeding seems to be more likely when tissue injury occurs in areas rich in fibrinolytic system activators such as prostatic, nasal, and oral mucosal surfaces (63). Although recurring mutations are not found in a large number of patients with other coagulation disorders, Ashkenazi Jews have three common mutations that account for factor XI deficiency. Defective processing of messenger RNA (type I), expression of a truncated protein (type II), or expression of a protein with reduced clotting activity owing to an amino acid substitution (type III) have been described. Patients with the lowest factor XI plasma activity and a clinical bleeding disorder are most often type II/III compound heterozygotes. Sixty-six of 72 alleles in a population of heterozygotes and homozygotes were found to be either type II or III in this population (64).

Factor XI activation on subendothelial tissue (65) or on the surface of platelets (66) is enhanced by binding to high-molecular-weight kininogen, but thrombin-induced activation is not. Thrombin generated early in the physiologic response to injury has been found to activate factor XI in vitro in a reaction requiring dextran sulfate. Thrombin activation of factor XI does proceed in the presence of large amounts of thrombin in vitro, so its physiologic significance is not known (67). Platelet factor XI activity is found in platelet α granules, and the factor XI level found is independent of the plasma level, suggesting a role for local synthesis. Because factor XI appears to be needed for normal hemostasis under some conditions, it is likely that it can be activated by mechanisms not dependent on contact activation pathways.

Factor IX

Activation of factor XII, prekallikrein, and factor XI can occur in the absence of calcium, but activation of factor IX and other vitamin K–dependent protease factors (factors VII and X, prothrombin, and protein C) requires calcium as the physiologic divalent cation. Vitamin K–dependent coagulation factors are differentiated according to their posttranslational modification with γ-carboxyglutamic acid residues at their amino termini. The vitamin K–dependent coagulation factor, protein C, and the vitamin K–dependent cofactor, protein S, have several calcium ion–binding sites where pairs of carboxyglutamic acid residues are located. Calcium binding or a protein conformation induced by calcium binding is responsible for the binding of these factors to the cell surface or phospholipid vesicles.

Factor IX can be activated by factor XIa or by the complex of factor VIIa and tissue factor (68). Studies on the level of prothrombin fragments in the plasma of patients with factor VII deficiency show that basal levels of these molecular fragments, which are caused by the presence of factor Xa, increase when factor VII deficiency is corrected. This observation suggests a physiologic role of the tissue factor–VIIa complex in basal hemostasis (69).

Factor X activation in vitro requires either phospholipid or a platelet or endothelial cell surface in the presence of the complex of thrombin-modified factor VIII, calcium, and factor IXa. Factor VII is also a substrate for factor IX. Studies of the level of factor VIIa in the plasma of patients with severe hemophilia B have shown that the level of factor VIIa is 0.33 ± 0.15 ng/ml, compared with the 4.34 ± 1.57 ng/ml of healthy persons and 2.69 ± 1.52 in patients with severe hemophilia A. This observation suggests that factor VIIa levels in plasma are regulated by the availability of factor IXa (70).

Platelet secretory granules contain β-amyloid protein precursor, which contains a Kunitz-like inhibitor domain and can inhibit factor XIa (71). This juxtaposition of protease and inhibitor may regulate factor IX activation in some circumstances.

Factor IX deficiency, hemophilia B, can be a severe bleeding disorder of lifelong spontaneous bleeding in joints and soft tissues. More than 600 molecular defects have been identified in patients with hemophilia B. The pattern of recurring mutations in different families suggests that there are "hot spots" in the gene.

Factor VIII—von Willebrand Factor

The bleeding defect in patients with severe factor VIII deficiency is clinically indistinguishable from that in severe factor IX deficiency. Factor VIII circulates in a complex with von Willebrand factor, which is synthesized in endothelial cells. The portion of the complex specified by the X chromosome gene is designated factor VIII or factor VIII:C (for coagulant). Von Willebrand factor is synthesized in endothelial cells, and its gene is on chromosome 12. Von Willebrand factor is essential for normal platelet adhesion and a normal bleeding time (Chapter 15). Patients with a low level of von Willebrand factor in the plasma, such as patients with a low level of or abnormal factor VIII, have a prolonged PTT and reduced factor VIII activity in a specific coagulation factor assay. This occurs because the factor VIII molecule must form a complex with von Willebrand factor to circulate in plasma. Purified recombinant factor VIII associates with von Willebrand factor in vivo (72) and is more rapidly cleared from the circulation in the absence of von Willebrand factor (73).

Deficiency of von Willebrand factor protein or abnormal function of the von Willebrand factor molecule is present in von Willebrand disease. Laboratory evidence of mild, autosomal dominant von Willebrand disease is present in 1% of the healthy population and rarely is a cause of hemorrhage (74). High plasma levels of von Willebrand factor or high levels of factor VIII:C have been thought to be either a marker or a risk factor for a tendency toward thrombosis (75). Deficiency of a plasma activity that reduces the molecular weight of von Willebrand multimers has been detected in the plasma of some patients with thrombotic thrombocytopenic purpura (TTP) and not in plasmas from patients with hemolytic uremic syndrome (76,77). Patients with TTP often have blocking activity to this metalloproteinase activity in normal plasma. The multimer pattern of plasma normalizes in some but not all patients receiving plasma therapy. This finding indicates replacement of normal multimerase activity. Large von Willebrand factor multimers favor shear-induced platelet aggregation that leads to microvascular thrombosis. The thrombosis accounts for some of the clinical features of this disease. Solvent-detergent–treated plasma lacks the high-molecular-weight forms of von Willebrand factor that are present in normal plasma and has been used in plasmapheresis of patients with TTP (78).

Thrombin-modified factor VIII is necessary for the optimal rate of activation of factor X in the presence of phospholipid, calcium, and activated factor IX. It is likely that thrombin-modified factor VIII is associated with the surface of platelets and facilitates the interaction of activated factor IX and surface-associated factor X (53). Thrombin potentiates the clotting activity of factor VIII but also degrades factor VIII after prolonged exposure in vitro. The same degradation of factor VIII in vivo probably occurs when there is excessive intravascular generation of thrombin in DIC.

Factor VII

Extrinsic coagulation is initiated by exposure of tissue factor at the site of blood vessel injury. Tissue factor is a transmembrane protein that cannot usually be detected on the surface of endothelial cells but is readily found on the surface of fibroblasts in the media of larger blood vessels. Tissue factor can be expressed by endothelial cells in culture in response to interleukin-1, and tissue factor messenger RNA is found in monocytes during endotoxemia (79). Factor VII in plasma binds to tissue factor, and a portion of the bound factor VII is activated. Trace proteases at the site of cellular injury may be sufficient to generate enough factor VIIa to activate small amounts of factor X. Factor Xa or factor IXa could act in an amplification loop to convert factor VII to factor VIIa. Factor VIIa and factor VII may compete for tissue factor; thus administration of VIIa may act by displacing the zymogen (80).

Most physiologic coagulation is thought to be initiated through the extrinsic or tissue factor–factor VIIa pathway, despite the low plasma concentration of factor VII (approximately 10 nmol/L) in plasma (Fig. 22.1). After activation of factor VII at the site of blood vessel injury, a series of coagulation reactions precede thrombin generation. These intermediate steps increase the number of ways in which the reaction can be regulated or amplified. The complexity of the regulation of the coagulation response probably reflects the need for control of clot generation in response to diverse stimuli, including vessel trauma and inflammation (Fig. 22.2).

Tissue factor pathway inhibitor is efficient in shutting off the tissue factor pathway once small amounts of factor Xa and a hemostatic response have been generated. In the presence of calcium, tissue factor pathway inhibitor binds to the complex of tissue factor, factor VIIa, and factor Xa on a phospholipid vesicle surface or on the surface of a cell and neutralizes both factor Xa and the factor VIIa–tissue factor complex (81) (Fig.

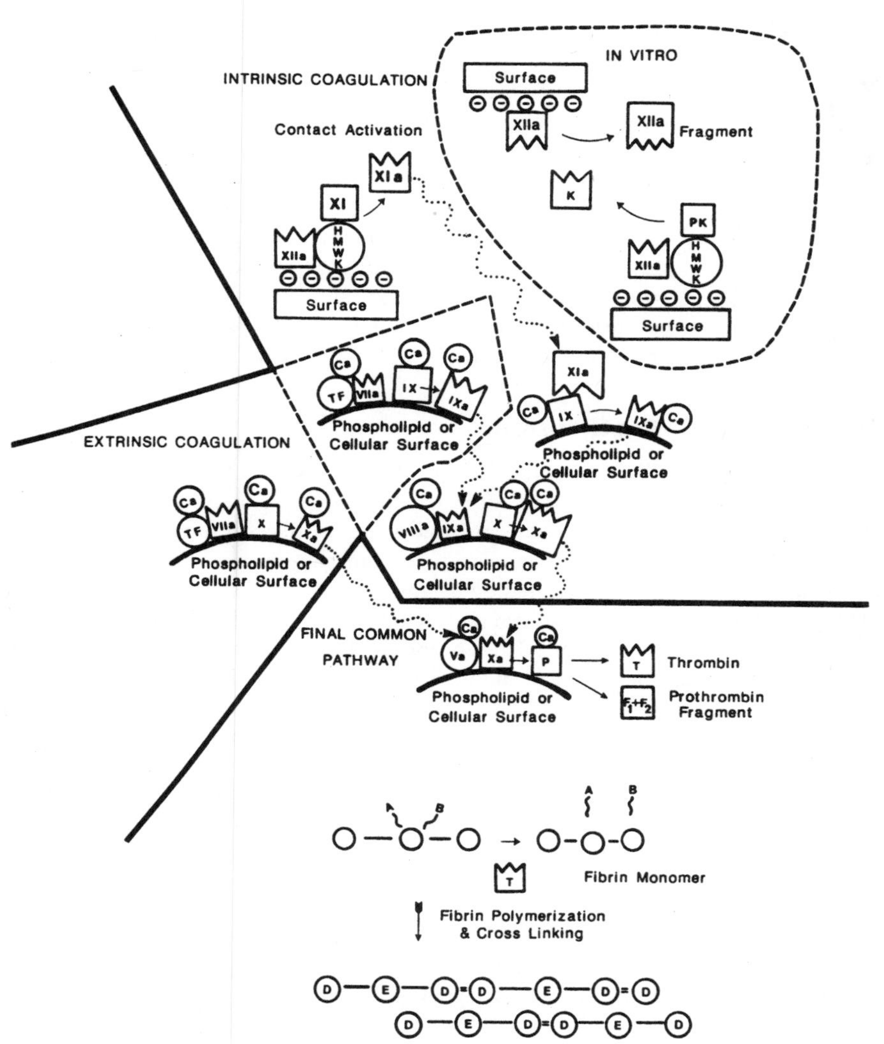

FIGURE 22.1. Generation of coagulation proteases on cellular surfaces and in solution. Factor XIIa is thought to appear after autocatalytic activation of factor XII on a negatively charged surface. Kallikrein converts surface bound factor XII to factor XIIa in an amplification cycle (not shown). Activation of factor XI in the presence of cofactors and a negatively charged surface is shown on the *left.* In vitro generation of factor XIIa fragments through the action of kallikrein is shown in the *upper right inside dashed lines.* These factor XIIa fragments can activate prekallikrein and lead to further amplification of factor XII activation. The mechanism for factor VII activation is not known. The diagram does not show thrombin modification of factors V and VIII or the possible role of thrombin in activation of factor XI. Regulation of the levels of factor Va and factor VIIIa by the protein C and S system also is not shown. Thrombin converts fibrinogen to fibrin; cleaves to factors V, VIII, and XIII; binds to platelets and endothelial cells; and converts protein C to activated protein C when bound to thrombomodulin on the surface of endothelial cells. Crossover of intrinsic and extrinsic pathways is shown in the region enclosed in *dashed lines on the left.* In the final steps of coagulation, thrombin cleaves two peptides, A and B, from fibrinogen. This is followed by polymerization and cross-linking of fibrin. *PK,* prekallikrein; *HMWK,* high-molecular-weight kininogen; *P,* prothrombin; *T,* thrombin; *TF,* tissue factor.

22.2). Tissue factor pathway inhibitor is released from the surface of endothelial cells after intravenous administration of heparin.

Bleeding with factor VII deficiency can be severe, but some patients with levels of factor VII as low as 1% to 2% have very little bleeding (82). Although at least some factor VII is needed for hemostasis, the complex of tissue factor and activated factor VII has a catalytic efficiency for factor X activation approximately 50-fold lower than that of the complex of factor IXa, factor VIIIa, and phospholipid (53). This in vitro observation may explain why the extrinsic pathway is not sufficient in the absence of the full function of the intrinsic pathway in patients with hemophilia A or B. Tissue pathway inhibitor also may dampen the extrinsic pathway and limit the hemostatic response in patients with impaired hemostasis due to deficiencies in the intrinsic systems.

Factor VIIa does not appear to have much activity in triggering coagulation in the absence of tissue factor. Recombinant factor VIIa given to patients with factor VIII inhibitors has been effective in stopping bleeding (83) and restores hemostasis to patients who have factor IX deficiency. Recipients have not had evidence of systemic activation of the coagulation system. Small amounts of tissue factor expressed at a site of injury may be already saturated with factor VII when factor VIIa is given to patients with hemophilia A or B who have inhibitors. The mechanism for activating the coagulation system may involve displacing zymogen factor VII or activation of factor X through tissue factor–independent pathways.

Plasma level of factor VII correlate with the risk of arterial thrombosis, but not all studies have shown a strong association independent of cholesterol level (84). The finding that a truncated form of tissue factor in complex with VIIa activates factor X but does not allow activation of factor VII by factors Xa or IXa has led to development of a simple PT-based assay for factor VIIa in plasma. Factor VIIa levels are elevated in patients with acute thrombosis (85) and normalize with warfarin therapy. It

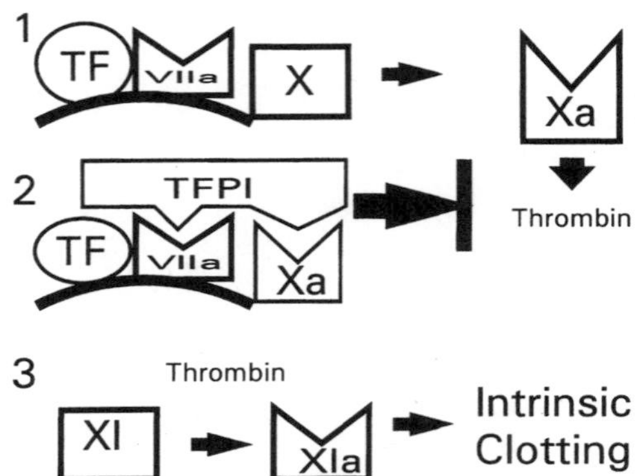

FIGURE 22.2. Tissue factor pathway inhibitor and interactions of extrinsic and intrinsic clotting. *Step 1,* activated factor VIIa is generated on the surface of a cell when tissue factor is expressed after injury. A small amount of activated factor X (factor Xa) is produced and eventually leads to production of thrombin through the final common pathway of coagulation. *Step 2,* tissue factor pathway inhibitor binds to the complex of factors VIIa, factor Xa, and tissue factor in the presence of calcium. This inhibitor blocks further production of factor Xa through the extrinsic pathway. *Step 3,* thrombin produced after the brief activation of the extrinsic pathway activated factor XI at the site of tissue injury. Factor XIa triggers intrinsic coagulation, and the initial response is amplified. Thrombin activation of factor XIa has not been shown to be important in vivo but can occur under some conditions in vitro.

is not known whether a high factor VII level in the plasma of patients at risk of coronary artery disease reflect high levels of factor VIIa.

Final Common Pathway—Factor X

Factor X, once activated by either the intrinsic or the extrinsic pathway, is able to generate further activation of factor VII in a positive-feedback reaction. Factor Xa activates prothrombin rapidly in vitro in a complex with thrombin-modified factor V, phospholipid vesicles on the platelet membrane surface, and calcium ions (53). Deficiency of factor X is most commonly associated with a mild or moderate clinical bleeding but patients with AL amyloidosis have been found susceptible to bleeding associated with even moderate factor X deficiency (86).

Factor V

Thrombin-modified factor V is a cofactor necessary for activation of prothrombin by factor Xa, calcium ions, and phospholipid vesicles or cellular surfaces. Thrombin-modified factor V has specific sites for binding to the platelet surface and for interacting with activated factor X. As much as 10% of the plasma factor V activity can be released from washed platelets after stimulation with ADP (87). Severe factor V deficiency can cause spontaneous intracerebral bleeding in infants. The bleeding that occurs with combined factor V and factor VIII deficiency is typically mild or moderate. A deficiency of the intracellular platelet protein multimerin, which is associated with low levels of platelet factor V, has been described in which the person with the disorder has a normal level of plasma factor V yet still has clinically significant bleeding (88). This observation suggests the importance of coagulation factors delivered by platelets to the site of injury. Acquired deficiency of factor V occurs in patients who receive bovine thrombin and develop alloantibodies to bovine thrombin and autoantibodies to human factor V (89).

The most common congenital condition predisposing to thrombosis in later life is found in persons whose plasma clotting times do not increase as expected when activated protein C is added to plasma. This phenomenon is due to replacement of arginine by glutamine at amino acid residue 506 in factor V in the heterozygous or homozygous state. This alteration of the protease recognition site blunts the coagulation inhibition that the protein C–protein S pathway provides (90).

Prothrombin

When vitamin K–dependent coagulation factors other than prothrombin are activated, the enzyme generated is anchored to the cell or phospholipid vesicle surface through binding of the carboxyglutamic acid–rich amino terminus. Thrombin in solution, generated by prothrombin activation, is free to react with its many substrates, including platelets, fibrinogen, factor VII, and factor XIII. Thrombin also binds to thrombomodulin on the surface of endothelial cells. This complex is a potent activator of protein C, but thrombin no longer has avidity for fibrinogen. Prothrombin deficiency is most commonly associated with a mild or moderate clinical bleeding disorder. Inactivated prothrombin genes in mice cause defective vascular development that may be due to the role of thrombin in signaling to vascular cells (52).

Fibrinogen—Factor XIII

Cleavage of fibrinopeptides A and B from fibrinogen generates fibrin monomer, which rapidly polymerizes to form fibrin. Fibrin is cross-linked by factor XIIIa. Patients with homozygous fibrinogen deficiency have a bleeding disorder of variable severity. Patients with abnormal fibrinogens can have delayed clot lysis and may have arterial and venous thrombosis (91). Patients with congenital or acquired factor XIII deficiency may have a severe bleeding disorder without abnormalities on clinical coagulation screening tests, and common polymorphisms are associated with venous thrombosis (92,93). Bleeding from the umbilical stump has been described in infants with factor XIII deficiency or congenital afibrinogenemia. Thrombin activates a carboxypeptidase activity, thrombin-activable fibrinolytic activity, that blunts fibrinolytic activity by alteration of fibrin cofactor activity in generation of plasmin. Thrombin-activable fibrinolytic activity provides a link between coagulation system activation and down-regulation of the fibrinolytic pathway (94).

COAGULATION INHIBITION

Protein C and Protein S

Protein C is activated by thrombin bound to thrombomodulin on the surface of endothelial cells. Activated protein C degrades thrombin-modified factors VIII and V in the presence of its protein S, calcium ion, and phospholipid. Thrombin-modified factor V bound to the platelet surface is less susceptible to degradation than is thrombin-modified factor V in solution. Deficiency of either protein C or protein S may lead to a thrombotic disorder, but as many as 0.31% of healthy blood donors have laboratory evidence of protein C deficiency without previous thrombosis (95). The functional activity of protein S in plasma is regulated by C4b binding protein that circulates in complex with approximately 60% to 70% of plasma protein S. In vitro testing shows that free protein S (not in complex with C4b binding protein) is the only physiologically active molecule. Some familial forms of protein S deficiency manifest as normal levels of total protein S but low levels of free protein.

The protein C pathway is important in physiologic coagulation inhibition. Patients who lack either protein C or protein S activity or who have resistance to activated protein C due to factor V polymorphism (90) have a moderately elevated risk of thrombosis. The importance of natural inhibitors of coagulation in regulating the procoagulant and inflammatory response in patients with gram-negative sepsis was found in a clinical trial of recombinant activated protein C. Constant infusion of this medication reduced mortality 19% compared with the placebo arm. Improvement in the clinical status of patients was paralleled by reduction in the immunologic measurement of plasma D-dimers (96). Down-regulation of thrombomodulin on the surface of endothelial cells in sepsis may reduce endogenous activated protein C in plasma, and replacement protein C may limit thrombin generation with coagulation system activation and may limit monocyte production of inflammatory cytokines. The importance of this anticoagulant pathway has been shown in mice with knock-out genes. Mice with inactivated thrombomodulin die in utero before the cardiovascular system develops, and mice with inactivated protein C genes die of coagulopathy (97, 98).

Antithrombin III

Antithrombin III is the principal inhibitor of factors IXa, Xa, and XIa and thrombin. Heparin binds to antithrombin III in plasma, produces a conformational change in the arginine-serine sequence of antithrombin III recognized by proteases and a 1,000-fold faster reaction rate that results in inhibition by means of formation of protease–antithrombin III complexes. A critical pentasaccharide sequence of heparin can produce this conformational change and is in clinical trials as a substitute for heparin (99). In vivo, heparin-like substances on the vascular endothelium appear to have the same role. Homozygous antithrombin III deficiency is not compatible with life, and heterozygous deficiency is a cause of a predisposition to venous thromboembolic disease. Some of these patients are found resistant to the in vitro anticoagulant effect of heparin and may have recurrent thrombosis during heparin treatment. Congenital antithrombin III deficiency is managed with oral anticoagulants for long-term prophylaxis. Heparin therapy and antithrombin III replacement have been used in these patients for prevention of thrombosis in pregnancy and for management of anticoagulation after surgical procedures. The interaction of antithrombin III with a number of proteases in coagulation pathways probably accounts for the effects of antithrombin III on the inflammatory response and survival of baboons challenged with *Escherichia coli* (100). Acquired deficiency of antithrombin III in DIC has been managed with antithrombin III concentrates. In many small studies, the coagulopathy has been shown to improve, but an effect on survival has been difficult to demonstrate (101). The incidence of thromboembolic phenomena is much higher in hereditary antithrombin III deficiency than in acquired forms.

Tissue Factor Pathway Inhibitor and Other Protease Inhibitors Important for Hemostasis

Tissue factor pathway inhibitor (TFPI) has been shown to inhibit the complex of factor Xa and factor VIIa–tissue factor (81). Tissue factor pathway inhibitor circulates at a concentration of 89 ng/ml, but plasma levels can increase 1.5- to 6.5-fold in response to heparin. Tissue factor pathway inhibitor can be synthesized by endothelial cells (102). A tissue homologue of TFPI, called *TFPI2* or *placental protein 5,* is present in the placenta and circulates in the plasma of pregnant women (103). Like their homologue, aprotinin, these inhibitors are slow, tightly binding, reversible inhibitors. Decreased levels of TFPI have been found in patients with sepsis, and recombinant TFPI can decrease the mortality of endotoxin infusion in baboons (104). Activation of coagulation in humans with experimental endotoxemia is inhibited by TFPI (105). Mice with inactivated TFPI genes die in utero (106). Factor VIIa in plasma is only slowly neutralized by antithrombin III with or without heparin, but factor VIIa in complex with tissue factor is readily neutralized by antithrombin III and heparin (107). The importance of the tissue factor pathway in regulating hemostasis has been shown in experiments in which depletion of plasma TFPI in a rabbit model of hemophilia A shortened the cuticle bleeding time (108). No congenital deficiency of TFPI has been found in patients with recurrent venous or arterial thrombosis, however. Levels of TFPI are elevated in patients with solid tumors (109).

Heparin cofactor II, protein C inhibitor, protein Z–dependent factor Xa inhibitor, α_2-macroglobulin, C1 inhibitor, and α_1-antitrypsin all may have a role in regulating coagulation under conditions such as DIC or shock when levels of protease inhibitors are depleted by consumption and when production is decreased because of organ dysfunction. Other mechanisms of inhibition of anticoagulation include phospholipid-binding proteins such as annexin V. Antiphospholipid antibodies inhibit binding of annexin V to phospholipid, and this mechanism is a potential mechanism for the thrombogenic effect (110).

FIBRINOLYTIC SYSTEM

Plasminogen activation by tissue plasminogen activator is the physiologically important mechanism for generation of plasmin for clot lysis. Plasminogen also is a substrate for prekallikrein and urokinase, but the prekallikrein pathway appears less important in vivo. Plasminogen conversion to plasmin through tissue plasminogen activator is most efficient on the surface of fibrin. The fibrin clot is digested at the exposed coiled structure connecting the D and E domains, the carboxy terminus of the γ chain, and the amino terminus of the α and β chains. Small E and DD/E fibrin degradation products are released from the fibrin clot, as are large cross-linked fibrin degradation products that may exceed the molecular weight of fibrinogen. Small amounts of fibrin degradation products in the circulation of hospitalized patients who have recently had an infection or undergone a surgical procedure appear to have little effect on hemostasis. Large amounts of fibrin degradation products, which appear in DIC or in the course of thrombolytic therapy, may have an inhibitory effect on bleeding time and results of coagulation screening tests and may contribute to bleeding complications in these patients. Plasmin degrades platelet glycoprotein IIb/IIIa in vitro (111).

Heterozygous deficiency of plasminogen is associated with recurrent venous thromboembolic disease. Activation of fibrinolysis with pharmacologic doses of tissue plasminogen activator, urokinase, or streptokinase causes substantial fibrinogenolysis. Fibrin degradation products are differentiated from fibrinogen degradation products by the presence of factor XIIIa cross-linked degradation products in serum or plasma as detected with immunologic tests.

Plasminogen activator inhibitor-1 and α_2-antiplasmin are inhibitors that regulate the fibrinolytic system. Congenital deficiency of PAI-1 has been shown to be a cause of hyperfibrinolytic bleeding. In a patient with undetectable PAI-1, the euglobulin clot lysis time was slightly shortened, but no circulating fibrin degradation products were detected (112). Patients with PAI-1 deficiency have undergone surgical procedures without need for plasma replacement therapy when antifibrinolytic therapy with ϵ-aminocaproic acid or tranexamic acid is used to prevent activation of plasminogen. A patient with reduced but measurable plasma and platelet PAI-1 had cessation of fibrinolytic bleeding with infusion of plasma (113). Deficiency of α_2-antiplasmin is associated with hyperfibrinolytic bleeding (114). A patient with this deficiency was supported through surgery without excess bleeding when plasma replacement was given. Data from in vitro experiments have indicated that α_2-antiplasmin activity is not preserved after solvent-detergent treatment of plasma. This findings raises concern about use of this product for replacement therapy (39). High expression of annexin II, a phospholipid-binding protein that acts to increase the effect of tissue plasminogen activator on plasmin on cell surfaces, is present in patients with acute promyelocytic leukemia and may contribute to bleeding among these patients (115).

CLINICALLY USEFUL COAGULATION SCREENING TESTS

Although hospitalized patients with acquired defects in hemostasis or thrombosis may have complex processes involving both deficient production and rapid destruction of coagulation factors, readily available screening tests often help to determine an approach to transfusion support. Appropriate transfusion support of patients with congenital bleeding disorders (see Chapters 28 and 31) frequently requires the use of specific coagulation factor assays for monitoring therapy.

The PTT, PT, thrombin time, fibrinogen, and immunologic assays for cross-linked fibrin degradation products can all be

TABLE 22.2. PLASMA CONCENTRATION, LEVELS RECOMMENDED FOR SURGICAL SUPPORT, AND CIRCULATORY PROPERTIES OF SELECTED COAGULATION AND FIBRINOLYTIC PROTEINS

Protein	Plasma Concentration (mg/L)	Biologic $t_{1/2}$ (h)	Recommended Level for Surgery	Intravascular Fraction (%)	Yield (%)
Fibrinogen	2,800 (116)	99 ± 3 (117)	1 g/L (117)	72 (116)	
Prothrombin	130 (118)	73 ± 7 (118)	40–50% (119)	58 (118)	
Factor V	68 (120)	12 (121), 36 (122)	10–30% (121)		83 (122)
Factor X	12 (123)	33 (124)	10–40% (124)		51 (125)
Factor VII	0.5 (126)	5 (82)	10–20% (82)		100 (82)
Factor VIII	0.24 (127)	13 ± 3 (128)	30–100% (129)		80 (130) 100 (131)
Factor IX	5 (132)	23 ± 2 (133)	20–60% (129)	22 (133)	24–54 (133)*
Factor XI	6 (134)	61 (135)	20–80% (135)		100 (135)
Factor XIII	29 (136)	282 (137)	10% (92)		50 (137)
Von Willebrand factor	6 (138)	20–40 (139)	20–50% (140)		73 (141)
Plasminogen	208 (142)	53 ± 6 (142)			
α_2-Antiplasmin	70 (143)	63 ± 8 (144)			
Tissue plasminogen activator	0.005 (144)	0.055 α, 0.43 β (145)			
Urokinase-like plasminogen activator	0.0012 (146)	1.01 (146)			
Plasminogen activator inhibitor-1	0.026 (113)				
Antithrombin III	150 (147)	65 ± 6 (148)			
Protein C	2.5 ± 0.9 (149)	7.4 − 7.8 (150)			
Protein S	26 ± 5 (151)				

Data from references shown in parentheses. The biologic half-life in hours is determined by the late-phase (β half-life) disappearance of coagulation factor activity or protein after early equilibration of intravascular and extravascular protein compartments (α half-life) has occurred. The level recommended for surgery includes the upper and lower limits of the target level after therapy. The levels required for replacement therapy of fibrinogen and factor XIII are not well defined. The intravascular portions of the administered dose of fibrinogen, prothrombin, and factor IX were determined with radiolabeled proteins. Yields of coagulation factors are defined as the percentage of the administered dose in plasma immediately after transfusion.

performed on a single tube of blood obtained in sodium citrate anticoagulant. The PTT is measured by means of adding a silicate (or another reagent with negatively charged surfaces) and phospholipid to anticoagulated plasma. After an incubation time to generate factor XIa, calcium is added, and the clotting time is recorded either mechanically or by means of a change in the optical density of the plasma sample when fibrin polymerization occurs. To measure PT, calcium and tissue factor (usually a rabbit brain extract or human recombinant tissue factor containing a complex of tissue factor and lipid) are added to the plasma sample, and the clotting time is recorded.

Fibrinogen concentration and thrombin time are measured by means of recording the clotting time of plasma after addition of commercially available bovine thrombin. In the thrombin time test, the thrombin is dilute so that the test is sensitive to inhibitors of the enzymatic activity or of fibrin polymerization thrombin, including fibrin degradation produces, because clot formation is the end point of the assay. In the kinetic method for fibrinogen quantitation, thrombin is added in excess so that the clotting time is proportional to the concentration of fibrinogen in the sample. High concentrations of fibrin degradation products in plasma can cause falsely low kinetic fibrinogen levels by inhibiting fibrin polymerization. Immunologic and protein assays of total clottable plasma fibrinogen can differ from those determined kinetically in samples with high levels of fibrin degradation products.

Immunologic tests for fibrin degradation products are commercially available. These tests are performed with latex beads coated with either antibodies to fibrin degradation products or monoclonal antibodies to a specific cross-linked fibrin degradation product, referred to as *D-D-dimer.* The test for D-D-dimer can be done on citrated plasma, because the monoclonal antibody does not react with fibrinogen in plasma. Other tests for fibrin degradation products are performed on serum from which the cross-reacting fibrinogen has been removed with the clot. The D-D-dimer is a sensitive indicator for activation of fibrinolysis in DIC. However, D-D-dimer is not present in plasma in primary fibrinogenolysis with prostate cancer, for example. Patients treated with thrombolytic therapy may have ex vivo fibrinogenolysis if fibrinolytic system inhibitors are not added to the sample collection tubes.

Abnormalities in PTT, PT, and thrombin time can be caused by deficiency of the factor or factors measured or by the presence of coagulation inhibitors (lupus-like anticoagulant, heparin, fibrin or fibrinogen degradation products, or antibodies to specific coagulation factors). If the abnormal PT and PTT persist after the plasma is mixed with an equal volume of normal pooled plasma, the prolonged clotting time (at least in part) is caused by the presence of coagulation inhibitors. Correction of PT and PTT to normal indicates single or multiple coagulation factor deficiencies. For example, if there is a complete lack of factor VIII in the patient sample, the factor VIII level in the mix of patient plasma and normal pooled plasma will be 0.5 U/ml, and the PTT on the mixture will be normal.

The appropriate sequence of screening tests differs for critically ill patients with acquired bleeding defects and for patients who are being evaluated for possible mild congenital disorders. Late-stage defects with hypofibrinogenemia and delayed fibrin polymerization from degradation products are common among critically ill patients, whereas intrinsic system defects and platelet function abnormalities are common congenital disorders. Patients with absence of α_2-antiplasmin, PAI-1, or factor XIII have excessive bleeding despite normal screening tests. Clot solubility in 5 mmol/L urea is abnormal in factor XIII deficiency, and patients with α_2-antiplasmin deficiency or PAI-1 deficiency have short clot lysis times.

Plasma levels of coagulation factors and their half-lives after transfusion are shown in Table 22.2. The use of the screening tests for diagnosis of acquired bleeding disorders is illustrated by the typical screening test profiles in Table 22.3. Diagnosis of and therapy for acquired and congenital bleeding disorders are discussed in Chapters 28 and 31.

TABLE 22.3. PROFILE OF HEMOSTATIC SCREENING TESTS

Test	Hemophilia A or B or Other Intrinsic System Deficiency or Inhibitor	Von Willebrand Disease	Severe Acute DIC	Heparin	Warfarin	Final Common Pathway Inhibitor or Deficiency	Factor VII Deficiency or Inhibitor	Hypos or Dysfbrinogenemia	Chronic Liver Disease
Platelet count	Normal	Normal	Low	Normal	Normal	Normal	Normal	Normal	Normal or low
Fibrinogen (kinetic method)	Normal	Normal	Low	Normal	Normal	Normal	Normal	Low or Normal	Normal or low
Thrombin time	Normal	Normal	Prolonged	Prolonged	Normal	Normal	Normal	Prolonged	Normal or prolonged
Reptilase time	Normal	Normal	Prolonged	Normal	Normal	Normal	Normal	Prolonged	Normal or prolonged
Prothrombin time	Normal	Normal	Prolonged	Normal or prolonged	Prolonged	Prolonged	Prolonged	Prolonged or Normal	Prolonged
Partial thromboplastin time	Prolonged	Normal or prolonged	Normal or prolonged	Prolonged	Prolonged	Prolonged	Normal	Normal or prolonged	Normal or prolonged

DIC, disseminated intravascular coagulation.
The testing sequence should differ for patients with suspected congenital bleeding disorders and critically ill patients with acquired bleeding defects. Coagulation defects involving the later stages of the coagulation cascade, including hypofibrinogenemia and delayed fibrin polymerization, are common among patients with acquired defects. Intrinsic system defects are common in congenital disorders. Patients with absence of α_2-antiplasmin, plasminogen activator inhibitor-1, or factor XIII have bleeding without any abnormality of prothrombin time, partial thromboplastin time, or fibrinogen level. Clot solubility in 5 mol/L urea is abnormal in patients with factor XIII deficiency. Patients who lack α_2-antiplasmin or plasminogen activator inhibitor-1 have a short euglobulin clot lysis time.

SUMMARY

Coagulation enzymes and cofactors are conveniently grouped into the intrinsic contact-activated system (factors XII, XI, IX, and VIII) and the extrinsic system (factor VII and tissue factor). The final common pathway consists of factor Xa, factor V, prothrombin, fibrinogen, and factor XIII. There are several ways in which activation of extrinsic clotting can stimulate the intrinsic system. Intrinsic coagulation factors in turn may regulate levels of factor VIIa in plasma. Factor V resistance to protein C degradation or deficiency of protein C, protein S, and antithrombin III can be found in patients with a predisposition to thrombosis, although patients with congenital TFPI deficiency have not been identified. The principal enzyme of the fibrinolytic system is plasminogen. When activated by tissue plasminogen activator on a fibrin surface, plasmin digests fibrin, and fibrin degradation products are released. Clinically useful coagulation tests include PTT, PT, thrombin time, fibrinogen level, and an immunologic assay for fibrin degradation products.

REFERENCES

1. Doweiko JP, Nompleggi DJ. Role of albumin in human physiology and pathophysiology. *JPEN J Parenter Enteral Nutr* 1991;15: 207–211.
2. Haupt H. Chemistry and clinical significance of human plasma proteins. *Behring Inst Mitt* 1990;86:1–66.
3. Code of Federal Regulations. 21CFR 640.34. Washington, DC. US Government Printing Office.
4. Horowitz B, Bonomo R, Prince AM, et al. Solvent/detergent-treated plasma: a virus-inactivated substitute for fresh frozen plasma. *Blood* 1992; 79:826–831.
5. Prusiner SB. Neurodegenerative diseases and prions. *N Engl J Med* 2001;1516–1526.
6. Peters T. Serum albumin. *Adv Protein Chem* 1985;37:161–245.
7. Takeda Y, Reeve EB. Studies of metabolism and distribution of albumin with autologous I131-albumin in healthy men. *J Lab Clin Med* 1963;61:183–202.
8. Quinlan GJ, Margarson MP, Mumby S, et al. Administration of albumin to patients with sepsis syndrome: a possible beneficial role in plasma thiol repletion. *Clin Sci* 1998;95:459–465.
9. Sort P, Navasa M, Arroyo V, et al. Effects of intravenous albumin on renal impairments and mortality in patients with cirrhosis and spontaneous bacterial peritonitis. *N Engl J Med* 1999;341:403–409.
10. Fliser D, Zurbruggen I, Mutschler E, et al. Coadministration of albumin and furosemide in patients with the nephrotic syndrome. *Kidney Int* 1999;55:629–634.
11. Shoham Z, Weissman A, Barash A, et al. Intravenous albumin for the prevention of severe ovarian hyperstimulation syndrome in an in vitro fertilization program: a prospective, randomized, placebo-controlled study. *Fertil Steril* 1994;62:137–142.
12. Messori A, Rampazzo R, Scroccaro G, et al. Efficacy of hyperimmune anti-cytomegalovirus immunoglobulins for the prevention of cytomegalovirus infection in recipients of allogeneic bone marrow transplantation: a meta-analysis. *Bone Marrow Transplant* 1994;13: 163–167.
13. Falagas ME, Snydman DR, Ruthazer R, et al. Cytomegalovirus immune globulin (CMVIG) prophylaxis is associated with increased survival after orthotopic liver transplantation. The Boston Center for Liver Transplantation CMVIG Study Group. *Clin Transplant* 1997; 11:432–437.
14. Centers for Disease Control. Post-exposure prophylaxis of hepatitis B. *MMWR Morb Mortal Wkly Rep* 1984;33:285–290.
15. Centers for Disease Control. Recommendations for protection against viral hepatitis. *MMWR Morb Mortal Wkly Rep* 1985;34: 313–324,329–335.
16. Centers for Disease Control. Rabies prevention—United States; *MMWR Morb Mortal Wkly Rep* 1984;33:393–402,407–408.
17. Kurtzman G, Frickhofen N, Kimball J, et al. Pure red-cell aplasia of 10 years duration due to persistent parvovirus B19 infection and its cure with immunoglobulin therapy. *N Engl J Med* 1989;321: 519–523.
18. Hartwell EA. Use of Rh immune globulin. *Am J Clin Pathol* 1998; 110:281–292.
19. Buckley RH, Schiff RI. The use of intravenous immune globulin in immunodeficiency diseases. *N Engl J Med* 1991;325;110–117.
20. Chapel HM, Lee M, Hargreaves R, et al. Randomized trial of intravenous immunoglobulin as prophylaxis against infection in plateau-phase multiple myeloma. *Lancet* 1994;343:1059–1063.
21. Weeks JC, Tierney MR, Weinstein MC. Cost effectiveness of prophylactic intravenous immune globulin in chronic lymphocytic leukemia. *N Engl J Med* 1991;325:81–86.
22. National Institute of Child Health and Human Development Intravenous Immunoglobulin Clinical Trial Study Group. Intravenous immunoglobulin for the prevention of bacterial infections in children with symptomatic human immunodeficiency virus infection. *N Engl J Med* 1991;325:73–80.
23. Saint-Marc T, Touraine JL, Berra N. Beneficial effects of intravenous immunoglobulins in AIDS. *Lancet* 1992;340:1347.
24. Wolff SN, Fay JW, Herzig RH, et al. High-dose weekly intravenous immunoglobulin to prevent infections in patients undergoing autologous bone marrow transplantation or severe myelosuppressive therapy: a study of the American Bone Marrow Transplant Group. *Ann Intern Med* 1993;118:937–942.
25. Sullivan KM, Storek J, Kopecky JK, et al. A controlled trial of long-term administration of intravenous immunoglobulin to prevent late infection and chronic graft-versus-host disease after marrow transplantation. *Biol Blood Marrow Transplant* 1996;2:44–53.
26. Blanchette V, Imbach P, Andrew M, et al. Randomized trial of intravenous immunoglobulin G, intravenous anti-D, and oral prednisone in childhood acute immune thrombocytopenic purpura. *Lancet* 1994; 344:703–707.
27. Mouthon L, Kaveri SV, Spalter SH, et al. Mechanisms of action of intravenous immune globulin in immune-mediated diseases. *Clin Exp Immunol* 1996;104:3–9.
28. Fischer P, Uttenreuther-Fischer. Kawasaki disease: update on diagnosis, treatment, and a still controversial etiology. *Pediatr Hematol Oncol* 1996;13:487–501.
29. Hahn AF, Bolton CF, Zochodne D, et al. Intravenous immunoglobulin treatment in chronic inflammatory demyelinating polyneuropathy: a double-blind, placebo-controlled, cross-over study. *Brain* 1996;119: 1067–1077.
30. Bril V, Ilse WK, Pearse R, et al. Pilot trial of immunoglobulin versus plasma exchange in patients with Guillain-Barré syndrome. *Neurology* 1996;46:100–103.
31. Valensise H, Vaquero E, De Carolis C, et al. Normal fetal growth in women with antiphospholipid syndrome treated with high-dose intravenous immunoglobulin (IVIG). *Prenat Diagn* 1995;15: 509–517.
32. Cherin P, Piette JC, Wechsler B, et al. Intravenous gamma globulin as first line therapy in polymyositis and dermatomyositis: an open study in 11 adult patients. *J Rheumatol* 1994;21:1092–1097.
33. Dalakas MC, Sonies B, Dambrosia J, et al. Treatment of inclusion-body myositis with IVIG: a double-blind, placebo-controlled study. *Neurology* 1997;48:712–716.
34. Crenier L, Ducobu J, des Grottes JM, et al. Low response to high-dose intravenous immunoglobulin in the treatment of acquired factor VIII inhibitor. *Br J Haematol* 1996;95:750–753.
35. van der Graaf F, Koedam JA, Bouma BM. Inactivation of kallikrein in human plasma. *J Clin Invest* 1983;71:149–158.
36. Agostini A, Lijnen HR, Pixley RA, et al. Inactionation of factor XII active fragment in normal plasma: predominant role of C1-inhibitor. *J Clin Invest* 1983;73:1542–1549.
37. Agostoni A, Cicardi M. Hereditary and acquired C1-inhibitor defi-

ciency: biological and clinical characteristics in 235 patients. *Medicine (Baltimore)* 1992;71:206–215.

38. Schmidt EW, Rasche B, Ulmer WT, et al. Replacement therapy for α-1-protease inhibitor deficiency in PiZ subjects with chronic obstructive lung disease. *Am J Med* 1988;84(suppl 6A):63–69.
39. Mast AE, Standanlick JE, Lockett JM, et al. Solvent/detergent-treated plasma has decreased antitrypsin activity and absent antiplasmin activity. *Blood* 1999;94:3922–3927.
40. Levi M, ten Cate H. Disseminated intravascular coagulation. *N Engl J Med* 1999;341:586–592.
41. Spector I, Corn M, Ticktin HE. Effect of plasma transfusion on the prothrombin time and clotting factors in liver disease. *N Engl J Med* 1966; 275:1032–1037.
42. Makris M, Greaves M, Phillips WS, et al. Emergency oral anticoagulant reversal. *Thromb Haemost* 1997;77:477–480.
43. Tawes RL Jr, Sydorak GR, DuVall TB. Autologous fibrin glue: the last step in operative hemostasis. *Am J Surg* 1994;168;120–122.
44. Martinowitz U, Schulman S, Horoszowski H, et al. Role of fibrin sealants in surgical procedures on patients with hemostatic disorders. *Clin Orthop* 1996;328:65–75.
45. McCarthy PM. Fibrin glue in cardiothoracic surgery. *Transfus Med Rev* 1993;7:173–179.
46. Weiss HJ, Turitto VT, Baumgartner HR. Role of shear rate and platelets in promoting fibrin formation on rabbit subendothelium: studies utilizing patients with quantitative and qualitative platelet defects. *J Clin Invest* 1986;78:1072–1082.
47. EPISTENT Investigators. Randomised placebo-controlled and balloon-angioplasty–controlled trial to assess safety of coronary stenting with use of platelet glycoprotein-IIb/IIIa blockade. *Lancet* 1998;352: 87–92.
48. The EPILOG Investigators. Platelet glycoprotein IIb/IIa receptor blockade and low-dose heparin during percutaneous coronary revascularization. *N Engl J Med* 1997;336:1689–1696.
49. Yusuf S. Clopidogrel in unstable angina to prevent recurrent ischemic events (CURE). Program and Abstracts of the 50th Annual Scientific Session of the American College of Cardiology, March 18–21, 2001.
50. Van der Velden P, Giles AR. A detailed morphological evaluation of the evolution of the haemostatic plug in normal, factor VII and factor VIII deficient dogs. *Br J Haematol* 1988;70:345–355.
51. Kahn ML, Nakanishi-Matsui M, Shapiro MJ, et al. Protease activated receptors 1 and 4 medicate activation of human platelets by thrombin. *J Clin Invest* 1999;103:879–888.
52. Sun WY, Witte DP, Degen JL, et al. Prothrombin deficiency results in embryonic and neonatal lethality in mice. *Proc Natl Acad Sci U S A* 1998;95:7597–7602.
53. Mann KG, Nesheim ME, Church WR, et al. Surface dependent reactions of the vitamin K–dependent enzyme complexes. *Blood* 1990; 76:1–16.
54. Collen D. Basic and clinical aspects of fibrinolysis and thrombolysis. *Blood* 1990;78:3114–3124.
55. Gailani D, Broze GJ Jr. Factor XII–independent activation of factor XI in plasma: effects of sulfatides on tissue factor–induced coagulation. *Blood* 1993;82:813–819.
56. Scott CF, Colman RW. Fibrinogen blocks the autoactivation and thrombin-mediated activation of factor XI on dextran sulfate. *Proc Natl Acad Sci U S A* 1992;89:11189–11193.
57. Alving BM, Hojima Y, Pisano JJ, et al. Hypotension associated with prekallikrein activator (Hageman-factor fragments) in plasma protein fraction. *N Engl J Med* 1978;299:66–70.
58. Scott CF, Brandwein H, Whitbread J, et al. Lack of clinically significant contact system activation during platelet concentrate filtration by leukocyte removal filters. *Blood* 1998;92:616–622.
59. Cyr M, Eastlund T, Blais C Jr, et al. Bradykinin metabolism and hypotensive transfusion reactions. *Transfusion* 2001;41:136–150.
60. Boisclair MD, Lane DA, Philippou H, et al. Mechanisms of thrombin generation during surgery and cardiopulmonary bypass. *Blood* 1993; 82:3350–3357.
61. Burman JF, Chung HI, Lane DA, et al. Role of factor XII in thrombin generation and fibrinolysis during cardiopulmonary bypass. *Lancet* 1994;344:1192–1193.
62. Currimbhoy Z, Vinciguerra V, Palakavongs P, et al. Fletcher factor deficiency and myocardial infarction. *Am J Clin Pathol* 1976;65: 970–974.
63. Bolton-Maggs PHB, Patterson DA, Wensley RT, et al. Definition of the bleeding tendency in factor XI deficient kindreds. *Thromb Haemost* 1995;73:194–202.
64. Hancock JF, Wieland K, Pugh RE, et al. A molecular genetic study of factor XI deficiency. *Blood* 1991;77:1942–1948.
65. Wiggins RC, Bouma BN, Cochrane CC, et al. Role of HMWK in surface binding and activation of coagulation factor XI and prekallikrein. *Proc Natl Acad Sci U S A* 1977;74:4636.
66. Gailani D, Ho D, Sun MF, et al. Model for a factor IX activation complex on blood platelets. *Blood* 2001;97:3117–3122.
67. Wuillemin WA, Mertens K, ten Cate H, et al. Thrombin-mediated activation of endogenous factor XI in plasma in the presence of physiologic amounts of glycosaminoglycans occurs only with high concentrations of thrombin. *Br J Haematol* 1996;92:466–472.
68. Bajaj SP, Rapaport SI, Russell WA. Determination of the rate-limiting step in the activation of factor IX by factor XIa and by factor VIIa/ tissue factor. *Biochemistry* 1983;22:4047–4053.
69. Bauer KA, Mannucci PM, Gringeri A, et al. Factor IXa–factor VIIa–cell surface complex does not contribute to the basal activation of the coagulation mechanism in vivo. *Blood* 1992;79:2039–2047.
70. Wildgoose P, Nemerson Y, Hansen LL, et al. Measurement of basal levels of factor VIIa in hemophilia A and B patients. *Blood* 1992;80: 25–28.
71. Smith RP, Higuchi DA, Broze GJ Jr. Platelet coagulation factor XIa-inhibitor, a form of Alzheimer amyloid precursor protein. *Science* 1990;24:1126–1128.
72. Giles AR, Tinlin S, Hoogendoorn H, et al. In vivo characterization of recombinant factor VIII in a canine model of hemophilia A (factor VIII deficiency). *Blood* 1988;72:335–339.
73. Brinkhous KM, Sandberg H, Carris JB, et al. Purified human factor VIII procoagulant protein: comparative hemostatic response after infusions into hemophilic and von Willebrand disease dogs. *Proc Natl Acad Sci U S A* 1985;82:8752–8756.
74. Sadler JE, Gralnick HR. Commentary: a new classification for von Willebrand disease. *Blood* 1994;84:676–679.
75. Kyrle PA, Minar E, Hirschl M, et al. High plasma levels of factor VIII and the risk of recurrent venous thromboembolism. *N Engl J Med* 2000;343:457–462.
76. Furlan M, Robles R, Galbusera M, et al. von Willebrand factor–cleaving protease in thrombotic thrombocytopenic purpura and the hemolytic-uremic syndrome. *N Engl J Med* 1998;339:1578–1584.
77. Tasi HM, Lian ECY. Antibodies to von Willebrand factor–cleaving protease in acute thrombotic thrombocytopenic purpura. *N Engl J Med* 1998;339:1585–1594.
78. Harrison CN, Lawrie AS, Iqbal A, et al. Plasma exchange with solvent/ detergent-treated plasma of resistant thrombotic thrombocytopenic purpura. *Br J Haematol* 1996;94:756–758.
79. Franco RF, deJonge E, Dekkers PEP, et al. The in vivo kinetics of tissue factor messenger RNA expression during human endotoxemia: relationship to activation of coagulation. *Blood* 2000;96:554–559.
80. van't Veer C, Golden NJ, Mann KG, Inhibition of thrombin generation by the zymogen factor VII. *Blood* 2000;95:1330–1335.
81. Rapaport SI, Rao VM. Initiation and regulation of tissue factor–dependent blood coagulation. *Arterioscler Thromb* 1992;12:1111–1121.
82. Marder VJ, Schulman NR. Clinical aspects of congenital factor VII deficiency. *Am J Med* 1964;37:182–194.
83. Hay CRM, Negrier C, Ludlam CA. The treatment of bleeding in acquired hemophilia with recombinant factor VIIa. *Thromb Haemost* 1997;78:1463–1467.
84. Meade TW, Brozovic M, Chakrabarti RR, et al. Haemostatic function and ischaemic heart disease: principal results of the Northwick Park Heart Study. *Lancet* 1986;2:533–537.
85. Morrissey JH, Macik BG, Neuenschwander PR, et al. Quantitation of activated factor VII levels in plasma using a tissue factor mutant selectively deficient in promoting factor VII activation. *Blood* 1993; 81:734–744.
86. Boggio L, Green D. Recombinant human factor VIIa in the manage-

ment of amyloid-associated factor X deficiency. *Br J Haematol* 2001; 112:1074–1075.
87. Vicic WJ, Lages B, Weiss HJ. Release of human platelet factor V activity is induced by both collagen and ADP and is inhibited by aspirin. *Blood* 1980;56:448–455.
88. Hayward CPM, Cramer EM, Kane WH, et al. Studies of a second family with the Quebec platelet disorder. *Blood* 1997;88:1243–1253.
89. Dorion RP, Hamati HF, Landis B, et al. Risk and clinical significance of developing antibodies inducted by topical thrombin preparations. *Arch Pathol Lab Med* 1998;122:887–984.
90. Simioni P, Prandoni P, Lensing AWA, et al. The risk of recurrent venous thromboembolism in patients with and $Arg^{508}\rightarrow$Gln mutation in the gene for factor V (factor V Leiden). *N Engl J Med* 1997;336: 399–403.
91. Galanakis DK. Inherited dysfibrinogenemia: emerging abnormal structure associations with pathologic and nonpathologic dysfunction. *Semin Thromb Hemost* 1993;19:386–395.
92. Kitchens CS, Newcomb TF. Factor XIII. *Medicine* 1979;58: 413–429.
93. Catto AJ, Kohler HP, Coore J, et al. Association of a common polymorphism in the factor XIII gene with venous thrombosis. *Blood* 1999;93:906–908.
94. Wang W, Boffa MB, Bajzar L, et al. A study of the mechanism of inhibition of fibrinolysis by activated thrombin–activable fibrinolysis inhibitor. *J Biol Chem* 1998;273:27176–27181.
95. Miletich J, Sherman L, Broze G Jr. Absence of thrombosis in subjects with heterozygous protein C deficiency. *N Engl J Med* 1987;317: 991–996.
96. Bernard GR, Vincent JL, Laterre PF, et al. Efficacy and safety of recombinant activated protein C for severe sepsis. *N Engl J Med* 2001; 344:699–709.
97. Healy A, Rayburn HB, Rosenberg RD, et al. Absence of the blood clotting protein regulator, thrombomodulin causes embryonic lethality in mice before development of a functional cardiovascular system. *Proc Natl Acad Sci U S A* 1995;68:291–296.
98. Jalbert LR, Rosen ED, Moons L, et al. Inactivation of the gene for anticoagulant protein C causes lethal perinatal consumptive coagulopathy in mice. *J Clin Invest* 1998;102:1481–1498.
99. Turpie AGG, Gallus AS, Hoek JA. A synthetic pentasaccharide for the prevention of deep-vein thrombosis after total hip replacement. *N Engl J Med* 2001;344:619–625.
100. Minnema MC, Chang ACK, Jansen PM, et al. Recombinant human antithrombin III improves survival and attenuates inflammatory responses in baboons lethally challenged with *Escherichia coli*. *Blood* 2000;95:1117–1123.
101. White B, Perry D. Acquired antithrombin deficiency in sepsis. *Br J Haematol* 2001;112:26–31.
102. Novotny WF, Brown SG, Miletich JP, et al. Plasma antigen levels of the lipoprotein-associated coagulation inhibitor in patient samples. *Blood* 1991;78:387–393.
103. Kisiel W. Evidence that a second human tissue factor pathway inhibitor (TFPI-2) and human placental protein 5 are equivalent. *Blood* 1994;84:4384–4385.
104. Creasey AA, Chang ACK, Feigen L, et al. Tissue factor pathway inhibitor reduces mortality from *Escherichia coli* septic shock. *J Clin Invest* 1993;91:2850–2860.
105. Jonge E, Dekkers PEP, Creasey AA, et al. Tissue factor pathway inhibitor dose-dependently inhibits coagulation activation without influencing the fibrinolytic and cytokine response during human endotoxemia. *Blood* 2000;95:1124–1129.
106. Huang ZF, Higuchi D, Lasky N, et al. Tissue factor pathway inhibitor gene disruption produces intrauterine lethality in mice. *Blood* 1997; 90:944–951.
107. Rao LVM, Nordfang O, Hoang AD, et al. Mechanism of antithrombin III inhibition of factor VIIa/tissue factor activity on a cell surface. *Blood* 1995;85:121–129.
108. Hedner U, Erhardtsen E. Future possibilities in regulation of the extrinsic pathway: rfviia and TFPT. *Ann Med* 2000;32[Suppl 1]: 68–72.
109. Iversen N, Lindahl AK, Abildgaard U. Elevated TFPI in malignant disease: relation to cancer type and hypercoagulation. *Br J Haematol* 1998;102;9889.
110. Rand JH, Wu XX, Andree HAM, et al. Antiphospholipid antibodies accelerate plasma coagulation by inhibiting annexin V binding to phospholipids. *Blood* 1998;92:1652–1660.
111. Pasche B, Ouimet H, Francis S, et al. Structural changes in platelet glycoprotein IIb/IIIa by plasmin: determinants and functional consequences. *Blood* 1994;83:404–414.
112. Dieval J, Nguyen G, Gross S, et al. A lifelong bleeding disorder associated with a deficiency of plasminogen activator inhibitor type I. *Blood* 1991;77:528–532.
113. Lee MH, Vosburgh E, Anderson K, et al. Deficiency of plasma plasminogen activator inhibitor 1 results in hyperfibrinolytic bleeding. *Blood* 1993;81:2357–2362.
114. Shahian DM, Levine JD. Open-heart surgery in a patient with heterozygous α_2-antiplasmin deficiency. *Chest* 1990;97:1488–1490.
115. Menell JA, Caesarman GM, Jacovina AT, et al. Annexin II and bleeding in acute promyelocytic leukemia. *N Engl J Med* 1999;340: 994–1004.
116. Collen D, Tytgat CN, Claeys H, et al. Metabolism and distribution of fibrinogen. *Br J Haematol* 1972;22:681–700.
117. Mammen EF. Fibrinogen abnormalities. *Semin Thromb Hemost* 1983; 9:1–9.
118. Rouvier J, Collen D, Swart ACW, et al. Prothrombin metabolism in healthy subjects and in two patients with congenital hypothrombinemia. In: Hemker HC, ed. *Prothrombin and related coagulation factors.* Leiden, The Netherlands: Leiden University Press, 1975: 167–182.
119. Mammen EF. Factor II abnormalities. *Semin Thromb Hemost* 1983; 9:13–16.
120. Tracy PB, Giles AR, Mann KC, et al. Factor V (Quebec): a bleeding diathesis associated with a qualitative platelet factor V deficiency. *J Clin Invest* 1984;14:1221–1228.
121. Mellinger EJ, Duckert F. Major surgery in a subject with factor V deficiency. *Thromb Diath Haemorrh* 1971;25:438–446.
122. Webster WP, Roberts HR, Penick CD. Hemostasis in factor V deficiency. *Am J Med* Sci 1964;248:194–202.
123. Fair DS, Plow EF, Edgington TS. Combined functional and immunochemical analysis of normal and abnormal human factor X. *J Clin Invest* 1979;64:884–893.
124. Roberts HP, Lechler E, Webster WP, et al. Survival of transfused factor X in patients with Stuart disease. *Thromb Diath Haemorrh* 1968;13:305–313.
125. Biggs R, Denson KWE. The fate of prothrombin and factors VIII, IX and X transfused to patient deficient in these factors. *Br J Haematol* 1963;9:532–547.
126. Bajaj SP, Rapaport SL, Brown SF. Isolation and characterization of human factor VII. *J Biol Chem* 1981;256:253–259.
127. Rotblat F, O'Brien DP, O'Brien FJ, et al. Purification of human factor VIII:C and its characterization by western blotting using monoclonal antibodies. *Biochemistry* 1985;24:4294–4300.
128. Weiss AE, Webster WP, Strike LE, et al. Survival of transfused factor VIII in hemophilic patients treated with epsilon aminocaproic acid. *Transfusion* 1976;16:209–214.
129. Levine PH. Clinical manifestations and therapy of hemophilias A and B. In: Colman RW, Hirsh J, Marder VJ, et al., eds. *Hemostasis and thrombosis: basic principles and clinical practice.* Philadelphia: JB Lippincott, 1987:97–111.
130. Biggs R. Plasma concentrations of factor VIII and factor IX and treatment of patients who do not have antibodies directed against these factors. In: Biggs R, ed. *The treatment of hemophilia A and B and von Willebrand's disease.* Oxford: Blackwell Scientific, 1978:110–126.
131. Allain JP, Verrcust F, Soulier JP. In vitro and in vivo characterization of factor VIII preparations. *Vox Sang* 1980;38:68–80.
132. Osterud B, Bouma BN, Griffin JH. Human blood coagulation factor IX. *J Biol Chem* 1978;253:5946–5951.
133. Smith KJ, Thompson AR. Labeled factor IX kinetics in patients with hemophilia-B. *Blood* 1981;58:625–629.
134. Saito H, Goldsmith GH Jr. Plasma thromboplastin antecedent (PTA,

factor XI): a specific and sensitive radioimmunoassay. *Blood* 1977; 50:377–385.
135. Nossel HL, Niemetz J, Mibashan RS, et al. The measurement of factor XI (plasma thromboplastin antecedent). *Br J Haematol* 1966; 12:133–144.
136. Skrzynia C, Reisner HM, McDonagh J. Characterization of the catalytic subunit of factor XIII by radioimmunoassay. *Blood* 1982;60: 1089–1095.
137. Miloszewski K, Losowsky MS. The half-life of factor XIII in vivo. *Br J Haematol* 1970;19:685–690.
138. Chopek MW, Girma JP, Fujikawa K, et al. Human von Willebrand factor: a multivalent protein composed of identical subunits. *Biochemistry* 1986;25:3146–3155.
139. Bennet B, Ratnoff OD. Studies on the response of patients with chronic hemophilia to transfusion with concentrates of antihemophilic factor. *J Clin Invest* 1972;51:2593–2601.
140. Holmberg L, Nilsson IM. von Willebrand's disease. *Eur J Haematol* 1992;48:127–141.
141. Over J, Sixma JJ, Marijke H, et al. Survival of ^{125}iodine-labeled factor VIII in normals and patients with classic hemophilia. *J Clin Invest* 1978;38:223–234.
142. Collen D, Tytgat G, Claeys H, et al. Metabolism of plasminogen in healthy subjects. *J Clin Invest* 1972;51:1310–1318.
143. Collen D, Wiman B. Turnover of antiplasmin, the fast-acting plasmin inhibitor of plasma. *Blood* 1979;53:313–324.
144. Rijken DC, Juhan-Vague I, DeCock F, et al. Measurement of human tissue type plasminogen activator by a two-site immuonoradiometric assay. *J Lab Clin Med* 1983;101:274–280.
145. Seifried E, Tanswell P, Rijken DC, et al. Pharmacokinetics of antigen and activity of recombinant tissue-type plasminogen activator after infusion in healthy volunteers. *Arzneimittelforschung* 1988;38: 418–422.
146. Kohler M, Sen S, Miyashita C, et al. Half-life of single-chain urokinase-type plasminogen activator (scu-PA) and two-chain urokinase-type plasminogen activator (tcu-PA) in patients with acute myocardial infarction. *Thromb Res* 1991;62:75–81.
147. Murano G, Williams L, Miller-Anderson M, et al. Some properties of antithrombin III and its concentration in human plasma. *Thromb Res* 1980;18:259–262.
148. Carlson TH, Simon TL, Atencio AC. In vivo behavior of human radioiodinated antithrombin III: distribution among three physiologic pools. *Blood* 1985;66:13–19.
149. Ikeda K, Stenflo J. A radioimmunoassay for protein C. *Thromb Res* 1985;39:297–306.
150. Marlar RA, Sills RH, Groncy PK, et al. Protein C survival during replacement therapy in homozygous protein C deficiency. *Am J Hematol* 1992;41:24–31.
151. Griffin JH, Gruber A, Fernandez JA. Reevaluation of total, free, and bound protein S and C4b-binding protein levels in plasma anticoagulated with citrate or hirudin. *Blood* 1992;79:3203–3211.

Rossi's Principles of Transfusion Medicine, Third Edition, edited by Toby L. Simon, Walter H. Dzik, Edward L. Snyder, Christopher P. Stowell, and Ronald G. Strauss. Lippincott Williams & Wilkins, Philadelphia © 2002.

23

PREPARATION OF PLASMA DERIVATIVES

WILLEM G. VAN AKEN

Medicinal products derived from plasma constitute important therapeutic and preventive modalities for clinical medicine. In this chapter the principles of collecting the source material (i.e., blood and plasma) and the methods used for the separation and purification of plasma proteins are described. The various measures to decrease the risk of transmission of blood-borne viruses by plasma derivatives are discussed, and an outline of quality assurance of the manufacturing process is presented. The clinical use of albumin is reviewed, taking into account the controversy over the use of albumin and substitutes thereof. Lastly, economic and logistic tradeoffs of some plasma derivatives are discussed.

Current transfusion practitioners strive to provide the blood component or plasma derivative best suited to a patient's needs. This demands a thorough knowledge of the clinical situations that require special blood components or derivatives, as well as of the sources these are derived from, the manufacturing processes, and their proper use.

Plasma contains more than 700 different proteins, usually categorized according to their function as transport proteins (notably albumin), immunoglobulins, lipoproteins, complement factors, coagulation factors, and proteinase inhibitors. There are large numbers of plasma proteins that are chemically well characterized but whose functions are still unknown. The concentration of each protein within individual groups varies considerably; for instance, among the various transport proteins, albumin concentrations range from 35 to 55 g/l, whereas transcobalamin II, which transports vitamin B_{12}, is present only in trace amounts (0.004 mg/l). Most coagulation factors and complement factors are present in even smaller concentrations.

Annually, about 30 million liters of plasma are processed worldwide through an industrial process called fractionation, which involves a complex sequence of extraction, purification, virus inactivation, and formulation steps, ultimately providing a variety of stable plasma derivatives for clinical use (Table 23.1).

PROCUREMENT OF HUMAN PLASMA

Plasma can be obtained by centrifugation of whole blood and by plasmapheresis. Depending on the separation and storage conditions, four types of plasma are distinguished: fresh frozen plasma, liquid plasma, source plasma, and recovered plasma (Table 23.2). In many countries with organized transfusion services, almost all (>95%) transfusions are given in the form of cellular blood components derived from donations of whole blood. This yields plasma that can be recovered and transfused directly or processed into plasma derivatives such as coagulation factor concentrates, albumin, and immune globulins. When plasma is the driving force for collection, apheresis is the most efficient method for collection. In the United States (and to a lesser extent in most other countries) about 75% of the plasma used for fractionation is collected by plasmapheresis, predominantly from paid donors.

W.G. van Aken: Director of Products and Medical Affairs, Sanguin Blood Supply Foundation, Amsterdam, The Netherlands.

TABLE 23.1. CLINICALLY USED PLASMA PRODUCTS

Plasma Product	Preparations	Indications (Usage)
Albumin		
Human serum albumin	20–25% solution for intravenous injection	Severe acute hypoproteinemia Exchange transfusion in neonates Adult respiratory distress syndrome
Plasma protein fraction	4.5–5% solution for intravenous injection	Shock syndromes Severe burns Therapeutic plasma exchange
Immunoglobulins		
Multispecific (normal) Immune serum globulin Immune globulin intravenous	Freeze-dried or in solution (16%) for intramuscular injection	Hypo-/Agammaglobulinemia Prophylaxis of infectious diseases (hepatitis A) Hypo-/Agammaglobulinemia Idiopathic thrombocytopenia Kawasaki syndrome
Specific (hyperimmune)	Freeze dried or in solution for intravenous injection (6%)	Prevention of:
Cytomegalovirus (CMV) immune globulin		CMV infection in immuno-suppressed individuals
Hepatitis B (HBV) immune globulin		HBV infection
Pertussis immune globulin		Whooping cough infection
Rabies immune globulin		Rabies infection
Rho (D) immune globulin		Hemolytic disease of the newborn and Rhesus sensitization in other situations
Tetanus immune globulin		Tetanus infection
Vaccinia immune globulin		Smallpox infection
Varicella immune globulin		Chickenpox infection
Coagulation Proteins		
Factor VIII	Freeze dried, for intravenous injection (potency data vary for manufacturers)	Hemophilia A
Factor IX complex		Hemophilia B, factor VII-, factor X, factor II-deficiency, coumarin overdose
Factor IX		Hemophilia B
Factor VII		Factor VII-deficiency
Factor XIII		Factor XIII-deficiency
von Willebrand factor		von Willebrand disease
Cryoprecipitate		Hemophilia A von Willebrand disease Fibrinogen deficiency
Activated factor IX complex/factor VIII by-passing activity		Factor VIII inhibitor
Fibrin sealant	Freeze dried, for topical application	Wound healing
Protease Inhibitors		
Antithrombin III	Freeze dried, for intravenous injection (potency data vary for manufacturers)	Antithrombin III-deficiency
α-1-proteinase inhibitor		Proteinase inhibitor deficiency
Cl-esterase inhibitor		Hereditary angioneurotic edema

TABLE 23.2. TYPES OF PLASMA FOR PREPARATION OF COMPONENTS

Name	Collection Method	Storage Condition
Fresh frozen plasma (FFP)	Whole-blood donation	Separated and frozen within 6 hours at −18°C or lower
Liquid plasma	Whole-blood donation	Separated within 26 days
Source plasma	Plasmapheresis	Frozen at −20°C
Recovered plasma	Whole-blood donation	Separated but storage conditions not defined

Plasma used for fractionation must meet certain requirements, which are formulated by national and international regulatory agencies. Requirements for viral safety, which are the same for all types of plasma, include screening of individual donations for markers of hepatitis B virus (HBV), human immunodeficiency virus (HIV), and hepatitis C virus (HCV) (1). Although in some countries testing of donor blood for anti-HBc, anti–human T-lymphotropic virus (HTLV) I/II, and alanine aminotransferase (ALT) is mandatory, the significance of these tests for viral safety of plasma is controversial (2). Recently nucleic acid amplification technology (NAT) for blood-borne viruses like HIV, HCV, and Parvovirus B19 in plasma (or plasma pools) has been introduced in a number of countries, some of which use these tests also for screening and releasing cellular blood components (3).

The quality of plasma depends on certain donor characteristics as well as the conditions of plasma collection, processing, and storage (4). Criteria for donor selection may pertain to the level of factor VIII–coagulant (factor VIII), the protein content, and the amount of antibodies to specific viruses in plasma. The content of factor VIII in donors with blood group O is 20% to 25% lower than in donors with other blood groups. Factor VIII is found to be increased when plasma from donors above the age of 45 years is compared to random plasmapheresis donors (4). Administration of desmopressin, which induces a 2 to 6 times increment in the factor VIII level, has been used in plasmapheresis donors but, because of ethical concerns about donor premedication, it has ultimately not been adopted for routine use.

To guarantee a proper concentration and spectrum of specific antibodies against pathogenic bacteria and viruses in the plasma pool (and consequently in the final product), it may be necessary to apply selection of donors. The composition and content of specific antibodies are dependent on the epidemiologic history of the donor population as well as on various vaccination programs. To ensure that the spectrum of antibody specificities is sufficiently broad, a minimum of 1,000 donors must be included in each plasma pool for fractionation. For the preparation of specific immunoglobulins such as anti-Rh(D) immune globulin, plasma is collected through apheresis from donors with high antibody titers.

Due to activation of the coagulation system during blood collection, some of the labile coagulation factors in donor plasma may decrease. To avoid this the following measures are used: successful venipuncture, sufficient flow of blood so that bleeding is completed within 12 minutes, effective and continuous mixing of blood with anticoagulant, and immediate stripping of the collection tubing (4). Although citrate-phosphate-dextrose (CPD) and acid-citrate-dextrose (ACD) are the most commonly used citrate-based anticoagulants for the collection of blood and plasma, the activity of factor VIII in plasma is better preserved with heparin or "half-strength citrate." For practical reasons this has, however, not been implemented.

Because whole blood stored at 4°C starts to lose factor VIII activity shortly after collection, it is recommended that separation of plasma be started as soon as possible. Furthermore, the number of contaminating cells in plasma, which may release proteolytic enzymes, should be lowered as much as possible. This guarantees that the largest von Willebrand factor (vWF) multimers are kept intact (5). Because delays in the processing of plasma are usually better controlled and kept brief for apheresis plasma, its quality in terms of the yield of clotting factors is higher than that of recovered plasma. Furthermore, the gradual mixing of anticoagulant and plasma during apheresis prevents the loss of factor VIII due to a drop in pH, which occurs during the initial phase of the collection of whole blood.

The separation method for plasma must be designed to prevent the introduction of microorganisms. Sterility of the starting plasma is usually not achieved. For the safe pooling of plasma units from multiple donors it is necessary that the process is designed to keep the microbial load in the starting plasma pool as low as possible before plasma enters into the fractionation process. In the final aseptic filling process all usual and necessary preventive and control measures are taken to ensure sterility at the level of the final product.

Freezing and thawing of plasma are of particular importance to preserve certain activities (e.g., factor VIII in cryoprecipitate). It is therefore essential to use appropriate end-point temperatures and controlled temperature changes during the freeze-thaw process. Source plasma and fresh frozen plasma are best suited for the preparation of the complete spectrum of plasma derivatives, whereas plasma from outdated units of whole blood (i.e., liquid plasma) is only valuable for the preparation of immune globulins and albumin.

METHODS OF PLASMA FRACTIONATION

The methods used for the separation and purification of human plasma proteins (Table 23.3) are based on the following principles: (a) differential solubility of proteins, (b) differential interaction of plasma proteins with solid media, and (c) differential interaction with physical yields.

The solubility of proteins is primary determined by their charge and isoelectric point, and furthermore by their size, composition, and conformation, as well as by the physical and chemical nature of their environment. Of the various ways to induce changes in protein solubility, precipitation by ethanol in the presence of low pH was initially the principal protein separation method for large-scale plasma fractionation. The cold ethanol method developed by Cohn et al. (6) during World War II, with subsequent modifications, is worldwide still the primary process for the preparation of the so-called *bulk* plasma proteins (i.e., albumin and immune globulins). To complement ethanol fractionation, chromatographic techniques are used nowadays for the purification of plasma proteins such as coagulation factors and protease inhibitors.

TABLE 23.3. METHODS OF (LARGE-SCALE) PLASMA PROTEIN FRACTIONATION

- Differential solubility
  - Cryoprecipitation
  - Salting-out with neutral salts or amino acids
  - Neutral polymer precipitation
  - Organic solvent-aqueous systems
  - Soluble anionic precipitants
- Differential interaction with solid media
  - Generalized adsorption onto surfaces
  - Ion exchange (including polyelectrolyte interaction) chromatography
  - Immune affinity chromotography
  - Hydrophobic interaction chromatography
  - Ultrafiltration
  - Charged membrane interaction
  - Adsorption membrane interactions
  - Gel filtration
- Differential interaction with physical fields
  - Centrifugal techniques
  - Electrophoretic techniques (limited scale)
  - Differential thermal denaturation

Cold Ethanol Fractionation

The method of Cohn et al. (6) uses five variables to obtain differential solubility of proteins in ethanol-water mixtures (Fig. 23.1). These variables include ethanol concentrations ranging from 8% to 40%, pH levels between 4.5 and 7.4, temperature ranges from −5° to −7°C, ionic strength differentials from 0.14 to 0.01, and protein concentrations from 5.1% at the start to 0.8% at later stages.

The fractionation process can call for precipitation of all undesired proteins with the desired protein(s) remaining in solution, or it can call for the precipitation of the desired protein(s) with all others left in solution. With each change in ethanol concentration or pH, different protein fractions are obtained (Table 23.4). Although continuous-flow processing under automatic control is occasionally used, the discontinuous method, using stirred batch tanks, has remained the dominant mode of operation in many institutions.

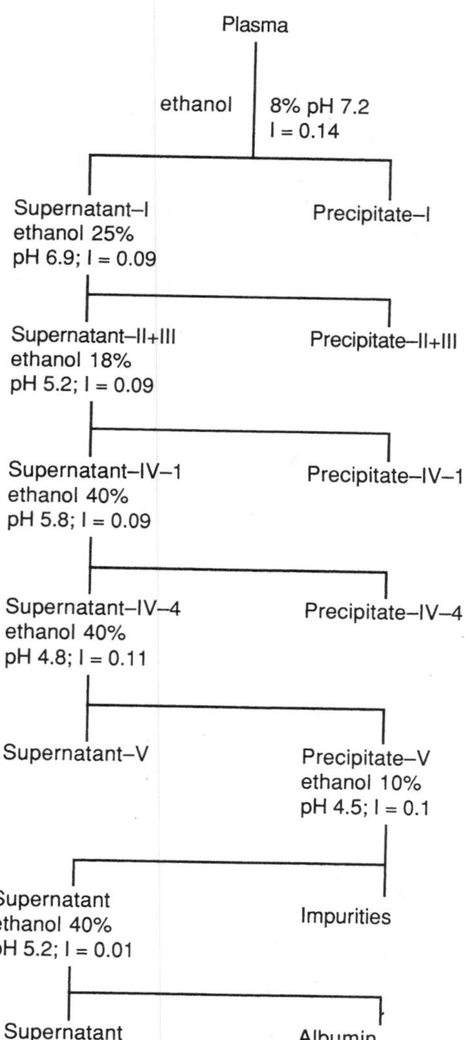

FIGURE 23.1. Plasma fractionation using ethanol, according to Cohn et al. This scheme represents one of the currently used variations of the original methods described by Cohn et al. (Cohn EJ, Gurd FRN, Surgenor DM, et al. A system for the separation of the components of human blood. Qualitative procedures for the separation of the protein components of human plasma. *J Am Chem Soc* 1950;72:465–474, with permission.)

TABLE 23.4. COHN FRACTIONATION METHOD AND DISTRIBUTION OF PLASMA PROTEINS

Fraction	% Ethanol	pH	Proteins
I	8–10	7.2	Fibrinogen, fibronectin, factor VIII, complement factors C1q, C1r and C1s
II + III	25	6.9	Factors II, V, VII, IX and X, fibrinogen, Immunoglobulins G, A and M, α- and β-globulins, β-lipoproteins, plasminogen
IV-1	18	5.2	Antithrombin III, α-1-proteinase inhibitor, complement components, immunoglobulin M, ceruloplasmin, α-lipoprotein, albumin
IV-4	40	5.8	Transferrin, haptoglobin, ceruloplasmin, α- and β-globulins, α-lipoprotein, albumin
V	40	4.8	Albumin, α- and β-globulins

Most manufacturers use cryoprecipitation as the first step in plasma fractionation to obtain the factor VIII–vWF complex. Several other coagulation factors (such as factor IX) and protease inhibitors (e.g., C1-esterase inhibitor) may be separated from cryosupernatant plasma by chromatography before it is processed by ethanol fractionation (7). Centrifugation or filtration harvests plasma fractions precipitated during cold ethanol fractionation. The removal of ethanol can be accomplished by freeze-drying or by ultrafiltration, which is faster and consumes less energy. Finally, the product (albumin) is pasteurized by heating for 10 hours at 60°C. The advantages of this fractionation system are that the process is suited to large-scale production and is performed batch-wise, which assures traceability. The precipitating agent, ethanol, can easily be removed during the formulation of the product. Furthermore, the low temperature required and the ethanol inhibit bacterial growth. Ethanol is inexpensive and, over the years, derivatives prepared in this manner have been extremely safe for clinical use. However, recovery of proteins is incomplete and biologic functions of some labile proteins may be destroyed by ethanol.

Precipitation by glycine or polyethylene glycol, which is also based on differential solubility and precipitation of proteins, is occasionally used for the preparation of a variety of plasma proteins (e.g., fibrinogen, factor VIII, immunoglobulin G [IgG], and albumin) (8).

Differential Interaction with Solid Media

Affinity and ion-exchange chromatography are purification processes that involve differential interaction with solid media. Ac-

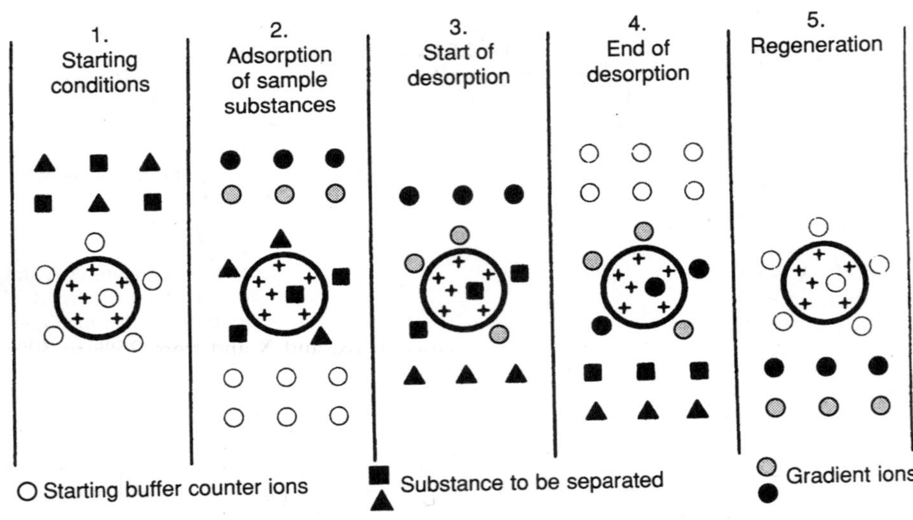

FIGURE 23.2. Principles of the ion-exchange procedure. Stage 1 shows the ion exchanger in equilibriation with its counterions. Sample substances are about to enter the ion-exchange bed. In stage 2, the counterions have been exchanged for sample substances. After this absorption, a gradient is applied. Desorption of one sample species occurs at stage 3. This substance is exchanged for counterions in the eluting buffer and is, therefore, eluted from the ion exchanger. At stage 4, the remaining sample substance is exchanged for gradient ions and eluted, after which regeneration begins. The gradient ions are exchanged for counterions in stage 5, and the exchanger is, thus, regenerated and ready for reuse. (From Pharmacia LKB Biotechnology AB, Uppsala, Sweden, with permission.)

cording to the forces responsible for adsorption, three categories of solid-phase reagents can be distinguished: (a) ion-exchange chromatography based on charge interactions, (b) affinity chromatography, based on biochemical interactions, and (c) immunoaffinity chromatography, using highly bioselective interactions (7). In addition, less well-characterized adsorbents, such as aluminum hydroxide and charged depth filters, are used to remove contaminating (lipo) proteins.

An ion exchanger consists of an insoluble matrix with covalently bound charged groups at the surface that are associated with mobile counterions. The latter can be exchanged reversibly with other ions of the same charge without altering the matrix (Fig. 23.2). Plasma proteins that carry the same charge as the counterions will be bound to an ion-exchange column. Unbound substances can be washed out from the exchanger bed with an appropriate buffer solution. Substances are eluted separately from the column as dictated by their different binding affinities at set conditions. The affinity can be controlled by varying the ionic strength and pH of the applied buffer. In ion-exchange chromatography, either the substance of interest can be bound or contaminants can be adsorbed, allowing the protein to be purified to pass through the column. Generally, when the protein of interest is not abundant, it is useful to adsorb the desired protein(s) because this allows a greater degree of purification. Instead, for purification processes such as used for manufacturing immune globulins, which are present in a relatively high concentration, the fraction of interest is not bound and is recovered in the breakthrough (9).

Ion-exchange chromatography is used for the purification of factor VIII and factor IX concentrates, the α_1-proteinase inhibitor, and as an adjunct to cold ethanol fractionation in the manufacture of albumin and IgG.

Affinity chromatography is a method of separation that uses biospecific immobilized molecules (ligands) covalently attached to an inert support matrix in such a way that the ligand retains its specific binding affinity for the substance of interest (i.e., specific plasma proteins) (10) (Fig.23.3). For the development of ligands that are specific for one particular protein, phage display technology and combinatorial chemistry may be used. The matrix support and the ligand must carry a well-defined pore size configuration and be accessible to the protein in question without causing protein denaturation. Methods are available for selectively desorbing the bound substances in an active form after washing away material that did not adsorb. Examples of large-scale purification by affinity chromatography are the preparation of antithrombin III or fibrinogen, using a heparin-coated matrix, and plasminogen by immobilized lysin (11). In some centers a

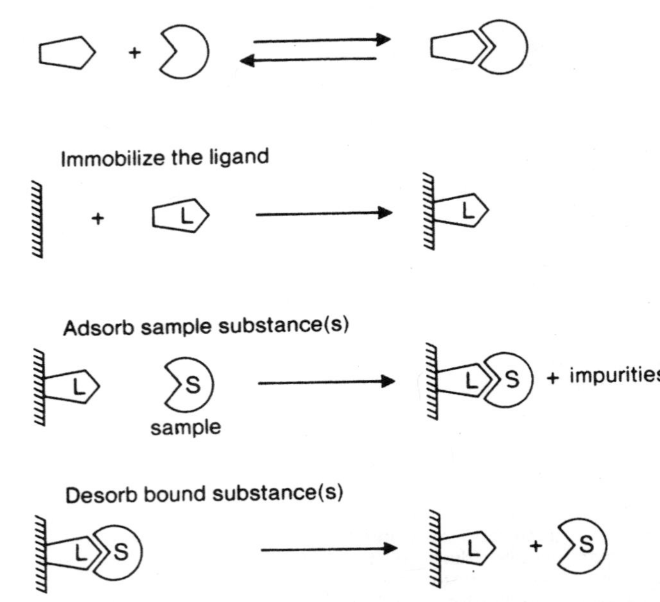

FIGURE 23.3. Principles of affinity chromotography. (From Pharmacia LKB Biotechnology AB, Uppsala, Sweden, with permission.)

heparin-coated matrix is also used in the preparation of highly purified factor IX concentrates.

Immunoaffinity chromatography involves the binding to a solid phase of a monoclonal antibody, which reacts with the protein, such as factor VIII or factor IX, to be purified (12). Alternatively, the antibody is directed to a closely associated protein (e.g., vWF), which itself is complexed with the product protein (factor VIII). After immunoaffinity chromatography, traces of monoclonal antibody protein, which may leach from the solid phase, and toxic chemicals used for desorption of the protein, are removed by binding of the protein of interest to an affinity or ion-exchange chromatography matrix.

The advantages of using chromatography for (plasma) protein purification are the selectivity and the relatively high yield, which is due to the mild conditions for the processing. There are some limitations that may notably affect its use for large-scale purification of plasma proteins. The processing volume is much larger than for ethanol fractionation because chromatographic methods can be applied only when dilute protein solutions are used. Bacterial growth, for which protein solutions provide excellent conditions, needs to be controlled. Plasma fractions with a high lipid content can cause clogging of chromatographic systems. Leaching of (degraded) ligand from the column may require additional steps to separate lost ligand from the target protein. Sanitation of chromatographic carriers, necessary to allow reuse notably when the costs of ligands and matrices are high, requires harsh conditions that can be detrimental to the chromatographic column (13).

The third methodology in this category, ultrafiltration, is used mainly for concentration of purified plasma proteins and for buffer exchange or the removal of precipitating substances such as ethanol.

Differential Interaction with Physical Fields

Of the methods based on differential interaction with physical fields, only thermal denaturation has been used in the past by some manufacturers for large-scale albumin preparation.

Fractionation for Coagulation Factor Concentrates

In every fractionation system, the most labile proteins—coagulation factors—are the first to be isolated. Cryoprecipitation, the rapid freezing and thawing of pooled plasma in a controlled way, generally is the first step in factor VIII production because of the purification and concentration obtained, the simplicity of the process, and because all other plasma proteins are kept intact in the cryosupernatant plasma. Although many studies have been performed to analyze the influence of various conditions on the recovery and purity of factor VIII in cryoprecipitate, the process is still not completely understood. It is generally agreed, however, that both freezing and thawing of plasma should proceed rapidly to obtain optimal factor VIII recovery and purity (14). Cryoprecipitation, which usually yields 50% of the factor VIII activity initially present in starting plasma, leads to a 20-fold purification and a five- to ten-fold increase in the concentration of factor VIII. Upon further processing using immunoaffinity chromatography, high-purity factor VIII concentrate with specific activity of at least 1,000 IU/mg protein is obtained (15). Because this purification step induces substantial additional losses of factor VIII, there is a clear tradeoff between yield and purity (16).

Ion-exchange chromatography, using 2-diethylaminoethanol (DEAE)-Sephadex, is used for the production of coagulation factors of the prothrombin complex concentrate (PCC) (17). Because of the low isoelectric point (pI 4.1 to 4.6), these vitamin K–dependent coagulation factors show a high affinity for anion exchangers at physiologic pH. Recovery of the various coagulation factors after desalting of the DEAE-Sephadex ranges from 50% to 70% for factors II, IX, and X and from 25% to 30% for factor VII, compared with the starting activity in the cryosupernatant plasma. The specific activity in PCC is about 10 IU/mg protein, except for factor VII, which is lower. High-purity factor IX–concentrate is prepared by affinity-chromatography using heparin-Sepharose or immunoaffinity chromatography (16).

Fibrinogen, which is recovered from cryoprecipitate or side fractions of factor VIII processing, can be supplied as a freeze-dried product either for infusion as fibrinogen or as part of a fibrin sealant used for wound healing.

Fractionation for Antiproteases

Antithrombin III, α_1-proteinase inhibitor (α_1-antitrypsin), and C1-esterase inhibitor are examples of antiproteases that are available for clinical use in patients with congenital or acquired deficiencies of these antiproteases. The marked affinity of antithrombin III for heparin is used to accomplish its purification by affinity chromatography on immobilized heparin. α_1-Proteinase, which inactivates leukocyte proteases like elastase, is concentrated in Cohn fraction IV (18). Another antiprotease, C1-esterase inhibitor, is recovered from plasma by anion exchange chromatography similar to that used for the preparation of PCC (19).

Plasma Fractionation for Immunoglobulins

Immunoglobulin G is usually extracted from pooled normal plasma or hyperimmune plasma by Cohn fractionation. Most centers start preparing with fraction II and III followed by further purification of fraction II that consists almost exclusively of immunoglobulins. The conditions for precipitation must be controlled carefully to avoid coprecipitation of proteolytic enzymes, which can lead to fragmentation of the IgG molecule (20). During the final processing, fraction II precipitate may contain some aggregated IgG and prekallikrein activator, which upon intravenous injection may give rise to anaphylactoid reactions (21). Immune globulins prepared by this method can therefore be given only intramuscularly.

For the preparation of IgG for intravenous infusion, Cohn fraction II is treated in a variety of ways, of which the most successful approaches include (a) gentle enzymatic degradation of the immunoglobulin molecule using pepsin (22), (b) chemical modification of the base molecule using β-propriolactone (23), (c) concentration at conditions of low pH or treatment with polyethylene glycol (24).

The IgG preparations that are currently available for clinical use consist predominantly of intact 7S molecules, possess opsonic activity but lack anticomplementary activity, and once injected have a half-life exceeding 14 days.

POTENTIAL DISEASE TRANSMISSION

Blood transfusion is a vehicle for transmission of several infectious diseases (1). With the advent of plastic disposable equipment and the sterile preparation of anticoagulant and additive solutions, febrile reactions attributable to pyrogens no longer pose a problem. When blood has been left standing at temperatures above 4°C, plasma occasionally yields the growth of cryophilic organisms such as pseudomonads, coliforms, and achromobacters.

Correct or not, the most feared adverse effect of the transfusion of plasma derivatives is the transmission of viral diseases. Patients treated with plasma protein concentrates are exposed to approximately 10,000 donors for each lot produced. If treated repeatedly, a patient could be exposed to millions of donors during a lifetime. Apart from the risk of transmitting viruses through the "open window" stage of an infection, there is also the possibility of exposure to the one donor in a million who is the carrier of a rare virus. Of the viruses that have been detected in plasma, HCV, HBV, HIV, and, in some regions, the hepatitis δ agent have caused severe disease in the past. In addition, hepatitis A virus (HAV) and human Parvovirus B19 have been found to be transferred by blood and blood products. Prions, the putative causative agent of transmissible spongiform encephalopathies such as Creutzfeldt Jakob disease have recently become a matter of concern (25).

Common viruses, such as cytomegalovirus and Epstein-Barr virus, and the HTLV type I are transmitted by blood cells but not by plasma (26,27). Such viruses are unstable outside the cell and must be transferred directly from cell to cell (1). As a consequence they pose no risk to plasma products. *Treponema pallidum* (syphilis) is inactivated during freezing. Bacteria and parasitic infections, such as malaria and trypanosomes, are not a risk with plasma products that have been sterile filtered.

The plasma pools used for the large-scale production of plasma derivatives presumably contain protective antibodies to many endemic viruses, which may neutralize viruses in occasionally viremic plasma donations. This is the reason why in the past some manufacturers have added small amounts of anti-hepatitis B immune globulin to products from pooled plasma to diminish the likelihood of hepatitis B transmission (28).

Measures to Decrease Infectivity

Four complementary approaches are used to decrease the risk of viral transmission by plasma products. They are: (a) suitability of donors, (b) testing of donations and plasma pools, (c) viral inactivation and removal during manufacturing, and (d) strict adherence to current Good Manufacturing Practices (cGMP). In addition, continued clinical and laboratory surveillance of the recipient population is critical to demonstrate viral safety and signal the entry of new viruses into the blood supply. These measures are discussed in Chapters 48, 66, and 68. Apart from specific methods for the removal and inactivation of viruses, the manufacturing process of plasma fractionation itself reduces the infectivity of viruses. Shifts in pH, high concentrations of alcohol, and (freeze) drying, which are part of the fractionation process, cause viral inactivation to some degree (29). Residual virus particles may become concentrated in precipitates that are not used for therapeutic preparations. During cold ethanol fractionation, most of the recoverable virus is found either in fraction I or in fraction III, a waste fraction containing a mixture of α- and β-globulins. The former conditions, combined with the possibility that neutralizing antibodies are concentrated in fraction II, explain the apparent safety of immune globulin preparations. Thus, there have been no reports of HBV or HIV transmission after the intramuscular or intravenous injection of immune globulins. Transmission of HCV by polyvalent immune globulins for intravenous use and anti-Rh(D) immune globulin has been described, but only for specific lots (28a).

To increase the removal or inactivation of viruses from final products, a variety of methods (Table 23.5) are being used (29). The selection of the method for inactivation and removal of viruses depends on the size and stability of the protein being prepared, the method(s) of purification, and the nature and titer of viruses that are of concern. The potency of various methods to eliminate specific viruses is usually expressed in terms of the logarithm of the reduction in infectivity, which is measured on a laboratory scale where the manufacturing conditions are mimicked as closely as possible. The need for this validation procedure can be illustrated by heat treatment for the inactivation of viruses in plasma products. When heat is employed for virus inactivation, proteins are first lyophilized to remove water. Alternatively stabilizers like amino acids, sugars, and citrate are added to the (intermediate) product to maintain the biologic function of labile proteins. Because such procedures and substances also stabilize viruses, it is necessary to determine the degree of virus inactivation in model studies. Furthermore the robustness of the

TABLE 23.5. METHODS TO DECREASE INFECTIVITY OF PLASMA PRODUCTS

- Physical inactivation
  - Heat treatment
    - Wet (pasteurization)
    - Steam
    - Dry
  - Light (ultraviolet)
- Physical removal
  - Chromatography
    - Hydrophobic interaction
    - Polyelectrolytes
    - Affinity chromatography
  - Partitioning during fractionation
- Chemical inactivation
  - Solvent or detergent
  - Ethanol
  - Immune neutralization
- Combinations
  - β-Propiolactone and ultraviolet

inactivation method, specifically the effect of (small) variations in factors such as moisture content, pH, protein content, and temperature, needs to be validated. For a product to be safe the process must remove or inactivate virus infectivity to a much greater extent than the level in the starting material.

Some techniques are effective against enveloped viruses but do not inactivate nonenveloped viruses (29). It is therefore advantageous to combine methods that are complementary to one another to enlarge the spectrum of viruses covered as well as the total quantity of virus that is inactivated. In addition, maintenance of protein structure and function should be evaluated. There have been instances in which treated product was found to be immunogenic following pasteurization (30).

The introduction of virus inactivation steps reduces the yield of product, requires extensive validation studies and continuous monitoring, and therefore, not surprisingly, comes with a price.

Methods of Virus Inactivation

Heating of albumin solutions for at least 10 continuous hours at 60°C (pasteurization) in the presence of sodium caprylate or N-acetyltryptophanate, has been successful in preventing transmission of hepatitis viruses and HIV for more than 40 years. Unfortunately, most plasma proteins undergo denaturation and aggregation when heated in the liquid state to the same degree.

Approaches to the viral inactivation of coagulation factor concentrates include heating of the product in the presence of stabilizers, in the lyophilized state ("dry heat"), or under humidified conditions (31). Heating of factor VIII in solution at 60°C for 10 hours in the presence of mixtures of sugars and amino acids, or at 80°C for 72 hours in the lyophilized state, produces favorable results with respect to inactivation of HBV, HCV, and HIV. A higher level of virus inactivation can be achieved by dry heat treatment at relatively high moisture content ("steam treatment") (32).

Several chemical agents (Table 23.5), which were previously used to sterilize viral vaccines, are used for the sterilization of plasma products. Mixtures of organic solvent (0.3% tri[n-butyl] phosphate) and nonionic detergent (1% Tween 80 or Triton X-100) cause disruption of the lipid membrane of enveloped viruses which can no longer bind to and infect cells (33). Because lipids are not essential components of plasma derivatives, this so-called solvent-detergent method effectively discriminates between the proteins to be preserved and the lipid-enveloped viruses that are rendered noninfectious. The safety of the solvent-detergent method with respect to enveloped viruses such as HBV, HCV, and HIV has been demonstrated in numerous clinical studies (29).

Low pH, such as pH 4 treatment, either alone or in the presence of small quantities of pepsin, is applied during the manufacturing of immune globulins to inactivate a number of enveloped viruses (34). This method is, however, not suitable for most other proteins which are denatured upon exposure to acidic conditions.

New viral inactivation methods applied to protein products such as ultraviolet light irradiation, polymer-linked iodine, and psoralen have been developed with the objective of broader viral coverage, improved complementation to existing methods, and reduced costs (35). Current experience with these methods is limited and clinical results are awaited.

Methods of Virus Removal

Ethanol fractionation and chromatography each contribute to reducing viral contamination of (intermediate) products, although elimination of viruses is not complete (36). In every step of the fractionation process a certain quantity of viruses will precipitate. Chromatography can remove both enveloped and nonenveloped viruses to variable degrees, depending on the type of chromatography. The log reduction factors are usually in the order of 1 to 3 for ion exchange chromatography and may reach 3 to 6 for very specific steps such as affinity chromatography. The success of virus removal is influenced by factors such as the composition of the buffers used, intermediate wash steps, and the protein composition of the preparation. Sanitation of resins and equipment between runs is performed to reduce the risk of contamination by viruses, which tend to stick to resins. Some resins withstand harsh chemical (e.g., alkaline or acid pH) or physical treatment (e.g., autoclaving) to inactivate viruses.

Nanofiltration can remove viruses based on size while permitting flow-through of the desired protein (37). Effective removal requires that the diameter of the virus exceed the pore size of the filter. Adsorption of viruses to the filter surface may also contribute to their removal. Several studies have demonstrated the efficiency of removing enveloped and nonenveloped viruses in the presence of plasma proteins by using appropriate membranes (38).

QUALITY ASSURANCE OF PLASMA FRACTIONATION

In most countries the preparation of plasma products is governed by the same regulatory considerations that are applied to drugs. Manufacturers are required to obtain manufacturing licenses, which must cover the method of preparation and product characteristics. To obtain a license, it is necessary to comply with cGMP. The guidelines for cGMP have been published by national regulatory agencies, such as the Food and Drug Administration in the United States, and by various international organizations such as the World Health Organization (WHO), the Commission of the European Communities, and the Pharmaceutical Inspection Convention.

The concept of GMP, which was born in the 1970s, emphasizes that end-product testing alone is not sufficient to guarantee the quality of a pharmaceutical product. Precise definition of the manufacturing process is required. The pharmaceutical manufacturer must demonstrate that the production process does what it is intended to do. Detailed cGMP requirements for aseptic processing have been published since 1984. Other guidelines are related to organization and personnel, premises, equipment, production and process controls, packaging and labeling, records, and reports (see Chapter 68).

Good documentation is required for the definition and control of production and processes. This avoids the risk of error inherent in oral communication, ensures the instruction of personnel in the procedures concerned, and permits investigation and tracing of defective products. In addition, the system of product documentation must be able to reconstruct the history of each batch of product from the use and disposal of starting materials to the packaging and release of the finished product.

Current Good Manufacturing Practices should be distinguished from quality control, which documents the sampling, specification, and testing of (half) products and source materials and defines the appropriate release procedures. Quality control ensures that necessary, relevant tests are carried out, and that materials are not released for use and products are not released for sale or supply until the quality has been judged satisfactory.

The critical purpose of these organizational measures is to guarantee that the final product—once it is available—will be subjected to as many tests as necessary to ensure its quality. These tests verify the identity, potency, and purity of the product. Testing throughout the shelf life monitors product stability. Detailed regulations are described in the Code of Federal Regulations (part 640), WHO reports, WHO requirements, and product monographs in pharmacopeias. Most of the products derived from plasma also require specific tests that evaluate their unique properties. Testing of the final product includes variables such as protein content and composition, sterility, pyrogenicity, abnormal toxicity, particulate contamination, and solubility. For specific products, it also may be necessary to test characteristics such as molecular size distribution, potency, the presence or level of specific antibodies, and prekallikrein activator content.

PLASMA COMPONENTS USED IN CLINICAL MEDICINE

Albumin

Albumin (molecular weight of 6.7 kd) is the single most abundant of all plasma proteins, its concentration ranging normally from 35 to 50 g/l. It is exclusively synthesized in the liver at a rate of 0.2 g/kg body weight per day. A healthy adult has approximately 4.2 g/kg of body weight of exchangeable albumin, which turns over at a rate of about 8% per day. About 40% of this albumin is present intravascularly and constitutes 80% of the total plasma colloid osmotic pressure. The exchange between the intravascular pool and the interstitial space, which normally amounts to 5% of the intravascular pool per hour, may increase up to three-fold during major vascular surgery and septicemia. Due to the large number of negative charges (and the large number of molecules in plasma) albumin has a vast capacity to bind compounds such as bilirubin and fatty acids, hormones like thyroxine, cortisol, and aldosterone, and a variety of drugs (e.g., warfarin, phenytoin, sulphonamides) (39). The capacity to bind bilirubin explains why albumin infusion protects infants with hyperbilirubinemia against bilirubin toxicity (kernicterus).

Low serum albumin concentrations occur in various disease states and may be due to leakage, renal excretion, increased metabolism, and insufficient synthesis in the liver, or combinations of these. Increased capillary permeability, such as occurs in severely burned patients, allows protein to leak into the extravascular fluid. Proteinuria due to nephrotic syndrome and conditions associated with protein-losing enteropathy, which involve predominantly the loss of albumin, may cause hypoalbuminemia. Furthermore, conditions such as extensive surgery, small bowel gastrointestinal disease, sepsis, trauma, alcoholism, and malignancy may lead to decrease of the serum albumin level due to a combination of decreased synthesis and increased vascular permeability (40). However, although the albumin level is reduced in a variety of conditions, it does not necessarily imply that hypoalbuminemia is always harmful. In the absence of data from controlled randomized clinical trials, there is continuous debate about the proper indications of colloids versus crystalloids and the dosage of albumin supplement.

Albumin is available for clinical use in different forms: as a 20% to 25% solution in distilled water, as a 5% solution in saline, and in the form of a plasma protein fraction (PPF), which is a 5% protein solution composed of 88% albumin and 12% α- and β-globulins. These preparations have a physiologic pH and a sodium content of approximately 145 ± 15 mEq/l. They are treated with heat for 10 hours at 60°C to inactivate bloodborne viruses. The PPF or a 5% albumin solution is used in the initial treatment of hemorrhagic shock and hypovolemic shock caused by burns. It is also used as a primer for the pump in cardiopulmonary bypass (40) and as a replacement for plasma exchanged during therapeutic plasmapheresis.

Adverse reactions to albumin are very rare. Circulatory overload can occur when the infusion rate is too fast. In the past, rapid infusion of the PPF has produced hypotension attributable to the presence of prekallikrein activator (41). In the products used currently, the level of this potentially hypotensive agent seems to be below the threshold required to produce adverse effects.

A recent metaanalysis of 30 randomized controlled trials that compared crystalloids with colloids in critically ill patients with hypovolemia from trauma or surgery, with burns, or with hypoalbuminemia found increased mortality in patients treated with colloids (42). Although for each patient category the risk of death in the albumin group was higher than in the comparison group, the pooled difference in mortality in patients treated with albumin was 6% (95% confidence interval, 3% to 9%) higher than in patients not given albumin. A plausible mechanism for this difference was, however, not provided. The authors of this study recommended that the use of human albumin in critically ill patients should be reviewed and that it should not be used outside the context of randomized, controlled trial. The design of this systematic review and the recommendations have been severely criticized (43) for a number of reasons. The quality of the evidence put forward was questioned, because part of the mortality data was not peer reviewed. The majority of the studies that were included in the final analysis had very small patient numbers and lacked homogeneity in terms of study design, cohort of patients, quantity of albumin given, and controls used. In addition, the end points of many studies were hemodynamic variables rather than mortality. Most studies included in the metaanalysis were published before 1990 and a significant minority before 1980 when albumin preparations were less pure than at present. Notwithstanding this critique the use of albumin in various countries has decreased significantly following the publication of the report.

Clotting Factor Concentrates

See Chapter 31.

Immunoglobulins

See Chapter 24.

Plasma Protease Inhibitors

Human plasma contains a number of proteins capable of inhibiting the proteases produced during activation of coagulation, and of fibrinolytic, complement, and kallikrein pathways, as well as the proteases released from leukocytes and platelets. Studies in patients with specific deficiencies of these protease inhibitors have provided evidence for their potential usefulness in therapy. Currently, three protease inhibitors derived from plasma have undergone (limited) clinical testing: antithrombin III, C1-esterase inhibitor, and α_1-antitrypsin.

Antithrombin III

Antithrombin III is the major inhibitor of thrombin and factor X^a and also inhibits, to a lesser extent, factors IX^a, XI^a, and XII^a. Its ability to bind to heparin markedly enhances its inhibitory effect on these coagulation enzymes (44). Congenital deficiencies or defects of antithrombin III occur in about 1 in 5,000 people and usually are associated with a thrombotic tendency (45). Deficiency states also occur in a variety of diseases, although the association with venous thrombosis is not always clear. Antithrombin III purified from plasma by affinity chromatography on heparin agarose has been used successfully in patients with congenital antithrombin III deficiency (46), whereas in acquired deficiency the complexity of the clinical condition in many patients makes it difficult to establish definite indications. Although it has been used in patients with acute hepatic dysfunction or surgery in cirrhotic patients, and in acute intravascular coagulation when heparin is contraindicated (47), further clinical evidence is awaited before these indications can be considered established.

C1-Esterase Inhibitor

C1-Esterase inhibitor inhibits the action of C1-esterase on its natural substrate's complement components, C2 and C4. A deficiency of this protease inhibitor is the underlying biochemical defect in hereditary angioneurotic disease, a dominantly inherited disorder characterized by recurrent attacks of nonhistamine edema localized in subcutaneous tissues and mucosa of the alimentary and respiratory tracts. The transfusion of C1-esterase inhibitor concentrate (or fresh frozen plasma) is effective as an emergency treatment for glottal edema (48).

α_1-Antitrypsin

The α_1-antitrypsin concentrate has been prepared and currently is tested clinically in patients with α_1-antitrypsin deficiency, an autosomal genetic defect characterized by an increased risk for the development of emphysema (49). Treatment attempts to raise lung α_1-antitrypsin levels to concentrations that protect against neutrophil elastase activity. Although preliminary results look promising (50), further studies must be done.

ECONOMIC AND LOGISTIC TRADEOFFS

The emergence of the acquired immunodeficiency syndrome and, subsequently, hepatitis C as major risks in blood transfusion has made product safety a top priority. The application of viral inactivation methods, together with donor screening, has greatly improved the safety of blood products. Although it seems logical to assume that high purity of blood products is beneficial, economic and social pressures demand that this is demonstrated before implementation of most protocols. Because high-technology products are expensive, the increased costs must be balanced against health care savings that result from improved product safety.

Until a few years ago, in many countries the demand for factor VIII has been the driving force for the collection of plasma. Following the introduction of recombinant factor VIII, the demand for plasma-derived factor VIII concentrates has dropped and in some countries patients are treated exclusively with recombinant products. Despite this change in the use of plasma for fractionation the demand for plasma is increasing, predominantly because of the tendency to use more immune globulins and also due to yield losses during the manufacturing process which are caused by viral inactivation procedures and sophisticated purification steps (51).

Recombinant Deoxyribonucleic Acid Technology and the Manufacture of Plasma Derivatives

The ability of genetic engineering to isolate specific genes of human origin responsible for the production of distinct proteins and the ability to transfer these nucleic acid strands into cell culture systems and microorganisms for the economic production of the desired proteins has provided new ways to prepare plasma products. The derivatives produced by recombinant deoxyribonucleic acid (rDNA) technology which are clinically used include factor VIII, factor IX, and factor VIIa, while recombinant albumin, vWF, antithrombin III, and α_1-antitrypsin are still to be tested clinically.

Cloning a specific DNA sequence first requires the construction of a library of DNA sequences that are complementary to the messenger ribonucleic acid in a given tissue. Then, either of the methods for screening the library can be used to identify and isolate a specific complementary DNA: antigenic identification, using monoclonal antibodies raised against purified plasma protein; or hybridization, using oligonucleotide probes derived from amino acid sequences of the protein of interest (52).

For the expression of recombinant factor VIII, the complementary DNA is placed in an expression vector next to a suitable promotor sequence in conjunction with enhancer sequences known to increase transcription. Such recombinant bacteria as *Escherichia coli* are suitable for manufacturing small proteins, but they are not equipped for the synthesis of a large and complex protein such as factor VIII (53). The vector described earlier was transfected into mammalian cells that began to secrete factor VIII. Attempts to optimize the production of the recombinant factor VIII in the culture medium led to the discovery that supplementation with vWF stabilizes the secreted factor VIII. An alternative approach is to transfect cells that express factor VIII with a vWF expression plasmid. The coexpression of vWF does not alter significantly the synthesis, processing, and secretion of factor VIII but remarkably enhances the recovery of the clotting protein. The expression level for factor VIII still is low for reasons that are not entirely clear. There is some evidence to suggest that retention of factor VIII by basic proteins within the endoplasmic reticulum play a role.

Two biologically active, full-length recombinant and one B-domain–restricted factor VIII products are presently on the market after extensive clinical testing. More recently B-domain–deleted recombinant factor VIII has become available for clinical use. The in vivo recovery and half-life are similar to those of plasma-derived factor VIII. The products are effective in preventing and treating hemorrhagic episodes in patients with hemophilia A (54). The application of rDNA technology has led to the cloning and expression of other important plasma proteins, some of which (e.g., factor IX) are used routinely while others are in the stage of clinical evaluation.

SUMMARY

Techniques that exploit the physicochemical differences among plasma proteins are used to isolate and purify plasma derivatives for clinical use. Cold ethanol fractionation, as developed by Cohn et al. (6) and subsequently modified by others, continues to be the primary method. Immunoglobulins and clotting factor concentrates have established indications, and other derivatives, such as antithrombin III, are being evaluated. The problem of disease transmission is coming under control, and a number of measures to decrease the infectivity of plasma derivatives are currently being used. The manufacturing of plasma proteins by rDNA technology is in some instances an alternative, as is demonstrated by recombinant factor VIII, factor IX, and factor VIIa products, which are licensed and available for clinical use.

REFERENCES

1. Goodnough LT, Brecher ME, Kanter MH, et al. Transfusion medicine. *N Engl J Med* 1999;340:438–447, 525–533.
2. Barbara J. Surrogate tests. *Vox Sang* 2000;78[Suppl 2]:63–65.
3. Nucleic acid amplification testing of blood donors for transfusion-transmitted infectious disease. Report of the interorganizational task force on nucleic acid amplification testing of blood donors. *Transfusion* 2000;40:143–159.
4. Myllyla G. Factors determining quality of plasma. *Vox Sang* 1998; 74[Suppl 2]:507–511.
5. Mannucci PM, Lattuada A, Ruggeri ZM. Proteolysis of von Willebrand factor in therapeutic plasma factor VIII concentrates. *Blood* 1994;83: 3018–3027.
6. Cohn EJ, Gurd FRN, Surgenor DM, et al. A system for the separation of the components of human blood. Qualitative procedures for the separation of the protein components of human plasma. *J Am Chem Soc* 1950;72:465–474.
7. Foster PR. Fractionation, blood plasma fractionation. In: Kirk RE, Othmer DF, Bickford, et al. *Kirk-Othmer encylopedia of chemical technology,* 4th ed. London: John Wiley and Sons, 1994:990–1021.
8. Curling JM, ed. *Methods of plasma protein fractionation.* London: Academic Press, 1980.
9. Falkreden L, Lundblad G. Ion exchange and polyethylene glycol precipitation of immunoglobulin G. In: Curling JM, ed. *Methods of plasma protein fractionation.* London: Academic Press, 1980:93–105.
10. Anonymous. *Ion exchange chromatography principles and methods.* Uppsala, Sweden: Pharmacia Orebro, 1979:1–112.
11. Miller-Andersson M, Borg H, Andersson LOA. Purification of antithrombin III by affinity chromatography. *Thromb Res* 1974;4: 439–452.
12. Zimmerman TS. Purification of factor VIII by monoclonal antibody affinity chromatography. *Semin Hematol* 1988;25[Suppl 1]:25–26.
13. Morgenthaler JJ. New developments in plasma fractionation and virus inactivation. *Vox Sang* 2000;78[Suppl 2]:217–221.
14. te Booy MP, Riehorst W, Faber A, et al. Affinity purification of plasma proteins: characterisation of six affinity matrices and their application for the isolation of human factor VIII. *Thromb Haemost* 1989;61: 234–237.
15. Hrinda ME, Huang C, Tarr GC. Preclinical studies of a monoclonal antibody–purified factor IX, mononine. *Semin Hematol* 1991; 28[Suppl 6]:6–14.
16. Horowitz B, Lippin A, Chang MY, et al. Preparation of anti-hemophilic factor and fibronectin from human plasma cryoprecipitate. *Transfusion* 1984;24:357–362.
17. Chandra S, Brummelhuis HGJ. Prothrombin complex concentrates for clinical use. *Vox Sang* 1981;41:257–273.
18. Wewers T, Casolaro MA, Sellers SE, et al. Replacement therapy for α_1-antitrypsin deficiency associated with emphysema. *N Engl J Med* 1987;316:1055–1062.
19. Harrison RA. Human C1 inhibitor: improved isolation and preliminary structural characterization. *Biochemistry* 1983;22:5001–5007.
20. Vogelaar EF, deBoer-van den Berg MAG, Brummelhuis HGJ, et al. Contributions to the optimal use of human blood. IV. Quantitative analysis of the immunoglobulin isolation. *Vox Sang* 1974;27:193–206.
21. Alving BM, Tankersley DL, Mason BL, et al. Contact-activated factors: contaminants of immunoglobulin preparations with coagulant and vasoactive properties. *J Lab Clin Med* 1980;96:334–346.
22. Morell A, Schhrch B, Ryser D. In vivo behaviour of γ-globulin preparations. *Vox Sang* 1980;38:272–283.
23. Stephan W. Undegraded human immunoglobulin for intravenous use. *Vox Sang* 1975;28:422–437.
24. Colomb MG, Dronet C, Law DTS, et al. Structural and biological properties of three intravenous immunoglobulin preparations. In: Morell A, Nydegger UE, eds. *Clinical use of intravenous immunoglobulins.* London: Academic Press, 1986:27–36.
25. Bradley R. BSE transmission studies with particular reference to blood. *Dev Biol Stand* 1999;99:35–40.
26. Donegan E, Lee H, Operskalski EA, et al. Transfusion transmission of retroviruses: human T-lymphotropic virus types I and II compared with human immunodeficiency virus (HIV) type 1. *Transfusion* 1994; 34:478–483.
27. Bowden RA, Sayers M. The risk of transmitting cytomegalovirus infection by fresh frozen plasma. *Transfusion* 1990;36:762–763.
28. Brummelhuis HGJ, Over J, Duivis-Vorst CC. Elimination of hepatitis B transmission by (potentially) infectious plasma derivatives. *Vox Sang* 1983;45:205–214.

28a. Yap PL. The viral safety of intravenous immunoglobulin. *Clin Exp Immunol* 1996;104[Suppl 1]:35–42.

29. Horowitz B, Ben-Hur E. Strategies for viral inactivation. *Curr Opin Hematol* 1995;2:484–492.
30. Gilles JGG, Jacquemin MG, Saint-Remy JMR. Factor VIII inhibitors. *Thromb Haemost* 1997;78:641–646.
31. Suomela H. Inactivation of viruses in blood and plasma products. *Tranfus Med Rev* 1993;7:42–57.

32. Mannucci PM. Modern treatment of hemophilia. *Thromb Haemost* 1993;70:17–23.
33. Horowitz B. Specific inactivation of viruses which can potentially contaminate blood products. *Dev Biol Stand* 1991;75:43–52.
34. Omar A, Kempf C, Immelmann A, et al. Virus inactivation by pepsin treatment at pH 4 of IgG solutions: factors affecting the rate of virus inactivation. *Transfusion* 1996;36:868–872.
35. Pamphilon D. Viral inactivation of fresh frozen plasma. *Br J Haematol* 2000;109:680–693.
36. Chandra S, Cavanaugh JE, Lin CM, et al. Virus reduction in the preparation of intravenous immune globulin: in vitro experiments *Transfusion* 1999;39:249–257.
37. Troccoli NM, McIver J, et al. Removal of viruses from human intravenous immune globulin by 35 nm nanofiltration. *Biologicals* 1998;26: 321–329.
38. Burnouf-Radosewich P, Appourchaux P, Huaart JJ, et al. Nanofiltration, a new specific virus elimination method applied to high-purity factor IX and factor XI concentrates. *Vox Sang* 1994;67:132–138.
39. Burtis CA, Ashwood ER, eds. *Amino acids and proteins. Textbook of clinical chemistry,* 2nd ed. Philadelphia: W.B. Saunders, 1994: 700–704.
40. Alexander MR, Alexander B, Mustion AL. Therapeutic use of albumin. *JAMA* 1982;274:831–835.
41. Alving BM, Hojima Y, Pisano JJ, et al. Hypotension associated with prekallikrein activator in plasma protein fraction. *N Engl J Med* 1978; 229:66–70.
42. Cochrane Injuries Group Albumin Reviewers. Human albumin administration in critically ill patients: systematic review of randomized controlled trials *BMJ* 1998;317:235–240.
43. Bell E. The dud sigar? Cochrane collaboration and the saga of human albumin. *Adverse Drug React Rev* 1999;18:149–163.
44. Hirsh J. Heparin. *N Engl J Med* 1991;324:1565–1574.
45. Bock SC. Antithrombin III, genetics, structure and functions. In: Hoyer LW, Drohan WN, eds. *Recombinant technology in hemostasis and thrombosis.* New York: Plenum Publishing, 1991:25–47.
46. Menache D. Replacement therapy in patients with hereditary antithrombin III deficiency. *Semin Hematol* 1991;28:31–38.
47. Fourrier F, Chopin C, Huart JJ et al. Double-blind, placebo-controlled trial of antithrombin III concentrates in septic shock with disseminated intravascular coagulation. *Chest* 1993;104:882–888.
48. Visentin DE, Yang WH, Karsh J. C1-esterase inhibitor transfusions in patients with hereditary angioedema. *Ann Allergy Asthma Immunol* 1998;80:457–461.
49. Wewers T, Casolaro MA, Sellers SE, et al. Replacement therapy for α_1-antitrypsin deficiency associated with emphysema. *N Engl J Med* 1987;316:1055–1062.
50. Hubbard RC, Brantly ML, Sellers, SE, et al. Anti-neutrophil-elastase defenses of the lower respiratory tract in α_1-antitrypsin deficiency directly augmented with an aerosol of α_1-antitrypsin. *Ann Int Med* 1989; 111:206–212.
51. van Aken WG. The potential impact of recombinant factor VIII on hemophilia care and the demand for blood and blood products. *Transfus Med Rev* 1997;11:6–14.
52. Pavirani A, Mauline P. Advances in biotechnology of factor VIII. In: Seghatchian MJ, Savidge GF, eds. *Factor VIII–von Willebrand factor.* Boca Raton, FL: CRC Press, 1989:26–39.
53. Kaufman RJ, Wasley LC, Dorner AJ. Synthesis, processing and secretion of recombinant human factor VIII expressed in mammalian cells. *J Biol Chem* 1988;263:6352–6362.
54. Lee C. Recombinant clotting factors in the treatment of hemophilia. *Thromb Haemost* 1999;82:516–524.

24

IMMUNOGLOBULINS IN CLINICAL MEDICINE

URS E. NYDEGGER
PAUL J. MOHACSI

The worldwide annual use of polyclonal polyspecific intravenous immune globulin (IVIG) prepared from healthy blood donor plasma pools currently approaches an estimated 40 tons. Treatment with IVIG attempts to reconstitute deficient function and may be enhanced with hyperimmunoglobulins and monoclonal antibody therapy. In contrast to the more locally produced and active cytokines, immunoglobulins appear throughout our bodies, are abundant in the blood stream, and represent about one-fourth of total plasma protein concentration. They are synthesized not by the liver, as are most other proteins, but by B lymphocytes and plasma cells. The synthesis rate can proceed at a rate of as much as 2,000 molecules per second per single B lymphocyte and can produce as much as 30 ng of IgG per B cell.

The function of immunoglobulins is reflected in their structure, with the recognition site for antigens found at the outer tips of two branches. The effector part is endowed with the capacity to activate complement and to bind to Fc receptors. Once bound to a cognate antigen, the resulting complex expresses different functions depending principally on its size and solubility (1). Antibodies can fix the antigen to lymphoid tissues for the prolonged periods required for antigen recognition, or they can present the antigen to monocyte-macrophages in the reticuloendothelial system for removal and disposal. Immunoglobulin molecules consist of paired polypeptide chains: two heavy (H) chains and two light (L) chains, each containing a constant region shared by different clones and a variable (V) region (i.e., a region that differs from one antibody specificity to the next). In contrast to the constant region genes, almost every B cell expresses a different pair of heavy- and light-chain variable region genes, a diversity that is generated during B cell development by somatic recombination at the DNA level of three major building blocks: V_H (variable), D (diversity), and J_H (joining) segments. Each block has several genes, which recombine and thus create diversity, enhanced by imprecise joining and the incorporation of untemplated nucleotides at the join (junctional diversity). The affinity of the antigen-antibody interaction is subsequently improved by somatic hypermutation of the rearranged genes followed by further rounds of selection, a process known as affinity maturation.

Intravenous immune globulin contains a repertoire of antibodies that in the donor's plasma have undergone selection, resulting in availability for the recipient of therapeutic and prophylactic antibodies with high efficiency. The response to infusion proceeds by isotype switch that generates antibodies of the same specificity but of different structure as IgG, IgA, or IgE. Such a switch confers on the humoral immune response a tremendous versatility; inasmuch as IgM is present primarily in the blood stream, IgG is distributed to interstitial fluids as well, and IgA serves as the protective antibody for mucosal surfaces. Switching involves intrachromosomal recombination in regions of tandem repeats (i.e., switch regions) that brings the fully as-

U.E. Nydegger: Department of Cardiology, Swiss Cardiovascular Center, University Hospital, Bern, Switzerland.
P.J. Mohacsi: Clinical Cardiovascular Surgery, University Hospital, Bern, Switzerland.

TABLE 24.1. SYNOPSIS OF INTERNATIONALLY AVAILABLE IV IMMUNE GLOBULIN PREPARATIONS (PART II)

Product	Octapharma Novartis	BPL —	BPL —	Griffois —	Alpha —	Alpha —	Biagini —	ISI Biagnini	LFB —	Finnish Red Cross	Human —	CSL —
Name(s)	OCTAGAM	Viagam-S	Viagam liquid	Alphaglobin Flebogamma	Venoglobulin S	Venoglobulin S	Blevin	Isivin	Tegeline	—	Humaglobin	Intragam
	—	—	—	Spain	5%	10%	—	—	—	—	—	—
Manufactured in Process	Austria	UK	UK		US	US	Italy	Italy	France	Finland	Hungary	Australia
	Cohn	Cohn	Cohn	Cohn	Cohn	Cohn	Cohn	Cohn	Cohn	Cohn	Cohn	Cohn/ Column
	pH4	Ion exchange	Ion exchange	PEG	PEG	PEG	Ion exchange	pH4	pH4/pepsin	pH4/pepsin	PEG	—
	—	—	pH4 Incub	—	—	—	—	—	—	—	—	—
Plasma source	Aus/Ger/US	USA	USA	US/EC	US	US	Italian	Italian	French	Finnish	Hungary	Australia
Type	7s	7s	7s	7s	7s	7s	7s	7s	7s	7s	7s	7s
Form	liquid	powder	liquid	liquid	liquid	liquid	powder	powder	powder	liquid	powder	liquid
Viral inactivation	SD/pH4	S/D	SD/pH4	Pasteurized	SD/pH4	SD/pH4	SD	SD/pH4	pH4	SD/Nanofiltr.	Heat	Unknown
Concentration	5%	5%	5%	5%	5%	10%	5%	5%	3–12%	5%	5%	6%
Half-life (days)	28	—	21	36—65	33.5 + / − 7	—	24	24	24	—	22	—
% IgG	>99	>98	100	>99	<>99	—	—	99	>97	—	>95	21–42
IgG1 %	63	51.7	56	69.7	69.7	—	—	62—70	58.8	—	68	—
IgG2 %	28.5	40.9	38	28.13	28.2	—	—	20–24	34.1	—	29	—
IgG3 %	6.3	6.4	5.4	1.32	1.3	—	—	8.6–9.4	5.4	—	1	—
IgG4 %	2.7	1	0.6	0.87	0.9	—	—	3.8–4.2	1.7	—	2	—
% Monomers	>92	93.3	95	—	>94	—	—	0	—	—	—	>90
% Dimers	>7%	—	3.5	—	—	—	—	100	—	—	—	—
IgA (mg/mL)	<0.1	5	5	<0.05	<0.008	—	0.1	0.118	0.85	—	<0.05	—
IgM (mg/mL)	<0.1	<0.1	—	<0.1	<0.1	—	<0.1	0.1	<0.1	—	—	—
Sodium (mg/mL)	0.01	5.9	119 mmol/???	—	—	—	9	8.5	2	—	—	—
Sugar/stabilizer	Maltose	Sucrose	Sucrose	d-Sorbitol	d-Sorbitol	d-Sorbitol	Sucrose	Sucrose	Sucrose	—	Glucose/glycine	Maltose
Osmolarity	>250 <350	340	400	—	300	330	—	450—600	—	—	>240	—
Albumin content	none	20	2 g/5g vial	—	1.3	2.6	none	none	—	—	—	none
pH	5.5–6.0	6.6	4.9	5.4	5.2–5.8	—	6.8	7	—	—	7.0	4.25
Anti-A	1:1	—	—	—	1:8	—	low	01:04	—	—	1:64	—
Anti-B	1:1	—	—	—	1:8	—	low	01:04	—	—	1:64	—
Anti-D	ND	—	—	—	—	—	low	—	—	—	—	—
Storage	Room temp.	Room temp.	Refrigerate	Room temp. Refrig. in Spain	Room temp.	Refrigerate	Room temp.	Room temp.	Room temp.	Room temp.	Refrigerate	Refrigerate
Solubility	—	—	—	—	—	—	—	—	—	—	—	—
Max. infusion rate	3 ml/min	3 ml/min	3 ml/min	—	0.08 ml/kg/min	0.05 ml/kg/min	—	—	0.067 ml/kg/min	—	0.01 ml/kg	4 ml/min
Registration notes	Worldwide	UK	UK	Spain, Port., UK Germ., Switz.	USA	USA	Italy	Italy	France	Finland	Hungary	PanPacific

All information is derived from manufacturer's sales brochures and package inserts.
Spaces without information: does not mean that these tests had not been performed.
SD = Solvent Detergent; Past. = Pasteurization

The quality of IMIG and IVIG depends on good manufacturing practice and quality control of each production batch, as well as on blood donor selection and screening for transfusion-transmitted viral diseases.

It is important to consider the source plasma used for purification of IgG. Antibody specificities directed at a spectrum of pathogenic microorganisms found in the final IMIG or IVIG product largely reflect the specificities present in the donating individuals. The pooling of single donations ensures that antibody specificities found in most donors will be well represented in the final product. Low-titer, less common antibodies and those that are highly concentrated in only a few donors will become diluted out in the pools. Infectious material has become rare under modern requirements for any source plasma. Source plasma for IVIG comes from both paid and noncompensated donors.

Immunoglobulins are hydrophobic and tend to adhere to surfaces during purification. Aggregated IgG molecules are common in purified IMIG preparations and make up 10% to 20% of the total protein. Dimer formation is reversible, but higher order polymers are stable and will cause serious side effects if infused inadvertently. The preparation method of IMIG or IVIG must be chosen to give high yields (50% to 70%) of a highly purified preparation. An information chart of 24 important IVIG preparations is given in Table 24.1.

Stringent requirements for IVIG have been set by the World Health Organization (WHO) and the committee for proprietary medicinal products (CPMP; http://eudraportal.eudra.org/). More than 90% of total protein must be monomeric IgG with intact Fab and Fc functions; the subclasses 1–4 of IgG must be present at the same ratio as found in normal plasma; the half-life after infusion must be the same as the half-life of normal IgG; no complement-activating IgG polymers can be present.

The main purification methods and procedures required to achieve intravenous tolerance are the following: Cohn fractionation in the cold after admixture of alcohol, pH4/pepsin treatment, β-propiolactone, sulfitolysis, affinity chromatography with 2-diethylaminoethanol (DEAE)-Sephadex, ion exchange, and polyethylene glycol (PEG) precipitation (Table 24.1).

As with other plasma products, contamination of IMIG and IVIG with infectious agents is a real possibility. Until 1980 it was generally believed that IMIG and IVIG obtained by Cohn's method could not transmit viruses. This has been confirmed with regard to human immunodeficiency virus (HIV). It was noted in 1983, however, that patients with immunodeficiency who received an experimental series of IVIG were developing hepatitis. Subsequently donors were tested for the presence of hepatitis C virus (HCV) antibodies. Nevertheless, HCV transmission with one special IVIG preparation was documented later (6), but it has not recurred since 1994. However, this very same study demonstrated a lack of transmission of hepatitis G virus (GBV-C) RNA by contaminated IVIG, because this viral material was not detected in the recipients up to 1 year after administration. The difficulty of interpreting and extending such findings to the overall danger of transmission is evident, because the reports are restricted to very few cases and to few preparations. Therefore preclinical endeavors to further increase safety have recently been extended to the search for genetic material for HCV in IVIG (7); studies using the polymerase chain reaction technique found that HCV RNA was detectable in the starting fraction of Cohn Fraction II paste, but not in the final IVIG preparation.

Seventeen different commercially available IMIG and IVIG preparations were analyzed for the presence of anti-HIV in the 1980s. Most materials were positive by antigen-binding assay for anti-HIV; on Western blot, 10 of 12 commercial lots were also positive for antibodies against glycoprotein (GP) 24 and GP 41 (8,9). These findings did not indicate infectivity, because no recipients, including patients with common variable immunodeficiency who have received IMIG or IVIG on a regular basis, have developed acquired immunodeficiency syndrome. Anti-HIV antibodies are now identified to help neutralize infectivity (10).

Continuous improvement of purification and viral inactivation-removal by major manufacturers in the preparation of IMIG and IVIG has occurred; thus, nanofiltered, proline/isoleucine- and nicotinamide-stabilized products were tested on healthy volunteers for tolerance before market launch (11). Some methods of preparation inherently contribute to inactivation of other viruses as well. Pepsin treatment at pH 4 abolished the infectivity of several enveloped viruses (12), and pasteurization or S-sulfonation completely inactivated viruses of the *Flavivirus* family, to which the hepatitis C virus belongs (13). Nanofiltration constitutes a further step to remove infectious material, adding a fourth safety level (11).

CLINICAL INDICATIONS FOR IMMUNE GLOBULIN PROPHYLAXIS AND THERAPY

The steadily increasing use of IMIG and IVIG should be continuously monitored to ensure that usage agrees with accepted indications; transfusion of large doses of IVIG to patients not really in need has created a shortage in the recent past. An updated summary of current indications related to either infectious diseases or immune disorders is found in Table 24.2.

Intravenous Immune Globulin in Bacterial Infectious Disease

Infectious diseases require immunoglobulins with antigen specificity that confers specific antibody reactivity on previously nonimmune individuals. Schedules, dosages, and routes of administration of immunoglobulin differ. Physicians should be familiar with the available IMIG preparations used in prophylaxis of infectious diseases: hepatitis A*; non-A, non-B hepatitis; hepatitis B*; rubella; rubeola; varicella zoster*; tick encephalitis virus*; rabies*; tetanus*; diphtheria*; and rhesus isoimmunization.* (IMIG preparations marked by an asterisk are in the form of hyperimmunoglobulins, in which the content of specific antibodies may be several logarithms higher than in standard immunoglobulin preparations.) The intramuscular route may be sufficient for preexposure prophylaxis, but to prevent an outbreak in exposed individuals an intravenous preparation may be needed. For antiinfectious immunoglobulins, donors with high titers are a source for antibody-enriched plasma, but with anti-

TABLE 24.2. LABELED AND NONLABELED INDICATIONS FOR IV IMMUNE GLOBULIN TRANSFUSIONS (PART I)

Condition	Dose Recommended	May Be Combined With	Priority
Primary Symptomatic Immunodeficiency States			
Humoral Immunodeficiency States (>3 bacterial infections of respiratory, intestinal, or urinary tract per annum)			
Adults: continued treatment of childhood antibody deficiency syndrome; hyper-IgM syndrome; common variable immunodeficiency of adults			
Children: Bruton agammaglobulinemia			
Prematures <1500 g: severe combined immunodeficiency; ataxia teleangiectasia; immunodeficiency with dwarfism; X-chromosomal-linked lymphoproliferative syndrome	Infusions to reach minimal serum IgG levels of >6 g/l: 300 mg/kg every 4 wk	Antibiotics only in case of severe bacterial infection	Initial treatment
Secondary Immunodeficiency States			
Adults: clinically manifest antibody deficiency in presence of malignant lymphoma, myeloma, or after intense plasmapheresis treatment			
Children: bacterial sepsis secondary to immunosuppressive treatment; HIV infection in newborns and small infants; hypogammaglobulinemia with protein-losing enteropathy; nephrotic syndrome or burns	300–400 mg/kg (adults) 400–500 mg/kg (children) Once or repeated according to clinical presentation HIV-infected children: every 3 to 4 wk	Antibiotics in case of infection	High
Postplasmapheresis syndrome	Once 300 mg/kg to reach serum conc. of 6 g/l	Prophylaxis of infections	High

LABELED AND NONLABELED INDICATIONS FOR IV IMMUNE GLOBULIN TRANSFUSIONS (PART II)

Condition	Dose Recommended	May Be Combined With	Priority
Graft and Transplantation			
Cytomegaloviral disease after organ transplantation	Special protocols	Ganciclovir	
Bone marrow	IVIG with known titer of specific anti-CMV antibody: 550 mg/kg/wk from 14 to +180 days (autologous bone marrow transplant, only <100 d) Children: special protocol		
Kidney	Polyspecific IVIG 20 g/kg/d Only if recipient is CMV negative		
Liver	With HBsAg-positive recipient during the anhepatic phase: anti-HBsAg-hyperimmunoglobulin Therapy: 20 g/d × 3d polyspecific IgG		
Heart	Only if recipient CMV negative and donor CMV positive: polyspecific IVIG 20 g/d/ × 3d		
Lung and heart	Hyperimmune anti-CMV		
Immunopathologic Diseases			
Acute ITP	400 mg/kg/d × 3–5d		Second-level treatment after steroids[a]
Posttransfusion ITP	400 mg/kg/d × 3–5d		Initial treatment
Neonatal alloimmune	In some cases 1 g once	Compatible platelet transfusion	Depends on clinical situation
ITP of systemic lupus erythematosus	Depending on platelet concentration and bleeding tendency	Cytoxan azathioprin steroids	Second-level treatment
HIV-related ITP	Depending on clinical course	E.g., preparation for splenectomy	Efficient only during therapy
Chronic relapsing ITP	According to clinical presentation	Splenectomy	Preparation for splenectomy
Toxic epidermiolysis syndrome	400 mg/kg/d × 3–5d		First (to be confirmed on a larger scale)

[a]Only in response to vaccination.
IgM, immunoglobulin M; IgG, immunoglobulin G; HIV, human immunodeficiency virus; IVIG, intravenous immune globulin; CMV, cytomegalovirus; HBsAg, hepatitis B surface antigen; ITP, idiopathic thrombocytopenic purpura.

RhD plasma, RhD-negative donors must repeatedly be boosted and may donate as much as 15 l/yr. It is difficult to determine the gram/liter concentration of specific antibody against complex antigens, because more than one specificity may help to kill a given virus. International standard preparations acknowledged by WHO need to be lyophilizable and sent around the world for comparison of titer strength in different countries. With monoclonal antibodies, the requirement is less stringent, because quantification is possible on a gram/liter basis in 100% of the molecules contained in such preparations carrying the same (i.e., monoclonal) specificity.

In diseases with hypogammaglobulinemia in which specific antibodies are insufficiently synthesized, resulting in more than three bacterial respiratory, intestinal, or urinary tract infections per annum, IVIG infusions must be administered on a regular basis. Patients with antibody deficiencies against several different strains of microorganisms are being treated with IVIG. There is no acceptable alternative therapy to immunoglobulin in patients with primary immunodeficiency diseases. For that reason, these patients are among those who should receive the highest priority in the use of IVIG. With the availability of IVIG, there has been a reduction in the morbidity associated with antibody deficiency and bacterial infections. The use of these preparations has dramatically improved the lives of patients, restoring many, if not most of them, to full and productive lives.

Premature newborns, physiologically immunodeficient, provide a natural test of IVIG efficiency in bacterial infection. Because IVIG crosses the placenta from 32 weeks of gestation on (14), both mother and fetus can be passively immunized if a premature birth is anticipated. The controversy as to use of IVIG at birth in preterm infants weighing <1500 grams has waned. There is a formal indication for all preterm infants at risk for infectious disease. Intravenous immune globulin is efficient in prophylaxis against respiratory syncytial virus infection in children with bronchopulmonary dysplasia and for HIV-positive children at risk for recurrent bacterial infections (15). As a clinical implication of basic research, it was observed recently that anti-HIV immune globulin may be protective against HIV infection in vaginally challenged macaques (16). In addition, neutralizing monoclonal antibodies protected newborn offspring of orally challenged macaques; shortly after birth, anti-HIV antibody–infused macaques became resistant to subsequent oral challenge. These studies provided proof that an appropriate serum antibody response may reduce the risk of infection at mucosal surfaces as well (10). A note of caution arises because in such experimental studies the viral challenge is usually timed to match the experimental peak serum antibody level, a situation which may not occur in the nonexperimental clinical situation. Neutropenic newborn rats infected with type III group B streptococci normalized their cytopenia after being treated with IVIG. Hyperimmunoglobulin anti–group B streptococcal IVIG was more effective than standard IVIG, indicating that a specific bacterial antibody can be a critical neutropenia-sparing component in IVIG.

Defects of single IgG subclasses may result in decreased serum antimicrobial activity. The subclass-restricted immune response to some of the major pathogenic agents is summarized in Table 24.3; effective passive immunization by IMIG or IVIG requires a complete set of IgG subclasses.

Despite improvements in antimicrobial drugs and supportive care given to normogammaglobulinemic patients, the morbidity and mortality associated with infectious diseases remain significant. In fact, *Streptococcus pneumoniae* is the most commonly identified bacterial cause of meningitis, otitis media, and community acquired pneumonia, and it is a frequent cause of bacteremia. Multidrug-resistant pneumococci, resistant to penicillin,

TABLE 24.3. PREVALENCE OF HUMAN ANTIBODY RESPONSE TO SELECTED BACTERIAL AND VIRAL ANTIGENES FOR IGG SUBCLASSES AND LIGHT CHAINS

	IgG Subclass[a]				Light Chain[a]	
	1	2	3	4	κ	λ
Bacterial						
H. influenzae B	(+)	++	—	—	+	(+)
S. pneumoniae 3	(+)	+++	—	—	(+)	+
N. meningitidis C	—	—	—	—	+	(+)
Tetanus toxoid	+++	+	—	—		
Viral						
Rubella	+	+	+++	(+)		
Hepatitis B virus	+++	0	+++	(+++)[a]		
HIV	+++ pol	gag[b]	gag	gag		
Polio	0	+	+++	0		
Herpes	0	+	+++	0		
Other						
Rhesus D antigen	+++	0	+++	0		

[a]Only in response to vaccination.
[b]Formed against gag and/or pol gene products.
(+), weak; 0, sought for but not found; —, not investigated.

cefotaxime, meropenem, erythromycin, and trimethoprim-sulfamethoxazole, are common and increasing. A need for conjugate vaccines, immunostimulatory DNA (3), and IVIG containing specific antibodies against these organisms is clear.

In search for novel adjunctive therapies, IVIG has been used to treat and prevent a number of infectious diseases in adults. In fact, the serum bactericidal activity (SBA) is assured by multiple factors such as specific antibodies, complement, lactoferrin, lysozyme, and fibronectin. It is used as an index of adequacy of antimicrobial therapy in several infections in different clinical settings. Furthermore, decreased SBA has been associated with increased susceptibility to the subsequent development of infections, whereas increased activity has been found to correlate with favorable clinical outcome. SBA appears to be a sensitive criterion to evaluate the effect of IVIG administration in preventing infections. Overall, the patient's own specific IgG might be destroyed by enzymes found in the infectious focus, such as in empyema (17). Proteases from *S. pneumoniae* and *Pseudomonas aeruginosa* also degrade IgG, and granulocyte elastase-like activity may attack C3b bound to surfaces, resulting in inactivation of complement-mediated opsonization. Free circulating bacterial surface antigens, such as the polyribosyl phosphate of *Haemophilus influenzae* and the galactosylα-(1,3)Gal epitopes of enterobacteriaceae, may absorb free antibody before it can become an opsonin. The opsonizing process may be disturbed at the very beginning by circulating non–complement activating IgA, which comes to block initiation of complement-mediated immune effector mechanisms. All or part of these phenomena may favor hematogenous bacterial dissemination of an organism despite the presence of functional antibacterial antibodies.

Administration of specific antimicrobiologic antibodies must be considered in patients normally not suffering from hypogammaglobulinemia. In a number of detailed studies, 150 severely injured patients requiring long-term artificial ventilation (18) and 329 surgical patients were studied, and a lower incidence of postoperative infection after standard immunoglobulin treatment was found (19). Studies in Athens on 21 patients receiving IVIG showed fewer pneumonias, non–catheter-related infections, and a significantly better SBA than 18 patients receiving placebo; in this study all patients suffered from an injury severity score between 16 and 50 (20). Such a study design is excellent, because patients were carefully selected for study entry from a group of 196, and they received the dosage of 1g/kg per day. In multiple myeloma, substantial amounts of intact or fragmented IgG or both are produced, but these are functionally ineffective and may inhibit other immune responses. Thus, patients with multiple myeloma are prone to recurrent infections predominantly caused by *S. pneumoniae* and *H. influenzae;* some patients with paraproteinemia are given IVIG electively and acquire fewer infections. In these patients, IVIG provides replacement of specific antimicrobial IgG with subsequent reduction of clinical infectious disease.

Intravenous Immune Globulin in Sepsis

A number of studies have demonstrated that IVIG can improve outcome in sepsis-related conditions (21). Antibodies cross-reactive to the core region of endotoxin lipopolysaccharide (LPS) are often depressed in sepsis. Endotoxin–core reactive antibody appears to be stable in all normal human plasma. This has made it possible to harvest hyperimmune plasma by regular plasmapheresis of a selected panel of high-titre volunteer donors: the isolated hyperimmune IgG was highly protective in an animal model of *Escherichia coli* sepsis (22). Treatment of sepsis outbreaks is now being reappraised using endotoxin-core antibodies (23).

Although monoclonal antibodies against endotoxin (24) do not convincingly reduce mortality in patients with septic shock (25), a human immunoglobulin preparation (Pentaglobin) containing IgM antibodies against endotoxin has reduced the levels of endotoxin in septic patients (26). IgM may be the most clinically effective antibody in gram-negative sepsis.

That IVIG preparations enriched with IgM are superior to normal IVIG for sepsis might be due to the IgM component that contains bactericidal antibodies to the O-specific side chain of the LPS (27): three IgG products from different manufacturers and one IgM-enriched product were tested and anti-LPS antibodies were seen in both isotypes G and M, in the former more particularly against LPS of a rough mutant. This study, for the first time, has extracted LPS from a large array of clinically infective *E. coli, Salmonella minnesota,* and *S. typhimurium* to study specificity of potentially therapeutic antibodies.

More aggressive therapeutic regimens in the future will help to return septic patients to disease-free status. Blockade of C5a low–molecular-weight anaphylatoxin using specific anti-C5a antibody therapy is an option (28). Another approach was recently chosen by Glauser et al. in Lausanne in search of new therapeutic targets for the management of septic shock. They have developed a mouse model in which lethal peritonitis is induced by cecal ligation and puncture. The deadly effect of this invasive procedure is mediated by macrophage migration inhibitory factor (MIF), a critical septic shock inducer. Anti-MIF antibody served to protect tumor necrosis factor (TNF)-α knock-out mice, thus identifying a new target for therapeutic intervention (29). Finally, septic patients have been plasma exchanged and plasma filtered to expedite removal of endotoxin, along with biochemical markers of inflammation, cytokines, and organ dysfunction (30). In the latter study, plasmafiltration caused a significant attenuation of the acute-phase response in sepsis. There was no significant difference in mortality compared to a randomized control group. But the intervention might improve the quality of life of survivors and spare use of antibiotics (18,20). Treatment, in combination with antimicrobial therapy, may bring greater improvement.

Intravenous Immune Globulin in Immune-mediated Disease

A special feature of alloimmune and autoimmune diseases is the potential to affect virtually any system or organ of the body. If IVIG is efficacious in such different diseases as neurologic, hematologic, endocrinologic, and others, there may be a common denominator among mechanisms. Accepted indications for IVIG are the following: replacement in (a) primary and (b) secondary immunodeficiency diseases, such as in B-cell lymphoproliferative disorder, (c) pediatric AIDS and (d) allogeneic bone marrow transplantation, (e) Kawasaki disease, (f) Guillain-Barré syndrome, (g) chronic inflammatory demyelinating polyneuropathy, (h) myasthenia gravis, and (i) dermatomyositis. The hematologic indications (31) are as follows: (j) immune thrombocytopenic purpura (ITP), (k) pure red blood cell aplasia, and (l) alloimmune-mediated thrombocytopenias. Further strong possibilities underscored by ongoing clinical studies are (m) systemic vasculitides, (n) recurrent pregnancy loss, (o) prevention of neonatal sepsis, (p) infections in polytraumatized patients and in patients after surgery, and (q) solid organ posttransplantation-immunomodulation. Most of these indications were anticipated with observations of single cases favorably responding to IVIG. This was followed by the classic sequence of the four phases of clinical studies. The CPMP directs the more interested reader to its core, defined by the European Pharmacopoeia Monograph 0918.

Will the list of formal indications continue to grow? An answer to this question is linked to whether the plasma fractionation industry is willing to sponsor further clinical studies that focus on more precise selection of subgroups of patients sharing common immunopathogenetic features likely to respond to IVIG. Many years of study on immune complex–mediated diseases (such as systemic lupus erythematosus (SLE), rheumatoid arthritis, and ankylosing spondylitis) now thought to be refractory to IVIG will be required. Thrombocytopenia and secondary myelofibrosis and/or cerebritis accompanying SLE seem to respond, and animal experiments of abrogation of experimental SLE with IVIG show benefit, suggesting there may be a role for IVIG in these diseases. The most active group in search of a definite SLE patient population to respond to IVIG is the one of Shoenfeld et al. in Israel. They have published recent evidence that IVIG treatment has a high response rate among selected patients with SLE, and that a combination of clinical manifestations, clinical laboratory findings positive for antibodies against DNA, and complement levels may help predict who among SLE patients will benefit from IVIG treatment (32). In leukocytoclastic vasculitis, IVIG may be helpful for patients in whom the disease process leads to ulceration (33).

History shows that conceptual design of a clear mechanism may lead to successful clinical trials of IVIG. Thus, two bleeding patients with autoantibodies against clotting factor VIII responded to IVIG (34), because the intrinsic regulation of the antibody network failed and could be reconstituted by IVIG. The mechanism of action is due to inhibition of the pathogenetic autoantibody by therapeutic IVIG.

As with infectious diseases the search to help an additional number of autoimmune patients with IVIG therapy might open a new chapter using IgM-enriched preparations, because it has been found that the IgM isotype plays an important role in control of IgG autoreactivity (35). Substituting defective IgM with IgM from healthy donors therefore might constitute an additional rationale currently being pursued in clinical studies. An IgM-enriched immunoglobulin preparation was a more potent down-regulator of an in vitro alloantigen-induced proliferation in the mixed lymphocyte reaction than a pure 7S IVIG. Therefore, some studies now claim that IgM-enriched IVIG might exert a greater therapeutic potential than regular IVIG preparations (36), an idea that awaits further proof.

Intravenous Immune Globulin in Neurologic Disorders

A significant increase in evidence-based medical indications has occurred during the last 5 years in the field of neurologic indications. Guillain-Barré syndrome, myasthenia gravis, dermatomyositis, and polymyositis have been labeled indications. Intravenous immune globulin has replaced plasma exchange therapy in most of them. There has been substantial progress in explaining the disease mechanisms. It appears that autoantibodies to ganglioside GM antigen on Schwann cells are a major disease-inducing factor, which becomes inhibited by antiidiotypic antibodies. Intravenous immune globulin also modulates the levels of proinflammatory cytokines in these diseases (37), selectively reducing TNF-α and interleukin-1, the levels of which can be correlated with disease severity. In dermatomyositis, IVIG therapy restores intramuscular capillaries by blocking the antibody-dependent formation of C5b-9 and the terminal membrane attack complex of complement that mediates endothelial cell damage. The response of patients with chronic inflammatory demyelinating polyneuropathy to IVIG might reflect additional factors than Fc receptor blockade (38).

Intravenous Immune Globulin in Cardiovascular Diseases

The single most important indication for IVIG in cardiovascular disease today is Kawasaki disease, a children's illness. It is also known as Kawasaki syndrome or mucocutaneous lymph node syndrome. Kawasaki disease and acute rheumatic fever are the two leading causes of acquired heart disease in children in the Western world. About 80% of the afflicted patients are younger than 5 years, slightly more frequently boys and amongst those of Asian ancestry, but it can occur in every racial and ethnic group. More than 1,800 cases of Kawasaki disease are diagnosed annually in the United States. At the Bern Center we recorded seven cases last year. In as many as 20% of the children with Kawasaki disease the heart is affected, more prominently the coronary arteries which can form aneurysms, thrombosis, and stasis. Other changes include myocarditis, arrhythmias, and valvular dysfunction. It is now standard therapy to administer IVIG early in the disease course even in cases in which the heart is not (yet) affected. If Kawasaki disease is triggered by viruses, such as has been observed after parvovirus infection, the IVIG may act through neutralizing Parvovirus B19–specific antibodies. However, in most children suffering from this syndrome the etiology remains unknown, and IVIG must be given early in conjunction with aspirin for at least 10 days to prevent the development of coronary artery aneurysms. Dosage should be 1.6 to 2.0 g/kg, administered in divided doses over 2 to 5 days, or 2 g/kg per day as a single dose.

Second, atherosclerosis in adults might be selected for clinical studies in the immediate future, mainly because our knowledge on the pathogenesis of this condition is improving. Atherosclerosis is increasingly thought of, at least in part, as an inflammatory disease in which the CD40/CD40L system plays a crucial part (39). Inflammatory conditions, independent of an identifiable infectious trigger, are mostly associated with cytokine release and complement activation, both of which respond favorably to IVIG (see later). The most convincing rationale to administer IVIG to recipients at risk for atherosclerosis comes from the observation that SandoglobulinR-injected mice deficient in apolipoprotein E (by the knock-out procedure), and therefore at high risk for cholesterol-induced atherosclerosis, had fewer fibrofatty lesions induced by a fatty protein diet (40). Although still unclear at this stage, the mechanisms addressed in this study purport down-regulation of autoantibody production against oxidized low-density lipoprotein, modulation of T cell functions in plaques, as well as control of complement activation and cytokine production (41).

Third, nonischemic idiopathic dilated cardiomyopathy (IDC), a major reason for heart transplantation, has recently been ascribed to the presence of autoantibodies reacting against cardiac cellular proteins. Rabbits developed the clinical entity of IDC after being immunized with sequences of the β1-adrenoreceptor against which autoantibodies were also found in humans, that is, in many patients suffering from IDC. Because certain authors advocate immunoadsorption regimens for removal of anti β1-adrenoreceptor autoantibodies, it is reasonable to administer IVIG to such patients on the assumption of antiidiotypic inhibition (42,43).

Fourth, inflammation of the myocardium is a condition of serious clinical importance with inflammatory etiologies ranging as widely as viral myocarditis, Chagas disease, and AIDS, and noninfectious causes, including posttransplant cardiac rejection. Progress in microtechnology in this field has recently allowed for cardiac catheterization via the right carotid artery in inbred mice. In such an animal experiment, it has been shown that autoimmune inflammation of the heart resulted in significant cardiac dysfunction, leading to significant fibrosis, expression of ventricular atrial natriuretic factor, as well as to a decrease in myosin heavy chainα consistent with phenotypic alterations (mRNA and Northern blot analysis). Again, within the framework of antiinflammatory potency, it is reasonable to try IVIG infusions in such patients with myocarditis (44). However, it has to be kept in mind that the diagnosis, even using new Dallas criteria, remains difficult. Moreover, only a small group of patients develop clinically overt myocarditis. It can be assumed that a considerable percentage of patients undergo unrecognized or nonovert myocarditis, resulting only partially in clinically overt IDC. Initial efforts to abrogate the development of cardiac dilation and dysfunction in patients with inflammatory myocarditis with immunosuppressive therapy were unsuccessful. When children with or without cellular inflammation shown by endomyocardial biopsy were treated with IVIG, significant improvement was noted in left ventricular function. In a recent study, the role of IVIG in the therapy of adults with recent onset of IDC or acute myocarditis was studied in ten patients hospitalized with New York Heart Association (NYHA) class III to IV heart failure, left ventricular ejection fraction <0.40, and symptoms for <6 months. At the time of diagnosis they were treated with IVIG and there was clinical and laboratory improvement: left ventricular ejection fraction improved by 17 ejection fraction units. The authors feel it warranted to evaluate the effectiveness of IVIG by randomized, multicenter trials (45). At least, virally induced myocarditis (46) might be worth a try for IVIG.

Finally, Hack et al. in the Netherlands have recently found both activated complement fragments and C-reactive protein in infarcted, but not in normal, myocardium of patients who had died after acute myocardial infarction. Because both components have also been found in human atherosclerotic vessels, they hypothesized that direct damage of endothelial cells and cardiomyocytes is mediated by complement activation (47) known to be down-regulated by IVIG as well as IgM-enriched IVIG (48).

Intravenous Immune Globulin in Organ Transplantation and Other New Aspects

Intravenous immunoglobulin has demonstrated efficacy in the modulation of alloantibodies that are significant barriers to solid organ transplantation. This form of therapy also appears to have a positive effect on prolonging long-term allograft survival in the treatment of allograft rejection. Clinical evidence has shown that IVIG can also modulate autoimmune vasculitic disorders with reversal of inflammatory events. As more sophisticated analysis of IVIG mechanisms of action become available, ideal patients for this therapy will be more easily identified. At present, the absence of prospective, controlled trials demonstrating clinical efficacy is a significant limitation in decision making about the use of IVIG in organ transplantation. Thus, by inference from theoretic reasoning, we have been able to successfully add IVIG and IgM-enriched IgG, together with the complement-inhibiting C1-esterase inhibitor preparation, to the therapeutic regimen of a group O man who 40 months ago accidentally received a B-type allogeneic heart (49). Of course, the multiplicity of therapeutic measures applied (plasma exchange, extracorporeal immunoabsorption, standard immunosuppressive regimens), means that the single measure which helped this patient to survive and adapt to his B-type heart cannot be identified. The reduction of anti-HLA alloreactivity is now acknowledged to respond to IVIG. This has served as a background to prime patients for cardiac transplantation (50). Should xenotransplantation see its day sometime in the future, IVIG would certainly, on the basis of its immunomodulatory potential, be a component of therapeutic strategy (51). It has been reasoned recently that xenoreactive natural antibodies (XNA), to which anti-galactose-$\alpha_{1\text{-}3}$-galactose (diGal) belong, are potent complement activators. Combined removal by plasma exchange and immunoabsorption, and inhibition, perhaps of XNA V-region specific nature by transfusion of IVIG, could add to the vision that during the time that the graft is in place in the "absence" of XNA, the endothelial cells would have time to heal in and recover from the trauma of having been exposed to relative hypothermia and low oxygen tensions. In addition to plain polyspecific, polyclonal IVIG, anti-μ-chain monoclonal antibodies (MAbs) could boost reduction of XNA levels (52). A five-agent graft-versus-host disease prophylaxis program consisting of cyclosporine, methotrexate, antithymocyte globulin, IgM-enriched IVIG, and metronidazole was given to 48 recipients of unrelated donor marrow and was effective (53).

The cytomegalovirus (CMV) hyperimmunoglobulins (CytoGam by MedImmune or Cytotect by Biotest) are used both prophylactically or therapeutically. Although some transplantation centers switched over to ganciclovir therapy alone, antiviral synergy might occur between ganciclovir and CMV hyperimmunoglobulins. In transplanted patients, CMV may be a risk factor for transplant vasculopathy. Some centers use a combination of the two therapeutic principles: specific antiviral antibody and virucidal synthetic nucleoside analogues (54). Prophylactic schedules may impose the use of IVIG rather than IMIG even in preexposure prophylaxis, such as in the prophylaxis of CMV disease in renal or bone marrow transplant recipients. Dosages and timing of administration may vary. In the postexposure situation, "the sooner the better" is an appropriate attitude. However, preexposure intramuscular prophylaxis must be given 2 to 3 days before the exposure, because maximal serum levels of specific antibodies are reached only 48 to 96 hours after injection.

Although the use of IVIG in bone marrow transplantation has declined, it is still prescribed to replace efficient antibody production in the prophylaxis of bacterial infections. It is also used to replace antibodies in patients who have received transplants for severe immunodeficiency syndromes, as well as in matched, unrelated-donor transplant patients taking intensely immunosuppressive preparative regimens. Some physicians use IVIG for graft-versus-host disease as a last measure, even though evidence for this use is lacking. Because CMV remains a threat in transplant rejection and vasculopathy, CMV hyperimmunoglobulins are given in 73% of the heart centers in Germany (55). The prophylactic use has been analyzed in a metaanalysis finding reduced numbers of CMV infections. The analysis, however, could not conclude that CMV hyperimmunoglobulins are better than polyspecific polyclonal IVIGs also containing anti-CMV (56).

The list of indications for IVIG continues to evolve. Two recent studies, both serving as possible starting points for further confirmatory or double-blind prospective studies, demonstrate this. The first is from the field of ophthalmology, where IVIG has been useful to arrest and resolve chronic conjunctivitis in ten patients with biopsy-proven progressive cicatricial pemphigoid affecting the eyes (57). The other comes from Saurat et al. in Geneva, demonstrating that Fas-mediated apoptotic keratinocyte death in the severe adverse drug reaction of toxic epidermal necrolysis is dampened by Fas-blocking antibodies contained within IVIG (58). The authors concluded that IVIG may also prove useful in the treatment of other diseases that are due to Fas-mediated tissue destruction, including graft-versus-host disease, Hashimoto thyroiditis, and fulminant hepatitis (58).

Animal antibodies against human lymphocytes also constitute a series of therapeutic IVIG preparations, which are used for patients having received allogeneic transplanted organs. The two major preparations (ATG-Fresenius, ATGAM, and thymoglobulin) follow the principle of OKT3 monoclonal antibody, to bind to lymphocytes cell surface markers, thereby producing cell lysis or inactivation. Both are elicited in the rabbit, the first being available in liquid, the second in lyophilized form. The human thymocytes used to immunize the rabbits have been tested for the absence of transfusion-transmitted viruses; the preparations obtained from the rabbits are sterile in this respect. When such preparations are used to treat transplant rejection, they are combined with agents that act in synergistic fashion to provide the potency, avoidance of side effects, convenience of administration, and cost appropriate for the individual patient.

MONOCLONAL ANTIBODIES, PHAGE DISPLAY TECHNOLOGY, AND FUSION PROTEINS

Introduction of Mabs into therapeutic medicine emerged during the last decade, although they were discovered in the mid-1970s by Kohler and Milstein. In the early 1980s, the consensus was that polyclonal polyspecific IVIG preparations would best be spiked by single specificities of Mabs, but this assumption was redeemed by using Mabs in pure form (59). The adverse reactions encountered in the original clinical studies with formation of human antimouse antibodies with consequently diminished serum half-life has now been overcome by development of chimeric and, even better, humanized Mabs, of which the only portion stemming from the mouse remains the hypervariable region recognizing the antigen (Fig. 24.2).

Currently, a whole array of preparations is coming onto the market, each one introduced upon demonstration of its efficacy. How far the engineering of antibody molecules will go depends on our capacity to produce designer molecules or immunoglobulin-based fusion proteins which combine the Fc region from mouse antibody with a cytokine or the ectodomain of a cell-surface receptor or adhesion molecule. Such hybrid molecules possess the properties of the antibody Fc domain, as well as the ligand of interest. One of the major interests of such fusion proteins would be a relatively long half-life compared to plain cytokines. For example for interleukin-10:Fc, it is 31 hours. The phage display technology, by which bacteriophages containing the relevant gene for the production of the specific antigen-interacting antibody residue are transfected to bacteria which produce large quantities of "antibodies," is a future technology (4,5). In Zurich, Hanes has been able to apply ribosome display, a technology for the in vitro selection and evolution of very large protein libraries to selection and evolution of single-chain antibody fragments (scFvs) from a large synthetic library (60). The so-obtained scFvs expressed high affinity and specificity due to accumulation of point mutations. The Hanes group was able to mimic the process of antibody generation and affinity maturation with a synthetic library in a cell-free system in a few days, obtaining molecules with higher affinities than most natural antibodies. In addition, plants have considerable potential for the production of biopharmaceutical proteins. In 1989, functional antibodies could be produced for the first time in transgenic plants. Since then, a considerable amount of effort has been invested in developing plants for antibody (or "plantibody") production. Many of the plantibodies might have potential applications for human and animal health care, a topic that has recently been updated elsewhere (61). Such technologies could one day be used to produce patient-specific drugs able to target the very specific protein which makes a given patient sick (5). Very–high-affinity Mabs, therapeutic antibody fragments with prolonged in vivo half-lives, bispecific fusion proteins for selective cancer chemotherapy, as well as anti-IgE for asthma therapy are future potential developments. Some Mabs currently used in clinical trials are shown in Table 24.4.

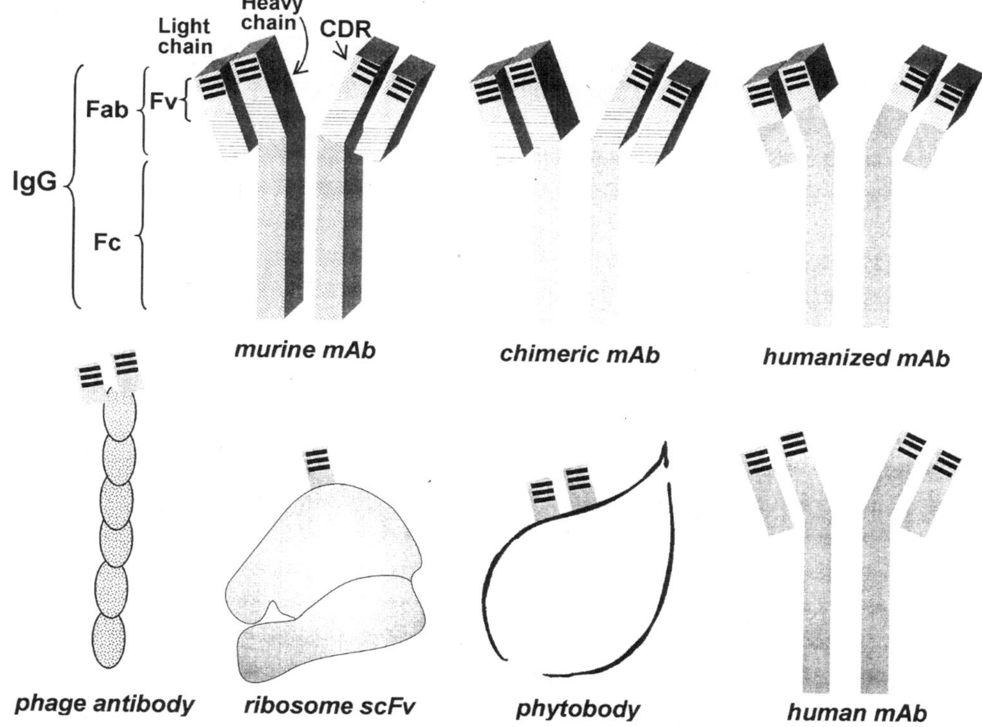

FIGURE 24.2. Certain interactions between biologic molecules can be highly specific. A good example is the interaction between a hormone and its receptor or between an antibody and its antigen. The latter example is sketched on this figure whereby only the Y-shaped pictures are true antibodies with antigen-recognizing and effector parts. The latter portion has also been termed the business end of the antibody, because this Fc fragment, upon binding of the Fab parts to antigen, activates complement and binds to Fc receptors. Thus, phage, ribosome scFv, and phytobodies have no such intact double-chain Fc fragment. However, such "antibodies" may be used to neutralize the antigen without inflammatory consequences or to bring toxins to the reactive site. (Van Uden J, Raz E. Introduction to immunostimulatory DNA sequences. *Springer Semin Immunopathol* 2000;22:1–9; Hanes J, Schaffitzel C, Knappik A, et al. Picomolar affinity antibodies from a fully synthetic naive library selected and evolved by ribosome display. *Nat Biotechnol* 2000;18:1287–1292; Giddings G, Allison G, Brooks D, et al. Transgenic plants as factories for biopharmaceuticals. *Nat Biotechnol* 2000;18:1151–1155, with permission.)

The many promising approaches might work best if combined with other prophylactic and therapeutic regimens. Thus, Mabs may kill lymphoma cells through a variety of different mechanisms. Radioimmunoconjugates or immunotoxins kill cells through emission of particles or the internalization of toxins brought to the cancer cell by the Mab. The example of Mab therapy in lymphoma has been updated recently (62). The treatment of autoimmune diseases with Mab is under development. At least nine different CD4 Mabs have been investigated in this respect (63) but further studies are needed.

MECHANISMS OF ACTION OF IVIG

Intravenous immune globulin (IVIG) should generally be used when a plausible mechanism of action can be determined.

Mechanisms of Action in Infectious Disease

As mentioned above, SBA measured in vitro is a composite action of a large number of antiinfectious agents in mammal serum samples. Most of these are invading organism–nonspecific, such as complement, lysozyme, lactoferrin, and fibrinonectin. There are IgM and IgG that constitute organism-specific sentinels, because specific antibodies belonging to these isotypes recognize the pathogenic organism in question. The immune system, with its sophisticated helper cell and cytokine algorithm, can enhance specific immune defense, whereas the nonspecific defenders are hypersynthesized only under the auspices of an acute phase reaction triggered by certain invaders more than by others. Binding of specific antibody to the infectious agents results in their decreased growth rate (bacteriostasis) and/or in removal by lysis (bacteriolysis, virolysis) and/or phagocytosis (opsonophagocytosis). The ratio of antigen to antibody (1) is important and influences the efficacy of the removal of the infectious agent. Proteins of the complement system as well as phagocyte receptors participate in efficient opsonization and phagocytosis, complement and natural antibodies in general constituting links between innate and adaptive immunity playing a role in the early handling by the host of antigen reaching its blood (65). Whereas natural antibodies are contained in IVIG, the host complement

TABLE 24.4. MONOCLONAL AND ENGINEERED ANTIBODIES FOR HUMAN THERAPY

Generic Name	Trade Name	Company	Makeup	Biological Activity	Therapeutic Promise
Trastuzumab	Herceptin	Roche	Recombinant, humanized mab	Binds to human epidemermal growth factor receptor 2 (HER2)	Breast cancer
Basiliximabum	Simulect	Novartis	Chimeric humanised mab (IgG1K)	Interleukin-2 receptor antagonist (α-CD25)	Immunosuppressive regimens
Daclizumab	Zenaprax	Roche	Recombinant humanized mab anti-Tac	Interleukin-2 receptor antagonist (α-CD25)	Antiinflammatory/antirejection therapy in transplantation
Abciximab	ReoPro	Lilly	Fab fragment of chimeric mab 7E3	Binds to glycoprotein lib/IIIa on human platelets	Prophylaxis of thrombosis
Muromonoabum	Orthoclone	Janssen-Cilag	Murine mag IgG2α	Reacts against CD3, a pan–T-cell marker	Prevents organ rejection
Rituximab			Chimeric (IDEC-C2B8)	Reacts against CD20	Low-grade follicular B-cell lymphomas
Gemtuzumab	Mylotarg	Wyeth-Ayerst (American Home Products), Celltech	Humanized mab-linked to calicheamicin isloted from a bacterium in caliche clay, Texas soil	Reacts against CD33, a glycoprotein commonly expressed by myeloid leukemic cells	Antibody-targeted chemotherapy with calicheamicin, a potent antitumor antibiotic
Infliximab			Chimeric humanized anti-TNFα	Inhibits the effects of TNFα	Rheumatoid arthritis

TNF, tumor necrosis factor; mab, monoclonal antibody.

could be substituted only by transfusions of fresh-frozen plasma. Depending on the strain of bacteria or the type of virus, the infectious target also may be lysed. Thus, the patient might suffer from release of bacterial products and of a deranged homeostasis of cytokines. In contrast, a terminal complement component deficiency, such as deficiency of C7, would affect neutrophilic granulocyte-mediated killing of certain strains of bacteria (such as type V group B streptococci) only minimally, but certainly would greatly impair killing of *Neisseria*. Neutrophil complement receptor 3 and either complement receptor 1 or FcR III optimize phagocytosis (1).

In the last 5 years, further advances have been achieved in our knowledge of Fc receptors (FcRs), mainly in the recognition of their genetic makeup. In fact, FcRs are a key to IVIG action, not only in antiinfectious but also autoimmune defense. Because the opsonophagocytosis phenomenon is so central to the action of IVIG, coincubation assays of bacteria, phagocytes, and IVIG now are a general requirement to prove the efficacy of IVIG; as yet, in vitro studies remain insufficient for the prediction of clinical efficacy (Table 24.5). The antiviral activity of IVIG is based on the virucidal capacity of specific antiviral, neutralizing antibodies, the subclass composition (Table 24.3), and complement-activating capacity, all of which may have decisive effects on their protective and nonprotective capacities.

Mechanisms of Action in Autoimmune Disease

Because IgM and IgG isotype antibodies are located at the crossroads of the immune response, their capacity to distinguish between self and nonself is so important that its failure results in overt autoimmune disease. Intravenous immune globulin, taken from thousands of apparently healthy donors, substitutes for regulatory antibodies to correct a deregulated system. The immunomodulatory effects of IVIG are Fc dependent and V region dependent, but also may be separated into early effects that occur within hours or days, and late effects noted well beyond the half-life of infused IVIG. Evidence for the ability of IVIG to transiently down-regulate the function of Fc receptors on splenic macrophages come from the following observations: (a) administration of IVIG results in a decrease in the clearance of anti-D–coated autologous red blood cells in vivo; (b) peripheral blood monocytes from IVIG-treated patients with ITP exhibit a decreased ability to form rosettes with IgG-coated red blood cells in vitro; (c) antibodies against Fcγ RIII (CD16) show similar effects to those of IVIG in patients with ITP; (d) anti-D IgG induces an increase in platelet counts in RhD-positive ITP patients; and (e) infusion of Fc fragments of IgG induces an increase in platelet counts in patients with ITP. Alternatively, FcγRIIB, the only IgG receptor in B cells, may be involved. This receptor contains a cytoplasmic inhibitory motif (immune receptor tyrosine-based inhibition motif [ITIM]), which when brought in proximity to receptors containing a specific activation motif, inhibits cell activation through the latter (64). The common feature of receptors as members of the inhibitory class is their ability to attenuate activation signals initiated by other receptors that are often of the immune receptor tyrosine-based activation motif (ITAM) class. An expanding family of immune inhibitory receptors can be identified by a consensus amino acid sequence, ITIM. IgG immune complexes were recognized as potent inhibitory ligands demonstrating that B cell activation could be attenuated by low-affinity interacting immune com-

TABLE 24.5. EFFICACY ASSESSMENT OF IV IMMUNOGLOBULIN PREPARATIONS FOR THEIR ANTIMICROBIAL CAPACITY

Technical Approach	Details of Procedure	Information Provided
Radioimmunoassay ELISA Antigen neutralization	Test antibody content against defined bacteria or viruses Test residual infectivity or toxicity of microbes or microbial toxins	Quantitative information about content of specific IgG; permits distinction between polyvalent and hyperimmune globulin; allows definition of antitoxic potency toward microbial products
Opsonophagocytic assay; chemilluminescence	Coincubation of bacterium with phagocytes in presence or absence of immunoglobulin	Opsonic activity or specific antibodies contained in IMIG or IVIG
Antibody-mediated cell-mediated (ADCC)	Killing of viruses in presence or absence of IMIG or IVIG and complement	Antiviral potency of preparation
Animal protection experiments	Infect laboratory animals (monkeys, rats, mice) with definite numbers of bacteria; protect previously with injections of IMIG or IVIG	Model for efficacy of passive immunization
Clinical studies in man	Prophylactic in high-risk or therapeutic in established infection; placebo-controlled and prospective whenever possible	Final proof of efficacy or futility of transfusion of IMIG or IVIG

ELISA, enzyme-linked immunosorbent assay; IMIG, intramuscular immune globulin; IVIG, intravenous immune globulin.

plexes. A molecular basis for this was suggested with the cloning of two genes for murine low-affinity IgG Fc receptors, now referred to as FcγRIIB and FcγRIII. The relevance of these interactions in IVIG therapy is that their infusion results in the formation of small immune complexes of idiotype-antiidiotype, which in turn bind to the Fc receptor apparatus. In addition, IgG inhibits antibody responses through Fc-independent mechanisms, most likely by masking antigenic epitopes without abolition of T cell priming (66). The fractional rate of catabolism is determined by the plasma concentration of IgG. Some experts believe that the acceleration of the rate of IgG catabolism is a plausible unifying explanation for the beneficial action of high doses of exogenous IgG in antibody-mediated autoimmune disorders (67). Studies with H2-deficient mice, corresponding in humans to HLA deficiency, revealed the mechanism by which plasma IgG concentrations regulate the rate of IgG catabolism. Mutant mice that had extremely low serum levels of IgG and immunization did not evoke a sustained increase in serum IgG, but IgM responses were normal. The low serum level of IgG in these mutant mice is attributed to the loss of a previously unrecognized transport receptor for IgG, present also on human placenta, FcRn. Normally, IgG entering cells is protected from catabolism by binding to FcRn, this receptor originally being identified in neonatal intestinal epithelium (and is therefore called FcRn, for Fc receptor of the neonate). In states of hypergammaglobulinemia, this receptor is saturated, permitting the degradation of IgG to occur in proportion to its total concentration in plasma. The IgG FcRn is found in many adult tissues, including skin, muscle, and intestine. Its high level of expression in vascular endothelial cells suggests that these cells are a major site of IgG catabolism (68). FcRn on placenta could be a selective entry door to the fetal side with respect to maternal anti-A/B antibodies (69). Such models advocate clinical trials using moderate instead of high doses of IVIG. Kazatchkine et al. in Paris has shown that IVIG induces cell death in human monocytic and lymphoblastoid cell lines and CD40-activated normal human B lymphocytes in vitro, and that cell death is associated with nucleosomal cleavage of cellular DNA and the expression of phosphatidylserines on the cell surface, an early event of apoptosis occurring before membrane disruption. They have demonstrated that IVIG-induced apoptosis of lymphocytes is dependent on Fas and on activation of the caspase family of proteases. They further showed the presence of anti-Fas antibodies in IVIG that can efficiently induce apoptosis upon affinity purification (70), confirming similar studies performed in Geneva, Switzerland (58).

The members of the TNF receptor superfamily and their ligands are critical regulators of immune responses. They can be divided into two groups: death receptors to which the above-mentioned Fas and nondeath receptors to which also the afore-mentioned CD40 belong. Mice or humans deficient in CD40 or CD40 ligand lack germinal centers and high-affinity IgG antibodies to T cell–dependent antigens but have augmented IgM production. Drugs, in addition to IVIG, that inhibit such receptors, as well as the newly identified BAFF (B cell activating factor) and APRIL (A proliferation inducing ligand) receptors of the TNF superfamily, may be useful for combined treatments not only for autoimmune diseases but also for B lymphoid malignancies (71). Other Fc-mediated mechanisms of IVIG therapy may depend on their ability to bind activated C3b and C4b, and deflect the activated complement to innocuous targets. V region–dependent mechanisms include the capacity of this portion of IgG in infused IVIG to interact with complementary V regions on the patients' autoantibodies, resulting in neutralization of circulating autoantibody activity and modulation of antibody synthesis by B cells endowed with surface immunoglobulins carrying the relevant idiotype at their surface. Interactions between IVIG and lymphocytes produce long-term suppression of autoantibody-secreting clones or selective stimulation of B- and T-cell clones that express antigen receptors. V region–dependent changes in network structure and function after IVIG infusion are evidenced by the restoration of normal spontaneous fluctuations in autoantibody titers. The ability of IVIG to interact with idiotypes and V regions of autoantibodies is based on the observation that $F(ab')_2$ fragments of IVIG neutralize the functional activity of autoantibodies or prevent their antigen binding or both; it is also based on the observation that autoantibodies specifically become retained on affinity chromatography columns of $F(ab')_2$ fragments of IVIG. Furthermore autoantibodies retained on IVIG coupled to affinity columns are selective for certain idiotypes expressed by the autoantibodies of a given individual. Finally, IVIG does not contain detectable antibodies against allotypes that are most commonly expressed in the $F(ab')_2$. Patients who spontaneously recover from autoimmune disease, healthy individuals >65 years, and multiparous women can be the sources of plasma with high antiidiotypic activity (72). Pools of IVIG also may express high antiidiotypic activity against autoantibodies because of the synergistic effect of mixing antibodies from different individuals (73).

Intravenous immune globulin also is known to interact with bacterial superantigens (74). For example, TNF becomes released to exacerbate experimental autoimmune encephalomyelitis in laboratory animals. Superantigens also can stimulate a large fraction of the nonsensitized T-cell population, which accounts for the central and peripheral neural damage found in autoimmune and virus-induced demyelinating diseases. They are, in part, mediated by proinflammatory cytokines produced by neuroantigen-specific helper cells and might respond to IVIG.

SIDE EFFECTS

The adverse effects of modern preparations of IVIG are rare. They are classified according to the mechanisms by which they arise or by the distinction between immediate and later effects. Most effects are mild, transient, and related to the speed of the infusion (75). The immediate or anaphylactoid reactions occur rarely and include flushing, malaise, hypotension, dyspnea, back pain, nausea, vomiting, or diarrhea. Dramatic side effects occur almost exclusively in previously untreated agammaglobulinemic patients with chronic infections. Milder reactions are seen in patients with Guillain-Barré syndrome, who respond to a reduction in the infusion rate. Selective IgA deficiency constitutes a risk for IVIG preparations that contain up to 1 mg IgA per gram of IgG (Table 24.1). Salama et al. have recently developed a test using the DiaMed gel perfusion system, which should easily identify patients sensitized to IgA (76). In patients with preexisting renal insufficiency, high-dose treatment with IVIG may lead to a transient increase in serum creatinine and to further impairment of renal function. Therefore, dialysis-dependent renal insufficiency is a contraindication for IVIG. Thrombosis after IVIG therapy might occur as a consequence of increased serum viscosity but reports of the occurrence have diminished, probably because physicians are now cautious with patients at risk. Volume overload and acute lung injury are also rare side effects (77).

The issue of hemolysis after IVIG therapy still remains unsettled but is certainly of minor importance, because so much material has been infused without anti-A/B antibodies having become well-known culprits. This is different when infusing anti-D hyperimmunoglobulins for treatment of ITP (78); this is not recommended for Rh(D)-negative individuals. Care should be taken when new preparations are introduced to the market, even if appropriately registered by official committees. In fact, the development of IgM- or IgA-enriched preparations, with demonstration of their efficacy in animal models followed by subsequent introduction to human use, must only be allowed under strict clinical surveillance and within the framework of Investigational New Drug or Drug Under Intensive Surveillance programs by the FDA or European Agency for the Evaluation of Medicinal Products (EMEA), respectively.

Side effects coming from transmission of infectious agents have become rare. To our knowledge, no preparation has been accused during the last 5 years for any of the transfusion-associated viral diseases. There is concern that IVIG might induce iatrogenic Creutzfeldt-Jakob disease (iCJD). It is unknown if IVIG transmits PrP^{Sc}, a human prion that is a transmissible pathogen for Creutzfeldt-Jakob disease. The risk of acquisition of CJD or vCJD from these preparations is felt to be very low (see Chapter 54).

ACKNOWLEDGMENTS

The authors kindly acknowledge the Katharina Huber Foundation, the Swiss National Foundation for Scientific Research, as well as Thierry Carrel, M.D., for continuous support.

REFERENCES

1. Nydegger UE. Immune complexes. In: Delves PJ, Roitt IM, eds. *Encyclopedia of immunology*, 2nd ed. London: Academic Press, 1998: 1220–1225.
2. Roux KH, Greenspan NS. Monitoring the formation of soluble immune complexes composed of idiotype and anti-idiotype antibodies by electron microscopy. *Mol Immunol* 1994;31:599–606.
3. Van Uden J, Raz E. Introduction to immunostimulatory DNA sequences. *Springer Semin Immunopathol* 2000;22:1–9.
4. Winter G, Griffiths AD, Hawkins RE, et al. Making antibodies by phage display technology. *Ann Rev Immunol* 1994;12:433–455.
5. Voorberg J, van den Brink EN. Phage display technology: a tool to explore the diversity of inhibitors to blood coagulation factor VIII. *Semin Thromb Hemost* 2000;26:143–150.
6. Berger A, Doerr HW, Sharrer I, et al. Follow-up of four HIV-infected individuals after administration of hepatitis C virus and GBV-C/hepatitis G virus–contaminated intravenous immunoglobulin: evidence for HCV but not for GBH-C/HGV transmission. *J Med Virol* 1997;53: 25–30.
7. Chandra S, Cavanaugh JE, Lin CM, et al. Virus reduction in the preparation of intravenous immune globulin: in vitro experiments. *Transfusion* 1999;39:249–257.
8. Gocke DJ, Raska K Jr, Pollack W, et al. HTLV III antibody in commercial immunoglobulin. *Lancet* 1986;1:37–38.
9. Steel P. HTLV III antibodies in human immune gammaglobulin [Letter]. *JAMA* 1986;255:609.

10. Nabel GJ, Sullivan NJ. Antibodies and resistance to natural HIV infection. *N Engl J Med* 2000;343:17:1263–1265.
11. Andresen I, Kovarik JM, Spycher M, et al. Product equivalence study comparing the tolerability, pharmacokinetics, and pharmacodynamics of various human immunoglobulin-G formulations. *J Clin Pharmacol* 2000;40:722–730.
12. Kempf C, Jentsch P, Poirier B, et al. Virus inactivation during production of intravenous immunoglobulins. *Transfusion* 1991;31:423–427.
13. Novak T, Gregersen J-P, Klockmann U, et al. Virus safety of human immunoglobulins: efficient inactivation of hepatitis C and other human pathogenic viruses by the manufacturing procedure. *J Med Virol* 1992;36:209–216.
14. Morell A, Sidioropoulos D, Hermann U, et al. IgG subclasses and antibodies to group B streptococci, pneumococci, and tetanus toxoid in preterm neonates after intravenous infusion of immunoglobulin to the mothers. *Pediatr Res* 1986;20:933–936.
15. Robinson RF, Nahata MC. Respiratory syncytial virus (RSV) immune globulin and palivizumab for prevention of RSV infection. *Am J Health Syst Pharm* 2000;57:259–264.
16. Mascola JR, Stiegler G, VanCott TC, et al. Protection of macaques against vaginal transmission of a pathogenic HIV-1/SIV chimeric virus by passive infusion of neutralizing antibodies. *Nature Medicine* 2000; 6:207–210.
17. Waldvogel FA, Vaudaux P, Lew PD, et al. Deficient phagocytosis secondary to breakdown of opsonic factors in infected exudates. In: Rossi F, Patriarcha P, eds. *Biochemistry and function of phagocytes.* London: Plenum Press, 1982:603–610.
18. Glinz W, Grob PJ, Nydegger UE, et al. Polyvalent immunoglobulins for prophylaxis of bacterial infections in patients following multiple trauma. A randomized, placebo-controlled study. *Intensive Care Med* 1985;11:288–294.
19. The Intravenous Immunoglobulin Collaborative Study Group. Prophylactic intravenous administration of standard immune globulin as compared with core-lipopolysaccharide immune globulin in patients at high risk of postsurgical infection. *N Engl J Med* 1992;327:234–240.
20. Douzinas EE, Pitaridis MT, Louris G, et al. Prevention of infection in multiple trauma patients by high-dose intravenous immunoglobulins. *Crit Care Med* 2000;28:8–15.
21. Pilz G, Appel R, Krezuzer E, et al. Comparison of early IgM-enriched immunoglobulin vs polyvalent IgG administration in score-identified postcardiac surgical patients at high risk for sepsis. *Chest* 1997;111: 419–426.
22. Hodgson JC, Barclay GR, Hay LA, et al. Prophylactic use of human endotoxin-core hyperimmune gammaglobulin in colostrum-deprived, gnotobiotic lambs challenged orally with *E. coli. FEMS Immunol Med Microbiol* 1995;11:171–180.
23. Barclay GR. Endotoxin-core antibodies: time for a reappraisal? *Intensive Care Med* 1999;25:427–429.
24. Gore DC, Sutherland G. Gut gavage with antiendotoxin antibodies reduces the liberation of tumor necrosis factor after hemorrhage/resuscitation. *Crit Care Med* 2000;28:2425–2428.
25. Greenman RI, Schein RHH, Martin MH, et al. A controlled clinical trial of E5 murine monoclonal IgM antibody to endotoxin in the treatment of gram-negative sepsis. *JAMA* 1991;266:1079–1102.
26. Behre G, Schedel I, Nentwig B, et al. Endotoxin concentration in neutropenic patients with suspected gram-negative sepsis: correlation with clinical outcome and determination of anti-endotoxin core antibodies during therapy with polyclonal immunoglobulin M–enriched immunoglobulins. *Antimicrob Agents Chemother* 1992;36:2139–2146.
27. Trautmann M, Held TK, Susa M, et al. Bacterial lipopolysaccharide (LPS)-specific antibodies in commercial human immunoglobulin preparations: superior antibody content of an IgM-enriched product. *Clin Exp Immunol* 1998;111:81–90.
28. Czermak BJ, Sarma V, Person CL, et al. Protective effects of C5a blockade in sepsis. *Nature Medicine* 1999;5:788–793.
29. Calandra T, Echtenacher B, Le Roy D, et al. Protection from septic shock by neutralization of macrophage inhibitory factor. *Nature Medicine* 2000;6:164–170.
30. Reeves JH, Butt WW, Shann F, et al. Continuous plasmafiltration in sepsis syndrome. Plasmafiltration in sepsis study group. *Crit Care Med* 1999; 27:2096–2104.
31. Nydegger UE, Hauser SP. Use of intravenous immunoglobulins in haematological disorders. *Clin Immunotherapy* 1996;5:465–485.
32. Levy Y, Sherer Y, Ahmed A, et al. A study of 20 SLE patients with intravenous immunoglobulin—clinical and serological response. *Lupus* 1999;8:705–712.
33. Ong CS, Benson EM. Successful treatment of chronic leukocytoclastic vasculitis and persistent ulceration with intravenous immunoglobulin. *Br J Dermatol* 2000;143:447–449.
34. Sultan Y, Kazatchine MD, Maisonneuve P, et al. Anti-idiotypic suppression of autoantibodies to factor VIII (antihemophilic factor) by high-dose intravenous gammaglobulin. *Lancet* 1984;2:765–768.
35. Nachbaur D, Herold M, Gächter A, et al. Modulation of alloimmune response in vitro by an IgM-enriched immunoglobulin preparation (Pentaglobin). *Immunology* 1998;94:279–283.
36. Poynton CH, Jackson S, Fegan C, et al. Use of IgM enriched intravenous immunoglobulin (Pentaglobin) in bone marrow transplantation. *Bone Marrow Transplant* 1992;9:451–457.
37. Sharief MK, Zingram DA, Swash M, et al. IV immunoglobulin reduces circulating pro-inflammatory cytokines in Guillain-Barré syndrome. *Neurology* 1999;52:1833–1838.
38. Stangel M, Toyka KV, Gold R. Mechanisms of high-dose intravenous immunoglobulins in demyelinating diseases. *Arch Neurol* 1999;56: 661–663.
39. Phipps RP. Atherosclerosis: the emerging role of inflammation and the CD40-CD40L ligand system. *Proc Natl Acad Sci U S A* 2000;97: 6930–6932.
40. Nicoletti A, Kaveri S, Caligiuri G, et al. Immunoglobulin treatment reduces atherosclerosis in apo E knockout mice. *J Clin Invest* 1998; 102:910–918.
41. Rewald E. Antifibrotic tendency as complement to inflammatory burnout? Six year IVIG treatment in a case with atherosclerosis and chronic hepatitis C. *Transfus Sci* 1999;21:3–5.
42. Mueller J, Wallukat G, Dandel M, et al. Immunoglobulin adsorption in patients with idiopathic dilated cardiomyopathy. *Circulation* 2000; 101:385–391.
43. Felix SB, Staudt A, Dorffel WV, et al. Hemodynamic effects of immunoadsorption and subsequent immunoglobulin substitution in dilated cardiomyopathy: three-month results from a randomized study. *J Am Coll Cardiol* 2000;35:1590–1598.
44. Stull LB, DiIulio NA, Yu M, et al. Alterations in cardiac function and gene expression during autoimmune myocarditis in mice. *J Mol Cell Cardiol* 2000;32:2035–2049.
45. McNamara DM, Rosenblum WE, Janosko KM, et al. Intravenous immune globulin in the therapy of myocarditis and acute cardiomyopathy. *Circulation* 1997;95:2476–2478.
46. Hufnagel G, Pankuweit S, Richter A, et al. The European study of epidemiology and treatment of cardiac inflammatory diseases (ESETCID). First epidemiological results. *Herz* 2000;5:279–285.
47. Lagrand WK, Visser CA, Hermens WT, et al. C-reactive protein as a cardiovascular risk factor. *Circulation* 1999;100:96–102.
48. Rieben R, Roos A, Muizert Y, et al. Immunoglobulin M–enriched human intravenous immunoglobulin prevents complement activation in vitro and in vivo in a rat model of acute inflammation. *Blood* 1999; 93.942–951.
49. Mohacsi P, Rieben R, Sigurdsson G, et al. Successful management of a B-type cardiac allograft into an O-type man with 3½-year clinical follow-up. *Transplantation,* 2001;72:1328–1330.
50. John R, Lietz K, Burke E, et al. Intravenous immunoglobulin reduces anti-HLA alloreactivity and shortens waiting time to cardiac transplantation in highly sensitized left ventricular assist device recipients. *Circulation* 1999;100:II229–235.
51. Magee JC, Collins BH, Harland RC, et al. Immunoglobulin prevents complement-mediated hyperacute rejection in swine-to-primate xenotransplantation. *J Clin Invest* 1995;96:2404–2412.
52. Bach FH, Auchincloss H, Robson RC. Xenotransplantation. In: Bach FH, Auchincloss H Jr, eds. *Transplantation immunology.* New York: Wiley-Liss, 1995:305–338.
53. Zander AR , Zabelina T, Kroeger N, et al. Use of a five-agent GVD

prevention regimen in recipients of unrelated donor marrow. *Bone Marrow Transplant* 1999;23:889–893.
54. Valentine HA, Gao SZ, Mednon SG, et al. Impact of prophylactic immediate posttransplant ganciclovir on development of transplant atherosclerosis: a post hoc analysis of a randomized, placebo-controlled study. *Circulation* 1999;100:61–66.
55. Arbeitsgruppe Thorakale Organtransplantation der Deutschen Gesellschaft für Kardiologie. Herztransplantation. Nachsorge und Rehabilitation. *Z Kardiol* 1996;85:67–77.
56. Glowacki LS, Smaill FM. Use of immune globulin to prevent symptomatic cytomegalovirus disease in transplant recipients. A metaanalysis. *Clin Transplant* 1994;8:10–18.
57. Foster CS, Ahmed AR. Intravenous immunoglobulin therapy for ocular cicatricial pemphigoid. *Ophthalmology* 1999;106:2136–2143.
58. Viard I, Wehrli PH, Bullaini R, et al. Inhibition of toxic epidermal necrolysis by blockade of CD95 with human intravenous immunoglobulin. *Science* 1998;282:490–493.
59. Breedveld FC. Therapeutic monoclonal antibodies. *Lancet* 2000;355: 735–740.
60. Hanes J, Schaffitzel C, Knappik A, et al. Picomolar affinity antibodies from a fully synthetic naive library selected and evolved by ribosome display. *Nat Biotechnol* 2000;18:1287–1292.
61. Giddings G, Allison G, Brooks D, et al. Transgenic plants as factories for biopharmaceuticals. *Nat Biotechnol* 2000;18:1151–1155.
62. Coiffier B. Monoclonal antibodies in the treatment of non-Hodgkin's lymphoma patients. *Haematologica* 1999;84:14–18.
63. Kalden JR, Breedveld FC, Burkhardt H, et al. Immunological treatment of autoimmune disease. *Adv Immunol* 1998;68:333–418.
64. Ravetch JV, Lanier LL. Immune inhibitory receptors. *Science* 2000; 290:84–88.
65. Ochsenbein AF, Zinkernagel RM. Natural antibodies and complement link innate and acquired immunity. *Immunol Today* 2000;21:624–629.
66. Karlsson MCI, Wernersson S, De Stahl TD, et al. Efficient IgG-mediated suppression of primary antibody responses in Fcg receptor-deficient mice. *Proc Natl Acad Sci U S A* 1999;96:2244–2249.
67. Yu Z, Lennon VA. Mechanisms of intravenous immune globulin therapy in antibody-mediated autoimmune diseases. *New Engl J Med* 1999; 340:227–228.
68. Gehtie V, Ward ES. FcRn: the MHC class I–related receptor that is more than an IgG transporter. *Immunol Today* 1997;18:592–598.
69. Hari Y, von Allmen EC, Boss GM, et al. The complement-activating capacity of maternal IgG antibodies to blood group A in paired mother/child serum samples. *Vox Sang* 1998;74:95–100.
70. Prasad NKA, Papoff G, Zeuner A, et al. Therapeutic preparations of normal polyspecific IgG (IVIG) induce apoptosis in human lymphocytes and monocytes: a novel mechanism of action of IVIG involving the Fas apoptotic pathway. *J Immunol* 1998;161:3782–3790.
71. Laabi Y, Strasser A. Lymphocyte survival-ignorance is BLys. *Science* 2000;289:883–884.
72. Dietrich G, Algiman M, Sultan Y, et al. Selection of the expressed B cell repertoire by infusion of normal immunoglobulin G in a patient with autoimmune thyroiditis. *Eur J Immunol* 1993;23:2945–2950.
73. Nguyen NG, Rieben R, Carrel T, et al. Anti-A ABO-histoblood group antibody binding in plain versus mixtures of O-type and A-type serum (in preparation).
74. Brocke S, Gaur A, Piercy CH, et al. Induction of relapsing paralysis in experimental autoimmune encephalomyelitis by bacterial superantigen. *Nature* 1993;365:642–644.
75. Nydegger UE, Sturzenegger M. Adverse effects of intravenous immunoglobulin therapy. *Drug Saf* 1999;21(3):171–185.
76. Salama A, Schwind P, Schönhage K, et al. Rapid detection of antibodies to IgA molecules using the particle gel immunoassay (ID-PaGIA). *Vox Sang* 2001;81:45–48.
77. Rizte A, Gorson KC, Kenney L, et al. Transfusion-related acute lung injury after the infusion of IVIG. *Transfusion* 2001;41:264–268.
78. Gaines AR. Acute onset hemoglobinemia and/or hemoglobinuria and sequelae following Rho(D) immune globulin intravenous administration in immune thrombocytopenic purpura patients. *Blood* 2000;95: 2523–2529.

Rossi's Principles of Transfusion Medicine, Third Edition, edited by Toby L. Simon, Walter H. Dzik, Edward L. Snyder, Christopher P. Stowell, and Ronald G. Strauss. Lippincott Williams & Wilkins, Philadelphia © 2002.

CASE 24A

UNEXPECTED THROMBOCYTOPENIA BEFORE SURGERY

CASE HISTORY

A 41-year-old African-American woman, with pelvic pain before and after menstrual periods for 3 months and menorrhagia for 2 years, was found to have a 5-cm complex left adnexal mass by ultrasonography. She gave a history of menses lasting 5 to 7 days with heavy bleeding, but denied easy bruising, bleeding, or epistaxis. There was no bleeding with a right breast biopsy for a benign nodule 3 years previously. She was scheduled for laparoscopic biopsy and possible oophorectomy and referred for a hematology consultation.

The medical history was negative for pregnancy. The patient had had a breast biopsy in 1995 which revealed a benign tumor. Peptic ulcer disease was diagnosed in 1998, and the patient had been taking 20 mg of omeprazole daily since that time. The patient had also been taking 325 mg of ferrous sulfate daily for the past several months.

The family history was positive for diabetes in her father and cancer of unknown type in her mother; both died in Africa. The patient has a brother and sister who are well. There was no family history of anemia or a blood disorder.

The review of systems was noncontributory.

The social history was negative for smoking or alcohol intake. The patient works as a nurse's aide.

The physical examination was negative for petechiae on the oral mucosa or cutaneous bruising. There was no lymphadenopathy or hepatosplenomegaly.

The laboratory showed a hemoglobin level of 9.8 g/dl with a mean corpuscular volume of 83.9 fl and a red cell distribution width of 20.9. The platelet count was 66,000/μl. The peripheral blood smear showed hypochromic microcytes. A bone marrow biopsy showed normal megakaryocyte numbers, but iron stores were absent.

The patient was told that no therapy was needed but that her platelet count should be checked during the week prior to surgery. At that point, the platelet count was found to be 37,000/μl, although the hemoglobin level had increased to 11.1 g/dl. The results of a test for the presence of an anti-platelet antibody were positive, confirming the clinical impression of immune thrombocytopenic purpura (ITP). The patient was called to the outpatient clinic and given intravenous immune globulin (IVIG) at a dose of 1 g/kg per day on 2 separate days. The platelet count was 105,000/μl prior to the second IVIG infusion. On the day of surgery, 2 days later, the platelet count was 181,000/μl. Blood loss was minimal during surgery. An endometrioma was removed without difficulty and oophorectomy was not done. The patient's platelet count increased to 451,000/μl on the third postoperative day (7 days after the start of IVIG). She was discharged, to be seen by her gynecologist for follow-up.

DISCUSSION

This woman with a gynecologic problem had the complications of iron deficiency anemia and ITP. Her platelet count continued to fall as the surgery date approached. Surgery was needed in the near future for a mass of unknown significance, which may have been contributing to increased blood loss during menses. At first her platelet count was felt to be adequate for surgery. Patients with thrombocytopenia due to increased platelet destruction, as in ITP, typically have better hemostasis at a particular count than would be expected when thrombocytopenia is due to depressed platelet production, presumably because the bone marrow is releasing younger, larger platelets in an attempt to correct the decreased platelet mass. However, as this patient's platelet count continued to fall, her physicians correctly decided that therapy was needed to ensure adequate hemostasis for surgery.

Intravenous immune globulin was an ideal choice in this situation. It has a fast onset, few side effects, and produces a response which is sufficiently sustained to cover surgery and the postoperative recovery period. Corticosteroids are more toxic and can increase complications of surgery. If the thrombocytopenic episode is short lived, as in this case, no further treatment may be needed. When immune thrombocytopenia becomes chronic and platelet counts are at a level at which hemostasis could be compromised (e.g., below 20,000/μl), other treatment modalities might need to be considered (see Chapter 27), but two-thirds of patients will continue to respond to IVIG. Because this disease can be self-limited, it is possible that one course of treatment will be all that is needed. In this case, the response was vigorous. The prior iron deficiency might account for the particularly high platelet count postoperatively. Endometriosis is not typically associated with thrombocytopenia, but the balance of platelet production and clearance could be affected by resulting inflammation.

Intravenous immune globulin toxicity is generally limited, particularly in young individuals, but headache, a migraine syndrome, or volume overload may occur. More serious side effects such as thrombosis, renal failure, and anaphylaxis are rare. In addition, this product has been free of viral transmission since 1994. It is costly, but because this case involved a short-term use to prepare for surgery, it was probably cost-effective because surgery could proceed on schedule. This treatment is particularly useful in children, for medical emergencies, during pregnancy, or to prepare for splenectomy. It is also recommended for patients who are refractory to other forms of therapy for ITP.

An alternative treatment would have been the intravenous administration of anti-D (WinRho). Anti-D is an effective therapy for ITP among Rh-positive individuals who have intact spleens. Anti-D treatment for ITP can be successful using 1,000 times less protein than that used with IVIG therapy (see Chapter 27). Physicans treating ITP patients with anti-D must anticipate some hemolysis during the week after therapy.

Case contributed by Toby L. Simon, M.D., Tricore Reference Laboratories, Albuquerque, NM; and Kenneth J. Smith, M.D., Emory University School of Medicine, Atlanta, GA.

REFERENCES

1. Bussel JB, Kimberly RP, Inman RD, et al. Intravenous γglobulin treatment of chronic idiopathic thrombocytopenic purpura. *Blood* 1983;62: 480–486.
2. Fehr J, Hoffman V, Keppeler U. Transient reversal of thrombocytopenia in idiopathic thrombocytopenic purpura by high dose intravenous immunoglobulin. *N Engl J Med* 1982;306:1254–1258.

25

PLASMA TRANSFUSION AND ALTERNATIVES

PEARL TOY

Previous chapters in this subsection described the coagulation mechanism, plasma composition, plasma collection, preparation of plasma derivatives, and immunoglobulins. This chapter describes the various plasma products available, the indications for their use, and the associated risks.

FRESH-FROZEN PLASMA

Fresh-frozen plasma (FFP) contains all plasma proteins, including all coagulation factors. To prepare FFP, a unit of whole blood from a single donor is centrifuged and the plasma separated from the red blood cells. The separated plasma is placed in a freezer within 8 hours of collection and stored at or below −18°C for 1 year, or stored at or below −65°C for 7 years. Prior to transfusion, FFP is thawed at 30° to 37°C and stored for 24 hours or less at 1° to 6°C (1). One bag contains approximately 200 to 250 ml. Larger volumes of "jumbo" FFP (approximately 400 to 600 ml) prepared by plasmapheresis from a single donor are available in some locations. The apheresis-prepared FFP has a lower percentage of anticoagulant (10% versus 20%) and less glucose than FFP (see Chapter 45).

ALTERNATIVES TO FFP

Plasma alternatives to FFP exist. Other plasma products from single donors include liquid plasma, thawed plasma, and cryoprecipitate-reduced plasma. These products have normal amounts of factors II, VII, IX, and X and can be used instead of FFP, for example, in patients requiring warfarin reversal or in liver disease (2). Unlike FFP, after whole blood collection and separation from red blood cells, liquid plasma is not frozen but is stored at 1° to 6°C for up to 5 days after expiration of the red blood cells (1). Thawed plasma (i.e., thawed FFP) is also stored at 1° to 6°C for up to 5 days (1). Both liquid and thawed plasma may have decreased amounts of the factors V and VIII because these factors are labile at 1° to 6°C. Cryoprecipitate-reduced plasma is the supernatant remaining after removal of cryoprecipitate and thus has reduced amounts of fibrinogen and factor VIII. It is stored at or below −18°C for up to 12 months from the original collection (1).

Other alternatives to allogeneic plasma exist. Crystalloid, colloid solutions containing albumin or plasma protein fraction, hydroxyethyl starch, and dextran are preferable to FFP for volume replacement. When both red blood cells and plasma are needed, whole blood should be given if available. For nutritional support, amino acid solutions and dextrose are available. Before elective surgery associated with a predicted significant blood loss, autologous whole blood donation is an alternative to allogeneic red blood cells and plasma.

SOLVENT DETERGENT TREATED PLASMA

Solvent detergent treated plasma (S/D plasma) is plasma pooled from approximately 2,500 donors. Lipid-enveloped viruses such as human immunodeficiency virus (HIV), hepatitis B virus (HBV), and hepatitis C virus (HCV) are inactivated by treatment with solvents and detergents (3). Hepatitis A virus and

P. Toy: Department of Laboratory Medicine, University of California San Francisco, San Francisco, California.

human Parvovirus B19 lack lipid envelopes and are not inactivated. The risk per unit from single donors is negligible but is a concern in pooled product such as S/D plasma. S/D plasma contains neutralizing antibodies, but the Parvovirus B19 antibody content may not always be sufficient to prevent transmission of the disease. A patient with myasthenia gravis who underwent plasma exchange developed a clinical illness due to Parvovirus B19 infection after the infusion of S/D plasma (4). Patients who are susceptible to parvovirus infection are pregnant women, patients with sickle cell disease, hemolytic anemias, or are immunosuppressed. Parvovirus screening with removal of high-titer units is now being added to the manufacturing process.

S/D plasma is standardized with respect to coagulation factors and appears comparable to FFP in treating multiple coagulation deficiencies. It lacks the largest von Willebrand multimers and thus resembles cryoprecipitate-reduced plasma. Because of this, S/D plasma appeared to be uniquely suitable for patients with thrombotic thrombocytopenic purpura (TTP) who receive plasma as their major blood component. However, S/D plasma has reduced protein S activity compared with FFP. When used as 50% to 100% replacement fluid for plasma exchange, three patients were reported to develop deep vein thromboses (5).

As an alternative to pooled products, some blood centers release FFP which has been "donor retested." The unit is held until the donor returns for testing at a later date (up to 6 months later). There is a Food and Drug Administration–approved label for such units.

GUIDELINES FOR THE USE OF PLASMA

Because of the increase in FFP use associated with decreased availability of whole blood, the National Institutes of Health (NIH) held a consensus conference on the use of FFP in 1984 (2). Many conclusions of the panel still hold, while others need to be updated. The panel found no justification for the use of FFP as a volume expander or as a nutritional source because safer therapies exist; this remains true. The panel recommended the use of FFP for reversal of warfarin effect, treatment of TTP, treatment of selected congenital plasma protein deficiencies, and massive blood transfusion, recommendations that still hold. However, since the conference, safe and purified products have become available for antithrombin III (ATIII) deficiency, immunoglobulin deficiency, and factor IX deficiency, and these products have replaced the use of FFP for these conditions.

The NIH consensus conference thus described broad and general guidelines for the use of plasma. Detailed practice guidelines were not described. In 1994, the College of Pathologists developed more specific guidelines on the use of FFP and other blood products (6), and these will be discussed in the ensuring sections.

MAJOR INDICATIONS FOR PLASMA

Liver Disease

Coagulopathy in patients with liver disease results from impairments in clotting and fibrinolytic systems, as well as from reduced numbers and function of platelets (7). Treatment is necessary for bleeding or prophylaxis prior to an invasive procedure. Current options available to treat the coagulopathy include vitamin K, plasma, cryoprecipitate, exchange plasmapheresis, and platelet transfusions. Vitamin K corrects decreased synthesis of clotting factors due to vitamin K deficiency associated with biliary obstruction, bacterial overgrowth, or malnutrition. Vitamin K, however, does not correct coagulopathy due to parenchymal liver injury. Plasma transfusion is the mainstay for such coagulopathy.

Bleeding Risk During Invasive Procedures in Liver Disease

Invasive procedures performed in these patients include liver biopsy, thoracentesis, paracentesis, placement of invasive vascular lines, and others. A widely held belief is that a coagulopathy predisposes a patient to bleeding. However, the search for a level of prothrombin time (PT) associated with increased bleeding during invasive liver biopsy has not been successful in several studies in the last two decades (8–12). One study of 177 patients with liver disease found no increased bleeding in patients with mild hemostatic abnormalities (defined as PTs and partial thromboplastin times [PTTs] 1.1 to 1.5 times the midrange of normal levels) compared with patients with normal PTs and PTTs (11). Although coagulation tests did not predict bleeding, factors that predicted bleeding included malignancy (10,11), age, sex, and the number of passes (10). Despite the unsuccessful search for a dangerous level of PT, it is still recommended that if the PT is 4 to 6 seconds prolonged, FFP should be given to bring the PT to less than 4 seconds prolonged (13). In addition, it is recommended that if the PT is greater than 6 seconds prolonged, other biopsy methods should be tried (13).

The level at which thrombocytopenia or prolonged bleeding time become contraindications to percutaneous liver biopsy vary. One study of 87 patients (14) found that those patients with a platelet count below 60,000/mm^3 were significantly more likely to bleed after percutaneous liver biopsy than those with platelet counts above this value. A survey of mostly U.S. centers showed a preference for platelet counts above 50,000/mm^3, while other countries prefer higher levels (15). Platelet function may be abnormal in liver disease, and increased bleeding has been reported after liver biopsy in patients with a prolonged bleeding time (16). The practice of measuring bleeding time before liver biopsy is much more common in Asia than in the United States (73% versus 36%) (15).

For thoracentesis and paracentesis, mild hemostatic abnormalities in patients with liver disease also did not increase the risk of bleeding (17,18), but a creatinine level from 6 to 14 mg/dl did increase the risk of bleeding (17). For placement of invasive vascular lines, a study of intensive care patients receiving arterial, pulmonary artery, and central venous lines found low rates of bleeding even without correction of coagulation abnormalities before the procedure. Rates of bleeding were closely related to the experience of the physician placing the lines (19).

Fresh-Frozen Plasma Transfusion in Liver Disease

Large volumes of plasma, 12 to 20 ml/kg, are needed to improve the PT, and even this volume will not correct the PT in all cases

(20). Furthermore, coagulation factors such as factor VII have a short half-life, so plasma must be transfused just prior to the procedure and repeated every 8 to 12 hours if needed. Alternatively, a continuous plasma infusion at a rate adjusted to the PT has been used. Cryoprecipitate may be useful for severe coagulopathy associated with hypofibrinogenemia.

Patients Undergoing Invasive Procedures

Prothrombin time data from multiple studies are difficult to combine or compare because the studies used different measurements. Guidelines for plasma infusion have suggested PT cutoff at 3 to 4 seconds prolongation or 1.5 times the midpoint of normal range. The problem is that these measurements may not be reproducible among laboratories and may vary within the same laboratory with different batches of reagents. The international normalized ratio (INR), while documented to be useful in standardizing PT prolongation due to warfarin, has not been studied for standardization of the coagulopathy of liver disease, which is more complicated than the coagulopathy induced by warfarin.

At our hospital, we use the following approach. With each change in batch PT reagent, we test the plasma of 30 current patients with liver disease for PT and levels of factors II, VII, IX, and X. Because individual factor levels of 30% are hemostatic in vivo, we select the PT level in seconds at which all patients have 30% or more of each of the factors tested. We consider this PT level safe regarding bleeding risk for invasive procedures.

Thus, the evidence for supporting the use of FFP prior to liver biopsy in patients with mild coagulopathy is unconvincing. If bleeding does occur and red blood cell transfusion is required, a dilutional coagulopathy can develop quickly because the patient has preexisting lower levels of coagulation factors. Thus, patients should be observed carefully after biopsy, especially those with liver malignancy, and FFP considered along with red blood cells should significant bleeding occur.

Exchange plasmapheresis has been useful in selected perioperative patients whose severe coagulopathies fail to correct with plasma transfusion and who have coexistent severe fluid overload (21).

Warfarin Reversal

Warfarin blocks the synthesis of fully active factors II, VII, IX, and X by blocking the vitamin K–dependent carboxylation of the precursors of these factors. Long-term oral anticoagulation with warfarin is used for patients with nonvalvular atrial fibrillation, venous thromboembolic disease, ischemic heart disease, mural thrombi, and mechanical heart valves.

If the patient is not bleeding and the INR is below 5, merely decreasing or stopping warfarin may suffice (22). The best dose and route for administering vitamin K to reverse warfarin is still under study and depends on the clinical situation (23). If there is time and vitamin K is needed, the oral route may suffice. Low-dose vitamin K can decrease the INR without completely reversing anticoagulation and without impairing long-term anticoagulation. Several studies have reported on the use of 1 to 2.5 mg of oral or 0.5 to 1 mg of intravenous vitamin K for partial reversal of warfarin anticoagulation (24–26). In a study of oral vitamin K, a mean single dose of 5 mg orally in preprocedure patients with initial mean INR of 2.6 was successful, while a mean single dose of 10 mg orally was successful in excessively anticoagulated patients with mean pre–vitamin K INR of 8.4. The administration of these single oral doses of vitamin K_1 was safe and effective in partially reversing anticoagulant therapy without disrupting the daily maintenance dose of warfarin (25).

The fastest reversal is by the intravenous route. In a study of asymptomatic or mildly hemorrhagic patients on warfarin with INR >7.0, patients were randomized to receive 0.5 mg, 1 mg, or 2 mg of intravenous vitamin K (27). Among 18 patients with INR between 7.0 and 9.5, 0.5 mg intravenous vitamin K successfully reduced the INR to 2 to 4 at day 1 in 67% of cases. In six more severely overanticoagulated patients with INR over 9.5, even 2 mg intravenous vitamin K failed to achieve an INR below 4.0 on day 1, suggesting that these patients may need a repeat dose if there is time or plasma transfusion in an emergency.

Plasma transfusion is indicated in patients for emergency reversal of oral anticoagulation if they are bleeding significantly or must undergo an invasive procedure and cannot wait for warfarin reversal by vitamin K within 12 to 24 hours. The dose of FFP is 10 to 15 ml/kg (22).

Dilutional Coagulopathy

When a patient bleeds, whole blood containing red blood cells, plasma, and platelets are lost. If the loss is replaced with red blood cells only (packed red blood cells, cell-saver red blood cells), the plasma proteins and platelets will be diluted and their concentrations will fall. Acute normovolemic dilution is a good experimental model as whole blood is removed and replaced by red blood cells and crystalloid/colloid without platelets or coagulation factors. Using such a model, when one-third of the blood volume was lost, the hematocrit and fibrinogen concentration fell to two-thirds of the baseline level (28). If coagulation factor levels were 100% before blood loss, a reduction to two-thirds, or 66%, would not increase the risk of bleeding. Thus, small blood volume losses can be replaced with red blood cells without concomitant plasma or platelet transfusion.

However, in massive transfusion, when a patient bleeds one blood volume or more, dilution is more severe. Intensive plasmapheresis without plasma replacement is a good model to study the hemostatic changes as whole blood is lost, replaced by red blood cells and no plasma. In patients who underwent 1- to 1.5-volume plasma exchanges, Urbaniak (29) found that fibrinogen levels were reduced to one-third of the preexchange level. Coagulation factors that are distributed in both intravascular and extravascular compartments were reduced less (e.g., factor IX), presumably as a result of equilibration. Fibrinogen is an essential coagulation factor and in patients with fibrinogen concentrations below 300 mg/dl, 1 to 1.5 volume exchanges would probably dilute the fibrinogen concentration below the hemostatic level of 100 mg/dl. Prothrombin time and activated PTT are highly variable in the diagnosis of increased surgical bleeding in massive transfusion (30). In a study of massively transfused trauma patients, Leslie and Toy (31) found consistent prolongation of the PT and activated PTT in patients who had been replaced 1 to 1.5 volumes with only red blood cells. Platelet counts were reduced to below 50,000/μl in patients replaced 1.5 volumes or more with platelet-free products (whole blood, red blood cells, cell-saver red blood cells).

From the above studies, plasma and platelet replacement may be necessary in patients who bleed one or more blood volumes replaced by red blood cells. Transfusion of plasma and platelets to prevent bleeding due to dilutional coagulopathy should be based on the patient's preexisting hemostatic competence, the surgical procedure, the amount of blood lost, and the amount of expected blood loss. Several special situations are worth mentioning. In hypothermic patients, normalization of clotting requires both rewarming and clotting factor repletion (32). Infants, children, and small adults have blood volumes smaller than the 70-kg adult patient, and massive transfusion must be based on their individual estimated blood volume. In pediatric open heart operations, ultrafiltration concentrates the hematocrit, plasma proteins, and fibrinogen and attenuates the dilutional coagulopathy associated with cardiopulmonary bypass in infants. In patients with preexisting low levels of coagulation factors, such as patients with cirrhosis, dilution associated with less than one blood volume of bleeding can reduce coagulation factors to below hemostatic levels.

Whole blood contains most coagulation factors, and massive transfusion with whole blood is not associated with dilutional coagulopathy. It should be used for massive transfusion if available.

Thrombotic Thrombocytopenic Purpura and Hemolytic Uremic Syndrome

Patients with the microangiopathic diseases TTP and hemolytic uremic syndrome (HUS) develop fever, thrombocytopenia, microangiopathic anemia, and ischemia of various organs. Platelet aggregates in the circulation in TTP produce ischemia or infarction in the brain. In the closely related HUS, ischemia is predominantly renal. In adults, TTP and HUS are probably the same disease. Without treatment, most of these patients die, but with plasma exchange 70% to 85% of patients achieve complete remission (33).

The pathophysiology of TTP/HUS has been elucidated (34). Unusually large von Willebrand factor (vWF) multimers released by the endothelium are usually cleaved by a protease into normal circulating vWF multimers. In TTP/HUS, excessive release of unusually large multimers from perturbed endothelial cells or interference with protease breakdown results in the presence of unusually large vWF multimers in the circulation. These multimers bind platelets and cause platelet aggregates that produce ischemia or infarction in various organs.

Plasma exchange accomplishes two purposes in these diseases. Firstly, the unusually large vWF multimers are removed and, secondly, normal protease is restored in the replacement plasma given. To remove the unusually large vWF multimers, the standard of practice is daily removal of 3 to 4 liters of plasma. Preliminary studies in Italy suggest that these multimers can also be removed by cascade filtration that removes plasma macromolecules, such as vWF and fibrinogen, and the remaining autologous plasma returned to the patient (35). To restore protease that cleaves unusually large vWF multimers, plasma is given as the replacement fluid. FFP is the standard product used. Cryopoor plasma has been advocated for refractory TTP, and its efficacy is being studied in a large randomized trial (33). S/D plasma eliminates the risk of lipid-enveloped viruses. However, the product has reduced protein S activity and may increase the risk of hypercoagulable complications. In three patients with TTP who received 50% to 100% S/D plasma as replacement fluid for plasma exchange, all developed low protein S levels and deep vein thrombosis (5).

Deficiencies of Specific Hemostatic or Anticoagulant Proteins

Plasma contains many proteins (e.g., anticoagulant proteins such as protein S, protein C, and ATIII). FFP has been used to correct deficiencies of these proteins. FFP can be used as a replacement source for patients with congenital deficiencies of factor II, V, VII, X, XI, or XIII to treat active bleeding or to prevent surgical blood loss. Plasma also has been used to treat deficiencies of the anticoagulant proteins such as congenital ATIII deficiency if ATIII concentrates are not available. Plasma can also be used for the treatment of congenital deficiencies of protein C in patients with coumadin skin necrosis, neonatal purpura fulminans, impending surgery, pregnancy, or ongoing thrombosis. Fresh-frozen plasma has been used for similar indications in patients with congenital protein S deficiency. Hematology consultation should be obtained in these cases (36).

Disseminated Intravascular Coagulation

Disseminated intravascular coagulation (DIC) is a relatively common syndrome characterized by increased generation of thrombin and increased consumption (and thus depletion) of coagulation factors and platelets. Patients with DIC can develop microvascular thrombosis, bleeding, or both. Disseminated intravascular coagulation always occurs in response to a primary pathologic process (for example, acute leukemia, burns, trauma, sepsis, obstetric catastrophe, or malignancy), although the initiating process is not always apparent. Consequently, therefore, the treatment strategies in DIC are directed primarily at reversing the underlying cause of the syndrome. Plasma, cryoprecipitate, and platelets can serve, however, as adjunctive therapy when depletion of coagulation factors and platelets has resulted in bleeding or in an overwhelming risk of bleeding (see Chapter 28). Activated protein C concentrate reduces mortality in severe sepsis but may be associated with more bleeding (37).

RISKS OF PLASMA THERAPY

The risks of plasma products from single donors are the same as the risks of any single-donor whole blood donation with exceptions. Because plasma is not a cellular product, plasma should not transmit cytomegalovirus and should not cause graft-versus-host disease. Because plasma from donors with red blood cell antibodies is not used for transfusion, ABO-compatible plasma does not cause hemolytic transfusion reactions except in rare cases in which the patient has red blood cell polyagglutination. Donor-retested plasma is collected from donors who have tested negative for viral disease markers on two separate occasions and thus may carry a lower risk for those diseases. Nucleic acid–inactivated plasma from single donors is being studied and should eliminate nucleic acid–containing pathogens.

The most severe reaction to plasma, anaphylaxis, is characterized clinically by wheezing, flushing, hypotension, and substernal chest pain (38,39). This reaction usually can be traced to class-specific anti–immunoglobulin A (IgA) formed as a consequence of previous transfusion in an IgA-deficient recipient. Nevertheless, some of the most severe anaphylactic reactions can occur in susceptible patients (with IgA deficiency) after transfusion of very small volumes of blood or plasma. Anaphylactic reactions have also been reported in patients who lack haptoglobin and have formed antibody to haptoglobin (40). Patients who have only mild reactions (e.g., pruritus or urticaria) may be treated with diphenhydramine 50 mg by mouth 1 hour before transfusion and 50 mg after the start of the transfusion. Treatment of severe allergic reactions should include airway and cardiopulmonary support, epinephrine in sufficient amounts to relieve wheezing and hypotension, intravenous antihistamines (e.g., 25 mg diphenhydramine), and a potent steroid (i.e., methylprednisolone, 40 mg).

Antileukocyte antibody reactions are common in persons who receive multiple transfusions and generally are mild, producing fever in the sensitized recipient of any blood component containing neutrophils. Noncardiogenic pulmonary edema, transfusion-related acute lung injury (TRALI), is an uncommon but well-recognized complication of plasma transfusion that is related to antileukocyte antibodies present in the donor, invariably a multiparous woman (41). Transfused lipids may also have a role (42). Alveolar and interstitial edema result in impaired gas exchange and hypoxemia. A syndrome very similar to adult respiratory distress syndrome may result. Efforts always should be made to identify donors of plasma or blood that has produced these reactions. Donors whose plasma has been implicated in an TRALI reaction should not serve as donors of FFP and platelets in the future; blood from these individuals may, however, be used to prepare red blood cells.

REFERENCES

1. *Standards of the American Association of Blood Banks,* 20th ed. Bethesda: American Association of Blood Banks, 2000.
2. NIH Consensus Conference. Fresh frozen plasma: indications and risks. *JAMA* 1985;253:551–553.
3. Klein HG, Dodd RY, Dzik WH, et al. Current status of solvent/detergent-treated frozen plasma. *Transfusion* 1998;38:102–107.
4. Koenigbauer UF, Eastlund T, Day JW. Clinical illness due to Parvovirus B19 infection after infusion of solvent/detergent-treated pooled plasma. *Transfusion* 2000;40:1203–1206.
5. Flamholz R, Jeon HR, Baron JM, et al. Study of three patients with TTP exchanged with solvent/detergent-treated plasma: is its decreased protein S activity clinically related to their development of deep venous thrombosis? *J Clin Apheresis* 2000;15:169–172.
6. College of American Pathologists Practice Guidelines Development Task Force. Practice parameter for the use of fresh-frozen plasma, cryoprecipitate, and platelets. *JAMA* 1994;271:777–781.
7. Kaul V, Munoz SJ. Coagulopathy of liver disease. *Curr Treat Options Gastroenterol* 2000;3:433–438.
8. Ewe K. Bleeding after liver biopsy does not correlate with indices of peripheral coagulation. *Dig Dis Sci* 1981;26:388–393.
9. Piccinino F, Sagnelli E, Pasquale G, et al. Complications following percutaneous liver biopsy. A multicenter retrospective study on 68,276 biopsies. *J Hepatol* 1986;2:165–173.
10. McGill DB, Rakela J, Zinsmeister AR, et al. A 21-year experience with major hemorrhage after percutaneous liver biopsy. *Gastroenterology* 1990; 99:1396–1400.
11. McVay PA, Toy PTCY. Lack of increased bleeding after liver biopsy in patients with mild hemostatic abnormalities. *Am J Clin Pathol* 1990; 94:747–753.
12. Dillon JF, Simpson KJ, Hayes PC. Liver biopsy bleeding time: an unpredictable event. *J Gastroenterol Hepatol* 1994;9:269–271.
13. Grant A, Neuberger J. Guidelines on the use of liver biopsy in clinical practice. *Gut* 1999;45:IV1–IV11.
14. Sharma P, McDonald GB, Banaji M. The risk of bleeding after percutaneous liver biopsy: relation to platelet count. *J Clin Gastroenterol* 1982; 4:451–453.
15. Sue M, Caldwell SH, Dickson RC, et al. Variation between centers in technique and guidelines for liver biopsy. *Liver* 1996;16:267–270.
16. Boberg KM, Brosstad F, Egeland T, et al. Is a prolonged bleeding time associated with an increased risk of hemorrhage after liver biopsy? *Thromb Haemost* 1999;81:378–381.
17. McVay PA, Toy PTCY. Lack of increased bleeding after paracentesis and thoracentesis in patients with mild coagulation abnormalities. *Transfusion* 1991;31:164–171.
18. Friedman EW, Sussman II. Safety of invasive procedures in patients with the coagulopathy of liver disease. *Clin Lab Haematol* 1989;11: 199–204.
19. DeLoughery TG, Liebler JM, Simonds V, et al. Invasive line placement in critically ill individuals: do hemostatic defects matter? *Transfusion* 1996;36:827–831.
20. Spector MD, Corn M, Ticktin HE. Effect of plasma transfusions on the prothrombin time and clotting factors in liver disease. *N Engl J Med* 1966;275:1032–1037.
21. Munoz SJ, Ballas SK, Moritz MJ, et al. Perioperative management of fulminant and subfulminant hepatic failure with therapeutic plasmapheresis. *Transplant Proc* 1989;21:3535–3536.
22. Macig GB, Wang P. Management of warfarin-induced bleeding. In: Alving BM, ed. *Blood components and pharmacologic agents in the treatment of congenital and acquired bleeding disorders.* Bethesda: American Association of Blood Banks, 2000:215–236.
23. Kearon C, Hirsh J. Management of anticoagulation before and after elective surgery. *N Engl J Med* 1997;336:1506–1511.
24. Shetty H, Backhouse G, Bentley DP, et al. Effective reversal of warfarin-induced excessive anticoagulation with low dose vitamin K. *Thromb Haemost* 1992;67:13–15.
25. Wentzien TH, O'Reilly RA, Kearns PJ. Prospective evaluation of anticoagulant reversal with oral vitamin K while continuing warfarin therapy unchanged. *Chest* 1998;114:1546–1550.
26. Crowther M, Donovan D, Harrison L, et al. Low-dose oral vitamin K reliably reverses over-anticoagulation due to warfarin. *Thromb Haemost* 1998;79:1116–1118.
27. Hung A, Singh S, Tait RC. A prospective randomized study to determine the optimal dose of intravenous vitamin K in reversal of over-warfarinization. *Br J Haematol* 2000;109:537–539.
28. Laks H, Handin RI, Martin V, et al. The effects of acute normovolemic hemodilution on coagulation and blood utilization in major surgery. *J Surg Res* 1976;20:225–230.
29. Urbaniak SJ. Intensive plasma exchange—effects on haemostasis. In: Collins JA, ed. *Massive transfusion in surgery and trauma.* New York: Alan Liss, 1982.
30. Murray D, Pennell B, Olson J. Variability of prothrombin time and activated partial thromboplastin time in the diagnosis of increased surgical bleeding. *Transfusion* 1999;39:56–62.
31. Leslie SD, Toy PTCY. Laboratory hemostatic abnormalities in mas-

sively transfused patients given red blood cells and crystalloid. *Am J Clin Pathol* 1991;96:770–773.
32. Gubler KD, Gentilello LM, Hassantash SA, et al. The impact of hypothermia on dilutional coagulopathy. *J Trauma* 1994;36:847–851.
33. Rock G, Porta C, Bobbio-Pallavicini E. Thrombotic thrombocytopenic purpura treatment in year 2000. *Haematologica* 2000;85:410–419.
34. Moake HL. Studies on pathophysiology of TTP. *Semin Hematol* 1997; 34:83–89.
35. Bruni R, Giannini G, Lercari G, et al. Cascade filtration of TTP: an effective alternative to plasma exchange with cryodepleted plasma. *Transfus Sci* 1999;21:193–199.
36. Alving BM. Beyond hemophilia and von Willebrand diseases: treatment of patients with other inherited coagulation factor and inhibitor deficiencies. In: BM Alving, ed. *Blood components and pharmacologic agents in the treatment of congenital and acquired bleeding disorders.* Bethesda: American Association of Blood Banks, 2000:341–354.
37. Bernard GR, Vincent JL, Laterre PF, et al. Efficacy and safety of recombinant human activated protein C for severe sepsis. *N Engl J Med* 2001;344:699–709.
38. Schmidt AP, Taswell F, Gleich GJ. Anaphylactic transfusion reactions associated with anti-IgA antibody. *N Engl J Med* 1969;280:188–193.
39. Vyas GN, Perkins HA. Anti-IgA in blood donors [Letter]. *Transfusion* 1975;16:289.
40. Koda Y, Watanabe Y, Soejima M, et al. Simple PCR detection of haptoglobin gene deletion in anhaptoglobinemic patients with antihaptoglobin antibody that causes anaphylactic transfusion reactions. *Blood* 2000;95:1138–1143.
41. Popovsky MA, Moore SB. Diagnostic and pathogenetic considerations in transfusion-related acute lung injury. *Transfusion* 1985;25:573–577.
42. Silliman CC, Paterson AJ, Dickey WO, et al. The association of biologically active lipids with the development of transfusion-related acute lung injury—a retrospective study. *Transfusion* 1997;37:719–726.

Rossi's Principles of Transfusion Medicine, Third Edition, edited by Toby L. Simon, Walter H. Dzik, Edward L. Snyder, Christopher P. Stowell, and Ronald G. Strauss. Lippincott Williams & Wilkins, Philadelphia © 2002.

CASE 25A

DANGER IN TREATING THE NUMBERS

CASE HISTORY

Mr. D. is a 66-year-old man who underwent coronary revascularization and mitral valve reconstruction in 1987. He did well for several years, but in 2001 he developed recurrent ischemic chest pain and heart failure. A cardiac catheterization demonstrated progression of atherosclerosis and occlusion of his bypass grafts. He was referred for repeat coronary bypass grafting and possible valve replacement. His preoperative evaluation was done as an outpatient.

His medications included warfarin (Coumadin) 5 mg/d orally, which he took because of chronic atrial fibrillation. He also took nitrates and digoxin. Mr. D. lives at home with his wife. He is a retired salesman. On the day prior to admission he omitted his usual warfarin dose on the instruction of his physician.

He was admitted to the hospital on the morning of his surgery. At the beginning of surgery his blood pressure was 140/78, pulse 100, and respiratory rate 12. His PO_2 on 100% oxygen was 427 mmHg at 9:10 AM. His prothrombin time (PT) was 14.8 seconds (normal range 11.5 to 13.0 seconds). The prolongation of the PT was presumed to be due to residual effect of warfarin. He was therefore given two units of fresh-frozen plasma (FFP) to "correct" the prolonged PT. The FFP was given in the operating room over 30 minutes.

Within 30 to 45 minutes of completion of the FFP, the anesthesiologist noted that the patient's oxygen saturation, measured on a finger oximeter, had declined. An arterial blood gas sample drawn at 12:50 PM showed a PO_2 of 41 mm Hg while the patient was receiving 100% oxygen from the ventilator. Evaluation of his airway showed copious secretions, and his lungs had quickly become "stiff" with increased fluid. Three repeat blood gas measurements drawn within the next 10 minutes all showed the same severe depression of oxygen content. The PCO_2 had risen to 60 mm Hg due to decreased lung compliance and difficulty ventilating the patient.

The diagnosis of transfusion-associated acute lung injury (TRALI) was strongly suspected, and it was decided to proceed with the planned surgery because this would result in the use of cardiopulmonary bypass. Shortly after initiation of bypass, an arterial blood gas sample drawn at 13:28 PM showed the PO_2 equal to 457 mm Hg with a PCO_2 of 35 mm Hg. During the next several hours the patient was given injections of corticosteroids, histamine blockers, and prostaglandins, without apparent effect on the pulmonary secretions. The cardiac bypass grafts were completed and the patient's mitral valve replaced with a prosthetic valve. He was given transfusions of packed red blood cells to increase his oxygen carrying capacity in expectation of a low oxygen saturation at the end of cardiopulmonary bypass. An extracorporeal membrane oxygenator was prepared as a backup in case his pulmonary function proved inadequate once bypass ended.

With the cardiac surgery completed it was time to come off bypass. During the 45 minutes prior to end of bypass, the patients pulmonary secretions appeared to decrease spontaneously. At 18:14 PM an arterial blood gas measurement, drawn off bypass and while the patient was receiving 100% oxygen, showed a PO_2 equal to 52 mm Hg. Inhalation therapy with nitric oxide was tried with no improvement in oxygenation. An intraaortic blood pump was placed.

Attempts to close the chest and suture the sternum resulted in a further decline in the oxygen saturation of the blood due to physical compression of the lungs. For this reason, it was decided to leave the chest open with the sternal spreader clamps in place (Fig. 25A.1B).

The patient was transferred to the cardiac surgery intensive care unit, and over the the next 48 hours he gradually improved. On postoperative day 2 the chest was closed, and on day 3 the intraaortic balloon pump was removed. His subsequent hospital course was prolonged and complicated by pulmonary and mediastinal infection, which responded to antibiotic therapy. He was discharged on warfarin and diuretics.

DISCUSSION

This case represents a dramatic example of TRALI—one of the leading serious noninfectious hazards of blood transfusion. The actual incidence of TRALI remains unknown, although the number of cases reported in the literature has increased dramatically. TRALI has become recognized as a leading cause of transfusion-related morbidity in the United Kingdom's Serious Hazards of Transfusion reporting program. Clarke et al. found that 46 of 2,430 platelet transfusions (2%) were associated with severe respiratory reactions over a 2-year period in a general hospital (1). There is ample reason to believe that TRALI may be significantly under-diagnosed. A recent study found that FFP donated by women with a history of three or more pregnancies resulted in significantly lower oxygen extraction compared with control FFP. In 4 of 100 patients a clinical pulmonary transfusion reaction was noted (2). In the case report presented here, the donors of the FFP were females. Evaluation of their plasma

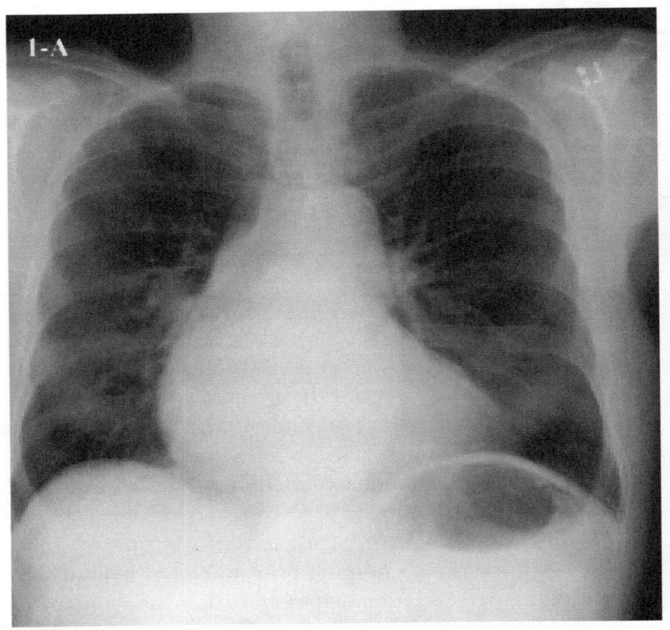

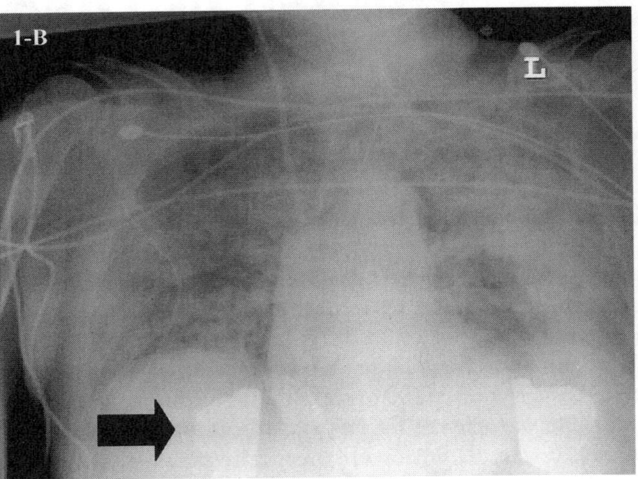

A B

FIGURE 25A.1. **A** shows the patient's chest radiograph prior to the FFP. **B,** taken postoperatively, shows extensive pulmonary edema as a result of TRALI. Note that the sternal spreader clamps have been left in place to keep the chest cage open and decrease lung compliance *(arrow).*

showed evidence of HLA antibodies, which presumably reacted with the HLA antigens of the recipient.

The real issue in this case, however, centers on the indication for the FFP that precipitated the TRALI. My experience in hospitals has taught me that large numbers of units of FFP are given to "correct" mild prolongations of the PT, especially prior to invasive bedside procedures. A review of the literature on this topic shows that there is no evidence that such transfusions are of any value (3). Indeed, many clinicians misinterpret a PT that is outside the range of normal to mean that a coagulopathy exists. This is no more true than that a hemoglobin value just below the normal range represents a clinically important anemia. The threshold value at which an elevated PT indicates abnormal coagulation represents a PT corresponding to approximately 30% residual coagulation factors. This PT value differs in different hospitals depending on the reagents used in each laboratory. In our hospital, the value is between 16.5 and 17 seconds as shown in Figure 25A.2.

Figure 25A.2 demonstrates a second point: transfusions given to patients with mild prolongations of the PT do not improve

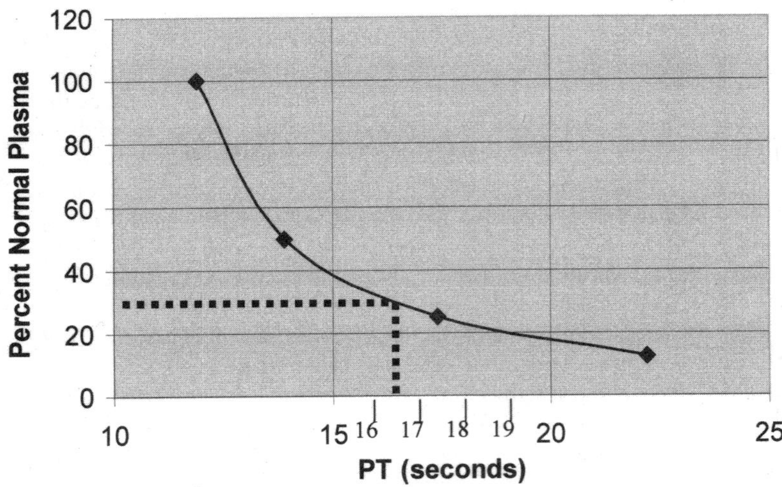

FIGURE 25A.2. Relationship between the level of coagulation factors expressed as a percent of normal *(y-axis)* and the PT *(x-axis).* The dotted line corresponds to the level of factors needed for normal hemostasis. Note that the relationship between factor levels and PT is exponential, not linear.

the laboratory test result! This is because the relationship of the coagulation levels to the PT is not linear, but rather is exponential. Thus, patients with mild prolongation of the PT are on the "steep" portion of the curve, and the increase in coagulation levels induced by a usual dose of FFP will change the PT by only tenths of a second. Much more education of clinicians is needed about that risk-to-benefit ratio of using FFP to treat patients with mild prolongations of the PT.

Case contributed by Walter H. Dzik, M.D., Massachusetts General Hospital, Boston, MA.

REFERENCES

1. Clarke G, Podlosky L, Petrie L, et al. Severe respiratory reactions to random donor platelets: an incidence and nested case control study. *Blood* 1994;84[Suppl]:465a(abst).
2. Palfi M, Berg S, Ernerudh J, et al. A controlled randomized study on transfusion related acute lung injury. *Vox Sang* 2000;78:S1(abst).
3. Dzik W. The use of blood components prior to invasive bedside procedures: a critical appraisal. In: Mintz PD, ed. *Transfusion therapy: clinical principles and practice.* Bethesda: American Association of Blood Banks, 1999:151–169.

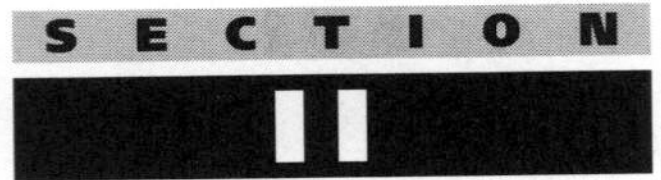

CLINICAL PRACTICE

PART I

Medical Patient

26

AUTOIMMUNE HEMOLYTIC ANEMIA AND PAROXYSMAL NOCTURNAL HEMOGLOBINURIA

THOMAS P. DUFFY

T.P. Duffy: Department of Internal Medicine, Yale University School of Medicine, New Haven, Connecticut.

Autoimmune hemolytic anemia (AIHA) and paroxysmal nocturnal hemoglobinuria (PNH) represent a group of disorders characterized by accelerated red blood cell destruction. The first is secondary to the presence of autoantibodies directed against self-antigens on red blood cells. The second is characterized by increased sensitivity of red blood cells to complement-mediated lysis. The first description of an autoimmune hemolytic disorder was Donath and Landsteiner's description in 1904 of three cases of paroxysmal cold hemoglobinuria (PCH). Dameshek and Schwartz created the first experimental model of immune hemolytic anemia (IHA) in 1938 by inducing hemolytic anemia in guinea pigs following the injection of heterologous antierythrocyte antibodies. In 1943, Dacie and Mollison showed that patients with acquired hemolytic anemia had an intrinsic factor (presumably an antibody) that caused increased red blood cell destruction. The introduction of the antiglobulin test in 1945 by Coombs et al. permitted the identification of the immune etiology of AIHA and established the foundation of immunohematology. Its subsequent application in patients with acquired hemolytic anemia by Boorman et al. and Loutit and Mollison in 1946 firmly established the importance of red blood cell autoantibodies in the pathogenesis of AIHA. Subsequent refinement of the antiglobulin test permitted detection of immunoglobulin classes and complement components on the red blood cell membrane, and dissection of the pathophysiology of the different forms of AIHA resulting from the different immune sensitizations (1). Paroxysmal nocturnal hemoglobinuria was first described in 1882, and since that time several hundred cases have been reported. This complement-mediated hemolytic anemia has its origin in the absence of a whole class of membrane-based proteins which include those responsible for protection of cells from random complement activation.

AUTOIMMUNE HEMOLYTIC ANEMIAS CLASSIFICATION

AIHAs are divided into warm and cold autoantibody types based on the temperatures at which the antibodies maximally react with red blood cells in vitro. Warm autoantibodies are more reactive at 37°C than at lower temperatures, whereas cold autoantibodies react optimally at 0° to 5°C and less strongly at higher temperatures. These two principal types are further subdivided into primary, or idiopathic, forms and secondary forms which are associated with an underlying disorder (Table 26.1).

Lymphoproliferative disorders are present in about half of the secondary warm and cold AIHAs with systemic lupus erythematosus (SLE) and other autoimmune disorders accounting for a majority of the remaining warm types. Transient, acute cold hemolytic anemias are often seen in association with infections, especially mycoplasmal pneumonia and infectious mononucleosis. The proportion of warm versus cold AIHA (20% to 80%) varies widely in reported series (2). This variation reflects the type of patient population studied and the particular interest and location of the investigators. As patients with assumed idiopathic etiology are observed over time, the likelihood of recognition of an associated or secondary disease increases.

A third category comprises drug-induced IHA. The drug-induced antibodies, usually of warm type, are directed against the ingested drug or its metabolites bound to the red blood cell membrane or to a combined drug–red blood cell membrane antigen. In IHA, the antibody can have a drug or its metabolite as the target antigen or, as with α-methyldopa, induce the forma-

TABLE 26.1. CLASSIFICATION OF AUTOIMMUNE HEMOLYTIC ANEMIA

Warm Autoantibody Type
Idiopathic
 Secondary: lymphoma, chronic lymphocytic leukemia, hairy cell leukemia, systemic lupus erythematosus, other autoimmune disorders, ovarian tumors, chronic inflammatory disorders

Cold Autoantibody Type
Cold hemagglutinin disease
 Idiopathic
 Secondary
  Transient (acute): *Mycobacterium pneumoniae* infection, infectious mononucleosis, other infections
  Chronic: lymphoreticular malignancies
Paroxysmal cold hemoglobinuria
 Idiopathic
 Secondary: viral and other infections, syphilis

Drug-induced Immune Hemolytic Anemia
Drug adsorption (hapten) type, e.g., penicillin
Drug-dependent antibody type (also referred to as immune complex), e.g., second-or third-generation cephalosporins
Autoimmune induction type, e.g., α-methyldopa
Nonimmunological adsorption of protein, e.g., cephalothin

tion of red blood cell autoantibodies in a fashion analogous to classic AIHA, with hemolysis persisting even in the absence of the offending drug.

EPIDEMIOLOGY

Autoimmune hemolytic anemias are relatively uncommon, with an incidence of 1 in 80,000 to 100,000 individuals. The warm autoantibody type is the most common. In a study of 347 patients (3), this type accounted for 70.3%; cold agglutinin syndrome, 15.6%; PCH, 1.7%; and drug-induced IHA, 12.4%. A lower percentage of warm-type autoantibodies was reported in a study of 865 cases in which warm-type autoantibodies were found in 41%, cold-type in 32%, drug-induced in 18%, PCH in 2%, and mixed warm and cold types in 7% (4). Mixed AIHA with features of both warm- and cold-type autoantibodies has been found in 6% to 8% in several series of patients (5). Autoimmune hemolytic anemia affects all ages, with the peak incidence of idiopathic disease in the fourth and fifth decades. Secondary AIHA reflects the age distribution of the underlying disease; lymphoproliferative disorders affect an older age group, whereas SLE involves younger patients. Women have a higher incidence of both idiopathic AIHA and secondary AIHA associated with SLE and other autoimmune disorders.

ETIOLOGY

The development of the autoantibodies results from a breakdown of immunoregulation, possibly determined by genetic factors as seen in the inbred NZB mouse model (6). The loss of suppressor T-cell regulation of autoantibody production and presence of overactive B cells lead to the emergence of autoantibodies. Infection, inflammatory disorders, or drugs often serve as triggers to initiate this process. Viral infections also trigger the onset of AIHA by dramatically increasing the ability of macrophages to phagocytose antibody-coated erythrocytes (7). Patients with warm-type AIHA sometimes have antinuclear and antiphospholipid antibodies without clinical manifestations of SLE, or may have symptoms of hemolysis before autoimmune disease is evident. In some instances, red blood cell autoantibodies are cross-reacting with red blood cell antigens. In the cold autoantibody type occurring with mycoplasmal pneumonia, cross-antigenicity between the mycoplasmal cell wall and the I antigen on the red blood cell membrane has been suggested (8). Because I antigens on cells may be receptors for attachment of mycoplasma, the mycoplasma may alter the I antigen to render it more immunogenic (9). There is, however, little evidence that red blood cell antigens have been significantly altered to induce immune responses, because eluted antibodies react equally well with normal red blood cells. Eluted red blood cell autoantibodies also have been shown to react with the patient's red blood cells years later, making it unlikely that a drug, virus, or bacteria had altered the red blood cells during the hemolytic episodes (10).

The lymphoproliferative disorders associated with AIHA represent a wide spectrum of disease, which includes chronic lymphocytic leukemia, Hodgkin and non–Hodgkin lymphoma, hairy cell leukemia, large granular lymphocytosis, angioimmunoblastic lymphoma, and Castleman disease. Chronic infections such as subacute bacterial endocarditis and inflammatory states such as ulcerative colitis may be complicated by warm-type AIHA. Interferon-α treatment in large doses may also give rise to a warm-type AIHA. Familial cases have been reported (11). More than 30 cases have been recorded in association with both benign and malignant ovarian neoplasms (12). Infection is a common antecedent to AIHA in children.

PATHOPHYSIOLOGY

The destruction of red blood cells occurs by intravascular, extravascular, and cell-mediated mechanisms. The reticuloendothelial system (mononuclear phagocytic system) in the spleen and, to a lesser degree, the liver is responsible for extravascular destruction of red blood cells. Immunoglobulin G (IgG)–coated red blood cells in warm-type AIHA are sequestered primarily in the spleen where vascular anatomy greatly enhances red blood cell interactions with macrophages. The IgG-coated red blood cells bind to macrophages by specific membrane receptors for the Fc portion of IgG, subclasses IgG1 and IgG3 (13), and phagocytosis of the entire red blood cell by the macrophage sometimes follows. More commonly, there is removal of only a portion of the red blood cell membrane with creation of a microspherocyte released back into the circulation. These altered cells, with a decreased surface area–to-volume ratio, have a greatly shortened lifespan because of their loss of plasticity and increased osmotic fragility (14). These cells are eventually destroyed as their flow is obstructed within the microcirculation, particularly in the spleen; microspherocytes in the peripheral blood indicates ongoing hemolysis. Enhanced function of the mononuclear-phagocytic system and an increase in Fc monocyte receptors also contribute to red blood cell destruction in AIHA (15).

Macrophages have IgG Fc receptors for only IgG1 and IgG3 (16); therefore the quantity and type of Ig on the red blood cell surface influences the degree of hemolysis. Red blood cells coated with IgG1 alone or in combination with IgG2 or IgG4 require an average of 2,000 molecules of IgG per red blood cell to stimulate phagocytosis and rosette formation in vitro, whereas an average of only 230 molecules of IgG3 per red blood cell are required for monocyte binding (17). Removal of red blood cells is further accelerated when complement is also present on the red blood cell membrane. Only IgG1 and IgG3 are efficient in activating complement. Because two IgG molecules in close proximity are required to bind C1q and activate the complement system (18), there must be a sufficient number of antibody molecules and antigenic sites for complement attachment. Once C1 is bound, C4 and C2 are activated to form C3 convertase, which then cleaves C3 and C3b. Several hundred molecules of C3b bind to the red blood cell membrane by the action of a single C3 convertase enzyme complex (19). Macrophages have receptors for C3b and iC3b (inactivated C3b), referred to as CR1 and CR3, respectively (20). The IgG Fc and complement receptors act together to enhance binding of red blood cells coated with both IgG and complement. Removal of IgG-coated red blood cells with or without complement occurs primarily in the spleen. When large amounts of IgG are present on the red blood cell, the liver also participates in their clearance (13). The spleen functions as a "fine" filter, the liver a "coarse" filter, of sensitized red blood cells in AIHA.

Autoimmune hemolytic anemia has also been associated with IgA and IgM warm autoantibodies (21). IgA-sensitized red blood cells are removed by the same splenic process as are IgG-coated red blood cells. Receptors for IgA have been demonstrated on mononuclear phagocytes. Intravascular hemolysis, observed in AIHA associated with IgA autoantibodies, is mediated by the binding of C5b-9 complexes to bystander red blood cells independent of C3 activation (22). IgM autoantibodies have been shown to agglutinate or hemolyze normal red blood cells and enzyme-treated red blood cells (3) and to sensitize red blood cells with or without fixing complement. Using anti-IgM antiglobulin serum in the direct antiglobulin test (DAT), IgM has been detected on the red blood cells of 8% of patients with warm AIHA, always associated with either IgG, IgA and C3, IgG and C3, or C3. By applying the more sensitive enzyme-linked antiglobulin test, IgM was found on the red blood cells of 38% of patients with AIHA whose DAT results were positive for IgG (23). Using the AutoAnalyzer, cell-bound IgM was found in 73% of patients with IgG-positive DAT results (24). Several cases of AIHA with warm-reacting IgM autoantibodies in association with cell-bound C3d have been reported. In one series of children, IgM was detected on the red blood cells by a radioimmune assay when the DAT result was negative (25). Severe hemolytic anemia, with or without the presence of IgG, has been noted in patients with warm-reactive IgM autoantibodies exhibiting specificity for sialidase-sensitive red blood cell antigen determinants, En^a, Pr, and Wr^b (26,27).

The quantity of the antibody on the red blood cell is not always an indicator of the presence or severity of hemolysis, because the interaction of several variables determines the rate of hemolysis. These include the IgG subclass, simultaneous presence of other immunoglobulin classes, affinity of the antibody, activation and presence of cell-bound complement, number of receptors on macrophages for IgG and complement, and chemical and physical characteristics of the antigens on the red blood cell membrane. Although there is overlap in the amount of IgG antibody on the red blood cells of patients with or without hemolytic anemia, patients with hemolytic anemia, on average, have more IgG molecules on their red blood cells (28). Patients whose red blood cells are coated with IgA and IgM in addition to IgG are more likely to have hemolysis than those whose red blood cells are coated with IgG alone (29). The presence or quantity of IgG3 on the red blood cell may not distinguish patients with hemolytic anemia from those without hemolytic anemia, but IgG3 is more commonly associated with hemolytic anemia (30). The presence of autologous IgM may also determine the autoreactivity of IgG in AIHA.

AUTOANTIBODIES AND SPECIFICITY

In a report of 2,000 cases of warm-type AIHA, IgG was found alone in 64% and in association with complement in 33% of cases (31). IgA or monomeric IgM autoantibodies were each found in about 1% of patients with warm-type AIHA and were frequently accompanied by complement. Warm-type autoantibodies are usually polyclonal, but there can be restrictions in their Gm allotype and/or light-chain type (32,33). By far the most frequent subclass of IgG warm-type autoantibody is IgG1, which is found in most patients with warm-type AIHA (31). Immunoglobulin G1 has been found in the majority of patients with AIHA with or without hemolysis, as well as in blood donors with positive DAT results; IgG3 alone has been found in only 3% of patients and in combination with other subclasses in 5% (34). Immunoglobulin G1 was often the only subclass identified on the red blood cell. Immunoglobulin G1 was associated with other subclasses in 37% of patients with AIHA and in 12.5% of those without AIHA. The percentage of patients with IgG3 alone was approximately the same for patients with and without AIHA, being 6.3% and 6.6%, respectively. Immunoglobulin G3 was found in only 2.6% of healthy blood donors and in association with other subclasses in 22% of patients with AIHA (35).

Initially most red blood cell autoantibodies were thought to be directed to antigens of the Rh system based on weak or negative reactivity with Rh_{null} red blood cells (lacking determinants of the Rh complex) and on the observation that some red blood cell autoantibodies react preferentially with defined Rh antigens such as e, E, or C. It is now appreciated that absent or weak reactivity of autoantibodies with Rh_{null} red blood cells does not always signify specificity to an Rh complex determinant, because Rh_{null} red blood cells also have other membrane abnormalities including a lack of LW and Fy, a marked decrease of U and to a lesser extent Ss, and glycophorin B levels that are 30% of normal. Eluates nonreactive with Rh_{null} cells were shown to contain anti-LW or anti-U reactivity (36,37). Many patients with AIHA have autoantibodies that react equally well with Rh_{null} red blood cells and red blood cells with normal phenotypes, indicating specificity to antigens outside of the Rh system. The target of these autoantibodies in selected patients include among others Wr^b, En^a, Ge, A, B, and antigens within the Kell and Kidd blood group systems (38).

The specificity of autoantibodies in the past has been largely determined by serologic techniques. More recently, immunochemical methods have been applied to elucidate better the autoantigens or epitopes in the red blood cell membrane reactive with autoantibodies. In addition to Rh antigens, membrane protein band 4.1 (39), band 3 (40), and glycophorin have been identified as targets for some red blood cell autoantibodies.

Another source of confusion is that autoantibodies sometimes have specificity for an antigen such as E, even though the red blood cells from which they are eluted are negative for E (41). These antibodies are most likely reacting with an antigen on the red blood cell, which is present in larger amounts on E-positive red blood cells and are termed mimicking antibodies, because they seem to be alloantibodies with anti-E specificity. Autoantibodies also may mimic alloantibodies when the corresponding antigen on the patient's red blood cell is weak or absent. When the patient is in remission and no longer has the serum antibody, the red blood cells can be shown to contain normal amounts of the red blood cell antigen. Furthermore, the stored autoantibody from the patient can be shown later to react with the patient's red blood cells. This phenomenon has been shown to occur with Rh, LW, Kell, Duffy, Kidd, and En[a] (42). A naturally occurring IgG autoantibody has been demonstrated in the sera of healthy persons that is specific for a senescent red blood cell antigen that appears as the red blood cell ages and is a degradation product of band 3 (43). A case of AIHA associated with autoantibodies to stored red blood cells has been reported in which the autoantibody was inhibited by a synthetic senescent red blood cell antigen (44). Some autoantibodies have been shown to react more strongly with immature red blood cells than with mature red blood cells.

Autoantibodies have been noted after transfusion (45), sometimes weeks to months after a delayed transfusion reaction. Alloimmunization has been suggested as a stimulant for autoantibody formation usually not accompanied by hemolysis.

Autoantibodies to phospholipids have been demonstrated on the red blood cell membrane and may account for the Coombs-positive hemolytic anemia found in some patients with primary antiphospholipid syndrome or antiphospholipid syndrome secondary to SLE (46). Eluates were shown to contain IgG with anticardiolipin reactivity. Antiphospholipid antibodies directed to the red blood cell membrane may explain the finding of IgG and complement on the red blood cells of some patients with SLE.

A population of IgG molecules was identified on the red blood cells of DAT-positive healthy blood donors that reacted with IgG anti–red blood cell autoantibody but not with the red blood cell membrane. Radiolabeled IgG autoantibodies in eluates prepared from IgG DAT-positive blood donors and adsorbed using nonhuman and human red blood cells with common and rare phenotypes contained several populations of autoantibodies (47). Some were bound to human red blood cells of common Rh phenotypes, and another, in addition to binding to Rh red blood cells, also was bound to Rh_{null} red blood cells. Approximately 30% of the IgG in the eluates was not adsorbed. Subsequent studies showed that some of the nonadsorbable IgG in the eluates had autoantiidiotypic-like reactivity in that it was able to agglutinate red blood cells sensitized with $F(ab')_2$ prepared from alloanti-D sera (48). Further studies are required to determine whether this antibody reacts with the epitope or with Fab of the red blood cell autoantibody. Autoantiidiotypic antibodies to red blood cell autoantibodies have been described in NZB mice with AIHA, suggesting that the idiotype-antiidiotype network affects immune regulation. The demonstration of autoidiotype antibodies in healthy blood donors with positive DAT results and their absence in DAT-positive patients with AIHA suggests these autoantibodies have a protective effect.

CLINICAL FEATURES

The clinical picture of warm-type AIHA is highly variable. Most patients seek treatment for symptoms attributable to anemia, such as fatigue, palpitations, and shortness of breath, but occasionally massive hemolysis manifested by hemoglobinemia, hemoglobinuria, and profound anemia is seen at onset with secondary AIHA. The associated illness often dominates the clinical picture. Autoimmune hemolytic anemia, however, may precede by months or even years the development of a disease such as SLE. Physical findings in idiopathic AIHA are related to the degree of anemia and include pallor, resting tachycardia, and mild jaundice; fever may be present in AIHA. The spleen is usually only moderately enlarged. When there is massive splenomegaly, an underlying lymphoproliferative disorder should be considered. The degree of anemia is variable and depends partly on the compensatory capacity of the bone marrow to respond to the increased rate of red blood cell destruction. Reticulocytopenia accompanying significant shortening of red blood cell survival is particularly threatening.

LABORATORY FEATURES

Peripheral blood smears show microspherocytes, polychromasia, and nucleated red blood cells. The presence of spherocytes indicates ongoing red blood cell destruction. Rosettes of red blood cells around white blood cells and erythrocytes are seen in a buffy-coat preparation; erythrophagocytosis by circulating monocytes is sometimes present. Bone marrow examination reveals erythroid hyperplasia, as well as increased numbers of lymphocytes or plasma cells in patients who have underlying lymphoproliferative or collagen vascular diseases. Flow cytometry of the bone marrow sometimes identifies a clonal population of lymphocytes even when morphologic evidence of lymphoma is not evident. The reticulocyte count is usually elevated, above the normal level of 1.5% to 2%; the red blood cell mean corpuscular volume is often increased to a macrocytic range. Superimposed folate deficiency can dampen or even eliminate the compensatory reticulocytosis. A rare patient will have persistent reticulocytopenia caused by inadequate bone marrow response or hemolytic destruction of erythroid precursors within the marrow. Unconjugated bilirubin is usually, but not always, elevated, and urinary urobilinogen is increased. Serum haptoglobin levels are reduced or absent. With severe hemolysis, hemoglobinemia, hemoglobinuria, and urine hemosiderin can be present. Mild leukocytosis (predominantly neutrophilia) is usually seen, sometimes with thrombocytosis. Neutropenia and thrombocytopenia, however, are occasionally found. The combination of autoimmune thrombocytopenia and AIHA is referred to as Evans syndrome, usually a complication of a lymphoproliferative or collagen vascular disease. If hemolysis is equivocal, a red blood cell survival study using chromium-51–labeled red blood cells or measuring endogenous carbon monoxide production provides needed information. The role of the spleen in the hemolytic process can be assessed during the course of the red blood cell survival study by comparing isotope uptake between liver and spleen; predominantly splenic uptake anticipates a favorable response to splenectomy.

Antiglobulin Tests

The diagnosis usually depends on the demonstration of a positive DAT result, indicating the presence of immunoglobulin or complement components or both on the red blood cell surface. A positive DAT result is sometimes seen without hemolysis. The DAT is performed by the addition of an antiglobulin serum to washed red blood cells, leading to agglutination when the antibody or complement or both is present on the red blood cell surface. A broad-spectrum antiglobulin reagent that contains antibodies for IgG immunoglobulins and complement components is recommended. When the test is positive, antiglobulin reagents specific for IgG or C3 are used to determine the presence of IgG or complement on the red blood cell. The anticomplement reagent should recognize the complement fragment C3d, which remains on the red blood cell surface. In special situations, antisera specific for IgA and IgM is used to demonstrate their role in the rare cases of AIHA caused by these Ig types. By the use of anti-IgG and anti-C3 antisera, three basic patterns of sensitization are observed: IgG alone, IgG plus C3, or C3 without detectable immunoglobulin. In several series of patients with warm-type AIHA, the frequency of IgG alone ranged from 18% to 64%; that of IgG plus C3, from 34% to 65%; and that of complement alone, from 10% to 33% (31, 49).

The indirect antiglobulin test (i.e., red blood cell antibody screen) detects free serum antibody. This test is performed by incubating a patient's serum with compatible washed donor red blood cells at 37°C. The donor red blood cells are then washed and incubated with an antiglobulin reagent to detect any serum antibodies that have adhered to the donor cells. The presence of free serum autoantibody depends on the dissociation constant of the autoantibody. It is rare to find a positive indirect test result in the absence of a positive DAT result; a positive DAT result is not infrequently accompanied by a negative indirect antibody screen. By using enzyme-treated donor red blood cells, however, autoantibodies have been demonstrated in the serum of patients with AIHA who had negative DAT results. Care must be taken in interpreting the finding of a positive indirect antiglobulin test result, because it may represent an alloantibody stimulated by previous transfusion or pregnancy. These alloantibodies must be identified by adsorption studies to ensure compatible red blood cells when transfusions are needed.

Negative DAT Results in Patients with Warm-type AIHA

A small number of patients have clinical AIHA but negative DATs. They usually respond to steroid therapy, with improvement of their hemolytic anemia similar to that of patients with positive antiglobulin tests. The frequency of DAT-negative AIHA has been reported in 2% and 4% of cases, but is probably much lower when more sensitive serologic techniques for cell-bound antibody are used. The manually performed DAT requires about 300 to 500 molecules of IgG per cell, based on quantitative studies of IgG red blood cell autoantibodies (50). Using an antibody consumption test, small amounts of IgG antibody were found on the red blood cells of some patients with DAT-negative hemolytic anemia (50). Immunoglobulin G was also detected on the red blood cells of some patients who had the complement-alone pattern (51). Using an enzyme-linked antiglobulin test and a radioimmune assay, 158 patients with AIHA had red blood cells with 200 or fewer molecules of IgG per cell. Two hundred molecules of IgG per cell was the threshold in this laboratory for a positive DAT result (52). A significant correlation between small increases of cell-bound immunoglobulins and hemolysis was shown in the 25% of patients with evidence for immune-mediated hemolysis. Several of these patients had complement and small amounts of IgA and IgM in association with the IgG. A sensitive radioactive antiglobulin test detected IgG in four of six cases of DAT-negative AIHA (53). IgG was also detected on the red blood cells of 13 of 20 patients whose DAT results were positive for only C3. As few as 70 molecules of IgG per red blood cell were measured using a radiolabeled, purified staphylococcal protein A assay (54). Immunoglobulin G was detected on the red blood cells of three of nine patients with DAT-negative AIHA. A two-stage immunoradiometric assay using radiolabeled staphylococcal protein A was described (55). In this assay, red blood cells were initially incubated with unlabeled antiglobulin serum. If red blood cell autoantibodies were present, the antiglobulin antibodies would bind to the autoantibodies and be detected in the next stage with radiolabeled staphylococcal protein A. A simpler and more readily available test that does not quantitate but is capable of detecting small amounts of autoantibody below the threshold of the DAT is the Polybrene test (56). Polyvalent cation hexadimethrine bromide (Polybrene) reduces the electrostatic repulsive charges on the red blood cells, permitting the cells to come closer together. Antibodies from one cell can then cross-link another cell, leading to agglutination that will remain after neutralization of Polybrene with a citrate resuspending solution. In a study comparing these sensitive tests, no one assay detected all patients having small quantities of IgG (57). Detection is increased with a combination of tests (e.g., Polybrene and an enzyme-linked antiglobulin test or flow cytometry). Even with these sensitive techniques, an antibody sometimes cannot be detected in patients suspected of having AIHA. Using a gel test with anti-IgA, these DAT-negative AIHA cases are often demonstrated to be mediated by IgA autoantibodies.

Positive DAT Results in Patients without Hemolytic Anemia

The frequency of positive DAT results was 1 in 14,000 healthy blood donors in one study (58). A much higher frequency of 1 in 1,000 also has been reported, although many of the DATs were only weakly reactive. The subclass of IgG on the red blood cell in these DAT-positive healthy blood donors is mainly IgG1. Immunoglobulin G3 was found in only one donor. Complement alone (C3d and C4d) was found in approximately 45% of healthy blood donors. With sensitive techniques, small amounts of C3d and both C3d and C4d have been found on all normal red blood cells. The quantity of C3d as measured by radioimmunoassay ranged from 50 to 160 molecules per cell, which is below the amount detectable by conventional antiglobulin tests. The presence of these complement fragments on normal red blood cells is thought to represent continuing low-grade activation of the complement system. The DAT for complement should be performed on freshly collected ethylenediaminetetraacetic acid-preserved blood, because the amount of C3d and C4d on the red blood cell increases when clotted blood is refrigerated (59).

Positive DAT results for IgG are frequently found in patients receiving α-methyldopa and are usually not associated with hemolysis. C3d has been found on the red blood cells of children with falciparum malaria (60). In two recent studies, the frequency of positive DAT results in patients with acquired immunodeficiency syndrome (AIDS) was found to be 18% and 21%, respectively (61,62). In another series, 85% of patients with AIDS were found to have positive DAT results (63). Red blood cell sensitization was attributable to varying combinations of IgG, IgM, and complement, as well as each alone. Eluates from these cells did not show anti–red blood cell activity. Positive DAT results were thought to be attributable to immune complexes attached to the red blood cell via the CR1 receptor. In the same study, red blood cell CR1 receptor activity correlated inversely with a positive DAT result. Red blood cells from these DAT-positive patients had increased osmotic fragility; which has also been found in patients with SLE and circulating immune complexes, low red blood cell CR1 activity, and positive DAT results (64). On the other hand, several cases of hemolytic anemia have been noted in AIDS and human immunodeficiency virus-related diseases in which red blood cell destruction was mediated by red blood cell autoantibodies (65). Some of these cases had reticulocytopenia despite erythroid hyperplasia of the bone marrow.

Concomitant Warm-type and Cold-type AIHA

Patients have been reported with both warm autoantibody AIHA and cold agglutinin disease (66). The DAT shows both IgG and C3. The cold agglutinin titer is usually high, being greater than 1:1,000 at 4°C, and the thermal amplitude of the cold agglutinin is above 30°C. Eluates from these patients' red blood cells contain an IgG warm-type autoantibody. In other cases of mixed-type AIHA, the titer of IgM cold agglutinins at 4°C was less than 64, and the cold agglutinins reacted with red blood cells at 30°C or higher. In these patients, exposure to cold did not increase hemolysis, and treatment with glucocorticoids was effective. Hemolytic anemia tends to be severe, having a chronic course with intermittent exacerbations. In most instances, patients respond to glucocorticoids, splenectomy, or cytotoxic agents. Lymphoma and SLE are frequently associated disorders.

AUTOIMMUNE HEMOLYTIC ANEMIA IN CHILDREN

Autoimmune hemolytic anemia in children is either an acute, transient, self-limited disease or a prolonged chronic disorder, with the former much more common. The peak incidence is in the first 4 years of life, particularly with transient disease, which often follows well-defined viral illnesses. Patients usually recover in less than 3 months. The DAT detects only complement in the majority of these patients. Donath-Landsteiner (D-L) antibodies associated with PCH are present in some patients, but in others no antibody is found. Autoimmune hemolytic anemia of the cold hemagglutinin type is unusual. The response to glucocorticoids is rapid and constant, but their necessity may be questioned in transient self-limited cases.

Children with chronic prolonged hemolytic anemia tend to be older, and the onset is more insidious. The DAT usually shows IgG or IgG and complement. Hemolytic anemia may be intermittent or persistent for months or years and has a variable response to glucocorticoids. The hemolytic anemia is controlled in some patients by splenectomy. The overall mortality in one study of patients with chronic disease was 11.2% (67).

TREATMENT

Transfusion

Treatment with glucocorticoids usually leads to stabilization and improvement. Because the intravascular blood volume is typically normal in these patients, the decision to transfuse is based solely on the need to increase the oxygen-carrying capacity of the blood. Transfusions should be reserved for those patients at risk because of underlying heart disease, cerebrovascular ischemia, or life-threatening anemia; care must be taken to avoid producing pulmonary edema by transfusing red blood cells in elderly anemic individuals whose plasma volume is already increased. Simultaneous administration of diuretics should prevent this complication. Polymerized bovine hemoglobin has been successfully used to maintain adequate oxygenation in a patient with severe AIHA; heightened research in this field is occurring to identify means of transfusion which dispense with the encumbrances of typing and cross-matching blood (68).

The major problem with transfusion is the difficulty of cross-matching, because the autoantibody may result in a positive antibody screening test and an apparently incompatible cross-match. Unless the patient has an antibody with specificity for a defined blood group, it may be difficult to find a donor whose blood will give compatible test results. Red blood cells from the patient should be used to adsorb the autoantibody from the patient's serum, which can be done only in a patient who has not received a transfusion within the past 3 months. The adsorbed serum then can be tested for the presence of an alloantibody. A masked alloantibody is the major concern. The patient's red blood cells also should be saved for subsequent adsorptions, should further transfusions be required. The most compatible blood should be given.

The patient is slowly given red blood cells in suspension and closely monitored for signs of increased hemolysis. The transfused red blood cells are usually destroyed as rapidly as the patient's own red blood cells unless the patient has responded to glucocorticoids. The notion that blood transfusion should be avoided because of the high incidence of alloimmunization and worsening of hemolysis has been refuted (69). No alloantibodies related to the transfusion developed in 53 patients with decompensated AIHA who received blood, nor had any of the patients an increased rate of hemolysis. Despite this observation, transfusion should be reserved for only those patients with life-threatening anemia; conversely, no patient should be deprived of transfusions when severe anemia complicates AIHA.

Glucocorticoids

The patient is immediately given a short-acting glucocorticoid. The initial dose of prednisone is usually 60 mg/d, given in three divided doses, for the first 10 to 14 days. The majority of patients will have marked improvements, with decreased hemolysis and stabilization, followed by a rise in hematocrit. At this time, prednisone is consolidated to a single morning dose and reduced by 10 mg/wk until a dose of 40 mg/d is reached. If clinical improvement is still sustained at this dose, the prednisone is then reduced by decrements of 5 mg weekly until 20 mg/d is reached. At this time, the dose can be further reduced by decrements of 2.5 mg weekly, depending on the clinical response. In some patients the dose cannot be further reduced because of increasing hemolytic activity, and these patients continue to receive 15 to 20 mg/d. To reduce the side effects of glucocorticoids, an alternate-day regimen can be tried. Patients who require more than 20 mg/d to control their hemolytic anemia after 2 to 3 months of treatment should be considered for splenectomy or other treatment.

Approximately 70% of patients show improvement with prednisone treatment, with 15% to 20% going into complete remission, which allows prednisone to be discontinued. Others require less than 20 mg/d to control their disease. About 10% of patients have little or no response to the initial high doses of prednisone. In these patients, higher doses of prednisone in the range of 80 to 100 mg/d can be tried. Another option is to use pulse steroid therapy, giving high-dose dexamethasone (Decadron), 40 mg for 4 days monthly (70). The patient is then placed back on a maintenance level of prednisone, which is reduced according to the clinical response.

Several mechanisms have been proposed for the beneficial effect of prednisone. Its most immediate action is to decrease red blood cell destruction by interfering with monocyte–red blood cell interactions in the spleen and liver (71). A later action is a reduction of the autoantibody. Prednisone also may act by decreasing the binding affinity of the autoantibody for red blood cell antigens.

Splenectomy

Splenectomy is considered in a patient who either has not initially responded to high doses of glucocorticoids or subsequently requires more than 15 to 20 mg/d for control of the hemolytic disease. The decision for splenectomy should be delayed until the patient has had an adequate trial of prednisone (usually 1 to 2 months). The exception is patients with little or no improvement when receiving high doses of prednisone (60 mg/d or more) for 2 to 3 weeks, in whom splenectomy is performed sooner. Based on a large number of reports, approximately two-thirds of patients will show a complete or partial response to splenectomy. Unfortunately, some patients relapse months or years after splenectomy. In most patients the dose of prednisone can be reduced or even discontinued after splenectomy. The response to splenectomy is significantly better in patients with idiopathic AIHA than in secondary cases; splenectomy in the latter must be recommended cautiously (72).

Splenectomy removes the major site of red blood cell destruction in warm-type AIHA, as well as a site for antibody production (as in autoimmune thrombocytopenic purpura) (73). Patients may show a decrease, no change, or an increase in cell-bound antibody (74). The morbidity and mortality from splenectomy are low; laparoscopic removal of spleens is now common with shortened postoperative recovery. Pneumococcal vaccine is recommended before splenectomy but also may be of value afterward (75). Postsplenectomy thrombocytosis may occur and persist chronically with the complication of thrombosis; pulmonary embolism may be a cause of death in splenectomized patients with AIHA.

Immunosuppressive Therapy

Cytotoxic drugs are also effective (76). They should be reserved for patients who have not responded to glucocorticoids and splenectomy or who are poor surgical risks for splenectomy. A favorable response to a cytotoxic drug allows reduction of the steroid dose. The drug is tapered and discontinued if there has been little or no response by 4 to 6 months. The most commonly used cytotoxic agents are azathioprine (1 to 2 mg/kg per day), cyclophosphamide (1 to 2 mg/kg per day), and chlorambucil (0.1 to 0.2 mg/kg per day). Intravenous cyclophosphamide, which has been shown to be effective in the treatment of lupus nephritis, also may be of benefit in AIHA. The dosage schedule is 0.5 to 1 g/m^2 of body surface area given at 1-to 3-month intervals, depending on the clinical response, bone marrow tolerance, and leukocyte nadir (no less than 2,000 $cells/mm^3$). The initial dose is 500 mg/m^2. The drug is administered in 1 hour, followed by 24 hours of hydration to ensure frequent voiding to reduce bladder toxicity. White blood cell counts must be closely monitored. Colony-stimulating factor administration helps reverse leukopenia postchemotherapy. The long-term use of these drugs is associated with an increased risk of subsequent neoplasia. Cyclophosphamide can cause alopecia, sterility, hemorrhagic cystitis, and bladder cancer.

Other Treatments

Other forms of treatment that have had variable success include danazol, cyclosporine, antilymphocyte or antithymocyte globulin, vinblastine-loaded platelets, and plasmapheresis. Cyclosporine, 4 mg/kg per day, has been used in AIHA with some success (77). Patients should be closely monitored for renal toxicity. Intravenous γ-globulin is effective less than in ITP (78). The usual dose is 400 mg/kg per day for 5 days, followed by single doses as needed. One rationale is that blocking the Fc receptors on macrophages within the reticuloendothelial system prevents trapping of IgG-coated red blood cells. Another therapeutic strategy is selectively injuring macrophages by exposing them to transfused platelets sensitized with IgG platelet antibodies and loaded with vincristine (79). Danazol, a synthetic androgen, also has been effective (80). The initial dose is 600 to 800 mg/d, tapered to 400 mg/d once the patient has a clinical response. Side effects include mild masculinization and cholestatic jaundice. Patients with persistent hemolysis should be given 1 mg of folic acid daily. Plasmapheresis is only a temporizing maneuver in the treatment of AIHA because this intervention is only weakly effective in reducing the level of IgG autoantibody in the plasma.

COLD AUTOANTIBODY TYPE

Cold-type autoantibodies react most strongly with red blood cells at 0° to 5°C but achieve clinical significance when their thermal range of reactivity extends to 28° to 31°C or higher. These are the temperatures encountered in the microvasculature of the skin, particularly in the distal extremities, ears, and the tip of the nose. Cold autoantibody types account for 15% to 25% of AIHA in most series (3,31). There are two basic types of cold autoantibody hemolytic anemia: cold hemagglutinin disease and PCH. Both require complement for red blood cell destruction and cause intravascular and extravascular hemolysis of varying degrees.

COLD HEMAGGLUTININ DISEASE

In 1903, Landsteiner demonstrated that the red blood cells of an animal could be agglutinated by its sera at temperatures near 0°C. In 1926, Landsteiner and Levine showed that the sera from most healthy persons agglutinated autologous red blood cells at 0°C. At about this time, Iwai and Mei-Sai reported two patients with Raynaud phenomenon. In one patient, impedance of blood flow was demonstrated in vitro; in the other, sludging of blood flow, resulting from autoagglutination of red blood cells, was observed in the nail bed capillaries at low temperatures. In the 1950s, the association between cold autoantibodies and hemolytic anemia was established. Schubothe introduced the term "cold agglutinin disease" to distinguish this disorder from paroxysmal hemoglobinuria.

Cold hemagglutinin disease occurs in a transient or chronic form. The transient form occurs with mycoplasmal pneumonia or infectious mononucleosis, primarily affecting adolescents or young adults. The antibody is usually IgM and polyclonal. Chronic cold agglutinin disease usually affects persons older than 50 years of age (81). The majority of these patients have no underlying illness identified; the remainder have lymphoproliferative disorders, including chronic lymphocytic leukemia, hairy cell leukemia, lymphomas, and Waldenström macroglobulinemia.

Although most patients with chronic idiopathic disease have IgM monoclonal cold agglutinins, a clinical picture of Waldenström macroglobulinemia or lymphoma develops in very few (82). Flow cytometry may identify a monoclonal B-cell population in some of these patients without other evidence for lymphoma.

Cold Agglutinins and Specificity

Cold agglutinins are most often reactive with the Ii blood group system. The Ii antigens are carbohydrates closely related to the ABO and Lewis blood groups and are present on red blood cells as glycoproteins (9,83). At birth, cord (neonatal) red blood cells express large amounts of i. During the first 18 months after birth, the proportion of i antigen decreases, and the expression of I antigen increases. Most individuals predominantly express I on their mature red blood cells, but rarely cells express only the i antigen. During maturation of a red blood cell, I antigen is formed by the action of a branching enzyme on the red blood cell glycoprotein. With repeated phlebotomy, the i reactivity of red blood cells of healthy individuals has been shown to increase, suggesting that increased i reactivity was inversely related to the bone marrow transit time (84). Reticulocytes express large amounts of i and reduced amounts of I. When the glycoprotein bearing the Ii antigens is extracted from the red blood cell membrane, both anti-I and anti-i react with their respective antigens at 37°C (85). This indicates that conformational changes in the red blood cell membrane induced by cold are required for the expression of the Ii antigens.

The autoantibody in patients with idiopathic chronic cold hemagglutinin disease (CCHAD) or CCHAD associated with lymphoid malignancy is usually monoclonal IgM. The specificity of monoclonal IgM with κ-light chains is usually directed against the I antigen (86), whereas IgM cold agglutinins with λ-light chains are usually directed against the i antigen and only rarely against the I antigen (87). Monoclonal antibodies with IgA or IgG cold agglutinins occasionally have been reported (88). Cold agglutinins associated with *Mycoplasma pneumoniae* pneumonia and infectious mononucleosis are IgM and polyclonal (89). Cold agglutinins associated with mycoplasmal infections are usually reactive with the I antigen (8), whereas in infectious mononucleosis the IgM cold agglutinin is often reactive with the i antigen (89). Approximately one-third of the cold agglutinins with anti-i specificity are cryoprecipitable. Some patients with infectious mononucleosis and angioimmunoblastic lymphadenopathy have a cold-reacting nonagglutinating IgG anti-i and an IgM anti-IgG that agglutinate IgG-coated red blood cells in the cold (90).

Other specificities of cold hemagglutinins have been occasionally observed in patients with cold hemagglutinin disease. Targets for cold hemagglutinins include Pr; Gd, Sa, Lud, and Fl, which are related to Pr; Vo biochemically related to Ii; and A, B, type IIH, Lewis, M-like, P, D, IA, IP, I^T, I^TP, and Ju (31). Determination of specificity is generally not necessary in clinical practice.

Pathophysiology

The hemolytic potential of cold agglutinins depends on their titer and ability to fix complement on red blood cells in vivo (91). Temperatures in the superficial blood vessels of the distal extremities range from 28° to 31°C, depending on the ambient temperature. Lower temperatures occur with extremes of cold. Patients who have cold agglutinins capable of reacting with red blood cells in the range of 28° to 31°C will have ongoing hemolysis at ordinary room temperatures, whereas those patients with antibodies that react at a lower thermal range may have episodes of hemolysis only on cold exposure. The thermal amplitude of the antibody, which is the highest temperature at which agglutination is still visible, usually correlates with the titer of cold agglutinin. Hemolytic anemia, however, has been reported in patients with low titers of IgM cold agglutinins that have a high thermal range (92).

At sites of lower temperature, IgM cold agglutinins react with red blood cells and bind C1. Only a single molecule of IgM is required to bind C1 and initiate the activation of the classic complement pathway (19). C1 sequentially activates C4 and C2, which bind to the red blood cell and form a C3 convertase enzyme complex. As the blood returns to the warmer temperatures within the body, cold agglutinins dissociate from the red blood cell membrane, but complement activation continues. C3 convertase cleaves C3 to C3b and C3a. A single bound C3 convertase enzyme complex can cleave several hundred molecules of C3 to C3b, many of which bind to the red blood cell membrane. Circulating red blood cells coated with C3b and iC3b are trapped predominantly in the liver, where they are bound to the CR1 and CR3 complement receptors, respectively, on the membranes of hepatic macrophages (19). This interaction of red blood cells with macrophages results in binding, sphering, and phagocytosis of red blood cells. The complement sequence goes to completion on some red blood cells, resulting in lytic destruction and intravascular hemolysis. The human red blood cell is relatively resistant to complement-mediated lysis because of regulatory proteins in the serum and on the red blood cell membrane (19).

Patients with chronic cold agglutinin disease develop a population of red blood cells with a normal survival (93). These resistant cells are coated with C3d that blocks further uptake of complement and develop as a result of the interaction of C3b-coated red blood cells with the CR1 complement receptors on macrophages. C3b is degraded to iC3b by factor I with factor H and Cr1 as cofactors. Subsequently, iC3b undergoes a second cleavage by factor I, leading to the formation of C3dg, which is further cleaved into C3d by trypsin-like enzymes. Because receptors on macrophages do not recognize these breakdown products of C3b, the red blood cells are released from the liver. A substantial number of C3b-coated red blood cells initially cleared by the liver are released back into the circulation as C3d-coated red blood cells by this mechanism (13,94).

Hemolysis secondary to cold agglutinin disease may also be exaggerated with any acute phase reaction that leads to an increase in complement production; infection frequently precipitates increased hemolysis in chronic cold agglutinin disease (95).

Clinical Features

Patients with chronic cold agglutinin disease often present with symptoms of chronic anemia. Episodes of acute hemolysis occur after cold exposure, manifested by hemoglobinemia and hemoglobinuria. Patients may note acrocyanosis of their distal extremities, nose, ears, and chin on cold exposure. Livedo reticularis, a sky-blue mottling of the skin of the extremities, is a result of agglutinated red blood cells impeding blood flow in the capillary bed. Some patients experience Raynaud phenomenon. Rarely, a patient develops a vascular occlusion, usually of a distal extremity, which is precipitated by prolonged exposure to cold. Patients with IgA monoclonal cold agglutinins manifest acrocyanosis but no hemolysis, because IgA does not activate the classic complement pathway. The course of patients with idiopathic chronic cold agglutinin disease is characterized by either chronic anemia or episodes of hemolysis, depending on the thermal amplitude of the cold agglutinin. In a few patients this progresses to a malignant lymphoproliferative disease. Features of malignant lymphoma may overshadow cold agglutinin disease. A very large spleen should suggest malignant lymphoma; flow cytometry may demonstrate a monoclonal B cell population with the light-chain restriction of the circulating IgM agglutinin.

In acute transient cold agglutinin disease, most often associated with *M. pneumoniae* pneumonia or infectious mononucleosis, hemolytic anemia appears in the second or third week of the illness; this interval between the acute illness and the subsequent bout of hemolysis leads to significant under-recognition of this phenomenon. Cold agglutinin disease rarely has been observed in association with chickenpox and infectious diseases other than the ones noted (96). The hemolysis in these disorders can be severe, resulting in significant hemoglobinuria and transient renal failure. Hemolytic anemia usually subsides spontaneously in 1 to 2 weeks, with the hematocrit quickly returning to normal. Patients may experience acrocyanosis, especially in a cold room. The spleen may be modestly enlarged.

Laboratory Features

The first indication that a patient might have cold agglutinins sometimes comes from the laboratory or blood bank after the observation of autoagglutination of the patient's red blood cells at room temperature. Blood smears show polychromasia, agglutinated red blood cells and, at times, spherocytes. The reticulocyte count and index are usually elevated. Clumping of red blood cells may lead to errors in calculating red blood cell indices because of autoagglutination. An elevated mean corpuscular volume that corrects to normal on heating the blood sample is good evidence for a cold agglutinin. Slight increases in unconjugated bilirubin and hemoglobinuria are sometimes present, especially after hemolytic episodes. Urine hemosiderin is often present.

Antiglobulin Tests

The DAT in patients with cold agglutinin disease shows C3 and, more specifically, C3d. When the DAT is performed, the red blood cells should be washed thoroughly at 37°C, because a small amount of cold agglutinin will interfere with the test. When cold agglutinins are being assayed, the red blood cells are separated from serum or plasma at 37°C so that cold agglutinin does not remain adsorbed to the red blood cell membrane. Normal donor cells warmed to 37°C are added to dilutions of the patient's plasma, which is also prewarmed to 37°C. Tubes are incubated at 37°C, then incubated at 4°C for at least 30 minutes to 1 hour. Agglutination occurring at cold temperatures should be reversible at 37°C. Healthy persons have low titers of IgM cold agglutinins that usually do not exceed a titer of 1:64 at 4°C. The specificity of these cold agglutinins is almost always anti-I.

Patients who have pathologic cold agglutinins usually have titers at 4°C of 1:1,000 or more in saline (97). When the cold agglutinin titer is less than 1:1,000, a thermal amplitude test can be performed. The patient's serum is initially tested against normal cells suspended in saline at 20°C. If negative, it is unlikely that cold agglutinins are causing the hemolytic anemia. If positive, a test is performed at 30°C in albumin; a positive test indicates that the cold agglutinin is of clinical importance (Table 26.2).

TABLE 26.2. AUTOIMMUNE HEMOLYTIC ANEMIA

Type	DAT	Serum Antibody	Antibody Specificity
Warm autoantibody type	IgG IgG+ C3d C3d[a]	Serum Ab in −50% with untreated red cells	Rh complex antigens in the majority; others include LW, U, Wr^b, En^a, Kidd, Kell, Ge
Cold auto-agglutinin type	C3d	Pathologic cold agglutinins a. 1:1000 at 4°C b. Positive at 30°C in albumin	Mainly I, also i and Pr
Paroxysmal cold hemoglobinuria	C3d	Biphasic hemolysin Ab reacts with red blood cell in cold; hemolysis occurs at 37°C in presence of complement (fresh serum)	

[a] IgG can be detected on red blood cells apparently coated with C3d alone by more sensitive techniques; warm-reacting IgM antibodies also may fix complement to red blood cells.
IgG, immunoglobulin G; IgM, immunoglobulin M.

Treatment

In most patients with chronic hemagglutinin disease, anemia is mild and treatment is largely symptomatic. Patients are advised to keep warm (particularly extremities). Large amounts of ice-cold beverages should be avoided. Because of the increased red blood cell turnover, folic acid 1 mg/d should be given. In patients with more severe hemolytic anemia, chlorambucil or cyclophosphamide is given, and in some patients this results in decreased titers of cold agglutinins and less hemolysis (98). Glucocorticoids and splenectomy generally are not effective, with some important exceptions. Prednisone was shown to be beneficial in patients with low titers of IgM cold agglutinins having high thermal amplitudes and in patients with IgG cold agglutinins (99). In the latter group, splenectomy was also effective. Plasmapheresis may provide temporary amelioration of hemolysis (100). α-Interferon therapy has been given to patients with severe cold agglutinin disease with variable results (101). CD20 monoclonal antibodies have been successful in treatment of some patients with cold agglutinin disease (102); flow cytometry of the bone marrow may identify a target for this effective and relatively innocuous immunotherapy.

Transfusion should be reserved for patients whose cardiovascular or cerebrovascular systems are significantly compromised by the degree of anemia. Washed red blood cells are preferable, to avoid supplying additional complement components to a patient whose low complement levels may be limiting the rate of hemolysis. The donor red blood cells should be warmed to body temperature, and the patient should be kept warm during the transfusion. If compatibility testing is performed using prewarmed techniques, difficulties are usually not encountered.

Because acute cold agglutinin disease associated with infection is self-limited, the best treatment is supportive therapy and judicious inaction. If the hemolysis is severe, these patients should be well hydrated to maintain renal blood flow. Acute renal failure occasionally occurs in the setting of severe hemolysis.

PAROXYSMAL COLD HEMOGLOBINURIA

A rare form of AIHA, PCH is characterized by the sudden onset of severe hemolysis particularly after infection. Children are most commonly affected. The disorder was first characterized by Donath and Landsteiner in 1904. They demonstrated the bithermic nature of this hemolysis, which they attributed to an initial sensitizing cold-reacting autohemolysin and a subsequent lytic warm-reacting serum factor. The biphasic laboratory test for PCH carries their names. In the first part of this century, PCH was most often associated with congenital syphilis and appeared as a chronic disorder with acute episodes of hemolysis precipitated by cold exposure, hence the term "paroxysmal cold hemoglobinuria." Today, PCH most often is encountered as an acute transient hemolytic anemia in children after a variety of infections with little if any cold exposure (103).

Pathophysiology

The D-L autohemolysin is an IgG autoantibody that reacts with red blood cells at reduced temperatures in the extremities and fixes the earlier components of complement (see Cold Hemagglutinin Disease). As blood returns to warmer temperatures within the body, complement activation continues. Some cells are coated with C3b and cleared by the liver and spleen, whereas others are lysed by the terminal components of complement.

The D-L antibody in patients with the acute transient form of the disease seldom binds to the red blood cell in vitro at temperatures higher than 20°C. However, hemolysis occurs in these patients even when they are not exposed to the cold, indicating that the D-L antibody is able to react with red blood cells at higher temperatures in vivo. The explanation for this paradox is not known. Patients with chronic PCH usually experience hemolysis only when exposed to the cold, similar to patients with chronic cold agglutinin disease.

In most patients the D-L antibody is IgG with anti-P specificity (104). The P antigen is a globoside. The D-L antibodies are inhibited by globoside and Forssman glycolipids, which are widespread in microorganisms (105). The D-L antibody, therefore, may represent an immunologic response to cross-reacting antigens present in microorganisms.

Paroxysmal cold hemoglobinuria is reported to be associated with a wide variety of infections, including measles (and measles vaccination), mumps, cytomegalovirus, infectious mononucleosis, chickenpox, mycoplasmal pneumonia, and *Haemophilus influenzae, Klebsiella pneumoniae,* and *Escherichia coli* infections. Frequently, the cause of the preceding illness is not identified.

Clinical Features

An acute attack typically occurs during the time a patient is recovering from a recent upper respiratory tract infection. Attacks are characterized by the sudden onset of shaking chills, back and leg pain, and abdominal cramps. Fever often follows and can be as high as 40°C. Fresh urine passed after the onset of symptoms usually contains hemoglobin. The attack may not be associated with any obvious cold exposure. The constitutional symptoms usually subside within a few hours. Cold urticaria may accompany an attack.

Attacks of PCH can be severe and life threatening. Most patients recover in a few days to several weeks without recurrence. Transient renal failure secondary to hemolysis develops in an occasional patient.

Laboratory Features

The hemoglobin level can be quite low. Reticulocytopenia can occur initially, but reticulocytosis subsequently develops. Leukopenia is followed by leukocytosis. Unconjugated bilirubin is increased. Hemoglobinemia and hemoglobinuria can be present. Serum complement levels are usually depressed during an acute attack. Peripheral blood smears show autoagglutination of red blood cells, polychromasia, nucleated red blood cells, spherocytes, and erythrophagocytosis involving monocytes or neutrophils or both.

The DAT result is positive for C3d. The D-L antibody is detected by the biphasic D-L test. The patient's serum is mixed with donor red blood cells and fresh normal serum as a source of complement. The mixture is incubated at 4°C, then warmed to 37°C. Hemolysis will occur when the D-L antibody is present. In some instances, the sera of patients with cold agglutinin disease may give false-positive results when the cold agglutinin has the property of a monophasic cold hemolysin. The frequency of false-positive results is greatly increased if enzyme-treated cells are used in the D-L test, making a control for monophasic lysis essential. False-positive results appear in only 2% of cold agglutinin sera when untreated red blood cells were used in the D-L test (106). A low titer of the D-L antibody may be present for several weeks to months after an episode of PCH (Table 26.2).

Treatment

Paroxysmal cold hemoglobinuria is usually a self-limiting illness, with recovery within a few days or a week. Patients are usually treated symptomatically by being kept warm. When transfusion is needed, P-positive red blood cells can be given and are unlikely to precipitate hemolysis, provided the blood is warm (104). Glucocorticoids and splenectomy are usually not effective. Glucocorticoids are often given empirically and, when given, should be tapered as quickly as possible. Although syphilis is rarely a cause today, it should be excluded in patients with chronic PCH. Patients with chronic idiopathic PCH should be advised to avoid cold and usually do not require any specific treatment.

DRUG-INDUCED IHA

Several drugs can produce a positive DAT result and, in some patients, hemolytic anemia. Drug-induced IHA has been reported in 12.4% and 18% of patients with AIHA (3). The first description of drug-induced, immune-mediated cytopenia was by Ackroyd (107) in 1949, who described thrombocytopenic purpura after allylisopropylacetyl carbamide (Sedormid) administration. In 1953, Snapper et al. (108) reported a patient with pancytopenia, hemolytic anemia, and a positive DAT result who was receiving mephenytoin. In 1956, Harris (109) reported hemolytic anemia recurring in patients after they received a second course of stibophen used in the treatment of schistosomiasis.

Three mechanisms by which drugs induce IHA have been described (110): drug adsorption (hapten), immune complex (innocent bystander), and induction of autoantibody. A fourth mechanism, nonimmunologic adsorption of proteins to the red blood cells, produces a positive DAT result but not hemolytic anemia. The so-called immune complex mechanism, which has accounted for the majority of reported cases of drug-induced IHA, is presently thought in most instances not to be mediated by circulating drug-antidrug immune complexes that bind nonspecifically to red blood cells, but to a specific interaction of a drug, the antibody, and red blood cells.

Evidence for this drug-dependent mechanism is provided by the studies (111), showing that quinidine-induced antibodies in the presence of quinidine were bound to the platelet through the Fab region or antigen-binding site and not through the Fc region of the antibody, as would be expected for binding of immune complexes. In studies on tolmetin-dependent, antibody-associated hemolytic anemia, the antidrug antibody in the presence of the drug was bound to the red blood cell through the Fab region (112). Drug-dependent antibodies react with a certain cell line (red blood cell, platelet, or white blood cell) and may recognize well-defined specific cell membrane antigens (113).

Types of drug-induced IHA will be discussed as (a) a drug adsorption mechanism, (b) a drug-dependent antibody mechanism, (c) an autoimmune induction mechanism, and (d) a nonimmunologic adsorption of protein (Table 26.3). The situation may be more complicated because some drugs may create hemolytic anemia via multiple mechanisms simultaneously in the same patient; diagnostic tests must be pursued with this in mind.

TABLE 26.3. DRUG-INDUCED IMMUNE HEMOLYTIC ANEMIA

Drug adsorption (e.g., penicillin)	IgG C3d[a]	Ab reacts with drug-coated; eluates react only with drug-coated red blood cells	Moderate degree of hemolysis, usually extravascular mechanism
Drug-dependent antibody type (e.g., cefotetan)	C3d	Ab + drug + red blood cell → sensitization, agglutination or hemolysis of red cells; Ab is IgG or IgM; eluate is negative	Abrupt onset of severe intravascular hemolysis; renal failure
Autoimmune induction (e.g., α-methyldopa)	IgG	Autoantibodies against red blood cell; eluate reacts with red blood cell	Mild-to-moderate degree of extravascular type hemolysis

[a]Present in approximately 40% of penicillin-induced immune hemolytic anemia.
IgG, immunoglobulin G; IgM, immunoglobulin M.

Drug Adsorption Mechanism

In the drug adsorption mechanism, drug-induced antibodies react with a drug already firmly bound to the red blood cell membrane. Penicillin is a prototype of drugs that produce IHA by this mechanism (114). Penicillin is covalently bound to red blood cell membrane protein and is not removed by washing the cells. Penicillin can be demonstrated on the red blood cells of 30% of patients receiving 1.2 to 2.5 million U/d and of all patients receiving 10 million U/d (114). Penicillin on these red blood cells does no harm if immune sensitization does not occur. Approximately 3% of patients receiving massive doses of intravenous penicillin in the range of 10 million U/d continuously for several days eventually will have a positive antiglobulin test result, but hemolytic anemia is rare. For hemolytic anemia to develop, intravenous doses of 10 million U or more over several days are necessary. Although IgM antibodies directed against the benzylpenicilloyl determinant of penicillin develop in approximately 90% of patients who receive penicillin, these antibodies are usually not involved in the pathogenesis of hemolytic anemia (115). The antibody involved is the IgG directed against the benzylpenicilloyl determinant or other metabolites of penicillin. The onset of hemolytic anemia is usually after 7 days of treatment but may be sooner in patients who have been previously immunized to penicillin. The mechanism of red blood cell damage is largely extravascular, occurring mainly in the spleen. The degree of hemolysis is usually mild to moderate.

The DAT shows IgG or occasionally IgG and complement (110). The indirect antiglobulin test result is negative unless donor cells coated with penicillin are used. Similarly, eluates from the patient's red blood cells react only with penicillin-coated donor red blood cells. The finding of a positive DAT result by itself does not dictate discontinuing the drug unless there is evidence for hemolysis. Once the drug is stopped, the hemolytic anemia abates within a few days. Prednisone is usually not required to control the hemolytic anemia, because the disease is self-limited. Penicillin antibodies can cross-react with cephalothin-treated red blood cells, and antibodies against cephalothin can cross-react with penicillin-coated red blood cells (116). Although cephalothin also binds strongly to the red blood cell membrane, it rarely causes hemolytic anemia. Other drugs that induce hemolytic anemia by this mechanism include tolbutamide, tetracycline, and streptomycin (117).

Drug-dependent Antibody Mechanism

In this mechanism (formerly termed immune complex/innocent bystander mechanism), a drug is thought to bind transiently with proteins on the red blood cell membrane to form an immunogen that stimulates production of an antibody (118). The demonstration of the antibody in vitro requires the presence of a free drug or its metabolites on red blood cells. For some drug-dependent antibodies, reactivity occurs only with red blood cells of a specific blood group. In previously sensitized patients, only a small quantity of the drug is required to initiate hemolysis. Hemolysis is abrupt and can be severe, causing massive hemoglobinemia and hemoglobinuria. Renal failure develops in approximately one-third of patients (3). Other complications include shock and disseminated intravascular coagulation.

All drugs should be discontinued until the responsible drug can be determined in the laboratory. Hemolysis usually disappears within a few hours or days. Patients should be closely observed for renal failure. The drug-dependent antibodies can persist for years, placing patients at great risk if again exposed to the responsible drug. Drug-induced autoantibodies, which also may be present, rapidly disappear within a few days after stopping the drug.

The responsible antibody may be IgG or IgM and is capable of activating complement. The DAT shows only C3d. In many cases the responsible drug is recognized by the antibody only when it is associated with a specific blood group antigen. In such cases, the drug and its antibody will not react with red blood cells lacking the specific antigen. Drug-dependent antibodies associated with rifampicin, nitrofurantoin, and dexchlorpheniramine have been shown to react with cells rich in I antigen (119, 120). Drug-dependent antibodies associated with thiopental and nomifensine are reactive with adult but not cord red blood cells (121). Drug-dependent antibodies in a patient with chlorpropamide-induced hemolytic anemia were detected only with Jk^a+

red blood cells (122). In some patients with drug-dependent IHA caused by nomifensine, the serum did not react with red blood cells in the presence of the parent drug but did react with red blood cells in the presence of urine, which contained the ex vivo antigen-metabolite (123). An ex vivo antigen-metabolite was also required to detect drug-dependent antibodies in a case of IHA caused by diclofenac (124). In cases of suspected drug-dependent IHA that are negative with the parent drug, it is important to test with ex vivo antigens-metabolites present in urine or serum collected from volunteers or patients after ingestion of the drug (125).

Many drugs have been reported to cause drug-dependent IHA, examples include second- and third-generation cephalosporins. In a patient receiving cefotaxime, severe intravascular hemolysis developed, which showed in vitro characteristics of drug-dependent and drug adsorption mechanisms (126). In a patient treated with cefotetan in whom hemolytic anemia and fatal renal failure developed, the serum contained antibodies that reacted with cefotetan-treated red blood cells, antibodies that reacted only with untreated red blood cells in the presence of the drug, and drug-independent autoantibodies (127). Both drug adsorption and drug-dependent antibodies were associated with ceftazidime-induced IHA (128). A case of sulindac-induced IHA was associated with a drug-dependent antibody having no blood group specificity (129). A patient receiving both suprofen and tolmetin (nonsteroidal antiinflammatory drugs) had severe intravascular hemolysis and renal failure. There were drug-dependent antibodies to both. Autoantibodies also were present (130). Phenacetin (131) and carbimazole (132) also have been associated with drug-dependent antibodies and autoantibodies.

Autoimmune Induction Mechanism

α-Methyldopa induces a positive antiglobulin test result in 11% to 36% of patients after 3 to 6 months of therapy (133). The incidence of a positive DAT result seems to correlate with the drug dose. The DAT results were positive in 11% of patients taking 1 g/d or less, 19% in those taking 1 to 2 g/d, and 36% in those taking more than 2 g/d (133). However, hemolytic anemia develops in less than 1%. On second exposure to the drug, the interval for the development of a positive DAT result is again 3 to 6 months, thus differing from the usual anamnestic immune response.

The positive DAT result shows IgG and occasionally IgG and complement (110). The indirect antiglobulin test is also positive, especially in those patients with hemolytic anemia. Eluates from patient's red blood cells as well as serum antibody do not require the drug to react with the red blood cell. The antibody specificity is to antigens related to the Rh complex (134). This conclusion is supported by the observation of Bakemeier et al. that antibodies associated with α-methyldopa AIHA recognize a 34-kd polypeptide and a 37- to 55-kd glycoprotein, which seem to be members of the Rh family (134).

The mechanism by which α-methyldopa induces AIHA is unknown. It has been proposed that α-methyldopa alters the red blood cell membrane to form neoantigens recognized as foreign, but there is little evidence to support this concept. α-Methyldopa causes an increase in lymphocyte cyclic adenosine monophosphate, which may inhibit suppressor T cells (135) and lead to overproduction of red blood cell autoantibodies. However, Garratty et al. (136) were unable to confirm α-methyldopa depression of suppressor cell function. α-Methyldopa–induced red blood cell autoantibodies rarely produce hemolytic anemia. Although impaired reticuloendothelial function has been demonstrated in patients receiving α-methyldopa (137), this cannot by itself explain the infrequency of immune hemolysis in these patients.

The degree of hemolysis is usually mild to moderate, and anemia develops gradually. Hemolysis usually regresses within a few days after the drug is stopped but may continue for several weeks to months. Generally no treatment is necessary. Glucocorticoids may shorten the period of recovery but are usually not required. A positive DAT result is not by itself an indication to discontinue α-methyldopa unless there is evidence of hemolytic anemia. The DAT result may remain positive for months to years after discontinuation of α-methyldopa. Other drugs that may induce hemolytic anemia by this mechanism include levodopa (138), mefenamic acid (139), and procainamide (140).

Nonimmunologic Adsorption of Protein

A small number (5%) of patients receiving cephalothin eventually have positive antiglobulin test results because of nonspecific adsorption of serum proteins (110). The DAT result becomes positive after a few days of treatment. Albumin, fibrinogen, complement, and immunoglobulins are detected on the red blood cell membrane (141). As noted earlier, cephalothin can produce hemolytic anemia by the drug adsorption mechanism, but this is unusual (142).

Red blood cells treated in vitro with the chemotherapeutic agent cisplatin can adsorb IgG nonimmunologically and produce a positive DAT result (143). Several cases of hemolytic anemia associated with cisplatin treatment have been reported, but in only one were antibodies to cisplatin demonstrated (144). Conceivably, nonimmunologic binding of IgG was responsible for the positive DAT results, whereas other unknown mechanisms may have caused that anemia.

PAROXYSMAL NOCTURNAL HEMOGLOBINURIA

Paroxysmal nocturnal hemoglobinuria is a rare acquired hemolytic anemia with protean manifestations that have their shared origin in the absence of an essential anchoring protein for many cell membrane–based molecules on the surface of hematopoietic elements.

Clinical Features and Biology

Clinical Picture and Course

Mild to moderate anemia is the most frequent initial clinical sign (Table 26.4). Complement-mediated intravascular hemolysis and hemoglobinuria can create the double insult of iron deficiency and hemolytic anemia. Passage of dark, hemoglobin-con-

TABLE 26.4. CLINICAL FEATURES AND DIAGNOSIS OF PAROXYSMAL NOCTURNAL HEMOGLOBINURIA

Signs and symptoms	Anemia, hemoglobinuria, thrombosis, infection
Age at onset	25–45 years
Laboratory findings	Moderate pancytopenia; elevated reticulocyte count, lactic dehydrogenase and bilirubin; hemosiderinuria; iron deficiency
Confirmatory tests	Flow cytometry for DAF and MIRL; positive acidified serum and sucrose hemolysis tests
Survival	Averages >10 years from diagnosis with cure possible with marrow transplantation
Complications	Venous thrombosis (especially hepatic vein); infection; aplastic anemia; acute leukemia

DAF, delay accelerating factor; MIRL, membrane inhibitor reactive lysis.

taining urine upon arising is the initial symptom in only a minority of cases. Chronic low-grade hemolysis is punctuated by hemolytic crises that are precipitated by infection, drug administration, transfusions, and other stresses (145). Adults 25 to 45 years of age are most frequently affected, although no age group is free of its involvement. Physical findings are related to anemia; some patients have mild splenomegaly (146). The course of the disease varies greatly, with 50% of patients surviving more than 15 years (145); interventions such as bone marrow transplantation now offer the possibility for cure of the disorder. Fatalities most frequently result from thrombotic and infectious complications. Hepatic and portal veins are often the sites of atypical thrombosis in this disorder (147). Paroxysmal nocturnal hemoglobinuria often occurs against the backdrop of aplastic anemia with this relationship contributing to theories regarding the etiology of the disorder (148). It may also evolve into aplastic anemia or acute nonlymphocytic leukemia (149).

Etiology

Paroxysmal nocturnal hemoglobinuria results from a somatic mutation in the X-linked phosphatidylinositol glycan (PIG)-A gene in a hematopoietic stem cell line; more than one hundred mutations in the gene have been described with the most common a "frameshift" mutation (150). The PIG-A gene product contributes to the construction of the glycosylphosphatidylinositol (GPI) anchor protein which constitutes the cytosolic tail of numerous transmembrane cell surface proteins. Almost 100 different GPI-anchored proteins have been identified, helping to explain the many manifestations of PNH. The deficit in two GPI-based molecules (decay-accelerating factor [CD55 or DAF] and membrane inhibitor of reactive lysis [CD59 or MIRL]) results in an inability to inactivate complement on the red blood cell surface leading to hemolysis. A deficiency of a urokinase plasminogen activator receptor on the surface of monocytes has been suggested as contributing to the thrombophilic complications of PNH (145).

The appearance and persistence of the PNH clone(s) in aplastic anemia has suggested that the PIG-A− cells possess a selective advantage over PIG-A+ cells. The correlation of PNH with immunologically-mediated aplastic anemia supports the hypothesis that the altered PNH clone escapes an immune-mediated assault leading to aplastic anemia. An interaction between certain GPI-anchored proteins and the immune system may be crucial for PNH pathogenesis. Affected cells may be advantaged to survive some injury sustained by the normal progenitors, consistent with the hypothesis of immune escape (151,152).

Pathogenesis

The increased sensitivity to C′ of blood cells from patients with PNH is the result of the PIG-A membrane defect, and the C′ system itself is normal (153). Red blood cells of patients with PNH exhibit augmented binding of C3 (145) and increased sensitivity to lysis by the C5b-9 membrane attack complex (MAC), as do PNH platelets, granulocytes, and some lymphocytes.

The biochemical lesion in PNH is deficiency of PIG-anchored proteins in the affected cell membranes. Two of these are important C′-regulating proteins: decay-accelerating factor (DAF; CD55), which inactivates C3b convertase complex (154), and MIRL (CD59), which inactivates MAC (155). C′ sensitivity varies inversely with levels of membrane expression of these proteins (156). Lymphoblastoid cell lines developed from patients with PNH express the PNH defect and are incapable of synthesizing PIG core substance, although they produce messenger RNA for PIG-anchored proteins. The specific abnormality in PNH is deficiency of uridine diphosphate-glucose-*N*-acetyl: phosphatidylinositol-α-1, 6-*N*-acetylglucosaminyltransferase (157). A kindred has been described in which there is a hereditary deficiency of MIRL (CD59). A single member of this kindred, born to cousins, is homozygous for MIRL deficiency and expresses a PNH phenotype (158).

The nature of the thrombotic tendency in PNH is incompletely understood (145). Paroxysmal nocturnal hemoglobinuria platelets are partially activated by sublethal C′-mediated damage, and this activation may predispose to thrombosis (159). However, because the clotting in PNH is principally venous (145, 147), the absent urokinase receptor may be important in decreasing the fibrinolytic system in resorbing venous clots (160). Thrombocytopenia in PNH is attributable more to defective synthesis than excessive consumption in clotting.

Diagnosis

Paroxysmal nocturnal hemoglobinuria may be diagnosed by demonstration of chronic intravascular hemolysis attributable to C′-sensitive cells (deficient in PIG-anchored proteins) in the blood. Paroxysmal nocturnal hemoglobinuria should be considered in cases of hemolytic anemia with a negative DAT, aplastic anemia, and poorly understood pancytopenia or iron deficiency; hemolytic transfusion reactions in the face of a negative immunologic evaluation should also raise consideration of PNH. Atypical thromboses, leukopenia, and thrombocytopenia are subtle signs of PNH.

Laboratory Findings

Most patients with PNH have a packed cell volume of less than 30%, and many exhibit hypochromic, microcytic indices because of iron deficiency (146). Reticulocytosis may be blunted because of the attendant iron deficiency. Elevated levels of serum bilirubin and lactic dehydrogenase are usual; haptoglobin levels are always reduced or absent. Virtually all patients have chronic hemosiderinuria, and absence of this finding should call the diagnosis into question. Granulocytopenia (<1.5 × 10^9/l) is common (146). The majority of patients also have mild thrombocytopenia (<150 × 10^9/l), with some platelet counts less than 50 × 10^9/l (146). The bone marrow cellularity varies from aplastic to hypercellular with erythroid hyperplasia. Maturation of bone marrow precursors is usually normal, but iron stores are characteristically reduced or absent.

TABLE 26.5. MANAGEMENT OF PAROXYSMAL NOCTURNAL HEMOGLOBINURIA

Hematinics	Folic acid supplementation: *cautious* iron replacement
Androgens	Minority of patients have dramatic reduction in anemia
Corticosteroids	One-half to two-thirds of patients benefit from alternate-day therapy; heparin is used for acute episodes but may sometimes increase hemolysis: thrombolytic agents may be useful in hepatic vein thrombosis
Transfusions	For refractory symptomatic anemia or to abort or avert an acute hemolytic crisis; washed or frozen deglycerolized cells should be used

Confirmatory Tests

Several serologic tests demonstrate the C′ sensitivity of PNH red blood cells. The acidified serum (Ham) test and the sucrose hemolysis test have been the standard confirmatory tests required for specific diagnosis (145,146,161). More recently a variety of monoclonal antibodies that recognize the PIG-anchored proteins deficient in PNH have become available.

Serologic Tests

In the acidified serum test, PNH red blood cells, but not normal cells, are lysed by normal human serum acidified to pH 6.5. With appropriate controls this test is specific for PNH, but it is more time-consuming and technically difficult than the sucrose hemolysis test (161). It rarely gives false-positive results in cases of hereditary erythrocyte multinuclearity with a positive acidified serum test (HEMPAS) or when intense spherocytosis is present (162). In the sucrose hemolysis test, PNH red blood cells are lysed by C′ components nonspecifically deposited on surfaces in solutions of low ionic strength. This test produces greater degrees of hemolysis than the acidified serum test, and values of 5% hemolysis or less are considered nonspecific and nondiagnostic (161). These tests are complementary and should be performed in parallel if there is a high suspicion of PNH. Although the sucrose hemolysis test is more sensitive, it may fail to detect PNH in some patients whose cells do not exhibit increased sensitivity to C5-C9 membrane attack complex and whose acidified serum tests give positive results (161).

Immunophenotyping

Monoclonal antibodies have been developed to DAF (CD55) and to several other determinants on PIG-anchored proteins. These include MIRL (CD59), FcγRIII (CD16), and CD48 (163,164). PIG-anchored proteins are expressed on a portion of PNH B cells, and a panel of monoclonal antibodies that detect CD55, CD59, and CD48 can be used to test for PNH (164). Unlike traditional serologic tests, immunophenotyping may be applied to patients with PNH who develop aplastic anemia or are otherwise so heavily transfused as to have a low percentage of native PNH red blood cells. A rapid microtyping card test based on antibodies to CD55 and CD59 has been developed (165). An improved method for the detection of PNH cells utilizes the selective binding of the protein aerolysin to GPI anchors; this is an important adjunct because no single monoclonal antibody can be used with confidence to diagnose PNH (166).

Pharmacologic and Surgical Treatment

Hematinics

Chronic hemolysis in PNH often produces iron and folic acid deficiency, which may worsen anemia. Patients with PNH should receive supplemental folic acid. Iron therapy carries some risk of exacerbating hemolysis because of production of a cohort of C′-sensitive red blood cells (167). Administration of oral iron is usually not accompanied by severe acute hemolysis and may be sufficient to offset urinary losses. However, when iron loss is more severe, some patients lose as much as 20 mg per day (167), and parenteral iron administration can become necessary. A severe acute hemolytic response to iron therapy often can be prevented by corticosteroid administration (167) (Table 26.5).

Androgens

A minority of patients with PNH respond to treatment with androgens (168). These drugs may function by decreasing hemolysis or by increasing red blood cell production. Methyltestosterone, parenteral preparations, and synthetic steroids (including danazol) all have been effective in some patients but they have serious side effects, including cholestatic jaundice and peliosis hepatis, and predispose to progressive hepatic venous thrombosis. Because the response to androgens cannot be predicted, a trial of fluoxymesterone (10 to 30 mg/d) or oxymetholone (10 to 50 mg/d) is worthwhile, but these drugs should be discontinued if no response has occurred in 6 to 8 weeks (168).

Corticosteroids

Steroids suppress hemolysis in the majority of patients with PNH. The onset of action generally occurs within hours, and 57% to 67% of patients respond to therapy with moderate-dose alternate-day oral prednisone (168,169). The mechanism of steroid action is uncertain. They may reduce C′ activation by the alternate pathway, but red blood cells of patients with PNH who are taking prednisone are no less sensitive to C′-mediated lysis in standard in vitro tests. Generally, prednisone doses of 20 to 60 mg/d are required to suppress hemolysis. Corticosteroids may be given daily for a limited time to achieve an immediate effect. However, their side effects, particularly predisposition to infection in patients already compromised by granulocytopenia, can be toxic. Corticosteroids should be prescribed for prolonged periods only on an alternate-day schedule and should be discontinued if they are ineffective after a trial of 2 to 4 weeks.

Splenectomy

There are potential hazards of surgical procedures in patients with PNH but, with careful attention to anesthetic and surgical technique, surgery can be accomplished with safety (170). Splenectomy is usually not useful in PNH. In some patients, however, splenectomy reduces the anemia associated with PNH. This procedure is worth considering in patients with myelofibrosis-associated PNH.

Erythropoietin and Cytokines

Biologic agents have been used in a few patients with PNH. Although erythropoietin levels are usually elevated in patients with PNH, chronic anemia in patients with PNH sometimes responds to erythropoietin at doses between 50 and 500 U/kg given three times weekly (171). Filgrastim (granulocyte colony–stimulating factor) administration led to recovery or protection from infection of two patients with PNH subject to repeated bacterial infection, and granulocyte colony–stimulating factor administration produced increased expression of PIG-anchored FcγRIII expression on their leukocytes (172). The use of these agents in the routine care of patients with PNH remains to be defined but offers the hope of decreased demand for transfusion therapy and better outcomes to infectious episodes.

Bone Marrow Transplantation

Clinical cures of PNH by allogeneic or syngeneic bone marrow transplantation have been increasingly reported, and expression of normal levels of PIG-anchored proteins on circulating blood cells of a transplanted patient with PNH has been directly demonstrated (173). Allogeneic or syngeneic transplantation seems to be very effective for patients with PNH in whom aplastic anemia has supervened. Allogeneic transplants can restore normal bone marrow function in about 50% of patients with PNH (174). The recent demonstration of a population of normal (DAF+ and CD59+) primitive (CD34+ and CD38+) cells in the bone marrow of patients with PNH suggests the possibility of selecting normal stem cells for autologous transplantation.

Anticoagulants and Thrombolytic Agents

Patients with PNH have a marked tendency for repeated venous thromboses (147), requiring aggressive use of anticoagulants. Warfarin should be given as soon as such a complication is recognized. Heparin therapy is required for hepatic venous thrombosis and has been used without incident in many patients with PNH, although heparin does precipitate hemolytic episodes in some individuals (168). Low–molecular-weight heparin may be more useful for both the inhibition of hemolysis and the prevention of thrombosis in PNH (175). Streptokinase has been used successfully to treat hepatic venous thrombosis (176).

Transfusion

Indications

Red blood cell transfusions are sometimes required for relief of symptoms in PNH when hemolysis produces anemia that cannot be corrected by the therapeutic maneuvers discussed above. Additionally, hypertransfusion to a packed cell volume of 35% to 40% can abort acute hemolytic crises refractory to corticosteroids (168).

Choice of Blood Components

Red Blood Cells

Transfusion of whole blood to patients with PNH can initiate hemolysis and worsen anemia. Infused plasma can increase C′ levels, whereas whole blood and red blood cells contain white blood cell fragments that can be immunogenic and result in C′ activation (177). Therefore, washed cells have been recommended and many transfusion services follow this practice. Sirchia and Zanella have presented evidence that white blood cell fragments are the element most likely to initiate hemolysis during transfusion of patients with PNH, and they advocate the use of blood components leukocyte reduced by filtration (178).

It seems clear that many patients with PNH tolerate infusion of whole blood or red blood cells without ill effects, but the proportion of patients with PNH who may experience increased hemolysis is not clear. The use of blood components leukocyte reduced by filtration seems to be safer, and the use of washed or frozen deglycerolized cells avoids the problem altogether.

Platelet Concentrates

Thrombocytopenia is common in patients with PNH and can be severe ($<20 \times 10^9$/l) enough to require platelet transfusion for surgery or for bleeding after trauma. Platelet preparations should be leukocyte reduced by filtration. The possibility of a hemolytic episode should be anticipated but can be treated with corticosteroids or hypertransfusion. Patients with PNH are likely to have had many red blood cell transfusions and to have developed platelet alloimmunization. HLA-matched or cross-matched platelet concentrates are sometimes required.

Special Situations

Pregnancy

Many successful pregnancies have occurred in women with PNH. Two-thirds had a successful outcome, but maternal death occurs in ~10% of PNH-affected pregnancies. Mothers often experience accelerated hemolysis and venous thrombosis (179). Increased red blood cell transfusion is usually necessary, and some authors advocate prophylaxis against venous thrombosis in patients who are bedridden and possibly also in the peripartum period (180). Because of multiple maternal red blood cell transfusions, hemolytic disease of the newborn is frequent (181).

Extensive Elective Surgery

When extensive surgery is planned for a patient with PNH, the possibility of severe hemolysis should be anticipated. An exchange transfusion can be performed before the operation. The precaution prevents hemolysis and provides the surgeon and anesthetist with a more stable patient (170).

Disseminated Intravascular Coagulation

Disseminated intravascular coagulation seems to be a rare direct complication of PNH (182). When asymptomatic, it has been treated with simple observation (182) or with blood component support. Additional special measures have not been required on account of PNH, and cryoprecipitate and platelet concentrates have been tolerated without accelerated hemolysis being noted.

Myelofibrosis

As many as 50% of patients with primary myelofibrosis exhibit red blood cell membrane defects of PNH and some suffer from thrombotic complications (183). These patients have bone marrow failure contributing to their anemia, in addition to hemolysis, and sometimes have substantial transfusion requirements. Contrary to the usual finding of iron deficiency, such patients can develop transfusion-related hemosiderosis.

Acute Leukemia

Paroxysmal nocturnal hemoglobinuria evolves into acute myelocytic leukemia (AML) in 2% to 4% of patients (184). Leukemia apparently develops in the PNH clone, and there is cytogenetic evidence of clonal evolution (185). Complete remissions can be induced with antileukemic therapy, and in these patients there has been no evidence of PNH during remission (186). Reports of patients with PNH who develop AML do not indicate increased complications referable to the PNH defect, despite the need for intensive transfusion support. In fact, in one patient who did not undergo induction chemotherapy for AML, complications of PNH decreased during the course of the leukemia (187).

Aplastic Anemia

Paroxysmal nocturnal hemoglobinuria may evolve from or into aplastic anemia (188). Development of this complication is compatible with prolonged survival with treatment similar to that prescribed for uncomplicated cases of PNH (189). Paroxysmal nocturnal hemoglobinuria–associated aplastic anemia may be successfully treated by bone marrow transplantation.

SUMMARY

Autoimmune hemolytic anemia is divided into warm and cold autoantibody types and may be idiopathic (primary) or associated with another disease (secondary). It also may be drug induced. The DAT is an important laboratory marker but may produce negative results in patients with anemia and positive results in patients without anemia. Transfusion frequently requires autoadsorption studies. Glucocorticoids and splenectomy are primary treatments, although immunosuppressive drugs and other treatments are also used. The cold autoantibody type of AIHA is either acute or CCHAD or PCH. Drug-induced hemolytic anemia involves drug adsorption, a drug-dependent antibody, or autoantibody induction mechanisms.

Paroxysmal nocturnal hemoglobinuria is an uncommonly diagnosed hemolytic anemia that arises from a somatic mutation of pluripotent hematopoietic stem cells. Hemolysis results from increased sensitivity to C′ produced by deficiency of the PIG-anchored proteins, including DAF and MIRL, in the red blood cell membrane. The acidified serum test, the sucrose hemolysis test, and immunophenotyping of blood cells are used for diagnosis. Various therapies including transfusion have been used, and a variety of complications may ensue.

REFERENCES

1. Mack P, Freedman J. Autoimmune hemolytic anemia: a history. *Transfus Med Rev* 2000;14:223–233.
2. Sokol RJ, Hewitt S, Stamps BK. Autoimmune haemolysis: an 18-year study of 865 cases referred to a regional transfusion centre. *BMJ* 1981;282:2023–2027.
3. Petz LD, Garratty G. Acquired immune hemolytic anemias. New York: Churchill Livingstone, 1980:29.
4. Sokol RJ, Hewitt S, Stamps BK. Autoimmune haemolysis: mixed warm and cold antibody type. *Acta Haematol* 1983;69:266–274.
5. Kajii E, Miura Y, Ikemoto S. Characterization of autoantibodies in mixed-type autoimmune hemolytic anemia. *Vox Sang* 1991;60: 45–52.
6. Theofilopoulos AN, Dixon FJ. Murine models of systemic lupus erythematosus. *Adv Immunol* 1985;37:269.
7. Meite M, Leonard S, Idrissi ME, et al. Exacerbation of autoantibody-mediated hemolytic anemia by viral infection. *J Virol* 2000;74: 6045–6049.
8. Janney FA, Lee LT, Howe C. Cold hemagglutinin cross-reactivity with *Mycoplasma pneumoniae. Infect Immun* 1978;22:29–33.
9. Feizi T. The monoclonal antibodies of cold agglutinin syndrome. *Med Biol* 1980;58:123–127.
10. Witebsky E. Acquired hemolytic anemia. *Ann N Y Acad Sci* 1965; 124:462–464.
11. Pirofsky B. Hereditary aspects of autoimmune hemolytic anemia: a retrospective analysis. *Vox Sang* 1968;14:334–347.
12. Cobo F, Pereira A, Nomdedeu B, et al. Ovarian dermoid cyst–associated autoimmune hemolytic anemia: a case report with emphasis on pathogenic mechanisms. *Am J Clin Pathol* 1996;105:567–571.
13. Schreiber AD, Frank MM. Role of antibody and complement in the immune clearance and destruction of erythrocytes. II. Molecular nature of IgG and IgM complement-fixing sites and effects of their interaction with serum. *J Clin Invest* 1972;52:583–589.
14. LoBuglio AF, Cotran RS, Jandl JH. Red cells coated with immunoglobulin G: binding and sphering by mononuclear cells in man. *Science* 1967;158:1582–1585.
15. Fries LF, Brickman CM, Frank MM. Monocyte receptors for the Fc portion of IgG increase in number in autoimmune hemolytic anemia

and other hemolytic states and are decreased by glucocorticoid therapy. *J Immunol* 1983;131:1240–1245.
16. Huber H, Douglas SD, Musbacher S, et al. IgG subclass specificity of monocyte receptor sites. *Nature* 1971;229:419–420.
17. Zupanska B, Brojer E, Thomson EE, et al. Monocyte-erythrocyte interaction in autoimmune haemolytic anaemia in relation to the number of erythrocyte-bound IgG molecules and subclass specificity of autoantibodies. *Vox Sang* 1987;52:213–218.
18. Freedman J, Semple JW. Complement in transfusion medicine. In: Garratty G, ed. *Immunobiology of transfusion medicine.* New York: Marcel Dekker Inc, 1994:403–434.
19. Frank MH. The complement system. In: Samter M, Talmage DW, Frank MM, et al., eds. *Immunologic diseases,* 4th ed. Boston: Little, Brown and Company, 1988:203–232.
20. Berger M, Gaither TA, Frank MM. Complement receptors. *Clin Immunol Rev* 1981–1982;1:471–545.
21. Clark DA, Dessypris EN, Jenkins DE Jr, et al. Acquired immune hemolytic anemia associated with IgA erythrocyte coating: investigation of hemolytic mechanisms. *Blood* 1984;64:1000–1005.
22. Salama A, Bhakdi S, Mueller-Eckhardt C. Evidence suggesting the occurrence of C3-independent intravascular immune hemolysis. *Transfusion* 1987;27:49–53.
23. Sokol RJ, Hewitt S, Booker DJ, et al. Enzyme linked direct antiglobulin tests in patients with autoimmune haemolysis. *J Clin Pathol* 1985; 38:912–914.
24. Hsu TCS, Rosenfield RE, Burkart P, et al. Instrumented PVP-augmented antiglobulin tests. II. Evaluation of acquired hemolytic anemia. *Vox Sang* 1974;26:305–325.
25. Salama A, Mueller-Eckhardt M. Autoimmune haemolytic anaemia in childhood associated with non-complement binding IgM autoantibodies. *Br J Haematol* 1987;65:67–71.
26. Arndt P, Clarke A, Domen R, et al. Two cases of severe warm type autoimmune hemolytic anemia associated with IgM anti-Ena and anti-Pr. *Transfusion* 1991;31:28S(abst).
27. Dankbar DT, Pierce SR, Issitt PD, et al. Fatal intravascular hemolysis associated with auto anti-Wr^b. *Tranfusion* 1987;27:534(abst).
28. Garratty G, Nance SJ. Correlation between in vivo hemolysis and the amount of red cell–bound IgG measured by flow cytometry. *Transfusion* 1990;30:617–621.
29. Sokol RJ, Hewitt S, Booker DJ, et al. Red cell autoantibodies, multiple immunoglobulin classes, and autoimmune hemolysis. *Transfusion* 1990;30:714–717.
30. Engelfriet CP, von dem Borne AEG, Beckers DO, et al. Immune destruction of red cell. In: Bell CA, ed. *A seminar on immune-mediated cell destruction.* Washington, DC: American Association of Blood Banks, 1981:93–103.
31. Engelfriet CP, Beckers ThAP, van't Veer MB, et al. Recent advances in immune haemolytic anemia. In: Hollan SR, ed. *Recent advances in haematology.* Budapest: Akademia Kiado, 1982:235–251.
32. Leddy JP, Bakemeier RF. Structural aspects of human erythrocyte autoantibodies. I. L chain types and electrophoretic dispersion. *J Exp Med* 1965;121:1–17.
33. Litwin SD, Balaban S, Eyster ME. Gm allotype preference in erythrocyte IgG antibodies of patients with autoimmune hemolytic anemia. *Blood* 1973;42:241–246.
34. Garratty G. Factors affecting the pathogenicity of red cell auto- and alloantibodies. In: Nance SJ, ed. *Immune destruction of red blood cells.* Arlington, VA: American Association of Blood Banks, 1989:109.
35. Garratty G. Target antigens for red-cell-bound autoantibodies. In: Nance SJ, ed. *Clinical and basic science aspects of immunohematology.* Arlington, VA: American Association of Blood Banks, 1991:33.
36. Celano MJ, Levine P. Anti-LW specificity in autoimmune acquired hemolytic anemia. *Transfusion* 1967;7:265–268.
37. Marsh WL, Reid ME, Scott EP. Autoantibodies of U blood group specificity in autoimmune haemolytic anaemia. *Br J Haematol* 1972; 22:625–629.
38. Issitt PD, Pavone BG, Goldfinger D, et al. Anti-Wr^b and other autoantibodies responsible for positive direct antiglobulin tests in 150 individuals. *Br J Haematol* 1976;34:5–18.
39. Wakui H, Imai H, Kobayashi R, et al. Autoantibody against erythrocyte protein 4.1 in a patient with autoimmune hemolytic anemia. *Blood* 1988;72:408–412.
40. Victoria EJ, Pierce SW, Branks MJ, et al. IgG red blood cell autoantibodies in autoimmune hemolytic anemia bind to epitope on red blood cell membrane band 3 glycoprotein. *J Lab Clin Med* 1990;115:74–88.
41. Issitt PD, Zellner DC, Rolih SD, et al. Autoantibodies mimicking alloantibodies. *Transfusion* 1977;17:531–538.
42. Garratty G. Autoimmune hemolytic anemia. In: Garratty G, ed. *Immunobiology of transfusion medicine.* New York: Marcel Dekker Inc, 1994:499–500.
43. Kay MMB. Cellular and molecular biology of senescent cell antigen. In: Garratty G, ed. *Immunobiology of transfusion medicine.* New York: Marcel Dekker Inc, 1994:173–198.
44. Arndt P, O'Hoski P, McBride J, et al. Autoimmune hemolytic anemia associated with an antibody reacting preferentially with "old" red cells. *Transfusion* 1989;29:48S.
45. Ness PM, Shirey RS, Thoman SK, et al. The differentiation of delayed serologic and delayed hemolytic transfusion reactions: incidence, long-term serologic findings, and clinical significance. *Transfusion* 1990;30:688–693.
46. Sthoeger Z, Sthoeger D, Green L, et al. The role of anticardiolipin autoantibodies in the pathogenesis of autoimmune hemolytic anemia in systemic lupus erythematosus. *J Rheumatol* 1993;20:2058–2061.
47. Masouredis SP, Branks MJ, Garratty G, et al. Immunospecific red cell binding of iodine 125-labeled immunoglobulin G erythrocyte autoantibodies. *J Lab Clin Med* 1987;110:308–317.
48. Masouredis SP, Branks MJ, Victoria EJ. Antiidiotypic IgG crossreactive with Rh alloantibodies in red cell autoimmunity. *Blood* 1987;70: 710–715.
49. Petz LD, Garratty G. *Acquired immune hemolytic anemias.* New York: Churchill Livingstone, 1980:193.
50. Gilliland BC. Coombs-negative immune hemolytic anemia. *Semin Hematol* 1976;13:267–275.
51. Sokol RJ, Hewitt S, Booker DJ, et al. Small quantities of erythrocyte-bound immunoglobulins and autoimmune haemolysis. *J Clin Pathol* 1987;40:254–257.
52. Bodensteiner D, Brown P, Skikne B, et al. The enzyme-linked immunosorbent assay: accurate detection of red blood cell antibodies in autoimmune hemolytic anemia. *Am J Clin Pathol* 1983;79:182–185.
53. Schmitz N, Dijibey I, Kretschmer V, et al. Assessment of red cell autoantibodies in autoimmune haemolytic anaemia of warm type by a radioactive anti-IgG test. *Vox Sang* 1981;41:224–230.
54. Yam P, Petz LD, Spath P. Detection of IgG sensitization of red cells with ^{125}I staphylococcal protein A. *Am J Hematol* 1982;12:337–346.
55. Salama A, Mueller-Eckhardt C, Bhakdi S. A two-stage immunoradiometric assay with ^{125}I-staphylococcal protein A for the detection of antibodies and complement on human blood cells. *Vox Sang* 1985; 48:239–245.
56. Owen I, Hows J. Evaluation of the manual hexadimethrine bromide (Polybrene) technique in the investigation of autoimmune hemolytic anemia. *Transfusion* 1990;30:814–818.
57. Garratty G, Postoway N, Nance S, et al. Detection of IgG on red cells of patients with suspected direct antiglobulin test negative autoimmune hemolytic anemia (AIHA). In: *Book of abstracts from the International Society of Blood Transfusion/American Association of Blood Banks Joint Congress.* Arlington, VA: American Association of Blood Banks, 1990:87(abst).
58. Gorst DW, Rawlinson VI, Merry AH, et al. Positive direct antiglobulin test in normal individuals. *Vox Sang* 1980;38:99–105.
59. Garratty G, Petz LD. The significance of red cell bound complement components in development of standards and quality assurance for the anti-complement components of antiglobulin sera. *Transfusion* 1976;16:297–306.
60. Abdalla S, Weatherall DJ. The direct antiglobulin test in *P. falciparum* malaria. *Br J Haematol* 1982;51:415–425.
61. Toy PT, Reid ME, Burns M. Positive direct antiglobulin test associated with hyperglobulinemia in acquired immunodeficiency syndrome (AIDS). *Am J Hematol* 1985;19:145–150.
62. Zon LI, Arkin C, Groopman JE. Haematologic manifestations of

the human immune deficiency virus (HIV). *Br J Haematol* 1987;66: 251–256.
63. Inada Y, Lange M, McKinley GF, et al. Hematologic correlates and the role of erythrocyte CR1 (C3b receptor) in the development of AIDS. *AIDS Res* 1986;2:235–247.
64. Inada Y, Kamiyama M, Kanemitsu T, et al. Relationships between C3b receptor (CR1) activity or erythrocytes and positive Coombs tests. *Ann Rheum Dis* 1986;45:367–372.
65. Telen MJ, Roberts KB, Bartlett JA. HIV-associated autoimmune hemolytic anemia: report of a case and review of the literature. *J Acquir Immune Defic Syndr* 1990;3:933–937.
66. McCann EL, Shirey RS, Kickler TS, et al. IgM autoagglutinins in warm autoimmune hemolytic anemia: a poor prognostic feature. *Acta Haematol* 1992;88:120–125.
67. Habibi B, Homberg JC, Schaison G, et al. Autoimmune hemolytic anemia in children. *Am J Med* 1974;56:61–69.
68. Mullon J, Giacoppe G, Clagett C, et al. Brief report: transfusions of polymerized bovine hemoglobin in a patient with severe autoimmune hemolytic anemia. *N Engl J Med* 2000;342:1638–1643.
69. Salama A, Berghöfer H, Mueller-Eckhardt C. Red blood cell transfusion in warm-type autoimmune haemolytic anaemia. *Lancet* 1992; 340:1515–1517.
70. Meyer O, Stahl D, Beckhove P, et al. Pulsed high-dose dexamethasone in chronic autoimmune haemolytic anaemia of warm type. *Br J Haematol* 1997;98:860–862.
71. Rosse WF. Quantitative immunology of immune hemolytic anemia. II. The relationship of cell-bound antibody to hemolysis and the effect of treatment. *J Clin Invest* 1971;50:734–743.
72. Akpek G, McAneny D, Weintraub L. Comparative response to splenectomy in Coombs-positive autoimmune hemolytic anemia with or without associated disease. *Am J Hematol* 1999;61:98–102.
73. Karpatkin S, Strick N, Siskind GW. Detection of splenic anti-platelet antibody synthesis in idiopathic autoimmune thrombocytopenic purpura (ATP). *Br J Haematol* 1972;23:167–176.
74. Allgood JW, Chaplin H. Idiopathic acquired autoimmune hemolytic anemia: a review of forty-seven cases treated from 1955 through 1965. *Am J Med* 1967;43:254–273.
75. Graffner H, Gullstrand P, Hallberg T. Immunocompetence after incidental splenectomy. *Scand J Haematol* 1982;28:369–375.
76. Worlledge S. Immune haemolytic anaemias. In: Hardesty RM, Weatherall DS, eds. *Blood and its disorders.* Oxford: Blackwell Science, 1974:714.
77. Hershko C, Sonnenblick M, Ashkenazi J. Control of steroid-resistant autoimmune haemolytic anaemia by cyclosporine. *Br J Haematol* 1990;76:436–437.
78. Flores G, Cunningham-Rundles C, Newland AC, et al. Efficacy of intravenous immunoglobulin in the treatment of autoimmune hemolytic anemia: results in 73 patients. *Am J Hematol* 1993;44:237–242.
79. Ahn YS, Harrington WJ, Byrnes JJ, et al. Treatment of autoimmune hemolytic anemia with Vinca-loaded platelets. *JAMA* 1983;249: 2189–2194.
80. Pignon J-M, Poirson E, Rochant H. Danazol in autoimmune haemolytic anaemia. *Br J Haematol* 1993;83:343–345.
81. Schubothe H. The cold hemagglutinin disease. *Semin Hematol* 1996; 3:27–47.
82. Evans RS, Baxter E, Gilliland BC. Chronic hemolytic anemia due to cold agglutinins: a 20-year history of benign gammopathy with response to chlorambucil. *Blood* 1973;42:463–470.
83. Feizi T. Immunochemistry of the Ii blood group antigens. In: Mohn JF, Plunkett RW, Cunningham RK, et al., eds. *Human blood groups.* Basel: S Karger, 1977:164–171.
84. Hellman RS, Giblett ER. Red cell membrane alternation associated with "marrow stress." *J Clin Invest* 1965;44:1730–1736.
85. Rosse WG, Lauf PK. Reaction of cold agglutinins with I antigen solubilized from human red cells. *Blood* 1970;36:777–784.
86. Harboe M, van Furth R, Schubothe H, et al. Exclusive occurrence of K chains in isolated cold haemagglutinins. *Scand J Haematol* 1965; 2:259–266.
87. Pruzanski W, Cowan DH, Parr DM. Clinical and immunochemical studies of IgM cold agglutinins with lambda type light chains. *Clin Immunol Immunopathol* 1974;2:234–245.
88. Costea N, Yakulis V, Heller P. Light-chain heterogeneity of cold agglutinins. *Science* 1966;152:1520–1521.
89. Rosenfield RE, Schmidt RJ, Calvo RC, et al. Anti-i, a frequent cold agglutinin in infectious mononucleosis. *Vox Sang* 1965;10:631–634.
90. Roelcke D. Sialic acid–dependent red blood cell antigens. In: Garratty G, ed. *Immunobiology of transfusion medicine.* New York: Marcel Dekker Inc, 1994:69–95.
91. Jaffe CJ, Atkinson JP, Frank MM. The role of complement in the clearance of cold agglutinin–sensitized erythrocytes in man. *J Clin Invest* 1976;58:942–949.
92. Schreiber AD, Herskovitz BS, Goldwein M. Low-titer cold hemagglutinin disease. *N Engl J Med* 1977;297:1490–1494.
93. Evans RS, Turner E, Bingham M. Chronic hemolytic anemia due to cold agglutinins: the mechanism of resistance of red cells to C′ hemolysis by cold agglutinins. *J Clin Invest* 1967;46:1461–1474.
94. Lachmann PJ, Pangburn MK, Oldroyd RG. Breakdown of C3 after complement activation. Identification of a new fragment, C3g, using monoclonal antibodies. *J Exp Med* 1982;156:205–216.
95. Ulvestad E, Berentsen S, Bo K, et al. Clinical immunology of chronic cold agglutinin disease. *Eur J Haematol* 1999;63:259–266.
96. Friedman HD, Dracker RA. Cold agglutinin disease after chicken pox. An uncommon complication of a common disease. *Am J Clin Pathol* 1992;97:92–96.
97. Petz LD, Garratty G. Acquired immune hemolytic anemias. New York: Churchill Livingstone, 1980:213–223.
98. Hippe E, Jensen KB, Olesen H, et al. Chlorambucil treatment of patients with cold agglutinin syndrome. *Blood* 1970;35:68–72.
99. Silberstein LE, Berkman EM, Schreiber AD. Cold hemagglutinin disease associated with IgG cold-reactive antibody. *Ann Intern Med* 1987; 106:238–242.
100. Andrzejewski C Jr, Cault E, Briggs M, et al. Benefit of a 37°C extracorporeal circuit in plasma exchange therapy for selected cases with cold agglutinin disease. *J Clin Apheresis* 1988;4:13–17.
101. Hillen HFP, Bakker SJL. Failure of interferon-α-2b therapy in chronic cold agglutinin disease [Letter]. *Eur J Haematol* 1994;53: 242–243.
102. Lee EJ, Kueck B. Rituxan in the treatment of cold agglutinin disease [Letter]. *Blood* 1998;92:3490–3491.
103. Sokol RJ, Hewitt S, Stamps BK. Autoimmune haemolysis associated with Donath-Landsteiner antibodies. *Acta Haematol* 1982;68:268–277.
104. Worlledge SM, Rousso C. Studies of the serology of paroxysmal cold hemoglobinuria (PCH) with special reference to its relationship with P blood group system. *Vox Sang* 1965;10:293–298.
105. Schwarting GA, Kundu SK, Marcus DM. Reaction of antibodies that cause paroxysmal cold hemoglobinuria (PCH) with globoside and Forrsman glycosphingolipids. *Blood* 1979;53:186–192.
106. Garratty G, Nance S, Arndt P, et al. Positive direct monocyte monolayer assays associated with positive Donath Landsteiner tests. *Transfusion* 1989;29:49S.
107. Ackroyd JF. The pathogenesis of thrombocytopenic purpura due to hypersensitivity to Sedormid (allyisopropyl-acetylcarbamide). *Clin Sci* 1949;7:249–283.
108. Snapper I, Marks D, Schwartz L, et al. Hemolytic anemia secondary to Mesantoin. *Ann Intern Med* 1953;39:619–623.
109. Harris JW. Studies on the mechanism of drug-induced hemolytic anemia. *J Lab Clin Med* 1956;47:760–775.
110. Petz LD, Garratty G. *Acquired immune hemolytic anemias.* New York: Churchill Livingstone, 1980:267–304.
111. Christie DJ, Muller PC, Aster RH. Rab-mediated binding of drug-dependent antibodies to platelets in quinidine- and quinine-induced thrombocytopenia. *J Clin Invest* 1985;75:310–314.
112. Jordan JV, Smith ME, Reid DM, et al. A tolmetin-dependent antibody causing severe intravascular hemolysis binds to erythrocyte band 3 and requires only the $F(ab)_2$ domain to react. *Blood* 1985;66[Suppl]: 104a(abst).
113. Salama A, Mueller-Eckhardt C. On the mechanisms of sensitization

and attachment of antibodies to RBC in drug-induced immune hemolytic anemia. *Blood* 1987;69:1006–1010.
114. Levine B, Redmond A. Immunochemical mechanisms of penicillin induced Coombs positivity and hemolytic anemia in man. *Int Arch Allergy Appl Immunol* 1967;31:594–606.
115. Garratty G, Petz LD. Drug-induced immune hemolytic anemia. *Am J Med* 1975;58:398–407.
116. Petz LD. Immunologic cross-reactivity between penicillins and cephalosporins. A review. *J Infect Dis* 1978;137[Suppl]:74–79.
117. Gilliland BC. Drug-induced autoimmune and hematologic disorder. *Immunol Allergy Clin North Am* 1991;11:525–553.
118. Salama A, Mueller-Eckhardt C. Immune-mediated blood cell dyscrasias related to drugs. *Semin Hematol* 1992;29:54–63.
119. Duran-Suarez JR, Martin-Vega C, Argelagues E, et al. Red cell I antigen as immune complex receptor in drug-induced hemolytic anemias. *Vox Sang* 1981;41:313–315.
120. Pereira A, Sanz C, Cervantes F, et al. Immune hemolytic anemia and renal failure associated with rifampicin-dependent antibodies with anti-I specificity. *Ann Hematol* 1991;63:56–58.
121. Habibi B, Basty R, Chodez S, et al. Thiopental-related immune hemolytic anemia and renal failure. *N Engl J Med* 1985;312:353–355.
122. Sosler SD, Behzad O, Garratty G, et al. Acute hemolytic anemia associated with a chlorpropamide-induced apparent autoanti-JK[a]. *Transfusion* 1984;24:206–209.
123. Salama A, Mueller-Eckhardt C. The role of metabolite-specific antibodies in nomifensine-dependent immune hemolytic anemia. *N Engl J Med* 1985;313:469–474.
124. Salama A, Göttsche B, Mueller-Eckhardt C. Autoantibodies with drug- or metabolite-dependent antibodies in patients with diclofenac-induced immune haemolysis. *Br J Haematol* 1990;77:546–549.
125. Cunha PD, Lord RS, Johnson ST, et al. Immune hemolytic anemia caused by sensitivity to a metabolite of etodolac, a nonsteroidal anti-inflammatory drug. *Transfusion* 2000;40:663–668.
126. Shulman IA, Arndt PA, McGehee W, et al. Cefotaxime-induced immune hemolytic anemia due to antibodies reacting in vitro by more than one mechanism. *Transfusion* 1990;30:263–266.
127. Arndt PA, Leger RM, Garratty G. Serology of antibodies to second- and third-generation cephalosporins associated with immune hemolytic anemia and/or positive direct antiglobulin tests. *Transfusion* 1999;39:1239–1246.
128. Chambers LA, Donovan LM, Kruskall MS. Ceftazidime-induced hemolysis in a patient with drug-dependent antibodies reactive by immune complex and drug adsorption mechanisms. *Am J Clin Pathol* 1991;95:393–396.
129. Angeles ML, Reid ME, Yacob UA, et al. Sulindac-induced immune hemolytic anemia. *Transfusion* 1994;34:255–258.
130. van Duk BA, Barrera Rico P, Hoitsma A, et al. Immune hemolytic anemia associated with tolmetin and suprofen. *Transfusion* 1989;29: 638–641.
131. Hart MN, Mesara BW. Phenacetin antibody cross-reactive with autoimmune erythrocyte antibody. *Am J Clin Pathol* 1969;52:695–701.
132. Salama A, Northoff H, Burkhardt H, et al. Carbimazole-induced immune haemolytic anaemia: role of drug-red blood cell complexes for immunization. *Br J Haematol* 1988;68:479–482.
133. Carstairs KC, Breckenridge A, Dollery CT, et al. Incidence of a positive direct Coombs test in patients on α-methyldopa. *Lancet* 1966; 2:133–134.
134. Bakemeier RF, Leddy JP. Erythrocyte autoantibody association with α-methyldopa: heterogeneity of structure and specificity. *Blood* 1968; 32:1–14.
135. Kirtland HH, Mohler DN, Horwitz DA. Methyldopa inhibition of suppressor-lymphocyte function. A proposed cause of autoimmune hemolytic anemia. *N Engl J Med* 1980;302:825–832.
136. Garratty G, Arndt P, Prince HP, et al. The effect of methyldopa and procainamide on suppressor cell activity. *Br J Haematol* 1993; 84:310–315.
137. Kelton JG. Impaired reticuloendothelial function in patients treated with methyldopa. *N Engl J Med* 1985;313:596–600.
138. Lindstrom FD, Lieden G, Engstrom MS. Dose-related levodopa-induced haemolytic anaemia. *Ann Intern Med* 1977;86:298–300.
139. Scott GL, Myles AB, Bacon PA. Autoimmune haemolytic anaemia and mefenamic acid therapy. *Br J Med* 1968;3:534–535.
140. Kleinman S, Nelson R, Smith L, et al. Positive direct antiglobulin tests and immune hemolytic anemia in patients receiving procainamide. *N Engl J Med* 1984;311:809–812.
141. Spath P, Garratty G, Petz LD. Studies on the immune response to penicillin and cephalothin in humans. II. Immunohematologic reactions to cephalothin administration. *J Immunol* 1971;107:860–869.
142. Gralnick HR, McGinnis MH, Elton W, et al. Hemolytic anemia associated with cephalothin. *JAMA* 1971;217:1193–1197.
143. Zeger G, Smith L, McQuiston D, et al. Cisplatin-induced nonimmunologic adsorption of immunoglobulin by red cells. *Transfusion* 1988; 28:493–495.
144. Getaz EP, Beckley S, Fitzpatrick J, et al. Cisplatin-induced hemolysis. *N Engl J Med* 1980;302:334–335.
145. Rosse W. Paroxysmal nocturnal hemoglobinuria as a molecular disease. *Med* 1997;76:63–93.
146. Forman K, Sokol RJ, Hewitt S, et al. Paroxysmal nocturnal hemoglobinuria: a clinicopathological study of 26 cases. *Acta Haematol* 1984; 71:217–226.
147. Peytremann R, Rhodes RS, Harmann RC. Thrombosis in paroxysmal nocturnal hemoglobinuria (PNH) with particular reference to progressive, diffuse hepatic venous thrombosis. *Ser Haematol* 1972;5: 115–136.
148. Rosse WF. Hematopoiesis and the defect in paroxysmal nocturnal hemoglobinuria. *J Clin Invest* 1997;100:953–954.
149. Harris JW, Koscick R, Lazarus HM, et al. Leukemia arising our of paroxysmal nocturnal hemoglobinuria. *Leuk Lymphoma* 1999;32: 401–426.
150. Nafa K, Bessler M, Castro-Malaspina H, et al. The spectrum of somatic mutations in the PIG-A gene in paroxysmal nocturnal hemoglobinuria includes large deletions and small duplications. *Blood Cells Mol Dis* 1998;24:370–384.
151. Young NS, Maciejewski JP. Genetic and environmental effects in paroxysmal nocturnal hemoglobinuria: this little *PIG-A* goes "Why? Why? Why?" *J Clin Invest* 2000;106:637–641.
152. Benz EJ Jr. Clonal variation, autoimmunity, and neoplasia: an ecology lesson from paroxysmal nocturnal hemoglobinuria. *Ann Intern Med* 1999;131:467–468.
153. Sun X, Funk CD, Deng C, et al. Role of decay-accelerating factor in regulating complement activation on the erythrocyte surface as revealed by gene targeting. *Proc Natl Acad Sci U S A* 1999;96: 628–633.
154. Nicholson-Weller A, March JP, Rosenfeld SI, et al. Affected erythrocytes of patients with paroxysmal nocturnal hemoglobinuria are deficient in the complement regulatory protein, decay accelerating factor. *Proc Natl Acad Sci U S A* 1983;80:5066–5070.
155. Holguin MH, Fredrick LR, Bernshaw NJ, et al. Isolation and characterization of a membrane protein from normal human erythrocytes that inhibits reactive lysis of the erythrocyte of paroxysmal nocturnal hemoglobinuria. *J Clin Invest* 1989;84:7–17.
156. Wilcox LA, Ezzell JL, Bernshaw NJ, et al. Molecular basis of the enhanced susceptibility of the erythrocytes of paroxysmal nocturnal hemoglobinuria to hemolysis in acidified serum. *Blood* 1991;78: 820–829.
157. Hillmen P, Bessler M, Mason PJ, et al. Specific defect in N-acetylglucosamine incorporation in the biosynthesis of the glycosylphosphatidylinositol anchor in cloned cell lines from patients with paroxysmal nocturnal hemoglobinuria. *Proc Natl Acad Sci U S A* 1993;90: 5272–5276.
158. Motoyama N, Okada N, Yamashina M, et al. Paroxysmal nocturnal hemoglobinuria due to heredity nucleotide deletion in the HRF20 (CD59) gene. *Eur J Immunol* 1992;22:2669–2673.
159. Ninomiya H, Kawashima Y, Hasegawa Y, et al. Complement-induced procoagulant alteration of red blood cell membranes with microvesicle formation in paroxysmal nocturnal haemoglobinuria (PNH): implication for thrombogenesis in PNH. *Br J Haematol* 1999;106:224–231.
160. Ploug M, Plesnar T, Ronne E, et al. The receptor for urokinase-type plasminogen activator is deficient on peripheral leukocytes in patients

with paroxysmal nocturnal hemoglobinuria. *Blood* 1992;79: 1147–1455.
161. Jenkins DE Jr. Diagnostic tests for paroxysmal nocturnal hemoglobinuria. *Ser Haematol* 1972;5:24–41.
162. Rosse WF, Logue GL, Adams J, et al. Mechanisms of immune lysis of the red cells in hereditary erythroblastic multinuclearity with a positive acidified serum test and paroxysmal nocturnal hemoglobinuria. *J Clin Invest* 1974;53:31–43.
163. Hillmen P, Hows JM, Luzzatto L. Two distinct patterns of glycosylphosphatidylinositol (GPI) linked protein deficiency in the red cells of patients with paroxysmal nocturnal haemoglobinuria. *Br J Haematol* 1992;80:399–405.
164. Schubert J, Alvarado M, Uciechowski P, et al. Diagnosis of paroxysmal nocturnal haemoglobinuria using immunophenotyping of peripheral blood cells. *Br J Haematol* 1991;79:487–492.
165. Nilsson B, Hagstrom U, Englund A, et al. A simplified assay for the specific diagnosis of paroxysmal nocturnal hemoglobinuria: detection of DAF (CD55)- and HRF20 (CD50)-erythrocytes in microtyping cards. *Vox Sang* 1993;64:43–46.
166. Brodsky RA, Mukhina GL, Li S, et al. Improved detection and characterization of paroxysmal nocturnal hemoglobinuria using fluorescent aerolysin. *Am J Clin Pathol* 2000;114:459–466.
167. Rosse WF, Gutterman LA. The effect of iron therapy in paroxysmal nocturnal hemoglobinuria. *Blood* 1970;36:559–565.
168. Harrington WJ Sr, Kolodny L, Horstman LL, et al. Danazol for paroxysmal nocturnal hemoglobinuria. *Am J Hematol* 1997;54: 149–154.
169. Issaragrisil S, Piankijagum A, Tank-Naitrisorana Y. Corticosteroid therapy in paroxysmal nocturnal hemoglobinuria. *Am J Med* 1987; 25:77–83.
170. Braren V, Jenkins DE Jr, Phythyon JM, et al. Perioperative management of patients with paroxysmal nocturnal hemoglobinuria. *Surg Gynecol Obstet* 1981;153:515–520.
171. Stebler C, Tichelli A, Dazzi H, et al. High-dose recombinant human erythropoietin for treatment of anemia in myelodysplastic syndromes and paroxysmal nocturnal hemoglobinuria: a pilot study. *Exp Hematol* 1990;18:1204–1208.
172. Ninomiya H, Muraki Y, Shibuya K, et al. Induction of Fc γ R-III (CD16) expression on neutrophils affected by paroxysmal nocturnal hemoglobinuria by administration of granulocyte colony–stimulating factor. *Br J Haematol* 1993;84:497–503.
173. Perez-Oteyza J, Roldan E, Brieva JA, et al. Expression of phosphatidylinositol anchored membrane proteins in paroxysmal nocturnal haemoglobinuria after bone marrow transplantation. *Bone Marrow Transplant* 1992;10:297–299.
174. Saso R, Marsh J, Cevreska L, et al. Bone marrow transplants for paroxysmal nocturnal haemoglobinuria. *Br J Haematol* 1999;104: 392–396.
175. Ninomiya H, Kawashima Y, Nagasawa T. Inhibition of complement-mediated haemolysis in paroxysmal nocturnal hemoglobinuria by heparin or low–molecular weight heparin. *Br J Haematol* 2000;109: 875–881.
176. Sholar PW, Bell WR. Thrombolytic therapy for inferior vena cava thrombosis in paroxysmal nocturnal hemoglobinuria. *Ann Intern Med* 1985;103:539–541.
177. Rosse WF. Transfusion in paroxysmal nocturnal hemoglobinuria. To wash or not to wash? *Transfusion* 1989;29:663–664.
178. Sirchia G, Zanella A. Transfusion of PNH patients [Letter]. *Transfusion* 1990;30:479.
179. Payne PR, Holt JM, Neame PB. Paroxysmal nocturnal haemoglobinuria parturition complicated by presumed hepatic vein thrombosis. *J Obstet Gynecol Br Commonwealth* 1968;75:1066–1068.
180. De Gramont A, Krulik M, Debray J. Paroxysmal nocturnal hemoglobinuria and pregnancy. *Lancet* 1987;1:868.
181. Jackson GH, Noble RS, Maung ZT, et al. Severe haemolysis and renal failure in a patient with paroxysmal nocturnal haemoglobinuria. *J Clin Pathol* 1992;45:176–177.
182. Boklan BF, Palakavongs P, Conway JD, et al. Disseminated intravascular coagulation in paroxysmal nocturnal hemoglobinuria. *N Y State J Med* 1977;77:1942–1943.
183. Kuo C, Van Voolen GA, Morrison AN. Primary and secondary myelofibrosis its relationship to "PNH-like defect." *Blood* 1972;40: 875–880.
184. Devine DV, Gluck WL, Rosse WF, et al. Acute myeloblastic leukemia in paroxysmal nocturnal hemoglobinuria: evidence of evolution from the abnormal paroxysmal nocturnal hemoglobinuria clone. *J Clin Invest* 1987;79:314–317.
185. Shichishima T, Terasawa T, Hashimoto C, et al. Discordant and heterogeneous expression of GPI-anchored membrane proteins on leukemic cells in patient with paroxysmal nocturnal hemoglobinuria. *Blood* 1993;8:1855–1862.
186. Krause JR. Paroxysmal nocturnal hemoglobinuria and acute nonlymphocytic leukemia: a report of three cases exhibiting different cytologic types. *Cancer* 1983;51:2078–2082.
187. Jenkins DE Jr, Hartmann RC. Paroxysmal nocturnal hemoglobinuria terminating in acute myeloblastic leukemia. *Blood* 1969;33:274–282.
188. Dunn DE, Tanawattanacharoen P, Boccuni P, et al. Paroxysmal nocturnal hemoglobinuria cells in patients with bone marrow failure syndromes. *Ann Intern Med* 1999;131:401–408.
189. Noji H, Shichishima T, Ishikawa S, et al. Effective treatment combining antithymocyte globulin, cyclosporine, and granulocyte colony–stimulating factor for atypical paroxysmal nocturnal hemoglobinuria accompanied by bone marrow hypoplasia. *Rinsho Ketsueki* 1999;40:240–243.

Rossi's Principles of Transfusion Medicine, Third Edition, edited by Toby L. Simon, Walter H. Dzik, Edward L. Snyder, Christopher P. Stowell, and Ronald G. Strauss. Lippincott Williams & Wilkins, Philadelphia © 2002.

27

MANAGEMENT OF IMMUNE THROMBOCYTOPENIA

THEODORE E. WARKENTIN

Thrombocytopenia can be caused by platelet underproduction, sequestration, hemodilution, or destruction. In this chapter, we explore the problem of immune platelet destruction.

T.E. Warkentin: Hamilton Regional Laboratory Medicine Program, Hamilton Health Sciences Corporation, Hamilton, Ontario, Canada.

GENERAL TESTS TO INVESTIGATE THROMBOCYTOPENIA

Immune thrombocytopenia is characterized by a shortened platelet life span caused by platelet-antibody interactions. Several indirect clues suggest a shortened life span, such as a rapid decrease in platelet count or severe thrombocytopenia in a patient with normal megakaryocyte numbers. Radioactive markers sometimes are needed to establish the existence of a shortened platelet survival time (see Chapter 14).

Complete Blood Cell Count and Blood Film

Platelets usually are quantitated during a complete blood cell count with a particle counter. A normal platelet count usually is 150 to 400 × 10^9/L, although the reference range may be lower in Mediterranean populations (125 to 300 × 10^9/L) that have larger-sized platelets. The platelet count usually remains fairly stable throughout a normal human life span (1). An exception occurs during pregnancy, when the platelet count decreases somewhat, perhaps owing to increased plasma volume (hemodilution). An elevated platelet count also is normal 10 to 14 days after a major surgical procedure (postoperative thrombocytosis, 250 to 1,000 × 10^9/L) before return to preoperative baseline by 3 weeks after the operation (2). Thus a platelet count of only 190 × 10^9/L 10 days after an operation on a patient with dyspnea who had received postoperative heparin prophylaxis could represent pulmonary embolism complicating heparin-induced thrombocytopenia (HIT).

A useful general rule is that isolated thrombocytopenia usually is caused by increased platelet destruction, whereas bicytopenia or pancytopenia usually is attributable to marrow dysfunction, hypersplenism, or hemodilution. Isolated, severe thrombocytopenia (platelet count less than 20 × 10^9/L) often indicates platelet destruction by autoantibodies, alloantibodies, or drug-dependent immunoglobulin G (IgG) antibodies. Such severe thrombocytopenia, however, occasionally occurs in patients with HIT (3) or septicemia, although platelet count nadirs are typically more than 20 × 10^9/L in these disorders characterized by in vivo platelet activation by IgG antibodies or thrombin, respectively. Examining a blood film is important to exclude pseudothrombocytopenia (spurious thrombocytopenia resulting from antibodies that cause ex vivo platelet agglutination) and to suggest various nonimmune causes of thrombocytopenia, such as toxic leukocytes indicating infection or fragmented red blood cells suggesting microangiopathic hemolysis. In contrast, immune thrombocytopenia usually is characterized by reduction in platelet numbers with otherwise unremarkable morphologic features, unless the thrombocytopenia is secondary to a disorder such as lymphoma.

Platelet Size, Platelet RNA, and Plasma Glycocalicin

A particle counter also is used to determine average platelet size, or mean platelet volume (MPV), which usually ranges from 7.0 to 10.5 fl. Disorders of increased platelet destruction usually are characterized by large platelets, and MPV ranges from 10 to 15 fl. Normal-sized or small platelets are common in disorders of underproduction or sequestration of platelets. Results of one study suggested that modal platelet size (highest peak of the platelet size histogram) is better than MPV in differentiating platelet destruction from underproduction in children (4).

Young platelets contain residual amounts of RNA, which can be detected by means of flow cytometric analysis of platelets labeled with either thiazole orange or auramine-O. However, such quantitation of reticulated platelets has not gained the acceptance that red blood cell reticulocyte assays have. One problem is that thiazole orange also labels platelet-dense granules nonspecifically.

Levels of glycocalicin (a soluble proteolytic product of platelet glycoprotein Ib [GP Ib]) are increased in patients with increased platelet destruction. Because of factors such as platelet count, renal function, disease-related proteolysis, and technical considerations, this assay is used predominantly for research (5).

Bone Marrow Examination

Disorders of increased platelet destruction are characterized by normal or increased numbers of megakaryocytes in the bone marrow. Sometimes examination of the marrow yields enough information to determine the cause of the thrombocytopenia, such as myelodysplasia or megaloblastic anemia.

Measurement of Platelet Life Span

Measurement of the life span of platelets is the definitive test for classifying the cause of thrombocytopenia. Indium 111 is the radiolabel of choice because of its high labeling efficiency and efficient range of γ emissions. Indium 111 is not released from platelets by antiplatelet autoantibodies. Three patterns of platelet survival can be observed, as follows: (a) normal platelet recovery (60% to 75%) and a normal survival time (7 to 10 days) characterize thrombocytopenia caused by underproduction; (b) a markedly reduced platelet life span (sometimes only hours) is found in patients with thrombocytopenia caused by increased platelet destruction; and (c) reduced platelet recovery (as low as 10% to 30%) with a normal or near-normal platelet survival time confirms the diagnosis of thrombocytopenia caused by increased platelet sequestration (hypersplenism). Platelet life span studies are not often performed, however, because physicians usually infer the mechanism of the thrombocytopenia from the clinical situation.

PLATELET-ANTIBODY ASSAYS

There are two broad categories of platelet-antibody assays—classic platelet-associated IgG assays and newer assays that specify the protein target of the antibody (protein-specific assays).

Classic Platelet-associated Immunoglobulin G Assays

Measurement of platelet-associated IgG (PAIgG) has been widely available for 25 years. Unfortunately, these assays have limited diagnostic usefulness. A positive assay result does not differentiate immune from nonimmune thrombocytopenia (6). These assays can help detect either surface-associated immunoglobulin or complement by means of direct binding of a labeled antiimmunoglobulin probe or total platelet-associated IgG measured after platelet lysis.

Direct Binding Assays for Platelet Surface Immunoglobulin G

In direct binding assays, binding of a labeled antiimmunoglobulin probe to the platelet surface is quantitated. The antiimmunoglobulin probe is labeled with radioisotope, fluorescent marker, or an enzyme. In the assay, the labeled probe (e.g., anti-IgG, anti-IgM, or anticomplement) is incubated with the washed test platelets. The unbound probe is washed away, and the amount bound to the platelets is measured (6). Although these assays are simple, a disadvantage is that platelet membranes nonspecifically adsorb proteins, including the labeled probe. However, there is a more fundamental problem: even monoclonal antiimmunoglobulin probes despite their low nonspecific binding to platelet membranes cannot help differentiate immune from nonimmune thrombocytopenic disorders (6). This type of assay can be diagnostically useful, however, in special situations, such as detecting a drug-dependent increase in platelet surface-bound IgG in the presence of patient serum (7).

Total Platelet-associated Immunoglobulin G

The total amount of IgG, from both the interior and the surface of platelets, can be measured as total PAIgG (6). The test platelets are washed and counted, and the platelet membranes are lysed with either detergent or repeated freezing and thawing. The total amount of PAIgG in soluble form can be measured with any technique used to measure fluid-phase IgG, such as nephelometry or immunoradiometric assay. However, the limited diagnostic value of this assay is not surprising given that less than 1% of PAIgG is bound to the platelet surface.

Protein-specific Platelet-Antibody Assays

The diagnostic usefulness of platelet-antibody assays has increased dramatically with the introduction of various protein-specific assays that help identify the platelet protein target of antibodies with either monoclonal antibodies or electrophoretic techniques.

Monoclonal Antibody Assays

Various monoclonal antibody–based assays can be used to detect platelet antibodies. Perhaps most widely used is the monoclonal antibody–immobilization of platelet antigen (MAIPA) assay. An improved modified MAIPA assay (8) is shown in Figure 27.1A. A technically simpler assay is the antigen capture enzyme immunoassay, in which anti–platelet glycoprotein monoclonal antibodies interact with detergent-solubilized platelet samples (Fig. 27.1B), rather than intact platelets (7,9).

Simplicity and relatively high diagnostic specificity are advantages of these assays, especially for the antigen capture assay. In addition to investigation of autoimmune thrombocytopenia, these assays can be adapted for study of alloimmune disorders with a panel of platelet glycoproteins of known alloimmune phenotype or of drug-induced thrombocytopenia through demonstration of drug-dependent binding of antibody to platelet glycoproteins (7). A disadvantage, however, is that they help detect only antibodies that bind to platelet proteins captured with the monoclonal antibody, so a large number of monoclonal reagents are needed. These assays also can give false-negative results if the patient antibody binds to the same epitope recognized by the monoclonal antibody. Some human sera contain antibodies that recognize murine IgG, which is why the modified MAIPA and antigen capture assays are preferred to the original MAIPA (8).

Immunoprecipitation

In immunoprecipitation, patient serum or plasma is allowed to interact with labeled platelet membrane (10). The test platelets are isolated and washed, and the proteins on the platelet surface are either radiolabeled with iodine 125 or tagged with nonradioactive biotin. Either the patient's platelets are used (direct immunoprecipitation), or patient serum or plasma is mixed with target platelets (indirect immunoprecipitation). The proteins are then solubilized by addition of detergent, and the antibody-protein complex is precipitated by addition of an antiimmunoglobulin bound to a solid phase (e.g., immobilized staphylococcal protein A). The labeled protein-antibody complexes are washed, and the platelet proteins are separated by means of sodium dodecyl sulfate–polyacrylamide gel electrophoresis with detection by means of autoradiography or use of enzyme-conjugated streptavidin. The target antigen is identified according to its electrophoretic mobility.

Immunoprecipitation offers advantages over immunoblotting because the antibody can bind to native platelet proteins. In particular, this technique has allowed detection of clinically significant antibodies against previously unrecognized platelet proteins, such as anti-Gov^{a} alloantibodies on a 175-kd glycosylphosphatidylinositol-anchored protein (11). The main disadvantage of immunoprecipitation is technical difficulty. In addition, not all platelet proteins are optimally-labeled (e.g., GP IV, GP VI, GP IX).

Immunoblotting (Western Blotting)

In immunoblotting, patient serum is allowed to interact with platelet proteins that have been electrophoretically separated and then immobilized onto a solid phase (nitrocellulose paper). The test serum is added and after washing, binding of patient antibody (either IgG or IgM) to specific protein bands is ascertained with a labeled antiimmunoglobulin. Although immunoblotting offers the advantage of simplicity and the opportunity to store the immobilized proteins for long periods, a major disadvantage is that protein antigens are denatured in this method. Even normal serum can contain antibodies that react with certain denatured internal platelet proteins (e.g., vinculin, talin), making interpretation difficult.

Tests for Heparin-induced Thrombocytopenia

Special tests are required to detect the antibodies that cause HIT. These assays are classified as platelet activation or as platelet factor 4 (PF4)–dependent antigen assays (12).

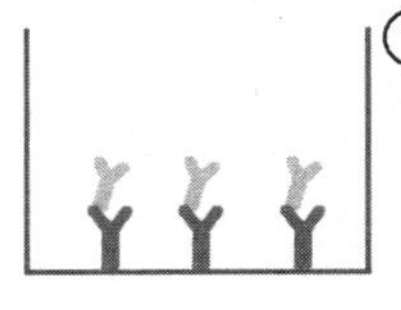
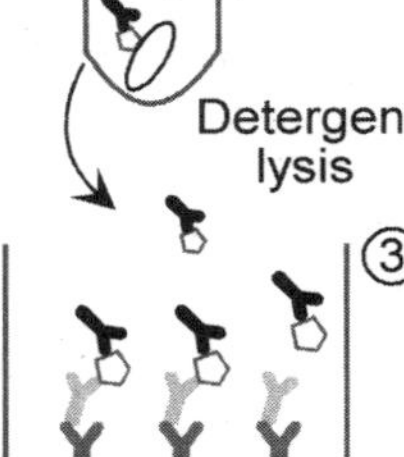
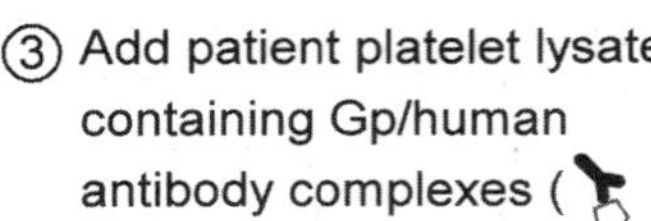

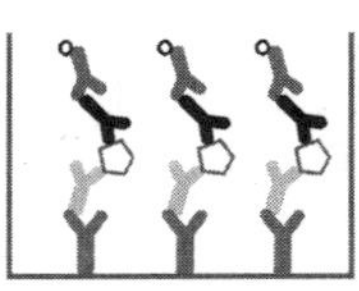

FIGURE 27.1. Modified monoclonal antibody–immobilization of platelet antigen (*MAIPA*) assay and antigen capture (*AC*) assay. "Direct" versions of both assays are shown, that is, the patient's platelets are tested for the presence of platelet glycoprotein (*GP*)–bound autoantibodies. (In indirect assays, the patient's serum or plasma is added to target platelets to detect the presence of serum or plasma anti–platelet glycoprotein antibodies.) **A:** In the MAIPA assay, the anti-glycoprotein monoclonal antibodies are added to washed intact patient platelets before detergent lysis (8). **B:** In the antigen capture assay, the patient's platelets are washed then lysed, and only later is anti-glycoprotein monoclonal antibody added (9). However, both assays resemble each other in the final stages (steps *4* and *5*). A relative advantage of the antigen capture assay is that platelets can be stored after initial washing and lysis. This means the assay can be performed later in batches. However, the early platelet lysis step also means that the antigen capture assay may detect antibodies against "internal" platelet antigens that may not be clinically pathogenic. *MoAb,* monoclonal antibody; *OD,* optical density.

Platelet Activation Assays

Heparin-induced thrombocytopenia antibodies have potent heparin-dependent, platelet-activating properties. Aggregation of platelets (prepared as citrate-anticoagulated platelet-rich plasma) by patient plasma detected with conventional platelet aggregometry once was a widely used assay for HIT; however, the sensitivity of this assay is relatively low for detecting HIT antibodies. In contrast, assays performed with washed platelets that have been resuspended in calcium-containing buffer, such as the platelet serotonin release assay (SRA) or heparin-induced platelet activation test, are both sensitive and specific for detecting clinically significant HIT antibodies (13). However, these assays are not widely available, because they are technically demanding, require careful platelet donor selection, and require a panel of strong and weak positive serum controls. Heparin-induced thrombocytopenia serum and plasma has a characteristic activation profile—platelet activation at therapeutic but not high heparin concentrations.

Platelet Factor 4 and Heparin Enzyme Immunoassay

In 1992, Amiral et al. (14) identified PF4 and heparin complexes as the antigen of HIT. Both commercial and in-house antigen assays based on enzyme immunoassay (EIA) methods have since become available. An intriguing feature of the HIT antigen is that certain polyanions other than heparin render PF4 antigenic. This is the basis of the PF4-polyvinylsulfonate EIA for HIT antibodies, available commercially in the United States since March 1999.

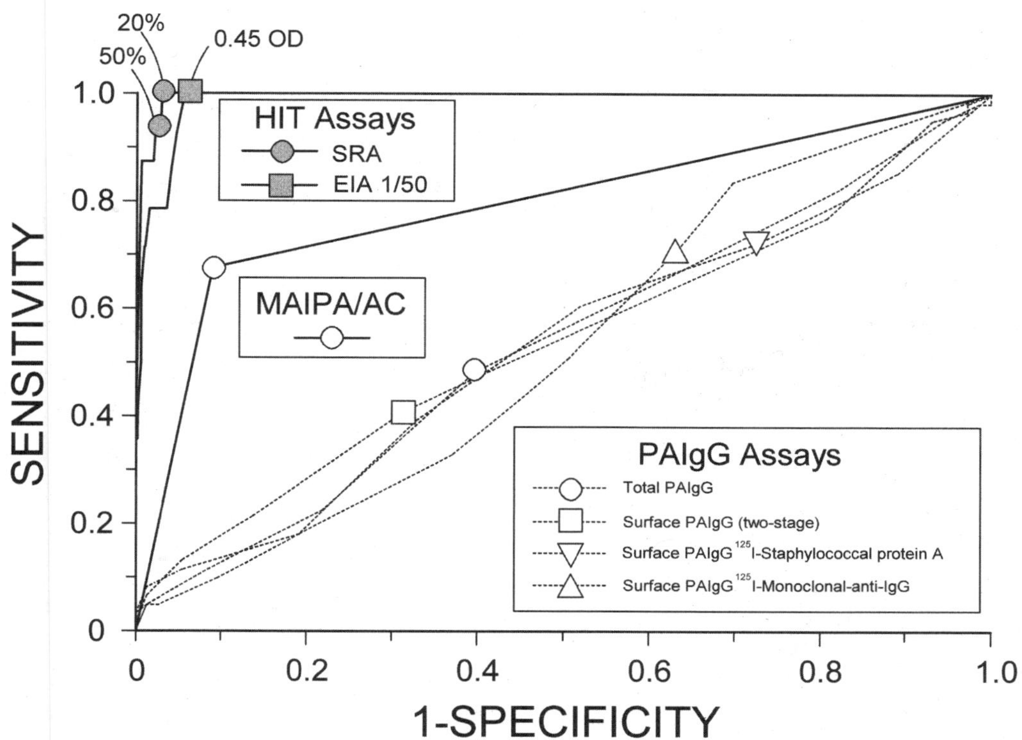

FIGURE 27.2. Operating characteristics of various platelet-antibody assays. The operating characteristics (sensitivity-specificity tradeoffs at various diagnostic cutoffs between positive and negative results) show that assays for heparin-induced thrombocytopenia (HIT) are diagnostically useful (high sensitivity and specificity) (2,13). The data for the HIT assays show two diagnostic cutoffs (20% and 50% serotonin release) for the serotonin release assay, and one diagnostic cutoff (0.45 optical density units) for the platelet factor 4–heparin enzyme immunoassay EIA (performed with serum at 1/50 dilution). In contrast, the modified monoclonal antibody–immobilization of platelet antigen (MAIPA) assay and antigen capture tests have moderate usefulness for diagnosis of autoimmune thrombocytopenia (high specificity but low to moderate sensitivity) (9), whereas conventional assays for platelet-associated immunoglobulin G (PAIgG) have minimal diagnostic value (6); that is, sensitivity is similar to 1-specificity. *Open symbols,* diagnostic cutoff actually used for each assay. The data used for the MAIPA, antigen capture, and PAIgG assays are from published sources (6,9). (From Warkentin TE. Laboratory testing for heparin-induced thrombocytopenia. *J Thromb Thrombolysis* 2001;10:S35–S45, with permission.)

Diagnostic Usefulness of Platelet-Antibody Assays

Figure 27.2 compares the operating characteristics (sensitivity-specificity trade-offs) for three types of platelet-antibody assays. Classic PAIgG assays provide limited diagnostic information (6), whereas the newer protein-specific platelet-antibody assays have moderate sensitivity and relatively high specificity for immune thrombocytopenia (9). Both the antigen and washed-platelet activation assays are useful for diagnosis of HIT (12,13).

PLATELET GENOTYPING

Serologic assays are generally reliable for detecting platelet alloantibodies. However, one disadvantage of antibody-based analysis is that there may not be sufficient platelets available from a patient with severe thrombocytopenia (e.g., posttransfusion purpura [PTP]) to allow determination of the reciprocal platelet alloantigen phenotype (15). Molecular techniques provide a reliable alternative to serologic phenotyping. Genomic DNA is used to determine the corresponding platelet alloantigen genotype. Sufficient DNA is readily available from a number of sources, including a small amount of peripheral blood. Molecular techniques also are useful in the evaluation of suspected neonatal alloimmune thrombocytopenia (NAT). Analysis of fetal cells (obtained by means of amniocentesis, chorionic villus sampling, or sampling of fetal blood) can help determine whether a fetus is at risk of this complication. Small amounts of fetal tissue can be studied (e.g., 5 to 10 ml of amniotic fluid), because the technique of polymerase chain reaction (PCR) greatly amplifies the fetal genomic DNA. The possibility of significant maternal DNA contamination of a fetal sample can be assessed with the forensic technique of variable-number tandem repeat analysis of the sample. The result is compared with the maternal profile to prove nonmaternal origin (16).

Polymerase Chain Reaction and Restriction Fragment Length Polymorphism

For all platelet alloantigen polymorphisms but one ($Pen^{a/b}$), the single base substitution responsible for the change in the expressed amino acid is associated with a restriction endonuclease recognition site (15). Accordingly, restriction fragment length polymorphism (RFLP) analysis was the first DNA-based genotyping assay developed to detect platelet alloantigens. Polymerase chain reaction–RFLP is a reliable but comparatively labor-intensive technique. In this method, a portion of the gene is PCR amplified. It contains both the platelet alloantigen gene polymorphism and another invariant region containing the same restriction site. When the amplified fragment is subjected to restriction enzyme digestion and separated by means of agarose gel electrophoresis, the position and number of fragments indicate the platelet antigen genotype. The invariant region always is cut by the enzyme regardless of the platelet alloantigen genotype and thus provides a means to assess the performance of the restriction enzyme. In this way, the platelet alloantigen genotype can be assessed accurately. One limitation is the possibility that another yet uncharacterized polymorphism within the amplified fragment could confound the genotyping, as has been seen for the *Msp* I site near Pl^{A2} (17).

Polymerase Chain Reaction and Oligonucleotide Dot Blotting

In this technique, the PCR-amplified fragment is blotted onto two nylon membranes, each of which is subsequently analyzed with a complementary oligonucleotide probe (usually approximately 20 bp in size) specific for either platelet allele. Stringency conditions are set so that the oligonucleotide binds only when there is 100% complementarity. The assay relies on the ability to differentiate a single nucleotide mismatch. However, like PCR-RFLP, this technique has the limitation that another polymorphism in the region of the oligonucleotide probe affects binding and can give a false-negative result. Therefore this assay is not suitable to assess the Tu^a (Ca^a) polymorphism because of the substitution of the degenerate nucleotide of the codon containing the wild-type polymorphism (18). The main advantage is that the assay can be readily semiautomated to allow simultaneous studies of many samples.

Allele-specific Polymerase Chain Reaction

For both RFLP and oligonucleotide dot-blotting analysis, the PCR is used to amplify a region of DNA containing the polymorphism. An alternative is the now widely used technique of allele-specific PCR in which one of the primers is specific for the particular allele to be amplified (19). With primers in which the allelic polymorphism is positioned at the 3′ end of the oligonucleotide, efficient amplification occurs only when the primer is 100% complementary to the genomic sequence. The only prerequisite is that *Taq* polymerase must be used for the PCR, because this enzyme does not repair single-base mismatches at the 3′ end of the primers that occur when the mismatch is present. Thus with each allele-specific primer with a common universal primer in separate reactions, amplification occurs only if the allele is present. The advantage of this method is that the PCR product is visualized directly in agarose gels to determine the genotype. A possible problem, however, is that absence of a signal can mean either that the genotype is absent or that the assay failed technically. (This is not a problem with PCR-RFLP, in which one of three predictable patterns based on one of the three allelic combinations, a/a, a/b, or b/b, invariably is seen.) One way to avoid such false-negative results with allele-specific PCR is to include with each mix an additional pair of primers designed to amplify a ubiquitous gene (usually human growth hormone) to provide the necessary internal control to show that the DNA was present. Again, allele-specific PCR can be used when unknown polymorphism occurs within the primer region. Unlike the situation for the previous two techniques discussed, however, single-base-pair mismatches have little effect on allele-specific PCR the farther they are from the 3′ end of the primer. The only theoretic concern is polymorphism in the position of the degenerate base of the next-to-last codon complementary to the primer (usually, the second or third nucleotide from the 3′ end of the allele-specific primer), which can cause a failure in PCR amplification regardless of a homologous match at the terminal nucleotide of the primer.

Real-time Polymerase Chain Reaction

Real-time PCR has improved both the speed and accuracy of genotyping (20). The use of glass microcapillary tubes and the addition of two specifically designed hybridization probes tagged with fluorescent dyes to the PCR mixture allow direct determination of the platelet genotype without gel electrophoresis or restriction enzymes, and in a single reaction. One hybridization probe, the donor, is tagged with a dye (fluorescein) and when excited with a light source emits light at a specific wavelength. The other probe, the acceptor, is tagged with a different dye. It straddles the single nucleotide polymorphism of interest and is 100% homologous to one of the platelet alleles. The acceptor probe usually is one nucleotide away from the donor probe in a head-to-tail arrangement; that is, the dyes are juxtaposed. The energy emitted by the dye of the donor probe is transferred to the adjacent dye of the acceptor probe, which emits light at a different wavelength. The intensity of the second light emitted is proportional to the amount of double-stranded DNA present. Unbound donor probe in the mixture can be excited but cannot transfer energy to the acceptor probe. At the end of the PCR, the platelet genotype is determined by means of melting curve analysis. Because the acceptor probe straddles the polymorphism and is 100% homologous to one of the alleles, the melting curve has a different temperature midpoint (T_m) depending on whether a mismatch is present. A properly designed acceptor probe can have as much as 5° to 8°C. difference in T_m between the two platelet alleles. In all, three melting curves are seen, one for each polymorphism, as is a composite melting curve when the heterozygous situation is present (20). The advantage of fluorescence-based real-time PCR with melting curve analysis is that the PCR product is measured directly and no further manipulation is required. Any additional polymorphism in the region of the acceptor probe is detected in the melting curve analysis. Because glass microcapillary tubes are used, thermal cycling usually is 40 minutes or less. Because the DNA can be obtained in less than 45 minutes, a platelet genotype can be determined within 2 hours of specimen collection.

PATHOPHYSIOLOGY OF IMMUNE PLATELET DESTRUCTION

Immune thrombocytopenia results from antibody-mediated platelet destruction. The IgG-sensitized platelets are phagocytosed by the monocytes and macrophages of the reticuloendothelial system. Reticuloendothelial cells are located throughout the body but are concentrated in the spleen, liver, lungs, and bone marrow. Pathogenic antibodies usually bind to platelets through the Fab termini, usually against specific autoantigen or alloantigen epitopes. Sometimes the target antigen is produced by a drug or drug metabolite. The result is a ternary complex that involves IgG Fab, drug, and a specific region on a platelet glycoprotein. Heparin-induced thrombocytopenia is an exception to these generalizations: although HIT antibodies bind to PF4-heparin complexes through the Fab termini, the Fc moieties of IgG interact with platelet FcγIIa receptors and produce platelet activation.

The rate of platelet destruction is determined by the quantity and subclass distribution of IgG on the platelet, the amount of complement, and the efficiency of reticuloendothelial clearance. The severity of thrombocytopenia reflects the balance between the rate of platelet destruction and the compensatory marrow thrombopoiesis.

IDIOPATHIC (IMMUNE) THROMBOCYTOPENIC PURPURA

Idiopathic thrombocytopenic purpura (ITP), also known as primary (auto)immune thrombocytopenic purpura, is a common disorder characterized by accelerated platelet destruction caused by platelet-reactive autoantibodies. It is defined as isolated thrombocytopenia with no clinically apparent associated conditions or other explanation such as human immunodeficiency virus (HIV) infection, systemic lupus erythematosus (SLE), lymphoproliferative disorders, myelodysplasia, hypogammaglobulinemia, drug-induced thrombocytopenia, alloimmune thrombocytopenia, or congenital or hereditary thrombocytopenia (21). Until recently, ITP was essentially a diagnosis of exclusion, but newer platelet-antibody assays now allow detection of platelet glycoprotein–reactive autoantibodies in at least 75% of patients with ITP with good diagnostic specificity (9, 22).

Pathogenesis

The basic pathogenesis of ITP was defined by Harrington et al. 50 years ago (23). They showed that ITP plasma infused into healthy volunteers caused acute severe thrombocytopenia. The platelet-destroying plasma factor was later shown to be IgG, although in some patients, IgM and IgA antibodies may be pathogenic. The immune target of the autoantibodies usually is one of the two major platelet glycoprotein complexes, with GP IIb/IIIa implicated more often than GP Ib/IX (9,22). Other less common autoantigen targets include GP Ia/IIa and, possibly, nonprotein targets such as glycosphingolipids.

The spleen is an important site of antibody production and is the dominant organ that clears IgG-sensitized platelets in most patients. The antibodies bind to platelets by way of their Fab termini and can cause binding of complement in vitro. However, in vivo complement-mediated platelet lysis has never been proved and seems unlikely on the basis of normal plasma β-thromboglobulin levels (a marker of platelet lysis) in patients with ITP (24). Megakaryocyte injury by autoantibodies decreases platelet production in some patients (22).

A fundamental research problem in ITP is to understand the relation between pathogenic platelet-reactive autoantibodies and measured PAIgG. Doubt regarding the pathogenic significance of elevated PAIgG levels was raised by the observation that even nonimmunoglobulin proteins, such as albumin, are elevated on platelets of patients with ITP (25). Results of subsequent investigations suggested that elevated PAIgG and albumin levels in ITP and other disorders with increased platelet turnover are caused by increased endocytosis of these plasma proteins into platelet α granules, which occurs either in megakaryocytes or mature platelets (26,27). Electron microscopic examination and immunogold labeling of IgG show increased amounts of IgG within the α granules as well as the open canalicular system and platelet surface of patients with ITP (28).

The fundamental cause of autoantibody formation in ITP is not known. Light-chain restriction of platelet-reactive antibodies suggests a clonal or oligoclonal origin of autoantibodies in chronic ITP (22). Further, the autoepitopes involved may be fairly narrow in scope (autoantigen hot spots).

Clinical and Laboratory Features

Patients are arbitrarily considered to have chronic ITP when thrombocytopenia has lasted more than 6 months. Although chronic ITP can occur at any age and in both sexes, women between 30 and 50 years of age are affected most often (female to male ratio, approximately 3:1). This condition usually is asymptomatic, or the symptoms and signs are limited to bleeding. If clinical evaluation reveals weight loss, fever, lymphadenopathy, hepatomegaly or splenomegaly, other diagnoses should be considered. Some physicians perform routine screening for thyroid disease (21), because both hyperthyroidism and hypothyroidism are associated with ITP.

The onset of bleeding symptoms typically is insidious. Mucocutaneous bleeding is the hallmark of ITP and manifests as purpura (petechiae, ecchymosis), epistaxis, menorrhagia, and oral mucosal and gastrointestinal bleeding. Aspirin ingestion can cause bleeding in a patient who otherwise has no symptoms. Idiopathic thrombocytopenic purpura can be life threatening; for example, spontaneous intracranial hemorrhage occurs secondary to severe thrombocytopenia. The risk of fatal bleeding is substantially higher among elderly patients with ITP (29). On the other hand, many patients even with severe thrombocytopenia have minimal or no bleeding, possibly because of the presence of small numbers of young, reticulated platelets with enhanced α-granule release to platelet agonists (30).

The complete blood cell count usually reveals isolated thrombocytopenia, although microcytic anemia can indicate iron deficiency in patients with chronic bleeding. The MPV usually is increased, although some patients with severe ITP can have a normal or even low MPV. The bone marrow examination shows normal or increased megakaryocyte numbers. The bleeding time usually is elevated only when the platelet count is less than 30 $\times$ 10^9/L. An elevated bleeding time with a high platelet count rarely is caused by autoantibodies that interfere with platelet glycoprotein function. Approximately 15% to 25% of patients with otherwise typical ITP have a positive result of an antinuclear antibody test, usually low titer. These patients generally do not have a different clinical outcome than do patients with negative antinuclear antibody results (31). Direct platelet-antibody assays that entail use of monoclonal antibody–based assays are more sensitive than are indirect assays with patient serum or plasma (~75% versus 50% sensitivity) (22).

Treatment Overview

The principles of treatment of adults with ITP are based on the following considerations:

1. Most patients with ITP have hyperfunctional platelets associated with an increased MPV. Thus many patients do not need treatment despite the existence of moderate or even severe thrombocytopenia.
2. The goal of treatment is to achieve a safe platelet count, not necessarily a normal count. The presence of petechiae might be helpful in assessing the need for treatment of a patient with minimal bleeding. Prophylactic platelet transfusions are rarely indicated in the management of ITP. Although a transient increase in platelet count usually can be achieved (32), the benefits of a short-lived increase in a chronic disorder are doubtful. Platelet transfusions are indicated in the care of patients with life-threatening bleeding (see later).
3. Most adults have chronic ITP; the rate of spontaneous remission is estimated to be only 5% (21). Thus the long-term risks of treatment must be balanced against the long-term risks of life-threatening bleeding. Most adults are not cured by a prolonged course of prednisone but often develop significant morbidity from this agent. Splenectomy offers a good chance for a long-term cure of ITP and avoids the long-term toxicity of medical therapy.
4. The first-line therapies of glucocorticoids and splenectomy fail in approximately 10% to 15% of cases. For these patients, the treatment options are less satisfactory. It is important to exclude an accessory spleen in these patients. Numerous alternative treatments are available, including danazol, vinca alkaloids, cyclophosphamide, azathioprine, intravenous immune globulin (IVIG), antirhesus globulin (anti-D), and cyclosporine, among others.
5. Patients should avoid drugs that interfere with platelet function, particularly aspirin, nonsteroidal antiinflammatory agents, and alcohol.

First-line Therapy

Glucocorticoids

Glucocorticoids improve platelet survival in ITP by reducing both reticuloendothelial phagocytic activity and synthesis of pathogenic autoantibodies. Glucocorticoids also may reduce capillary leakiness, an observation that could explain the reduction in bleeding that sometimes precedes the increase in platelet count.

The standard initial dosage of prednisone is 1 mg/kg per day, usually given until the platelet count has increased to safe values. Regardless of the response, tapering usually is started on the fourteenth day of therapy, if not sooner. Two prospective studies (33, 34) compared conventional and lower-dose prednisone therapy (1 mg/kg versus 0.25 mg/kg per day in one trial, 1.5 mg/kg versus 0.5 mg/kg per day in the other). There was no significant difference in remission at 6-month follow-up evaluation. In the larger study (34), however, the higher-dose regimen showed a trend to a higher rate of complete remission (46% versus 35%) as well as higher platelet counts at 14-day follow-up evaluation (77% versus 51% having a platelet count more than 50 $\times$ 10^9/L).

In a small trial (35), prednisone (1 mg/kg per day) resulted in short- and long-term outcomes at least as good as that achieved with either IVIG or the combination of both treatments. Whether repeated use of anti-D as initial therapy provides better outcome than conventional first-line therapy is under investigation.

Very large doses of glucocorticoids, such as pulse methylprednisolone (1 g over 30 minutes once daily for 3 days) and intermittent high-dose dexamethasone, have been used to manage ITP with variable results (36). Comparative trials with standard-dose prednisone are lacking.

At least two-thirds of patients attain safe platelet counts (minimum, 30 $\times$ 10^9/L) within 1 to 2 weeks of receiving glucocorticoids. Most responders achieve platelet counts greater than 100 to 150 $\times$ 10^9/L. However, ITP in adults usually is a chronic disorder, and most patients have a relapse of thrombocytopenia either during tapering of prednisone, or even months or years after discontinuation of the drug (37).

Overall, approximately 30% of patients are in complete remission (normal platelet count) soon after stopping prednisone, and another 20% are in partial remission (platelet count, 50 to 150 $\times$ 10^9/L) (33,34,38,39). Thus approximately one-half of patients who receive prednisone have a safe platelet count during the early follow-up period after stopping the drug. Patients with shorter duration of bleeding symptoms are more likely to respond favorably (39). For patients who suffer relapse of thrombocytopenia after initial complete remission, an additional course of prednisone can be effective (38).

Results of studies with longer follow-up periods indicate that the continuing risk of relapse among adult patients with initial complete remission is substantial. For example, one study (38) showed that only 29% of adult patients who entered complete remission remained in remission 4 years later. In summary, only approximately 10% to 15% of adult patients with ITP who receive prednisone have a durable remission. Consequently, most need either long-term medical treatment or splenectomy.

Common adverse effects of prednisone occurring among 5% to 20% of patients treated include facial swelling, weight gain, and behavioral changes (21,39). Less common (1% to 5%) but important complications include infection, myopathy, hyperglycemia, psychosis, hypertension, and hypokalemia. Osteonecrosis, most commonly involving the femoral head, occurs as a late side effect in approximately 5% of patients who undergo prolonged therapy. This complication sometimes occurs after intensive short-term glucocorticoid therapy (40).

Splenectomy

Splenectomy frequently is successful because for most patients the spleen is the major site of both autoantibody production and platelet destruction. Complete remission occurs in approximately 75% of patients within 4 to 6 weeks after splenectomy (39,41). In these complete responders, normal platelet counts are reached within 7 days in 90% and within 6 weeks in 98% of patients; spontaneous remission rarely is encountered thereafter. In a further 5% to 10% of patients, partial remission is achieved. Of the remaining nonresponders, some now benefit from low doses of prednisone.

Features associated with a higher probability of response to splenectomy include a previous response to glucocorticoids (41) or IVIG (42), younger age (41), and predominantly splenic clearance of platelets, as shown with radionuclide platelet imaging techniques (43). However, splenectomy results in complete or partial remission among at least 50% of patients who lack one or more of these favorable prognostic features. Unlike those who undergo glucocorticoid therapy, patients with longer duration of thrombocytopenia are not less likely to respond to splenectomy (39). The risk of thrombocytopenic relapse after complete postsplenectomy remission is low (approximately 10% to 15% at 10 years).

Laparascopic splenectomy is an increasingly popular surgical approach to management of ITP. The results are similar to those of open splenectomy (44). A concern is that residual spleen tissue (accessory spleens) may be present more frequently than with open splenectomy. (Accessory spleens are found in approximately 20% of patients undergoing open splenectomy for ITP.) Regardless of the technique used, careful intraoperative searching for accessory spleens is important to reduce the risk of postsplenectomy failure or relapse of ITP.

The presence of residual accessory spleen should be considered when splenectomy fails, including patients with relapse of ITP months or years postoperatively (45). Postsplenectomy blood film changes (e.g., Howell-Jolly bodies) do not necessarily eliminate the possibility of a residual accessory spleen. Approximately 10% to 50% of patients with postsplenectomy relapse have accessory spleens detected with sensitive radionuclide imaging, such as heat-damaged red blood cells labeled with technetium 99m (45) or indium 111–labeled platelets. Approximately two thirds achieve partial or complete remission after removal of the accessory spleen, which can be performed by means of open or laparoscopic technique.

Perioperative morbidity after splenectomy is less than 10%. The most frequent complications are pleuropulmonary (pneumonia, subphrenic abscess, pleural effusion) in 4% of patients, major bleeding in 1.5%, and thromboembolism in 1%. Morbidity is probably even lower when laparoscopic splenectomy is performed by an experienced surgeon. Perioperative mortality is less than 1%. The major long-term risk is overwhelming postsplenectomy infection (OPSI), although this is rare in appropriately immunized adult patients who have undergone splenectomy for ITP.

Perioperative management of splenectomy involves (a) optimizing the platelet count before surgery; (b) vaccination to minimize risk of OPSI, and (c) prevention of thromboembolism. Adequate perioperative hemostasis usually can be achieved with preoperative high-dose IVIG or glucocorticoids. Sometimes despite these measures, patients have thrombocytopenia at splenectomy. However, most of these do not have excessive bleeding; therefore platelet transfusions should not be given prophylactically but only for suspected perioperative bleeding. The risk of fatal OPSI in adults who have undergone splenectomy (prevaccination era) was estimated at 1 death per 1,000 to 1,500 patient-years (46). All patients should be vaccinated with polyvalent pneumococcal vaccine, quadrivalent meningococcal polysaccharide vaccine, and *Haemophilus influenzae* type b vaccine (47). If possible, the vaccines should be given at least 2 weeks before the planned splenectomy, because effectiveness may be blunted after splenectomy. Paradoxically, postoperative thromboembolism is the most common cause of postoperative mortality; thus, for patients with delayed postoperative mobilization, prophylactic low-molecular-weight heparin should be considered when the platelet count is recovering.

Long-term Management: Second-line Therapy

Approximately 10% to 15% of patients with ITP do not have a durable response to prednisone followed by splenectomy. The large number of therapies that have been used for these treatment failures attests to the difficulty in caring for such patients.

Danazol

Danazol is an attenuated androgen with mild virilizing effects that can be used to treat men and nonpregnant women. There is evidence its mechanism of action is counteracting the effects of estrogens on reticuloendothelial cells (estrogens increase Fc receptor numbers and the rate of clearance of IgG-sensitized red blood cells). Danazol decreases the number of monocyte IgG Fc receptor (48). Usually, 400 to 800 mg is administered daily in divided doses, although some physicians use low doses (50 mg/d). A response usually occurs within 2 months, although when low doses are used, as long as 6 months may be needed.

Danazol appears to produce a sustained increase in platelet count in approximately 30% to 40% of treated patients. The response rate may be higher among patients with associated rheumatologic disorders (49). Danazol usually must be continued to maintain the platelet count, although the physician should attempt periodically to decrease the dose.

Danazol is generally well tolerated. The most frequent adverse effects are fluid retention, nausea, amenorrhea, and liver dysfunction. Rarely encountered side effects include peliosis of the liver and spleen, headache, increased fibrinolysis, and mild virilization. Fetal damage precludes use during pregnancy. In rare instances, idiosyncratic thrombocytopenia is caused by danazol.

Vinca Alkaloids

Vinca alkaloids (vincristine, vinblastine) can produce generally short-lived increases in platelet count in approximately 65% of patients (50). These drugs bind to platelet microtubules and so might work by being delivered to, and thereby inhibiting, reticuloendothelial macrophages. Because other reticuloendothelial inhibiting agents (IVIG, anti-D) have similar short-term efficacy with less toxicity, vinca alkaloids are now rarely used to treat patients with ITP. Side effects include neutropenia, alopecia, and peripheral neuropathy.

Cyclophosphamide, Azathioprine

Cyclophosphamide and azathioprine have similar immunosuppressive activity, clinical efficacy, and toxicity. Cyclophosphamide is an alkylating agent, whereas azathioprine is metabolized to 6-mercaptopurine, a purine antimetabolite. Either drug as a single agent at a dose of 1 to 2 mg/kg per day has been used to treat patients with refractory ITP. The dose is decreased if leukopenia develops. It usually takes a minimum of 2 to 4 weeks before a response to either agent occurs, and sometimes treatment must be given for 3 to 6 months before a response is seen. Cyclophosphamide also has been given in intermittent pulses (1.0 to 1.5 g/m^2 every 4 weeks by rapid intravenous infusion) (51). Cyclophosphamide sometimes is combined with other cytotoxic agents in a regimen resembling antineoplasia therapy.

Approximately two-thirds of patients have some platelet count response to either cyclophosphamide or azathioprine; however, only approximately 20% to 30% have complete remission that persists after the drug is stopped. Both agents cause myelosuppression and alopecia and carry a long-term risk of secondary neoplasia and infertility. Acute leukemia has been reported after use of cyclophosphamide for chronic ITP (52). Animal studies suggest that intermittent treatment may be less leukemogenic than is daily administration. Cyclophosphamide also can cause hemorrhagic cystitis and hepatic toxicity.

Intravenous Immune Globulin

High-dose IVIG has been used to manage ITP since 1981 (53). Prepared by means of ethanol precipitation of pooled plasma followed by a technique to minimize IgG self-aggregation, monomeric IgG is stabilized with sugar. Thus more than 95% of IVIG consists of monomeric IgG. Immunoglobulin G aggregates, IgA, and other contaminants constitute a negligible fraction. The IgG possesses both Fab and Fc activities required for antigen neutralization and reticuloendothelial cell interaction, respectively, and has the expected half-lives and subclass distribution of human IgG.

Reticuloendothelial blockade probably explains the efficacy of IVIG in the management of ITP, but suppression of autoantibody synthesis also has been postulated (54). Treatment with high-dose IVIG increases serum IgG concentration twofold to fourfold, a level that blocks clearance of radiolabeled, IgG-sensitized red blood cells. Monomeric IgG is in equilibrium with the Fc receptors on the reticuloendothelial cells, and even though the binding affinity of these Fc receptors for monomeric IgG is low, the high plasma IgG concentration results in receptor occupancy. However, this reticuloendothelial blockade theory cannot explain the occasional long-term response to IVIG treatment, nor can it account for the observation that Fc-depleted immunoglobulin preparations can be effective in the management of ITP. Thus immune suppression by IVIG can occur, either through poorly defined nonspecific effects of large amounts of IgG in reducing antibody synthesis, or perhaps by specific interaction of certain IgG molecules (antiidiotype antibodies) within the IVIG preparation against the Fab regions of the pathogenic autoantibodies.

In a small, randomized trial, IVIG was not superior to prednisone as initial therapy for adult ITP (35). Intravenous immune globulin is very expensive (55). Thus use of this agent usually is limited to patients with ITP in whom a rapid increase in platelet count is needed, as for emergency treatment of a patient who is bleeding or have severe thrombocytopenia or for preoperative preparation.

The usual dose of IVIG is 2 g/kg, given either as 0.4 g/kg for 5 consecutive days or as 1 g/kg given twice, either 1 or 2 days apart. One trial showed no difference between one dose of 1 g/kg and two doses 1 day apart (56). Thus one approach is to give 1 g/kg as a single dose and to repeat the dose 2 days later if no significant platelet count increase has occurred. This may avoid unnecessary use of a second dose. To minimize acute side effects, the infusion is given over at least 4 to 8 hours, as tolerated. Several preparations are available, although there is no evidence that any offers a major advantage over another.

Intravenous immune globulin increases the platelet count to more than 50×10^9/L in approximately 80% of adult patients with chronic ITP, usually beginning within 1 to 3 days of the start of treatment. In more than half of the responders, platelet count becomes normal. Unfortunately, the response usually is transient. Peak platelet count usually occurs 5 to 10 days after the start of treatment and returns to baseline within 2 to 4 weeks. There is no difference in response among patients of differing ABO or Rh groups.

Although long-lasting complete remission after a single course of IVIG for chronic ITP in adults is uncommon, repeating treatments a few weeks apart results in complete or partial remission without need for further IVIG in approximately one-third of patients (56). Of the remaining patients, approximately one-half continue to respond to ongoing maintenance therapy, and one-half experience refractoriness. However, the high cost and limited availability of IVIG generally preclude use of this agent in maintenance therapy for chronic ITP.

Use of IVIG is relatively safe. Common but usually mild side effects, which occur among 15% to 75% of patients, include headache, backache, nausea, flushing, and fever (21). These can be controlled by temporarily stopping or reducing the rate of infusion. Premedication with acetaminophen, antihistamine, or glucocorticoids can be helpful. Chest pain, hypertension, hypotension, bronchospasm, and laryngeal edema are described, but are uncommon. Other rare side effects include hemolysis caused by ABO alloantibodies within the IVIG, acute cryoglobulinemic nephropathy in rheumatoid factor-positive recipients, and aseptic meningitis (21). High-dose IVIG also has been associated with acute myocardial infarction (57) and thrombotic stroke, particularly in elderly patients. Because IVIG is prepared from pooled plasma from thousands of donors, there is the potential for infection, but the product has been free from transmission of disease since 1994 (see Chapter 24).

Anti-Rhesus Globulin (Anti-D)

Like IVIG, the mechanism of action of anti-D is believed to be reticuloendothelial blockade, which probably occurs through occupancy of the reticuloendothelial cell Fc receptors by the IgG-sensitized red blood cells. The result is less platelet clearance. Thus the therapy is ineffective in the treatment of Rhesus [Rh_0(D)]–negative persons. Further support for this mechanism of action is the observation that plasma containing high-titer anti-c alloantibodies also can increase the platelet count of patients with ITP whose red blood cells bear this Rhesus system alloantigen. Anti-D usually is ineffective in the treatment of patients who have undergone splenectomy (58).

A total dose of 25 to 75 μg/kg usually is given over 2 to 5 days. A well-studied regimen is to administer 25 μg/kg of anti-D intravenously over 3 to 5 minutes and to administer the same dose 2 days later if no or only a minimal platelet count response has occurred (56,58). Small intermittent maintenance doses have been given to responding patients, possibly obviating splenectomy.

The likelihood of response is similar to that of IVIG, and likewise the increase in platelet count following anti-D treatment usually is transient (2 to 4 weeks), although long-term remissions sometimes occur. The peak platelet count tends to be lower with anti-D than with IVIG, but the time to reach peak platelet count often is longer; therefore a greater interval between maintenance injections may be possible with anti-D (59). Some patients who do not respond to IVIG respond to anti-D, and vice versa. Costs associated with use of anti-D in the United States are approximately 35% to 60% less than with use of IVIG (55).

The only clinically important adverse effect of anti-D is alloimmune hemolysis. Usually only a positive result of a direct antiglobulin test (100% of patients) and a decrease in hemoglobin level (<20 g/L) occurs. However, in at least 1 of 1,000 recipients, life-threatening acute intravascular hemolysis necessitates transfusion or even hemodialysis (60). Such patients have usually received the U.S. Food and Drug Administration–approved dose of 50 μg/kg, and the explanation for the severe hemolysis is unknown. Although current anti-D preparations are considered pathogen free, the theoretic risk of transmitting infection is illustrated by the epidemic of hepatitis C during 1978 and 1979 in Ireland. It affected young mothers who received perinatal anti-D contaminated with this virus from a single infected donor (61). Current availability of solvent-detergent anti-D should make the risk of infection negligible. Table 27.1 compares IVIG and anti-D.

Miscellaneous Treatments

Other treatments (21) with anecdotal, at least transient, benefit for some patients with ITP include: interferon-alfa, cyclosporine, Fc-receptor-blocking or B-lymphocyte-depleting monoclonal antibodies, and others (colchicine, dapsone, protein A immunoadsorption, plasmapheresis). Initial promising results of interferon-alfa-2b for refractory ITP have not been confirmed. Responses, when they occur, are generally transient, and a few patients appear to have worse thrombocytopenia and bleeding (62). In contrast, this agent usually increases the platelet count of patients with isolated thrombocytopenia caused by chronic hepatitis C infection (63).

Cyclosporine selectively inhibits adaptive immune responses by blocking T-cell-dependent biosynthesis of lymphokines, particularly interleukin-2, at the level of messenger RNA transcription. Several different groups have reported at least transient benefit to this drug in the care of both adults and children with refractory ITP (64). Experimental treatments with Fc-receptor-blocking monoclonal antibody or the humanized B-lymphocyte depleting monoclonal antibody rituximab (65) have been used

TABLE 27.1. COMPARISON OF HIGH-DOSE INTRAVENOUS IMMUNE GLOBULIN (IVIG) AND ANTI-D FOR MANAGEMENT OF IMMUNE THROMBOCYTOPENIC PURPURA (ITP)

Characteristic	High-Dose IVIG	Anti-D (Anti-Rhesus Globulin)
Side effects	Common: headache, hypertension, fever and chills Rare: hemolysis, renal failure, myocardial infarction, stroke	Common: mild hemolysis Rare: severe hemolysis necessitating transfusion or hemodialysis
Response rate	~80%	~80%
Response duration	Usually transient	Usually transient
Pattern of platelet increase	Faster increase, higher peak, shorter duration of response	Slower increase, lower peak, longer duration of response
Influence of ABO, Rh type	No influence	Only D-positive patients respond
Influence of splenectomy	Unknown	Minimal response in patients without a spleen
Suitability for emergency management of ITP	Recommended	Not recommended

successfully to manage severe immune-mediated thrombocytopenia.

Special Treatment Situations

Emergency Treatment of a Bleeding Patient

Any patient with ITP who has life-threatening bleeding needs immediate platelet transfusion (5 to 10 $\times$ 10^{11} platelets, or approximately 5 to 10 units). The patient then should receive IVIG (1 g/kg) over 4 to 6 hours to block the reticuloendothelial system and then receive more platelet transfusions (66). Some physicians use continuous infusions of IVIG and platelets for this situation (67). Other treatments (e.g., glucocorticoids) to achieve longer-term control of thrombocytopenia should be started simultaneously.

Preparation for Invasive Procedures

High-dose IVIG usually is the treatment of choice of severely thrombocytopenic patients with ITP who need urgent surgery or an invasive procedure. Timing of prophylactic platelet transfusion when deemed necessary should be aimed for when maximal hemostasis is required, because any increment in platelet count is very transient. For situations in which at least 2 or 3 days are available before the planned procedure, less expensive and equally effective options include glucocorticoids or anti-D.

Idiopathic (Immune) Thrombocytopenic Purpura in Pregnancy

Thrombocytopenia during pregnancy usually is not caused by ITP. Rather, a benign condition known as *incidental* or *gestational thrombocytopenia* is the most likely cause. It occurs in approximately 5% of pregnancies at term. Newborns of mothers with incidental thrombocytopenia are not at increased risk of neonatal thrombocytopenia (68). The second most likely cause of thrombocytopenia is pregnancy-induced hypertension (pre-eclampsia). Pre-eclampsia occurs in approximately 10% of pregnancies and causes thrombocytopenia in one-fourth of affected mothers. Pre-eclampsia is associated with increased maternal and fetal morbidity and mortality. Secondary causes of immune thrombocytopenia that can occur in young women, such as SLE or HIV infection, should also be considered in the clinical context.

Although relatively uncommon, ITP in pregnancy is an important disorder because of the treatment implications for the mother as well as the possibility of fetal-neonatal thrombocytopenia caused by transplacental passage of IgG antiplatelet autoantibodies (passive autoimmune thrombocytopenia). Fetuses of mothers with ITP were often routinely delivered by means of cesarean section. However, this procedure usually is not performed today for two reasons. First, the frequency of severe fetal thrombocytopenia (platelet count less than 20 $\times$ 10^9/L) is known to be quite low (approximately 4%) (69). Second, there is no evidence that cesarean section leads to less intracranial or other bleeding than does vaginal delivery.

Many pregnant women with ITP do not need specific treatment. However, if the platelet count decreases to levels less than 20 to 50 $\times$ 10^9/L or if there is evidence of impaired hemostasis on clinical evaluation, treatment should be given. There are two major treatment options—intermittent high-dose IVIG and low-dose prednisone. Because of risks of use of prednisone during pregnancy (teratogenicity in the first trimester, preeclampsia in the second and third trimesters), IVIG usually is the therapy of choice for ITP in pregnancy (1 g/kg every 2 to 4 weeks, depending on the platelet count response). At delivery, patients thrombocytopenic should not be subjected to a potentially dangerous hemostatic insult such as epidural analgesia. If the patient has received glucocorticoids, consideration should be given to increasing the dose at delivery. Otherwise, no special steps are taken. Platelet transfusions are almost never needed at delivery.

There are no reliable ways to predict fetal thrombocytopenia. Even the severity of maternal thrombocytopenia is not predictive (indeed, women cured of ITP with splenectomy can bear infants with passive autoimmune thrombocytopenia). Results of maternal platelet-antibody tests also are not helpful. Although it is possible to determine the fetal platelet count by means of fetal cord sampling (cordocentesis), this procedure causes morbidity or mortality in 1% to 2% of fetuses sampled. Consequently, many physicians would not perform this procedure on pregnant patients with ITP. Fetal scalp sampling during labor can be used to obtain the fetal platelet count, but falsely low platelet counts are frequently obtained, and this procedure is now rarely performed.

At our center, pregnant patients with ITP are followed with frequent platelet counts (every few weeks, depending on the platelet count). Testing for antiphospholipid antibodies (lupus anticoagulant and anticardiolipin antibodies) is performed because this can be an indication for treatment, especially if previous miscarriages have occurred (70). If therapy for maternal thrombocytopenia is needed, we prefer IVIG. It is possible, although unproven, that glucocorticoids or IVIG improves fetal platelet count. Splenectomy occasionally may be appropriate during the second trimester, if the mother has severe, refractory thrombocytopenia (less than 10 $\times$ 10^9/L) (21).

Unless cesarean section is needed for unrelated obstetric indications, spontaneous vaginal delivery is recommended for mothers with ITP. An immediate fetal umbilical vein platelet count is obtained at delivery. Relatively severe neonatal thrombocytopenia ($<50 \times 10^9$/L) should be aggressively managed, usually with IVIG or glucocorticoids. It is important to recognize that the platelet count of a newborn infant with passive autoimmune thrombocytopenia decreases, and the platelet count nadir is reached 2 to 5 days after delivery (71). A daily platelet count should be obtained until a normal platelet count is documented.

ACUTE IDIOPATHIC (IMMUNE) THROMBOCYTOPENIC PURPURA OF CHILDHOOD

Acute ITP of childhood is a relatively common, generally self-limited, immune thrombocytopenic disorder with a peak incidence between 2 and 6 years of age. Boys and girls are equally affected. Most children (80% to 90%) with acute ITP recover completely within 6 months, but the others have persistent thrombocytopenia. It is likely that acute ITP of childhood is a transient autoimmune disorder, because anti–platelet glycoprotein antibodies usually are detected (72).

The typical clinical manifestations are bleeding and bruising that follow a viral infection by a few weeks. The mortality is approximately 0.4%; most deaths are caused by intracranial hemorrhage. Laboratory abnormalities include isolated thrombocytopenia and normal or increased MPV. A bone marrow examination usually is not performed on a child with typical clinical features of ITP, but it is indicated if unexpected clinical or laboratory findings exist. Normal or increased numbers of megakaryocytes are observed. Sometimes, morphologically distinct lymphoid cells, called *hematogones,* constitute up to one half of the marrow cells and may cause confusion with acute leukemia (73). These nonneoplastic cells have the surface immunophenotypic profile of immature lymphocytes.

Treatment

Acute ITP in children usually is a benign disease. Deaths are rare. It would be difficult to perform a clinical trial that would prove statistically that any treatment could prevent death, even if the treatment were highly effective. For this reason, clinical trials have focussed on the time to increase the platelet count to safe levels.

Blanchette et al. (74) showed that either oral prednisone or high-dose IVIG was more effective than no therapy. A subsequent randomized trial by these investigators (75) involving patients with severe acute ITP (platelet count less than 20×10^9/L) showed that high-dose IVIG was more effective at increasing the platelet count than was oral prednisone (4 mg/kg per day with tapering) or anti-D (25 μg/kg on two consecutive days). On the basis of the results of this study and on other data (53,74), high-dose IVIG is the recommended initial therapy for severe acute ITP. Oral prednisone or an additional dose of IVIG (75) is added if the platelet count remains less than 20×10^9/L 48 hours after initial treatment. It appears that lower doses of IVIG (e.g., 250 to 500 mg/kg per day for 2 days rather than the standard 1 g/kg per day) may be similarly effective in the management of childhood ITP (76).

Even higher doses of glucocorticoids (e.g., intravenous methylprednisolone at 30 mg/kg per day for 3 days or oral methylprednisolone 30 to 50 mg/kg per day for 7 days) also rapidly increase the platelet count in children with acute severe ITP (77). Combined treatment with IVIG and pulse methylprednisolone may be indicated in the care of the few children with severe thrombocytopenia judged to be at high risk of intracranial hemorrhage (78).

CHRONIC IDIOPATHIC (IMMUNE) THROMBOCYTOPENIC PURPURA OF CHILDHOOD

Approximately 10% to 20% of children with ITP eventually have chronic ITP, defined as a platelet count less than 100×10^9/L for more than 6 months. As many as one-third of children who meet this definition can still enter late spontaneous remission, sometimes as long as 5 to 10 years after diagnosis. Chronic ITP in children is an autoimmune disorder and resembles adult chronic ITP.

Treatment

Some patients have no symptoms despite marked thrombocytopenia. These children probably should not receive treatment. For children with symptoms, options include long-term or intermittent administration of glucocorticoids, maintenance IVIG or anti-D injections, splenectomy, administration of vinca alkaloids, and use of immunosuppressive agents (79).

Intravenous immune globulin (2 g/kg over 2 to 5 days) increases the platelet count of most children with chronic ITP (53,79). Because of the higher risk of OPSI among children who have undergone splenectomy, repeated courses of IVIG have been used to defer or to prevent splenectomy on children with chronic ITP. Most patients respond favorably to maintenance IVIG with long-term complete or partial remissions that persist after treatment, or they maintain adequate hemostasis with intermittent injections of IVIG. Unfortunately, approximately 25% of patients become refractory to treatment. Cost-effectiveness analysis shows lesser cost for young children (younger than 6 years of age) treated with maintenance IVIG rather than splenectomy (80). Low-dose, alternate-day glucocorticoid therapy may improve the results of maintenance IVIG.

Anti-D is effective in increasing the platelet count of most children with chronic ITP (59,81). The benefit usually is transient; the median duration of benefit is approximately 3 weeks. The usual absence of tachyphylaxis means that anti-D can be considered splenectomy-sparing maintenance therapy (81). However, anti-D is generally ineffective for patients who have undergone splenectomy and have refractory ITP (81).

Splenectomy sometimes is performed on children with chronic ITP who cannot be maintained on low-dose maintenance glucocorticoids, IVIG, or anti-D therapy. Because of the high probability of a cure (approximately 70%), some physicians perform splenectomy before instituting potentially toxic immunosuppressive therapy. However, because children are at high risk of postsplenectomy sepsis, because of the possibility of late spontaneous remission of ITP, and because of the efficacy of intermittent maintenance therapy with IVIG or anti-D, splenectomy rarely is performed on very young children with chronic ITP. Patients must receive polyvalent pneumococcal and meningococcal vaccination and, particularly, *H. influenzae* type b vaccination, preferably before the splenectomy (47).

Results of use of immunosuppressive agents (azathioprine or cyclophosphamide) and vinca alkaloids to treat children with chronic ITP are variable and based on uncontrolled studies (79). Pulse methylprednisolone has been used to treat children with chronic ITP. In one series (82), approximately one half of the patients maintained platelet counts of more than 50×10^9/L for a minimum of 1 month after a 3-day course of methylprednisolone. Further evaluation of the benefits and complications of repeated administration of this treatment is needed. Occasional children with chronic ITP refractory to splenectomy have been reported to benefit from cyclosporine (64). Danazol can be tried in the treatment of adolescent patients.

SECONDARY IDIOPATHIC (IMMUNE) THROMBOCYTOPENIC PURPURA

Systemic Lupus Erythematosus and Antiphospholipid Antibody Syndromes

Systemic lupus erythematosus and antiphospholipid antibody syndrome (APLAS) are autoimmune disorders complicated by thrombocytopenia in 15% to 25% of patients. Mechanisms of thrombocytopenia include platelet glycoprotein–reactive autoantibodies, β_2-glycoprotein I–containing and other platelet-reactive immune complexes, and hypersplenism, among others. Whether antibody-induced platelet activation in vivo contributes to thrombosis in SLE or APLAS is uncertain.

Various thrombocytopenic syndromes occur. Sometimes the thrombocytopenia is chronic, resembling ITP, and is the predominant clinical manifestation of SLE or APLAS (83). Sometimes patients with even mild thrombocytopenia have platelet dysfunction and prolonged bleeding. Thrombocytopenia complicated by antiphospholipid antibodies carries increased risk of thrombotic, rather than bleeding, complications (84). These patients often have livedo reticularis or acrocyanosis that can progress to digital necrosis (85). Acute, severe thrombocytopenia can be prominent in patients with severe multisystem exacerbation of SLE (83) or the catastrophic APLAS (86). In rare instances, patients with SLE have an illness that closely resembles thrombotic thrombocytopenic purpura (TTP) or hemolytic uremic syndrome (HUS). These patients often are treated with plasma exchange (87).

Treatment

Thrombocytopenia associated with SLE is managed similarly to ITP, except that we recommend danazol be tried before splenectomy. Glucocorticoids are used as initial therapy. Many patients are highly sensitive to glucocorticoids, and thus thrombocytopenia may reoccur during tapering of prednisone. Steroid maintenance should be considered especially if this treatment controls other aspects of SLE. The role of glucocorticoids in APLAS-associated thrombocytopenia is less clear. As have others (88), we have seen patients have progressive ischemic necrosis of digits during glucocorticoid therapy.

Splenectomy probably is as effective in achieving platelet count remission in SLE and APLAS as it is in ITP (89). Some physicians first try danazol (an attenuated androgen) for several weeks or months in doses of 200 to 1,200 mg/d (49) before considering splenectomy. For patients with disease refractory to danazol and splenectomy, more aggressive therapies such as high-dose IVIG, azathioprine, intermittent pulse cyclophosphamide (90), plasmapheresis synchronized with pulse intravenous cyclophosphamide (91), and cyclosporine (92) can be tried.

Human Immunodeficiency Virus—associated Idiopathic (Immune) Thrombocytopenic Purpura

Thrombocytopenia occurs in approximately 10% to 15% of persons with asymptomatic HIV infection and 30% to 40% of patients with acquired immunodeficiency syndrome (AIDS). Besides immune platelet destruction, there are many other ways that infection with HIV can cause thrombocytopenia (93), including impaired platelet production secondary to HIV infection of megakaryocytes, drug-induced myelosuppression (commonly zidovudine, ganciclovir, and trimethoprim-sulfamethoxazole), HIV-associated thrombotic microangiopathy, hypersplenism, and marrow infiltration by tumor or opportunistic infections. Platelet kinetic studies have shown a complex interaction of impaired platelet production, increased platelet destruction, and predominant splenic platelet sequestration and destruction (94).

Immune platelet destruction may be related to antibodies that cross-react with GP IIb/IIIa or GP Ib/IX complexes (95). Immune complexes containing IgM antiidiotype antibodies against anti–GP IIIa may explain the paradox of high levels of platelet-bound IgG and IgM but low levels of serum platelet-reactive antibodies in HIV-associated ITP (96).

The occurrence of isolated immune thrombocytopenia does not necessarily indicate increased risk of progression to a more advanced stage of HIV infection. Particularly if they are children, patients with HIV-associated thrombocytopenia may not even have helper-T-cell lymphopenia. Sometimes thrombocytopenia disappears spontaneously.

Treatment

Anti-HIV therapy, as with zidovudine, often increases the platelet count in patients with HIV-associated thrombocytopenia (97). For patients whose condition is refractory to zidovudine, interferon-alfa has been reported to be effective. Highly active antiretroviral therapy, typically consisting of two nucleoside analogues in conjunction with an HIV protease inhibitor or a non-nucleoside reverse transcriptase inhibitor, has improved survival among patients with HIV infection. Such regimens also increase the platelet count of patients with thrombocytopenia in inverse proportion to the reduction in HIV viral load (98).

Many patients have no or minimal bleeding and do not need specific therapy for HIV-associated thrombocytopenia. For patients with symptomatic thrombocytopenia, however, the treatment approach is similar to therapy for classic ITP, because most patients respond to conventional medical treatments (glucocorticoids, IVIG, anti-D), at least transiently (59,99). Splenectomy appears to be at least as effective in achieving long-term remission of HIV-associated thrombocytopenia as it is in the management of primary ITP (100). Splenectomy also does not accelerate, and may even reduce, the rate of progression to AIDS among persons with HIV infection.

Neoplasia-associated Idiopathic (Immune) Thrombocytopenic Purpura

Immune thrombocytopenia can precede or accompany neoplastic disorders, especially lymphoproliferative syndromes (101). Decreased platelet survival and the presence of platelet-reactive autoantibodies (102) have been found. In general, the thrombocytopenia represents less of a risk to the patient than does the underlying malignant disease, and the first step is management of the underlying disorder. Sometimes the thrombocytopenia resolves as the tumor responds to treatment, but at other times, it necessitates the therapy used to manage chronic ITP (glucocorticoids followed by splenectomy). In one study, 30% of patients with ITP and Hodgkin's disease responded to glucocorticoids, whereas 75% benefited from splenectomy (101).

Transplantation-associated Idiopathic (Immune) Thrombocytopenic Purpura

Severe persistent thrombocytopenia despite recovery of red and white blood cells is relatively common after allogeneic or autologous bone marrow or peripheral blood transplantation. Autoimmune thrombocytopenia has been implicated in some patients. Later-onset thrombocytopenia following bone marrow, stem cell, or solid-organ transplantation that responds to glucocorticoids, IVIG, and splenectomy also has been attributed to autoimmune and even alloimmune thrombocytopenia (103). However, while considering immune-mediated thrombocytopenia, the physician also should suspect other, more common explanations for thrombocytopenia in these patients, including infection, organ rejection, or use of drugs that increase platelet destruction (e.g., antilymphocyte globulin) or that cause bone marrow suppression (azathioprine, sulfamethoxazole-trimethoprim). Approximately 2% of recipients of solid-organ transplants have HUS within the first year after transplantation (104).

DRUG-INDUCED IMMUNE THROMBOCYTOPENIA

Drugs can produce several immune-mediated thrombocytopenic disorders (105–107) (Table 27.2). The most common is HIT, which paradoxically is associated with increased risk of thrombosis but not of bleeding. In contrast, many other drugs in rare instances cause severe thrombocytopenia and bleeding, a syndrome called *drug-induced immune thrombocytopenic purpura* (DITP) to emphasize its clinical resemblance to acute ITP. Some drugs cause atypical clinical signs and symptoms (e.g., abciximab-induced thrombocytopenia) or trigger an illness that resembles TTP or HUS (Table 27.2).

Heparin-induced Thrombocytopenia

Heparin-induced thrombocytopenia is a relatively common, IgG-mediated, adverse reaction to heparin that has a strong association with venous and arterial thrombosis (2,3,108). Heparin-induced thrombocytopenia can be considered a clinicopathologic syndrome; that is, the diagnosis is made most reliably on both clinical and serologic grounds (109). Thus HIT antibody formation without thrombocytopenia or other abnormalities is not HIT, whereas HIT antibody formation accompanied by an otherwise unexplained 50% or greater postoperative decrease in platelet count (even if the platelet count remains greater than 150×10^9/L) or complicated by skin lesions at heparin injection sites (108) are examples of HIT syndrome. Indeed, the thrombocytopenia usually is much less severe in HIT (3) than in DITP (110) or abciximab-induced thrombocytopenia (111) (Fig.

TABLE 27.2. DRUG-INDUCED IMMUNE THROMBOCYTOPENIC SYNDROMES

Syndrome and Drug	Comment
Heparin-induced thrombocytopenia	Prothrombotic reaction caused by heparin-dependent platelet-activating IgG antibodies that recognize platelet factor 4-heparin complexes. Caused less often by low-molecular-weight heparin than by unfractionated heparin.
Drug-induced immune thrombocytopenic purpura (DITP)	Prohemorrhagic reaction caused by IgG antibodies that recognize drug (or drug metabolite) bound to platelet glycoprotein (GP). Patients have severe thrombocytopenia and mucocutaneous bleeding.
Quinine	Quinine-dependent anti-GP IIb/IIIa and GP Ib/IX IgG implicated. Drug is widely available (e.g., tonic water, filler in illicit drugs).
Quinidine	Antibodies usually distinct from quinine-dependent antibodies.
Rifampin	Rifampin-dependent anti-GP IIb/IIIa and GP Ib/IX IgG implicated.
Sulfa antibiotics	Occurs in ~1 of 25,000 patients receiving trimethoprim-sulfamethoxazole.
Vancomycin	Vancomycin-dependent anti-GP IIb/IIIa IgG.
Iodinated contrast medium	Severe thrombocytopenia begins after radiologic procedure.
Acetaminophen	IgG recognizes metabolite of acetaminophen.
Many others	See published lists (105, 106) and website (106).
Atypical DITP	
Abciximab	Abrupt onset of moderately severe thrombocytopenia (platelet count nadir, ~$15–35 \times 10^9$/L) perhaps by naturally occurring anti-ligand-induced binding site (LIBS) antibodies.
Gold	Thrombocytopenia can persist for many months after gold therapy is stopped.
Measles-mumps-rubella vaccine	Transient autoimmune thrombocytopenia (anti-GP IIb/IIIa) that occurs a few weeks after vaccination (resembles childhood acute immune thrombocytopenic purpura).
DITP: hapten mechanism	Indicates that IgG recognizes drug that remains bound to platelet surface even after platelet washing.
Penicillin	Not well-established.
Drug-induced TTP or HUS	
Ticlopidine	Estimated frequency, 1/2,000–1/5,000.
Clopidogrel	Estimated frequency, 1/20,000.
Quinine	Quinine-dependent IgG against platelets and other cells found.
Cyclosporine	May be pathogenic factor in transplantation-associated TTP/HUS.
Others	See text.

TTP, thrombotic thrombocytopenic purpura; HUS, hemolytic uremic syndrome.

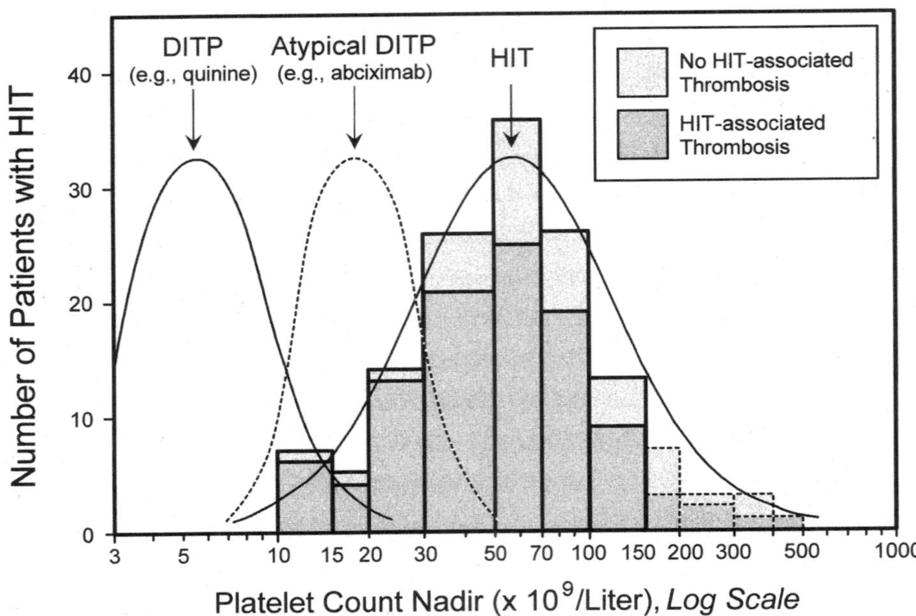

FIGURE 27.3. Severity of thrombocytopenia in various drug-induced immune thrombocytopenic disorders. Platelet counts are typically less than 20 × 10^9/L in patients with typical drug-induced thrombocytopenia, such as that caused by quinine, sulfa antibiotics, or rifampicin (110). In contrast, for approximately 85% of patients with heparin-induced thrombocytopenia (HIT), the platelet count nadir is between 20 and 150 × 10^9/L (3). Atypical thrombocytopenia caused by platelet fibrinogen receptor inhibitors such as abciximab (ReoPro) typically gives a platelet count of 10 to 50 × 10^9/L. The data to construct the HIT curve have been published previously (3,112).

27.3). Another contrast from DITP is that even when severe thrombocytopenia occurs in HIT, petechiae and other bleeding typically are not observed (108). Indeed, even the one uncommon, though characteristic, hemorrhagic complication of HIT (bilateral adrenal hemorrhage) is caused by thrombosis (adrenal hemorrhagic necrosis secondary to adrenal vein thrombosis) (108).

The target antigen recognized by HIT antibodies consists of a multimolecular complex between PF4 (a platelet α-granule protein of the CXC family of chemokines) and heparin (14, 113). The HIT antibodies bind to one or more PF4 regions that have undergone conformational modification through binding to heparin. The formation of the antigen is somewhat nonspecific, because PF4 can be rendered antigenic by binding to other polyanions, such as pentosan polysulfate or polyvinyl sulfonate. At least 12 to 14 saccharide units are needed for heparin to form the antigen complex with PF4. This may explain why low-molecular-weight heparin preparations are less immunogenic than is unfractionated heparin and are less likely to cause HIT (2). Although low-molecular-weight heparin does sometimes cause HIT, it is likely that very small heparin preparations (e.g., synthetic anti–factor Xa–binding pentasaccharide) or specially engineered heparins (e.g., highly-sulfated heparin moieties bridged with nonsulfated spacer regions) do not cause HIT.

Figure 27.4 illustrates several possible mechanisms to explain the intense thrombin generation that occurs in HIT (114,115). These include the formation of procoagulant, platelet-derived microparticles (116) that result from cell signaling triggered by clustering of platelet Fc receptors. Recent data suggest that in situ formation of IgG-PF4-heparin complexes on the platelet surface leads to platelet activation (117). In vivo platelet activation is suggested by expression of P selectin by circulating platelets in HIT as well as by increased levels of circulating microparticles. Tissue factor expression by endothelium or monocytes activated by HIT antibodies that recognize PF4 bound to surface glycosaminoglycans are other possible procoagulant events.

Marked in vivo thrombin generation helps explain several clinical features of HIT, including its association with venous and arterial thrombosis (hypercoagulable state), the occurrence of decompensated disseminated intravascular coagulation with low fibrinogen levels in approximately 5% of patients, and the potential for deep venous thrombosis (DVT) to progress to venous limb gangrene, particularly in patients treated with warfarin (114). This syndrome results from impaired procoagulant-anticoagulant balance: warfarin-induced protein C depletion leads to microvascular thrombosis caused by ongoing intense thrombin generation. Patients with warfarin-induced venous gangrene typically have a supratherapeutic international normalized ratio (INR), usually more than 4.0. The explanation is a concomitant severe decrease in factor VII that parallels the decrease in protein C. The importance of in vivo thrombin generation in HIT provides a rationale for current consensus recommendations that an agent that reduces thrombin generation or directly inactivates thrombin be used for the management of this syndrome (109).

The frequency of HIT varies among different patient populations. For example, orthopedic surgical patients are more likely than cardiac surgical patients to have HIT, even though the latter group is more likely to form HIT antibodies (13). Medical patients appear to have HIT less often that do surgical patients (118).

Management of Heparin-induced Thrombocytopenia–associated Thrombosis

Results of prospective and retrospective studies (2,112,118) indicate that approximately 50% to 75% of patients with HIT have

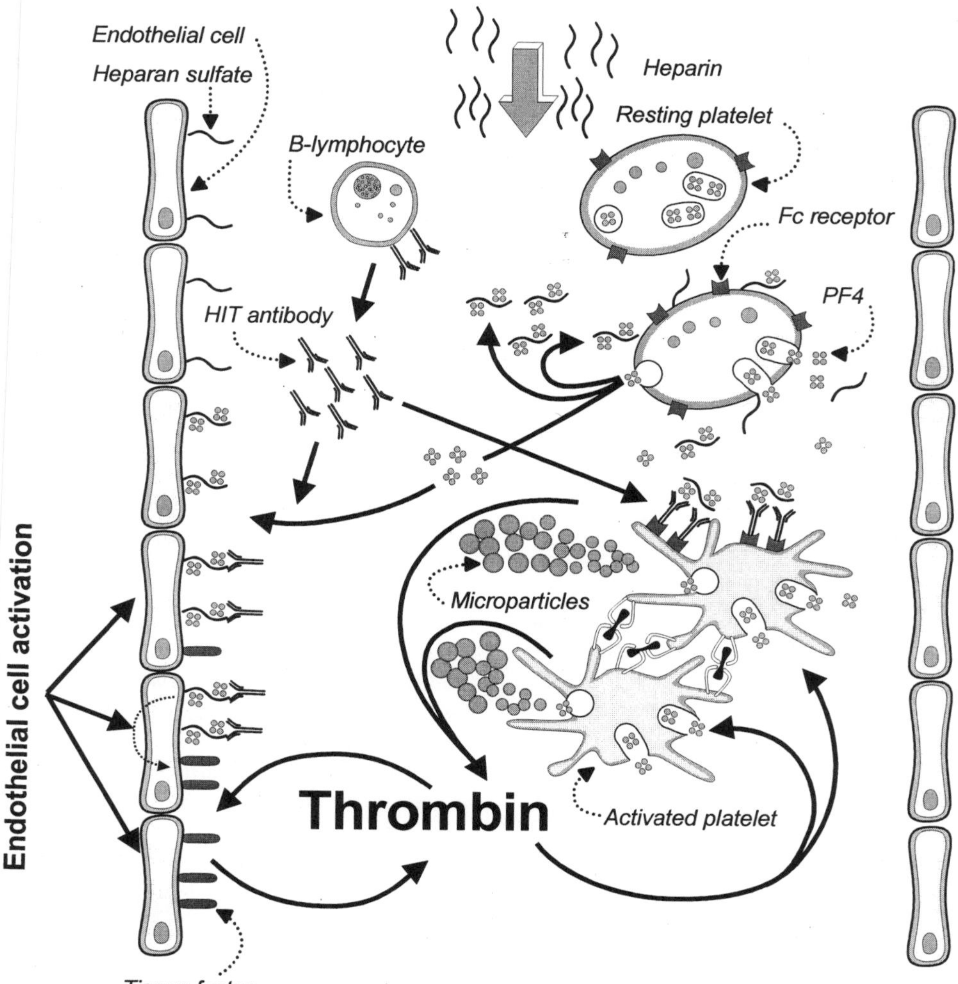

FIGURE 27.4. Pathogenesis of heparin-induced thrombocytopenia (HIT). Fc receptor-mediated platelet activation (with formation of procoagulant, platelet-derived microparticles) and endothelial cell activation (with expression of tissue factor) lead to increased thrombin generation in HIT. *PF4,* platelet factor 4. (From Warkentin TE, Kelton JG. Thrombocytopenia due to platelet destruction and hypersplenism. In: Hoffman R, Benz EJ Jr, Shattil SJ, et al., eds. *Hematology: basic principles and practice,* 3rd ed. New York: Churchill Livingstone, 1999:2138–2154, with permission.)

new, progressive, or recurrent thrombosis. Thus the need for an alternative anticoagulant is a common issue in the care of these patients.

Danaparoid sodium (Orgaran) is a mixture of anticoagulant glycosaminoglycans with predominant anti–factor Xa activity that decreases thrombin generation in patients with HIT (119). A randomized trial showed a higher thrombosis resolution rate among patients treated with danaparoid and warfarin than among those treated with dextran and warfarin, especially for patients with severe thrombosis (92% versus 33%; $P < .001$) (120). Although as many as 40% of HIT serum samples show in vitro cross-reactivity with danaparoid (enhanced platelet activation in the presence of danaparoid), this effect is substantially weaker than with unfractionated or low-molecular-weight heparin and is not predictive of adverse outcome (120). Danaparoid usually is given without previous in vitro testing for cross-reactivity. The success rate is high (approximately 90%), as defined by platelet count recovery without new thrombosis (120,121). The anticoagulant effect of danaparoid is monitored with a chromogenic anti–factor Xa assay, which must be performed with a standard curve prepared with danaparoid. The target range is generally 0.5 to 0.8 anti–factor Xa U/ml although we sometimes aim for levels of 1.0 U/ml or higher in the treatment of patients with severe thrombosis. Most patients achieve therapeutic levels with conventional dosing (Table 27.3). We advocate anticoagulant monitoring for very small or large patients, patients with renal failure, and patients with life- or limb-threatening HIT. Danaparoid does not interfere with INR measurements. This is an advantage in the care of patients with venous thromboembolism in whom overlapping warfarin anticoagulation usually is

TABLE 27.3. MANAGEMENT OF HEPARIN-INDUCED THROMBOCYTOPENIA: PROTOCOLS FOR DANAPAROID, LEPIRUDIN, AND ARGATROBAN

Danaparoid
For rapid therapeutic anticoagulation (IV infusion)
Loading dose[a]: 2,250 U bolus (1,500 U if <50 kg; 3,000 U if 75–90 kg; 3,750 U if >90 kg) followed by 400 U/h for 4 h, then 300 U/h for 4 h
Maintenance[b]: 150 to 200 U/h to maintain antifactor Xa levels between 0.5 and 0.8 IU/mL[c]

Lepirudin (Recombinant Hirudin)
For rapid therapeutic anticoagulation (IV infusion)
Loading dose: 0.4 mg/kg bolus IV
Maintenance: 0.15 mg/kg/h IV with adjustments to maintain aPTT 1.5 to 2.5 times the median of the normal laboratory range

Argatroban
For rapid therapeutic anticoagulation (IV infusion)
Initial dose: 2 μg/kg per minute
Maintenance: Above initial dose adjusted to maintain aPTT 1.5 to 3.0 times the initial baseline value (not to exceed 100 s)

[a]All bolus doses are based on 750 U ampule availability.
[b]If preferred, after initial bolus, danaparoid can be given by the subcutaneous route (generally, 1,500 U every 8–12 h).
[c]If antifactor Xa levels are not available, danaparoid can still be given safely to most patients, because there is a high probability of achieving the target anticoagulant range with this regimen, and bleeding complications are uncommon. However, monitoring is recommended for very small and large patients, patients with renal failure, and patients with life- or limb-threatening thrombosis.
aPTT, activated partial thromboplastin time.

performed after resolution of thrombocytopenia. Danaparoid is approved therapy for HIT in the European Union, Canada, and elsewhere. In the United States, it is approved only for prophylaxis of DVT; however, the predominant use of this agent in the United States is off-label management or prevention of HIT-associated thrombosis.

Lepirudin (Refludan) is a hirudin derivative manufactured by means of recombinant technology. Two prospective cohort studies (122,123) of lepirudin with a prespecified dosing schedule for the management of HIT-associated thrombosis (Table 27.3) (with historical controls for comparison) led to approval of this agent in the United States, Canada, and the European Union for treatment of patients with HIT-associated thrombosis. Metaanalysis (115) of these two studies showed that a subtherapeutic activated partial thromboplastin time (aPTT) ratio (<1.5) was associated with increased risk of thrombosis, whereas a therapeutic aPTT ratio above the therapeutic range (>2.5) was associated with increased bleeding without further reduction in antithrombotic efficacy. However, even for patients within the target therapeutic range, the risk of bleeding was significantly greater than that among historical controls (relative risk approximately 3).

The anticoagulant effect of lepirudin can be simply monitored with aPTT. Lepirudin is renally excreted, and should not be used to treat patients with renal failure because there is substantial risk of overdosing, and no antidote exists. The half-life of lepirudin is short (approximately 1.3 hours) in patients with normal renal function. This is an advantage if bleeding occurs or cessation of anticoagulation is needed because of an invasive procedure. A high proportion of patients develop anti-hirudin antibodies, which occasionally results in a paradoxic increase in the anticoagulant effects of the drug (perhaps through reduced renal clearance). Thus ongoing aPTT monitoring is recommended during lepirudin treatment, even if initial anticoagulation is stable.

Argatroban (Novastan) is a small-molecule, direct thrombin inhibitor approved in the United States for the management and prevention of HIT-associated thrombosis (Table 27.3) (124). Advantages of argatroban include its short half-life (40-50 min) as well as its hepatic route of metabolism. No dosage adjustments are needed for patients with moderate renal failure, although dose reduction is needed in the presence of hepatic insufficiency. Anticoagulant monitoring is easily performed with aPTT. Unfortunately, argatroban also prolongs the INR, which means that the target INR may be as high as 6.0 to 8.0 (depending on the assay reagent) during overlapping anticoagulation with oral anticoagulants.

There are several important contraindications to therapy for acute HIT, including warfarin monotherapy, low-molecular-weight heparin, and prophylactic platelet transfusion (125). Warfarin therapy can lead to acute depletion of protein C, which can cause microvascular thrombosis in HIT and lead to venous limb gangrene (114). However, once thrombocytopenia has resolved, it is safe to overlap warfarin with one of the agents that can reduce thrombin generation in HIT (danaparoid, lepirudin, argatroban). Thus warfarin is the usual antithrombotic drug for longer-term management of thrombosis. Use of low-molecular-weight heparin is contraindicated because of a high risk of treatment failure (approximately 50% of patients have further thrombocytopenia or thrombosis) (125). Prophylactic platelet transfusion is relatively contraindicated because even patients with severe thrombocytopenia do not usually have evidence of hemostatic dysfunction, such as petechiae, and platelet transfusions may contribute to increase risk of thrombosis (125).

Management of Isolated Heparin-induced Thrombocytopenia

Isolated HIT is defined as HIT recognized because of thrombocytopenia without evidence of HIT-associated thrombosis (112). Unfortunately, simply stopping administration of heparin or substituting warfarin for heparin is inadequate treatment of these patients. In a large retrospective cohort study (112), we found the risk of thrombosis among these patients to be approximately 10% at 2 days, 40% at 7 days, and 53% at 30-day follow-up evaluations. Other investigators (126) with a similar approach subsequently found a 38% rate of thrombotic events despite stopping administration of heparin. The frequency of thrombosis surprisingly was not any lower in the subgroup of patients for whom heparin was stopped fairly promptly (<48 hours) after the onset of thrombocytopenia than it was among patients with later cessation of heparin (45 versus 34%; $P = .26$). Two prospective cohort studies in Germany showed a thrombosis rate of 6% per day before administration of lepirudin was started after the serologic confirmation of HIT (115).

For patients believed to have isolated HIT, our approach is to discontinue heparin, to start administration of an alternative rapidly acting anticoagulant, and to screen for subclinical DVT by means of compression ultrasonography (approximately 50% of patients are shown to have DVT with this approach) (127). Whether or not thrombosis is found, we usually give therapeutic-dose anticoagulation (Table 27.3) to these patients (127). This is because prophylactic-dose anticoagulation appears to have a higher failure rate than does therapeutic-dose anticoagulation (121). Further, argatroban was approved in therapeutic doses for prevention of thrombosis in the care of patients with HIT (124). After platelet count recovery, we reconfirm the absence of venous thrombosis before discharge. For patients found at initial or follow-up imaging to have venous thrombosis, overlapping warfarin anticoagulation is begun for longer-term antithrombotic control (127). This approach has not been prospectively evaluated.

Reexposure to Heparin in a Patient with a History of Heparin-induced Thrombocytopenia

Patients who have circulating HIT antibodies can have an abrupt decrease in platelet count if heparin is administered. However, the risk of such abrupt-onset HIT on reexposure to heparin is restricted to the first few months after use of heparin. This is because HIT antibodies begin to decline after heparin is discontinued, and usually they are no longer detectable by the 3-month follow-up evaluation (128). Under exceptional circumstances (e.g., need to perform heart or vascular surgery), it is reasonable to readminister heparin to a patient with previous HIT, provided that HIT antibodies are no longer detectable with a sensitive and reliable assay (e.g., platelet serotonin release assay or PF4-dependent EIA) (128). Interestingly, such patients usually do not form HIT antibodies after the brief reexposure to heparin. Nevertheless, it seems prudent to limit the heparin reexposure to the operation itself and to use an alternative anticoagulant for perioperative anticoagulation.

Typical Drug-induced Immune Thrombocytopenia

The clinical criteria supporting a diagnosis of DITP are (a) thrombocytopenia that occurs during drug treatment and that is corrected completely after discontinuation of the drug; (b) the implicated drug was the only one used when thrombocytopenia occurred, or platelet count recovery occurred or persisted despite continuation or reintroduction of the other drugs used; (c) other causes of thrombocytopenia are excluded; and (d) reexposure to the implicated agent resulted in recurrent thrombocytopenia (106). For reasons of patient safety, drug reexposure is rarely performed deliberately, but sometimes the outcome of unintentional reexposure can provide important diagnostic information (e.g., recurrent thrombocytopenia following ingestion of tonic water suggests quinine-induced thrombocytopenia). Meeting all four criteria provides definite evidence of causation, whereas meeting the first three criteria suggests a probable cause (106).

Thrombocytopenia typically begins abruptly and is severe, most patients having a platelet count less than 20×10^9/L (110). Although the interval between starting the drug and development of thrombocytopenia usually is 1 or 2 weeks, occasionally it can be several months or even longer after administration of the drug is started. Sometimes, thrombocytopenia persists for several weeks even after the drug is stopped, possibly because some of the IgG antibodies formed have drug-independent platelet reactivity.

Although many dozens of drugs have been implicated as causing DITP, convincing evidence to support a causal relation exists for relatively few drugs (105–107). A website lists the supporting evidence for the drugs claimed to cause DITP (http://moon.ouhsc.edu/jgeorge) (106). The risk of DITP is approximately 1 case in 1,000 for quinine and 1 in 25,000 for sulfamethoxazole-trimethoprim (129). Quinine is present in certain beverages (e.g., tonic water) and consequently patients may not be aware of exposure.

The pathogenesis of DITP involves formation of a ternary complex involving a platelet glycoprotein (usually, the GP IIb/IIIa complex, less often GP Ib/IX), drug (or drug metabolite), and the Fab terminus of IgG (7,130,131). Such a mechanism has been invoked for quinine, quinidine, sulfonamide, rifampin, vancomycin, and pentamidine, among others. Unlike the mechanism of HIT, the platelet Fc receptors are not involved (132). Further, the drug does not function as a hapten; that is, drug-dependent IgG does not bind to platelets that have been washed after pretreatment with the implicated drug (107). Limited evidence of a hapten mechanism of DITP has been suggested only for penicillin; that is, penicillin-dependent IgG binds to platelets that have been washed after pretreatment with penicillin (107).

Treatment

In a case of suspected DITP, as many drugs as possible should be discontinued. If further drug treatment is necessary, an immunologically non-cross-reactive substitute should be prescribed. Platelet transfusions should be given to patients with life-threatening bleeding. High-dose IVIG, 1 g/kg given over 6 to 8 hours for 2 consecutive days, usually is effective. Glucocorticoids are relatively ineffective in the management of this condition (110).

Atypical Drug-induced Immune Thrombocytopenic Purpura

Abciximab-induced Thrombocytopenia

Abciximab (c7E3, ReoPro) is a humanized chimeric Fab fragment of a murine monoclonal antibody (7E3) directed against GP IIb/IIIa. It is used to prevent restenosis after coronary angioplasty. Approximately 0.5% of patients have moderate or severe thrombocytopenia (platelet count nadir, 10 to 50×10^9/L) within several hours of treatment with this drug (Fig. 27.3). Perhaps surprisingly, given the degree of thrombocytopenia and use of a major platelet glycoprotein inhibitor, most patients do not have petechiae or bleeding (111), although fatal bleeding episodes have been reported. Platelet transfusions and IVIG should be given to bleeding patients, although the efficacy remains unestablished. The mechanism of thrombocytopenia is uncertain, although the abrupt onset of severe thrombocytopenia suggests an immune pathogenesis, perhaps by naturally occurring anti-GP IIb/IIIa antibodies that recognize conformational modifications of GP IIb/IIIa induced by abciximab, that is, ligand-induced binding sites. For approximately one third of patients with apparent thrombocytopenia, examination of the blood film shows platelet clumping. This finding suggests pseudothrombocytopenia caused by ex vivo platelet clumping has been caused by abciximab (133). Such patients are not at risk of bleeding and do not need treatment.

Drug-induced Autoimmune Thrombocytopenia

Approximately 1% to 3% of patients treated with gold have thrombocytopenia that sometimes can persist for weeks or months despite cessation of the drug, thus the disorder resembles chronic ITP (134). It remains uncertain whether this is true drug-induced autoimmune thrombocytopenia or is caused by gold-dependent IgG antibodies that are slowly released from tissues. Procainamide and α-methyldopa also may cause autoimmune thrombocytopenia. In extremely rare instances, measles-mumps-rubella vaccination causes an acute ITP-like illness in which anti-GP IIb/IIIa IgG is formed (135).

Drug-induced Thrombotic Thrombocytopenic Purpura and Hemolytic Uremic Syndrome

In rare instances, drugs cause thrombotic microangiopathy that closely resembles TTP or HUS. Paradoxically, such platelet-mediated thrombotic disorders can even be caused by the antiplatelet agents ticlopidine (136) and clopidogrel (137). Ticlopidine-induced TTP is estimated to occur in 1 in 2,000 to 5,000 patients who receive this drug after coronary stenting. The characteristic onset is between 1 and 8 weeks after administration of the drug is started. Clopidogrel-induced TTP occurs in approximately 1 in 20,000 recipients, generally within the first 2 weeks of treatment. Autoantibodies to von Willebrand factor–cleaving metalloproteinase have been identified in these patients and may contribute to the pathogenesis (138).

Other drugs that cause an illness that resembles HUS include quinine (139), antineoplastic chemotherapy (e.g., mitomycin C, cisplatin, bleomycin), immunosuppressive agents (e.g., cyclosporin, FK506 [tacrolimus]), and miscellaneous drugs (penicillamine, penicillin) (105). Because some of the medical conditions leading to use of these drugs can be associated with microangiopathic blood film changes (neoplasia, organ rejection, graft versus host disease, vasculitis), causal relations to the various drugs listed can be problematic.

Treatment

The mortality of drug-induced TTP is high. Early recognition and discontinuation of the drug are essential. Response to plasma exchange has been observed. Many physicians also give glucocorticoids, although the efficacy remains unproven. Specific therapy for drug-induced HUS (dialysis, plasmapheresis, glucocorticoids) is individualized depending on the clinical situation.

ALLOIMMUNE THROMBOCYTOPENIA

Alloantigens are genetically determined molecular variations of proteins or carbohydrates that can be recognized immunologically by some healthy persons. Exposure to alloantigens occurs during pregnancy, transfusion, or transplantation. If alloantibodies form against platelet alloantigen targets, alloimmune thrombocytopenia can result from platelet clearance mediated by the reticuloendothelial system. Five alloimmune thrombocytopenic disorders have been described (Table 27.4) (140), the most common being NAT.

TABLE 27.4. THE FIVE ALLOIMMUNE THROMBOCYTOPENIC SYNDROMES

Classic alloimmune thrombocytopenic syndromes
Neonatal alloimmune thrombocytopenia
Posttransfusion purpura
Other alloimmune thrombocytopenic syndromes
Passive alloimmune thrombocytopenia
Transplantation-associated thrombocytopenia
Platelet transfusion refractoriness

From Warkentin TE, Smith JW. The alloimmune thrombocytopenic syndromes. *Transfus Med Rev* 1997;11:296–307, with permission.

Alloantigens

More than 20 platelet alloantigens have been identified (140–142). Table 27.5 classifies the platelet alloantigens by glycoprotein localization and gene frequency, the latter divided into public and private (or low frequency, arbitrarily less than 0.02). More than one-half of the alloantigens that have been identified are located on one of the two glycoproteins that constitute the GP IIb/IIIa complex (platelet fibrinogen receptor). One of these alloantigens, usually called Pl^{A1} in North America, is located on GP IIIa. It is responsible for most alloimmune thrombocytopenia in white populations, including almost all patients with severe alloimmune thrombocytopenia. The other major platelet glycoprotein complex (GP Ib/IX, von Willebrand factor–binding complex) rarely is implicated in alloimmune thrombocytopenia. However, the GP Ia/IIa complex (platelet collagen receptor), which bears the $Br^{a/b}$ ($Zav^{a/b}$) alloantigen system, is a relatively common cause of moderately severe alloimmune thrombocytopenia (143). The $Gov^{a/b}$ alloantigen system (144) has been shown to be a relatively common cause of alloimmune thrombocytopenia that like $Br^{a/b}$ tends not to be very severe (144).

Immunogenetics and Frequency of Alloimmune Thrombocytopenia

The Pl^{A1} alloantigen is far more immunogenic than is its corresponding allele, Pl^{A2}. For example, consider the frequency of NAT caused by either anti-Pl^{A1} or anti-Pl^{A2} alloantibodies in relation to the genotype frequency of Pl^{A1} (0.85) and Pl^{A2} (0.15). A homozygous Pl^{A2} (Pl^{A1}-negative) woman, representing approximately 2% (0.15 × 0.15) of the population, would have an 85% probability of being exposed to the Pl^{A1} alloantigen during pregnancy. In contrast, a homozygous Pl^{A1} woman, approximately 72% (0.85 × 0.85) of the population, would have a

TABLE 27.5. PLATELET ANTIGENS CLASSIFIED ACCORDING TO GLYCOPROTEIN LOCATION AND GENE FREQUENCY

Platelet-specific Alloantigen (Alternative Nomenchlature)	GP GP	Gene Frequency Among White Persons	NAT	PTP	PAT	TAT	PTR
GP IIb/IIIa: public (gene frequency >0.02)							
$P1^{A1}$ (HPA-1a, Zw^a)	IIIa	0.85	++	++	+	+	(+)
$P1^{A2}$ (HPA-1b, Zw^b)	IIIa	0.15	+	+	–	–	(+)
Bak^a (HPA-3a, Lek^a)	IIb	0.61	+	+	–	–	(+)
Bak^b (HPA-3b)	IIb	0.39	?	+	–	–	(+)
Pen^a (HPA-4a, Yuk^b)	IIIa	>0.99	+	+	–	–	(+)
GP IIb/IIIa: private low-frequency (arbitrarily, gene frequency <0.02)							
Pen^b (HPA-4b, Yuk^a)	IIIa	<0.01	+	–	–	–	–
Tu^a (HPA-6b, Ca^a)	IIIa	0.003	+	–	–	–	–
Mo^a (HPA-7b)	IIIa	0.001	+	–	–	–	–
Sr^a (HPA-8b)	IIIa	<0.003	+	–	–	–	–
Max^a (HPA-9b)	IIb	0.003	+	–	–	–	–
La^a (HPA-10b)	IIIa	<0.01	+	–	–	–	–
Gro^a (HPA-11b)	IIIa	<0.001	+	–	–	–	–
Va^a	IIb/IIIa	<0.002	+	–	–	–	–
Oe^a	IIIa	<0.005	+	–	–	–	–
GP Ia/IIa: public							
Br^b (HPA-5a, Zav^b)	Ia	0.89	+	?	–	–	(+)
Br^a (HPA-5b, Zav^a, Hc^a)	Ia	0.11	++	+	+	+	(+)
Sit^a (HPA-13b)	Ia	0.0025	+	–	–	–	–
GP Ib/IX: public							
Ko^b (HPA-2a)	Ibα	0.89	–	–	–	–	?
Ko^a (HPA-2b, Sib^a)	Ibα	0.11	+	?	–	–	(+)
GP Ib/IX: private							
Iy^a (HPA-12b)	1bβ	0.002	+	–	–	–	–
CD109: public							
Gov^a	CD109	0.53	+	?	–	–	–
Gov^b	CD109	0.47	+	–	–	–	(+)
GP38							
Dy^a	38kd	<0.01	+	–	–	–	–
Platelet-nonspecific alloantigens							
ABO			–	–	–	–	++
HLA			–	–	–	–	++

GP, glycoprotein; NAT, neonatal alloimmune thrombocytopenia; PTP, posttransfusion purpura; PAT, passive alloimmune thrombocytopenia; TAT, transplantation-associated alloimmune thrombocytopenia; PTR, platelet transfusion refractoriness.

++, relatively common; +, established but rare; –, not reported; (+), probable association, but definitive link inconclusive; ?, possible association but not established.

Modified from Warkentin TE, Smith JW. The alloimmune thrombocytopenic syndromes. *Tranfus Med Rev* 1997;11:296–307, with permission.

15% probability of being exposed to the Pl^{A2} alloantigen during pregnancy. If both alloantigens were equally immunogenic, one would expect anti-Pl^{A2} to occur approximately 6 times more often than anti-Pl^{A1}: $(0.72 \times 0.15)/(0.02 \times 0.85) = 6.4$. However, the opposite is actually observed: anti-Pl^{A1} is far more common than anti-Pl^{A2} (Table 27.6). In a study of 348 cases of suspected NAT (143), only one case caused by anti-Pl^{A2} antibodies was found, compared with 144 cases of proven or suspected NAT caused by anti-Pl^{A1}. Thus the observed ratio of NAT caused by anti-Pl^{A2}/anti-Pl^{A1} (1:144, or 0.007) is almost 1,000 times less than predicted with the theoretic ratio (6.4).

Immunogenetics is a major factor determining alloimmunization against Pl^{A1}. There is a strong association between formation of anti-Pl^{A1} and HLA-DRB3*0101 and HLA-DQB1*0201 (odds ratio, 25 and 40, respectively) (145). In contrast, no HLA association exists for immunization against Pl^{A2} (147). Thus it appears that persons with certain HLA genotypes are much more likely to generate an alloimmune response when GP IIIa bears the leucine$_{33}$ substitution that determines the Pl^{A1} phenotype.

Overall, on the basis of the observed allelic frequencies, the expected theoretic ratio of NAT for anti-Br^a, compared with anti-Br^b, should be approximately 8 (Table 27.6). A similar ratio

TABLE 27.6. OBSERVED FREQUENCIES OF NEONATAL ALLOIMMUNE THROMBOCYTOPENIA (NAT) AND POSTTRANSFUSION PURPURA (PTP) IN RELATION TO EXPECTED (THEORETIC) FREQUENCY OF THE P1$^{A1/A2}$, BR$^{a/b}$, AND BAK$^{a/b}$ ALLOANTIGEN SYSTEMS

Target Alloantigen	Percentage of Pregnancies at Theoretic Risk of NAT[a] (Descending Order)	Observed Cases of NAT[b]	Observed Cases of PTP[c]
Bak^b	14.5	0	0
P1^{A2}	10.8	0	11
Bak^a	9.3	1	6
Br^a	8.7	6	3
P1^{A1}	1.9	44	76
Br^b	1.1	0	3

Note the lack of correlation between the theoretic and observed risk of NAT.
[a]Percentage of pregnancies at theoretic risk of NAT for a given target alloantigen is determined as follows: $x(1 - x)^2 \times 100$, where x is the gene frequency of the target alloantigen.
[b]Data are from Mueller-Eckhardt et al. (143) and represent serologic investigations using a defined protocol over an 18-month period ending June 30, 1988.
[c]Data are from McFarland (15,146) and include only those cases in which one platelet-specific alloantibody was detected.
NAT, neonatal alloimmune thrombocytopenia; PTP, posttransfusion purpura.
From Warkentin TE, Smith JW. The alloimmune thrombocytopenic syndromes. *Transfus Med Rev* 1997;11:296–307, with permission.

(47:3, or 15.7) has been observed. However, although the expected and observed ratios are similar (contrast the Pl^{A1}/A2 system), a role for immunogenetics and alloimmunization exists also for the Br$^{a/b}$ system (148).

Severity of Alloimmune Thrombocytopenia

In general, the severity of thrombocytopenia is greater for alloimmune thrombocytopenia that involves the GP IIb/IIIa complex, compared with the GP Ia/IIa complex (Table 27.7; 140,143,146,149). Because there are approximately 20 times more GP IIb/IIIa molecules compared with GP Ia/IIa complexes (40,000 versus 2,000), this suggests that greater numbers of alloantibodies binding to the more numerous GP IIb/IIIa receptors results in greater platelet destruction.

Neonatal Alloimmune Thrombocytopenia

Neonatal alloimmune thrombocytopenia is a transient but potentially life-threatening thrombocytopenic disorder limited to

TABLE 27.7. SEVERITY OF THROMBOCYTOPENIA BY PLATELET COUNT NADIRS ($\times 10^9$/L) IN RELATION TO TARGET GLYCOPROTEIN FOR VARIOUS ALLOIMMUNE THROMBOCYTOPENIC SYNDROMES

Glycoprotein	NAT	PTP	PAT	TAT
GP IIb/IIIa				
P1A1 (IIIa)	17 (n = 81)	6 (n = 43)	8 (n = 9)	8 (n = 4)
P1A2 (IIIa)	9 (n = 2)	5 (n = 4)	—	—
Bak$^{a/b}$ (IIb)	10 (n = 5)	3 (n = 4)	—	—
Pen$^{a/b}$ (IIIa)	13 (n = 7)	6 (n = 1)	—	—
Mean	16	6	8	8
GP Ia/IIa				
Br^a	44 (n = 48)	26 (n = 1)	35 (n = 1)	43 (n = 1)
Br^b	35 (n = 5)	—	—	—
Mean	43	26	35	43

The data show that alloimmune thrombocytopenic syndromes that involve GP IIb/IIIa are more likely to cause severe thrombocytopenia than are those involving GP Ia/IIa. The data are combined for alloimmune thrombocytopenic syndromes involving either allele of the Bak$^{a/b}$ and Pen$^{a/b}$ alloantigen systems, whereas the data are shown separately for the alleles of the P1$^{A1/A2}$ and Br$^{a/b}$ systems.
NAT, neonatal alloimmune thrombocytopenia; PTP, posttransfusion purpura; PAT, passive alloimmune thrombocytopenia; TAT, transplantation-associated alloimmune thrombocytopenia.
Data from Warkentin TE, Smith JW. The alloimmune thrombocytopenic syndromes. *Transfus Med Rev* 1997;11:296–307 and Brunner-Bolliger S, Kiefel V, Horber FF, et al. Antibody studies in a patient with acute thrombocytopenia following infusion of plasma containing anti-P1A1. *Am J Hematol* 1997;56:119–121.

fetal and neonatal life. It is caused by maternal IgG alloantibodies that cross the placenta and cause premature destruction of platelets bearing paternally derived platelet alloantigens (analogous to hemolytic disease of the newborn). Neonatal alloimmune thrombocytopenia occurs in approximately 1 to 1.5 per 1,000 live births (150).

Approximately 75% of cases in a white population are caused by fetomaternal incompatibility for the platelet-specific alloantigen, Pl^{A1}, and 20% by Br^{a} (143). Other alloantigens implicated in NAT, including private alloantigens identified in only one or a few families (e.g., Tu^{a}/Ca^{a}, Mo^{a}), are shown in Table 27.5. In oriental populations, anti-Pen^{b} is more common than is anti-Pl^{A1}. Although HLA or ABO alloantibodies have been claimed to cause NAT, it is more likely that undetected platelet-specific alloantibodies or another diagnosis causes the thrombocytopenia (151).

The typical clinical manifestation of NAT is isolated severe thrombocytopenia in an otherwise healthy neonate, especially if fetomaternal incompatibility involves an alloantigen on the GP IIb/IIIa complex (Table 27.6). Petechiae are found in 90%, gastrointestinal tract hemorrhage in 30%, and hemoptysis, hematuria, and retinal bleeding in fewer than 10% of patients. Approximately 15% of patients have intracranial hemorrhage (143). The thrombocytopenia usually resolves within 1 to 3 weeks. Serious sequelae of fetal and neonatal intracranial bleeding include hydrocephalus, porencephalic cysts, and epilepsy. First-born offspring constitute approximately one-half of patients. This suggests that unlike the situation for hemolytic disease of the newborn, sensitization can occur early during the first pregnancy (143). Subsequent affected siblings usually have thrombocytopenia to a similar or greater extent, an observation used to emphasize preventive treatment in subsequent pregnancies.

Laboratory investigation of possible NAT involves three steps. First, there must be a high index of suspicion. Isolated thrombocytopenia in an otherwise well infant must be assumed NAT until proved otherwise. The second step is to type maternal platelets to see whether the mother lacks certain platelet alloantigens that often are associated with alloimmune thrombocytopenia; for example, maternal homozygous $Pl^{A2}/^{A2}$ (or Pl^{A1}-negative) status confers risk of NAT caused by anti-Pl^{A1} alloantibodies. The third step is to determine whether the mother has antiplatelet alloantibodies in her serum. Sometimes, no alloantibodies can be detected in maternal serum despite severe neonatal thrombocytopenia. Indeed, for approximately one-fourth of Pl^{A1}-negative mothers with infants believed to have had NAT, anti-Pl^{A1} alloantibodies cannot be detected (143). The potential for low-incidence platelet-specific alloantigens to explain fetomaternal incompatibility means that maternal serum should be tested against paternal platelets whenever possible. There remains debate as to whether titer of alloantibodies predicts severity of fetal thrombocytopenia.

Neonatal Treatment

The optimal treatment of a neonate in whom NAT is suspected because of severe thrombocytopenia is to increase the platelet count urgently to safe levels, even before serologic confirmation of the diagnosis. In some centers (e.g., the National Blood Service in the United Kingdom), Pl^{A1}- and Br^{a}-negative platelets can be obtained on request. These should be effective for more than 95% of patients (152). When matched platelets are not available, washed and irradiated maternal platelets should be given to the neonate. These platelets are obtained by means of pheresis and are washed to remove the maternal alloantibodies. Irradiation is performed to prevent graft versus host disease caused by maternal lymphocytes. In an emergency, immediate administration of random donor platelets may be of some benefit to a bleeding infant. Giving high-dose IVIG to the neonate increases the platelet count of approximately 65% of patients (153). This treatment should be combined with maternally derived platelets. Glucocorticoids are not recommended.

Prenatal Management

Approximately one-half of the time, NAT is suspected during the prenatal period, usually because the mother previously bore an affected infant, although the diagnosis sometimes is suggested in utero when fetal ultrasonography shows cerebral hemorrhage, hydrocephalus, or hydrops fetalis (152). One tenet of management is that thrombocytopenia in a subsequently affected offspring is generally as severe as, or more severe than, a previously affected sibling. Neonatal alloimmune thrombocytopenia caused by anti-Pl^{A1} alloantibodies is more likely to cause fetal morbidity and mortality than that caused by anti-Br^{a} alloantibodies and usually requires more aggressive treatment. When the father is known to be heterozygous for the implicated alloantigen (a situation that occurs approximately 25% and 20% of the time for NAT involving the $Pl^{A1}/^{A2}$ and $Br^{a/b}$ systems, respectively), prenatal fetal typing (usually performed with genetic methods) is important, because it identifies the homozygous infant who is not at risk, obviating further treatment. For pregnancies at risk, general advice to the mother includes avoiding aspirin and nonsteroidal antiinflammatory medications (152).

Two general approaches have been taken to manage pregnancies at high risk of severe NAT (152,154): regular administration of high-dose IVIG, repeated in utero platelet transfusions, or both. The initial step is to obtain a fetal platelet count by means of percutaneous umbilical blood sampling, generally starting at 20 to 24 weeks of gestation. Because of the risk of fetal exsanguination, maternal platelets should be on hand for transfusion if the fetal platelet count is shown to be less than $50 \times 10^9/L$ (154). Intravenous immune globulin is given at a dosage of 1 g/kg per week starting within 1 week of documentation of fetal thrombocytopenia. Fetal blood sampling is repeated 4 to 6 weeks later; if no response is seen, glucocorticoid salvage treatment (prednisone, 60 mg/d) is started (154). However, not all fetuses respond to this approach.

Another approach, which has been used in certain European centers, involves regular intrauterine platelet transfusions by means of percutaneous umbilical blood sampling, including a short time before delivery. This approach has led to good outcome in situations in which previous siblings were severely affected (155). Each fetal platelet transfusion carries risk of fetal hemorrhage and death (156) that likely depends on the experience of the fetomaternal unit. There is no consensus on which approach is preferred.

Regardless of the antenatal management, there is consensus that delivery should be by means of elective cesarean section, performed as soon as fetal maturity is documented. The main reason for this mode of delivery is that it allows an organized, multidisciplinary approach to the peripartum care of the newborn. This approach includes urgent determination of the cord platelet count, provision of washed, irradiated maternal platelets and, usually, the use of high-dose IVIG (1 g/kg per day for 2 consecutive days) to control severe neonatal thrombocytopenia.

Posttransfusion Purpura

Posttransfusion purpura is a very rare disorder that typically manifests as severe thrombocytopenia and bleeding that begin 5 to 10 days after blood product transfusion (usually red blood cell concentrates) (146,157). In 95% of cases, elderly women are affected. This finding suggests that alloimmune sensitization occurred during a pregnancy. The observation that previous blood transfusions can be sensitizing explains why, in rare instances, men have PTP. Although the thrombocytopenia usually lasts 1 to 4 weeks, the duration can be as short as 3 days to as long as 4 months or more. The platelet count usually is less than 10×10^9/L (Table 27.6). Mucocutaneous and postoperative wound bleeding is common, and approximately 5% to 10% of patients die. Because effective treatments are available (see later), it is important to diagnose PTP promptly to minimize morbidity and mortality.

Pathogenesis

Invariably, high-titer, platelet-specific alloantibodies are found in the patient's serum or plasma. Although platelet-specific alloantibodies are causative, the pathogenesis remains obscure, and the conundrum is why autologous platelets are destroyed. Three major hypotheses have been proposed to explain the pathogenesis of PTP, as follows:

1. Immune complex platelet destruction. Autologous platelets are destroyed by immune complexes consisting of alloantibodies that interact with allogeneic platelet antigens.
2. Conversion of antigen-negative to antigen-positive platelets. Soluble allogeneic platelet antigens bind onto autologous platelets, rendering them susceptible to alloimmune destruction.
3. Cross-reaction between alloantibodies and antigen-positive and antigen-negative platelets (pseudospecificity). The pathogenic alloantibodies recognize the autologous platelet determinants and the foreign alloantigen. Taaning and Tønnesen (158) reported that panreactive anti-GP IIb/IIIa antibodies are readily detected during, but not after, an episode of PTP. In contrast, alloantibody reactivity usually persists for several years.

Although the Pl^{A1} alloantigen has been implicated most often, other alloantigens reported to cause PTP include Pl^{A2}, Bak^a, Bak^b, Pen^a, and Br^a. Often, more than one type of platelet-specific alloantibody can be identified in the patient's serum. As in NAT, the HLA-DR3 antigen is found in most Pl^{A1}-negative patients with PTP.

Treatment

High-dose IVIG was first reported to be effective in the management of PTP in 1983, and it remains the treatment of choice. More than 90% of patients respond, attaining a platelet count greater than 100×10^9/L in an average of 4 days (159). Although some physicians also give glucocorticoids, this agent probably does not influence the course of disease and should be considered adjunctive rather than primary therapy. In rare instances, splenectomy may be considered for a patient with disease refractory to IVIG, glucocorticoids, and compatible platelet transfusion.

Random-donor platelets should not be administered; they usually are destroyed quickly, and they can cause febrile or even anaphylactoid reactions (158). The efficacy of Pl^{A1}-negative platelet transfusions (for patients with PTP caused by anti-Pl^{A1} alloantibodies) is uncertain. Some reports indicate lack of benefit (160). Red blood cells should be washed (161) or filtered (160) before administration to remove contaminating platelet antigens. For a patient who has recovered from PTP, future precautions usually include avoidance of incompatible blood products in the future (only autologous, washed, or platelet alloantigen-compatible red blood cells are given, or platelet alloantigen-compatible plasma or platelet products are given). However, PTP does not necessarily recur even if incompatible blood is given, possibly because residual high-titer platelet alloantibodies immediately clear the alloantigens. Patients with a history of PTP must not donate blood because their plasma can trigger passive alloimmune thrombocytopenia.

Passive Alloimmune Thrombocytopenia

Passive alloimmune thrombocytopenia is characterized by abrupt onset of thrombocytopenia within a few hours after transfusion of a blood product (140). It is caused by the passive transfer of platelet-reactive alloantibodies in the blood product that rapidly clear the incompatible recipient platelets. Protein-specific platelet-antibody studies confirm that the alloantibodies bind to the recipient's platelets. However, although the alloantibody can be detected in the donor's plasma, it is not detectable in the recipient's plasma. This finding suggests that almost 100% of the transfused alloantibody binds soon after transfusion (149, 162). Only two alloantigens (Pl^{A1} and Br^a) have been implicated in this syndrome. In general, the severity of bleeding parallels the degree of thrombocytopenia; thus spontaneous mucocutaneous bleeding occurs in patients with severe thrombocytopenia caused by anti-Pl^{A1} alloantibodies. The duration of thrombocytopenia is generally less than 1 week, unlike that of PTP. It is important to investigate suspected PAT, because the risk that numerous recipients can develop this syndrome means that the implicated blood donor must not donate blood in the future.

Tranplantation-associated Alloimmune Thrombocytopenia

In rare instances, alloimmune mechanisms explain thrombocytopenia that occurs in the setting of transplantation of peripheral blood progenitor cells, bone marrow, or solid organs.

Bone Marrow Transplantation

Panzer et al. (163) described a 32-year-old man with chronic myeloid leukemia who had severe thrombocytopenia (platelet count, 17×10^9/L) beginning 18 months after allogeneic marrow transplantation from his HLA-matched sister. High-dose IVIG gave transient increases in platelet count, and persisting remission followed splenectomy. Antibodies with anti-Pl^{A1} specificity were eluted from the patient's platelets. This led to further investigations, which showed that a small number of residual, nonneoplastic lymphoid cells of host origin produced anti-Pl^{A1} alloantibodies against the Pl^{A1}-positive platelets formed by donor-derived megakaryocytes. Thus host versus donor alloimmune thrombocytopenia resulted from mixed chimerism, in which residual host lymphoid cells derived from a Pl^{A1}-negative individual developed an alloimmune response against platelets derived from the engrafted Pl^{A1}-positive marrow.

A similar situation attributable to anti-Br^a alloantibodies after allogeneic marrow transplantation for chronic myeloid leukemia has been reported (164). However, in this patient, anti-Br^a alloantibodies were detectable both before and after transplantation, and the early posttransplantion thrombocytopenia (which also responded transiently to high-dose IVIG treatment) gradually improved as elutable anti-Br^a alloantibodies became more difficult to detect.

Alloimmune thrombocytopenia may have played a role in two cases of transfusion-refractory thrombocytopenia associated with an increase in titer of anti-Pl^{A1} alloantibodies (compared with the pretransplantation state) that developed after autologous peripheral blood cell transplantation performed for metastatic carcinoma of the breast. However, these reports are not conclusive, because it is difficult to differentiate a PTP-like illness (which implies destruction of engrafted autologous donor marrow-derived platelets) from typical posttransplantation platelet transfusion refractoriness (165).

Solid-organ Transplantation

In rare instances, immunocompetent lymphoid cells within a transplanted solid organ cause alloimmune thrombocytopenia in the recipient of the organ. A dramatic scenario was reported by West et al. (166). All three organ recipients (two of a kidney, one of a liver) had severe thrombocytopenia and bleeding within 5 to 8 days after transplantation from a multiparous female organ donor with a normal platelet count who had sustained a subarachnoid hemorrhage. The two recipients of renal transplants had thrombocytopenia refractory to high-dose IVIG and platelet transfusions. One of these patients died, but the other recovered after splenectomy performed 50 days after transplantation. The recipient of the liver transplant had organ rejection, which was accompanied by correction of the platelet count when he received a new liver allograft. Anti-Pl^{A1} alloantibodies were detected in the organ donor and posttransplant (but not pretransplant) recipient serum. These cases illustrate that passenger immunocompetent lymphoid cells occasionally induce severe alloimmune thrombocytopenia when introduced into an alloincompatible environment.

TABLE 27.8. GENERAL CAUSES OF PLATELET TRANSFUSION REFRACTORINESS, LISTED IN PROBABLE DESCENDING ORDER OF FREQUENCY

Nonimmune mechanisms
Septicemia, fever, disseminated intravascular coagulation, amphotericin B therapy, hypersplenism, fixed platelet count requirements in severe thrombocytopenia
Platelet-nonspecific alloantibodies
HLA alloantibodies
ABO alloantibodies
Platelet-specific alloantibodies
Drug-dependent antibodies (e.g., vancomycin)
Platelet-reactive autoantibodies

Modified from Warkentin TE, Smith JW. The alloimmune thrombocytopenic syndromes. *Transfus Med Rev* 1997;11:296–307, with permission.

Platelet Transfusion Refractoriness

Platelet transfusion refractoriness (PTR), which is failure to achieve the expected platelet increment after two consecutive platelet transfusion episodes, has several explanations (Table 27.8; see Chapter 18). Nonimmune, patient-dependent factors are probably the most important, which means that poor platelet count recoveries can persist even when HLA alloimmunization is prevented with leukocyte-depleted blood products (167) and HLA- or ABO-compatible platelets are given.

There is anecdotal evidence that platelet-specific alloantibodies sometimes cause PTR. However, prospective studies have shown that this is a relatively infrequent occurrence. For example, Novotny et al. (168) found that even when HLA alloantibody formation was largely prevented with blood products filtered before storage, platelet-specific alloantibodies at most explained 4 of 79 (5%) of cases of PTR. There are occasions, however, on which the transfusion service needs to provide HLA- and platelet-specific antigen-compatible platelet products to treat certain patients with PTR (169).

SUMMARY

A variety of platelet-antibody and other assays have improved the ability of the clinician to make an accurate diagnosis of immune thrombocytopenia in many diverse clinical settings that can involve pathogenic autoantibodies, alloantibodies, and drug-dependent antibodies. The treatment decisions that arise depend on several factors, including the nature of the specific diagnosis, the expected prognosis, and the presence of clinically evident bleeding or thrombosis.

REFERENCES

1. Brecher G, Schneiderman M, Cronkite EP. The reproducibility and constancy of the platelet count. *Am J Clin Pathol* 1953;23:15–26.
2. Warkentin TE, Levine MN, Hirsh J, et al. Heparin-induced thrombocytopenia in patients treated with low-molecular-weight heparin or unfractionated heparin. *N Engl J Med* 1995;332:1330–1335.

3. Warkentin TE. Heparin-induced thrombocytopenia: a ten-year retrospective. *Annu Rev Med* 1999;50;129–147.
4. Niethammer AG, Forman EN. Use of the platelet histogram maximum in evaluating thrombocytopenia. *Am J Hematol* 1999;60:19–23.
5. Beer JH, Büchi L, Steiner B. Glycocalicin: a new assay the normal plasma levels and its potential usefulness in selected diseases. *Blood* 1994;83:691–702.
6. Kelton JG, Murphy WG, Lucarelli A, et al. A prospective comparison of four techniques for measuring platelet-associated IgG. *Br J Haematol* 1989;71:97–105.
7. Visentin GP, Wolfmeyer K, Newman PJ, et al. Detection of drug-dependent, platelet-reactive antibodies by antigen-capture ELISA and flow cytometry. *Transfusion* 1990;30:694–700.
8. Kiefel V. The MAIPA assay and its applications in immunohaematology. *Transfus Med* 1992;2:181–188.
9. Warner MN, Moore JC, Warkentin TE, et al. A prospective study of protein-specific assays used to investigate idiopathic thrombocytopenic purpura. *Br J Haematol* 1999;104:442–447.
10. Smith JW, Hayward CPM, Warkentin TE, et al. Investigation of human platelet alloantigens and glycoproteins using non-radioactive immunoprecipitation. *J Immunol Methods* 1993;158:77–85.
11. Smith JW, Hayward CPM, Horsewood P, et al. Characterization and localization of the Gova/b alloantigens to the glycosylphosphatidylinositol-anchored protein CDw109 on human platelets. *Blood* 1995; 86:2807–2814.
12. Warkentin TE. Laboratory testing for heparin-induced thrombocytopenia. *J Thromb Thrombolysis* 2001;10:S35–S45.
13. Warkentin TE, Sheppard JI, Horsewood P, et al. Impact of the patient population on the risk for heparin-induced thrombocytopenia. *Blood* 2000;96:1703–1708.
14. Amiral J, Bridey F, Dreyfus M, et al. Platelet factor 4 complexed to heparin is the target for antibodies generated in heparin-induced thrombocytopenia [letter]. *Thromb Haemost* 1992;68:95–96.
15. McFarland JG. Platelet and neutrophil alloantigen genotyping in clinical practice. *Transfus Clin Biol* 1998;5:13–21.
16. Denomme GA, Waye JS, Burrows RF, et al. The prenatal identification of fetal compatibility in neonatal alloimmune thrombocytopenia using amniotic fluid and variable number of tandem repeat (VNTR) analysis. *Br J Haematol* 1995;91:742–746.
17. Unkelbach K, Kalb R, Breitfeld C, et al. New polymorphism on platelet glycoprotein IIIa gene recognized by endonuclease Msp I: implications for PlA typing by allele-specific restriction analysis. *Transfusion* 1994;34:592–595.
18. Wang R, McFarland JG, Kekomaki R, et al. Amino acid 489 encoded by a mutational hot spot on the β_3 integrin chain: the CA/TU human platelet alloantigen system. *Blood* 1993;82:3386–3391.
19. Skogen B, Bellissimo DB, Hessner MJ, et al. Rapid determination of platelet alloantigen genotypes by polymerase chain reaction using allele-specific primers. *Transfusion* 1994;34:955–960.
20. Nauck MS, Gierens H, Nauck MA, et al. Rapid genotyping of human platelet antigen 1 (HPA-1) with fluorophore-labelled hybridization probes on the LightCycler. *Br J Haematol* 1999;105:803–810.
21. George JN, Woolf SH, Raskob GE, et al. Idiopathic thrombocytopenic purpura: a practice guideline developed by explicit methods for the American Society of Hematology. *Blood* 1996;88:3–40.
22. McMillan R. Autoantibodies and autoantigens in chronic immune thrombocytopenic purpura. *Semin Hematol* 2000;37:239–248.
23. Harrington WJ, Minnich V, Hollingsworth JW, et al. Demonstration of a thrombocytopenic factor in the blood of patients with thrombocytopenic purpura: 1951 *J Lab Clin Med* 1990;115:636–645.
24. Han P, Turpie AGG, Genton E. Plasma β-thromboglobulin: differentiation between intravascular and extravascular platelet destruction. *Blood* 1979;54:1192–1196.
25. Kelton JG, Steeves K. The amount of platelet-bound albumin parallels the amount of IgG on washed platelets from patients with immune thrombocytopenia. *Blood* 1983;62:924–927.
26. George JN. Platelet IgG: measurement, interpretation, and clinical significance. *Prog Hemost Thromb* 1991;10:97–106.
27. Hughes M, Hayward CPM, Horsewood P, et al. Measurement of endogenous and exogenous alpha-granular platelet proteins in patients with immune and nonimmune thrombocytopenia. *Br J Haematol* 1999;106:762–770.
28. Hughes M, Webert K, Kelton JG. The use of electron microscopy in the investigation of the ultrastructural morphology of immune thrombocytopenic purpura platelets. *Semin Hematol* 2000;37: 222–228.
29. Cohen YC, Djulbegovic B, Shamai-Lubovitz O, et al. The bleeding risk and natural history of idiopathic thrombocytopenic purpura in patients with persistent low platelet counts. *Arch Intern Med* 2000; 160:1630–1638.
30. Rinder HM, Tracey JB, Recht M, et al. Differences in platelet alpha-granule release between normals and immune thrombocytopenic patients and between young and old platelets. *Thromb Haemost* 1998; 80:457–462.
31. Vantelon JM, Godeau B, André, C, et al. Screening for autoimmune markers is unnecessary during follow-up of adults with autoimmune thrombocytopenic purpura and no autoimmune markers at onset. *Thromb Haemost* 2000;83:42–45.
32. Carr JM, Kruskall MS, Kaye JA, et al. Efficacy of platelet transfusions in immune thrombocytopenia. *Am J Med* 1986;80:1051–1054.
33. Mazzucconi MG, Francesconi M, Fidani P, et al. Treatment of idiopathic thrombocytopenic purpura (ITP): results of a multicentric protocol. *Haematologica* 1985;70:329–336.
34. Bellucci S, Charpak Y, Chastang C, et al. Low doses v conventional doses of corticoids in immune thrombocytopenic purpura (ITP): results of a randomized clinical trial in 160 children, 223 adults. *Blood* 1988;71:1165–1169.
35. Jacobs P, Woods L, Novitzky N. Intravenous gammaglobulin has no advantages over oral corticosteroids as primary therapy for adults with immune thrombocytopenia: a prospective randomized clinical trial. *Am J Med* 1994;97:55–59.
36. Warner M, Wasi P, Couban S, et al. Failure of pulse high-dose dexamethasone in chronic idiopathic immune thrombocytopenia. *Am J Hematol* 1997;54:267–270.
37. Stasi R, Stipa E, Masi M, et al. Long-term observation of 208 adults with chronic idiopathic thrombocytopenic purpura. *Am J Med* 1995; 98:436–442.
38. DiFino SM, Lachant NA, Kirshner JJ, et al. Adult idiopathic thrombocytopenic purpura: clinical findings and response to therapy. *Am J Med* 1980;69:430–442.
39. Pizzuto J, Ambriz R. Therapeutic experience on 934 adults with idiopathic thrombocytopenic purpura: multicentric trial of the Cooperative Latin American Group on Hemostasis and Thrombosis. *Blood* 1984;64:1179–1183.
40. Mankin HJ. Nontraumatic necrosis of bone (osteonecrosis). *N Engl J Med* 1992;326:1473–1479.
41. Coon WW. Splenectomy for idiopathic thrombocytopenic purpura. *Surg Gynecol Obstet* 1987;164:225–229.
42. Law C, Marcaccio M, Tam P, et al. High-dose intravenous immune globulin and the response to splenectomy in patients with idiopathic thrombocytopenic purpura. *N Engl J Med* 1997;336:1494–1498.
43. Najean Y, Rain JD, Billotey C. The site of destruction of autologous 111In-labelled platelets and the efficiency of splenectomy in children and adults with idiopathic thrombocytopenic purpura: a study of 578 patients with 268 splenectomies. *Br J Haematol* 1997;97:547–550.
44. Marcaccio MJ. Laparoscopic splenectomy in chronic idiopathic thrombocytopenic purpura. *Semin Hematol* 2000;37:267–274.
45. Facon T, Caulier MT, Fenaux P, et al. Accessory spleen in recurrent chronic immune thrombocytopenic purpura. *Am J Hematol* 1992;41: 184–189.
46. Styrt B. Infection associated with asplenia: risks, mechanisms, and prevention. *Am J Med* 1990;88:5N–33N.
47. Centers for Disease Control and Prevention. Recommendations of the Advisory Committee on Immunization Practices (ACIP). Use of vaccines and immune globulins in persons with altered immunocompetence. *MMWR Morb Mortal Wkly Rep*1993;42:(RR-4):1–18.
48. Schreiber AD, Chien P, Tomaski A, et al. Effect of danazol in immune thrombocytopenic purpura. *N Engl J Med* 1987;316:503–508.
49. Blanco R, Martinez-Taboada VM, Rodriguez-Valverde V, et al. Successful therapy with danazol in refractory autoimmune thrombocyto-

penia associated with rheumatic diseases. *Br J Rheumatol* 1997;36: 1095–1099.
50. Facon T, Caulier MT, Wattel E, et al. A randomized trial comparing vinblastine in slow infusion and by bolus i. v. injection in idiopathic thrombocytopenic purpura: a report on 42 patients. *Br J Haematol* 1994;86:678–680.
51. Reiner A, Gernsheimer T, Slichter SJ. Pulse cyclophosphamide therapy for refractory autoimmune thrombocytopenic purpura. *Blood* 1995;85:351–358.
52. Krause JR. Chronic idiopathic thrombocytopenic purpura (ITP): development of acute non-lymphocytic leukemia subsequent to treatment with cyclophosphamide. *Med Pediatr Oncol* 1982;10:61–65.
53. Imbach P, Barandun S, d'Appuzo V, et al. High-dose intravenous gammaglobulin for idiopathic thrombocytopenic purpura in childhood. *Lancet* 1981;1:1228–1231.
54. Smiley JD, Talbert MG. Southwestern Internal Medicine Conference: high-dose intravenous gammaglobulin therapy: how does it work? *Am J Med* Sci 1995;309:295–303.
55. Sandler SG, Novak SC, Roland B. The cost of treating immune thrombocytopenic purpura using intravenous Rh immune globulin versus intravenous immune globulin. *Am J Hematol* 2000;63: 156–158.
56. Godeau B, Lesage S, Divine M, et al. Treatment of adult chronic autoimmune thrombocytopenic purpura with repeated high-dose intravenous immunoglobulin. *Blood* 1993;82:1415–1421.
57. Elkayam O, Paran D, Milo R, et al. Acute myocardial infarction associated with high dose intravenous immunoglobulin for autoimmune disorders: a study of four cases. *Ann Rheum Dis* 2000;59:77–80.
58. Bussel JB, Graziano JN, Kimberly RP, et al. Intravenous anti-D treatment of immune thrombocytopenic purpura: analysis of efficacy, toxicity, and mechanism of effect. *Blood* 1991;77:1884–1893.
59. Scaradavou A, Woo B, Woloski BMR, et al. Intravenous anti-D treatment of immune thrombocytopenic purpura: experience in 272 patients. *Blood* 1997;89:2689–2700.
60. Gaines AR. Acute onset hemoglobinemia and/or hemoglobinuria and sequelae following Rho(D) immune globulin intravenous administration in immune thrombocytopenic purpura patients. *Blood* 2000;95: 2523–2529.
61. Kenny-Walsh E, for the Irish Hepatology Research Group. Clinical outcomes after hepatitis C infection from contaminated anti-D immune globulin. *N Engl J Med* 1999;340:1228–1233.
62. Stern SCM, Asagba GO, Hegde UM. Prolonged thrombocytopenia following alpha-interferon for refractory immune thrombocytopenic purpura. *Clin Lab Haematol* 1994;16:183–185.
63. Garcia-Suárez J, Burgaleta C, Hernanz N, et al. HCV-associated thrombocytopenia: clinical characteristics and platelet response after recombinant α2b-interferon therapy. *Br J Haematol* 2000;110: 98–103.
64. Emilia G, Messora C, Longo G, et al. Long-term salvage treatment by cyclosporin in refractory autoimmune haematological disorders. *Br J Haematol* 1996;93:341–344.
65. Ratanatharathorn V, Carson E, Reynolds C, et al. Anti-CD20 chimeric monoclonal antibody treatment of refractory immune-mediated thrombocytopenia in a patient with chronic graft-versus-host disease. *Ann Intern Med* 2000;133:275–279.
66. Baumann MA, Menitove JE, Aster RH, et al. Urgent treatment of idiopathic thrombocytopenic purpura with single-dose gammaglobulin infusion followed by platelet transfusion. *Ann Intern Med* 1986; 104:808–809.
67. Chandramouli NB, Rodgers GM. Prolonged immunoglobulin and platelet infusion for treatment of immune thrombocytopenia. *Am J Hematol* 2000;65:85–86.
68. Burrows RF, Kelton JG. Incidentally detected thrombocytopenia in healthy mothers and their infants. *N Engl J Med* 1988;319:142–145.
69. Burrows RF, Kelton JG. Pregnancy in patients with idiopathic thrombocytopenic purpura: assessing the risks for the infant at delivery. *Obstet Gynecol Surv* 1993;48:781–788.
70. Caruso A, De Carolis S, Di Simone N. Antiphospholipid antibodies in obstetrics: new complexities and sites of action. *Hum Reprod Update* 1999;5:267–276.
71. Burrows RF, Kelton JG. Low fetal risks in pregnancies associated with idiopathic thrombocytopenic purpura. *Am J Obstet Gynecol* 1990;163: 1147–1150.
72. Winiarski J. Mechanisms in childhood idiopathic thrombocytopenic purpura. *Acta Paediatr Suppl* 1998;424:54–56.
73. Longacre TA, Foucar K, Crago S, et al. Hematogones: a multiparameter analysis of bone marrow precursor cells. *Blood* 1989;73:543–552.
74. Blanchette VS, Luke B, Andrew M, et al. A prospective randomised trial of high-dose intravenous immunoglobulin G (IVIgG), oral prednisone and no therapy in childhood acute immune thrombocytopenic purpura. *J Pediatr* 1993;123:989–995.
75. Blanchette V, Imbach P, Andrew M, et al. Randomised trial of intravenous immunoglobulin G, intravenous anti-D, and oral prednisone in childhood acute immune thrombocytopenic purpura. *Lancet* 1994; 344:703–707.
76. Warrier I, Bussel JB, Valdez L, et al. Safety and efficacy of low-dose intravenous immune globulin (IVIG) treatment for infants and children with immune thrombocytopenic purpura. *J Pediatr Hematol Oncol* 1997;19:197–201.
77. Albayrak D, İslek İ, Kalayci AG, et al. Acute immune thrombocytopenic purpura: a comparative study of very high oral doses of methylprednisolone and intravenously administered immune globulin. *J Pediatr* 1994;125:1004–1007.
78. Gereige RS, Barrios NJ. Treatment of childhood acute immune thrombocytopenic purpura with high-dose methylprednisolone, intravenous immunoglobulin, or the combination of both. *P R Health Sci J* 2000;19:15–18.
79. Tarantino MD. Treatment options for chronic immune (idiopathic) thrombocytopenia purpura in children. *Semin Hematol* 2000; 37[Suppl 1]:35–41.
80. Hollenberg JP, Subak LL, Ferry JJ Jr, et al. Cost-effectiveness of splenectomy versus intravenous gamma globulin in treatment of chronic immune thrombocytopenic purpura in childhood. *J Pediatr* 1988; 112:530–539.
81. Andrew M, Blanchette VS, Adams M, et al. A multicenter study of the treatment of childhood chronic idiopathic thrombocytopenic purpura with anti-D. *J Pediatr* 1992;120:522–527.
82. de Principe, Menichelli A, Mori PG, et al. Phase II trial of methylprednisolone pulse therapy in childhood chronic thrombocytopenia. *Acta Haematol* 1987;77:226–230.
83. Miller MH, Urowitz MB, Gladman DD. The significance of thrombocytopenia in systemic lupus erythematosus. *Arthritis Rheum* 1983; 26:1181–1186.
84. Love PE, Santoro SA. Antiphospholipid antibodies: anticardiolipin and the lupus anticoagulant in systemic lupus erythematosus (SLE) and in non-SLE disorders. *Ann Intern Med* 1990;112:682–698.
85. Naldi L, Locati F, Marchesi L, et al. Cutaneous manifestations associated with antiphospholipid antibodies in patients with suspected primary antiphospholipid syndrome: a case-control study. *Ann Rheum Dis* 1993;52:219–222.
86. Triplett DA, Asherson RA. Pathophysiology of the catastrophic antiphospholipid syndrome (CAPS). *Am J Hematol* 2000;65:154–159.
87. Nesher G, Hanna VE, Moore TL, et al. Thrombotic microangiopathic hemolytic anemia in systemic lupus erythematosus. *Semin Arthritis Rheum* 1994;24:165–172.
88. Davies GE, Triplett DA. Corticosteroid-associated blue toe syndrome: role of antiphospholipid antibodies. *Ann Intern Med* 1990;113: 893–895.
89. Hakim AJ, Machin SJ, Isenberg DA. Autoimmune thrombocytopenia in primary antiphospholipid syndrome and systemic lupus erythematosus: the response to splenectomy. *Semin Arthritis Rheum* 1998;28: 20–25.
90. Boumpas DT, Barez S, Klippel JH, et al. Intermittent cyclophosphamide for the treatment of autoimmune thrombocytopenia in systemic lupus erythematosus. *Ann Intern Med* 1990;112:674–677.
91. Hanly JG, Hong C, Zayed E, et al. Immunomodulating effects of synchronised plasmapheresis and intravenous bolus cyclophosphamide in systemic lupus erythematosus. *Lupus* 1995;4:457–463.
92. Manger K, Kalden JR, Manger B. Cyclosporin A in the treatment of

systemic lupus erythematosus: results of an open clinical study. *Br J Rheumatol* 1996;35:669–675.
93. Coyle TE. Hematologic complications of human immunodeficiency virus infection and the acquired immunodeficiency syndrome. *Med Clin North Am* 1997;81:449–470.
94. Cole JL, Marzec UM, Gunthel CJ, et al. Ineffective platelet production in thrombocytopenic human immunodeficiency virus-infected patients. *Blood* 1998;91:3239–3246.
95. Bettaieb A, Fromont P, Louache F, et al. Presence of cross-reactive antibody between immunodeficiency virus (HIV) and platelet glycoproteins in HIV-related immune thrombocytopenic purpura. *Blood* 1992;80:162–169.
96. Nardi M, Karpatkin S. Antiidiotype antibody against platelet anti-GPIIIa contributes to the regulation of thrombocytopenia in HIV-1-ITP patients. *J Exp Med* 2000;191:2093–2100.
97. Landonio G, Cinque P, Nosari A, et al. Comparison of two dose regimens of zidovudine in an open, randomized, multicentre study for severe HIV-related thrombocytopenia. *AIDS* 1993;7:209–212.
98. Aboulafia DM, Bundow D, Waide S, et al. Initial observations on the efficacy of highly active antiretroviral therapy in the treatment of HIV-associated autoimmune thrombocytopenia. *Am J Med Sci* 2000; 320:117–123.
99. Jahnke L, Applebaum S, Sherman LA, et al. An evaluation of intravenous immunoglobulin in the treatment of human immunodeficiency virus–associated thrombocytopenia. *Transfusion* 1994;34:759–764.
100. Lord RVN, Coleman MJ, Milliken ST. Splenectomy for HIV-related immune thrombocytopenia: comparison with results of splenectomy for non-HIV immune thrombocytopenic purpura. *Arch Surg* 1998; 133:205–210.
101. Sonnenblick M, Kramer MR, Hershko C. Corticosteroid responsive immune thrombocytopenia in Hodgkin's disease. *Oncology* 1986;43: 349–353.
102. Berchtold P, Harris JP, Tani P, et al. Autoantibodies to platelet glycoproteins in patients with disease-related immune thrombocytopenia. *Br J Haematol* 1989;73:365–368.
103. Jillella AP, Kallab AM, Kutlar A. Autoimmune thrombocytopenia following autologous hematolpoietic cell transplantation: review of literature and treatment options. *Bone Marrow Transplant* 2000;26: 925–927.
104. Singh N, Gayowski T, Marino IR. Hemolytic uremic syndrome in solid-organ transplant recipients. *Transpl Int* 1996;9:68–75.
105. Warkentin TE, Kelton JG. Thrombocytopenia due to platelet destruction and hypersplenism. In: Hoffman R, Benz EJ Jr, Shattil SJ, et al., eds. *Hematology: basic principles and practice,* 3rd ed. New York: Churchill Livingstone, 1999:2138–2154.
106. George JN, Raskob GE, Shah SR, et al. Drug-induced thrombocytopenia: a systematic review of published case reports. *Ann Intern Med* 1998;129:886–890.
107. Aster RH. Drug-induced immune thrombocytopenia: an overview of pathogenesis. *Semin Hematol* 1999;36[Suppl 1]:2–6.
108. Warkentin TE. Clinical picture of heparin-induced thrombocytopenia. In: Warkentin TE, Greinacher A, eds. *Heparin-induced thrombocytopenia,* 2nd ed. New York: Marcel Dekker, 2001:43–86.
109. Warkentin TE, Chong BH, Greinacher A. Heparin-induced thrombocytopenia: towards consensus. *Thromb Haemost* 1998;79:1–7.
110. Pedersen-Bjergaard U, Andersen M, Hansen PB. Drug-induced thrombocytopenia: clinical data on 309 cases and the effect of corticosteroid therapy. *Eur J Clin Pharmacol* 1997;52:183–189.
111. Dasgupta H, Blankenship JC, Wood GC, et al. Thrombocytopenia complicating treatment with intravenous glycoprotein IIb/IIIa receptor inhibitors: a pooled analysis. *Am Heart J* 2000;140:206–211.
112. Warkentin TE, Kelton JG. A 14-year study of heparin-induced thrombocytopenia. *Am J Med* 1996;101:502–507.
113. Greinacher A, Pötzsch B, Amiral J, et al. Heparin-associated thrombocytopenia: isolation of the antibody and characterization of a multimolecular PF4-heparin complex as the major antigen. *Thromb Haemost* 1994;71:247–251.
114. Warkentin TE, Elavathil LJ, Hayward CPM, et al. The pathogenesis of venous limb gangrene associated with heparin-induced thrombocytopenia. *Ann Intern Med* 1997;127:804–812.
115. Greinacher A, Eichler P, Lubenow N, et al. Heparin-induced thrombocytopenia with thromboembolic complications: meta-analysis of two prospective trials to assess the value of parenteral treatment with lepirudin and its therapeutic aPTT range. *Blood* 2000;96:846–851.
116. Hughes M, Hayward CPM, Warkentin TE, et al. Morphological analysis of microparticle generation in heparin-induced thrombocytopenia. *Blood* 2000;96:188–194.
117. Newman PM, Chong BH. Heparin-induced thrombocytopenia: new evidence for the dynamic binding of purified anti-PF4-heparin antibodies to platelets and the resultant platelet activation. *Blood* 2000; 96:182–187.
118. Lee DP, Warkentin TE. Frequency of heparin-induced thrombocytopenia. In: Warkentin TE, Greinacher A, eds. *Heparin-induced thrombocytopenia,* 2nd ed. New York: Marcel Dekker, 2001:87–121.
119. Warkentin TE. Limitations of conventional treatment options for heparin-induced thrombocytopenia. *Semin Hematol* 1998;35[Suppl 5]:17–25.
120. Chong BH, Magnani HN. Danaparoid for the treatment of heparin-induced thrombocytopenia. In: Warkentin TE, Greinacher A, eds. *Heparin-induced thrombocytopenia,* 2nd ed. New York: Marcel Dekker, 2001:323–347.
121. Farner B, Eichler P, Kroll H, et al. A comparison of lepirudin and danaparoid for the treatment of heparin-induced thrombocytopenia. *Thromb Haemost* 2001;85:950–957.
122. Greinacher A, Völpel H, Janssens U, et al. Recombinant hirudin (lepirudin) provides safe and effective anticoagulation in patients with heparin-induced thrombocytopenia: a prospective study. *Circulation* 1999;99:73–80.
123. Greinacher A, Janssens U, Berg G, et al. Lepirudin (recombinant hirudin) for parenteral anticoagulation in patients with heparin-induced thrombocytopenia. *Circulation* 1999;100:587–593.
124. Lewis BE, Wallis DE, Berkowitz SD, et al. Argatroban anticoagulant therapy in patients with heparin-induced thrombocytopenia. *Circulation* 2001;103:1838–1843.
125. Hirsh J, Warkentin TE, Shaughnessy SG, et al. Heparin and low-molecular-weight heparin: mechanisms of action, pharmacokinetics, dosing, monitoring, efficacy, and safety. *Chest* 2001; 119[Suppl 1]: 64S–94S.
126. Wallis DE, Workman DL, Lewis BE, et al. Failure of early heparin cessation as treatment for heparin-induced thrombocytopenia. *Am J Med* 1999;106:629–635.
127. Warkentin TE. Heparin-induced thrombocytopenia: yet another treatment paradox? *Thromb Haemost* 2001;85:947–949.
128. Warkentin TE, Kelton JG. Temporal aspects of heparin-induced thrombocytopenia. *N Engl J Med* 2001;344:1286–1292.
129. Kaufman DW, Kelly JP, Johannes CB, et al. Acute thrombocytopenic purpura in relation to the use of drugs. *Blood* 1993;82:2714–2718.
130. Christie DJ, van Buren N, Lennon SS, et al. Vancomycin-dependent antibodies associated with thrombocytopenia and refractoriness to platelet transfusion in patients with leukemia. *Blood* 1990;75: 518–523.
131. Pereira J, Hidalgo P, Ocqueteau M, et al. Glycoprotein Ib/IX complex is the target in rifampicin-induced immune thrombocytopenia. *Br J Haematol* 2000;110:907–910.
132. Smith ME, Reid DM, Jones CE, et al. Binding of quinine and quinidine-dependent drug antibodies to platelets is mediated by the Fab domain of the immunoglobulin G and is not Fc dependent. *J Clin Invest* 1987;79:912–917.
133. Sane DC, Damaraju LV, Topol EJ, et al. Occurrence and clinical significance of pseudothrombocytopenia during abciximab therapy. *J Am Coll Cardiol* 2000;36:75–83.
134. Adachi JD, Bensen WG, Kassam Y, et al. Gold-induced thrombocytopenia: 12 cases and a review of the literature. *Semin Arthritis Rheum* 1987;16:287–293.
135. Nieminen U, Peltola H, Syrjala MT, et al. Acute thrombocytopenic purpura following measles, mumps and rubella vaccination: a report on 23 patients. *Acta Paediatr* 1993;82:267–270.
136. Bennett CL, Weinberg PD, Rozenberg-Ben-Dror K, et al. Thrombotic thrombocytopenic purpura associated with ticlopidine: a review of 60 cases. *Ann Intern Med* 1998;128:541–544.

137. Bennett CL, Connors JM, Carwile JM, et al. Thrombotic thrombocytopenic purpura associated with clopidogrel. *N Engl J Med* 2000;342:1773–1777.
138. Tsai HM, Rice L, Sarode R, et al. Antibody inhibitors to von Willebrand factor metalloproteinase and increased binding of von Willebrand factor to platelets in ticlopidine-associated thrombotic thrombocytopenic purpura. *Ann Intern Med* 2000;132:794–799.
139. Gottschall JL, Neahring B, McFarland JG, et al. Quinine-induced immune thrombocytopenia with hemolytic uremic syndrome: clinical and serological findings in nine patients and review of literature. *Am J Hematol* 1994;47:283–289.
140. Warkentin TE, Smith JW. The alloimmune thrombocytopenic syndromes. *Transfus Med Rev* 1997;11:296–307.
141. Santoso S, Kiefel V. Human platelet-specific alloantigens: update. *Vox Sang* 1998;74[Suppl 2]:249–253.
142. Smith JW, Horsewood P, McCusker PJ, et al. Severe neonatal alloimmune thrombocytopenia due to a novel low-frequency alloantigen, Dya. *Blood* 1998;90[Suppl 1]:180a(abst).
143. Mueller-Eckhardt C, Kiefel V, Grubert A, et al. 348 cases of suspected neonatal alloimmune thrombocytopenia. *Lancet* 1989;1:363–366.
144. Berry JE, Murphy CM, Smith GA, et al. Detection of Gov system antibodies by MAIPA reveals an immunogenicity similar to the HPA-5 alloantigens. *Br J Haematol* 2000;110:735–742.
145. L'Abbé, D, Tremblay L, Filion M, et al. Alloimmunization to platelet antigen HPA–1a (Pl^{A1}) is strongly associated with both HLA-DR3 *0101 and HLA-DQB1*0201. *Hum Immunol* 1992;34:107–114.
146. McFarland JG. Posttransfusion purpura. In: Popovsky MA, ed. *Transfusion reactions.* Bethesda, MD: American Association of Blood Banks, 1996:205–227.
147. Kuippers RWAM, von dem Borne AEGK, Kiefel V, et al. Leucine33-proline33 substitution in human platelet glycoprotein IIIa determine HLA-DRw52a(Dw24) association of the immune response against HPA-1a (Zwa/Pl^{A1}) and HPA-1b (Zwb/Pl^{A2}). *Hum Immunol* 1992;34:253–256.
148. Semana G, Zazoun T, Alizadeh M, et al. Genetic susceptibility and anti-human platelet antigen 5b alloimmunization: role of HLA Class II and TAP genes. *Hum Immunol* 1996;46:114–119.
149. Brunner-Bolliger S, Kiefel V, Horber FF, et al. Antibody studies in a patient with acute thrombocytopenia following infusion of plasma containing anti-Pl^{A1}. *Am J Hematol* 1997;56:119–121.
150. Blanchette VS, Johnson J, Rand M. The management of alloimmune neonatal thrombocytopenia. *Baillieres Clin Haematol* 2000;13:365–390.
151. Taaning E. HLA antibodies and fetomaternal alloimmune thrombocytopenia: myth or meaningful. *Transfus Med Rev* 2000;14:275–280.
152. Ouwehand WH, Smith G, Ranasinghe E. Management of severe alloimmune thrombocytopenia in the newborn. *Arch Dis Child Fetal Neonatal Ed* 2000;82:F173–F175.
153. Massey GV, McWilliams NB, Mueller DG, et al. Intravenous immunoglobulin in treatment of neonatal alloimmune thrombocytopenia. *J Pediatr* 1987;111:133–135.
154. Bussel JB, Berkowitz RL, Lynch L, et al. Antenatal management of alloimmune thrombocytopenia with intravenous γ-globulin: a randomized trial of the addition of low-dose steroid to intravenous γ-globulin. *Am J Obstet Gynecol* 1996;174:1414–1423.
155. Murphy MF, Waters AH, Doughty HA, et al. Antenatal management of fetomaternal alloimmune thrombocytopenia: report of 15 affected pregnancies. *Transfus Med* 1994;4:281–292.
156. Silver RM, Porter TF, Branch DW, et al. Neonatal alloimmune thrombocytopenia: antenatal management. *Am J Obstet Gynecol* 2000;182:1233–1238.
157. Kunicki TJ, Beardsley DS. The alloimmune thrombocytopenias: neonatal alloimmune thrombocytopenic purpura and post-transfusion purpura. *Prog Hematol* 1989;9:203–232.
158. Taaning E, Tønnesen F. Pan-reactive platelet antibodies in post-transfusion purpura. *Vox Sang* 1999;76:120–123.
159. Mueller-Eckhardt C, Kiefel V. High-dose IgG for post-transfusion purpura: revisited. *Blut* 1988;57:163–167.
160. Win N, Matthey F, Slater GP. Blood components: transfusion support in post-transfusion purpura due to HPA-1a immunization. *Vox Sang* 1996;71:191–193.
161. Gabriel A, LaBnigg A, Kurz M, et al. Post-transfusion purpura due to HPA-1a immunization in a male patient: response to subsequent multiple HPA-1a-incompatible red-cell transfusions. *Transfus Med* 1995;5:131–134.
162. Warkentin TE, Smith JW, Hayward CPM, et al. Thrombocytopenia caused by passive transfusion of anti-glycoprotein Ia/IIa alloantibody (anti-HPA-5b). *Blood* 1992;79:2480–2484.
163. Panzer S, Kiefel V, Bartram CR, et al. Immune thrombocytopenia more than a year after allogeneic marrow transplantation against donor platelets with anti-Pl^{A1} specificity: evidence for a host-derived immune reaction. *Br J Haematol* 1989;71:259–264.
164. Bierling P, Pignon JM, Kuentz M, et al. Thrombocytopenia after bone marrow transplantation caused by a recipient origin Br^a alloantibody: presence of mixed chimerism 3 years after the graft without hematologic relapse. *Blood* 1994;83:274–279.
165. Roy V, Verfaillie CM. Refractory thrombocytopenia due to anti-PLA1 antibodies following autologous peripheral stem cell transplantation: case report and review of literature. *Bone Marrow Transplant* 1996;17:115–117.
166. West KA, Anderson DR, McAlister VC, et al. Alloimmune thrombocytopenia after organ transplantation. *N Engl J Med* 1999;341:1504–1507.
167. The Trial to Reduce Alloimmunization to Platelets Study Group. Leukocyte reduction and ultraviolet B irradiation of platelets to prevent alloimmunization and refractoriness to platelet transfusions. *N Engl J Med* 1997;337:1861–1869.
168. Novotny VMJ, van Doorn R, Witvliet MD, et al. Occurrence of allogeneic HLA and non-HLA antibodies after transfusion of prestorage filtered platelets and red cells: a prospective study. *Blood* 1995;85:1736–1741.
169. Kekomäki S, Volin L, Koistinen P, et al. Successful treatment of platelet transfusion refractoriness: the use of platelet transfusions matched for both human leucocyte antigens (HLA) and human platelet alloantigens (HPA) in alloimmunized patients with leukaemia. *Eur J Haematol* 1998;60:112–118.

CASE 27A

A DIAGNOSIS YOU DON'T WANT TO MISS

CASE HISTORY

A 59-year-old, otherwise healthy man was admitted to the hospital because of acute onset of chest pain. The diagnosis was unstable angina due to coronary artery disease. Treatment included intravenous heparin for 1 week, and coronary artery bypass graft surgery was scheduled for hospital day 7. On the morning of the scheduled operation, a preoperative coagulation screen revealed a platelet count of 60 $\times$ $10^3/\mu l$ with normal prothrombin time and activated partial thromboplastin time. The rest of the complete blood cell count and the results of preoperative chemistry tests were normal. The platelet count had been normal at 237 $\times$ $10^3/\mu l$ on admission, but additional platelet counts were not available. To prepare the patient for surgery, 12 units of platelets were administered immediately before the operation, and the grafting procedure was performed. Heparin was administered according to the usual protocol during cardiopulmonary bypass and was reversed with protamine. However, soon after the surgery, the patient's legs became cold and pulseless, and severe renal failure ensued. The patient was found to have bilateral, extensive thrombosis in the femoral and renal arteries. Despite attempts to manage the thrombosis, both lower extremities had to be amputated, and the patient needed lifelong hemodialysis. The cause of thrombosis, established with a positive result of a heparin-induced platelet aggregation assay (1), was heparin-induced thrombocytopenia (HIT).

DISCUSSION

Heparin-induced thrombocytopenia is a diagnosis that you do not want to miss. As illustrated in this case, the main concern is the high risk of thrombosis that occurs with HIT, which often leads to permanent disability or death. Heparin-induced thrombocytopenia develops in approximately 3% of all patients exposed to heparin, and thrombosis develops in one-third or more of these patients. Given the large number of patients exposed to heparin, HIT is a common occurrence. Despite thrombocytopenia, bleeding complications are not common in HIT.

An important point illustrated by this case is that platelet transfusions are contraindicated in the acute setting of HIT, because they can precipitate or extend thrombosis. The thrombosis and thrombocytopenia are caused by platelet activation by the HIT antibody bound to heparin and platelets. Transfusing platelets into a patient with acute HIT adds fuel to the fire in that the transfused platelets can become activated by the HIT antibody, increasing the risk of thrombosis. Another point illustrated by this case is that thrombosis in HIT tends to be unusually extensive, which helps account for the high morbidity and mortality among patients with HIT-associated thrombosis.

To prevent these complications, platelet counts should be followed for all patients during heparin exposure. Heparin-induced thrombocytopenia should be suspected when the platelet count decreases 50% or more from baseline. As shown in Figure 27A.1,in patients with HIT exposed to heparin for the first time, the platelet count begins to decrease 4 to 20 days after initiation of heparin exposure, most commonly between days 5 and 12 with the median on day 10. In patients who have been sensitized to heparin in the past, platelet counts may decrease within the first 3 days or even hours after reexposure to heparin. In both scenarios, platelet count decreases progressively until it reaches a nadir, which is variable, but averages approximately 50 $\times$ $10^3/\mu l$ (range, 20 $\times$ 10^3 to 150 $\times$ $10^3/\mu l$). The platelet count characteristically does not decrease any further. A common mistake is to conclude that a patient does not have HIT because the platelet count does not continue to decrease to less than 50 $\times$ 10^3 to 100 $\times$ $10^3 \mu l$ despite continued heparin exposure.

In patients who have HIT for the first time, the nadir is reached approximately 5 days after the onset of the decline, although this timing is variable. In previously sensitized patients, the nadir can be reached as soon as the first day or two after heparin reexposure. After heparin is discontinued, the platelet count starts to increase after 2 to 3 days and usually returns to normal within 4 to 10 days. However, recovery occasionally takes as long as 25 days.

Thrombosis in HIT usually occurs when patients have thrombocytopenia. However, thrombosis can occur with a normal platelet count. Thrombotic skin lesions also can occur with normal platelet counts in HIT, particularly at subcutaneous heparin injection sites. Therefore HIT also can be suspected when a patient treated with heparin has a normal platelet count but has thrombosis or skin lesions.

Errors in interpreting results of laboratory tests for HIT should be avoided. Platelet aggregation is the least sensitive of the assays. A negative test result does not exclude the possibility of HIT with certainty. Even with the most sensitive tests, seroto-

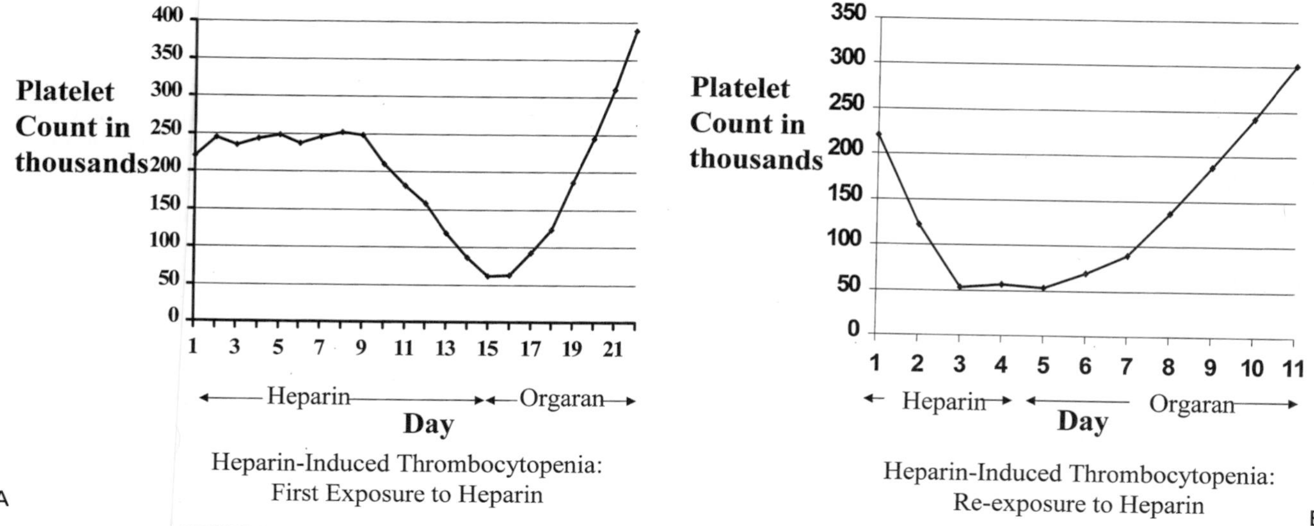

FIGURE 27A.1. A: Development of thrombocytopenia in a typical patient with heparin-induced thrombocytopenia (HIT) after first exposure to heparin. **B:** The more rapid onset of thrombocytopenia in a patient with HIT on re-exposure to heparin. The anamnestic immune response causes a more rapid onset of thrombocytopenia among previously sensitized persons.

nin release and platelet factor 4 enzyme-linked immunosorbent assays, occasional false-negative results occur. A negative assay result should not be relied on exclusively. In addition, when patients tell their physicians they believe they have a history of HIT, a common mistake is to immediately request an HIT test to verify the diagnosis. However, HIT antibodies disappear, often quickly, after heparin is discontinued. A negative HIT test result once the patient is not being treated with heparin cannot be considered informative regarding a history of HIT. If the patient is being treated with heparin and a serotonin release or platelet aggregation assay is being performed, the laboratory must be notified, because heparin must be removed from the sample before testing. Use of HIT tests to screen patients taking heparin who have no symptoms is not recommended, because some patients develop the HIT antibody without having clinical HIT, particularly as a result of bypass surgery. It is not known whether such patients are at risk of thrombocytopenia or thrombosis.

Several alternative anticoagulants are now available for the management of HIT. These include danaparoid (Orgaran), hirudin (lepirudin [Refludan], desirudin [Revasc]), and argatroban. Perhaps because of unfamiliarity with these new anticoagulants or owing to their expense, a common mistake is to initiate warfarin immediately after discontinuation of heparin when the diagnosis of HIT is made. Warfarin has precipitated venous limb gangrene when used as the sole anticoagulant in the acute setting of HIT, apparently because of a rapid decrease in protein C combined with the hypercoagulable HIT state. Warfarin should be avoided initially. If it is used, an immediate-acting alternative anticoagulant, such as hirudin, danaparoid, or argatroban, should be used with it until warfarin is therapeutic. Low-molecular-weight heparin (LMWH) is associated with a lower incidence of HIT than is unfractionated heparin. However, the cross-reactivity of the HIT antibody against LMWH is high enough that now that alternatives are available (2–5), LMWH is contraindicated for patients with HIT.

Coronary artery bypass operations on HIT patients are difficult, because no suitable alternative anticoagulant has been established in this setting. Orgaran has been used but is associated with bleeding owing to its long half-life and the lack of a reversal agent. Hirudin has been used in Germany, but the monitoring test (ecarin clotting time) is not readily available in the United States. Argatroban has not yet been used for bypass operations on humans. There is no reversal agent for hirudin or argatroban, although the half-lives of these agents are short if renal or liver function is normal. One option for nonurgent bypass procedures is to defer surgery until the HIT antibody is no longer detectable with laboratory tests. Another option is to use platelet inhibitors with heparin during bypass to prevent HIT-induced thrombosis, including iloprost (an analogue of prostacyclin) or to use prostaglandin E_1. Heparin exposure in these situations is strictly limited to the required intraoperative dose.

In summary, platelet count should be followed for patients being treated with heparin, so that if HIT develops, the diagnosis can be made promptly. Heparin-induced thrombocytopenia carries high risk of thrombosis, and HIT with thrombosis has a high mortality. Although HIT does not invariably reoccur when a patient is reexposed to heparin, heparin should be permanently discontinued in the care of patients with HIT. This includes heparin flushes and use of heparin-coated catheters (special arrangements are made for patients who need bypass surgery). Platelet transfusions should be avoided in the acute setting of HIT. Patients with HIT often are treated with danaparoid, hirudin, or argatroban. Warfarin should not be used as the sole anticoagulant in HIT, and LMWH is contraindicated.

Case contributed by Elizabeth Van Cott, M.D., Massachusetts General Hospital, Boston, MA.

REFERENCES

1. Calaitges JG, Liem TK, Spadone D, et al. The role of heparin-associated antiplatelet antibodies in the outcome of arterial reconstruction. *J Vasc Surg* 1999;29:779–786.
2. D'Ambra MN, Avery EG, Willsey DB, et al. A novel treatment regimen for heparin induced thrombocytopenia: PGE1/dipyridamole in cardiopulmonary bypass patients with anti-heparin-PF4 (HIT) antibodies. *Anesth Analg* 2001;92:SCA8.
3. Greinacher A. Antigen generation in heparin-associated thrombocytopenia: the nonimmunologic type and the immunologic type are closely linked in their pathogenesis. *Semin Thromb Hemost* 1995;21:106–116.
4. Warkentin TE. Heparin-induced thrombocytopenia: IgG-mediated platelet activation, platelet microparticle generation, and altered procoagulant/anticoagulant balance in the pathogenesis of thrombosis and venous limb gangrene complicating heparin-induced thrombocytopenia. *Transfus Med Rev* 1996; 10:249–258.
5. Warkentin TE, Chong BH, Greinacher A. Heparin-induced thrombocytopenia: towards consensus. *Thromb Haemost* 1998;79:1–7.

28

BLEEDING FROM ACQUIRED COAGULATION DEFECTS AND ANTITHROMBOTIC THERAPY

THOMAS J. RAIFE
STEPHAN B. ROSENFELD
STEVEN R. LENTZ

Acquired disorders of hemostasis can occur in association with specific clinical conditions or arise spontaneously in otherwise healthy patients. Unlike inherited coagulation disorders, acquired coagulation disorders often occur among adult patients, although they may manifest at any age. Bleeding symptoms can vary from mild bruising and mucosal bleeding to prolonged postoperative bleeding and severe hemorrhage (1). If the patient does not have a history of serious hemostatic challenge such as surgery or trauma, it may be difficult to differentiate an acquired coagulation defect from an undiagnosed congenital disorder such as mild hemophilia or von Willebrand disease. Management of acute bleeding in patients with acquired coagulation disorders requires prompt recognition of the specific hemostatic defect. The initial laboratory evaluation should usually include the prothrombin time (PT), activated partial thromboplastin time (PTT), thrombin time, fibrinogen level, and platelet count. For most patients, bleeding time is not recommended, because the sensitivity and specificity are poor, particularly in hospitalized patients. A relatively new hemostatic assay, platelet function analysis (PFA-100), is receiving increasing attention as a more informative alternative to bleeding time (2).

The acquired coagulation defects discussed in this chapter and their characteristic effects on laboratory tests of hemostasis are summarized in Table 28.1. Congenital disorders of coagulation are considered in Chapter 31, and hemostatic support in the perioperative setting and in solid-organ transplantation are reviewed in Chapters 42 and 43.

LIVER DISEASE

Pathophysiology

Liver disease and liver transplantation are associated with multiple hemostatic defects, including quantitative and qualitative

T.J. Raife: Department of Pathology, University of Iowa College of Medicine, Iowa City, Iowa.
S.B. Rosenfeld and S.R. Lentz: Department of Internal Medicine, University of Iowa College of Medicine, Iowa City, Iowa.

TABLE 28.1. LABORATORY TESTS OF HEMOSTASIS IN PATIENTS WITH ACQUIRED COAGULATION DEFECTS

Disorder	PT	PTT	TT	Fibrinogen	Platelet Count
Liver disease	↑	(↑)	↑	(↓)	(↓)
Vitamin K deficiency or warfarin therapy	↑	↑	N	N	N
Disseminated intravascular coagulation	↑	↑	↑	↓	↓
Inhibitor to factor VIII (acquired hemophilia)	N	↑	N	N	N
Acquired von Willebrand syndrome	N	(↑)	N	N	N
Inhibitor to factor V	↑	↑	N	N	N
Acquired factor X deficiency	↑	↑	N	N	N
Lupus anticoagulant	(↑)	(↑)	N	N	N
Heparin therapy	N	↑	↑	N	N
Direct thrombin inhibitor therapy	↑	↑	N	N	N
Fibrinolytic therapy	↑	↑	↑	↓	N

PT, prothrombin time; PTT, activated partial thromboplastin time, TT, thrombin time.
↑, increased; ↓, decreased; N, normal; parentheses, mild or variable effect.

abnormalities of coagulation factors, thrombocytopenia, and platelet dysfunction. The liver produces most of the soluble components of the coagulation pathways and many of the regulatory proteins, including factors II, V, VII, IX, X, XI, XII, and XIII, prekallikrein, high-molecular-weight kininogen, plasminogen, α_2-macroglobulin, antiplasmins, antithrombin III, protein C, and protein S (1,3). Factor VIII, the factor deficient in patients with classic hemophilia, also is produced by the liver. However, plasma levels of factor VIII are determined by release of von Willebrand factor (vWF) from endothelium, and the level may be elevated, rather than decreased, in patients with liver disease. The liver also plays a key role in clearance of activated coagulation factors and fibrinolytic fragments that interfere with hemostatic mechanisms. Marked liver dysfunction therefore can lead to bleeding from impaired biosynthesis of several hemostatic factors combined with failed clearance of inhibitory factors.

In both acute and chronic liver disease, the extent of hepatocellular damage generally correlates with the magnitude of the hemostatic defect, as assessed with laboratory tests and clinical bleeding. In acute hepatitis, plasma levels of the vitamin K–dependent factors II, VII, IX, and X are quantitatively decreased. Deficiency of factor VII may precede that of other factors because of its short (6 hour) biologic half-life. Levels of factor IX may be less depressed than those of other vitamin K–dependent factors (4). Levels of factor V, which is not vitamin K dependent, also may be decreased in acute hepatitis, but this is a variable finding. In contrast, the level of factor V is considered a reliable indicator of hepatic synthetic function in patients with chronic hepatitis (3). Levels of fibrinogen often are elevated in acute hepatitis as part of the acute-phase response. In chronic hepatitis, levels of fibrinogen are typically normal or mildly decreased. Severe hypofibrinogenemia (fibrinogen level less than 100 mg/dl) from synthetic impairment is indicative of end-stage liver disease and thus is a sign of a poor prognosis (3).

Biosynthesis of dysfunctional hemostatic proteins also contributes to the bleeding diathesis of liver disease. Vitamin K utilization may be impaired, resulting in production of dysfunctional, noncarboxylated vitamin K–dependent factors. Both abnormal fibrinogens (dysfibrinogenemia) and accumulation of fibrin degradation products (FDP) may impair coagulation. The level of FDP in plasma may increase from both impaired hepatic clearance and increased production due to disseminated intravascular coagulation. Dysfibrinogenemia due to abnormal post-translational processing of fibrinogen is common in chronic active hepatitis and hepatic cirrhosis. The abnormal fibrinogens produced have been shown to have antithrombin activity and to impair fibrin polymerization, which may result in formation of fibrin clots with impaired structural integrity (5). Fibrin degradation products also impair fibrin polymerization and can be a major cause of excessive bleeding in chronic liver disease.

Thrombocytopenia and platelet dysfunction are important components of the hemostatic deficit in patients with liver disease. Portal hypertension with resultant splenomegaly and sequestration of platelets is the primary cause of thrombocytopenia in chronic liver disease (3,4). In acute viral hepatitis, thrombocytopenia usually is modest. Even when the platelet count is normal, platelet-dependent hemostatic mechanisms may be defective (6).

Laboratory Features

The PT is generally the most sensitive laboratory screening test for coagulation defects in liver disease (Table 28.2). Prothrombin time is used to monitor the tissue factor (extrinsic) coagulation pathway, which is particularly sensitive to decreased levels of factor VII. Because of its short half-life, factor VII is a reliable indicator of hepatic synthesis of vitamin K–dependent hemostatic factors. The PTT and thrombin time also may be prolonged owing to deficiencies of other coagulation factors and inhibitory effects of dysfunctional fibrinogens and FDP. When thrombin time is prolonged despite normal levels of fibrinogen and minor elevations of FDP, dysfibrinogenemia should be suspected. In acute hepatitis, the fibrinogen level usually is normal, but it may be elevated when there is an acute-phase response. A significant decline in plasma fibrinogen level occasionally is

TABLE 28.2. HEMOSTATIC DEFECTS ASSOCIATED WITH LIVER DISEASE

Laboratory Abnormality	Cause
Increased PT	Decreased production of coagulation factors, impaired utilization of vitamin K, decreased clearance of FDP
Increased PTT	Decreased production of coagulation factors, impaired utilization of vitamin K, decreased clearance of FDP
Increased thrombin time	Decreased production of fibrinogen, dysfibrinogenemia, decreased clearance of FDP, fibrinolysis
Decreased fibrinogen	Decreased production of fibrinogen, dysfibrinogenemia, decreased clearance of FDP, fibrinolysis
Decreased platelet count	Splenic sequestration, consumption

PT, prothrombin time; PTT, activated partial thromboplastin time; FDP, fibrin degradation products.

caused by decreased hepatic production, but this generally occurs only when liver disease is severe.

Prolonged clotting times usually correct to normal or near normal when the patient's plasma is mixed 1:1 with normal plasma. Levels of individual vitamin K–dependent coagulation factors II, VII, IX, and X as well as factor V, which is not vitamin K dependent, often are decreased in liver disease. In contrast, levels of factor VIII, which are regulated by vWF, typically are normal or elevated. It usually is not necessary to measure levels of individual coagulation factors in the care of most patients with liver disease. However, measurement of the individual factors V, VII, and VIII can be useful in the care of some patients to help differentiate vitamin K deficiency (in which factor VII level is decreased, whereas levels of factors V and VIII are normal), synthetic liver dysfunction (in which levels of factors V and VII are decreased, but factor VIII level is normal or elevated), and consumption of coagulation factors (in which levels of all three factors may be decreased).

Management of Bleeding

Bleeding associated with severe liver disease can be a major clinical challenge for which surgical, pharmacologic, and transfusion support may be needed. Because the hemostatic defect invariably includes deficiency of coagulation factors, often with coexisting thrombocytopenia, transfusion of plasma and platelets is the mainstay of therapy. Although published data are conflicting regarding the risk of bleeding from invasive procedures on patients with liver failure, transfusion of plasma or platelets is recommended before biopsy or surgery when the PT is prolonged more than 3 seconds or the platelet count is less than 50×10^3 to $70 \times 10^3/\mu l$, respectively (4).

A typical starting dose of plasma is 15 ml/kg body weight, doses ranging up to 30 ml/kg in severe liver disease (4). The hemostatic benefit of plasma transfusion often is quite transient, necessitating frequent dosing, which can precipitate problems of volume overload. The PT may be used to monitor efficacy and to determine requirements for repeated administration of plasma. The PT may remain prolonged by as much as 3 seconds despite hemostatically adequate levels of vitamin K–dependent factors. It often is difficult to correct such mild elevations in PT, and attempts to do so may consume large quantities of plasma without success. This difficulty may be related to the short half-life of factor VII, the poor recovery of factor IX from transfused plasma, the rapid loss of transfused clotting factors into third-space fluid, or other factors. Prolongation of the PT more than 6 seconds may result from a severe deficiency of a single coagulation factor but more often indicates the presence of moderate deficiencies of several factors.

Solvent-detergent–treated plasma is a virally attenuated plasma product that can be used for coagulation factor replacement in the care of patients with liver disease. Compared with untreated plasma, this product contains similar concentrations of the major procoagulant hemostatic factors but is deficient in certain regulatory factors, including protein C and protein S. The use of solvent-detergent–treated plasma has been associated with thrombotic and hemorrhagic complications in a small number of liver transplantation procedures. Therefore its use in this setting should be undertaken with caution.

Fibrinogen levels seldom are decreased enough from liver dysfunction to cause major bleeding. However, severe hypofibrinogenemia (fibrinogen level less than 100 mg/ml) present in a patient with active bleeding should be managed with cryoprecipitate. Each unit of cryoprecipitate contains 150 to 250 mg of fibrinogen. Empiric doses in adults typically begin with 10 to 15 units, which in the absence of accelerated consumption should increase the plasma concentration of fibrinogen 50 to 75 mg/dl (1).

Active bleeding in a patient with a platelet count less than $50 \times 10^3/\mu l$ generally should be managed with platelet transfusion. As with plasma transfusion, several physiologic factors diminish the recovery of transfused platelets (5). The degree to which qualitative platelet abnormalities contribute to bleeding in liver failure is controversial (6).

Vitamin K sometimes is used to manage the coagulopathy of liver disease. The effectiveness of vitamin K often is poor, however, and even if shortening of the PT is achieved, clinical bleeding may not be controlled. Another nontransfusional therapy sometimes used to control bleeding in liver disease is administration of desmopressin acetate (1-deamino-[8-D-arginine]-vasopressin; DDAVP), which stimulates release of vWF and possibly factor VIII from storage sites in endothelial cells. Plasma levels of factor VIII and vWF usually are elevated in liver disease, however, so the value of desmopressin acetate is uncertain, and its utility has not been rigorously tested (7).

Prothrombin complex concentrates, which contain vitamin K–dependent coagulation factors, have been used to manage bleeding in patients with liver disease. Several studies have documented serious thromboembolic complications in this setting, however, and use of these agents has fallen out of favor. It is likely that activated factors present in these concentrates, combined with impaired hepatic clearance, contribute to the observed thrombotic complications (4).

When liver disease is complicated by disseminated intravascular coagulation (DIC), brisk systemic fibrinolysis may result in uncontrolled bleeding. In this circumstance, antifibrinolytic agents may be of benefit. ε-Aminocaproic acid has been shown to improve postsurgical bleeding in the presence of liver disease, but its use also has been associated with thromboembolic complications (1). In one study, administration of recombinant factor VIIa (NovoSeven) was found beneficial to patients with bleeding from liver failure complicated by DIC (8).

VITAMIN K DEFICIENCY

Pathophysiology

Vitamin K comprises a group of fat-soluble vitamins available from many dietary sources and from gastrointestinal flora. Because there are two independent sources of vitamin K, deficiency solely from inadequate dietary absorption or inadequate production by gastrointestinal flora is rare. Deficiency usually arises from disruption of both sources (4).

Vitamin K is a coenzyme in the hepatocellular pathway that synthesizes coagulation factors II, VII, IX, and X as well as the regulatory factors protein C and protein S. Vitamin K is required for the γ-carboxylation of several amino terminal glutamyl residues during posttranslational processing of these proteins. The carboxylated glutamyl residues provide negative charge densities that allow formation of ionic bridges between the factors and phospholipid surfaces, and they facilitate protein-protein interactions between coagulation factors (5). The ability of the vitamin K–dependent clotting factors to assemble on anionic phospholipid surfaces, such as platelet membranes, is essential for normal hemostasis. In conditions of vitamin K deficiency, plasma levels of vitamin K–dependent coagulation factors are quantitatively decreased, and production of dysfunctional noncarboxylated factors also contributes to impairment of hemostasis.

Hemorrhagic Disease of the Newborn

Hemorrhagic disease of the newborn is a postnatal bleeding disorder caused by inadequate production of vitamin K–dependent coagulation factors. A transient physiologic decrease in coagulation factors normally occurs during the newborn period owing to synthetic limitations of the immature liver. In the presence of maternal or newborn vitamin K deficiency, plasma concentrations of the vitamin K–dependent factors can decline to levels inadequate to maintain hemostasis. Bleeding in hemorrhagic disease of the newborn can be severe and can include melena, intracranial hemorrhage, bleeding from circumcision, generalized ecchymosis, and intramuscular hemorrhage. Factors that predispose to hemorrhagic disease of the newborn include prematurity, delayed bacterial colonization of the gastrointestinal tract, liver disease, inadequate maternal or infant vitamin K intake, and prenatal exposure to coumarin or anticonvulsant drugs. Because breast milk is a poor source of vitamin K, postnatal deficiency of vitamin K may be more severe among breast-fed infants who do not receive vitamin K supplementation (1).

The PT is invariably prolonged in hemorrhagic disease of the newborn, and it is the primary guide to therapy. Levels of individual vitamin K–dependent factors are decreased, often more severely in activity assays than in antigenic assays. Levels of fibrinogen and factors V and VIII are usually within the normal reference range, as is the platelet count (1). Treatment relies on administration of vitamin K in the form of vitamin K_1 (phytonadione). Intramuscular injection of 0.5 to 1 mg of vitamin K_1 usually produces normal neonatal levels of vitamin K–dependent factors within 24 hours. In cases of severe hemorrhage, transfusion of plasma should be given along with vitamin K_1. Treatment with vitamin K_1 may be less effective in the care of premature infants because of liver immaturity. Administration of very large doses of vitamin K_1 to neonates can produce hemolysis, hyperbilirubinemia, and kernicterus.

Prophylactic administration of vitamin K_1 to newborns (1 mg parenterally or 2 mg orally) diminishes the transient decrease in vitamin K–dependent factors during the newborn period and thereby prevents hemorrhagic disease of the newborn. This practice, which is mandated by law in many countries, accounts for the rarity of the disorder in the developed world. In countries where vitamin K is not routinely provided and breast-feeding is the main source of infant nutrition, hemorrhagic disease of the newborn remains a serious public health problem.

Other Causes of Vitamin K Deficiency

Malabsorption syndromes, including celiac disease, sprue, inflammatory bowel disease, and parasitic infestations, can impair absorption of dietary vitamin K. Absorption of vitamin K also can be impaired in severe biliary stasis or after ingestion of bile acid–sequestering resins. Ingestion of high doses of aspirin, high doses of vitamin E, or warfarin or another coumarin is a common cause of vitamin K deficiency, either from decreased absorption or vitamin K antagonism (1). Antibiotic therapy contributes to vitamin K deficiency by inhibiting the synthetic capability of vitamin K–producing bacteria. Certain antibiotics, such as cephalosporins that contain an *N*-methylthiotetrazole ring, interfere directly with vitamin K activity. The combination of inadequate dietary intake of vitamin K and use of broad-spectrum antibiotics is an insidious cause of vitamin K deficiency among hospitalized patients.

Treatment

Depending on the severity of vitamin K deficiency, a single oral dose of 5 to 10 mg of vitamin K_1 may restore adequate levels of vitamin K–dependent coagulation factors within 24 hours. Larger doses may be needed by patients with severe deficiency, particularly that associated with warfarin or another coumarin. In cases of ingestion of warfarin-like rodent poisons, doses of vitamin K_1 up to 100 mg daily (orally or parenterally) may be needed because of the potent vitamin K antagonistic effects and extremely long biologic half-lives of these poisons. Oral or subcutaneous administration is preferred, because intravenous administration has been associated in rare instances with anaphylaxis. If emergency reversal (within 24 hours) of the bleeding diathesis is needed, transfusion of fresh frozen plasma may be necessary. Plasma should be given in quantities sufficient to increase levels of vitamin K–dependent factors to 30% to 50% of normal. A typical initial dosage of plasma is 15 ml/kg of body weight.

DISSEMINATED INTRAVASCULAR COAGULATION

Pathophysiology

Disseminated intravascular coagulation is a syndrome of diverse causation characterized by pathologic activation of procoagulant and fibrinolytic pathways. Systemic activation of these pathways causes two seemingly paradoxic clinical problems—tissue injury due to disseminated microvascular thrombosis and hemorrhage caused by consumption of coagulation factors and accelerated fibrinolysis. Some patients, such as those with DIC caused by meningococcemia, may experience severe thrombosis of the skin and other organs but have little clinical evidence of bleeding. Other patients with DIC may have bleeding from surgical sites, severe ecchymosis, and diffuse oozing from phlebotomy sites and mucosal surfaces. Still other patients may have clinical manifestations of both thrombosis and hemorrhage.

Disseminated intravascular coagulation usually is a secondary phenomenon, and the clinical entities that underlie its development are impressively diverse. They include obstetric accidents, intravascular hemolysis, sepsis, viral illnesses, crush injuries, burns, head injuries, autoimmune and inflammatory disorders, malignant disease, exposure to toxins, and use of medications. The most common causes of DIC in the developed world are obstetric accidents and infection. Worldwide, venomous snakebite is estimated to be among the most common causes of DIC (9).

Disseminated intravascular coagulation often occurs in patients who have features of systemic inflammatory response syndrome. In this syndrome, pathologic processes evoke the production of inflammatory mediators that stimulate aberrant expression of procoagulant tissue factor and release of plasminogen activators from endothelial cells (9,10). Tissue factor initiates thrombin production, and plasminogen activators generate plasmin, which mediates fibrinolysis. Thrombin has many prothrombic functions, including stimulation of platelet aggregation, activation of coagulation factors V and VIII, and cleavage of fibrinogen to fibrin monomer, which polymerizes to form fibrin matrices. Generation of thrombin in the systemic circulation can lead to diffuse microvascular deposition of fibrin, which is considered one of the most devastating features of DIC (11). Under normal circumstances, thrombin is localized to sites of vascular injury by the thrombomodulin–protein C anticoagulant system, but this regulatory system is impaired in patients with DIC because of down-regulation of thrombomodulin and consumption of protein C (12,13). Plasmin proteolytically cleaves both fibrin clots (fibrinolysis) and soluble fibrinogen (fibrinogenolysis). Therefore generation of plasmin in the systemic circulation causes proteolytic consumption of fibrinogen and accumulation of FDP that interfere with normal hemostatic mechanisms. Both of these effects of plasmin contribute to bleeding in DIC.

Another important cause of bleeding in DIC is thrombocytopenia. Platelet activation and aggregation occur during formation of microvascular thrombi, and the resulting platelet aggregates are removed from the circulation. Consumption of platelets in DIC can be extremely rapid, overwhelming the capability of the bone marrow to replenish the circulating pool of platelets. In addition, partial activation of platelets and accumulation of FDP can produce a functional defect in platelets that remain in the circulation.

Clinical Features

Disseminated intravascular coagulation syndromes compose a clinical spectrum of disorders with acute and chronic manifestations. In fulminant acute DIC, thrombosis and hemorrhage may produce multiple organ failure that manifests as renal, pulmonary, hepatic, cutaneous, and central nervous system dysfunction. Metabolic instability, hypotension, fever, proteinuria, and hypoxia are common. Hematologic signs include generalized ecchymosis, petechiae, or skin necrosis and bleeding or oozing from mucosal surfaces, venipuncture sites, and surgical sites. In patients with bacterial sepsis due to meningococcemia, the appearance of rapidly progressing retiform skin lesions indicates a poor prognosis. The skin lesions in these patients are caused by widespread thrombosis of dermal and subdermal vessels (14). The thrombotic diathesis of DIC also can include substantial large-vessel thrombosis (11).

Chronic DIC reflects low-grade systemic activation of hemostatic pathways and is associated most frequently with underlying vascular disease, autoimmune disorders, chronic inflammatory disorders, malignant disease, or chronic liver disease. Because hemostatic compensatory mechanisms usually keep pace with consumption, hemorrhagic complications may be less prominent than thrombotic complications unless there is severe thrombocytopenia. Clinical manifestations are variable and may include deep venous thrombosis or migratory thrombophlebitis as well as epistaxis and ecchymosis (9,10).

Laboratory Features

Many laboratory tests have been developed to aid in the diagnosis of DIC. These tests include assays for activated coagulation factors, specific activation fragments of coagulation factors, complexes of hemostatic factors with inhibitors, fibrin monomer, and various products of fibrin degradation (15). Although these assays offer the potential to refine the diagnostic criteria and pathophysiologic understanding of DIC syndromes, a more commonly available set of laboratory tests suffices in most clinical circumstances.

If acute DIC is suspected, the initial laboratory evaluation should include the PT, PTT, platelet count, thrombin time, measurement of fibrinogen concentration, and a test for FDP or D-dimer. Collectively these assays provide correlative data that reflect the degree of depletion of hemostatic factors and the extent of fibrinolytic activity. The PT and PTT are used to assess the collective function of coagulation factors and with the platelet count and fibrinogen level provide an indication of available hemostatic resources. Thrombin time reflects the kinetics of fibrin polymerization and is influenced by the concentration of fibrinogen and the presence of inhibitory FDP.

Because fibrinogen concentration increases during the acute-phase response, it may be normal or elevated in early DIC despite increased consumption. A low or decreasing fibrinogen level in combination with other coagulation abnormalities is strong evidence of DIC. Levels of FDP and D-dimer almost always are elevated in DIC because of accelerated fibrinolysis. Whereas FDP levels reflect both fibrinolysis and fibrinogenolysis, D-dimer level indicates only products of fibrinolysis and therefore is a more specific indicator of fibrin formation (11). It is important to remember, however, that these tests do not differentiate the systemic fibrinolysis of DIC and localized fibrinolysis, which occurs normally after trauma or surgical procedures. Therefore the results of tests for FDP and D-dimer must be interpreted in conjunction with the fibrinogen level and results of other hemostatic assays.

In chronic DIC, low-grade consumption of coagulation factors is partially compensated by increased hepatic synthesis, and levels of fibrinogen and factor VIII often are elevated owing to chronic inflammation. The PT and PTT may be normal or even shortened. Increased FDP and D-dimer levels are of particular value in the diagnosis of chronic DIC (10,11).

Treatment

Definitive management of DIC requires control of the triggering pathologic process. Management of bleeding and thrombosis in DIC is an important adjunctive measure that can be life or organ saving and can provide time for definitive therapy, such as antimicrobial therapy, surgery, or cancer treatment, to become effective. Prevention of ischemic organ injury is of paramount concern. Other supportive measures include volume enhancement, oxygenation, and correction of hypotension to improve microcirculation (10,15).

The use of heparin in DIC highlights the dilemma of managing a disorder that simultaneously produces thrombotic and hemorrhagic diatheses. Although it may be counterintuitive for clinicians to consider using an anticoagulant such as heparin in the face of pathologic bleeding, the devastating consequences of systemic thrombosis make heparin a rational agent to manage DIC. Moreover, by slowing consumption of coagulation factors, heparin may improve the bleeding diathesis. Heparin inhibits thrombin activity and slows the consumptive process while reducing microvascular fibrin deposition (15). Heparin has been found to prevent complications of DIC in certain syndromes, such as DIC associated with acute promyelocytic leukemia or solid tumors, but its value in the management of DIC in other clinical settings is less certain (11). When used, heparin often is initiated at a relatively low dosage (e.g., 8 U/kg per hour by means of continuous intravenous infusion) and titrated according to the hemostatic response. Declining levels of FDP and D-dimer, increasing levels of fibrinogen, and shortening of the PTT demonstrate the efficacy of heparin in slowing consumption of coagulation factors and decreasing fibrin formation.

The practice of transfusion of platelets and fibrinogen-containing blood products in the care of patients with DIC has generated concern about feeding the fire of systemic thrombosis, which could theoretically lead to increased systemic fibrin deposition and FDP accumulation with perpetuation of thrombosis and bleeding (11). This theoretic concern has not been borne out in clinical practice, however, and replacement of platelets, fibrinogen, and other coagulation factors can be life saving for some patients with severe bleeding (9,10). In the absence of major bleeding, it is reasonable to restrict transfusion support to blood products that contain minimal amounts of fibrinogen, such as packed red blood cells, platelet concentrates, and volume expanders. For patients with active bleeding or impending biopsy and laboratory evidence of severe consumption of fibrinogen (fibrinogen level less than 100 mg/dl) or other coagulation factors (PT greater than 1.5 times control value), transfusion of cryoprecipitate (0.2 unit/kg) or plasma (15 ml/kg) is indicated (9,10). It is important to remember that some patients who have definitive laboratory evidence of DIC may not have clinically significant thrombosis or hemorrhage. Such patients may not need any specific therapy other than management of the underlying process triggering DIC.

When bleeding associated with DIC is refractory to heparin and transfusion therapy, antifibrinolytic agents such as ϵ-aminocaproic acid are occasionally used. Inhibition of fibrinolysis can exacerbate fibrin deposition in DIC, however. The result is severe thrombotic complications. Antifibrinolytic agents should therefore be reserved for life-threatening hemorrhage and probably should be used only in conjunction with heparin (11).

The continuing development and commercial production of new hemostatic agents has led to several new products that may prove useful for management of DIC. These new products include proteins such as antithrombin III, protein C, activated protein C, and tissue factor pathway inhibitor, as well as small molecules that directly inhibit thrombin or factor Xa. Antithrombin III is a serine protease inhibitor that irreversibly inactivates thrombin, factor Xa, and other coagulation factors. Heparin is a cofactor for antithrombin III, and if antithrombin III becomes depleted in DIC, the effectiveness of heparin anticoagulation may be limited. Antithrombin III has been reported to be beneficial as an adjunctive to heparin therapy for DIC when its levels are depleted to less than 70% of normal (16,17). Protein C is an anticoagulant agent that inhibits thrombin production by inactivating factors Va and VIIIa. Protein C and activated protein C have shown efficacy in clinical trials of DIC associated with bacterial sepsis (18,19). Combination therapy with protein C and antithrombin III was reported successful in the treatment of a patient with severe coagulopathy (20). Tissue factor pathway inhibitor is a regulatory factor that inactivates tissue factor complexed with factor Xa. Concentrates of tissue factor pathway inhibitor were found beneficial in a clinical trial involving patients with sepsis and DIC (21). These new agents, as well as others in development, offer the promise for improved management of DIC.

COAGULATION FACTOR INHIBITORS

Normal blood plasma contains several proteins that inhibit activated coagulation factors. These natural coagulation factor inhibitors include antithrombin III, heparin cofactor II, α_1-antitrypsin, α_2-macroglobulin, C1 esterase inhibitor, plasminogen activator inhibitors, and tissue factor pathway inhibitor (22).

They function to limit the extent of hemostatic and fibrinolytic reactions and thereby localize thrombi to sites of vascular injury.

Unlike natural coagulation factor inhibitors, pathologic inhibitors usually are immunoglobulins that bind directly to coagulation factors and either inhibit their activity or increase their clearance. Pathologic inhibitors, also known as circulating anticoagulants, can be present in an immunologic response to coagulation factor therapy in patients with hereditary hemophilia. They also can arise spontaneously as autoantibodies in patients without a history of abnormal hemostasis (22,23). Patients who experience spontaneous development of inhibitors of coagulation factor VIII often have a severe bleeding diathesis and are said to have *acquired hemophilia.* Spontaneous inhibitors of other coagulation factors are encountered less frequently but also can cause abnormal bleeding. When the presence of a coagulation factor inhibitor is suspected, it is essential to differentiate an inhibitor of a specific coagulation factor, which often predisposes to bleeding, and a nonspecific inhibitor, such as a lupus anticoagulant, which can predispose to thrombosis rather than bleeding.

TABLE 28.3. MANAGEMENT OF ACUTE BLEEDING EPISODES IN PATIENTS WITH ACQUIRED FACTOR VIII INHIBITORS

Low-inhibitor level (<10 Bethesda units)
Desmopressin acetate (DDAVP)
Human factor VIII concentrate
Recombinant human factor VIII
High inhibitor level (>10 Bethesda units)
Porcine factor VIII concentrate
Prothrombin complex concentrate
Activated prothrombin complex concentrate
Recombinant human factor VIIa
Plasmapheresis, followed by human factor VIII concentrate or recombinant human factor VIII (if inhibitor level <30 Bethesda units)
Adjunctive measures
Immobilization
Compression
Avoidance of aspirin and other antiplatelet agents
ε-Aminocaproic acid therapy (if bleeding is mucosal)

Factor VIII Inhibitors (Acquired Hemophilia)

Acquired hemophilia is a rare disorder caused by the spontaneous development of an autoantibody inhibitor of coagulation factor VIII. The annual incidence has been estimated to be approximately one case per million persons (23,24). Autoantibodies to factor VIII are present mainly in adults. They can arise in the postpartum period or in association with other immunologic disorders such as systemic lupus erythematosus, rheumatoid arthritis, inflammatory bowel disease, or lymphoproliferative disorders. Approximately 50% of cases occur among elderly patients without an underlying medical condition.

The characteristic clinical manifestation of acquired hemophilia is the appearance of pathologic hemorrhage in a patient with no history of abnormal bleeding. Patients may have rapidly enlarging ecchymosis, soft-tissue hematoma, gross hematuria, hemarthrosis, or gastrointestinal bleeding. Bleeding can be severe and life threatening. Because of the lack of history of a bleeding disorder, the presence of an inhibitor may not be recognized before surgical procedures. In some instances, the diagnosis is made only after the patient experiences excessive postoperative bleeding (23).

The presence of a circulating inhibitor to factor VIII can be readily detected in the hemostasis laboratory. Typically, the PTT is prolonged, and it does not correct to the normal reference range when repeated on a 1:1 mixture of the patient's plasma with normal plasma. Occasionally, the 1:1 mixture must be incubated for up to 2 hours to allow the inhibitor to completely inactivate factor VIII before PTT is measured. The PT usually is normal. Factor VIII activity level is low (often less than 10% of normal), but levels of other coagulation factors (such as IX, XI, and XII) are normal. If several coagulation factors are affected, the presence of a nonspecific inhibitor (lupus anticoagulant) should be suspected. The diagnosis of the presence of a specific factor VIII inhibitor is confirmed by means of quantitative assay of inhibitor level (often expressed in Bethesda units) (25).

The course of acquired hemophilia is variable. In some cases, such as those that manifest in the postpartum period, the inhibitor may disappear spontaneously within weeks to months (26). In other cases, the inhibitor may persist for many years. In patients with active bleeding, the immediate goal of treatment is to control acute hemorrhage (Table 28.3). Invasive procedures, intramuscular injections, and the use of antiplatelet agents should be avoided if possible. If the bleeding is mucosal, an antifibrinolytic agent such as ε-aminocaproic acid should be given.

If the inhibitor level is low (<10 Bethesda units), large doses of human factor VIII (starting dose of 100 to 150 U/kg, followed by continuous infusion of 10 U/kg per hour) can be given to overwhelm the inhibitor. Many clinicians prefer to use recombinant human factor VIII, rather than plasma-derived factor VIII concentrates, to minimize exposure to numerous blood donors (23). Factor VIII levels should be measured frequently to assess the response to treatment; the usual goal of factor VIII replacement in the care of a patient with active bleeding is to maintain a factor VIII activity level more than 50% of normal.

Patients with very low inhibitor levels (<3 Bethesda units) may respond to desmopressin acetate, which acts by stimulating release of endogenous vWF and factor VIII from endothelial storage sites. Desmopressin acetate can be administered either intravenously or nasally, and the dose can be repeated every 24 hours for up to 3 days. Side effects of desmopressin acetate include fluid retention and hyponatremia. Therefore this drug should not be used to treat elderly patients with a history of cardiovascular disease. Use of desmopressin acetate for more than three doses may result in loss of its hemostatic effectiveness due to depletion of vWF factor from storage sites (7).

If the inhibitor level is high (>10 Bethesda units), the likelihood of achieving a therapeutic response to human factor VIII is low, and alternative treatments should be considered. Plasmapheresis may be used to immediately decrease the plasma level of a circulating inhibitor to allow successful treatment with human factor VIII (22). This approach usually is not successful if the inhibitor level is greater than 30 Bethesda units. Some patients may respond well to porcine factor VIII concentrate (starting dose of 50 to 100 U/kg), because most acquired inhibitors have low cross-reactivity with porcine factor VIII. However, continuous or repeated use of porcine factor VIII may result in the development of inhibitors of porcine factor VIII, which may limit therapeutic options for management of future episodes of bleeding. Other therapeutic options for management of acute bleeding in patients with acquired hemophilia include prothrombin complex concentrates, activated prothrombin complex concentrates (also called factor VIII inhibitor bypassing concentrates), and recombinant factor VIIa. These products contain activated coagulation factors that appear to bypass factor VIII–dependent clotting reactions. Because the goal of therapy is to bypass rather than replace factor VIII, it is not necessary to measure factor VIII levels when using these products. It is important to differentiate prothrombin complex concentrates, which contain factor VIII bypassing activity, and highly purified plasma-derived factor IX concentrates or recombinant factor IX (e.g., BeneFix), which cannot be used to bypass factor VIII inhibitors.

Long-term treatment of patients with acquired factor VIII inhibitors should be directed toward eradication of the inhibitor. Although some inhibitors may disappear spontaneously, even after many years, a trial of immunosuppressive therapy should be considered for most patients. Some patients may respond to glucocorticoids alone (23). Other immunosuppressive treatments include cyclophosphamide, azathioprine, and intravenous immune globulin (IVIG) and antibodies against antibody producing leukocytes. Only a small number of patients respond, however. If the inhibitor level has not decreased substantially within 3 months, immunosuppressive therapy probably should be discontinued.

Lupus Anticoagulants

Lupus anticoagulants are autoantibodies that nonspecifically inhibit phospholipid-dependent coagulation reactions in vitro. Although first recognized in patients with systemic lupus erythematosus, nonspecific inhibitors are actually encountered more frequently in patients without lupus (27). Lupus anticoagulants can be induced by certain medications, including procainamide, hydralazine, quinidine, and chlorpromazine (28) or can be present in association with human immunodeficiency virus infection (29). Lupus anticoagulants also may arise spontaneously in patients who are otherwise healthy.

Lupus anticoagulants represent a subset of a larger group of autoantibodies that recognize phospholipid-protein complexes (30). These antiphospholipid autoantibodies can be detected in the laboratory as lupus anticoagulants or anticardiolipin antibodies or by means of a variety of assays used to detect binding of antibodies to anionic phospholipids or phospholipid-associated proteins such as β_2-glycoprotein I or prothrombin. Antiphospholipid antibodies usually are either immunoglobulin G (IgG) or IgM. Other immunoglobulin classes are rare. Lupus anticoagulants often prolong the PTT, but rarely prolong the PT. The PTT usually does not correct completely to normal when the patient's plasma is mixed 1:1 with normal plasma, but correction in mixing studies can be observed with lupus anticoagulants of low titer or low avidity. Some lupus anticoagulants may not prolong either the PTT or PT. Several alternative clotting assays, including the dilute Russell viper venom time and kaolin clotting time, have been developed as high-sensitivity screening tests for lupus anticoagulants. Whether or not the PTT or one of the alternative assays is used to detect the lupus anticoagulant, a confirmatory test should be performed to establish that the inhibitor is phospholipid dependent.

Paradoxically, although lupus anticoagulants prolong clotting time in vitro, they often are associated clinically with thrombosis rather than with bleeding (30). Thrombotic events in patients with lupus anticoagulants can be either venous, such as deep venous thrombosis and pulmonary embolism, or arterial, such as myocardial infarction, stroke, and peripheral arterial occlusion. A syndrome of severe microvascular thrombosis resulting in acute multiple organ failure (catastrophic antiphospholipid antibody syndrome) has been described in some patients (31). In addition to thrombosis, patients with lupus anticoagulants may experience pregnancy loss, thrombocytopenia, neurologic symptoms, and livedo reticularis (30). The mechanisms by which lupus anticoagulants predispose to these clinical conditions are poorly understood (27).

Individual patients with antiphospholipid antibodies may have positive results of laboratory tests for lupus anticoagulants, anticardiolipin antibodies, or both (Fig. 28.1). However, none of the results of currently available laboratory tests for antiphospholipid antibodies are predictive with certainty of which patients are at increased risk of clinical complications. It is likely that only a subset of individuals with abnormal test results are actually predisposed to thrombosis. There is growing evidence, however, that patients with lupus anticoagulants, either with or without anticardiolipin antibodies, may be at higher risk of thrombotic complications than are those with isolated anticardiolipin antibodies (32).

Identification of a lupus anticoagulant in a bleeding patient is important for several reasons. First, because most lupus anticoagulants do not cause a bleeding diathesis (with the rare exception of those associated with severe thrombocytopenia or hypoprothrombinemia; see later), a search for another abnormality of hemostasis should be undertaken. Second, recognition that prolongation of PTT is caused by a lupus anticoagulant may

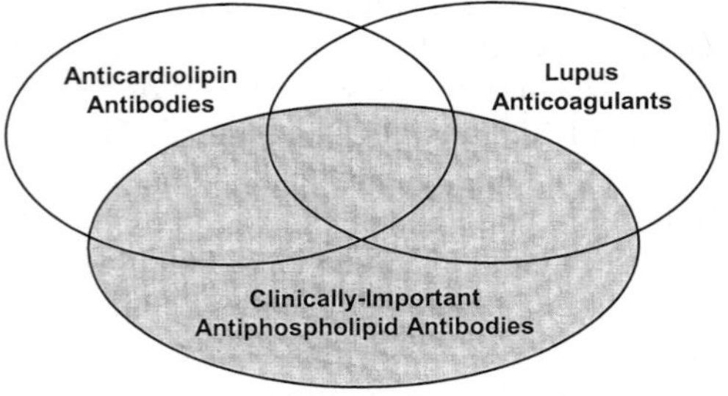

FIGURE 28.1. Antiphospholipid antibodies. (Modified from Lentz SR. Hypercoagulable states and cerebrovascular disease. In: Gilman S, ed. *MedLink neurology.* San Diego, CA: Arbor Publishing, 2001, with permission.)

prevent inappropriate transfusion of plasma and other blood products. Third, all patients with lupus anticoagulants should be considered at high risk of thrombosis, particularly in the settings of surgery, trauma, or pregnancy.

Patients with lupus anticoagulants may have coexistent autoimmune thrombocytopenia. The thrombocytopenia often is mild but can be associated with abnormal bleeding if the platelet count decreases to less than $50 \times 10^3/\mu l$. Another circumstance in which lupus anticoagulants may be directly associated with increased risk of bleeding, rather than thrombosis, is hypoprothrombinemia-lupus anticoagulant syndrome. Patients with this syndrome appear to have an autoantibody inhibitor that causes accelerated clearance of prothrombin from plasma (33). The PT typically is prolonged out of proportion to the PTT. The diagnosis can be confirmed with a specific assay for prothrombin (factor II) activity or antigen. A prothrombin level less than 20% of normal can produce severe hemorrhage. Management of bleeding in such patients is challenging. Transfusion of plasma may be ineffective. Treatment options for acute bleeding include IVIG and recombinant factor VIIa (34,35). Immunosuppressive therapy with glucocorticoids or danazol may be effective long-term management (36).

In patients with venous or arterial thrombosis, anticoagulant therapy with heparin followed by long-term anticoagulation with warfarin usually is indicated. The presence of a lupus anticoagulant may interfere with monitoring of heparin by means of PTT, and alternative monitoring methods such as factor Xa inhibition assays may be needed to measure heparin level. An alternative is to use a fixed dose of low-molecular weight heparin without laboratory monitoring. Lupus anticoagulants can influence the international normalized ratio (INR) in patients treated with warfarin. For such patients, it may be necessary to monitor warfarin therapy by measuring the level of a specific vitamin K–dependent factor (such as factor II or X) or by using an alternative assay such as prothrombin-proconvertin time (37).

Acquired von Willebrand Disease

Autoantibody inhibitors of vWF can arise spontaneously in previously healthy persons or occur in association with neoplastic, rheumatologic, or hematologic disorders. As many as 50% of patients have monoclonal gammopathy or a lymphoproliferative disorder (38). The clinical manifestations of acquired von Willebrand disease are similar to those of congenital von Willebrand disease. Symptoms may vary from mild cutaneous and mucosal bleeding (ecchymosis, epistaxis, gingival hemorrhage, or menorrhagia) to severe, life-threatening hemorrhage. The diagnosis should be suspected when a patient has a prolonged bleeding time or a prolonged PFA-100 closure time. The PTT may be prolonged or normal. The diagnosis is confirmed with the finding of abnormally low vWF functional activity (ristocetin cofactor assay). Levels of vWF antigen and factor VIII also may be depressed. The inhibitor typically causes rapid clearance of vWF from the circulation, and inhibitory activity usually cannot be found in the patient's plasma with mixing studies.

Management of bleeding in patients with vWF inhibitors can be difficult. As for patients with other bleeding disorders, invasive procedures, intramuscular injections, and the use of antiplatelet agents should be avoided if possible. For patients with an underlying hematoproliferative disorder, treatment with chemotherapeutic or cytoreductive agents can lead to resolution of the long-term bleeding diathesis (38). For patients with acute bleeding, therapeutic options include desmopressin acetate or infusion of factor VIII concentrates that contain large quantities of vWF (e.g., Humate-P, Koate-DVI, or Alphanate). Although these partially purified factor VIII concentrates are derived from pooled plasma, they are subjected to viral attenuation procedures during processing, so the risk of virus transmission is considered low. Highly purified factor VIII concentrates or recombinant human factor VIII cannot be used, because these products generally contain little or no vWF. Purified vWF concentrates are available in Europe. Cryoprecipitate can be given as a source of vWF, but its use is discouraged because of a greater risk of exposure to blood-borne pathogens. Replacement therapy may be only transiently effective, because of the short half-life of vWF due to excessive clearance from the circulation. Antifibrinolytic agents such as ε-aminocaproic acid may be beneficial, particularly in the care of patients with mucosal bleeding. A recent report suggests that treatment with recombinant factor VIIa may be efficacious in the care of some patients with vWF inhibitors (39). Administration of high-dose IVIG (2 g/kg over 2 to 5 days) may result in a rapid increase in vWF level. Administration of IVIG every 3 weeks may be effective in controlling chronic bleeding (40).

Inhibitors of Factor V

Autoantibody inhibitors of factor V may arise in patients after surgery, transfusions, or antibiotic therapy. Most cases have been reported in patients exposed to topical hemostatic agents, such as bovine thrombin or fibrin glue, that contain trace amounts of bovine factor V. The inhibitor presumably arises as an alloantibody to bovine factor V that cross-reacts with human factor V (41). Inhibitors to factor V may be present after a single exposure to fibrin glue, but reexposure appears to increase the likelihood of inhibitor development (42). Both PT and PTT typically are prolonged and do not correct to normal when the tests are performed on a 1:1 mixture of patient's plasma with normal plasma. The thrombin time also may be prolonged owing to the presence of a coexisting inhibitor to bovine thrombin. The diagnosis can be confirmed with a quantitative assay of factor V inhibitor level. The clinical manifestations are quite variable, ranging from apparently normal hemostasis to severe hemorrhage, possibly because of differential effects of the inhibitor on plasma and platelet pools of factor V. Treatment options for acute bleeding are limited. Some patients may respond to transfusion of platelets, immunoadsorption, or plasmapheresis (43). In most patients, the inhibitor disappears within weeks to months, and immunosuppressive therapy does not appear to influence the time course of the disease.

Acquired Factor X Deficiency

Acquired deficiency of factor X can occur in patients with primary amyloidosis. The deficiency arises from accelerated clearance of factor X from the circulation due to adsorption of factor

X to amyloid fibrils (44). Both PT and the PTT are prolonged, but unlike the situation in patients with circulating inhibitors, PT and PTT usually correct to normal when performed on a 1:1 mixture of the patient's plasma with normal plasma. The hemostatic defect in these patients is multifactorial. In addition to factor X deficiency, patients with amyloidosis may have excessive fibrinolysis and amyloid infiltration of blood vessels. Management of bleeding in such patients is difficult. Replacement therapy in the form of fresh frozen plasma or prothrombin complex concentrate often is ineffective, and antifibrinolytic agents such as ϵ-aminocaproic acid are of limited benefit.

Other Coagulation Factor Inhibitors

Autoantibody inhibitors of other coagulation factors are rarely encountered. Like inhibitors of factor V, inhibitors of prothrombin prolong both PT and PTT. Like inhibitors of factor VIII, inhibitors of factors IX or XI prolong only the PTT. Specific factor and inhibitor assays can be performed to differentiate the type of inhibitor present. Depending on the inhibitor, management options for bleeding episodes include fresh frozen plasma, prothrombin complex concentrates, factor IX concentrates, or recombinant factor VIIa. Adjunctive treatment with antifibrinolytic agents such as ϵ-aminocaproic acid also may be beneficial.

Inhibitors of factor XIII do not affect either PT or PTT. Specific assays of fibrin stabilization, such as the urea clot lysis assay, are necessary to identify these inhibitors (45). In patients with acute bleeding, large doses of cryoprecipitate or factor XIII concentrate can be given to try to overwhelm the inhibitor, but this approach may have limited effectiveness.

ACQUIRED PLATELET FUNCTION DISORDERS

Acquired disorders of platelet function are much more common than are congenital platelet abnormalities. Acquired platelet dysfunction can be caused by drugs such as aspirin, medical conditions such as chronic renal insufficiency, or procedures such as cardiopulmonary bypass. The risk of bleeding among patients with acquired platelet dysfunction is variable and unpredictable, and abnormal bleeding may occur only in the presence of additional hemostatic defects (46). Diagnostic tests of platelet function include bleeding time and PFA-100. Although useful for screening, these tests lack specificity, and they cannot be used to predict bleeding risk. The bleeding time may be prolonged owing to abnormalities of cutaneous connective tissue, and both bleeding time and results of PFA-100 may be abnormal in the presence of anemia (hematocrit <30%) or thrombocytopenia (platelet count $<100 \times 10^3/\mu l$). Formal platelet aggregation testing can be useful in the evaluation of selected patients.

Drug-induced Platelet Dysfunction

A large number of drugs and medications have been reported to impair platelet function (Table 28.4). Among the most frequently encountered are aspirin, nonsteroidal antiinflammatory drugs, and newer antiplatelet agents such as ticlopidine, clopidogrel, and abciximab. Aspirin produces platelet dysfunction by irreversibly inactivating platelet cyclooxygenase (47). Inactivation of cyclooxygenase causes deficient synthesis of thromboxane A_2, which normally strengthens the platelet aggregation response by provoking release of platelet granules. The influence of aspirin on platelet function can be demonstrated in the laboratory by abnormal platelet aggregation responses to epinephrine, adenosine diphosphate, arachidonic acid, or low concentrations of collagen or thrombin (46). Because the effects on platelets are irreversible, platelet dysfunction may persist for as long as 7 days after aspirin is discontinued. Most other nonsteroidal antiinflammatory drugs also inhibit the activity of platelet cyclooxygenase, but the inhibition is reversible, and platelet function usually returns to normal within 24 hours when the drug is discontinued. Nonsteroidal antiinflammatory drugs that selectively inhibit cyclooxygenase-2, such as celecoxib or rofecoxib, appear to have little effect on platelet cyclooxygenase (48). The risk of clinical bleeding caused by aspirin or other nonsteroidal antiinflammatory agents is generally low, particularly in the absence of other hemostatic abnormalities. However, ingestion of these drugs can increase the risk of serious bleeding among patients who also have additional hemorrhagic risk factors. If severe hemorrhage due to defective platelet function is suspected, transfusion of platelets can rapidly restore normal hemostasis. Because the risk of serious bleeding is generally low, however, platelet transfusion should not be given prophylactically.

TABLE 28.4. EXAMPLES OF DRUGS THAT CAUSE IMPAIRMENT OF PLATELET FUNCTION

Aspirin	Dextrans
Nonsteroidal antiinflammatory drugs	Nitroglycerin
	Isosorbide dinitrate
Ticlopidine	Nitroprusside
Clopidogrel	Propranolol
Abciximab	Nifedipine
Eptifibatide	Verapamil
Tirofiban	Diltiazem
β-Lactam antibiotics	Antidepressants
Prostacyclin	Phenothiazines
Dipyridamole	Ethanol

Ticlopidine and clopidogrel inhibit platelet function by disrupting interactions of platelets with adenosine diphosphate and fibrinogen. Because the effects of these drugs on platelets persists for many days, it is recommended that they be discontinued at least 10 days before invasive procedures (49). Other adverse effects of ticlopidine and clopidogrel include neutropenia and thrombotic thrombocytopenic purpura (49,50).

Abciximab is the prototype of a relatively new class of antiplatelet drugs that directly block the binding of fibrinogen to its platelet receptor, glycoprotein IIb/IIIa (integrin αIIbβ3). Other drugs in this class include eptifibatide and tirofiban. These agents are indicated for use in the management of acute coronary syndromes and often are given in conjunction with other antithrombotic agents such as heparin (51). Management of bleeding in patients receiving glycoprotein IIb/IIIa antagonists may be complicated by the development of acute thrombocytopenia (platelet count less than $50 \times 10^3/\mu l$), which occurs in as many as 5% of patients. The antiplatelet effects of eptifibatide and tirofiban are transient and usually resolve within a few hours of discontinuation in patients with normal renal function (52). Abciximab has an extended biologic half-life because of its high affinity for glycoprotein IIb/IIIa. The antiplatelet effects can therefore persist for several days (52). In cases of severe bleeding, platelet transfusions are an effective approach to control hemorrhage in either the presence or the absence of thrombocytopenia.

Other drugs that can impair platelet function include β-lactam antibiotics, prostacyclin, dipyridamole, dextrans, cardiovascular drugs such as nitroglycerin, nitroprusside, propranolol, quinidine, and calcium channel blockers, antidepressant and antipsychotic medications, and ethanol. The antiplatelet effects of β-lactam antibiotics are generally apparent only in patients receiving large parenteral doses of penicillins or cephalosporins. The frequency of clinically important bleeding in patients taking β-lactam antibiotics appears low, however, and is not predicted with bleeding time or other laboratory tests of platelet function (46). Prostacyclin and dipyridamole inhibit platelet aggregation by elevating the intracellular concentration of cyclic adenosine monophosphate. Infusion of dextran inhibits platelet aggregation and enhances fibrinolysis through multiple mechanisms (53). Nitrovasodilators (nitroglycerin, isosorbide dinitrate, and nitroprusside) inhibit platelet function through nitric oxide–dependent mechanisms. Both tricyclic antidepressants and selective serotonin reuptake inhibitors can alter platelet function, but the risk of serious clinical bleeding appears low (54). Phenothiazines such as chlorpromazine, promethazine, and trifluoperazine have been reported to have mild antiplatelet effects (55). Consumption of ethanol can produce platelet dysfunction and thrombocytopenia and may contribute to clinical bleeding in patients with alcoholic liver disease (46).

Uremia

Chronic renal insufficiency is associated with both hemorrhagic and thrombotic manifestations (56). The primary hemostatic abnormality in uremia is thought to be a defect in platelet function, but the pathophysiologic mechanism of the platelet function defect remains poorly understood. Both dialyzable and nondialyzable substances may contribute to the defect. As in many other acquired disorders of platelet function, the clinical importance of platelet dysfunction in uremia is uncertain (46). In general, abnormalities of bleeding time or platelet aggregation responses do not correlate with the severity of renal insufficiency or the degree of bleeding.

Management of bleeding in uremia is directed by the clinical circumstances rather than the results of laboratory tests of platelet function. Many patients with chronic renal failure do not have significant problems with bleeding despite a prolonged bleeding time and abnormal platelet aggregation responses. If bleeding is encountered in a patient with uremia, other potential causes of defective hemostasis should be considered. Coexisting anemia may contribute to a bleeding propensity, and patients with acute bleeding may benefit from transfusion of red blood cells or treatment with erythropoietin to maintain a hematocrit greater than 30%. Patients with uremia may be unusually sensitive to anticoagulants or antiplatelet medications such as aspirin, which should be discontinued if possible. Intensive dialysis may be effective in correcting abnormal platelet function and diminishing acute bleeding, but the benefit often is transient (57). Transfusion of cryoprecipitate may partially correct the hemorrhagic diathesis of uremia. Transfusion of platelets is not recommended in the absence of thrombocytopenia (platelet count $<50 \times 10^3/\mu l$), because uremic plasma has been found to induce dysfunction in normal platelets (46). Treatment with desmopressin acetate has been recommended for management of bleeding in uremia, but controlled clinical trials have not been performed (7). Conjugated estrogens and estradiol, given either orally or transdermally, have been advocated for long-term management of uremic bleeding (58).

Cardiopulmonary Bypass

Abnormal platelet function is a frequent cause of bleeding in patients undergoing cardiopulmonary bypass. The risk of perioperative bleeding varies depending on the type of surgical procedure, the age of the patient, preoperative renal function, and the duration of bypass (59). Previous exposure to antiplatelet agents and other antithrombotic medications may increase the risk of bleeding.

The platelet defect caused by cardiopulmonary bypass is thought to result from activation of platelets within the extracorporeal circulation. Platelet activation is stimulated by numerous mediators, including thrombin generated from activation of the intrinsic and extrinsic coagulation pathways, mechanical stress, complement activation, hypothermia, and exposure of platelets to the blood-air interface (55). Partial activation and degranulation lead to desensitization of residual circulating platelets. The severity of platelet dysfunction correlates with the duration of bypass. Platelet function abnormalities usually resolve within 5 hours but can persist for 24 hours or longer after complicated surgery (60). Bleeding from platelet dysfunction often is exacerbated by thrombocytopenia caused by hemodilution and consumption of platelets. Consumption of coagulation factors, increased fibrinolytic activity, and inadequate neutralization of heparin with protamine sulfate also can contribute to bleeding.

Management of bleeding associated with cardiopulmonary bypass is generally based on clinical considerations rather than results of laboratory tests. Results of tests of platelet function, such as bleeding time or PFA-100, are abnormal in almost all patients and are not predictive of perioperative blood loss (60). Routine prophylactic administration of plasma or platelets is discouraged (59). In the setting of excessive perioperative or early (within 24 hours) postoperative bleeding, however, platelet transfusions may be indicated even when the platelet count exceeds $100 \times 10^3/\mu l$. The use of desmopressin acetate has been advocated to decrease blood loss, particularly in high-risk patients (7). The protease inhibitor aprotinin, which inhibits activation of platelets by thrombin and plasmin, is used at some centers in the care of patients at high risk.

ANTITHROMBOTIC THERAPY

Use of antithrombotic drugs has increased in recent years because of growing recognition of the efficacy of these medications for the prevention and management of venous thromboembolism, embolic stroke, and other thrombotic disorders. Although warfarin, heparin, and aspirin continue to be the most commonly prescribed antithrombotic medications, several new antithrombotic drugs are making their way into routine clinical use. These new drugs include low-molecular-weight heparin, direct thrombin inhibitors, fibrinolytic agents, ticlopidine, clopidogrel, and platelet glycoprotein IIb/IIIa antagonists (61). The most important complication of all these medications is bleeding. In this section, the management of bleeding associated with warfarin, heparin, low-molecular-weight heparin, direct thrombin inhibitors, and fibrinolytic therapy is considered. Management of bleeding associated with antiplatelet medications is discussed earlier (see Drug-induced Platelet Dysfunction).

Warfarin

Warfarin and other oral anticoagulants produce their antithrombotic effects by inhibiting the hepatic synthesis of vitamin K–dependent coagulation factors. Vitamin K becomes oxidized to vitamin K epoxide during γ-carboxylation of coagulation factors II, VII, IX, and X. Warfarin inhibits cyclic regeneration of active vitamin K by blocking the action of vitamin K epoxide reductase and vitamin K reductase (62). In the absence of adequate concentrations of active vitamin K, hepatic production of vitamin K–dependent coagulation factors is limited, and the factors produced have decreased procoagulant activity owing to hypocarboxylation. The anticoagulant effect of warfarin can be overcome by administration of vitamin K1, which can be converted to the active form of vitamin K by an alternative, warfarin-insensitive reductase (62).

Clinical response to warfarin is influenced by many factors, including diet, patient compliance, hereditary factors, liver dysfunction, and interactions with other medications. Numerous drugs influence the pharmacokinetics of warfarin by altering its absorption or metabolic clearance or by altering the production of vitamin K by intestinal flora. As a rule, any change in medication regimen, including nonprescription medications and dietary supplements that contain vitamin K, should be presumed to have an effect on the anticoagulant response to warfarin.

The most common laboratory method for monitoring the anticoagulant effect of warfarin is PT. Because the response of the PT to depletion of vitamin K–dependent coagulation factors is highly variable when measured in different laboratories, the INR has been widely adopted as a method to standardize monitoring of oral anticoagulant therapy. The INR compares the ratio of the patient's PT to the mean PT of a group of healthy persons. The ratio is adjusted for the sensitivity of the PT reagent used in each laboratory. The target therapeutic INR for most indications is 2.0 to 3.0, although different therapeutic ranges are recommended for some indications (62).

The risk of major bleeding among patients undergoing chronic warfarin therapy has been estimated to be 1% to 5% per year (63). The risk of bleeding is influenced by the intensity and duration of anticoagulation, the age of the patient, and the simultaneous use of other antithrombotic drugs. Intensity of anticoagulation is probably the most important risk factor for hemorrhage, particularly when the INR is greater than 5.0 (63). Clinical conditions that may increase the risk of hemorrhage include hypertension, cerebrovascular disease, heart disease, renal insufficiency, and a history of gastrointestinal bleeding. The risk of hemorrhagic complications due to warfarin therapy decreases when patients are enrolled in coordinated programs for management of anticoagulation (64).

Reversal of the anticoagulant effects of warfarin can be achieved through discontinuation of warfarin, administration of vitamin K_1, or transfusion of plasma or prothrombin complex concentrates. Management should be guided by the degree of elevation of the INR and the presence or absence of clinical bleeding (Table 28.5). Minor or moderate elevation of the INR (above the therapeutic target but less than 9.0) in the absence of bleeding often can be managed safely by decreasing or omitting several doses of warfarin until the INR approaches the therapeutic range. Major elevation of the INR (>9.0), even in the absence of clinically evident bleeding, should be managed by means of discontinuation of warfarin and administration of vitamin K_1 (2.5 to 5.0 mg orally). In the care of patients with active bleeding, administration of plasma or prothrombin complex concentrates may be life saving. Recombinant factor VIIa also may be effective in the treatment of such patients (65).

Several approaches can be used to manage warfarin anticoagulation for patients who need elective surgery (66). For many patients, a reasonable approach is to discontinue warfarin 4 to 5 days before surgery and begin heparin or a low-molecular-weight heparin along with warfarin in the postoperative period. Heparin or low-molecular-weight heparin can then be discontin-

TABLE 28.5. GUIDELINES FOR REVERSAL OF WARFARIN ANTICOAGULATION

INR	Bleeding	Recommendation
<5.0	None	Decrease or discontinue warfarin
	Minor	Discontinue warfarin Consider vitamin K_1 (2.5 mg orally)
	Major	Discontinue warfarin Vitamin K_1 (10 mg parenterally)[a] Consider fresh frozen plasma (15 ml/kg)
5.0–9.0	None	Discontinue warfarin
	Minor	Discontinue warfarin Vitamin K_1 (2.5 mg orally)
	Major	Discontinue warfarin Vitamin K_1 (10 mg parenterally)[a] Fresh frozen plasma (15 ml/kg)
>9.0	None	Discontinue warfarin Vitamin K_1 (2.5 to 5.0 mg orally)
	Minor	Discontinue warfarin Vitamin K_1 (2.5 to 5.0 mg orally) Consider fresh frozen plasma (15 ml/kg)
	Major	Discontinue warfarin Vitamin K_1 (10 mg parenterally) Fresh frozen plasma (15 ml/kg) Consider prothrombin complex concentrate

[a]For parenteral administration, vitamin K_1 can be given subcutaneously or by means of slow intravenous infusion. Intravenous administration of vitamin K_1 produce an anaphylactic reaction in rare instances.
INR, international normalized ratio.

ued when the INR returns to the target therapeutic range. Patients who need major surgery urgently (within 24 hours) should receive plasma (15 ml/kg) and vitamin K_1 (2.5 to 5 mg orally or parenterally).

Heparin

The antithrombotic effect of heparin is mediated by its ability to potentiate the inhibition of activated coagulation factors by antithrombin III. In the presence of heparin, antithrombin III irreversibly inactivates thrombin, factor Xa, and to a lesser extent, other coagulation factors. Heparin often is administered intravenously, although it also may be given subcutaneously. When heparin is administered by means of intravenous infusion, the onset of its anticoagulant action is rapid.

Weight-based dosing of heparin appears to improve clinical outcome for patients with venous thromboembolism (67). A common dosing schedule is an intravenous bolus dose of 80 U/kg followed by 18 U/kg per hour by means of continuous infusion. The dosage then is adjusted to maintain a therapeutic PTT. The therapeutic range may vary between laboratories that use different reagents for measuring the PTT. Therapeutic ranges should be established for each laboratory by comparing PTT values with heparin levels by means of either a protamine titration method or an anti–factor Xa assay (67). In many laboratories, prolongation of PTT to a value 1.5- to 3.0-fold higher than the control value corresponds to a therapeutic heparin level. For certain indications, such as cardiopulmonary bypass surgery, higher doses of heparin are needed and monitoring is performed with activated clotting time rather than PTT.

The main side effect of heparin therapy is hemorrhage. In clinical studies of heparin administered for short-term management of venous thromboembolism, rate of major bleeding has ranged from zero to 7% (63). In some patients, bleeding is exacerbated by thrombocytopenia or platelet dysfunction. Because heparin has a short biologic half-life of approximately 1 hour, the primary approach to management of bleeding is discontinuation of heparin. Among patients with therapeutic levels of heparin, recovery from the anticoagulant effects can be expected within 2 hours after discontinuation of heparin infusion. In cases of major hemorrhage, or when very large doses of heparin have been given (e.g., for cardiopulmonary bypass or through a medication error), protamine sulfate should be administered.

Protamine sulfate is a strongly basic protein that neutralizes the anticoagulant effects of heparin within minutes. It is given by means of slow intravenous injection. The recommended dose of protamine sulfate is 1.0 mg for every 100 units of heparin remaining in the patient, which can be calculated according to the 60-minute half-life of heparin. For example, a patient receiving 1,000 units of heparin per hour by means of continuous intravenous infusion should be given enough protamine to neutralize all of the heparin administered within the last hour (1, 000 units) plus half of the heparin administered in the preceding hour (500 units) plus one fourth of the heparin administered in the previous hour (250 units). Therefore the total dose of protamine sulfate would be 17.5 mg. Protamine sulfate itself has a weak anticoagulant effect, and overdosage may exacerbate bleeding.

Low-molecular-weight Heparin

Low-molecular-weight heparins are derived from heparin by means of chemical or enzymatic fragmentation (67). Several formulations of low-molecular-weight heparin, including ardeparin, dalteparin, enoxaparin, and tinzaparin, and are available for prevention or management of venous thromboembolism, unstable angina, and other indications. Danaparoid sodium is not derived from heparin, but it is a mixture of glycosaminoglycans that resemble low-molecular-weight heparin. Although danaparoid sodium is considered a heparinoid, its effects are similar to those of low-molecular-weight heparin.

Compared with unfractionated heparin, low-molecular-weight heparin has less inhibitory activity against thrombin and greater relative inhibitory activity against factor Xa. Low-molecular-weight heparin produces a more predictable anticoagulant response than does unfractionated heparin, reflecting better bioavailability, longer half-life, and dose-independent clearance (67). These properties allow subcutaneous administration of low-molecular-weight heparin once or twice a day, usually without laboratory monitoring. Because low-molecular-weight heparin is cleared through the renal route, dosages may have to be adjusted for patients with renal insufficiency.

A large number of randomized clinical trials have shown that low-molecular-weight heparin is at least as safe and effective as unfractionated heparin for many indications (67). A metaanalysis showed a trend toward fewer instances of major hemorrhage among patients receiving low-molecular-weight heparin compared with those receiving unfractionated heparin for management of deep venous thrombosis (68). The incidence of heparin-induced thrombocytopenia is lower with low-molecular-weight heparins than with unfractionated heparin (see Chapter 27).

Despite the apparently favorable safety profile of low-molecular-weight heparin, bleeding remains a serious side effect. In clinical trials of low-molecular-weight heparin for management of venous thromboembolism, the rate of occurrence of major bleeding has ranged from zero to 3% (63). Epidural bleeding and spinal hematoma have been reported among patients receiving low-molecular-weight heparin concurrently with spinal or epidural anesthesia (69). Management of bleeding is complicated by the long half-life of these medications. Unlike those of unfractionated heparin, the anticoagulant effects of low-molecular-weight heparin cannot be reversed completely with administration of protamine sulfate, and there are no alternative methods to effectively correct the hemostatic defect. Therefore management of bleeding relies on local measures and prompt discontinuation of low-molecular-weight heparin.

Direct Thrombin Inhibitors

In an attempt to overcome the limitations of heparin and low-molecular-weight heparin, several new anticoagulants have been developed that directly inhibit the activity of thrombin (61).

These direct thrombin inhibitors include desirudin, lepirudin, bivalirudin, and argatroban. Because the direct thrombin inhibitors are structurally unrelated to heparin, one major indication for their use is in the management of heparin-induced thrombocytopenia. These agent also are being evaluated for use in prophylaxis of deep venous thrombosis, cardiopulmonary bypass surgery, and the management of acute coronary syndromes.

Most of the direct thrombin inhibitors are administered parenterally and are monitored with PTT. They have short half-lives (<2 hours) when given by means of intravenous infusion. Because lepirudin, desirudin, and bivalirudin are cleared renally, the half-life may be prolonged dramatically in renal failure. Clearance of argatroban is not influenced by renal impairment but may be decreased in the presence of hepatic dysfunction. The risk of bleeding among patients receiving direct thrombin inhibitors appears dose dependent (70). Management of bleeding relies on prompt discontinuation of the drug.

Fibrinolytic Agents

Pharmacologic lysis of fibrin thrombi is a commonly used strategy for management of acute myocardial infarction. It also is used in selected cases of stroke, peripheral arterial occlusion, and venous thromboembolism (71). Most fibrinolytic agents in clinical use are plasminogen activators, which include streptokinase, anistreplase, urokinase, and recombinant forms of tissue plasminogen activator such as alteplase and reteplase. Plasminogen activators produce thrombolysis by converting plasminogen to plasmin, which then degrades fibrin into soluble FDP. Fibrinolytic agents can be administered systemically by means of intravenous infusion or be delivered in proximity to sites of thrombi by means of catheter-directed approaches. Contraindications to the use of fibrinolytic therapy include recent hemorrhagic stroke or major surgery, prolonged cardiopulmonary resuscitation, uncontrolled hypertension, and active gastrointestinal bleeding (72).

In addition to producing therapeutic lysis of pathologic thrombi, fibrinolytic agents may generate plasmin in the systemic circulation. The result is bleeding from lysis of hemostatic plugs at surgical sites and other locations (72). Bleeding, therefore, is a major complication of fibrinolytic therapy. Because circulating plasmin degrades fibrinogen, hypofibrinogenemia can contribute to bleeding. The extent of systemic fibrinogenolysis varies with different fibrinolytic agents and different routes of administration (71). Laboratory abnormalities associated with the use of fibrinolytic agents include decreased fibrinogen, decreased plasminogen, prolonged thrombin time, and decreased euglobulin clot lysis time. These laboratory values, however, are poorly predictive of bleeding risk (72).

The risk of major hemorrhage associated with fibrinolytic therapy is influenced by the age of the patient and concomitant use of additional antithrombotic agents such as heparin, direct thrombin inhibitors, or antiplatelet agents. In the absence of invasive procedures or simultaneous heparin therapy, management of acute myocardial infarction with fibrinolytic agents generally is associated with a low incidence of major bleeding (<5%). Intracranial hemorrhage is a rare but potentially devastating complication of fibrinolytic therapy. In large clinical trials of streptokinase, anistreplase, or alteplase for management of acute coronary ischemia, the incidence of intracranial hemorrhage has ranged from 0.2% to 0.8% (72).

Bleeding that occurs in association with fibrinolytic therapy often can be managed by means of discontinuing infusion of the plasminogen activator and replacing fibrinogen with transfusion of cryoprecipitate (0.2 unit/kg). The goal of transfusion therapy with cryoprecipitate is to maintain a plasma fibrinogen level greater than 100 mg/dl. Adjunctive treatment with antifibrinolytic agents such as ε-aminocaproic acid or aprotinin may be beneficial when rapid reversal of bleeding is desired.

REFERENCES

1. Grosset A, Rodgers GM. Acquired coagulation disorders. In: Lee GR, Foerster J, Lukens J, et al., ed. *Wintrobe's clinical hematology,* 10th ed. Baltimore: Williams & Wilkins, 1999:1733–1780.
2. Mammen EF, Comp PC, Gosselin R, et al. PFA-100 system: a new method for assessment of platelet dysfunction. *Semin Thromb Hemost* 1998;24:195–202.
3. Joist JH, George JN. Hemostatic abnormalities in liver and renal disease. In: Colman R, W, Hirsh J, Marder V, et al., ed. *Hemostasis and thrombosis,* 4th ed. Philadelphia: Lippincott Williams & Wilkins, 2001: 955–973.
4. Martinez J, Barsigian C. Coagulopathy of liver failure and vitamin K deficiency. In: Loscalzo J, Schafer A, ed. *Thrombosis and hemorrhage,* 2nd ed. Baltimore: Williams & Wilkins, 1998:987–1004.
5. Thompson AR, Harker LA. Acquired abnormalities of coagulation. In: Thompson AR, Harker LA, ed. *Manual of hemostasis and thrombosis,* 3rd ed. Philadelphia: FA Davis Co, 1988:115–128.
6. Violi F, Leo R, Vezza E, et al. Bleeding time in patients with cirrhosis: relation with degree of liver failure and clotting abnormalities. Coagulation Abnormalities in Cirrhosis Study Group. *J Hepatol* 1994;20: 531–536.
7. Mannucci PM. Desmopressin (DDAVP) in the treatment of bleeding disorders: the first 20 years. *Blood* 1997;90:2515–2521.
8. Chuansumrit A, Chantarojanasiri T, Isarangkura P, et al. Recombinant activated factor VII in children with acute bleeding resulting from liver failure and disseminated intravascular coagulation. *Blood Coagul Fibrinolysis* 2000;11:S101–S105.
9. Williams E. Disseminated intravascular coagulation. In: Loscalzo J, Schafer A, ed. *Thrombosis and hemorrhage,* 2nd ed. Baltimore: Williams & Wilkins, 1998:963–985.
10. Selighsohn U. Disseminated intravascular coagulation. In: Beutler E, Lichtman MA, Coller BS, et al., ed. *Williams hematology,* 6th ed. New York: McGraw–Hill, 2001:1677–1695.
11. Bick RL. Disseminated intravascular coagulation: pathophysiological mechanisms and manifestations. *Semin Thromb Hemost* 1998;24:3–18.
12. Taylor FB Jr, Chang A, Esmon CT, et al. Protein C prevents the coagulopathic and lethal effects of *Escherichia coli* infusion in the baboon. *J Clin Invest* 1987;79:918–925.
13. Lentz SR, Sadler JE. The molecular basis of thrombomodulin function. In: Giddings JC, ed. *Thrombin, thrombomodulin, and the control of hemostasis.* Austin, TX: RR Landes, 1994:91–120.
14. Piette WW. The differential diagnosis of purpura from a morphologic perspective. *Adv Dermatol* 1994;9:3–23.
15. Feinstein DI, Marder VJ, Colman RW. Consumptive thrombohemorrhagic disorders. In: Colman RW, Hirsh J, Marder VJ, et al., ed. *Hemostasis and thrombosis,* 4th ed. Philadelphia: Lippincott Williams & Wilkins, 2001:1197–1233.

16. Balk R, Emerson T, Fourrier F, et al. Therapeutic use of antithrombin concentrate in sepsis. *Semin Thromb Hemost* 1998;24:183–194.
17. Levi M, de Jonge E, van der Poll T, et al. Novel approaches to the management of disseminated intravascular coagulation. *Crit Care Med* 2000;28:[Suppl 9]:S20–S24.
18. Ettingshausen CE, Veldmann A, Beeg T, et al. Replacement therapy with protein C concentrate in infants and adolescents with meningococcal sepsis and purpura fulminans. *Semin Thromb Hemost* 1999;25: 537–541.
19. Bernard GR, Vincent JL, Laterre PF, et al. Efficacy and safety of recombinant human activated protein C for severe sepsis. *N Engl J Med* 2001; 344:699–709.
20. Favier R, Deschamps A, Belhocine R, et al. Simultaneous administration of antithrombin III and protein C concentrate in infants and adolescents with meningococcal sepsis and purpura fulminans. *Hematol Cell Ther* 1998;40:67–70.
21. Abraham E. Tissue factor inhibition and clinical trial results of tissue factor pathway inhibitor in sepsis. *Crit Care Med* 2000;28:[Suppl 9]: S31–S33.
22. Sallah S. Inhibitors to clotting factors. *Ann Hematol* 1997;75:1–7.
23. Lusher JM. Inhibitor antibodies to factor VIII and IX: management. *Semin Thromb Hemost* 2000;26:179–188.
24. Bossi P, Cabane J, Ninet J, et al. Acquired hemophilia due to factor VIII inhibitors in 34 patients. *Am J Med* 1998;105:400–408.
25. Kasper M. Laboratory diagnosis of factor VIII inhibitors. In: Kessler C, ed. *Acquired hemophilia,* 2nd ed. Princeton, NJ: Excerpta Medica, 1995:9–23.
26. Michiels JJ. Acquired hemophilia A in women postpartum: clinical manifestations, diagnosis, and treatment. *Clin Appl Thromb Hemost* 2000;6:82–86.
27. Bick RL, Baker WF. Antiphospholipid syndrome and thrombosis. *Semin Thromb Hemost* 1999;25:333–350.
28. Bell WR, Boss GR, Wolfson JS. Circulating anticoagulant in the procainamide-induced lupus syndrome. *Arch Intern Med* 1977;137: 1471–1473.
29. Cohen AJ, Philips TM, Kessler CM. Circulating coagulation inhibitors in the acquired immunodeficiency syndrome. *Ann Intern Med* 1986; 104:175–180.
30. Triplett DA. Protean clinical presentation of antiphospholipid-protein antibodies (APA). *Thromb Haemost* 1995;74:329–337.
31. Asherson RA, Cervera R, Piette JC, et al. Catastrophic antiphospholipid syndrome. Clinical and laboratory features of 50 patients. *Medicine* 1998;77:195–207.
32. Ginsberg JS, Wells PS, Brilledwards P, et al. Antiphospholipid antibodies and venous thromboembolism. *Blood* 1995;86:3685–3691.
33. Bajaj SP, Rapaport SI, Barclay S, et al. Acquired hypoprothrombinemia due to non-neutralizing antibodies to prothrombin: mechanism and management. *Blood* 1985;65:1538–1543.
34. Pernod G, Arvieux J, Carpentier PH, et al. Successful treatment of lupus anticoagulant-hypoprothrombinemia syndrome using intravenous immunoglobulins. *Thromb Haemost* 1997;78:969–970.
35. Holm M, Andreasen R, Ingerslev J. Management of bleeding using recombinant factor VIIa in a patient suffering from bleeding tendency due to a lupus anticoagulant-hypoprothrombinemia syndrome. *Thromb Haemost* 1999;82:1776–1778.
36. Williams S, Linardic C, Wilson O, et al. Acquired hypoprothrombinemia: effects of danazol treatment. *Am J Hematol* 1996;53:272–276.
37. Moll S, Ortel TL. Monitoring warfarin therapy in patients with lupus anticoagulants. *Ann Intern Med* 1997;127:177–185.
38. Veyradier A, Jenkins CSP, Fressinaud E, et al. Acquired von Willebrand syndrome: from pathophysiology to management. *Thromb Haemost* 2000;84:175–182.
39. Ciavarella N, Schiavoni M, Valenzano E, et al. Use of recombinant factor VIIa (NovoSeven) in the treatment of two patients with type III von Willebrand's disease and an inhibitor against von Willebrand factor. *Haemostasis* 1996;26:[Suppl 1]:150–154.
40. Federici AB, Stabile F, Castaman G, et al. Treatment of acquired von Willebrand syndrome in patients with monoclonal gammopathy of uncertain significance: comparison of three different therapeutic approaches. *Blood* 1998;92:2707–2711.
41. Ortel TL, Charles LA, Keller FG, et al. Topical thrombin and acquired coagulation factor inhibitors: clinical spectrum and laboratory diagnosis. *Am J Hematol* 1994;45:128–135.
42. Banninger H, Hardegger T, Tobler A, et al. Fibrin glue in surgery: frequent development of inhibitors of bovine thrombin and human factor V. *Br J Haematol* 1993;85:528–532.
43. Knobl P, Lechner K. Acquired factor V inhibitors. *Baillieres Clin Hematol* 1998;11:305–318.
44. Furie B, Voo L, McAdam KP, et al. Mechanism of factor X deficiency in systemic amyloidosis. *N Engl J Med* 1981;304:827–830.
45. Egbring R, Kroniger A, Seitz R. Factor XIII deficiency: pathogenic mechanisms and clinical significance. *Semin Thromb Hemost* 1996;22: 419–425.
46. George JN, Shattil SJ. Acquired disorders of platelet function. In: Hoffman R, Benz EJ Jr, Shattil SJ, et al., ed. *Hematology: basic principles and practice,* 3rd ed. New York: Churchill Livingstone, 2000:2172–2186.
47. Roth GJ, Stanford N, Majerus PW. Acetylation of prostaglandin synthase by aspirin. *Proc Natl Acad Sci U S A* 1975;72:3073–3076.
48. Patrignani P, Sciulli MG, Manarini S, et al. COX-2 is not involved in thromboxane biosynthesis by activated human platelets. *J Physiol Pharmacol* 1999;50:661–667.
49. Sharis PJ, Cannon CP, Loscalzo J. The antiplatelet effects of ticlopidine and clopidogrel. *Ann Intern Med* 1998;129:394–405.
50. Wood AJ. Thrombotic thrombocytopenic purpura and clopidogrel: a need for new approaches to drug safety. *N Engl J Med* 2000;342: 1824–1826.
51. Bhatt DL, Topol EJ. Current role of platelet glycoprotein IIb/IIIa inhibitors in acute coronary syndromes. *JAMA* 2000;284:1549–1558.
52. Tcheng JE. Clinical challenges of platelet glycoprotein IIb/IIIa receptor inhibitor therapy: bleeding, reversal, thrombocytopenia, and retreatment. *Am Heart J* 2000;139:S38–S45.
53. Strauss RG. Volume replacement and coagulation: a comparative review. *J Cardiothorac Anesth* 1988;2:24–32.
54. de Abajo FJ, Jick H, Derby L, et al. Intracranial haemorrhage and use of selective serotonin reuptake inhibitors. *Br J Clin Pharmacol* 2000; 50:43–47.
55. George JN, Shattil SJ. The clinical importance of acquired abnormalities of platelet function. *N Engl J Med* 1991;324:27–39.
56. Sagripanti A, Barsotti G. Bleeding and thrombosis in chronic uremia. *Nephron* 1997;75:125–139.
57. Couch P, Stumpf JL. Management of uremic bleeding. *Clin Pharm* 1990;9:673–681.
58. Sloand JA, Schiff MJ. Beneficial effect of low-dose transdermal estrogen on bleeding time and clinical bleeding in uremia. *Am J Kidney Dis* 1995;26:22–26.
59. Despotis GJ, Goodnough LT. Management approaches to platelet-related microvascular bleeding in cardiothoracic surgery. *Ann Thorac Surg* 2000;70[Suppl 2]S20–S32.
60. Lasne D, Fiemeyer A, Chatellier G, et al. A study of platelet functions with a new analyzer using high shear stress (PFA100™) in patients undergoing coronary artery bypass graft. *Thromb Haemost* 2000;84: 794–799.
61. Hirsh J, Weitz JI. New antithrombotic agents. *Lancet* 1999;353: 1431–1436.
62. Hirsh J, Dalen JE, Anderson DR, et al. Oral anticoagulants: mechanism of action, clinical effectiveness, and optimal therapeutic range. *Chest* 1998;114[Suppl 5]:445S–469S.
63. Levine MN, Raskob G, Landefeld S, et al. Hemorrhagic complications of anticoagulant treatment. *Chest* 1998;114[Suppl 5]:511S–523S.
64. Ansell JE. Anticoagulation management clinics for the outpatient control of oral anticoagulants. *Curr Opin Pulm Med* 1998;4:215–219.
65. Erhardtsen E, Nony P, Dechavanne M, et al. The effect of recombinant factor VIIa (NovoSeven) in healthy volunteers receiving acenocoumarol to an international normalized ratio above 2.0. *Blood Coagul Fibrinolysis* 1998;9:741–748.

66. Kearon C, Hirsh J. Management of anticoagulation before and after elective surgery. *N Engl J Med* 1997;336:1506–1511.
67. Hirsh J, Warkentin TE, Raschke R, et al. Heparin and low-molecular-weight heparin: mechanisms of action, pharmacokinetics, dosing considerations, monitoring, efficacy, and safety. *Chest* 1998;114[Suppl 5]: 489S–510S.
68. Rodger M, Bredeson C, Wells PS, et al. Cost-effectiveness of low-molecular-weight heparin and unfractionated heparin in treatment of deep vein thrombosis. *CMAJ* 1998;159:931–938.
69. Llau JV. Safety of neuraxial anesthesia in patients receiving perioperative low-molecular-weight heparin for thromboprophylaxis. *Chest* 1999;116:1843–1844.
70. Anand S. Direct thrombin inhibitors. *Haemostasis* 1999;29[Suppl S1]: 76–78.
71. Weitz JI, Stewart RJ, Fredenburgh JC. Mechanism of action of plasminogen activators. *Thromb Haemost* 1999;82:974–982.
72. Marder VJ. Thrombolytic therapy. In: Hoffman R, Benz EJ Jr, Shattil SJ, et al., ed. *Hematology: basic principals and practice,* 3rd ed. New York: Churchill Livingstone, 2001:2056–2074.

CASE 28A

IT SEEMED LIKE A MAGIC POTION

CASE HISTORY

A 13-month-old boy had acute onset of jaundice, clay-colored stools, dark urine, and elevated results of liver function tests. Physical examination revealed slight hepatomegaly and splenomegaly, lethargy, and jaundice without bruising or spontaneous bleeding. The child weighed 9.7 kg. Initial laboratory testing showed an alkaline phosphatase level of 615 U/L; aspartate aminotransferase, 3,080 U/L; alanine aminotransferase, 3,279 U/L; γ-glutamyl transpeptidase, 310; and bilirubin, 9.3 mg/dL (total) and 7.7 mg/dL (direct). The result of a hepatitis B surface antigen test was negative, as were those of tests for antibodies to hepatis A and C viruses, cytomegalovirus, Epstein-Barr virus, and toxoplasma. Results of a toxic screen test were negative. A presumptive diagnosis of viral hepatitis (uncertain virus) was made. The patient was admitted to the hospital for observation and received vitamin K (2 mg intravenously on two occasions).

Over the next several days, progressive fulminant hepatic failure developed that was characterized by hypoglycemia, profound jaundice, severe coagulopathy, and increasing lethargy. The decision was made to proceed with segmental liver transplantation with the boy's mother as the donor. On the day before the operation, the prothrombin time (PT) increased to 34 seconds (normal value, 11 to 13 seconds). After infusion of fresh frozen plasma FFP (100 ml at 25 ml/h), the PT improved from 34 seconds to 23 seconds. Then 30 μg/kg (300 μg) of recombinant factor VIIa (NovoSeven; Novo Nordisk Pharmaceuticals, Princeton, NJ) was injected intravenously over 15 minutes. The PT promptly corrected from 23 to 13.5 seconds, and factor VII concentration increased from less than 1% to 42% (Table 28A.1). After infusion of recombinant factor VIIa, at a time when the PT was 13.5 seconds, an arterial catheter and a central venous catheter were placed in preparation for transplantation. The operation was performed without complications with an anhepatic time of 60 minutes and an estimated blood loss of 400 ml. During the operation, 9 hours after the initial dose of recombinant factor VIIa, the PT gradually increased from 13.5 to 25 seconds. A second infusion of 300 μg resulted in prompt correction of the PT to 15.1 seconds. Pathologic examination of the resected liver showed panlobular parenchymal degeneration consistent with fulminant viral hepatitis. The patient needed no fresh frozen plasma after surgery and was discharged from intensive care on the third postoperative day.

DISCUSSION

Patients undergoing liver transplantation often have profound acquired derangements of coagulation. In addition to depressed hepatic synthesis of coagulation factors, patients with terminal liver disease have elevated levels of fibrin degradation products, increased fibrinolysis, and decreased defenses against disseminated intravascular coagulation. Those with chronic liver disease often have splenomegaly and thrombocytopenia, engorged veins of the portal collateral circulation, and poor tissue turgor from chronic malnutrition. This patient had abnormalities typical of fulminant hepatic failure. The case was further complicated by the patient's small size. Blood volume management is difficult for pediatric patients, and the technical challenges of liver transplantation in small patients are considerable.

All coagulation factors except factor VIII are synthesized in the liver. However, each coagulation factor has its own natural biologic half-life in the circulation. The shorter the half-life, the greater is the demand for synthesis of the factor. Factor VII has the shortest half-life of all— only 7 hours. Thus the liver must maintain a high rate of synthesis of factor VII. In the setting of impaired hepatic function, the level of factor VII decreases to the lowest levels of all coagulation factors. The PT is dramatically prolonged in the setting of liver disease, because the PT assay is particularly sensitive to factor VII levels. Many clinicians incorrectly believe that PT is prolonged to an equal degree by an equivalent deficiency of factors II, V, VII, or X or fibrinogen. The PT is actually more sensitive to deficiencies of factor VII than to any other coagulation factor. Thus the PT is greatly prolonged in patients with fulminant liver disease and undergoes dramatic correction after infusion of recombinant factor VIIa. Correction of PT with recombinant factor VIIa should not be mistakenly considered to represent correction of hemostasis.

Recombinant factor VIIa has been licensed for the treatment of patients with hemophilia who have inhibitors. Bernstein et al. (1) described their experience with recombinant factor VIIa in the treatment of ten adult patients with chronic cirrhosis and moderate prolongation of PT. After injection of 20 μg/kg recombinant factor VIIa, the PT normalized for 6 hours. The short biologic half-life of factor VII means that the effect of injected recombinant factor VIIa does not last long. There has been little experience with use of this agent in the care of patients awaiting liver transplantation. Kalicinski et al. (2) described the use of recombinant factor VIIa immediately before liver transplantation in the care of two patients with fulminant hepatic failure. The patient in this case was younger than those patients and had more severe coagulopathy. As shown in Table 28A.1, this case documents how infusion of 30 μg/kg recombinant factor VIIa affects levels of coagulation factors.

Cases such as this one suggest that recombinant factor VIIa will become part of the supportive care of pediatric patients with

TABLE 28A.1. COAGULATION VALUES DURING HOSPITAL COURSE

Date	Platelet Count (no./L)	Fibrinogen Level (mg/dl)	PT (s)	aPTT (s)	Coagulation Factor Level (%)				Comment
					II	V	X	VII	
5 days before operation	142,000	138	16.0	34	8	38	8	2	No bleeding
2 days before operation	60,000	142	22.5	47	8	39	7	1	Mild bleeding around catheter site
1 day before operation	73,000	85	34.1	83				<1	Skin bleeding
Immediately before operation	69,000	75	23.1	43				<42	Preinfusion rVIIa
Immediately before operation	68,000	46	13.5	32					Postinfusion rVIIa
During operation	53,000	84	25.0	96.6					Preinfusion rVIIa
During operation	31,000	115	15.1	70.3					Postinfusion rVIIa
In recovery room	39,000	141	13.7	37.8					
Postoperative day 1	43,000	197	13.2	32.2					
Postoperative day 2	44,000		13.5	28.7					

PT, prothrombin time; aPTT, activated partial thromboplastin time; rVIIa, recombinant factor VIIa.

fulminant hepatic failure who are awaiting liver transplantation. While patients are being considered for transplantation, infusion of recombinant factor VIIa can result in a substantial correction of the factor VII deficiency that accompanies liver failure but still allow the transplantation team to monitor levels of other liver-dependent coagulation factors, such as factors X, V, or II, as an index of the need for transplantation. Thus risk of severe coagulopathy or procedure-related bleeding can be decreased among patients awaiting the decision for transplantation. This therapy also may reduce the risk of and avoid large volume infusions of fresh frozen plasma. The substantial correction of coagulation resulting from the use of recombinant factor VIIa immediately before and during transplantation operations is expected to decrease intraoperative bleeding, but this has not yet been studied in clinical trials. A particular advantage of recombinant factor VIIa in the care of pediatric patients is the small volume of fluid needed to correct the factor VII deficiency. In this patient, the PT was corrected by the injection of only 0.5 ml of recombinant factor VIIa. Unfortunately, recombinant factor VIIa is very expensive; use in the care of adults would require thousands of dollars of treatment per day. Thus much more clinical study is needed so that this new "magic potion" can be used appropriately.

Case contributed by Walter H. Dzik, M.D., Massachusetts General Hospital, Boston, MA.

REFERENCES

1. Bernstein DE, Jeffers L, Erhardtsen E, et al. Recombinant factor VIIa corrects prothrombin time in cirrhotic patients: a preliminary study. *Gastroenterology* 1997;113:1930–37.
2. Kalicinski P, Kaminski A, Drewniak T, et al. Quick correction of hemostasis in two patients with fulminant liver failure undergoing liver transplantation by recombinant activated factor VII. *Transplant Proc* 1999; 31:378–379.

PART II
Pediatric Obstetric, Congenital

29

FETAL AND NEONATAL HEMATOPOIESIS

ROBERT D. CHRISTENSEN
MARTHA C. SOLA

The purpose of hematopoiesis in the fetus differs from that in the adult. The primary function of hematopoiesis in adults is to produce sufficient hemic cells to balance hemic cellular losses. In contrast, in the fetus constant growth and dramatic physiologic changes necessitate a system with other functions. For example, the remarkable rate of somatic growth in the fetus and neonate and the resultant need to constantly increase blood volume necessitate an extraordinary hematopoietic effort, assessed as daily cell production per kilogram of body weight. In addition, the relatively low oxygen tensions but high metabolic rates of fetal tissues require a system of oxygen delivery fundamentally different from that in adults. Moreover, the sterile intraamniotic environment and consequently the low demand for the antimicrobial actions of neutrophils change markedly at birth. The extrauterine environment demands a constant and lifelong need for the antimicrobial actions of neutrophils. These issues are summarized in Table 29.1.

The hematopoietic system of a fetus and neonate must be sufficiently plastic to accommodate many marked changes and dichotomies. It has been speculated that improved familiarity with developmental hematopoietic regulation improves interpretation of postnatal hematologic data and enhances appreciation of the granulocytopoietic, erythropoietic, and thrombopoietic capacities and limitations of prematurely delivered neonates. Cytopenia certainly is common in neonatal intensive care units (NICUs). Neutropenia occurs in 5% to 8% of patients in NICUs (1), thrombocytopenia in 25% to 30% (2), and anemia in perhaps as many as 50% (3) at some time before discharge home. The prevalence of cytopenia among patients in NICUs is related to gestational age. The prevalence is higher among those delivered at the earliest gestational ages. Transfusion is the only means of managing severe cytopenia among neonates, but alternatives to repeated transfusions should emerge as more is learned about developmental hematopoiesis.

Developmental hematopoiesis can be viewed as occurring in three anatomic stages—mesoblastic, hepatic, and myeloid. Mesoblastic hematopoiesis occurs in extraembryonic structures, principally the yolk sac, and begins between the 16th and 19th days of gestation. By about 6 weeks of gestation, the extraembryonic sites of hematopoiesis begin to ablate and hepatic hematopoiesis is initiated. By the 10th to 12th week, mesoblastic hematopoiesis ceases, and a small amount of hematopoiesis is evident in the bone marrow. In humans, it seems that the clavicle is the first bone to develop a marrow cavity (4). The first cells present in the developing marrow space have macrophage surface markers and phenotypes, These are followed by myeloperoxidase-positive cells with the characteristics of neutrophils. However, the liver remains the predominant hematopoietic organ until the last trimester of pregnancy.

The anatomic site of hematopoiesis does not simply transfer

R.D. Christensen and M.C. Sola: Division of Neonatology, Department of Pediatrics, University of Florida College of Medicine, Gainesville, Florida.

TABLE 29.1. INHERENT DIFFERENCES IN HEMATOPOIETIC SYSTEMS OF THE FETUS, NEONATE, AND ADULT

Fetus

Exists in a sterile environment. Until near term, does not generally need an antibacterial defense system.

Must produce a neutrophil reserve in preparation for extrauterine life.

Fetal hematocrit and blood platelet concentration increase only slightly from 20 weeks to term, whereas blood volume increases approximately ten fold. Thus erythrocyte and platelet production must be extremely rapid during this period to keep pace with the rapid expansion of blood volume.

Neonate

At birth, the fetus moves from a sterile into a non sterile environment and must have a neutrophil reserve already developed to survive in this environment.

At birth, oxygen delivery to tissues markedly increases, as PaO_2 increases from 27 to >90 mm Hg. This effectively shuts off erythropoietin production. Consequently, erythropoiesis temporarily ceases, eventuating in the physiologic anemia of infancy.

Rapid growth and blood volume expansion continue. However, platelet concentration does not change, and platelet production is very rapid during this period.

Adult

The rapid somatic growth and blood volume expansion of infancy and childhood cease. Thus the previous need to accelerate hematopoiesis to keep pace with somatic growth ends.

The neutrophil system must continue to be responsive to rapid increases in demand for cells.

Blood platelet concentration and hematocrit remain relatively constant throughout healthy life.

from yolk sac to liver to bone marrow (5). Rather, each organ subsequently houses distinct hematopoietic populations. For example, at 18 to 20 weeks of gestation, more than 85% of the cells in the fetal liver are erythroid, and few neutrophils are present. At the same time, fewer than 40% of the cells within the bone marrow are erythroid, and most are neutrophils. The mechanisms responsible for the changing anatomic sites of hematopoiesis and for the differences in hemic cells produced in the mesoblastic, hepatic, and myeloid sites have not been determined. Regardless of gestational age or anatomic location, production of all hematopoietic tissues begins with pluripotent cells capable of both self-renewal and clonal maturation into all blood cell lineages. Progenitor cells differentiate under the influence of hematopoietic growth factors, which include those listed in Table 29.2.

GRANULOCYTOPOIESIS

A traditional view is that neutrophil production, like hematopoiesis in general, begins in the yolk sac and moves to the liver and spleen and finally to the bone marrow. However, recent results of studies of human fetuses do not support this concept. Specifically, the human yolk sac contains no neutrophils—its hematopoietic activity is limited to erythropoiesis and production of a small number of macrophages (5). Similarly, the human fetal liver produces few, if any, neutrophils. The few neutrophils found in photomicrographic sections of human fetal liver are not arranged in clusters of hematopoietic nests but are widely separated and found surrounding the blood vessels, as if they were carried in by the circulation, not produced in the organ. Moreover, the spleen is not a granulocytopoietic organ in human

TABLE 29.2. HEMATOPOIETIC GROWTH FACTORS

Growth Factors	Molecular Mass (kd)	Chromosomal Location	Principal Target Cell
Erythropoietin	30.4	7q11–22	CFU-E, fetal BFU-E
Colony-stimulating factors			
G-CSF	18.8	17q11.2–21	CFU-G
GM-CSF	14.4	5q23–31	All CFC
M-CSF	26 (dimer)	1p13–21	CFU-M
SCF	15–20 (dimer)	12q2–24	Primitive CFC
Interleukins			
IL-1α	17	2q13	Primitive CFC, hepatocyte, macrophage
IL-1β	17	2q13	Primitive CFC, hepatocyte, macrophage
IL-2	15–20	4q26–27	T cell
IL-3	14–15	5q23–31	All CFC
IL-4	16–20	5q23–31	T cell, B cell
IL-5	13.2 (dimer)	5q23–31	CFO-EOS
IL-6	20.8	7p21–24	Primitive CFC
IL-7	25	8q12–13	B cell
IL-8	8–10	4	Neutrophil, endothelial cell
IL-9	16	5q31–32	BFU-E, primitive CFC
IL-10	23	1	Macrophage, lymphocyte
IL-11	22	19q13	Primitive CFC, BFU-MK, CFU-MK
IL-12	70–75		T cell, NK cell, macrophage
Thrombopoietin	35	3q26–28	BFU-MK, CFU-MK

CFO-EOS, eosinophil colony-forming unit; BFU-E, primitive erythroid progenitor; G-CSF, granulocyte colony-stimulating factor; CFU-G, granulocyte colony forming unit; GM-CSF, granulocyte-macrophage colony-stimulating factor; CFC, colony-forming cells; M-CSF, macrophage colony-stimulating factor; SCF, stem cell factor; IL, interleukin; BFU-MK, primitive megakaryocyte progenitor; CFU-MK, mature megakaryocyte progenitor; NK, natural killer.

fetuses, as it is in rodents (6). No granulocytopoietic nests are found in human fetal spleen, and the neutrophils within it are mostly mature and evenly dispersed. This finding suggests they were carried there in the blood, not produced locally.

Where, then, do neutrophils originate in the human fetus? The first neutrophils are present approximately 5 weeks after conception and are clustered in the periaortic tissue. These first fetal neutrophils contain myeloperoxidase, and they mature into cells with band and segmented nuclei, but beyond these features, any differences or similarities between them and the neutrophils of adults have not been reported (7). The function of these cells in the fetus and the explanation for this location of origin are unclear. The fetal bone marrow space begins to develop approximately 8 weeks after conception (Figs. 29.1, 29.2). The space is lined by osteoclast-like cells with cell-surface characteristics of macrophages. These cells appear to core-out the space from the primitive cartilage. Eight to ten weeks after conception, the bone marrow space progressively enlarges, but no neutrophils are present within the space until 10.5 to 11 weeks (4) (Fig. 29.3). The first neutrophils in the marrow do not have band or segmented nuclei, but they contain myeloperoxidase and express the cell surface characteristics of myeloblasts and promyelocytes. From 14 weeks to term, the most common cell type in the fetal bone marrow space is the neutrophil, although the marrow space is

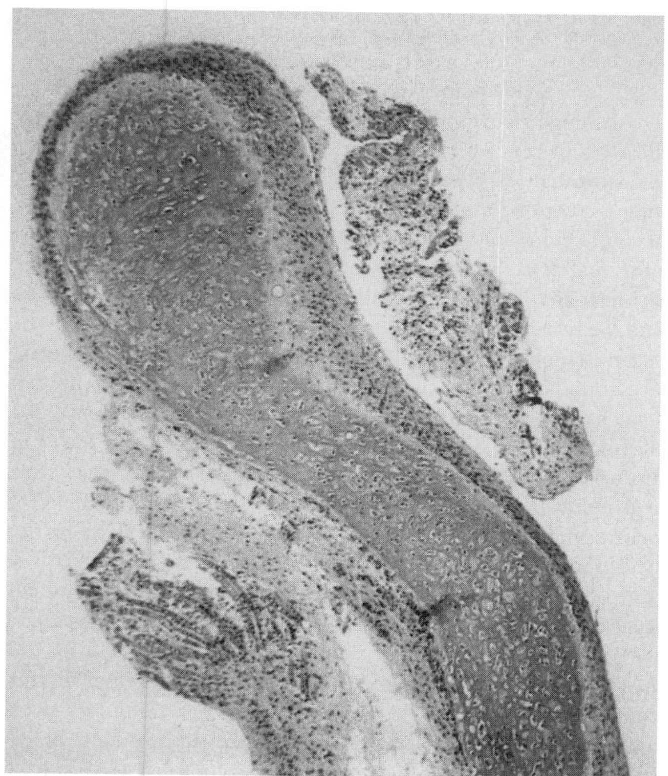

FIGURE 29.1. Clavicle approximately 7 weeks after conception, before any marrow space is present. In the human fetus, the first bone to contain a developing marrow space is the clavicle, followed closely by the other long bones. (Hematoxylin and eosin stain; original magnification, ×100).

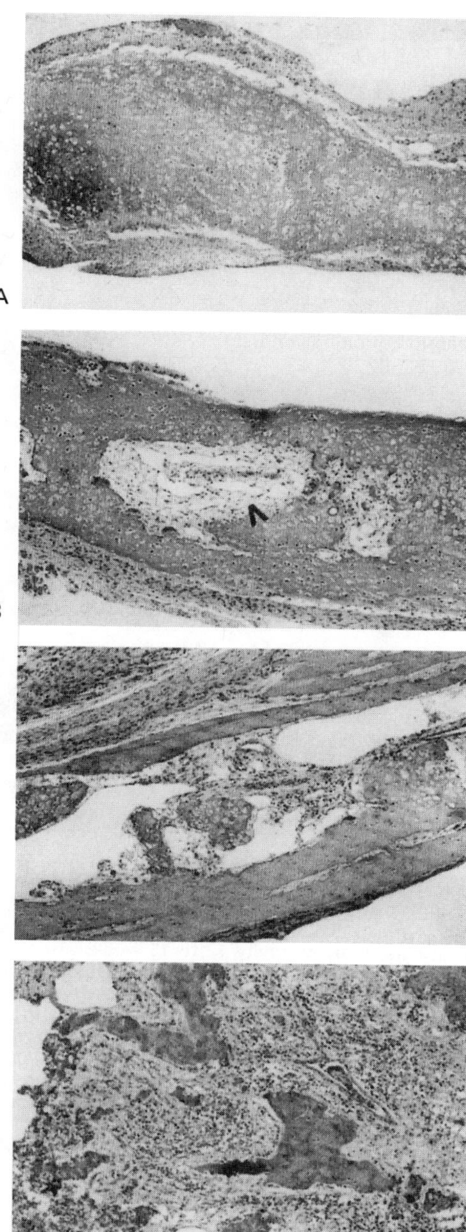

FIGURE 29.2. Photomicrographs of clavicles 6 to 14 weeks after conception (Hematoxylin and eosin stain; original magnification, ×100). **A:** Six weeks after conception. Clavicles at this stage consist of primitive cartilage and contain no marrow cavity and no myeloperoxidase positive cells. **B:** Nine weeks after conception. Clavicles at this stage have the beginning of a marrow cavity (*arrowhead*) but no myeloperoxidase positive cells. **C:** Eleven weeks after conception. Clavicles at this stage have an elongated marrow cavity and small hematopoietic islands of myeloperoxidase positive cell in the marrow space. **D:** Fourteen weeks after conception. Spiculation has begun, and the volume of hematopoietic marrow has begun to increase. (Modified from Slayton WB, Li Y, Calhoun DA, et al. The first appearance of neutrophils in the human fetal bone marrow cavity. *Early Hum Dev* 1998;53:129–144, with permission.)

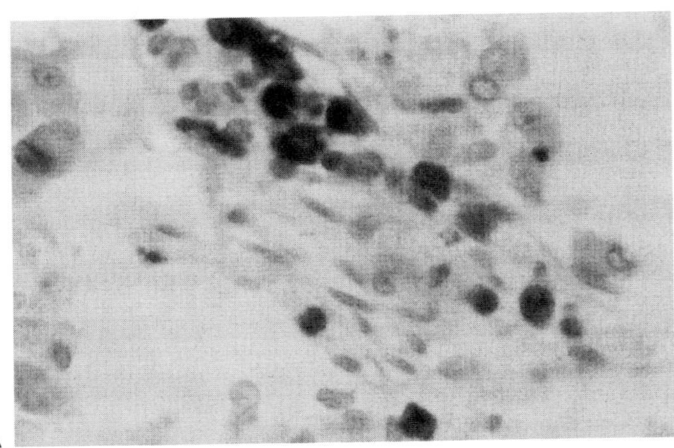
A

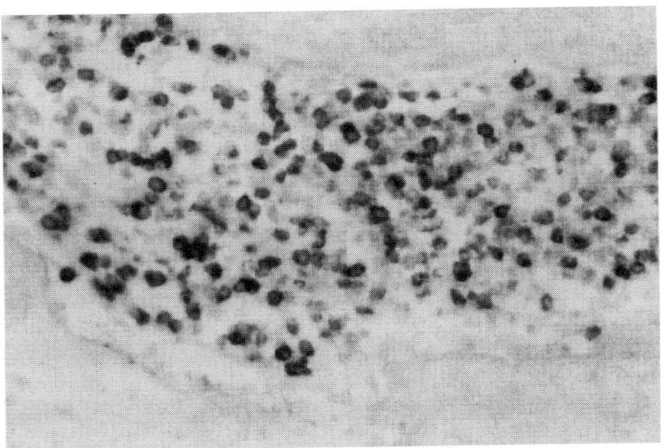
B

FIGURE 29.3. Appearance and subsequent expansion of neutrophils within the clavicular marrow cavity 12 to 15 weeks after conception. **A:** At 12 weeks of gestation a small number of myeloperoxidase-positive cells are present in the developing marrow cavity. Many of these cells have the morphologic appearance of neutrophils with segmented or band nuclei and they appear in discrete clusters within the marrow cavity. (Myeloperoxidase stain; original magnification, ×400.) **B:** At 15 weeks, clavicles have a marrow cavity that contains numerous myeloperoxidase-positive cells. (Original magnification, ×200.) (Modified from Slayton WB, Li Y, Calhoun DA, et al. The first appearance of neutrophils in the human fetal bone marrow cavity. *Early Hum Dev* 1998;53: 129–144, with permission.)

not nearly so densely packed with cells as it becomes in older children and adults (4,7).

Macrophages are crucial to fetal morphogenesis, because they aid in shaping of organs and scavenging debris and apoptotic cells. Although neutrophils and macrophages have a common progenitor cell, the discordant temporal appearance of neutrophils and macrophages in the fetus and the divergence of their anatomic locations are striking (8). Recent observations have cast doubt on long-held theories about the origins of macrophages in the human fetus. For example, it was believed that macrophages form from precursor cells in the bone marrow and mature through a progression of cell types from monoblast to promonocyte to monocyte, which then migrate to various tissues and differentiate into macrophages. Observations of human fetuses do not support this origin of macrophages. First, macrophages appear in the yolk sac, liver, lung, and brain long before the bone marrow cavity has been formed. Second, promonocytes and monocytes are absent in the yolk sac and liver, but macrophages are present there nevertheless. Thus the macrophages in the yolk sac may develop directly from stem cells without passing through a monocyte stage. It is not clear whether these primitive macrophages migrate from the yolk sac to populate the lungs, liver, brain, and other organs (9).

The mechanisms that regulate neutrophil production during human fetal development are not clear. Granulocyte colony-stimulating factor (G-CSF) and macrophage colony-stimulating factor (M-CSF) are present in developing fetal bone as early as 6 weeks after conception and in the fetal liver as early as 8 weeks (10). Granulocyte-macrophage colony stimulating factor (GM-CSF) is widely distributed in fetal tissues, including pulmonary epithelium, and is involved in pulmonary homeostasis. Stem cell factor messenger RNA (mRNA) is present in the yolk sac, liver, and bone marrow at the earliest stages of their respective development (5). No changes in mRNA concentrations of these factors or of their specific receptors or in the concentrations of proteins, judged with immunohistochemical staining, appear to constitute the signal for production of neutrophils. Thus the precise signals that initiate the production of macrophages and neutrophils in the embryo and fetus are not known. It is curious that the actions of G-CSF, M-CSF, GM-CSF, and stem cell factor are not limited to hematopoiesis in the fetus and neonate. Receptors for all of these factors are located in distinct areas of the fetal central nervous system and gastrointestinal tract, where their patterns of expression change with development. Important undefined developmental roles clearly exist for these factors that are beyond those known for hematopoiesis.

Although neutrophil production in the bone marrow space clearly is present by 14 weeks of gestation, the blood of the fetus, even through 20 weeks, contains few neutrophils. Forestier et al. (11) reported that fetuses at 20 weeks of gestation had a mean absolute blood neutrophil concentration of only 190/μl, a range of 0 to 490/μl, and a mode concentration of zero (11). Despite the near absence of circulating neutrophils in the first trimester, and the relative scarcity (by adult standards) of neutrophils in the second trimester, progenitor cells with the capacity to generate neutrophils in vitro (CFU-GM) are abundant in the early human fetal liver, bone marrow, and blood (12–17). In rodents, the number of CFU-GM per gram of body weight is far fewer in animals delivered prematurely than in those delivered at term and is lower in term animals than in adults. The quantity of neutrophilic progenitor cells per gram of body weight in the developing human fetus has not been reported (18). Thus it is not clear whether, as in experimental animals, preterm human infants have a relatively small supply of granulocytic progenitors. The venous blood of adults contains approximately 20 to 300 CFU-GM per milliliter. In contrast, the blood of term infants contains approximately 2,000 CFU-GM per milliliter. Even higher concentrations are present in the blood of infants delivered prematurely. The high concentrations of CFU-GM in fetal blood, however, do not necessarily indicate a large total body quantity of CFU-GM. It is likely that a significant percentage of fetal CFU-GM are in the circulation (16).

When fetal CFU-GM are cultured in vitro in the presence

of recombinant G-CSF they undergo maturation into colonies of neutrophils. Fetal CFU-GM often clonally mature into larger colonies and contain more cells than do CFU-GM obtained from the bone marrow of adults (19). The physiologic role of G-CSF includes up-regulation of neutrophil production. This appears to be the case for the fetus and neonate as well as for the adult. Thus the low quantities of circulating and storage neutrophils in the midtrimester human fetus may be due in part to low production of G-CSF. Supporting this hypothesis are observations of poor production of G-CSF by cells of human fetal origin (19,20). Monocytes isolated from the blood of adults produce G-CSF when stimulated with a variety of inflammatory mediators, such as bacterial lipopolysaccharide or interleukin-1. In contrast, monocytes isolated from the umbilical cord blood of preterm infants and from the liver and bone marrow of aborted fetuses up to 24 weeks of gestation generate only small quantities (10 to 100 times less per cell) of G-CSF protein and mRNA after lipopolysaccharide or interleukin-1 stimulation (19,20). Despite the poor capacity to generate G-CSF, it appears that G-CSF receptors on the surface of neutrophils of newborn infants are equal in number and affinity to those on adult neutrophils.

Thus relatively few neutrophils are present in the human embryo and early fetus, and neutrophil production is a relatively minor component of hematopoiesis in the midtrimester fetus. On this basis, one might anticipate that neonates delivered extremely prematurely would be at high risk of serious bacterial infection. Indeed, of all the risk factors for neonatal infection analyzed in the national collaborative study on neonatal infections, premature birth had the strongest correlation.

ERYTHROPOIESIS

Production of erythrocytes requires a constant supply of amino acids, lipids, iron, specific vitamins, and trace nutrients (21). Limitations in any of these can thwart production. However, the rate of erythrocyte production is regulated not by any of these substances but rather by the concentration of erythropoietin. Erythropoietin is an 18.4-kd glycoprotein that binds to specific receptors on the surface of erythroid precursors and various other cells and supports their clonal maturation (21,22). In the human fetus, erythropoietin is produced by a surprising variety of cells, including cells of monocyte-macrophage origin in the liver (23, 24). The absence of erythropoietin or its receptor, as has been produced in murine knock-out models, leads to profound anemia and fetal death on approximately embryonic day 13 (25, 26). Postnatally erythropoietin is produced almost exclusively by peritubular cells of the kidney, with a small amount produced by neuronal and glial cells in the central nervous system. Although some erythropoietin production occurs in the fetal kidney, it is minimal. Anephric fetuses have normal serum erythropoietin concentrations and hematocrits (27). The factors that regulate the switch of erythropoietin production from the liver to the kidney are not known. However, some investigators have suggested that among preterm neonates a developmental delay in this switch is responsible for the relatively low concentrations of circulating erythropoietin in the common hyporegenerative anemia known as *anemia of prematurity* (28).

It has become clear that the actions of erythropoietin in the human fetus are widespread. Erythropoietin receptors have been documented on the surface of cells within a surprising variety of nonhematopoietic fetal tissues, including intestinal villi, endothelium, mesangium, smooth muscle, placenta, and neurons (23, 24,29,30). Erythropoietin has an antiapoptotic effect on several of these cells types in vitro. Erythropoietin also occurs in relatively high concentration in human amniotic fluid, colostrum, and milk—fluids that are swallowed in large amounts by the fetus and neonate (31). A healthy midtrimester human fetus may swallow 200 to 300 ml of amniotic fluid per kilogram of body weight per day. With an amniotic fluid erythropoietin concentration of 200 mU/ml, the fetus would swallow approximately 60,000 mU/kg a day—an amount that if given systemically to a neonate would have a marked erythropoietic effect. Erythropoietin receptors are present along the villous border of the fetal and neonatal intestine (Fig. 29.2) (23,31). It appears that erythropoietin in amniotic fluid, colostrum, and human milk is not absorbed into the circulation and has no systemic effect but acts locally in the intestine as a trophic and antiapoptotic factor. Erythropoietin in amniotic fluid, colostrum, and milk tends to resist digestive conditions present in the fetal and neonatal gastrointestinal tract (31,32).

Erythropoietin is present, in concentrations of 20 to 50 mU/ml, in the spinal fluid of neonates. Markedly greater spinal fluid concentrations of erythropoietin are seen after perinatal asphyxia, and this erythropoietin appears to be derived within the brain as opposed to crossing the blood-brain barrier (33,34). Further evidence that erythropoietin does not cross the blood-brain barrier in neonatal humans includes the observation that neonates treated with recombinant erythropoietin do not have elevated erythropoietin concentrations in their spinal fluid (34). The spinal fluid of adults generally has an erythropoietin concentration lower than the lower limit of detectability (33,34).

The biologic roles of erythropoietin and erythropoietin receptors in the fetal and neonatal intestinal tract and central nervous system are not known. One potential function for erythropoietin in the fetal brain is as a neuroprotectant (35). This postulate is supported by the observations that erythropoietin production increases in the brain during fetal hypoxia, and that recombinant erythropoietin protects neurons in tissue culture from hypoxemic damage and does so by diminishing apoptosis, which is analogous to the function it has in erythropoiesis.

Culture of bone marrow cells in tissue culture has added to the understanding of erythropoietic regulation. When bone marrow cells are placed in semisolid media culture systems for 5 to 7 days, the erythropoietin-sensitive precursors (CFU-E) clonally mature into clusters containing 30 to 100 normoblasts (36). Erythroid-specific progenitors that are less well differentiated than CFU-E, and hence more primitive cells, are called *burst-forming units-erythroid* (BFU-E). Twelve to 14 days after bone marrow cells are placed in semisolid culture systems, BFU-E have developed into large clusters of normoblasts, each containing 200 to more than 10,000 normoblasts. Burst-forming units-erythroid from human fetuses respond in a slightly different manner than do BFU-E isolated from adults. Specifically,

BFU-E of fetal origin generally develop into erythroid clones more rapidly and generally develop substantially more normoblasts than do BFU-E of adult origin (37,38). Also, BFU-E from adult bone marrow require a combination of erythropoietin plus another factor, such as interleukin-3 or GM-CSF, to clonally mature, whereas many fetal BFU-E mature in the presence of erythropoietin alone (37,38).

Tissues must receive a constant supply of oxygen. The development of oxygen-carrying proteins has increased the ability of blood to transport oxygen. Combination of oxygen and its dissociation from hemoglobin are accomplished without expenditure of metabolic energy (39). Hemoglobin consists of iron-containing heme groups and globin, a protein moiety. An interaction between heme, globin, and 2,3-diphosphoglycerate (also called 2,3-bisphosphoglycerate) gives hemoglobin its unique properties in the reversible transport of oxygen. Hemoglobin is a tetrameric molecule composed of two pairs of polypeptide chains, each encoded by a different family of genes; the α-like globin genes on chromosome 16 and the β-like globin genes on chromosome 11. The main hemoglobin of normal adults (HbA) is made up of one pair each of α and β chains ($\alpha_2\beta_2$). Six distinct hemoglobins can be detected within the erythrocytes of the human embryo, fetus, child, and adult—Gower-1, Gower-2, Portland, fetal hemoglobin (HbF), and the adult hemoglobins HbA and HbA_2. The time of appearance and quantitative relations among the hemoglobins are determined by complex developmental processes that are not well defined.

Human embryos have the slowly migrating hemoglobins Gower-1, Gower-2, and Portland. The ζ chains of Hb Portland and Gower-1 are structurally similar to α chains. Both Gower hemoglobins contain a unique polypeptide chain, the ε chain. Gower-1 Hb has the structure $\zeta_2\epsilon_2$ and Gower-2, $\alpha_2\epsilon_2$. Portland Hb has the structure $\zeta_2\gamma_2$. Four to eight weeks after conception, the Gower hemoglobins predominate, but by 12 to 14 weeks, they are no longer detected.

Fetal hemoglobin contains γ chains in place of the β chains of HbA and are represented as $\alpha_2\gamma_2$. The resistance of HbF to denaturation by strong alkali usually is used in its quantitation. After the eighth postconceptional week, HbF is the predominant hemoglobin. At 24 weeks of gestation, it constitutes 90% of total hemoglobin. Thereafter a gradual decline in HbF occurs, so that at birth the average is 70% of the total. Synthesis of HbF decreases rapidly postnatally, and by 6 to 12 months of age only a trace is present. Fetal hemoglobin is heterogeneous because of two types of γ chains synthesis of which is directed by two sets of genes. The chains differ at position 136 in the presence of either a glycine (Gγ) or an alanine (Aγ) residue. In the neonate, the relative proportion of Gγ to Aγ chain is 3:1.

Trace quantities of HbA can be detected in embryos. Thus it is possible to make an early prenatal diagnosis of major β-chain hemoglobinopathy. Prenatal diagnosis is based on techniques used to examine the rates of synthesis of β chains or the structure of newly synthesized β chains or on molecular techniques from sampling the chorionic villus tissue or amniotic fluid. Gene deletion disorders, such as α-thalassemia, can be detected with the same methods.

At 24 weeks of gestation, approximately 5% to 10% of hemoglobin in a fetus is HbA. Thereafter a steady increase follows, so that at term, the proportion of HbA averages 30%. By 1 year of age, the normal adult hemoglobin pattern appears. The minor adult hemoglobin component (HbA_2) contains δ chains and has the structure $\alpha_2\delta_2$. It is seen only when significant amounts of HbA are present. At birth, less than 1% of HbA_2 is present, but by 12 months, the normal level of 2% to 4% is attained. Throughout life the normal ratio of HbA to HbA_2 is approximately 30:1.

In the fetus and neonate, the rates of synthesis of γ and β chains and the amounts of HbA and HbF are inversely related. This has been attributed to a switch mechanism, but the developmental processes that direct the switch from predominantly γ-chain synthesis in utero to predominantly β-chain synthesis after birth are unclear. Primitive erythrocyte progenitors undergoing clonal maturation in culture (BFU-E) predominantly generate HbF. This may be the basis for the increased levels of HbF that occur in anemia with severe erythropoietic stress. Alternative explanations involve more basic genetic regulators in the DNA sequences that flank the hemoglobin gene complexes.

Because hemoglobins containing ε chains are normally present only very early in intrauterine life, they are largely of theoretic interest. Small amounts of the Gower hemoglobins have been detectable in a few neonates with trisomy 13. Increased levels of Hb Portland have been found in cord blood of stillborn infants with homozygous α-thalassemia.

The normal adult level of HbA_2 (2.4% to 3.4%) is seldom altered. Levels of HbA_2 exceeding 3.4% are found in most persons with the β-thalassemia trait and in those with megaloblastic anemia secondary to vitamin B_{12} and folic acid deficiency. Decreased HbA_2 levels are found in those with iron deficiency anemia and thalassemia (40).

THROMBOPOIESIS

Platelets were described in the early part of the nineteenth century, but it was not until 1882 that their role in hemostasis was recognized. The origin of platelets from megakaryocytes was reported in 1906 (41), and since then the study of mechanisms responsible for platelet production has focused on megakaryocytes. The megakaryocyte compartment in the bone marrow consists of two pools of cells (42). One is composed of cells that are morphologically unrecognizable but are committed to the megakaryocyte lineage. These cells, the megakaryocyte progenitors, retain a high proliferative capacity and ultimately determine the number of megakaryocytes in the bone marrow. The other pool consists of nondividing cells that are morphologically recognizable as megakaryocytes and undergo endoreduplication or endomitosis, a process in which the ploidy of the cell increases without cellular division.

Progenitor cells committed to the megakaryocyte lineage can be identified by two methods—a culture system, in which they are identified by their ability to form megakaryocyte colonies, and immunologic staining, which allows characterization according to the specific antigens expressed on their membranes. With these methods, two different megakaryocyte progenitor cells have been identified; the burst-forming unit megakaryocyte (BFU-MK), which constitutes the most primitive megakaryocyte progenitor (43,44), and a later progenitor known as the colony-forming unit megakaryocyte (CFU-MK) (42,45). In cul-

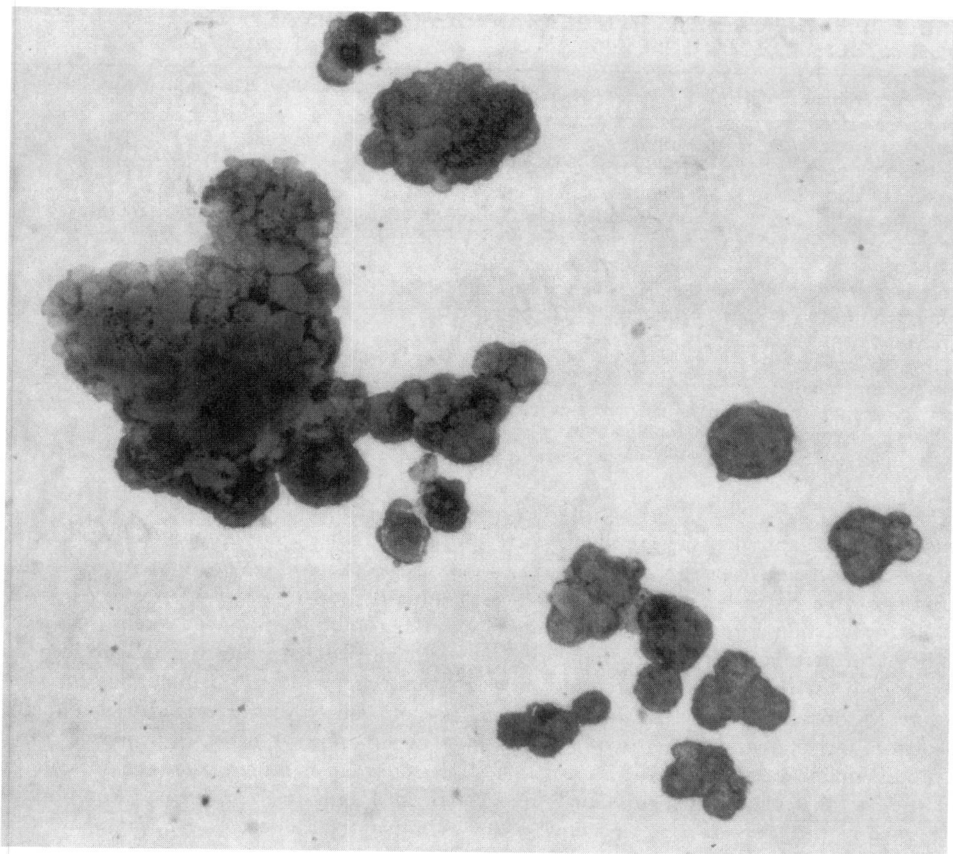

FIGURE 29.4. Photomicrograph shows a megakaryocyte colony derived from a megakaryocyte progenitor (CFU-MK) from the bone marrow of a thrombocytopenic preterm neonate. (Original magnification, ×400). Light-density mononuclear cells isolated from the bone marrow were cultured in a collagen-based serum-free media with 50 ng/ml of recombinant human thrombopoietin. After fixation, the colonies were stained with a monoclonal antibody against glycoprotein IIb/IIIa to allow accurate identification of megakaryocytes.

ture, CFU-MK–derived colonies are smaller (3 to 50 cells per colony) and primarily unifocal (Fig. 29.4), whereas BFU-MK–derived colonies are larger (>50 cells per colony) and have multiple foci of development. When immunologically phenotyped, CFU-MKs express CD34 and HLA-DR, whereas BFU-MKs express CD34 but not HLA-DR.

There are no differences between fetal and adult megakaryocyte progenitors in immunologic profiles of the expression of CD34 and HLA-DR (46). However, fetal BFU-MK–derived colonies are significantly larger than adult BFU-MK–derived colonies and usually are composed of only one or two foci of development. Adult BFU-MK–derived colonies are multifocal (46). In addition, a unique megakaryocyte progenitor present in fetal bone marrow has an unusually high proliferative potential and gives rise to very large unifocal colonies (>300 cells) (47). This cell, not found in adult bone marrow cultures, may represent a more primitive megakaryocyte progenitor. The development of miniaturized assay systems to study megakaryocyte progenitors has made it possible to study these cells in the peripheral blood of neonates. With these techniques, it has been shown that preterm neonates (24 to 36 weeks) have higher circulating concentrations of all megakaryocyte progenitors than do term neonates (48).

Unlike their progenitors, megakaryocytes have no proliferative abilities but undergo a complex maturational process. Through this process, they evolve from small, mononuclear cells to very large, polyploid cells easily recognized in the bone marrow as mature megakaryocytes (49,50). The modal ploidy is 16N in normal adult bone marrow (51).

In the human fetus, megakaryocytes are first detected in the circulatory system at 8 weeks of gestation, and the first platelets appear at 5 weeks (52). Compared with the megakaryocytes of adults, fetal megakaryocytes are smaller at all stages of maturation. Their ploidy distribution is shifted to the left with a higher proportion of immature megakaryocytes (53–55). The modal ploidy in the bone marrow of near-term fetuses is 8N (56).

Umbilical cord blood has higher concentrations of circulating megakaryocytes than does adult blood. As in the fetus, cord blood megakaryocytes are considerably smaller than adult circulating megakaryocytes (57). "Adult-size" megakaryocytes appear by 2 years of age, but the evolution of the process of megakaryocytopoiesis in the first year of life is poorly understood because of the lack of normal bone marrow specimens. Because large megakaryocytes generate more platelets than do small megakaryocytes, it is reasonable to assume that neonatal megakaryocytes produce fewer platelets than do their adult counterparts. The

TABLE 29.3. DIFFERENCES IN MEGAKARYOCYTOPOIESIS BETWEEN NEONATES AND ADULTS

Characteristic	Neonates	Adults
Serum thrombopoietin concentration	Higher	Lower
MK progenitors	Higher concentration in cord blood	Lower concentration in peripheral blood
BFU-MK	Generate larger, unifocal colonies	Generate smaller, multifocal colonies
Response of MK progenitors to recombinant thrombopoietin	More sensitive	Less sensitive
MK size and ploidy	Smaller, lower ploidy (modal ploidy = 8N)	Larger, higher ploidy (modal ploidy = 16N)

MK, megakaryocyte; BFU, burst forming unit.

normal platelet counts of fetuses and neonates probably are maintained by the increased proliferative potential of the fetal megakaryocyte progenitors (Table 29.3).

The process of platelet production and release is one of the less well understood steps of thrombopoiesis. Two main theories have been proposed to explain the formation of platelets from megakaryocytes. Some investigators hypothesize that small buds, proplatelets, are formed from megakaryocytes and then released as platelets (58,59), a process mainly occurring in the bone marrow. Others have hypothesized that platelets are principally released from megakaryocytes in the lungs as a consequence of shear forces, a theory supported by the observation that circulating megakaryocytes are more abundant in the lungs than in other organs (60,61).

Thrombopoietin is the recently discovered physiologic regulator of platelet production. Fluorescence in situ hybridization studies have shown the gene that encodes thrombopoietin has been localized to the long arm of human chromosome 3 (62). Thrombopoietin mRNA is expressed primarily in liver and to a lesser extent in other tissues, including kidney and bone marrow stromal cells (63). In vitro, thrombopoietin acts as a potent stimulator of all stages of megakaryocyte growth and develop-

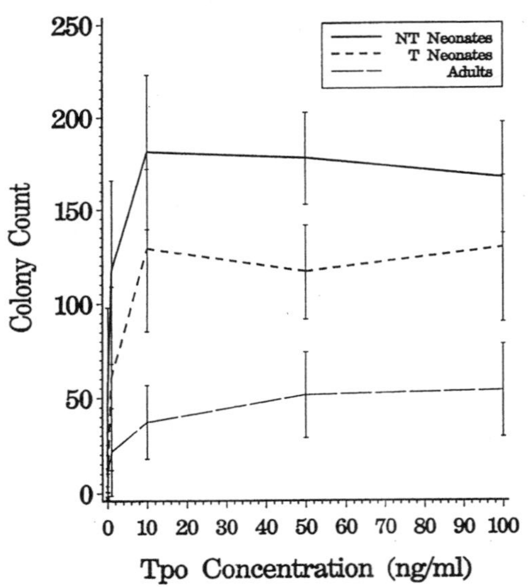

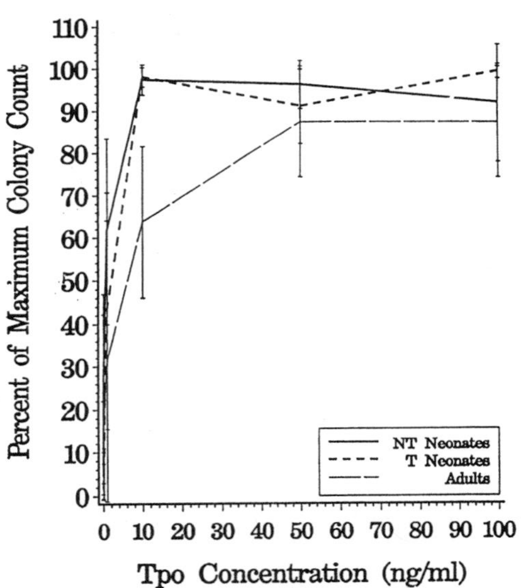

FIGURE 29.5. A: Dose response to recombinant thrombopoietin of megakaryocyte progenitors obtained from the bone marrow of neonates with thrombocytopenia (*T*), neonates without thrombocytopenic (*NT*), and healthy adults. The marrow obtained from neonates generated approximately three times more colonies (per 10^5 low density cells) than the marrow obtained from adults. **B:** In a percentage of maximal colony count versus recombinant thrombopoietin concentration curve, the curves for the neonates with thrombocytopenia and those without thrombocytopenia reached a plateau at 10 ng/ml, compared with 50 ng/ml for the adults. This indicates that megakaryocyte progenitors from neonates are more sensitive to recombinant thrombopoietin in vitro than are their adult counterparts. (From Sola MC, Du Y, Hutson AD, et al. Dose-response relationship of megakaryocyte progenitors from the bone marrow of thrombocytopenic and non-thrombocytopenic neonates to recombinant thrombopoietin. *Br J Haematol* 2000;110:449–453, with permission.)

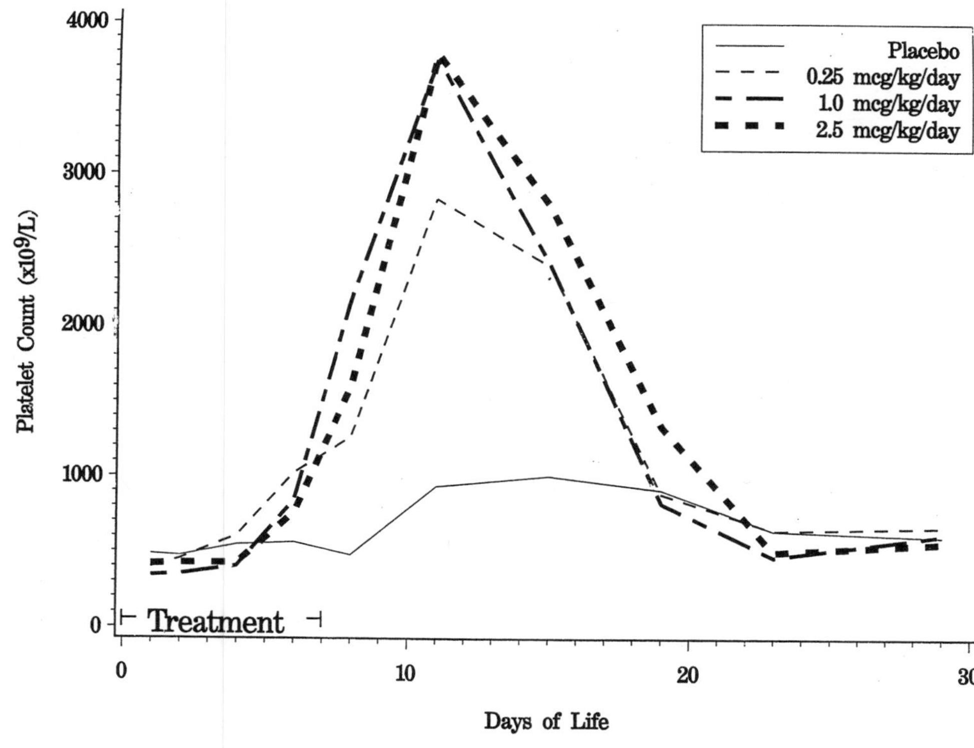

FIGURE 29.6. Dose-response of polyethylene glycol (PEG)–rHuMGDF (a truncated form of rTpo) on the blood platelet concentration in newborn rhesus monkeys, demonstrating the sensitivity of megakaryocyte progenitors of neonates to rTpo in vivo. The monkeys received daily subcutaneous injections of placebo or PEG-rHuMGDF at doses of 0.25, 1.00, or 2.50 μg/kg a day for 7 days. Each *line* represents the average platelet counts of the two monkeys in each treatment group sampled on study days 2, 4, and 6 and then twice weekly until day 28. The peripheral platelet count increased on day 6 of treatment, peaked on day 11, and returned to baseline by day 23. The two higher doses generated similar increases in platelet count. (From Sola MC, Christensen RD, Hutson AD, et al. Pharmacodynamics, pharmacokinetics and safety of administering pegylated recombinant megakaryocyte growth and development factor to newborn rhesus monkeys. *Pediatr Res* 2000;47:208–214, with permission.)

ment (64). It also plays a role in platelet activation, mostly priming the platelets to the aggregatory effect of other agonists (65). Thrombopoietin and thrombopoietin receptor knock-out mice models have been generated (66,67). These mice have megakaryocyte and blood platelet concentrations only 10% to 15% those of control mice. The results of these studies confirm the speculation that thrombopoietin is a primary regulator of platelet production and prove that alternative pathways exist for megakaryocytopoiesis.

Much attention has been directed to the effects of thrombopoietin on other hematologic cell types. In vitro, thrombopoietin alone stimulates the proliferation and survival of erythroid, myeloid, and multipotential progenitors (68). Thrombopoietin also enhances erythropoietin-induced erythroid burst formation, an effect mediated by its ability to inhibit apoptosis of erythroid progenitors (69).

Results of several studies with animals have confirmed the role of thrombopoietin as a potent stimulator of platelet production. The recombinant human full-length thrombopoietin molecule (rTpo) and a recombinant human polypeptide that contains the receptor-binding N-terminal domain of thrombopoietin (rHuMGDF) have been the subject of several studies. When injected into normal animals, rTpo and rHuMGDF induce marked thrombocytosis (70,71). Administered to animals exposed to myelosuppressive chemotherapy, rHuMGDF not only is able to ameliorate the associated thrombocytopenia but also accelerates red blood cell and neutrophil recovery (72,73).

Several phase I and II trials with human subjects have demonstrated the efficacy of rTpo and rHuMGDF as stimulators of platelet production in adults without thrombocytopenia (74) and in patients with chemotherapy-induced thrombocytopenia (75,76). However, the appearance of thrombocytopenia secondary to antithrombopoietin antibodies in a small number of patients receiving rHuMGDF (77) led to the interruption of all clinical studies in which this formulation was being used. The recombinant full-length thrombopoietin molecule is still undergoing phase II and phase III testing, and new peptides with thrombopoietin-like activity are being developed (78).

Little is known about the role of thrombopoietin or the theoretic benefits of administration of rTpo to neonates. Recombinant thrombopoietin certainly supports the growth of megakaryocyte colonies from the blood or bone marrow of neonates (Fig. 29.4). Bone marrow progenitors from neonates are more sensitive to rTpo than are progenitors from adults in vitro (Fig. 29.5) (79). Similarly, newborn rhesus monkeys are highly sensitive to rTpo in vivo (Fig. 29.6) and respond to lower doses (per kilogram body weight) than those required in adult rhesus monkeys to achieve a similar effect (80). Megakaryocyte progenitors from healthy neonates or those born preterm with thrombocytopenia seem to be more sensitive to rTpo than are progenitors from term neonates (81). Whether rTpo or other thrombopoietin-mimetic peptides will be clinically useful as an alternative to platelet transfusion in the care of neonates with thrombocytopenia remains to be determined.

SUMMARY

Neutropenia, anemia, and thrombocytopenia are relatively common problems in the NICU. These forms of cytopenia stem from multiple etiologic factors, and they involve many different kinetic mechanisms. However, all types of cytopenia in the NICU are more prevalent among those of shortest gestation and smallest birth weight. It is proposed that this relation is the result of gestational age-linked developmental differences in hematopoietic regulation. Transfusion currently is the only therapy available for patients in a NICU who have severe and prolonged cytopenia. As more is learned about human fetal hematopoieses, perhaps alternatives to transfusion will emerge. To a certain extent, this process has already begun, because treatments such as recombinant erythropoietin and administration of rG-CSF have been used in neonatology. Much remains to be accomplished, such as more precise definition of which neonates with cytopenia will benefit from treatment with recombinant hematopoietic growth factors, better methods for dosing and monitoring such treatments, and more precise means of identifying the risks and benefits of such treatments.

REFERENCES

1. Christensen, RD, Calhoun DA, Rimsza LM. A practical approach to evaluating and treating neutropenia in the neonatal intensive care unit. *Clin Perinatol* 2000;27:577–602.
2. Sola MC, Del Vecchio A, Rimsza LM. Evaluation and treatment of thrombocytopenia in the neonatal intensive care unit. *Clin Perinatol* 2000;27:655–679.
3. Ohls RK. Evaluation and treatment of anemia in the neonate. In: Christensen RD, ed. *Hematologic problems of the neonate.* Philadelphia: WB Saunders, 2000:137–170.
4. Slayton WB, Li Y, Calhoun DA, et al. The first appearance of neutrophils in the human fetal bone marrow cavity. *Early Hum Dev* 1998; 53:129–144.
5. Yoder MC. Embryonic hematopoiesis. In: Christensen RD, ed. *Hematologic problems of the neonate.* Philadelphia: WB Saunders, 2000:3–19.
6. Calhoun DA, Li, Y, Braylan R, et al. Assessment of the contribution of the spleen to granulocytopoiesis and erythropoiesis of the mid-gestation human fetus. *Early Hum Dev* 1996; 46:217–227.
7. Charboard P, Tavian M, Humeau L, et al. Early ontogeny of the human marrow from long bones: an immunohistochemical study of hematopoiesis and its micro-environment. *Blood* 1996;78:4109–4119.
8. Kelemen E. Macrophages are the first differentiated blood cells formed in human embryonic liver. *Exp Hematol* 1980;8:996–1000.
9. Yoder MC, Hiatt K. Engraftment of embryonic hematopoietic cells in conditioned newborn recipients. *Blood* 1997;89:2176–2183.
10. Slayton WB, Juul SE, Calhoun DA, et al. Hematopoiesis in the liver and marrow of human fetuses at 5 to 16 weeks postconception: quantitative assessment of macrophage and neutrophil populations. *Pediatr Res* 1998;43:774–782.
11. Forestier F, Daffos F, Galacteros F, et al. Hematological values of 163 normal fetuses between 18 and 30 weeks of gestation. *Pediatr Res* 1986; 20:342–346.
12. Christensen RD, Rothstein G. Pre- and postnatal development of granulocytic stem cells in the rat. *Pediatr Res* 1984;18:599–602.
13. Migliaccio G, Migliaccio A, Petti S, et al. Human embryonic hemopoiesis: kinetics of progenitors and precursors underlying the yolk-sac-liver transition. *J Clin Invest* 1986;78:51–60.
14. Christensen RD, Harper TE, Rothstein G. Granulocyte-macrophage progenitor cells in term and preterm neonates. *J Pediatr* 1986;109: 1047–1051.
15. Christensen RD. Circulating pluripotent hematopoietic progenitor cells in neonates. *J Pediatr* 1987;110:622–626.
16. Christensen RD. Developmental changes in pluripotent hematopoietic progenitors (CFU-GEMM). *Early Hum Dev* 1988;16:195–205.
17. Broxmeyer H, Hangoc G, Cooper S, et al. Growth characteristics and expansion of human umbilical cord blood and expansion in adults. *Proc Natl Acad Sci U S A* 1992;89:4109–4113.
18. Ohls RK, Li Y, Abdel-Mageed A, et al. Neutrophil pool sizes and granulocyte colony-stimulating factor production in human mid-trimester fetuses. *Pediatr Res* 1995;37:806–811.
19. Schibler KR, Liechty KW, White WL, et al. Production of granulocyte colony-stimulating factor in vitro from monocytes from preterm and term neonates. *Blood* 1993;82:2269–2289.
20. Cairo M, Suen Y, Knoppel E, et al. Decreased G-CSF and IL-3 production and gene expression from mononuclear cells of newborn infants. *Pediatr Res* 1992;31:574–578.
21. Lai PH, Everette R, Wang FF, et al. Structural characterization of human erythropoietin. *J Biol Chem* 1986;261:3116–3121.
22. Bunn H, Gu J, Huang L, et al. Erythropoietin: a model system for studying oxygen-dependent gene regulation. *J Exp Biol* 1998;201: 1197–1201.
23. Juul SE, Yachnis AT, Christensen RD. Tissue distribution of erythropoietin and erythropoietin receptor in the developing human fetus. *Early Hum Dev* 1998;52:235–249.
24. Juul SE, Yachnis AT, Rojiani AM, et al. Immunohistochemical localization of erythropoietin and its receptor in the developing human brain. *Pediatr Dev Pathol* 1999;2:142–158.
25. Wu H, Liu X, Jaenisch R, et al. Generation of committed erythroid BFU-E and CFU-E progenitors does not require erythropoietin or the erythropoietin receptor. *Cell* 1995;83:59–67.
26. Wu H Lee SH, Gao J, et al. Inactivation of erythropoietin leads to defects in cardiac morphogenesis. *Development* 1999;126:3597–3605.
27. Widness HA, Kulhavy JC, Johnson KJ, et al. Clinical performance of an in-line point-of-care monitor in neonates. *Pediatrics* 2000;106: 497–504.
28. Dame C, Juul SE. The switch from fetal to adult erythropoiesis. In: Christensen RD, ed. *Hematologic problems of the neonate.* Philadelphia: WB Saunders, 2000:27:507–526.
29. Morishita E, Masuda S, Nagao M, et al. Erythropoietin receptor is expressed in rat hippocampal and cerebral cortical neurons, and erythropoietin prevents in vitro glutamate-induced neuronal death. *Neuroscience* 1997:76:105–116.
30. Juul SE, Anderson DK, Ki Y, et al. Erythropoietin and erythropoietin receptor in the developing human central nervous system. *Pediatr Res* 1998;43:40–49.
31. Juul SE, Zhao Y, Dame JB, et al. Origin and fate of erythropoietin in human milk. *Pediatr Res* 2000;48:600–667.
32. Kling PJ, Sullivan TM, Roberts RA, et al. Human milk as a potential enteral source of erythropoietin. *Pediatr Res* 1998;43:216–221.
33. Juul SE, Harcum J, Li Y, et al. Erythropoietin is present in the cerebrospinal fluid of neonates. *J Pediatr* 1997;130:428–430.
34. Juul SE, Stallings SA, Christensen RD. Erythropoietin in the cerebrospinal fluid of neonates who sustained CNS injury. *Pediatr Res* 1999; 46:543–547.
35. Dame C, Juul SE, Christensen RD. The biology of erythropoietin in the central nervous system and its neurotrophic and neuroprotective potential. *Biol Neonate* 2001;79:228–235.
36. Holbrook ST, Christensen RD, Rothstein G. Erythroid colonies derived from fetal blood display different growth patterns from those derived from adult marrow. *Pediatr Res* 1988;24:605–608.
37. Emerson SG, Thomas S, Ferrara JS, et al. Developmental regulation of erythropoiesis by hematopoietic growth factors: analysis on populations of BFU-E from bone marrow, peripheral blood, and fetal liver. *Blood* 1989;74:49–55.
38. Valtieri M, Gabbianelli M, Pelosi E, et al. Erythropoietin alone induces erythroid burst formation by human embryonic but not adult BFU-E in unicellular serum-free culture. *Blood* 1989;74:460–470.
39. Bard H. Hemoglobin synthesis and metabolism during the neonatal period. In: Christensen RD, ed. *Hematologic problems of the neonate.* Philadelphia: WB Saunders, 2000: 365–388.
40. Harthoorn-Lasthuizen EJ, Lindemans J, Langenhuijsen MM. Influence of iron deficiency anaemia on haemoglobin A2 levels: possible consequences for beta-thalassaemia screening. *Scand J Clin Lab Invest* 1999; 59:65–70.

41. Wright JH. The origin and nature of the blood plates. *Boston Med Surg J* 1906;154:643–645.
42. Mazur EM, Hoffman R. Human megakaryocyte progenitors. In: Golde DW, ed. *Hematopoiesis.* New York: Churchill Livingstone, 1984:133.
43. Long MW, Gragowski LL, Heffner CH, et al. Phorbol diesters stimulate the development of an early murine progenitor cell: the burst-forming unit–megakaryocyte. *J Clin Invest* 1985;76:431–438.
44. Briddell RA, Brandt JE, Straneve JE, et al. Characterization of the human burst-forming unit–megakaryocyte. *Blood* 1989;74:145–151.
45. Mazur EM, Hoffman R, Bruno E. Regulation of human megakaryocytopoiesis: an in vitro analysis. *J Clin Invest* 1981;68:733–741.
46. Zauli G, Valvassori L, Capitani S. Presence and characteristics of circulating megakaryocyte progenitor cells in human fetal blood. *Blood* 1993; 81:385–390.
47. Bruno E, Murray LJ, DiGiusto R, et al. Detection of a primitive megakaryocyte progenitor cell in human fetal bone marrow. *Exp Hematol* 1996;24:552–558.
48. Murray NA, Roberts IAG. Circulating megakaryocytes and their progenitors (BFU-MK and CFU-MK) in term and pre-term neonates. *Br J Haematol* 1995;89:41–46.
49. Williams N, Levine RF. The origin, development and regulation of megakaryocytes. *Br J Haematol* 1982;52:173–180.
50. Levine RF, Hazzard KC, Lamberg JD. The significance of megakaryocyte size. *Blood* 1982;60:1122–1131.
51. Tomer A, Harker LA, Burstein SA. Flow cytometric analysis of normal human megakaryocytes. *Blood* 1988;71:1244–1252.
52. Kelemen E, Calvo W, Fliedner TM. *Atlas of human hemopoietic development.* Berlin: Springer-Verlag,1979:51.
53. Allen Graeve JL, de Alarcon PA. Megakaryocytopoiesis in the human fetus. *Arch Dis Child* 1989;64:481–484.
54. Hegyi E, Nakazawa M, Debili N, et al. Developmental changes in human megakaryocyte ploidy. *Exp Hematol* 1991;19:87–94.
55. De Alarcon PA, Graeve JLA. Analysis of megakaryocyte ploidy in fetal bone marrow biopsies using a new adaptation of the Feulgen technique to measure DNA content and estimate megakaryocyte ploidy from biopsy specimens. *Pediatr Res* 1996;39:166–170.
56. Ma DC, Sun YH, Chang KZ, et al. Developmental change of megakaryocyte maturation and DNA ploidy in human fetus. *Eur J Haematol* 1996;57:121–127.
57. Levine RF, Olson TA, Shoff PK, et al. Mature micromegakaryocytes: an unusual developmental pattern in term infants. *Br J Haematol* 1996; 94:391–399.
58. Choi ES, Nichol JL, Hokom MM, et al. Platelets generated in vitro from proplatelet-displaying human megakaryocytes are functional. *Blood* 1995;85:402–413.
59. Cramer EM, Norol F, Guichard J, et al. Ultrastructure of platelet formation by human megakaryocytes cultured with the Mpl ligand. *Blood* 1997;89:2336–2346.
60. Kaufman RM, Airo R, Pollack S, et al. Circulating megakaryocytes and platelet release in the lung. *Blood* 1965;26:720–731.
61. Levine RF, Eldor A, Shoff PK, et al. Circulating megakaryocytes: delivery of large numbers of intact, mature megakaryocytes to the lungs. *Eur J Haematol* 1993;51:233–246.
62. Foster DC, Sprecher CA, Grant FJ, et al. Human thrombopoietin: gene structure, cDNA sequence, expression, and chromosomal localization. *Proc Natl Acad Sci U S A* 1994;91:13023–13027.
63. Sungaran R, Markovic B, Chong BH. Localization and regulation of thrombopoietin mRNA expression in human kidney, liver, bone marrow and spleen using in situ hybridization. *Blood* 1997;89:101–107.
64. Debili N, Wendling F, Katz A, et al. The Mpl-ligand or thrombopoietin or megakaryocyte growth and differentiative factor has both direct proliferative and differentiative activities on human megakaryocyte progenitors. *Blood* 1995;86:2516–2525.
65. Chen J, Herceg-Harjacek L, Groopman JE, et al. Regulation of platelet activation in vitro by the c-Mpl ligand, thrombopoietin. *Blood* 1995; 86:4054–4062.
66. De Sauvage F, Carver-Moore K, Luoh S, et al. Physiological regulation of early and late stages of megakaryocytopoiesis by thrombopoietin. *J Exp Med* 1996;183:651–656.
67. Gurney AL, Carver-Moore K, de Sauvage FJ, et al. Thrombocytopenia in c-mpl-deficient mice. *Science* 1994;265:1445–1447.
68. Yoshida M, Tsuji K, Ebihara Y, et al. Thrombopoietin alone stimulates the early proliferation and survival of human erythroid, myeloid and multipotential progenitors in serum-free culture. *Br J Haematol* 1997; 98:254–264.
69. Ratajczak MZ, Ratajczak J, Marlicz W. Recombinant human thrombopoietin (Tpo) stimulates erythropoiesis by inhibiting erythroid progenitor cell apoptosis. *Br J Haematol* 1997;98:8–17.
70. Harker LA, Hunt P, Marzec UM, et al. Regulation of platelet production and function by megakaryocyte growth and development factor in nonhuman primates. *Blood* 1996;87:1833–1844.
71. Harker LA, Marzec UM, Hunt P, et al. Dose-response effects of pegylated human megakaryocyte growth and development factor on platelet production and function in nonhuman primates. *Blood* 1996;88: 511–521.
72. Grossmann A, Lenox J, Ren HP, et al. Thrombopoietin accelerates platelet, red blood cell, and neutrophil recovery in myelosuppressed mice. *Exp Hematol* 1996;24:1238–1246.
73. Neelis KJ, Qingliang L, Thomas GR, et al. Prevention of thrombocytopenia by thrombopoietin in myelosuppressed rhesus monkeys accompanied by prominent erythropoietic stimulation and iron depletion. *Blood* 1997;90:58–63.
74. Vadhan-Raj S, Murray LJ, Bueso-Ramos C, et al. Stimulation of megakaryocyte and platelet production by a single dose of recombinant human thrombopoietin in patients with cancer. *Ann Intern Med* 1997; 126:673–681.
75. Basser RL, Rasko JEJ, Clarke K, et al. Randomized, blinded, placebo-controlled phase I trial of pegylated recombinant human megakaryocyte growth and development factor with filgrastim after dose-intensive chemotherapy in patients with advanced cancer. *Blood* 1997;89: 3118–3128.
76. Vadhan-Raj S, Verschraegen CF, Bueso-Ramos C, et al. Recombinant human thrombopoietin attenuates carboplatin-induced severe thrombocytopenia and the need for platelet transfusions in patients with gynecologic cancer. *Ann Intern Med* 2000;132:364–368.
77. Yang L, Xia Y, Li J, et al. The appearance of anti-thrombopoietin antibody and circulating thrombopoietin-IgG complexes in a patient developing thrombocytopenia after the injection of PEG-rHuMGDF. *Blood* 1999;94[Suppl 1]:681a(abst).
78. Cwirla SE, Balasubramanian P, Duffin DJ, et al. Peptide agonist of the thrombopoietin receptor as potent as the natural cytokine. *Science* 1997;276:1696–1699.
79. Sola MC, Du Y, Hutson AD, et al. Dose-response relationship of megakaryocyte progenitors from the bone marrow of thrombocytopenic and non-thrombocytopenic neonates to recombinant thrombopoietin. *Br J Haematol* 2000;110:449–453.
80. Sola MC, Christensen RD, Hutson AD, et al. Pharmacodynamics, pharmacokinetics and safety of administering pegylated recombinant megakaryocyte growth and development factor to newborn rhesus monkeys. *Pediatr Res* 2000;47:208–214.
81. Murray NA, Watts TL, Roberts IAG. Endogenous thrombopoietin levels and effect of recombinant human thrombopoietin on megakaryocyte precursors in term and preterm babies. *Pediatr Res* 1998;43: 148–151.

30

HEMOLYTIC DISEASE OF THE FETUS OR NEWBORN: TREATMENT AND PREVENTION

ARTHUR W. BRACEY
KENNETH J. MOISE, JR.

Hemolytic disease of the newborn (HDN) is a pathologic condition that results in accelerated destruction of erythrocytes in the fetus and newborn. This disease is associated with intrinsic red blood cell (RBC) abnormalities (membrane defects, enzymopathies) and acquired disorders (infections, alloimmunization to RBC antigens) (Table 30.1). This chapter focuses on immune-mediated HDN, the most common form of the disorder. Despite important advances in prevention and therapy, immune HDN remains an important clinical problem some 50 years after elucidation of its mechanisms.

A.W. Bracey: Department of Clinical Pathology, University of Texas Medical School, and Transfusion Service, St. Luke's Episcopal Hospital, Houston, Texas.

K.J. Moise, Jr: Division of Maternal-Fetal Medicine, University of North Carolina at Chapel Hill, Chapel Hill, North Carolina.

HISTORY

Hemolytic disease of the newborn was first described by a French midwife in 1609. Diamond and colleagues (1) are credited with recognizing that hydrops fetalis, neonatal jaundice, and neonatal anemia are clinical syndromes that have a common mechanism. Hallmark studies of RBC antigens by Landsteiner and Weiner (2) produced an antibody in guinea pigs injected with rhesus (Rh) RBCs, indicating that HDN is associated with an immune response to RBC antigens. The antibodies raised in those experiments, recognizing the LW antigen, reacted with 85% of human RBCs, thereby allowing serologic definition of the Rh system, because anti-LW reacts primarily with Rh(D)-positive individuals. Subsequent advances in immunohematology, including the development of the antiglobulin method by Coombs, Mourant, and Fischer, allowed more widespread assessment of neonatal anemia with blood typing. Levine et al. (3) showed that the serum of Rh-negative mothers who deliver anemic infants contains a factor (anti-D) that is incompatible with the RBCs of

TABLE 30.1. CATEGORIES OF HEMOLYTIC DISEASE OF THE NEWBORN

Immune
Alloimmune: Rh disease
Isoimmune: ABO
Maternal autoimmune hemolytic anemia

Congenital Red Blood Cell Defects
Enzyme deficiencies: glucose-6-phosphate dehydrogenase, pyruvate kinase
Red blood cell membrane defects: hereditary elliptocytosis, hereditary spherocytosis, pyropoikilocytosis
Hemoglobinopathies: hemoglobin H, hemoglobin S

Acquired Red Blood Cell Defects
Related to infections such as congenital syphilis, toxoplasmosis, cytomegalovirus, rubella, *Coxsackie B* sepsis, and *Escherichia coli* sepsis

anemic infants. Subsequent serologic evaluation of Rh-positive mothers of anemic newborns, such as Mrs. Kell, led to the discovery of many of the RBC antigens known to modern immunohematology.

SEROLOGIC AND CLINICAL FEATURES

Development of immune HDN requires (a) maternal immunization against paternal antigens on RBCs that either passed from the fetus into the maternal circulation or that were present in previous transfusions (b) and fetal-neonatal inheritance of the stimulating antigen. Rarely, preformed antibodies against autoantigens or high-frequency antigens not expressed on maternal RBCs will contribute to RBC injury in the fetus and neonate.

To cause HDN, the implicated antibody must be able to cross the placental barrier, allowing injury of fetal RBCs. Antibody moves from the mother to the placenta via a one-way active transport process that depends on an interaction between immunoglobulin and synciotrophoblast Fc receptors. Only immunoglobulin G (IgG)-class immunoglobulins can be transported via this mechanism, so HDN is limited to IgG antibodies. Within the IgG subclasses, only IgG1 and IgG3 antibodies are transportable. The subclass distinction is also important in phagocytic interaction, only IgG1 and IgG3 being able to bind macrophage Fc receptors.

Hemolytic disease of the newborn manifests in a variety of ways, ranging from clinically imperceptible states to the most severe form of the disease, referred to as hydrops fetalis, which frequently causes death in utero. In the affected fetus or newborn, clinical manifestations are caused either by the hypoxic effects of anemia or by toxic effects attributable to metabolites that result from hemoglobin degradation. The principal adaptive response to fetal anemia is expansion of fetal erythropoiesis which, in severe cases, leads to the syndrome of erythroblastosis fetalis. The hydropic fetus has massive tissue edema and hypoproteinemia, which result in scalp edema, ascites, and pleural effusions. In erythroblastosis fetalis, the widespread increase in extramedullary hematopoiesis in the liver, spleen, and other organs is believed to impinge on the portal and umbilical venous systems, causing portal hypertension. The placenta becomes swollen and poorly perfused. Hepatic dysfunction leads to hypoproteinemia, which further enhances the edema. In utero, the fetus is protected from the deleterious effects of bilirubin metabolites by maternal metabolism of the products of heme-porphyrin breakdown. Soon after birth, however, the plasma content of unconjugated bilirubin can reach levels high enough to interfere with the development of the newborn.

ABO Disease

ABO incompatibility between the mother and fetus is common, accounting for the most prevalent form of HDN. With respect to ethnic groups, the prevalence of maternal-newborn ABO incompatibility ranges from 31% in whites to 50% in Asians. Fortunately, ABO HDN is a relatively mild disorder in most instances. A number of factors combine to minimize the impact of maternal-fetal ABO incompatibility. First, ABO antigens are weakly expressed on RBCs in utero and in the neonate. The predominant immunoglobulin class of anti-A and anti-B antibodies found in group B and group A mothers is IgM, which cannot be transported across the placenta. ABO maternal-fetal incompatibility involving group O mothers, whose sera contain more harmful IgG anti-A and anti-B, is limited to 15% of pregnancies. Widespread expression of ABO antigens on fetal tissue causes absorption of ABO antibodies, reducing the impact on RBCs. Fetal plasma may also contain soluble ABO blood group substances capable of neutralizing antibodies. Because of these protective features, only 10% of ABO-incompatible newborns require therapy (4).

Typically, ABO HDN causes mild postpartum jaundice, which is detected 24 hours after delivery and can be managed without RBC transfusion; in very rare cases, however, hemolysis severe enough to cause hydrops has been reported (5). Unlike in non-ABO HDN, the firstborn is at risk for significant hemolysis, because the anti-ABO antibodies are developed before pregnancy. Antepartum and postpartum serologic tests are poor predictors of ABO hemolytic disease. The result of the direct antiglobulin test (DAT) is positive in only 20% to 40% of ABO-incompatible maternal-fetal pairs. In infants with a positive DAT result, the test does not differentiate newborns with clinical hemolysis from unaffected newborns. Only 10% of the DAT-positive, ABO-incompatible maternal-fetal pairs studied by Desjardins and associates (6) developed clinically significant ABO hemolytic disease. Of the infants with clinically significant hemolysis, 80% had a positive DAT result. The eluate was positive in all but one of the remaining affected infants. When sensitive serologic techniques such as heat eluates are used to evaluate ABO incompatibility, most tests of ABO-incompatible newborns will yield positive results despite the low incidence of clinical disease. In severe cases, maternal birth history can be important in predicting the severity of ABO HDN. Katz et al. (7) reported a recurrence rate of 88%; 62% of the affected patients required therapy for ABO HDN. Careful assessment of the newborn is the key to managing ABO-incompatible maternal-fetal pairings. Intrapartum monitoring for ABO HDN has

TABLE 30.2. MOST COMMON ALLOANTIBODIES ASSOCIATED WITH HEMOLYTIC DISEASE OF THE NEWBORN (excluding anti-D)

Antibody	Incidence (%)	HDN Severity	Titer Predictive?
Anti-K1[a]	28.5	Mild-severe	No
Anti-E	18.2	Mild-severe	Yes
Anti-c	7.5	Mild-severe	Yes
Anti-C	6.1	Mild	Yes
Anti-Fy[a]	7.1	Mild	No
Anti-M	4.5	Mild	No
Anti-Jk[a]	1.9	Mild	No

[a]Suppresses colony-forming units of erythrocytes (CFU-E).
HDN, hemolytic disease of the newborn.

no role except in rare mothers with a history of severe anemia secondary to ABO HDN during a previous pregnancy.

Non-ABO Disease

The RBC membrane contains numerous antigen systems capable of expressing hundreds of antigens. Genetic disparity among individuals leads to the risk of maternal alloimmunization against paternal antigens not expressed on maternal RBCs. A list of the antibodies other than anti-D most commonly associated with HDN is included in Table 30.2. In identifying the fetus at risk for HDN, RBC serology plays a key role. Early approaches for managing HDN relied heavily on serology for fetal monitoring. After the introduction of more direct measures of fetal status, the role of serology diminished. The appropriate use of serology in fetal monitoring for HDN is addressed in a subsequent section.

Of the many non-ABO RBC antigens, Rh(D) antigen is the most immunogenic. In a large series of women screened before the implementation of routine Rh immune globulin (RhIg) prophylaxis, anti-D accounted for 48% to 65% of the antibodies detected (Table 30.3) (8). More recent studies reflect the impact of RhIg prophylaxis on decreasing the relative frequency of anti-D as a cause of HDN. In a study of women of childbearing age admitted to a large hospital over a 2.5-year interval in central New York, anti-D accounted for 18.4% of all antibodies detected. Similarly, in a Swedish blood donor population, anti-D accounted for 19% of the antibodies (9). These data confirm the importance of anti-D as a persistent contributor to fetal and neonatal pathology despite widespread use of RhIg immunoprophylaxis.

A number of factors combine to make Rh(D) sensitization a frequently severe form of HDN. Maternal antibodies against Rh(D) are typically IgG and, therefore, able to cross the placenta and bind fetal RBCs. In clinical practice, IgG subclasses of anti-D are those associated with phagocyte binding and hemolytic injury: IgG1 only, 9 of 44 (20.4%); IgG3 only, 1 of 44 (2.3%); IgG1 and IgG3, 34 of 44 (77.3%) (10). After primary sensitization occurs, secondary exposure during subsequent pregnancies often leads to increased production of anti-D, as revealed by high maternal titers of IgG anti-D in these women. On fetal RBCs, the Rh(D) antigen is fully expressed, occurring in a quantity second only to that of ABO antigens. The RBCs of a heterozygous fetus contain a large number of D antigens (10,000 copies), providing ample sites for IgG binding and allowing sufficient interaction with monocyte receptors to induce phagocytosis.

Other than Rh(D), the RBC antigens most likely to cause severe HDN are c and E of the rhesus system and K1 of the Kell system. Currently, anti-K1 is the most common antibody encountered in women in the United States, accounting for 22% of the antibodies detected. Most women with anti-K1 have been

TABLE 30.3. IRREGULAR ANTIBODIES IN FIVE SERIES OF PATIENTS, 1967–1996

Antibody	Polesky (1967)	Queenan (1969)	Pepperell (1977)	Filbey (1995)	Geifman-Holtzman (1996)
D	1,864 (63.1%)	304 (48.3%)	958 (65.3%)	159 (19.0%)	101 (18.4%)
E	80 (2.7%)	34 (5.3%)	64 (4.7%)	5 (6.1%)	77 (14.0%)
C	448 (15.2%)	34 (5.3%)	9 (0.6%)	36 (4.3%)	26 (4.7%)
Cw	4 (0.14%)	—	—	10 (1.2%)	1 (0.2%)
c	68 (2.3%)	12 (1.9%)	59 (4.0%)	38 (4.5%)	32 (5.8%)
e	2 (0.07%)	3 (0.4%)	6 (0.04%)	1 (0.1%)	—
K1	93 (3.1%)	30 (4.7%)	34 (2.3%)	48 (5.7%)	12 (22%)
Duffy	17 (0.6%)	12 (1.9%)	8 (0.5%)	26 (3.1%)	31 (5.6%)
MNS	45 (1.5%)	20 (3.1%)	18 (1.2%)	35 (4.2%)	26 (4.7%)
Kidd	7 (0.2%)	7 (1.1%)	2 (0.14%)	10 (1.2%)	8 (1.5%)
Lutheran	—	3 (0.4%)	—	13 (1.6%)	7 (1.3%)
P1	27 (0.9%)	15 (2.3%)	129 (8.8%)	48 (5.7%)	1 (0.2%)
Lewis	94 (3.2%)	51 (8.1%)	174 (11.9%)	241 (28.8%)	113 (20.5%)
I	13 (0.4%)	15 (2.3%)	—	—	5 (0.9%)
Others	194 (6.6%)	90 (14.3%)	1 (0.07%)	120 (14.4%)	1 (0.2%)
Total	2,956	630	1,467	836	550
Blood samples	43,000	18,378	72,138	110,765	37,506
Duration	7 y	8 y	10 y	12 y	2.5 y
Location	Minnesota	New York	Australia	Sweden	New York

immunized by previous transfusions. The relatively low prevalence of K1 in the general population (9% in whites) limits this incompatibility as a contributor to HDN. Conversely, antibodies against Rh determinants c and E were present in 19.8% of antibody-positive samples in the aforementioned New York series (8).

Alloantibodies other than anti-D, if not detected on the initial maternal visit, can pose a diagnostic challenge, because repeat antibody screening is not recommended in Rh(D)-positive mothers, owing to the very low incidence of alloimmunization (11). Fortunately, many antigens outside the Rh and Kell systems are poorly immunogenic or unlikely to cause severe hemolysis, so clinically important hemolytic disease involving RBC antigen systems other than Rh and Kell is fairly uncommon. There is no significant benefit associated with the use of exquisitely sensitive antibody screening methods. Mothers who have undergone multiple transfusions (e.g., for thalassemia or sickle cell disease) require serial antibody screening irrespective of their Rh(D) antigen status, because RBC alloantibodies are frequently found in this population.

PROPHYLAXIS

Fetal RBCs frequently pass into the maternal circulation. A fetomaternal hemorrhage of as little as 0.1 ml of Rh(D)-positive RBCs can cause sensitization of unprotected Rh-negative mothers (12). Rh(D) antigens are fully expressed on fetal RBCs as early as 4 weeks of gestation (13). Although, theoretically, Rh(D) alloimmunization can occur very early in pregnancy, the risk of fetomaternal hemorrhage and RBC alloimmunization increases during gestation, the highest risk occurring during delivery. Fetal RBCs are found in the peripheral blood in 0.4% of women at 28 to 30 weeks and in 1.8% of women at 30 to 39 weeks of gestation (14). In up to 50% of ABO-compatible mothers, fetal cells are found immediately after labor. Before routine Rh(D) prophylaxis was available, anti-D was formed by 6 months after the first pregnancy in 4.3% to 9.0% of the Rh(D)-negative mothers tested; by the end of the second pregnancy with an Rh(D)-positive fetus, as many as 17% of Rh(D)-negative mothers had anti-D in their serum (15).

After observing alteration of immunization in the presence of a passive antibody (16) and noting the natural protective effect of ABO incompatibility against HDN, investigators theorized that anti-D antibody might have a protective effect (17). In 1961, Finn et al. (18) reported the initial trial involving the prevention of Rh hemolytic disease. Subsequently, large trials conducted in the United States by Freda et al. and in the United Kingdom by the Medical Research Council (MRC) confirmed that the passive administration of RhIg could prevent Rh alloimmunization (19). A dose of 20 μg of RhIg per ml of Rh(D)-positive RBCs is effective in preventing Rh(D) sensitization. The exact mechanism of protection afforded by passive anti-D administration remains unknown. Hypothetical mechanisms include antigen alteration by steric changes in conformation after antibody binding, interference with host processing of the D antigen secondary to antibody blocking, and antiidiotype feedback inhibition (20).

By 1968, RhIg had been licensed in the United States and made available to the general public for Rh prophylaxis. After routine administration of RhIg postpartum, the alloimmunization rate of multiparous mothers fell from historic levels of 18.4 per 100,000 births in the United Kingdom to 1.3 per 100,000 births by 1992. Freda et al. (19) reported that, in U.S. patients, the incidence of alloimmunization in Rh(D)-negative mothers had decreased from 14% in 1960 to <2% by 1974. Bowman (21) attributed persistent Rh(D) alloimmunization failures to Rh(D) exposure related to antepartum fetomaternal bleeding, which occurs in normal pregnancy as a consequence of maternal-fetal vascular interaction. These researchers further reduced the incidence of Rh(D) alloimmunization in Rh(D)-negative mothers from 1.2% to 0.2% by giving RhIg antepartum (21). Administration of RhIg after 28 to 32 weeks of pregnancy and in the postpartum interval is now routinely practiced. According to the Centers for Disease Control's Birth Defects Monitoring Program, the incidence of Rh HDN in 1986, after routine antepartum prophylaxis was recommended, was 10.6 per 10,000 total births; this incidence exceeds the expected optimal rate of 3.1 per 10,000 total births, assuming that antenatal and postnatal RhIg prophylaxis has a failure rate of 0.2% (22). The infrequent but continued prevalence of Rh(D) HDN may be attributed to system-based problems, including medical error and poor access to medical care.

Rh Immune Globulin

Rh immune globulin is prepared from plasma pools by means of the Cohn acid-alcohol fractionation technique. The processing method typically inactivates infectious agents but, in a small number of European preparations, transmission of hepatitis C virus (HCV) was observed after RhIg administration before screening for anti-HCV became routine. Additional measures, including viral inactivation and nucleic acid screening, have been added to enhance the safety profile of RhIg. As produced today, RhIg should pose a risk only for the transmission of non-lipid-coated viruses, including Parvovirus B19. To eliminate the risk of transmitting this virus, screening is performed with nucleic acid methodology. Some manufacturers also filter plasma pools used for RhIg preparation to eliminate non-lipid-coated viruses. Millions of doses of virally inactivated plasma products have been administered worldwide, and there have been no reports of disease transmission.

In early studies, fractionated anti-D was radiolabeled with Iodine-125 to allow determination of RBC-bound antibody as a means defining the anti-D content in microgram quantities. Since then, manufacturers have converted from radiometric anti-D quantitation to methods that employ automated hemagglutination. An anti-D dose is expressed in either μg/ml or IU/ml (1 μg/ml = 5 IU). The first generation of RhIg products was prepared exclusively for intramuscular injection owing to the possible development of complement activation attributable to Ig aggregates formed as a byproduct of plasma processing. More recently, an intravenous preparation has also been licensed. The preparations are equally effective in Rh(D) prophylaxis. When administered, the intravenous preparation causes less patient discomfort, perhaps offering a significant advantage when large doses, requiring multiple vials, are needed. However, the added cost of the intravenous preparation is a disadvantage. Overall, when used as recommended RhIg is well tolerated, with few reports of serious adverse events.

Indications

All Rh(D)-negative women should be treated at 28 weeks of pregnancy and in the postpartum interval if the newborn is Rh(D) positive. Additional indications include invasive procedures capable of disrupting the maternal-fetal blood barrier and traumatic obstetric complications (Table 30.4).

Practice varies with respect to the eligibility of Rh(D)-positive, weak-D (also referred to as D^u) mothers for RhIg immunoprophylaxis. Neither the American Society of Clinical Pathologists nor the American College of Obstetricians and Gynecologists recommends the use of RhIg in weak-D mothers. However, rare cases of Rh(D)-related HDN in Rh(D)-positive mothers are reported, including at least two reports of fatal HDN (23), prompting some to recommend that RhIg be used for weak D because of partial D status. In most Rh(D)-positive, weak-D mothers, the RBCs express the complete Rh(D) antigen and, therefore, these women are not at risk for forming anti-D. There are at least six classes of Rh(D)-positive, partial-D phenotypes, as determined by serologic assay, for example, Rh(D) variant VI. Gene rearrangements (n = 22) and point mutations (n = 9) responsible for partial-D status have been reported after molecular analysis of the Rh(D) gene (24). Partial-D mothers are at risk for alloimmunization to the subcomponent of the Rh(D) antigen missing from their RBCs. Further work is needed to clarify the optimal immunoprophylaxis for partial-D pregnancies.

TABLE 30.4. INDICATIONS FOR USE OF Rh IMMUNE GLOBULIN

- Amniocentesis
- Antepartum (routine at 28 weeks)
- Chorionic villus sampling
- Ectopic pregnancy
- Immune thrombocytopenic purpura
- Obstetric complications
  - Abdominal trauma
  - Abruptio placentae
  - Antepartum vaginal bleeding
  - Death in utero
  - External cephalic version
  - Manual removal of placenta
  - Placenta previa
  - Threatened abortion
  - Trophoblastic disease or neoplasm
- Percutaneous umbilical blood sampling
- Postpartum (infant must be Rh positive)
- Termination of pregnancy
- Transfusion of Rh-positive blood

Modified from Hartwell EA. Use of Rh immune globulin: ASCP practice parameter. American Society of Clinical Pathologists. *Am J Clin Pathol* 1998;110:281–292, with permission.

The U.S. study was limited with regard to access to study subjects, so a 72-hour interval between the injection of Rh(D)-positive RBCs and the administration of RhIg became the upper limit of the exposure time evaluated for Rh immunoprophylaxis. Subsequent trials revealed that treatment with RhIg for up to 13 days after exposure to Rh-positive cells confers protection against alloimmunization to Rh(D) (25). Rh immune globulin should be routinely administered within 72 hours after delivery, documented fetomaternal bleeding, or the onset of any condition that increases the risk of fetomaternal bleeding (Table 30.4). If RhIg prophylaxis is not initiated within 72 hours of exposure, it should be given anyway, because it may be efficacious at more distant intervals after exposure to Rh(D)-positive RBCs.

Dosage

In the United States, the typical dose of RhIg administered at 28 weeks of gestation and postpartum is 300 μg or 1,500 IU (Table 30.5). The dose is equivalent for intramuscular and intravenous RhIg preparations. In the United Kingdom, RhIg dose recommendations differ, the MRC recommending treatment with 100 μg or 500 IU. This lower dose was adopted to conserve RhIg resources. Most fetomaternal hemorrhages are small in volume. According to the MRC, a hemorrhage of >4 ml (the U.K. standard dose limit) of fetal RBCs occurs in 0.7% of cases. The volume of fetal bleeding exceeds 15 ml (the U.S. standard dose limit) in 0.3% of cases. Thus, in both systems, additional dosing of RhIg above the 100- or 300-μg threshold is limited to a small population of mothers.

Accurate screening for large-volume fetomaternal bleeding is a critical element of effective RhIg prophylaxis. During the postpartum interval and when a clinical condition associated with excessive blood loss develops, all Rh-negative women should be screened with a method capable of detecting excessive fetomaternal hemorrhage. Early investigators noted that conversion of the maternal Rh(D) type from negative to positive (Rh weak D) is associated with a large-volume fetomaternal hemorrhage. This method detects 85% of fetomaternal hemorrhages of >30 ml, while RBC rosette screening with Rh(D)-positive indicator cells coated with anti-D detects 100% of these simulated hemorrhages (26). Therefore, the rosette method has supplanted the postpartum Rh(D), weak-D antiglobulin-based phenotype study as the preferred method for detecting excessive postpartum hemorrhage.

When the fetal screen yields a positive result, an assay must be done to quantitate the volume of fetal bleeding. Classic studies by Kleihauer et al. (27) reported a differential solubility for fetal hemoglobin (HbF) versus adult hemoglobin (HbA). Assessment of fetomaternal hemorrhage with this technique is complicated by several factors. All normal control subjects have a small number of F cells. The F-cell content is increased in pregnancy, and some individuals have increased expression of HbF throughout adulthood. Even without these challenging conditions, the assay can be imprecise. The College of American Pathologists' laboratory proficiency survey program shows wide variation in samples with a known fetal RBC content. Newer methods using flow cytometry to detect RBCs that contain hemoglobin F or

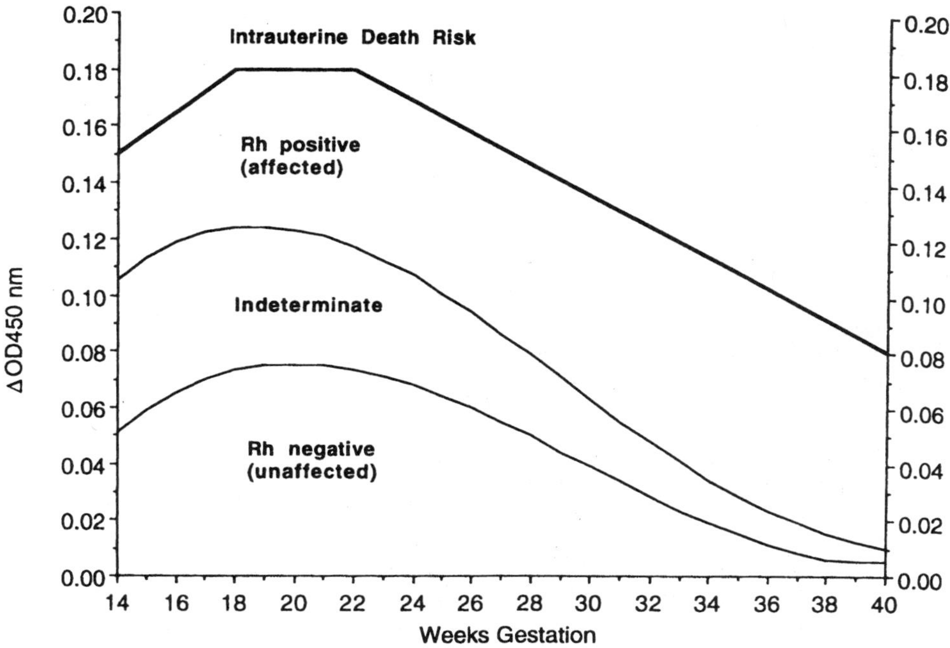

FIGURE 30.1. Queenan curve for amniotic fluid bilirubin (ΔOD_{450}) levels. Rh, rhesus.

of the fetal hemolytic process. To follow trends in the ΔOD_{450} values, serial procedures are undertaken at 10-day to 2-week intervals and are continued until delivery. An increasing value that reaches the 80th percentile of zone 2 on the Liley curve or that enters the "intrauterine transfusion" zone of the Queenan curve necessitates investigation by means of fetal blood sampling. After 37 weeks of gestation, fetal lung maturity can also be assessed; if the lungs are mature, induction of labor can be considered in lieu of another amniocentesis. A lecithin/sphingomyelin (L/S) ratio of $\geq$2.0 should be used instead of the FLM-TDX test, because the latter would be falsely elevated due to excess bilirubin. Early in the course of treatment, Rh phenotype testing of the patient's partner will reveal a heterozygosity in approximately 50% of cases. Because the other Rh antigens (C/c, E/e) are inherited in a closely linked fashion, antisera to these antigens can be employed, along with gene frequency tables based on race, to determine the paternal zygosity at the RhD locus. In the case of a heterozygous RhD paternal phenotype (Fig. 30.2), amniocentesis be can routinely done, using the polymerase chain reaction (PCR), to determine the fetal blood type. Nevertheless, this technique yields false-negative results in up to 1.5% of cases (48), primarily because of rearrangements in the RhD gene. To reduce such errors, most labs now require that a sample of paternal blood be sent with the amniotic fluid. By checking the paternal blood (the source of the fetal RhD gene) with the same primers used on the amniotic fluid, one can verify that a gene rearrangement is not a potential source of error. If the paternity is unknown or if the patient's partner is not available, a repeat maternal antibody titer should be obtained 4 to 6 weeks after the first one. If a four-fold increase in the antibody titer is noted, an RhD-negative fetal result is questionable. The physician should consider performing another amniocentesis to evaluate the ΔOD_{450} or sampling the fetal blood to determine the fetal RhD status using serologic techniques (Fig. 30.2).

Fetal Blood Sampling

Ultrasonographically directed fetal blood sampling (also called percutaneous umbilical blood sampling, cordocentesis, and funipuncture) allows direct access to the fetal circulation to obtain important laboratory data such as the fetal blood type, hematocrit, direct Coombs result, reticulocyte count, and total bilirubin level. Although fetal hematocrit levels based on gestational age are published in the literature, most authorities would consider a fetal hematocrit of <30% to indicate fetal anemia. In general, an immobile segment of the umbilical cord near the insertion into the placenta is targeted under continuous ultrasonographic guidance. The cord insertion site at the fetal umbilicus should be avoided, because vagal innervation is thought to be present at this site, increasing the likelihood of fetal bradycardia. Also, Weiner et al. (49) noted that puncture of the midsegment of the umbilical cord was associated with a 2.5-fold higher incidence of fetal bradycardia compared with puncture at the placental insertion site. The vessel of interrogation should be the umbilical vein instead of one of the umbilical arteries. In one series of 750 diagnostic or therapeutic cordocenteses, the incidence of fetal bradycardia was 21% with puncture of the umbilical artery but only 3% with umbilical venous puncture. Several authors have conjectured that this may be due to spasm of the muscularis of the umbilical artery. Fetal loss rates of 1% to 2% have been reported with this procedure.

Serial fetal blood samplings have been proposed as one

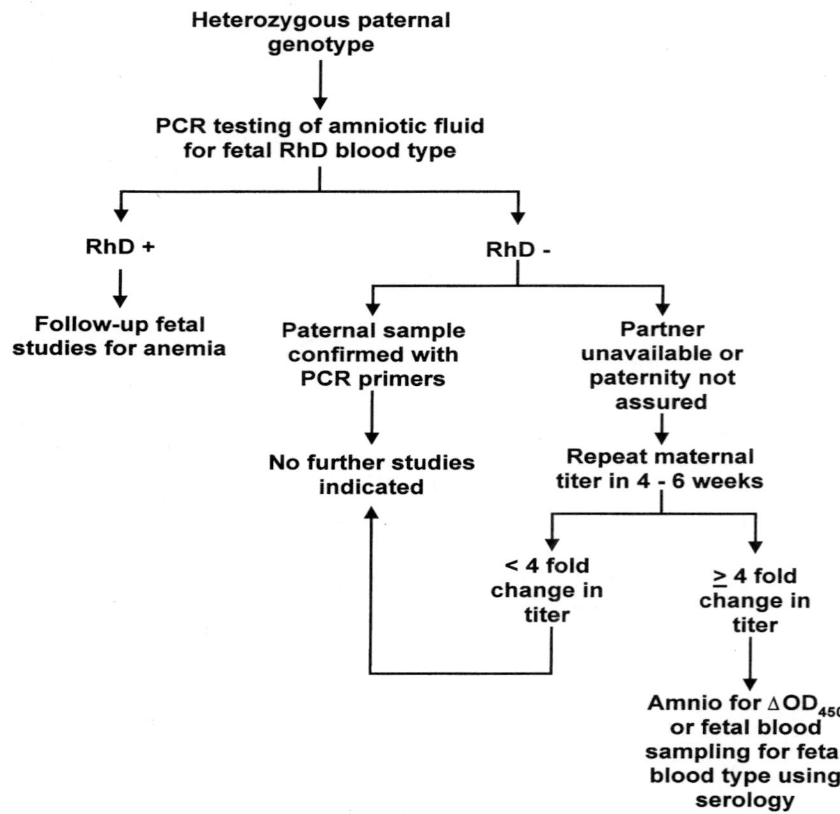

FIGURE 30.2. Management of the heterozygous paternal genotype. ΔOD_{450}, amniotic fluid bilirubin levels; PCR, polymerase chain reaction; Rh, rhesus.

method for following up alloimmunized pregnancies after a critical maternal titer has been reached (50). At most centers, however, fetal blood sampling is usually reserved for patients with elevated ΔOD_{450} values at amniocentesis or elevated Doppler velocities in the fetal middle cerebral artery. The fetal risk can also be lessened if blood is available for intrauterine transfusion (IUT) at the time of fetal blood sampling. If fetal anemia is detected, IUT is initiated.

Clinical Management

Use of the different diagnostic tools varies based on whether the mother has previously had an affected fetus or infant (Fig. 30.3).

First Affected Pregnancy

An antibody screen should be obtained at the first prenatal visit in all pregnancies. If an antibody associated with HDN is detected, a titer should be determined in the antiglobulin phase. During the first affected pregnancy, maternal titers are followed every 2 to 4 weeks. Once a critical value (usually 32) is reached, amniocentesis is performed every 10 days to 2 weeks for ΔOD_{450} determination. Paternal typing for the RhD antigen should be performed; if the result is positive, phenotype testing is then undertaken. If the paternal phenotype is heterozygous, an amniotic fluid sample obtained at the time of the first amniocentesis can be evaluated to determine the fetal RhD status. If the fetus is RhD negative and if simultaneous testing of paternal blood confirms the PCR results, no further testing is warranted. If the paternal phenotype is homozygous or the fetus is RhD positive on PCR testing, serial amniocentesis should be continued. If the ΔOD_{450} increases to 80% in zone 2 of the Liley curve or to a value in the IUT zone of the Queenan curve, fetal blood sampling should be performed with blood readied for IUT if the fetal hematocrit is <30%. If no increase in the ΔOD_{450} values occurs, the last amniocentesis should be performed at 37 weeks of gestation. If the L/S ratio is mature, labor can be induced at 39 weeks of gestation in lieu of another amniocentesis.

Previously Affected Fetus or Infant

In general, due to an anamnestic maternal antibody response resulting from entry of fetal cells into the maternal circulation at delivery, subsequent pregnancies will involve a greater severity of fetal and neonatal hemolytic disease. After the first affected gestation, maternal titers are not helpful in following up the degree of fetal anemia. With a heterozygous paternal phenotype, an amniocentesis can be performed after 15 weeks of gestation to determine the fetal RhD status. In approximately 50% of such cases, the fetus is unaffected and further testing can be omitted. If the fetus is RhD positive by PCR or there is a homozygous paternal phenotype, serial amniocenteses for ΔOD_{450} using the Queenan curve or middle cerebral artery Doppler velocity assessment at 18 weeks of gestation is initiated. Assessment is repeated at 2-week intervals. If the ΔOD_{450} value rises into

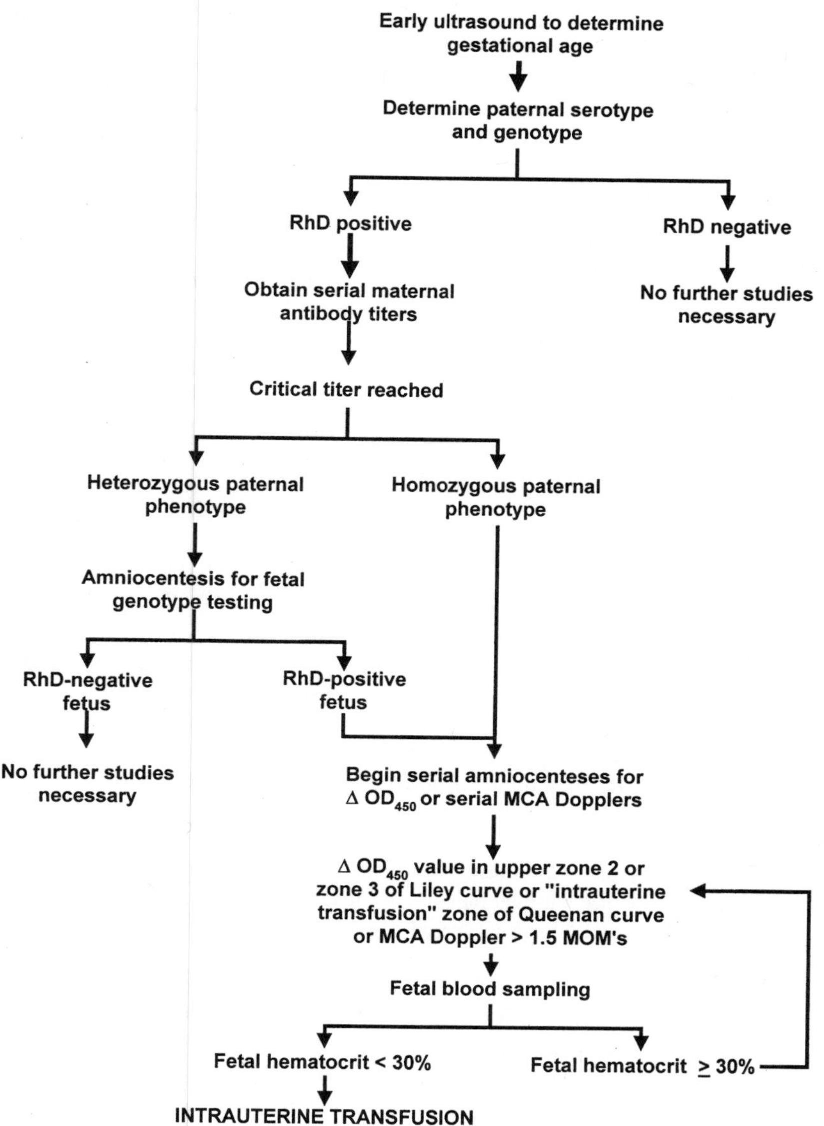

FIGURE 30.3. Flow chart showing a plan for managing the first affected pregnancy. ΔOD_{450}, amniotic fluid bilirubin levels; MCA, middle cerebral artery; MOMs, multiples of the median; Rh, rhesus.

the IUT zone of the Queenan curve or if Doppler ultrasonography shows that the blood velocity in the middle cerebral artery is >1.5 multiples of the median (MOMs), fetal blood sampling is performed with blood readied for IUT for a fetal hematocrit of <30%.

Intrauterine Transfusion

History

The first successful treatment of hemolytic disease of the fetus was described by Liley, in 1963, when he introduced the technique of intraperitoneal transfusion (IPT) (51). No further technical modifications occurred until 1981. In that year, Rodeck et al. (52) described intravascular transfusion (IVT) of the fetus with a needle directed into chorionic plate vessels, as visualized through a fetoscope. In 1982, a group in Denmark reported IVT of a fetus by means of umbilical venous puncture under ultrasonographic guidance (53). By 1986, two schools of thought had emerged regarding the optimal method for IVT. A group at Yale recommended an exchange technique similar to that used to treat HDN in the neonate (54). A second group, at Mt. Sinai Medical Center in New York, championed direct IVT (55). As more experience was gained with the two techniques, direct IVT became more widely adopted by many centers because it took less time. Because of interest in IVT, IPT has been virtually abandoned by most centers that treat RBC alloimmunization.

Method of Transfusion

Before the advent of IVT, it was generally accepted that the hydropic fetus was unable to absorb RBCs effectively from its peritoneal cavity after IPT (56). Although no randomized studies have been undertaken to compare results of IPT to those of IVT, a case-control study demonstrated only a slight improvement in the survival rate of the nonhydropic fetus but almost doubling of the survival rate of the hydropic fetus when IVT was employed (57). In addition, fewer neonatal exchange transfusions were required, and the stay in the intensive care nursery was shorter in the IVT group. Intraperitoneal transfusion, however, remains a practical method for delivering RBCs to the nonhydropic fetus when the umbilical cord or intrahepatic umbilical vein is hard to access. Blood infused into the peritoneal reservoir will be absorbed via the diaphragmatic lymphatic vessels over a 7- to 10-day period. Bowman (58) proposed a formula for calculating the IPT volume (ml) that has withstood the test of time. The volume of RBCs to be infused is calculated by subtracting 20 from the gestational age (in weeks) and multiplying this number by a factor of 10. For example, a 30-week-old fetus would receive 100 ml of blood for IPT (30 wk $-$ 20 $=$ 10 $\times$ 10 $=$ 100 ml).

Serial hematocrits from fetuses transfused with IVTs alone reveal a marked decline, of approximately 1% per day, between procedures (55). To avoid this problem, we evaluated whether a combined IPT-IVT technique would result in a more stable fetal hematocrit between transfusions (59). Our technique involved administering enough packed RBCs (hematocrit 75% to 85%) by means of an IVT to achieve a final fetal hematocrit of 35% to 40%. To attain this goal, we periodically measured the fetal hematocrit during the IVT. A standard IPT was then undertaken. We hypothesized that the intraperitoneal infusion of blood would serve as a reservoir, allowing slow absorption of RBCs between procedures. Four transfusion techniques were compared in 19 fetuses. Combined direct IVT-IPT achieved a more stable fetal hematocrit than direct IVT alone, resulting in decline of 0.01% and 1.14% per day, respectively, between transfusions. Use of the combined approach allows more prolonged intervals between procedures and, therefore, can reduce the total number of procedures necessary.

Red Blood Cells for Transfusion

Red blood cells for IUT must undergo the same rigorous testing as for any allogenic donation. In addition, RBCs from a donor who is seronegative for cytomegalovirus (CMV) are preferred. For enhancing the level of 2,3-diphosphoglycerate (2,3-DPG; also known as 2,3-bisphosphoglycerate), a fresh unit is superior to stored blood. In the United Kingdom, standards require that RBCs used for IUT have a shelf life of less than 5 days. A recent review noted that six cases of graft-versus-host reaction have been reported in infants undergoing IUT (60). Bohm et al. (61) proposed that this reaction was due to the induction of immune tolerance to engrafting lymphocytes that gain entry into the fetal circulation through large-volume IUTs. The British Blood Transfusion Task Force (62) and the American Association of Blood Banks (63) recommend that RBC units for IUT undergo γ-irradiation to prevent graft-versus-host reaction. In addition, leukocyte reduction is a requirement in the United Kingdom; although not routinely practiced in the United States, this technique is often used to reduce the risk of CMV and is likely to be universally accepted in the near future.

Although not practiced at many centers, maternal blood donation is an excellent source of RBCs for IUT. Such donation is well tolerated. In 21 patients at our center, up to six units per patient were harvested for IUT (64). In all cases, supplementation with prenatal vitamins, folate, and ferrous sulfate prevented maternal anemia. No serious maternal or fetal effects were noted. Moreover, the psychologic benefit to the patient cannot be overstated. Patients often profess guilt because their immune system is rejecting their fetus. Maternal donation helps ameliorate these feelings. Other theoretic advantages to using maternal blood include a decreased risk of sensitization to new RBC antigens, a longer half-life owing to the fresh source of cells, and a decreased risk of transmitting viral agents. Vietor et al. (65) investigated the source of new RBC antibodies in 91 patients undergoing 280 IUTs. Twenty-four (26%) of the women developed new antibodies. In 14 cases, the source of the sensitizing antigen could be determined; in 3 (20%) of these 14 cases, donor RBCs carried the involved antigen. Therefore, it would appear that, in 5% of cases, use of maternal blood as the source of RBCs for IUT would prevent the development of new anti-RBC antibodies. Only one investigation has compared the fetal effects of maternal versus donor RBCs for IUT (66). Seventy-six IUTs using maternal blood were compared to 213 IUTs using donor RBCs. The rate of decline was statistically less in the maternal RBC group, but this difference did not manifest until after 33 weeks of gestation. In addition, infants who received maternal blood required fewer neonatal transfusions (mean, 0.38 versus 1.48) than infants who received donor cells. The authors conjectured that this finding could be related to increased maternal reticulocytosis after repeated maternal donations. Such reticulocytosis would result in a younger population of RBCs that would exhibit a longer half-life in the fetus. They concluded that maternal RBCs are preferred over donor RBCs because the maternal cells may decrease the total number of IUTs necessary for treating a particular fetus. To date, no study has compared maternal versus donor RBCs with respect to the risk of fetal viral infection.

In a maternal blood donation program, if IUTs are likely to be needed, the patient can donate a unit of RBCs after the first trimester. The unit can be separated into two smaller aliquots and refrigerated for up to 42 days. If not used by the end of that time, the unit can then be frozen for use later in the pregnancy. Although this approach may negate some of the advantages of a fresher unit (see above), these units can be used to supplement maternal donations later in the gestation, when a single unit of maternal cells may yield an insufficient volume for performing an optimal IUT. Patients should be given additional iron therapy (324 mg of ferrous sulfate twice daily), as well as additional folate (1 mg daily). Additional pregnancy-related considerations include positioning the patient in the left lateral recumbent position during blood donation and replacing the donated volume with isotonic intravenous fluids. Fetal monitoring during the procedure is unnecessary (67). A standard volume of 450 $\pm$ 45 ml is drawn, because subsequent washing and packing will markedly reduce the final volume available for IUT. The maternal blood requires some additional processing before it can be used for IUT. The blood is washed several times to remove the offending antibody. Because the mother and fetus will share HLA antigens at many loci, the possibility of a graft-versus-host reaction is higher when blood from an unrelated donor is used.

Thus, irradiation with 2,500 Gy of external beam radiation is imperative. Use of maternal blood is controversial in patients who are positive for CMV antibody. Dormant CMV is known to reside in the polymorphonuclear leukocytes. Both leukodepletion and washing are effective mechanisms for preventing the transmission of CMV (68). In our program, all RBC units for IUT are leukocyte-reduced to minimize the risk of CMV transmission. For this reason, we proceed with the use of maternal CMV-seropositive blood after carefully counseling the patient.

How Much to Transfuse

The end point for an IUT varies considerably, most centers using a target hematocrit to decide when a transfusion is completed. Advocates of direct IVT will usually transfuse until a final value of 50% to 65% is reached. This will allow for a reasonable interval between procedures, based on a projected decline in hematocrit of 1% per day. However, in transfusing the fetus, one should be cautious about raising the hematocrit to nonphysiologic values. Welch et al. (69) demonstrated that a marked increase in whole blood viscosity is associated with fetal hematocrits above 50%. Centers that use a combined technique will generally aim for a final target hematocrit of 35% to 40% for the intravascular portion of the procedure.

Several authors have proposed formulas for calculating the volume of RBCs to be transfused. In the formula introduced by Mandelbrot and associates (70), the initial step involves calculating the fetoplacental volume (ml) from the ultrasonographic estimate of the fetal weight in grams (1.046 + fetal weight in g × 0.14). The volume (ml) to be transfused is then calculated with the following formula:

$$V_{transfused} = V_{fetoplacental} \times (Hematocrit_{final} - Hematocrit_{initial}) \times Hematocrit_{transfused\ blood}$$

in which $V_{transfused}$ is the volume of RBCs (ml) to be given during the IVT, $V_{fetoplacental}$ is the combined blood volume (ml) in the fetus and placenta, $Hematocrit_{final}$ is the target fetal hematocrit (%) desired at the conclusion of the IVT, $Hematocrit_{initial}$ is the fetal hematocrit at the start of the IVT, and $Hematocrit_{transfused}$ blood is the hematocrit (%) of the donor unit of RBCs used for the IVT. For example, if a fetus weighs 1,000 g determined by ultrasonography, the estimated fetoplacental volume would be 140 ml (1.046 + 1000 = 1001.46 × 0.14 = 140). Assuming that the hematocrit of the donor unit of RBCs is 80%, that the desired final fetal hematocrit is 40%, and that the fetal hematocrit is 20% at the start of the IVT, a volume of 35 ml would be needed to achieve the desired final fetal hematocrit of 40% ([140 × (40 − 20)] / 80 = 35).

Giannina et al. (71) proposed a simpler method of calculating the volume of packed RBCs needed for IUT. Assuming that the donor unit has a hematocrit of approximately 75%, they calculated a series of transfusion coefficients for raising the initial fetal hematocrit to a desired final value (Table 30.9). The operator simply multiplies the coefficient by the ultrasonographically estimated fetal weight to achieve the final desired fetal hematocrit. In the example described in the preceding paragraph, one would multiply the fetal weight (in this case, 1,000 g) by 0.04 (the coefficient used to raise the hematocrit by 20%), thereby determining that a volume of 40 ml would be needed in order to obtain the desired final fetal hematocrit of 40%. When tested prospectively, Mandelbrot's equation and Giannina's technique yielded similar results, but both methods overestimated the final fetal hematocrit by 8%.

After the first IUT, subsequent procedures are scheduled at 14-day intervals until suppression of fetal erythropoiesis is noted on a Kleihauer-Betke stain or a fetal cell stain using flow cytometry. Suppression usually occurs by the third IUT. Thereafter, the interval for repeat procedures can be based on the decline in hematocrit for the individual fetus, usually being 3 to 4 weeks.

TABLE 30.7. INDICATIONS FOR EXCHANGE TRANSFUSION[a]

Infants With Hemolytic Disease That Is Otherwise Uncomplicated

Anemia (hematocrit <45%), a positive Coombs test result, and an increase of >0.5 mg/dl/h in the serum bilirubin concentration

In ABO disease, an increase of >1.0 mg/dl/per hour in the serum bilirubin concentration

Reduced bilirubin-binding capacity, as indicated by the salicylate saturation index or HBABA dye-binding capacity, if available

A serum bilirubin concentration of ≥20 mg/dl at any time

A serum bilirubin concentration of >15 mg/dl for >36 h; dye-binding capacity not available

Infants With Or Without Hemolytic Disease

Serum bilirubin concentration of >20 mg/dl

Clinical factors that may suggest exchange transfusion at lower serum bilirubin concentrations include:

- Prematurity
- Sepsis
- Hypoxia and acidosis (present or past)
- Hypoproteinemia or use of a drug that competes for bilirubin-binding sites
- Evidence of reduced binding capacity (using binding tests noted above)
- A bilirubin concentration close to the exchange level for >36h

[a]From Poland RL, Ostrea EM Jr. Neonatal hyperbilirubinemia. In: Klaus MH, Fanaroff AA, eds. *Care of the high-risk neonate*, 4th ed. Philadelphia: WB Saunders, 1993:313, with permission.
HBABA, 2-(4′-hydroxybenzeneazo)benzoic acid.

The Severely Anemic Fetus

The fetus that is severely anemic at 18 to 24 weeks of gestation may have difficulty adapting to acute correction of its anemia. Monitoring of the umbilical venous pressure during IVT is useful in such cases (72). An increase of >10 mm Hg predicts fetal death within 24 hours after transfusion with a sensitivity of 80%. Radunovic et al. (73) noted a 37% mortality within 72 hours of IVT in fetuses with severe anemia and hydrops. These authors recommended that, in the severely anemic fetus, the increase in the final posttransfusion hematocrit after IVT should not exceed 25% or a four-fold increase from the pretransfusion value. At our center, we use the umbilical venous pressure to determine when to conclude an IVT in a very anemic fetus in the early second trimester. This pressure is periodically evaluated, and the procedure is concluded when the change in pressure approaches 10 mm Hg. A second IVT is performed within 48 hours to bring the fetal hematocrit into the normal range, and a third procedure is scheduled for 7 to 10 days later. Thereafter, repeat transfusions are undertaken on the basis of fetal hematocrits and cell stains.

Outcome

Overall survival after IUT varies with the center, its degree of experience, and the presence of hydrops fetalis. An overview of the literature shows an overall survival of 84% (74). After the first IUT, the survival rate is one-fourth lower for fetuses who were hydropic during IUT than for those who were nonhydropic (70% versus 92%, respectively).

With regard to the sick fetus, enhanced survival and its relationship to the long-term outcome have been addressed in two investigations. Using a two-sample analysis, Janssens et al. (75) failed to find a correlation between either the presence of hydrops or the number of IUTs and a poor neonatal neurologic outcome. Using a multivariate analysis, our group could find no relationship between global neonatal developmental scores and the number of IUTs, the lowest fetal hematocrit, or the presence of hydrops. These data are useful in counseling the couple that has a severely anemic fetus. The couple can be reassured that more than 90% of surviving infants can be expected to have a normal neurologic outcome even if hydrops fetalis is present during the first IUT.

Fetal Physiologic Effects of IVT

After IVT, acute changes in blood volume and viscosity result in extensive changes in the fetal cardiovascular system. Acute increases in both the umbilical venous pressure and blood flow have been documented (76–78). After decreasing by as much as 25% (78), the fetal cardiac output begins to return to pretransfusion levels within 2 hours after IVT (79), reaching a normal level approximately 24 hours after the procedure (80). One likely explanation for these hemodynamic alterations is that the cardiac afterload increases markedly because of a rapid rise in the blood viscosity. The fetus responds with a decreased stroke volume, which leads to a reduced cardiac output, increased right atrial and umbilical venous pressures, and decreased heart rate (78).

The fetal circulation also responds to this increased afterload by undergoing generalized vasodilation. Pulsed Doppler assessment of the umbilical and fetal femoral, renal, and cerebral vessels has revealed an overall decrease in vascular resistance (81, 82). An increase in both fetal vasodilator prostaglandins and atrial natriuretic peptide has been documented after IVT and probably contributes to the lowered resistance (83–87).

Clinically significant alterations in the fetal metabolism also occur because of IVT. Both the umbilical venous pH and the base excess undergo a decrease, while the carbon dioxide partial pressure increases acutely after the procedure (88). This change is probably due to the acidic pH of the transfused blood. Acute correction of this exogenous source of acidosis may be achieved through rapid equilibration across the placenta. The oxygen dissociation curve of HbF favors the uptake of oxygen in the placenta. Therefore, replacing fetal RBCs with adult cells at the time of transfusion may adversely affect oxygen delivery to the fetal tissues. Soothill et al. (89) compared the blood gas values of fetuses transfused with adult-type hemoglobin-containing RBCs with the blood gas values of control subjects. The transfused fetuses had a lower umbilical artery pH, a greater base deficit, and higher umbilical venous oxygen partial pressure. The authors postulated that an increased uteroplacental blood flow may be one compensatory mechanism for preventing hypoxia of the fetal tissues. An increased fetal plasma 2,3-DPG concentration has also been documented, and it may serve as another compensatory mechanism that improves the release of oxygen (90). However, overall fetal growth and well-being does not appear to be affected. Although fetuses affected by severe hemolytic disease tend to be small for their gestational age, IUT results in catch-up fetal growth (91).

Nasrat et al. (92) demonstrated a potential risk for iron overload in Rh-alloimmunized fetuses undergoing transfusion. These authors described plasma ferritin levels indicative of iron overload in several fetuses. Severe fetal hemolytic anemia leads to elevated iron stores, which further increase in a manner that is directly correlated with the volume of RBCs transfused. Neonatal cholestasis and hepatitis related to severe intrahepatic iron deposition after fetal transfusion have been reported (93).

TREATMENT OF THE NEWBORN

Management of Hyperbilirubinemia

After delivery, the neonate is routinely evaluated for anemia and hyperbilirubinemia. The Apgar scoring system is an effective means of assessing a newborn's clinical status in the early postpartum interval. The Apgar score reflects signs and symptoms associated with neonatal anemia, for example, color, tachypnea, tachycardia, and lethargy. Careful clinical evaluation is essential, because serologic data are often poor predictors of the severity of anemia except for anti-D incompatibility. Routine testing of cord blood is unnecessary but, in clinically jaundiced neonates, cord hemoglobin and bilirubin measurements are important for determining the presence of HDN. Comparison of maternal and neonatal ABO and Rh(D) status, along with assessment of a DAT using cord or infant blood, can help determine whether anemia is due to an immune etiology. The reticulocyte count and, more recently, measurement of the serum erythropoietin levels are also useful for differentiating hyporegenerative anemia from hemolytic states (94). When secondary to anti-K1, HDN causes both hemolytic RBC injury and suppression of erythroid precursors (39).

Once HDN has been diagnosed, blood transfusion is rarely the first choice of therapy except in newborns known to be at risk for severe immune HDN in whom more than 90% of the RBCs circulating at delivery may have originated from donors as a result of repeated IUT. Hydropic neonates require urgent resuscitation including intermittent positive pressure ventilation and relief of hydrothorax and hydroperitoneum, which may interfere with lung expansion. Neonates with critically low hemoglobin levels must be treated promptly with a direct or exchange transfusion of RBCs, taking care to prevent volume overload. If severe HDN is a possible outcome, a maternal blood sample should be used to select compatible RBCs before delivery.

Postpartum RBC degradation accounts for 80% of the bilirubin produced by the newborn (95). During the postpartum interval, the mother and placenta no longer metabolize bilirubin for the infant. The neonate's ability to process bilirubin is limited for a finite interval, pending maturation of hepatic catabolic and excretory pathways. The circulating RBC mass is increased, and RBC survival is reduced. These factors contribute to the high prevalence of postpartum jaundice. In newborns with physiologic jaundice, the bilirubin levels commonly peak at 5 to 6 mg/dl. Immune hemolysis further compounds the postpartum bilirubin load. Serum bilirubin levels of >17 mg/dl or jaundice developing within 24 hours after birth is pathologic, mandating evaluation for hemolysis or an alternative cause.

Unconjugated bilirubin is the principal deleterious by-product of postpartum hemolysis. When present in excessive amounts it precipitates in the newborn's basal ganglia, causing neuron dysfunction and death. Bilirubin alters cellular metabolism by inhibiting mitochondrial enzymes, DNA synthesis, and protein metabolism, as well as inducing DNA-strand breakage. Kernicterus is the clinical syndrome caused by the pathologic effect of indirect bilirubin on the central nervous system. The manifestations of kernicterus range from nerve deafness to advanced disease associated with severe brain damage, mental retardation, spasticity, athetoid movements, and death. Subtle end effects of kernicterus include extrapyramidal disorders, gaze disturbance, and deafness, which may not be apparent until after the first year of life. Unconjugated bilirubin levels of >20 mg/dl increase the incidence of kernicterus to 10%, while levels of >30 mg/dl increase the incidence to 50%. On the basis of these findings, early intervention is recommended to maintain bilirubin concentrations of <20 mg/dl.

Phototherapy

With milder forms of HDN, phototherapy is typically the initial method for bilirubin management. Approximately 60% of newborns develop visible jaundice. Phototherapy is an effective means of increasing bilirubin catabolism related to photooxidation and photoisomer formation, yielding ready excretable, water-soluble bilirubin metabolites. Phototherapy is typically initiated in term neonates if their bilirubin concentration increases 0.5 mg/dl per day or if their total bilirubin concentration exceeds 10, 12, or 14 mg/dl at less than 12, 18, and 24 hours of life, respectively. Because of the low prevalence of kernicterus, as well as the reevaluation of previous large studies concerning the efficacy of exchange transfusion in preventing this condition, some experts have suggested that the traditional bilirubin treatment thresholds be lowered (96). However, neonates with hemolysis are considered at heightened risk, and recent revised guidelines do not apply to intervention in these patients. An international survey detected great variation in the management of hyperbilirubinemia by means of exchange transfusion (97).

Transfusion Criteria

Exchange transfusion is indicated when phototherapy fails. The criteria used to assess the need for exchange transfusion include the bilirubin level, hemoglobin level, and clinical status (Table 30.7). A controlled trial demonstrated the efficacy of exchange transfusion in preventing kernicterus when the serum bilirubin concentration was maintained below 20 mg/dl. Either an absolute concentration of 20 mg/dl or a bilirubin increment of 5 mg/dl per day (>10 mg/dl per day for ABO HDN) is the usual threshold for exchange transfusion. Birth weight is considered, because immature infants are at increased risk. The transfusion threshold also stratifies newborns according to clinically defined factors known to increase the risk of kernicterus such as acidosis and hyperosmolarity (97).

Data for assessing hemoglobin as a determinant of the need for transfusion have been less rigorously analyzed. Normally, cord blood hemoglobin values range from 13.7 to 20 g/dl. The published values recommended for initiating an exchange transfusion range from 10.5 to 14.8 g/dl. A cord blood hemoglobin of <10 g/dl is a generally accepted value for initiating an RBC exchange. Fortunately, because of advances in intrauterine monitoring and transfusion therapy, life-threatening anemia (i.e., hemoglobin 4 to 6 g/dl or lower) is rarely encountered.

Postpartum transfusion decisions are complicated by physiologic adaptation from intrauterine to extrauterine life. The hemoglobin level gradually declines postpartum and, in full-term

TABLE 30.8. COMPLICATIONS OF EXCHANGE TRANSFUSIONS[a]

Vascular
Embolization of air or thrombi
Thrombosis

Cardiac
Arrhythmias
Volume overload
Cardiac arrest

Electrolytic
Hyperkalemia
Hypernatremia
Hypocalcemia
Acidosis

Coagulative
Overheparinization
Thrombocytopenia

Infectious
Bacteremia
Hepatitis
Cytomegalovirus

Other
Mechanical injury to donor cells
Necrotizing enterocolitis
Hypothermia
Hypoglycemia

[a]From Poland RL, Ostrea EM Jr. Neonatal hyperbilirubinemia. In: Klaus MH, Fanaroff AA, eds. *Care of the high-risk neonate*, 4th ed. Philadelphia: WB Saunders, 1993:315, with permission.

infants, typically reaches a nadir of 8.8 to 11.5 g/dl by the sixth week. A more precipitous, or steeper, decline in the postpartum hemoglobin level necessitates an evaluation for hemolysis. Unfortunately, there have been no well-designed, randomized trials designed to substantiate existing transfusion thresholds, based on the hemoglobin level, in infants with hemolytic disease. In these cases, the decision to transfuse must take account of the newborn's clinical status, as well as pertinent laboratory data.

Exchange Transfusion

Simple or booster transfusion of RBCs is not typically considered for newborns with ongoing hemolysis. In hemolytic states, exchange transfusion is the method of choice, because the exchange removes incompatible RBCs, preventing a further increase in bilirubin levels. Exchange transfusion is also an effective way of eliminating bilirubin bound to albumin. A double-volume exchange decreases the incompatible RBC content by 87%; in contrast, bilirubin removal is less efficient, reducing the content by 45%. The choice of donor blood for an exchange transfusion depends on the underlying cause of HDN. In cases of Rh alloimmunization, ABO-compatible, Rh-negative blood is used. In cases of ABO incompatibility, washed type O, Rh-specific blood cells are used. These cells are reconstituted with type AB plasma (and thus do not contain the anti-A or anti-B antibody). In cases involving atypical antibodies, one must obtain donor blood that is compatible with maternal serum as shown by antiglobulin phase cross-matching. The volume of donor blood needed for an exchange transfusion is twice the blood volume of a newborn (2 × 85 ml/kg = 170 ml/kg). It has become common practice to use packed RBCs of the appropriate ABO and Rh type that are compatible with the maternal serum (depending on the cause of HDN) and that are reconstituted with type AB (or other compatible) plasma, to attain the desired hematocrit (usually 45% to 55% in newborns).

Exchange transfusion has become less common since the introduction of IUT methods. Traditionally, the threshold for exchange has been twice the original blood volume. It is important that institutional procedures are reviewed by the personnel who perform those transfusions and that competency programs are in effect. The infant should be immobilized and continuously monitored for blood pressure, pulse, and respiratory rate. Infants whose condition is unstable should undergo aggressive treatment of hypoxia and acid-base disturbances before an exchange transfusion is undertaken. Blood access for such a transfusion is typically gained by inserting a 5, 6, or 8 French catheter, with a three-way stopcock attached to the end, through the umbilical vein, through the ductus venosus, and into the inferior vena cava above the diaphragm or right atrium. The catheter should be tested to ensure a free flow of blood. Radiographic or ultrasonographic confirmation of catheter placement is then obtained. An initial sample is drawn to check the hemoglobin and bilirubin levels. The exchange transfusion should be performed slowly, over 60 to 90 minutes; 5- to 10-ml volumes of blood are exchanged by initially extracting newborn blood and then replacing it with an equal volume of donor blood. Intermittent measurement of the central venous pressure is helpful, but care must be taken to avoid introducing air during this process. If reduction of the bilirubin concentration is a primary goal, intravenous infusion of albumin (1 g/kg) can increase the efficiency of bilirubin extraction by 40% (98).

In 106 patients evaluated over a 15-year interval, exchange transfusion was associated with a mortality of 2% (99). Serious complications developed in 12% of the patients. Indeed, this method involves a number of potential complications, including embolism, vasospasm, thrombosis, infarction, cardiac dysrhythmias, volume overload, electrolyte imbalance, bleeding, and infection (Table 30.8). Its indications must be determined carefully in light of the inherent risks. Newly trained clinicians must be especially careful; they have generally had little experience with this procedure because of the dramatic decrease in pregnancy-related Rh sensitization since the advent of RhIg prophylaxis.

TABLE 30.9. TRANSFUSION COEFFICIENT FOR CALCULATING TRANSFUSION VOLUME

Target Increase in Fetal Hematocrit	Transfusion Coefficient
10%	0.02
15%	0.03
20%	0.04
25%	0.05
30%	0.06

Blood Requirements

Rigorous analysis of optimal component preparation for neonatal exchange transfusion has not been done. In light of the metabolic derangements associated with exchange transfusion, some neonatologists recommend that fresh blood be used for exchange transfusion of the anemic newborn. This approach would minimize the impact of metabolic derangements and RBC potassium leakage, would improve overall survival, and would optimize the immediate oxygen delivery characteristics. Nevertheless, controlled trials to support this approach have not been done. The maternal blood sample should be used for pretransfusion serologic tests because the pathologic antibodies are derived from the mother. In cases of ABO HDN, the transfused RBCs should be group O. The whole blood should be reconstituted to a hematocrit of 50% by adding group AB fresh-frozen plasma. After initial serum screening, one may continue to select crossmatch-compatible units or may administer units that are negative for the antigen that is causing the hemolytic anemia.

Owing to reports of sickling crises in hypoxic infants transfused with blood from donors heterozygous for hemoglobin A and hemoglobin S (HbAS), blood for exchange transfusion must be negative for hemoglobin S (sickle cell trait). Red blood cells for use in exchange transfusion must also be made CMV-safe by means of leukocyte reduction and must undergo irradiation. Because fresh whole blood is generally not available, thawed fresh-frozen plasma is used to reconstitute whole blood (target hematocrit, 50%). The platelet content of the reconstituted component is not a concern, provided that the newborn's platelet count is not seriously compromised.

CONCLUSION

In HDN, maternal IgG antibodies cross the placental barrier, causing hemolysis of fetal RBCs, usually related to the Rh, ABO, or Kell blood groups. Although HDN can be fatal, advances in diagnosis, treatment, and prevention have made it increasingly controllable. Diagnostic modalities include maternal assays, ultrasonography, amniocentesis, and fetal blood sampling. Antenatal treatment consists of in utero transfusion and prophylaxis with anti-D. Postpartum management includes treatment of hyperbilirubinemia, usually by means of phototherapy, and performance of simple or exchange blood transfusion for correction of anemia. With these methods, the mortality and morbidity of HDN has been greatly reduced during the past half century. Because a utilization gap remains, however, physicians who treat women in their childbearing years should be aware of HDN and its diagnosis and management.

REFERENCES

1. Diamond LK, Blackfan KD, Baty JM. Erythroblastosis fetalis and its association with universal edema of the fetus, icterus gravis neonatorum and anemia of the newborn. *J Pediatr* 1932;1:269–277.
2. Landsteiner K, Weiner AS. An agglutinable factor in human blood recognized by immune sera for rhesus blood. *Proc Soc Exp Biol Med* 1940;43:223.
3. Levine P, Vogel P, Katzin EM, et al. Pathogenesis of erythroblastosis fetalis: statistical evidence. *JAMA* 1941;116:825–827.
4. Dufour DR, Monoghan WP. ABO hemolytic disease of the newborn: a retrospective analysis of 254 cases. *Am J Clin Pathol* 1980;73:369–373.
5. Gilja BK, Shah VP. Hydrops fetalis due to ABO incompatibility. *Clin Pediatr* 1988;27:210–212.
6. Desjardins L, Blajchman MA, Chintu C, et al. The spectrum of ABO hemolytic disease of the newborn infant. *Pediatrics* 1979;95:447.
7. Katz MA, Kanto WP Jr, Korotkin JH. Recurrence rate of ABO hemolytic disease of the newborn. *Obstet Gynecol* 1982;59:611–614.
8. Geifman-Holtzman O, Wojtowycz M, Kosmas E, et al. Female alloimmunization with antibodies known to cause hemolytic disease. *Obstet Gynecol* 1997;89:272–275.
9. Shanwell A, Sallander S, Bremme K, et al Clinical evaluation of a solid-phase test for red cell antibody screening of pregnant women. *Transfusion* 1999:39:26–31.
10. Garner SF, Gorick BD, Lai WYY et al. Prediction of severity of hemolytic disease of the newborn. *Vox Sang* 1995;68:169–176.
11. ACOG Practice Bulletin. Prevention of RhD alloimmunization. *Int J Gynaecol Obstet* 1999;66:63–70.
12. Zipursky A, Israels LG. The pathogenesis and prevention of Rh immunization. *CMAJ* 1967;97:1245–1257.
13. Keith L, Danis RP, Berger GS. Clinical experience with the prevention of Rh isoimmunization. A historical comparative analysis. *Am J Reprod Immunol Microbiol* 1984;5:84–89.
14. Bowman J, Pollock JM. Failures of intravenous Rh immune globulin. *Transfus Med Rev* 1987;1:101–112.
15. Mollison PL. *Blood transfusion in clinical medicine,* 10th ed. Oxford: Blackwell Science, 1997:359.
16. Smith T. Active immunity produced by so-called balanced or neutral mixtures of diphtheria toxin and antitoxin. *J Exp Med* 1909;11:241.
17. Nevanlinna HR, Vainio T. The influence of mother-child ABO incompatibility on Rh immunization. *Vox Sang* 1956;1:26–36.
18. Finn R, Clarke CA, Donohoe WTA, et al. Experimental studies on the prevention of Rh haemolytic disease. *BMJ* 1961;1:1486.
19. Freda VJ, Gorman JG, Pollack W, et al. Prevention of Rh hemolytic disease—ten years' clinical experience with Rh immune globulin. *N Engl J Med* 1975;292:1014–1016.
20. Contreras M, de Silva. The prevention and management of hemolytic disease of the newborn. *J R Soc Med* 1994;57:256–258.
21. Bowman JM. Antenatal suppression of Rh alloimmunization. *Clin Obstet Gynecol* 1991;34:296–303.
22. Chavez GF, Mulinare J, Edmonds LD. Epidemiology of Rh hemolytic disease of the newborn in the United States. *JAMA* 1991;265: 3270–3274.
23. Mayne KM, Allen DL, Bowell PJ. 'Partial D' women with anti-D alloimmunization in pregnancy. *Clin Lab Haematol* 1991;13:239–244.
24. Avent ND, Reid ME. The Rh blood group system: a review. *Blood* 2000;95:375–387.
25. Samson D, Mollison PL. Effect on primary Rh immunization of delayed administration of anti-Rh. *Immunology* 1975;28:349–357.
26. Sebring ES, Polesky HF. Detection of fetal maternal hemorrhage in Rh immune globulin candidates. *Transfusion* 1982;22:468–471.
27. Kleihauer E, Braun H, Betke K. Demonstration von fetalem Hamoglobin in den Erythrocyten eines Blutausstrichs. *Klin Wochenschr* 1957; 35:637–638.
28. Davis BH, Olsen S, Bigelow NC, et al. Detection of fetal red cells in fetomaternal hemorrhage using a fetal hemoglobin antibody by flow cytometry. *Transfusion* 1998;38:749–756.
29. Bromilow IM, Duguid JKM. Measurement of feto-maternal haemorrhage: a comparative study of three Kleihauer techniques and two flow cytometry methods. *Clin Lab Haematol* 1992;19:137–142.
30. Tavassoli M. Embryonic and fetal hemopoiesis: an overview. *Blood Cells* 1991;17:269–281.
31. Wu H, Liu X, Jaenisch R, et al. Generation of committed erythroid BFU-E and CFU-E progenitors does not require erythropoietin or the erythropoietin receptor. *Cell* 1995;83:59–67.
32. Campbell J, Wathen N, Lewis M, et al. Erythropoietin levels in amniotic fluid and extraembryonic coelomic fluid in the first trimester of pregnancy. *Br J Obstet Gynaecol* 1992;99:974–976.
33. Bergstrom H, Nilsson LA, Nilsson L, et al. Demonstration of Rh antigens in a 38-day-old fetus. *Am J Obstet Gynecol* 1967;99:130–133.
34. Toivanen P, Hirvonen T. Antigens Duffy, Kell, Kidd, Lutheran and Xga in fetal red cells. *Vox Sang* 1973;24:372–376.
35. Medvinsky A, Dzierzak E. Definitive hematopoiesis is autonomously initiated by the AGM region. *Cell* 1996;86:897–906.
36. Moritz KM, Lim GB, Wintour EM. Developmental regulation of erythropoietin and erythropoiesis. *Am J Physiol* 1997;273: R1829–R1844.
37. Nicolaides KH, Soothill PW, Clewell WH, et al. Fetal haemoglobin measurement in the assessment of red cell isoimmunisation. *Lancet* 1988;1:1073–1075.
38. Moise KJ, Perkins JT, Sosler SD, et al. The predictive value of maternal serum testing for detection of fetal anemia in red blood cell alloimmunization. *Am J Obstet Gynecol* 1995;172:1003–1009.
39. Vaughan IL, Manning M, Warwick RM, et al. Inhibition of erythroid progenitor cells by anti-Kell antibodies in fetal alloimmune anemia. *N Engl J Med* 1998;338:798–803.
40. Nicolaides KH, Fontanarosa M, Gabbe SG, et al. Failure of ultrasonographic parameters to predict the severity of fetal anemia in rhesus isoimmunization. *Am J Obstet Gynecol* 1988;158:920–926.
41. Oepkes D, Meerman RH, Vandenbussche FP, et al. Ultrasonographic fetal spleen measurements in red blood cell-alloimmunized pregnancies. *Am J Obstet Gynecol* 1993;169:121–128.
42. Roberts AB, Mitchell JM, Pattison NS. Fetal liver length in normal and isoimmunized pregnancies. *Am J Obstet Gynecol* 1989;161:42–46.
43. Bahado-Singh R, Oz U, Deren O, et al. Splenic artery Doppler peak systolic velocity predicts severe fetal anemia in rhesus disease. *Am J Obstet Gynecol* 2000;182:1222–1226.
44. Mari G, for the Collaborative Group for Doppler Assessment of the Blood Velocity in Anemic Fetuses. Noninvasive diagnosis by Doppler ultrasonography of fetal anemia due to maternal red-cell alloimmunization. *N Engl J Med* 2000;342:9–14.
45. Liley AW. Liquor amnii analysis in the management of pregnancy complicated by rhesus sensitization. *Am J Obstet Gynecol* 1961;82: 1359–1370.
46. Nicolaides KH, Rodeck CH, Mibashan RS, et al. Have Liley charts outlived their usefulness? *Am J Obstet Gynecol* 1986;155:90–94.

47. Queenan JT, Tomai TP, Ural SH, et al. Deviation in amniotic fluid optical density at a wavelength of 450 nm in Rh-immunized pregnancies from 14 to 40 weeks' gestation: a proposal for clinical management. *Am J Obstet Gynecol* 1993;168:1370–1376.
48. Van den Veyver IB, Subramanian SB, Hudson KM, et al. Prenatal diagnosis of the RhD fetal blood type on amniotic fluid by polymerase chain reaction. *Obstet Gynecol* 1996;87:419–422.
49. Weiner CP, Wenstrom KD, Sipes SL, et al. Risk factors for cordocentesis and fetal intravascular transfusion. *Am J Obstet Gynecol* 1991;165: 1020–1025.
50. Weiner CP, Williamson RA, Wenstrom KD, et al. Management of fetal hemolytic disease by cordocentesis. I. Prediction of fetal anemia. *Am J Obstet Gynecol* 1991;165:546–553.
51. Liley AW. Intrauterine transfusion of foetus in haemolytic disease. *BMJ* 1963;2:1107–1109.
52. Rodeck CH, Kemp JR, Holman CA, et al. Direct intravascular fetal blood transfusion by fetoscopy in severe Rhesus isoimmunisation. *Lancet* 1981;1:625–627.
53. Bang J, Bock JE, Trolle D. Ultrasound-guided fetal intravenous transfusion for severe rhesus haemolytic disease. *BMJ* 1982;284:373–374.
54. Grannum PA, Copel JA, Plaxe SC, et al. In utero exchange transfusion by direct intravascular injection in severe erythroblastosis fetalis. *N Engl J Med* 1986;314:1431–1434.
55. Berkowitz RL, Chitkara U, Goldberg JD, et al. Intrauterine intravascular transfusions for severe red blood cell isoimmunization: ultrasound-guided percutaneous approach. *Am J Obstet Gynecol* 1986;155: 574–581.
56. Lewis M, Bowman JM, Pollock J, et al. Absorption of red cells from the peritoneal cavity of an hydropic twin. *Transfusion* 1973;13:37–40.
57. Harman CR, Bowman JM, Manning FA, et al. Intrauterine transfusion-intraperitoneal versus intravascular approach: a case-control comparison. *Am J Obstet Gynecol* 1990;162:1053–1059.
58. Bowman JM. The management of Rh-isoimmunization. *Obstet Gynecol* 1978;52:1–16.
59. Moise KJ Jr, Carpenter RJ Jr, Kirshon B, et al. Comparison of four types of intrauterine transfusion: effect on fetal hematocrit. *Fetal Ther* 1989;4:126–137.
60. Harte G, Payton D, Carmody F, et al. Graft versus host disease following intrauterine and exchange transfusions for rhesus haemolytic disease. *Aust N Z J Obstet Gynaecol* 1997;37:319–322.
61. Bohm N, Kleine W, Enzel U. Graft-versus-host disease in two newborns after repeated blood transfusions because of rhesus incompatibility. *Beitr Pathol* 1977;160:381–400.
62. British Committee for Standards in Haematology, Blood Transfusion Task Force. Guidelines on γ-irradiation of blood components for the prevention of transfusion-associated graft-versus-host disease. *Transfus Med* 1996;6:261–271.
63. Vengelen-Tyler V, ed. *Technical manual of the American Association of Blood Banks,* 13th ed. Bethesda: American Association of Blood Banks, 1999.
64. Gonsoulin WJ, Moise KJ Jr, Milam JD, et al. Serial maternal blood donations for intrauterine transfusion. *Obstet Gynecol* 1990;75: 158–162.
65. Vietor HE, Kanhai HH, Brand A. Induction of additional red cell alloantibodies after intrauterine transfusions. *Transfusion* 1994;34: 970–974.
66. El-Azeem SA, Samuels P, Rose RL, et al. The effect of the source of transfused blood on the rate of consumption of transfused red blood cells in pregnancies affected by red blood cell alloimmunization. *Am J Obstet Gynecol* 1997;177:753–757.
67. Herbert WN, Owen HG, Collins ML. Autologous blood storage in obstetrics. *Obstet Gynecol* 1988;72:166–170.
68. Pamphilon DH, Rider JR, Barbara JA, et al. Prevention of transfusion-transmitted cytomegalovirus infection. *Transfus Med* 1999;9:115–123.
69. Welch R, Rampling MW, Anwar A, et al. Changes in hemorheology with fetal intravascular transfusion. *Am J Obstet Gynecol* 1994;170: 726–732.
70. Mandelbrot L, Daffos F, Forestier F, et al. Assessment of fetal blood volume for computer-assisted management of in utero transfusion. *Fetal Ther* 1988;3:60–66.
71. Giannina G, Moise KJ Jr, Dorman K. A simple method to estimate the volume for fetal intravascular transfusion. *Fetal Diagn Ther* 1998; 13:94–97.
72. Hallak M, Moise KJ Jr, Hesketh DE, et al. Intravascular transfusion of fetuses with rhesus incompatibility: prediction of fetal outcome by changes in umbilical venous pressure. *Obstet Gynecol* 1992;80: 286–290.
73. Radunovic N, Lockwood CJ, Alvarez M, et al. The severely anemic and hydropic isoimmune fetus: changes in fetal hematocrit associated with intrauterine death. *Obstet Gynecol* 1992;79:390–393.
74. Schumacher B, Moise KJ Jr. Fetal transfusion for red blood cell alloimmunization in pregnancy. *Obstet Gynecol* 1996;88:137–150.
75. Janssens HM, de Haan MJ, van Kamp IL, et al. Outcome for children treated with fetal intravascular transfusions because of severe blood group antagonism. *J Pediatr* 1997;131:373–380.
76. Weiner CP, Pelzer GD, Heilskov J, et al. The effect of intravascular transfusion on umbilical venous pressure in anemic fetuses with and without hydrops. *Am J Obstet Gynecol* 1989;161:1498–1501.
77. Nicolini U, Talbert DG, Fisk NM, et al. Pathophysiology of pressure changes during intrauterine transfusion. *Am J Obstet Gynecol* 1989; 160:1139–1145.
78. Moise KJ Jr, Mari G, Fisher DJ, et al. Acute fetal hemodynamic alterations after intrauterine transfusion for treatment of severe red blood cell alloimmunization. *Am J Obstet Gynecol* 1990;163:776–784.
79. Rizzo G, Nicolaides KH, Arduini D, et al. Effects of intravascular fetal blood transfusion on fetal intracardiac Doppler velocity waveforms. *Am J Obstet Gynecol* 1990;163:1231–1238.
80. Copel JA, Grannum PA, Green JJ, et al. Fetal cardiac output in the isoimmunized pregnancy: a pulsed Doppler-echocardiographic study of patients undergoing intravascular intrauterine transfusion. *Am J Obstet Gynecol* 1989;161:361–365.
81. Mari G, Moise KJ Jr, Deter RL, et al. Flow velocity waveforms of the umbilical and cerebral arteries before and after intravascular transfusion. *Obstet Gynecol* 1990;75:584–589.
82. Mari G, Moise KJ Jr, Deter RL, et al. Flow velocity waveforms of the vascular system in the anemic fetus before and after intravascular transfusion for severe red blood cell alloimmunization. *Am J Obstet Gynecol* 1990;162:1060–1064.
83. Weiner CP, Robillard JE. Effect of acute intravascular volume expansion on human fetal prostaglandin concentrations. *Am J Obstet Gynecol* 1989;161:1494–1497.
84. Kingdom JC, Ryan G, Whittle MJ, et al. Atrial natriuretic peptide: a vasodilator of the fetoplacental circulation? *Am J Obstet Gynecol* 1991; 165:791–800.
85. Panos MZ, Nicolaides KH, Anderson JV, et al. Plasma atrial natriuretic peptide in human fetus: response to intravascular blood transfusion. *Am J Obstet Gynecol* 1989;161:357–361.
86. Robillard JE, Weiner C. Atrial natriuretic factor in the human fetus: effect of volume expansion. *J Pediatr* 1988;113:552–555.
87. Weiner CP. Nonhematologic effects of intravascular transfusion on the human fetus. *Semin Perinatol* 1989;13:338–341.
88. Nicolini U, Santolaya J, Fisk NM, et al. Changes in fetal acid base status during intravascular transfusion. *Arch Dis Child* 1988;63:710–714.
89. Soothill PW, Nicolaides KH, Rodeck CH, et al. The effect of replacing fetal hemoglobin with adult hemoglobin on blood gas and acid-base parameters in human fetuses. *Am J Obstet Gynecol* 1988;158:66–69.
90. Soothill PW, Lestas AN, Nicolaides KH, et al. 2,3-Diphosphoglycerate in normal, anaemic and transfused human fetuses. *Clin Sci* 1988;74: 527–530.
91. Roberts A, Grannum P, Belanger K, et al. Fetal growth and birthweight in isoimmunized pregnancies after intravenous intrauterine transfusion. *Fetal Diagn Ther* 1993;8:407–411.
92. Nasrat HA, Nicolini U, Nicolaidis P, et al. The effect of intrauterine intravascular blood transfusion on iron metabolism in fetuses with Rh alloimmunization. *Obstet Gynecol* 1991;77:558–562.
93. Lasker MR, Eddleman K, Toor AH. Neonatal hepatitis and excessive hepatic iron deposition following intrauterine blood transfusion. *Am J Perinatol* 1995;12:14–17.

94. Denner PA, Rhine WD, Stevenson DO. Neonatal jaundice-what now? *Clin Pediatr* 1995;34:103–107.
95. Schwoebel A, Sakraida S. Hyperbilirubinemia: new approaches to an old problem. *J Perinat Neonatal Nurs* 1997;11:78–97.
96. Newman TB, Maisels MJ. Evaluation and treatment of jaundice in the term newborn: a kinder, gentler approach. *Pediatrics* 1992;89: 809–818.
97. Hansen T. Therapeutic approaches to neonatal jaundice: an international survey. *Clin Pediatr* 1996;35:309–316.
98. Odell G, Cohen S, Gordes E. Administration of albumin in the management of hyperbilirubinemia by exchange transfusion. *Pediatrics* 1962;30:613–621.
99. Jackson JC. Adverse events associated with exchange transfusion in healthy and ill newborns. *Pediatrics* 1997;99:E7.

Rossi's Principles of Transfusion Medicine, Third Edition, edited by Toby L. Simon, Walter H. Dzik, Edward L. Snyder, Christopher P. Stowell, and Ronald G. Strauss. Lippincott Williams & Wilkins, Philadelphia © 2002.

CASE 30A

NEW TREATMENT FOR AN OLD PROBLEM

CASE HISTORY

Baby "P" is a 35-week-gestation baby girl born with jaundice and anemia. Her mother is 30 years old, gravida 5, para 2, aborta 3, with a history of two previous pregnancies that ended in fetal demise in El Salvador.

Prenatal testing showed mother to be immune to rubella, nonreactive for syphilis antibody, negative for hepatitis B surface antigen, and negative for evidence of infection with gonorrhea or chlamydia. Mother is group A, Rh negative but had never received anti-D prophylaxis. Her antibody screen is positive, and antibody identification demonstrates anti-D reacting 3+ at the antiglobulin phase of testing.

During the pregnancy, the mother received care at another hospital. Her anti-D was reported to have reacted to a dilution of 1 to 16 at some point during the pregnancy. Serial amniocenteses were done and the optical density measured at 450 nm placed the pregnancy in the high region of zone 2 on a Liley graph, indicating a pregnancy at high risk for hemolytic disease of the newborn (HDN). She was admitted to our hospital on the day of delivery and after evaluation the baby was delivered by cesarean section. The initial Apgar scores were 8 and 9, indicating a very viable newborn.

Newborn's Physical Examination

The baby's oxygen saturation on admission to the intensive care nursery was 100% on room air. She was in no acute distress and was hemodynamically stable. The anterior fontanel was open and flat, and the child had no dysmorphic features. The palate was intact. The baby was jaundiced but the physical examination was otherwise not remarkable. In particular there was no obvious evidence of edema, congestive heart failure, or organomegaly.

Initial Laboratory Data

The initial hematocrit was 29.5% with a platelet count of 216,000/μl, white blood cell count 12,400/μl, total bilirubin 6.5 mg/dl with direct bilirubin of 0.9 mg/dl, total protein 5.1 g/dl, and albumin 2.5 g/dl. The peripheral blood smear is shown in Figure 30A.1. The baby's blood group was found to be group A, Rh positive (probable R_2/r). The direct antiglobulin test was 4+ reactive with anti-immunoglobulin G (IgG) and nonreactive with anti-C3. An eluate of the baby's cells showed anti-D.

Hospital Course

Because of the blood grouping details, the initial anemia, high bilirubin, and peripheral smear, the patient underwent an emergency double–blood volume exchange transfusion at 10:00 PM as treatment of HDN. The postexchange hematocrit was 49%, platelet count was 43,000/μl, but the total bilirubin was found to be higher at 11 mg/dl. The baby was placed under phototherapy. By the next morning the bilirubin was still elevated and later that day was found to rise to 15 mg/dl (Fig. 30A.2).

Because of the rising bilirubin, the patient was then treated with an infusion of intravenous immune globulin (IVIG) in order to decrease the pace of hemolysis. With continued phototherapy, the baby's bilirubin began to decrease, and a second blood exchange was not needed. The platelet count rose to 140,000/μl. On the fourth day of life, phototherapy was discontinued. A rebound bilirubin was measured at 10.3 mg/dl, but the patient continued to improve.

DISCUSSION

Although HDN due to anti-D has become an infrequent complication of pregnancy in the developed world, it remains a seri-

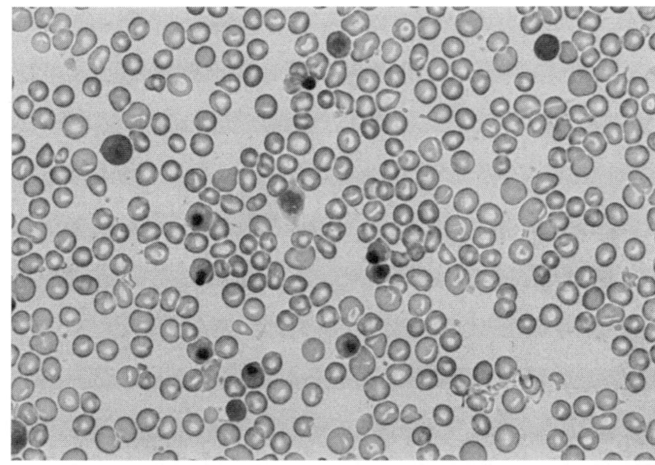

FIGURE 30A.1. Peripheral blood smear in a newborn baby with HDN due to anti-D. Note the marked polychromasia and the frequent nucleated red blood cells.

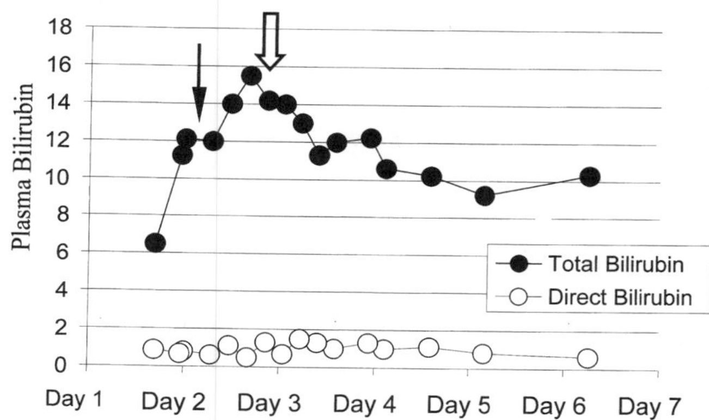

FIGURE 30A.2. Course of bilirubin levels during management of HDN for the first few days of life. The exchange transfusion is indicated by the *solid arrow*. The infusion of IVIG is indicated by the *open arrow*.

ous problem in nations where mothers do not have access to anti-D prophylaxis. As illustrated by this case, hemolysis in HDN due to anti-D can be significant. This is not only because mothers can make high-titer anti-D, but also because the D antigen is well expressed on the red blood cell of the developing fetus. As a result of the maternal history, the prenatal blood group serology testing, amniotic fluid analysis, and prenatal ultrasonography, the diagnosis was not a surprise to the clinicians. The newborn's initial anemia and a rising bilirubin level are classic signs of poor prognosis in HDN and demand intervention to prevent excessively high bilirubin levels, which can result in permanent neurologic damage.

Exchange transfusion remains a classic therapy for HDN. However, the treatment carries considerable risk. A review of 140 exchange transfusions among 106 neonates found that hypocalcemia was a common serious morbidity: more than 34% of infants had documented hypocalcemia during exchange. One in 20 infants demonstrated electrocardiographic changes, and one had a cardiac arrest. Among a subset of 25 ill neonates, 12% experienced severe complications (including two deaths) attributed to transfusion (1).

This case illustrates the use of IVIG as a newer adjunct to exchange transfusion therapy. Intravenous immune globulin was used in this case to prevent the need for a second exchange transfusion. The mechanism by which IVIG interferes with hemolysis due to anti-D is not known. Nevertheless, two recent nonblinded randomized clinical trials provide testimony to its potential value as a new treatment for this old problem. In one study conducted in Argentina researchers randomized 40 affected babies into two groups: one group received IVIG at 800 mg/kg per day for 3 days plus phototherapy, while the other group received just phototherapy (2). They found that babies treated with IVIG had fewer transfusions, shorter lengths of stay, less evidence for hemolysis, and lower elevations of the bilirubin. A second study was conducted in Turkey and randomized 116 affected babies to receive either high-dose IVIG (1,000 mg/kg over 4 hours at the time of diagnosis) plus phototherapy or to receive phototherapy alone (3). Exchange blood transfusion was required in the management of 22 of 58 (38%) babies receiving phototherapy alone, but was required in only 8 of 58 babies (14%) who received both IVIG and phototherapy. The IVIG-treated babies also received a shorter duration of phototherapy and had a shorter length of stay in hospital.

Case contributed by Walter H. Dzik, M.D., Massachusetts General Hospital, Boston, MA.

REFERENCES

1. Jackson JC. Adverse events associated with exchange transfusion in healthy and ill newborns. *Pediatrics* 1997;99:E7.
2. Voto LS, Sexer H, Ferreiro G, et al. Neonatal administration of high-dose intravenous immunoglobulin in rhesus hemolytic disease. *J Perinat Med* 1995;23:443–451.
3. Alpay F, Sarici SU, Okutan V, et al. High-dose intravenous immunoglobulin therapy in neonatal immune haemolytic jaundice. *Acta Paediatr* 1999;88:216–219.

31

CONGENITAL DISORDERS OF CLOTTING PROTEINS AND THEIR MANAGEMENT

JEANNE M. LUSHER

HEMOPHILIA

Hemophilia A (factor VIII deficiency) and hemophilia B (factor IX deficiency) are inherited disorders of coagulation that have many features in common. Both are inherited as X-linked recessive traits and thus affect males almost exclusively. There are, however, some reports of hemophilia A and B in females, presumably due to extreme lyonization, inheritance of a gene for hemophilia from both parents, or a new mutation. The genes for factor VIII and factor IX are on the long arm of the X chromosome in band Xq28 and Xq27, respectively. Clinically, hemophilia A and B are indistinguishable, with bleeding into joints and soft tissues being characteristic of both. Laboratory screening tests are the same in both disorders as well. Persons with hemophilia A or B characteristically have normal values for prothrombin time, platelet count, and template bleeding time but have a greatly prolonged activated partial thromboplastin time (APTT). The two disorders can be distinguished by performance of assays for factor VIII and factor IX coagulant activity.

In hemophilia A, factor VIII coagulant activity is deficient or abnormal, whereas other components of the factor VIII system (von Willebrand factor [vWF] and vWF antigen [vWF:Ag]) are normal. In general, clinical severity is correlated with the degree of factor VIII deficiency. Persons with severe hemophilia have $<1\%$ (<0.01 IU/ml) factor VIII activity, while those with 1% to 5% of normal factor VIII activity are classified as moderate. Severely affected persons have spontaneous bleeding into joints and soft tissues. Those with factor VIII values of $>5\%$ to 40% (>0.05 to <0.40 IU/ml) have clinically mild disease, usually bleeding only with surgery or trauma (1). The degree of factor VIII deficiency is fairly constant in individuals, and in affected members in the same kindred. "Normal" is 1 IU/ml of factor VIII (100%), as defined by the current World Health Organization International Standard for Plasma Factor VIII (as distributed by the National Institute for Biological Standards and Control, Potters Bar, Hertfordshire, U.K.) (1).

Hemophilia B (Christmas disease) is characterized by subnormal factor IX activity. Depending on the genetic defect, factor IX deficiency may reflect a quantitative or qualitative abnormality in the factor IX molecule. Several different subtypes of hemophilia B have been described. In fact, genotype heterogeneity is quite marked, with almost every family with hemophilia B having its own unique mutation (2). Hemophilia B is far less common than hemophilia A, accounting for approximately 15% to 20% of cases of hemophilia. As in hemophilia A, clinical severity is correlated with the degree of factor IX deficiency, with those with factor IX levels of $\leq 1\%$ generally having spontaneous bleeding into joints and soft tissues.

Hemophilia is worldwide in distribution and affects all racial groups. The incidence of hemophilia in the United States is approximately 1 in 5,000 males (3); this condition affects at least 20,000 persons in the United States alone. Results of a U.S. epidemiologic survey indicated that $\sim 43\%$ of hemophiliacs are severe, with 26% classified as moderate, and 31% as mild (3). The Haldane hypothesis predicts that one-third of all individuals with an X-linked lethal disorder should represent new mutations. In past times, the one-third of hemophilia chromosomes present in males would be lost from the population due to the early death of severely affected males. Because the frequency of the disease is in equilibrium, these lost hemophilic alleles could be assumed to be replaced by an equal number of new mutations (4). Whereas most affected adult males have a family history of hemophilia, approximately 30% of newly diagnosed infants have no family history of the disorder.

Neither factor VIII nor factor IX crosses the placenta; thus

J.M. Lusher: Department of Pediatrics, Wayne State University School of Medicine; and Division of Hematology—Oncology, Children's Hospital Michigan, Detroit, Michigan.

the diagnosis of hemophilia A or B can be made at birth from a sample of cord blood drawn from a vessel on the fetal side of the placenta. The blood should be collected in citrate (1:10 dilution) and sent immediately to the laboratory for a factor VIII or IX assay.

The diagnosis of hemophilia also can be made in utero by direct mutation testing or DNA-linkage analysis, on a chorionic villus biopsy sample obtained as early as 10 weeks of pregnancy, or from amniotic fluid cells at 16 to 18 weeks and analysis of DNA (5).

Although a large number of mutations in the factor VIII and factor IX genes have been described (2,4–6), an inversion in the factor VIII gene accounts for roughly 45% of cases of severe (not mild or moderate) hemophilia A (7,8). Thus, the search for inversions of factor VIII should be considered as the first DNA diagnostic option in a person or a family with severe hemophilia A (4). The inversion mutation can be detected by Southern blot using a blood sample from a person with hemophilia A or from a possible carrier, or using fetal or chorionic villus cells. Interestingly, the majority of de novo factor VIII inversion mutations have been found to originate in male germ cells from the maternal grandfather (6).

Treatment of Hemostatic Abnormalities in Hemophilia

Blood Component Therapy

In general, if a person with a hereditary defect in coagulation is bleeding and treatment is judged to be indicated, the person should receive an intravenous injection of the clotting factor he or she lacks. Until the mid-1960s, whole normal plasma (fresh plasma or fresh-frozen plasma [FFP]) was the only preparation that could be used to treat factor VIII or factor IX deficiency. Then, in 1965, Pool et al. (9) described a simple method for concentrating factor VIII in the form of a cold-insoluble precipitate (cryoprecipitate). By the late 1960s, the availability of cryoprecipitates had revolutionized the treatment of hemophilia A and made possible elective surgery and outpatient treatment of bleeding episodes.

Cryoprecipitates, prepared from single units of plasma, contain approximately 50% of the factor VIII activity, vWF, and fibrinogen, as well as factor XIII, of the starting unit of plasma. Thus, for purposes of calculation, a single bag of cryoprecipitate contains, on average, 100 IU of factor VIII and 0.2 g of fibrinogen in a volume of 8 to 10 ml. Although largely replaced by lyophilized factor VIII concentrates in the 1970s and 1980s and recombinant factor VIII (rfVIII) concentrates in the 1990s, cryoprecipitates are still used in many parts of the world to treat persons with severe or moderately severe hemophilia A. Additionally, until the use of 1-deamino, 8-D-arginine vasopressin (desmopressin [DDAVP]) became widespread in the 1980s, cryoprecipitates were regarded as the treatment of choice for all persons with von Willebrand disease (vWD). Today, even for treatment of bleeding in severe and variant forms of vWD, cryoprecipitates have been largely replaced by certain plasma-derived lyophilized factor VIII concentrates (Aventis Behring GmbH's Humate-P, Alpha's Alphanate SD, and Bayer's Koate-DVI), which are rich in the higher–molecular-weight multimers of vWF. These products are not only effective in vWD, but are preferred over cryoprecipitates because of greater viral safety (each of them is virally attenuated). Cryoprecipitates also can be used for the treatment of bleeding in persons with hypofibrinogenemia, afibrinogenemia, or dysfibrinogenemia.

Disadvantages of cryoprecipitates over commercially prepared concentrates include (a) a slightly increased risk of bloodborne viral disease transmission (particularly hepatitis C virus [HCV]), (b) a required storage temperature of <20° to <30°C, and (c) marked variation in the factor VIII and vWF content of preparations.

By 1970, methods of fractionation had been developed to produce concentrates of both intermediate-purity factor VIII and prothrombin complex concentrate (PCC), the latter of which contain the vitamin K–dependent clotting factors (II, VII, IX, and X) as well as proteins C and S. The availability of these lyophilized concentrates quickly led to home treatment (self-infusion) programs throughout the United States and abroad. For the first time, persons with hemophilia were not totally dependent on family members, hospital personnel, and emergency rooms. Bleeding episodes could be treated more promptly, less time was lost from work or from school, and the incidence of progressive chronic musculoskeletal disease was decreased. However, it soon became apparent that there was a price to be paid for the use of these very convenient lyophilized factor VIII and IX concentrates. By the mid-1970s, it was clear that many persons with hemophilia had developed hepatitis and had persisting alterations of liver function (10–13). Some had progressed to cirrhosis. As many as 90% of hemophiliacs became seropositive to hepatitis B surface antigen (14). Because of this serious complication, in 1980 Hyland Laboratories developed and introduced a factor VIII concentrate (Hemofil T) that was heated in the dry state for 72 hours at 60°C. Studies in chimpanzees suggested that this method of heating destroyed hepatitis viruses; however, when Hemofil T was infused into previously untreated children with hemophilia, 84% developed non-A, non-B hepatitis, as evidenced by elevations in alanine aminotransferase (14).

In the early 1980s, the first cases of acquired immunodeficiency syndrome (AIDS) in persons with hemophilia were noted, and as the number of AIDS cases continued to rise, it was apparent that this too was being transmitted by blood and blood products, including clotting factor concentrates (15). It is now known that approximately 90% of persons who received factor VIII concentrates and 55% of those who received PCCs prepared in the United States between 1979 and 1984 became seropositive for human immunodeficiency virus (HIV). Fortunately, HIV proved to be heat labile (16). Although the dry heating method used in production of Hyland's Hemofil T did not prevent non-A, non-B hepatitis, it did seem to destroy HIV. Thus, by late 1984 almost all hemophiliacs in the United States were receiving dry heat–treated concentrates. Additionally, by the spring of 1985, mandatory screening of all blood and plasmapheresis donors for HIV seropositivity was in place. These measures greatly improved the safety of plasma-derived factor VIII and factor IX concentrates in terms of HIV transmission.

In an attempt to produce safer products, manufacturers of

plasma-derived clotting factor concentrates developed a variety of new methods during the late 1980s. These newer methods were aimed at killing viruses more effectively and improving purity (10,17). In addition to dry heating, viral attenuation methods included solvent-detergent treatment (which kills viruses by disrupting lipid viral envelopes), heating in an aqueous solution (pasteurization), vapor (steam) treatment, and heating in a suspension in an organic solvent. Although such viral attenuation methods were thought to eliminate HIV, sporadic instances of seroconversion to HIV were reported between 1985 and 1987. Analysis of these cases indicated that 14 of 18 seroconversions worldwide (including a cluster of 7 in western Canada reported in late 1987) were attributable to one method of dry heating that used a temperature of 60°C for 30 hours (18). This method of heating was thus abandoned in favor of higher temperatures for longer periods of time.

In addition to better viral attenuated products, factor VIII concentrates purified by using murine monoclonal antibodies and immunoaffinity chromatography became commercially available in 1987 (19). Several logs of virus were eliminated in the purification process. These monoclonal antibody–purified products are further virally attenuated by pasteurization (in the case of Aventis Behring GmbH's Monoclate P) or by solvent-detergent treatment (in the case of Baxter Hyland-Immuno's Hemofil M and the American Red Cross' Monarc-M).

Viral Safety

In terms of replacement therapy, viral safety is of paramount importance. None of the commercially available plasma-derived products in current use has been implicated in any case of seroconversion to HIV or HCV. In addition to improved donor screening methods and much better viral attenuation methods for plasma-derived products (20), for well over a decade hepatitis B vaccination has been recommended for all hepatitis B–seronegative hemophiliacs. However, sporadic outbreaks of other blood-borne viral diseases in the 1980s and 1990s were cause for concern. These included HCV transmission by intravenous immunoglobulin, hepatitis A in 88 hemophilic recipients of solvent-detergent–treated factor VIII concentrate, and transmission of human Parvovirus B19 by pasteurized, vapor-treated, and solvent-detergent–treated concentrates. Human Parvovirus B19 (which can cause severe anemia in immunocompromised hosts) and hepatitis A virus are non–lipid-enveloped viruses, which are resistant to most viral inactivation techniques (11,20). Some worried that other pathogenic viruses with features similar to human Parvovirus B19 and hepatitis A virus might exist. Although there have been no documented instances of transmission of Creutzfeldt-Jacob disease (21) or new variant Creutzfeldt-Jacob disease, the mere possibility of such transmission has been cause for further concern among hemophilic patients and their physicians. Thus the use of safer alternatives to blood products such as rfVIII and desmopressin (see below) has had considerable appeal.

Product Purity

Although theoretically a purer product (containing only factor VIII or factor IX) would seem preferable, there are only two situations in which there is evidence that purer is better. In HIV-infected hemophiliacs, several published studies have shown that cellular immunity was better preserved in those receiving monoclonal antibody–purified factor VIII concentrates than in those receiving intermediate purity factor VIII concentrates, although none of the studies showed a difference in the appearance of clinical endpoints of HIV disease (20).

The only other situation in which purer is definitely better is in the case of those patients with hemophilia B who are at an increased risk of thrombotic disease (see below), because the high-purity factor IX preparations are considerably less thrombogenic than crude PCCs.

Product Cost and Usage in the United States

All of the newer factor VIII concentrates are very expensive, especially when compared with the dry-heated factor VIII concentrates that were the mainstay of treatment in the United States from 1985 through 1987. Throughout 1987, most hospital pharmacies purchased dry-heat–treated factor VIII concentrates for 7 to 9 cents per factor VIII unit. By the spring of 1988, costs had increased dramatically, to 65 cents per factor VIII unit for monoclonal antibody–purified factor VIII concentrate. Although the currently available plasma-derived factor VIII concentrates vary considerably in terms of cost, rfVIII products are even higher per unit price. The same is true of factor IX concentrates. The high-purity plasma-derived factor IX concentrates, and rfIX are much more expensive than are PCCs. Despite this the majority (80% to 85%) of factor VIII and factor IX concentrates used in the United States in 2000 and 2001 are rfVIII and rfIX concentrates; in fact, if there were greater availability of rfVIII concentrates, usage would no doubt be even higher.

Recombinant Factor VIII

As noted earlier, despite improved methods of donor screening, and improved methods of viral attenuation of plasma-derived clotting factor concentrates since the mid-1980s, the transmission of certain blood-borne viruses remains a concern. Thus recombinant clotting factor concentrates have had great appeal. After a series of landmark papers in *Nature* in 1984 in which scientists at the Genetics Institute and Genentech described the molecular cloning of a complementary DNA (cDNA)-encoding human factor VIII (23) and the expression of human factor VIII from recombinant DNA clones (24) scale-up, purification, and standardization were rapidly accomplished. Prelicensure clinical trials in humans began in 1987, and three companies' rfVIII products are now licensed in the United States. Baxter Hyland-Immuno's Recombinate was licensed by the U.S. Food and Drug Administration (FDA) in December 1992, and Bayer's Kogenate was licensed in February 1993. Baxter's rfVIII is made in Chinese hamster ovary (CHO) cells (transfected with the gene for human factor VIII), whereas Bayer's rfVIII is produced in baby hamster kidney (BHK) cells. In patients with hemophilia A, both of the original, "first-generation" full-length rfVIII products have demonstrated the same pharmacokinetics and clinical effectiveness as plasma-derived factor VIII products (25,

26). However, both contain human serum albumin, which is added as a stabilizer and is the major component of these rfVIII concentrates.

Although the early appearance of inhibitor antibodies to factor VIII in both companies' trials of previously untreated patients (PUPs) raised some concern, as the trials progressed it became apparent that neither product was any more antigenic than plasma-derived factor VIII. The PUP trials with Kogenate (27) and Recombinate (28) measured inhibitor assays every 3 months, which was more frequent than in older studies of plasma-derived factor VIII. Many of the inhibitors detected in the two rfVIII PUP trials occurred after relatively few exposures to rfVIII; many were low titer and transient and might well have been missed entirely had inhibitor assays not been done as frequently as every 3 months (29).

Despite the cost of rfVIII, many patients (especially those who are HIV seronegative) now have been switched from plasma-derived to rfVIII, because of the added margin of viral safety. However, despite their excellent record of safety and increased usage, there was concern among some that human serum albumin was in these rfVIII products (and was, in fact, the major component in the final products) and *might* transmit a blood-borne disease.

The "next generation" of rfVIII products being developed includes truncated molecules. Because the heavily glycosylated B domain seemed to be dispensable for the hemostatic activity of factor VIII (30), a B-domain–deleted form of factor VIII was developed (31,32). This much smaller molecule is secreted more efficiently by CHO cells, is less prone to proteolytic degradation, and no serum albumin is needed for stabilization of the final product. Genetics Institute's B-domain–deleted (BDD) rfVIII began to be tested in clinical trial in humans in early 1993 and proved to be effective and safe (33). It was licensed by the FDA in the spring of 2000. This product, unlike Kogenate and Recombinate, contains no human albumin as a stabilizer; although albumin is used during manufacture (none is detectable in the final product, however). B-domain–deleted rfVIII (ReFacto) has proven to be effective in a wide variety of situations (acute bleeding episodes, prophylaxis, home treatment, surgery, etc.), is safe, and is well tolerated (34).

In the PUP study with BDD rfVIII, 33 of 101 PUPs (all severely affected) developed inhibitors to factor VIII after a median of 12 exposure days. Seventeen of the 33 patients who developed an inhibitor had peak values of <5 Bethesda units (BU), while 16 had peak values of ≥ 5 BU. Eight of the 33 inhibitors were transient, disappearing despite "on demand" (as necessary, for bleeding episodes) treatment with BDD rfVIII. Twelve additional patients (most high-responder inhibitor patients) had a good response to immune tolerance induction (ITI) with BDD rfVIII, with their latest inhibitor titers being negative (34). These results are very similar to those seen with the two full-length rfVIII preparations (35). In PUPs, inhibitor development follows a typical pattern; the highest risk is within the first 20 exposure days to FVIII. In each similarly conducted, prospective PUP study, approximately one-third are high-titer inhibitors (usually defined as ≥ 10 BU), and two-thirds are low-titer inhibitors (<10 BU). Roughly one-third (usually low-titer inhibitors) are transient.

The only "problem" with BDD rfVIII is that usual, one-stage (APTT-based) factor VIII assays give roughly 50% of expected values in the recipient's plasma (33,34,36,37). There are marked differences in the phospholipid requirement in the assay of BDD rfVIII compared to the other factor VIII preparations. Thus, if one is monitoring factor VIII levels in a patient with hemophilia A who is receiving BDD rfVIII, one-stage factor VIII assays will appear to be lower than expected (calculated). On the other hand, chromogenic substrate assays, although infrequently done in U.S. clinical laboratories, will give expected recovery values. Also, if one uses a small test vial of BDD rfVIII as the factor VIII standard in the one-stage assay, results will be as expected. Small test vials of BDD rfVIII (prepared by National Institute for Biological Standards and Control [NIBSC] in the United Kingdom) are available for this purpose.

Another "second generation" rfVIII product is Bayer's Kogenate FS, which is a full-length rfVIII preparation but is formulated with sucrose, rather than human serum albumin. As with Bayer's original rfVIII preparation, Kogenate, this new product is produced by transfected BHK cells. Modifications to the purification process were made in order to eliminate the need for the addition of albumin during purification. A solvent-detergent step has also been added during purification. Kogenate FS entered prelicensure clinical trials in North America, Europe, and Japan in 1996; all trial data demonstrated Kogenate FS to be safe and effective (38). This product was licensed by the FDA in 2000.

Dosage and Administration of Factor VIII

Factor VIII concentrates are routinely used for treating acute bleeding episodes in persons with moderate or severe hemophilia A. The most common indications for treatment are acute hemarthrosis and intramuscular bleeding. Such events should be treated promptly to prevent or reduce complications (such as chronic joint disease) and to minimize the need for additional infusion of clotting factor (Table 31.1). In addition, factor VIII concentrates are often used for prophylaxis (to prevent bleeding), for surgical coverage, and for ITI in persons with factor VIII inhibitors.

In calculating the dose, it can be assumed that 1 IU of factor VIII/kg of body weight will raise the patient's factor VIII level by 2% (0.02 IU/ml). Thus, if the patient's baseline factor VIII level is 0.01 IU/ml, a dosage of 20 IU/kg would be expected to raise the level to 40% (0.40 IU/ml). The half-life of factor VIII is 10 to 12 hours but may be less than this if the recipient is febrile, is bleeding extensively, has a factor VIII inhibitor, or is a small child.

The author's recommended dosage for various types of bleeding are given in Table 31.1. It should be noted that the need for additional doses and for adjunctive forms of treatment (e.g., an antifibrinolytic agent) (39) varies depending on the location, nature, and extent of the bleeding episode.

Serious, life-threatening bleeding into the central nervous system or intraoperative and postoperative bleeding should be treated with a continuous infusion of factor VIII. After an initial bolus of 40 to 50 IU/kg (which will raise the patient's factor VIII level to 80% to 100%), a continuous infusion should be

TABLE 31.1. HEMOPHILIA A—RECOMMENDED DOSAGES OF FACTOR VIII[a]

Type Of Bleeding	Dose (U/kg)	Dosage Factor VIII (U/kg) Repeat Dosing	Other Treatment
Acute hemarthrosis			Ice packs, non–weight-bearing sling, or light-weight splint may be helpful; rarely, joint aspiration
Early	10	Seldom necessary	
Late	20	20 every 12 hours	
Intramuscular hemorrhage	20–30	20 every 12 hours (often several days of treatment required)	Non-weight-bearing; complete bed rest for iliopsoas hemorrhage
Life-threatening situations	50	25–30 every 8–12 hours OR (Preferably) as a continuous infusion (3–4 U/kg/hr)	
Intracranial hemorrhage			
Major surgery			
Major trauma			
Tongue or neck bleeding with potential airway obstruction			
Severe abdominal pain	20–40	20–25 every 12 hours	
Tongue and mouth lacerations	20	20 every 12 hours	An antifibrinolytic agent (tranexamic acid or ϵ-aminocaproic acid), sedation, nothing by mouth in small child; local application of oradhesive gauze may be beneficial for gum bleeding
Extractions of permanent teeth	20	20 every 12 hours; however, often not necessary in uncomplicated extractions	Antifibrinolytic agent beginning 1 day preoperatively; continue 7–10 days
Painless spontaneous gross hematuria	None	None	Increased fluids orally; corticosteroids and/or factor VIII are used by some

[a]Refers to viral-attenuated plasma-derived factor VIII or recombinant factor VIII.
In persons who have mild hemophilia A, DDAVP (desmopressin) is the treatment of choice rather than factor VIII concentrates, except for life-threatening bleeding.
These situations should be treated in a comprehensive hemophilia center. If the patient is first seen in another hospital, the hemophilia center should be contacted, and the patient should be transferred after emergency treatment is given at the local hospital.

started. An initial rate of 3 to 4 IU/kg per hour should be subsequently adjusted as indicated by the recipient's factor VIII level. In general, a rate of 2 IU/kg per hour will achieve a factor VIII level of 25%; 3 IU/kg per hour will yield a 50% level; and 4 IU/kg per hour will result in a 75% level. However, these levels should not be assumed, and daily monitoring should be performed.

Prophylactic treatment may be indicated in an attempt to interrupt a vicious cycle of rebleeding into a particular "target joint." For such secondary prophylaxis, factor VIII concentrates are generally given in a dosage of 15 to 20 IU/kg every other day or three times a week. This is generally continued for a period of 2 to 6 months.

Primary Prophylaxis

Chronic hemophilic arthropathy, resulting from repeated bleeding into joints, is the major cause of morbidity in persons with severe hemophilia. In those whose factor VIII or IX levels are less than 0.01 IU/ml, bleeding episodes occur approximately 30 to 35 times per year (40). Primary prophylaxis, which is aimed at preventing spontaneous hemarthroses, was begun in Malmö, Sweden, over 30 years ago (40,41). Now, all boys with severe hemophilia seen at the Malmö center start prophylaxis when they are 1 to 2 years old. The regimen used for severe hemophilia A is 25 to 40 IU of factor VIII/kg of body weight given every other day; for hemophilia B, 25 to 40 IU/kg of factor IX is given twice weekly. Although venous access may be a problem in younger children, central venous catheters (e.g., PORT-A-CATH) are often used. With such devices the risk of bleeding or infection is generally low but must be considered. The results of such primary prophylaxis in Sweden have been excellent (40, 41), prompting others to adopt this practice. In early 1994 the U.S. National Hemophilia Foundation's Medical and Scientific Advisory Council recommended that primary prophylaxis be considered optimal treatment for children with severe hemophilia A or B (42).

Desmopressin

Desmopressin ([DDAVP], produced by Ferring Pharmaceuticals in Malmö, Sweden, and distributed by Aventis Behring GmbH in the United States) is the treatment of choice for persons with mild or moderate hemophilia A, whenever an approximately three-fold increase in factor VIII is sufficient to control bleeding. This synthetic agent effects a rapid two- to ten-fold (average of three-fold) increase in factor VIII and an average two-fold increase in vWF:Ag and ristocetin cofactor (RCoF). The recommended dosage is 0.3 μg/kg intravenously (43). If repeated doses are given in rapid succession, many (but not all) persons have tachyphylaxis (a diminishing response). This is thought to reflect a depletion of the storage sites for factor VIII and vWF. Desmopressin is remarkably free of undesirable side effects. In most persons, side effects are limited to facial flushing and a feeling of facial warmth. The antidiuretic properties of the drug seldom cause a problem. However, if repetitive doses of desmopressin are used along with large amounts of intravenous fluids, fluid and electrolyte balance must be carefully monitored to avoid hyponatremia and water intoxication. This precaution is particularly important in infants and small children and in elderly patients. In fact, when desmopressin is given to small children, fluid intake during the next 18 hours should be limited to avoid the possibility of water intoxication (44). Several formulations of desmopressin are available (45). The highly concentrated intranasal spray (Stimate Nasal Spray) is ideally suited for outpatient and home use (45,46). For patients weighing <50 kg, one spray (in one nostril) is recommended, while for those weighing >50 kg, two sprays (one in each nostril) should be given. The metered dose pump delivers 0.1 ml (150 μg of desmopressin) per actuation.

Antifibrinolytic Agents

ε-Aminocaproic acid (Amicar) and tranexamic acid (Cyklokapron) are antifibrinolytic agents that inhibit plasminogen activation. These agents are useful adjuncts in certain situations, to prevent lysis of a clot that has already formed as a result of specific replacement therapy. Antifibrinolytic agents are particularly useful in the control of bleeding in the oral cavity (e.g., extraction of permanent teeth, lacerations of the tongue and mouth, and oral surgery) (47).

The recommended dosage of ε-aminocaproic acid is 75 mg/kg every 4 to 6 hours orally. That of tranexamic acid is 25 mg/kg every 6 to 8 hours. For invasive dentistry, antifibrinolytic therapy should be started the evening before the procedure and be continued for 7 to 10 days.

Swedish investigators (48) have demonstrated that transfusion requirements and postoperative bleeding after oral surgery in patients with hemophilia can be significantly reduced by the use of a tranexamic acid mouthwash in addition to systemic antifibrinolytic treatment. The mouthwash is prepared from 10% tranexamic acid for injection, diluted with sterile water. Sindet-Pederson et al. (48) recommend the use of 10 ml of 4.8% tranexamic acid solution for 2 minutes four times daily.

Hepatitis B Vaccine

In view of the risk, albeit very slight, of posttransfusion hepatitis, all persons with hemophilia (mild, moderate, or severe), as well as all children in general, should be immunized against hepatitis B. Although all units of blood or plasma collected must be tested for hepatitis B surface antigen, such testing may not be 100% effective in screening out all units that might transmit hepatitis B, and the risk is multiplied substantially in the case of plasma-derived clotting factor concentrates in which plasma from 2,500 to 20,000 plasma donors is used to produce a single lot of concentrate. Vaccination against hepatitis B (with recombinant hepatitis B vaccine) should begin as soon as a diagnosis of hemophilia has been made.

Hepatitis A Vaccine

Hepatitis A vaccine is also available, and is recommended for children (or any seronegative persons) with hemophilia (49). It can be given subcutaneously (49) as well as intramuscularly.

Avoidance of Drugs that Can Cause Platelet Dysfunction

Certain drugs, aspirin in particular, induce platelet dysfunction that can aggravate the bleeding tendency in persons with hemophilia (or another underlying abnormality of hemostasis). Joint or soft-tissue bleeding is often painful. If aspirin or an aspirin-containing compound is taken to relieve pain, the bleeding tendency may worsen, and a vicious cycle may ensue. This effect of aspirin is caused by an irreversible inhibition of platelet cyclooxygenase, which inhibits prostaglandin synthesis. Thus, aspirin and all aspirin-containing compounds should be avoided by people who have underlying coagulation disorders. Acetaminophen is a good alternative to relieve mild pain or temperature elevation. Other drugs that induce platelet dysfunction include antihistamines, phenothiazines, and nonsteroidal antiinflammatory agents such as indomethacin and ibuprofen (Motrin).

Concentrates Currently Available for the Treatment of Hemophilia B

Until late 1990, intermediate-purity PCCs were the mainstay of treatment for persons with hemophilia B. They contain the vitamin K–dependent clotting factors II, VII, IX, and X, as well as proteins C (50) and S. Now, in addition to PCC, there are two licensed high-purity plasma-derived factor IX concentrates and one licensed rfIX concentrate.

Thromboembolic Complications Associated with PCCs

In addition to nonactivated factors II, VII, IX, and X, PCCs contain some of these in activated form as well. This occasionally results in disseminated intravascular coagulation (DIC) or thromboembolic complications in recipients of PCCs or both. The risk of DIC and thromboembolism is greatest in recipients who have sustained crush injuries or extensive soft-tissue bleeding, or who have undergone orthopedic surgery and are immobile. In such situations, thromboplastic materials are released into the circulation. The risk is also enhanced in persons with hepatocellular disease, because clotting intermediates are not optimally cleared from the circulation, and antithrombin III levels are often low (13,51).

The actual degree of risk is not known. However, for a time many followed the 1975 recommendations of the International

Committee on Thrombosis and Haemostasis to add heparin to reconstituted PCC just before use (5 ml of heparin per 1 ml of reconstituted PCC), especially in high-risk situations such as orthopedic surgery or crush injuries in patients with hemophilia B; however, there is no evidence that this lessened the risk of thrombosis. It seems likely that a greater awareness of potential complications has resulted in more appropriate use of PCCs (often with use of high-purity factor IX concentrates rather than PCC).

Prothrombin complex concentrates which are currently licensed for use in the United States include Baxter Hyland-Immuno's Bebulin VH, Bayer's Kogenate 80, and Alpha Therapeutic Corporation's Profilnine SD.

Coagulation Factor IX Concentrates

In view of the thrombogenic potential of PCC, there was an obvious need for high-purity factor IX concentrates. The first of these, Alpha Therapeutic Corporation's Alphanine (now Alphanine SD), was licensed by the FDA on December 31, 1990. Shortly thereafter, Aventis Behring GmbH's Mononine was licensed. In 1997 Genetics Institute's rfIX, BeneFix, was licensed (see below). These so-called *coagulation factor IX concentrates* are considerably more expensive than PCC; however, they are far less thrombogenic (52). These high-purity virally attenuated factor IX concentrates and rfIX concentrates are recommended for use in neonates and children, in persons with hemophilia B undergoing surgery (particularly orthopedic surgery), in those with crush injuries or large intramuscular hemorrhages, in those with hepatocellular dysfunction, and in anyone with a history of thrombotic problems after receiving PCCs (i.e., in any high-risk situation for thrombosis or DIC)—in fact, they are the preferred products for anyone with hemophilia B.

Recombinant Factor IX

Factor IX was successfully cloned in the early 1980s (at approximately the same time as factor VIII) (53). Prelicensure clinical trials with Genetics Institute's rfIX began in 1995; the product was licensed in the United States in February 1997. The CHO cell line used in its manufacture is cotransfected with a human rfIX cDNA expression plasmid and a cDNA expression plasmid that encodes an engineered form of the paired amino acid–cleaving enzyme (PACE), which improves the processing efficiency of profactor IX expressed in CHO cells (54). No albumin is used, and no human plasma, animal plasma, or animal-derived protein is used in its manufacture or purification (55).

Dosage and Administration of Factor IX

Because factor IX is a smaller molecule than factor VIII and diffuses from extravascular to intravascular sites, a larger dose must be given to achieve the same concentration in the circulation. Whereas a dose of factor VIII of 1 IU/kg will raise the serum factor VIII level by 0.02 IU/ml (2%), the same dose of (plasma-derived) factor IX will raise the circulating factor IX level by only 0.01 IU/ml (1%). As in the case of factor VIII deficiency, in hemophilia B the recommended dosage for treatment of bleeding depends on the nature and severity of the bleeding episode (Table 31.2). In general, the circulating level of factor IX required to achieve hemostasis is somewhat less than that for factor VIII. For most situations, dosages should be calculated to raise the factor IX level to 0.2 IU/ml (20%). However, as shown in Table 31.2, larger doses are recommended for treatment of serious, life-threatening bleeding episodes and for surgery.

In the case of Genetics Institute's rfIX (BeneFix), lower recoveries are frequently seen and may be as low as 50% of expected recovery in some persons (54). The difference in recovery is due to a simple difference in the posttranslational modification of rfIX, namely, the differences in sulfation of tyrosine 155 and phosphorylation of serine 158, residues which play a role in the clearance of factor IX (54). Thus, it is recommended that one use a somewhat larger dose of BeneFix than one would of a plasma-derived factor IX product. The product package insert recommends the following calculation of dosage: number of factor IX units required = body weight (kg) × desired factor IX increase (%) × 1.2. However, one should be aware that there are wide variations in recovery among individuals. Infants and children tend to have lower recovery rates than adults (55).

Surgery in Persons with Hemophilia B

Through the 1980s many hemophilia centers avoided elective surgery (particularly orthopedic surgery) in persons with hemophilia B because of the risk of DIC and thromboembolic complications. As noted earlier, the risk is greatest in persons undergoing extensive orthopedic surgery on the lower extremities, because there is release of thromboplastic materials into the circulation and the patient is likely to be immobile. Now that less thrombogenic plasma-derived factor IX preparations (coagulation factor IX concentrates such as Mononine and AlphaNine SD), and rfIX (BeneFix) are available, these should be used during and after surgery.

Treatment of Hemophiliacs with Inhibitors

Approximately 20% to 35% of persons with severe hemophilia A develop inhibitor antibodies to factor VIII. A lesser percentage (1% to 3%) of persons with severe hemophilia B develop factor IX inhibitors. In certain individuals whose severe hemophilia B results from a large deletion, frameshift mutation, or stop codon in the factor IX gene, inhibitor antibody development may be accompanied by severe allergic reactions (even anaphylaxis) whenever a factor IX–containing product is infused (56,57).

The presence of an inhibitor does not increase the likelihood of bleeding, but it does make the treatment of bleeding more difficult. Many hemophiliacs with inhibitors are called *high responders,* having a marked increase in inhibitor concentration after exposure to factor VIII. These patients are particularly difficult to treat (58).

Most inhibitors occur early in life, after relatively few exposures to factor VIII or factor IX (median in various prospective trials has been 9 to 12 exposure days). As noted earlier, roughly one-half are high-titer inhibitors, while the remainder are low-titer inhibitors (≤10 BU). Approximately one-third of inhibitors (usually low-titer inhibitors) are transient (59, 60).

TABLE 31.2. HEMOPHILIA B—RECOMMENDED DOSAGE SCHEDULE

Type Of Bleeding	Initial Dose Of High-Purity Factor IX (U/kg)	Repeated Doses Of Factor IX (IX U/kg)	Other Treatment
Acute Hemarthrosis In Person With			
Mild hemophilia B	15	None	
Early, in severe hemophilia B	20	None	Seldom necessary
Late (pain, swelling, limitation of motion), in severe hemophilia B	30	20–25 every 12 h	Ice packs; non–weight-bearing; a sling may be useful
Intramuscular Hemorrhage			
In person with mild hemophilia B	15	10–15 every 12 h	
In severe hemophilia B	30–40	30 every 12 h	Non–weight-bearing; complete bed rest for iliopsoas hemorrhage
Life-Threatening Situations Intracranial hemorrhage Major trauma Tongue or neck bleeding with potential airway obstruction	50	20–25 every 12 h OR As a continnous infusion	
Severe Abdominal Pain			
In mild hemophilia B	15	10 every 12 h	
In severe hemophilia B	40	20 every 12 h	
Tongue And Mouth Lacerations, Extraction Of Permanent Teeth			
In mild hemophilia B	15	10 every 12 h	An antifibrinolytic agent (EACA or tranexamic acid), continue 7–10 days
In severe hemophilia B	30	20 every 12 h; however, may not be necessary in uncomplicated extractions	An antifibrinolytic agent (EACA or tranexamic acid), continue 7–10 days; oradhesive gauze may be helpful for gum bleeding
Painless Spontaneous Gross Hematuria	None	None	Increased Fluids Orally; Corticosteroids And/Or Factor IX Used By Some

High-purity (coagulation factor IX) concentrates are the preferred products for most of the above situations.
These situations should be treated in a comprehensive hemophilia center. If the patient is first seen in another hospital, the hemophilia center should be contacted, and the patient should be transferred after emergency treatment is given at the local hospital.

The management of patients with inhibitors has two important aspects. The first is treatment for bleeding, and the second involves attempts to eliminate the inhibitor.

Treatment of Bleeding Episodes in Patients with Inhibitors

Bleeding in so-called *low-responder* patients with inhibitors often can be treated with factor VIII concentrates in usual or somewhat increased dosages, because anamnestic responses are minimal and hemostatic levels of factor VIII, therefore, can be achieved. However, other approaches must be used in high responders. The choice of treatment depends on several variables: the patient's inhibitor concentration, whether or not he is naive to plasma-derived products, the degree of cross-reactivity of the inhibitor to porcine factor VIII, the nature and extent of bleeding, product availability, and the experience and preference of the medical personnel involved.

Prothrombin Complex Concentrates

Prothrombin complex concentrates and activated PCCs (APCCs) have been extensively used for the treatment of bleeding in patients with inhibitors since 1972 and until recently have been the mainstay of treatment for joint and soft-tissue bleeding. They can be used in both factor VIII and factor IX inhibitor patients. The so-called *nonactivated* or *standard* PCCs have been largely replaced by the purposely activated products (APCCs), Baxter Hyland-Immuno's FEIBA-VH and Nabi's Autoplex T. Although they are not always effective, there is no readily available laboratory test for monitoring the recipient, and no one has demonstrated convincingly how they work (58, 59), many still use APCCs. The recommended dose is 50 to 75 IU/kg (50 to 75 factor VIII correctional units [FECUs] of Autoplex per kg and 50 to 75 FEIBA IU/kg). If necessary, this dosage can be repeated for a total of three or four doses. However, the use of frequent repetitive doses should be avoided. If a patient's bleeding fails to respond to three or four doses it is unlikely that additional doses will be effective, and there is a slight risk of myocardial infarction (51).

In each of three controlled trials conducted in the late 1970s and early 1980s, a single dose of PCC was judged effective in roughly 50% of episodes of joint bleeding. Autoplex was also effective in 50% of episodes, whereas FEIBA was somewhat more effective (64%) when compared with Immuno's nonactivated PCC (61). No more recent controlled trials with these products have been conducted.

Porcine Factor VIII Concentrates

Factor VIII inhibitors exhibit varying degrees of species specificity. Most human factor VIII inhibitors destroy human factor VIII to a greater degree than factor VIII from another species. Polyelectrolyte (PE) porcine factor VIII (Hyate:C) is a highly purified freeze-dried porcine factor VIII concentrate that has a much lower incidence of side effects than the older porcine preparations that were largely abandoned in the 1960s. Polyelectrolyte porcine factor VIII was licensed in the United States in 1986 for life- and limb-threatening emergencies. It is produced by Ipsen Biopharm in Wrexham, Wales, and is available in the United States through Ipsen, Inc.

Kernoff (62) demonstrated that patients whose antihuman factor VIII inhibitor concentration is less than 50 BUs generally respond well to PE porcine factor VIII. The recommended starting dose is 50 to 100 IU/kg, with the subsequent dosage determined by monitoring the recipient's factor VIII level. This product has been used extensively in the United Kingdom and elsewhere in Europe and in the United States over the past two decades. Side effects are generally mild (although anaphylaxis has been reported on rare occasions) and can be minimized by giving 100 mg of hydrocortisone with the first injection (62). However, many physicians no longer give hydrocortisone unless the patient has a history of allergic reactions to Hyate:C. Some recipients develop transient thrombocytopenia; however, this is less severe than with the older porcine preparations used in the 1960s.

Polyelectrolyte porcine factor VIII, unlike PCCs and APCCs, permits the measurement of factor VIII levels in the recipient. This product has never been reported to transmit blood-borne viruses. It has proved life saving in many serious situations. The author and her colleagues have used PE porcine factor VIII in children with traumatic intracranial hemorrhages and in several surgical emergencies with excellent results (58).

Plasma-derived Human Factor VIII Concentrates and Recombinant Factor VIII

Some physicians prefer to use human factor VIII concentrates in the treatment of serious life-threatening bleeding episodes or surgical emergencies in patients with factor VIII inhibitors. However, human factor VIII is more likely to be effective if the patient's inhibitor concentration is quite low (<5 BU), than if it is higher.

Recombinant Factor VIIa

Hedner et al. at Novo Nordisk (Copenhagen, Denmark) have developed a recombinant factor VIIa (rVIIa [NovoSeven]) that has been successful in maintaining hemostasis during and after surgery in many patients with high-titer factor VIII and factor IX inhibitors. It also has been used with clinical success in both hemophilic and nonhemophilic patients with inhibitors who had life-threatening bleeding episodes (59,63), as well as in patients with acute joint bleeding, muscle bleeding, and mucocutaneous hemorrhages (64–66). Monroe et al. demonstrated that concentrations of factor VIIa much higher than those found normally in the circulating blood are able to mediate a tissue factor–independent conversion of factor X to factor Xa on a phospholipid surface (67). The same investigators showed that rfVIIa binds to activated platelet surfaces with a low affinity. Thrombin formation was detected in the absence of factor VIII or factor IX when rfVIIa was added in concentrations 50 nmol/L or greater (68). These findings indicate that rfVIIa in concentrations of ≥50 nmol/L may be able to compensate for the absence of factor VIII or factor IX or both in vitro, and are consistent with the clinical experiences using rfVIIa in hemophilia patients with inhibitors.

Since the first human patient was successfully treated with rfVIIa (NovoSeven), during and following open synovectomy (69,70), a large number of clinical trials with rfVIIa have been conducted. These included pharmacokinetic studies (which documented the short half-life of the product, of 2 to 3 hours) (71), dose-finding studies (72), home treatment studies (73), and a U.S. surgical study (74). In most of these studies, as well as in the large compassionate use database with rfVIIa, it has been given by intravenous bolus injections. The drug was licensed for use in the United States in March 1999. The recommended dose is 90 μg/kg of body weight per dose, with repeat dosing (if necessary) given every 2 to 3 hours for the first 24 hours (or more), with increasing intervals of 3 to 6 hours thereafter. However, the clearance rate varies among individuals, with some children less than 15 years of age having three times the clearance rate achieved in adults (75).

Several investigators have tried giving rfVIIa by continuous infusion; however, results have been variable, with breakthrough bleeding being reported in some individuals. Thus, optimal dosage and administration have not been completely worked out as of April 2001. In small trials, some have found greater success with a single, large (140 to 270 μg/kg) dose for controlling acute hemarthrosis or soft-tissue bleeding. Additionally, each of several studies have demonstrated that early treatment with rfVIIa gives a higher success rate, with fewer doses being required (59–65).

Use of rfVIIa in Hemophilia B Patients with Inhibitors and Severe Allergic Reactions

In those persons (usually infants and young children) who have severe hemophilia B and develop an inhibitor, roughly 40% to 50% will have severe allergic reactions (including anaphylactic shock) when infused with any factor IX-containing product (plasma, plasma-derived factor IX concentrates or rfIX) (56,57). While a few such patients have been desensitized to factor IX, for the majority of hemophilia B patients who have had severe allergic reactions to factor IX-containing products, rfVIIa is regarded to be the treatment of choice.

Staphylococcal Protein A Immunoabsorption of Inhibitor Antibodies

Although available in a few centers, the use of staphylococcal protein A immunoabsorption columns (to rapidly reduce a very–high-titer factor VIII or factor IX inhibitor) is not often used. In view of the availability of "bypassing" agents such as APCC and rfVIIa, which work as well in patients with high-titer inhibitors, there is not often a need to rapidly reduce an inhibitor titer in a bleeding patient. They are, however, used on occasion in order to decrease an inhibitor titer in a patient in preparation for certain immune tolerance regimens, such as the Malmö regimen.

Attempts to Suppress or Eradicate Inhibitors: Immune Tolerance Regimes

In the 1970s, Brackmann (76) at the University of Bonn, Germany, designed a regimen for the induction of immune tolerance to factor VIII. The original "Bonn protocol," although often successful, used very large and very frequent doses of both factor VIII and APCC (FEIBA) during a period of many months or even years. The Bonn protocol never gained widespread popularity elsewhere, because it was very costly and very demanding of the patient and physician. However, in the 1980s other investigators began reporting success with modifications of the Bonn regimen that involve smaller doses of factor VIII given at less frequent intervals (58). Ewing et al. (77) at Orthopaedic Hospital in Los Angeles had considerable success with a regimen consisting of a daily infusion of factor VIII of 50 IU/kg, and others have reported suppression of inhibitors in a high percentage of patients given factor VIII at 25 IU/kg on alternate days (78) or two or three times a week. Yet other groups reported an enhancement of immune tolerance with the addition of intravenous γ-globulin or immunosuppressive agents or both (79,80).

Although even these modifications of the Bonn regimen are costly and require good venous access and patient compliance (and a guaranteed supply of factor VIII), it now seems that such approaches may suppress many inhibitors completely and may convert other high responders to low responders. Observations to date indicate that timing is extremely important in the use of an immune tolerance regimen. Optimally, it should begin as soon as possible after a patient is demonstrated to have a high-titer inhibitor. Predictors of success include a low level (<10 BU) of factor VIII inhibitor when ITI is begun, beginning the ITI regimen within 6 months of inhibitor detection, and use of a high dose of factor VIII (≥100 IU/kg per day).

Although many physicians treating hemophiliacs now institute an ITI regimen in an attempt to suppress or eradicate factor VIII inhibitors, the success rate is poorer when ITI is attempted in hemophilia B patients with inhibitors (roughly 50% success versus 85% success in hemophilia A with inhibitors). The success rate is even poorer in children with hemophilia B who have had severe allergic reactions as well as a factor IX inhibitor, and there have been approximately 12 reported cases of nephrotic syndrome with ITI in such patients (81).

VON WILLEBRAND DISEASE

First described by the Finnish physician Dr. Erik von Willebrand in 1924, vWD is characterized by mucous membrane bleeding, excessive bruising, excessive bleeding during and after surgery or invasive dental procedures, and an autosomal dominant mode of inheritance. Von Willebrand disease is the most common of the hereditary coagulation disorders. The incidence of vWD in the United States is estimated to be between 0.82% and 1.6% of the population. Clinical severity varies greatly, and many affected individuals have minimal symptoms unless challenged by surgery. A number of subtypes of vWD have been described; the more common of these will be discussed below.

The basic defect is in vWF, a large multimeric plasma glycoprotein (GP) that supports the adhesion of platelets to the vascular subendothelium. Von Willebrand factor is normally present in plasma in multimers of up to 20 million daltons. The highest–molecular-weight multimers are the most important hemostatically. Von Willebrand factor circulates as a complex with factor VIII and protects factor VIII from rapid proteolytic degradation, as well as transporting it to sites of active hemostasis.

Von Willebrand factor is synthesized in endothelial cells and megakaryocytes and is stored in organelles (in Weibel-Palade bodies of endothelial cells and in granules of platelets). The gene for vWF is located on the short arm of chromosome 12 (82). Von Willebrand factor levels are influenced by a number of things, including ABO blood type (83), with the lowest levels being found in persons of blood group O and the highest in those with blood group AB. There also may be an effect of Lewis (Le) blood group and secretor genes because Le (a− b−) and Le (a− b+) group O individuals have vWF levels about 90% lower than Le(a+ b−)individuals (84). Additionally, the hormonal changes accompanying pregnancy will increase the levels of vWF, factor VIII, and fibrinogen.

Von Willebrand factor is released from its storage sites in a regulated manner after stimulation by certain agonists, including thrombin, histamine, and the calcium ionophore A23187 (85). It is thought that the physiologic function of the regulated pathway is to create a high local concentration of large vWF multimers to enhance platelet adhesion at sites of vascular injury (86). A second, unregulated "constitutive" pathway, with a continuous release of lower–molecular-weight multimers, may provide the vWF needed for binding factor VIII in the circulating plasma (87).

Von Willebrand disease results from a quantitative or qualitative deficiency of vWF. If vWD is suspected, a battery of tests should be performed. Screening tests such as the APTT and bleeding time may or may not be abnormal, especially in persons with mild vWD. More specific tests include quantitation of vWF:Ag by an immunoelectrophoretic assay (the Laurell technique) or by an enzyme-linked immunosorbent assay, an RCoF assay as a measure of vWF activity, a factor VIII assay, and multimeric analysis of vWF using sodium dodecyl sulfate (SDS) agarose gel electrophoresis.

In view of accumulating new data, in 1994 the Subcommittee on von Willebrand Factor of the ISTH endorsed a revised classification of vWD (88). This revised classification was intended to reflect differences in pathophysiologic mechanisms that lead to particular disease phenotypes. Type I vWD is the most common form. It is characterized by a prolonged bleeding time and proportionately low levels of vWF:Ag, vWF activity, and factor VIII. Multimeric analysis of the patient's vWF reveals that all sizes of vWF multimers are present. In type I vWD, vWF levels are subnormal, but the vWF produced is structurally and functionally normal.

Type II variants are characterized by structurally and functionally abnormal vWF (88). On SDS agarose gel electrophoresis the hemostatically important high–molecular-weight multimers of vWF are lacking. In vWD type IIA, a genetic mutation in the A2 domain produces a vWF that is unusually susceptible to proteolysis after secretion (or even prevents its secretion). Patients may have normal or only slightly reduced vWF and factor VIII levels but may have a loss in the high– and intermediate–molecular-weight multimers of vWF in plasma. Affected individuals usually have a mild-to-moderate bleeding tendency and generally have a poor response to desmopressin.

In vWD type IIB, missense mutations in the A1 domain results in a heightened affinity of vWF binding to platelets (specifically, to platelet GP 1b/IX). In type IIB, the patient's vWF spontaneously binds to platelets and is extremely sensitive to the reagent ristocetin. Affected individuals often have mild thrombocytopenia caused by in vivo platelet aggregation, and on ex vivo testing, their platelets aggregate with very low concentrations of ristocetin (enhanced ristocetin-induced platelet aggregation [RIPA]) which do not normally produce a response. On SDS agarose gel electrophoresis, the highest–molecular-weight multimers are absent (88).

Von Willebrand disease type IIN (for Normandy) is an uncommon but interesting variant. It is characterized by a mutation in vWF which prevents the binding of factor VIII but does not interfere with platelet adhesion. Thus, uncomplexed factor VIII is rapidly degraded in the circulation, resulting in low levels of factor VIII, mimicking hemophilia A (89).

In vWD type III, patients have a severe bleeding tendency and very low levels of vWF and factor VIII. The latter two may be undetectable, and the bleeding time is prolonged. In addition to severe mucous membrane bleeding, patients may bleed into joints and soft tissues. Type III is thought to result from a doubly heterozygous state or a homozygous state. It seems that most cases of vWD type III are caused by deletions, nonsense, missense, and frame shift mutations in the vWF gene (84).

Type I vWD is by far the most common of the types of vWD, accounting for at least 80% of cases. The type II variants account for 10% to 15%, whereas type III is relatively rare.

Treatment of vWD

Treatment will be determined by the type of vWD. For persons with type I vWD, the treatment of choice is desmopressin (43, 45,46). When given intravenously in a dosage of 0.3 μg/kg, the drug will effect a rapid two- to ten-fold increase in vWF activity and vWF:Ag, and a near normalization of the bleeding time. Although the magnitude of response varies among individuals, the response to desmopressin in a given individual is generally consistent over time (i.e., three-fold increases in vWF activity and vWF:Ag on one occasion are likely to be duplicated during retreatment at a later date). It is thus important to give a patient with vWD a test dose of desmopressin to confirm responsiveness and to determine the magnitude of the response. Tachyphylaxis is much less of a problem in persons with vWD than in those with mild hemophilia A (90).

Because the effectiveness of desmopressin is attributable to the rapid release of vWF from storage sites, desmopressin will be ineffective in patients with type III vWD, who have nothing in storage to be released. In patients with type IIA vWD, desmopressin may be effective and should be tried. However, in type IIB, most consider desmopressin to be contraindicated, because the release of the functionally abnormal vWF produces in vivo platelet aggregation and a rapid drop in platelets and is hemostatically ineffective (86,91).

Although desmopressin is generally given intravenously to hospitalized patients, the highly concentrated intranasal spray formulation (Stimate) is ideal for home use. It provides excellent bioavailability of the drug and effects an increase of vWF similar to that obtained with an intravenous dose of 0.2 μg/kg desmopressin. The compression metered spray pump delivers 0.1 ml (150 μg) of solution per spray. The dose for children and adolescents is one spray; for adults a spray is given in each nostril. This highly concentrated intranasal spray is particularly useful for the treatment of menorrhagia and for prophylaxis before invasive dentistry or other minor surgery (45).

Replacement therapy with a plasma-derived intermediate-purity factor VIII concentrate rich in vWF is still needed in certain situations. For those with vWD type I whose responses to desmopressin are not sufficient (e.g., for major surgery), a clotting factor concentrate containing the higher–molecular-weight multimers of vWF (such as Aventis Behring GmbH's Humate-P (86,92), Alpha's Alphanate, or Bayer's Koate-DVI), should be given. In children younger than 2 years and in persons with histories of myocardial infarction or stroke, it is probably best to avoid the use of desmopressin to prevent any possible complications (44). For persons with vWD types 2B and 3, Humate-P (or other concentrates rich in the hemostatically important high–molecular-weight multimers of vWF) should be given for the treatment of serious bleeding episodes or for surgical prophylaxis. This also applies to those with type IIA who do not have an adequate response to desmopressin.

The optimal replacement therapy for vWD corrects both the vWF defect (quantitatively and qualitatively) and the factor VIII concentration. Because most commercial factor VIII concentrates do not contain the hemostatically important high–molecular-weight multimers of vWF, several investigators have conducted comparative studies of various products in patients with severe vWD. Humate-P was found to be most effective (86,92, 93). This pasteurized concentrate is thought to be safer than cryoprecipitate, which is not viral inactivated. For the treatment of severe bleeding or for surgical coverage in a patient with vWD type III, a dosage of 40 to 60 IU/kg factor VIII twice daily is recommended (94).

Other agents that may be useful include the antifibrinolytic drugs, ϵ-amino caproic acid and tranexamic acid, and oral contraceptive agents. For the treatment of minor mucosal bleeding, particularly in patients with mild vWD, an antifibrinolytic drug may suffice. Antifibrinolytic agents also should be used in conjunction with desmopressin or Humate-P for invasive dental procedures, tonsillectomy, or other bleeding in the oral cavity. As is true for all coagulopathies, persons with vWD should avoid aspirin, all aspirin-containing compounds, and other drugs that interfere with platelet function.

OTHER INHERITED DISORDERS OF COAGULATION

Although rare hereditary deficiencies of all the other known coagulation factors have been described, these deficiency states seem to be heterogeneous. Thus, not all affected families with a particular factor deficiency have the same degree of bleeding tendency. Because no specific clotting factor concentrates are licensed and available in the United States for use in these relatively rare deficiency states, the treatment of choice for bleeding in most of them is still plasma (solvent-detergent–treated or donor-retested) or cryoprecipitate. In general, the level required to achieve hemostasis is relatively low and thus can be attained by plasma in a dosage of 10 ml/kg. Once hemostasis has been achieved, continued treatment is seldom necessary (95). However, plasma (plasma here refers to either solvent-detergent–treated FFP or donor-retested FFP) (96) and cryoprecipitates have the disadvantages of potential viral contamination, volume overload, and allergic reactions.

Bleeding in persons with congenital afibrinogenemia or hypofibrinogenemia should be treated with cryoprecipitate in a dosage of four bags/10 kg of body weight. Cryoprecipitate contains approximately 200 mg of fibrinogen per bay, or "unit." (Because of the long half-life of fibrinogen, replacement therapy is generally given every 3 to 4 days.) Although seldom necessary, additional doses of two bags/10 kg can be given every 3 to 4 days.

In hereditary deficiencies of factors II (prothrombin), VII, or X, plasma or PCC can be used. For serious, life-threatening bleeding, PCC should be used to achieve higher levels of the missing factor. For factor V deficiency (which is usually symptomatic in homozygotes), plasma should be given. Novo Nordisk's rfVIIa (NovoSeven) is the treatment of choice for factor VII deficiency. Deficiencies of the "contact factors," factor XII (Hageman factor), prekallikrein (Fletcher factor), and high–molecular-weight kininogen (Fitzgerald factor), are rarely associated with clinical bleeding and thus do not require treatment. Although the hemorrhagic tendency in factor XI deficiency is also usually mild, on occasion excessive bruising, epistaxis, menorrhagia, and postoperative bleeding have been observed. The half-life of transfused factor XI is 60 to 80 hours. Although a factor XI concentrate is produced in England, it is not licensed for use in the United States. Fresh-frozen plasma infused at the rate of 10 to 20 ml/kg per day usually provides sufficient factor XI to maintain hemostasis. The APTT or the specific assay for factor XI or both should be used to monitor treatment.

Congenital deficiency of factor XIII (fibrin-stabilizing factor) is a rare disorder characterized by umbilical bleeding in neonates, excessive bruising, and delayed wound healing (97,98). In others, epistaxis, gingival or musculoskeletal bleeding, and severe intracranial hemorrhage after minor trauma have been reported. Only homozygous individuals with no detectable factor XIII activity have bleeding manifestations. The prothrombin time, APTT, and thrombin time are normal in factor XIII deficiency. However, the diagnosis can be made by testing for clot solubility in 5 mol urea (95). Clots formed in the presence of factor XIII deficiency are soluble in 5 mol urea or 1% monochloroacetic acid (normal plasma clots remain insoluble for 24 hours). (A more accurate assay to detect very low levels of factor XIII is available in a few highly specialized laboratories [e.g., Dr. Diane Nugent's laboratory at the Children's Hospital of Orange County, California]). Low concentrations of factor XIII (approximately 0.01 to 0.05 IU/ml of plasma) are sufficient for adequate hemostasis. Because the half-life of factor XIII is long, prophylactic therapy with factor XIII concentrates can be given with a monthly dosage of 250 IU in children and 500 IU in adults (98). Aventis Behring GmbH's Fibrogammin, although not licensed in the United States, is available on a clinical trial basis for patients with severe factor XIII deficiency. If it is not readily available for some reason, a single infusion of plasma of 5 to 10 ml/kg usually will provide effective therapy for bleeding episodes.

SUMMARY

Hemophilia A (factor VIII deficiency) and hemophilia B (factor IX deficiency) are clinically indistinguishable, sex-linked coagulopathies that affect approximately 20,000 persons in the United States. Hemophilia A is the more common of the two and accounts for 80% of the cases. In the past, the treatment of hemophilia with plasma-derived products resulted in extremely high rates of hepatitis and HIV seroconversion. However, improved donor screening tests and newer viral attenuation and purification methods have resulted in much safer plasma-derived factor VIII and factor IX concentrates. Recombinant factors VIII and IX concentrates are also available. Although the currently available plasma-derived factor VIII concentrates seem to be safe in terms of both hepatitis and HIV, one cannot be absolutely sure of the viral safety of these products, because certain non-lipid-enveloped viruses such as human Parvovirus B19 can still be transmitted by them. The majority of factor VIII and factor IX used in the United States is now recombinant (DNA-derived).

Desmopressin is considered the treatment of choice for bleeding in patients with vWD type I, with plasma-derived factor VIII concentrates rich in the high–molecular-weight multimers of vWF being used in those with type II variants and type III vWD. Fresh-frozen plasma (either solvent-detergent–treated or donor-retested) and cryoprecipitates are still used to treat many of the rare coagulation factor deficiencies.

REFERENCES

1. White GC II, Rosendaal F, Aledort LM, et al. Definitions in hemophilia. Recommendation of the Scientific Subcommittee on Factor VIII and Factor IX of the Scientific and Standardization Committee of the International Society on Thrombosis and Haemostasis. *Thromb Haemost* 2001;85:860.
2. Giannelli F, Green PM, Sommer SS, et al. Haemopihlia B. Database

of point mutations and short additions and deletions—8th edition. *Nucleic Acids Res* 1998;26:265–268.
3. Soucie JM, Evatt B, Jackson D. Occurrence of hemophilia in the United States. The hemophilia surveillance system project. *Am J Hematol* 1998;59:288–294.
4. Peake I. The molecular basis of haemophilia A. *Haemophilia* 1998;4: 346–349.
5. Ljung RCR. Prenatal diagnosis of haemophilia. *Baillieres Clin Haematol* 1996;9:243–257.
6. Rossiter JP, Young M, Kimberland ML, et al. Factor VIII gene inversions causing severe hemophilia A originate almost exclusively in male germ cells. *Hum Mol Genet* 1994;3:1035–1039.
7. Lakich D, Kazazian HH Jr, Antonarakis SE, et al. Inversions disrupting the factor VIII gene are a common cause of severe hemophilia A. *Nat Genet* 1993;5:238–241.
8. Antonarakis SE, Rossiter JP, Young M, et al. Factor VIII gene inversions in severe hemophilia A: results of an international consortium study. *Blood* 1995;86:2206–2212.
9. Pool JG, Shannon AE. Production of high potency concentrates of antihemophilic globulin in a closed bag system: assay in vitro and in vivo. *N Engl J Med* 1965;273:1443–1447.
10. Kasper CK, Lusher JM, and the Transfusion Practices Committee. Recent evolution of clotting factor concentrates for hemophilia A and B. *Transfusion* 1993;33:422–434.
11. Lee CA. Transfusion-transmitted disease. *Baillieres Clin Haematol* 1996;9:369–394.
12. Gerety RJ, Aronson DL. Plasma derivatives and viral hepatitis. *Transfusion* 1982;22:347–351.
13. Menach D. Prothrombin complex concentrates: clinical use. *Ann N Y Acad Sci* 1981;370:747–756.
14. Colombo M, Mannucci PM, Carnelli V, et al. Transmission of non-A, non-B hepatitis by heat-treated factor VIII concentrate. *Lancet* 1985; 2:1–4.
15. Centers for Disease Control. Update: acquired immunodeficiency syndrome (AIDS) in persons with hemophilia. *MMWR* 1984;33: 589–592.
16. McDougal JS, Martin LS, Cort SP, et al. Thermal inactivation of the acquired immunodeficiency syndrome virus, human T lymphotropic virus-III/lymphadenopathy associated virus, with special reference to antihemophilic factor. *J Clin Invest* 1985;76:875–877.
17. Lusher JM, Salzman P. The Monoclate study group. Viral safety and inhibitor development associated with factor VIII C ultrapurified from plasma in hemophiliacs previously unexposed to FVIII:C concentrates. *Semin Hematol* 1990;27:1–7.
18. Centers for Disease Control. Safety of therapeutic products for hemophilia patients. *MMWR* 1988;37:441–444, 449–450.
19. Zimmerman TS. Purification of factor VIII by monoclonal antibody affinity chromatography. *Semin Hematol* 1988;25[Suppl 1]:25–26.
20. Mannucci PM. Viral safety of plasma-derived and recombinant products used in the management of haemophilia A and B. *Haemophilia* 1995;1[Suppl 1]:14–20.
21. Brown P, Rohwer RG, Dunstan BC, et al. The distribution of infectivity in blood components and plasma derivatives in experimental models of transmissible spongiform encephalopathy. *Transfusion* 1998;38: 810–816.
22. Houston F, Foster JD, Chong A, et al. Transmission of BSE by blood transfusion in sheep. *Lancet* 2000;356:999–1000.
23. Toole JJ, Knopf JL, Wozney JM, et al. Molecular cloning of a cDNA encoding human antihaemophilic factor. *Nature* 1984;312:342–347.
24. Wood WI, Capon DJ, Simonsen CC, et al. Expression of active human factor VIII from recombinant DNA clones. *Nature* 1984;312: 330–337.
25. Schwartz RS, Abildgaard CF, Aledort LM, et al. Human recombinant DNA-derived antihemophilic factor (factor VIII) in the treatment of hemophilia A. *N Engl J Med* 1990;323:1800–1805.
26. Morfini M, Longo G, Messori A, et al. Pharmacokinetic properties of recombinant factor VIII compared with a monoclonally purified concentrate (Hemofil M). *Thromb Haemost* 1992;68:433–435.
27. Lusher JM, Arkin S, Abildgaard CF, et al., The Kogenate Previously Untreated Patients Study Group. Recombinant factor VIII for the treatment of previously untreated patients with hemophilia A. Safety, efficacy and development of inhibitors. *N Engl J Med* 1993;328: 453–459.
28. Bray G, Gomperts E, Courter S, et al. A multicenter study of recombinant factor VIII (Recombinate): safety, efficacy and inhibitor risk in previously untreated patients with hemophilia A. *Blood* 1994;83: 2428–2435.
29. Lusher JM, Abildgaard CF, Arkin S, et al. Human recombinant DNA-derived antihemophilic factor in the treatment of previously untreated patients with hemophilia A: final report on a hallmark clinical investigation. *Am J Hematol (in press).*
30. Toole JJ, Pittman DD, Orr EC, et al. A large region (=95 kDa) of human factor VIII is dispensable for in vitro procoagulant activity. *Proc Natl Acad Sci U S A* 1986;83:5939–5942.
31. Mikaelsson M, Eriksson B, Lin P, et al. Manufacturing and characterization of a new B-domain deleted recombinant factor VIII, r-VIII SQ. *Thromb Haemost* 1993;69:1205.
32. Sandberg A, Brandt J, Alin P, et al. Glycosylation pattern of a B-domain-deleted recombinant factor VIII molecule (r-VIII-SQ). *Thromb Haemost* 1995;73:1214.
33. Lusher JM. Recombinant clotting factor concentrates. *Baillieres Clin Haematol* 1996;9:291–303.
34. Lusher JM, Lee C, Kessler CM, et al. Safety, efficacy and inhibitor development in persons with severe hemophilia A treated with a "second generation" B-domain deleted recombinant FVIII concentrate (BDDrFVIII) *(manuscript submitted).*
35. Scharrer I , Bray GL, Neutzling O. Incidence of inhibitors in haemophilia A patients—a review of recent studies of recombinant and plasma-derived FVIII concentrates. *Haemophilia* 1999;5:145–154.
36. Mikaelsson M, Oswaldsson Y, Sandberg H. Influences of phospholipids on the assessment of factor VIII activity. *Haemophilia* 1998;4: 646–650.
37. Sandberg H, Almstedt A, Brandt J, et al. Structural and functional characteristics of the B-domain-deleted recombinant factor VIII protein, r-VIII SQ. *Thromb Haemost* 2001;85:93–100.
38. Abshire TC, Brackmann HpH, Scharrer I, et al., and the International Kogenate FS Study Group. Sucrose formulated recombinant human antihemophilic factor VIII is safe and efficacious for treatment of hemophilia A in home therapy: results of a multicenter, international clinical investigation. *Thromb Haemost* 2000;83:811.
39. Montgomery RR, Gill JC, Scott JP. Hemophilia and von Willebrand disease. In: Nathan DG, Orkin SH, eds. *Nathan and Oski's hematology of infancy and childhood,* 5th ed. Philadelphia: W.B. Saunders, 1998: 1631–1659.
40. Berntorp E. Methods of haemophilia care delivery: regular prophylaxis versus episodic treatment. *Haemophilia* 1995;1[Suppl 1]:3–7.
41. Nilsson IM, Berntorp E, Lofqvist T, et al. Twenty-five years experience of prophylactic treatment in severe haemophilia A and B. *J Intern Med* 1992;232:25–32.
42. National Hemophilia Foundation. Medical and Scientific Advisory Council (MASAC) recommendations concerning prophylaxis. Medical Bulletin 193, Chapter Advisory 197. New York: The National Hemophilia Foundation, 1994.
43. Mannucci PM. Desmopressin (DDAVP) for treatment of disorders of hemostasis. *Prog Hemost Thromb* 1986;8:19–45.
44. Lusher JM. Myocardial infarction and stroke: is the risk increased by desmopressin? In: Mariani G, Mannucci PM, Cattaneo M, eds. *Desmopressin in bleeding disorders. NATO ASI series A: life sciences.* New York: Plenum Press, 1993;42:347–353.
45. Nilsson IM, Lethagen S. Current status of DDAVP formulations and their use. In: Lusher JM, Kessler CM, eds. *Hemophilia and von Willebrand's disease in the 1990s.* Amsterdam: Excerpta Medica, 1991: 443–453.
46. Lusher JM, Miller E, Wiseman C, et al. Use of highly concentrated intranasal spray formulation of desmopressin in persons with congenital bleeding disorders. In: Mariani G, Mannucci PM, Cattaneo M, eds. *Desmopressin in bleeding disorders. NATO ASI series A: life sciences.* New York: Plenum Press, 1993:317–324.
47. Reid WO, Lucase ON, Francisco S, et al. The use of ϵ-amino caproic

acid in the management of dental extractions in the hemophiliac. *Am J Med Sci* 1964;248:184–188.
48. Sindet-Pederson S, Ingerslev J, Ramstrom G, et al. Management of oral bleeding in haemophiliac patients [Letter]. *Lancet* 1988;2:566.
49. Ragni M, Lusher JM, Koerper M, et al. Safety and immunogenicity of subcutaneous hepatitis A vaccine in children with haemophilia. *Haemophilia* 2000;2:98–103.
50. Menach, D. Factor IX concentrates. *Thromb Diath Haemorrh* 1975; 33:600–605.
51. Lusher JM. Thrombogenicity associated with factor IX complex concentrates. *Semin Hematol* 1991;28[Suppl 6]:3–5.
52. Kim HC, McMillan CW, White GC, et al. Factor IX using monoclonal immunoaffinity technique: clinical trials in hemophilia B and comparison to prothrombin complex concentrates. *Blood* 1992;79:568–575.
53. Anton DS, Austen DEG, Brownlee GG. Expression of active human clotting factor IX from recombinant DNA clones in mammalian cells. *Nature* 1985;315:683–685.
54. White GC II, Beebe A, Nielsen B. Recombinant factor IX. *Thromb Haemost* 1997;78:261–265.
55. Shapiro, A, Abshire T, Gill J, et al. Recombinant FIX (rFIX) in the treatment of previously untreated patients (PUPs) with severe or moderately severe hemophilia. *Blood* 1998;92:356a.
56. Thorland EC, Drost JB, Lusher JM, et al. Anaphylactic response to factor IX replacement therapy in haemophilia B patients: complete gene deletions confer the highest risk. *Haemophilia* 1999;5:101–105.
57. Warrier I, Ewenstein BM, Koerper MA, et al. Factor IX inhibitors and anaphylaxis in hemophilia B. *J Pediatr Hematol Oncol* 1997;19:23–27.
58. Lusher JM. F VIII inhibitors. Etiology, characterization, natural history and management. *Ann N Y Acad Sci* 1987;509:89–102.
59. Lusher JM. Inhibitors in young boys with haemophilia A and B. *Baillieres Clin Haematol* 2000;13:457–468.
60. Lusher JM. First and second generation recombinant clotting factor concentrates—results of controlled clinical trials. *Semin Thromb Hemost (in press).*
61. Lusher JM. Controlled clinical trials with prothrombin complex concentrates. *Prog Clin Biol Res* 1984;150:227–290.
62. Kernoff PBA. Porcine factor VIII: preparation and use in treatment of inhibitor patients. *Prog Clin Biol Res* 1984;150:207–224.
63. Hedner U, Feldstedt M, Glazer S. Recombinant FVIIa in hemophilia treatment. In: Lusher JM, Kessler CM, eds. *Hemophilia and von Willebrand's disease in the 1990s.* Amsterdam: Elsevier Science, 1991: 283–292.
64. Lusher JM. Recombinant activated Factor VII for treatment of intramuscular hemorrhages: a comparison of early vs. late treatment. *Blood Coagul Fibrinolysis* 1998;9[Suppl l]:111–114.
65. Lusher JM. Early treatment with recombinant Factor VIIa results in greater efficacy with less product. *Eur J Haematol* 1998;71:7–10.
66. Key NS, Aledort LM, Beardsley D, et al. Home treatment of mild to moderate bleeding episodes using recombinant factor VIIa (Novoseven) in haemophiliacs with inhibitors. *Thromb Haemost* 1998;80:912–918.
67. Monroe DM, Hoffmann M, Liver JA, et al. Platelet activity of high-dose factor VIIa is independent of tissue factor. *Br J Haematol* 1997; 99:542–547.
68. Kjalke M, Monroe DM, Hoffmann M, et al. High-dose factor VIIa restores platelet activation and total thrombin generation in a model system mimicking hemophilia A or B conditions. *Thromb Haemost* 1999;[Suppl]:303.
69. Hedner U, Glazer S, Pingel K, et al. Successful use of recombinant factor VIIa in patients with severe haemophilia A during synovectomy. *Lancet* 1988;2:1193.
70. Hedner U, Ingerslev J. Clinical use of recombinant FVIIa. *Transfus Sci* 1998;19:163–176.
71. Lindley CM, Sawyer WT, Macik G, et al. Pharmacokinetics and pharmacodynamics of recombinant factor VIIa. *Clin Pharmacol Ther* 1994; 55:638–648.
72. Lusher JM, Roberts HR, Davignon G, et al., and the rFVIIa Study Group. A randomized, double-blind comparison of two dosage levels of rFVIIa in the treatment of joint, muscle and mucocutaneous haemorrhages in persons with haemophilia A with and without inhibitors. *Haemophilia* 1998;4:790–798.
73. Key NS, Aledort LM, Beardsley D, et al. Home treatment of mild to moderate bleeding episodes using recombinant factor VIIa (Novoseven) in haemophiliacs with inhibitors. *Thromb Haemost* 1998;80:912–918.
74. Shapiro AD, Gilchrist GS, Hoots WK, et al. Prospective, randomized trial of two doses of rFVIIa in haemophilia patients with inhibitors undergoing surgery. *Thromb Haemost* 1998;80:773–778.
75. Hedner U, Kristensen HI, Berntorp E, et al. Pharmacokinetics of rFVIIa in children. In: Uri Martinowitz, ed. Abstracts of the XXIII International Congress of the World Federation of Hemophilia, The Hague, Netherlands, 17–21 May 1998. *Haemophilia* 1998;4:no. 3(abst).
76. Brackmann HH. Induced immune tolerance in Factor VIII inhibitor patients. *Prog Clin Biol Res* 1986;150:181–195.
77. Ewing NP, Sanders NL, Dietrich SL, et al. Induction of immune tolerance to factor VIII in hemophiliacs with inhibitors. *JAMA* 1988;259: 65–68.
78. van Leeuwen EF, Mauser-Bunschoten EP, van Kijken PJ, et al. Disappearance of factor VIII:C antibodies in patients with haemophilia A upon frequent administration of factor VIII in intermediate or low dose. *Br J Haematol* 1986;64:291–297.
79. Zimmerman R, Kommerell B, Harenberg J, et al. Intravenous IgG for patients with spontaneous inhibitor to factor VIII. *Lancet* 1985;1: 273–274.
80. Nilsson IM, Berntorp E, Zetterfall O. Induction of immune tolerance in patients with hemophilia and antibodies to factor VIII by combined treatment with intravenous IgG, cyclophosphamide and factor VIII. *N Engl J Med* 1988;318:947–950.
81. Ewenstein B, Takemoto C, Warrier I, et al. Nephrotic syndrome as a complication of immune tolerance in hemophilia B. *Blood* 1997;89: 115–116.
82. Mancuso DI, Tuley EA, Westfield LA, et al. Structure of the gene for human von Willebrand factor. *J Biol Chem* 1989;264:19514–19527.
83. Gill JC, Endres-Brooks J, Bauer PJ, et al. The effect of ABO blood group on the diagnosis of von Willebrand disease. *Blood* 1987;69: 1691–1695.
84. Sadler JE, Matsushita T, Dong Z, et al. Molecular mechanism and classification of von Willebrand disease. *Thromb Haemost* 1995;74: 161–166.
85. Sporn LA, Marder VJ, Wagner DD. Von Willebrand factor released from Weibel-Palade bodies binds more avidly to extracellular matrix than that secreted constitutively. *Blood* 1987;69:1531–1534.
86. Lethagen S. Von Willebrand's disease. Pathogenesis and clinical aspects. *Crit Rev Oncol Hematol* 1993;15:1–11.
87. Wagner DD, Marder VJ. Biosynthesis of von Willebrand protein by human endothelial cells: processing steps and their intracellular location. *J Cell Biol* 1984;99:2123–2130.
88. Sadler JE. A revised classification of von Willebrand disease. *Thromb Haemost* 1994;71:520–525.
89. Mauzrier C. Von Willebrand disease masquerading as haemophilia A. *Thromb Haemost* 1992;67:391–396.
90. Mannucci PM, Bettega D, Cattaneo M. Patterns of development of tachyphylaxis in patients with haemophilia and von Willebrand disease after repeated doses of desmopressin (DDAVP). *Br J Haematol* 1992; 82:87–93.
91. Holmberg L, Nilsson IM, Borge L, et al. Platelet aggregation induced by 1-deamino-8-D-arginine vasopressin (DDAVP) in type IIB von Willebrand's disease. *N Engl J Med* 1983;309:816–821.
92. Mannucci PM, Tenconi PM, Castaman G, et al. Comparison of four virus-inactivated plasma concentrates for treatment of severe von Willebrand disease: a cross-over randomized trial. *Blood* 1992;79: 3130–3137.
93. Lethagen S, Berntorp E, Nilsson IM. Pharmacokinetics and hemostatic effect of different factor VIII/von Willebrand factor concentrates in von Willebrand's disease type III. *Ann Hematol* 1992;65:253–259.
94. Holmberg L, Nilsson IM. Von Willebrand's disease. *Eur J Haematol* 1992;48:127–141.

95. Colman RW, Hirsh J, Marder VJ, et al., eds. *Hemostasis and thrombosis: basic principles and clinical practice,* 2nd ed. Philadelphia: JB Lippincott, 1987.
96. National Hemophilia Foundation. *MASAC resolution concerning plasma transfusion alternative.* New York: The National Hemophilia Foundation, 1998.
97. McDonagh J. Structure and function of factor XIII. In: Colman RW, Hirsh J, Marder VJ, et al., eds. *Hemostasis and thrombosis: basic principles and clinical practice,* 2nd ed. Philadelphia: JB Lippincott, 1987: 289–300.
98. Losowsky MS, Miloszewski KJA. Annotation: factor XIII. *Br J Haematol* 1977;37:1–5.

Rossi's Principles of Transfusion Medicine, Third Edition, edited by Toby L. Simon, Walter H. Dzik, Edward L. Snyder, Christopher P. Stowell, and Ronald G. Strauss. Lippincott Williams & Wilkins, Philadelphia © 2002.

32

MANAGEMENT OF CONGENITAL HEMOLYTIC ANEMIAS

BRUCE I. SHARON
GEORGE R. HONIG

The congenital hemolytic anemias comprise a heterogeneous group of intrinsic red blood cell abnormalities that may be conveniently classified as disorders of hemoglobin (hemoglobinopathies and thalassemia syndromes), red blood cell enzyme–deficiency disorders, and abnormalities of the red blood cell membrane and cytoskeleton. In patients affected with any of these conditions, red blood cell transfusions may be indicated to compensate for the decreased oxygen-carrying capacity associated with the underlying anemia but, in addition, pathophysiologic consequences unique to each of these disorders may lead to other indications for transfusion. The hemoglobin-related abnormalities have special significance in clinical transfusion medicine, and particular emphasis is devoted to this group of disorders.

HEMOGLOBINOPATHIES AND THALASSEMIAS

The hemoglobinopathies are characterized by structural changes affecting the protein globin portion of the hemoglobin molecule, resulting from deoxyribonucleic acid (DNA) mutations in the corresponding globin genes. Most forms of thalassemia, on the other hand, are characterized by the production of diminished quantities of globin chains that are structurally normal. In certain globin-gene disorders, the molecular defect produces both a quantitative and a qualitative abnormality; examples include hemoglobin (Hb) E (a β-globin abnormality) and Hb Constant Spring (an α-globin abnormality). This discussion on hemoglobin disorders focuses on sickle cell disease and the α and β thalassemias.

B.I. Sharon and G.R. Honig: Department of Pediatrics, University of Illinois College of Medicine and University of Illinois Hospital, Chicago, Illinois.

Sickle Cell Disease

Epidemiology

The geographic distribution of the sickle globin (β^S) gene in the Old World is shown in Figure 32.1. The greatest concentration of individuals carrying this gene is localized in central West Africa, where the gene frequency for sickle hemoglobin (HbS) may be as high as 0.14. Appreciable numbers of affected individuals have also been identified in other parts of equatorial Africa, the Mediterranean, and parts of the Saudi Arabian peninsula and India. This distribution substantially coincides with regions that historically have had endemic falciparum malaria. Ample epidemiologic evidence suggests that the β^S gene was subject to positive selection pressure because of the survival advantage that it confers in heterozygous individuals who are infected by the malarial parasite. In the New World, the β^S gene arrived as a result of the importation of slaves from Africa; in North America its gene frequency is approximately 0.04 to 0.05 among those of African descent. (Thus, approximately 10% of American blacks are sickle heterozygotes.)

Molecular and Cellular Pathophysiology

The fundamental defect in sickle cell disease is the substitution of thymine for adenine in the sixth codon of the gene for the β-globin chain, leading to a replacement of glutamic acid by valine at this site. In contrast to normal hemoglobin tetramers, HbS has an altered surface charge that promotes the formation of lengthy polymeric chains (gelation) when in the deoxygenated state. The oxygen affinity of dilute, unpolymerized HbS is similar to that of normal hemoglobin. However, the oxygen affinity of concentrated HbS solutions is decreased (1), thereby representing a further stimulus for molecular polymerization.

Once a critical nucleation step has been achieved, the polymerization process may quickly progress to form rapidly lengthening fibers, which can further organize into filaments and even

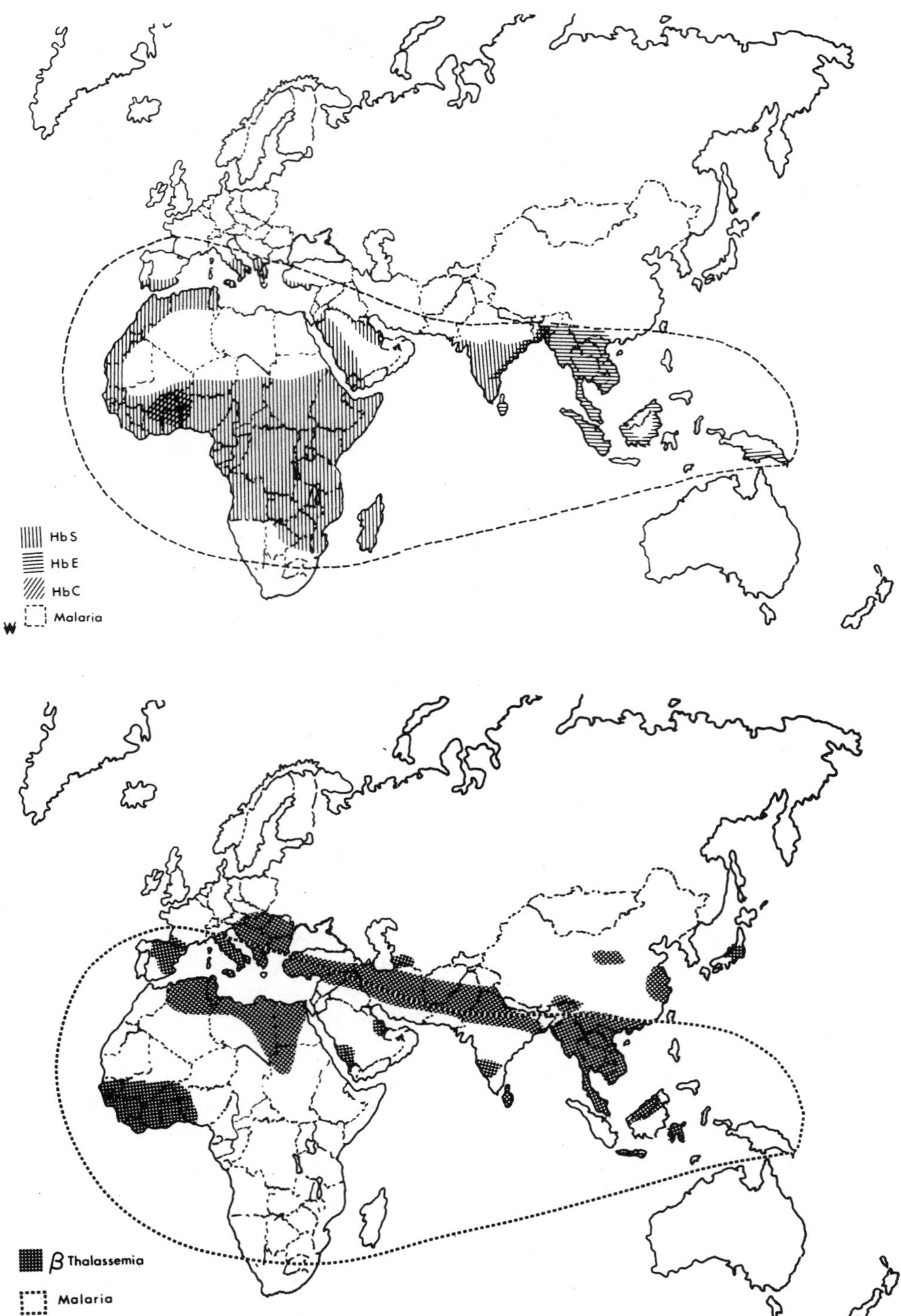

FIGURE 32.1. The geographic distribution of hemoglobins S, C, and E *(upper panel)* and β thalassemia *(lower panel)*. The regions where falciparum malaria was formerly endemic are also indicated. (From Honig GR, Adams JG III. *Human hemoglobin genetics.* Vienna: Springer-Verlag, 1986:238, with permission.)

thicker strands. At the cellular level, this is reflected by the conversion of normal, deformable, biconcave red blood cells to rigid, highly viscous erythrocytes with the characteristic sickle shape. For the most part, the process of sickle hemoglobin gelation and erythrocyte sickling is a reversible one, but after repeated cycles these cells may become irreversibly sickled cells (ISCs). These ISCs maintain an abnormal sickled shape even in the absence of HbS polymerization and are probably a consequence of cumulative red blood cell membrane damage sustained during repeated sickle-unsickle cycles. Irreversibly sickled cells are much more rigid than biconcave red blood cells and have a much shorter life span, thus appreciably contributing to the hemolytic anemia that is characteristic of this disorder. Curiously, there is no close correlation between the percentage of circulating ISCs in an individual and the clinical severity of the disease.

As the process of sickling progresses and an increasing number of cells assume the sickle shape and become rigid, blood viscosity rises sharply. This change causes a marked delay in the transit of blood through the microvasculature, which in turn leads to increased oxygen extraction at the local tissue level. The resultant decrease in hemoglobin oxygen saturation further increases the propensity toward sickling, thus completing a self-propagating cycle.

A critical determinant for the initiation of the sickling process is the intraerythrocytic concentration of deoxygenated HbS (deoxy-HbS). As the concentration of deoxy-HbS rises, the delay time (i.e., the time required to achieve a critical minimum polymer nucleus) diminishes exponentially, approximately on the order of the 15th to 30th magnitude (2). Several genetic and cellular (erythrocyte) modulators of disease severity have been proposed and are reviewed below (3,4). Some act by altering the intraerythrocytic concentration of HbS, whereas others exert their effect through unrelated and, in some cases, undetermined mechanisms.

Genetic factors that contribute most importantly to the severity of sickle cell disease include the concurrence of a thalassemia, β^0 or β^+ thalassemia, or any of a number of other hemoglobin abnormalities including HbC, HbD, HbO, and syndromes of hereditary persistence of fetal hemoglobin (HPFH) (see Sickle Cell Syndromes).

Other genetic determinants of the clinical expression of sickle cell disease appear to be related to the DNA "background" upon which the sickle mutation is found. The β-globin gene cluster is located on the short arm of chromosome 11 and contains the β-, δ-, and γ-globin genes, whose globin chain products, in combination with α chains, form hemoglobins A, A_2, and F, respectively. The DNA "haplotype" of a given region is defined by the local array of restriction endonuclease fragment–length polymorphisms. Three major DNA haplotypes have been described for the African β^S-globin region (5), and it appears that at least certain measures of sickle cell disease severity may correlate with the different DNA haplotypes, probably in large part because of the differences they mediate in fetal hemoglobin (HbF) expression. Despite the influence that these genetic factors may have on the expression of sickle cell disease, they clearly are not the sole determinants of disease severity. Individuals with apparently identical globin genotypes can vary markedly in their clinical courses.

A variety of erythrocyte-related factors have also been implicated as possible modulators of disease severity (3,4). They include the erythrocyte levels of 2,3-diphosphoglycerate (2,3-DPG; also known as 2,3-bisphosphoglycerate) or adenosine triphosphate, glucose-6-phosphate dehydrogenase (G6PD) deficiency, calcium or zinc deficiency, the ISC count, the degree of intraerythrocytic polymerization of deoxy-HbS, and the degree of cellular dehydration (3,4).

Increasingly, the role of extra-erythrocytic factors in the vasoocclusive process is being appreciated. Sickle red blood cells have increased adherence to vascular endothelium (6), and this property appears to have a strong correlation with the severity of vasoocclusive disease (7). Nitric oxide is an important vasodilator that is synthesized by the vascular endothelium (8), and low levels in sickle cell disease may contribute to the pathophysiology of complications such as acute chest syndrome (ACS) and stroke (9,10). Elevated plasma homocysteine levels, probably related to folic acid deficiency, appear to be associated with an increased risk of stroke (11). Various clinical findings in young children with sickle cell disease, including early onset of dactylitis, severity of anemia, and presence of leukocytosis, appear to be predictive for disease severity (12,13).

Mechanisms of Anemia

The anemia of sickle cell (HbSS) disease is characterized by increased peripheral destruction of the HbS-containing red blood cells. Progressive membrane damage to these spiny, brittle, poorly deformable erythrocytes is further intensified by secondary changes, including alterations in membrane lipid composition and oxidant damage. Erythrocyte production is substantially increased, in partial compensation for the rapid peripheral destruction. However, compensation is incomplete because of the rightward shift of the oxygen-hemoglobin binding curve that results from deoxy-HbS polymerization. The red blood cell life span in patients with sickle cell disease is approximately 5 to 20 days. Sickle cell complications, including acute splenic sequestration crisis (ASSC) and aplastic crisis, may intensify the anemia (see Clinical Features). In addition, other conditions common in sickle cell patients may contribute to anemia, including fever or infection or both, immune hemolysis, G6PD deficiency, and folic acid deficiency.

Sickle Cell Syndromes

Because of the prevalence of other α- and β-globin mutations within the African sickle cell population, sickle cell disease is a heterogeneous group of disorders. In each individual syndrome, the primary determinants of sickling are the intracellular concentration of HbS and the propensity of other nonsickle globins present within the cell to participate in the polymerization process. Fetal hemoglobin is virtually totally resistant to incorporation into sickle globin polymers, whereas both adult hemoglobin (HbA) and HbC participate to some degree in this process. However, patients with HbSC disease have a higher percentage of HbS in their erythrocytes than do individuals with sickle cell trait (HbAS). In addition, HbSC erythrocytes have a membrane defect that leads to intracellular dehydration, causing a further

TABLE 32.1. HEMATOLOGIC VALUES ASSOCIATED WITH COMMON SICKLE CELL SYNDROMES IN ADULTS

Hemoglobin Genotype	Hemoglobin Concentration (g/dl)	Mean Cell Volume (fL)	Hb F (%)
Hb AA (normal)[a]	12–18	80–100	1
Hb AS[a]	12–16	82–92	1
Hb SS	6.5–9.5	80–98	2–20
Hb S/β^0 thalassemia	6.0–12.5	63–88	1.4–20
Hb S/β+ thalassemia	6.5–14.0	62–84	1–15
Hb SC	8.5–12	82–92	1–8
Hb S/HPFH[b]	7–18	75–89	15–85
Hb SS/α-thal trait	7.5–10	60–80	5–20

[a]No associated clinical disease; included for comparison.
[b]Hereditary persistence of fetal hemoglobin.

increase in the intraerythrocytic hemoglobin concentration (14). Because of both these factors, HbSC erythrocytes are far more likely to undergo sickling than are HbAS cells. As would be predicted from these differences, the relative expected disease severity is: HbSS, HbS/β^0 thalassemia > HbSC, HbS/β^+ thalassemia > HbS/HPFH > HbAS. Concomitant α thalassemia in individuals with HbSS disease does not appear to impose a significant change in the frequency of pain crises. However, some forms of chronic organ damage may be increased in this disorder because of higher hemoglobin levels, which could lead to increased blood viscosity (15). Characteristic hematologic indices of some of the important sickle syndromes are shown in Table 32.1.

Clinical Features

At birth, infants with homozygous sickle cell disease (HbSS) are clinically and hematologically normal because of the predominance of HbF during this period. During the ensuing several months, as the percentage of HbF naturally declines, anemia and other hematologic abnormalities become increasingly apparent. Susceptibility to clinical sequelae of sickle cell disease typically begins at 3 to 6 months of age. The hallmark clinical expressions of sickle cell disease are acute sickle cell "crises."

Acute Sickle Cell Crises

Acute Pain Crisis These episodes, which are believed to result from vasoocclusion, account for the majority of hospitalizations of sickle cell patients in the United States. Pain crises may involve practically any area of the body but most often are musculoskeletal or soft tissue in origin. These episodes may be brought on by a variety of initiating conditions, including fever, infection, acidosis, and hypoxia, but frequently there is no identifiable precipitant. Occasionally, pain crises may be so severe as to be unresponsive to high-dose narcotic analgesia, and they may occur with great enough frequency to be debilitating and severely disruptive of school or work. Acute dactylitis ("hand-foot syndrome") involves the distal extremities and characteristically occurs in infancy. Frequently, this complication represents the initial identifiable clinical event in children with sickle cell disease.

Acute Splenic Sequestration Crisis In patients with sickle cell disease, repetitive microocclusive events occur in the spleen throughout early childhood, so that by adulthood the spleen is often "autoinfarcted" and lacks any appreciable blood circulation. Prior to reaching this state, and primarily in early childhood, the spleen is subject to acute obstruction by sickle cells in the efferent circulation. In about one-half of reported cases, there was an antecedent history of infectious illness. Splenic sequestration is a rapidly progressive and potentially fatal process. The clinical course may progress from a state of relative well-being to circulatory shock within just a few hours. Upon admission, the hemoglobin concentration may be as low as 2 g/dl. Forewarning of family members to seek medical attention promptly and the rapid institution of vigorous resuscitation measures, including transfusion, are critical in reducing fatalities from this complication. The period of risk for acute splenic sequestration is typically prolonged until the early adult years in patients with the milder sickle syndromes (e.g., HbSC and HbS/β^+ thalassemia).

Aplastic Crisis This complication typically occurs in children of an age and antecedent history similar to those of children who experience splenic sequestration. Aplastic crisis is a transient, self-limited condition but is not without risk, because profound degrees of anemia may result, with hemoglobin concentrations as low as 2 to 3 g/dl. A human parvovirus has been found to be etiologic in most, if not all, cases (16). This virus is also responsible for the development of aplastic episodes in other congenital hemolytic anemias.

Stroke

In addition to the pain episodes that apparently result from vasoocclusion, patients with sickle cell disease may also experience major, in some cases catastrophic, ischemic events. Sickle vasoocclusion in the cerebral circulation may cause cerebrovascular accidents, producing hemiplegia, seizures, and coma or death. In children, strokes usually are caused by cerebral infarction, whereas subarachnoid or cerebral hemorrhages become more prevalent with advancing age. Over two-thirds of strokes in patients with sickle cell disease occur during childhood, and approximately 8% to 11% of children with sickle cell disease suffer from stroke (17). In the absence of further intervention, approximately two-thirds of sickle cell patients with stroke will have a recurrent episode, usually within 3 years (17). Functional recovery after a first stroke is variable, and subsequent episodes may produce additional and frequently more devastating sequelae. The acute mortality in adult patients is especially high and may approach 50%. Acute cerebral events that produce focal neurologic deficits lasting less than 24 to 48 hours—transient ischemic attacks (TIAs)—may be a harbinger of stroke in these patients.

Acute Chest Syndrome

The clinical picture of ACS includes fever, cough, chest pain, hypoxia, and pulmonary infiltrates visible on the chest radiograph. Regardless of whether the primary pathophysiologic process is pulmonary vasoocclusion or pneumonia, the clinical picture is often similar. Especially in young children, one complication may be associated with the other.

Among those patients with an infectious etiology of ACS, the most common pathogens are *Chlamydia pneumoniae, Mycoplasma pneumoniae,* and respiratory syncytial virus. Pulmonary fat embolism, presumably caused by infarction of bone during a vasoocclusive event, is another important cause of ACS (18).

Sickling in the Liver

Sickling in the liver produces sharp right upper quadrant abdominal pain, hyperbilirubinemia, and other abnormal liver function values. The clinical picture often resembles that seen in acute cholelithiasis. Because asymptomatic gallstones are coincidentally seen in approximately one-half of all young adult patients with sickle cell disease, it is important to distinguish between the two conditions to avoid unnecessary cholecystectomy.

Priapism

Prolonged, painful, and unwanted penile erection occurs in up to 89% of male patients with sickle cell disease (19) and results from impaired venous outflow from the corpora cavernosa. Common clinical pictures include erection lasting only a few hours, which may be only moderately painful with no long-term sequelae, or prolonged erection, which often results in severe pain, difficulty in urination, and impotence.

Hematuria

Patients with sickle cell disease may experience episodes of gross hematuria, often in association with renal papillary necrosis. If hematuria is sufficiently severe or prolonged, it may intensify the degree of anemia.

Chronic Effects of Sickle Cell Disease

Chronic organ damage from sickle cell disease may produce an additional spectrum of disease manifestations.

Cardiac Effects Cardiomegaly, especially left ventricular hypertrophy, most often reflects chronic anemia, but may also result from sickle cardiomyopathy. Even though the coronary circulation is a site of high oxygen extraction, the incidence of myocardial infarction is diminished in sickle cell patients. Apparently, the short transit time through the coronary circulation is less than the delay time for sickling.

Pulmonary Effects Chronic lung disease with ventilation-perfusion mismatch or reduction in lung volume may result from repeated or severe episodes of pneumonia or pulmonary infarction.

Hepatobiliary Effects Cholelithiasis occurs in approximately 40% to 50% of patients with sickle cell disease by the time they reach young adulthood, but in the majority of cases it is asymptomatic and does not require surgery unless there is biochemical or radiologic evidence of biliary obstruction.

Renal Effects The renal medulla is a hypertonic, acidotic environment that readily encourages intravascular sickling. Beginning in early childhood, intrarenal ischemia leads to an impaired ability to concentrate urine maximally (hyposthenuria). Infrequently, patients with sickle cell disease may also develop nephrotic syndrome and overt renal failure. Their anemia may also worsen in the face of frank renal failure.

Skeletal Effects Sickle cell–induced infarction of the vertebral bodies causes a "fishmouth" appearance of the vertebrae on radiographic examination. Aseptic necrosis of the femoral heads produces Legg-Perthes–like radiographic changes and occurs particularly frequently in adults with HbSC disease.

Dermal Effects Adolescent and adult sickle cell patients are prone to develop leg ulcers, usually in the anterior tibial region or adjacent to the medial malleolus. When severe, leg ulcers adversely affect mobility, employability, and overall quality of life.

Ophthalmic Effects Patients with sickle cell disease are at increased risk for retinal disease, which may occur in a variety of forms. Nonproliferative lesions, which frequently can be identified by direct ophthalmoscopic examination, are usually not severe. Proliferative retinopathy occurs primarily in adolescent or older patients with HbSC or HbS/β^+ thalassemia (20) and can progress to blindness; indirect ophthalmoscopy and fluorescein angiography may be required to detect the characteristic retinal vascular changes.

Constitutional Effects of Sickle Cell Disease

Patients with sickle cell disease are subject to two major adverse constitutional effects: increased morbidity from infection and impaired growth and development. These patients have impaired host defense function with increased susceptibility, particularly to bacterial infections. In the absence of intervention, young children with sickle cell disease are at increased risk for pneumococcal infections, with a frequency approximately 400 times that in normal children, and *Haemophilus influenzae* infections occur at about 2 to 4 times the usual rate. Both the absolute and relative risks of those infections have undoubtedly declined substantially with the advent of vaccines specific for them, but they nonetheless continue to pose a significant threat. In addition, bouts of infection are considerably more severe and protracted in patients with sickle cell disease, compared to normal individuals. In the growth of children with sickle cell disease, weight gain is characteristically affected more than height, and the degree of impairment correlates well with the overall severity of the sickle cell disorder. Sexual maturation may also be delayed.

Transfusion Therapy in Sickle Cell Disease

The chronic anemia of sickle cell disease is usually well tolerated, but during intercurrent illnesses red blood cell transfusions may be required. Transfusions may also be indicated in order to limit or prevent vasoocclusive complications, either acute or chronic. As indicated in Table 32.2, some of the complications of sickle cell disease are characterized by both anemia and vasoocclusive manifestations. In general, for complications in which anemia is the predominant concern, traditional transfusion goals such as adequate hemoglobin concentration are appropriate. In contrast, for complications in which sickle cell vasoocclusion is the

TABLE 32.2. ACUTE AND CHRONIC COMPLICATIONS OF SICKLE CELL DISEASE THAT MAY REQUIRE TRANSFUSION BECAUSE OF ANEMIA OR VASOOCCLUSION

	Anemia	Anemia and Vasoocclusion	Vasoocclusion
Acute	Aplastic crisis	Acute chest syndrome Acute splenic sequestration Acute papillary necrosis Sepsis	Stroke Priapism Intractable pain crisis
Chronic	Pregnancy Hematuria Chronic renal failure Cardiac failure	Surgery Pregnancy, high-risk	Skin ulcer Prophylaxis for: Stroke Splenic sequestration Angiography Intractable pain

overriding concern, the primary objective of red blood cell transfusion is to achieve a favorable balance between the relative concentrations of normal and sickle red blood cells.

Aplastic Crisis

Because the life span of sickle red blood cells is only 5 to 20 days, any temporary cessation of erythrocyte production will lead to severe anemia within a short time. On the other hand, aplastic crisis is characteristically self-limited, and spontaneous recovery usually occurs within a few days of onset. Decisions regarding transfusion must take into account the patient's clinical status as well as the hemoglobin concentration and any evidence of recovery, as reflected by the reticulocyte count. When possible, an early decision about transfusion may help to diminish the period of mandatory close observation and shorten the hospital stay. In some cases, a bone marrow aspirate evaluation may be helpful by providing an estimate of the expected time to recovery of erythropoiesis. Transfusion to or near baseline hemoglobin levels is sufficient, and under such circumstances there need not be concern that transfusion will delay the recovery from bone marrow aplasia.

Transfusion in Patients with Sickle Cell Vasoocclusion

The purpose of transfusion in the management of sickle cell vasoocclusion is to diminish the likelihood of intravascular sickling through the dilution and replacement of the recipient's sickle cells by transfused, nonsickleable cells. Clinical experience has shown that vasoocclusion is unlikely to occur with mixtures of AA (normal) and SS (sickle) cells if the relative concentration of HbS-containing cells is less than 30% to 40%. This finding is supported by in vitro data from Lessin et al. (21), who showed that the relative resistance to flow of mixtures of AA and SS red blood cells rose sharply when the proportion of SS cells exceeded 40%. Schmalzer et al. (22) showed that at a fixed concentration of sickle cells (H_S/H_T or H_S alone, where H_T is the total hematocrit and H_S is the hematocrit of sickle cells), the viscosity (η) rose with the hematocrit (H_T), owing to the addition of AA cells (Figs. 32.2 and 32.3). These authors also showed that deoxygenation does not change the viscosity of AA cells but causes appreciable increases in the viscosity of SS cells, especially at higher hematocrits (Fig. 32.2). The rise in viscosity was steepest with higher H_S values, and at fixed absolute (H_S) or relative (H_S/H_T) concentrations of sickle cells the effective oxygen delivery (H_T/η) (22) declined when H_T rose through the physiologic range (20% to 40%) (Fig. 32.4). This effect, too, was more pronounced with higher H_S (or H_S/H_T). These results indicate that in suspensions of normal cells (H_S or H_S/H_T = O), as H_T rises, the benefit provided by increased oxygen-carrying capacity is nearly equally offset by the adverse effect of increased viscosity, so that the effective oxygen delivery remains nearly constant (Fig. 32.4). On the other hand, in the presence of sickle cells (higher H_S or H_S/H_T), the effect upon viscosity predominates and a net decrease in the effective oxygen delivery results. These data strongly emphasize the rheologic advantages of exchange

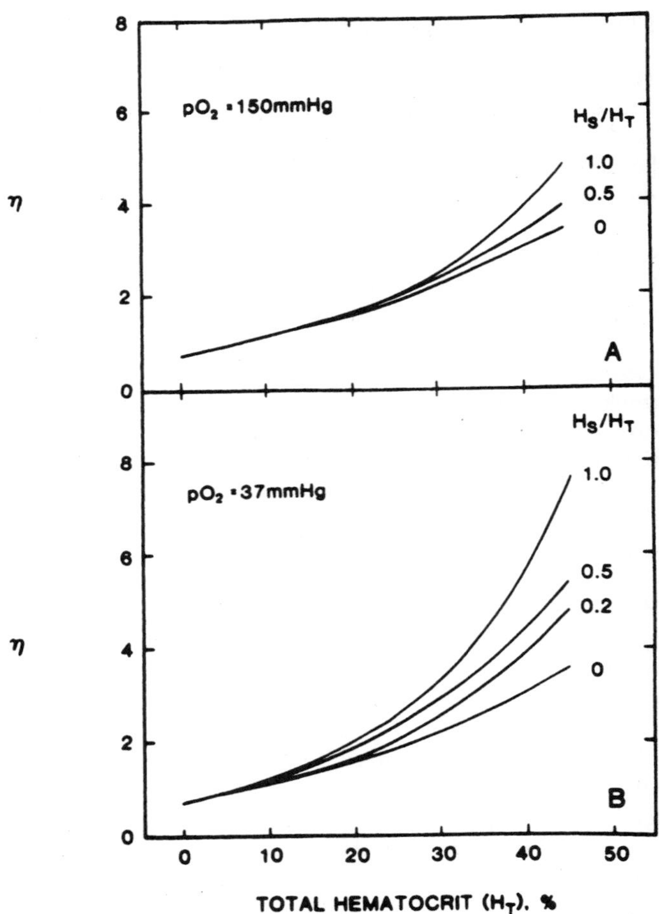

FIGURE 32.2. The rise of viscosity (η) with H_T at given proportions of sickle cells to total cells (H_S/H_T) in the suspension. (See text for definition of terms.) **A,** Oxygenated cell suspensions. **B,** Deoxygenated suspensions. (From Schmalzer EA, Lee JO, Brown AK, et al. Viscosity of mixtures of sickle and normal red blood cells at varying hematocrit levels. *Transfusion* 1987;27:228–233, with permission.)

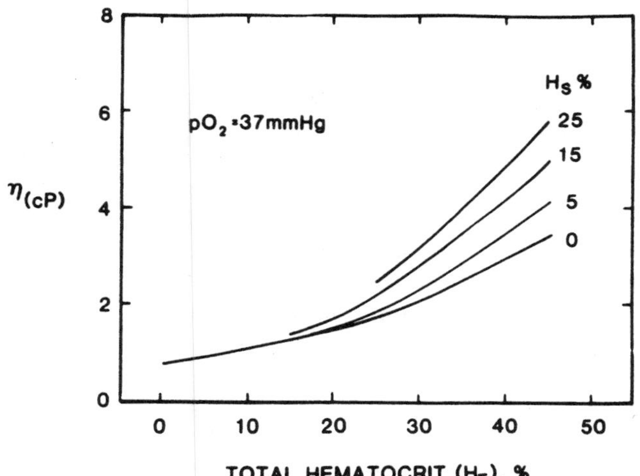

FIGURE 32.3. The data from Figure 32.2 *(lower)* replotted to show the rise in viscosity (η) with H_T at various hematocrit levels of sickle cells (H_S). (From Schmalzer EA, Lee JO, Brown AK, et al. Viscosity of mixtures of sickle and normal red blood cells at varying hematocrit levels. *Transfusion* 1987;27:228–233, with permission.)

transfusion over simple transfusion when used in the management of patients with sickle cell vasoocclusion. Either type of transfusion produces relative enrichment of normal over sickle cells, but the exchange method has the added benefits of rapidly diminishing H_S and limiting the rise in H_T. Both effects are helpful in reducing viscosity and improving oxygen delivery to tissues (Fig. 32.4).

The distribution of HbS among the erythrocytes significantly influences the overall likelihood of sickling. For example, in mixtures of AA and SS erythrocytes the SS cells fully retain the capacity to sickle, whereas AA cells, of course, lack any potential to sickle. Similarly, in HbSC disease or other clinically significant compound heterozygous condition, each HbS-containing cell retains the potential to sickle under suitable physiologic conditions. When planning transfusions for managing sickle vasoocclusion in individuals with compound heterozygous conditions, it is therefore most prudent not to focus on the percentage of the HbS, but rather to consider the percentage of cells that are sickleable. For example, if the recommendation for a particular indication in HbSS disease is to achieve a HbS concentration of 30%, it should be reinterpreted in HbSC disease to mean that transfusion should achieve 30% sickleable cells (yielding approximately 15% HbS) or an HbA concentration of 70%.

Stroke

A primary element in the acute therapy of stroke in patients with sickle cell disease is exchange transfusion to limit further intracerebral sickling. At a minimum, a single-volume exchange should be performed, with the aim of achieving an HbS concentration of approximately 30%. In more severe cases, a greater level of protection may be desirable during the acute phase; a double-volume exchange would be expected to reduce the level of HbS to approximately 10%.

The recurrence rate of stroke in sickle cell patients is high. Chronic transfusion to maintain the HbS concentration below 30% to 40% has been effective in reducing the incidence and severity of recurrent neurologic events (23). However, this beneficial effect may be temporary, lasting only for the duration of transfusion therapy. For example, the incidence of recurrence is reduced to less than 10% during transfusion therapy but increases again within 1 year after the cessation of transfusions (24). The appropriate duration of therapy, therefore, remains a vexing clinical question. Prolonged transfusion therapy lasting 3 years or longer is likely to result in arteriographic improvement (23) or at least will halt radiologically detectable disease progression, but it is unclear when, or even if, transfusion therapy can be safely discontinued.

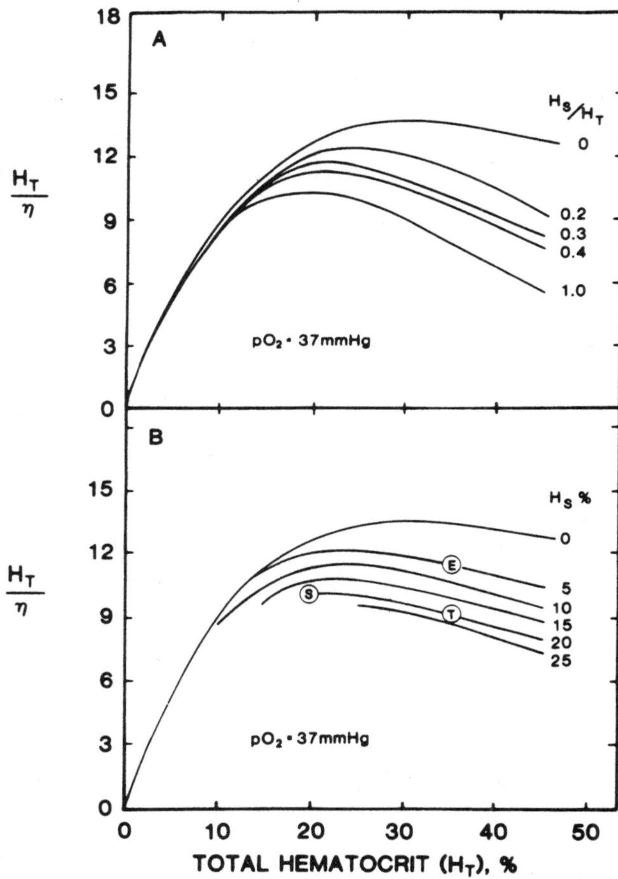

FIGURE 32.4. The H_T/η ratio for suspensions containing mixtures of AA and SS cells. **A,** Increasing H_S/H_T ratios cause a lowering of the H_T/η curve. **B,** The same data as in A is plotted with constant levels of H_S. The relative merits of simple versus exchange transfusion can be analyzed by using the curves for H_T/η **(B)** to illustrate a hypothetical patient. *Point S* represents a patient with sickle cell disease with H_T = H_S = 20% before transfusion treatment. After simple transfusion to raise the H_T to 35%, *Point S* moves along the same H_T/η curve (H_S = 20%) to *Point T,* and there is a drop of about 11% in oxygen delivery (H_T/η). However, if an exchange transfusion is carried out to lower the H_T level of the patient to 5%, although the H_T is raised to 35% with AA cells, the result would be at *Point E,* where the H_T/η is 11% more than at *Point S* and about 23% more than at *Point T.* (From Schmalzer EA, Lee JO, Brown AK, et al. Viscosity of mixtures of sickle and normal red blood cells at varying hematocrit levels. *Transfusion* 1987;27:228–233, with permission.)

The following management of stroke is advised. The acute exchange transfusion aims to achieve rapid reduction of circulating sickle cells to less than 30%. If cerebral angiography is planned, a further decrease of HbS to 20% should be achieved. Chronic transfusion therapy to maintain the HbS concentration at less than 30% is advised for at least 3 to 5 years. Usually, this requires packed red blood cell transfusions of 10 to 15 ml/kg every 2 to 4 weeks. Transfusion therapy should be monitored by hemoglobin electrophoresis for determination of the percentage of HbA and HbS, as well as hemoglobin and reticulocyte determinations. If frequent electrophoretic measurements are impractical, it may be possible to estimate an individual's transfusion requirement with reasonable accuracy by measuring the reticulocyte count and hemoglobin level after the patient's individual pattern has been established (25). Currently, there are insufficient data to determine the desirability of continuing transfusions indefinitely. Weighing the potential risks and benefits of long-term transfusion requires individualized decisions based upon such factors as recurrence of neurologic symptoms while receiving transfusion therapy and complications resulting from transfusions, such as hepatitis, alloimmunization, and iron overload. Because there is no close correlation between cerebral arteriographic findings, stroke severity, or risk of recurrence, cerebral arteriography may be of limited usefulness. In order to diminish the transfusion load, it may be preferable to relax the transfusion criteria after 5 years and maintain the level of HbS at less than 50% (26).

All these treatment considerations unfortunately underscore a great deficiency in the attempt to prevent stroke in sickle cell patients—they are designed to prevent a second stroke, but ignore the considerable morbidity that occurred as a result of the first event. Is there a reliable means to identify patients prospectively who are at high risk for developing a first stroke, so that they can be offered prophylactic therapy? Children with elevated cerebral blood flow velocity, as measured by transcranial Doppler (TCD) ultrasonography, have an increased risk for developing stroke during the several years following abnormal studies. On the basis of this screening method, the Stroke Prevention Trial in Sickle Cell Anemia ("STOP") tested the hypothesis that regular prophylactic transfusions in patient with abnormal TCD findings could prevent a first stroke (27). A total of 1,934 children ages 2 to 16 years were screened using TCS, and 206 were found to have abnormal results. Of 130 children who were deemed suitable for the study, 63 patients were randomly assigned to receive regular transfusions designed to maintain the concentration of HbS at less than 30%, and 67 patients were assigned to receive standard care (no transfusions). During the course of the trial, ten patients dropped out of the transfusion group, and two patients assigned to standard care transferred to the transfusion group. After a follow-up period of up to 30 months, there were ten cerebral infarctions and one intracerebral hematoma in the standard care group, compared with one infarction in the transfusion group. Because of the obvious benefit afforded by prophylactic transfusion, this study was terminated early in order to allow patients in the standard care group to elect to receive regular transfusions.

Despite these promising results, many questions remain unanswered. That regular transfusions are highly effective in preventing stroke is hardly surprising. The crucial question is, what is the sensitivity and specificity of TCD in identifying patients who are at risk for stroke? Unfortunately, this study does not provide all the data necessary to make such a determination. The incidence of stroke in the large number of patients who had normal TCD results was not reported. In the course of this study, 11 of 67 standard care patients (16%) developed intracerebral complications; if prophylactic transfusion is recommended for this entire group, then many will have received this costly and hazardous therapy unnecessarily. Because this study extended over a relatively brief period, it is reasonable to presume that a considerable number of additional patients would have incurred a stroke during a longer observation period. Even so, the number of patients who would be destined to receive unnecessary regular transfusions on the basis of abnormal TCD results remains disconcertingly high. Only about one-half of the patients eligible to receive prophylactic transfusions actually received them, raising questions about the acceptability of the TCD screening approach in the target population. As in the standard approach (prophylactic transfusion only after a first stroke), the necessary duration of regular transfusions remains to be determined.

Priapism

Because conservative treatment with intravenous hydration and analgesia is frequently unsuccessful, red blood cell transfusion should be considered first-line therapy for patients who require hospitalization for priapism. In milder cases of very recent onset, simple transfusions of packed red blood cells may be given. Seeler (28) obtained satisfactory results by transfusing sufficient packed red blood cells to double the hemoglobin concentration. In more severe or prolonged cases (those lasting longer than 6 to 12 hours), a single-volume exchange transfusion should be strongly considered. If this is successful, relief of pain may occur within a day, but complete detumescence may take several days or even weeks. If this approach is unsuccessful, a surgical shunt between the corpora cavernosa and corpus spongiosum may relieve the circulatory obstruction. If surgery is required, an exchange transfusion will prepare the patient for anesthesia and surgery (see Special Indications for Transfusion). Local treatment, with aspiration of the corpora cavernosa followed by irrigation with an epinephrine solution, has proven to be effective, and may obviate the need for transfusion (29).

Acute neurologic events, including seizure and stroke, have been reported in children who have undergone partial exchange transfusion for priapism (35,36), and the association between the two has been termed the ASPEN syndrome (association of sickle cell disease, priapism, exchange transfusion, and neurologic events) (30). This complication frequently begins with acute onset of severe headache. The etiology of these neurologic complications is not well understood, but hyperviscosity or high HbS percentage do not appear implicated; many of the affected patients were found to have previously undetected vascular abnormalities of the cerebral circulation.

Acute Pain Crisis

Red blood cell transfusions may be indicated for the treatment of severe or protracted episodes of acute pain crisis or for the prevention of frequent recurrences. When severe acute pain crisis is unresponsive to the standard therapy of intravenous hydration and analgesia, exchange transfusion designed to lower the HbS to less than 40% to 50% may produce relief. Debilitating cycles of frequent pain crises may be arrested by regular courses of transfusion that maintain the HbS at less than 40% to 50%. However, this approach is associated with a high risk of recurrence when the transfusions are stopped.

Skin Ulcer

When local measures are unsuccessful in the management of severe ulcers, a transfusion program lasting several months often achieves satisfactory results (31).

Acute Splenic Sequestration Crisis

Children with classic ASSC often arrive in hypovolemic shock with peripheral circulatory failure. Prompt transfusion with either whole blood or packed red blood cells is essential. Whole blood, if immediately available, is preferable in order to restore simultaneously intravascular volume and red blood cell oxygen-carrying capacity. If any delay is expected, volume resuscitation can be initiated with crystalloid solution followed by packed red blood cells. The volume of red blood cell transfusions should be sufficient to restore baseline hemoglobin levels. One or 2 days following transfusion, splenomegaly will typically diminish and the hemoglobin will spontaneously rise, indicating resolution and liberation of formerly sequestered blood cells into the circulation.

In contrast to the typical, rapidly progressive course of ASSC, subacute, minor episodes may be seen, especially in children with chronic hypersplenism. A single transfusion of packed red blood cells sufficient to double the hemoglobin concentration will often permanently correct the severe hematologic changes seen in young children with chronic hypersplenism. If splenectomy is being considered to avert recurrence of ASSC or hypersplenism, a limited transfusion program of 1 year may resolve the disease process and avoid surgery. At the least, transfusion may stave off surgery until the patient reaches an age when splenectomy would pose less risk of sepsis. As in other long-term transfusion programs intended to prevent sickle vasoocclusion, the HbS concentration should be maintained at less than 30% to 40%. Vigilance against recurrence of sequestration must be maintained even during the period of transfusion, for repeated episodes have been reported with HbS concentrations as low as 14% to 16% (32).

Acute Chest Syndrome

Red blood cell transfusions may be necessary for the treatment of this complication if it is associated with significant hypoxemia. In critical situations, a single-volume exchange transfusion is recommended, because this approach poses no risk of volume overload and achieves a rapid replacement of sickle cells with normal red blood cells. In less urgent situations, simple transfusions are usually satisfactory.

Acute Papillary Necrosis

Significant urinary blood loss due to acute papillary necrosis, in patients with sickle cell disease as well as those with sickle cell trait, may require transfusions for correction of anemia. It is unclear whether transfusion accelerates healing of the renal papillae in these patients.

Sepsis and Other Severe Illness

Sepsis may hinder erythropoiesis, as well as accelerate hemolysis. In severe infections, the red blood cell T cryptantigen may be exposed, leading to red blood cell polyagglutination (33). Transfusions may be indicated in sickle cell patients with sepsis in order to improve oxygen-carrying capacity and to prevent widespread sickling that might result from associated hypoxia or acidosis.

Special Indications for Transfusion in Sickle Cell Patients

Pregnancy

Pregnancy poses special risks to the mother with sickle cell disease and to her fetus. Potential maternal complications include an increased frequency of painful vasoocclusive crises, worsening of anemia, increased infection (especially urinary tract infections), toxemia, and death. The fetus is at increased risk for growth retardation, premature birth, stillbirth, and spontaneous abortion. In mothers with HbSS disease, maternal complications and fetal death occur most frequently in the third trimester, whereas fetal death is more frequent in the first trimester in mothers with HbSC disease (34). As recently as 1971, Fort et al. (35) reported an overall maternal death rate of more than 6% and an infant perinatal mortality rate of approximately 45% in mothers with sickle cell disease. These authors concluded that measures should be taken to prevent pregnancies in these women, including sterilization or abortion. Since 1972, the maternal death rate has been less than 2% and the perinatal death rate has been less than 25% in pregnancies not managed with prophylactic hypertransfusion (34).

Recommendations for the prenatal care of the mother with sickle cell disease have included prophylactic transfusion at the onset of pregnancy or at the beginning of the third trimester, prophylactic transfusion only in those pregnancies considered high risk, or obstetric management without transfusion. Many of the earlier studies of transfusion in pregnant women with sickle cell disease are difficult to evaluate because of differences in design and the use of historic controls.

The most informative study to date is that of Koshy et al. (36). In this prospective study, 72 pregnant women with sickle cell disease were randomly assigned to receive either prophylactic red blood cell transfusions or only therapeutically indicated transfusions for defined medical or obstetric emergencies. Those patients assigned to prophylactic transfusions received an average of 12 units of packed cells during the course of pregnancy, while nearly one-half of the controls received an average of only 6.5 units. When patients with high-risk factors (i.e., multiple gestation or a history of previous perinatal mortality) were excluded, there were no significant differences in maternal and fetal outcome between the prophylactic transfusion and control groups, except (as might be expected) that the number of pain crises in the prophylactic transfusion group was significantly reduced.

These findings suggest that prophylactic transfusion therapy may be unnecessary, and better avoided, in pregnant women with sickle cell disease who lack underlying high-risk factors. Whether prophylactic transfusions might be beneficial in high-risk patients could not be ascertained by this study, and this may be difficult to determine because of the large number of study patients required to achieve statistically significant results (34).

Surgery

The patient with sickle cell disease is at increased risk for perioperative complications including sudden death, pulmonary infarction, infection, and pain crisis. Changes in regional perfusion, accidents of anesthesia (e.g., aspiration, difficulty in intubation, etc.), or a variety of surgical circumstances may alter oxygenation, hydration, temperature, or acid-base balance and lead to localized or generalized sickle cell vasoocclusion.

Some studies have reported favorable surgical results without the use of prophylactic transfusion. Homi et al. (37) avoided transfusion throughout the entire perioperative period in 137 of 200 sickle cell patients who underwent surgery with general anesthesia. In the remaining patients transfusions were given either to restore the hemoglobin to baseline levels or to combat anticipated or actual blood loss. Six patients died, all during the postoperative period. Detailed transfusion information related to these fatalities was not provided, but five of the six patients had undergone emergency surgery and were in poor physical condition preoperatively. In a nonrandomized study of 66 patients with sickle syndromes (50 HbSS, 13 HbSC, 3 HbS/β thalassemia) who underwent 82 surgical procedures, no major differences in perioperative morbidity and mortality were seen, regardless of whether transfusions were given preoperatively, intraoperatively, postoperatively, or not at all (38).

Other groups routinely employed elective preoperative transfusion with good results. Janik and Seeler (39) described 32 patients with HbSS disease who underwent 46 operations following preparative packed red blood cell transfusions of 15 to 20 ml/kg, designed to raise the hematocrit to a minimum of 36%. The posttransfusion level of HbS was between 32% and 55%. In this series, there was no reported morbidity or mortality. Prophylactic exchange transfusions designed to achieve hematocrit values of more than 35% and HbA concentrations of more than 40% were administered in another study of 42 patients with sickle cell disease (40). There were no reported deaths, and postoperative complications were infrequent and unremarkable; there were no apparent cases of vasoocclusive crisis or pulmonary embolus. Preoperative exchange transfusions have also been given successfully to patients with sickle cell disease prior to vitreoretinal surgery in order to diminish the risk of anterior segment ischemia (41).

The Preoperative Transfusion in Sickle Cell Disease Study Group has provided the most comprehensive comparison of conservative and aggressive transfusion regimens. In 1995, this group reported results from a prospective study of 551 patients (a total of 604 operations), some of whom were randomly assigned to one of these two transfusion regimens (42). The aggressive transfusion regimen was intended to achieve a HbS concentration of 30% or less, while the conservative transfusion regimen sought to attain a minimum hemoglobin concentration of 10g/dl. Although some overlap existed in the hematologic features of the two groups, data were analyzed on an intent-to-treat basis. Cholecystectomies, and otolaryngologic and orthopedic procedures accounted for more than three-fourths of the operations performed. A serious or life-threatening complication, most commonly ACS, was experienced by about 20% of the patients in each group. The aggressively transfused group used twice as many red blood cell units and had twice the alloimmunization rate, in comparison with the conservatively managed group.

The study group reported a subset of 364 patients who underwent cholecystectomy, using either traditional (58% of patients) or laparoscopic techniques (42% of patients) (43). In this study, 110 patients were randomized to receive aggressive preoperative transfusion, 120 patients were randomized to conservative transfusion, 37 patients were nonrandomly assigned no transfusion, and 97 patients were nonrandomly assigned transfusion. Among all groups combined, the total complication rate was 39%, and sickle cell events occurred in 19%. However, patients who were nonrandomly assigned to receive no transfusion had a sickle cell complication rate of 32%. Patients who underwent laparoscopic procedures had longer anesthesia time but shorter duration of hospitalization, compared with those who had an open abdominal procedure. The incidence of complications did not differ between these two groups.

In a review of 118 patients who underwent elective tonsillectomy and adenoidectomy or myringotomy, and who were randomly assigned either conservative or aggressive preoperative transfusion protocols, the study group found no major differences in complication rates (44). About one-third of all patients experienced serious, nontransfusion-associated complications.

In all these reports, the study group concluded that a conservative preoperative transfusion regimen had equivalent efficacy to an aggressive transfusion regimen in preventing perioperative complications. Furthermore, the conservative transfusion regimen was associated with one-half the transfusion-associated complications. Therefore, a conservative preoperative transfusion approach was advocated. However, other interpretations of the data should be considered as well. For example, because of the overlap in percentage of HbS achieved between the aggressively and conservatively transfused groups, the two groups may not have differed from each other sufficiently to produce clinically distinct outcomes. Also, the aggressively transfused group may not have been transfused intensely enough to provide adequate physiologic protection from sickle cell events. The experience from Duke University supports the latter hypothesis: a very low complication rate was experienced by sickle cell patients there who were preoperatively transfused to mean hemoglobin values of 11.2 g/dl and an average of 21% HbS (45).

Based upon all these results, the following guidelines would seem to be appropriate for most sickle cell patients who are undergoing surgery:

1. The most critical aspect of perioperative management is meticulous anesthetic and surgical care, avoiding hypoxemia, dehydration, acidosis, and hypothermia.
2. Preoperative red blood cell transfusions are warranted when prolonged general anesthesia is used or anticipated (i.e., when

there is reasonable likelihood that local anesthesia will prove to be inadequate). For uncomplicated minor procedures in which brief inhalation anesthetic is used (e.g., some dental procedures), transfusion is seldom necessary.

3. The specific method of transfusion—regular or partial exchange—is not as important as the hematologic end point. A preoperative HbS of 30% to 40% and hemoglobin concentration in an intermediate range (11 to 13 g/dl) are desirable, based upon empirical clinical experience and data cited previously. Special surgical situations characterized by low regional blood flow, especially if in a critical anatomic site (e.g., major cardiac, orthopedic, or neurosurgery), may warrant even more aggressive preoperative transfusion. The choice of the method of transfusion largely depends upon the clinical circumstance. When surgery is urgent, a single-volume exchange transfusion (60 to 70 ml/kg) will rapidly achieve the hematologic goal, but when sufficient time is available prior to elective surgery, repeated regular transfusions over 2 to 4 weeks can be employed, with the attendant benefits of greater technical ease, lower procedural risk, and possibly a lower overall transfusion requirement.
4. In the various compound heterozygous sickle syndromes (with the exception of HbS/β^0 thalassemia, which has a hemoglobin pattern similar to that of HbSS disease) it is safest not to monitor the percentage of HbS per se, but to consider the percentage of sickleable cells.
5. In most circumstances no special measures need to be taken in the preoperative management of patients with sickle cell trait. A possible exception is for patients requiring open heart surgery (46) because of the risk that circulatory stasis might induce sickling in sickle cell–trait erythrocytes. In addition, prophylactic transfusion may well be appropriate for patients with sickle cell trait who will be undergoing orthopedic surgery requiring prolonged tourniquet application, although this view is not universally held (46).

Angiography

Cerebral or coronary angiography in patients with sickle cell disease should be performed only after prophylactic transfusion has achieved an HbS concentration of less than 20% and with adequate hydration (47). Intravenous urography may be performed without preparative transfusion, but vigorous hydration should be maintained both before and after the procedure.

Donor Selection and Transfusion-related Complications in Patients with Sickle Cell Disease

Alloimmunization

Sensitization to transfused red blood cell antigens (alloimmunization) may lead to an inconvenient and costly delay or even a life-threatening inability to find compatible blood. In addition, significant alloimmunization in patients with sickle cell disease may result in delayed hemolytic transfusion reactions (DTHRs) that are often serious and occasionally even lethal. Whenever there is a prolonged or repeated requirement for transfusion, it is prudent to obtain a full red blood cell antigen profile of the recipient before transfusion therapy is initiated. This information will be very useful later if alloimmunization is suspected.

Studies of adult and pediatric patients who have been transfused suggest that the overall risk of alloimmunization in sickle cell disease is about 20% to 30%. Many of these studies, however, were retrospective and did not examine the patients' transfusion histories prior to the study.

Patients who are frequently transfused appear to be somewhat more likely to develop alloantibodies than those who receive infrequent transfusions. Chronically transfused patients who develop alloantibodies often appear to do so early in their transfusion courses (48) and are also more likely to develop multiple alloantibodies. In this regard, patients with sickle cell disease appear to be similar to the population at large: there is a subpopulation of "hyperresponders" who readily become alloimmunized, but the majority are nonresponders in spite of numerous transfusions (49). Approximately one-half to two-thirds of alloantibodies identified in patients with HbSS disease have been directed at antigens of the Rh blood group system, and the majority of these are anti-Rh(E). Anti-Kell (K) and anti-Kidd (Jk^a and Jk^b) antibodies account for approximately 20% of alloantibodies in transfused patients with sickle cell disease (49). Lewis antibodies account for up to one-third of alloantibodies, but as in the general population these are generally regarded as "naturally occurring" and do not appear to be clinically significant.

The impact of racial differences between donors and recipients on the rates of alloimmunization of patients with HbSS disease has been examined in several studies. Overall, approximately 20% to 30% of transfused patients with sickle cell disease become alloimmunized, in comparison with 5% to 10% of thalassemia patients who are transfused in the United States (50). The increased incidence of alloimmunization in patients with sickle cell disease has been attributed to the greater disparity in race and red blood cell phenotypic profile that exists between typical blood donors and sickle cell recipients, in comparison with other recipients (50,51). In many urban centers, the blood donor pool is often 90% to 95% white (50,51), and these donors often possess a variety of Rh, Duffy, Kell, and Kidd antigens that are less frequently found in black patients (52). Orlina et al. (51) calculated that a black recipient has a 33% chance of compatibility for these antigens from a black donor pool, in comparison with an only 3% chance of compatibility with the typical urban donor pool of 90% white and 10% black. However, 70% to 80% of blacks are Fy(a − b −), whereas more than 99% of whites are positive for one or both antigens, yet the frequency of Duffy alloimmunization in transfused sickle cell patients is only 15% or less (49). When the blood donor and recipient belong to different racial groups, the risk of alloimmunization depends not only on whether the two populations have different frequencies of blood group antigens but also on the intrinsic antigenicity of each blood group antigen.

Previous recommendations have included selecting donors (a) according to an extended red blood cell antigen profile, so that compatibility is achieved for Kell and secondary Rh group antigens (i.e., C and E), (b) according to race, and (c) to no special extent other than the standard $Rh_0(D)$ and ABO groups.

If any special preselection of donors is performed, it should be maintained on a regular basis, because hyperresponders often become immunized after only 10 to 20 transfusions. Under most circumstances, it is not cost effective or feasible to preselect red blood cell donors for sickle cell patients. Routine donors are usually acceptable. If a patient with sickle cell disease has clinically significant alloantibodies, then specific compatibility testing must, of course, be performed. Because of the existence of hyperresponders, it may be advisable to match as closely as possible all individuals who have developed one or more alloantibodies. In such cases, the search for compatible blood may be hastened by screening units obtained from same-race donors (50).

Delayed Hemolytic Transfusion Reaction

This complication is due to acute destruction of transfused red blood cells beginning several days after transfusion. It is typically caused by an alloantibody to a blood group antigen produced in anamnestic fashion in a previously sensitized patient. Clinically, DHTR is characterized by fever and a precipitous drop in hemoglobin, often to levels lower than those which existed prior to transfusion. Hemoglobinuria is often seen, due to intravascular hemolysis. Delayed hemolytic transfusion reaction has distinctive features when present in patients with sickle cell disease, and thus it may even constitute a unique syndrome in this setting (53). It occurs in about 5% to 20% of regularly transfused patients with sickle cell disease, an incidence considerably higher than that seen in other multiply transfused populations (54). Pain is commonly experienced by sickle cell patients with DHTR and it may be readily confused with that from vasoocclusive crisis. Marked reticulocytopenia is occasionally seen, and this may contribute to the anemia. When DHTR is suspected, serial hemoglobin electrophoreses may be a useful means to document alloimmune hemolysis, by showing a rapid fall in donor cell–derived HbA. However, although hemolysis of donor red blood cells is typically the principal concern, destruction of autologous cells can occur as well through a phenomenon that has been referred to as "bystander hemolysis" (55). In this process, antigen-negative red blood cells are destroyed by autoantibodies with an indeterminate specificity, or by deposition of antigen-antibody complexes on red blood cell membranes, causing complement activation and lysis of red blood cells. These reactions are an especially serious threat, because this potentially life-threatening complication is not always prevented by the use of phenotypically matched blood. In the face of a DHTR, additional transfusion should be avoided whenever possible in order to prevent exacerbation of the hemolytic process.

Blood from Sickle Cell Trait Donors for Patients without Sickle Cell Disease

The oxygen-carrying capacity of HbAS blood is comparable to that of normal (HbAA) blood, and in the great majority of general, elective transfusion settings, HbAS blood may be transfused without any untoward consequence. However, this blood should be avoided in neonates (especially ventilator-dependent premature infants), in patients with severe cardiopulmonary illness or shock, and in those who require high-volume blood transfusions (e.g., in cases of severe acute hemorrhage). All of these conditions may be associated with hypoxemia and acidosis severe enough to cause sickling, of sickle trait erythrocytes. Leukocyte-reduction fillers often are unsuccessful, and HbAS erythrocytes sometimes hemolyze during the process of deglycerolization (56). *Accordingly, red blood cells destined for leukoreduction or frozen storage should be screened to detect, and possibly eliminate, sickle cell trait–containing units.*

Because HbAS blood is acceptable for routine transfusion into individuals without sickle cell disease, there should be no objection to using autologous transfusion in patients with sickle cell trait, as long as none of the risk factors cited above is present (57).

Blood from Sickle Cell Trait Donors for Patients with Sickle Cell Disease

Blood obtained from donors with sickle cell trait is undesirable for use in patients with sickle cell disease, primarily because the resultant mixture of HbSS and HbAS cells will obfuscate hemoglobin electrophoresis results generally used to monitor the progress of transfusion therapy. In addition, in nearly all sickle cell conditions requiring transfusion therapy there is a danger of progressive sickling. As noted above, even HbAS blood can sickle under severely unfavorable physiologic conditions and thus should be avoided.

Hepatitis

In those individuals for whom chronic or repeated transfusion appears likely, immunization with hepatitis B vaccine is recommended. Patients with sickle cell disease have been shown to respond normally to the vaccine (Heptavax-B).

Thalassemias

Epidemiology

The frequency of thalassemia genes in world populations is surprisingly high, with the thalassemias in aggregate representing the most prevalent of all known genetic diseases (58). Occasional individuals with thalassemia have been observed in native populations in virtually all areas of the world where they have been sought, but most cases are concentrated within a broad subtropical "thalassemia belt" extending from Western Europe to Southeast Asia (Fig. 32.1). Within this region there are areas with especially high frequencies of thalassemia genes, with as many as 50% of some populations having one or more forms of thalassemia.

The characterization in recent years of the underlying mutations of the thalassemia syndromes has added considerably to our understanding of the population genetics of these disorders. In general, each of the geographic areas with a high prevalence of thalassemia, particularly the β form, has a characteristic and often unique group of thalassemia mutations. In most of these populations, a small number of mutations account for most of the observed cases. These mutations probably arose independently in each population, and they achieved high frequency because of strong selective pressure. There is considerable information suggesting that resistance to falciparum malaria is the selective force responsible for the high frequency of thalassemia. One line of evidence in support of this hypothesis is the geographic concurrence of the "thalassemia belt" and the areas where malaria was formerly endemic (Fig. 32.1). This relationship is particularly striking in the "micromapping" of contiguous geographic areas discordant for the presence of endemic malaria. Other evidence in support of the "malaria hypothesis" includes the observation that *Plasmodium falciparum* grows poorly in erythrocytes containing elevated levels of HbF (59) and that oxidative changes known to occur in thalassemic erythrocytes inhibit parasite growth (60).

Molecular Basis for the Thalassemia Syndromes

More than 100 distinct thalassemia mutations are now known. A summary of the major categories of these molecular abnormalities is shown in Table 32.3; a detailed description is given elsewhere (61). In spite of the considerable diversity of forms and sites of mutations in the globin genes, as well as the variety of mechanisms by which they lead to inhibition of globin-chain synthesis, the clinical phenotypes of most forms of thalassemia are remarkably similar (see below). For most clinical purposes, therefore, the identification of the specific mutations of thalassemia patients is of little importance. However, for prenatal diagnosis, and because of the potential for ameliorating the effects of thalassemia genes, this information may eventually assume fundamental significance.

Pathophysiology

The pathogenesis of most of the symptomatic forms of thalassemia follows a similar mechanism. The pathogenesis of homozygous β thalassemia ("Cooley's anemia") serves as a representative example.

Bone marrow erythroid cells of affected individuals exhibit a diminution or absence of hemoglobin β-chain synthesis. Although this defect is partially compensated for by an increase in the synthesis of HbF γ chains, a major disparity nevertheless exists between α-chain and non-α-chain synthesis (Fig. 32.5), with α-chain synthesis occurring in considerable excess. The deficiency of β and γ chains results in severe underhemoglobinization of the red blood cells because of insufficient quantities of HbA ($\alpha_2\beta_2$) or HbF ($\alpha_2\gamma_2$).

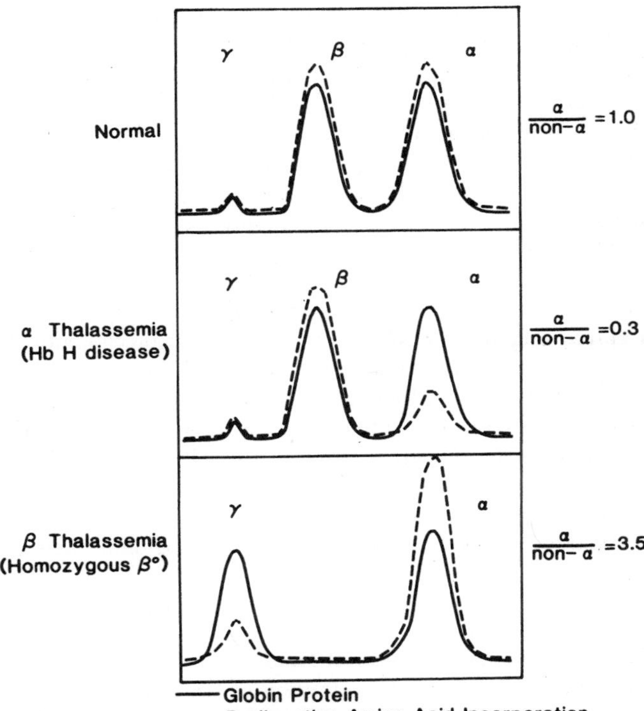

FIGURE 32.5. Synthesis of globin chains by erythroid cells from a normal individual *(top)*, a patient with α thalassemia *(middle)*, and a patient with severe β^0 thalassemia *(bottom)*. (From Honig GR, Adams JG III. *Human hemoglobin genetics.* Vienna: Springer-Verlag, 1986, with permission.)

TABLE 32.3. EXAMPLES OF MOLECULAR ABNORMALITIES OF THALASSEMIA GENES

1. Globin gene deletions, partial or complete
2. Nucleotide substitutions in the promoter regions, which inhibit globin-gene transcription
3. Nucleotide substitutions or deletions at splice-junction sites, which prevent the formation of normal globin messenger RNA (mRNA)
4. Nucleotide substitutions in the coding segments or introns, which result in abnormally spliced globin mRNA
5. Nucleotide substitutions in the transcription-termination signal region, which result in the formation of abnormal globin mRNA
6. Nucleotide substitutions in translation-initiation codons, which inhibit mRNA translation
7. Nucleotide deletions or insertions that result in the formation of premature termination codons
8. Nucleotide substitutions in the translation-termination codons, producing extended-length globin chains
9. Mutations that produce highly unstable globin chains, which undergo rapid degradation within the erythrocytes

The excess of uncombined α chains that accumulate in the red blood cells of these patients is also responsible for other deleterious effects. Uncombined α subunits are unstable and precipitate within erythrocytes. This process, which is accompanied by oxidation of heme iron, releases superoxide ions, which in turn inflict oxidative damage on the red blood cell (62). In severe forms of β thalassemia, the latter process results in destruction of a major fraction of erythroid cells, even before they are released from the bone marrow, producing what has been termed "ineffective erythropoiesis." In compensation for this process, these patients develop an enormous expansion of their bone marrow, a change that produces characteristic bony deformities most apparent in the skull and face. The resulting anemia in the most severe forms of homozygous β thalassemia (β^0) is incompatible with long-term survival unless periodic transfusions are given.

Compound Heterozygous Forms

In geographic areas with high frequencies of thalassemia, both α- and β-thalassemia alleles may coexist in the same population, and both types of abnormalities may therefore occur in the same individual. Surprisingly, the combination of homozygous β^0 thalassemia with concomitant α thalassemia produces a clinically mild form of Cooley's anemia (63). The most plausible explanation for the ameliorative effect of the α thalassemia in such individuals is that a more nearly normal balance is achieved between α-chain and β-chain synthesis and that the harmful series of events described above is suppressed.

Hemoglobin E, an abnormal hemoglobin prevalent in Southeast Asia, produces thalassemia-like hematologic effects, possibly by two separate mechanisms. First, HbE is an unstable variant and may undergo β-chain loss by intracellular precipitation or degradation or both. Second, the HbE mutation produces an aberrant splicing site, leading to a decreased production of β^E messenger RNA (mRNA) (64). Large series of patients with the compound heterozygous combination of HbE and β^0 thalassemia have been reported (65). This syndrome has variable expression, with more severely affected individuals requiring periodic transfusions to maintain adequate hemoglobin levels.

Homozygous β Thalassemia (Cooley's Anemia)

Clinical Features and Natural History

The clinical and hematologic features of the major forms of β thalassemia are summarized in Table 32.4. Because the molecular abnormalities that cause these disorders are within or in close proximity to the β-globin genes, the onset of expression of β thalassemia occurs some months after birth when HbF is replaced by HbA. Affected infants are therefore normal at birth, and evidence of the disease first appears by the middle or end of the first year. Anemia gradually develops, accompanied by progressive enlargement of the liver and spleen and cardiovascular changes related to congestive heart failure. A large fraction of the cardiac output is shunted through the hypertrophied bone marrow of untransfused thalassemia patients and this change contributes to an expansion of the plasma volume, resulting in increasing hemodilution and worsening cardiac failure. The size of the spleen and the liver in these patients, prior to the introduction of modern transfusion methods, progressed to a massive degree, primarily because of reticuloendothelial cell proliferation. Hyperexpanded marrow also results in a thinning of cortical bone, predisposing these children to fractures. Craniofacial bone deformities are variable in degree but often severe, frequently resulting in considerable malocclusion due to maxillary hyperplasia. In the absence of transfusion support, children with severe β thalassemia succumb to the effects of anemia and heart failure within the first years of life. Milder forms of β thalassemia are accompanied by a slower rate of progression and correspondingly longer survival.

Transfusion Therapy for Patients with β Thalassemia

The earliest transfusion regimens for patients with β thalassemia consisted of administering mainly whole blood as infrequently as possible and only when severe anemia developed (65). This form of management protected these children from early death due to progressive heart failure but did not mitigate the full expression of the disease. With the development of outpatient transfusion programs, most centers in the United States turned to the regular use of packed red blood cell transfusions and generally sought to maintain hemoglobin levels in the range of

TABLE 32.4. CLINICAL AND HEMATOLOGIC FEATURES OF THE MAJOR FORMS OF β THALASSEMIA

Type	Hemoglobin Findings	Hematologic Changes	Clinical Features
Heterozygous			
β^+ (severe) (high A_2)	A_2, 3.5–7.5% F, 1–6%	Erythrocyte microcytosis and hypochromia; mild to moderate anemia	Possible splenomegaly and mild icterus
β^- (mild) (high A_2)	A_2, 3.5–7.5%	Erythrocyte microcytosis and hypochromia; mild or absent anemia	Usually none
β silent carrier	A_2 and F, normal (F-containing cells sometimes detectable by slide elution test)	Hematologically normal	None
δβ (high F)	A_2, normal or low F, 5–20%	Erythrocyte microcytosis and hypochromia; mild or absent anemia	Usually none
Homozygous			
β^+	F, 30–95%	Markedly abnormal red blood cell morphology with microcytosis and hypochromia, nucleated red blood cells; severe anemia	Pallor, jaundice, bone deformities with abnormal facies, hepatosplenomegaly, usually transfusion-dependent
β^-	F, 40–80%	Poikilocytosis, anisocytosis, target cells; moderate anemia	Pallor, hepatosplenomegaly, jaundice; transfusions not usually required
δβ (high F)	F, 100%	Poikilocytosis, anisocytosis, hypochromia, microcytosis; mild to moderate anemia	Mild jaundice, hepatosplenomegaly usually present

6 to 8 g/dl. A critical turning point in the approach to the transfusion management of β thalassemia patients came in 1964, when reports by Schorr and Radel (66) and by Wolman (67) compared the clinical status of patients whose hemoglobin levels had been maintained at different levels. The principal finding was that children with thalassemia fared better if their hemoglobin levels were maintained above 8 g/dl. Compared with other β thalassemia patients, the group with a high hemoglobin level exhibited more normal growth, a lesser extent of liver and spleen enlargement, less bony deformity and orthodontic abnormalities, and a considerably lower frequency of cardiac enlargement. Although these patients had received a larger number of transfusions and had correspondingly higher levels of iron stores, their considerably improved clinical status demonstrated that, at least in younger children, the hemoglobin level was more important than iron overload as a determinant of clinical status (67).

The findings from these studies led rapidly to the introduction of transfusion regimens that sought to maintain higher hemoglobin levels, usually higher than 9.5 or 10 g/dl. This approach, frequently referred to as "hypertransfusion," usually consists of packed red blood cell transfusions of about 20 ml/kg, given whenever the patient's hemoglobin falls below the targeted level. Importantly, once these patients are fully transfused, the blood requirement to maintain them on the hypertransfusion regimen is no greater than that needed to maintain patients at a lower hemoglobin level (68). Immediate posttransfusion hemoglobin levels typically average 14 g/dl, returning to baseline after 3 to 6 weeks. Hypertransfusion is also accompanied by a reduction in gastrointestinal absorbance of iron (69). The rate of iron accumulation can therefore be lessened while maintaining a more desirable hemoglobin level.

In addition to improved clinical status, the correction of anemia by hypertransfusion also exerts a suppressive effect on the erythropoietic drive that causes bone marrow hypertrophy. The bony abnormalities, which in the past were so characteristic of this disease, are now entirely preventable (70), and these patients now experience no increased risk of fractures. In addition, the bone marrow suppressive effect of hypertransfusion prevents the release of the deformed, short-lived Cooley's anemia erythrocytes and delays the onset of hypersplenic changes, permitting splenectomy to be safely postponed until an older age.

Appropriately transfused patients with Cooley's anemia gradually experience increasing splenomegaly due to reticuloendothelial proliferation. Although this process is considerably delayed by hypertransfusion, it cannot be totally prevented. The development of hypersplenism shortens the transfusion interval and increases transfusion requirements. Piomelli and Loew (71) have suggested that a packed red blood cell transfusion requirement of more than 200 ml/kg per year in these patients is usually an indication for splenectomy.

Propper et al. (72) have proposed a transfusion regimen for Cooley's anemia that maintains the hematocrit above 35%, but this "supertransfusion" approach is no longer recommended (58). Indeed, moderate transfusion regimens, which target a baseline hemoglobin level of 9 to 10 g/dl, appear to offer the best combination of preventing the long term adverse consequences of anemia and excessive erythropoiesis, while minimizing iron accumulation (73).

Individuals with heterozygous β thalassemia ordinarily have no unusual need for transfusions. An exception is during pregnancy, when women with thalassemia trait often develop more severe anemia (74) and occasionally require transfusion support (75).

α *Thalassemia*

Wasi et al. (65), in summarizing their experience in Thailand with a large number of patients with HbH disease (Table 32.5), showed that this syndrome often produced Cooley's anemia–like changes, with anemia, bony deformities, and splenomegaly. However, these changes appear to reflect, in part, the effects of infections and other environmental factors superimposed upon the genetic abnormality. HbH disease in the United States generally exhibits a relatively mild thalassemia intermedia–like syndrome and seldom requires blood transfusion except during surgery.

The hydrops fetalis form of α thalassemia, in which α-chain synthesis is totally lacking, has until recent years been invariably fatal, the infants surviving no longer than a few hours after birth.

A few recent examples have been reported of such infants who received vigorous resuscitative measures, including transfusions at birth, with survival beyond the neonatal period (76). This syndrome is characterized by the production almost exclusively of homotetramers of γ and β chains (Table 32.5). These abnormal hemoglobins have virtually no physiologically useful oxygen-transporting capacity because of their very high oxygen affinity. Infants who survive are therefore at great risk of developing hypoxic encephalopathy during the neonatal period and are totally dependent on transfused red blood cells throughout their lives.

Effects and Management of Chronic Transfusion Therapy

Hemosiderosis

Each unit of packed red blood cells contains approximately 250 mg of iron. Unfortunately, physiologic mechanisms for the elimination of excess iron are lacking. Signs of clinical toxicity often become apparent when total body iron reaches 400 to 1,000 mg/kg of body weight, and levels in excess of this are potentially lethal (77).

Once reticuloendothelial sites of iron storage become saturated, parenchymal deposition increases and tissue damage ensues. The primary targets of iron toxicity are the liver, pancreas and other endocrine organs, and heart. Hepatotoxicity, expressed initially by fibrosis and subsequently cirrhosis, is the most common early manifestation of transfusion-related iron overload. Cardiac toxicity, causing cardiomyopathy and arrhythmia, has been the most frequent cause of death in chronically transfused patients.

When faithfully administered, treatment with daily subcutaneous deferoxamine has been shown to arrest or even reverse hepatic (78) and cardiac (79) iron toxicity in thalassemia patients, especially when started early in the course of transfusion therapy. This drug has also been effective in patients with sickle

TABLE 32.5. CLINICAL AND HEMATOLOGIC FEATURES OF α THALASSEMIA

Form of α Thalassemia	Genotype	Hemoglobin Findings		Hematologic Changes	Clinical Features
		Newborn	Adults		
Silent carrier	αα/α−	1–2% Hb γ_4 (Bart's)	No abnormality	Usually no abnormality; mild microcytosis may be present	Clinically normal
α-Thalassemia trait	αα/−− or α−/α−	2–10% Hb γ_4	No abnormality	Red red cell microcytosis and hypochromia with mildly abnormal morphology; anemia mild or absent	Usually normal
Hb H disease	α−/−−	20–30% Hb γ_4	5–25% Hb H (β_4); may be traces of Hb γ_4	Moderately severe anemia with marked anisopoikilocytosis and microcytosis; red blood cell inclusion bodies demonstrable by supravital staining	Pallor, jaundice hepatosplenomegaly; cholelithiasis occurs commonly in adults
Hydrops fetalis	−−/−−	80% Hb γ_4, with the remainder Hb β_4 and Hb Portland ($\zeta_2\gamma_2$)	—	Severe anemia, markedly abnormal erythrocyte morphology with anisopoikilocytosis, hypochromia, and pronounced erythroblastemia	Massive hepatosplenomegaly, generalized edema with ascites and pleural and pericardial effusion; nearly all are stillborn or die shortly after birth

cell anemia (80). Deferoxamine is usually prescribed in a daily dose of 50 to 75 mg/kg of body weight, administered subcutaneously over 8 to 12 hours (usually overnight) via a portable infusion pump. Unfortunately, this agent is costly and, because of the parenteral route of administration and the special measures required to use the pump, is cumbersome to administer. The infusion may also be painful, especially for children. Not surprisingly, compliance is often poor, thus limiting the effectiveness of this therapy.

The most practical measurement of body iron stores is the serum ferritin concentration, which is in equilibrium with storage iron up to a level of approximately 4,000 μg/l (77). However, in the face of a high body iron burden, and in a variety of disease states (e.g., acute inflammatory conditions, hepatocellular damage), the serum ferritin loses its reliability as a marker for the total body iron burden. The hepatic iron concentration determined from liver biopsy specimens is an excellent indicator of total body iron stores in patients with thalassemia major (81). Despite the relative difficulty in obtaining such specimens, this method is recommended for the reliable measurement of the total amount iron stored in the body (82). A superconducting quantum interference device (SQUID) susceptometer measures body iron noninvasively and produces results equivalent to those obtained by liver biopsy, but his method is not widely available (82).

The transfusion regimen employed for the long-term management of chronically transfused patients can significantly affect the rate of iron accumulation. In sickle cell patients who require protracted courses of transfusion, exchange procedures can considerably decrease the rate of accumulation (83). Transfusion regimens intended to achieve this goal for chronically transfused patients with thalassemia are summarized below.

Young Red Blood Cells for Transfusions

Piomelli et al. (84) first proposed the use of red blood cell preparations enriched with a younger cell population ("neocytes") for chronic transfusion therapy. The lower density of less mature erythrocytes provides the means for the preparation of such red blood cell concentrates. The potential advantages that accrue from the use of "neocytes" include a longer transfusion interval and a correspondingly lower rate of iron accumulation (Fig. 32.6).

Two major studies have described the results of transfusion with these young cell–enriched red blood cell concentrates. Cohen et al. (85) transfused six thalassemia patients over a 3-year period, using red blood cells comprising approximately the upper 57% of each blood unit. Blood requirements needed to maintain a hemoglobin level above 9 g/dl in these patients decreased an average of 15.8% with use of the young red blood cell preparations. This small improvement involved an 84% increase in cost, compared with the use of frozen red blood cell units. In addition, despite the reduced transfusion requirements achieved by this approach, the patients in this study were exposed to approximately 50% more donors.

Marcus et al. (86) conducted a prospective double-blind study of 48 transfusion-dependent thalassemia patients. Half of them received young red blood cell concentrates derived from the 50%-less-dense fraction of blood units, and the other half received standard blood transfusions. Each patient was studied

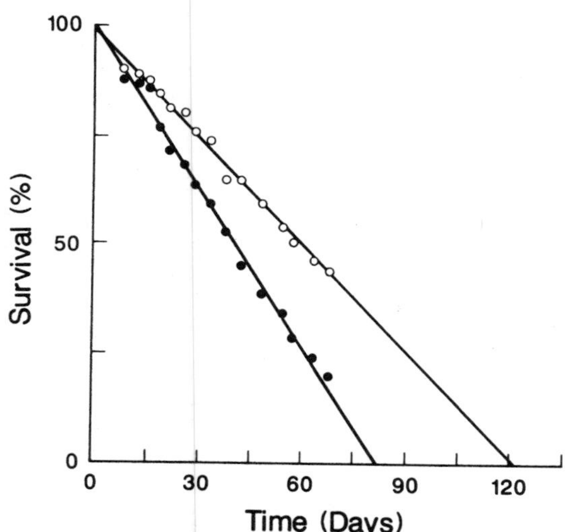

FIGURE 32.6. Survival of younger and older red blood cell fractions from a standard blood unit. The packed red blood cells from the unit were centrifuged for an additional 30 minutes, and the upper half of the cells was transferred to a separate bag. The cells from the upper fraction were tagged with ^{14}C-labeled diisopropyl fluorophosphate (DFP) *(solid circles)*, and those from the lower fraction were tagged with ^{3}H-DFP *(open circles)*, and the cells were reinfused into the donor for the survival study. Similar results were obtained when the radioactive tagging of the two cell fractions was reversed. (From Hammer G, Orlina A, Honig G, unpublished results.)

for a period of 15 months. Unfortunately, this study failed to reveal any reduction in blood consumption in the patients given the young red blood cell preparations, nor was any difference seen in their transfusion interval or rate of decline in hemoglobin values. These investigators concluded that the expense, time, and increased exposure to donors could not be justified by the results obtained.

Berdoukas et al. (87) described a somewhat different approach to young red blood cell transfusion methodology that appears promising. This regimen uses conventional red blood cell units as part of an exchange transfusion. The patient is connected to a continuous flow cell separator. The most dense, oldest red blood cell fraction is removed from the patient and discarded; the lighter cell fractions are returned to the patient, supplemented by donor red blood cells. Using this approach, Berdoukas et al. observed a 42% increase in the transfusion interval, a 25% reduction in the rate of fall of the hemoglobin concentration, and a 29% reduction in red blood cell consumption.

Patients maintained on this transfusion regimen required transfusions at 7- to 8-week intervals, with the red blood cell exchange process itself lasting 90 to 120 minutes. This transfusion method achieved a high degree of satisfaction with both patients and families, and there was strong pressure to continue this form of therapy. However, in spite of these gratifying results and the presumed decrease in iron accumulation that could be expected, this approach does impose substantial costs and increased risks. Adequate venous access and anticoagulation is required for the procedure, and despite the decrease in total red blood cell consumption, patients are exposed to approximately 50% more donors. Moreover, this procedure was estimated to cost approximately 50% more than conventional transfusion programs. In spite of these concerns, this approach to young cell transfusion appears to be the only one that may have practical value in patient management.

ERYTHROCYTE ENZYME ABNORMALITIES

Enzyme-mediated metabolic pathways in the red blood cell function to maintain the hemoglobin and the cell membrane in a reduced state. These objectives are accomplished primarily through the reactions linked to the pentose phosphate shunt and, for metabolic energy requirements, through the glycolytic pathway. Many enzyme deficiencies in these metabolic pathways have been described. The majority are inherited as autosomal recessive abnormalities. Two exceptions—G6PD deficiency and phosphoglycerate kinase deficiency—are transmitted in an X-linked recessive mode.

Glucose-6-phosphate dehydrogenase deficiency is prevalent in the same geographic areas in which there is a high frequency of hemoglobin disorders (Fig. 32.1). In common with many of the hemoglobinopathies and thalassemia syndromes, hemizygous carriers of G6PD abnormalities are more resistant to falciparum malaria. Two common clinical forms of G6PD deficiency are the African variant, designated Gd^{A-}, and the Mediterranean variant, $Gd^{Mediterranean}$. Both are characterized by an accelerated age-dependent decrease in red blood cell G6PD activity. In the red blood cells of affected males or homozygous females with the African Gd^{A-} variant, there is a comparatively slow decline in enzyme activity with age, so that only a minority of cells, the most senescent, are substantially lacking in enzyme activity. The $Gd^{Mediterranean}$ variant has much less enzyme activity, and in affected males even newly released reticulocytes have a substantial deficiency in enzyme activity; the mature circulating erythrocytes are essentially devoid of measurable G6PD activity.

Glucose-6-phosphate dehydrogenase catalyzes the initial step in the pentose phosphate shunt pathway, which is essential in the mature red blood cell for the regeneration of reduced nicotinamide adenine dinucleotide phosphate (NADPH) from nicotinamide adenine dinucleotide phosphate (NADP). The reduced form is a required cofactor for the enzyme glutathione reductase, which together with glutathione peroxidase protects the hemoglobin, the supporting structures, and the enzymes of the red blood cell against oxidative damage. In the face of G6PD deficiency, erythrocytes may be extremely vulnerable to oxidant stress, which may result from exposure to certain drugs, chemicals, and infectious agents. During periods of oxidant stress, the hemoglobin may undergo intracellular precipitation to form Heinz bodies. These precipitates, which become associated with the cell membrane, are normally removed in the spleen, but in the process the cell may become damaged and undergo rapid destruction.

Both the African and the Mediterranean types of G6PD deficiency are associated with little or no hematologic abnormality under normal circumstances. In individuals with the African variant, only a comparatively small fraction of circulating red blood cells are significantly deficient in G6PD at any given time, and even though severe hemolysis and anemia may result from an episode of oxidative stress, the process is typically self-limited. The younger population of red blood cells that remains after hemolysis has occurred retains a higher level of enzyme activity, and these cells are thus relatively protected from further oxidative challenge. In individuals with the Mediterranean variant, all of the circulating erythrocytes are severely G6PD deficient and hence susceptible to oxidant challenge. Patients with this variant are at risk for acute, life-threatening hemolysis if exposed to a significant oxidant challenge. Transfusions may be lifesaving during episodes of acute hemolysis.

Pyruvate kinase (PK) deficiency occurs most often in northern Europeans and is the most prevalent enzyme deficiency disorder affecting the glycolytic pathway. Impaired synthesis of adenosine triphosphate in PK-deficient red blood cells results in potassium depletion, intracellular dehydration, and impaired passage of the erythrocytes through the spleen. Premature destruction ensues in the spleen, liver, or bone marrow, resulting in variable degrees of anemia. In severe forms of the disease, splenectomy may ameliorate the degree of hemolysis, but ongoing transfusion support may nevertheless be required to maintain an adequate hemoglobin level in these patients.

DISORDERS OF THE RED BLOOD CELL MEMBRANE

The primary functions of the red blood cell membrane are to maintain the structural integrity of the cell and to regulate cation transport and permeability. The most prevalent of the red blood cell membrane disorders include hereditary spherocytosis (HS) and hereditary elliptocytosis (HE). Rarer membrane-related disorders include a group of hereditary stomatocytosis syndromes and hereditary pyropoikilocytosis. Hereditary spherocytosis predominates in individuals of northern European extraction, whereas HE has been found in numerous population groups. There are numerous variants of each of these disorders, and in most cases inheritance follows an autosomal dominant pattern.

The extent of hemolysis in HS and HE varies considerably among the different variants. In some cases hemolysis is fully compensated and barely perceptible, whereas in more severe forms anemia may be pronounced. The underlying defects in these disorders are structural abnormalities of the red blood cell membrane cytoskeleton, but this alone is not the direct cause of hemolysis. Rather, the misshapen cells have impaired deformability and difficulty in traversing the splenic circulation, and undergo destruction within the spleen. Accordingly, splenectomy is frequently effective in ameliorating the hemolysis and the anemia, especially in HS.

Prior to splenectomy, patients with these hemolytic disorders are also at risk of developing acute episodes of aplasia accompanied by reticulocytopenia and a rapid fall in hemoglobin levels. These episodes typically follow a trivial viral illness, and they have been linked to the same parvovirus agent that causes aplastic episodes in patients with sickle cell disease (16). During these aplastic crises, as in sickle cell disease, red blood cell transfusions may be required to sustain life.

REFERENCES

1. Sunshine HR, Hofrichter J, Ferrone FA, et al. Oxygen binding by sickle hemoglobin polymers. *J Mol Biol* 1982;158:251–273.
2. Hofrichter J, Ross PD, Eaton WA. A physical description of hemoglobin S gelation. In: Hercules JI, Cottam GL, Waterman MR, et al., eds. Proceedings of the symposium on molecular and cellular aspects of sickle cell disease. DHEW publication (NIH) 76-1007. Bethesda: US Department of Health, Education, and Welfare, 1976:185–224.
3. Steinberg MH, Hebbel RP. Clinical diversity of sickle cell anemia: genetic and cellular modulation of disease severity. *Am J Hematol* 1983; 14:405–416.
4. Embury SH. The clinical pathophysiology of sickle cell disease. *Annu Rev Med* 1986;37:361–376.
5. Pagnier J, Mears JG, Dunda-Belkhodja O, et al. Evidence for the multicentric origin of the sickle cell hemoglobin gene in Africa. *Proc Natl Acad Sci U S A* 1984;81:1771–1773.
6. Bunn HF. Mechanisms of disease: pathogenesis and treatment of sickle cell disease. *N Engl J Med* 1997;337:762–769.
7. Hebbel RP, Boggaerts MAB, Eaton JW, et al. Erythrocyte adherence to endothelium in sickle-cell anemia. *N Engl J Med* 1980;302:992–995.
8. Aslan M, Thornley-Brown D, Freeman BA. Reactive species in sickle cell disease. *Ann N Y Acad Sci* 2000;899:375–391.
9. Stuart MJ, Setty BN. Sickle cell acute chest syndrome: pathogenesis and rationale for treatment. *Blood* 1999;94:1555–1560.
10. French JA II, Kenny D, Scott JP, et al. Mechanisms of stroke in sickle cell disease: sickle erythrocytes decrease cerebral blood flow in rats after nitric oxide synthase inhibition. *Blood* 1997;89:4591–4599.
11. Houston PE, Rana S, Sekhsaria S, et al. Homocysteine in sickle cell disease: relationship to stroke. *Am J Med* 1997;103:192–196.
12. Platt OS, Brambilla DJ, Rosse WF, et al. Mortality in sickle cell disease—life expectancy and risk factors for early death. *N Engl J Med* 1994;330:1639–1644.
13. Miller ST, Sleeper LA, Pegelow CH, et al. Prediction of adverse outcomes in children with sickle cell disease. *N Engl J Med* 2000;342: 83–89.
14. Ballas SK, Larner J, Smith ED, et al. The xerocytosis of Hb SC disease. *Blood* 1987;69:124–130.
15. Steinberg MH, Embury SH. α-Thalassemia in blacks: genetic and clinical aspects and interactions with the sickle hemoglobin gene. *Blood* 1986;68:985–990.
16. Saarinen UM, Chorba TL, Tattersall P, et al. Human Parvovirus B19–induced epidemic acute red cell aplasia in patients with hereditary hemolytic anemia. *Blood* 1986;67:1411–1417.
17. Powars D, Wilson B, Imbus C, et al. The natural history of stroke in sickle cell disease. *Am J Med* 1978;65:461–471.
18. Vichinsky EP, Neumayr LD, Earles AN, et al. Causes and outcomes of the acute chest syndrome in sickle cell disease. *N Engl J Med* 2000; 342:1855–1865.
19. Mantadakis E, Don Cavender J, Rogers Z, et al. Prevalence of priapism in children and adolescents with sickle cell anemia. *J Pediatr Hematol Oncol* 1999;21:518–522.
20. Kimmel AS, Magargal LE, Maizel R, et al. Proliferative sickle cell retinopathy under age 20: a review. *Ophthalmic Surg* 1987;18:126–128.
21. Lessin LS, Kurantsin-Mills J, Klug PP, et al. Determination of rheologically optimal mixtures of AA and SS erythrocytes. *Blood* 1977;50[Suppl 1]:111.
22. Schmalzer EA, Lee JO, Brown AK, et al. Viscosity of mixtures of sickle and normal red cells at varying hematocrit levels. *Transfusion* 1987; 27:228–233.
23. Russel MO, Goldberg HI, Hodson A, et al. Effect of transfusion therapy on arteriographic abnormalities and on recurrence of stroke in sickle cell disease. *Blood* 1984;63:162–169.
24. Wilimas J, Goff JR, Anderson HR, et al. Efficacy of transfusion therapy for 1 to 2 years in patients with sickle cell disease and cerebrovascular accidents. *J Pediatr* 1980;96:205–208.
25. Quattlebaum TG, Pierce MM. Estimates of need for transfusions during hypertransfusion therapy in sickle cell disease. *J Pediatr* 1986;109: 456–459.
26. Cohen AR, Martin MB, Silber JH, et al. A modified transfusion pro-

gram for prevention of stroke in sickle cell disease. *Blood* 1992;79: 1657–1661.
27. Adams RJ, McKie VC, Hsu L, et al. Prevention of a first stroke by transfusions in children with sickle cell anemia and abnormal results on transcranial Doppler ultrasonography. *N Engl J Med* 1998;339: 5–11.
28. Seeler RA. Intensive transfusion therapy for priapism in boys with sickle cell anemia. *J Urol* 1973;110:360–361.
29. Mantadakis E, Ewalt DH, Don Cavender J, et al. Outpatient penile aspiration and epinephrine irrigation for young patients with sickle cell anemia and prolonged priapism. *Blood* 2000;95:78–82.
30. Siegel JF, Rich MA, Brock WA. Association of sickle cell disease, priapism, exchange transfusion and neurological events: ASPEN syndrome. *J Urol* 1993;150:1480–1482.
31. Charache S, Lubin B, Reid CD. Management and therapy of sickle cell disease. NIH publication 84-2117. Bethesda: US Department of Health and Human Services, 1984.
32. Kinney TR, Ware RE, Schultz WH, et al. Long-term management of splenic sequestration in children with sickle cell disease. *J Pediatr* 1990; 117:194–199.
33. Weisz-Carrington P. *Principles of clinical immunohematology.* Chicago: Year Book, 1986:183.
34. Powars DR, Sandhu M, Niland-Weiss J, et al. Pregnancy in sickle cell disease. *Obstet Gynecol* 1986;67:217–228.
35. Fort AT, Morrison JC, Berreras L, et al. Counseling the patient with sickle cell disease about reproduction: pregnancy outcome does not justify the maternal risk! *Am J Obstet Gynecol* 1971;111:324–327.
36. Koshy M, Burd L, Wallace D, et al. Prophylactic red-cell transfusions in pregnant patients with sickle cell disease. *N Engl J Med* 1988;319: 1447–1452.
37. Homi J, Reynolds J, Skinner A, et al. General anesthesia in sickle cell disease. *BMJ* 1979;1:1599–1601.
38. Bischoff RJ, Williamson A, Dalali MJ, et al. Assessment of the use of transfusion therapy perioperatively in patients with sickle cell hemoglobinopathies. *Ann Surg* 1988;207:434–438.
39. Janik J, Seeler RA. Perioperative management of children with sickle hemoglobinopathy. *J Pediatr Surg* 1980;15:117–120.
40. Morrison JC, Whybrew WD, Bucovaz ET. Use of partial exchange transfusion preoperatively in patients with sickle cell hemoglobinopathies. *Am J Obstet Gynecol* 1978;132:59–63.
41. Jampol LM, Green JL, Goldberg MF, et al. An update on vitrectomy surgery and retinal detachment repair in sickle cell disease. *Arch Ophthalmol* 1982;100:591–593.
42. Vichinsky EP, Haberkern CM, Neumayr L, et al. A comparison of conservative and aggressive transfusion regimens in the perioperative management of sickle cell disease. Preoperative Transfusion in Sickle Cell Disease Study Group. *N Engl J Med* 1995;333:206–213.
43. Haberkern CM, Neumayr LD, Orringer EP, et al. Cholecystectomy in sickle cell anemia patients: perioperative outcome of 364 cases from the National Preoperative Transfusion Study. Preoperative Transfusion in Sickle Cell Disease Study Group. *Blood* 1997;89:1533–1542.
44. Waldon P, Pegelow C, Neumayr L, et al. Tonsillectomy, adenoidectomy, and myringotomy in sickle cell disease: perioperative morbidity. Preoperative Transfusion in Sickle Cell Disease Study Group. *J Pediatr Hematol Oncol* 1999;21:129–135.
45. Adams DM, Ware RE, Schultz WH, et al. Successful surgical outcome in children with sickle hemoglobinopathies: the Duke University experience. *J Pediatr Surg* 1998;33:428–432.
46. Eichhorn JH. Preoperative screening for sickle cell trait [Editorial]. *JAMA* 1988;259:907.
47. Stockman JA, Nigro MA, Mishkin MM, et al. Occlusion of large cerebral vessels in sickle-cell anemia. *N Engl J Med* 1972;287:846–849.
48. Blumberg N, Ross K, Avila E, et al. Should chronic transfusions be matched for antigens other than ABO and $Rh_0(D)$? *Vox Sang* 1984; 47:205–208.
49. Alarif L, Castro O, Ofosu M, et al. HLA-B35 is associated with red cell alloimmunization in sickle cell disease. *Clin Immunol Immunopathol* 1986;38:178–183.
50. Vichinsky EP, Earles A, Johnson RA, et al. Alloimmunization in sickle cell anemia and transfusion of racially unmatched blood. *N Engl J Med* 1990;322:1617–1621.
51. Orlina AR, Sosler SD, Koshy M. Problems of chronic transfusion in sickle cell disease. *J Clin Apheresis* 1991;6:234–240.
52. Sosler SD, Jilly BJ, Saporito C, et al. A simple, practical model for reducing alloimmunization in patients with sickle cell disease. *Am J Hematol* 1993;43:103–106.
53. Petz LD, Calhoun L, Shulman IA, et al. The sickle cell hemolytic transfusion reaction syndrome. *Transfusion* 1997;37:382–392.
54. Garratty G. Severe reactions associated with transfusion of patients with sickle cell disease [Editorial]. *Transfusion* 1997;37:357–361.
55. King KE, Shirey RS, Lankiewicz MW, et al. Delayed hemolytic transfusion reactions in sickle cell disease: simultaneous destruction of recipients' red cells. *Transfusion* 1997;37:376–381.
56. Vengelen-Tyler V, ed. *Technical manual of the American Association of Blood Banks,* 13th ed. Arlington, VA: American Association of Blood Banks, 1999:180.
57. Romanoff, ME, Woodward DG, Bullard WG. Autologous blood transfusion in patients with sickle cell trait. *Anesthesiology* 1988;68:820–821.
58. Olivieri N. Medical progress: the β-thalassemias. *N Engl J Med* 1999; 341:99–109.
59. Pasvol G, Weatherall DJ, Wilson RJM. Effects of foetal haemoglobin on susceptibility of red cells to *Plasmodium falciparum*. *Nature* 1977; 270:171–173.
60. Friedman MJ. Oxidant damage mediates red cell resistance to malaria. *Nature* 1979;280:245–247.
61. Honig GR, Adams JG III. *Human hemoglobin genetics.* Vienna: Springer-Verlag, 1986.
62. Rachmilewitz EA. Denaturation of the normal and abnormal hemoglobin molecule. *Semin Hematol* 1974;11:441–462.
63. Furbetta M, Tuveri T, Rosatelli C, et al. Molecular mechanism accounting for milder types of thalassemia major. *J Pediatr* 1983;103: 35–39.
64. Orkin SH, Kazazian HH Jr, Antonarakis SE, et al. Abnormal RNA processing due to the exon mutation of β^E-globin gene. *Nature* 1982; 300:768–769.
65. Wasi P, Na-Nakorn S, Pootrakul S, et al. α- and β-Thalassemia in Thailand. *Ann N Y Acad Sci* 1969;165:60–82.
66. Schorr JB, Radel E. Transfusion therapy and its complications in patients with Cooley's anemia. *Ann N Y Acad Sci* 1964;119:703–708.
67. Wolman IJ. Transfusion therapy in Cooley's anemia: growth and health as related to long-range hemoglobin levels. *Ann N Y Acad Sci* 1964; 119:736–747.
68. Gabutti V, Piga A, Nicola P, et al. Haemoglobin levels and blood requirements in thalassaemia. *Arch Dis Child* 1982;57:156–158.
69. Cavill I, Worwood M, Jacobs A. Internal regulation of iron absorption. *Nature* 1975;256:328–329.
70. Piomelli S, Danoff SJ, Becker MH, et al. Prevention of bone malformations and cardiomegaly in Cooley's anemia by early hypertransfusion regimen. *Ann N Y Acad Sci* 1969;165:427–436.
71. Piomelli S, Loew T. Management of thalassemia major (Cooley's anemia). *Hematol Oncol Clin North Am* 1991;5:557–569.
72. Propper RD, Button LN, Nathan DG. New approaches to the transfusion management of thalassemia. *Blood* 1980;55:55–60.
73. Cazzola M, Borgna-Pignatti C, Locatelli F, et al. A moderate transfusion regimen may reduce iron loading in β-thalassemia major without producing excessive expansion of erythropoiesis. *Transfusion* 1997;37: 135–140.
74. Schuman JE, Tanser CL, Peloquin R, et al. The erythropoietic response to pregnancy in β-thalassaemia minor. *Br J Haematol* 1973;25: 249–260.
75. Hocking IW, Ibbotson RN. The effect of the β thalassaemia trait on pregnancy with particular reference to its complications and outcome. *Med J Aust* 1966;2:397–400.
76. Singer ST, Styles L, Bojanowski J, et al. Changing outcome of homozygous α-thalassemia: cautious optimism. *J Pediatr Hematol Oncol* 2000; 22:539–542.
77. Gordeuk VR, Bacon BR, Brittenham GM. Iron overload: causes and consequences. *Annu Rev Nutr* 1987;7:485–508.
78. Maurer HS, Lloyd-Still JD, Ingrisano C, et al. A prospective evaluation

of iron chelation therapy in children with severe β-thalassemia. *Am J Dis Child* 1988;142:287–292.
79. Wolfe L, Olivieri N, Sallan D, et al. Prevention of cardiac disease by subcutaneous deferoxamine in patients with thalassemia major. *N Engl J Med* 1985;312:1600–1603.
80. Cohen AR, Schwartz E. Excretion of iron in response to deferoxamine in sickle cell anemia. *J Pediatr* 1978;92:659–662.
81. Angelucci E, Brittenham GM, McLaren CE, et al. Hepatic iron concentration and total body iron stores in thalassemia major. *N Engl J Med* 2000;343:327–331.
82. Olivieri NF, Brittenham GM. Iron-chelating therapy and the treatment of thalassemia. *Blood* 1997;89:739–761.
83. Porter JB, Huehns ER. Transfusion and exchange transfusion in sickle cell anemias, with particular reference to iron metabolism. *Acta Haematol* 1987;78:198–205.
84. Piomelli S, Seaman C, Reibman J, et al. Separation of younger red cells with improved survival in vivo: an approach to chronic transfusion therapy. *Proc Natl Acad Sci U S A* 1978;75:3474–3478.
85. Cohen AR, Schmidt JM, Martin MB, et al. Clinical trial of young red cell transfusions. *J Pediatr* 1984;104:865–868.
86. Marcus RE, Wonke B, Bantock HM, et al. A prospective trial of young red cells in 48 patients with transfusion-dependent thalassemia. *Br J Haematol* 1985;60:153–159.
87. Berdoukas VA, Kwan YL, Sansotta ML. A study on the value of red cell exchange transfusion in transfusion dependent anaemias. *Clin Lab Haematol* 1986;8:209–220.

Rossi's Principles of Transfusion Medicine, Third Edition, edited by Toby L. Simon, Walter H. Dzik, Edward L. Snyder, Christopher P. Stowell, and Ronald G. Strauss. Lippincott Williams & Wilkins, Philadelphia © 2002.

CASE 32A

A DELAYED HEMOLYTIC TRANSFUSION REACTION RUN AMOK

CASE HISTORY

A 29-year-old woman from the Middle East with sickle cell disease and hereditary persistence of fetal hemoglobin (HbF) experienced a seizure and was found to have a 7-cm mass in the left cerebral ventricle. She was started on phenytoin and dexamethasone and over the next few weeks had no recurrence of the seizures. The patient traveled by plane via Frankfort to the United States for workup and therapy for the brain mass. On departure she was asymptomatic, but during the 7-hour flight from Frankfort she became increasingly uncomfortable.

Upon admission to the hospital, she was found to have abdominal pain, rash, and fever (102°F). Her hematocrit had dropped from 34.1% several days prior to admission (the patient had brought along a copy of her records) to 23.4% with a reticulocyte count of 13.2%. Her medical history was significant for only three relatively mild hemolytic crises and four uncomplicated vaginal deliveries, presumably because of the protective effect of HbF. She had never traveled by air before. The differential diagnosis on admission included hypersensitivity reaction to phenytoin, gastroenteritis, and sickle cell crisis. Phenytoin was replaced with valproic acid and a dexamethasone taper was begun. The fever and rash began to subside, but abdominal pain persisted, the hematocrit continued to fall to 20.7%, and her LDH was 849 U/L. Her clinical course is shown in Figure 32A.1. She received three units of red blood cells, which brought her hematocrit to 30.5%. The hematocrit rose to 35.1% over the next 5 days but decreased thereafter at an accelerating pace. Between day 15 and day 18, the hematocrit fell from 31.3% to 17.0% with a reticulocyte count of 6.8%; the LDH was 1,419 U/L, the total bilirubin was 2.9 mg/dl, and the direct bilirubin was 2.0 mg/dl. The patient was again febrile and complaining of leg pain. Two units of red blood cells were given over the next 24 hours with a resulting hematocrit of 14.4%; the LDH was now 1,914 U/L, the total bilirubin was 9.0 mg/dl, and the direct bilirubin was 6.2 mg/dl. Additional red blood cell transfusions were ordered.

On admission, the blood bank workup demonstrated the presence of anti-e and anti-Jk^a. A sample drawn the day before the hematocrit began to fall precipitously demonstrated a new anti-Fy^a. A sample drawn after the two-unit transfusion contained yet another new alloantibody, an anti-M which was reactive at 37°C and antiglobulin phase with anti-IgG (i.e., had an IgG component). The direct antiglobulin test was consistently negative.

At the time that the new anti-M was found and the staff began requesting additional units of difficult-to-find red blood cells, a transfusion medicine physician saw the patient and suggested the diagnosis of sickle cell hemolytic transfusion reaction syndrome. He recommended hydration, high-dose steroids, and withholding additional red blood cell transfusions. The patient's hematocrit fell as low as 11.2%, but thereafter it began to increase and was 22.7% at the time of discharge on gabapentin, a prednisone taper, and weekly erythropoietin injections.

A month later the patient was admitted with a hematocrit of 26.6% for embolization and resection of the intraventricular mass, which proved to be a meningioma. She was transfused with three units of blood that she had donated between the two admissions and which had been stored in the liquid state. She was discharged with a hematocrit of 26.3% and no neurologic sequelae.

DISCUSSION

Approximately a week following transfusion for sickle cell crisis, this patient developed a delayed hemolytic transfusion reaction (DHTR) with the production of a new alloantibody, anti-Fy^a (and perhaps anti-M), and accelerated destruction of red blood cells. The (re)appearance of a new alloantibody following transfusion does not generally cause hemolysis; hence, the designation delayed *serologic* transfusion reaction. Typically a new alloantibody is demonstrated in the serum or in an eluate, often as an incidental finding by the transfusion service. Accelerated red blood cell destruction is less commonly observed (i.e., delayed *hemolytic* transfusion reaction). Even in DHTR, hemolysis is usually limited and may be clinically apparent only by early requirement for retransfusion, low-grade fever, or a mild elevation in bilirubin levels.

In patients with sickle cell disease, however, DHTRs occasionally run amok and are associated with dramatic reactions, with marked hemolysis and apparent worsening of sickle cell crisis following transfusion. In sickle cell hemolytic transfusion reaction (HTR) syndrome (1) hemolysis may be delayed or acute, but characteristically the hematocrit is lower following allogeneic red blood cell transfusion than it was before. Note that in this patient the hematocrit went from 17.0% to 14.4% after transfusion of two units of red blood cells, and she had an apparent painful relapse of sickle cell crisis. Suppressed erythro-

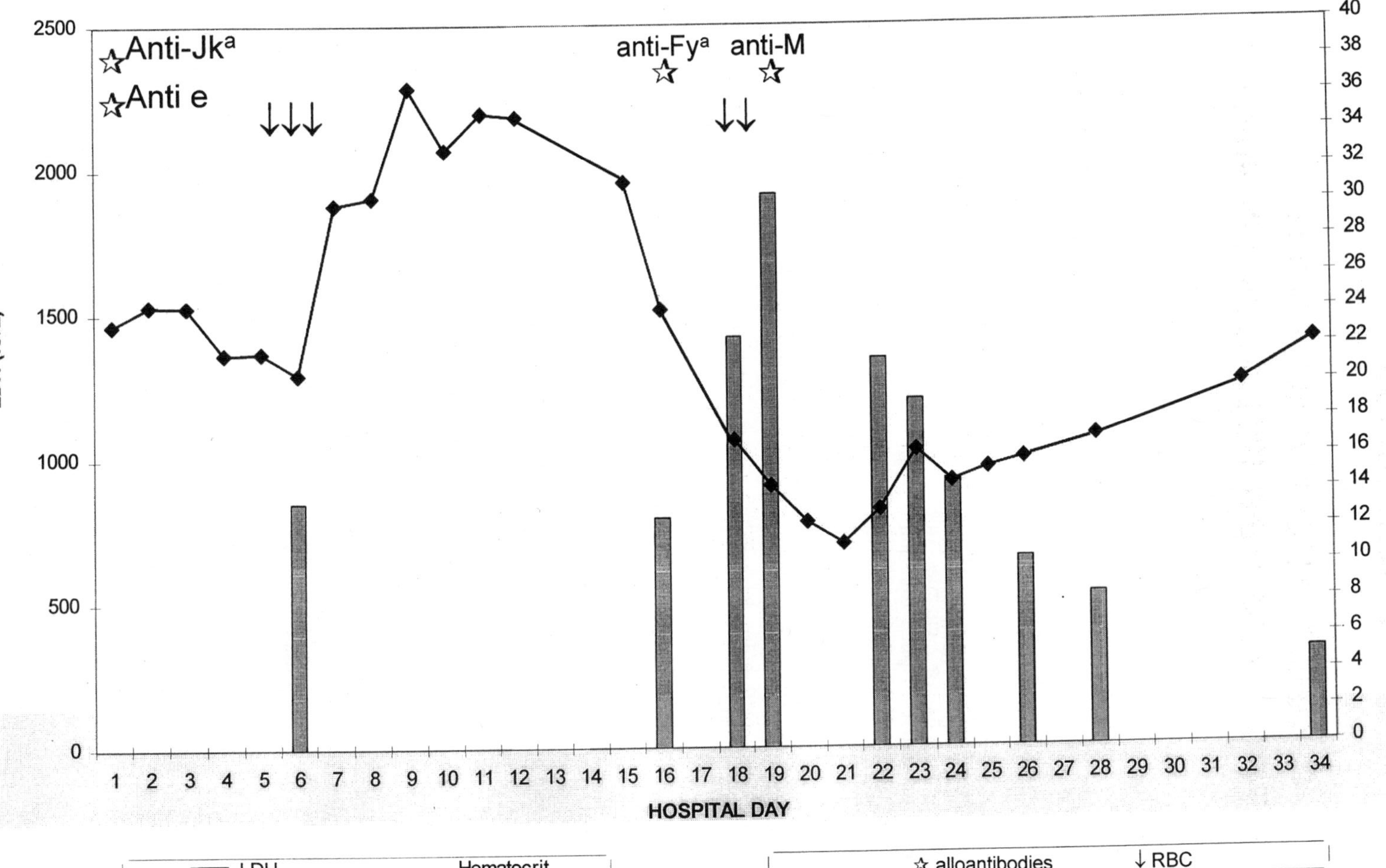

FIGURE 32A.1. Hospital Course. The *line* represents hematocrit and the *bars* LDH levels. Each *arrow* represents one unit of red blood cells transfused and each *star* shows when the indicated alloantibody was detected. Note that the hematocrit is lower after the two-unit transfusion than before.

poiesis may contribute to the marked drop in hematocrit after transfusion in sickle cell HTR syndrome. These patients characteristically exhibit inappropriately low reticulocyte levels at the time of acute hemolysis, as did this patient (i.e., 6.8% at a time when the hematocrit was 17.0%). Another factor contributing to the plummeting hematocrit may be *hyperhemolysis,* the destruction of autologous red blood cells as well as those transfused (2). Two mechanisms have been proposed for hyperhemolysis, the development of a red blood cell autoantibody or bystander hemolysis. In the latter, antigen-antibody complexes activate complement, to which sickle cells are particularly sensitive. Further transfusion serves only to exacerbate hemolysis in this situation. For this reason, it is important to withhold red blood cell transfusion. High-dose steroid therapy has also been used successfully. After such an episode, some patients will be transfused again without incident, but others will exhibit hyperhemolysis with subsequent red blood cell transfusions.

The characteristic serologic findings in sickle cell HTR syndrome include the presence of multiple red blood cell alloantibodies and, occasionally, autoantibodies as well. The finding of a new alloantibody, particularly in an eluate, is also typical. However, the serologic findings do not always explain the hemolytic reaction. Hemolysis of antigen-negative transfused units has been observed and, in a few patients with brisk hemolysis, no alloantibodies could be demonstrated at all (1). In this patient, new alloantibodies were identified 2 days before and immediately after the transfusions associated with hyperhemolysis. The direct antiglobulin test was not reactive, however, possibly due to rapid hemolysis of antigen-positive red blood cells.

This patient recovered from her hyperhemolytic crisis only to be faced with the problem of requiring cranial surgery for what was suspected to be a highly vascular tumor. Even in the absence of hyperhemolysis, she posed a significant challenge to the transfusion service to find sufficient units of blood compatible with anti-e, anti-Jk^a, anti-Fy^a, and anti-M. Fewer than 1 in 1,000 Rh(D)-positive donors would lack all four antigens, and only 1 or 2 per 1,000 would lack e, Jk^a, and Fy^a. One option would have been to find units via the American Rare Donor Program. Another solution, in theory, would have been to determine her siblings' phenotypes. Unfortunately, not only were two of her three siblings out of the country, but they both had sickle cell disease.

Finding compatible donor units presented a formidable task, so autologous blood was an obvious alternative. The patient was given recombinant human erythropoietin and, once her hematocrit exceeded 27%, began a program of preoperative autologous blood donation. Her donations were scheduled to occur within 35 days of surgery because it is difficult to freeze and thaw sickle cells without extensive hemolysis. Even red blood cells from sickle cell heterozygotes form a jelly-like mass and hemolyze if hypertonic saline is used for deglycerolizing (3). The usual qualifying criterion of a predonation hematocrit of 34% was waived in this situation given the extenuating circumstances and that she was a young woman who had exhibited no evidence of coronary insufficiency at hematocrits as low as 11%. This patient's autologous units were successfully stored in liquid form and transfused without incident during her tumor resection.

Case contributed by Christopher P. Stowell, M.D., Ph.D., Massachusetts General Hospital, Boston, MA.

REFERENCES

1. Petz LD, Calhoun L, Shulman IA, et al. The sickle cell hemolytic transfusion reaction syndrome. *Transfusion* 1997;37:382–392.
2. King KE, Shirey RS, Lankiewicz MW, et al. Delayed hemolytic transfusion reactions in sickle cell disease: simultaneous destruction of recipient's red cells. *Transfusion* 1997;37:376–381.
3. Meryman HT, Hornblower M. Freezing and deglycerolizing sickle trait red blood cells. *Transfusion* 1976;16:627–632.

33

NEONATAL RED BLOOD CELL, PLATELET, PLASMA, AND NEUTROPHIL TRANSFUSIONS

RONALD G. STRAUSS

Many aspects of hematopoiesis are incompletely developed in preterm infants. This lack of development diminishes the capability to produce red blood cells (RBCs), platelets, and white blood cells, such as neutrophils, particularly during the stress of life-threatening illnesses such as sepsis, severe pulmonary dysfunction, necrotizing enterocolitis, and immune cytopenia. Similarly, hepatic function is immature, and the result is low levels of plasma clotting proteins. Premature birth also can be complicated by serious medical problems accompanied by phlebotomy blood losses, bleeding, hemolysis, and consumptive coagulopathy. Thus preterm infants begin life with quantities of blood cells and clotting proteins that are barely adequate and, very importantly, with a diminished ability to compensate for the complications of prematurity. These circumstances lead to the need for blood component transfusions.

To illustrate, premature infants, most frequently those with birth weight less than 1.0 kg, are given numerous RBC transfusions early in life owing to several interacting factors. Infants delivered before 28 weeks of gestation (birth weight <1.0 kg) are born before the bulk of iron transport through the placenta from mother to fetus has occurred and before the marked erythropoietic activity of fetal marrow has begun during the third trimester. Hence preterm infants of very low birth weight enter extrauterine life with low iron stores and a small circulating mass of RBCs. Soon after preterm birth, severe respiratory disease can lead to repeated blood sampling for laboratory studies and consequently to replacement RBC transfusions. As a final factor, preterm infants are unable to mount an effective erythropoietin response to decreasing numbers of RBCs, and this diminished compensation contributes to the need for RBC transfusions.

The physiology of hematopoiesis in the fetus and newborn is discussed in detail in Chapter 29, as are clotting proteins in Chapter 31. Accordingly, only the aspects of physiology and pathophysiology that pertain to neonatal transfusion medicine are included here. The emphasis is on transfusion management during the first several weeks after birth.

RED BLOOD CELL TRANSFUSION

Pathophysiology of Anemia of Prematurity

During the first weeks of life, all infants experience a decline in the number of circulating RBCs caused both by physiologic factors and, in sick premature infants, phlebotomy blood losses. In healthy term infants, the nadir blood hemoglobin value rarely falls to less than 9 g/dl at an age of approximately 10 to 12 weeks (1). Among preterm infants, this decline occurs at an earlier age and is more pronounced in severity. Mean hemoglobin concentration decreases to approximately 8 g/dl in infants of 1.0 to 1.5 kg birth weight and to 7 g/dl in infants weighing less than 1.0 kg (2). Because this postnatal decrease in hemoglobin level is universal and is well tolerated by term infants, it is commonly called *physiologic anemia of infancy.* However, in

R.G. Strauss: Departments of Pathology and Pediatrics, University of Iowa College of Medicine, and DeGowin Blood Center, University of Iowa Hospitals and Clinics, Iowa City, Iowa.

preterm infants, this marked decline in hemoglobin frequently is exacerbated by phlebotomy blood losses and may be associated with symptomatic anemia that necessitates RBC transfusions, making anemia of prematurity unacceptable as a purely "physiologic" event.

Physiologic factors that influence erythropoiesis and the biologic characteristics of erythropoietin are critical in the pathogenesis of anemia of prematurity. Growth is extremely rapid during the first weeks of life, and RBC production by neonatal bone marrow must increase commensurately or circulating RBCs are diluted within the expanding blood volume. The circulating life span of neonatal RBCs in the bloodstream is shorter than that of adult RBCs. In addition, a key clinical factor is the need for repeated blood sampling to monitor the condition of critically ill neonates. The most premature infants, who are the most critically ill and have the smallest blood volumes, need the most frequent blood sampling. Another important reason that the nadir hemoglobin values of premature infants are lower than those of term infants is that premature infants have a relatively diminished erythropoietin plasma level in response to anemia (3,4). Although anemia provokes erythropoietin production in premature infants, the plasma levels achieved are lower than those of older persons with comparable degrees of anemia. When related quantitatively, increasing erythropoietin levels and decreasing blood hemoglobin concentrations correlate weakly (4). This relatively ineffective erythropoietin response limits compensation for anemia in the newborn caused by rapid growth and RBC loss due to procedures and conditions such as phlebotomy, clinical bleeding, and hemolysis.

Erythroid progenitor cells of premature infants are quite responsive to recombinant erythropoietin (5). Thus inadequate production of erythropoietin is a major cause of physiologic anemia—not a subnormal response of erythroid progenitors to this growth factor. The mechanisms responsible for diminished erythropoietin plasma levels in premature neonates are only partially understood. One mechanism of apparent importance is the reliance of premature infants on the liver, rather than kidney, as the primary site of erythropoietin production during the first several weeks of life (6,7). This dependency on hepatic production of erythropoietin is important because the liver is less sensitive to anemia and tissue hypoxia than is the kidney (6). This accounts for the relatively ineffective erythropoietin response of fetuses and neonates to decreasing RBC counts. The switch to renal erythropoietin is not complete until after birth and is timed from conception, not from birth; that is, it is not accelerated by preterm delivery. Abnormal pharmacokinetics are another mechanism that may contribute to low plasma erythropoietin levels in preterm infants because plasma levels are a balance of production (input) and metabolism (clearance). Data about human infants suggest that low plasma erythropoietin levels are caused at least in part by increased clearance of plasma erythropoietin and greater volume of distribution in neonates than in adults—a situation in which rapid removal from plasma accentuates the problem of diminished erythropoietin production (8).

Red Blood Cell Transfusion Practices

Red blood cell transfusions are given to maintain the hematocrit at a level judged best for the clinical condition of the infant.

TABLE 33.1. GUIDELINES FOR SMALL-VOLUME RED BLOOD CELL TRANSFUSIONS GIVEN TO INFANTS

Maintain >40%–45% hematocrit (Hct) for severe[a] cardiopulmonary disease
Maintain >30%–35% Hct for moderate[a] cardiopulmonary disease
Maintain >30%–35% Hct for major[a] surgery
Maintain >20%–30% Hct for infants whose anemia is stable, especially if the following are present:
Unexplained[a] breathing disorders
Unexplained[a] poor growth

[a]Must be defined locally. For example, "severe" pulmonary disease may be defined as requiring mechanical ventilation with >0.35 FiO_2 and "moderate" as less intensive assisted ventilation.

General guidelines acceptable to most neonatologists are listed in Table 33.1. However, many aspects of neonatal RBC transfusion therapy are controversial. This lack of consistency stems from incomplete knowledge of the cellular and molecular biologic mechanisms of erythropoiesis during the perinatal period, of the physiologic effects of neonatal anemia, and of the infant's response to RBC transfusions. Although in some instances the value of RBC transfusions is clear (e.g., to manage anemia that has caused congestive heart failure), in others it is not (e.g., to correct irregular patterns of heart or respiratory rates). Because clearly established indications for neonatal RBC transfusions based on results of controlled scientific studies do not exist, it is important that pediatricians critically evaluate the guidelines in Table 33.1 and apply them in light of neonatal practice at their respective institutions. To assist in this task, the rationale for each of the guidelines in Table 33.1 is discussed (9–11).

Maintain Hematocrit Greater than 40% to 45% for Severe Cardiopulmonary Disease

In neonates with severe respiratory or cardiac disease, defined as that necessitating administration of relatively large quantities of oxygen and continuous ventilator support, it is customary to maintain the hematocrit at greater than 40% (blood hemoglobin greater than 13 g/dl). Proponents believe that transfusion of RBCs containing adult hemoglobin, with its superior interaction with 2,3-diphosphoglycerate (2,3-DPG; also known as 2,3-bisphosphoglycerate) and better oxygen off-loading than infant RBCs containing fetal hemoglobin, is likely to improve oxygen delivery throughout the period of diminished cardiopulmonary function. Although this practice is widely recommended, little evidence is available to establish its efficacy, to define its optimal use (the best hematocrit for each degree of cardiopulmonary dysfunction), or to document the risk. In a study of 10 infants with severe (oxygen-dependent) bronchopulmonary dysplasia, physiologic end points improved (systemic oxygen transport increased and oxygen use decreased) after small-volume RBC transfusions were given. However, blood hemoglobin levels were not predictive of which infants benefited from the RBC transfusions (12).

Maintain Hematocrit Greater than 30% to 35% for Moderate Cardiopulmonary Disease

Although more information is needed to define the precise indication for and benefits of RBC transfusions (hematocrit or measurement of tissue oxygenation) for infants with heart and lung disorders, it is logical to presume that infants with moderate degrees of cardiopulmonary dysfunction need less vigorous RBC transfusion support than do those with severe disease. A lower hematocrit is suggested for infants with only moderate degrees of cardiopulmonary disease (Table 33.1).

Maintain Hematocrit Greater than 30% to 35% for Major Surgery

The need to achieve a specific hematocrit preoperatively and to maintain a desired value during a surgical procedure has been controversial for years in the care of patients of all ages. For many years, a minimum hematocrit of 30% (10 g/dl hemoglobin) was preferred. Acceptance of much lower values has been encouraged, particularly for patients able to compensate for anemia. Results of definitive studies are not available to establish the optimal hematocrit for neonates facing major surgery. It seems reasonable, however, to maintain an hematocrit greater than 30% because of the limited ability (albeit, not absent) of the neonatal heart, lungs, and blood vessels to compensate for anemia, the inferior off-loading of oxygen due to diminished interaction between fetal hemoglobin and 2.3-DPG, and developmental impairment of neonatal renal, hepatic, and neurologic function to withstand the stress of major surgery in the face of marked anemia.

Maintain Hematocrit Greater than 20% to 30% for Symptomatic Anemia

Neonates in stable condition with a low hematocrit do not need RBC transfusions unless they have clinical problems presumed to be related to the degree of anemia present. Proponents of RBC transfusion therapy for symptomatic anemia believe that the low RBC mass contributes to tachypnea, dyspnea, apnea, tachycardia, bradycardia, feeding difficulties, and lethargy and that these problems can be alleviated by RBC transfusion (9–11). When a sick premature infant has anemia and severe apnea together, it is tempting to believe that transfusion of RBCs may increase oxygen delivery to the respiratory center of the brain and decrease the number of apneic spells. In support, RBC transfusions were shown to diminish irregular breathing patterns and episodes of bradycardia in preterm infants with anemia when the mean hematocrit was increased from 27% to 36% (13). Other investigators found no benefit of RBC transfusions in improving breathing patterns (14). Similarly, some neonatologists consider poor weight gain an indication for RBC transfusions, particularly when the hemoglobin concentration is less than 10 g/dl (hematocrit <30%) and if other signs of distress are evident (e.g., tachycardia, dyspnea, weak suck, less vigorous cry, and diminished physical activity). In support, Stockman and Clark (15) investigated the effects of RBC transfusion on weight gain in a study with premature infants in relatively stable condition. They found increased weight gain after transfusion to be associated with a low pretransfusion hematocrit and a posttransfusion decrease in metabolic rate (measured by oxygen consumption). They recommended RBC transfusions to manage unexplained growth failure only in the care of infants with clinical manifestations of anemia. In agreement, Blank et al. (16) found no benefit to small-volume RBC transfusions given to apparently well premature infants to maintain a hemoglobin level greater than 10 g/dl. Results of a study by Ross et al. (17) supported RBC transfusions only for infants with symptoms. Factors that helped identify infants who benefited from RBC transfusions included pretransfusion tachycardia (>153 beats/min), presence of apnea or bradycardia necessitating intervention, and elevated blood lactate level.

Red Blood Cell Product to Transfuse

Most RBC transfusions are given to preterm infants as small-volume transfusions (10 to 20 ml/kg body weight) of RBCs suspended either in citrate-phosphate-dextrose-adenine solution at a hematocrit of approximately 70% or in extended storage media (additive solution AS-1, AS-3, AS-5) at a hematocrit of approximately 60% (Table 33.2). Some centers prefer to centrifuge RBC aliquots before transfusion to prepare a uniformly packed RBC concentrate (hematocrit >80%) (18). Most RBC transfusions are infused slowly over 2 to 4 hours. Because of the small quantity of extracellular fluid (RBC storage media) infused very slowly with small-volume transfusions, particularly when the hematocrit is increased by means of centrifugation, the type of anticoagulant and preservative solution in which the RBCs are suspended is unlikely to pose risk for most premature infants (19). Accordingly, the traditional use of relatively fresh RBCs (<7 days of storage) has been challenged by the idea of repeatedly using a dedicated unit (or part of a unit) of stored RBCs for each infant in efforts to diminish the high donor exposure rates among infants who undergo numerous transfusions. Neonatologists who object to prescribing stored RBCs and insist on transfusing fresh RBCs generally raise the following three objections: (a) the increase in the level of potassium in the plasma, (b) the decrease in the level of RBC 2,3-DPG (both of which occur during extended storage), and (c) the possible risks of use of additives such as mannitol and the relatively large amounts of glucose (dextrose) and phosphate present in extended-storage preservative solutions. Although these concerns are legitimate for large-volume (≥25 ml/kg) transfusions, particularly when infusion is rapid, they do not apply to small-volume transfusion for the following reasons.

After 42 days of storage in extended storage medium (AS-1, AS-3, AS-5) at a hematocrit of approximately 60%, extracellular ("plasma") potassium levels in RBC units approximate 50 mEq/L (0.05 mEq/ml), a value that at first glance seems alarmingly high. Simple calculations, however, show the actual dose of bioactive potassium transfused (ionic potassium in the extracellular fluid) is small. An infant weighing 1 kg given a 15-ml/kg transfusion of RBCs stored in extended storage medium and centrifuged to packed RBCs at a hematocrit of approximately 80% receives 3 ml of extracellular fluid containing only 0.15 mEq of potassium to be infused slowly. Even if RBCs are not packed

TABLE 33.2. FORMULATION OF ANTICOAGULANT-PRESERVATIVE SOLUTIONS IN BLOOD COLLECTION SETS

Constituent	CPDA	AS-1	AS-3	AS-5
Volume (ml)	63[a]	100[b]	100[b]	100[b]
Sodium chloride (mg)	None	900	410	877
Dextrose (mg)	2,00	2,200	1,100	900
Adenine (mg)	17.3	27	30	30
Mannitol (mg)	None	750	None	525
Trisodium citrate (mg)	1,660	None	588	None
Citric acid (mg)	206	None	42	None
Sodium phosphate (monobasic) (mg)	140	None	276	None

[a]Approximately 450 ml of donor blood is drawn into 63 ml of citrate-phosphate-dextrose-adenine (CPDA) solution. One unit of red blood cells (hematocrit, ~l70%) is prepared by means of centrifugation and removal of most plasma.
[b]When additive solution AS-1 or AS-5 is used, 450 ml of donor blood is first drawn into 63 ml of CPD, which is identical to CPDA except it contains 1,610 mg dextrose per 63 ml and has no adenine. When AS-3 is used, donor blood is drawn into CP2D, which is identical to CPD except it contains double the amount of dextrose. After centrifugation and removal of nearly all plasma, red blood cells are resuspended in 100 ml of the additive solution (AS-1, AS-3 or AS-5) at a hematocrit of approximately 55% to 60%.

but are removed directly from the blood bag and are infused at a hematocrit of 60%, the potassium dose is only 0.3 mEq. The potassium concentration of RBCs stored in citrate-phosphate-dextrose-adenine solution at a hematocrit of approximately 70% approximates 70 to 80 mEq/L after the 35 days of permitted storage, and the dose of potassium infused with a 15-ml/kg transfusion to a one-kg infant is 0.3 to 0.4 mEq. These doses are quite small when compared to the usual daily $K+$ requirement of 2 to 3 mEq/kg and have been shown in clinical studies not to cause hyperkalemia, whether packed RBCs (20,21) or unmodified RBCs (22-24) were transfused (Table 33.3).

By 21 days of storage, 2,3-DPG is totally depleted from RBCs as reflected by a P_{50} value that decreases from approximately 27 mm Hg in fresh blood to 18 mm Hg in stored RBCs at the time of outdate. Owing to the effects of high fetal hemoglobin levels in neonatal RBCs, the 18 mm Hg value of RBCs transfused after maximum storage corresponds to the expectedly low P_{50} value obtained from the blood of many healthy preterm infants at birth. Thus both older stored RBCs and RBCs from infants have a similarly reduced ability to off-load oxygen compared with fresh adult RBCs. However, older adult RBCs in units of blood bank RBCs provide an advantage over the infant's own RBCs because 2,3-DPG and the P_{50} of transfused adult RBCs (but not endogenous infant RBCs) increase rapidly after transfusion. When studied in the setting of small-volume (15 ml/kg) RBC transfusion, 2,3-DPG levels were maintained in infants given stored RBCs (20).

The quantity of additives present in RBCs stored in extended storage media is unlikely to be dangerous for neonates given small-volume transfusions (~15 ml/kg) (19). Regardless of the type of suspending solution, the quantity of additives is quite small in the clinical setting in which a neonate would receive a single, small-volume transfusion of RBCs over 2 to 4 hours. With AS-1 and AS-3 RBCs as examples (Table 33.4), the dose of extended storage medium additives transfused during a typical small-volume RBC transfusion is estimated to be far less than levels believed to be toxic (19). This assumption was proved correct in clinical studies in which infants received one or more RBC transfusions (20,21,25). Thus there is no information to document failure to metabolize or excrete additives by preterm infants given multiple transfusions; that is, there is no evidence of cumulative toxicity.

TABLE 33.3. SMALL-VOLUME RED BLOOD CELL TRANSFUSIONS GIVEN AS STORED RED BLOOD CELLS TO LIMIT DONOR EXPOSURE WITHOUT CAUSING APPARENT ADVERSE EFFECTS

Reference	Solution	Storage (d)	Dose (ml/kg)	Hematocrit (%)[a]	Transfusions[b]	Donors[b]
22	CPDA	≤35	15	75	5.6	2.1
23	CPDA	≤35	13	68–75	6.0	2.0
24	NR	≤35	15	NR	5.6	4.9
20	AS-1	≤42	15	85	3.5	1.2
21	AS-3	≤42	15	85	3.6	1.3

[a]Hematocrit of transfused red blood cells.
[b]Mean number per infant.
CPDA, citrate-phosphate-dextrose-adenine; NR, not reported; AS, additive solution.

TABLE 33.4. QUANTITY (TOTAL mg/kg) OF ADDITIVES INFUSED DURING A TRANSFUSION OF 15 mL/kg AS-1 OR AS-3 RED BLOOD CELLS AT A HEMATOCRIT OF 60%

Additive	AS-1	AS-3	Toxic Dose[a]
Sodium chloride	42	7.5	137 mg/kg per day
Dextrose	129	23	240 mg/kg per hour
Adenine	0.6	0.6	15 mg/kg per dose
Citrate	9.8	12.6	180 mg/kg per hour
Phosphate	2.0	5.6	>60 mg/kg per day
Mannitol	33	0	360 mg/kg per day

[a]The accuracy of toxic dose is difficult to predict for transfusions to individual infants because infusion rates generally are slow, allowing metabolism and distribution of additives from blood into extravascular sites. In addition, dextrose, adenine and phosphate enter red blood cells and are somewhat sequestered and not immediately "available" in the extracellular solution. Potential toxic doses from Luban NLC, Strauss RG, Hume HA. Commentary on the safety of red blood cells preserved in extended storage media for neonatal transfusions. *Transfusion* 1991;31:229–235.

Many neonatal intensive care centers have embraced the concept of transfusing stored RBCs, rather than fresh, to diminish donor exposure. The reported experience from five studies is presented in Table 33.3. In these reports, stored RBCs were transfused safely, without increased hyperkalemia or acidosis and in most instances with donor exposure decreased more than 50% from that observed with transfusions of fresh blood (20–24). To compare the effects of transfusing RBCs stored for varying lengths of time, results of two studies of AS-3 RBCs (21,26) are combined and presented in Table 33.5. Of the 120 AS-3 RBC transfusions given, RBCs for 78 (65%) were stored 1 through 21 days and for 42 (35%) were stored 22 through 42 days. In comparisons of pretransfusion versus posttransfusion laboratory results for these two groups (<22 days versus ≥22 days), no statistically significant differences were found that could be related to the length of storage (Table 33.5). Thus RBCs from one donor stored up to 42 days can safely provide all RBCs needed by most individual preterm infants (20,21,26).

Approach to Anemia of Prematurity

For most infants with a birth weight less than 1.0 kg, anemia of prematurity is severe and necessitates therapy. Red blood cell transfusion or administration of recombinant erythropoietin plus iron are possibilities. For decades, RBC transfusion has been the standard of care, and in my view continues to be so. The caveat is that allogeneic donor exposure be minimized by transfusing RBCs stored as long as permitted (e.g., 42 days for extended-storage anticoagulant-preservative solutions). At the University of Iowa DeGowin Blood Center, preterm infants who need RBC transfusions are assigned to dedicated units of RBCs suspended in extended-storage (42-day) solutions. At the time

TABLE 33.5. MEAN CHANGE IN BLOOD CHEMISTRY LEVELS DURING RED BLOOD CELL TRANSFUSIONS

	Days of Storage[a]	
Value	1 to 21 (n = 78)	22 to 42 (n = 42)
Hematocrit (%)	+12 ± 5	+12 ± 4
Glucose (mg/dl)	−12 ± 24	−16 ± 28
Lactate (mmol/L)	−0.6 ± 1.1	−0.2 ± 0.3
pH	0.00 ± 0.08	0.00 ± 0.06
Calcium (mg/dl)	−0.1 ± 0.5	0.0 ± 0.8
Sodium (mEq/L)	+0.3 ± 4.6	−0.4 ± 4.7
Potassium (mEq/L)	+0.2 ± 0.8	+0.2 ± 0.6

Change (Δ ± SD) is posttransfusion value minus pretransfusion value.
Statistical tests used were *t* test for pH, sodium, potassium, and glucose (normal distribution) and Wilcoxon rank sum test for hematocrit, calcium, and lactate (abnormal distribution).
No statistically significant differences were found (*P* values all >.05) comparing 1 to 21 days versus 22 to 42 days of storage.
From Strauss RG, Burmeister LF, Johnson K, et al. Feasibility and safety of AS-3 red blood cells for neonatal transfusions. *J Pediatr* 2000;136:215–219 and Strauss RG, Burmeister LF, Johnson K, et al. Randomized trial assessing feasibility and safety of biological parents as red blood cell donors for their preterm infants. *Transfusion* 2000;40:450–456, with permission.

the first RBC transfusion is ordered, one-half of a freshly collected unit (stored ≤7 days) is dedicated to a preterm infant with a birth weight of 1.0 kg or less. The rest of the unit can be assigned to another infant. Thus one complete unit can serve two very-low-birth-weight infants simultaneously. Larger infants may be assigned to only one-third or one-fourth of a unit, depending on anticipated RBC needs. When RBC transfusions are ordered, aliquots are removed sterilely and issued (18). Although units are used throughout 42 days of storage, once a unit has been stored 14 days, it has become relatively aged (14 of its 42 storage days have lapsed), and no new preterm neonates are assigned to it. This plan has been demonstrated to be cost-effective (27).

Low plasma erythropoietin levels are a major pathogenetic factor in anemia of prematurity. Clonogenic erythroid progenitors from neonates respond well to erythropoietin in vitro. When given in sufficient doses to human infants, erythropoietin and iron effectively stimulate erythropoiesis in vivo, evidenced in many clinical studies by increased blood reticulocyte and RBC counts. However, the primary goal of erythropoietin therapy is to reduce the number of RBC transfusions, and in this regard, the efficacy of erythropoietin has not been convincingly demonstrated (28). Results of at least 22 controlled studies of the efficacy of erythropoietin in reducing the number of RBC transfusions to manage anemia of prematurity have been published (28, 29), but the relevance of many of the findings to contemporary neonatal transfusion practice is debated (9).

A metaanalysis was conducted on the controlled clinical studies of the efficacy of erythropoietin in the management of anemia of prematurity published between 1990 and 1999. Two major conclusions emerged from the metaanalysis (29). First, the controlled trials of erythropoietin to manage anemia of prematurity differed from one another in several ways and consequently produced markedly variable results that cannot be adequately explained. Until the reasons for variation are understood, it is premature to make firm recommendations regarding the clinical use of erythropoietin to manage anemia of prematurity. Second, although erythropoietin was efficacious in significantly reducing RBC transfusion needs, the magnitude of the effect of erythropoietin on reducing the total RBC transfusions needed by neonates throughout their initial hospitalization was relatively small. For example, in the multicenter trial by Shannon et al. (30), significantly fewer RBC transfusions were given to erythropoietin-treated infants than to placebo-treated controls (1.1 transfusions per infant versus 1.6 transfusions per infant, respectively) during the study period, but erythropoietin exerted only a modest effect on overall RBC transfusion needs (4.4 transfusions per erythropoietin-treated infant versus 5.3 per placebo-treated infant).

Recombinant erythropoietin plus iron offers an alternative to—or a therapy to be combined with—RBC transfusions for anemia of prematurity. However, those wishing to prescribe erythropoietin for management of anemia in very-low-birth-weight infants are in a dilemma. Relatively large preterm infants or those in stable condition who have been shown to respond best to erythropoietin plus iron are given relatively few RBC transfusions with today's conservative practices. Accordingly they have little need for erythropoietin to avoid transfusions. Extremely small preterm infants, who are sick and have the greatest need for RBC transfusions soon after birth, have not consistently responded to erythropoietin plus iron—again causing one to question the efficacy of erythropoietin. In my view, the lack of definitive information regarding the efficacy and potential toxicity of erythropoietin and iron preclude this treatment as part of routine neonatal care. Erythropoietin and iron should be prescribed only with the understanding and consent of the parents that it is a therapy that lacks universal acceptance and that because both erythropoietin and iron often are given in relatively high doses, the therapy carries with it uncertain long-term effects.

PLATELET TRANSFUSION

Pathophysiology of Neonatal Thrombocytopenia

Blood platelet counts of 150×10^9/L or more are present in normal fetuses (≥17 weeks of gestation) and neonates. Lower platelet counts indicate potential problems. Preterm infants commonly have thrombocytopenia (e.g., in one neonatal intensive care unit, 22% of infants had platelet counts less than 150×10^9/L) (31). Blood platelet counts less than 100×10^9/L pose significant clinical risks. In one study, results for infants with birth weights less than 1.5 kg and a platelet count less than 100×10^9/L were compared with those for control infants of similar size who did not have thrombocytopenia (32). The bleeding time was prolonged when platelet counts were less than 100×10^9/L, and platelet dysfunction was suggested by bleeding times disproportionately long for the degree of thrombocytopenia present. The incidence of intracranial hemorrhage was 78% among infants with thrombocytopenia and a birth weight less than 1.5 kg versus 48% for infants of similar size without thrombocytopenia. Moreover, the extent of hemorrhage and neurologic morbidity was greater among infants with thrombocytopenia (32).

Although many pathogenetic mechanisms likely are involved in these sick neonates, accelerated platelet destruction frequently is implicated by shortened platelet survival time, increased level of platelet-associated immunoglobulin G, increased platelet volume, normal number of marrow megakaryocytes, and an inadequate response to platelet transfusions (31,33). Another mechanism that contributes to neonatal thrombocytopenia is diminished platelet production. This is evidenced by decreased numbers of clonogenic megakaryocyte progenitors and relatively low levels of thrombopoietin in response to thrombocytopenia compared with the response of children and adults with thrombocytopenia (34–36). Reminiscent of the situation with erythropoietin and anemia of prematurity (erythropoietin produced but at levels inappropriately low for the degree of anemia), thrombopoietin is produced by preterm infants with thrombocytopenia but at relatively low levels.

Recommendations for Platelet Transfusion during Infancy

Prophylactic platelet transfusion to prevent bleeding in preterm neonates has been studied systematically (37). However, no ran-

TABLE 33.6. GUIDELINES FOR PLATELET TRANSFUSIONS GIVEN TO INFANTS

Maintain >50 to >100 × 10^9/L platelets for significant[a] bleeding
Maintain >50 × 10^9/L platelets for invasive procedures
Maintain >20 × 10^9/L platelets for prophylaxis (clinically stable[a])
Maintain >50 to >100 × 10^9/L platelets for prophylaxis (clinically unstable[a])

[a]Must be defined locally. For example, consider bleeding site and extent, degree of prematurity, and underlying medical condition.

domized clinical trials of therapeutic platelet transfusions have been reported as treatment of infants with thrombocytopenia who are bleeding. Although the relative risks of different degrees of thrombocytopenia in various clinical settings during infancy remain largely unanswered, it seems logical to transfuse platelets into infants with thrombocytopenia. Guidelines are presented in Table 33.6.

Two firm indications for therapeutic platelet transfusion are either to control hemorrhage that has already occurred or to prevent it from complicating an invasive procedure. Little disagreement exists over using a blood platelet count of 50 × 10^9/L as a minimum transfusion trigger in these instances. However, platelet transfusions are given more liberally by some physicians to control bleeding that occurs during infancy at higher platelet counts (between 50 and 100 × 10^9/L) or to diminish either the threat of or worsening of intracranial hemorrhage in high-risk preterm infants whenever the platelet count is less than 100 × 10^9/L (32). No data exist to clearly establish the efficacy of platelet transfusion at these relatively high blood platelet levels.

Prophylactic platelet transfusions can be given to infants either to prevent bleeding when severe thrombocytopenia poses a risk of spontaneous hemorrhage or to maintain the presence of a relatively normal platelet count to prevent the infant from slipping into high-risk situations caused by progressing thrombocytopenia. Regarding the first circumstance, most experts agree that it is reasonable to give platelets to any infant with a blood platelet count less than 20 × 10^9/L because spontaneous hemorrhage is a risk at this platelet count. Severe thrombocytopenia occurs most commonly among sick infants who because of the illness receive medications that can compromise the function of their already diminished number of platelets. Because these factors are more pronounced in extremely preterm infants, some neonatologists favor prophylactic platelet transfusion whenever the platelet count falls to less than 50 × 10^9/L, or even to less than 100 × 10^9/L, in critically ill infants (32).

The need to maintain a completely normal platelet count (150 × 10^9/L) or even higher in preterm infants without bleeding is unproved. It can place infants at risk due to platelet donor exposure. Intracranial hemorrhage occurs commonly among sick preterm infants. Although neither a causative role for thrombocytopenia nor a therapeutic benefit for platelet transfusion has been established in this disorder, it seems logical to presume thrombocytopenia is a risk factor (38). In a randomized trial designed to address this issue, transfusion of platelets whenever the platelet count decreased to less than the normal value of 150 × 10^9/L (which maintained the average platelet count greater than 200 × 10^9/L) was compared with transfusion of platelets only when the platelet count decreased to the relatively severe thrombocytopenic level of less than 50 × 10^9/L (37). The authors did not detect a difference in the incidence of intracranial hemorrhage (28% versus 26% in the two groups) (37). Thus there is no documented benefit to transfusion of "prophylactic platelets" to maintain a completely normal platelet count in preterm infants versus transfusion of "therapeutic platelets" in response to thrombocytopenia when it actually occurs.

Platelet Product to Transfuse

The ideal goal of platelet transfusions in the care of many infants with thrombocytopenia is to increase the low pretransfusion platelet count to a posttransfusion count greater than 50 × 10^9/L and for sick preterm infants to more than 100 × 10^9/L. This can be achieved consistently by means of infusion of 5 to 10 ml/kg of unmodified platelet concentrates (withdrawn from a unit of platelets collected originally by means of either centrifugation of fresh units of whole blood or automated plateletpheresis and direct transfusion). Platelet concentrates should be infused as rapidly as the overall condition allows, certainly within 2 hours.

Routinely reducing the volume of platelet concentrates for infants by means of additional centrifugation steps is both unnecessary and unwise, unless a specific reason exists to do so. The method of reduction and the efficacy of platelet transfusions after reduction must be validated locally to ensure the quantity and quality of platelets remaining after modification. Transfusion of 10 ml/kg platelet concentrate, taken directly from the unit and transfused, provides approximately 10 × 10^9 platelets. If the blood volume of an infant is 70 ml/kg body weight, the platelet dose of 10 ml/kg increases the platelet count 143 × 10^9/L above the pretransfusion baseline. With modest thrombocytopenia, a 5 ml/kg dose may be sufficient. This calculated increment is consistent with the actual increment achieved after this dose as reported in clinical studies (37). In general, 5 to 10 ml/kg is not an excessive transfusion volume even for sick infants, if the intake of other intravenous fluids, medications, and nutrients is monitored and adjusted.

In the selection of platelet units for transfusion, it is desirable for the infant and the platelet donor to be of the same ABO blood group. It is important to minimize repeated transfusions of group O platelets to group A or B recipients, because large quantities of passive anti-A or anti-B can lead to hemolysis. This should be easily avoided, with the exception of a directed-donor situation in which the infant is forced to receive platelet transfusions from an out-of-group donor. Proven methods exist to reduce the volume of platelet concentrates when truly warranted (many transfusions anticipated in which several doses of passive anti-A or anti-B may lead to hemolysis or failure to respond to a transfusion of 10 ml/kg of unmodified platelet concentrate). However, additional processing should be performed with great care because of probable platelet loss, clumping, and dysfunction caused by the additional handling.

Approach to the Care of Infants with Thrombocytopenia

Thrombocytopenia exists wherever the blood platelet count is less than 150 × 10^9/L. Every infant with thrombocytopenia needs an evaluation—if nothing more than a repeated complete blood cell count and a review of the medical history and physical examination. Definitive management of thrombocytopenia depends on the underlying disorder and is beyond the scope of this discussion (see Chapter 27). Correction of the thrombocytopenia per se by means of platelet transfusions is based on maintaining a blood platelet count deemed appropriate for the infant's clinical condition (Table 33.6).

There are no alternatives to platelet transfusion in the care of neonates with thrombocytopenia. Recombinant thrombopoietin (c-Mpl ligand or megakaryocyte growth and differentiation factor) and interleukin-11 are promising agents. However, neither is recommended for use during infancy, and both have potential toxicities that can preclude their use in the care of sick preterm infants. Thrombopoietin has broad actions on the early precursors of all three major lineages in the bone marrow and may produce effects in excess of those expected on megakaryocytes and platelets, and interleukin-11 may cause anemia. Clearly they must not be prescribed in the treatment of infants, except in experimental settings with parental consent.

PLASMA TRANSFUSION

Pathophysiology of Neonatal Clotting Proteins

Hemostasis in a neonate is quantitatively and qualitatively different from that in an older child or adult, and the risk exists of either serious hemorrhage or thrombosis. Although a comprehensive discussion of hemostasis is presented in Chapters 22 and 31, a few important facts about neonatal clotting proteins are summarized before issues of plasma transfusion are addressed.

Maternal clotting factors do not cross the placenta, and fetal levels depend on endogenous production. Clotting proteins are synthesized by the fetus beginning in the first trimester, concentrations gradually increasing throughout gestation (39). At birth, the mean levels of the contact factors (factors XII and XI, prekallikrein, and high-molecular-weight kininogen) are approximately 40% to 50% of adult values in term infants and approximately 30% to 40% of adult values in preterm infants. The vitamin K–dependent factors (II, VII, IX, and X) are present at approximately 40% to 50% of adults value in term infants and approximately 20% to 50% of adult value in preterm infants. Strikingly low levels are present in very immature neonates. Neonatal levels of factors VIII and XIII and fibrinogen are comparable with adult levels, although the level of factor XIII can be quite low in some infants at birth. The natural anticoagulant proteins (antithrombin III and proteins C and S) are 30% to 50% of adult values. Fibrinolysis is less well studied but probably is diminished to a considerable degree because the plasminogen level is moderately low.

Plasma Transfusion Practices

Guidelines for neonatal transfusion of fresh frozen plasma (FFP) are presented in Table 33.7. Clotting time is prolonged in infants compared with that of older children and adults because of developmental deficiency of clotting proteins. Fresh frozen plasma should be transfused only after reference to normal values accepted for the birth weight and age of the infant. The indications for transfusion of FFP into neonates include reconstitution of RBC concentrates to simulate whole blood for use in massive transfusions (e.g., exchange transfusion, extracorporeal membrane oxygenation, or cardiovascular surgery) and management of disseminated intravascular coagulation with bleeding, hemorrhage from vitamin K deficiency, and bleeding or thrombosis in congenital factor deficiency when more specific treatment (purified and virus-inactivated factor concentrate) is unavailable or the diagnosis of a specific factor deficiency has not been made.

TABLE 33.7. GUIDELINES FOR PLASMA TRANSFUSIONS GIVEN TO INFANTS

High risk of bleeding due to acquired deficiency of clotting proteins
Exchange transfusion
Extracorporeal membrane oxygenation
Cardiac bypass surgery
Disseminated (consumptive) coagulation
Bleeding due to congenital clotting protein deficiency
Bleeding due to vitamin K deficiency
Thrombosis due to anticoagulant protein deficiency

Dose depends on severity of the deficiency, but a satisfactory starting dose is 10 to 15 ml/kg body weight of fresh frozen plasma.

The use of prophylactic transfusion of FFP to prevent intraventricular hemorrhage in premature infants is not recommended. Use of FFP as a suspending agent to adjust the hematocrit of RBC concentrates before small-volume RBC transfusion should be discouraged because FFP offers no apparent medical benefit over the use of sterile solutions for this purpose. Similarly, the use of FFP in partial exchange transfusion for the management of neonatal hyperviscosity syndrome (erythrocytosis) is unnecessary, because safer colloid solutions are available. In the treatment of bleeding infants, cryoprecipitate often is considered an alternative to FFP because of its small volume. However, cryoprecipitate contains only fibrinogen and factors VIII and XIII. It is not effective for managing the more extensive clotting factor deficiencies that are commonly encountered—despite the desirability of a small infusion volume. Finally, concerns have been raised over the theoretic risks of use of plasma treated by the solvent-detergent method. These risks include pooling of multiple-donor units and exposure to residual chemicals. This product has been transfused with apparent safety in many parts of the world, but experience is limited in the United States. Each physician and institution must make local decisions regarding selection of plasma treated by the solvent-detergent method or conventional FFP.

NEUTROPHIL TRANSFUSION

Pathophysiology of Neonatal Neutropenia

Neonates are unusually susceptible to severe bacterial infection, and multiple abnormalities of neonatal body defenses contribute. Blood neutrophils from infants have both quantitative and qualitative abnormalities related to the increased incidence, morbidity, and mortality of bacterial infection. These abnormalities include absolute and relative neutropenia, diminished chemotaxis, abnormal adhesion and aggregation, defective cellular orientation and receptor capping, decreased deformability, inability to alter membrane potential during stimulation, imbalances of oxidative metabolism, and a diminished ability to withstand oxidant stress (40).

Neutropenia can occur during fulminant bacterial infection. Because physiologic neutrophilia occurs soon after birth, it is quite unusual for the absolute blood neutrophil count to decrease to less than 2 × 10^9/L during the first week of life. Although an abnormally low neutrophil count can occur in neonates with disorders as diverse as sepsis, asphyxia, and maternal hypertension, suspicion of severe bacterial infection must always be high whenever relative neutropenia (blood neutrophil count <2 × 10^9/L) occurs in a sick neonate. The mechanisms responsible for abnormal neonatal granulopoiesis are only partially defined. One factor is that the postmitotic marrow neutrophil storage pool (metamyelocytes and mature, segmented neutrophils) is inadequate during fulminant infection. The neutrophil storage pool accounts for 26% to 60% of all nucleated cells in the bone marrow of normal neonates, whereas neonates with sepsis may have a storage pool numbering less than 10% of nucleated marrow cells. Thus they have severely diminished marrow neutrophil reserves (41). Second, storage pool neutrophils are released at an excessively rapid and apparently poorly regulated rate from the marrow during stress. Third, committed (clonogenic) neutrophil precursors in neonatal marrow are fewer in neonates than in older patients, and most of these cells are actively proliferating even when studied at an apparently basal state (41,42). Thus neonatal bone marrow functions at capacity and is unable to either rapidly expand production or release stored neutrophils to meet the increased demands of infection. Results of studies of cytokines involved in granulopoiesis, such as granulocyte colony-stimulating factor (G-CSF) and granulocyte-macrophage colony-stimulating factor (GM-CSF), are controversial and are discussed later. Fetal and neonatal hematopoiesis is discussed in Chapter 29.

Neutrophil Transfusion Practices

Because both quantitative and qualitative abnormalities of neonatal neutrophils have been reported, neutrophil transfusions have been used to control neonatal sepsis whether or not neutropenia is present. Neutrophil transfusions generally were given to neonates with fulminant sepsis and relative neutropenia (neutrophil count less than 2 to 3 × 10^9/L during the first week of life or <1.0 × 10^9/L thereafter). The results of six controlled studies are presented in Table 33.8. Encouraging is that four (43–46) of the six controlled studies (43–48) showed significant benefit from neutrophil transfusion.

Unfortunately, neutrophil transfusion has not provided a satisfactory solution to neonatal sepsis, and it is used infrequently for several reasons. Although neutrophil transfusion is efficacious for some infants with neutropenia and fulminant sepsis, only neutrophil concentrates obtained by means of automated leukapheresis for transfusion have demonstrated effectiveness (49). The controlled trials contain scientific flaws (49), and in many instances, conventional supportive care with antibiotics seemed equally efficacious (Table 33.8). Each institution must assess its own experience with neonatal sepsis. If nearly all infants survive without apparent long-term morbidity when treated only with antibiotics, neutrophil transfusions are unnecessary, and attention should be focused on prompt diagnosis and optimal antibiotic therapy. If the outcome of standard therapy is not optimal, alternative therapies must be considered to improve the outlook. If neutrophil transfusion is to be used, the transfusions must be given optimally—in a dose of at least 1 × 10^9 neutrophils per kilogram of infant body weight, and the neutrophils must be collected by means of automated leukapheresis (49).

Approach to the Care of Infants with Sepsis and Neutropenia

Neonatologists do not regularly prescribe neutrophil transfusion for infants whose condition is septic. The proper role of neutrophil transfusion has not been definitively established with controlled clinical trials. Moreover, preparation of neutrophil con-

TABLE 33.8. SIX CONTROLLED TRIALS OF NEONATAL NEUTROPHIL TRANSFUSION

		No. of Neonates		No. of Neonates	
Reference	Randomized	Transfusion	Survival Rate (%)	No Transfusion	Survival Rate (%)
44	No	20	90[a]	18	28
43	Yes	7	100[a]	9	11
	No[b]	—	—	10	100
45	Yes	13	100[a]	10	60
46	Yes[a]	21	95[a]	14	64
47	Yes	12	58	13	69
48	Yes	4	50	5	40
	No	—	—	11	91

[a]Survival rate of infants who underwent transfusion was significantly better than that of infants who did not.
[b]Infants who did not undergo transfusion were not randomized because all had adequate bone marrow storage pools.
Expanded version of study reported earlier (45).

centrates by means of leukapheresis can be cumbersome and expensive. Accordingly, alternative therapies have been suggested. However, the efficacy of these treatments has not been clearly established, the risks are only partially defined, and the therapies must be studied extensively before they are widely accepted. Two alternative therapies that have been suggested are intravenous immune globulin (IVIG) and myeloid cytokines (G-CSF or GM-CSF).

Most studies evaluating prophylactic IVIG to prevent neonatal infection have shown either little or only modest benefit, whereas several therapeutic studies have shown a benefit to adding IVIG to antibiotics (50). Metaanalysis of studies of prophylactic use of IVIG has shown only minimum benefit, whereas therapeutic IVIG had unequivocal benefit (50). Overall, data are insufficient to justify the use of IVIG as a standard of care of all preterm neonates to prevent or manage sepsis. However, it seems reasonable to give "physiologic" doses of IVIG (0.3 to 0.4 g/kg) to very-low-birth-weight newborns in septic condition. These infants are likely to have hypogammaglobulinemia as a result of extremely premature birth, that is born before major placental transport of immunoglobulin G has taken place.

To date, properly designed clinical studies of recombinant myeloid growth factors given to human neonates are limited, and firm recommendations cannot be made for use of these agents. In a controlled study, 42 neonates with presumed bacterial sepsis recognized within the first 3 days of life were randomly assigned to receive three doses of either G-CSF or a placebo (51). Granulocyte colony-stimulating factor induced a significant increase in blood neutrophil count, an increase in the bone marrow neutrophil storage pool, and an increase in expression of neutrophil membrane C3bi, the last being an indication of enhanced functional capability. Similarly, in a controlled study of GM-CSF, 20 premature neonates were designated within 72 hours of birth to receive either GM-CSF or a placebo for 7 days (52). Granulocyte-macrophage colony-stimulating factor increased the blood neutrophil count, the bone marrow neutrophil storage pool, and C3bi receptor expression. Neonates receiving GM-CSF also had an increase in blood monocyte and platelet counts. Neither study was designed to assess efficacy for the prevention or management of infection.

A few randomized clinical trials have been conducted to assess the efficacy of G-CSF and GM-CSF, but a clear clinical benefit has not been documented. In a study of G-CSF, 20 infants with neutropenia and sepsis received either G-CSF (10 μg/kg a day) or placebo for 3 days (53). Acknowledging that the number of study subjects was too small for definitive conclusions, G-CSF did not significantly lessen the severity of illness or decrease the morbidity or mortality of sepsis. In a study of GM-CSF, preterm infants received either GM-CSF (8 μg/kg a day) or placebo for the first 28 days of life in an attempt to reduce the incidence of infection (54). Although GM-CSF was well tolerated and significantly increased blood leukocyte count, it did not significantly decrease the infection rate. In another study of GM-CSF, 75 neonates of less than 32 weeks' gestation were randomized to receive either GM-CSF (10 μg/kg subcutaneously for 5 days beginning within 72 hours of birth) or to a control group (55). Neonates with evidence of infection were not enrolled. Prophylactic GM-CSF completely abolished neutropenia, whereas neutropenia (blood neutrophil count $<1.7 \times 10^9$/L) occurred in 41% of controls ($P < .001$), 18% of controls having a neutrophil count less than 1.0×10^9/L ($P = .01$). Despite elimination of neutropenia, blood culture–positive sepsis occurred in 31% of GM-CSF neonates versus 46% of controls (not statistically different) (55). Therefore although myeloid growth factors are promising in many respects, firm guidelines cannot be offered at this time regarding the proper role of these agents in the management of neonatal neutropenia or sepsis.

There is no universally accepted role for neutrophil transfusion, IVIG, or myeloid growth factors as a standard of practice for the management of neonatal sepsis. Until more information becomes available, it seems reasonable to manage fulminant sepsis in neonates with neutropenia (blood neutrophil counts $<2 \times 10^9$/L during the first week of life or $<1 \times 10^9$/L thereafter) as follows. For infants born before 30 weeks of gestation, give one dose of 500 μg/kg of IVIG to correct possible hypogammaglobulinemia plus 5 μg/kg of G-CSF or 10 μg GM-CSF on 3 consecutive days. For infants born at 30 weeks of gestation or after, give 5 μg/kg of G-CSF or 10 μg GM-CSF on 3 consecutive days. This therapy should be adjunctive to optimal antibiotic and supportive care, and it must be given with parental consent and the understanding that its efficacy and potential toxicity are not completely understood. As a case in point, some neonates in septic condition have high blood levels of endogenous G-CSF. It has been cautioned that adding additional exogenous recombinant G-CSF offers no benefit (56). If cells for neutrophil transfusion can be collected by means of automated leukapheresis and transfused promptly, it is reasonable to include transfusion in the therapy plan for infants in whom neutropenia is not reversed within 12 hours or so of the beginning of antibiotic, IVIG, and G-CSF or GM-CSF therapy.

ACKNOWLEDGMENT

Supported by National Institute of Health grants P01 HL46925 and RR00059.

REFERENCES

1. Strauss RG. Current issues in neonatal transfusions. *Vox Sang* 1996; 51:1–9.
2. Stockman JA. Anemia of prematurity: current concepts in the issue of when to transfuse. *Pediatr Clin North Am* 1986;33:111–128.
3. Brown MS, Phibbs RH, Garcia JF, et al. Postnatal changes in erythropoietin levels in untransfused premature infants. *J Pediatr* 1983;103: 612–617.
4. Brown MS, Garcia JF, Phibbs RH, et al. Decreased response of plasma immunoreactive erythropoietin to "available oxygen" in anemia of prematurity. *J Pediatr* 1984;105:793–798.
5. Rhondeau SM, Christensen RD, Ross MP, et al. Responsiveness to recombinant human erythropoietin of marrow erythroid progenitors from infants with "anemia of prematurity." *J Pediatr* 1988;112: 935–940.
6. Zanjani ED, Ascensao JL, McGlave PB, et al. Studies in the liver to kidney switch of erythropoietin production. *J Clin Invest* 1981;67: 1183–1188.
7. Dane C, Fahnenstich H, Freitag P, et al. Erythropoietin mRNA expression in human fetal and neonatal tissue. *Blood* 1998;92:3218–3225.

8. Widness JA, Veng-Pedersen P, Peters C, et al. Erythropoietin pharmacokinetics in premature infants: developmental, nonlinearity, and treatment effects. *J App Physiol* 1996;80:140–148.
9. Strauss RG. Managing the anemia of prematurity: red blood cell transfusions versus recombinant erythropoietin. *Transfus Med Rev* 2001;15:213–223.
10. Strauss RG. Red blood cell transfusion practices in the neonate. *Clin Perinatol* 1995:22:641–655.
11. Ramasethu J, Luban NL. Red blood cell transfusions in the newborn. *Semin Neonatol* 1999:4:5–16.
12. Alverson DC, Isken VH, Cohen RS. Effect of booster blood transfusions on oxygen utilization in infants with bronchopulmonary dysplasia. *J Pediatr* 1988;113:722–726.
13. Joshi A, Gerhardt T, Shandloff P, et al. Blood transfusion effect on the respiratory pattern of preterm infants. *Pediatrics* 1987;80:79–85.
14. Keyes WG, Donohur PK, Spivak JL, et al. Assessing the need for transfusion of premature infants and role of hematocrit, clinical signs and erythropoietin level. *Pediatrics* 1989;84:412–418.
15. Stockman JA, Clark DA. Weight gain: a response to transfusion in selected preterm infants. *Am J Dis Child* 1984;138:828–835.
16. Blank JP, Sheagren TG, Vajaria J, et al. The role of RBC transfusion in selected preterm infants. *Am J Dis Child* 1984;138:831–837.
17. Ross MP, Christensen RD, Rothstein G, et al. A randomized trial to develop criteria for administering erythrocyte transfusions to anemic preterm infants 1 to 3 months of age. *J Perinatol* 1989;9:246–250.
18. Strauss RG, Villhauer PJ, Cordle DG. A method to collect, store and issue multiple aliquots of packed red blood cells for neonatal transfusions. *Vox Sang* 1995;68:77–81.
19. Luban NLC, Strauss RG, Hume HA. Commentary on the safety of red blood cells preserved in extended storage media for neonatal transfusions. *Transfusion* 1991;31:229–235.
20. Strauss RG, Burmeister LF, Johnson K, et al. AS-1 red blood cells for neonatal transfusions: a randomized trial assessing donor exposure and safety. *Transfusion* 1996;36:873–878.
21. Strauss RG, Burmeister LF, Johnson K, et al. Feasibility and safety of AS-3 red blood cells for neonatal transfusions. *J Pediatr* 2000;136:215–219.
22. Liu EA, Mannino FL, Lane TA. Prospective, randomized trial of the safety and efficacy of a limited donor exposure transfusion program for premature neonates. *J Pediatr* 1994;125:92–96.
23. Lee DA, Slagel TA, Jackson TM, et al. Reducing blood donor exposures in low birth weight infants by the use of older, unwashed packed red blood cells. *J Pediatr* 1995;126:280–286.
24. Wood A, Wilson N, Skacel P, et al. Reducing donor exposure in preterm infants requiring multiple blood transfusions. *Arch Dis Child* 1995;72:F29–F33.
25. Goodstein MH, Locke RG, Wlodarczyk D, et al. Comparison of two preservation solutions for erythrocyte transfusions in newborn infants. *J Pediatr* 1993;123:783–788.
26. Strauss RG, Burmeister LF, Johnson K, et al. Randomized trial assessing feasibility and safety of biological parents as red blood cell donors for their preterm infants. *Transfusion* 2000;40:450–456.
27. Hilsenrath P, Nemechek J, Widness JA, et al. Cost-effectiveness of a limited donor blood program for neonatal RBC transfusions. *Transfusion* 1999;39:938–943.
28. Widness JA, Strauss RG. Recombinant erythropoietin in the treatment of the premature newborn. *Semin Neonatol* 1998;3:163–171.
29. Vamvakas EC, Strauss RG. Meta-analysis of controlled clinical trials studying the efficacy of recombinant human erythropoietin in reducing blood transfusions in the anemia of prematurity. *Transfusion* 2001;41:406–415.
30. Shannon KM, Keith JF III, Mentzer WC, et al. Recombinant human erythropoietin stimulates erythropoiesis and reduces erythrocyte transfusions in very-low-birth-weight preterm infants. *Pediatrics* 1995;95:1–8.
31. Castle V, Andrew M, Kelton J, et al. Frequency and mechanism of neonatal thrombocytopenia. *J Pediatr* 1986:108:749–755.
32. Andrew M, Castle V, Saigal S, et al. Clinical impact of neonatal thrombocytopenia. *J Pediatr*1987;110:457–464.
33. Castle V, Coates G, Kelton JG, et al. ^{111}In-oxine platelet survivals in thrombocytopenic infants. *Blood* 1987;70:652–656.
34. Murray NA, Roberts IA. Circulating megakaryocytes and their progenitors in early thrombocytopenia in preterm neonates. *Pediatr Res* 1996;40:112–119.
35. Wolber EM, Dame C, Fahnenstich H, et al. Expression of the thrombopoietin gene in human fetal and neonatal tissues. *Blood* 1999:94:97–105.
36. Sola MC, Calhoun DA, Hutson AD, et al. Plasma thrombopoietin concentrations in thrombocytopenic and nonthrombocytopenic patients in a neonatal intensive care unit. *Br J Haematol* 1999;104:90–92.
37. Andrew M, Vegh P, Caco C, et al. A randomized trial of platelet transfusions in thrombocytopenic premature infants. *J Pediatr* 1993;123:285–291.
38. Lupton BA, Hill A, Whitfield MF, et al. Reduced platelet count as a risk factor for intraventricular hemorrhage. *Am J Dis Child* 1988;142:1222–1224.
39. Reverdiau-Moalic P, Delahousse B, Brody G, et al. Evolution of blood coagulation activators and inhibitors in the healthy human fetus. *Blood* 1996;88:900–908.
40. Rosenthal J, Cairo MS. Neonatal myelopoiesis and immunomodulation of host defenses. In: Petz LD, Swisher SN, Kleinman S, et al., eds. *Clinical practice of transfusion medicine,* 3rd ed. New York: Churchill Livingstone, 1995;685–704.
41. Christensen RD, MacFarlane JL, Taylor NL, et al. Blood and marrow neutrophils during experimental group B streptococcal infection: quantification of the stem cell, proliferative, storage and circulating pools. *Pediatr Res* 1982;16:549–554.
42. Erdman SH, Christensen RD, Bradley PP, et al. Supply and release of storage neutrophils: a developmental study. *Biol Neonate* 1982;41:132–137.
43. Christensen RD, Rothstein G, Anstall HB, et al. Granulocyte transfusions in neonates with bacterial infection, neutropenia and depletion of mature marrow neutrophils. *Pediatrics* 1982;70:1–6.
44. Laurenti F, Ferro R, Isacchi G, et al. Polymorphonuclear leukocyte transfusion for the treatment of sepsis in the newborn infants. *J Pediatr* 1981;98:118–123.
45. Cairo MS, Rucker R, Bennetts GA, et al. Improved survival of newborns receiving leukocyte transfusions for sepsis. *Pediatrics* 1984;74:887–892.
46. Cairo MS, Worcester C, Rucker R, et al. Role of circulating complement and polymorphonuclear leukocyte transfusion in treatment and outcome in critically ill neonates with sepsis. *J Pediatr* 1987;110:935–941.
47. Baley JE, Stork EK, Warkentin PI, et al. Buffy coat transfusions in neutropenic neonates with presumed sepsis: a prospective, randomized trial. *Pediatrics* 1987;80:712–720.
48. Wheeler JC, Chauvenet AR, Johnson CA, et al. Buffy coat transfusions in neonates with sepsis and neutrophil storage pool depletion. *Pediatrics* 1987;79:422–425.
49. Strauss RG, Current status of granulocyte transfusions to treat neonatal sepsis. *J Clin Apheresis* 1989;5:25–29.
50. Jenson HB, Pollock BH. Meta-analyses of the effectiveness of intravenous immune globulin for prevention and treatment of neonatal sepsis. *Pediatrics* 1997;99:E2.
51. Gillan ER, Christensen RD, Suen Y, et al. A randomized, placebo-controlled trial of recombinant human granulocyte colony-stimulating factor administration in newborn infants with presumed sepsis: significant induction of peripheral and bone marrow neutrophilia. *Blood* 1994;84:1427–1433.
52. Cairo MS, Christensen R, Sender LS, et al. Results of a phase I/II trial of recombinant human granulocyte-macrophage colony-stimulating factor in very low birthweight neonates: significant induction of circulatory neutrophils, monocytes, platelets, and bone marrow neutrophils. *Blood* 1995;86:2509–2515.
53. Schibler KR, Osborne KA, Leung LY, et al. A randomized, placebo-controlled trial of granulocyte colony-stimulating factor administration to newborn infants with neutropenia and clinical signs of early-onset sepsis. *Pediatrics* 1998;102:6–13.

54. Cairo MS, Agosti J, Ellis R, et al. A randomized, double-blind, placebo-controlled trial of prophylactic recombinant human granulocyte-macrophage colony-stimulating factor to reduce nosocomial infections in very low birth weight neonates. *J Pediatr* 1999;134:64–70.
55. Carr R, Modi N, Dore CJ, et al. A randomized, controlled trial of prophylactic granulocyte-macrophage colony-stimulating factor in human newborns less than 32 weeks gestation. *Pediatrics* 1999;103:796–802.
56. Calhoun DA, Lunoe M, Du Y, et al. Granulocyte colony-stimulating factor serum and urine concentrations in neutropenic neonates before and after intravenous administration of recombinant granulocyte colony-stimulating factor. *Pediatrics* 2000;105:392–397.

Rossi's Principles of Transfusion Medicine, Third Edition, edited by Toby L. Simon, Walter H. Dzik, Edward L. Snyder, Christopher P. Stowell, and Ronald G. Strauss. Lippincott Williams & Wilkins, Philadelphia © 2002.

PART III

Oncology Patients

34

TRANSFUSION SUPPORT FOR THE ONCOLOGY PATIENT

MARGOT S. KRUSKALL

BLOOD COMPONENTS IN THE ONCOLOGIC SETTING

A substantial portion of blood products transfused at medical centers go to patients with solid tumor or hematologic malignant disease. These products are used to combat effects of the primary illness and to manage complications of chemotherapy, radiation therapy, surgery, and transplantation. The care of patients with cancer can be multifaceted and resource intense, and blood transfusions are an integral part of this complexity. The purpose of this chapter is to consider aspects of blood component transfusions that are unique or challenging from the standpoint of the oncology patient. Particular attention is paid to situations that affect the choice of blood component or blood type or result in important or unique risks or complications in the setting of cancer.

RED BLOOD CELL TRANSFUSIONS

Indications

Anemia is a common complication in oncology when the disease involves the bone marrow and even more frequently when the

M.S. Kruskall: Division of Laboratory and Transfusion Medicine, Beth Israel Deaconess Medical Center, and Departments of Pathology and Medicine, Harvard Medical School, Boston, Massachusetts.

treatment—chemotherapy, radiation therapy, or transplantation—affects bone marrow progenitor cell growth. Transfusion of red blood cells is given for the same indications used in the general patient population—improvement in oxygen delivery to the tissues. And as in other patient populations, there exists no evidence that increasing the hematocrit far above the level needed to forestall symptoms of tissue hypoxia is of any particular value in the care of patients with cancer.

ABO Blood Group System: Typing and Choice of Components

For most patients with cancer, no specific limitations or considerations apply to compatibility testing of red blood cells outside of conventional practices. However, the ABO blood group system occasionally presents interesting problems for recipients of allogeneic bone marrow transplants. Unlike that of solid-organ transplants, survival of hematopoietic progenitor cell grafts does not require that the ABO blood groups of the donor and of the recipient be identical. Therefore in the posttransplantation period, the recipient typically maintains two identifiable populations of red blood cells either transiently or permanently. When ABO disparity exists, the ABO grouping may reflect that of the donor or that of the recipient or be mixed (microchimerism). In addition, preexisting incompatible donor and recipient isoagglutinins may persist for weeks after transplantation. Three potential sources of antibody exist in the transplantation setting—mature immunized donor lymphocytes transfused with the marrow or organ, donor lymphocytes that engraft and mature after transplantation, and immunized recipient lymphocytes. Donor-derived red blood cell antibodies can cause or contribute to hemolytic anemia after bone marrow transplantation owing to destruction of recipient red blood cells, especially in the setting of marrow T-cell depletion or suppression (Fig. 34.1). Fortunately, severe hemolysis is unusual (1). In rare situations, hemolysis can be fatal. Such cases appear to be more likely to occur when peripheral blood stem cells are transplanted, possibly because they contain relatively larger numbers of B and T lymphocytes than do bone marrow sources (2). Disappearance of donor antibodies in the recipient heralds lifelong tolerance to the old host blood group (3). Where antibodies originate in the recipient, their presence after transplantation can contribute to delayed engraftment and impaired production of red blood cells. Their disappearance correlates with improved donor cell erythropoiesis.

In either form of ABO-incompatible bone marrow transplantation, the net effects of reduced erythropoiesis or red blood cell hemolysis or both result in higher volumes of red blood cell transfusion in the posttransplantation period than in ABO-compatible transplantation. In one study of patients undergoing bone marrow transplantation for aplastic anemia, the median use of red blood cells during the first 13 weeks was 4.5 units for ABO-matched transplants, 11.0 units for minor incompatibilities (the donor had antibodies to recipient red blood cells), and 17.5 units for major incompatibilities (the recipient had antibodies to the donor red blood cells) (4).

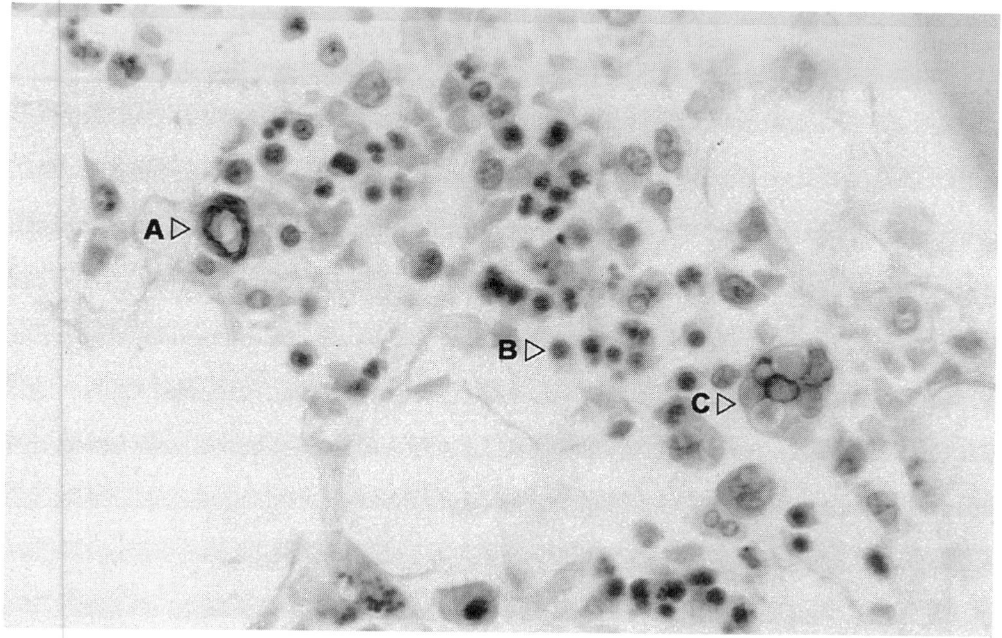

FIGURE 34.1. Recipient red blood cell destruction in minor-mismatch bone marrow transplantation. This bone marrow biopsy section from a group A patient who received a group O marrow transplant has been stained with a mouse anti-human blood group A antibody. The recipient's group A type is evident from the stained endothelial cells (*arrow A*). The nucleated red blood cell precursors are unstained and are presumably donor-derived group O cells (*arrow B*). Intracellular, phagocytosed, group A red blood cells are evident (*arrow C*). (From Benjamin R, Zubair A. Erythrophagocytosis after an ABO-mismatched stem cell transplant. *Transfusion* 2001;41:1463, with permission).

TABLE 34.1. RED CELL AND PLASMA TRANSFUSIONS IN THE HEMATOPOIETIC STEM CELL TRANSPLANT RECIPIENT, IN RELATION TO DONOR AND RECIPIENT ABO BLOOD GROUPS

Recipient Blood Group	Donor Blood Group			
	O	A	B	AB
O	C	M	M	M
A	m	C	Mm	M
B	m	mM	C	M
AB	m	m	m	C

C, compatible transplant; M, major incompatibility; m, minor incompatibility; mM, two-way (major and minor) incompatibility.

These incompatibilities also complicate the selection of blood for transfusion in the care of recipients of allogeneic transplants. In the setting of a major incompatibility, when the recipient has anti-A or anti-B directed against donor red blood cell epitopes, the use of recipient type red blood cells is necessary until the antibody has disappeared (Tables 34.1 and 34.2) (5). For minor incompatibilities, when the donor's antibody is the possible source of complication, the donor red blood cell type can be used immediately, but recipient type plasma and platelets are necessary until recipient red blood cells disappear. Two-way incompatibilities require attention to both sets of problems. Use of group O red blood cells and AB plasma (and platelets when possible) is indicated until the respective recipient antibodies and cells have disappeared. These choices may be important not only to survival of the graft and prevention of hemolysis but also to morbidity and mortality. A report has described increased risk of multiple organ failure and infection among patients receiving ABO-incompatible (major or minor) plasma transfusions (6).

Alloimmunization to Red Blood Cell Antigens

Patients being treated for cancer, especially those being treated for hematologic malignant disease and other illnesses with high-dose chemotherapy and hematopoietic progenitor cell transplantation, should be quite immunosuppressed, and the development of alloantibodies may be expected to be suppressed as well. However, non-ABO red blood cell alloantibodies do occasionally appear in the posttransfusion period. The incidence of antibody formation in bone marrow transplantation, for example, has been reported to be 2% to 8% (7). It is curious that antibody formation to red blood cell epitopes (other than ABO) may occur more frequently if the graft is an ABO mismatch, possibly because this scenario leads to a generally exaggerated immune response (8).

Autologous Blood Transfusion

Autologous blood collection is for the most part not relevant in the setting of cancer operations, in which the preoperative time often is intentionally short and in which larger than expected and unpredictable blood needs may exist perioperatively and later in the course of therapy. However, concerns about the immunomodulatory effects of allogeneic blood transfusion on the rate of cancer progression (see later in Chapter) have inspired modest interest in the use of these techniques in limited circumstances. For example, preoperative collection of autologous blood has been reported in the situation of a slowly progressing tumor, such as prostate cancer (9). The intraoperative

TABLE 34.2. TRANSFUSION PROTOCOL

Transplant	Time Period	Choice Of Blood Group		
		Red Blood Cells	Plasma	Platelets
Major incompatibility	Preparative regimen	Recipient	Donor	Donor
	Transplantation period			
	Recipient antibodies still present	Recipient	Donor	Donor
	Recipient antibodies gone	Donor	Donor	Donor
Minor incompatibility	Preparative regimen	Donor	Recipient	
	Transplantation period			Recipient
	Recipient cells still present	Donor	Recipient	Recipient
	Recipient cells gone	Donor	Donor	Donor
Two-way (major and minor) incompatibility	Preparative regimen	Group O	Group AB	
	Transplantation period			Group AB
	Recipient antibodies still present	—	Group AB	Group AB
	Recipient antibodies gone	—	Donor	Donor
	Recipient cells still present	Group O	—	—
	Recipient cells gone	Donor	—	—

technique of acute normovolemic hemodilution also has been advocated for radical prostatectomy. A randomized trial comparing preoperative collection versus hemodilution showed equivalent effects with regard to the sparing of allogeneic transfusions, and hemodilution was less expensive (10). However, some authors have questioned the need for blood transfusion at all in this operation (11).

Intraoperative autologous blood salvage during tumor resection has tempted some investigators. Unfortunately, tumor cells can be identified readily in shed blood (12) and are not separated by filtration or centrifugation. Thus a theoretic risk of hematogenous dissemination of cancer has been raised and has not been put to rest in small observational studies the results of which suggest no increase in the rate of occurrence of metastatic disease after surgery (13). High doses of radiation (50 Gy) have been used under experimental conditions to demonstrate the elimination of proliferative cells in vitro (14). This may have value in clinical settings, although the irradiation time (up to 10 minutes) adds logistic complexity to the procedure.

Leukoreduction of Red Blood Cell Components

Use of leukoreduced red blood cell components is desirable in oncology to forestall alloimmunization to HLA and other antigens. In addition to the implications for choice of organ donor, prevention of this problem is essential for platelet transfusion support (see later). Furthermore, leukoreduction prevents many other white blood cell–associated problems that may be particularly severe in immunosuppressed patients, such as transmission of cytomegalovirus (CMV; see later) and febrile transfusion reactions. Many countries have already adapted universal leukoreduction policies. The United States is in transition—more than 20% of red blood cells were subjected to leukoreduction in 1999 (15). As of this writing, most red blood cells from major blood suppliers are subjected to leukoreduction.

PLATELET TRANSFUSION

Indications

Platelet transfusion is specifically indicated in the management of microvascular bleeding associated with thrombocytopenia and thrombopathy. Most platelet transfusions administered in the oncologic setting, however, are given prophylactically because of a specific platelet count less than which the risk of bleeding is likely to be increased. This practice has its origin in older studies of patients with leukemia that showed the value of platelets in reducing bleeding in general (16) and life-threatening central nervous system and pulmonary hemorrhage in particular (17). A clear relation between the frequency and severity of bleeding and platelet count can be demonstrated (18). Unfortunately, this does not translate to a discrete threshold platelet count at which risk increases. Many confounding variables, including underlying anatomic lesions prone to bleeding, fever, and use of invasive procedures, play into the likelihood of hemorrhage in individual patients (19).

Data from studies with humans suggest that if the confounding factors could be eliminated, very low platelet counts could be tolerated without bleeding. For example, in a study of fecal blood loss in 20 patients with severe aplastic anemia, the platelet count at which spontaneous bleeding occurred (>5 ml/24 h) was less than 10×10^9/L. Only in patients with counts less than 5×10^9/L was gastrointestinal hemorrhage (>20 ml/24 h) significant and predictable (20). These experimental data are supported by other work by these authors demonstrating that only a small fixed volume of platelets per day is needed to repair endothelial injuries and prevent spontaneous bleeding (21). With these data and supportive results of clinical trials, some groups have proposed that a threshold for prophylactic platelet transfusion in the care of patients in otherwise stable condition without signs of bleeding, could be as low as 5×10^9/L (20, 22). However, the need to consider patient-specific variables has led most recent studies and practice guidelines to focus on a more conservative limit of 10 to 20×10^9/L (23). One study showed that the lower trigger of 10×10^9/L leads to no increased risk of bleeding compared with 20×10^9/L and reduces platelet resource utilization one-third (24). The prophylactic threshold for platelet transfusion may have to be higher in certain higher-risk situations, such as surgery, in which a more appropriate trigger is 50×10^9/L, and tumors in which the risk of bleeding is higher owing to features of the tumor, such as aggressive growth, necrosis, or location.

Single-donor (Apheresis) versus Multiple-donor Platelets

Platelet transfusion prepared from donated whole blood necessitates pooling of several components, usually four to ten donated products, to provide a sufficient number of cells, typically more than 3.5×10^{11} for therapeutic efficacy in adults. Such pools can be from platelet concentrates, as in the United States with platelet-rich plasma separated from whole blood, or platelet buffy coats, as in Europe. An alternative, automated apheresis technology, has allowed collection from single donors of full therapeutic doses. Sometimes enough platelets are collected that the product can be split for use in two or three separate transfusions. Although strong polar positions had been taken in the past concerning whether apheresis components were better suited to oncology, the differences between the two camps have narrowed over time. They relate to the following factors.

Number of Donors

The risk of transfusion-transmitted infection increases as the number of donor exposures increases, although the relation may not be strictly linear. For example, the risk of hepatitis tends to plateau with increased numbers of blood transfusions (25). As the stringency of donor testing increases and the risk of transfusion-transmitted disease such as hepatitis and human immunodeficiency virus infection have fallen, the importance of number of donor exposures has decreased. In addition, because the average oncology patient receives dozens, sometimes hundreds, of red blood cell and plasma transfusions in addition to platelets, a reduction in platelet donor exposures has less of an effect on overall risk.

Platelet Quality

Concentrates differ from apheresis components in terms of anticoagulant-preservative solution (citrate-phosphate-dextrose-adenine in the former, acid citrate dextrose in the latter), rapidity of exposure to these chemicals (immediately in the former, measured ratio in the latter), and centrifugation conditions. These and other features contribute to measurable differences in expression of glycoprotein Ib (reduced in platelet concentrates) and P selectin (increased in concentrates) (26). However, no study has been able to draw a clinical correlation between these data and reduced survival or function of concentrates after transfusion.

White Blood Cell Content and Reaction Risk

Use of pooled concentrates is associated with a higher proportion of febrile reactions in recipients, and this is not entirely eliminated with poststorage filtration (27). These reactions are related to the accumulation of white blood cell–derived cytokines during storage before collection (28). Use of newer filters that allow removal of white blood cells in the hours immediately after collection may decrease the risk of reactions so that it is similar to that for leukoreduced apheresis products, from which white blood cells are removed during collection.

Risk of Alloimmunization

Risk of formation of HLA alloantibodies increases with the number of allogeneic white blood cell exposures. Therefore pooled concentrates should pose a bigger problem. However, leukoreduction levels the playing field. After leukoreduction, apheresis and pooled concentrates have been shown to have equivalent low risk of alloimmunization in recipients (29).

Considering all this information, apheresis platelets do not appear to offer any advantage over pooled concentrates except in the situation in which an antigen-matched donor (HLA or platelet specific) is being sought.

Choice of ABO and Rh Blood Group

Platelets carry modest amounts of ABH antigens, both intrinsic to the red blood cell membrane and adsorbed from the plasma. The use of platelets without regard to ABO type can substantially reduce the outdating of wasted components (from 19% to 5.5% in one study). However, 50% of platelets issued for patients with group O blood are likely to be incompatible (30). In most patients receiving ABO incompatible platelets, the effect on posttransfusion increments is minimal although measurable—a 23% reduction in one study (31). Frank clinical refractoriness can occur in the occasional patient with higher titers of anti-A or anti-B (32). Such refractoriness can be exacerbated when the donor platelets have a high A or B antigen density. In a study conducted in Japan, 7% of donors were of this high-expression phenotype—some with 20-fold more blood group antigen—apparently because of increased activity of the relevant glycosyl transferase (33). Repeated exposure to ABO-incompatible platelets appears to hasten the appearance of alloimmune refractoriness caused by HLA and platelet antibodies (30). Some authors have suggested that ABO-incompatible transfusions be limited to short time intervals and restricted to recipients with low-titer isoagglutinins and that compatible transfusions be chosen for heavier platelet support (30).

Although platelets do not carry Rh glycoproteins, a small number of contaminating donor red blood cells are always present in platelet components. Such red blood cells may be sufficient to immunize an Rh-negative recipient. This appears to be true even of immunosuppressed oncology patients, although the incidence is probably lower than among healthy persons (34). Prevention of immunization to the D antigen is of particular importance to women before and throughout their childbearing years. It also may be valuable to protect all children (boys as well as girls) because of their long potential life span and later need for transfusions. The volume of red blood cells in a platelet concentrate should be no more than 0.5 ml. It should be no more than 2 ml in an apheresis component. That is, such products do not look visibly contaminated with red blood cells (35). When it is desirable to prevent alloimmunization, a dose of 250 IU (50 μg) intravenous anti-D immune globulin suffices to prevent immunization (36). Because a patient receiving platelets usually has thrombocytopenia even after transfusion, an immune globulin that can be administered intravenously rather than intramuscularly is desirable.

Leukoreduction of Platelet Components

Leukoreduced platelets for transfusion are desirable in oncology, both to prevent alloimmunization to HLA and other white blood cell antigens and to reduce the risk of transfusion reactions, to which oncology patients, who undergo frequent transfusions, are particularly prone.

Adverse Reactions and Complications

A common reaction to transfusion of platelets is chills or frank rigors, often but not always accompanied by fever (27). These symptoms are particularly frequent among oncology patients in part because most patients receiving platelets come from this population. Although the precise pathophysiologic mechanism of the reaction is not understood, donor white blood cells are clearly involved. Removal of white blood cells decreases the frequency of reactions (37), especially if the leukoreduction occurs soon after product collection (38). Concentrations of cytokines such as interleukin-6, which are released by white blood cells during storage at room temperature, have been correlated with the occurrence and frequency of symptoms (28,39). The reaction can be interrupted by means of discontinuing the transfusion. For severe rigors, intravenous administration of 25 to 50 mg meperidine provides rapid relief (40). Meperidine also can be administered prophylactically immediately before platelet transfusion. The effect is good on patients who have recurrent reactions. In most instances, the symptoms can be avoided by use of prestorage leukoreduced platelet components. Washing a leukocyte-rich component immediately before transfusion to remove supernatant plasma also can prevent problems.

Also frequent is a positive result of a direct antiglobulin test (direct Coombs test) in a patient who has received out-of-group platelet transfusions (41). Frank hemolysis in this setting, although reported, is very rare. However, the risk may be higher with apheresis platelets, as opposed to platelet pools, if the single donor has a high titer of anti-A or anti-B. In a pool of platelet concentrates, the volume of plasma from each individual donor is less than 50 ml, as opposed to 300 ml in an apheresis component (42). The use of ABO identical or plasma-compatible platelet components may be desirable from this vantage point, although it is not always feasible owing to the short storage life and small size of typical platelet inventories.

Refractoriness to Platelet Transfusions

Progressive, intermittent or abrupt deterioration in the effectiveness of platelet transfusion, measured with the absolute or corrected platelet count increment, is one of the most common, difficult, and life-threatening aspects of oncologic care. A number of variables affect the 1-hour posttransfusion platelet count. (Table 34.3) (43,44). The establishment of alloimmune-mediated refractoriness is based on ruling out other etiologic factors and on the presence of HLA or, less frequently, platelet-specific or ABH-specific antibodies.

Management of refractoriness can be extremely difficult. It is valuable to know the patient's class I HLA typing results. Many programs perform this test routinely for a patient about to begin a regimen likely to cause transfusion-dependent thrombocytopenia. Selection of HLA-matched platelets is complex because of extensive polymorphism in the class I HLA antigens to which platelet cytotoxic antibodies are directed. To improve the potential donor pool, most strategies allow transfusion of partially mismatched donations, according to the Duquesnoy grading system (Table 34.4; Fig. 34.2) (45). However, as many as 30% of transfusions may have poor results, possibly because of unrecognized incompatible donor antigens or concomitant nonimmune clinical factors. The use of platelet cross-matching (46) or a combination of both HLA selection and platelet cross-matching (47) may improve this situation. Incorporation of HLA antibody specificity (or probable specificity, because in many patients multiple antibodies are present and identification of individual target specificities is difficult) also can increase the number of possibly compatible donors (48). Strategies to attempt to reduce the antibody titer or otherwise impede the immune process, including splenectomy, administration of steroids, plasmapheresis, use of high-dose intravenous immune globulin, and massive platelet transfusion, have had little or no effect in most cases (49). In emergencies, administration of the antifibrinolytic agent ϵ-aminocaproic acid by the oral or the intravenous route has been reported to control bleeding and blood use (50).

Prevention of primary alloimmunization is more straightforward. Alloimmunization to HLA epitopes is fostered by contaminating white blood cells in platelets and other cellular components. Transfusion of leukoreduced components prevents this primary immunization (29). Exclusive use of leukoreduced cellular components in patients never before exposed to blood or foreign tissue antigens can effectively forestall HLA alloimmunization. Unfortunately, the same is not true of patients previously immunized, for example by previous pregnancy or transfusion. For them the value of leukocyte reduction is uncertain, because platelet epitopes themselves or residual levels of white blood cells appear sufficiently stimulatory to invoke an anamnestic response (51). This problem speaks to the importance of prevention and is an important benefit of universal leukoreduction.

TABLE 34.3. CAUSES OF PLATELET TRANSFUSION–REFRACTORY THROMBOCYTOPENIA AMONG ONCOLOGY PATIENTS

Nonimmune causes
- Splenomegaly
- Venoocclusive disease of the liver
- Microangiopathy (thrombotic thrombocytopenic purpura, hemolytic uremic syndrome)
- Amphotericin B
- Bleeding
- Fever
- Disseminated intravascular coagulation

Immune causes
- HLA alloantibodies
- Platelet-specific alloantibody
- ABO incompatible platelet transfusions[a]
- Idiopathic thrombocytopenic purpura

[a] In a recipient with a high-titer ABO antibody.

TABLE 34.4. HLA-MATCH GRADES FOR PLATELET COMPONENTS

Grade	Criterion
A	All 4 antigens of the donor identical to those of the recipient
B1U	Only 3 antigens detected in the donor; all present in the recipient
B1UX	Of the 4 identified donor antigens, 3 identical to recipient; one cross-reactive with recipient
B2U	Only 2 antigens detected in the donor; both present in the recipient
B2UX	Only 3 antigens detected in the donor; 2 identical with the recipient and one cross-reactive
B2X	Of the 4 identified donor antigens, 2 identical with the recipient, and 2 cross-reactive
C	One donor antigen not present in recipient and not cross-reactive with recipient
D	Two donor antigens not present in recipient and not cross-reactive with recipient

Matching involves the comparison of class I (A and B) antigens of the donor and recipient.
From Duquesnoy RJ, Filip DJ, Rodey GE, et al. Successful transfusion of platelets "mismatched" for HLA antigens to alloimmunized thrombocytopenic patients. *Am J Hematol* 1977;2:219–226, with permission.

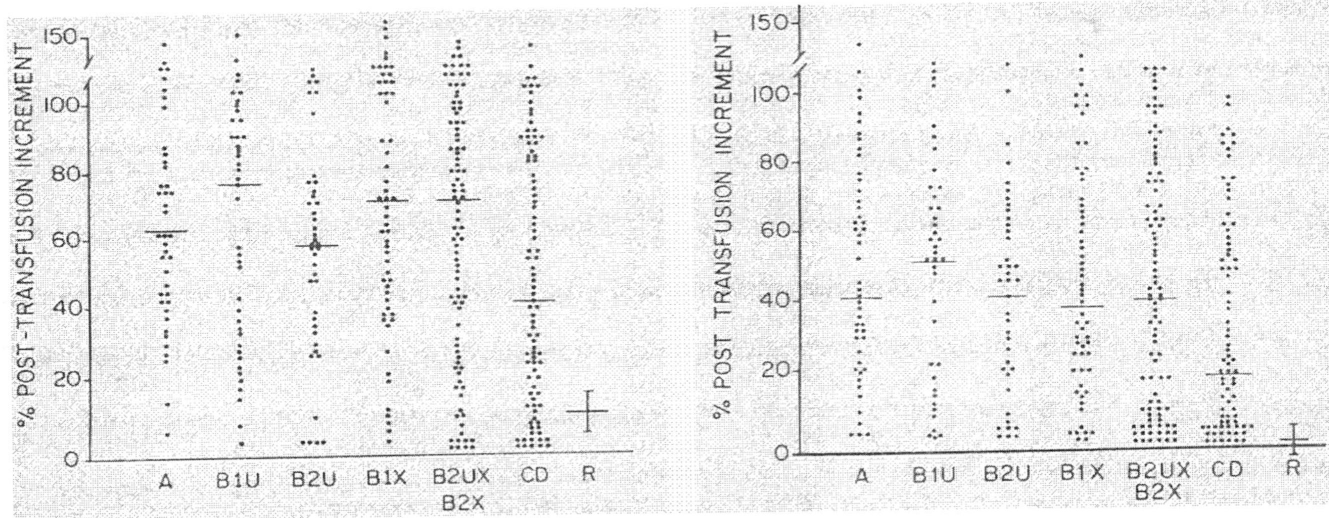

FIGURE 34.2. Platelet increments in alloimmunized patients 1 hour (*left*) and 24 hours (*right*) after transfusion of apheresis platelets from HLA-matched donors (match grades A through D; Table 34.4). *Horizontal bar,* median response. *R,* pooled random platelets. *Horizontal bar* is mean ± 1 SD. (From Duquesnoy RJ, Filip DJ, Rodey GE, et al. Successful transfusion of platelets "mismatched" for HLA antigens to alloimmunized thrombocytopenic patients. *Am J Hematol* 1977;2:219–226, with permission).

GRANULOCYTE TRANSFUSION

Indications

Bacterial and fungal infections following chemotherapy-induced neutropenia can be a life-threatening problem in oncologic care. Transfusion of allogeneic granulocytes may be useful to patients with severe neutropenia (<500 neutrophils per microliter of blood) with a documented infection that is not responding to antibiotics. Daily production of neutrophils in a healthy human without infection is 6×10^{10} cells/day, and the need for these cells increases twofold to threefold with infection. A transfused dose of 1×10^{11} granulocytes per square meter of body surface can increase the blood cell count of a patient 1,000 to 2,000 cells/μl (52). However, this number of cells until recently could be obtained only from donors with chronic myelogenous leukemia (CML). Cells of CML also were of value because granulocyte precursors were transfused, and the half-life of such youthful cells could be 1 day or more, as opposed to the 6-hour circulation period of mature granulocytes. In a few recipients, prolonged white blood cell recoveries over many weeks ensued owing to transient allografts of the CML granulocyte precursors. The risk of transfusion-associated graft versus host disease and other consequences of transfusion of leukemic cells made this approach unappealing, and alternatives to increasing white blood cell yields from healthy donors have been pursued instead.

Typical granulocyte collection protocols involve leukapheresis with the administration of hydroxyethyl starch to promote red blood cell sedimentation and separation from the buffy coat coupled with administration of steroids to the donor to increase neutrophil demargination. However, total yields are rarely greater than 2 to 3×10^{10} granulocytes, often without measurable postdonation increases in the recipient's white blood cell count. It has been difficult to demonstrate dramatic, or even uniform, response to granulocyte transfusions, although the disappearance of fever could be shown to correlate with the number of white blood cells transfused. Because of these poor results and improved antibiotic regimens for neutropenia, interest in granulocyte transfusion remained limited until recently.

The availability of the recombinant human cytokine granulocyte colony-stimulating factor (G-CSF) appears to have the potential to reinvigorate granulocyte transfusion. After a single subcutaneous injection into a healthy blood donor, a dose-dependent increase in peripheral blood neutrophils occurs, reaching a maximum at 12 hours. The increase is caused by release of bone marrow reserves and acceleration of neutrophil maturation. If such a treated donor undergoes leukapheresis, collection yields of 4 to 10×10^{10} cells are typical, often tenfold higher than could have occurred with steroids alone. Collections of this size lead to increments in granulocyte count of 2 to 5×10^3/μl in the recipient (53). Improved posttransfusion white blood cell survival of donor G-CSF–stimulated granulocytes also occurs because mobilized immature precursors are collected, analogous to the phenomenon in CML granulocyte donors. Granulocyte colony-stimulating factor also inhibits apoptosis of white blood cells, adding to their life span, and enhances their phagocytic ability (54).

The optimal schedule for cytokine administration and collection is still under consideration. Most popularly studied is a regimen of 300 to 600 μg G-CSF (5 to 10 μg/kg) plus 8 mg dexamethasone 12 hours before collection. This regimen can be used for a single-time donation, or donation can be repeated for a donor willing to undergo serial daily collections. Side effects in donors are common but mild, including bone pain, headaches, fluid retention, and myalgia. Steroids may contribute insomnia to this mix (54).

Precautions, Adverse Reactions, and Complications

Granulocytes for transfusions usually contain red blood cells and therefore should be matched to ABO blood group and be crossmatch compatible with the recipient. A daily transfusion regimen is necessary during the period of infection and neutropenia. Approximately one-third of recipients may be expected to have fever and chills at least once during this course (53). In a recipient with HLA-directed alloantibodies, neutrophil increments often are reduced, and complications due to leukoagglutination, such as pulmonary insufficiency, also appear. The severity of pulmonary complications is magnified by concomitant use of amphotericin (55). The use of HLA-compatible donors sometimes is necessary. Unmatched components are far less likely to be effective, as has been demonstrated by the absence of indium-labeled white blood cell migration to sites of infection in alloimmunized recipients of nonmatched components (56). Granulocyte transfusions from randomly picked (non-HLA-matched) donors frequently lead to HLA, red blood cell, and platelet alloimmunization (57). This risk must be considered in the care of patients headed for later allogeneic transplantation or intensive platelet support (58). Because most patients into whom this component is transfused can be considered immunosuppressed, granulocytes should be γ-irradiated before transfusion to protect the recipient from transfusion-associated graft versus host disease (59). Finally, the risk of CMV infection increases in association with granulocyte transfusion (60). Donors should be screened and have negative serologic results when time and circumstances allow.

INTRAVENOUS IMMUNE GLOBULIN

Indications

Intravenous immune globulin (IVIG) has become part of the pharmaceutical armamentarium in the care of heavily alloimmunized oncology patients, especially in transplantation. After bone marrow transplantation, the risk of infection in the recipient lasts up to 6 months after autologous bone marrow transplantation and up to 9 months if allogeneic marrow is used (61). This risk is due not only to neutropenia, which usually resolves with marrow recovery in a matter of weeks, but also to other effects of treatment on the immune system, including impaired function of B lymphocytes. Cytomegalovirus infection is one serious infection risk in this setting. It is notorious for particularly severe morbidity, including interstitial pneumonitis, and mortality. Both CMV hyperimmune globulin and IVIG prevent CMV disease. Both have some degree of efficacy when coupled with antiviral agents such as ganciclovir, in the management of established infection (62). Intravenous immune globulin, however, has become a standard of care in bone marrow transplantation, because, in keeping with its myriad effects on the immune system, it has other beneficial effects on transplant recipients, including preventing other infections, decreasing acute graft versus host disease, and interrupting autoimmune complications associated with transplantation (63). The net result, a reduction in transplantation-related complications, translates in many studies to reduced overall mortality (64,65). The mechanism accounting for the reduced incidence of graft versus host disease remains uncertain, but it may involve inhibition of donor B and T cells, interference with cytokine production, or protection against intestine-derived bacteria and their toxins.

The optimal dosage of IVIG for prophylaxis is under study. A schedule of 500 mg/kg weekly for 13 weeks then monthly through the end of the first year after transplantation, or 12 g/kg total dose, appears as effective as higher-dose regimens (1,000 mg/kg) at curtailing infection (66). Treatment with IVIG generally is unnecessary beyond 90 days after transplantation in the absence of hypogammaglobulinemia (61). Amelioration of graft versus host disease appears to be correlated with higher serum levels of immunoglobulin G. The benefit is lessened with regimens (e.g., 250 mg/kg per dose) that result in lower levels (67). Intravenous immune globulin has been used successfully to manage posttransplantation immune-mediated cytopenia (68, 69).

Precautions, Adverse Reactions, and Complications

Intravenous immune globulin usually is well tolerated by patients, including oncology patients. However, thrombotic events, including stroke, myocardial infarction, and deep venous thrombosis, have been linked to use of this agent, possibly owing to an increase in plasma viscosity or platelet activation induced by the immune globulin (70). A particular concern in this regard is hepatic venoocclusive disease, a syndrome of hepatomegaly, ascites, and hyperbilirubinemia associated with narrowing or complete occlusion of hepatic venules. In one study involving patients randomized to receive either IVIG or no treatment, 5 of 82 in the IVIG group had fatal venoocclusive disease whereas none of 88 control patients did (71). Also relevant to oncology patients is the warning that IVIG, especially brands prepared with sucrose as a stabilizer, may cause acute renal failure when given in high doses to patients with underlying kidney disease, sepsis, or the presence of a paraprotein (J.S. Epstein, K.C. Zoon, *personal communication,* 1999). Thus close observation of the treated patient is necessary.

The presence of IVIG can lead to the appearance of unexpected antibodies against red blood cells, most commonly due to anti-A/B, anti-D, and anti-Kell (72). For the most part, the antibody titers in the components are low, and the problems associated with passive transfusion appear to be largely limited to a positive result of a direct Coombs test or detection in serum without clinical sequelae. Frank hemolysis is rare (73). Platelet and granulocyte antibodies can be identified, also apparently without clinical consequences (74). Intravenous immune globulin can contain antibodies to viral agents of importance to oncology patients. In the early 1990s, anti–hepatitis C virus (HCV) was present in pooled donor material (75). Patients who received transfusions with IVIG regularly underwent seroconversion due to this passive transfer without necessarily being infected with HCV. This phenomenon has proved diagnostically challenging; scattered outbreaks of true hepatitis C have been associated with a few lots of IVIG before 1995, the unintended consequence of the screening of source plasma donors for hepatitis C virus antibodies (76). The U.S. Food and Drug Administration now requires that HCV antibody–positive donors be removed from the plasma pools to be used for IVIG manufacture. Additional steps, including nucleic acid detection and virus inactivation strategies have been incorporated. However, no screening is done for anti-hepatitis A virus, anti–hepatitis B core, anti-hepatitis B surface antigen, or anti-CMV. These antibodies can cause confusion if the passive nature of their appearance in a recipient's blood after use of IVIG is not considered.

SPECIAL TRANSFUSION-ASSOCIATED PROBLEMS OF ONCOLOGY PATIENTS

Transfusion-associated Graft versus Host Disease

Graft versus host disease is a nearly 100% fatal complication of blood transfusion. It is of particular importance to patients with cancer, because both the underlying illness, especially Hodgkin's disease, and the effects of treatment, especially high-dose chemotherapy in preparation for autologous or allogeneic transplantation, increase the risk of this syndrome (77). Potent new immunosuppressive agents also are to blame, particularly the synthetic purine analogues 2-chlorodeoxyadenosine (cladribine) and fludarabine. Both are used increasingly to manage lymphoma and chronic lymphocytic leukemia, cause marked reductions in the number of CD4 lymphocytes, and carry increased risk of transfusion-associated graft versus host disease, even though the underlying disease may not (78). The syndrome has a fatality rate of almost 100%. A diagnosis of leukemia may increase the risk of transfusion-associated graft versus host disease, although the mortality is lower (79).

Transfusion from HLA haplotype homozygous donors places the recipient at risk. In one study, the estimated risk of pairing an HLA-homozygous donor with a one haplotype–matched heterozygous recipient was between 1 in 17,600 and 1 in 39,000 transfusions (80). This donor characteristic may be of particular importance in the care of patients with cancer receiving HLA-compatible platelets, because HLA haplotype homozygous donors, who have fewer unique antigens, make better match grades and are therefore more likely to be a part of this donor population. The use of family members as compatible platelet donors skews the odds in favor of such pairings. Fortunately, other factors, such as the number of white blood cells in the component and the age of the component at transfusion, often militate against development of the syndrome.

Prevention of transfusion-associated graft versus host disease necessitates γ-irradiation of blood components intended for recipients at risk with a minimum of 2,500 rad (25 Gy) (Table 34.5). An alternative approach to selective irradiation of blood components for patients at risk is to irradiate the entire blood supply in use at an institution. This approach has become increasingly popular at centers with unique or disproportionately large oncology services, because of the logistic challenges of identifying patients at risk. Components with white blood cell contents less than 1×10^6 are rarely associated with transfusion-associated graft versus host disease. The move to universal leukoreduction is likely to reduce the risk and incidence of transfusion-associated graft versus host disease. However, because of variability in residual leukocyte counts, leukoreduction is a less reliable approach to the prevention of transfusion-associated graft versus host disease and should not be relied on as an alternative to γ-irradiation.

TABLE 34.5. PATIENTS FOR WHOM CELLULAR BLOOD COMPONENTS SHOULD BE TREATED WITH GAMMA IRRADIATION

Recipients with hematologic malignant disease
Hodgkin's disease
Non-Hodgkin's lymphoma
Acute myelocytic leukemia
Acute lymphocytic leukemia
Recipients of allogeneic bone marrow transplants
Recipients of autologous bone marrow transplants
Recipients treated with purine analogues, such as fludarabine
Recipients of haplotype-homozygous HLA-compatible apheresis platelets

Transfusion-transmitted Disease

The immunosuppressed state of many oncology patients puts them at unique risk of a few transfusion-transmitted infections that are largely, and safely, overlooked in the general population.

Cytomegalovirus

Cytomegalovirus infection, of almost no clinical consequence to immunocompetent persons, can have profound implications in recipients of bone marrow transplants, including pneumonia, esophagitis and other gastrointestinal disorders, and delayed engraftment of neutrophils and platelets (81). Both seronegative and seropositive recipients are at risk. Seronegative patients can contract infection from seropositive or infected bone marrow donation or from transfusion of seropositive or infected blood components (82). Seropositive patients experience frequent reactivations of disease in the setting of the accompanying immunosuppression of the primary oncologic illness and its management. Compounding this is an apparent facilitating effect of acute graft versus host disease in recipients of allogeneic transplants. Graft versus host disease may function as do other immunologic stimuli in reactivating latent viruses (83). Another explanation, although hypothetical, is that a second-strain infection occurs in seropositive patients. In antibody-positive patients, the use of seronegative blood transfusions does not reduce the risk of CMV infection (84). An incidence as high as 79% speaks to the importance of reactivation as an etiologic factor (85).

For CMV-negative recipients of transplants from CMV-negative donors, CMV-negative blood is an effective preventive approach. The requirement for serologically screened blood poses interesting medical and logistic questions. Many, often most, adult blood donors have CMV antibodies, but the meaning of this finding in relation to predicted infectivity of the blood component is uncertain. Not every seropositive donor is necessarily infectious at the time of donation; however, over time the virus can be found with polymerase chain reaction amplification in peripheral blood mononuclear cells in all antibody-positive donors. To make matters worse, many antibody-negative donors harbor the virus (86). Thus the certainty of providing blood free of CMV risk by means of serologic screening is not absolute. A number of clinical trials have established the use of leukoreduction as an equivalent approach to screening for seronegative donors. Particularly pivotal was a large, multicenter, randomized trial of bone marrow recipients who received either seronegative or leukocyte-reduced components. Although bedside filtration, a less-than-optimal leukoreduction technique, was used in this study, the authors found the rates of posttransfusion CMV infection in the two arms were statistically equivalent (87). Although a specific threshold white blood cell count less than which a component is noninfectious has not been established, current U.S. standards for leukoreduction ($<5 \times 10^6$ cells per component transfused) appears satisfactory and equivalent to CMV antibody–negative blood as a source of "CMV-safe" components. At present, this requires that hospitals using nonleukoreduced components establish specific transfusion protocols for patients at risk. As the move to universally leukoreduced blood components in many parts of the world, including the United States, progresses, the need for these logistics should become moot.

Parvovirus B19

Parvovirus B19 infects erythroid precursors and can cause erythroid hypoplasia and even pure red blood cell aplasia in susceptible persons. The clinical manifestations are especially obvious in persons with high rates of red blood cell destruction but also can occur in persons with compromised bone marrow, such as oncology patients. Isolated cases of transfusion-transmitted Parvovirus B19 infection have been reported, including one in a recipient of a bone marrow transplant. In this case, the patient received platelets from an actively infected donor. The consequence was transfusion-dependent chronic anemia and reticulocytopenia that lasted until after the patient was treated with two courses of IVIG (88).

Chagas Disease

Trypanosoma cruzi infection is a zoonosis spread by means of insect bite. The resulting disease in humans is characterized by cardiac disease (arrhythmia and cardiac failure), gastrointestinal problems (megaesophagus and megacolon), and neurologic complications (encephalopathy and seizures). The disease is widespread in Latin America, where 18 million persons have the infection, and transfusion-transmitted disease is a major problem in this part of the world (89). More than 100,000 persons with the infection live in North America. Only a few cases have been reported in North America, but they involve patients with oncologic diagnoses such as leukemia (90) and Hodgkin's disease (91). The likelihood of transfusion-associated disease is related to the immune status of the patient and to parasite load. Leukoreduction eliminates a proportion of parasites (92). Other approaches for screening donors by history or blood test are under investigation but not yet implemented in North America.

Transfusion-associated Immunomodulation

Allogeneic blood transfusion has an incompletely understood but influential role in immune modulation of the recipient, and this may be of particular importance to patients with cancer. A beneficial effect of allogeneic blood transfusions before renal transplantation on the outcome of organ survival has been upheld in numerous studies. Reduction in the recurrence rate of Crohn's disease also has been observed (93). Unfortunately, the same postulated mechanisms that may aid solid organ transplantation, including inactivation of alloreactive lymphocyte clones, development of antiidiotype antibodies, and development of suppressor T cells, are likely to have adverse implications for patients with malignant disease in terms of more rapid growth of disease and rate of metastasis.

Numerous investigators have attempted to use retrospective clinical studies to explore the effect of perioperative blood transfusions on patients with cancer. The results have been mixed. A fastidious metaanalysis of 60 such observational studies showed that a sizable portion of the apparent increased relative risk of tumor recurrence associated with transfusion in many clinical studies was due to overlooked or incompletely analyzed confounding variables (94). In contrast, in animal models, an early but compelling case for an untoward effect has been presented. In rabbits, for example, allogeneic blood transfusion, in particular the white blood cell fraction, enhances tumor growth (95,96). This effect is ameliorated if the white blood cells are removed before but not after storage of the blood component in advance of the transfusion. Thus the effect may be due to white blood cells themselves or to accumulation of cytokines and other bioactive, white blood cell–derived substances in blood components during storage.

The effect of transfusion therapy on cancer remains uncertain. Although data from studies with animals suggest an effect exists, the influence may be very small and therefore difficult to measure in comparison with other factors (97). This controversy will probably be satisfactorily resolved only with prospective, randomized clinical trials or, in countries that have already moved to total leukoreduction, with observational trials with historical controls. The impending move to universal leukoreduction of blood components may render this issue moot. The exception is the residual question of the timing of leukoreduction. Poststorage removal may not be as effective as prestorage efforts if accumulation of bioactive white blood cell materials in the component supernatant during storage is a factor in the immunomodulatory effect (98).

SUMMARY

Blood transfusion is a cornerstone of cancer care. Use of transfusion requires attention to nuances specific for oncology patients. Blood transfusion into recipients of bone marrow transplants must respect the chimeric state of the recipient and the presence of residual incompatible donor or recipient ABO antibodies. Platelet transfusion requires close monitoring for identification and care of patients whose condition is refractory. Granulocyte transfusion therapy may become more relevant for patients with neutropenia with the advent of G-CSF for donor collection. Intravenous immune globulin is used frequently in the care of bone marrow recipients to protect against and manage CMV and other infections. Special problems of oncology patients include transfusion-associated graft versus host disease, which can be prevented with γ-irradiation of all cellular blood components before transfusion into patients at risk. Some transfusion-transmitted diseases are particularly problematic in cancer care, including CMV infection. Immunosuppressed patients are vulnerable to other rare disorders, such as Chagas disease and Parvovirus B19 infections. Transfusion-associated immunomodulation may have particular importance to patients with cancer, although effects are difficult to discern from other clinical factors. Donor white blood cells play key roles in a number of these problems, including alloimmunization, CMV infection, transfusion-associated graft versus host disease, and immune modulation. Universal leukoreduction of blood products is likely to reduce or eliminate many of these risks.

REFERENCES

1. Greeno EW, Perry EH, Ilstrup SJ, et al. Exchange transfusion the hard way: massive hemolysis following transplantation of bone marrow with minor ABO incompatibility. *Transfusion* 1996;36:71–74.
2. Bolan CD, Childs RW, Procter JL, et al. Massive immune hemolysis after allogeneic peripheral blood stem cell transplantation with minor ABO incompatibility. *Br J Haematol* 2001;112:787–795.
3. Wernet D, Mayer G. Isoagglutinins following ABO-incompatible bone marrow transplantation. *Vox Sang* 1992;62:176–179.
4. Wulff JC, Santner TJ, Storb R, et al. Transfusion requirements after HLA-identical marrow transplantation in 82 patients with aplastic anemia. *Vox Sang* 1983;44:366–374.
5. Lasky LC, Warkentin PI, Kersey JH, et al. Hemotherapy in patients undergoing blood group incompatible bone marrow transplantation. *Transfusion* 1983;23:277–285.
6. Benjamin RJ, McGurk S, Ralston MS, et al. ABO incompatibility as an adverse risk factor for survival after allogeneic bone marrow transplantation. *Transfusion* 1999;39:179–187.
7. Abou-Elella AA, Camarillo TA, Allen MB, et al. Low incidence of red cell and HLA antibody formation by bone marrow transplant patients. *Transfusion* 1995;35:931–935.
8. de la Rubia J, Arriaga F, Andreu R, et al. Development of non-ABO RBC alloantibodies in patients undergoing allogeneic HPC transplantation: is ABO incompatibility a predisposing factor? *Transfusion* 2001; 41:106–110.
9. Toy PTCY, Menozzi D, Strauss RG, et al. Efficacy of preoperative donation of blood for autologous use in radical prostatectomy. *Transfusion* 1993;33:721–724.
10. Ness PM, Bourke DL, Walsh PC. A randomized trial of perioperative hemodilution versus transfusion of preoperatively deposited autologous blood in elective surgery. *Transfusion* 1992;32:226–230.
11. Goh M, Kleer CG, Kielczewski P, et al. Autologous blood donation prior to anatomical radical retropubic prostatectomy: is it necessary? *Urology* 1996;49:569–574.
12. Hansen E, Wolff N, Knuechel R, et al. Tumor cells in blood shed from the surgical field. *Arch Surg* 1995;130:387–393.
13. Valbonesi M, Bruni R, Lercari G, et al. Autoapheresis and intraoperative blood salvage in oncologic surgery. *Transfus Sci* 1999;21:129–139.
14. Hansen E, Knuechel R, Altmeppen J, et al. Blood irradiation for intraoperative autotransfusion in cancer surgery: demonstration of efficient elimination of contaminating tumor cells. *Transfusion* 1999;39: 608–615.
15. National Blood Data Resource Center. Comprehensive report on blood collection and transfusion in the United States in 1999. Bethesda, MD: National Blood Data Resource Center, 2001:1–35.
16. Higby DJ, Cohen E, Holland JF, et al. The prophylactic treatment of thrombocytopenic leukemic patients with platelets: a double blind study. *Transfusion* 1974;14:440–446.
17. Han T, Stutzman L, Cohen E, et al. Effect of platelet transfusion on hemorrhage in patients with acute leukemia. *Cancer* 1966;19: 1937–1942.
18. Gaydos LA, Freireich EJ, Mantel N. The quantitative relation between platelet count and hemorrhage in patients with acute leukemia. *N Engl J Med* 1962;266:905–909.
19. Rebulla P, Finazzi G, Marangoni F, et al. A multicenter randomized trial of the threshold for prophylactic platelet transfusions in adults with acute myeloid leukemia. *N Engl J Med* 1997;337:1870–1875.
20. Slichter SJ, Harker LA. Thrombocytopenia: mechanisms and management of defects in platelet production. *Clin Haematol* 1978;7:523–538.
21. Hanson SR, Slichter SJ. Platelet kinetics in patients with bone marrow hypoplasia: evidence for a fixed platelet requirement. *Blood* 1985;66: 1105–1109.
22. Gmur J, Burger J, Schanz U, et al. Safety of stringent prophylactic platelet transfusion policy for patients with acute leukemia. *Lancet* 1991;338:1223–1226.
23. Schiffer CA, Anderson KC, Bennett CL, et al. Platelet transfusion for patients with cancer: clinical practice guidelines of the American Society of Clinical Oncology. *J Clin Oncol* 2001;19:1519–1538.
24. Wandt H, Frank M, Ehninger G, et al. Safety and cost effectiveness of a 10×10^9/L trigger for prophylactic platelet transfusions compared with the traditional 20×10^9/L trigger: a prospective comparative trial in 105 patients with acute myeloid leukemia. *Blood* 1998;91: 3601–3606.
25. Alter HJ, Purcell RH, Holland PV, et al. Donor transaminase and recipient hepatitis: impact on blood transfusion service. *JAMA* 1981; 246:630–634.
26. Sloand E, Yu M, Klein HG. Comparison of random-donor platelet concentrates prepared from whole blood units and platelets prepared from single-donor apheresis collections. *Transfusion* 1996;36:955–959.
27. Chambers LA, Kruskall MS, Pacini DG, et al. Febrile reactions following platelet transfusions: the effect of single versus multiple donors. *Transfusion* 1990;30:219–221.
28. Heddle NM, Klama L, Singer R, et al. The role of the plasma from platelet concentrates in transfusion reactions. *N Engl J Med* 1994;331: 625–628.
29. Trial to Reduce Alloimmunization to Platelets (TRAP) Trial Study Group. Leukocyte-reduction and UV-B irradiation of platelets to prevent alloimmunization and refractoriness to platelet transfusions. *N Engl J Med* 1997;337:1861–1869.
30. Carr R, Hutton JL, Jenkins JA, et al. Transfusion of ABO-mismatched platelets leads to early platelet refractoriness. *Br J Haematol* 1990;75: 408–413.
31. Duquesnoy RJ, Anderson AJ, Tomasulo PA, et al. ABO compatibility and platelet transfusions of alloimmunized thrombocytopenic patients. *Blood* 1979;54:595–599.
32. Brand A, Sintnicolaas K, Claas FHJ, et al. ABH antibodies causing platelet transfusion refractoriness. *Transfusion* 1986;26:463–466.
33. Ogasawara K, Ueki J, Takenaka M, et al. Study on the expression of ABH antigens on platelets. *Blood* 1993;82:993–999.
34. Baldwin ML, Ness PM, Scott D, et al. Alloimmunization to D antigen and HLA in D-negative immunosuppressed oncology patients. *Transfusion* 1988;28:330–333.
35. Vengelen-Tyler V. *Technical manual,* 13th ed. Bethesda, MD: American Association of Blood Banks, 1999.
36. Lee D, Contreras M, Robson SC, et al. Recommendations for the use of anti-D immunoglobulin for Rh prophylaxis. *Transfus Med* 1999;9: 93–97.
37. Mangano MM, Chambers LA, Kruskall MS. Limited efficacy of leukopoor platelets for prevention of febrile transfusion reactions. *Am J Clin Pathol* 1991;95:733–738.
38. Sarkodee-Adoo CB, Kendall JM, Sridhara R, et al. The relationship between the duration of platelet storage and the development of transfusion reactions. *Transfusion* 1998;38:229–235.
39. Muylle L, Wouters E, Peetersmans ME. Febrile reactions to platelet transfusion: the effect of increased interleukin 6 levels in concentrates

prepared by the platelet-rich plasma method. *Transfusion* 1996;36: 886–890.
40. Friedlander M, Noble WH. Meperidine to control shivering associated with platelet transfusion reaction. *Can J Anaesth* 1989;36:460–462.
41. Shanwell A, Ringdén O, Wiechel B, et al. A study of the effect of ABO incompatible plasma in platelet concentrates transfused to bone marrow transplant recipients. *Vox Sang* 1991;60:23–27.
42. Larsson LG, Welsh VJ, Ladd DJ. Acute intravascular hemolysis secondary to out-of-group platelet transfusion. *Transfusion* 2000;40:902–906.
43. Bishop JF, Matthews JP, McGrath K, et al. Factors influencing 20-hour increments after platelet transfusion. *Transfusion* 1991;313:392–396.
44. Bishop JF, McGrath K, Wolf MW, et al. Clinical factors influencing the efficacy of pooled platelet transfusions. *Blood* 1988;71:383–387.
45. Duquesnoy RJ, Filip DJ, Rodey GE, et al. Successful transfusion of platelets "mismatched" for HLA antigens to alloimmunized thrombocytopenic patients. *Am J Hematol* 1977;2:219–226.
46. Kickler TS. The challenge of platelet alloimmunization: management and prevention. *Transfus Med Rev* 1990;4[Suppl 1]:8–18.
47. Moroff G, Garratty G, Heal JM, et al. Selection of platelets for refractory patients by HLA matching and prospective crossmatching. *Transfusion* 1992;32:633–640.
48. Petz LD, Garratty G, Calhoun L, et al. Selecting donors of platelets for refractory patients on the basis of HLA antibody specificity. *Transfusion* 2000;40:1446–1456.
49. Wuest DL. Transfusion and stem cell support in cancer treatment. *Hematol Oncol Clin North Am* 1996;10:397–429.
50. Bartholomew JR, Salgia R, Bell WR. Control of bleeding in patients with immune and nonimmune thrombocytopenia with aminocaproic acid. *Arch Intern Med* 1989;149:1959–1961.
51. Sintnicolaas K, van Marwijk Kooij M, van Prooijen HC, et al. Leukocyte depletion of random single-donor platelet transfusions does not prevent secondary human leukocyte antigen-alloimmunization and refractoriness: a randomized prospective study. *Blood* 1995;85:824–828.
52. Freireich EJ. White cell transfusion born again. *Leuk Lymphoma* 1994; 11[Suppl 2]:161–165.
53. Price TH, Bowden RA, Boeckh M, et al. Phase I/II trial of neutrophil transfusions from donors stimulated with G-CSF and dexamethasone for treatment of patients with infections in hematopoietic stem cell transplantation. *Blood* 2000;95:3302–3309.
54. Price TH. The current prospects for neutrophil transfusions for the treatment of granulocytopenic infected patients. *Transfus Med Rev* 2000;14:2–11.
55. Wright DG, Robichaud KJ, Pizzo PA, et al. Lethal pulmonary reactions associated with the combined use of amphotericin B and leukocyte transfusions. *N Engl J Med* 1981;304:1185–1189.
56. Dutcher JP, Schiffer CA, Johnston GA, et al. Alloimmunization prevents the migration of transfused indium-111-labeled granulocytes to sites of infection. *Blood* 1983;62:354–360.
57. Pegels JG, Bruynes ECE, Engelfriet CP, et al. Serological studies in patients on platelet- and granulocyte-substitution therapy. *Br J Haematol* 1982;52:59–68.
58. Schiffer CA, Aisner J, Daly PA, et al. Alloimmunization following prophylactic granulocyte transfusion. *Blood* 1979;54:766–774.
59. Weiden PL, Zuckerman N, Hansen JA, et al. Fatal graft-versus-host disease in a patient with lymphoblastic leukemia following normal granulocyte transfusions. *Blood* 1981;57:328–332.
60. Hersman J, Meyers JD, Thomas ED, et al. The effect of granulocyte transfusions on the incidence of cytomegalovirus infection after allogeneic marrow transplantation. *Ann Intern Med* 1982;96:149–152.
61. Sullivan KM. Secondary immunodeficiencies and stem cell transplantation: issues of administration and safety of intravenous immunoglobulin. *Clin Ther* 1996;18[Suppl B]:126–136.
62. Zikos P, van Lint MT, Lamparelli T, et al. A randomized trial of high dose polyvalent intravenous immunoglobulin (HDIgG. vs. cytomegalovirus (CMV. hyperimmune IgG in allogeneic hemopoietic stem cell transplants (HSCT). *Haematologica* 1998;83:132–137.
63. Gale RP, Winston D. Intravenous immunoglobulin in bone marrow transplantation. *Cancer* 1991;15[Suppl]:1451–1453.
64. Winston DJ, Ho WG, Lin CH, et al. Intravenous immune globulin for prevention of cytomegalovirus infection and interstitial pneumonia after bone marrow transplantation. *Ann Intern Med* 1987;106:12–18.
65. Sullivan KM, Kopecky KJ, Jocom J, et al. Immunomodulatory and antimicrobial efficacy of intravenous immunoglobulin in bone marrow transplantation. *N Engl J Med* 1990;232:705–712.
66. Feinstein LC, Seidel K, Jocum J, et al. Reduced dose intravenous immunoglobulin does not decrease transplant-related complications in adults given related donor marrow allografts. *Biol Blood Marrow Transplant* 1999;5:360–378.
67. Abdel-Mageed A, Graham-Pole J, Del Rosario MLU, et al. Comparison of two doses of intravenous immunoglobulin after allogeneic bone marrow transplants. *Bone Marrow Transplant* 1999;23:929–932.
68. Khouri IF, Ippoliti C, Gajewski J, et al. Neutropenias following allogeneic bone marrow transplantation: response to therapy with high-dose intravenous immunoglobulin. *Am J Hematol* 1996;52:313–315.
69. Klumpp TR, Block CC, Caliguri MA, et al. Immune-mediated cytopenia following bone marrow transplantation: case reports and review of the literature. *Medicine* 1992;71:73–83.
70. Go RS, Call TG. Deep venous thrombosis of the arm after intravenous immunoglobulin infusion: case report and literature review of intravenous immunoglobulin–related thrombotic complications. *Mayo Clin Proc* 2000;75:83–85.
71. Wolff SN, Fay JW, Herzig RH, et al. High-dose weekly intravenous immunoglobulin to prevent infections in patients undergoing autologous bone marrow transplantation or severe myelosuppressive therapy: a study of the American Bone Marrow Transplant Group. *Ann Intern Med* 1993;118:937–942.
72. Garratty G. Problems associated with passively transfused blood group alloantibodies. *Am J Clin Pathol* 1998;109:769–776.
73. Okubo S, Ishida T, Yasunaga K. Hemolysis after intravenous immune globulin therapy: relation to IgG subclasses of red cell antibody. *Transfusion* 1990;30:436–438.
74. Klumpp TR, Herman JH, Mangan KF, et al. Lack of transmission of neutrophil and platelet antibodies by intravenous immunoglobulin in bone marrow transplant patients. *Transfusion* 1994;34:677–679.
75. Dodd LG, McBride JH, Gitnick GL, et al. Prevalence of non-A, non-B hepatitis/hepatitis C virus antibody in human immunoglobulins. *Am J Clin Pathol* 1992;97:108–113.
76. Yap PL. Intravenous immunoglobulin and hepatitis C virus: an overview of transmission episodes with emphasis on manufacturing data. *Clin Ther* 1996;18[Suppl B]:43–58.
77. Anderson KC, Weinstein HJ. Transfusion-associated graft-versus-host disease. *N Engl J Med* 1990;323:315–321.
78. Briz M, Cabrera R, Sanjuan I, et al. Diagnosis of transfusion-associated graft-versus-host disease by polymerase chain reaction in fludarabine-treated B-chronic lymphocytic leukaemia. *Br J Haematol* 1995;91: 409–411.
79. Leitman SF, Holland PV. Irradiation of blood products: indications and guidelines. *Transfusion* 1985;25:293–300.
80. Wagner FF, Flegel WA. Transfusion-associated graft-versus-host disease: risk due to homozygous HLA haplotypes. *Transfusion* 1995;35: 284–291.
81. Sayers MH, Anderson KC, Goodnough LT, et al. Reducing the risk for transfusion-transmitted cytomegalovirus infection. *Ann Intern Med* 1992;116:55–62.
82. Meyers JD, Flournoy N, Thomas ED. Risk factors for cytomegalovirus infection after human marrow transplantation. *J Infect Dis* 1986;153: 478–488.
83. Rinaldo CRJr, Hirsch MS, Black PH. Activation of latent viruses following bone marrow transplantation. *Transplant Proc* 1976;8: 669–672.
84. Miller WJ, McCullough J, Balfour HH Jr, et al. Prevention of cytomegalovirus infection following bone marrow transplantation: a randomized trial of blood product screening. *Bone Marrow Transplant* 1991; 7:227–234.
85. Rubie H, Attal M, Campardou AM, et al. Risk factors for cytomegalovirus infection in BMT recipients transfused exclusively with seronegative blood products. *Bone Marrow Transplant* 1993;11:209–214.
86. Larsson S, Söderberg-Nauclér C, Wang FZ, et al. Cytomegalovirus DNA can be detected in peripheral blood mononuclear cells from all

seropositive and most seronegative healthy blood donors over time. *Transfusion* 1998;38:271–278.
87. Bowden RA, Slichter SJ, Sayers M, et al. A comparison of filtered leukocyte-reduced and cytomegalovirus (CMV) seronegative blood products for the prevention of transfusion-associated CMV infection after marrow transplant. *Blood* 1995;86:3598–3603.
88. Cohen BJ, Beard S, Knowles WA et al. Chronic anemia due to Parvovirus B19 infection in a bone marrow transplant patient after platelet transfusion. *Transfusion* 1997;37:947–952.
89. Moraes-Souza H, Bordin JO. Strategies for prevention of transfusion-associated Chagas' disease. *Transfus Med Rev* 1996;10:161–170.
90. Nickerson P, Orr P, Schroeder ML, et al. Transfusion–associated *Trypanosoma cruzi* infection in a non-endemic area. *Ann Intern Med* 1989; 111:851–853.
91. Grant IH, Gold JWN, Wittner M, et al. Transfusion–associated acute Chagas disease acquired in the United States. *Ann Intern Med* 1989; 111:849–851.
92. Moraes-Souza H, Bordin JO, Bardossy L, et al. Prevention of transfusion-associated Chagas' disease: efficacy of white cell-reduction filters in removing *Trypanosoma cruzi* from infected blood. *Transfusion* 1995; 35:723–726.
93. Bordin JO, Heddle NM, Blajchman MA. Biologic effects of leukocytes present in transfused cellular blood products. *Blood* 1994;84: 1703–1721.
94. Vamvakas EC. Perioperative blood transfusion and cancer recurrence: meta-analysis for explanation. *Transfusion* 1995;35:760–768.
95. Bordin JO, Bardossy L, Blajchman MA. Growth enhancement of established tumors by allogeneic blood transfusion in experimental animals and its amelioration by leukodepletion: the importance of the timing of the leukodepletion. *Blood* 1994;84:344–348.
96. Blajchman MA, Bardossy L, Carmen R, et al. Allogeneic blood transfusion-induced enhancement of tumor growth: two animal models showing amelioration by leukodepletion and passive transfer using spleen cells. *Blood* 1993;81:1880–1882.
97. Vamvakas EC, Blajchman MA. Deleterious clinical effects of transfusion-associated immunomodulation: fact or fiction? *Blood* 2001;97: 1180–1195.
98. Vamvakas EC, Blajchman MA. Prestorage versus poststorage white cell reduction for the prevention of the deleterious immunomodulatory effects of allogeneic blood transfusion. *Transfus Med Rev* 2000;14: 23–33.

Rossi's Principles of Transfusion Medicine, Third Edition, edited by Toby L. Simon, Walter H. Dzik, Edward L. Snyder, Christopher P. Stowell, and Ronald G. Strauss. Lippincott Williams & Wilkins, Philadelphia © 2002.

CASE 34A

FIRST THINGS FIRST

CASE HISTORY

Corey is a very bright 20-year-old man with acute myeloid leukemia in relapse. He was admitted to the hospital for what eventually turned out to be a 6-month hospitalization. During that time he received multiple doses of chemotherapy in order to achieve remission and his therapy was complicated by pulmonary aspergillosis and prolonged pancytopenia.

He first sought treatment and was diagnosed with acute leukemia 6 months before this admission. At that time he achieved a remission on the first cycle of induction chemotherapy and received three cycles of consolidation treatment using high-dose cytarabine. However, after only a brief period off treatment he relapsed and was admitted for this hospitalization.

At the time of admission he complained only of mild shortness of breath and his physical exam was otherwise not remarkable. There was no splenomegaly. His platelet count was 5,000/µl. A chest radiograph showed nodular lesions most consistent with recurrent aspergillosis.

Amphotericin B therapy was begun, which resulted in a fever to 103°F and a diffuse morbilliform rash. He received multiple courses of antibiotics and chemotherapy. During this stormy hospitalization, he had profound thrombocytopenia and received many infusions of platelet concentrates. Sometimes he got a reasonable platelet increment in response to transfusion, but other times he got no increment. The unpredictable nature of the response to platelets began to concern the nurses and the patient.

The patient has a large and supportive family, and the nurses encouraged them to donate platelets on the patient's behalf and to supplement platelet support from the general hospital inventory. The nurses later noted that they had hoped to find a few good donors among the family members. The patient became very focused on which donors gave him a better increment. He asked his family members to keep track of their donation numbers so that he could identify his response to their donations. Using a laptop computer at his bedside, he began keeping a "scorecard" of his platelet increments in an attempt to identify which donors' platelets he responded to best. After several weeks, he presented the following data to his doctors who in turn asked the blood bank to explain the results to the patient (Table 34A.1).

DISCUSSION

Patients often show varying degrees of platelet increment to different donors. Consistent platelet refractoriness can be due to either immunologic or nonimmunologic causes (1). Although much energy is spent looking for immune causes of refractoriness, nonimmune causes are probably more common. Nonimmune causes include splenomegaly, sepsis, diffuse endothelial activation perhaps mediated by inflammatory cytokines, graft-versus-host disease, drug reactions, disseminated intravascular coagulation, and direct platelet toxicity from drugs such as amphotericin B. Immune refractoriness can result from autoantibodies, drug-related antibodies (especially heparin, vancomycin, and cephalosporins), and alloantibodies to either HLA, ABO, or platelet-specific antigens.

Optimal platelet support for complicated and sick oncology patients such as Corey is often frustrating to everyone involved. Frequently no answer is found. Identification of the cause of platelet refractoriness is often so delayed that the patient recovers from the treatment that first caused the thrombocytopenia. Various algorithms for the evaluation and management of patients with suspected refractoriness have been published (2). The initial approach used at our hospital to respond to requests for matched platelets is shown in Figure 34A.1.

Corey's blood was tested for antibodies against HLA, but his percent reactive antibody (PRA) was zero. Using a commercially available enzyme immunoassay, Corey was found to have no antibodies to platelet-specific antigens. Because HLA antigens are generally more immunogenic than the platelet antigen sys-

TABLE 34A.1. PLATELET TRANSFUSION RESPONSES RECORDED BY THE PATIENT

Date	Donor's Initials	Platelet Increment
Dec 23	AS	38,000
Dec 28	JA	6,000
Jan 8	SI	14,000
Jan 13	PC	22,000
Jan 16	JS	22,000
Jan 21	DR	5,000
Jan 27	SI	16,000
Feb 5	RD	4,000
Feb 11	JP	18,000
Feb 13	RW	17,000
Feb 19	VW	13,000
Feb 19	BT	poor
Feb 25	JA	2,000
Feb 26	MM	3,000
Mar 11	SS	15,000

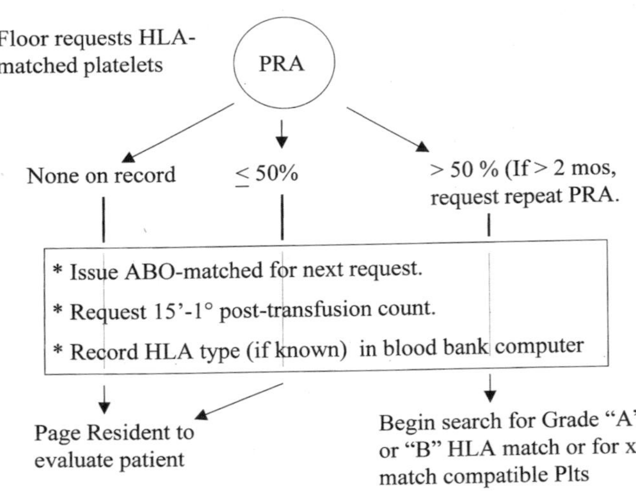

FIGURE 34A.1. Initial approach to requests for "matched platelets." The resident evaluation includes a checklist to identify potential nonimmunologic causes of refractoriness. Platelet serology is done only after ruling out nonimmune causes and ABO and HLA antibodies.

tems, this result did not surprise us. What did surprise us was that the problem was simply an ABO incompatibility.

The patient is group O. We used the data that the patient had given to us and rearranged it according to the ABO groups of the donors and found the results that follow.

Table 34A.2 shows that the patient responds poorly to group A, better to group B, and best to group O donors. The one exception seemed to be donor PC whom we found to be a group A_2! Group A_2 individuals do not strongly express A antigen on platelets (3), and this might account for the patient's good response to donor PC.

On March 18, we found his direct agglutinating titers of anti-A to be 1:128 and anti-B to be 1:32. Some young individuals are known to make very strong (high-titer) ABO antibodies. There is controversy regarding the exact role of ABO in platelet refractoriness. Nevertheless, in some patients ABO undoubtedly plays a role and should not be forgotten when evaluating a patient with inconsistent responses to transfused platelets. We reviewed

TABLE 34A.2. PLATELET RESPONSES ORDERED BY INCREMENT AND INCLUDING DONOR ABO

Platelet Increment	Date	Donor's Initials	ABO
38,000	Dec 23	AS	O
22,000	Jan 16	JS	O
22,000	Jan 13	PC	A
18,000	Feb 11	JP	B
17,000	Feb 13	RW	O
16,000	Jan 27	SI	B
15,000	Mar 11	SS	B
14,000	Jan 8	SI	B
13,000	Feb 19	VW	O
6,000	Dec 28	JA	A
5,000	Jan 21	DR	A
4,000	Feb 5	DR	A
3,000	Feb 26	MM	A
2,000	Feb 25	JA	A
poor	Feb 19	BT	A

the patient's own data with him, his physician, and the nurses and assigned him to receive only group O platelets.

In late March, a repeat bone marrow biopsy showed 90% blasts despite prior rounds of chemotherapy. Following this, he was given an experimental chemotherapy drug. He tolerated it well and showed a partial remission. By June he was well enough to be discharged to home with a white blood cell count of 10,100/μl and a platelet count 21,000/μl. His differential showed 35% blasts. He required parenteral nutrition at home and was not expected to survive his leukemia.

Case contributed by Walter H. Dzik, M.D., Massachusetts General Hospital, Boston, MA.

REFERENCES

1. Novotny VM. Prevention and management of platelet transfusion refractoriness. *Vox Sang* 1999;76:1–13.
2. Slichter SJ. Algorithm for managing the platelet refractory patient. *J Clin Apheresis* 1997;12:4–9.
3. Skogen B, Rossebo B, Husebekk A, et al. Minimal expression of blood group A antigen on thrombocytes from A_2 individuals. *Transfusion* 1988; 28:456–459.

35

HEMATOPOIETIC GROWTH FACTORS (CYTOKINES)

KAI HÜBEL
W. CONRAD LILES
DAVID C. DALE

Hematopoietic growth factor (HGF) is an inclusive term for the family of glycoproteins that regulate proliferation and differentiation of hematopoietic cells (1–5). Many of these factors also influence cell function. The nomenclature is somewhat confusing. The term *cytokine* sometimes is used as a synonym for HGFs, but it also is used as a broader term for the natural products of cells that influence functions of other cells. Some cytokines that function as HGFs are also called *interleukins* (ILs), regulatory factors produced by leukocytes that influence functions of other leukocytes. *Colony-stimulating factor* (CSF) is used in naming some cytokines that stimulate hematopoietic cells to grow in vitro in culture systems, such as granulocyte CSF (G-CSF), granulocyte-macrophage CSF (GM-CSF), and macrophage CSF (M-CSF). Another CSF, formerly called *multi-CSF,* is now most commonly called *IL-3.* The HGFs, their names, and principal functions are outlined in Table 35.1.

CELL BIOLOGY AND PHYSIOLOGY

The HGFs share some general structural features among themselves and with other cytokines, but each is the product of a different gene and has a distinctive amino acid sequence, secondary and tertiary structures, receptor-binding domain, and glycosylation site (6–8). Some HGFs, such as erythropoietin, are produced by relatively few cells at selected tissue sites (e.g., the juxtaglomerular cells of the kidney), whereas others, such as G-CSF, are produced almost ubiquitously by endothelial cells, fibroblast cells, and many other cell types. The factors governing production and secretion also vary substantially. The feedback regulation of erythropoietin in relation to tissue oxygenation is well characterized. The relations governing leukocyte production and deployment are less well understood. For example, complete absence of G-CSF leads to severe neutropenia (9,10), and neutrophilia attributable to stimulated production and secretion of this cytokine occurs with many acute inflammatory conditions and in some malignant diseases (11,12). Levels of G-CSF are elevated and severe neutropenia occurs in the presence of fever and infection (13,14). Assay systems for G-CSF are not yet sufficient, to determine whether there is a true direct feedback relation between plasma levels of G-CSF and blood neutrophil count or whether some product of the neutrophil governs production of this factor. Levels of other cytokines that influence neutrophil formation (e.g., IL-1 and IL-6) also increase with inflammation (14). In contrast, serum levels of GM-CSF, another factor that stimulates neutrophil formation, do not correlate with the presence of neutropenia or infection (13,14). Levels of thrombopoietin–megakaryocyte growth and development factor (Tpo/MGDF) vary inversely with platelet count, but many physiologic details of regulation of platelet levels are lacking (15,16). Better understanding of these relations requires improved immunoassay systems and more complete understanding of the pharmacokinetics and tissue binding of HGFs.

Proliferation, differentiation, and stimulation of hematopoi-

K. Hübel, W.C. Liles, and D.C. Dale: Department of Medicine, University of Washington, Seattle, Washington.

TABLE 35.1. HEMATOPOIETIC GROWTH FACTOR

Factor	Other Name	Cell Source	Chromosome Location	Function
Epo	Erythropoietin	Juxtaglomerular cells	7q	Stimulates erythrocyte formation and release from marrow
Tpo	Thrombopoietin, MGDF	Hepatocytes, renal and endothelial cells, fibroblasts	3q 27	Stimulates megakaryocyte proliferation and platelet formation
G-CSF	Granulocyte colony-stimulating factor; filgrastim; lenograstim	Endothelial cells, monocytes, fibroblasts	17q 11.2 q21	Stimulates formation and function of neutrophils
GM-CSF	Granulocyte-macrophage colony-stimulating factor	T lymphocytes, monocytes, fibroblasts	5q 23–31	Stimulates formation and function of neutrophils, monocytes, and eosinophils
M-CSF	Macrophage colony-stimulating factor; colony- stimulating factor-1 (CSF-1)	Endothelial cells, macrophages, fibroblasts	5q 33.1	Stimulates monocyte formation and function
IL-1 α and β	Endogenous pyrogen hemopoietin-1	Monocytes, keratinocytes, endothelial cells	2q 13	Proliferation of T, B, and other cells; induces fever and catabolism
IL-2	T-cell growth factor	T cells (CD4+, CD8+), large granular lymphocytes (NK cells)	4q	T-cell proliferation, antitumor and antimicrobial effects
IL-3	Multicolony-stimulating factor; mast cell growth factor	Activated T cells; large granular lymphocytes (NK cells)	5q 23–31	Proliferation of early hematopoietic cells
IL-4	B-cell growth factor; T-cell growth factor II; mast cell growth factor II	T cells	5q 23–31	Proliferation of B and T cells; enhances cytotoxic activities
IL-5	Eosinophil differentiation factor; eosinophil colony-stimulating factor	T cells	5q 23.3–q32	Stimulates eosinophil formation; stimulates T- and B-cell functions
IL-6	B-cell stimulatory factor 2; hepatocyte stimulatory factor	Monocytes, tumor cells, B and T cells, fibroblasts, endothelial cells	7p	Stimulates and inhibits cell growth; promotes B-cell differentiation
IL-7	Lymphopoietin 1; pro-B-cell growth factor	Lymphoid tissues and cell lines	8q 12–13	Growth factor for B and T cells
IL-11	Plasmacytoma stimulating activity	Fibroblasts, trophoblasts, cancer cell lines	19q 13.3–13.4	Stimulates proliferation of early hematopoietic cells; induces acute phase protein synthesis
IL-12	Natural killer cell-stimulating factor	Macrophages, B cells	5q 31–33; 3p 12–q13.2	Stimulates T-cell expansion and IFN-γ production; synergistically promotes early hematopoietic cell proliferation
LIF	Leukemia inhibitory factor	Monocytes and lymphocytes; stromal cells	22q	Stimulates hematopoietic differentiation
SCF	Kit ligand; steel factor	Endothelial cells; hepatocytes	4q11–q20	Stimulates proliferation of early hematopoietic cells and mast cells

MGDF, megakaryocyte growth and development factor; IL, interleukin; NK, natural killer.

etic cells occur through factor-specific cell surface receptors composed of dimers or trimers of transmembrane proteins (17). There are general structural similarities in the extracellular and intracellular domains of receptors for many HGFs, and there are common components to the receptors for some factors (e.g., a common β chain of the receptors for IL-3, IL-5, and GM-CSF). Specificity is caused by the unique. or private, components of the receptor for each factor. Receptor binding and cellular activation lead to conformational changes in the receptor, activation of intracellular kinases, and phosphorylation of specific proteins, which are transferred to the cell nucleus (17,18).

PHARMACOKINETICS AND PHARMACODYNAMICS

The pharmacologic properties of HGFs depend on the dose, route of administration, affinity of binding to receptors, and complex circulatory and distribution factors, as with other drugs. There are extensive pharmacokinetic and pharmacodynamic data on erythropoietin, G-CSF, and GM-CSF (the growth factors approved for clinical use) but relatively little data on the other factors.

Intravenously administered erythropoietin has a circulating half-life of 4 to 13 hours in patients with chronic renal failure and approximately 20% less in healthy volunteers (19). Therapeutically effective levels are maintained after a single intravenous or subcutaneous injection for at least 24 hours. An increase in reticulocyte counts occurs within 10 days if erythropoietin is given daily. Exogenous erythropoietin accelerates erythropoiesis, but detectable increases in hematocrit and hemoglobin level usually take approximately 2 weeks to develop (20).

Granulocyte colony-stimulating factor can be administered intravenously or subcutaneously. After intravenous administration, the elimination half-life is approximately 3.5 hours (21).

Blood levels are influenced by the neutrophil count, because neutrophils actively bind the injected drug (22). Granulocyte colony-stimulating factor both stimulates proliferation of neutrophil progenitors and mobilizes mature neutrophils from the bone marrow reserves. It increases blood neutrophils threefold to fourfold in hematologically healthy persons within 4 to 6 hours (23,24). As production increases, a sustained increase occurs if administration of G-CSF is continued (25). Granulocyte colony-stimulating factor accelerates neutrophil formation, which leads to an increased percentage of circulating band neutrophils with more deeply staining primary granules. These changes are similar to those commonly seen with bacterial infection.

Granulocyte-macrophage colony-stimulating factor can be administered intravenously or subcutaneously, but intravenous administration has been associated with toxicity that includes fever, dyspnea, and the adult respiratory distress syndrome (26, 27). These effects seem to be dose related and to occur less frequently with subcutaneous administration. Like G-CSF, GM-CSF stimulates neutrophil production and release of cells from the bone marrow (28). When given repeatedly for several days, GM-CSF increases total white blood cell count, including eosinophils and monocytes as well as neutrophils (29). Leukocyte count returns to the baseline level when administration of G-CSF or GM-CSF is discontinued (26–28).

Results of in vitro assays show that both G-CSF and GM-CSF influence the function of neutrophils (30,31). Both types of CSF "prime" neutrophils to increase their responsiveness to other stimulators of the neutrophil oxidative (respiratory) burst, such as opsonized particles or bacteria. Neutrophils and other leukocytes produced in vivo in response to G-CSF or GM-CSF stimulation in general have normal or increased, not decreased, responsiveness to exogenous stimulators of neutrophil function. The clinical significance of these findings is not clear. Substantial clinical data and numerous animal experiments indicate that neutrophils produced in vivo in response to these cytokines are capable of killing bacteria and accelerating recovery from bacterial infection (32).

The pharmacologic and physiologic properties of other HGFs are less well understood, but some generalizations are possible. The factors influencing the early phases of hematopoiesis tend to have multiple side effects, such as fever and flulike symptoms, and a narrower range of tolerable doses than do factors that influence the later phases of hematopoiesis. Examples of early factors with substantial side effects include IL-1, IL-2, IL-3, IL-4, and IL-6 and stem cell factor. The late-acting factors such as erythropoietin, G-CSF, GM-CSF, and M-CSF are much better tolerated (1–5).

CLINICAL APPLICATIONS

The use of erythropoietin for the management of anemia and to stimulate erythropoiesis for autologous transfusion therapy is described in Chapter 41. Chapter 20 describes the role of myeloid growth factors in granulocyte collection and transfusion. Most growth factors mentioned herein are investigational drugs with currently undefined roles in the management of neutropenia and thrombocytopenia. Only G-CSF and GM-CSF have been approved by the U.S. Food and Drug Administration for the management of neutropenia in specific clinical situations; however, in clinical practice they are used somewhat interchangeably. Despite a number of clinical trials, potential clinical indications for the use of IL-3, M-CSF, and Tpo/MGDF remain unclear.

In phase I and II studies involving patients with relapses of lymphoma, small-cell lung cancer, breast cancer, and ovarian cancer, administration of IL-3 at a dose of 5 to 10 μg/kg subcutaneously daily for 5 to 10 days accelerated recovery of neutrophil and platelet counts after chemotherapy. (33). Similar results did not occur when IL-3, administered either alone or in combination with other growth factors, was used in a similar manner for the treatment of patients with myelodysplastic syndromes, aplastic anemia, and other bone marrow disorders (33,34). At present, no results of phase III studies evaluating the role of IL-3 in human disease have been reported.

Clinical experience with M-CSF is relatively limited. Macrophage colony-stimulating factor has not been used for harvesting of hematopoietic stem cells, and only two reports describe the use of M-CSF in the setting of neutropenia after chemotherapy (35,36). To date, results of prospective, randomized, controlled trials of M-CSF for adjunctive management of infection have not been published.

Results of preliminary studies with animals suggest that Tpo/MGDF may be well tolerated. Preclinical data indicate that twofold to fivefold increases in platelet count do not lead to platelet aggregation or thrombotic events (15,16). Both the full-length molecule recombinant human thrombopoietin (rhTpo) and the truncated version of the molecule, polyethylene glycol–recombinant human megakaryocyte growth and development factor (PEG-rHuMGDF), have been evaluated in phase I and II clinical trials with healthy subjects and patients with cancer receiving myelosuppressive chemotherapy. Considerable data demonstrate the effectiveness of PEG-rHuMGDF in platelet stimulation, but the development of neutralizing antibodies and significant thrombocytopenia in some subjects has led to discontinuation of clinical trials (37–39). Recombinant human thrombopoietin appeared safe when administered to patients with acute myelogenous leukemia, but if used after a 7-day course of standard chemotherapy, the drug does not accelerate platelet recovery (40). However, rhTpo has been shown to reduce thrombocytopenia associated with nonmyeloablative chemotherapy (41). Results of studies indicate that rhTpo is effective in mobilizing peripheral blood stem cells (see later) (42). Further clinical investigation is needed to establish the role of Tpo/MGDF in clinical practice.

Use of Myeloid Growth Factors to Mobilize Peripheral Blood Stem Cells

For years it has been recognized that circulating hematopoietic progenitor cells are capable of forming hematopoietic colonies in vitro culture in systems and of repopulating the bone marrow after total ablation. These cells appear to function normally to sustain hematopoiesis and to allow expansion in states of hematopoietic stress.

Before the availability of HGFs, several investigators reported that the number of circulating hematopoietic progenitor cells increases during the recovery period after hematotoxic chemotherapy (43,44). It was subsequently learned that a similar response occurs in hematologically intact persons given HGFs (45, 46). Numerous studies have shown that the number of these progenitor cells, now generally called *peripheral blood stem cells* (PBSC) or *peripheral blood progenitor cells,* predictably increases in the blood as much as 100-fold during recovery from chemotherapy or 4 to 6 days after administration of HGF is begun (46–52). The quantity and quality of cells are sufficient for infusion of PBSC to be capable of rapidly replacing bone marrow transplantation for autologous reconstitution after myeloablative therapy (53). Peripheral blood stem cells are preferred because of the relative ease of procurement, more rapid restoration of blood counts compared with marrow infusion, and the possible recovery of these cells from patients who previously received intensive chemotherapy or radiation therapy and from patients with tumors involving the bone marrow (53).

An unexpected benefit of the development of support with PBSC came with the recognition that the transfusions accelerated recovery of platelet counts and obviated many platelet transfusions (48). This finding suggests that the persisting thrombocytopenia historically seen 3 to 6 weeks after conventional bone marrow transplantation is caused by the limited number or function of precursor cells infused rather than deficiencies in humoral or environmental factors.

The basic physiologic principles governing mobilization of PBSC are poorly understood. Granulocyte colony-stimulating factor and GM-CSF increase the number of circulating blood neutrophils. They also increase the number of circulating PBSC, but they do not proportionately increase the numbers of circulating promyelocytes, myelocytes, or metamyelocytes. Thus the increase in circulating early and late cells is a selective effect of these HGFs on the bone marrow. The kinetics of the response (delay of a few days before the increase in PBSC occurs) suggests that early hematopoietic cells may need to expand in numbers before they "spill over" into the blood. In primates, antibodies to the adherence protein VLA-4 can induce more rapid mobilization of PBSC than of HGFs. This finding suggests that expansion and spillover are an oversimplified mechanism (54). The increase in PBSC in the recovery phase from chemotherapy generally occurs when the marrow is still relatively hypocellular. This finding implies that marrow cell density is not the simple explanation for mobilization (43,44).

In the initial development of support with PBSC, many investigators questioned whether these cells are truly hematopoietic stem cells. Most of the cells collected and transfused after treatment with HGFs or chemotherapy undoubtedly are differentiated precursor cells. However, results of experiments with mice, dogs, and nonhuman primates as well as with humans support the contention that preparations of PBSC do contain long-lived precursor cells. Further studies may be needed to confirm these findings.

Technical Considerations

Quantitation

Peripheral blood stem cells are quantitated according to the cell surface expression of cluster determinant 34 (CD34) or granulocyte-macrophage colony-forming unit (CFU-GM) as measured with an in vitro colony-forming assay (47–52,55). Because the in vitro bioassay requires approximately 2 weeks to complete and is highly dependent on the expertise of the tissue culture laboratory, it is used largely for quality control and for research studies. Flow cytometric analysis for $CD34^+$ cells can be performed quickly and easily on the day of collection and is essential to determine the adequacy of collection of PBSC. Total mononuclear cell numbers also are useful. Cell numbers that usually correlate with engraftment are 4×10^8 or more mononuclear cells per kilogram, 2×10^6 or more $CD34^+$ cells per kilogram, and 2×10^5 or more CFU-GMs per kilogram. Because this antigen is expressed on cells that have differentiated beyond the colony-forming stage, the number of $CD34^+$ cells is tenfold greater than the required number of CFU-GMs (56).

Cytokine Doses

Currently, G-CSF is the cytokine most frequently used to mobilize PBSC. At doses of 5 μg/kg or less per day, the harvest of PBSC usually is inadequate. Doses of approximately 10, 16, 24, and 32 μg/kg per day have been used in clinical trials (46–52). Although the yield may be slightly increased at higher doses, the usual dose is 10 to 16 μg/kg per day. Granulocyte-macrophage colony-stimulating factor, IL-3, and stem cell factor (c-*kit* ligand) also mobilize PBSC but have greater side effects. The role of thrombopoietin is still uncertain (42). Combinations of G-CSF with each of these cytokines or with chemotherapy are under investigation at many centers. In general, it seems that a regimen of chemotherapy plus G-CSF (with or without a second cytokine) yields the greatest quantity of $CD34^+$ cells and allows for the fewest leukapheresis procedures, but there is not yet a standard approach. Cyclophosphamide, carboplatin, paclitaxel, etoposide, and ifosfamide are the chemotherapeutic agents that have been studied most extensively for mobilization and harvesting of PBSC.

Collection and Processing of Peripheral Blood Stem Cells

Currently, PBSC are collected and used for both autologous and allogeneic hematopoietic stem cell transplantation (53,56). Under these circumstances, the type and intensity of previous therapy affect collection of PBSC. Extensive previous treatment may render adequate collection difficult, if not impossible. Most collections are performed with techniques and equipment evaluated by committees of the American Association of Blood Banks, International Society for Cellular Therapy, and the American Society for Apheresis (57). When patients are treated with HGFs alone, collection usually is begun on treatment day 4. Four to 18 liters of blood are processed to separate predominately mononuclear cells, and the CD34+ cell collections of the first and succeeding days are counted to determine the total number of leukapheresis procedures to be performed.

Tumor Cell Contamination

Both bone marrow aspirated for transplantation and apheresis-collected PBSC may contain tumor cells. The number of contaminating cells seems to be determined according to bone marrow involvement, stage of disease, tumor type, and previous therapy (57–59). Previously untreated patients tend to have greater bone marrow reserves or mobilizable tumor cell burdens. Techniques for detecting tumor cells in these preparations are rapidly improving. It is unclear what the minimal tumor cell contamination must be to avoid the risk of tumor cell engraftment with PBSC mobilized by administration of HGFs.

Selection for Peripheral Blood Stem Cells

Because CD34 is a useful marker of early hematopoietic cells, several methods have been devised in which antibodies to CD34 are used for selective collection of PBSC (60). The goal is to select PBSC and eliminate tumor cells from the materials to be transfused. At present, these technologies do not eliminate all tumor cells completely but reduce the numbers markedly. Studies are in progress to determine the clinical advantage of these procedures.

Cryopreservation

Peripheral blood stem cells collected after treatment with HGFs usually are preserved by means of controlled rate freezing with 10% dimethyl sulfoxide (DMSO). Results of some studies suggest that HGFs may inhibit spontaneous apoptosis, but it is unclear whether this is clinically important for preservation of PBSC (56,57; see Chapter 36).

Clinical Trials of Growth Factor–Mobilized Peripheral Blood Stem Cells

Numerous uncontrolled trials and a few randomized-controlled clinical trials have shown the efficacy of HGF-mobilized PBSC to accelerate marrow recovery after intensive chemotherapy or myeloablative chemoradiation therapy (61,62). The results of these studies have established that administration of more than 4×10^6 $CD34^+$ PBSC per kilogram mobilized by G-CSF results in neutrophil recovery to more than 0.5×10^9/L and platelets to 20×10^5/L in approximately 10 to 12 days. These recovery times probably can be achieved without treating the recipient with HGFs after infusion of PBSC. These times for recovery with PBSC are considerably shorter than those after autologous bone marrow transplantation. Neutrophil and platelet counts recover to 0.5×10^9/L on approximately day 18 after treatment with PBSC without G-CSF or GM-CSF therapy and to 20×10^5/L on approximately day 20 or later after autologous bone marrow transplantation (53,56).

Other Considerations

Many laboratories are intensively studying the expansion of bone marrow cells and PBSC using in vitro incubation of the cells with a mix of growth factors, including stem cell factor, IL-3, IL-6, GM-CSF, G-CSF, and erythropoietin (63,64). This approach is a promising way to expand the number of differentiated progenitor cells for supportive care. It also may prove useful for providing undifferentiated and stem cell support if cells can be expanded without stimulating differentiation. Paralleling these efforts, many investigators are studying genetic alteration of PBSC mobilized by HGF administration with the intent to introduce therapeutically important genes into PBSC (65,66). This strategy may prove useful for the management of genetic, infectious, and malignant diseases. This work is still at an investigational stage.

Granulocyte Colony-Stimulating Factor and Granulocyte-Macrophage Colony-stimulating Factor for Neutropenia Associated with Chemotherapy and Hematopoietic Stem Cell Transplantation

For many years, the myelosuppressive effect of chemotherapy has been the dominant factor determining treatment doses and schedules in therapy for hematologic and nonhematologic malignant diseases (2–4). It is generally believed that recovery of blood leukocyte and platelet counts is delayed because of the time required for cell proliferation and differentiation as well as for the generation of endogenous factors regulating cell recovery. The potency of G-CSF and GM-CSF to stimulate recovery, and the effectiveness of prophylactic administration of G-CSF to stimulate recovery were easily recognized in the first clinical trials (2–4,23,27). In two randomized, controlled trials (67,68), the effectiveness of prophylactic administration of G-CSF was definitively demonstrated in the care of patients with small-cell lung cancer. In these studies, patients treated with cyclophosphamide, doxorubicin, and etoposide received either placebo or G-CSF at a dose of 5 μg/kg per day. The incidence of fever and documented infections was reduced in the G-CSF–treated group both in the first cycle and for the overall six cycles of treatment. Antibiotic use and days of hospitalization also decreased. The results of this trial have been replicated in a number of studies (69,70), and this same accelerating effect on the recovery of the blood neutrophil count has been demonstrated for GM-CSF (71). Randomized clinical trials also have shown that marrow recovery after bone marrow transplantation is accelerated by GM-CSF and G-CSF (56,72–74).

The results of these trials have led to a number of conclusions (71). Granulocyte colony-stimulating factor or GM-CSF effectively stimulates marrow recovery after chemotherapy for many malignant diseases, including myeloid and nonmyeloid leukemia. The greatest value is in the care of patients with sustained neutropenia, in which the likelihood of a febrile course is greater than 40%. In a patient with documented febrile neutropenia after one course of chemotherapy, the use of these factors to avoid infectious complications while maintaining dose intensity is generally indicated unless a dose-reduction strategy is more appropriate. With very intensive chemotherapy and anticipated prolonged neutropenia, CSF treatment is probably indicated in almost all cases. The use of G-CSF and GM-CSF in the management of myeloid malignant disease is still under investigation. It appears that these agents can be used safely to accelerate marrow recovery after chemotherapy, as in the management of nonmyeloid malignant disease (75).

The timing of administration G-CSF or GM-CSF is still under study. These factors usually are given after the completion of, not concomitantly with, chemotherapy. In addition to scheduling issues, uncertainty exists about optimal dosing. For GM-CSF, dosing may be limited by side effects. For G-CSF, the acceptable dose range is much broader, but evidence suggests that doses of more than 5 μg/kg per day do not significantly accelerate marrow recovery (76), and doses of less than 5 μg/kg per day may be effective.

Colony-Stimulating Factors for Idiosyncratic Drug-induced Neutropenia

A wide array of drugs induce transient neutropenia, presumably on an immune or toxic basis. The penicillins, sulfonamides, and antithyroid and psychotropic drugs often are implicated. With respect to treatment, the offending or presumably offending agent should be discontinued, and patients with a fever should be treated with broad-spectrum antibiotics (77). Numerous case studies have suggested that HGFs may accelerate bone marrow recovery in these conditions. However, the evidence is largely anecdotal, and practices differ considerably. The sickest patients with documented infections and delayed marrow recovery are the most likely to benefit from G-CSF or GM-CSF treatment.

Colony-stimulating Factors in the Management of Chronic Neutropenia

A wide array of conditions cause chronic neutropenia (77). The benefits and risks of long-term use of G-CSF or GM-CSF in the treatment of many of these patient are not yet known. For one group, patients with severe chronic neutropenia caused by congenital neutropenia (including Kostmann syndrome), idiopathic neutropenia, or cyclic neutropenia, the clinical benefit of long-term G-CSF therapy has been established (78). In a randomized, controlled trial involving patients with severe chronic neutropenia, the occurrences of fever, oropharyngeal ulcers, infections, hospitalization, and antibiotic use were all significantly reduced by means of long-term G-CSF treatment. The quality of life and activity profiles of these patients also improved. The principal side effect of G-CSF therapy is musculoskeletal pain early in the course of treatment. However, data from the Severe Chronic Neutropenia International Registry showed that 23 of 249 patients with congenital neutropenia treated with G-CSF had myelodysplasia or acute myelogenous leukemia within an average follow-up period of 4.5 years (79). Careful follow-up evaluation of patients receiving long-term CSF therapy is indicated.

Colony-Stimulating Factors in the Management of Nonneutropenic Infectious Disease

Considerable research efforts have been devoted to the possible use of CSFs as adjunctive therapy for nonneutropenic infectious conditions. To date, several phase I and II studies have had promising results, and large phase III trials are under investigation, or the results have been recently published. The rationale for these studies has been to enhance the number and functional activities of preformed neutrophils to promote recovery from or prevention of local or systemic infections. Prophylaxis of sepsis is a promising indication for the use of CSFs in the care of patients without neutropenia when the time point of risk of infection is known or can be anticipated, as in surgery, trauma, burn injury, or local infection.

In the management of pneumonia, resolution of infection depends on neutrophil function (80). In a double-blind, controlled, multicenter trial, 756 patients with community-acquired bacterial pneumonia were enrolled to receive intravenous antibiotics plus either G-CSF (300 μg/day for up to 10 days; n = 380) or placebo (n = 376) (81). Outcome measures included time to resolution of morbidity, 28-day mortality, length of stay, and occurrence of adverse events. A microbial cause of pneumonia was identified for 56% of patients, and an independent review group judged use of antimicrobial agents appropriate in the care of 98% of the patients. Administration of G-CSF increased the peripheral blood neutrophil count threefold, but time to resolution of morbidity, mortality, and length of hospitalization were not affected. However, the time of resolution of infiltrates was significantly more rapid in the G-CSF–treated group. Only one patient had empyema compared with six patients in the placebo group. Administration of G-CSF was safe and well tolerated, and the rate of development of sepsis-related organ failure and disseminated intravascular coagulopathy was significantly reduced among the recipients of G-CSF.

Because of a lack of neutrophilia in diabetes and impaired superoxide generation in neutrophils from patients with diabetes, G-CSF appears to be a reasonable candidate for adjunctive therapy in the management of severe foot infections in these patients. In a randomized, double-blind, placebo-controlled trial, 40 patients with insulin-dependent diabetic and foot infections were assigned to receive either G-CSF (n = 20) or placebo (n = 20) for 7 days (82). Both groups were treated with similar antibiotic and insulin regimens. After 7 days of G-CSF treatment, neutrophil superoxide production was significantly greater in the G-CSF group than in the placebo group. Administration of G-CSF was associated with significantly earlier eradication of pathogens, quicker resolution of cellulitis, shorter hospital stay, and shorter duration of antibiotic treatment. No patient treated with G-CSF needed surgery, whereas two recipients of placebo underwent amputation and two needed extensive débridement. These results await corroboration in a multicenter trial before adoption of use of G-CSF for this purpose in routine clinical practice.

Colony-stimulating factors may have therapeutic potential in the treatment of persons with human immunodeficiency virus (HIV). Granulocyte-macrophage colony-stimulating factor has been shown to partially correct HIV-1–mediated impairment in the ability of monocyte-derived macrophages to phagocytose *Mycobacterium avium* complex in vitro (83). In a study with 258 patients with HIV-1-infection and moderate neutropenia, G-CSF treatment significantly reduced the incidence of severe neutropenia and bacterial infection (84). Patients treated with G-CSF also had 54% fewer episodes of severe bacterial infection and needed 45% fewer days of hospitalization for management of bacterial infection than did the control group.

It has been well documented that GM-CSF can inhibit intracellular replication of bacteria or protozoa. Macrophages, which provide a protected environment for microorganisms against extracellular concentrations of antibiotics, are activated by GM-CSF to allow higher intracellular concentrations of certain antimicrobial agents (85). Small studies have shown beneficial effects of CSF therapy in the management of nonneutropenic infectious conditions. Patients with multiple trauma or patients undergoing major surgery may benefit from prophylactic administration of G-CSF (86,87). In a very small study, 24 patients with sepsis-induced granulocytopenia who did not respond to antibiotics were treated with low-dose G-CSF (75 μg/day) for 5 days (88). Leukocyte counts increased ninefold in 19 survivors, and 5 nonresponders died. Thus G-CSF may favorably modulate the host immune response during the "immune paralysis" of late sepsis.

Granulocyte Colony-stimulating Factor for Mobilization of Neutrophils in Granulocyte Transfusion Therapy

Granulocyte transfusion therapy would appear to be a rational approach to the management of severe bacterial and fungal infections in patients with prolonged neutropenia (89). Potential clinical efficacy, however, has long been limited by insufficient donor stimulation regimens and suboptimal leukapheresis techniques. Methodologic progress, in particular mobilization of neutrophils in healthy donors by means of administration of G-CSF, has greatly enhanced leukapheresis yields (90,91). Granulocyte transfusion therapy is discussed in detail in Chapter 20.

SUMMARY

The discovery and clinical development of HGFs have had great effect on the use of blood products in the supportive care of patients with many hematologic and malignant diseases. Hematopoietic growth factors are providing new opportunities for the provision of blood services, such as collection PBSC, autologous erythrocyte transfusion for elective surgical procedures, and G-CSF mobilization of neutrophils for granulocyte transfusion therapy.

REFERENCES

1. Metcalf D. The colony stimulating factors: discovery, development, and clinical applications. *Cancer* 1990;65:2185–2195.
2. Williams ME, Quesenberry PJ. Hematopoietic growth factors. *Hematol Pathol* 1992;6:105–124.
3. Petersdorf SH, Dale DC. The biology and clinical applications of erythropoietin and the colony-stimulating factors. *Adv Intern Med* 1994; 40:395–428.
4. Buchner T. Hematopoietic growth factors in cancer treatment. *Stem Cells* 1994;12:241–252.
5. Nemunaitis J. Biological activities of hematopoietic growth factors that lead to future clinical application. *Cancer Invest* 1994;12:516–529.
6. Kaushansky K. Structure-function relationships of the hematopoietic growth factors. *Proteins* 1992;12:1–9.
7. Osslund T, Boone T. Biochemistry and structure of filgrastim (R-metHuG-CSF). In: Morstyn G, Dexter TM, eds. *Filgrastim (r-metHuG-CSF) in clinical practice.* New York: Marcel Dekker, 1994:23–31.
8. Bazan JF. Haemopoietic receptors and helical cytokines. *Immunol Today* 1990;11:350–354.
9. Hammond WP, Csiba E, Canin A, et al. Chronic neutropenia: a new canine model induced by human granulocyte colony-stimulating factor. *J Clin Invest* 1991;87:704–710.
10. Lieschke GJ, Grail D, Hodgson G, et al. Mice lacking granulocyte colony-stimulating factor have chronic neutropenia, granulocyte and macrophage progenitor cell deficiency, and impaired neutrophil mobilization. *Blood* 1994;84:1737–1746.
11. Kawakami M, Tsutsumi H, Kumakawa T, et al. Levels of serum granulocyte colony-stimulating factor in patients with infections. *Blood* 1990; 76:1962–1964.
12. Dale DC. Neutrophilia. In: Williams WJ, ed. *Hematology,* 5th ed. New York: McGraw-Hill 1995:824–828.
13. Cebon J, Layton J, Maher D, et al. Endogenous haemopoietic growth factors in neutropenia and infection. *Br J Haematol* 1994;86:265–274.
14. Cebon J, Layton J. Measurement and clinical significance of circulating hematopoietic growth factor levels. *Curr Opin Hematol* 1994;1: 228–234.
15. Kaushansky K, Lok S, Holly RD, et al. Promotion of megakaryocyte progenitor expansion and differentiation by the c-Mpl ligand thrombopoietin. *Nature* 1994;369:568–571.
16. Hunt P, Hokom M, Dwyer E, et al. Megakaryocyte growth and development factor (MGDF) is a potent, physiological regulator of platelet production in normal and myelocompromised animals. *Blood* 1994; 84[Suppl 1]:390A(abst).
17. D'Andrea A. Cytokine receptors in congenital hematopoietic disease. *N Engl J Med* 1994;330:839–846.
18. Kirken RA, Rui H, Howard OM, et al. Involvement of JAK-family tyrosine kinases in hematopoietin receptor signal transduction. *Prog Growth Factor Res* 1994;5:195–211.
19. Egrie JC, Eschbach JW, McGuire T, et al. Pharmacokinetics of recombinant human erythropoietin (r-HuEPO) administered to hemodialysis (HD) patients. *Kidney Int* 1988;33:262(abst).
20. Erslev AJ. Erythropoietin. *N Engl J Med* 1991;324:1339–1344.
21. Layton J, Hockman H, Sheridan W, et al. Evidence for a novel in vivo control mechanism of granulopoiesis: mature cell-related control of a regulatory growth factor. *Blood* 1989;74:1303–1307.
22. Vincent ME, Foote MA, Morstyn G. Pharmacology of filgrastim (r-metHuG-CSF). In: Morstyn G, Dexter TM, eds. *Filgrastim (r-metHuG-CSF) in clinical practice.* New York: Marcel Dekker 1994: 33–50.
23. Demetri G, Griffin J. Granulocyte colony-stimulating factor and its receptor. *Blood* 1991;78:2791–2808.
24. Chatta GS, Price TH, Stratton JR, et al. Aging and marrow neutrophil reserves. *J Am Geriatr Soc* 1994;42:77–81.
25. Price TH, Chatta GS, Dale DC. The effect of recombinant granulocyte colony-stimulating factor (G-CSF) on neutrophil kinetics in normal human subjects. *Blood* 1992;80[Suppl 1]:350A(abst).
26. Gasson JC. Molecular physiology of granulocyte-macrophage colony-stimulating factor. *Blood* 1991;77:1131–1145.
27. Grant S, Heel R. Recombinant granulocyte-macrophage colony-stimulating factor (rGm-CSF): a review of its pharmacological properties and prospective role in the management of myelosuppression. *Drugs* 1992;43:516–560.
28. Aglietta M, Piacibello W, Sanavio F, et al. Kinetics of human hemopoietic cells after in vivo administration of granulocyte-macrophage colony stimulating factor. *J Clin Invest* 1989;83:551–557.
29. Dale DC, Liles WC, Llewellyn C, et al. Effects of granulocyte-macrophage colony-stimulating factor (GM-CSF) on neutrophil kinetics and function in normal human volunteers. *Am J Hematol* 1998;57:7–15.
30. Balazovich KJ, Almedia HI, Boxer LA. Recombinant human G-CSF and GM-CSF prime human neutrophils for superoxide production through different signal transduction mechanisms. *J Lab Clin Med* 1991;118:576–584.
31. Sullivan GW, Carper HT, Mandell GL. The effect of three human recombinant hematopoietic growth factors (granulocyte-macrophage colony-stimulating factor, and interleukin-3) on phagocyte oxidative activity. *Blood* 1993;81:1863–1870.
32. Dale DC, Liles WC, Summer WR, et al. Review: granulocyte colony-stimulating factor: role and relationships in infectious diseases. *J Infect Dis* 1995;172:1061–1075.
33. Mangi MH, Newland AC. Interleukin-3 in hematology and oncology: current state of knowledge and future directions. *Cytokines Cell Mol Ther* 1999;5:87–95.

34. Musto P, Sanpaolo G, D'Arena G, et al. Adding growth factors or interleukin-3 to erythropoietin has limited effects on anemia of transfusion-dependent patients with myelodysplastic syndromes unresponsive to erythropoietin alone. *Haematologica* 2001;86:44–51.
35. Nemunaitis J, Meyers JD, Buckner CD, et al. Phase I trial of recombinant human macrophage colony-stimulating factor in patients with invasive fungal infections. *Blood* 1991;78:907–913.
36. Nemunaitis J, Shannon-Dorcy K, Appelbaum FR, et al. Long-term follow-up of patients with invasive fungal diseases who received adjunctive therapy with recombinant human macrophage colony-stimulating factor. *Blood* 1993;82:1422–1427.
37. Vadhan-Raj S. Clinical experience with recombinant human thrombopoietin in chemotherapy-induced thrombocytopenia. *Semin Hematol* 2000;37[2 Suppl 4]:28–34.
38. Goodnough LT, DiPersio J, McCullough J, et al. Pegylated recombinant human megakaryocyte growth and development factor (PEG-rHuMGDF) increases platelet count and apheresis yields of normal platelet donors: initial results. *Transfusion* 1997;37[Suppl]:67S(abst).
39. Li J, Xia Y, Bertino A, et al. Characterization of an anti-thrombopoietin antibody that developed in a cancer patient following the injection of PEG-rHuMGDF. *Blood* 1999;94[Suppl 1]:51A(abst).
40. Kaushansky K. Use of thrombopoietic growth factors in acute leukemia. *Leukemia* 2000;14:505–508.
41. Kuter DJ. Future directions with platelet growth factors. *Semin Hematol* 2000;37[2 Suppl 4]:41–49.
42. Linker C. Thrombopoietin in the treatment of acute myeloid leukemia and stem-cell transplantation. *Semin Hematol* 2000;37[2 Suppl 4]: 35–40.
43. Richman CM, Weiner RS, Yankee RA. Increase in circulating stem cells following chemotherapy in man. *Blood* 1976;47:1031–1039.
44. To LB, Haylock DN, Kimber RJ, et al. High levels of circulating hematopoietic stem cells in very early remission from acute non-lymphocytic leukaemia and their collection and cryopreservation. *Br J Haematol* 1984;58:399–410.
45. Socinski MA, Cannistra SA, Elias A, et al. Granulocyte-macrophage colony-stimulating factor expands the circulating haemopoietic progenitor cell compartment in man. *Lancet* 1988;1:1194–1198.
46. Duhrsen U, Villeval JL, Boyd J. Effects of recombinant human granulocyte colony-stimulating factor on hematopoietic progenitor cells in cancer patients. *Blood* 1988;72:2074–2081.
47. Anderson KC. The role of the blood bank in hematopoietic stem cell transplantation. *Transfusion* 1992;32:272–285.
48. Sheridan WP, Begley CG, Juttner CA, et al. Effect of peripheral-blood progenitor cells mobilised by filgrastim (G-CSF) on platelet recovery after high-dose chemotherapy. *Lancet* 1992;339:640–644.
49. Elias AD, Ayash L, Anderson KC, et al. Mobilization of peripheral blood progenitor cells by chemotherapy and granulocyte-macrophage colony-stimulating factor for hematologic support after high-dose intensification for breast cancer. *Blood* 1992;79:3036–3044.
50. Weaver CH, Buckner DC, Longin K, et al. Syngeneic transplantation with peripheral blood mononuclear cells collected after the administration of recombinant human granulocyte colony-stimulating factor. *Blood* 1993;82:1981–1984.
51. Elias AD, Ayash L, Tepler I, et al. The use of G-CSF or GM-CSF mobilized peripheral blood progenitor cells (PBPC) alone or to augment marrow as hematologic support of single of multiple cycle high-dose chemotherapy. *J Hematother* 1993;2:377–382.
52. Dicke KA, Hood D, Hanks S. Peripheral blood stem cell collection after mobilization with intensive chemotherapy and growth factors. *J Hematother* 1994;3:141–144.
53. Bensinger WI, Martin PJ, Storer B, et al. Transplantation of bone marrow as compared with peripheral-blood cells from HLA-identical relatives in patients with hematologic cancers. *N Engl J Med* 2001;344: 175–181.
54. Papayannopoulou T, Nakamoto B. Peripheralization of hematopoietic progenitors in primates treated with anti-VLAy integrin. *Proc Natl Acad Sci U S A* 1993;90:9374–9378.
55. Eaves C. Peripheral blood stem cells reach new heights. *Blood* 1993; 82:1957–1959.
56. Singer JW, Nemunaitis J. Use of recombinant growth factors in bone marrow transplantation. In: Forman S, Blume K, Thomas ED, eds. *Bone marrow transplantation.* Boston: Blackwell Scientific Publications 1994:309–326.
57. Snyder EL, Anderson K, Silberstein L, et al. *Transfusion* medicine. In: *Hematology 1994: –the education program of the American Society of Hematology.* 96–106.
58. Shpall EJ, Jones RB. Release of tumor cells from bone marrow. *Blood* 1994;83:623–625.
59. Brugger W, Bross KJ, Glatt J, et al. Mobilization of tumor cells and hematopoietic progenitor cells into peripheral blood of patients with solid tumors. *Blood* 1994;83:636–640.
60. Berenson RJ, Bensinger WI, Hill RS, et al. Engraftment after infusion of CD34+ marrow cells in patients with breast cancer or neuroblastoma. *Blood* 1994; 83:623–625.
61. Schenkein DP, McCann J, Kanteti R, et al. A randomized trial of filgrastim (G-CSF) primed peripheral blood stem cells (PBSC) vs. bone marrow as a reconstitution source for high dose chemotherapy in patients with lymphoma and Hodgkin's disease: an interim clinical and molecular analysis. *Blood* 1994;84[Suppl 1]:204A(abst).
62. Schmitz N, Linch DC, Dreger P, et al. A randomized phase III study of filgrastim-mobilised peripheral blood progenitor cell transplantation (PBPCT) in comparison with autologous bone marrow transplantation (ABMT) in patients with Hodgkin's disease (HD) and non-Hodgkin's lymphoma (NHL). *Blood* 1994;84[Suppl 1]:204A(abst).
63. Srour EF, Brandt JE, Briddell RA, et al. Long-term generation and expansion of human primitive hematopoietic progenitor cells in vitro. *Blood* 1993;81:661–669.
64. Sato N, Sawada K, Koizumi K, et al. In vitro expansion of human peripheral blood CD34+ cells. *Blood* 1993;82:3600–3609.
65. Brenner MK, Rill DR, Holladay MS, et al. Gene marking to determine whether autologous marrow infusion restores long-term haemopoiesis in cancer patients. *Lancet* 1993;342:1134–1137.
66. Bauer TR, Schwartz BR, Liles WC, et al. Retroviral-mediated gene transfer of the leukocyte integrin CD18 into peripheral blood CD34+ cells derived from a patient with leukocyte adhesion deficiency type 1. *Blood* 1998;91:1520–1526.
67. Crawford J, Ozer J, Stoller R, et al. Reduction by granulocyte colony-stimulating factor of fever and neutropenia induced by chemotherapy in patients with small-cell lung cancer. *N Engl J Med* 1991;325: 164–170.
68. Trillet-Lenoir V, Green J, Manegold C, et al. Recombinant granulocyte colony-stimulating factor reduced the infectious complications of cytotoxic chemotherapy. *Eur J Cancer* 1993;29A:319–324.
69. Pettengell R, Gurney H, Radford J, et al. Granulocyte colony-stimulating factor to prevent dose-limiting neutropenia in non-Hodgkin's lymphoma: a randomized controlled trial. *Blood* 1992;80:1430–1436.
70. Lieschke GJ, Burgess A. Granulocyte colony-stimulating factor and granulocyte-macrophage colony-stimulating factor, parts I and II. *N Engl J Med* 1992;327:28–35,99–106.
71. Ozer H. American Society of Clinical Oncology recommendation for the use of hematopoietic colony-stimulating factors: evidence-based clinical practice guidelines. *J Clin Oncol* 1994;12:2471–2508.
72. Nemunaitis J, Rabinowe S, Singer J, et al. Recombinant granulocyte-macrophage colony-stimulating factor after autologous bone marrow transplantation for lymphoid cancer. *N Engl J Med* 1991;324: 1773–1778.
73. Advani R, Chao N, Horning S, et al. Granulocyte-macrophage colony-stimulating factor (GM-CSF) as an adjunct to autologous hematopoietic stem cell transplantation for lymphoma. *Ann Intern Med* 1992; 116:183–189.
74. Gisselbrecht C, Prentice HG, Bacigalupo A, et al. Placebo-controlled phase III trial of lenograstim in bone-marrow transplantation. *Lancet* 1994;343:696–700.
75. Estey E. Use of colony-stimulating factors in the treatment of acute myeloid leukemia. *Blood* 1994;83:2015–2019.
76. Toner GC, Laidlaw C, Millward MJ. Low versus standard dose G-CSF prophylaxis after chemotherapy: a randomized crossover comparison. *Blood* 1994;84[Suppl 1]:26A(abst).
77. Dale DC, Neutropenia. In: Williams WJ, et al. , *Hematology,* 5th ed. New York: McGraw-Hill 1995:815–824.

78. Dale DC, Bonilla MA, Davis MW, et al. A randomized controlled phase III trial of recombinant human G-CSF for treatment of severe chronic neutropenia. *Blood* 1993;81:2496–2502.
79. Freedman MH. Safety of long-term administration of granulocyte colony-stimulating factor for severe chronic neutropenia. *Curr Opin Hematol* 1997;4:217–224.
80. Smith JA. Neutrophils, host defense, and inflammation: a double-edged sword. *J Leukoc Biol* 1994;56:672–686.
81. Nelson S, Belknap SM, Carlson RW, et al. A randomized controlled trial of filgrastim as an adjunct to antibiotics for treatment of hospitalized patients with community-acquired pneumonia. *J Infect Dis* 1998; 178:1075–1080.
82. Gough A, Clapperton M, Rolando N, et al. Randomized placebo-controlled trial of granulocyte-colony stimulating factor in diabetic foot infection. *Lancet* 1997;350:855–859.
83. Kedzierska K, Mak J, Mijch A, et al. Granulocyte-macrophage colony-stimulating factor augments phagocytosis of *Mycobacterium avium* complex by human immunodeficiency virus type 1-infected monocytes/macrophages in vitro and in vivo. *J Infect Dis* 2000;181:390–394.
84. Mitsuyasu R. Prevention of bacterial infections in patients with advanced HIV infection. *AIDS* 1999;13[Suppl 2]:S19–S23.
85. Silverstein SC, Cao C, Rudin D, et al. Organic anion transporters promote the secretion of anionic antibiotics from cells of the J774 macrophage-like cell line. In: Van Furth R, ed. *Hematopoietic growth factors and mononuclear phagocytes.* Basel: Karger 1993:134–139.
86. Weiss M, Gross-Weege W, Schneider M, et al. Enhancement of neutrophil function by in vivo filgrastim treatment for prohylaxis of sepsis in surgical intensive care patients. *J Crit Care* 1995;10:21–26.
87. Schafer H, Hübel K, Bohlen H, et al. Perioperative treatment with granulocyte colony-stimulating factor (G-CSF) in patients with esophageal cancer stimulates granulocyte function and reduces infectious complications after esophagectomy. *Ann Hematol* 2000;79:143–151.
88. Endo S, Inada K, Inoue Y, et al. Evaluation of recombinant human granulocyte colony-stimulating factor (rhG-CSF) therapy in granulopoietic patients complicated with sepsis. *Curr Med Res Opin* 1994;13: 233–241.
89. Hubel K, Dale DC, Engert A, et al. Current status of granulocyte (neutrophil) transfusion therapy for infectious diseases. *J Infect Dis* 2001;183:321–328.
90. Hubel K, Dale DC, Engert A, et al. Use of G-CSF for granulocyte transfusion therapy. *Cytokines Cell Mol Ther* 2000;6:89–95.
91. Price TH, Bowden RA, Boeckh M, et al. Phase I/II trial of neutrophil transfusions from donors stimulated with G-CSF and dexamethasone for treatment of patients with infections in hematopoietic stem cell transplantation. *Blood* 2000;95:3302–3309.

Rossi's Principles of Transfusion Medicine, Third Edition, edited by Toby L. Simon, Walter H. Dzik, Edward L. Snyder, Christopher P. Stowell, and Ronald G. Strauss. Lippincott Williams & Wilkins, Philadelphia © 2002.

36

PROCESSING AND PRESERVATION OF HEMATOPOIETIC PROGENITOR CELLS

RONALD A. SACHER
SUSAN SORENSEN

Transplantation of allogeneic hematopoietic stem cells (HSC) is recognized therapy for hematologic diseases such as severe aplastic anemia and most forms of leukemia (1–3). The knowledge that bone marrow function can be restored by means of infusion of stem cells has led to widespread use of this treatment as autologous rescue from high-dose myeloablative chemoradiation therapy for lymphoma and some solid tumors (4,5). With the development of recombinant colony-stimulating factors (CSFs), it has become possible to mobilize large numbers of progenitor cells into the peripheral circulation. In the circulation they can be collected by means of apheresis and used for marrow rescue in place of, or in addition to, autologous bone marrow (6,7). Advances in cell separation technology are making it possible to engineer bone marrow and peripheral blood stem cell (PBSC) grafts so that specific cell populations can be isolated and infused. Incubation with certain cytokines and pharmacologic agents can induce in vitro proliferation of specific cell types while inhibiting expansion of others (8–11). These cells then can serve purposes other than conventional marrow replacement or rescue. They can be used for adoptive immunotherapy (8,12), as vehicles for gene therapy (13), and perhaps even to induce tolerance of an organ transplant from the same donor (14).

An expanding area of transfusion medicine and clinical laboratory technology is cellular processing and engineering. Laboratories concentrate, separate, isolate, purify, enrich, manipulate, preserve, quantitate, and assay cellular components such as bone marrow, peripheral blood, and umbilical cord blood.

R.A. Sacher and S. Sorensen: Hoxworth Blood Center, University of Cincinnati Medical Center, Cincinnati, Ohio.

SOURCES OF HEMATOPOIETIC PROGENITOR CELLS

The preferred source of allogeneic HSC customarily has been the bone marrow of related, usually sibling, donors who are human leukocyte antigen (HLA) identical at the A, B, and DR loci. An alternative and more practical source is the mobilized peripheral blood progenitor cells from these same donors. These cells can be collected from adults with minimal risk (15). Collection of PBSC from pediatric donors after mobilization has been performed without adverse effects (16). When such a match cannot be found, a number of less desirable options are available. Related donors mismatched at one or two HLA loci have been used, as have phenotypically matched unrelated volunteer donors (17).

Patients who do not qualify for allogeneic transplantation may be eligible to receive their own (autologous) bone marrow or PBSC after cytotoxic therapy and radiation. Although the peripheral blood of healthy persons contains fewer than 0.1% HSC, this number increases dramatically during recovery from cytotoxic therapy and even more so when recombinant CSFs such as granulocyte and granulocyte-macrophage CSF (G-CSF and GM-CSF) are administered (6). This allows collection of the circulating PBSC by means of apheresis techniques.

Another source of HSC is umbilical cord blood, which has been transplanted successfully from both related and unrelated donors (18,19). Most of the transplants of umbilical cord blood have been obtained from related siblings. Cord blood donated for allogeneic transplantation is, however, becoming more readily available and is a feasible alternative if a matched, unrelated donor is needed (19). Because of the limited volume of blood and the number of cells that can be acquired from this source, most recipients have been children. However, adults also have undergone successful transplantation with umbilical cord blood (9). The time to engraftment correlates with the number of nucleated cells administered. A great deal of experimental work is being done with ex vivo expansion of umbilical cord blood (20). Successful ex vivo expansion of the umbilical cord blood would improve the prospects for the use of cord blood as a source of unrelated HSC for adult patients. The availability and relative ease of collection of cord stem cells along with the reported decreased rate of graft versus host disease makes the unrelated umbilical cord blood transplantation an attractive option (18,19).

Fresh bone marrow, unlike other tissues and organs, is not generally taken from cadaveric donors for transplantation into waiting recipients. The patient must receive conditioning therapy for a number of days before the marrow infusion. It is highly improbable that a nonrelated donor would be a phenotypic HLA match for an intended recipient. Fetal bone marrow and liver are rich in HSC, but the usefulness of these cells is limited by ethical issues.

COLLECTION OF PROGENITOR CELLS

Bone marrow harvesting is a surgical procedure performed in an operating room. The donor receives general or regional anesthesia. Although the marrow donor customarily has remained in the hospital overnight, it is possible in many cases to perform the marrow harvest as an outpatient procedure with local anesthesia (21).

The marrow is taken from the posterior iliac crests with stainless steel beveled harvesting needles and glass or plastic syringes. In the original technique developed by Thomas and Storb (22), tissue culture medium and heparin are placed in stainless steel beakers for dilution and anticoagulation of the marrow. At the end of the harvest, the marrow is pressed through two stainless steel mesh screens, of 300 and 200 μm, to filter out most of the bone chips, clots, fat, and fibrin. The collection is then transferred to one or more sterile blood transfer packs and transported to the laboratory. The introduction of a disposable collection kit (Baxter Biotech, Deerfield, IL) made up of a filtered and capped plastic collection container with interlocking filters and transfer bags has modernized this procedure and decreased the risk of bacterial contamination. At least 1 L of marrow usually is needed to yield sufficient nucleated cells for an adult allogeneic recipient, especially if any processing is to be performed (23).

Peripheral blood stem cells are collected by means of apheresis, a process that does not necessitate hospitalization or anesthesia. That stem cells circulate has been known for many years. By stimulating the donor with either hematopoietic growth factors, or chemotherapy for autologous donation, the number of circulating stem cells can be increased (24). Peak counts usually are obtained 5 days after stimulation with G-CSF. This mobilization can even be achieved in healthy allogeneic donors with a 3-day course of G-CSF (25). This allows collection of an adequate number of PBSC, as quantitated by the presence of the CD34 antigen, in one or two apheresis procedures. Steady-state levels of circulating $CD34^+$ cells appear to predict which donor will respond best to G-CSF mobilization (5). Mobilized PBSC have a shorter engraftment time than do traditional bone marrow harvests (5). Because much of the morbidity and mortality of bone marrow transplantation is related to the length of time to engraftment, use of PBSC can dramatically reduce the length of stay in the hospital and thus the total cost of transplantation. A target level of $CD34^+$ cells or nucleated cells usually is calculated according to the weight of the recipient but is usually greater than 1×10^6/kg. Most transplant physicians prefer a dose of 5×10^6/kg. At this dose, there is prompt engraftment (25). For doses less than 5×10^6/kg the reported median number of days to an absolute neutrophil count greater than 5×10^9/L is 10 days, platelet recovery to more than 20×10^9/L occurring at 12 days (5). When the dose of PBSC is increased to more than 5×10^6 CD34/kg, the neutrophil median time to engraftment decreases to 9 days with platelet recovery at 10 days (5). However, there does not appear to be any advantage to CD34 doses greater than 8×10^6/kg in terms of time to engraftment (24–27). After collection the cells are cryopreserved and infused after the patient has undergone myeloablative therapy.

To collect the optimal number of PBSC, volumes of 9 to 24 L of blood or 2 to 5 times the patient's calculated blood volume may be processed with a commercially available cell separation device originally developed for plasmapheresis, leukapheresis, and platelet donation. Investigators have reported that the yield of $CD34^+$ cells increases continuously as more blood volumes were separated (27). Although up to five times the patient's blood volume can be safely processed and provide high numbers of progenitor cells, some patients may not be able to tolerate 5 or 6 hours connected to an apheresis machine. Therefore many patients need repeated collections on sequential days once the peripheral CD34 count has increased to acceptable levels for collection.

Harvesting of umbilical cord blood is the least invasive of all HSC collection techniques. The cord is clamped, and a 16-gauge needle from a standard blood donor set containing an anticoagulant (usually anticoagulant acid citrate dextrose formula A or citrate-phosphate-dextrose-adenine) is inserted into the umbilical vein. The volume of anticoagulant in the blood collection set is reduced to 23 ml to match the smaller volumes collected from the umbilical cord blood (28). Collection can be performed by the obstetrician with the placenta in situ or after delivery by a trained team in a location other than the delivery room. If cells are collected after delivery, the placenta can be suspended from a specially constructed frame to aid in drainage of the cord blood. The usual volume collected is less than 170 ml (28). After collection by means of gravity blood still in the placenta can be expressed by means of massage. A report of a device that applies pressure to the placenta in a funnel-like framework has shown increased yields in total volume and $CD34^+$ content (29). The time that the umbilical cord is clamped may affect the volume collected. Some physicians have raised concerns that early clamping may result in an adverse outcome for the neonate. In at least one study of term newborns, early clamping (within 30 seconds after delivery) showed a de-

TABLE 36.1. YIELD OF HEMATOPOIETIC PROGENITOR CELLS BY SOURCE

Source (Reference)	Volume (ml)	Total Nucleated Cells (× 10^9)	CFU-GM (× 10^5)	CD34 Positive (× 10^7)
Bone marrow	1,380 (22)	22.0 (22)	28.0 (24)	130.0 (22)
PBSC (not mobilized) (23)	10 L processed	10.0	2.5	NA
PBSC (chemotherapy mobilized) (23)	10 L processed	7.3	15.0	4.0
PBSC (chemotherapy and CSF mobilized) (23)	10 L processed	20.8	213.0	38.8
Umbilical cord blood (28)	121	1.3	1.9	1.3

CFU-GM, granulocyte-macrophage colony-forming unit; PBSC, peripheral blood stem cells; NA, not available; CSF, colony-stimulating factor.

crease of 1.2 g/dl in neonatal hemoglobin level, but no adverse clinical outcome was documented (30). Table 36.1 compares nucleated cells, granulocyte-macrophage colony-forming units (CFU-GMs), and CD34$^+$ cells yielded by these sources.

PROCESSING OF HEMATOPOIETIC CELLS

Cell Separation and Concentration

Bone marrow and umbilical cord blood and to a lesser extent PBSC are heterogeneous collections of cellular and noncellular components. Because the cells that lead to hematopoietic reconstitution exist among the mononuclear cells in the bone marrow and peripheral blood, other cell populations in the graft may be superfluous at best and detrimental at worst. Although collections of PBSC may consist of primarily mononuclear cells, most of the cells in the bone marrow and umbilical cord blood are mature red blood cells (RBCs) and granulocytes. Incompatible RBCs or plasma can induce a hemolytic transfusion reaction in recipients of allogeneic grafts, whereas granulocytes lysed by means of freezing and thawing may release enzymes that adversely affect the autologous patient. Other cells may carry surface antigens that can compete for monoclonal antibodies used for purging of autologous tumor cells. Platelets and plasma proteins also can cause clumping of progenitor cells after thawing (31).

In any of the situations described, the cell suspension must be manipulated to remove the undesirable material (Table 36.2). Plasma can be removed by means of centrifugation of the cell suspension in blood bags. Red blood cells can be depleted with a number of techniques (28,32). If hydroxyethyl starch is added and the graft is allowed to stand for 0.5 to 3 hours, the RBCs sediment and can be removed from the bone marrow bag. This technique has been reported to remove as many as 99% of erythrocytes (32). A somewhat less pure product results from centrifugation followed by removal of the buffy coat or white blood cell layer. The buffy coat can be further purified by means of layering onto a density gradient to isolate the mononuclear cells and remove almost all the RBCs.

Semiautomated and automated cell processing is performed with equipment available in most blood centers and transfusion medicine departments. In 1983, Gilmore et al. (33) described their separation technique performed with a Cobe 2991 cell washer, an instrument designed for washing and deglycerolizing RBCs. This method produced a buffy coat that contained approximately 75% of the nucleated cells with no enrichment for mononuclear cells. Other workers (34) devised a density gradient isolation technique performed with the same instrument. The gradient medium was pumped into the continuously revolving processing bag. With the centrifuge still turning, the cell suspension was slowly layered onto the gradient, after which the gradient and mononuclear cell layer were collected and washed.

Procedures for isolating mononuclear cells have been devised to be performed with cell separators such as the CS3000 (Baxter, Deerfield, IL) and Spectra (Cobe, Lakewood, CO) (35). These methods entail differential centrifugation to remove at least 95% of the RBCs while more than 75% of CFUs are recovered in a final product that contains more than 80% mononuclear cells. These are closed continuous flow systems that reduce the risk of bacterial contamination and reduce the processing time to approximately 1 hour, substantially less than with manual systems. If necessary, the graft can be further purified with a density gradient step (32). Intermittent flow devices such as the Haemonetics MCS also can be used. Counterflow centrifugal elutriation

TABLE 36.2. PROCESSING OF HEMATOPOIETIC PROGENITOR CELLS

- Cell separation and concentration
  - Plasma removal: Centrifugation
  - Red blood cell depletion
    - Sedimentation
    - Centrifugation
      - Buffy coat
      - Density gradient
    - Cell washer
    - Cell separator
- Purging
  - Allogeneic: T-cell depletion
  - Autologous: Tumor cell removal
- Cryopreservation and storage
  - Mechanical freezer
  - Liquid nitrogen
    - Liquid phase
    - Vapor phase
  - Refrigerated storage

is a more precise method of separating cells according to size. This procedure is most commonly used to remove allogeneic lymphocytes for prevention of graft versus host disease (see later).

Purging of Marrow and Peripheral Blood Stem Cells

To prevent adverse responses to administration of the assorted cell types present in unmanipulated marrow and stem cell grafts, various techniques have been developed for depleting or "purging" the undesirable cells before infusion (Table 36.3).

In allogeneic transplantation, it is hypothesized that graft versus host disease is the result of recruitment to various tissue and organ sites of host $CD4^+$ effector T lymphocytes by donor $CD8^+$ cytotoxic-suppressor cell T lymphocytes. The result is an immunologic response (36). The skin, liver, and gastrointestinal tract are most often affected, the reaction being especially severe in mismatched-related and matched-unrelated donation (37). Although various combinations of potent immunosuppressive drugs are available for prophylactic administration, use of these drugs does not always prevent this often fatal complication.

Removal of T lymphocytes from the allogeneic graft can prevent or reduce the severity of graft versus host disease. However, because other types of these cells seem necessary for marrow to engraft and to express antitumor or graft versus leukemia activity, removal can actually increase the incidence of graft failure and disease recurrence compared with the situation for unmanipulated allogeneic grafts (38). The critical number of T cells for the graft versus leukemia effect has not yet been determined. However, transplantation with a T-cell dose of 1×10^5/kg body weight allows engraftment and minimizes the severity of graft versus host disease (39). The T cells can be quantitated with cell surface markers and flow cytometry. It is not uncommon in a highly manipulated graft for the transplantation physician to request that a certain dose of T cells specifically be included in the graft. This is achieved by means of counting the number of T cells in the graft after processing and administering an "addback" of T cells to the patient to reach the total number of T cells desired by the transplantation physician. The addback usually is taken from the "waste" remaining after the graft is processed. This portion is assayed and a volume containing the number of T cells needed is infused into the patient. This addback technique has been used as an adjuvant in diseases such as acute lymphocytic leukemia, chronic myelogenous leukemia, aplastic anemia, and acute nonlymphocytic leukemia.

TABLE 36.3. PURGING METHODS FOR ALLOGENEIC AND AUTOLOGOUS BONE MARROW AND PERIPHERAL BLOOD STEM CELLS

Purging Method	Allogeneic	Autologous
Immunologic: Monoclonal antibodies	X	X
Complement	X	X
Immunotoxins	X	X
Magnetic microspheres	X	X
Immunoadsorption		
Negative selection	X	X
Positive selection	X	X
Lectin and E-rosetting	X	
Radioisotopes		X
Pharmacologic		
4-Hydroperoxycyclophosphamide		X
Mafosfamide		X
Etoposide		X
Methylprednisolone	X	X
Vincristine	X	X
Alkyl-lysophospholipids		X
L-leucyl-*l*-leucine methyl ester	X	
Other		
Elutriation	X	
Cytokine activation		X
Long-term culture		X
Hyperthermia		X
Freezing		X

Transfusion of collected T cells from the original donor to the patient after the patient has had a relapse is called *donor lymphocyte infusion.* The T cells can be collected from the donor by means of whole blood collection or apheresis, or the T cells can be allocated from the original bone marrow or PBSC harvest and frozen for future use. Donor lymphocyte infusion has been able to induce complete remission of chronic myelogenous leukemia, acute myelogenous leukemia, myelodysplastic syndrome, and multiple myeloma. It is most successful with chronic myelogenous leukemia. Approximately 65% of patients achieve complete remission in comparison with 25% of patients with acute myelogenous leukemia or myelodysplastic syndrome (40). Donor lymphocyte infusion has been used to manage multiple myeloma and has induced remission. However, the duration of the remission in these patients is variable. The risks of donor lymphocyte infusion are graft versus host disease and marrow suppression. The risk is minimized if treatment begins with a small dose that is increased if there is no response. Doses range from 0.1 to 11×10^8 mononuclear cells per kilogram (40). Donor lymphocyte infusion is most effective when administered early in the relapse.

Contamination of autologous bone marrow and PBSC with occult tumor cells has been shown to contribute to the higher rate of relapse in autologous bone marrow transplantation. Accordingly, there is interest in developing techniques for in vitro or in vivo removal of these cells (4). Historically, tumor cell purging has occurred in vitro by pharmacologic means or immunologic selection and binding of the malignant cells (41). Advantages to the development of in vivo purging would be the ability to collect an autologous graft with less tumor contamination. Use of this technique in animal models has resulted in complete remission if the tumor burden is low (4). Purging strategies also have been successfully combined with donor lymphocyte infusion and immunotherapy (4).

Pharmacologic Purging

The first attempts at tumor cell removal were based on the concept that certain chemicals are more toxic to rapidly dividing clonogenic leukemic cells than to the more slowly cycling uncommitted hematopoietic progenitor cells. The most commonly used agents were cyclophosphamide derivatives such as 4-hydroperoxycyclophosphamide and mafosfamide, although other chemotherapeutic drugs have been used, both singly and in combination (42,43). The cell suspension was incubated with the drug or drugs for the appropriate time and then washed and cryopreserved. This type of purging is relatively nonspecific and can lethally damage committed myeloid progenitors, often resulting in extended periods of neutropenia and thrombocytopenia with an accompanying increase in morbidity (44). Other chemotherapeutic drugs such as etoposide, vincristine, and glucocorticoids have been proposed for ex vivo purging, but because of risk of toxicity and damage to the stem cells, these are not in common use.

Pharmacologic purging of allogeneic grafts is not performed as frequently as are other methods of T-cell depletion because of the few agents that preferentially damage T cells. L-Leucyl-L-leucine methyl ester and methylprednisolone-vincristine seem to be particularly toxic to the $CD4^+$ subset of T lymphocytes (41,45).

Immunologic Purging

Early T-cell depletion techniques were based on the phenomenon by which T cells incubated with soybean lectin form rosettes around sheep RBCs (46). After rosetting, the T cells can be removed from the suspension by means of density gradient centrifugation. Although this technique is tedious and labor intensive, it is effective.

Certain cell surface markers have been identified that appear exclusively or predominately on certain tumor cells. Monoclonal antibodies to these markers have been used in various techniques to remove or destroy contaminating tumor cells. In complement-mediated immunologic purges, antibody-sensitized target cells are lysed after several incubations with complement (47, 48). This method can be effective in removing antigen-positive cells but is also extremely laborious and has variable efficacy. Different lots of complement can have substantially different levels of activity; many lots of reagent may have to be tested before an acceptable one is found.

Immunotoxin purging is performed with monoclonal antibodies linked to toxins such as the A chain of the ricin molecule or pseudomonal exotoxin. The antibody binds to the target cell, which is then poisoned by the attached toxin (49). Recent research has concentrated more on immunotherapy than on immunotoxic therapy.

A tumor-specific monoclonal antibody can be administered before collection of bone marrow at the time of mobilization. This agent also can be given after transplantation as an immunotherapeutic adjuvant. One antibody currently undergoing investigation is rituximab. This agent is an immunoglobulin G1 κ antibody that reacts with the CD20 antigen on normal and malignant B cells. Rituximab has been used to sensitize drug-resistant B cells to the cytotoxic effects of chemotherapeutic agents (4). The antibody does not affect the stem cell because it does not have the CD20 antigen. Alemtuzumab is another antibody that binds to the CD52 antigen and is currently undergoing investigation in the management of chronic lymphocytic leukemia (4).

An efficient technique for removal of targeted cells that does not adversely affect hematopoietic cells involves use of magnetic polymer microspheres bound to one or more monoclonal antibodies (50,51). The antibody-coated beads attach to the cells of interest during an incubation period, after which the cell suspension is exposed to a strong magnet. The magnet holds the cells that have bound to the beads, allowing the unbound cells to be removed from the suspension. This same technique can be used to bind $CD34^+$ cells or perform "positive selection" (see later).

As monoclonal antibodies to specific tumor antigens can be used to remove tumor cells from autologous bone marrow grafts, antibodies to T-cell antigens can be used to remove these cells in allogeneic transplantation (52–55). Methods have been developed in which antibodies to antigens such as CD3, CD4, CD5, CD6, and CD8 are used in conjunction with complement, immunotoxins, and magnetic microspheres to remove T cells from allogeneic grafts. Some protocols involve use of combinations of pharmacologic and immunologic purging agents in an attempt to increase tumor cell purging efficiency by attempting to remove heterogeneous populations of tumor cells from the marrow graft (54,56).

Positive Selection

Immature progenitor cells possess a surface marker (CD34) that gradually disappears as the hematopoietic cells mature and differentiate (57). If a patient's tumor cells do not contain this antigen, a more efficient method of preventing tumor cell reinfusion than either the "shotgun" approach of chemical purging or negative selection with "cocktails" of monoclonal antibodies would be isolation and infusion of only $CD34^+$ cells. Techniques that take advantage of the high affinity between avidin and biotin yield $CD34^+$ cells "positively" selected that have resulted in rapid engraftment (58). The $CD34^-$ cells that run through the column can be discarded, whereas the antigen-positive cells can be detached by means of agitation, collected, and cryopreserved. Selection of $CD34^+$ cells also can be performed with immunomagnetic beads. Several devices for this technique have been developed. The Isolex 300i produced by Nexell Therapeutics (Irvine, CA) has received U.S. Food and Drug Administration (FDA) approval for use in autologous processing of PBSC. The average $CD34^+$ cell recovery is approximately 50% with an average purity of 90%, which is higher than the percentage with techniques performed with avidin-biotin devices (59). Many clinicians have used immunogenic beads to harvest PBSC over several days and to positively select the collections until the desired $CD34^+$ dose per kilogram is achieved. Researchers have been interested in applying this technology to bone marrow harvesting as a method of T-cell depletion because it results in 3.7-log T-cell reduction (60). Using this technology on harvested bone marrow, however, results in a lower yield of $CD34^+$ cells of 39% (61). Factors that can affect the yield of $CD34^+$ cells include technical problems, cell clumping, and loading too many cells on the column, effectively overwhelming the binding sites (31,60). As the technology and specificity of techniques with monoclonal antibodies improve, this process will be applied both to allogeneic PBSC and bone marrow.

Mechanical Purging

Counterflow centrifugal elutriation can be used to separate cell populations by size. As the flow rate of the media through the centrifuge rotor increases, larger cells can be separated and collected. Because lymphocytes are significantly smaller than HSC, this technique is primarily used for lymphocyte removal as a means of T-cell depletion (32).

Other Purging Techniques

Bone marrow and to an even greater extent PBSC can be induced to generate cytotoxic effector cells when incubated with interleukin-2 for 24 hours or more (8,12). These cells are potent antitumor effectors both in vitro and in vivo. Studies with animals have shown that infusion of these activated cells followed by a course of intravenous interleukin-2 can reduce the incidence of disease recurrence. Clinical trials are underway to ascertain whether the same result occurs in human subjects with solid tumors or hematologic malignant disease. Other novel biologic purging strategies take advantage of differential sensitivities of tumor cells to infection with viruses and consequent generation of cell-mediated cytotoxicity (62).

Because tumor cells seem to be more sensitive than HSC to certain environmental conditions, purging techniques have been developed to take advantage of these differential sensitivities. Normal HSC survive both cryopreservation and hyperthermia better than do tumor cells (63). Culturing bone marrow from patients with chronic myelogenous leukemia for 7 days or more at 37°C generally results in a decrease in the number of cells positive for the Philadelphia chromosome. A number of patients have received transplants of autologous marrow from such long-term cultures with at least temporary disappearance of the Philadelphia chromosome–positive clone (64). Therapy with STI571 inhibits the Bcr-Abl tyrosine kinase that is a product of the Philadelphia chromosome and offers a new type of therapeutic intervention for chronic myelogenous leukemia (65).

Ex Vivo Expansion of Stem Cells and Immunotherapy

The ability of a cellular therapy laboratory to expand a limited number of $CD34^+$ cells to a larger population of cells that can be genetically manipulated and targeted for certain tumors is the future direction of stem cell transplantation. There are several advantages to the patient. The first is that only a small volume (100 to 200 ml) of mobilized peripheral blood has to be collected. Because the volume collected is small, in theory the amount of contamination of the graft by circulating malignant cells also is small. This technique will allow multiple treatments in the event of relapse. When the cells are expanded in vivo, greater numbers of stem cells can be administered. This method shortens the time to engraftment and therefore decreases the morbidity and mortality of the procedure.

Studies have shown that committed progenitor cells can be grown in stroma-free liquid culture with the addition of hematopoietic growth factors such as stem cell factor or c-*kit* ligand (11). The optimal combination of growth factors for such expansion has not been determined and is a focus of intense research. Whether the most primitive progenitor stem cells can be expanded is not known. An assay to detect the most primitive stem cell does not exist. The true test of the presence of the most primitive stem cell is its ability to engraft and replace the marrow in a host that has undergone myeloablation. Long-term culture-initiating cells (LTCIC) are cells that after culture for 5 weeks with stromal cells retain the ability to form CFUs. After culture in a semisolid medium, CFU cells form hematopoietic colonies. In the ex vivo expanded grafts, the number of LTCIC does not increase but appears to stay the same as it was originally (11,66). Whether expansion of committed progenitor cells without an increase in more primitive progenitor cells will support long-term engraftment also is unknown. It is possible that expansion may exhaust the primitive progenitor cells (67–69).

Ex vivo expansion of the more committed lineages, however, will allow the cell therapy laboratory of the future to design specific immunotherapy for a patient. The laboratory will be able to produce tumor cell vaccines, genetically modified T cells, and dendritic cells to target tumor antigens or viruses (70,71). Infusion of viral antigen-specific cytotoxic T cells targeting Epstein-Barr virus–associated lymphoma and Hodgkin's disease have shown responses but unfortunately no remissions (72,73). Cytomegalovirus-targeted T cells also have been shown to decrease viral load in the immunosuppressed renal transplant recipients in the immediately postoperative period (74).

Dendritic cells are specialized antigen-presenting cells. They couple the presentation of antigen with accessory molecules and the major histocompatibility complex to initiate a cellular immune response. These cells are able to capture exogenous antigens from dying cells for antigen presentation that would simply be phagocytized by a regular macrophage. Ex vivo expansion of dendritic cells may hold the most promise for immunotherapy that would reverse the anergy that appears to exist to tumor antigens in a given patient. The combination of large amounts of costimulatory accessory molecules with antigen presentation may make dendritic cells a potent producer of T cells vaccines to target tumor antigens. Malignant melanoma, a disease with a known immunologic response, is being targeted by many investigators using dendritic cell therapy (75,76).

Umbilical cord blood may be the best source of primitive stem cells for ex vivo expansion. Compared with bone marrow, umbilical cord blood contains a higher proportion of cells capable of differentiating into CFUs (77). In addition, the number of LTCIC in umbilical cord blood is greater than it is in bone marrow (78). Because of the higher proliferative potential of umbilical cord blood, it is a better target for gene therapy than are other sources of stem cells. Studies have shown that retrovirus-mediated gene transfer occurs more efficiently in umbilical cord blood than in adult bone marrow (79). Results of studies of the ability of an ex vivo expanded portion of an umbilical cord blood graft to shorten the time to engraftment have been disappointing (80). Fernandez et al. (20) used expanded cord blood along and unexpanded cord blood from a different donor in transplantation procedures on patients. The genetic difference in the grafts was expected to enable the researchers to determine which clone contributed the most to engraftment. Unfortunately, the preliminary reports did not show a significant contribution of the ex vivo expanded cells to early engraftment. The researchers speculate that the lack of improvement with expanded cells may be due to low numbers or a lack of ability of the expanded cells to migrate to the marrow after expansion.

STORAGE OF PROGENITOR CELLS

Transplantation of autologous bone marrow and PBSC as well as allogeneic umbilical cord blood requires a means of efficient preservation of HSC, sometimes for months or even years before transplantation. After the cell suspension has been concentrated and manipulated with the techniques described earlier, it is divided into a number of freezing bags to which an equal volume of a freezing solution, usually containing dimethyl sulfoxide (DMSO), is added. Although glycerol is the cryoprotectant of choice for freezing RBCs, it must be removed from the cells with serial washes in saline solution of varying concentrations. Because washing HSC suspensions after thawing usually results in an unacceptable loss of cells, it is preferable to use an agent that does not have to be removed during thawing. Dimethyl sulfoxide, a small molecule that easily traverses the cell membrane and does not have to be extracted from the cells before infusion, is a more appropriate cryopreservative in this setting. The standard freezing mixture contains 20% DMSO (final concentration, 10%), an isotonic saline or electrolyte solution, and a source of protein, usually autologous plasma or human serum albumin (81). Stiff et al. (82) modified the standard freezing technique to incorporate a low-molecular-weight fraction of hydroxyethyl starch (Pentastarch; McGaw Chemical, Irvine, CA) as an additional cryoprotectant. This modification makes it possible to use one-half the amount of DMSO (final concentration, 5%) with cell recovery and viability comparable with those of the standard method. A lower concentration of DMSO may be especially desirable when large volumes of thawed cells are infused because of the unpleasant side effects occasionally experienced during or after DMSO infusion (31,83,84).

Whichever cryoprotectant is used, the freezing rate seems to be important for viable cell recovery. A controlled rate of −1°C to −5°C per minute is described as optimal in most reports (81). Freezing is performed in the chamber of a programmable device into which liquid nitrogen is pumped to maintain the desired rate. When the freezing program is completed, the bags can be removed from the chamber and placed in a liquid nitrogen storage refrigerator in either the liquid or the vapor phase. Although liquid storage allows storage of all bags at a uniform temperature of −196°C, there is a risk of cross-contamination by microorganisms transmitted through the liquid (85). Hepatitis B was transmitted from the person with the index case to three other patients who had cells stored in the same freezer (85). With vapor phase storage, however, there is a gradual increase in temperature from the bottom to the top of the freezer, so bags at different levels are stored at different temperatures. One report described engraftment failure in a number of dogs that received transplants with bone marrow stored in the vapor phase (86). A further limitation of vapor phase freezing is that the small amount of liquid nitrogen in the freezer leaves little safety margin should the nitrogen source become depleted.

Some centers do not use a programmed freezer but instead place the cells into a mechanical freezer (−70°C to −80°C), either leaving them there until needed for infusion or transferring them to nitrogen storage when completely frozen (82). Although the storage of HSC at −80°C does not seem to cause obvious damage during short periods, there is some concern that complete cessation of enzymatic and metabolic activity does not occur until a temperature of −135°C has been reached (81).

Cryopreserved allogeneic bone marrow and umbilical cord blood have been transplanted successfully (87,88). Although fresh cells may be preferable to frozen because of the often substantial cell loss after thawing, the following factors are arguments in favor of storing allogeneic cells before beginning the patient's conditioning regimen:

1. The donor can become ill or otherwise unable to donate on the scheduled day.
2. The donor can refuse to donate.
3. The number of cells collected can be inadequate, necessitating an additional harvest on another day.
4. The collection can be contaminated with microorganisms.

Additional risks are related to the increasing number of transplants from unrelated volunteers who donate marrow at centers distant from the patient. These collections must be transported by courier, sometimes over a long distance and for many hours. Transportation problems can occur because of weather conditions or missed connections, causing extensive delays in delivery of the graft, which may then need processing. If bone marrow or PBSC were harvested from allogeneic donors and stored at the transplantation center before the start of the conditioning regimen, there would be no risk of donor unavailability at the required time.

Successful autologous transplantation with HSC after storage at refrigerator temperatures has been reported (89,90). Hematopoietic stem cells maintain their viability for several days if carefully stored. Most studies have used 4°C as the standard temperature for noncryopreserved storage. Some data support storage conditions in a liquid state, but the ideal conditions have not been described. Preti et al. (91) found a 33% loss of myeloid precursors during cryopreservation and thawing. When they looked at recovery of CFU-GM from the liquid stored samples, however, the investigators did not find a significant difference from the cryopreserved samples (91). They conducted a nonrandomized, retrospective comparison between 45 patients who received grafts stored in the liquid state (median 4 days of storage) and 54 patients who received cryopreserved marrow (median 69 days of storage). They did not find any statistically significant difference in time to engraftment in the two groups (91).

INFUSION

Cryopreserved cells seem to be less prone to injury when thawed rapidly (92). The bags of cell suspension usually are thawed at the bedside in a 37°C to 40°C water bath and immediately infused through a central venous catheter. The bag of cells may be hung and allowed to drip through an administration set, or the cell suspension can be withdrawn from the bag with a syringe and injected directly into the catheter port. Some centers thaw and dilute or wash the cell suspension to remove DMSO, because this agent has been implicated in infusion-related toxicity (93). Because of the fragility of the cells after thawing, any procedure must treat the cells gently and not subject them to vigorous shaking or centrifugation, which can cause the suspension to clump, which results in poor cell recovery. If any postthaw processing is anticipated, it is probably advisable to consider the addition of deoxyribonuclease either during freezing or during thawing to reduce the clumping caused by single-stranded DNA from the cells that did not survive the freeze-thaw process (94).

QUALITY ASSURANCE

Hematopoietic stem cells are biologic products. They therefore are subject to regulation by the FDA. Although the FDA has not begun licensing and inspecting laboratories that process HSC, it has clearly communicated its intent that it will regulate production of "extensively manipulated" products (95). Voluntary standards have been developed by two professional organizations in an effort to improve the quality of care of patients receiving the product and ensure the purity, potency, and the safety of the product. The American Association of Blood Banks and the Foundation for the Accreditation of Hematopoietic Cell Therapy both have published standards for the collection, processing, storage, and infusion of products (96,97). Both professional organizations offer on-site inspection and accreditation of laboratories acting in accordance with the published standards. Both systems emphasize the prevention of errors and an ongoing process of continuous quality improvement. This has become critical as processing techniques have become more complex.

As additional techniques are developed for HSC manipulation, there is additional risk of damaging the cells during processing. The following are the goals for every processing laboratory dealing with any HSC component:

1. There must be minimal loss of or damage to the hematopoietic progenitor cells. Adequate cells must remain after processing to anticipate complete engraftment in a reasonable amount of time.
2. The processing techniques must not put the component at risk of contamination with microorganisms. All procedures must be performed under aseptic conditions with appropriate assays for detection and identification of infectious agents.
3. Purging methods should be aimed at removal of sufficient target cells while allowing recovery of adequate numbers of HSC. Bioassays to determine numbers of residual target cells should be performed when available.

Quantitation of Progenitor Cells

After each step of HSC collection and processing, the laboratory should quantify the number of nucleated cells and mononuclear cells remaining in the collection. Most laboratories use an automated cell counting device because of the speed and accuracy of these devices. Manual cell counts also can be performed. The percentage of mononuclear cells can be determined by performing a differential count on a stained smear. The percentage of the original mononuclear cells recovered after each manipulation of the marrow should be calculated. Besides determining the number of nucleated cells and mononuclear cells remaining after each stage of processing, the laboratory also must examine the viability and function of these cells, especially when chemical agents that can damage HSC and target cells are used.

The ability of the viable cell membrane to exclude dyes such as trypan blue and erythrosin is the principle of the dye exclusion viability test (98,99). Although this is a simple technique, it cannot be used to differentiate healthy and functional cells from those that have been lethally damaged by purging agents.

A surrogate test for HSC is the CFU assay. This is a semisolid culture system containing various growth factors. It generates colonies from committed myeloid and erythroid hematopoietic progenitors. Although occasional reports have shown a correlation between the number of CFU-C cells and the number of days to engraftment (99,100), the results of the assay are generally used for qualitative assessment of the graft. Collections with very low numbers of CFU-C cells usually forecast later engraftment than do collections with high numbers. Although this assay conveys information about both function and numbers of progenitor cells, it requires a 2-week incubation period, making it worthless for immediate graft evaluation.

Other culture-based assays include pre-CFU assays, LTCIC culture assays and extended LTCIC assays (101). There are also models in which xenogenic immunodeficient animals (mice and sheep) are used as a host for human hematopoiesis (101). These are primarily research tools and not practical for the assessment of functional grafts.

Monoclonal antibodies to the CD34 antigen are being used in a standard test to evaluate HSC numbers. These antibodies are now commercially available. Bound to fluorescent dyes, these antibodies offer a rapid method of enumerating progenitor cells with a flow cytometer or fluorescence microscope (102,103). Because CD34 is present on both committed and uncommitted progenitor cells, it serves only as a surrogate marker for the pluripotent HSC. If antigens such as CD33 or CD38, which represent the more committed and differentiated progenitor cells, also are analyzed, the percentage of early progenitors can be calculated. Flow cytometry has become the standard of care for assessing the donor and the product. The procedure is fairly rapid, requiring approximately 1 hour of preparation time. Assessment of viability can be performed by means of propidium iodide exclusion at the same time as the CD34 enumeration. The flow cytometer can measure the size, granularity, and up to three fluorochromes to characterize a cell. Several different techniques are used to measure $CD34^{+}$ cells. Some use two antibodies, and some use one antibody (104). The gating strategy used by the operator also affects the yield. Even in laboratories using the same technique, there appears to be a great deal of variability in results. Because of this, the International Society for Hematotherapy and Graft Engineering (ISHAGE) developed recommendations for the performance of $CD34^{+}$ enumeration by means of flow cytometry with multiparameter techniques and a sequential gating strategy (104). Newer techniques are being evaluated with the ISHAGE guidelines as the standard. A technique of microvolume fluorometry was developed that in comparison studies with the standard method gave a good correlation with the reported ISHAGE method (105,106). This method has not been further pursued by the manufacturers.

Evaluation of Purging

Whether any purging method currently in use can remove an adequate number of clonogenic cells to prevent disease recurrence is not yet known. Techniques used to try to detect residual malignant cells include polymerase chain reaction (PCR) to amplify malignant genetic material to the level of detection, clonal assays, flow cytometry, and sensitive immunocytostaining techniques. The PCR involves the gene rearrangements and translocations identified in diseases such as multiple myeloma, breast cancer, and B-cell non-Hodgkin's lymphoma to detect residual tumor in the graft (107,108). The sensitivity of this technique is as low as 1 in 1 million normal cells. If a graft is purged from a PCR-positive state to a PCR-negative state, there is a correlation with relapse-free survival (109).

Because flow cytometry can be performed with multiple antibodies and physical characteristics of the cells, its sensitivity in detecting malignant cell populations can be increased. Flow cytometry has been used to detect contaminating breast cancer cells in a graft to a count as low as 1 in 10,000 nucleated cells (110). As different antibodies to cell surface markers are developed, the role of flow cytometry because of its speed and ease of use will continue to expand. Flow cytometry is currently the most practical technique for quantitation of T cells and T-cell subsets after T-cell depletion.

A variety of sophisticated cell culture and molecular techniques are either available or in development for detection of occult tumor cells in bone marrow and PBSC (111,112), but these are not easily adapted to a clinical laboratory setting. Cells from the grafts are plated with growth factors and examined after incubation at 37°C. This technique has been used to detect contaminating residual malignant cells in breast cancer (113), non-Hodgkin's lymphoma (108,114), leukemia (115), and neuroblastoma (116).

Immunocytochemical assays for identifying infrequently occurring tumor cells in marrow and PBSC grafts are performed with the immunoperoxidase staining method. This is based on a chemical reaction between a coloring agent and an enzyme. It has been used to detect residual breast cancer cells in PBSC (113) with a sensitivity of 1 tumor cell in 500,000 mononuclear cells.

As these new techniques for detection and quantification of residual target cells after marrow purging are introduced, it is critical that the laboratory take into account the limitations before using them as an absolute indicator of the efficacy of a particular purging method. There are differences in sensitivity and specificity between the various assay systems as well as great interlaboratory variability even with the same technique because of differences in monoclonal antibodies, serum and complement lot, and other reagents and materials.

Sterility Testing

Even if every effort is made to maintain sterility during collection and processing of HSC, there is a risk of contamination with microorganisms, especially when multiple manipulations are performed. Contamination can come from the skin or bloodstream of the patient or donor, improperly sterilized equipment and materials, environmental contaminants, or faulty handling of the graft. Studies of contamination of the grafts quote a 2% rate of contamination (117). Bacterial and fungal cultures should be performed after collection and at different stages of processing to determine whether any of the techniques or materials used are compromising the purity of the cells. Storage in liquid nitrogen can be a source of contamination of the product. One case of hepatitis B virus contamination of a freezer has been reported (85). The product also can be contaminated at the time of thawing. Studies have shown a correlation between organisms found in liquid nitrogen freezers and contamination of products (118, 119).

SUMMARY

Hematopoietic stem cells can be collected from bone marrow, peripheral blood, and umbilical cord blood. These cells are used to restore lymphohematopoietic function after myeloablative therapy for a number of malignant diseases and hematologic defects. Developments in molecular and cell biology have added other applications for treatment with HSC, such as gene therapy and adoptive immunotherapy. These advances in gene therapy will lead to the development of cellular engineering to produce targeted vaccines for immunologic therapy for malignant disease without the associated toxicities of conventional chemotherapy. Hematopoietic stem cells are a target for gene insertion and most likely will be the cells engineered to correct metabolic and hematologic genetic diseases caused by deletion of certain genes. Because cell therapy laboratories have experience in engineering bone marrow grafts, when ex vivo expansion of other primordial stem cells occurs, these laboratories will be able to apply their technical skills to the field of tissue grafting.

REFERENCES

1. Buchner T. Treatment of adult acute leukemia. *Curr Opin Oncol* 1997;9:18–25.
2. Kernan NA, Bartsch G, Ash RC, et al. Analysis of 462 transplantations from unrelated donors facilitated by the National Marrow Donor Program. *N Engl J Med* 1993;328:593–602.
3. Sobocinski KA, Horowitz MM, Rowlings PA, et al. Bone marrow transplantation 1994: a report from the International Bone Marrow Transplant Registry and the North American Autologous Bone Marrow Transplant Registry. *J Hematother* 1994;3:95–102.
4. Margolis J, Borrello I, Flinn I. New approaches to treating malignancy with stem cell transplantation. *Semin Oncol* 2000;27:5:524–530.
5. DiPersio JF, Khoury H, Haug J, et al. Innovations in allogeneic stem cell transplantation. *Semin Hematol* 2000;37[Suppl 2]:33–41.
6. Bensinger W, Singer J, Appelbaum F, et al. Autologous transplantation with peripheral blood mononuclear cells collected after administration of recombinant granulocyte stimulating factor. *Blood* 1993; 81:3158–3163.
7. Peters WP, Rosner G, Ross M, et al. Comparative effects of granulocyte macrophage colony stimulating factor (GM-CSF) and granulocyte colony stimulating factor (G-CSF) on priming peripheral blood progenitor cells for use with autologous bone marrow after high dose chemotherapy. *Blood* 1993;81:1709–1719.

8. Verma UN, Areman EM, Sacher RA, et al. In vitro activation of PBSCs with interleukin 2. In: Gee AP, Gross S, Worthington-White DA, eds. *Advances in bone marrow purging and processing: fourth international symposium.* New York: Wiley-Liss, 1994:245–255.
9. Perora AL, Stiff P, Jennis A, et al. Prompt and durable engraftment in two older adult patients with high risk chronic myelogenous leukemia (CML) using ex vivo expanded and unmanipulated unrelated umbilical cord blood. *Bone Marrow Transplant* 2000;[Suppl 2]:797–799.
10. Zucali JR, Suresh A, Tung F, et al. Cytokine protection of hematopoietic stem cells. In: Gee AP, Gross S, Worthington-White DA, eds. *Advances in bone marrow purging and processing: fourth international symposium.* New York: Wiley-Liss, 1994:207–216.
11. Brugger W, Scheding S, Ziegler B, et al. Ex vivo manipulation of hematopoietic stem and progenitor cells. *Semin Hematol* 2000; 37[Suppl 2]:42–49.
12. Charak BS, Areman EM, Dickerson SA, et al. A novel approach to immunomodulation of frozen human bone marrow with interleukin 2 for clinical application. *Bone Marrow Transplant* 1993;11:147–154.
13. Anderson WF. Human gene therapy. *Science* 1992;256:808–813.
14. Sykes M, Khan A, Sachs DH, et al. Bone marrow transplantation for the induction of tolerance. *Exp Hematol* 1994;22:1(abst).
15. Anderlini P, Trzepiorka D, Korbling M, et al. Blood stem cell procurement: donor safety issues. *Bone Marrow Transplant* 1992;21[Suppl 3]:35–39.
16. Verdeguer A, Bermudez M, de la Rubia J, et al. Allogeneic PBPC transplantation in children. *Cytotherapy* 1999;1:195–201.
17. Szydlo R, Goldman JM, Klein JP, et al. Results of allogeneic bone marrow transplants using donors other than HLA-identical siblings. *J Clin Oncol* 1997;15:1767–1777.
18. Rubinstein P, Carrier C, Scaradavou A, et al. Outcomes of 562 recipients of placental-blood transplants from unrelated donors. *N Engl J Med* 1998;339:1565–1577.
19. Banker JN, Davies SM, DeFor T, et al. Survival after transplantation of unrelated donor umbilical cord blood is comparable to that of HLA matched unrelated bone marrow: results of a matched pair analysis. *Blood* 2001;97:2957–2961.
20. Fernandez MN, Granena A, Millan I, et al. Evaluation of engraftment of ex-vivo expanded cord blood cells in humans. *Bone Marrow Transplant* 2000;25[Suppl 2]:561–567.
21. Dicke K, Hood D, Hanks S, et al. The efficiency of outpatient marrow harvesting under local anesthesia. *Exp Hematol* 1994;22:373(abst).
22. Thomas ED, Storb R. Technique for human marrow grafting. *Blood* 1970;36:507– 515.
23. Spitzer TR, Areman EM, Cirenza E, et al. The impact of harvest center on quality of marrows collected from unrelated donors. *J Hematother* 1994;3:65–70.
24. Kessinger A, Sharp JG. Mobilization of blood stem cells. *Stem Cells*1998;16[Suppl 1]:139–43.
25. deFabritis P, Iori AP, Mengarelli A, et al. CD34+ cell mobilization for allogeneic progenitor cell transplantation: efficacy of a short course of G-CSF. *Transfusion*2001;41:190–195.
26. Saba N, Abraham R, Keating A. Overview of autologous stem cell transplantation. *Crit Rev Oncol Hematol* 2000;36:27–48.
27. Bojko P, et al. Kinetic Study of CD34 cells during PBSC. *J Clin Apheresis* 1999;14:18–25.
28. Rubenstein P, Dobrila L, Rosenfield RE, et al. Processing and cryopreservation of placental/umbilical cord blood for unrelated bone marrow reconstitution. *Proc Natl Acad Sci U S A* 1995;92: 10119–10122.
29. Belvedere O, Feruglio C, et al. Increased blood volume and CD34+CD38-progenitor cell recovery using a novel umbilical cord blood collection system. *Stem Cells* 2000;18:245–251.
30. Bertolini F, Battaglia M, De Iulio C, et al. Placental blood collection: effects on newborns [letter]. *Blood* 1995;85:3361–3362.
31. Reiser M, Draube A, Scheid C, et al. High platelet contamination in progenitor cell concentrates results in significantly lower CD34+ yield after immunoselection. *Transfusion* 2000;40:178–181.
32. Areman E, Deeg HJ, Sacher RA eds. *Bone marrow and stem cell processing: a manual of current techniques.* Philadelphia: FA Davis Co 1992: 68–73.
33. Gilmore MJ, Prentice HG, Corringham RE, et al. Separation of mononuclear bone marrow cells using the COBE 2991 blood cell separator. *Vox Sang* 1983;45:294–302.
34. Jin N, Hill R, Segal G, et al. Preparation of red blood cell depleted marrow for ABO incompatible marrow transplantation by density gradient separation using the IBM 2991 blood cell processor. *Exp Hematol* 1987;15:93–98.
35. Areman EM, Cullis H, Spitzer T, et al. Automated processing of human bone marrow can result in a population of mononuclear cells capable of achieving engraftment following transplantation. *Transfusion* 1991;31:724–730.
36. Deeg HJ. Acute graft-versus-host disease. In: Deeg HJ, Klingemann HG, Phillips GL, eds. *A guide to bone marrow transplantation.* Berlin: Springer Verlag, 1988:86–97.
37. Champlin R, Lee K. T cell depletion to prevent graft versus host disease following allogeneic bone marrow transplantation. In: Areman E, Deeg HJ, Sacher RA, eds. *Bone marrow and stem cell processing: a manual of current techniques.* Philadelphia: FA Davis Co, 1992: 163–170.
38. Horowitz MM, Gale RP, Sondel PM, et al. Graft versus leukemia reactions after bone marrow transplantation. *Blood* 1990;75: 555–562.
39. Verdonck LF, de Gast GC, van Heugten HG, et al. A fixed low number of T cells in HLA identical allogeneic bone marrow transplantation. *Blood* 1990;75:776–780.
40. Baron F, Beguin Y. Adoptive immunotherapy with donor lymphocyte infusions after allogeneic HPC transplantation. *Transfusion* 2000;40: 468–476.
41. Areman E, Deeg HJ, Sacher RA, eds. *Bone marrow and stem cell processing: a manual of current techniques.* Philadelphia: FA Davis Co, 1992:218–291.
42. Kaiser H, Stuart RK, Brookmeyer R, et al. Autologous bone marrow transplantation in acute leukemia: a phase I study of in vitro treatment of marrow with 4 hydroperoxycyclophosphamide to purge tumor cells. *Blood* 1985;65:1504–1510.
43. Rizzoli V, Mangoni L. Pharmacological mediated purging with mafosfamide in acute and chronic myeloid leukemias. In: Gross SR, Gee AP, Worthington-White DA, eds. *Bone marrow purging and processing.* New York: Alan R. Liss, 1990:21–38.
44. Rowley SD, Piantadosi S, Marcellus DC, et al. Analysis of factors predicting speed of hematologic recovery after transplantation with 4 hydroperoxycyclophosphamide purged autologous bone marrow grafts. *Bone Marrow Transplant* 1991;7:183–191.
45. Blazar BR, Thiele DL, Vallera DA. Pretreatment of murine donor grafts with L-leucyl-L-leucine methyl ester: elimination of graft versus host disease without detrimental effects on engraftment. *Blood* 1990; 75:798–805.
46. Reisner Y, Kapoor N, Kirkpatrick D, et al. Transplantation for acute leukemia with HLA-A and -B nonidentical parental marrow cells fractionated with soybean agglutinin and sheep red blood cells. *Lancet* 1981;2:327–336.
47. Ramsay N, Lebien T, Nesbit M, et al. Autologous bone marrow transplantation for patients with acute lymphoblastic leukemia in second or subsequent remission: results of bone marrow treated with monoclonal antibodies BA-1, BA-2, and BA-3 plus complement. *Blood* 1985;66:508–513.
48. Ball ED, Mills LE, Cornwell GG III, et al. Autologous bone marrow transplantation for acute myeloid leukemia using monoclonal antibody-purged bone marrow. *Blood* 1990;75:1199–1206.
49. Ucken FM, Gajl Peczalska K, Meyers DE, et al. Marrow purging in autologous bone marrow transplantation for T lineage acute lymphoblastic leukemia: efficacy of ex vivo treatment with immunotoxins and 4-hydroperoxycyclophosphamide against fresh leukemic marrow progenitor cells. *Blood* 1987;69:361–366.
50. Gee AP, Lee C, Bruce KM, et al. Immunomagnetic purging and autologous transplantation in stage D neuroblastoma. *Bone Marrow Transplant* 1987;2[Suppl 2]:89–98.
51. Shimazaki C, Wisniewski D, Scheinberg DA, et al. Elimination of myeloma cells from bone marrow using monoclonal antibodies and magnetic immunobeads. *Blood* 1988;72:1248–1254.

52. Antin JH, Bierer BE, Smith BR, et al. Depletion of bone marrow T-lymphocytes with an anti-CD5 monoclonal immunotoxin (ST-1 immunotoxin): effective prophylaxis for graft versus host disease. In: Gross SR, Gee AP, Worthington-White DA, eds. *Bone marrow purging and processing.* New York: Alan R. Liss, 1990:207–215.
53. Martin PJ, Hansen JA, Torok-Storb B, et al. Effects of treating marrow with a CD3-specific immunotoxin for prevention of acute graft-versus-host disease. *Bone Marrow Transplant* 1988;3:437–444.
54. Lamb Jr LS, Gee AP, Hazlett LJ, et al. Influence of T cell depletion method on circulating (gamma-delta) T cell reconstitution and potential role in the graft-versus-leukemia effect. *Cytotherapy* 1999;1:7–19.
55. Shimazaki C, Inaba T, Murakami S, et al. Purging of myeloma cells from bone marrow using monoclonal antibodies and magnetic immunobeads in combination with 4-hydroperoxycyclophosphamide. In: Gross SR, Gee AP, Worthington-White DA, eds. *Bone marrow purging and processing.* New York: Alan R. Liss, 1990:311–319.
56. Shpall EJ, Anderson IC, Bast RC Jr, et al. Immunopharmacologic purging of breast cancer from bone marrow for autologous bone marrow transplantation. In: Gross SR, Gee AP, Worthington-White DA, eds. *Bone marrow purging and processing.* New York: Alan R. Liss, 1990:321–336.
57. Civin CI, Strauss LC, Brovall C, et al. Antigenic analysis of hematopoiesis, III: a hematopoietic progenitor cell surface antigen defined by a monoclonal antibody raised against KG 1a cells. *J Immunol* 1984; 133:157–161.
58. Stray KM, Corpuz S, Kalamasz D, et al. Purging tumor cells from bone marrow or peripheral blood using avidin biotin immunoadsorption. In: Gee AP, Gross S, Worthington-White DA, eds. *Advances in bone marrow purging and processing: fourth international symposium.* New York: Wiley-Liss, 1994:97–103.
59. Rowley SD, Loken M, Radich JF, et al. Isolation of CD34+ cells from blood stem cell components using the Baxter Isolex system. *Bone Marrow Transplant* 1998 21,1253–1262
60. G. A. Martin-Henao, M. Picon, Amill B, et al. Isolation of CD34+ progenitor cells from peripheral blood by use of an automated immunomagnetic selection system: factors affecting the results. *Transfusion* 2000:40:35–43
61. Olivero S, G Novakovitch, P Ladaique, et al. T cell depletion of allogenic bone marrow grafts: enrichment of mononuclear cells using the COBE Spectra cell processor, followed by immunoselection of CD34+ cells. *Cytotherapy* 1999;1:469–476.
62. Wu A, Mazumder A, Martuza RL, et al. Biological purging of breast cancer cells using an attenuated replication-competent herpes simplex virus in human hematopoietic cell transplantation. *Cancer Res* 2001; 61:3009–3015.
63. Allieri MA, Lopez M, Douay L, et al. Clonogenic leukemic progenitor cells in acute myelocytic leukemia are highly sensitive to cryopreservation: possible purging effect for autologous bone marrow transplantation. *Bone Marrow Transplant* 1991;7:101–105.
64. Barnett MJ, Eaves CJ, Phillips GL, et al. Successful autografting in chronic myeloid leukaemia after maintenance of marrow in culture. *Bone Marrow Transplant* 1989;4:345– 351.
65. Druker BJ, Sawyers CL, Kantarjian H, et al. Activity of a specific inhibitor of the BCR-ABL tyrosine kinase in the blast crisis of chronic myeloid leukemia and acute lymphoblastic leukemia with the Philadelphia chromosome. *N Engl J Med* 2001;344:1038–1042.
66. Henschler R, Brugger W, Luft T, et al. Maintenance of transplantation potential in ex vivo expanded CD34+ selected human peripheral blood progenitor cells. *Blood* 1994;84:2899–2903.
67. Peters SO, Kittler EL, Ramshaw HS, et al. Ex vivo expansion of murine marrow cells with interleukin-3 IL3, IL6, IL11, and stem cell factor leads to impaired engraftment in irradiated hosts. *Blood* 1996; 87:30–37.
68. Tisdale JF, Sellers SE, Agricola BA, et al, Gene marking studies indicate that ex vivo expansion of mobilized peripheral blood cells results in rapid initial engraftment but diminished long-term repopulating ability. *Blood* 1996;[Suppl]188:300(abst).
69. Uonemura Y, Ku H, Hirayama F, et al. Interleukin 3 or interleukin 1 abrogates the reconstituting ability of hematopoietic stem cells. *Proc Natl Acad Sci U S A* 1996;93:4040–4044.
70. Kleihauer A, Grigoleit U, Hebart H, et al. Ex vivo generation of human cytomegalovirus-specific cytotoxic T cells by peptide pulsed dendritic cells. *Br J Haematol* 2001;113:231–239.
71. Regn S, Raffegerst S, Chen X, et al. Ex vivo generation of cytoxic T lymphocytes specific for one or two distinct viruses for prophylaxis of patients receiving an allogeneic bone marrow transplant. *Bone Marrow Transplant* 2001;27:53–64.
72. Rooney CM, Smith CA, Ng CYC, et al. Infusion of cytotoxic T cells for the prevention and treatment of Epstein-Barr virus induced lymphoma in allogeneic transplant recipients. *Blood* 1998;92: 1549–1555.
73. Roskrow MA, Suzuki N, Gan YJ, et al. EBV-specific cytotoxic T lymphocytes for the treatment of patients with EBV positive relapsed Hodgkin's disease. *Blood* 1998;91;2925–2934.
74. Reusser P, Cathomas G, Attenhofer T, et al. Cytomegalovirus (CMV)–specific T cell immunity after renal transplantation mediates protection from CMV disease by limiting the systemic virus load. *J Infect Dis* 1999;180:247–253.
75. Thurner B, Haendle I, Roder C, et al. Vaccination with mage-3a1 peptide-pulsed mature, monocyte-derived dendritic cells expands specific cytotoxic T cells and induces regression of some metastases in advanced stage IV melanoma. *J Exp Med* 1999;190:1669–1678.
76. Nestle FO, Alijagic S, Gilleiet M, et al. Vaccination of melanoma patients with peptide-or tumor lysate-pulsed dendritic cells. *Nat Med* 1998:4:328–332.
77. Lu L, Xiao M, Shen RN, et al. Enrichment, characterization and responsiveness of single primitive CD34+ human umbilical cord blood hematopoietic progenitors with high proliferative and replating potential. *Blood* 1993;81;41–48.
78. Hows JM, Bradley BA, Marsh JCW, et al. Growth of umbilical cord blood in longterm haemopoietic cultures. *Lancet* 1991;340:73–76.
79. Moritz T, Kellerc DC, Williams DA. Human cord blood cells as targets for gene transfer: potential use in genetic therapies of severe combined immunodeficiency disease. *J Exp Med* 1993; 178:529–536.
80. Kogler G, Nurberger W, Fisher H, et al. Simultaneous cord blood transplantation of ex vivo expanded together with non expanded cells for high risk leukemia. *Bone Marrow Transplant* 1999;24:397–403.
81. Gorin NC. Cryopreservation and storage of stem cells. In: Areman E, Deeg HJ, Sacher RA, eds. *Bone marrow and stem cell processing: a manual of current techniques.* Philadelphia: FA Davis Co, 1992: 292–308.
82. Stiff PJ, Koester AR, Weidner MK, et al. Autologous bone marrow transplantation using fractionated cells cryopreserved in dimethylsulfoxide and hydroxyethyl starch without controlled rate freezing. *Blood* 1987;70:974–978.
83. Smith DM, Weisenburger DD, Bierman P, et al. Acute renal failure associated with autologous bone marrow transplantation. *Bone Marrow Transplant* 1987;2:196–201.
84. Keung YK, Lau S, Elkayam U, et al. Cardiac arrhythmia after infusion of cryopreserved stem cells. *Bone Marrow Transplant* 1994;14: 363–367.
85. Tedder RS, Zuckerman MA, Goldstone AQH, et al. Hepatitis B transmission from contaminated cryopreservation tank. *Lancet* 1995; 346;137–140.
86. Appelbaum FR, Herzig GP, Graw RG, et al. Study of cell dose and storage time on engraftment of cryopreserved autologous bone marrow in a canine model. *Transplantation* 1978;26:245–248.
87. Korbling M, Przepiorka D, Huh YO, et al. Allogeneic blood stem cell transplantation for refractory leukemia and lymphoma: potential advantage of blood over marrow allografts. *Blood* 1995;85: 1659–1665.
88. Wagner JE, Kernan NA, Broxmeyer HE, et al. Allogeneic umbilical cord blood transplantation: a report of results in 26 patients. *Blood* 1993; 82[Suppl]:86a(abst).
89. Burnett AK, Tansey P, Hill C, et al. Hematological reconstitution following high dose and supralethal chemoradiotherapy using stored non-cryopreserved autologous bone marrow. *Br J Haematol* 1983;54: 309–316.
90. Koppler H, Pfluger KH, Havemann K. Hematopoietic reconstitution

after high dose chemotherapy and autologous nonfrozen bone marrow rescue. *Ann Hematol* 1991;63:253–258.

91. Preti RA, Razis E, Ciavarella D, et al. Clinical and laboratory comparison study of refrigerated and cryopreseved bone marrow for transplantation. *Bone Marrow Transplant* 1994;13:253–260.
92. Mazur P. Theoretical and experimental effects of cooling and warming velocity on the survival of frozen and thawed cells. *Cryobiology* 1966; 2:181–192.
93. Beaujean F, Hartmann O, Kuentz M, et al. A simple, efficient washing procedure for cryopreserved human hematopoietic stem cells prior to reinfusion. *Bone Marrow Transplant* 1991;8:291–294.
94. Davis JM, Rowley SD. Treatment of density gradient separated cells with 4 hydroperoxycyclophosphamide, vincristine and methylprednisolone. In: Arema E, Deeg HJ, Sacher RA, eds. *Bone marrow and stem cell processing: a manual of current techniques.* Philadelphia: FA Davis Co, 1992:286–291.
95. Kessler DA, Siegel JP, Noguchi PD, et al. Regulation of somatic-cell therapy and gene therapy by the Food and Drug Administration. *N Engl J Med* 1993;16:1169–1173.
96. Menitove JE, ed. *Standards for hematopoietic progenitor cell services,* 2nd edition, Bethesda, MD: American Association of Blood Banks, 2000.
97. *Standards for hematopoietic progenitor cell collection, processing and transplantation.* Omaha, NE : Foundation for the Accreditation of Hematopoietic Cell Therapy, 1996.
98. Wilson AP. Cytotoxicity and viability assays. In: Freshney RI, ed. *Animal cell culture: a practical approach.* Washington, DC: IRL Press, 1986:183–216.
99. Spitzer G, Verma DS, Fisher R, et al. The myeloid progenitor cell: its value in predicting hematologic recovery after autologous bone marrow transplant. *Blood* 1980;55:317– 323.
100. Rowley SD, Zuehlsdoerf M, Braine HG, et al. CFU-GM content of bone marrow graft correlates with time to hematologic reconstitution following autologous bone marrow transplantation with 4-hydroperoxycyclophosphamide–purged bone marrow. *Blood* 1987;70: 271–275.
101. Verfaillie CM, Ploemacher T, Di Persio J, et al. Assays to determining hematopoietic stem cell content in blood or marrow grafts. *Cytotherapy* 1999;1:41–49.
102. Chen CH, Lin W, Shye S, et al. Automated enumeration of CD34 cells in peripheral blood and bone marrow. *J Hematother* 1994;3: 3–13.
103. Brecher ME, Sims L, Schmintz J., et al. North American multicenter study on flow cytometric enumeration of CD34+ hematopoietic stem cells. *J Hematother* 1996:5;227–236.
104. Sutherland DR, Anderson L, Kenney M, et al. The ISHAGE guidelines for CD34+ cell determination by flow cytometry. *J Hematother* 1996;3:213–226.
105. Read EJ, Kunitake ST, Carter CS, et al. Enumeration of CD34+ hematopoietic progenitor cells in peripheral blood and leukapheresis products by microvolume fluorimetry: a comparison with flow cytometry. *J Hematother* 1997:6:291–301.
106. Chapple P, Prince H M, et al. Comparison of three methods of CD34+ cell enumeration in peripheral blood: dual-platform ISHAGE protocol versus single-platform, versus microvolume fluorimetry. *Cytotherapy* 2000;2:371–376.
107. Negrin RS. Use of the polymerase chain reaction for the detection of tumor cell involvement of bone marrow and peripheral blood: implications for purging. *J Hematother* 1992;1:361–368.
108. Ladetto M, Sametti S, Donovan JW, et al. A validated real-time quantitative PCR approach shows a correlation between tumor burden and successful ex vivo purging in follicular lymphoma patients. *Exp Hematol* 2001;29:183–193.
109. Gribbon JG, Freedman AS, Neuberg D, et al. Immunologic purging of marrow assessed by PCR before autologous bone marrow transplantation for B-cell lymphoma. *N Engl J Med* 1991;325:1525–1533.
110. Leslie DS, Johnston WW, Daly L, et al. Detection of breast carcinoma cells in human bone marrow using fluorescence activated cell sorting and conventional cytometry. *Am J Clin Pathol* 1990;94:8–13.
111. Huang W, Sun GL, Li XS. Acute promyelocytic leukemia: clinical relevance of two major PNL-RAR" isoforms and detection of minimal residual disease by retrotranscriptase/polymerase chain reaction to predict relapse. *Blood* 1993;82:1264–1269.
112. Joshi SS, Kessinger A, Mann SL, et al. Detection of malignant cells in histologically normal bone marrow using culture techniques. *Bone Marrow Transplant* 1987;1:303– 310.
113. Ross AA, Cooper BW, Lazarus HM, et al. Detection and viability of tumor cells in peripheral blood stem cell collections from breast cancer patients using immunocytochemical and clonogenic assay techniques. *Blood* 1993;82:2605–2610.
114. Sharp JG, Joshi SS, Armitage JO, et al. Significance of detection of occult non-Hodgkin's lymphoma in histologically uninvolved bone marrow by a culture technique. *Blood* 1992;79:1074–1080.
115. Miller CB, Zenbauer BA, Piantadosi S, et al. Correlation of occult clonogenic leukemia drug sensitivity with relapse after autologous bone marrow transplantation. *Blood* 1991;78:1125–1131.
116. Thierry D, Validire P, Hardy M, et al. Long term bone marrow culture in metastatic neuroblastoma. *Eur J Cancer Clin Oncol* 1989; 25:167.
117. Padley D, Koontz F, Trigg ME, et al. Bacterial contamination rates following processing of bone marrow and peripheral blood progenitor cell preparations. *Transfusion* 1996;35:53–56.
118. Fountain D, Talston M, Higgins M, et al. Liquid nitrogen freezers: a potential source of microbial contamination of hematopoietic stem cell components. *Transfusion* 1997;37:585–590.
119. Webb IJ, Coral FS, Andersen JW, et al. Sources and sequelae of bacterial contamination of hematopoietic stem cell components. *Transfusion* 1996;36:782–788.

CASE 36A

WHERE AM I?

CASE HISTORY

A 58-year-old woman had a 2-week history of early satiety, increasing abdominal girth, and diffuse abdominal pain. The medical history included chronic glomerulonephritis, migraine headaches, and hypothyroidism. Computed tomography of the chest, abdomen, and pelvis showed an infiltrating abdominal mass involving a loop of small intestine. Results of fine-needle aspiration biopsy of the abdominal mass suggested a diagnosis of large-cell non-Hodgkin's lymphoma. This was confirmed by means of flow cytometry. Before chemotherapy was begun, the small intestine perforated, and the lesion was surgically repaired. Postoperative recovery was uneventful.

The patient was treated with five cycles of cyclophosphamide, doxorubicin, vincristine, and prednisone chemotherapy (CHOP) and had a good partial response with stable but residual disease. After the fifth cycle of CHOP, the patient was treated with rituximab and received granulocyte colony-stimulating factor to facilitate mobilization for proposed stem cell transplantation. Because of the chemotherapy treatments before stem cell collection, mobilization was poor. The peripheral blood CD34 count remained in the range of 11 to 14 cells/μl throughout leukapheresis. Because of the refractoriness of the disease, the patient's oncologist wanted to collect a full transplantation dose of stem cells (5×10^6 $CD34^+$ cells per kilogram), even though it would involve numerous collections and infusions. Eight leukapheresis sessions were needed to achieve a collection of 4.7×10^6 $CD34^+$ cells per kilogram. The peripheral stem cells were cryopreserved with 10% dimethyl sulfoxide (DMSO) and 10% donor plasma and stored in the vapor phase of liquid nitrogen.

The patient was admitted to the inpatient oncology unit for high-dose chemotherapy and autologous hematopoietic stem cell rescue. On admission, she had a white blood cell count of 3.2×10^9/L with 67% neutrophils and 27% lymphocytes, a hematocrit of 31%, and a platelet count of 93×10^9/L. On the day of stem cell infusion, the patient was hydrated and premedicated at 12:30 p.m. with 650 mg acetaminophen, and 20 mg dexamethasone administered orally. An intravenous line and pulse oximeter were placed.

The patient's previously collected peripheral stem cells were removed from liquid nitrogen and brought to the oncology unit on dry ice from the stem cell processing laboratory. At the bedside, the blood bank technologist thawed each bag of stem cells one at a time in a 37°C water bath. Immediately after thawing, an experienced oncology nurse infused the stem cells to the patient through a 170-μm filter at a rate of 20 to 30 ml/min. The patient was encouraged to use hard candies to mask any unpleasant taste of the DMSO.

DISCUSSION

Multiple cycles of chemotherapy, as was given in this case, often produce an inadequate response to mobilization of stem cells. It has been reported that among patients with Hodgkin's disease or non-Hodgkin's lymphoma who received mobilization chemotherapy and growth factors, each cycle of previous chemotherapy could result in a decrease of 0.2×10^6 $CD34^+$ cells per kilogram (1). To obtain sufficient stem cells in poorly mobilized patients, several collections may be needed. Accordingly, the final dose infused can be composed of several bags, each with relatively few $CD34^+$ stem cells but with a substantial volume of DMSO and with the potential for cumulative toxicity.

Dimethyl sulfoxide is the most commonly used cryopreservation agent for peripheral blood stem cell transplantation (2,3). The addition of DMSO to stem cells during rapid cooling prevents formation of intracellular ice crystals and dehydration injury and thereby reduces cellular damage associated with freezing. However, once stem cells are thawed, DMSO is considered toxic, especially after prolonged exposure at room temperature. To preserve cell viability, it is ideal for the hematopoietic stem cell components to be infused within 30 minutes of thawing. In practice, and as described for this case, stem cells often are thawed at the bedside and quickly infused into the patient.

Pure DMSO is colorless and odorless. It is converted to dimethyl sulfone ($DMSO_2$) and dimethyl sulfide ($DMSH_2$) in hepatic microsomes (4). Dimethyl sulfone has a longer half-life (72 hours) and is excreted by the kidney. Dimethyl sulfide has a shorter half-life (24 hours) and is expired through the lungs. Dimethyl sulfide is responsible for the garlic odor often noticed for several days after stem cell infusion.

CASE HISTORY, CONTINUED

The patient's vital signs and symptoms during stem cell infusion are shown in Table 36A.1. Five minutes after infusion of the first bag, the patient had mild wheezing and skin flushing. The infusion was stopped, and 50 mg diphenhydramine was given intravenously with almost immediate resolution of the symptoms. The infusion was restarted 10 minutes later with no further wheezing or flushing.

During infusion of the third bag, the patient reported severe

TABLE 36A.1. SIGNS AND SYMPTOMS DURING STEM CELL INFUSION

Time	Bag	Volume (ml)	Blood Pressure (mm Hg)	Pulse (Beats/Min)	Temperature (°)	Respiratory Rate (Breaths/Min)	Oxygen Saturation (%)	Reaction
Day 1								
13:25	1	50	122/68	69	96.8	18	100	Wheezing, flushing
13:55	2	75	122/64	62	96.8	18	100	
14:15	3	60	118/68	59	97.2	18	100	Nausea, vomiting
14:35	4	68	126/68	52	97.0	18	100	
14:58	5	59	118/62	54	96.8	18	100	
15:25	6	48	120/70	58	97.6	18	100	
15:33			60/palp	45	97.5	30	88	Nausea, vomiting, diaphoretic, and unresponsive
Day 2								
10:35	7	60	126/68	52	97.0	18	100	
10:58	8	50	118/62	54	96.8	18	100	

nausea, abdominal cramping, and feeling hot. She then had sudden projectile vomiting of approximately 200 ml of clear yellow fluid and said she did not feel well. The stem cell infusion was stopped, and the patient was treated with 16 mg ondansetron hydrochloride intravenously. After the attending oncologist, nurses, and patient discussed the situation, they decided to continue the stem cell infusion. The infusion was restarted at a slower rate of 2 to 3 ml/min and was well tolerated by the patient with no other episodes of wheezing, flushing, nausea, or emesis with infusion of the next two bags. However, during infusion of the sixth bag, the patient again had projectile vomiting and became diaphoretic and lethargic. Oxygen saturation decreased from 100% to 88%, but the patient's condition quickly improved to 96% with 2 L of oxygen through a nasal cannula. The blood pressure declined from 120/70 mm Hg to 60/palp with a decrease in heart rate from 58 to 45 beats/min. Soon after this episode, the patient became unresponsive. A cardiac arrest code was called as a precautionary measure. It was aborted when the patient awoke in response to a fluid challenge and regained full consciousness minutes later. When she awoke, the patient greeted the nurse with, "Where am I?" Cardiovascular and mental status stabilized fully in 40 minutes, after administration of supplemental fluids.

Because the patient had an adverse reaction to the infusion, all component labels were checked for the name and medical record number of the intended recipient, and these were found to be correct. Processing records were reviewed, and no evidence of errors or deviation in processing was found. Results of bacterial cultures of all the bags and the patient were negative. The next day, the two remaining bags of stem cells were thawed and washed to remove DMSO. The patient tolerated the infusion of these two units of washed stem cells without any complications.

DISCUSSION, CONTINUED

This 58-year-old woman with non-Hodgkin's lymphoma had severe nausea and projectile vomiting while receiving a peripheral blood stem cell infusion. Over 2 hours, the patient received a total of 360 ml of peripheral stem cells containing 36 ml of 10% DMSO. Several possibilities composed the immediate differential diagnosis according to the history and treatment regimen. These included intestinal obstruction, bacterial or viral gastroenteritis, migraine, increased intracranial pressure, cardiac arrhythmia, anaphylactic reaction, vasovagal reaction, stroke, fluid overload, and DMSO toxicity. However, the patient did not have many signs or symptoms compatible with most of these entities, and the most likely working diagnosis was acute DMSO toxicity.

Toxicity of DMSO accounts for most adverse reactions to cryopreserved stem cell infusion. The most common symptoms of DMSO toxicity after intravenous infusion include nausea, abdominal pain, and emesis. Most patients have some degree of nausea during infusion. Because of release of bradykinin and histamine by DMSO, various degrees of anaphylactoid reactions occur, such as flushing, hypotension, and bronchospasm. This type of reaction should and can be prevented or managed with an antihistamine. Infusion of DMSO also has been associated with cardiovascular toxicity, including bradycardia, heart block, and even cardiac arrest (5,6). There also have been reports of neurologic toxicity related to DMSO infusion, including peripheral neuropathy, transient global amnesia, and cerebral infarction (7). Severe or life-threatening reactions to DMSO are extremely rare, but deaths have been reported (8).

Toxicity of DMSO seems dose dependent and short-lived. In most cases, so that as many stem cells as possible can be infused, peripheral blood stem cells are not washed to remove DMSO, and patients receive a variable dose of DMSO with the peripheral blood stem cell infusion. The usual procedure is to start the infusion at a rate of 3 to 5 ml/min and to assess toxicity as the infusion continues and symptoms develop. It is generally better to continue the infusion at a slow rate rather than to stop or restart the infusion several times. If the patient has a severe reaction, it may be useful to wash the cells to remove DMSO, as was done in this case.

Case contributed by Yanyun Wu, M.D., Benjamin C. Calhoun, M.D., and Edward L. Snyder, M.D., Yale-New Haven Hospital, New Haven, CT.

REFERENCES

1. Haas R, Mohle R, Fruhauf S, et al. Patient characteristics associated with successful mobilizing and autografting of peripheral blood progenitor cells in malignant lymphoma. *Blood* 1994;83:3787–3794.
2. Snyder E, Haley NR, ed. *Hematopoietic progenitor cells: a primer for medical professionals.* Bethesda, MD: American Association of Blood Banks, 2000.
3. Rowley SD, Anderson GL. Effect of DMSO exposure without cryopreservation on hematopoietic progenitor cells. *Bone Marrow Transplant* 1993;11:389–393.
4. Egorin MJ, Rosen DM, Sridhara R, et al. Plasma concentrations and pharmacokinetics of dimethylsulfoxide and its metabolites in patients undergoing peripheral-blood stems-cell transplants. *J Clin Oncol* 1998; 16:610–615.
5. Zambelli A, Poggi G, Da Prada G, et al. Clinical toxicity of cryopreserved circulating progenitor cells infusion. *Anticancer Res* 1998;18: 4705–4708.
6. Alessandrino EP, Bernasconi P, Caldera D, et al. Adverse events occurring during bone marrow or peripheral blood progenitor cell infusion: analysis of 126 cases. *Bone Marrow Transplant* 1999;23: 533–537.
7. Hoyt R, Szer J, Grigg A. Neurological events associated with the infusion of cryopreserved bone marrow and/or peripheral blood progenitor cells. *Bone Marrow Transplant* 2000;25:1285–1287.
8. Zenhäusen R, Tobler A, Leoncini L, et al. Fatal cardiac arrhythmia after infusion of dimethyl sulfoxide-cryopreserved hematopoietic stem cells in a patient with severe primary cardiac amyloidosis and end-stage renal failure. *Ann Hematol* 2000;79:523–526.

37

HUMAN PROGENITOR CELL—AUTOLOGOUS TRANSPLANTATION

SCOTT D. ROWLEY
STUART L. GOLDBERG

The number of patients undergoing autologous or allogeneic hematopoietic stem cell (HSC) transplantation has grown rapidly over the last 2 decades. Registries have collected data on over 65,000 transplants, but this is believed to represent less than 50% of all transplants performed (1). In Europe alone, over 12,000 bone marrow and peripheral blood stem cell (PBSC) transplants are performed annually (2). Much of this increased activity derives from the widespread adoption of PBSCs as the primary source of HSCs for transplantation, a change driven by the more rapid engraftment parameters of PBSCs, with resulting lower morbidity, mortality, and costs. Also, the use of high-dose therapy with stem cell rescue has increased because of success in randomized trials of dose-intensive therapy in achieving durable remissions in common dose-responsive malignancies such as multiple myeloma (3), Hodgkin's disease (4), and non-Hodgkin's lymphoma (5). It has been 40 years since the discovery that cellular elements of the bone marrow protect against lethal irradiation (6). Transplantation science during this interval is notable for the development of antineoplastic conditioning regimens achieving effective tumor cell kill, immunomodulation regimens allowing allogeneic transplantation without fatal graft versus host reactions, and cryopreservation and ex vivo purging techniques facilitating autologous transplantation. The availability of hematopoietic growth factors and improved techniques for collection of hematopoietic progenitor and stem cells has decreased both regimen-related toxicity and the period of intensive medical support required, thereby decreasing the morbidity and overall cost of transplantation for individual patients. An understanding of the hematopoietic and immunologic systems has continued to develop, so that enriched populations of HSCs or immunologic effector cells may be isolated and manipulated ex vivo to generate "somatic cell therapy" products that differ in function from native bone marrow cells.

Historically, HSC transplantation was developed as a technique to deliver high doses of chemotherapy with or without radiation therapy. The collection, storage, and infusion of autologous HSCs were intended merely to alleviate the iatrogenic bone marrow failure of the high-dose chemo- and radiotherapy regimen used to treat the patient. The infusion of autologous HSCs, in contrast to allogeneic transplantation, conveys no direct antineoplastic benefit to the recipient. Autologous transplantation is, therefore, based on two considerations:

- The dose sensitivity of the disease being treated and the availability of dose-intense regimens capable of ablating this disease, and
- The ability to collect and successfully store adequate numbers of HSCs to allow rapid reconstitution of the bone marrow function.

S.D. Rowley and S.L. Goldberg: Blood and Marrow Transplant Program, Hackensack University Medical Center, Hackensack, New Jersey.

Although autologous HSC transplantation does not convey the immunologic graft versus disease effect achieved with allogeneic transplantation (Chapter 38), the corresponding lack of graft versus host disease and the avoidance of toxic immunosuppressive medications required after allogeneic transplantation allows the use of dose-intense therapy by older patients, including patients in their eighth decade of life as well as patients with comorbid conditions that might preclude allogeneic transplantation.

IMPORTANCE OF DOSE-INTENSITY AND DOSE-DENSITY IN THE MANAGEMENT OF MALIGNANCIES

Both the dose and combination of agents for chemotherapy are important in achieving cure of malignant diseases. Malignant diseases such as Hodgkin's disease, intermediate grade non-Hodgkin's lymphoma, and acute leukemia are potentially curable if multiple chemotherapy agents are administered in a regimen that allows the use of an effective dose of each agent. The importance of combining multiple chemotherapy agents is illustrated by the increase in cure rates for Hodgkin's disease treated with effective drugs in combination in contrast to similar drugs used singly or in sequence. The importance of dose is illustrated by the lack of further increase in the proportion of patients cured by the addition of more chemotherapeutic agents to a regimen if such addition requires a reduction of dose to avoid regimen-related toxicities. Thus, the combination of mechlorethamine, vincristine, prednisone, and procarbazine (MOPP) and doxorubicin, bleomycin, vinblastine, and dacarbazine (ABVD) in alternating schedules that doubles the number of drugs is no more effective than either regimen used alone in the treatment of Hodgkin's disease, because in combining these regimens the dose of the individual drugs is reduced by 50% by the alternate-cycle administration of each regimen. Frei et al. proposed that effectiveness of a chemotherapy regimen can be estimated by calculating the "summation dose intensity" that includes the amount of drug delivered over a period of time (7).

The curative treatment of other dose-responsive malignancies such as breast cancer is limited by the lower activity of the chemotherapy agents available and because almost all of the agents are myelosuppressive, requiring dose reduction to accommodate combination chemotherapy. However, even for breast cancer, the importance of dose density was demonstrated in 1981 by Bonadonna and Valagussa in a retrospective analysis of two of their clinical trials with cyclophosphamide, methotrexate, and 5-fluorouracil (5-FU) (8). They found that disease-free survival was longer for those patients who received a higher percentage of the intended dose of chemotherapy. This could reflect either the larger amount of drug delivered or that women who tolerated the drugs were also more likely to live longer. However, Wood et al. showed in a prospectively randomized trial that the delivery of higher doses resulted in a significantly better survival of women being treated for early breast cancer. This larger amount of chemotherapy delivered was better regardless if it was delivered in higher doses with fewer cycles or if an equivalent amount of chemotherapy was delivered in lower doses but over a longer period of time (9). The authors conclude that these data are consistent with either a dose-response effect or a threshold level of the dose or dose intensity. Therefore, it is still not known, at least for breast cancer treated in either the adjuvant setting or for metastatic disease, whether it is the intensity (e.g., one-time administration of high-dose chemotherapy) or the density (e.g., the amount of chemotherapy administered over a period of time) of the regimen that is more important. The results of randomized studies of dose-intense therapy (see Breast Cancer, below) are still awaiting final analysis.

The infusion of HSCs allows the administration of a dose-intense regimen without concern for the effects on hematopoiesis (myeloablative regimens). The importance of dose intensity instead of dose density for many diseases is demonstrated by randomized trials of autologous transplantation for diseases such as multiple myeloma (3), Hodgkin's disease (4), and non-Hodgkin's lymphoma (5)—these trials illustrate that dose-intense therapy is more effective than available nontransplant regimens delivered in multiple cycles over time. Attempts to deliver more chemotherapy using sequential (tandem) transplants have been limited by the nonmyeloid toxicity of the regimens used.

However, the infusion of HSCs has also been demonstrated to allow the administration of dose-dense nonmyeloablative regimens, potentially achieving a doubling of the amount of chemotherapy administered (10,11). The potential of this approach was most clearly illustrated by Petengell et al. who treated 25 patients with small cell lung cancer with multiple cycles of ifosfamide, carboplatin, and etoposide (ICE) chemotherapy (11). Peripheral blood stem cells were collected after each cycle of chemotherapy and used for the support of the following cycle. They were able to double the dose density, although only about 50% of the patients were able to complete the planned therapy. Five patients reverted to standard-dose therapy at median chemotherapy cycle four. Three patients died while on study (two of sepsis). Others reverted to standard-dose therapy because of prolonged cytopenias (two patients) and inability to collect cells or intolerance of dimethylsulfoxide (DMSO) (one patient each). One group treated 18 patients with sarcoma with high-dose ifosfamide and doxorubicin using a single PBSC collection split into multiple fractions and cryopreserved (10). They administered a median of 0.9×10^6 $CD34^+$ cells/kg with each cycle of therapy; the patients experienced a granulocyte count $<500/\mu l$ for a median of 4 days and a platelet count $<20{,}000/\mu l$ for a median of 2 days. The acceptability of cell support for dose-dense regimens is limited by the logistics of delivering cryopreserved cells in hospitals and offices without easy access to this technology.

TECHNIQUES OF AUTOLOGOUS HSC TRANSPLANTATION

Patient Eligibility for Autologous HSC Transplantation

Careful patient selection and timing of treatment are critical to the success of dose-intense therapy. Patients with bulky tumor masses and patients with chemotherapy-resistant malignancies are much less likely to achieve a durable control of malignancy even with the use of dose-intense regimens. The early introduction of dose-intense therapy in the treatment of a patient, before chemotherapy resistance and excessive chemotherapy-induced organ toxicity develop, is paramount. Therefore treatment algorithms incorporating HSC salvage strategies must be part of the initial therapeutic decisions for each patient with a disease possibly treatable by high-dose therapy. Patients being prepared for autologous transplantation will frequently undergo several cycles of chemotherapy intended to:

- Demonstrate the sensitivity of the disease to chemotherapy,
- Reduce the bulk of the disease before autologous transplantation, and
- Facilitate the collection of PBSCs (12).

Radiotherapy can be used to debulk large tumor masses but is, in general, reserved for administration after recovery from transplantation because of the deleterious effects of this treatment modality on the collection of PBSCs and the increase in organ toxicity within the treatment field with subsequent administration of chemotherapy (13). Radiotherapy used as consolidation therapy after autologous transplantation sometimes requires the infusion of additional HSCs to offset the bone marrow–suppressive effects of this therapy. This illustrates the need for comprehensive planning to assure reserve quantities of HSCs are available if needed.

Patients undergo a detailed evaluation to uncover any organ dysfunction that could preclude the safe administration of this therapy. Although HSC reinfusion rescues the patient from the hematologic toxicity of the conditioning regimen, the nonhematologic (organ) toxicity of dose-intense therapies remains. A retrospective review of 383 consecutive transplants noted factors predictive of early transplant-related mortality including an FEV_1 (forced expiratory volume in 1 second) less than 78% of predicted, serum creatinine greater than 1.1 mg/dl, and serum bilirubin greater than 1.1 mg/dl (14).

Current transplantation techniques using PBSCs minimize the period of neutropenia and the infection risk. Current mortality rates reported after autologous HSC transplantation are frequently less than 5%, although this risk increases somewhat for older patients (15). Because of this risk, patients undertaking dose-intense therapy, if possible, should be free of infection and have other comorbid conditions such as diabetes mellitus under optimal medical control.

Selection of Conditioning Regimen

Autologous HSC transplantation facilitates disease cure through the administration of dose-intensive regimens. Therefore, the conditioning regimen used should include drugs that are effective in the treatment of the particular malignancy and induce minimal nonhematopoietic organ damage at the myeloablative doses used for transplantation. Immunosuppression is not required for engraftment of autologous HSCs, so agents such as antithymocyte globulin or total body irradiation (TBI) are not necessary. Some regimens, such as high-dose melphalan for the treatment of patients with multiple myeloma and BCNU-based regimens for the treatment of lymphoma, are commonly used based on the results of multicenter phase III studies showing the tolerability of these regimens. Relapse is the major cause of failure of autologous HSC transplantation. Therefore, some transplant programs are exploring novel techniques to deliver yet more intensive conditioning to the regimen. One example of this is the addition of radiolabeled antibodies to a chemotherapy or TBI-based regimen to target specifically areas of tumor while sparing radiation-sensitive organs such as the liver, lung, and kidney (16). In one study 20 to 27 Gy of iodine 131-labeled anti-CD20 antibody was added to a conditioning regimen of etoposide (20 mg/kg) and cyclophosphamide (100 mg/kg). This resulted in a 77% complete response rate and a 68% 2-year probability of progression-free survival (PFS) for patients with relapsed non-Hodgkin's lymphoma (16). The 2-year PFS was almost double that previously experienced (36%) by similar patients treated with chemotherapy alone.

Selection of HSC Source

Peripheral blood stem cells have virtually replaced bone marrow as the HSC component for autologous transplantation and have shown benefit in phase III studies in allogeneic transplantation (17). The ease of collection and the rapid engraftment kinetics of PBSCs compared to bone marrow are widely recognized. Median times to achieve an absolute neutrophil count (ANC) $>500/\mu l$ are typically about 12 to 14 days, and platelet recovery is even faster (Table 37.1) (13,18–21). In one phase III study of 47 patients treated for germ cell tumor, rapid engraftment kinetics were achieved with PBSC transplantation. Although all patients received granulocyte colony–stimulating factor (G-CSF) after transplantation, and despite the small number of patients enrolled, the recipients of PBSCs achieved a neutrophil count of $>500/\mu l$ 1 day faster, and a sustained platelet count of $>20{,}000/\mu l$ 7 days faster than the patients receiving marrow (22). A similar trial for patients with non-Hodgkin's lymphoma or Hodgkin's disease reported faster platelet recovery (time to count $>20{,}000/\mu l$ of 16 versus 23 days) and faster granulocyte recovery (time to a neutrophil count $>500/\mu l$ of 11 versus 14 days) for recipients of PBSCs compared to recipients of bone marrow (23). The PBSC recipients also spent fewer days hospitalized and required fewer red blood cell and platelet transfusions.

There are also disadvantages to the use of PBSC components as a source of HSCs for autologous transplantation. These include the usual need for multiple days of collection, the current need for sophisticated flow cytometric analysis of the components to ensure adequacy of HSC content, the inability to collect adequate components from all patients, the (minimal) risks associated with administration of hematopoietic cytokines and the apheresis procedures, and the risks of infusion if the multiple components are cryopreserved. Bone marrow collection and infusion is available to patients for whom adequate PBSC component(s), defined by the number of $CD34^+$ cells collected (Chapter 36), cannot be harvested and stored.

The dose of $CD34^+$ cells in the PBSC component(s) required for infusion depends upon the intended treatment regimen. Lower doses of $CD34^+$ cells appear satisfactory for nonablative regimens (10,11). For example, one group infused 0.9×10^6 $CD34^+$ cells per cycle for patients treated with high-dose

TABLE 37.1. RELATIONSHIP BETWEEN MOBILIZATION SCHEME, DOSE OF CFU-GM OR CD34+ CELLS INFUSED, AND ENGRAFTMENT KINETICS AFTER AUTOLOGOUS PBSC TRANSPLANTATION

			Progenitor Cell Dose		Engraftment Kinetics	
Author	Patients	Therapy	CFU-GM × 10⁴/kg	CD34+ × 10⁶/kg	ANC >500/μl	Platelet >20,000/μl
Nademanee (18)	39	G-CSF	ND	6.2	10 (7–40)	15.5 (7–63)
Sheridan (19)	29	G-CSF	21.0	ND	6 (4–10)	11 (9–136)
Weaver (21)	692	Chemotherapy[a] G-CSF	30.8[b]	9.9[b]	9 (5–38)	9 (4–53+)
Bensinger (13)	124	Chemotherapy[a] G-CSF	ND	9.4	11 (4–20)	10 (6–65)

Shown are mean values for progenitor cell quantities infused and median values for time to achieve the particular end-point of engraftment.
CFU-GM, colony-forming unit–granulocyte-macrophage; PBSC, peripheral blood stem cell; ANC, absolute neutrophil count; ND, no data; G-CSF, granulocyte colony–stimulating factor.
[a]CFU-GM cultures performed on thawed cells.
[b]Shown are median values.

ifosfamide and doxorubicin (10). Despite an overall doubling of the ifosfamide dose in this phase I study, the median times between cycles did not progressively increase, indicating adequate bone marrow stores were maintained. For marrow-ablative regimens, increasingly higher $CD34^+$ doses result in greater likelihood of rapid recovery of peripheral blood cell counts (21). Patients who receive a dose of $CD34^+$ cells above an ill-defined threshold will engraft. At lower doses of $CD34^+$ cells there is considerable heterogeneity in engraftment speed, especially for platelet recovery, with some patients experiencing quick engraftment despite low doses of PBSCs. It is not known why this heterogeneity exists but it may reflect a weakness in the correlation between $CD34^+$ cells and the cells responsible for hematologic recovery or, more simply, a greater degree of error in the measurement of $CD34^+$ cells at the lower cell concentrations. As the dose of $CD34^+$ cells increases, the engraftment speed becomes more consistent for the population studied, although the median days of cytopenia and the minimum number of days is not affected (13,21). Several investigators showed more consistently rapid granulocyte and platelet engraftment for recipients of products containing a quantity of $CD34^+$ cells above a dose of about 2 to 3 $\times$ 10^6 per kilogram of recipient weight (24–26).

Many of the studies showing an advantage of autologous HSC transplantation over other (nontransplant) therapies used bone marrow as the source of HSCs. The duration of aplasia predicts the incidence of peritransplant mortality after autologous transplantation (27). Although this may reflect patient characteristics rather than graft characteristics, it is possible that use of PBSCs will result in yet a greater difference in the outcome of these therapies.

Expansion of Inadequate HSC Components

Hematopoietic stem cells are characterized by the ability to self-renew and to differentiate to mature blood cells. Collections of HSCs from the bone marrow or peripheral blood are termed "stem cells" despite the fact that they contain distinct populations of true HSCs and more differentiated progenitor cells with limited proliferative capacity. In vitro techniques to increase (expand) the numbers of HSCs in components that contain limited or inadequate numbers of HSCs are being developed with the hope that expansion of HSCs will allow simpler collection techniques or the administration of dose-intense therapy to patients from whom adequate marrow or PBSC components cannot be collected. These techniques have been used in phase I studies involving bone marrow, PBSCs, or umbilical cord blood cells (28). The results of these studies are encouraging, but clinical utility requires further study.

Tumor Cell Purging

Hematopoietic stem cell components are a complex mixture of cells, and many of these cell populations affect the outcome of allogeneic or autologous transplantation. The preponderance of evidence demonstrates that malignant cells contained in an HSC graft may be a cause of disease after transplantation. The transmission of malignant cells in an organ graft has been demonstrated in both HSC and solid organ (e.g., orthotopic heart, liver, or kidney) transplantation from living or cadaveric donors suffering from occult disease at the time the graft was harvested (29,30). These reports conclusively demonstrate that even very small quantities of malignant cells can engraft when infused into a properly conditioned host. It is not surprising, therefore, that relapse of disease can occur after autologous HSC transplantation for diseases involving or likely to involve the blood or bone marrow.

Tumor cell contamination (minimal residual disease [MRD]) of the component contributing to relapse after autologous HSC transplantation was demonstrated in studies involving the transplantation of genetically marked bone marrow cells from patients with acute or chronic leukemia or neuroblastoma (31–33). The level of marked cells detected after relapse was very low, and these studies cannot conclude that the cell inoculum was the sole source of malignant cells causing the disease relapse. Nor do these studies demonstrate that purging of tumor cells is necessary or effective. However, the implication of these studies, as with the solid organ transplant experience, is that the infusion of tumor-contaminated HSCs is detrimental to the recipient and purging, if without undue toxicity, may be beneficial to the subset of patients whose HSC components are contaminated by tumor cells. The unanswered question, therefore, is not whether the cell inoculum can be a source of posttransplant relapse but, rather, whether manipulation of the HSC component can affect this outcome.

It is generally accepted that collections of hematopoietic progenitor cells from the peripheral blood may contain fewer malignant cells than bone marrow collections. However, circulating malignant cells have been found for patients with neuroblastoma, breast cancer, and lymphoma (34). Despite the evidence cited above about the potential contribution of MRD to poor transplant outcome, no study to date in any malignant disease demonstrates a benefit from purging of HSC components intended for autologous transplantation. The hypothesis that purging may be beneficial for patients with B-cell malignancies such as chronic lymphocytic leukemia (CLL) or non-Hodgkin's lymphoma is supported by clinical reports from both the University of Nebraska Medical Center and Dana-Farber Cancer Institute transplant programs. The Nebraska program reported that 10 of 11 patients transplanted with marrow from which lymphoma cells could be cultured relapsed after transplantation compared with 2 of 13 patients who received "culture-negative" grafts (35). This group subsequently reported a four-fold greater PFS (57% versus 17%) for recipients of grafts with no detectable MRD (36). Only the assigned risk group and the presence of a positive culture from the HSC inoculum predicted for relapse in a subsequent randomized study conducted by this group comparing PBSCs and marrow as sources of HSCs (37).

The Dana-Farber transplant program reported similar differences in disease-free survival (DFS) based on the presence or absence of detectable MRD in trials involving antibody-mediated purging (38–40). In these studies, using sensitive polymerase chain reaction (PCR) techniques to monitor the presence of tumor cells before and after purging with monoclonal antibodies and complement, patients who had documented persistence of tumor cells had a significantly lower probability of DFS than patients who received components that were PCR negative after purging. The difference in DFS remains highly significant even after 10 years of follow-up (Kaplan-Meier estimate of DFS probability of 80% versus 10%) (41). These publications provide the strongest evidence to date that complete tumor cell purging (based on the most sensitive tumor cell detection assays available) is both necessary and beneficial. This group reported much less success in achieving PCR negativity in the purging of components from patients with mantle cell non-Hodgkin's lymphoma and a concomitant high relapse rate after transplantation for that disease (42). Although the number of patients transplanted for CLL was too small for definitive conclusions, the Dana-Farber group likewise suggested a higher probability of DFS for those patients who received PCR-negative HSC components (43).

These MRD detection techniques are surrogate markers for transplant outcome. It is, therefore, not surprising that other transplant programs have published contradictory reports. For example, one group reported relapses for three of four patients treated for follicular non-Hodgkin's lymphoma whose bone marrow components became PCR negative after purging with one antibody and complement but for only 11 of 25 patients who received PCR-positive marrow (44). A multivariate analysis to determine the risk of relapse for 24 patients with poor-prognosis non-Hodgkin's lymphoma transplanted with unpurged PBSCs by other investigators did not demonstrate any effect from tumor cell contamination on risk of relapse after transplantation (45). Yet these investigators did report that the persistence or return of tumor cells detected by molecular analysis into the blood or marrow after transplantation predicted for relapse in 81% of the patients, and that patients with detectable disease after transplantation experienced a 24-fold higher risk of relapse compared with patients who became and remained PCR negative.

An alternative explanation of the Nebraska and Dana-Farber Cancer Institute reports is that the detection of tumor in the graft with or without purging reflects the quantity of tumor cells in the component which, in turn, is proportional to the amount in the patient. Patients with higher body burdens of tumor are less likely to achieve a durable remission after HSC transplantation. Sharp et al., however, assigned patients with bone marrow involvement to PBSC transplantation, so the better PFS observed by them after PBSC transplantation does not support the contention that marrow contamination reflects overall body burden of tumor. Although many patients relapse at sites of previous disease, this could reflect preferential trafficking into previous sites of disease of malignant lymphocytes reintroduced with the HSC inoculum (46). Recurrence at previous sites of disease is not conclusive evidence that residual disease in the patient is the only source of relapse after autologous HSC transplantation. The discrepancy between the experiences of these various centers could reflect the importance of adequate purging, differences in patient selection, or the efficacy of the conditioning regimen. This discrepancy also illustrates the need for properly designed studies to directly address the benefit and toxicity of purging. A variety of purging agents have been tested in phase I and II studies. The numbers of patients estimated to be required for definitive phase III tests of purging efficacy has discouraged the conduct of these studies.

Cryopreservation of HSC Components

The primary difficulty in using HSC components to reduce the hematologic toxicity of dose-intense regimens is the necessity for cryopreservation. Three considerations apply. First, current cryopreservation techniques for PBSC components require cryopreservation of both the HSCs that account for about 1% of the nucleated cell population of the component and the mature blood cells that do not contribute to the recovery of bone marrow function after infusion. These mature cells both increase the volume of the component (thereby increasing the amount of cryoprotectant solution added) and appear to contribute to the postinfusion morbidity experienced by the recipient (47). Second, the recipient of cryopreserved HSC components may experience considerable toxicity from the dimethylsulfoxide used in the cryoprotectant solution that relates to the DMSO dose. Third, the cryopreservation of HSCs is technically difficult.

Long-term cryopreservation of cells using DMSO requires storage and shipping of cells at a temperature below − 135°C, generally using liquid nitrogen containers. The thawing of large numbers of bags of cells is usually performed by a skilled laboratory technologist at the patient's bedside.

A high incidence of generally mild, infusion-related morbidity with the reinfusion of cryopreserved cells has been reported by several centers (48–50). Dimethylsulfoxide has a variety of pharmacologic effects (51) that are compounded by the presence of lysed blood cells, foreign proteins from tumor cell purging procedures, or contaminants from nonpharmaceutical grades of reagents used by some laboratories in the processing. The LD_{50} values (amount of DMSO required to kill 50% of test animals) reported for intravenous infusion of DMSO are 3.1 to 9.2 g/kg for mice and 2.5 g/kg for dogs (52). The acute toxic dose of DMSO for humans has not been determined. If a large amount of cryopreserved material is to be infused (e.g., >1g DMSO/kg of patient weight), the infusion can be separated over 2 days to avoid complications from infusion of excessive amounts of DMSO. Because the osmolality of thawed bone marrow (with 10% DMSO) is about 1,800 mOsm/kg, central venous catheters are the preferred route of administration. The incidence of the more common reactions appears to be related to the volume of the product infused. The most dramatic toxicity is the rare anaphylactic reaction occurring during the initial administration of thawed cells. This appears to be an allergic reaction to DMSO or other components of the solution used for cryopreservation and, after resuscitation of the recipient, the remainder of the cells may be administered cautiously. Nonallergic, profound hypotension may result from the intravenous infusion of DMSO, presumably from histamine-induced vasodilation, especially for patients who were not adequately premedicated with appropriate antihistaminic medications such as diphenhydramine (51,52). Skin flushing, dyspnea, abdominal cramping, nausea, and diarrhea, reported to varying degrees after HSC infusion, can also all be attributed to DMSO-induced histamine release. These complaints resolve over a few hours and are treated symptomatically. Dimethylsulfoxide affects the cardiovascular system in a variety of ways. In a series of 82 patients who were premedicated with diphenhydramine, both increased blood pressure and decreased heart rate maximal about 1 hour after the completion of the marrow infusion were observed (48). A number of authors have noted cardiac arrest or high-degree heart block occurring during or immediately after the infusion of cryopreserved marrow or PBSCs (53,54). In two series, the incidence of bradycardia (heart rate <60 beats/min) was 48.8% and 65%, second-degree heart block was 9.7% and 24%, and complete (third-degree) heart block was 4.8% and 5.9% (53,54). In both reports, the median time of onset was about 3 hours after the completion of the infusion. In one series, the authors noted that the heart block was often episodic, occurring with episodes of emesis (53). In both series, the cardiac rhythm abnormalities resolved spontaneously within 24 hours of infusion. In contrast, another group found no cardiac rhythm changes in a prospective series of 29 patients (55). A slower overall infusion rate may have accounted for the lack of rhythm changes. Headache has been reported in up to 70% of recipients of cryopreserved cells (50), but other central nervous system complications are rare and generally related to the amount of DMSO infused. Two recipients who received HSC components containing a total of 225 ml and 120 ml, respectively, of DMSO developed reversible encephalopathy (56). The first patient underwent plasmapheresis with prompt improvement in mental status; the second patient recovered over 5 days without specific treatment. The weights of the patients were not cited in this report, but both patients probably received over 2 g DMSO per kilogram of body weight. The infusion of large quantities of poorly cryopreserved mature blood cells may cause renal failure (57). Seizures have been associated with the infusion of highly concentrated PBSC products, suggesting that freezing at very high cell concentrations is not an acceptable strategy to avoid large volumes of DMSO (47).

Posttransplant Support

Administration of hematopoietic growth factors may speed engraftment after allogeneic or autologous transplantation. A variety of growth factors are now available. Randomized studies of granulocyte-macrophage colony-stimulating factor (GM-CSF) or G-CSF administration after autologous HSC transplantation demonstrated that these hematopoietic cytokines speed granulocyte recovery, decrease the morbidity caused by the transplant procedure, and are associated with a smaller probability of relapse (58–60). But this has not consistently translated into earlier hospital discharge or reduced transplant cost. Administration of cytokines that primarily stimulate the proliferation of mature hematopoietic progenitor cells may not greatly affect the time to initial hematopoietic recovery after transplantation, although the subsequent rate of rise in peripheral blood counts is notably enhanced, suggesting that adequate numbers of cells at the appropriate maturational stage must be present before growth-regulatory effect from these cytokines can be obtained (61). Late administration of cytokine support (starting several days after HSC infusion) may be as effective as early administration while being less costly to the patient (62).

Complications of High-dose Therapy

The patient undergoing dose-intense therapy with autologous HSC transplantation experiences a period of bone marrow hypoplasia that can persist for days or (rarely, with PBSCs) weeks. During this time, the patient requires antibiotic and blood component support, but death from infection or hemorrhage is uncommon.

Common nonhematopoietic toxicity that is not life-threatening includes alopecia, sterility, and varying degrees of mucositis with concomitant mouth pain, inanition, and diarrhea. Rarely, mucositis compromises airway patency, and intubation of the patient is temporarily required for airway protection. Serious organ toxicity includes hepatic venocclusive disease (from high-dose regimens in general), interstitial pneumonitis (e.g., BCNU-induced), cardiomyopathy (e.g., cyclophosphamide-induced), and hemorrhagic cystitis (e.g., cyclophosphamide-induced). The risk of nonhematopoietic toxicity increases for older patients and for patients who previously received intensive chemotherapy regimens. For these patients, reduction of dose of the transplant conditioning regimen reduces toxicity but possibly increases risk of disease relapse.

The development of myelodysplasia or secondary leukemia is being increasingly reported for patients previously treated with autologous HSC transplantation, particularly for patients with the diagnosis of non-Hodgkin's lymphoma (63,64). The incidence of this complication appears to be small in patients treated for leukemia (64) but has been reported above 10% for patients treated for lymphoid malignancies (63).

Adjuvant Therapy with Autologous HSC Transplantation

The incidence of relapse after high-dose therapy leads to the conclusion that high-dose therapy with autologous HSC transplantation, although well tolerated and likely to prolong life, should be viewed as a platform for other approaches that may be effective in eliminating the MRD of patients destined to relapse after dose-intense therapy is administered. Additional or yet higher-dose chemotherapy or radiotherapy, unless directly targeted to the tumor target, increases the risks of nonhematopoietic toxicity and loss of patients from causes other than relapse. Immunologically based therapies are of interest in this regard and include administration of posttransplant cytokines (65), the addition of tumor-specific antibodies used before or after transplantation or both as an "in vivo purge,"(66) and the development of tumor-specific vaccines such as with tumor-antigen pulsed dendritic cells (DCs). Preliminary data of DC-derived cellular vaccines illustrate the potential promise of cell-based therapy of patients with multiple myeloma and other types of cancer, such as renal cell carcinoma, pancreatic or prostate cancer, and melanoma (67–69). Clinical studies of DC therapy for patients with multiple myeloma mostly use the autologous idiotype protein, which is unique to the malignant clone, as a tumor-associated antigen for DC pulsing (69,70–72). The treatment appeared to be well tolerated by patients with, if any, minor and transient side effects (72,73). After vaccination, idiotype-specific responses were observed, characterized by T cell-proliferative responses with cytokine release and the production of antiidiotype antibodies (70,73).

DISEASES

Acute Myelogenous Leukemia

Induction chemotherapy yields complete remission for most patients with acute myelogenous leukemia, but these patients will rapidly relapse without postinduction consolidation therapy. Randomized studies of consolidation regimens of varying intensity demonstrate that intensity is correlated with probability of durable remissions (74). The role of autologous or allogeneic HSC transplantation as intensive consolidation therapy for patients entering first remission has been explored in several randomized studies that assigned patients with available sibling donors to allogeneic transplantation and randomized other patients to autologous transplantation or nontransplant consolidation therapy (75–79). In general, autologous bone marrow transplantation has not proven to be more effective than nontransplant intensive consolidation chemotherapy (Table 37.2). In a study sponsored by the Eastern Cooperative Oncology Group (ECOG), patients assigned to allogeneic transplantation achieved a 43% DFS compared with 35% for patients assigned to chemotherapy and 35% for patients assigned to autologous transplantation using marrow cells purged ex vivo with a cyclophosphamide derivative (75). Overall survival (OS) was slightly but significantly higher for chemotherapy-treated patients because of the ability to rescue patients who relapsed, with subsequent autologous transplantation administered in second remission. However, only 54% of patients assigned to autologous transplantation in the ECOG-sponsored study received this treatment, raising the question of whether a difference could have been found with better compliance. Furthermore, transplant-related mortality was 14% for patients assigned to the autologous marrow transplant group, which is higher than would be expected for PBSC transplantation. In contrast, in one study the DFS at 7 years was 54% for recipients of autologous transplantation compared to 40% for recipients of chemotherapy ($P = 0.04$) (76). Another study demonstrated a significantly

TABLE 37.2. MULTICENTER RANDOMIZED STUDIES COMPARING AUTOLOGOUS MARROW TRANSPLANTATION TO INTENSIVE CONSOLIDATION CHEMOTHERAPY

	Probability of Event-Free Survival (%)		
Investigator	Allogeneic	Autologous	Chemotherapy
Zittoun (79)	55[a]	48	30 (4 year)[c]
Cassileth (75)	43	35	35 (4 year)
Burnett (76)	ND[b]	53[a]	40 (7 year)
Harousseau (77)	44	44	40 (4 year)
Ravindranath (78)	ND[b]	38	36 (3 year)

[a] Significantly different compared to chemotherapy treatment arm.
[b] ND; Allogeneic transplantation was not performed as part of this trial.
[c] Shown is the median duration of follow-up at time of analysis.

better DFS for recipients of allogeneic transplantation (48% versus 30%, P = 0.04) compared to recipients of chemotherapy. The probability of DFS for recipients of autologous bone marrow was intermediate, but not significantly different from either of the two other arms (79).

The role for autologous transplantation in the treatment of patients in first remission is not obvious, and questions remain about the selection of HSC source, value of ex vivo purging, and timing of transplantation relative to other cycles of postinduction consolidation.

A number of phase II studies of autologous transplantation for the treatment of patients with acute myelogenous leukemia in second or later remission have been published (80,81). Many of these studies reported survival probabilities of 35% or better, which is higher than what would be expected with standard chemotherapy regimens. Autologous HSC transplantation appears to be effective therapy for the patient with acute myelogenous leukemia in second complete remission.

Purging of tumor cells may be beneficial. In nonrandomized studies, patients who received marrow cells treated with chemotherapy agents were less likely to relapse after transplantation (82). Similarly, indirect laboratory assessments of purging efficacy suggest a benefit for patients who are treated with an aggressive purging technique (83,84). The role of purging has not been proven in randomized studies, nor has it been shown to be of benefit for recipients of PBSCs.

Acute Lymphoblastic Leukemia

Few adults with acute lymphoblastic leukemia (ALL) are currently cured with induction and consolidation regimens (85). Results have improved modestly with more intensive postremission chemotherapy and with tailoring of protocols in individuals with specific subsets of ALL. The performance of allogeneic bone marrow transplant in first remission is effective in some individuals (e.g., those with Philadelphia (Ph)1-positive ALL). There are few data, however, supporting the effectiveness of autologous HSC transplantation as currently performed in ALL despite its theoretic potential. Two published reports comparing autologous to allogeneic bone marrow transplantation reported DFS after autologous transplantation similar to that reported for patients undergoing less intense induction and maintenance chemotherapy (approximately 20% to 30%) (86,87). Investigators from the University of Minnesota and Dana-Farber transplant programs reported 56 recipients out of 214 adults alive and without disease at a median of 25 months after transplantation (86). Another group reported 3-year probability of DFS of 68% for recipients allocated to receive allogeneic transplantation from an HLA-matched sibling donor compared to 26% for recipients of autologous transplantation (87). The randomized addition of posttransplant interleukin-2 therapy after autologous transplantation did not improve the DFS. A similar matched pair study involving children transplanted in second remission reported a 9-year probability of DFS of 26% for patients undergoing autologous transplantation compared to 32% for similar patients treated with chemotherapy alone (88). In contrast, others reported a 1-year DFS of 50% for adult patients transplanted in first remission and 27% for patients in second or later remission using bone marrow with or without ex vivo purging (89).

Chronic Myelogenous Leukemia

Limited numbers of patients with chronic myelogenous leukemia in chronic phase or with more advanced disease have been treated with autologous HSC transplantation (90). In a large, single-center study of 73 patients, the survival of patients with chronic-phase disease who underwent transplantation did not differ from patients treated with interferon. Of patients with more advanced disease, 58% achieved a complete hematologic remission but only 10% achieved a complete cytogenetic response, and the median survival for this group of patients was only 5 months. Autologous HSC transplantation for this disease is, in general, limited to clinical research protocols.

Chronic Lymphocytic Leukemia

Aggressive treatment is less likely to be used in chronic lymphocytic leukemia because of its long natural history, indolent nature, and the advanced age of most patients (91). Although the disease responds to chemotherapy and radiotherapy initially, relapse is inevitable. The extensive infiltration of bone marrow by malignant lymphocytes has served to focus transplantation trials on allogeneic transplantation or autologous transplantation with HSC products collected in remission or purged ex vivo. Few clinical studies have been reported. Investigators from the M.D. Anderson Cancer Institute reported 6 of 11 patients treated with autologous marrow cells (seven purged ex vivo) surviving in remission up to 29 months after transplantation (92). Investigators at the Dana-Farber Cancer Institute reported a high complete remission response rate for 12 patients who received autologous bone marrow that had been purged with multiple monoclonal antibodies (93). Relapses are the most frequent source of late mortality; many attempts have been made to achieve a tumor-free cell inoculum (94). Currently, autologous HSC transplantation is limited to clinical research protocols.

Multiple Myeloma and Other Plasma Cell Diseases

Multiple myeloma is a malignancy of plasma cells with a median age at time of diagnosis of 65 years. The poor long-term survival of patients treated with standard-dose regimens led to the exploration of high-dose regimens with or without HSC support. In 1983, McElwain et al. reported the use of high-dose melphalan (140 mg/m^2) for nine patients with refractory myeloma and noted dramatic response (95). This led to a series of phase I and II studies of high-dose therapy with autologous bone marrow or PBSC support, and eventually to phase III studies comparing standard and high-dose regimens. In 1993 the French Myeloma Intergroup reported a large-scale (200 patients) randomized trial that demonstrated the superiority of high-dose therapy (3). Patients treated with high-dose therapy consisting of melphalan and TBI after four cycles of induction therapy showed higher complete response rates (22% versus 5%), median event-free survival (EFS) (27 months versus 18 months), and median OS

TABLE 37.3. RISK FACTORS FOR SURVIVAL AFTER AUTOLOGOUS TRANSPLANTATION FOR MULTIPLE MYELOMA

Event-Free Survival[a]			Overall Survival		
Variable	**RR**	**P**	**Variable**	**RR**	**P**
No change in chromosome 13	0.5	<.0001	No change in chromosome 13	0.4	<.0001
β2M ≤2.5 mg/l	0.7	<.0001	β2M ≤2.5 mg/l	0.6	<.0001
≤12 m therapy	0.7	<.0001	≤12 m Therapy	0.7	.0001
Sensitive disease	0.8	<.0001	CRP ≤4.0 mg/l	0.7	<.0002
Any 2nd transplant	0.8	.0004	Sensitive disease	0.8	.0002
Non-IgA	0.7	.002	Non-IgA	0.7	.002
Any CR	0.8	.002	Any 2nd transplant	0.04	<.0001

β-2-microglobulin, immunoglobulin A; CRP, C-reactive protein; CR, complete remission.
[a] From Desikan, R, Barlogie B, Sawyer J, et al. Results of high-dose therapy for 1000 patients with multiple myeloma: durable complete remissions and superior survival in the absence of chromosome 13 abnormalities. *Blood* 2000;95:4008–4010, with permission.

(60 months or longer versus 37 months). A matched pair analysis conducted by Southwest Oncology Group reached a similar conclusion (96). A benefit in overall survival could be gained even for patients who underwent delayed high-dose therapy (median survivals from time of diagnosis of 64 and 63 months), although the complete response rate and quality of life were not as good (97).

These studies, however, did not show a plateau in the survival probability curves, indicating that all patients will ultimately relapse and succumb to this disease. Molecular monitoring of bone marrow samples shows a high incidence of residual disease after autologous transplantation (98). The persistence or reappearance of clonal markers using sensitive detection techniques for patients who have achieved a clinical complete remission indicates relapse in the immediate future. Retrospective reviews of large numbers of patients have identified a number of risk factors for both disease progression and overall survival after high-dose chemotherapy and autologous transplantation (Table 37.3) (99).

One possible reason for relapse after autologous transplantation is the reintroduction of malignant cells with the cryopreserved HSC component. In a multicenter randomized study of enrichment of $CD34^+$ cells as a technique to purge $CD34^-$ cells including $CD34^-$ tumor cells from the HSC component (100), 131 patients with myeloma were enrolled, and all components were analyzed before and after processing by PCR determination assay using patient-specific immunoglobulin (Ig) gene primers. Clonal Ig sequences could be found in 42% of the study group and 30% of the control group. No tumor cells were detected in the apheresis collection for 14% of the study group and 21% of the control group. CD34 selection removed all detectable tumor cells for 11 of 24 of the study group patients whose components were positive; a median 3.1-log depletion was achieved by the processing. However, progression-free survivals at 1 year after transplantation did not differ between the two groups. $CD34^+$ cell enrichment is a nonselective tumor cell depletion technique; unless the malignant myeloma stem cells are $CD34^+$, these data indicate that reintroduction of tumor cells is not the primary cause of failure after autologous HSC transplantation.

Cytogenetic information is limited in multiple myeloma because the cells are mainly terminally differentiated B cells with low proliferative activity. Abnormal karyotypes are observed in only 30% to 50% of cases, but the rate is higher for relapsing patients (35% to 60%) than for newly diagnosed patients (20% to 35%) (101). The higher incidence of karyotypic abnormalities for relapsing patients presumably reflects an increased proliferative activity for previously treated patients. Flow cytometric analysis of chromosome number and fluorescence in situ hybridization (FISH) studies of interphase cells indicate the presence of cytogenetic abnormalities in 80% to 90% of patients.

A study of the karyotypes of 492 patients with myeloma undergoing autologous HSC transplantation found abnormalities in 133 (27%); 73 (55%) had three or more trisomes involving chromosomes 3, 5, 7, 9, 11, 15, 19, and 21; 57 had complete or partial loss of chromosome 13; and 38 had abnormalities of 1q, 33 involving 14q, 32 involving 1p, 21 involving 11q, and 20 involving 6q (102). Complete or partial deletions of chromosome 13 and 11q abnormalities were found more commonly in patients with stage III disease, low serum albumin levels, elevated serum creatinine levels, and IgA isotype.

This group subsequently reported that of 135 patients enrolled in a study of tandem autologous HSC transplantation, patients with normal cytogenetics had median event-free survival (EFS) and OS of 43 and 50 months or more, respectively (103). The EFS and OS for patients with abnormalities of chromosome 13 were 21 and 29 months; for patients with abnormalities involving 11q, 20 and 21 months; and for patients with abnormalities of both 13 and 11q, 11 and 12 months. The absence of chromosomal abnormalities was the single strongest prognostic factor associated with prolonged survival in this study.

Amyloidosis

Primary amyloidosis is a plasma cell dyscrasia in which clonal plasma cells in the bone marrow produce a monoclonal immunoglobulin protein. These M-protein light chains or light-chain fragments form insoluble fibrils that are deposited into the extracellular matrix of a variety of tissues, resulting in severe organ dysfunction and poor patient survival.

Randomized studies have shown that melphalan-based therapy can prolong the life of patients with primary amyloidosis (104). High-dose therapy with melphalan and autologous PBSC transplantation can induce a complete remission (105). Responders who achieve a complete disappearance of light-chain secretion are more likely to achieve reversal of underlying organ dysfunction (106). Multiorgan disease and cardiac dysfunction in specific predict a poor transplant outcome. In one study, the EFS was 60% for patients with cardiac involvement but 100% for patients with renal involvement and no evidence of cardiac dysfunction (105).

Waldenström's Macroglobulinemia

Waldenström's macroglobulinemia is an incurable lymphoproliferative disorder characterized by the production of IgM paraprotein. In a phase I/II study of autologous transplantation for the treatment of this plasma cell disease (107), seven patients (untreated or after first-line therapy) with symptomatic disease underwent two or three cycles of cytoreductive chemotherapy with collection (and purging) of PBSCs followed by autologous transplantation after conditioning with total body irradiation and high-dose cyclophosphamide. Engraftment was prompt, without any procedure-related deaths. A strong reduction or normalization of the bone marrow infiltration and serum IgM levels occurred in all evaluable patients, but immunofixation electrophoresis revealed persistent paraproteinemia in five. This pilot trial showed that high-dose radiochemotherapy with purged stem cells is effective and may improve patients' clinical courses. In the majority of cases, however, complete eradication of the disease does not appear to be possible with autologous HSC transplantation alone.

Lymphoma

The lymphomas represent a diverse group of hematologic malignancies arising from lymphoid tissues. They vary from the slowest to some of the fastest growing tumors. They also range from highly curable to essentially incurable. Approximately 60,000 new cases are diagnosed each year. The lymphomas are highly responsive to chemotherapy and radiation in most cases. These tumors exhibit a strong dose-response relationship, and the benefit of high-dose treatment with autologous stem cell rescue is well established for some categories of this disease.

Several high-dose chemotherapy regimens have been developed for the treatment of the lymphomas. Radiation-based regimens including cyclophosphamide with TBI and etoposide plus TBI have significant activity but frequently are difficult to administer in patients already exposed to radiotherapy. Popular chemotherapy regimens include cyclophosphamide, BCNU, and etoposide (CBV) and BCNU, etoposide, cytarabine, and melphalan (BEAM). However, no single chemotherapeutic regimen has emerged as a superior treatment.

Hodgkin's Disease

Many patients with Hodgkin's disease will achieve durable remissions with nontransplant chemotherapy with or without radiation therapy, and algorithms for staging and treatment of this disease are well defined. Dose-intense therapy with autologous transplantation should be considered for those patients who do not achieve a remission or who relapse after initial therapy and will succumb without aggressive therapy (4,108).

For patients who suffer a relapse after achieving a complete remission, the prognosis with conventional salvage therapy is directly related to the duration of the initial remission. The outcome for patients whose remissions lasted less than 1 year is dismal with standard-dose second-line treatments, and most experts concur that these patients are best treated with high-dose chemotherapy with stem cell rescue. Approximately 40% to 50% of patients with Hodgkin's disease who suffer a relapse within 1 year will achieve durable remissions after autologous HSC transplantation (109–111).

For patients whose first remission lasts more than 1 year, both conventional-dose chemotherapy and high-dose autologous stem cell therapy provide the possibility of durable second remissions (112). Two randomized trials comparing high-dose chemotherapy with conventional salvage treatment have been performed (4,113). These studies suggest similar overall long-term survival rates but possibly a greater disease-free survival rate for the transplant arms. A British national lymphoma trial compared high-dose BEAM-with-transplant with mini-BEAM salvage therapy. Accrual was terminated prematurely because patients refused randomization and requested the high-dose therapy. Patients who underwent autologous transplantation had statistically greater event-free and progression-free survival rates. Overall survival rates, however, were the same in both groups in this very small trial (4). A second German EBMT trial comparing standard-dose with high-dose treatment revealed improved time to treatment failure with the autologous arm but, again, overall survival in this slightly larger trial was not yet improved (113).

Patients with refractory Hodgkin's disease may achieve durable complete remissions with high-dose chemotherapy and stem cell rescue. Numerous series, including that from the Autologous Blood and Marrow Transplant Registry (ABMTR) demonstrate that high-dose treatment can overcome drug resistance in Hodgkin's disease. In the ABMTR analysis, patients were considered to have primary refractory Hodgkin's disease if they never achieved a complete remission. Following transplantation, the probability of 3-year progression-free survival was 38% with an overall survival rate of 50% (114). Results from an EBMT Registry analysis were similar to that in the American series. The European group reported an actuarial 5-year disease-free survival rate of 30% and an overall survival rate of 34% for patients with refractory Hodgkin's disease (115).

Low-grade Non-Hodgkin's Lymphoma

Low-grade non-Hodgkin's lymphoma, in general, exhibits a variable and prolonged natural course, with many patients not requiring treatment until symptoms or organ toxicity appear. Therefore, most of the experience with HSC transplantation has been in patients after initial relapse rather than at the time of initial diagnosis, avoiding the potential for morbidity and mortality of dose-intense therapy. Randomized studies comparing autologous HSC transplantation to other, nontransplant therapies for patients at time of initial treatment have not been reported. A number of phase II and registry data have been published (116–119). Although response rates are high, a continuing pattern of relapse has been observed with autologous transplant. One group reported a 68% complete remission rate for a single-center series of 100 patients with relapsed disease but, at a median of 4 years, a probability of failure-free survival of 44% with no plateau to the curve depicting probability of relapse (118). The Dana-Farber transplant program reported a series of 86 patients with advanced follicular lymphoma who underwent autologous bone marrow transplantation as part of initial therapy in a publication that raised the question about the necessity for and efficacy of tumor cell purging (40). Patients who received marrow products that were free of disease (based on a sensitive PCR detection technique for the t14; 18 abnormality commonly found in follicular non-Hodgkin's lymphoma) experienced a much lower rate of relapse than similar patients whose products contained detectable tumor after purging. However, no plateau to the curve depicting probability of relapse was reported. Patients who undergo allogeneic transplantation will experience a higher probability of transplant-related mortality but a lower risk of relapse after transplantation (120). The difference in relapse rates could result either from reintroduction of lymphoma cells in the HSC product or from the lack of a graft versus disease effect of autologous transplantation.

Small numbers of patients have undergone autologous HSC transplantation for aggressive non-Hodgkin's lymphoma after transformation from indolent non-Hodgkin's lymphoma (121). A large proportion of these patients achieved durable remissions, suggesting that this therapy should be considered for older patients or those lacking an allogeneic donor.

Aggressive Non-Hodgkin's Lymphoma

The standard of care for patients with B-cell non-Hodgkin's lymphoma in first "chemotherapy-sensitive" relapse is HSC transplantation (122–124). The success of this therapy reflects the extent and the responsiveness of the disease to chemotherapy at the time of transplantation (125,126). Relapse is the major cause of failure of autologous transplantation.

The role of high-dose chemotherapy with stem cell rescue in patients with chemotherapy-sensitive aggressive (intermediate or high-grade) lymphomas in relapse has become well established. The Parma trial randomized 109 patients in first chemotherapy-sensitive relapse after two cycles of salvage chemotherapy to either high-dose therapy or four additional cycles of conventional-dose treatment. The EFS at 5 years was superior for the group undergoing high-dose therapy compared with the group receiving standard-dose treatment (46% versus 12%, $P = 0.001$). The same superiority for transplant was true of 5-year overall survival (53% versus 32%, $P = 0.038$). Furthermore, it is notable that in the Parma trial no patients assigned to the conventional-dose salvage therapy could be rescued at the time of second relapse with a delayed transplant. Therefore, excessive pretransplant "debulking" therapy with or without delays in transplant timing should be avoided. This randomized trial, which confirmed previous phase II studies, conclusively demonstrated that transplantation therapy represents the treatment of choice for most patients with chemotherapy-sensitive first-relapsed aggressive non-Hodgkin's lymphoma (5).

Hematopoietic stem cell transplant may also be indicated for patients who respond slowly to initial therapy, have high-risk disease, are resistant to initial therapy, and are in relapse with chemotherapy-insensitive disease. The appropriate approach for patients who achieve less than a complete response or who exhibit a slow response to conventional induction therapy is not yet clear. In one small trial of 69 slow responders to CHOP chemotherapy (cyclophosphamide, doxorubicin, and vincristine along with prednisolone), the use of early transplant compared to five additional cycles of CHOP was not associated with an overall improvement in survival or EFS ($P < 0.10$) (127).

The International Prognostic Index (IPI) identifies patients with aggressive non-Hodgkin's lymphoma who have a high likelihood of relapse and poor overall survival with conventional first-line therapy (128). The French LNH-87 trial examined the role of consolidation transplantation for patients in first complete remission after standard-dose treatment (123,129). The initial analysis of this trial demonstrated no advantage gained by the addition of intensive consolidation. However, subsequent analysis that included only those patients with high-intermediate or high risk by the more restrictive criteria of the IPI, revealed a superior disease-free survival for those patients undergoing high-dose transplant (123). Similarly, the Italian Non-Hodgkin's Lymphoma Study Group showed no benefit to high-dose therapy with stem cell rescue in patients judged to be at high risk by virtue of tumor bulk or advanced-stage disease (130). However, a striking advantage in disease-free survival was noted when the 70 patients who qualified as high-intermediate or high risk based on the IPI were analyzed. In this subgroup, transplantation yielded a superior 6-year disease-free survival rate (87% versus 48%, $P = 0.008$). Autologous transplantation therapy is likely to be beneficial in patients with high-risk disease as measured by IPI.

Analysis of the ABMTR data showed that among 184 patients who had never achieved a complete remission with conventional therapy (primarily induction failures), 44% could achieve one after autologous bone marrow or PBSC transplantation. The probability of progression-free survival at 5 years after transplantation was 31%. Chemotherapy resistance, administration of multiple cycles of chemotherapy before transplantation, poor performance status at time of transplantation, older age, and the lack of use of consolidative radiotherapy before or after transplantation predicted poor outcome (131).

Patients with disease that is unresponsive to chemotherapy at the time of relapse have a low (about 15% to 20%) chance of achieving a long-term remission with high-dose therapy and stem cell rescue.

Mantle cell lymphoma is known for its unremitting clinical course when treated conventionally and has proven relatively resistant to high-dose treatment, especially when used as a salvage therapy (132). Incorporating high-dose therapy into the initial overall treatment plan, however, may be more likely to provide durable remissions. At M.D. Anderson Cancer Institute the results of using an intensive induction regimen followed by autologous transplantation have been encouraging (133). Among previously untreated patients, the EFS rate at 3 years was 72%.

Burkitt's lymphoma, Burkitt's-like lymphomas, and lymphoblastic lymphomas are eminently curable in most children. However, these high-grade non-Hodgkin's lymphomas are associated with relatively poor long-term survival rates in adults. Data from the European Bone Marrow Transplant Registry (EBMTR) suggests that disease status at the time of transplant is the most important predictor of outcome in patients with high-grade disease (126). For Burkitt's and Burkitt's-like lymphoma, the 3-year actuarial overall survival rate was 72% for patients transplanted during first complete remission, compared with 37% in those with chemotherapy-sensitive relapse, and 7% in patients with disease that is unresponsive to chemotherapy. For patients with lymphoblastic lymphoma, the 6-year actuarial survival rate ranged from 63% in patients who were in first complete remission to 15% in those who had resistant disease. Patients in second complete remission had an intermediate survival rate of 31% at 6 years. These results with transplantation are superior to conventional-dose salvage therapy.

Solid Tumors

Autologous transplantation for the treatment of solid tumors is less established, primarily because most malignancies do not exhibit the strong dose response to myelosuppressive chemotherapeutic agents. Exceptions are germ cell tumors and some pediatric malignancies such as neuroblastoma. Breast cancer, which at one point was the most frequent indication for autologous transplantation (134), is a subject of controversy pending the final analysis of randomized trials. Small cell lung cancer and ovarian carcinoma are being studied in clinical trials of autologous transplantation.

Breast Cancer

Approximately 180,000 women in the United States will develop this cancer each year and nearly 40,000 will die. Although disease confined to the breasts and the lymph nodes is curable with multimodality therapy (surgery, radiation, chemotherapy, and hormone manipulation), once breast cancer has spread to distant organs cure may not be possible. Adjuvant chemotherapy shows improved EFS for patients at high risk of developing metastatic disease. The experience of Bonadonna and others showing a dose response for this malignancy led investigators in the early 1990s to explore the use of dose-intense chemotherapy regimens for women with micrometastases involving ten or more axillary lymph nodes and in women with inflammatory breast cancer. Peters et al. treated 102 women with high-risk (≥10 axillary lymph nodes positive for disease) stage IIA, IIB, IIIA or IIIB cancer with four cycles of standard-dose CAF chemotherapy followed by high-dose STAMP-1 (cyclophosphamide, carmustine (BCNU), and cisplatin) chemotherapy with autologous stem cell rescue (135). The actuarial EFS for the study population at 2.5 years was 72%. Comparison to three historic or concurrent Cancer and Leukemia Group B adjuvant chemotherapy trials selected for similar patients showed an EFS at 2.5 years to be between 38% and 52%. The 3-year probability of progression-free survival was 65% for stage II and 60% for stage III patients for a review of over 5,000 transplants for breast cancer performed at U.S. transplant programs using outcomes data submitted to the North American ABMTR (134).

Several randomized trials performed to determine the role of high-dose chemotherapy for patients with ten or more involved axillary lymph nodes were recently closed to patient accrual. Interim analyses of the largest trials have been reported in abstract form.

- Preliminary analysis of the Netherlands Cancer Institute study's leading 284 patients (with the longest follow-up) showed a 3-year progression-free survival for the transplantation arm of 77% and for the conventional-dose arm of 62% (P = 0.009) (136). The overall survival with transplantation also compared favorably (89% versus 79%, P = 0.039). The high-dose arm, consisting of cyclophosphamide, thiotepa, and carboplatinum (STAMP-5 regimen) and PBSC support was well tolerated, with four deaths from transplant-related causes (<1%) compared with one death in the nontransplant group. The complete cohort of 885 patients will be analyzed in 2002.
- In contrast, preliminary results of a U.S. intergroup trial in which all patients received four cycles of standard-dose chemotherapy followed by randomization to transplantation using a conditioning regimen consisting of STAMP-1 with bone marrow, or PBSC support, or a single cycle of the same drugs at lower (but still above conventional) doses did not demonstrate a significant difference (137). At a median follow-up of 5.1 years, the EFS was 61% for the transplant group and 60% for the chemotherapy group. There were fewer relapses after transplantation (29% versus 39%) but more treatment-related deaths. Overall survival rates at 5 years were also similar. The lack of difference in the EFS to date was attributed to the 7.4% peritransplant mortality rate in the transplant arm as a result of pulmonary toxicity from the dose-intense conditioning regimen; this rate was much higher than observed in other studies.
- A Scandinavian study enrolled 575 women with high-risk breast cancer who were randomized between nine cycles of dose-intensive "tailored" chemotherapy with 5-fluorouracil, epirubicin, and cyclophosphamide (FEC) regimen versus three cycles of standard-dose FEC followed by transplantation using STAMP-5 and bone marrow infusion. With the median follow-up of only 23 months, the survivals of the two arms are equivalent at approximately 80% (138).
- An Italian trial for women with four or more involved axillary lymph nodes noted no overall survival advantage for high-dose therapy with 5-year progression-free survival rates of 76% for transplant recipients and 77% for standard adjuvant therapy recipients. Among younger patients (<36 years) there was a trend towards improved progression-free survival with transplantation (139).

The ABMTR data, single-institution studies, and historic case control trials have all suggested that transplantation might have a role for patients with high-risk breast cancer. Until there is formal analysis of the randomized studies noted above, the role of high-dose chemotherapy will be unknown.

Inflammatory breast cancer represents a unique clinical entity with a high propensity for both local and distant metastatic spread. Given the rarity of inflammatory breast carcinoma, no formal randomized trials have been performed in this disease. In one series 47 consecutive patients with stage IIIB inflammatory breast cancer were treated with standard-dose induction chemotherapy followed by high-dose chemotherapy and stem cell support (140). At 30 months, the Kaplan-Meier estimates of disease-free and overall survival from diagnosis were 57% and 59% respectively. At 4 years, the Kaplan-Meier estimate of disease-free survival and overall survival from diagnosis were 51%. In a multivariate analysis, the factors associated with better survival were favorable response to the initial neoadjuvant chemotherapy and receipt of tamoxifen.

Metastatic breast cancer is rarely curable, although some women will benefit from a more indolent course lasting years with responses to a variety of different regimens. A role of dose-intense therapy is not clear for this stage of this disease. The United States Intergroup Trial noted similar survival rates for one cycle of high-dose chemotherapy compared to 24 months of CMF (cyclophosphamide, methotrexate, and 5-fluorouracil) conventional-dose treatment (141). This trial, opened for accrual in 1990, registered 553 patients, of whom 513 were eligible to receive salvage chemotherapy. After receiving six cycles of induction treatment, patients were randomized to either a single transplant using the STAMP-5 regimen or maintenance chemotherapy with CMF for 18 months or until progression. Of the eligible patients, only 11% achieved a complete response and 47% had a partial response to initial salvage chemotherapy. Of the 296 patients eligible for randomization, only 199 were randomized. One hundred ten women were treated with transplant and 89 were treated with maintenance CMF. The 3-year overall survival rates were 32% for patients receiving transplant and 38% for patients receiving CMF. The 3-year progression-free survivals were 6% and 12% respectively. In summary, there were no differences in complete response rates, time to progression-free survival, 3-year progression-free survival, or 3-year overall survival in this analysis.

Germ Cell Tumors

Germ cell cancers are relatively uncommon diseases accounting for about 1% of all malignancies in (primarily adolescent and young) men. Germ cell tumors, highly curable with nontransplant therapies, are classified as seminomatous or nonseminomatous tumors.

Despite a propensity for metastatic spread, germ cell cancers are one of the most highly curable human malignancies. Over 60% of patients with high-risk disseminated disease will achieve durable responses after treatment with four cycles of cisplatin, etoposide, and bleomycin. Patients with refractory disease or who relapse after initial treatment can be effectively rescued with one or two cycles of dose-intense therapy.

Forty cisplatin-refractory patients were entered into a large multicenter phase II (ECOG-sponsored) trial of carboplatinum and etoposide, of whom 58% (22 patients) were able to proceed to a second cycle (142). Toxicity included five patients (13%) dying of treatment-related causes including infection, hemorrhage, and hepatic venoocclusive disease. All treatment-related deaths occurred during the first course of therapy. Nine patients (24%) achieved a complete response (including two patients after surgical resection of residual disease). Another eight patients achieved a partial response for an overall response rate of 45%. Three of the complete responses occurred after the first bone marrow transplant, and for four patients the partial response converted to complete response after the second bone marrow transplant. Five of the nine patients were alive and free of disease at a minimum follow-up of 18 months. A striking finding of this study was the poor outcome in patients with nonseminomatous primary mediastinal germ cell tumors. Eleven patients with this diagnosis were enrolled in this study and none obtained a durable complete remission.

The initial ECOG experience with multiple cycles of high-dose therapy has been replicated at single centers. The Memorial Sloan Kettering group treated 58 patients with refractory germ cell tumors with two cycles of high-dose carboplatin, etoposide, and cisplatin. Forty percent achieved a complete response, with a 2-year survival rate of 31%. Patients having pretreatment β-hCG values below 100 and those without retroperitoneal masses fared better (143).

The Indiana University group reported 25 patients who had relapsed following cisplatin-based regimens (144). Patients received one to two cycles of conventional-dose salvage, followed by two cycles of high-dose carboplatin and etoposide with stem cell support. At a median of 26 months of follow-up, 13 patients (52%) remain progression free. This very aggressive schedule resulted in one of the highest response rates noted to date. Based on this and other reports from this program, two cycles of dose-intense therapy with autologous transplantation is now considered to be standard for patients failing initial therapy.

Ovarian Carcinoma

Autologous transplantation for the treatment of ovarian carcinoma remains under active investigation, and promising results have been reported for some groups of women. A randomized study of high-dose chemotherapy for women with low amounts of residual tumor demonstrated a prolongation of DFS for women who received the dose-intense regimen (145). The median survival for these women was 22 months, compared to 11 months for women who received standard-dose chemotherapy ($P = 0.03$).

Other Diseases

Autoimmune Disorders

The improved safety of autologous PBSC transplantation encourages studies of dose-intense therapy in the treatment of nonmalignant diseases, including autoimmune disorders such as multiple sclerosis, scleroderma, systemic lupus erythematosus (SLE), and refractory rheumatoid arthritis. The hypothesis of currently ongoing studies is that dose-intense lymphoablative conditioning regimens will achieve prolonged remission or cure of these diseases by destruction of the clone of cells responsible for the disease. This hypothesis is supported by reports of remission of autoimmune diseases (e.g., rheumatoid arthritis, SLE) that existed as a comorbid condition for patients undergoing autologous or allogeneic transplantation (146,147), although this has not been a universal finding (148). The use of intensive chemoradiotherapy with HSC rescue offers an opportunity to deliver maximally tolerated immunosuppression. Factors that may influence the relative efficacy of this approach include the number and relative resistance to ablation of the responsible lymphoid effector populations and the nature and persistence of the relevant antigen against which the immune response is raised. Although lymphoid effectors are not well defined for these diseases, evidence points to the involvement of T and B lymphocytes. High-dose therapy followed by autologous HSC transplantation may allow the immune system to "reset" with control of the autoreactive lymphocytes. As with the treatment of malignant diseases, depletion of the unwanted lymphoid cell population from the HSC inoculum (purging) might be necessary for optimal clinical outcome. These nonmalignant diseases are debilitating, and appropriate patient selection is necessary so that the risks (morbidity and mortality) are appropriately balanced against the benefits (possibly, lack of progression instead of reversal of damage already incurred) of this therapy.

Some preliminary data on autologous transplantation for the treatment of autoimmune diseases have now been reported. Stabilization or improvement for patients undergoing autologous transplantation for multiple sclerosis has been reported (149). In a recent publication, seven patients with SLE were treated with autologous PBSC transplantation (150). All were refractory to conventional intensive immunosuppressive therapy and two had a creatinine clearance <30 ml/min. Treatment involved mobilization of PBSCs with cyclophosphamide 2 gm/m^2 followed by filgrastim; the PBSCs were depleted of lymphocytes by enrichment of $CD34^+$ cells. The dose-intense immunoablative regimen consisted of cyclophosphamide 50 mg/kg times four and antithymocyte globulin 90 mg/kg. At a median of 25 (12 to 40) months all patients were free of clinical signs of active SLE, suggesting that this approach may be more effective than conventional therapies in refractory SLE.

SUMMARY

Autologous HSC transplantation with dose-intense therapy is now a standard treatment for many diseases. Improved safety of this therapy has increased acceptance by patients and allowed its extension to older patients and those with comorbid diseases. The major failing is the difficulty in curing patients with advanced or refractory diseases. Posttransplant immunologic approaches now being studied may, however, be able to convert the minimal disease remaining after transplantation into a cure. Continued effort will determine if modifications of pretransplant conditioning regimens, choice of HSC source, ex vivo processing, or supplementation of the cell inoculum with other myeloid or lymphoid cells affects engraftment kinetics or immunologic reconstitution, and thereby enhances the therapeutic value of autologous transplantation for patients with malignant and nonmalignant diseases.

REFERENCES

1. Horowitz MM, Rowlings PA. An update from the International Bone Marrow Transplant Registry and the Autologous Blood and Marrow Transplant Registry on current activity in hematopoietic stem cell transplantation. *Curr Opin Hematol* 1997;4:395–400.
2. Gratwohl A, Hermans J, Baldomero H. Blood and marrow transplantation activity in Europe 1995. European Group for Blood and Marrow Transplantation. *Bone Marrow Transplant* 1997;19:407–419.
3. Attal M, Harousseau J-L, Stoppa A-M, et al. A prospective, randomized trial of autologous bone marrow transplantation and chemotherapy in multiple myeloma. *N Engl J Med* 1996;335:91–97.
4. Linch DC, Winfield D, Goldstone AH, et al. Dose intensification with autologous bone-marrow transplantation in relapsed and resistant Hodgkin's disease: results of a BNLI randomized trial. *Lancet* 1993;341:1051–1054.
5. Philip T, Guglielmi C, Hagenbeek A, et al. Autologous bone marrow transplantation as compared with salvage chemotherapy in relapses of chemotherapy-sensitive non-Hodgkin's lymphoma. *N Engl J Med* 1995;333:1540–1545.
6. Santos GW. History of bone marrow transplantation. *Clin Haematol* 1983;12:611–639.
7. Frei E, Elias A, Wheeler C, et al. The relationship between high-dose treatment and combination chemotherapy: the concept of summation dose intensity. *Clin Cancer Res* 1998;4:2027–2037.
8. Bonadonna B, Valagussa P. Dose-response effect of adjuvant chemotherapy in breast cancer. *N Engl J Med* 1981;304:10–15.
9. Wood WC, Budman DR, Korzun AH, et al. Dose and dose intensity of adjuvant chemotherapy for stage II, node-positive breast cancer. *N Engl J Med* 1994;330:1253–1259.
10. Bokemeyer C, Franzke A, Hartmann JT, et al. A phase I/II study of sequential, dose-escalated, high dose ifosfamide plus doxorubicin with peripheral blood stem cell support for the treatment of patients with advanced soft tissue sarcomas. *Cancer* 1997;80:1221–1227.
11. Pettengell R, Woll PJ, Thatcher N, et al. Multicyclic, dose-intensive chemotherapy supported by sequential reinfusion of hematopoietic progenitors in whole blood. *J Clin Oncol* 1995;13:148–156.
12. Moskovitz CH, Nimer SD, Zelenetz AD, et al. A 2-step comprehensive high-dose chemoradiotherapy second-line program for relapsed and refractory Hodgkin disease: analysis by intent to treat and development of a prognostic model. *Blood* 2001;97:616–623.
13. Bensinger W, Appelbaum F, Rowley S, et al. Factors that influence collection and engraftment of autologous peripheral-blood stem cells. *J Clin Oncol* 1995;13:2547–2555.
14. Goldberg SL, Klumpp TR, Magdalinski AJ, et al. Value of the pretransplant evaluation in predicting toxic day 100 mortality among blood stem cell and bone marrow recipients. *J Clin Oncol* 1998;16:3796–3802.
15. Kusnierz-Glaz CR, Schlegel PG, Wong RM, et al. Influence of age on the outcome of 500 autologous bone marrow transplant procedures for hematologic malignancies. *J Clin Oncol* 1997;15:18–25.
16. Press O, Eary JF, Gooley T, et al. A phase I/II trial of iodine-131-tositumomab (anti-CD20), etoposide, cyclophosphamide, and autologous stem cell transplantation for relapsed B-cell lymphomas. *Blood* 2000;96:2934–2942.
17. Bensinger WI, Martin PJ, Storer B, et al. Transplantation of bone marrow as compared with peripheral-blood cells from HLA-identical relatives in patients with hematologic cancers. *N Engl J Med* 2001;344:175–181.
18. Nadamanee A, Sniecinski I, Schmidt GM, et al. High-dose therapy followed by autologous peripheral-blood stem-cell transplantation for patients with Hodgkin's disease and non-Hodgkin's lymphoma using unprimed and granulocyte colony-stimulating factor–mobilized peripheral-blood stem cells. *J Clin Oncol* 1994;12:2176–2186.
19. Sheridan WP, Begley CG, To LB, et al. Phase II study of autologous filgrastim (G-CSF)-mobilized peripheral blood progenitor cells to restore hemopoiesis after high-dose chemotherapy for lymphoid malignancies. *Bone Marrow Transplant* 1994;14:105–111.
20. Sheridan WP, Begley CG, Juttner CA, et al. Effect of peripheral-blood progenitor cells mobilised by filgrastim (G-CSF) on platelet recovery after high-dose chemotherapy. *Lancet* 1992;339:640–644.
21. Weaver CH, Hazelton B, Birch R, et al. An analysis of engraftment kinetics as a function of the CD34 content of peripheral blood progen-

itor cell collections in 692 patients after the administration of myeloablative chemotherapy. *Blood* 1995;86:3961–3969.
22. Beyer J, Schwella N, Zingsem J, et al. Hematopoietic rescue after high-dose chemotherapy using autologous peripheral-blood progenitor cells or bone marrow: a randomized comparison. *J Clin Oncol* 1995;13: 1328–1335.
23. Schmitz N, Linch DC, Dreger P, et al. Randomised trial of filgrastim-mobilised peripheral blood progenitor cell transplantation versus autologous bone-marrow transplantation in lymphoma patients. *Lancet* 1996;347:353–357.
24. Haas R, Möhle R, Frühauf S, et al. Patient characteristics associated with successful mobilizing and autografting of peripheral blood progenitor cells in malignant lymphoma. *Blood* 1994;83:3787–3794.
25. Tricot G, Jagannath S, Vesole D, et al. Peripheral blood stem cell transplants for multiple myeloma: identification of favorable variables for rapid engraftment in 225 patients. *Blood* 1995;85:588–596.
26. Schwella N, Beyer J, Schwaner I, et al. Impact of preleukapheresis cell counts on collection results and correlation of progenitor-cell dose with engraftment after high-dose chemotherapy in patients with germ cell cancer. *J Clin Oncol* 1996;14:1114–1121.
27. Offner F, Schoch G, Fisher LD, et al. Mortality hazard functions as related to neutropenia at different times after marrow transplantation. *Blood* 1996;88:4058–4062.
28. Pecora AL. Progress in clinical application of use of progenitor cells expanded with hematopoietic growth factors. *Curr Opin Hematol* 2001;8:142–148.
29. Niederwieser DW, Appelbaum FR, Gastl G, et al. Inadvertent transmission of a donor's acute myeloid leukemia in bone marrow transplantation for chronic myelocytic leukemia. *N Engl J Med* 1990;322: 1794–1796.
30. Penn I. Donor transmitted disease: Cancer. *Transplant Proc* 1991;23: 2629–2631.
31. Brenner MK, Rill DR, Moen RC, et al. Gene-marking to trace origin of relapse after autologous bone-marrow transplantation. *Lancet* 1993; 341:85–86.
32. Rill DR, Santana VM, Roberts WM, et al. Direct demonstration that autologous bone marrow transplantation for solid tumors can return a multiplicity of tumorigenic cells. *Blood* 1994;84:380–383.
33. Deisseroth AB, Zu Z, Claxton D, et al. Genetic marking shows that Ph+ cells present in autologous transplants of chronic myelogenous leukemia (CML) contribute to relapse after autologous bone marrow in CML. *Blood* 1994;83:3068–3076.
34. Moss TJ, Ross AA. The risk of tumor cell contamination in peripheral blood stem cell collections. *J Hematotherapy* 1992;1:225–232.
35. Sharp JG, Joshi SS, Armitage JO, et al. Significance of detection of occult non-Hodgkin's lymphoma in histologically uninvolved bone marrow by a culture technique. *Blood* 1992;79:1074–1080.
36. Sharp JG, Kessinger A, Mann S, et al. Outcome of high-dose therapy and autologous transplantation in non-Hodgkin's lymphoma based on the presence of tumor in the marrow or infused hematopoietic harvest. *J Clin Oncol* 1996;14:214–219.
37. Vose JM, Sharp JG, Chan W, et al. High-dose chemotherapy (HDC) and autotransplant for non-Hodgkin's lymphoma (NHL): randomized trial of peripheral blood (PSCT) versus bone marrow (ABMT) and evaluation of minimal residual disease (MRD). *Proc Am Soc Clin Oncol* 1997;16:90a.
38. Gribben JG, Freedman AS, Neuberg D, et al. Immunologic purging of marrow assessed by PCR before autologous bone marrow transplantation for B-cell lymphoma. *N Engl J Med* 1991;325:1525–1533.
39. Gribben JG, Neuberg D, Freedman AS, et al. Detection by polymerase chain reaction of residual cells with the bcl-2 translocation is associated with increased risk of relapse after autologous bone marrow transplantation for B-cell lymphoma. *Blood* 1993;81:3449–3457.
40. Freedman AS, Gribben JG, Neuberg D, et al. High-dose therapy and autologous bone marrow transplantation in patients with follicular lymphoma during first remission. *Blood* 1996;88:2780–2786.
41. Gribben JG. Antibody-mediated purging. In Thomas ED, Blume KG, Forman SJ, eds. *Hematopoietic cell transplantation,* 2nd ed. Malden: Blackwell Science, 1999:207–216.
42. Anderson NS, Donovan JW, Borus JS, et al. Failure of immunologic purging in mantle cell lymphoma assessed by polymerase chain reaction detection of minimal residual disease. *Blood* 1997;90: 4212–4221.
43. Provan D, Bartlett-Pandite L, Zwicky C, et al. Eradication of polymerase chain reaction–detectable chronic lymphocytic leukemia cells is associated with improved outcome after bone marrow transplantation. *Blood* 1996;88:2228–2235.
44. Johnson PWM, Price CGA, Smith T, et al. Detection of cells bearing the t(14:18) translocation following myeloablative treatment and autologous bone marrow transplantation for follicular lymphoma. *J Clin Oncol* 1994;12:798–805.
45. Hardingham JE, Kotasek D, Sage RE, et al. Significance of molecular marker–positive cells after autologous peripheral-blood stem-cell transplantation for non-Hodgkin's lymphoma. *J Clin Oncol* 1995;13: 1073–1079.
46. Springer TA. Traffic signals for lymphocyte recirculation and leukocyte emigration: the multistep paradigm. *Cell* 1994;76:301–314.
47. Rowley SD, MacLeod B, Heimfeld S, et al. Severe central nervous system toxicity associated with the infusion of cryopreserved peripheral blood stem cell components. *Cytotherapy* 1999;1:311–317.
48. Davis JM, Rowley SD, Braine HG, et al. Clinical toxicity of cryopreserved bone marrow graft infusion. *Blood* 1990;75:781–786.
49. Stroncek DF, Fautsch SK, Lasky LC, et al. Adverse reactions in patients transfused with cryopreserved marrow. *Transfusion* 1991;31: 521–526.
50. Okamoto Y, Takaue Y, Saito S, et al. Toxicities associated with cryopreserved and thawed peripheral blood stem cell autografts in children with active cancer. *Transfusion* 1993;33:578–581.
51. David NA. The pharmacology of dimethyl sulfoxide 6544. *Ann Rev Pharmacol* 1972;12:353–374.
52. Willhite CC, Katz PI. Dimethyl sulfoxide. *J Appl Toxicol* 1984;4: 155–160.
53. Styler MJ, Topolsky DL, Crilley PA, et al. Transient high grade heart block following autologous bone marrow infusion. *Bone Marrow Transplant* 1992;10:435–438.
54. Keung Y-K, Lau S, Elkayam U, et al. Cardiac arrhythmia after infusion of cryopreserved stem cells. *Bone Marrow Transplant* 1994;14: 363–367.
55. Lopez-Jimenez J, Cervero C, Munoz A, et al. Cardiovascular toxicities related to the infusion of cryopreserved grafts: results of a controlled study. *Bone Marrow Transplant* 1994;13:789–793.
56. Dhodapkar M, Goldberg SL, Tefferi A, et al. Reversible encephalopathy after cryopreserved peripheral blood stem cell infusion. *Am J Hematol* 1994;45:187–188.
57. Smith DM, Weisenberger DD, Bierman P, et al. Acute renal failure associated with autologous bone marrow transplantation. *Bone Marrow Transplant* 1987;2:195–201.
58. Nemunaitis J, Rabinowe SN, Singer JW, et al. Recombinant granulocyte-macrophage colony-stimulating factor after autologous bone marrow transplantation for lymphoid cancer. *N Engl J Med* 1991; 324:1773–1778.
59. Gulati SC, Bennett CL. Granulocyte-macrophage colony-stimulating factor (GM-CSF) as adjunct therapy in relapsed Hodgkin disease. *Ann Intern Med* 1992;116:177–182.
60. Advani R, Chao NJ, Horning SJ, et al. Granulocyte-macrophage colony-stimulating factor (GM-CSF) as an adjunct to autologous hemopoietic stem cell transplantation for lymphoma. *Ann Intern Med* 1992; 116:183–189.
61. Brandt SJ, Peters WP, Atwater SK, et al. Effect of recombinant human granulocyte-macrophage colony-stimulating factor on hematopoietic reconstitution after high dose chemotherapy and autologous bone marrow transplantation. *N Engl J Med* 1988;318:869–876.
62. Bolwell BJ, Pohlman B, Andresen S, et al. Delayed G-CSF after autologous progenitor cell transplantation: a prospective randomized trial. *Bone Marrow Transplant* 1998;21:369–373.
63. Micallef IN, Lillington DM, Apostolidis J, et al.. Therapy-related myelodysplasia and secondary acute myelogenous leukemia after high-dose therapy with autologous hematopoietic progenitor-cell support for lymphoid malignancies. *J Clin Oncol* 2000;18:947–955.
64. Sobecks RM, Le Beau MM, Anastasi J, et al. Myelodysplasia and

acute leukemia following high-dose chemotherapy and autologous bone marrow or peripheral blood stem cell transplantation. *Bone Marrow Transplant* 1999;23:1161–1165.

65. Nagler A, Ackerstein A, Or R, et al. Immunotherapy with recombinant human interleukin-2 and recombinant interferon-α in lymphoma patients postautologous marrow stem cell transplantation. *Blood* 1997;89:3951–3953.
66. Magni M, DeNicola M, Devizzi L, et al. Successful in vivo purging of CD34-containing peripheral blood harvests in mantle cell and indolent lymphoma: evidence for a role of both chemotherapy and rituximab infusion. *Blood* 2000;96:864–869.
67. Timmerman JM, Levy R. Dendritic cell vaccines for cancer immunotherapy. *Annu Rev Med* 1999;50:507–529.
68. Hájek R, Butch AW. Dendritic cell biology and the application of dendritic cells to immunotherapy of multiple myeloma. *Med Oncol* 2000;17:2–15.
69. Reichardt VL, Okada CY, Liso A et al. Idiotype vaccination using dendritic cells after autologous peripheral blood stem cell transplantation for multiple myeloma—a feasibility study. *Blood* 1999;93: 2411–2419.
70. Titzer S, Christensen O, Manzke O, et al. Vaccination of multiple myeloma patients with idiotype-pulsed dendritic cells: immunological and clinical aspects. *Br J Haematol* 2000;108:805–816.
71. Wen YJ, Ling M, Bailey-Wood R, et al. Idiotypic protein-pulsed adherent peripheral blood mononuclear cell-derived dendritic cells prime immune system in multiple myeloma. *Clin Cancer Res* 1998; 4:957–962.
72. Lim SH, Bailey-Wood R. Idiotypic protein-pulsed dendritic cell vaccination in multiple myeloma. *Int J Cancer* 1999;83:15–22.
73. Cull G, Durrant L, Stainer C, et al. Generation of anti-idiotype immune responses following vaccination with idiotype-protein pulsed dendritic cells in myeloma. *Br J Haematol* 1999;107:648–655.
74. Cassileth PA, Lynch E, Hines JD, et al. Varying intensity of postremission therapy in acute myeloid leukemia. *Blood* 1992;79:1924–1930.
75. Cassileth PA, Harrington DP, Appelbaum FR, et al. Chemotherapy compared with autologous or allogeneic bone marrow transplantation in the management of acute myeloid leukemia in first remission. *N Engl J Med* 1998;339:1649–1656.
76. Burnett AK, Goldstone AH, Stevens RM, et al. Randomised comparison of addition of autologous bone-marrow transplantation to intensive chemotherapy for acute myeloid leukaemia in first remission: results of MRC AML 10 trial. *Lancet* 1998;351:700–708.
77. Harousseau JL, Cahn JY, Pignon B, et al. Comparison of autologous bone marrow transplantation and intensive chemotherapy as postremission therapy in adult acute myeloid leukemia. *Blood* 1997;90: 2978–2986.
78. Ravindranath Y, Yeager AM, Chang MN, et al. Autologous bone marrow transplantation versus intensive consolidation chemotherapy for acute myeloid leukemia in childhood. *N Engl J Med* 1996;334: 1428–1434.
79. Zittoun RA, Mandelli F, Willemze R, et al. Autologous or allogeneic bone marrow transplantation compared with intensive chemotherapy in acute myelogenous leukemia. *N Engl J Med* 1995;332:217–223.
80. Yeager AM, Kaizer H, Santos GW, et al. Autologous bone marrow transplantation in patients with acute nonlymphocytic leukemia, using ex vivo marrow treatment with 4-hydroperoxycyclophosphamide. *N Engl J Med* 1986;315:141–147.
81. Lenarsky C, Weinberg K, Petersen J, et al. Autologous bone marrow transplantation with 4-hydroperoxycyclophosphamide purged marrow for children with acute non-lymphoblastic leukemia in second remission. *Bone Marrow Transplant* 1990;6:425–429.
82. Gorin NC, Aegerter P, Auvert B, et al. Autologous bone marrow transplantation for acute myelocytic leukemia in first remission: a European survey of the role of marrow purging. *Blood* 1990;75: 1606–1614.
83. Rowley SD, Jones RJ, Piantadosi S, et al. Efficacy of ex vivo purging for autologous bone marrow transplantation in treatment of acute nonlymphoblastic leukemia. *Blood* 1989;74:501–506.
84. Miller CB, Zehnbauer BA, Piantadosi S, et al. Correlation of occult clonogenic leukemia drug sensitivity with relapse after autologous bone marrow transplantation. *Blood* 1991;78:1125–1131.
85. Copelan EA, McGuire EA. The biology and treatment of acute lymphoblastic leukemia in adults. *Blood* 1995;85:1151–1168.
86. Weisdorf DJ, Billett AL, Hannan P, et al. Autologous versus unrelated donor allogeneic marrow transplantation for acute lymphoblastic leukemia. *Blood* 1997;90:2962–2968.
87. Attal M, Blaise D, Marit G, et al. Consolidation treatment of adult acute lymphoblastic leukemia: a prospective, randomized trial comparing allogeneic versus autologous bone marrow transplantation and testing the impact of recombinant interleukin-2 after autologous bone marrow transplantation. BGMT Group. *Blood* 1995;86:1619–1628.
88. Borgmann A, Schmid H, Hartmann R, et al. Autologous bone-marrow transplants compared with chemotherapy for children with acute lymphoblastic leukaemia in a second remission: a matched-pair analysis. The Berlin-Frankfurt-Munster Study Group. *Lancet* 1995;346: 873–876.
89. Doney K, Buckner CD, Fisher L, et al. Autologous bone marrow transplantation for acute lymphoblastic leukemia. *Bone Marrow Transplant* 1993;12:315–321.
90. Khouri IF, Kantarjian HM Talpaz M, et al. Results with high-dose chemotherapy and unpurged autologous stem cell transplantation in 73 patients with chronic myelogenous leukemia: The MD Anderson experience. *Bone Marrow Transplant* 1996;17:775–779.
91. Rozman C, Montserrat E. Chronic lymphocytic leukemia. *N Engl J Med* 1995;333:1052–1057.
92. Khouri IF, Keating MJ, Vriesendorp HM, et al. Autologous and allogeneic bone marrow transplantation for chronic lymphocytic leukemia: preliminary results. *J Clin Oncol* 1994;12:748–758.
93. Rabinowe SN, Soiffer RJ, Gribben JG, et al. Autologous and allogeneic bone marrow transplantation for poor prognosis patients with B-cell chronic lymphocytic leukemia. *Blood* 1993;82:1366–1376.
94. Paulus U, Schmitz N, Viehmann K, et al. Combine positive/negative selection for highly effective purging of PBPC grafts: towards clinical application in patients with B-CLL. *Bone Marrow Transplant* 1997; 20:415–420.
95. McElwain TJ, Powles RL. High-dose intravenous melphalan for plasma-cell leukaemia and myeloma. *Lancet* 1983;2:822–824.
96. Barlogie B, Jagannath S, Vesole DH, et al. Superiority of tandem autologous transplantation over standard therapy for previously untreated multiple myeloma. *Blood* 1997;89:789–793.
97. Fermand JP, Ravaud P, Chevret S, et al. High-dose therapy and autologous peripheral blood stem cell transplantation in multiple myeloma: up-front or rescue treatment? Results of a multicenter sequential randomized clinical trial. *Blood* 1998;92:3131–3136.
98. Martinelli G, Terragna C, Zamagni E, et al. Molecular remission after allogeneic or autologous transplantation of hematopoietic stem cells for multiple myeloma. *J Clin Oncol* 2000;18:2273–2281.
99. Desikan R, Barlogie B, Sawyer J, et al. Results of high-dose therapy for 1000 patients with multiple myeloma: Durable complete remissions and superior survival in the absence of chromosome 13 abnormalities. *Blood* 2000;95:4008–4010.
100. Vescio R, Schiller G, Stewart AK, et al. Multicenter phase III trial to evaluate $CD34^+$-selected versus unselected autologous peripheral blood progenitor cell transplantation in multiple myeloma. *Blood* 1999;93:1858–1868.
101. Sawyer J, Waldron J, Jagannath S, et al. Cytogenetic findings in 200 patients with multiple myeloma. *Cancer Genet Cytogenet* 1995;82: 41–49.
102. Feinman R, Sawyer J, Hardin J, et al. Cytogenetics and molecular genetics in multiple myeloma. *Hematol Oncol Clin North Am* 1997; 11:1–25.
103. Tricot G, Barlogie B, Jagannath S, et al. Poor prognosis in multiple myeloma is associated only with partial or complete deletions of chromosome 13 or abnormalities involving 11q and not with other karyotype abnormalities. *Blood* 1995;86:4250–4256.
104. Kyle RA, Gertz MA, Greipp PR, et al. A trial of three regimens for primary amyloidosis: colchicine alone, melphalan and prednisone, and melphalan, prednisone, and colchicine. *N Engl J Med* 1997;336: 1202–1207.

105. Comenzo RL, Vosburgh E, Simms RW, et al. Dose-intensive melphalan with blood stem-cell support for the treatment of AL (amyloid light-chain) amyloidosis: survival and responses in 25 patients. *Blood* 1998;91:3662–3670.
106. Dember LM, Sanchorawala V, Seldin DC, et al. Effect of dose-intensive intravenous melphalan and autologous blood stem-cell transplantation on AL amyloidosis-associated renal disease. *Ann Intern Med* 2001;134:746–753.
107. Dreger P, Glass B, Kuse R, et al. Myeloablative radiochemotherapy followed by reinfusion of purged autologous stem cells for Waldenström's macroglobulinaemia. *Br J Haematol* 1999;106:115–118.
108. Sweetenham JW, Carella AM, Taghipour G, et al. High-dose therapy and autologous stem-cell transplantation for adult patients with Hodgkin's disease who do not enter remission after induction chemotherapy: results in 175 patients reported to the European Group for Blood and Marrow Transplantation. Lymphoma Working Party. *J Clin Oncol* 1999;17:3101–3109.
109. Chopra R, McMillan AK, Linch DC, et al. The place of high-dose BEAM therapy and autologous bone marrow transplantation in poor-risk Hodgkin's disease. A single-center eight-year study of 155 patients. *Blood* 1993;81:1137–1145.
110. Bierman PJ, Anderson JR, Freeman MB, et al. High-dose chemotherapy followed by autologous hematopoietic rescue for Hodgkin's disease patients following first relapse after chemotherapy. *Ann Oncol* 1996;7:151–156.
111. Yuen AR, Rosenberg SA, Hoppe RT, et al. Comparison between conventional salvage therapy and high-dose therapy with autografting for recurrent or refractory Hodgkin's disease. *Blood* 1997;89: 814–822.
112. Bonfante V, Santoro A, Viviani S, et al. Outcome of patients with Hodgkin's disease failing after primary MOPP-ABVD. *J Clin Oncol* 1997;15:528–534.
113. Schmitz N, Sextro M, Pfistner D, et al. High-dose therapy (HDT) followed by hematopoietic stem cell transplantation (HSCT) for relapsed chemosensitive Hodgkin's disease (HD): Final results of a randomized GHSG and EBMT trial (HD-R1). *Proc Am Soc Clin Oncol* 1999;18:2a.
114. Lazarus HM, Rowlings PA, Zhang MJ, et al. Autotransplants for Hodgkin's disease in patients never achieving remission: a report from the Autologous Blood and Marrow Transplant Registry. *J Clin Oncol* 1999;17:534–545.
115. Sweetenham JW, Taghipour G, Linch DC, et al. Thirty percent of adults patients with primary refractory Hodgkin's Disease (HD) are progression free at 5 years after high dose therapy (HDT) and autologous stem cell transplantation (ASCT): data from 290 patients reported to the EBMT. *Blood* 1996;88:486a.
116. Colombat P, Cornillet P, Deconinck E, et al. Value of autologous stem cell transplantation with purged bone marrow as first-line therapy for follicular lymphoma with high tumor burden: a GOELAMS phase II study. *Bone Marrow Transplant* 2000;26:971–977.
117. Rohatiner AZ, Johnson PW, Price CG, et al. Myeloablative therapy with autologous bone marrow transplantation as consolidation therapy for recurrent follicular lymphoma. *J Clin Oncol* 1994;12: 1177–1184.
118. Bierman PJ, Vose JM, Anderson JR, et al. High-dose therapy with autologous hematopoietic rescue for follicular low-grade non-Hodgkin's lymphoma. *J Clin Oncol* 1997;15:445–450.
119. Bociek G, Bierman P, Lynch J, et al. High-dose therapy with autologous hematopoietic stem cell transplantation for follicular non-Hodgkin's lymphoma: long-term results. *Proc Am Soc Clin Oncol* 1999;18: 3a.
120. Verdonck LF, Deffer AW, Lokhorst HM, et al. Allogeneic versus autologous bone marrow transplantation for refractory and recurrent low-grade non-Hodgkin's lymphoma. *Blood* 1997;90:4501–4505.
121. Williams CD, Harrison CN, Lister TA, et al. High-dose therapy and autologous stem-cell support for chemosensitive transformed low-grade follicular non-Hodgkin's lymphoma: a case-matched study from the European Bone Marrow Transplant Registry. *J Clin Oncol* 2001; 19:727–735.
122. Gianni AM, Bregni M, Siena S, et al. High-dose chemotherapy and autologous bone marrow transplantation compared with MACOP-B in aggressive B-cell lymphoma. *N Engl J Med* 1997;336:1290–1297.
123. Haioun C, Lepage E, Gisselbrecht C, et al. Benefit of autologous bone marrow transplantation over sequential chemotherapy in poor-risk aggressive non-Hodgkin's lymphoma: updated results of the prospective study LNH87-2. *J Clin Oncol* 1997;15:1131–1137.
124. Guglielmi C, Gomez F, Philip T, et al. Time to relapse has prognostic value in patients with aggressive lymphoma enrolled onto the Parma trial. *J Clin Oncol* 1998;16:3264–3269.
125. Vose JM, Anderson JR, Kessinger A, et al. High-dose chemotherapy and autologous hematopoietic stem-cell transplantation for aggressive non-Hodgkin's lymphoma. *J Clin Oncol* 1993;11:1846–1851.
126. Sweetenham JW, Pearce R, Taghipour G, et al. Adult Burkitt's and Burkitt-like non-Hodgkin's lymphoma—outcome for patients treated with high-dose therapy and autologous stem-cell transplantation in first remission or at relapse: results from the European Group for Blood and Marrow Transplantation. *J Clin Oncol* 1996;14: 2465–2472.
127. Verdonck LF, van Putten WL, Hagenbeek A, et al. Comparison of CHOP chemotherapy with autologous bone marrow transplantation for slowly responding patients with aggressive non-Hodgkin's lymphoma. *N Engl J Med* 1995;332:1045–1051.
128. Anonymous. A predictive model for aggressive non-Hodgkin's lymphoma. The International Non-Hodgkin's Lymphoma Prognostic Factors Project. *N Engl J Med* 1993;329:987–994.
129. Haioun C, Lepage E, Gisselbrecht C, et al. Comparison of autologous bone marrow transplantation with sequential chemotherapy for intermediate-grade and high-grade non-Hodgkin's lymphoma in first complete remission: a study of 464 patients. Groupe d'Etude des Lymphomes de l'Adulte. *J Clin Oncol* 1994;12:2543–2551.
130. Santini G, Salvagno L, Leoni P, et al. VACOP-B versus VACOP-B plus autologous bone marrow transplantation for advanced diffuse non-Hodgkin's lymphoma: results of a prospective randomized trial by the non-Hodgkin's Lymphoma Cooperative Study Group. *J Clin Oncol* 1998;16:2796–2802.
131. Vose JM, Zhang MJ, Rowlings PA, et al. Autologous transplantation for diffuse aggressive non-Hodgkin's lymphoma in patients never achieving remission: a report from the Autologous Blood and Marrow Transplant Registry. *J Clin Oncol* 2001;19:406–413.
132. Freedman AS, Neuberg D, Gribben JG, et al. High-dose chemoradiotherapy and anti-B-cell monoclonal antibody-purged autologous bone marrow transplantation in mantle-cell lymphoma: no evidence for long-term remission. *J Clin Oncol* 1998;16:13–18.
133. Khouri IF, Romaguera J, Kantarjian H, et al. Hyper-CVAD and high-dose methotrexate/cytarabine followed by stem-cell transplantation: an active regimen for aggressive mantle-cell lymphoma. *J Clin Oncol* 1998;16:3803–3809.
134. Antman KH, Rowlings PA, Vaughan WP, et al. High-dose chemotherapy with autologous hematopoietic stem-cell support for breast cancer in North America. *J Clin Oncol* 1997;15:1870–1879.
135. Peters WP, Ross M, Vredenburgh JJ, et al. High-dose chemotherapy and autologous bone marrow support as consolidation after standard-dose adjuvant therapy for high-risk primary breast cancer. *J Clin Oncol* 1993;11:1132–1143.
136. Rodenhuis S, Bontenbal M, Beex L, et al. Randomized phase III study of high-dose chemotherapy with cyclophosphamide, thiotepa and carboplatin in operable breast cancer with 4 or more axillary lymph nodes. *Proc Am Soc Clin Oncol* 2000;19:74a.
137. Peters W, Rosner G, Vredenburg J, et al. Updated results of a prospective randomized comparison of two doses of combination alkylating agents (AA) as consolidation after CAF in high-risk primary breast cancer involving ten or more axillary lymph nodes (LN): CALGB 9082/SWOG 9114/NCIC Ma-13. *Proc Am Soc Clin Oncol* 2001;20: 21a.
138. The Scandinavian Breast Cancer Study Group 9401. Results from a randomized adjuvant breast cancer study with high dose chemotherapy with CTCb supported by autologous bone marrow stem cells versus dose escaltated and tailored FEC therapy. *Proc Am Soc Clin Oncol* 1999;18:2a.
139. Gianni A, Bonadonna A. Five-year results of the randomized clinical

trial comparing standard versus high-dose myeloablative chemotherapy in the adjuvant treatment of breast cancer with >3 positive nodes (LN+). *Proc Am Soc Clin Oncol* 2001;20:21a.

140. Adkins D, Brown R, Trinkaus K, et al. Outcomes of high-dose chemotherapy and autologous stem-cell transplantation in stage IIIB inflammatory breast cancer. *J Clin Oncol* 1999;17:2006–2014.
141. Stadtmauer EA, O'Neill A, Goldstein LJ, et al. Conventional-dose chemotherapy compared with high-dose chemotherapy plus autologous hematopoietic stem-cell transplantation for metastatic breast cancer. Philadelphia Bone Marrow Transplant Group. *N Engl J Med* 2000;342:1069–1076.
142. Nichols CR, Andersen J, Lazarus HM, et al. High-dose carboplatin and etoposide with autologous bone marrow transplantation in refractory germ cell cancer: an Eastern Cooperative Oncology Group protocol. *J Clin Oncol* 1992;10:558–563.
143. Motzer RJ, Mazumdar M, Bosl GJ, et al. High-dose carboplatin, etoposide, and cyclophosphamide for patients with refractory germ cell tumors: treatment results and prognostic factors for survival and toxicity. *J Clin Oncol* 1996;14:1098–1105.
144. Broun ER, Nichols CR, Gize G, et al. Tandem high dose chemotherapy with autologous bone marrow transplantation for initial relapse of testicular germ cell cancer. *Cancer* 1997;79:1605–1610.
145. Cure H, Battista C, Guastalia J, et al. Phase III randomized trial of high-dose chemotherapy (HDC) and peripheral blood stem cell (PBSC) support as consolidation in patients (pts) with responsive low-burden advanced ovarian cancer (AOC): preliminary results of a GINECO/FNCLCC/SFGM-TC study. *Proc Am Soc Clin Oncol* 2001;20:4a.
146. Schachna L, Ryan PF, Schwarer AP. Malignancy-associated remission of systemic lupus erythematosus maintained by autologous peripheral blood stem cell transplantation. *Arthritis Rheum* 1998;41:2271–2272.
147. Snowden JA, Kearney P, Kearney A, et al. Long-term outcome of autoimmune disease following allogeneic bone marrow transplantation. *Arthritis Rheum* 1998;41:453–459.
148. Euler HH, Marmont AM, Bacigalupo A, et al. Early recurrence or persistence of autoimmune diseases after unmanipulated autologous stem cell transplantation. *Blood* 1996;88:3621–3625.
149. Fassas A, Anagnostopoulos A, Kazis A, et al. Peripheral blood stem cell transplantation in the treatment of progressive multiple sclerosis: first results of a pilot study. *Bone Marrow Transplant* 1997;20: 631–638.
150. Traynor AE, Schroeder J, Rosa RM, et al. Treatment of severe systemic lupus erythematosus with high-dose chemotherapy and haemopoietic stem-cell transplantation: a phase I study. *Lancet* 2000;356:701–707.

38

BLOOD AND MARROW TRANSPLANTATION

JAMES L. GAJEWSKI
YAN MA
CINDY IPPOLITI
RICHARD E. CHAMPLIN

PROCEDURE FUNDAMENTALS

Traditionally, blood and bone marrow transplantation has been considered a therapeutic means of providing hematopoietic support enabling the administration of dose-intensive chemotherapy and radiation therapy for treatment of malignancies (1–3). Recent advances, however, are transforming our perception of this therapy toward being a vehicle for cellular immunotherapy of cancer. The hematopoietic stem cells in the marrow produce the cellular elements of blood, including neutrophils, granulocytes, macrophages, erythrocytes, platelets, and both T and B lymphocytes (4). Pluripotent stem cells give rise to stem cells committed to a single line of differentiation. The transplantation of a few pluripotent stem cells can reconstitute hematopoiesis and immunity in appropriately prepared recipients. Donor-derived immunopoiesis after allogeneic blood and marrow transplantation gives therapeutic benefit by reducing the risk of relapse for some types of cancer (4–7). Indications for transplants are shifting from those solely performed for patients with neoplasms exhibiting a dose-dependent response to chemotherapy or irradiation or both to those patients with malignancies demonstrating a cellular immune responsiveness (7–10).

Donor sources of hematopoietic progenitors include (a) autologous transplants in which a patient serves as a self-donor of hematopoietic cells, (b) syngeneic transplants derived from a genetically identical twin donor, and (c) allogeneic transplants obtained from a donor genetically different from the intended recipient. Autologous and syngeneic transplants are associated with less risk because the cells will not be immunologically rejected or mediate an immunologic reaction. Allogeneic transplants have a greater rate of complications due to the potential for immunologic problems associated with graft versus host disease (GVHD). However, for patients with bone marrow involvement by their malignancy, this donor-derived immunosuppression is beneficial owing to a therapeutic graft versus malignancy effect. Typically, autologous transplants are used to provide hematopoietic cellular rescue for patients whose neoplasm exhibits sensitivity to high-dose chemotherapeutic preparative regimens in which the major toxicity is marrow aplasia.

In order to receive an autologous bone marrow or peripheral blood stem cell transplant, the patient must first undergo stem cell collection, followed by cryopreservation and storage of the bone marrow or peripheral blood progenitor cells. Collection

J.L. Gajewski and R.E. Champlin: Department of Blood and Marrow Transplantation, University of Texas—M.D. Anderson Cancer Center, Houston, Texas.

C. Ippoliti and Y. Ma: Department of Pharmacy, University of Texas—M.D. Anderson Cancer Center, Houston, Texas.

of either marrow or peripheral blood progenitor cells should optimally occur at a time when the bone marrow is normocellular and does not contain malignant cells. Subsequently the patient can receive intensive marrow-ablative chemotherapy or irradiation or both, followed by reinfusion of the previously cryopreserved marrow to restore hematopoiesis. With current techniques, marrow or peripheral blood progenitor cells can remain viable for at least 5 years after cryopreservation.

Progenitor cells capable of reconstituting hematopoiesis can be collected from the peripheral blood by repeated leukopheresis, as well as by multiple bone marrow aspirations from sites containing marrow with active hematopoiesis, such as the ilium. Circulating progenitor cells are rare in the peripheral blood, but can be increased following injections of hematopoietic growth factors such as granulocyte colony-stimulating factor (G-CSF) with or without concomitant use of mobilizing doses of cytoreductive chemotherapy (11–14). Combinations of chemotherapy and hematopoietic growth factors generally give an optimal yield of progenitor cells versus regimens only using hematopoietic growth factors (15). Peripheral blood progenitor cell collections are now largely replacing bone marrow harvesting procedures. Indeed, use of mobilized peripheral blood progenitor cells results in quicker recovery of granulocytes and platelets than does marrow transplantation (13,14,16). A major area of research involves development of systems for ex vivo expansion of hematopoietic progenitors from either blood or bone marrow. To date, this expansion has been impossible to achieve without also providing progenitor cell differentiation.

One major potential limitation of autologous transplantation is the possibility of tumor contamination of the collected bone marrow or peripheral blood. Initially, peripheral blood progenitors were believed to be a potential "tumor-free" source of stem cells for patients with bone marrow contaminated by malignant cells. It remains controversial if the level of contaminating malignant cells is less in the peripheral blood than in the marrow. A number of investigators are evaluating techniques to detect submicroscopic involvement by tumor (17,18). Data suggest that detection of marrow involvement by these techniques may be predictive of outcome (18). Approaches to selectively depleting occult malignant cells from the normal bone marrow cells prior to cryopreservation include ex vivo treatment with antitumor monoclonal antibodies, antibody-toxin conjugates, chemotherapy, physical techniques, or by gene therapy purging. An alternative method is to positively select the hematopoietic stem cells. CD34-positive cells represent less than 1% of the bone marrow but include the progenitors capable of reconstituting hematopoiesis. Highly enriched CD34 positively selected cells have been used for autologous bone marrow or blood stem cell transplants, resulting in a rapid hematologic recovery (19,20).

Historically the most frequent types of allogeneic bone marrow transplants performed have involved human lymphocyte antigen (HLA)-identical siblings. With family size decreasing, the possibility of having an identical HLA-matched sibling donor is decreasing. Partially HLA-matched family donors, closely matched unrelated donors, and related and unrelated umbilical cord blood donors are being increasingly used (21–25). The HLA system, as the major histocompatibility complex in humans, is the principal determinant of procedure risk (26). The HLA system is encoded by several closely linked genes located on the short arm of chromosome 6. They have been subdivided into class I loci, which includes HLA-A, -B, and -C, and class II loci, which includes HLA-DR, -DRW, -DQ, and -DP. Originally, the HLA genes were defined serologically using antisera obtained from multiparous women. Increasingly however, molecular technology is using either allele or sequence-specific oligonucleotide typing, and even complete sequencing to define specific antigens with far greater resolution than serotyping (27–29). Matching with higher-resolution molecular typing is reducing the risks of immunologic complications with unrelated allogeneic transplantation (30). Because HLA genotypically identical siblings also can develop immunologic complications with blood and marrow transplantation, the HLA system is apparently not the only mediator of immunologic complications in allogeneic transplantation. In HLA-identical sibling bone marrow transplants, GVHD must be due to mismatching of poorly defined minor histocompatibility antigens. The only easily identified minor histocompatibility antigen is the HY antigen (31). The chance of mismatching for these minor antigens should increase with increasing distance in the relationship between donor and recipient (32).

More intensive pretransplant immunosuppression is required for bone marrow and blood transplantation than is necessary to prevent rejection of solid organ allografts, such as kidney, liver, or heart. The preparative treatment administered prior to transplantation should ablate the recipient's immunity, including T-lymphocyte and natural killer cell function. Different bone marrow transplant preparative regimens have varying degrees of immunosuppression. The choice of preparative regimen depends on the immunocompetence of the recipient, the composition of the transplanted cells, and the HLA disparity between donor and recipient. Historically, bone marrow transplant preparative regimens for malignancies opted for maximal dose intensity. As evidence has emerged that allogeneic immunopoiesis is tumor suppressive and potentially tumoricidal, newer and less toxic preparative regimens have been developed with the sole goal of establishing donor immunopoiesis. Traditional immunologic theory has argued that donor T lymphocytes are necessary for engraftment, but recent theories are emerging that high-dose $CD34^+$ grafts can tolerize to establish engraftment (33,34). The donor-derived allogeneic cellular immunity thus becomes the primary therapeutic tool of the bone marrow transplant.

After the conditioning therapy is completed, the donor blood or bone marrow cells are infused intravenously. Allogeneic bone marrow transplants require approximately 1 to 5 $\times$ 10^8 nucleated cells/kg of recipient body weight to achieve engraftment, and allogeneic peripheral blood progenitor cell regimens require 3 to 4 $\times$ 10^6 $CD34^+$ cells/kg. Approximately 1 to 5 $\times$ 10^7 marrow cells/kg are sufficient for syngeneic or autologous transplants, with 1 to 2 $\times$ 10^6 CD34 peripheral blood progenitor $CD34^+$ cells/kg needed for autologous peripheral blood progenitor cell engraftment (10,20). Optimal outcomes may require higher doses (33–35). Bone marrow dosing criteria were developed prior to identifying CD34 as a surrogate marker for the pluripotent hematopoietic stem cell.

Engraftment of donor cells can be documented by recipient acquisition of donor-type cell surface antigens, chromosome markers, or by use of molecular tests such as DNA-restriction fragment-length polymorphisms, or by polymerase chain reactions of microsatellite regions. Chimerism status is most typically now ascertained by molecular technologies or cytogenetics. Use of red blood cell phenotyping in heavily transfused patients, however, has made this technology problematic, because the red blood cell phenotyping procedure may detect transfused red blood cells. If there is a cytogenetic abnormality to follow, patients should be tested by both standard cytogenetics and molecular testing techniques. Polymerase chain reaction testing may detect 1 in 1,000 to 1 in 100,000 cells. Interphase fluorescent in situ hybridization techniques (FISH) are probably not suitable tests for mixed chimeric status, particularly for chronic myelogenous leukemia (CML) in which the normal patient population is 10% positive. Cytogenetic cell technology, although usually thought to be less sensitive than molecular techniques, may occasionally detect tumor cells missed by molecular techniques. Cytogenetic testing forces cells to enter cell division so the metaphase can be analyzed, because tumor cells may be more prone to proliferation. Standard cytogenetics should still be used to follow patients with sex-mismatched donors or in recipients with known cytogenetic abnormalities. Following successful transplantation, cells of the recipient's reconstituted hematologic and immunologic systems are primarily derived from the donor's blood or bone marrow, although in some cases mixed chimerism occurs in which both donor- and recipient-derived cells are present in the recipient's circulation (36,37). Parenchymal cells of visceral organs and most mesenchymal cells remain of host origin. Endothelial cells within the vascular system may convert to donor origin (38).

CHOOSING THE DONOR

Related donor-recipient pairs that are mismatched for only one A, B, or DR HLA locus, or HLA phenotypically identical pairs, have had a higher incidence of acute GVHD. However, survival rates are similar to those of transplants between HLA-identical siblings with advanced-stage hematologic malignancies (21,39, 40). Use of unmodified bone marrow grafts from recipients mismatched for two or more loci have shown a high risk of graft rejection, GVHD, and other complications (41). However with the use of peripheral blood progenitor cells with a purified CD34 selection and an aggressive 4.5- to 5-log T-cell depletion, results with haploidentical transplants are dramatically improving (42, 43). Use of related and unrelated umbilical cord blood donation is increasing. Umbilical cord blood is harvested by drawing blood from the umbilical cord at time of delivery. Banks of unrelated cryopreserved umbilical cord blood have been established. Umbilical cord blood transplants have a lower risk of GVHD than do transplants with cells obtained from pediatric or adult donors. The cell numbers collected from cord blood are low, however, and use of umbilical cord blood donors is associated with a 20% graft failure risk in adults, with outcomes in leukemic patients ranging from 20% to 40% (44–47). A dose of 2×10^7 cord blood cells/kg is considered to be the minimal acceptable dose for a cord blood transplant. Studies are underway combining umbilical cord blood units, but this approach is far from the standard of care. Use of ex vivo expanded cord blood cells to augment the collected cells is currently under investigation.

Due to the tremendous polymorphism of the HLA loci, it is unlikely that a patient will be HLA identical with a randomly selected unrelated individual. More than 3.5 million individuals are now typed and available in worldwide registries. Human lymphocyte antigen gene frequencies vary considerably among racial groups, and linkage disequilibrium occurs such that some haplotypes do occur commonly, but approximately 50% of people have rare haplotypes. The incidence and severity of GVHD is higher in recipients of unrelated bone marrow grafts compared with transplants from HLA genotypically identical siblings. This is presumably related to greater genetic disparity with unrelated donors; these unrelated pairs are more likely to be mismatched for HLA variants and minor histocompatibility loci than are related donors.

The options for choice of a donor still depend on clinical circumstances. Unless a syngeneic or HLA genotypically identical sibling has an underlying risk of a genetic defect or viral infection and is in poor health, it is rare to choose an unrelated donor over a family donor. For CML it may be preferable to consider an HLA genotypically identical sibling donor over a syngeneic donor to take advantage of the superior outcome with a graft versus tumor effect. The choice between a partially matched family donor, unrelated donor, or umbilical cord blood is more problematic. The first issue in the decision-tree analysis is how good is the matching and what type of cell processing support is available. Related donors mismatched for two or more HLA-A, -B, or -DR antigens have reasonable success rates but only with aggressive T-cell depletion. To have a successful outcome with haploidentical bone marrow transplantation, the cell processing lab needs to have technology available to reduce T cells by 4 to 5 logs and still infuse greater than 6 million $CD34^+$ cells/kg. These transplants are associated with prolonged delayed immunoreconstitution and many posttransplant opportunistic infections. The advantage of related donors is that the donors are usually readily available. A 2- to 6-month search process is required to find an unrelated donor who most often can not be made immediately available. For the rare recipient of an unrelated graft, where there is a donor matched by high-resolution molecular techniques of HLA-A, -B, -C, -DR, and -DQ loci, equivalent survival to that reported in an HLA genotypically identical sibling transplant recipient has been observed. Umbilical cord blood can be obtained quickly; however, given the low numbers stored in cryopreservation banks it may be hard to find an appropriately matched unit. Multiple umbilical cord blood pooled from different donors should not be used for transplantation except in a clinical trial. Umbilical cord blood should be considered only if a cell dose is greater than about 2×10^7 cells/kg with documented viability. Given the small numbers of cells in umbilical cord blood samples, it has not been possible to do immunophenotyping of umbilical cord blood to establish a minimal $CD34^+$ cells/kg standard.

POTENTIAL COMPLICATIONS OF DOSE-INTENSIVE THERAPY WITH BONE MARROW TRANSPLANTATION

Intensive chemoradiotherapy and bone marrow transplantation is associated with many complications, including toxicity from the pretransplant conditioning regimen, infections due to granulocytopenia or posttransplant immunodeficiency, bleeding due to thrombocytopenic graft failure and, in the case of allogeneic transplants, transplant rejection and GVHD. Mortality as the result of the transplant ranges from 5% to 10% in autologous transplant recipients and varies from 10% to 50% in allogeneic transplants recipients depending on disease stage and donor matching.

Hematologic Toxicity

Blood and bone marrow transplantation patients typically develop profound pancytopenia lasting approximately 2 to 3 weeks until the transplanted hematopoietic progenitor cells restore hematopoiesis. During this period of pancytopenia patients are at risk for infectious complications. While GM-CSF and G-CSF have been shown to accelerate hematopoietic recovery, neither prevents the nadir of granulocytes. Neither factor positively affects (decreases) erythrocyte or platelet time to recovery. Because of the perceived low risk of red blood cell transfusions, erythropoietin has not been adequately studied in the bone marrow transplant setting. Interleukin-11 and recombinant human thrombopoietin have had limited efficacy trials but may hasten platelet recovery. Use of peripheral blood progenitor cells has recently been shown to produce more rapid recovery of hematopoiesis than has use of bone marrow transplants (14).

Organ Toxicity

Following blood and bone marrow transplantation, severe toxicity involving the liver, lung, heart, nervous system and, less frequently, other tissues may occur. Fatal hepatic venoocclusive disease occurs and is more common in older patients, patients with preexisting liver function abnormalities, active hepatitis B infections, and prior chemotherapy exposure. Preparative regimen-related pneumonitis and pulmonary hemorrhage is often difficult to distinguish from an infectious process. It is most common with preparative regimens containing 1,3-bis(2-chloroethyl)-1-nitrosourea (BCNU; carmustine) and in patients who have received transplants following mediastinal radiotherapy (48). If unexplained dyspnea and hypoxia occur 1 to 9 months posttransplant, this diagnosis must be considered. Bronchoscopy to rule out an infectious etiology, particularly viral etiology, must be done quickly. More frequently, this pneumonitis is associated with a diffuse alveolar hemorrhage (49–51). Early administration of high-dose steroids is necessary to avoid a fatal outcome, but steroids may compromise survival if this is a viral process. Recombinant activated factor VII has helped in our experience (52). Some patients develop obliterative bronchiolitis, a delayed form of respiratory failure due to obstructive terminal airway disease 6 months to 2 years posttransplant (53,54). This often results in recurrent pneumothorax and progressive respiratory insufficiency, which is often fatal. Its pathogenesis is poorly defined but typically occurs in patients with chronic GVHD and is usually not associated with a documented infection. No effective therapy has been reported. Cardiac toxicity is common with high-dose cyclophosphamide regimens. Central nervous system complications are relatively uncommon, but dementia or leukoencephalopathy can occur. Endocrine complications may develop but are generally not life-threatening. Hypothyroidism commonly occurs as a delayed complication 6 months to 2 years posttransplant (55). Intensive combined-modality therapy typically results in sterility for both males and females, although gonadal endocrine function and ejaculation are usually intact. Cataracts are a common delayed complication of total body irradiation (55). Bladder toxicity due to high-dose cyclophosphamide chemotherapy is a common problem and has been reported following other regimens (56–58). When associated with high-dose cyclophosphamide, this is probably mediated by acrolein, a metabolite of 4-hydroxycyclophosphamide that is toxic to transitional cell epithelium. Hemorrhagic cystitis may develop acutely or as a delayed complication weeks to months later. Mesna, a uroprotective agent that binds to acrolein, has been reported to reduce the risk of urinary toxicity from use of cyclophosphamide in bone marrow transplant patients without inhibiting its therapeutic effects (56,58). Hemorrhagic cystitis has also been observed with other agents and may also be due to viral infection, particularly adenoviruses (57). Initial treatment is always bladder irrigation. If that fails, carboprost, a prostaglandin E_2 inhibitor, which causes local vasoconstriction, has had some success. The other option is surgery to do cauterization or fulguration with formalin. Rarely, a cystectomy needs to be done.

Graft Rejection and Graft Versus Host Disease

For allogeneic transplant recipients, graft rejection may occur, mediated by host T lymphocytes or natural killer cells (59). Graft rejection from an HLA-identical donor is rare, except in patients with aplastic anemia. Patients receiving transplants from HLA-nonidentical donors and recipients of T lymphocyte-depleted transplants have a greater risk of rejection (60).

The more frequent problem with allogeneic transplants is GVHD. It results from engraftment of immunocompetent cells from the donor bone marrow which react against recipient tissues. Acute GVHD occurs within the first 100 days posttransplant, and chronic GVHD occurs after 100 days. The pathophysiology of acute GVHD is incompletely defined but is initiated by donor T lymphocytes reacting against disparate host antigens. A biopsy of the site of GVHD discloses cellular destruction and the absence of an inflammatory infiltrate, indicating a cytokine-mediated cell death (61). The incidence of GVHD is affected by several factors, including the degree of genetic disparity between the donor and recipient, patient age, donor age, and the nature and quantity of the transplanted cells (62). Besides HLA compatibility issues, donor factors include age, sex, parity if female, and number of transfusion exposures. Target organs typically include skin, liver, and the gastrointestinal tract. Moderate-to-severe acute GVHD occurs in 10% to 30% of HLA-identical transplant recipients, typically develops within 30 to 100 days, and is fatal in approximately one-half of affected patients. In HLA genotypically identical sibling transplant recipients, preliminary reports indicate the use of peripheral blood progenitor cells as the source of hematopoietic support may produce less acute GVHD due to quicker engraftment and less organ toxicity. Graft versus host disease is more frequent after HLA-mismatched transplants (14), and the incidence increases with recipient age. Most patients have received prophylactic posttransplant immunosuppressive treatment with either cyclosporine or tacrolimus, with either methotrexate or corticosteroids, for 3 to 6 months (63). Results with tacrolimus may be slightly improved compared with those of cyclosporine, but the principal benefit of tacrolimus is that the drug level is predictive of toxicity (63).

Depletion of T lymphocytes from the donor bone marrow or peripheral blood progenitor cells prior to transplantation is an alternative approach to GVHD prevention. The most common techniques include agglutination with lectins and E rosette depletion or treatment with anti-T-cell monoclonal antibodies (64–67). In vivo T-cell depletion can also be accomplished with anti-T-lymphocyte antibodies administered to the recipient in high doses (64). In T-cell depletion, the risk of graft failure due to rejection is increased, possibly due to the lack of a graft versus host effect abrogating residual immunocompetent host cells. Recipients of T-lymphocyte–depleted transplants also have a greater risk of leukemia relapse, indicating that marrow T lymphocytes may contribute to the beneficial graft versus leukemia (GVL) effect (66).

Patients who develop acute GVHD are generally treated with high-dose corticosteroids, such as methylprednisolone 2 mg/kg. Patients with steroid-resistant GVHD have a poor prognosis, although some respond to additional immunosuppressive therapy such as antithymocyte globulin. Newer T-cell suppressive agents or monoclonal antibodies targeting T cells are also being tried. There is considerable recent interest in the role of cytokines in the pathophysiology of GVHD. Interleukin-1 and tumor necrosis factor have been implicated, and cytokine blockade therapy may therefore be useful for prophylaxis or treatment of GVHD (67). Protection of the gastrointestinal tract is another approach that may help prevent GVHD (68).

Chronic GVHD affects approximately 25% of transplant recipients who survive longer than 6 months (69). Two-thirds of afflicted patients have preceding acute GVHD, but it develops de novo in one-third of patients. The incidence of chronic GVHD increases with recipient age. The risk of chronic GVHD may be increased in recipients who receive an allogeneic peripheral blood progenitor cell transplant (70). Chronic GVHD may develop in two forms, a limited form involving localized areas of the skin and an extensive form with generalized skin and multisystem involvement. Chronic GVHD has clinical manifestations similar to that observed in several rheumatologic and autoimmune disorders, such as progressive systemic sclerosis, systemic lupus erythematosis, Sjögren syndrome, and primary biliary cirrhosis. Chronic GVHD is a disease of disordered immunity; patients have a spectrum of immune-related abnormalities, including profound immunodeficiency, autoantibodies, and excessive nonspecific suppressor T-cell activity. Affected patients often die of infections. The limited form does not require therapy. The systemic form of chronic GVHD is more serious and responds poorly to treatment. Corticosteroids, antithymocyte globulin, and other immunosuppressive or cytotoxic agents are usually ineffective in advanced disease. Thalidomide has been effective in some patients (71). Photopheresis and psoralen and long-wave ultraviolet radiation (PUVA) therapy has been effective for patients with skin-only chronic GVHD (72).

Immunohematology Issues with Blood and Bone Marrow Transplantation

Peripheral blood and bone marrow transplant patients present several unique immunohematologic problems, because blood group barriers are routinely mismatched with this therapy (73). The inheritance of blood group antigens is independent of the HLA gene complex. Family members are often matched for blood groups whereas unrelated donors are selected primarily for HLA identity, cytomegalovirus (CMV) status, size, and age, and rarely for compatibility in blood type. The terminology used for this circumstance is major ABO incompatibility, in which the recipient possesses antibodies capable of reacting with red blood cell antigens on the surface of the donor's red blood cells (e.g., a group A donor and a group O recipient). Minor ABO incompatibility also exists when the donor possesses hemagglutinins capable of reacting with erythrocyte antigens on the recipients red blood cells (a group O donor and a group A recipient). At times, both major and minor ABO incompatibilities exist, such as a group B donor and a group A recipient. Initially, it was thought that ABO blood group incompatibility could result in both graft rejection and GVHD. Time and experience has largely dispelled this fear. Although in the early era of bone marrow transplant there was some evidence of delayed engraftment with major ABO incompatibility, use of growth factors and peripheral blood progenitors has made this less problematic (73).

Existence of a major and minor ABO incompatibility requires special processing of a fresh bone marrow allograft. With major ABO incompatibility the red blood cells need to be removed from the donor graft. Several closed systems exist to do this including sedimentation using hetastarch (74–78), a machine-based mononuclear cell concentration; or a more purified mononuclear cell separation such as is obtained with a Ficoll or Percoll separation. For the majority of donors and recipients of the same size, a machine mononuclear cell concentration suffices. This technique leaves a marrow product with a 3% to 4% hematocrit, and usually a normal adult can handle 10 to 30 ml of incompatible red blood cells with minor complications. Occasionally recipients have a severe transfusion reaction with just the minimal contact of donor red blood cells, particularly in patients with prior sensitization to donor red blood cells, such as in a mother-child transplant. The problems of blood group incompatibility occasionally extend beyond the ABO system. High titers to the minor red blood cell antigens in particular can be detected. Usually assessing an antibody screen with the donor-recipient is all that is warranted and felt to be more sensitive than a transplant crossmatch. However, when there is a possibility of prior sensitization, a transplant crossmatch should be considered to assess for possible hemolysis risk. Plasma exchange of the recipient was tried prior to red blood cell depletion technologies but had only marginal success in preventing a reaction with the marrow infusion.

With minor ABO incompatibility, there is risk of both immediate and delayed hemolysis with infusion of the bone marrow graft. The immediate hemolysis is usually an issue with large volumes of donor bone marrow into small recipients, such as a parent-child transplant or use of a group O donor with high titers. Group O donors usually have higher anti-A titers than anti-B titers. When there is such a large mismatch in size between donor and recipient or when the titers are excessively high (greater than 1,028), it would be reasonable and prudent to do a plasma separation of the marrow graft before infusion. If anti-A and anti-B titers cannot be obtained, plasma separation should always be done. The infusion of a minor ABO marrow graft can also be associated with a delayed hemolytic transfusion reaction (79–81). A delayed hemolytic transfusion reaction due to passenger lymphocytes occurs at approximately day 5 to 8 posttransplant when the lymphocytes start producing antibodies directed against recipient antigens. Gajewski et al. (80) and Hows et al. (79) previously reported that at times this type of delayed hemolytic transfusion reaction can develop into an episode of clinically significant hemolysis. Sometimes the amount of red blood cell hemolysis was far in excess of the recipient's estimated red blood cell volume. This type of reaction appears to be quite common in patients receiving cyclosporine without methotrexate for GVHD prophylaxis. As previously reported by Hows (79) and later documented by Gajewski (80), pretransplant red blood cell exchange did not prevent this problem from recurring.

Patients with major-minor ABO incompatibility should have the transplanted bone marrow processed by mononuclear cell concentration because of the need to remove both red blood cells and plasma. Because cell dose is essential to engraftment with a cord blood transplant, cord bloods are often cryopreserved with no red blood cell depletion. The risk of delayed hemolytic transfusion reactions with peripheral blood stem cells has been much less frequent than that seen following bone marrow transplants. This is surprising given that the number of B cells infused with the peripheral blood stem cell graft is probably 1 log greater than that infused with a marrow graft. The reasons for this could include that almost all patients are now receiving a short course of methotrexate for GVHD prophylaxis and possibly that there is a much greater T-cell infusion with the peripheral blood stem cell graft, which may also suppress B-cell function. Further study of this issue is currently in progress.

Peripheral blood stem cell collections present fewer immunohematologic problems following graft infusion, because the CD34$^+$ progenitors are collected as a mononuclear cell concentrate without contaminating red blood cells, plasma, or platelets. However, with major or major-minor ABO incompatibility, the pheresis operation should try to minimize the number of red blood cells collected. The rhesus (Rh) incompatibility is less of an issue unless prior sensitization is detected by the antibody screen.

TABLE 38.1. TRANSFUSION POLICY

Recipient	Donor	RBC Transfusion	Plasma & Platelet Transfusion
O	A	O	A or AB
O	B	O	B or AB
O	AB	O	AB
A	O	O	A or AB
A	AB	O, A	AB
A	B	O	AB
B	O	O	B or AB
B	AB	O, B	AB
B	A	O	AB
AB	A	O, A	AB
AB	B	O, B	AB
AB	O	O	AB

Management of ABO transfusion requirements should start at the initiation of the preparative regimen with infusion of blood found to be compatible with both the recipient's and the donor's tissues. In the case of a major-minor ABO incompatible graft, only group O red blood cells should be transfused. Platelet products should have plasma that, theoretically, is compatible with both donor and recipient. If there is the risk of incompatibility, the platelet products should be reduced to minimize antibody exposure. Only after the donor graft is firmly established should changes in this transfusion practice be initiated (Table 38.1).

Patients must be watched very closely with infusion of intravenous immune globulin. High-dose intravenous immune globulin preparations are not manufactured as ABO type specific. They usually contain high quantities of anti-A and this is thought to be a cause of hemolysis. Many transplant centers will not give immune globulin to group A patients.

With the use of nonmyeloablative transplants, posttransplant mixed chimeric states are occurring more frequently. The transfusion needs of these nonmyeloablative transplants remains to be studied, but there potentially is more risk for posttransplant hemolysis (82).

The instance of posttransplant thrombotic thrombocytopenia purpura (TTP) appears to be increasing. However, both passenger lymphocyte syndrome and immunoglobulin-mediated hemolysis make confirming TTP more difficult. The increased incidence of TTP possibly reflects the increase in posttransplant viral infections. Improved antifungal and antibacterial drugs have made infection with these pathogens less problematic, thus allowing more opportunity for viral infection (83). In this setting TTP is best managed by therapeutic plasma exchange. Further immunosuppression has not proven to be beneficial, although most people usually give high-dose steroids during these circumstances.

Infections

Both allogeneic and autologous bone marrow transplant recipients are predisposed to develop a number of infectious complications (84–91). During the immediate posttransplantation period, patients have granulocytopenia and a high incidence of bacterial and fungal infections. Mucosal herpes simplex infections are also common during this period but seldom disseminate; prophylactic treatment with acyclovir may decrease their incidence and may help prevent pulmonary hemorrhage. Viral gastroenteritis may also occur and may be confused with manifestations of GVHD (86). Patients receiving both allogeneic and autologous transplants need prophylaxis for pneumocystis pneumonia. Herpes zoster is common during the first several years posttransplantation, usually in just a single dermatome, although occasionally multiple dermatomes become involved and rarely a pneumonitis develops. Abdominal zoster infection appears as a severe subxiphoid abdominal pain. Treatment with high-dose intravenous acyclovir is beneficial in patients with disseminated disease, multiple dermatome zoster, and ocular zoster and is used to attempt to prevent dissemination in immunocompromised patients with localized involvement. The erratic absorption of oral acyclovir is responsible for its therapeutic benefits in bone marrow transplant patients. Valacyclovir and penciclovir are oral alternatives for patients with single-dermatome herpes zoster.

Disease caused by CMV remains one of the major complications of allogeneic bone marrow transplantation. Exogenous CMV infections can be acquired via blood product transfusions, although the widespread use of white blood cell filters has prevented much of this (84). Cytomegalovirus-seropositive recipients are at high risk for CMV disease from reactivation of latent endogenous infection. Factors important in the development of CMV disease include age, GVHD, posttransplant immunodeficiency, and drug- or radiation-related lung injury. For CMV-seronegative recipients, acquisition of CMV can be prevented by selecting blood products from CMV-seronegative donors. Several trials of high-dose immune globulin given posttransplant have reduced GVHD and may improve survival. Foscarnet or ganciclovir have not improved survival in bone marrow transplant patients with active CMV. The combination of ganciclovir and intravenous immune globulin has had limited effects in treating pneumonitis but may assist in treatment of CMV gastroenteritis. Ganciclovir has been studied as prophylaxis for CMV infection in seropositive recipients. Although this agent reduces the incidence of CMV infection, ganciclovir frequently produces granulocytopenia and its use has not been shown to improve survival. Rather than relying on growing CMV in tissue cultures, patients are now being screened with antigen testing or by molecular techniques using polymerase chain reaction. Early treatment of patients, often before CMV can grow in culture, has proven to be beneficial in several trials (83–87).

Respiratory syncytial virus (RSV) has been seen increasingly in patients posttransplant. It has been associated with diffuse alveolar hemorrhage but also occurs as interstitial pneumonitis (90,91). Screening for RSV antigens via a nasal wash and throat culture prior to admission helps prevent RSV-associated deaths. The use of digital chest radiographs has actually hurt the ability to detect early interstitial pneumonitis (88). Analog radiographs more clearly define interstitial pneumonitis. Hypoxemia and unexplained dyspnea with a normal radiograph must be aggressively evaluated in the bone marrow transplant patient.

Pneumocystis carinii infection most frequently occurs in patients with lymphoid malignancies, and prophylactic sulfamethoxazole-trimethoprim is indicated for bone marrow transplant recipients. For sulfonamide-allergic patients, pentamidine and atovaquone may be a substitute (91).

Fungal infections remain problematic after bone marrow transplant, and fluconazole has helped prevent a variety of fungal infections (90). Aspergillus, however, remains an almost incurable infection after bone marrow transplant.

Second Malignancies

The high-dose chemotherapy and radiation treatment regimens for bone marrow transplantation are potentially carcinogenic and may predispose to the development of secondary malignancies. Indeed, secondary malignancies occur, albeit rarely, after marrow transplantation. Cytogenetic abnormalities observed prior to cryopreserving autologous progenitor cells can expand clonally and cause acute myelogenous leukemia (AML) or myelodysplasia posttransplant (92). Solid tumors, particularly sarcomas and thyroid cancer, are more common in allogeneic transplant recipients receiving total body irradiation, but still the risk is only approximately 1 in 250 long-term survivors (93). Lymphoproliferative disorders related to Epstein-Barr infection occur due to spread via donor-derived B lymphocytes. This clinical scenario may occur, particularly in heavily immunosuppressed patients treated with intravenous antithymocyte globulin or anti-T-cell antibody therapy; or in HLA-mismatched or T cell-depleted transplants. These B-lymphocyte malignancies frequently respond to an allogeneic donor lymphocyte infusion (DLI) of T lymphocytes from the donor in a concentration of 1×10^5 CD 34+ cells/kg; many other similar types of tumors respond to rituximab (94,95).

RESULTS OF BONE MARROW TRANSPLANTATION FOR TREATMENT OF MALIGNANCY

Acute Myelogenous Leukemia

Although the best results of allogeneic bone marrow transplantation are achieved in patients in first remission, most centers are trying to limit transplantation to patients with a poor prognosis following standard chemotherapy. The rationale for the former approach includes treatment of patients with a relatively low burden of malignant cells prior to the development of resistant leukemia. But even patients with refractory AML have a 15% to 25% chance of long-term survival. The use of nonmyeloablative regimens has opened the option of allogeneic transplantation for patients up to 75 years of age, up from the prior limit of 55 years.

Several controlled trials comparing allogeneic bone marrow transplantation with combination chemotherapy have been reported in patients with AML in first remission. Each study has shown a significantly lower relapse rate in patients receiving bone marrow transplantation. However, marrow transplantation is more likely to be associated with fatal treatment-related complications than is chemotherapy (96–101). A recent Southwest Oncology Group (SWOG) trial did not show an advantage of transplantation over chemotherapy. The Medical Research Council (MRC) tenth trial, which stratified patients by cytogenetic risk groups, however, showed superior outcomes with autologous transplantation in high, intermediate, and poor prognostic groups. With an intention-to-treat analysis, better results were observed only in the intermediate prognostic group for the allogeneic transplant arm. The good prognostic group did well with any treatment. The poor prognostic group did poorly, in part, because four cycles of chemotherapy were given prior to transplant, and patients relapsed without ever getting a transplant.

Based on the age-dependent results of bone marrow transplantation, most data suggest that allogeneic bone marrow transplants from an HLA-identical sibling donor are indicated in children and young adults with AML in first remission. It is uncertain whether older adults should be treated with allogeneic bone marrow transplantation in first remission or receive postremission chemotherapy with marrow transplantation at the time of relapse. Recipients with only an unrelated donor, a family-mismatched donor, or a family-mismatched donor for two or more HLA-A, -B, -DR antigens should receive a transplant only after relapse unless there are associated poor risk factors, abnormal cytogenetics, or an antecedent hematologic disorder.

Autologous bone marrow transplantation has been evaluated as an approach to patients with AML who lack an HLA-identical donor. Procurement of the hematopoietic progenitors should occur only when the patient is in remission, with normal cytogenetics documented immediately prior to collection. For patients receiving autologous marrow transplants while in relapse, the major problem has been rapid relapse of leukemia; the median duration of remission has been 3 to 5 months, and less than 10% of patients survived 1 year. Better results have occurred with autologous marrow transplantation in patients in first or second remission. Approximately 20% to 40% of patients transplanted during second remission have achieved a longer than 2-year disease-free survival (102,103).

For relapsed AML patients lacking a sibling or syngeneic donor, whether to pursue an unrelated donor transplant, a haploidentical transplant, or an autologous transplant depends on circumstances. Autologous transplants should be considered only for patients in a well-established second remission with the harvested cells collected during remission. Because it often takes 2 to 6 months to identify an unrelated donor and procure a bone marrow sample, the patient's disease status must allow this lead time. Unrelated umbilical cord blood can be obtained more quickly, but for most normal size adults the graft failure rate is 20% or higher. Aggressively T-cell depleted haploidentical bone marrow transplant can salvage 20% to 30% of patients with relapsed AML.

Acute Lymphoblastic Leukemia

Conventional chemotherapy offers prolonged remission and even a cure for most children and many adults. Accordingly, transplant is not usually undertaken until after relapse. First remission transplantation should be considered for those with high-risk disease such as patients with t(4:15) or t(9:22) cytogenetics. Successful results of bone marrow transplants in first remission for these patients range from 30% to 60%, depending on patient age and donor type. The GVL effect may be less in acute lymphoblastic leukemia (ALL) than is observed in AML and CML. The rarity of allogeneic donor lymphocyte infusion restoring donor chimerism for relapses post–allogeneic transplant supports this observation. Patients with active leptomeningeal leukemia should have this complication treated prior to transplant, because few bone marrow transplant preparative regimens have agents that cross the blood-brain barrier in therapeutic doses (104–111).

Recurrent leukemia is a major problem in patients with ALL following bone marrow transplantation. Approaches to overcoming this problem include the use of high-dose fractionated radiation, high-dose cytarabine, etoposide, or other chemotherapeutic agents, and the use of posttransplant treatment. None of these approaches has been convincingly shown to reduce the relapse rate or to improve survival in controlled trials.

Despite the availability of a number of monoclonal antibodies to leukemia-associated antigens that are nonreactive with normal hematopoietic progenitors, autologous transplants have not been successful in ALL, even with in vivo purging. The majority of autologous transplants have resulted in long-term survival of 20% or less. Results in poor-risk patients have been even worse (112).

Chronic Myelogenous Leukemia

Allogeneic or syngeneic bone marrow transplantation is an effective treatment for CML, capable of producing long-term disease-free survival. Approximately 20% of syngeneic recipients transplanted during blast crisis have survived free of disease longer than 5 years, demonstrating that the intensive marrow-ablative therapy can eradicate even far-advanced disease in some patients. Better results have been reported for patients receiving allogeneic or syngeneic bone marrow transplantation while in the chronic phase, with an actuarial survival of 65% at more than 5 years. If the transplant is performed within 1 to 2 years of diagnosis from an allogeneic HLA genotypically identical sibling donor, survival is 80% to 90%. Although most patients have received high-dose cyclophosphamide and total body irradiation for the preparative regimen, the combination of busulfan and cyclophosphamide without radiotherapy is equally effective. Oral busulfan has been associated with erratic absorption. The new intravenous preparation does not have this adverse aspect and may be preferable to oral busulfan. Intravenous busulfan therapy has not been compared to total body irradiation plus cyclophosphamide. Overall results are dependent on the stage of the disease at the time of transplantation (113–117).

The alternatives to transplantation are interferon-α–based approaches and imatinib mesylate (Gleevec), a new type of tyrosine kinase inhibitor (118). Gleevec has been very successful in putting most patients into hematologic remission (118). These remissions, however, have not been durable in patients in accelerated or blast crisis, and the data with chronic-phase patients remain uncertain. Transplantation for CML is being done less often because of Gleevec, but the long-term benefits remain unclear. Gleevec is now being evaluated after transplantation for patients at high risk for relapse. Approximately 30% of newly diagnosed patients achieve a complete hematologic and cytogenetic remission if interferon-α is given in conjunction with cytarabine; median duration of survival exceeds 8 years among respondents. These data using interferon-α in patients with early chronic-phase CML have prompted some centers to delay the use of bone marrow transplantation in older adults for approximately 6 months to 1 year to allow for a trial of interferon.

Considerable data indicate that the high-dose preparative regimen does not completely eliminate all malignant cells in patients with CML and that an important GVL effect is necessary to prevent relapse. Most patients have small numbers of Philadelphia chromosome–positive cells identified by cytogenetics or by polymerase chain reaction analysis for the Bcr/Abl gene rearrangement (104). Many patients receiving unmodified transplants have remained in hematologic remission, and the Philadelphia chromosome–positive cells may spontaneously disappear in later analyses. In recipients of T cell-depleted bone marrow, however, >90% of patients with cytogenetic relapse progress to an overt clinical relapse (116). These data support the concept that the GVL effect is largely mediated by alloreactive T cells present in donor marrow. Infusion of donor T lymphocytes can ultimately salvage 90% of patients with CML relapsing in a chronic phase (117). Typically these cells are collected in one to two leukapheresis procedures (119). The optimal dose in HLA-identical siblings is 1×10^7 $CD34^+$ cells/kg recipient body weight. The response for conversion of patients to donor hematopoiesis takes about 3 to 4 months to 12 months. Patients typically become cytopenic 4 to 6 weeks after infusion of the donor lymphocytes. Graft versus host disease can occur with donor lymphocyte infusions and is a major risk if the donor is more of a mismatch from the patient than an HLA-identical sibling (120). The efficacy of this GVH effect is why CML has been particularly suited to the nonmyeloablative transplant, in which the preparative regimen's principal goal is to immunosuppress the recipient. Early data suggest nonmyeloablative approaches have had similar success rates to myeloablative for patients with CML (121).

Autologous transplants for CML involve collection and cryopreservation of bone marrow or peripheral blood stem cells during the chronic phase of the disease. Patients later receive intensive chemotherapy alone or combined with total body irradiation, and followed by reinfusion of cryopreserved autologous cells. The objective of this approach is to restore the early chronic phase and, if possible, diploid hematopoiesis. Because Philadelphia chromosome–positive cells are reinfused, cure is not possible (122). Gleevec may be the cause for this largely abandoned approach to be reconsidered (118).

Chronic Lymphocytic Leukemia

Chronic lymphocytic leukemia (CLL) is the most prevalent form of leukemia. It is a clonal disorder with accumulation of small lymphocytes of B-cell lineage. Although this disease has an indolent natural history, it is incurable with available treatments. Historically, few bone marrow transplants have been performed for this disease, because CLL primarily affects the elderly and the marrow is heavily involved with malignant cells, precluding autologous transplantation. High-dose cyclophosphamide, total body irradiation, and allogeneic bone marrow transplantation have been effective in producing prolonged disease-free survival in selected younger patients (123). This disease has been very sensitive to less intensive nonablative regimens using fludarabine-based regimens followed by allogeneic hematopoietic progenitors cells. It is also very responsive to donor lymphocytes for treatment of relapse after allogeneic bone marrow transplant. Chronic lymphocytic leukemia will typically persist for months after an allograft, particularly if the preparative regimen was nonmyeloablative. One should follow this disease for several months after an allograft before treating with a DLI. Measuring peripheral blood T-cell chimerism may be the preferred method of monitoring these patients (124).

LYMPHOID MALIGNANCIES

Lymphoma

Relapsed non-Hodgkin lymphoma is treatable with a syngeneic, allogeneic, or autologous bone marrow transplant (125). The Parma study was a randomized trial comparing standard salvage chemotherapy in first relapse of large cell lymphoma to standard chemotherapy plus autologous bone marrow transplant. This trial demonstrated a definitive advantage for patients receiving a bone marrow transplant. For large cell non-Hodgkin lymphoma, the best results have been noted in patients treated while in a second remission or during a relapse that is still responsive to chemotherapy, with results ranging from 20% to 60% long-term survival. Recently, encouraging results have been reported in patients receiving autologous transplants in partial remission after initial induction therapy for large cell lymphoma. Until recently, allogeneic bone marrow transplant was less preferred for large cell and immunoblastic lymphoma. For patients with marrow involvement or whose disease is refractory to standard chemotherapy, allogeneic bone marrow transplant can still salvage 33% of patients (126). Burkitt lymphoma and leukemia have not been responsive to an allogeneic GVL effect. Autologous bone marrow transplantation has been successful, but only when performed during first remission. For Burkitt lymphoma, preparative regimens should preferably contain cyclophosphamide. Mantle cell lymphoma, a recently described aggressive lymphoma, has proven very resistant to standard chemotherapy. Allogeneic bone marrow transplantation has accomplished a 90% survival when done during first remission and 30% for patients receiving transplants during relapse. Autologous bone marrow transplants have been successful with a 75% long-term remission rate when done during first remission. Beyond first remission, autologous bone marrow transplantation has been less disappointing (126).

Both autologous and allogeneic transplantation have been evaluated for patients with low-grade lymphoma. Low-grade lymphoid malignancies frequently have bone marrow involvement.

Purging techniques generally achieve approximately a 2- to 3-log reduction of malignant cells. These systems, however, cannot effectively deplete cells from patients with clinically involved bone marrow but may be successful for patients whose marrows are histologically in remission. Gribben et al. (17) reported significantly better disease-free survival in patients receiving autologous marrow who were successfully purged, free of evidence of residual lymphoma as evidenced by being free of the *bcl*-2 gene rearrangement by the polymerase chain reaction. Just like CLL, low grade lymphomas have proven very sensitive to allogeneic transplants. Results have shown 60% 5-year disease survival, even in refractory patients. The indolent nature of this disease allows donor lymphocyte infusions to be a treatment after relapse following allogeneic bone marrow transplantation. Allogeneic transplant is now the preferred option for low-grade lymphoma, given the difficulty in purging lymphoma cells from the marrow or peripheral blood. Just like with CLL, the fludarabine-based nonmyeloablative regimens have shown excellent results with this diagnosis. One recent report demonstrated 100% survival with the nonmyeloablative transplant approach. This group is slow to clear the malignant cells posttransplant. Clear-cut progress should be confirmed before a DLI is given (127–132).

Hodgkin Disease

High-dose chemotherapy and autologous bone marrow transplantation is an effective treatment for relapsed high-risk patients with Hodgkin disease (133,134). Treatment results have a complete remission rate of more than 50% to 80% and a 20% to 60% disease-free survival at 3 to 5 years. The most commonly used regimens involve a nitrosourea, alkylating agents, and etoposide. The doses employed have varied widely from center to center. Prognostic factors for response and survival after autologous bone marrow transplantation include age, performance status, disease stage at time of transplantation, number of extranodal sites, number of prior treatment regimens, and response to prior chemotherapy and radiation treatment. These factors are similar to prognostic factors for patients receiving salvage chemotherapy.

Allogeneic bone marrow transplantation has been associated with a treatment-related mortality in approximately 40% of patients. Relatively few allogeneic transplants have been performed in patients with Hodgkin disease. Studies in patients with advanced disease probably not suitable for autologous transplantation have a 15% to 20% salvage rate with HLA-matched sibling bone marrow transplant (134).

Multiple Myeloma

Because a randomized trial showed an advantage of autologous bone marrow transplantation over standard chemotherapy, autologous bone marrow transplantation is used increasingly to treat myeloma. The preparative regimen studied was high-dose melphalan. Although autologous transplants have been associated with prolonged survival, they rarely have produced a cure. Recently, autologous transplants have been studied for patients up to age 70 years. The patients most likely to benefit from autologous transplant are those who are treated for primary resistant disease or responding disease with low β2-microglobulin and lactic dehydrogenase levels within 1 year of diagnosis (135, 136).

Although autologous transplants have rarely been curative therapy, the prolongation of survival and event free survival has left little opportunity for allogeneic bone marrow transplantation. Approximately one-third of allogeneic transplant recipients survive for 1 to 3 years free of relapse. Allogeneic transplant has been shown to rescue patients after relapse following autologous bone marrow transplantation. Nonmyeloablative approaches are being studied extensively in these patients. Patients with poor prognostic features, such as any abnormality of chromosome 13, should be considered for allogeneic bone marrow transplantation very early in their treatment plans (137–139).

Pediatric Solid Tumors

Bone marrow transplantation may be particularly useful in the treatment of several pediatric tumors, such as neuroblastoma and Ewing sarcoma, which are highly sensitive to a number of chemotherapeutic agents and radiation yet have a poor prognosis in patients with advanced disease (140). Monoclonal antibodies to neuroblastoma-related antigens can be used to detect microscopic bone marrow involvement and to purge metastatic neuroblastoma cells from the marrow prior to cryopreservation. Gene-marking studies of autologous marrow demonstrate that malignant cells infused in the autotransplant can contribute to relapse.

Ewing sarcoma is another potential candidate tumor for autologous bone marrow transplantation. High-dose melphalan or cyclophosphamide and total body irradiation with autologous bone marrow transplantation can produce complete remissions in patients with relapsed Ewing sarcoma, but these responses are usually brief.

Breast Cancer

Treatment of breast cancer by autologous transplantation has been controversial. Most chemotherapeutic agents active against breast cancer exhibit a dose-dependent antitumor response. However, increasing dosage results in increased cytotoxicity. The maximal dosage of most agents is limited by myelosuppression. Dose escalation is possible, however, if followed by intravenous infusion of bone marrow or peripheral blood progenitors to regenerate hematopoiesis. The most effective high-dose chemotherapy regimens used with autologous marrow or blood stem cell transplantation include combinations of alkylating agents and related drugs, including cyclophosphamide, melphalan, thiotepa, carmustine, cisplatin, or carboplatin. Taxanes are now being studied in bone marrow transplant–preparative regimens. Studies in patients with chemotherapy-responsive metastatic breast cancer have documented that this approach significantly increases the complete remission rate to >50%. Preliminary results of several randomized trials have recently been published or presented at national meetings, sometimes with conflicting results. Part of the issue has been the short follow-up for 2 to 5 years. The Parma trial with the more rapidly growing large cell lymphoma did not become definitively positive until 7 years, so the breast cancer evaluation may require 10 or more years of follow-up to be conclusive. The majority of the adjuvant studies of autologous transplant have shown trends in favor of transplant with reduced relapsed risk, improved progression-free survival, and no impact on overall survival. For stage IV breast cancer, the trials have had mixed to largely negative results (141–146).

Other Solid Tumors

A similar approach with autologous bone marrow transplantation has been used for the treatment of other chemotherapy-responsive solid tumors in adults, including ovarian cancer, testicular and germ cell carcinomas, and small cell carcinoma of the lung.

Testicular carcinoma is a chemotherapy-responsive malignancy that is frequently cured using standard-dose cisplatin-based chemotherapy. Patients failing first- and second-line chemotherapy regimens have received high-dose chemotherapy and autologous bone marrow transplants. Response rates are high, and a minority has achieved long-term remissions; unfortunately, responses in most patients are usually of short duration.

Dose-intensive chemotherapy is being used increasingly for treating ovarian cancer. Like breast cancer, this tumor is sensitive to alkylating agents, platinum-based chemotherapy agents and taxanes, and topoisomerase I inhibitors. Transplants have not been used commonly in the adjuvant setting but have a role for patients with low-bulk disease after a second-look laparoscopy and for patients with chemotherapy-sensitive low-bulk, relapsed disease.

Recent work has demonstrated an allogeneic effect on renal cell carcinoma with 38% progression-free survival (147). Allogeneic bone marrow transplantation is also being reviewed for breast cancer (148).

FUTURE DIRECTIONS

Blood and bone marrow transplantation is at a crossroads. Increased regulatory pressures have been necessary because of the dissemination of this technology to the community. Payer pressures have dramatically increased financial risk to providers offering this procedure. Alternative drug therapies like Gleevec and trastuzumab (Herceptin) have much less difficulty showing efficacy in clinical trials (118). On the other hand, technology is rapidly coming to offer antigen-specific cellular therapies. This will potentially enable bone marrow transplantation to have the focus of a monoclonal antibody. The hematopoietic stem cells have also shown to have potential to heal heart and neural tissue ischemic damage. Time will determine if bone marrow transplantation will remain a rapidly growing therapy or be relegated to a minor chapter in the history of medicine.

REFERENCES

1. Thomas E, Storb R, Clift RA, et al. Bone marrow transplantation (first of two parts). *New Engl J Med* 1975;292:832–843.
2. Elias A, Armitage JO. Bone marrow transplantation. *New Engl J Med* 1994;331:617.
3. O'Reilly RJ. Allogeneic bone marrow transplantation: current status and future directions. *Blood* 1983;62:942–946.
4. Lum LG. The kinetics of immune reconstitution after human marrow transplantation. *Blood* 1987;69:369–380.
5. Fefer A, Cheever MA, Thomas ED, et al. Bone marrow transplantation for refractory acute leukemia in 34 patients with identical twins. *Blood* 1981;57:421–430.
6. Sullivan KM, Weiden PL, Storb R, et al. Influence of acute and chronic graft-versus-host disease on relapse and survival after bone marrow transplantation from HLA identical siblings as treatment of acute and chronic leukemia. *Blood* 1989;73:1720–1728.
7. Horowitz MM, Gale RP, Sondel PM, et al. Graft-vs.-leukemia reaction after bone marrow transplantation. *Blood* 1990;75:555–562.
8. Carella AM, Champlin R, Slavin S, et al. Mini-allografts: ongoing trials in humans [Editorial]. *Bone Marrow Transplant* 2000;25:345–350.
9. Khouri IF, Keating M, Korbling M, et al. Transplant-lite: induction of graft-versus-malignancy using fludarabine-based nonablative chemotherapy and allogeneic blood progenitor cell transplantation as treatment for lymphoid malignancies. *J Clin Oncol* 1998;16:2817–2824.
10. Childs R, Clave E, Contentin N, et al. Engraftment kinetics after nonmyeloablative allogeneic peripheral blood stem cell transplantation: full donor T-cell chimerism precedes alloimmune responses. *Blood* 1999b;94:3234–3241.
11. Appelbaum FR, Herzig GP, Graw RG, et al. Study of cell dose and storage time on engraftment of cryopreserved autologous bone marrow in a canine model. *Transplantation* 1978;26:245–248.
12. Korbling M, Huh YO, Durrett A, et al. Allogeneic blood stem cell transplantation: peripheralization and yield of primitive donor-derived hematopoietic progenitor cells ($CD34^+$ Thy- 1dim) and lymphoid subsets, and possible predictors of engraftment and graft-versus-host disease. *Blood* 1995;86:2842–2848.
13. Stadtmauer EA, Schneider CJ, Silberstein LE. Peripheral blood progenitor cell generation and harvesting. *Semin Oncol* 1995;22:291–300.
14. Bensinger WI, Martin PJ, Storer B, et al. Transplantation of bone marrow as compared with peripheral-blood stem cells from HLA-identical relatives in patients with hematologic cancers. *New Engl J Med* 2001;344:175–181.
15. Korbling M, Przepiorka D, Huh YO, et al. Allogeneic blood stem cell transplantation for refractory leukemia and lymphoma: potential advantages of blood over marrow allografts. *Blood* 1995;85:1659–1665.
16. Gajewski JL, Saliba R, Korbling M, et al. High doses of $CD34^+$ cells and chemomobilization are associated with a reduced progression rate after autologous PBSC transplantation for breast cancer in a phase III trial. ASCO 2001.
17. Gribben JG, Freedman AS, Neuberg D, et al. Immunologic purging of marrow assessed by PCR before autologous bone marrow transplantation for B-cell lymphoma. *New Engl J Med* 1991;325:1525–1533.
18. Vredenburgh JJ, Peters WP, Rosner G, et al. Detection of tumor cells in the bone marrow at stage IV breast cancer patients receiving high-dose chemotherapy: the role of induction chemotherapy. *Bone Marrow Transplant* 1995;16:815–821.
19. Berenson RJ, Bensinger WI, Hill RS, et al. Engraftment after infusion of $CD34^+$ marrow cells in patients with breast cancer or neuroblastoma. *Blood* 1991;77:1717–1722.
20. Shpall EJ, LeMaistre CF, Holland K, et al. A prospective randomized trial of buffy coat vs. CD34-selected autologous bone marrow support in high-risk breast cancer patients receiving high-dose chemotherapy. *Blood* 1997;90:4313–4320.

21. Beatty PG, Clift RA, Mickelson EM, et al. Marrow transplantation from related donors other than HLA-identical siblings. *New Engl J Med* 1985;313:765–771.
22. Gajewski J, Cecka M, Champlin R. Bone marrow transplantation utilizing HLA-matched unrelated marrow donors. *Blood Rev* 1990; 4:132–138.
23. Kernan NA, Bartsch G, Ash RC, et al. Retrospective analysis of 462 unrelated marrow transplants facilitated by the National Marrow Donor Program (NMDP) for treatment of acquired and congenital disorders of the lymphohematopoietic system and congenital metabolic disorders. *New Engl J Med* 1993;328:593–602.
24. Gluckman E, Rocha V, Boyer-Chammard A, et al. Outcome of cord blood transplantation from related and unrelated donors. Eurocord Transplant Group and the European Blood and Marrow Transplantation Group. *New Engl J Med* 1997;337:373–381.
25. Kurtzberg J, Laughlin M, Graham MC, et al. Placental blood as a source of hematopoietic stem cells for transplantation into unrelated recipients. *New Engl J Med* 1996;335:157–166.
26. Teraskai PI, McLelland J. Microdroplet assay of human serum cytotoxins. *Nature* 1964;204:988–1000.
27. Olerup O, Zetterquist H. HLA-DR typing by PCR amplification with sequence-specific primers (PCR-SSP) in 2 hours: an alternative to serological DR typing in clinical practice including donor-recipient matching in cadaveric transplantation. *Tissue Antigens* 1992;39: 225–235.
28. Buyse I, Decorte R, Cuppens H, et al. Rapid DNA typing of class II HLA antigens using the polymerase chain reaction and reverse dot blot hybridization. *Tissue Antigens* 1993;41:1–14.
29. Van Rood JJ, Jough B, Claas FHJ, et al. New facts on HLA genetics: are they relevant in bone marrow transplantation? *Semin Hematol* 1984;21:65–79.
30. Petersdorf EW, Gooley T, Anasetti C, et al. Optimizing outcome after unrelated marrow transplantation by comprehensive matching of HLA class I and II alleles in the donor and recipient. *Blood* 1998; 92:3515–3520.
31. Vogt MH, Goulmy E, Kloosterboer FM, et al. UTY gene codes for an HLA-B60-restricted human male-specific minor histocompatibility antigen involved in stem cell graft rejection: characterization of the critical polymorphic amino acid residues for T-cell recognition. *Blood* 2000;96:3126–3132.
32. Martin PJ. Increased disparity for minor histocompatibility antigens as a potential cause of increased GVHD risk in marrow transplantation from unrelated donors compared with related donors. *Bone Marrow Transplant* 1991;8:217.
33. Reisner Y, Martelli MF. Bone marrow transplantation across HLA barriers by increasing the number of transplanted cells. *Immunol Today* 1995;16:437–440.
34. Bacher-Lustig E, Rachamim N, Li HW, et al. Megadose of T cell-depleted bone marrow overcomes MHC barriers in sublethally irradiated mice. *Nat Med* 1995;1:1268–1273.
35. Handgretinger R, Schumm M, Lang P, et al. Transplantation of megadoses of purified haploidentical stem cells, *Ann N Y Acad Sci* 1999; 872:351–361.
36. Hill RS, Petersen FB, Storb R, et al. Mixed hematologic chimerism after allogeneic marrow transplantation for severe aplastic anemia is associated with higher risk of graft rejection and a lessened incidence of acute graft-versus-host disease. *Blood* 1986;67:811–816.
37. Sharabi Y, Abraham VS, Sykes M, et al. Mixed allogeneic chimeras prepared by a nonmyeloablative regimen: requirement for chimerism to maintain tolerance. *Bone Marrow Transplant* 1992;9:191–197.
38. Shi Q, Wu MH, Fujita Y, et al. Genetic tracing of arterial graft flow surface endothelialization in allogeneic marrow transplanted dogs. *Cardiovasc Surg* 1999;7:98–105.
39. Szydlo R, Goldman JM, Klein JP, et al. Results of allogeneic bone marrow transplants for leukemia using donors other than HLA-identical siblings. *J Clin Oncol* 1997;15:1767–1777.
40. Anasetti C. Transplantation of hematopoietic stem cells from alternate donors in acute myelogenous leukemia. *Leukemia* 2000;14:502–504.
41. Henslee-Downey PJ, Abhyankar SH, Parrish RS, et al. Use of partially mismatched related donors extends access to allogeneic marrow transplant. *Blood* 1997;89:3864–3872.
42. Aversa F, Tabilio A, Velardi A, et al. Treatment of high risk acute leukemia with T cell-depleted stem cells from related donors with one fully mismatched HLA haplotype. *New Engl J Med* 1998;339: 1186–1193.
43. Guinan EC, Boussiotis VA, Neuberg D, et al. Transplantation of anergic histoincompatible bone marrow allograft. *New Engl J Med* 1999;340:1704–1714.
44. Sanz GF, Saavedra S, Jimenez C, et al. Unrelated donor cord blood transplantation in adults with chronic myelogenous leukemia: results in nine patients from a single institution. *Bone Marrow Transplant* 2001;27:693–701.
45. Wagner JE, Rosenthal J, Sweetman R, et al. Successful transplantation of HLA-matched and HLA-mismatched umbilical cord-blood from unrelated donors: analysis of engraftment and acute graft-versus-host disease. *Blood* 1996;88:795–802.
46. Cairo MS, Wagner JE. Placental and/or umbilical cord blood: an alternative source of hematopoietic stem cells for transplantation. *Blood* 1997; 90:4665–4678.
47. Rubinstein P, Carrier C, Scaradavou M, et al. Outcome among 562 recipients of placental blood transplants from unrelated donors. *New Engl J Med* 1998;339:1565–1577.
48. Sobecks RM, Daugherty CK, Hallahan DE, et al. A dose escalation study of total body irradiation followed by high-dose etoposide and allogeneic blood stem cell transplantation for the treatment of advanced hematologic malignancies. *Bone Marrow Transplant* 2000;25: 807–813.
49. Robbins RA, Linder J, Stahl MG, et al. Diffuse alveolar hemorrhage in autologous bone marrow transplant recipients. *Am J Med* 1989; 87:511–518.
50. Mulder POM, Meinesz AF, de Vries EGE, et al. Diffuse alveolar hemorrhage in autologous bone marrow transplant recipients. *Am J Med* 1991;90:278–280.
51. Lewis ID, Defor T, Weisdorf DJ. Increasing incidence of diffuse alveolar hemorrhage following allogeneic bone marrow transplantation: cryptic etiology and uncertain therapy. *Bone Marrow Transplant* 2000; 26:539–543.
52. Hicks K, Peng D, Gajewski J. Successful treatment of diffuse alveolar hemorrhage after allogeneic bone marrow transplant with recombinant factor VIIa. (submitted- *Bone Marrow Transplant*)
53. Chan CK, Hyland RH, Hutcheon MA. Pulmonary complications following bone marrow transplantation. *Clin Chest Med* 1990;11: 323–332.
54. Alessandrino EP, Bernasconi P, Colombo A, et al. Pulmonary toxicity following carmustine-based preparative regimens and autologous peripheral blood progenitor cell transplantation in hematological malignancies. *Bone Marrow Transplant* 2000;25:309–313.
55. Sullivan KM, Mori M, Sanders J, et al. Late complications of allogeneic and autologous marrow transplantation. *Bone Marrow Transplant* 1992;10[Suppl 1]:127–134.
56. Sencer SF, Haake RJ, Weisdorf DJ. Hemorrhagic cystitis after bone marrow transplantation: risk factors and complications. *Transplantation* 1993;56:875–879.
57. Chen FE, Liang RHS, Lo JY, et al. Treatment of adenovirus-associated haemorrhagic cystitis with ganciclovir. *Bone Marrow Transplant* 1997; 20:997–999.
58. Shepherd JD, Pringle LE, Barnett MJ, et al. Mesna versus hyperhydration for the prevention of cyclophosphamide-induced hemorrhagic cystitis in bone marrow transplantation. *J Clin Oncol* 1991;9: 2016–2020.
59. Kernan NA, Flomenberg N, Dupont B, et al. Graft rejection in recipients of T-cell-depleted HLA-nonidentical marrow transplants for leukemia. Identification of host-derived antidonor allocytotoxic lymphocytes. *Transplantation* 1987;43:842–847.
60. Champlin RE, Passweg JR, Zhang MJ, et al. T-cell depletion of bone marrow transplants for leukemia from donors other than HLA-identical siblings: advantage of T-cell antibodies with narrow specificities. *Blood* 2000;95:3996–4003.
61. Champlin RE, Schmitz N, Horowitz MM, et al. Blood stem cells

compared with bone marrow as a source of hematopoietic cells for allogeneic transplantation. IBMTR Histocompatibility and Stem Cell Sources Working Committee and the European Group for Blood and Marrow Transplantation (EBMT). *Blood* 2000;95:3702–3709.

62. Ferrara JL, Deeg HJ. Graft-versus-host disease. *New Engl J Med* 1991; 324:667–674.
63. Schreiber SL, Crabtree GR. The mechanism of action of cyclosporin A and FK 506. *Immunol Today* 1992;13:136–142.
64. Hiscott A, McLellan DS. Graft-versus-host disease in allogeneic bone marrow transplantation: the role of monoclonal antibodies in prevention and treatment. *Br J Biomed Sci* 2000;57:163–169.
65. Kottaridis PD, Milligan DW, Chopra R, et al. In vivo CAMPATH-1H prevents graft-versus-host disease following nonmyeloablative stem cell transplantation. *Blood* 2000;96:2419–2425.
66. Mitsuyasu R, Champlin RE, Gale RP, et al. Treatment of donor bone marrow with monoclonal anti-T-cell antibody and complement for the prevention of graft-versus-host disease. *Ann Intern Med* 1986;105: 20–26.
67. Mathias C, Mick R, Grupp S, et al. Soluble interleukin-2 receptor concentration as a biochemical indicator for a graft-versus-host disease after allogeneic bone marrow transplantation. *J Hematother Stem Cell Res* 2000;9:393–400.
68. Hill GR, Ferrara JL. The primacy of the gastrointestinal tract as a target organ of acute graft-versus-host disease: rationale for the use of cytokine shields in allogeneic bone marrow transplantation. *Blood* 2000;95:2754–2759.
69. Sullivan KM, Agura E, Anasetti C, et al. Chronic graft-versus-host disease and other late complications of bone marrow transplantation *Semin Hematol* 1991;28:250–259.
70. Storek J, Gooley T, Sladak M, et al. Allogeneic peripheral blood stem cell transplantation may be associated with a high risk of chronic graft versus host disease. *Blood* 1997;90:4705–4709.
71. Vogelsang GB, Farmer ER, Hess AD, et al. Thalidomide for the treatment of chronic graft-versus-host disease. *New Engl J Med* 1992; 326:1055–1058.
72. Rosetti F, Zulian F, Dall'Amico R, et al. Extracorporeal photochemotherapy as single therapy for extensive, cutaneous, chronic graft-versus-host disease. *Transplantation* 1995;59:149–151.
73. Petz LD. Immunohematologic problems associated with bone marrow transplantation. *Transfus Med Rev* 1987;1:85–100.
74. Braine HG, Sensenbrener LL, Wright SK, et al. Bone marrow transplantation with major ABO blood group incompatibility using erythrocyte depletion of marrow prior to infusion. *Blood* 1982;60: 420–425.
75. Ho WG, Champlin RE, Feig SA, et al. Transplantation of major ABH incompatible bone marrow: gravity sedimentation of donor marrow. *Br J Haematol* 1984;57:155–162.
76. Dinsmore RE, Reich LM, Kapoor N, et al. ABH incompatible bone marrow transplantation: removal of erythrocytes by starch sedimentation. *Br J Haematol* 1984;54:441–449.
77. Warkentin PI, Hilden JM, Kersey JH, et al. Transplantation of major ABO-incompatible bone marrow depleted of red cells by hydroxyethyl starch. *Vox Sang* 1985;48:89–104.
78. Sniecinski I, Henry S, Ritchey B, et al. Erythrocyte depletion of ABO-incompatible bone marrow. *J Clin Apheresis* 1985;2:231–234.
79. Hows J, Beddow K, Gordon-Smith E, et al. Donor-derived red blood cell antibodies and immune hemolysis after allogeneic bone marrow transplantation. *Blood* 1986;67:177–181.
80. Gajewski JL, Petz LD, Calhoun L, et al. Hemolysis of transfused group O red blood cells in minor ABO-incompatible unrelated-donor bone marrow transplants in patients receiving cyclosporin without post-transplant methotrexate. *Blood* 1992;79:3076–3085.
81. Bolan CD, Childs RW, Procter JL, et al. Massive immune haemolysis after allogeneic peripheral blood stem cell transplantation with minor ABO incompatibility. *Br J Haematol* 2001;112:787–795.
82. Lapierre V, Oubouzar N, Auperin A, et al. Influence of the hematopoietic stem cell source on early immunohematologic reconstitution after allogeneic transplantation. *Blood* 2001;97:2580–2586.
83. Han CS, Miller W, Haake R, et al. Varicella zoster infection after bone marrow transplantation: incidence, risk factors and complications. *Bone Marrow Transplant* 1994;13:277–283.
84. Bowden RA, Slichter SJ, Sayers M, et al. A comparison of filtered leukocyte-reduced and cytomegalovirus (CMV) seronegative blood products for the prevention of transfusion-associated CMV infection after marrow transplant. *Blood* 1995;86:3598–3603.
85. Enright H, Haake R, Weisdorf D, et al. Cytomegalovirus pneumonia after bone marrow transplantation: risk factors and response to therapy. *Transplantation* 1993;55:1339–1346.
86. Goodrich JM, Bowden RA, Fisher L, et al. Ganciclovir prophylaxis to prevent cytomegalovirus disease after allogeneic marrow transplant. *Ann Intern Med* 1993;118:173–178.
87. Winston DJ, Ho WG, Bartoni K, et al. Ganciclovir prophylaxis of cytomegalovirus infection and disease in allogeneic bone marrow transplant recipients: results of a placebo-controlled, double-blind trial. *Ann Intern Med* 1993;118:179–184.
88. Goodrich JM, Mori M, Gleaves CA, et al. Early treatment with ganciclovir to prevent cytomegalovirus disease after allogeneic bone marrow transplantation. *New Engl J Med* 1991;325:1601–1607.
89. Whimbey E, Champlin RE, Couch RB, et al. Community respiratory virus infections among hospitalized adult bone marrow transplant recipients. *Clin Infect Dis* 1996;22:778–782.
90. Goodman JL, Winston DJ, Greenfield RA, et al. A controlled trial of fluconazole to prevent fungal infections in patients undergoing bone marrow transplantation. *New Engl J Med* 1992;326:845–851.
91. Souza JP, Boeckh M, Gooley TA, et al. High rates of *Pneumocystis carinii* pneumonia in allogeneic blood and marrow transplant recipients receiving dapsone prophylaxis. *Clin Infect Dis* 1999;29: 1467–1471.
92. Armitage JO. Myelodysplasia and acute leukemia after autologous bone marrow transplantation. *J Clin Oncol* 2000;18:945–946.
93. Curtis RE, Rowlings PA, Deeg HJ, et al. Solid cancers after bone marrow transplantation *New Engl J Med* 1997;336:897–904.
94. Benkerrou M, Durandy A, Fischer A. Therapy for transplant-related lymphoproliferative diseases. *Hematol Oncol Clin North Am* 1993;7: 467–475.
95. Fischer A, Blanche S, Le Bidois J, et al. Anti-B cell monoclonal antibodies in the treatment of severe B-cell lymphoproliferative syndromes following bone marrow and organ transplantation. *New Engl J Med* 1991;324:1451–1456.
96. Cassileth PA, Harrington DP, Appelbaum FR, et al. Chemotherapy compared with autologous or allogeneic bone marrow transplantation in the management of acute myeloid leukemia in first remission. *New Engl J Med* 1998;339:1649–1656.
97. Zittoun RA, Mandelli F, Willemze R, et al. Autologous or allogeneic bone marrow transplantation compared with intensive chemotherapy in acute myelogenous leukemia. *New Engl J Med* 1995;332:217–223.
98. Champlin RE, Ho WG, Gale RP, et al. Treatment of acute myelogenous leukemia: a prospective controlled trial of bone marrow transplantation versus consolidation chemotherapy. *Ann Intern Med* 1985; 102:285–291.
99. Reiffers J, Stoppa AM, Attal M, et al. Allogeneic vs. autologous stem cell transplantation vs. chemotherapy in patients with acute myeloid leukemia in first remission: the BGMT 87 study. *Leukemia* 1996;10: 1874–1882.
100. Mayer RJ, Davis RB, Schiffer CA, et al. Intensive postremission chemotherapy in adults with acute myeloid leukemia. Cancer and Leukemia Group B. *N Engl J Med* 1994;331:896–903.
101. Burnett AK, Goldstone AH, Steven RMF, et al. Randomised comparison of addition of autologous bone marrow transplantation to intensive chemotherapy for acute myeloid leukaemia in first remission: results of MRC AML 10 trial. UK Medical Research Council Adult and Children's Leukaemia Working Parties. *Lancet* 1998;351: 700–708.
102. Cassileth PA, Andersen J, Lazarus HM, et al. Autologous bone marrow transplant in acute myeloid leukemia in first remission. *J Clin Oncol* 1993;11:314–319.
103. Ball ED, Rybka WB. Autologous bone marrow transplantation for adult acute leukemia. *Hematol Oncol Clin North Am* 1993;7: 201–231.

104. Zhang MJ, Hoelzer D, Horowitz MM, et al. Long-term follow up of adults with acute lymphoblastic leukemia in first remission treated with chemotherapy of bone marrow transplantation: the acute lymphoblastic leukemia working committee. *Ann Intern Med* 1995;15: 428–431.
105. Martin TG, Gajewski JL. Allogeneic stem cell transplantation for acute lymphocytic leukemia in adults. *Hematol Oncol Clin North Am* 2000;15:97–120.
106. Forman SJ, Blume KG. Allogeneic bone marrow transplantation for acute leukemia. *Hematol Oncol Clin North Am* 1990;4:517–534.
107. Forman SJ, O'Donnell MR, Nadamanee AP, et al. Bone marrow transplantation for patients with Philadelphia chromosome–positive acute lymphoblastic leukemia. *Blood* 1987;70:587–588.
108. Sebban C, Lepage E, Vernant JP, et al. Allogeneic bone marrow transplantation in adult acute lymphoblastic leukemia in first complete remission: a comparative study. *J Clin Oncol* 1994;12:2580–2587.
109. Barrett AJ, Horowitz MM, Ash RC, et al. Bone marrow transplantation for Philadelphia chromosome–positive acute lymphoblastic leukemia. *Blood* 1992;79:3067–3070.
110. Kersey JH, Weisdorf D, Nesbit ME, et al. Comparison of autologous and allogeneic bone marrow transplantation for treatment of high risk refractory acute lymphoblastic leukemia in second remission. *New Engl J Med* 1987;317:461–467.
111. Sierra J, Radich J, Hansen JA, et al. Marrow transplants from unrelated donors for treatment of Philadelphia chromosome–positive acute lymphoblastic leukemia. *Blood* 1997;90:1410–1414.
112. Sallan SE, Niemeyer CM, Billett Al, et al. Autologous bone marrow transplantation for acute lymphoblastic leukemia. *J Clin Oncol* 1989; 7:1594–1601.
113. Thomas ED, Clift RA. Indications for marrow transplantation in chronic myelogenous leukemia. *Blood* 1989;73:861–864.
114. Goldman JM, Szdylo R, Horowitz MM, et al. Choice of pretransplant and timing of transplants for chronic myelogenous leukemia in chronic phase. *Blood* 1993;82:2235–2238.
115. Slattery JT, Clift RA, Buckner CD, et al. Marrow transplantation for chronic myelogenous leukemia: the influence of plasma busulfan levels on the outcome of transplantation. *Blood* 1997;89:3055–3060.
116. Barrett AJ, Mavroudis D, Tisdale J, et al. T cell-depleted bone marrow transplantation and delayed T cell add-back to control acute GVHD and conserve a graft-versus-leukemia effect. *Bone Marrow Transplant* 1998;21:543–551.
117. Drobyski WR, Hessner MJ, Klein JP, et al. T-cell depletion plus salvage immunotherapy with donor leukocyte infusions as a strategy to treat chronic-phase chronic myelogenous leukemia patients undergoing HLA-identical sibling marrow transplantation. *Blood* 1999;94:434–441.
118. Drucker BJ, Sawyers CL, Kantarjian H, et al. Activity of a specific inhibitor of the Bcr-Abl tyrosine kinase in the blast crisis of chronic myeloid leukemia and acute lymphoblastic leukemia with the Philadelphia chromosome. *New Engl J Med* 2001;344:1038–1042.
119. Kolb HJ, Mittermuller J, Clemm C, et al. Donor leukocyte transfusions for treatment of recurrent chronic myelogenous leukemia in marrow transplant patients. *Blood* 1990;76:2462–2465.
120. McGlave PB, Shu XO, Wen W, et al. Unrelated donor marrow transplantation for chronic myelogenous leukemia: 9 years experience of the national marrow donor program. *Blood* 2000;95:2219–2225.
121. Shimoni A, Giralt S, Khouri I, et al. Allogeneic hematopoietic transplantation for acute and chronic myeloid leukemia: non-myeloablative preparative regimens and induction of the graft-versus-leukemia effect. *Curr Oncol Rep* 2000;2:132–139.
122. Talpaz M, Kantarjian H, Liang J, et al. Percentage of Philadelphia chromosome (Ph)-negative and Ph-positive cells found after autologous transplantation for chronic myelogenous leukemia depends on percentage of diploid cells induced by conventional-dose chemotherapy before collection of autologous cells. *Blood* 1995;85:3257–3263.
123. Khouri IF, Keating MJ, Vriesendorp HM, et al. Autologous and allogeneic bone marrow transplantation for chronic lymphocytic leukemia: preliminary results. *J Clin Oncol* 1994;12:748–758.
124. Rondon G, Giralt S, Huh Y, et al. Graft-versus-leukemia effect after allogeneic bone marrow transplantation for chronic lymphocytic leukemia. *Bone Marrow Transplant* 1996;18:669–672.
125. Hale GA, Phillips GL. Allogeneic stem cell transplantation for the non-Hodgkin's lymphomas and Hodgkin's disease. *Cancer Treat Rev* 2000;26:411–427.
126. Van Besien KW, Mehra RC, Giralt SA, et al. Allogeneic bone marrow transplantation for poor-prognosis lymphoma: response, toxicity, and survival depend on disease histology. *Am J Med* 1996;100:299–307.
127. Freedman AS, Neuberg D, Gribben JG, et al. High-dose chemoradiotherapy and anti-B-cell monoclonal antibody purged autologous bone marrow transplantation in mantle-cell lymphoma: no evidence for long-term remission. *J Clin Oncol* 1998;16:13–18.
128. Van Besien K, Sobocinski K, Rowlings PA, et al. Allogeneic bone marrow transplantation for low-grade lymphoma. *Blood* 1998;92: 1832–1836.
129. Attal M, Socie G, Molina L, et al. Allogeneic bone marrow transplantation for refractory and recurrent follicular lymphoma: a case-matched analysis with autologous transplantation from the French Bone Marrow Transplant Group Registry data. *Blood* 1997;93:1120a.
130. Khouri I, Lee M-S, Palmer L, et al. Transplant-lite using fludarabine-cyclophosphamide and allogeneic stem cell transplantation for low grade lymphoma. *Blood* 1999;94:1553a.
131. Bierman PJ. Allogeneic bone marrow transplantation for lymphoma. *Blood Rev* 2000;14:1–13.
132. Nagler A, Slavin S, Varadi G, et al. Allogeneic peripheral blood stem cell transplantation using a fludarabine-based low intensity conditioning regimen for malignant lymphoma. *Bone Marrow Transplant* 2000; 25:1021–1028.
133. Reece DE. Evidence-based management of Hodgkin's disease; the role of autologous stem cell transplantation. *Cancer Control* 2000;7: 266–275.
134. Gajewski JL, Phillips GL, Sobocinski KA, et al. Bone marrow transplants from HLA-identical siblings in advanced Hodgkin's disease. *J Clin Oncol* 1996;14:572–578.
135. Vesole DH, Barlogie B, Jagannath S, et al. High-dose therapy for refractory multiple myeloma: improved prognosis with better supportive care and double transplants. *Blood* 1994;84:950–956.
136. Bensinger WI, Rowley SD, Demirer T, et al. High-dose therapy followed by autologous hematopoietic stem-cell infusion for patients with multiple myeloma. *J Clin Oncol* 1996;14:1447–1456.
137. Gahrton G, Tura S, Ljunhman P, et al. Allogeneic bone marrow transplantation in multiple myeloma. *New Engl J Med* 1991;325: 1267–1273.
138. Goldschmidt H, Egerer G, Ho AD. Autologous and allogeneic stem cell transplantation in multiple myeloma. *Bone Marrow Transplant* 2000;26[Suppl]:S25–26.
139. Zojer N, Konigsberg R, Ackermann J, et al. Deletion of 13q14 remains an independent adverse prognostic variable in multiple myeloma despite its frequent detection by interphase fluorescence in situ hybridization. *Blood* 2000;95:1925–1930.
140. Matthay KK, O'Leary MC, Ramsay NK, et al. Role of myeloablative therapy in improved outcome for high risk neuroblastoma: review of recent Children's Cancer Group results. *Eur J Cancer* 1995;31A: 572–575.
141. Chaos surrounds high-dose chemotherapy for breast cancer. *Lancet* 1999;353:1633.
142. Antman K, Ayash L, Elias A, et al. A phase II study of high-dose cyclophosphamide, thiotepa, and carboplatin with autologous marrow support in women with measurable advanced breast cancer responding to standard-dose therapy. *J Clin Oncol* 1992;10:102–110.
143. Peters WP, Ross M, Vredenburgh JJ, et al. High-dose chemotherapy and autologous bone marrow support as consolidation after standard-dose adjuvant therapy for high-risk primary breast cancer. *J Clin Oncol* 1993;11:1132–1143.
144. Stemmer SM, Cagnoni PJ, Shpall EJ, et al. High-dose paclitaxel, cyclophosphamide, and cisplatin with autologous hematopoietic progenitor-cell support: a phase I trial. *J Clin Oncol* 1996;14:1463–1472.

145. Antman KH, Rowlings PA, Vaughan WP, et al. High-dose chemotherapy with autologous hematopoietic stem-cell support for beast cancer in North America. *J Clin Oncol* 1997;15:1870–1879.
146. Stadtmauer EA, O'Neill A, Goldstein LJ, et al. Conventional-dose chemotherapy compared with high dose chemotherapy plus autologous hematopoietic stem-cell transplantation for metastatic breast cancer. *New Engl J Med* 2000;342:1069–1076.
147. Childs RW, Clave E, Tisdale J, et al. Successful treatment of metastatic renal cell carcinoma with nonmyeloablative allogeneic peripheral-blood progenitor-cell transplant: evidence for a graft-versus-tumor effect. *J Clin Oncol* 1999;17:2044–2049.
148. Ueno NT, Rondon G, Mirza NQ, et al. Allogeneic peripheral-blood progenitor-cell transplantation for poor risk patients with metastatic breast cancer. *J Clin Oncol* 1998;16:986–993.

Rossi's Principles of Transfusion Medicine, Third Edition, edited by Toby L. Simon, Walter H. Dzik, Edward L. Snyder, Christopher P. Stowell, and Ronald G. Strauss. Lippincott Williams & Wilkins, Philadelphia © 2002.

CASE 38A

BREAK ON THROUGH TO THE OTHER SIDE

CASE HISTORY

A.J. is a group O 23-year-old black man referred to us for therapy of leukemia. He originally presented with priapism as the chief complaint and was found to have a white blood cell (WBC) count of 690,000/μl. He was treated with emergency leukapheresis (lowering his WBC to 350,000/μl) and surgical shunting. A bone marrow and cytogenetic analysis were consistent with Philadelphia chromosome–positive chronic myelogenous leukemia (CML). His leukemic cells were found to be doubly positive for the Philadelphia chromosome, thus bearing an extra chromosome containing the Bcr/Abl gene rearrangement, which is considered a poor prognostic finding. He underwent initial chemotherapy with topotecan and cytosine arabinoside, with a partial response. Because of his youth, high-performance status, and the severity of his underlying disease, an allogeneic bone marrow transplantation (BMT) was planned. The patient was fortunate to have an HLA-matched sister who served as the donor.

Although A.J.'s sister was a perfect HLA match, she was blood group A, representing a major blood group incompatibility for her brother, who was group O. Because bone marrow harvests are unavoidably contaminated with large amounts red blood cells (RBCs), the incompatible RBCs were removed (reduced to less than 10 ml RBCs) prior to transplant to prevent acute hemolysis. We used a continuous flow cell separator (Fenwal CS-3000 Plus, Baxter Healthcare, Deerfield, IL) to not only deplete the marrow of RBCs, but also reduce the volume of the bone marrow product, with satisfactory recovery of progenitor cells.

Following conditioning with busulfan and cytoxan, A.J. underwent BMT, receiving 0.66×10^8 mononuclear cells per kg body weight. He received cyclosporin A as immunoprophylaxis for graft versus host disease. His immediate posttransplant course was complicated by mucositis that was severe enough to require parenteral nutrition and patient-adjusted dosing of morphine. He remained pancytopenic through day 20, when a bone marrow biopsy showed a hypocellular marrow. He was dependent on transfusions, receiving group O (recipient type) RBCs and group A (donor type) platelets. He was begun on granulocyte colony–stimulating factor (G-CSF) for persistent fevers and neutropenia. On day 22 he complained of right upper quadrant pain, had persistent low-grade fever, hepatosplenomegaly, and slightly elevated bilirubin. He was pancytopenic (WBC 100/μl, platelets 23,000/μl) and had mild diarrhea. There was no skin rash, although there was mild palmar erythema. Radiologic studies showed no evidence for venoocclusive disease of the liver. The signs and symptoms were attributed to an early engraftment syndrome rather than graft versus host disease.

By day 30 his blood counts began to improve, with WBC 500/μl, hematocrit 28%, and platelets 24,000/μl. A repeat bone marrow biopsy again showed hypocellularity but no evidence of leukemia. Cytogenetic examination showed normal female karyotype in 20 of 20 cells. Over the next several days he improved gradually. His fevers and mucositis abated, he was able to eat, and his medications were adjusted toward prevention of graft rejection. His bilirubin declined to normal levels and there was no evidence of graft versus host disease. Finally, on day 50, although still RBC transfusion dependent, he was discharged to home with a hematocrit of 29%, WBC 3,500 /μl, and platelets 40,000 /μl.

A.J.'s posthospitalization course is partially summarized in Figure 38A.1, showing that he was transfusion dependent over the first 9 months following BMT. His reticulocyte count remained consistently low (<0.5%), while his blood grouping "front typed" as group O (recipient type and transfusion type). Of particular note, his ABO "back type" showed persistence of anti-A, consistent with residual host-type isohemagglutinins. His back type also showed anti-B, which could have represented either donor or residual host-type isohemagglutinins. His WBC count and platelet count were low but adequate, and he did not require platelet transfusion support. A bone marrow examination 4 months posttransplant showed trilineage engraftment of donor type cells and no evidence of leukemia, but markedly reduced erythroid series.

DISCUSSION

A.J. experienced a stormy hospital course, but after discharge he was mostly troubled by dependence on RBC transfusions, receiving 48 RBC units over 9 months. His inadequate red blood cell production was considered to be due to persistent anti-A, preventing maturation of donor-type RBCs. Blood group A is expressed on both early and late progenitors, which is consistent with the bone marrow biopsy finding of a paucity of cells in the erythroid lineage. The ABO isohemagglutinin titers measured at several times are shown in Figure 38A.1. A trial of intravenous immune globulin (IVIG) (2 g/kg total) at approximately 4

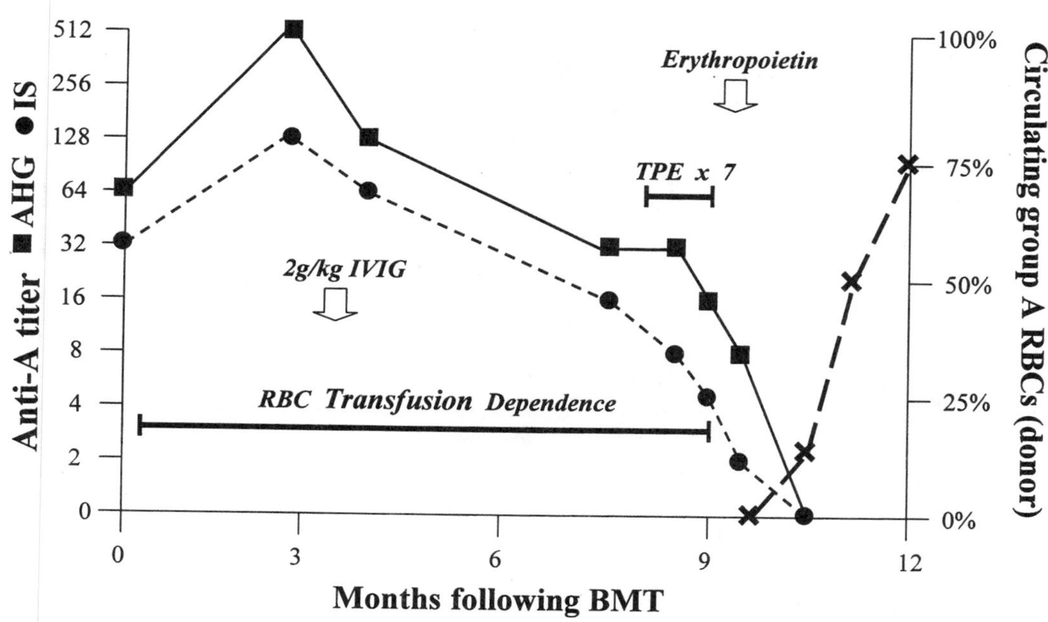

FIGURE 38A.1. One year post-BMT course. Anti-A titers are shown on the *left axis* as a function of time. Titers are shown as either immediate spin titers *(circles)* or antiglobulin phase titers *(squares)*. Estimates of the percentage of circulating red blood cells which were group A (donor origin) are shown on the *right axis* as a function of time. Therapeutic interventions such as plasmapheresis (TPE), intravenous immune globulin (IVIG), erythropoietin are indicated. The period of transfusion dependence is shown by the *horizontal black bar.*

months post-BMT had no apparent effect on his anti-A titers. At this point, because only 4 months had passed, his physicians elected to continue supporting him with group O RBCs in the hope that his host anti-A production would decrease spontaneously. However, more than 8 months after hospital discharge, A.J. remained RBC dependent with anti-A titers of 16 to 32 and no evidence of circulating group A RBCs. He underwent seven total plasma exchanges over 3 weeks and received erythropoietin injections in an attempt to further deplete his system of host anti-A, while stimulating production of donor erythropoiesis.

Coincident with the plasma exchanges and erythropoietin therapy, the anti-A titers declined, followed by appearance of group A RBCs in the circulation. Approximately 9 months following BMT, A.J.'s dependence on transfusion ended. Using gel card technology, we were able to easily demonstrate an increasing proportion of donor group A RBCs. With this method, agglutinated group A RBCs are trapped at the top of the resin, while nonagglutinated group O RBCs pass through the resin, collecting in a button at the bottom of the column. In Figure 38A.2, *column A* shows results obtained shortly after plasmapheresis when just a small proportion of group A RBCs were detectable. However, by 12 months *(column C),* almost all of the peripheral circulating RBCs were donor group A. These findings were corroborated in parallel by conventional tube methods. Just over a year after discharge, A.J.'s blood group (front and back typing) converted fully to donor type group A and a bone marrow biopsy at 1 year was read as normal, without evidence of leukemia. He remains in a good clinical state 2 years after transplant. Despite a difficult clinical course during the first year following his diagnosis, A.J. is in complete remission and enjoying life again.

FINAL COMMENT

ABO major–incompatible transplants may be complicated by delayed engraftment of RBCs. However, the majority of patients will convert to donor type within a few weeks to months without the need for special therapeutic interventions. Some retrospective studies have suggested that ABO incompatibility is an adverse risk factor for survival (1,2), while other studies suggest it is not an overall negative prognostic indicator (3). ABO incompatibility has not been shown to be independently associated with delayed WBC or platelet engraftment or increased risk of graft versus host disease (1,2,3). The use of plasmapheresis (4) and erythropoietin (5) have been reported previously as a means to promote donor erythropoiesis following ABO-incompatible BMTs. As can be seen in Figure 38A.1, a trial of IVIG did not appear to have an impact on A.J.'s anti-A and was unlikely to have played a role in promoting donor erythropoiesis. While the pretransplant antibody titer may correlate with the risk of RBC aplasia in major ABO-mismatched donor-recipient pairs,

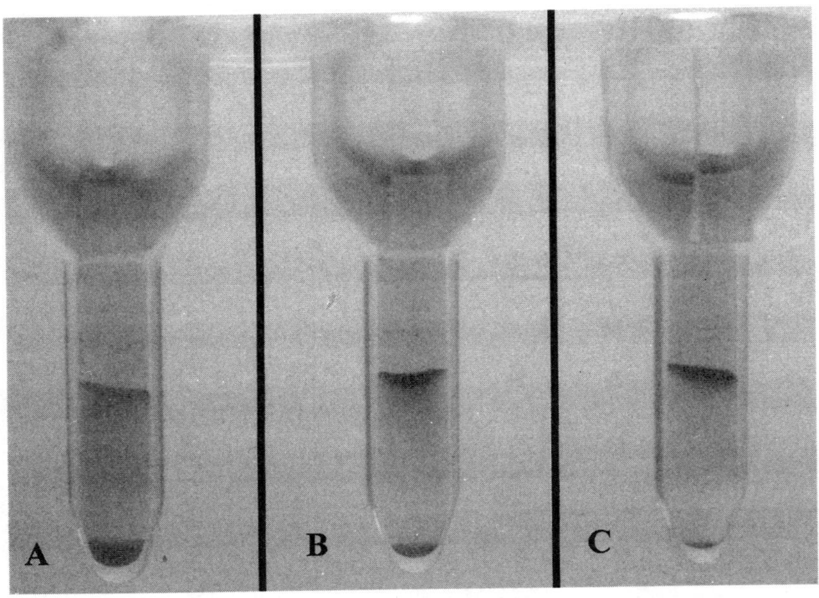

FIGURE 38A2. Gel card technology showing two populations of red blood cells. Buffered gel cards (Micro Typing Systems, Pampano Beach, Florida) were used. Washed patient red blood cells were added to the gel in the presence of standard blood grouping anti-A reagent. **A,** Ten months post-BMT, the gel shows a button of group O (nonreactive) cells and a small layer of trapped agglutinated group A red blood cells trapped at the top of the resin, estimated to represent 10% to 15% of the total red blood cell input. **B,** Eleven months post-BMT, the gel shows an increasing proportion (approximately 50%) of agglutinated group A red blood cells trapped at the resin surface. **C,** Twelve months post-BMT shows nearly complete conversion (approximately 75%) to group A cells and a much smaller group O button. Estimates were made based on visual comparison of artificially spiked mixtures of reagent group A and group O red blood cells.

A.J.'s pretransplant anti-A titers were only modestly elevated (Fig. 38A.1). Of note is the rise in anti-A titers above baseline which occurred several months following transplant, which indicated persistence of host antidonor antibody production. Because karyotype analysis and peripheral flow cytometry indicated essentially complete conversion to donor (female, XX) hematopoiesis, the anatomic distribution and regulation of these residual host anti-A-producing plasma cells is of particular interest from an immunologic perspective. Such a small relative proportion of anti-A-producing host B lymphocytes and plasma cells, in a hematopoietic environment composed predominantly of donor cells, suggests a state of functional residual host hematopoietic microchimerism. Whether these residual host cells are eventually deleted from the immune repertoire or are suppressed by regulatory mechanisms merits further study.

The deregulated tyrosine kinase activity of the Bcr/Abl fusion protein is the cause of malignant transformation in virtually all cases of CML. As a result of rational drug design strategies, the signal transduction inhibitor STI571 has emerged as an Abl-specific tyrosine kinase inhibitor. Under the product name Gleevec (Novartis, Basel, Switzerland) this drug has shown great therapeutic promise for patients with CML (6). Fortunately for A.J., this drug represents a treatment option should he relapse.

Case contributed by David Andrews, M.D., and Walter H. Dzik, M.D., Massachusetts General Hospital, Boston, MA.

REFERENCES

1. Benjamin RJ, McGurk S, Ralston MS, et al. ABO incompatibility as an adverse risk factor for survival after allogeneic bone marrow transplantation. *Transfusion* 1999;39:179–187.
2. Stussi G, Seebach L, Muntwyler J, et al. Graft-versus-host disease and survival after ABO-incompatible allogeneic bone marrow transplantation: a single-centre experience. *Br J Haematol* 2001;113:251–253.
3. Mielcarek M, Leisenring W, Torok-Storb B, et al. Graft-versus-host disease and donor-directed hemagglutinin titers after ABO-mismatched related and unrelated marrow allografts: evidence for a graft-versus-plasma cell effect. *Blood* 2000;96:1150–1156.
4. Worel N, Greinix HT, Schneider B, et al. Regeneration of erythropoiesis after related- and unrelated-donor BMT or peripheral blood HPC transplantation: a major ABO mismatch means problems. *Transfusion* 2000; 40:543–550.
5. Paltiel O, Cournoyer D, Rybka W. Pure red cell aplasia following ABO-incompatible bone marrow transplantation: response to erythropoietin. *Transfusion* 1993;33:418–421.
6. O'Dwyer ME, Druker BJ. Chronic myelogenous leukaemia—new therapeutic principles. *J Int Med* 2001;250:3–9.

39

ADOPTIVE IMMUNOTHERAPY

IAIN J. WEBB

Adoptive immunotherapy involves administration of functional immune cells to a patient for the management of disease. The treatment approaches currently in development can be classified into one of three broad categories, including allogeneic donor lymphocyte infusion (DLI), antigen-presenting cells, and antigen-specific or cytotoxic lymphocytes (CTL). The role of the immune system in preventing and responding to infections is well established and has led to the evaluation of adoptive immunotherapy to control infectious pathogens (1,2). Observations that allogeneic graft versus leukemia and graft versus tumor effects exist have precipitated interest in the use of adoptive immunotherapy to manage malignant disease.

With the development of allogeneic hematopoietic progenitor cell (HPC) transplantation and the subsequent discovery of the allogeneic graft versus leukemia effect, adoptive immunotherapy has been increasingly used to treat patients with hematologic malignant disease. Similar approaches are being developed for patients with solid tumors. Until recently, a large fraction of HPC transplantation at many centers was in support of high-dose chemotherapy administered to patients with solid tumors, including breast and ovarian cancer. Forty percent of all autologous transplants registered with the Autologous Blood and Marrow Transplant Registry of North America in 1995 were for breast cancer. However, after the release of data from randomized trials that showed no survival advantage, the use of high-dose chemotherapy to manage solid tumors decreased (3). Despite the lack of success in the autologous setting, investigators are increasingly optimistic concerning the possible use of similar strategies for allogeneic transplantation.

Novel immunotherapy approaches are being developed and are replacing much of the cell-processing laboratory procedures previously performed to support autologous peripheral blood stem cell transplantation. For example, preliminary reports have suggested that allogeneic peripheral blood stem cell components may produce a graft versus tumor effect in patients with solid tumors (4). In addition, dendritic cells, antigen-presenting cells commonly derived from peripheral blood collections, are increasingly being used as cancer vaccines (5,6). Other approaches in which lymphocytes are used as immunotherapeutic agents also are being evaluated.

ALLOGENEIC DONOR LYMPHOCYTES

Allogeneic bone marrow transplantation has been used for more than 40 years in support of myeloablative therapy for various malignant and nonmalignant disorders (7,8). In the first procedures, allogeneic bone marrow was infused in an attempt to provide HPCs for recovery of hematopoiesis in recipients of otherwise lethal doses of chemotherapy and radiation. Once it became clear that hematopoiesis could be reestablished with allogeneic cells, efforts were undertaken to find ways to minimize the toxicities associated with myeloablative therapy and to decrease the incidence and severity of graft versus host disease (GVHD), a major cause of morbidity and mortality among allograft recipients. Attempts to abrogate GVHD included introduction of T-cell depletion procedures and intensification of prophylactic immune suppression. It became evident that recipients of T-cell-depleted grafts were at higher risk of relapse (9) and that disease response often was associated with the occurrence of GVHD (10). Both of these observations supported the existence of a graft versus leukemia effect. Recent efforts have focused on improving the understanding of this phenomenon. The intent is to attempt to harness the graft versus leukemia effect while avoiding GVHD and to minimize toxicity while improving outcomes. Attempts have been made to minimize GVHD and non-GVHD toxicity at the time of HPC transplantation.

Options for the management of relapse of disease after allogeneic HPC transplantation are limited. Salvage chemotherapy rarely is effective in providing long-term remission and has considerable toxicity. Second transplantation procedures have a

I.J. Webb: Millennium Pharmaceuticals, Cambridge, Massachusetts.

markedly increased incidence of morbidity and mortality due to cumulative multiple organ system damage. In an attempt to exploit the immune system and its role in disease suppression, approaches entailing cellular therapy to manage and prevent relapse after DLI have been initiated.

Efficacy of Donor Lymphocyte Infusion in the Management of Relapses

Donor lymphocyte infusion is an effective method to induce a graft versus leukemia effect and is now commonly used to treat patients with hematologic malignant disease who have relapses after allogeneic bone marrow transplantation. Use of DLI can produce complete hematologic and cytogenetic response rates among more than 75% of patients with stable phase chronic myelogenous leukemia treated with DLI at the time of relapse (11,12).

As indicated in Table 39.1, the European Group for Blood and Marrow Transplantation (EBMT) documented DLI-induced complete remission in 54 patients with relapsed chronic myelogenous leukemia (11). A total of 87% of patients remained in remission 3 years after treatment. Grade II or greater GVHD developed in 41% of patients, as did myelosuppression in 34% of patients. These clinical features of GVHD were associated with the attainment of remission, suggesting a potential relation between GVHD and the graft versus leukemia effect of lymphocyte infusion.

Marked responses and complete remissions have occurred in a variety of other malignant hematologic diseases, including multiple myeloma, chronic lymphocytic leukemia, non-Hodgkin's lymphoma, myelodysplastic syndrome, and acute leukemia. Collins et al. (12) in 1997 reviewed the experience of 25 North American bone marrow transplantation programs. Aggregate reports revealed that complete responses occurred in 60% of patients with chronic myelogenous leukemia. The response rates were higher among patients with cytogenetic and chronic-phase relapse (75.7%) than among patients with accelerated-phase (33.3%) or blastic-phase (16.7%) relapse. A large number, 89.6% of patients, remained in complete remission 2 years after treatment. Complete remission was less common among patients with acute myelogenous leukemia (15.4% of 39 patients) and acute lymphocytic leukemia (18.2% of 11 patients). Two of four patients with myeloma who were available for evaluation and two of five with myelodysplasia also had complete remission. Among the patients with chronic myelogenous leukemia, response was more common if the disease was in the chronic phase or the patient had developed chronic GVHD after HPC transplantation. Responses were correlated with the development of acute and chronic GVHD after DLI infusion. Acute GVHD occurred in 60% and chronic GVHD in 60.7% of DLI recipients. In addition, 18.6% had pancytopenia, the second most common adverse effect of DLI.

Donor Lymphocyte Infusion and Novel Transplantation Approaches

Attempts to harness the graft versus leukemia effect while minimizing toxicity have included introduction of nonmyeloablative conditioning regimens as well as T-cell depletion in combination with DLI. One approach to overcoming the increased risk of relapse associated with T-cell depletion is to use DLI to treat patients in early stages of relapse. In a retrospective analysis of patients with chronic-phase chronic myelogenous leukemia treated with allogeneic bone marrow transplantation, outcomes were compared for 46 patients receiving T-cell-depleted grafts and 40 patients receiving standard immunosuppressive therapy (13). Both groups were eligible to receive DLI. All subjects were patients at one of two neighboring institutions and were treated during the same period. The two groups of patients received similar myeloablative regimens and had similar pretreatment characteristics. The incidence of grade II to IV acute (15% versus 37%, $P = .026$) and chronic GVHD (18% versus 42%, $P = .024$) was lower in the T-cell-depleted group, but the estimated 3-year probability of relapse was greater for this group. Twenty-three patients (20 in the T-cell-depleted group and 3 in the non-T-cell-depleted group) received and were available for evaluation

TABLE 39.1. RESPONSE TO DONOR LYMPHOCYTE INFUSION

Diagnosis	No. Of Pts. Evaluable	Complete Remission	Percentage Complete Remission
Chronic myelogenous leukemia			
All stages	75	54	72
Cytogenetic relapse	17	14	82
Hematologic relapse	50	39	78
Accelerated, blastic	8	1	12.5
Polycythemia vera	1	1	100
Acute myeloid leukemia	17	5	29
Myelodysplastic syndrome	4	1	5
Acute lymphoblastic leukemia	12	0	0
Total	109	61	56

From Kolb HJ, Schattenberg A, Goldman JM, et al. Graft-versus-leukemia effect of donor lymphocyte transfusions in marrow grafted patients. European Group for Blood and Marrow Transplantation Working Party Chronic Leukemia. *Blood* 1995;86:2041–2050, with permission.

of response to DLI. After DLI, 17 of 20 patients in the T-cell-depleted group and 2 of 3 patients in the non-T-cell-depleted group achieved complete remission. Overall survival 3 years after treatment was similar for the T-cell-depleted group and the non-T-cell-depleted group (72% versus 68%, respectively; $P = .38$). The results suggested that DLI can restore the graft versus leukemia effect decreased by T-cell depletion. Efforts are currently underway to develop strategies to minimize GVHD at the time of transplantation through the use of T-cell depletion of the HPC component while maximizing the graft versus leukemia effect through the administration of DLI at a later time.

Nonmyeloablative transplantation in conjunction with solid-organ transplantation has been reported. Spitzer et al. (14) described simultaneous transfer of allogeneic peripheral blood stem cells and a kidney into a patient with multiple myeloma and end-stage renal failure. The results in this case suggest that mixed chimerism after nonmyeloablative allogeneic HPC transplantation may lead to recipient tolerance of the transplanted solid organ.

Clinical trials at many transplantation centers have focused on methods to induce the graft versus leukemia effect without the high doses of chemotherapy or radiation therapy used in conventional myeloablative bone marrow transplantation. Nonmyeloablative conditioning regimens are being used to establish donor cell engraftment while significantly reducing morbidity and mortality after conventional allogeneic bone marrow transplantation (15). This approach is now being used to treat patients with hematologic malignant disease and certain solid tumors. Miniature allografts, however, commonly are associated with mixed chimerism, and this may predispose to relapse. Mixed chimerism can be converted to full donor chimerism by means of infusion of donor lymphocytes. Once donor cell engraftment has been achieved, patients often need adoptive immunotherapy with donor lymphocytes to induce or amplify a graft versus leukemia effect. It consequently is becoming standard practice to follow nonmyeloablative transplantation with DLI at a later date.

Evidence of a graft versus tumor response exists not only for hematologic malignant disease but also for solid tumors (16,17). In 1998, Ueno et al. (4) described a series of 10 patients with breast cancer who had received allogeneic peripheral blood stem cell transplants. These 10 patients received allografts from HLA-matched sibling donors, were in stable condition or responding to standard therapy, and had tumor infiltration of the liver or at least 20% tumor involvement of the bone marrow. Conditioning included cyclophosphamide, carmustine, and thiotepa. One patient, who had a complete response before therapy, remained in this condition after transplantation. Three patients had partial responses, and five patients had stable disease. There was evidence of a graft versus tumor response in two patients with progressive disease after transplantation. Two of four patients who had immunosuppression reduced had responses in the liver that included development of or exacerbation of GVHD.

Childs et al. (18) described a series of 19 patients with metastatic renal cell carcinoma who received nonmyeloablative peripheral blood stem cell transplants from sibling donors. Seventeen of the donors were fully HLA matched, and two were mismatched at one HLA locus. In addition to cyclosporine, the recipients of the mismatched grafts received antithymocyte globulin. After the tapering of cyclosporine, patients were eligible for DLI if they had stable or progressive disease that showed no evidence of grade II to IV GVHD. Responses were seen in 10 of the 19 patients (53%) a median of 4 months after transplantation. The likelihood of a response was significantly higher if GVHD was present. Although these novel transplantation strategies have been used in a limited number of patients and diseases, there is enough evidence of success to warrant further investigation and optimization of these strategies.

Toxicity of Donor Lymphocyte Infusion

Donor lymphocyte infusion commonly produces remission among patients with chronic myelogenous leukemia who have a relapse after bone marrow transplantation. Donor lymphocyte infusion, however, has significant complications. The two most common are pancytopenia and GVHD. In early reports, pancytopenia occurred in more than 50% of patients (19). The mechanism responsible for the development of pancytopenia is not understood, but the phenomenon may represent a form of transfusion-associated GVHD (20). In this clinical situation, the likelihood of pancytopenia is associated with the extent of donor chimerism in the recipient's bone marrow before DLI. This suggests that the donor lymphocytes are ablating the recipient's hematopoietic cells and that pancytopenia develops if adequate donor HPC function has not been established to maintain a normal peripheral blood cell count. The development of cytopenia is associated with response and occurs at a similar time after infusion. Pancytopenia can be prolonged and has been reported to cause death. In most cases, if cytopenia is recognized at an early stage, collection and administration of additional HPCs from the donor usually reverse it.

Initial studies of DLI showed a high incidence of acute GVHD (80%); however, subsequent studies showed a lower incidence of marked GVHD (40%) (11,19). Chronic GVHD occurs in a significant number of patients who do not have manifestations of acute GVHD. In part owing to the high incidence of GVHD, the mortality rate after DLI in early studies was as high as 22% (19).

Attempts have also been made to minimize the risk of GVHD by altering the dosing regimen for administration of DLI as well as by manipulating the DLI components themselves. Some groups have chosen to infuse serial doses of donor lymphocytes until response is achieved. At the Dana-Farber Cancer Institute, we have successfully used T-cell depletion of donor bone marrow as a means to abrogate GVHD. We have similarly depleted DLI of $CD8^+$ T cells in an attempt to decrease the incidence of GVHD while preserving the graft versus leukemia effect (21). Our approach has been to use serial incubations with anti-$CD6^+$ cell monoclonal antibodies and baby rabbit complement to deplete T cells from bone marrow (22–25) and serial incubations with anti-$CD8^+$ cell monoclonal antibodies and baby rabbit complement to deplete T cells from lymphapheresis collections. In a study with DLI depleted of $CD8^+$ cells, increasing numbers of $CD4^+$ cells were infused (21). Serial cohorts of patients received 0.3, 1.0, or 1.5×10^8 $CD4^+$ cells per kilogram. Disease responses after $CD4^+$ DLI were documented in

15 of 19 patients (79%) with a relapse of early-phase chronic myelogenous leukemia, 5 of 6 patients (83%) with a relapse of multiple myeloma, and 1 patient with myelodysplasia. Overall, 12 of 38 patients (32%) who could not be evaluated for toxicity had acute or chronic GVHD. However, 6 of 27 patients (22%) receiving 0.3×10^8 CD4 cells per kilogram had GVHD compared with 6 of 11 patients (55%) who received 1.0×10^8 or more CD4 cells per kilogram ($P = .07$). Neutropenia and thrombocytopenia developed in 7 patients who responded to DLI, but the response was transient in all but one patient. This patient had prolonged cytopenia, which resolved after infusion of additional bone marrow collected from the donor. Cytopenia and a cytogenetic response in the patients with chronic myelogenous leukemia occurred a median of 12 and 13 weeks, respectively, after treatment with DLI. Treatment-related mortality was low (3%); one death was related to infection in the setting of immunosuppression for GVHD. All patients in this trial who had GVHD had tumor regression, but the presence of GVHD was not required for patients to achieve a response, because 48% of responding patients never had evidence of GVHD. Because of the relatively low risk of toxicity associated with infusion of defined numbers of $CD4^+$ donor cells, further studies can be undertaken in the setting of persistent minimal residual disease to prevent relapse after allogeneic bone marrow transplantation.

The pathogenesis of the graft versus leukemia effect is poorly understood. The lymphocyte populations responsible for the graft versus leukemia effect, transfusion-associated GVHD, and post-HPC transplantation GVHD have not been determined. Depletion of either $CD6^+$ or $CD8^+$ T lymphocytes from donor bone marrow has been shown to prevent GVHD at the time of allogeneic transplantation (22,26), whereas $CD4^+$ cells have been implicated in the graft versus leukemia effect (27). Further experiments to identify the role of donor lymphocyte subpopulations in GVHD are necessary.

ANTIGEN-PRESENTING CELLS

T-cell activity depends on proper stimulation with the antigen presented to the T cell by accessory cells known as *antigen-presenting cells*. Among the most powerful accessory cells in presenting antigen are dendritic cells, isolation of which was first reported in 1973 by Steinman et al. (28–32). Dendritic cells can initiate responses to viral, bacterial, and tumor antigens (33). Originally isolated from the spleens of mice, dendritic cells were subsequently isolated from both lymphoid and nonlymphoid tissues. Dendritic cells also are present in the peripheral blood. These numbers can be increased with administration of cytokines known to mobilize dendritic cells (34,35).

In the cell-processing laboratory, mature mononuclear cells or $CD34^+$ cells can be cultured to produce dendritic cells (36). Apheresis usually is performed to collect leukocytes. Typically, CD34 cell selection or plastic adherence to enrich for monocytes is performed (37,38). Cells are then cultured with cytokines, usually granulocyte-macrophage colony-stimulating factor (GM-CSF) and interleukin-4 (IL-4). Tumor necrosis factor α or lymphocyte-conditioned medium can be added as a maturing agent. Dendritic cells can then be exposed to antigen and subsequently returned to the patient to boost T-cell activity. Dendritic cells may be exposed to synthesized peptides, proteins, tumor cell lysates, transduced with genetic material, or fused to whole tumor cells.

The correct route of administration for dendritic cells is uncertain at this time. Because of the capability of these cells to migrate, Fong et al. (39) reviewed the immune responses of 21 patients with prostate cancer who had received two intravenous, intradermal, or intralymphatic injections of antigen-pulsed dendritic cells. All patients had antigen-specific T-cell responses, but only the patients receiving intradermal or intralymphatic vaccination had responses with production of interferon-γ. These findings suggested these two routes may be superior.

An alternative strategy is to fuse dendritic cells to whole tumor cells. This approach has been used to develop therapeutic strategies for renal cell carcinoma, breast cancer. and ovarian cancer (5,6). Kugler et al. (5) reported their results in the care of a series of 17 patients with renal cell carcinoma who received vaccines composed of dendritic cells fused to whole tumor cells. The dendritic cells were cultured from adherent peripheral blood mononuclear cells collected from allogeneic HLA-mismatched blood donors. Cells were cultured in GM-CSF and IL-4. Tumor necrosis factor α was added for the last 2 days. Tumor cells were digested with collagenase and DNAse then electrofused to the dendritic cells. Patients received two vaccinations 6 weeks apart. Each vaccine was composed of 50 million dendritic cells fused to 50 million tumor cells. Responses occurred in 7 of the 17 patients (41%) a mean of 13 months after treatment. There were four complete responses, one mixed response, and two partial responses.

Gong et al. (6) evaluated autologous and allogeneic dendritic cells fused to ovarian cancer cells. These fused heterokaryons have been shown to express both the CA-125 tumor antigen and dendritic cell–associated costimulatory and adhesion molecules. Both the allogeneic and autologous dendritic cell fusion products expressed similar antigens and were capable of inducing cytolytic T-cell activity and lysis of autologous tumor cells by a class I major histocompatibility complex–restricted mechanism. Unlike systems in which immunotherapy components are produced with specificity against single or limited numbers of recognized tumor-associated antigens, this system produces components that may express and induce responses to important antigens that are currently not identified.

ANTIGEN-SPECIFIC LYMPHOCYTES

The ability of T cells to react in a targeted way has stimulated interest in isolating T cells from the body and expanding them to boost their numbers as a means of better combating the target, such as a pathogen or cancer (40). Several groups and companies have developed strategies for isolating T cells from patients with certain diseases and expanding them in vitro to use them for adoptive immunotherapy. In general, these strategies involve isolation, stimulation, and readministration of a patient's own harvested T cells. Thus the procedures depend on the types of T cells that already exist in vivo and that can be isolated from the patient. As such, several drawbacks exist, including the possibility that a high-specificity, highly effective T cell does not exist in the body or may not be isolated. These technologies are not able to differentiate T cells to potentially yield optimally reactive T cells. They also are not useful in the treatment of patients with poor thymic function or immunosuppressive disorders, in which the number and function of T cells can be markedly depressed.

Cytotoxic T lymphocytes recognize nonhost peptides expressed on the cell surface, in the context of HLA antigens (41). These cells typically are $CD8^+$ and destroy cells that bind antigen to class I HLA molecules. Attempts have been made to develop ex vivo systems to produce CTL clones that can recognize specific antigens on and then destroy cells infected by viruses, bacteria, parasites as well as malignant cells expressing antigens in excess or expressing abnormal antigens. These engineered CTL clones have been shown highly effective in animal models, and have been developed for use in the management of disease that affects humans. Clinical trials to manage Epstein-Barr virus (EBV) infection, cytomegalovirus infection, malaria, and solid tumors have been initiated.

Rooney and Heslop et al. (42–44) have reported the use of cytotoxic T cells to manage as well as to prevent EBV-associated lymphoma in recipients of allogeneic HPC transplants. In their strategy, donor-derived peripheral blood mononuclear cells were plated and stimulated with autologous lymphoblastoid cells to produce EBV-specific cytotoxic T cells. These polyclonal T-cell lines, composed of both CD4 and CD8 cells, were both safe and effective. In a study of the treatment of 39 patients at high risk receiving two to four infusions of EBV-specific T cells, there was evidence of the continued presence of the gene-marked EBV-specific T cells for as long as 38 months after infusion. Six patients with high levels of EBV DNA at entrance into the study had a 2- to 4-log decrease in viral DNA levels within 2 to 4 weeks after infusion. No cases of immunoblastic lymphoma developed in the patients receiving prophylaxis, whereas two patients who did not receive prophylaxis and had overt lymphoma responded to the T-cell infusions (44).

Approaches to the management of both cytomegalovirus and human immunodeficiency virus (HIV) infection have been developed (45–47). Efforts have included production of $CD8^+$ CTLs against cytomegalovirus- and HIV-1–related antigens. These CTLs can be safely infused, and the results of initial trials suggest they may have some efficacy. Other strategies have included production of $CD4^+$ T-cell clones by means of stimulation with CD3 and CD28 (48). Stimulation with both CD3 and CD28 has been shown more effective in eliciting cell proliferation than has stimulation with mitogens or with CD3 alone. In one approach, peripheral blood mononuclear cells are collected, then monocytes, macrophages, B cells, and CD8 cells are removed. The remaining CD4-enriched cells are cultured with beads coated with anti-CD3 and anti-CD28 antibodies. After activation, the beads are removed and the cells can be infused. This approach has been used to treat donors with HIV-1 infection and may be useful in cancer immunotherapy. In recipients with HIV-1 infection, CD3- and CD28-stimulated cells exhibited down-regulation of a coreceptor (CXCR-4) of viral entry, reducing the potential infectivity of these cells.

Although in their infancy, these novel graft engineering strategies offer great therapeutic potential. However, many questions have to be addressed concerning timing, dose, and route of administration. In addition, the isolation of antigens specifically associated with disease is critical to the success of cellular immunotherapy.

STANDARDS AND REGULATIONS

Principles of current good manufacturing practice and total quality management developed for hematopoietic progenitor cell components can be applied to adoptive immunotherapy components. In 1991, the fourteenth edition of American Association of Blood Banks (AABB) standards for blood banks and transfusion services was extended to include hematopoietic stem cells. In 1996, the AABB published separate standards for hematopoietic progenitor cells to expand and replace section Q of the standards for blood banks and transfusion services (49,50). These standards include sections concerning donor selection, component collection, processing, testing, labeling, storage, transportation, issue, infusion, and record keeping for hematopoietic progenitor cells, including autologous and allogeneic bone marrow, peripheral blood progenitor cells, and cord blood.

The Foundation for the Accreditation of Hematopoietic Cell Therapy (FAHCT) was formed in 1993 with programs for inspection and accreditation of HPC collection and processing facilities as well as transplantation programs. The FAHCT standards represent a consensus document of several organizations working together in the field of clinical conduct of hematopoietic progenitor cell transplantation, including the International Society for Hematotherapy and Graft Engineering, the American Society for Blood and Marrow Transplantation, and nine others (51). The U.S. Food and Drug Administration (FDA) is reviewing the regulation of HPC components and in February 1997 issued a comprehensive draft document concerning its approach to regulation (52). The FDA has not yet finalized its approach to the regulation of this rapidly developing field but as a first step has required that all cell- and tissue-processing facilities register and report their activities (53). The development of standardized procedures for quality control of hematopoietic stem cell products, similar to those currently in use for cellular blood components, will be required to assure the safety of myeloablative therapy, immune modulation, and gene therapy. The FDA has outlined good tissue practice to meet these goals (54).

SUMMARY

The role of adoptive immunotherapy is becoming more important as it is realized that an immune response is useful in the management of a variety of malignant conditions. Optimal protocols for the isolation of lymphocyte subsets and expansion of immune effector cells remain to be determined. There are numerous unanswered questions concerning dose and route of administration. The need to separate the toxic effects of GVHD and the beneficial effects of graft versus malignant disease is being appreciated and requires further research. In the future, the concept of high-dose chemotherapy may be replaced by more specific and less toxic immunotherapeutic interventions. This will occur as we achieve better understanding of the biologic characteristics of the cells involved in initiating and controlling malignant disease.

REFERENCES

1. Delves PJ, Roitt IM. The immune system, I. *N Engl J Med* 2000;343: 37–49.
2. Delves PJ, Roitt IM. The immune system, II. *N Engl J Med* 2000; 343:108–117.
3. Stadtmauer EA, O'Neill A, Goldstein LJ, et al. Conventional-dose chemotherapy compared with high-dose chemotherapy plus autologous hematopoietic stem-cell transplantation for metastatic breast cancer. Philadelphia Bone Marrow Transplant Group. *N Engl J Med* 2000; 342:1069–1076.
4. Ueno NT, Rondon G, Mirza NQ, et al. Allogeneic peripheral-blood progenitor-cell transplantation for poor-risk patients with metastatic breast cancer. *J Clin Oncol* 1998;16:986–993.
5. Kugler A, Stuhler G, Walden P, et al. Regression of human metastatic renal cell carcinoma after vaccination with tumor cell-dendritic cell hybrids. *Nat Med* 2000;6:332–336.
6. Gong J, Nikrui N, Chen D, et al. Fusions of human ovarian carcinoma cells with autologous or allogeneic dendritic cells induce antitumor immunity. *J Immunol* 2000;165:1705–1711.
7. Thomas ED, Lochte HLJ, Lu WC, et al. Intravenous infusion of bone marrow in patients receiving radiation and chemotherapy. *N Engl J Med* 1957;257:491–496.
8. Thomas ED, Storb R. Technique for human marrow grafting. *Blood* 1970;36:507–515.
9. Marmont AM, Horowitz MM, Gale RP, et al. T-cell depletion of HLA-identical transplants in leukemia. *Blood* 1991;78:2120–2130.
10. Horowitz MM, Gale RP, Sondel PM, et al. Graft-versus-leukemia reactions after bone marrow transplantation. *Blood* 1990;75:555–562.
11. Kolb HJ, Schattenberg A, Goldman JM, et al. Graft-versus-leukemia effect of donor lymphocyte transfusions in marrow grafted patients. European Group for Blood and Marrow Transplantation Working Party Chronic Leukemia. *Blood* 1995;86:2041–2050..
12. Collins RH, Jr., Shpilberg O, Drobyski WR, et al. Donor leukocyte infusions in 140 patients with relapsed malignancy after allogeneic bone marrow transplantation. *J Clin Oncol* 1997;15:433–444.
13. Sehn LH, Alyea EP, Weller E, et al. Comparative outcomes of T-cell-depleted and non-T-cell-depleted allogeneic bone marrow transplantation for chronic myelogenous leukemia: impact of donor lymphocyte infusion. *J Clin Oncol* 1999;17:561–568.
14. Spitzer TR, Delmonico F, Tolkoff-Rubin N, et al. Combined histocompatibility leukocyte antigen–matched donor bone marrow and renal transplantation for multiple myeloma with end stage renal disease: the induction of allograft tolerance through mixed lymphohematopoietic chimerism. *Transplantation* 1999;68:480–484.
15. Khouri IF, Keating M, Korbling M, et al. Transplant-lite: induction of graft-versus-malignancy using fludarabine-based nonablative chemotherapy and allogeneic blood progenitor-cell transplantation as treatment for lymphoid malignancies. *J Clin Oncol* 1998;16:2817–2824.
16. Ueno NT, Hortobagyi GN, Champlin RE. Allogeneic peripheral blood progenitor cell transplantation in solid tumors. *Cancer Treat Res* 1999; 101:133–156.
17. Bay JO, Choufi B, Pomel C, et al. Potential allogeneic graft-versus-tumor effect in a patient with ovarian cancer. *Bone Marrow Transplant* 2000;25:681–682.
18. Childs R, Chernoff A, Contentin N, et al. Regression of metastatic renal-cell carcinoma after nonmyeloablative allogeneic peripheral-blood stem-cell transplantation. *N Engl J Med* 2000;343:750–758.
19. Antin JH. Graft-versus-leukemia: no longer an epiphenomenon. *Blood* 1993;82:2273–2277.
20. Webb IJ, Anderson KC. Transfusion-associated graft-versus-host disease. In: Popovsky MA, ed. *Transfusion reactions*. Bethesda, MD: American Association of Blood Banks Press, 1996:185–204.
21. Alyea EP, Schlossman RL, Canning C, et al. CD8-depleted donor lymphocyte infusions mediate graft–versus–multiple myeloma effect. *Blood* 1996;88:258a(abst).
22. Soiffer RJ, Murray C, Mauch P, et al. Prevention of graft-versus-host disease by selective depletion of CD6-positive T lymphocytes from donor bone marrow. *J Clin Oncol* 1992;10:1191–1200.
23. Soiffer RJ, Ritz J. Selective T cell depletion of donor allogeneic marrow with anti-CD6 monoclonal antibody: rationale and results. *Bone Marrow Transplant* 1993;12:S7–S10.
24. Soiffer RJ, Fairclough D, Robertson M, et al. CD6-depleted allogeneic bone marrow transplantation for acute leukemia in first complete remission. *Blood* 1997;89:3039–3047.
25. Soiffer RJ, Mauch P, Fairclough D, et al. CD6+ T cell depleted allogeneic bone marrow transplantation from genotypically HLA nonidentical related donors. *Biol Blood Marrow Transplant* 1997;3:11–17.
26. Champlin R, Ho W, Gajewski J, et al. Selective depletion of $CD8^+$ T lymphocytes for prevention of graft-versus-host disease after allogeneic bone marrow transplantation. *Blood* 1990;76:418–423.
27. Faber LM, van Luxemburg-Heijs SAP, Veenhof WFJ, et al. Generation of $CD4^+$ cytotoxic T-lymphocyte clones from a patient with severe graft-versus-host disease after allogeneic bone marrow transplantation: implications for graft-versus-leukemia reactivity. *Blood* 1995;86: 2821–2828.
28. Steinman RM, Cohn ZA. Identification of a novel cell type in peripheral lymphoid organs of mice, I: morphology, quantitation, tissue distribution. *J Exp Med* 1973;137:1142–1162.
29. Steinman RM, Cohn ZA. Identification of a novel cell type in peripheral lymphoid organs of mice, II: functional properties in vitro. *J Exp Med* 1974;139:380–397.
30. Steinman RM, Lustig DS, Cohn ZA. Identification of a novel cell type in peripheral lymphoid organs of mice, III: functional properties in vivo. *J Exp Med* 1974;139:1431–1445.
31. Steinman RM, Adams JC, Cohn ZA. Identification of a novel cell type in peripheral lymphoid organs of mice, IV: identification and distribution in mouse spleen. *J Exp Med* 1975;141:804–820.
32. Steinman RM, Inaba K. Myeloid dendritic cells. *J Leukoc Biol* 1999; 66:205–208.
33. Roncarolo MG, Levings MK, Traversari C. Differentiation of T regulatory cells by immature dendritic cells. *J Exp Med* 2001;193:F5–F9.
34. Avigan D, Wu Z, Gong J, et al. Selective in vivo mobilization with granulocyte macrophage colony-stimulating factor (GM-CSF)/granulocyte-CSF as compared to G-CSF alone of dendritic cell progenitors from peripheral blood progenitor cells in patients with advanced breast cancer undergoing autologous transplantation. *Clin Cancer Res* 1999; 5:2735–2741.
35. Pulendran B, Banchereau J, Burkeholder S, et al. Flt3-ligand and granulocyte colony-stimulating factor mobilize distinct human dendritic cell subsets in vivo. *J Immunol* 2000;165:566–572.
36. Thurner B, Roder C, Dieckmann D, et al. Generation of large numbers of fully mature and stable dendritic cells from leukapheresis products for clinical application. *J Immunol Methods* 1999;223:1–15.
37. Bernhard H, Disis ML, Heimfeld S, et al. Generation of immunostimulatory dendritic cells from human CD34+ hematopoietic progenitor cells of the bone marrow and peripheral blood. *Cancer Res* 1995;55: 1099–1104.
38. Bender A, Sapp M, Schuler G, et al. Improved methods for the generation of dendritic cells from nonproliferating progenitors in human blood. *J Immunol Methods* 1996;196:121–135.
39. Fong L, Brockstedt D, Benike C, et al. Dendritic cells injected via different routes induce immunity in cancer patients. *J Immunol* 2001; 166:4254–4259.
40. Lanzavecchia A, Sallusto F. Dynamics of T lymphocyte responses: intermediates, effectors, and memory cells. *Science* 2000;290:92–97.
41. von Andrian UH, Mackay CR. Advances in immunology: T-cell function and migration—two sides of the same coin. *N Engl J Med* 2000; 343:1020–1033.
42. Rooney CM, Smith CA, Ng CY, et al. Use of gene-modified virus-

specific T lymphocytes to control Epstein-Barr virus–related lymphoproliferation. *Lancet* 1995;345:9–13.
43. Heslop HE, Ng CY, Li C, et al. Long-term restoration of immunity against Epstein-Barr virus infection by adoptive transfer of gene-modified virus-specific T lymphocytes. *Nat Med* 1996;2:551–555.
44. Rooney CM, Smith CA, Ng CY, et al. Infusion of cytotoxic T cells for the prevention and treatment of Epstein-Barr virus–induced lymphoma in allogeneic transplant recipients. *Blood* 1998;92:1549–1555.
45. Walter EA, Greenberg PD, Gilbert MJ, et al. Reconstitution of cellular immunity against cytomegalovirus in recipients of allogeneic bone marrow by transfer of T-cell clones from the donor. *N Engl J Med* 1995; 333:1038–1044.
46. Lieberman J, Skolnik PR, Parkerson GR, et al. Safety of autologous, ex vivo expanded human immunodeficiency virus (HIV) specific cytotoxic T-lymphocyte infusion in HIV-1 infected patients. *Blood* 1997; 90:2196–2206.
47. Brodie SJ, Lewinsohn DA, Patterson BK, et al. In vivo migration and function of transferred HIV-1–specific cytotoxic T cells. *Nat Med* 1999;5:34–41.
48. Levine BL, Cotte J, Small CC, et al. Large-scale production of $CD4^+$ T cells from HIV-1 infected donors after CD3/CD28 costimulation. *J Hematother* 1998;7:437–448.
49. Menitove JE, ed. *Standards for hematopoietic progenitor cells.* Bethesda, MD: American Association of Blood Banks, 1996.
50. Klein H, ed. *Standards for blood banks and transfusion services,* 17th ed. Bethesda, MD: American Association of Blood Banks, 1996.
51. Foundation for the Accreditation of Hematopoietic Cell Therapy. *Standards for hematopoietic progenitor cell collection, processing, and transplantation, North America.* Omaha, NE: Foundation for the Accreditation of Hematopoietic Cell Therapy, 1996.
52. Proposed approach to regulation of cellular and tissue-based products: availability and public meeting. *Federal Register* 1997;62:9721–9722.
53. Human cells, tissues, and cellular and tissue-based products: establishment registration and listing. *Federal Register* 2001:66:5447–5469.
54. Current good tissue practice for manufacturers of human cellular tissue-based products: inspection and enforcement. *Federal Register* 2001:66: 1508–1559.

Rossi's Principles of Transfusion Medicine, Third Edition, edited by Toby L. Simon, Walter H. Dzik, Edward L. Snyder, Christopher P. Stowell, and Ronald G. Strauss. Lippincott Williams & Wilkins, Philadelphia © 2002.

40

GENE THERAPY IN TRANSFUSION MEDICINE

DIANE S. KRAUSE

Gene therapy, the use of DNA that encodes or corrects a gene for medical therapy, is achieved by transfer of genetic material to a patient's cells. The specific manner by which gene therapy is performed varies significantly based on the disease to be treated, the gene to be inserted, the target cells of insertion, the vector used to transmit the gene, and the route of administration of the gene. This chapter discusses these variables as well as the current successes and challenges in the field of gene therapy.

Potential diseases that may be treated using gene therapy are listed in Table 40.1. It is hoped that the target diseases for gene therapy will eventually include most serious diseases for which the molecular etiology is well understood. Gene therapy may prove useful for gene replacement for congenital enzyme deficiencies or gene abnormalities. For treatment of cancer, gene therapy may be used to induce selective cancer cell death. Alternatively, cancer treatment could be achieved by using gene therapy to replace a missing tumor suppressor gene, to insert a chemotherapy drug-resistance gene selectively into normal cells, or to enhance the immunogenicity of cancer cells. It is also hoped that gene therapy will eventually be used to treat infectious diseases such as acquired immunodeficiency syndrome (AIDS).

GENE THERAPY AND TRANSFUSION MEDICINE

Transfusion medicine is the science of administering cells or other biologic materials (e.g., serum, isolated clotting factors) to treat patients. The growing field of gene therapy has impacted transfusion medicine on several levels.

First, gene therapy is introducing new biologicals for transfusion in the clinic setting. Because gene therapy often requires the infusion of either gene-modified cells or direct administration of viral vectors that contain the therapeutic gene, it falls within the purview of transfusion medicine. Like other blood products, the safety and efficiency of gene therapy agents must be optimized. Therefore, at the same time as a new gene therapy strategy is being developed in the research laboratory, quality control and infection control measures need to be developed for the clinical laboratory.

Second, novel technical manipulations are being developed for hematopoietic stem cells and the mature blood cells into which they differentiate. Hematopoietic cells have been excellent targets for gene therapy trials. They are easily accessed and may be incubated ex vivo with the vectors containing the genetic repair material. Their wide circulation suggests that hematopoietic cells may be used as gene delivery systems even for nonhematologic diseases, and autologous bone marrow or peripheral blood stem cell (PBSC) transplantation provides a relatively safe standard of care for some malignancies. Ideally, one needs only to infect the "stem" cells in order to get large-scale amplification and long-term expression of a transgene.

Third, gene therapy strategies are under development to treat several diseases that directly impact transfusion medicine, including hemoglobinopathies and clotting factor disorders. For example, hemophilia A, in which patients lack expression of functional clotting factor VIII, is likely to be one of the first

D.S. Krause: Department of Laboratory Medicine, Yale University School of Medicine, New Haven, Connecticut.

TABLE 40.1. DISEASES THAT MAY BE TREATED USING GENE THERAPY

Disease Type	Examples
Gene deficiency/mutation	Hemophilia Cystic fibrosis Thalassemia Severe combined immunodeficiency Gaucher disease Sickle cell anemia
Lack/mutation of tumor suppressor gene	Cancer
Autoimmune diseases	Rheumatoid arthritis
Infections	AIDS

AIDS, acquired immunodeficiency syndrome.

diseases to be treated successfully with gene therapy. This is partly because the factor VIII protein product can be produced by any cells in the body, not necessarily the normal site of production in the liver, as long as the protein is secreted into the circulation. Also, the levels of circulating factor VIII that are necessary to treat the disease need not be highly regulated as long as there is at least 5% of the normal physiologic level present.

VECTOR DESIGN

The many aspects that go into designing an ideal gene therapy vector are largely based on the specific disease to be treated, the target cells, and the therapeutic strategy. Three major questions that must be addressed are:

- What gene should be inserted?
- How should this be administered?
- What vector should be used?

What Gene Should Be Inserted?

Based on the disease to be treated, the gene that will be inserted can confer a variety of attributes. The gene can provide a functional form of a missing or defective gene, it can be a gene designed to give the cell in which it is expressed a survival advantage, or it can act as a suicide gene designed to kill the cell in which it is expressed. See Table 40.2 for examples of each of these gene insertion strategies. For inherited diseases in which there is a nonfunctional gene product, such as cystic fibrosis, gene therapy approaches are being taken to add a functional gene. Similarly, for inherited diseases in which a gene is missing, such as thalassemia, the gene for the fully functional protein product is inserted. For cancer, the genes to be inserted can take one of several different forms. For example, one could insert a suicide gene selectively into the cancer cells. An example of one such "suicide" gene is HSV-TK (herpes simplex virus–thymidine kinase) which can phosphorylate ganciclovir, which is then incorporated into the DNA, preventing its replication and thereby killing the cell. Alternatively, one could replace a missing or mutated p53 gene with the wild-type gene, which will restore normal apoptotic (cell death) machinery to the cell.

In addition to determining which gene to administer, the gene regulatory elements must be inserted in order to achieve target specificity. The process by which a gene is transcribed into messenger RNA (mRNA) and then translated into protein is controlled at multiple levels. Some genes will be therapeutic as long as they are present and the actual level does not need to be highly regulated (e.g., circulating level of clotting factor VIII in hemophilia or adenosine deaminase [ADA] levels). In contrast, other therapeutic genes, if expressed at either too high or too low a concentration, could be deleterious (e.g., β-globin). For another example, if diabetes is going to be treatable by gene therapy, then insulin must be produced in response to elevated circulating glucose levels and reduced when the glucose level falls below normal levels.

Multiple approaches have been taken in order to be able to control gene expression. The first is that the gene therapy vectors are being designed in order to infect only specific target cells, so that the transgene is not expressed in cells in which it will be deleterious. Secondly, research has been focused on designing the regulatory domains of the transgenes (the promoters) so that the gene is either regulated as it would normally be in the cell with a tissue specific promoter, or regulated by an inducible promoter. Every cell type in the body, although containing the same genomic DNA, presents a different pattern of gene expression. This process is controlled at multiple levels, the most common of which is the level of gene expression as controlled by the promoters, enhancers, and silencers of the gene in the specific context of the cell's nucleus. Promoters that are used only in specific cell types (e.g., the insulin promoter in pancreatic cells) are referred to as cell type–specific or tissue-specific promoters.

How Should the Gene Therapy Be Administered?

Gene therapy vectors can be applied to cells ex vivo and then transplanted back to the patient. Alternatively, viral vectors that have been tested to make sure that they are replication incompetent (incapable of replication) can be directly administered into the patient for infection of target cells in vivo. So far, most animal and human clinical trials have used ex vivo infection with retroviruses. This allows for selection of virally infected cells prior to use in order to guarantee vector insertion (1). The ex vivo approach minimizes infection of unintended cellular targets, and because the cells are washed free of unincorporated viral vector prior to infusion, this approach significantly decreases the potential risks of exposing the patient to large amounts of viral vector. Alternatively, the gene therapy vector can be administered directly to the patient. The direct administration of vector to the patient overcomes the difficulties of maintaining fully functional target cells ex vivo. However, because there can be risks associated with transgene expression in unintended host cells, it is critical that the vector administered in vivo have target specificity or have little toxicity if expressed by cell types other than the intended target tissue. This in vivo infection has mostly

TABLE 40.2. GENES USED IN CURRENT GENE THERAPY TRIALS

Gene Type	Disease	Gene	Vector	Target Cell
Replacement of missing or defective gene	Thalassemia	Beta-globin	Retrovirus	Hematopoietic stem cell
—	Sickle cell anemia	Beta-globin	Retrovirus	Hematopoietic stem cell
—	Severe combined immunodeficiency	Adenosine deamininase	Retrovirus	T lymphocyte
—	Cystic fibrosis	Cystic fibrosis conductance regulator (CFTR)	Adenovirus	Respiratory epithelial cell
	Hemophilia	Clotting factor VIII or IX	AAV	Hepatocyte
Survival advantage	Chemotherapy for multiple forms of cancer	Multiple drug resistance (MDR)	Retrovirus	Hematopoietic stem cell
Suicide gene	Graft-versus-host disease caused by allogeneic donor T lymphocytes	Thymidine kinase gene (kills cell when exposed to ganciclovir)	Retrovirus	Hematopoietic stem cell
	—	Cytosine deaminase (kills when exposed to 5FU)	Retrovirus	Hematopoietic stem cell

AAV, adeno-associated virus; 5FU, 5fluorouracil.

been used in clinical trials to treat patients with cystic fibrosis. Adenoviral vectors containing the gene that is mutated in cystic fibrosis (the ion channel protein called CFTR) are inhaled and then infect respiratory epithelial cells.

What Vector Should Be Used?

The ideal vector should have no toxicity to the patient, should not cause an immune response, should be able to hold a large amount of genetic information (large gene-carrying capacity), should have target specificity or the ability to program target specificity, should infect target cells with a high efficiency, should have controllable gene expression (persistent versus regulatable), and should have a controlled integration site that prevents nonspecific effects.

The choice of which vector to use will be affected by the level and longevity of expression desired. Depending on the application, some genes need to be expressed long term in the individual (e.g., replacement of a missing globin gene in thalassemia) and therefore must be incorporated into the genomic DNA of a cell population that will survive long term (the hematopoietic stem cell), and others may require only transient expression (e.g., induction of tumor cell death) for which adenoviral vectors can be useful. Each application requires the design of specific gene elements for insertion into specific vectors that will target appropriate levels of gene expression to the appropriate tissues.

Many research laboratories are developing strategies to optimize current vectors to meet the criteria for an ideal vector. Provided below is an overview of the advantages and remaining challenges to using each of the three most well-established vector systems being used in clinical trials—retroviruses, adeno-associated viruses, and adenoviruses. Table 40.3 summarizes the salient features of these viral vectors. Nonviral techniques that are under development for gene therapy will be discussed briefly as well.

SPECIFIC VIRAL VECTORS

A list of viral vectors and their receptors is given in Table 40.4.

Retroviruses

Retroviruses have an enveloped single-stranded RNA genome and are approximately 100 nm in diameter. They were the first gene therapy vectors to be used. For applications using retroviruses, the therapeutic gene is inserted between the two long terminal repeats (LTRs) at each end of the retroviral genome and replaces many of the normal viral genes (*gag, pol,* and *env*). By removing these genes, the virus will no longer be able to proliferate without special assistance. The LTRs play a role in incorporating the genes into the genomic DNA of the target cells and also are required for expression of the inserted genes. The maximal insert size for the expressed gene(s) is approximately 8 kb, which can be quite limiting because the coding region for many genes is longer than 8 kb, and often more than one gene (e.g., a therapeutic gene and a selectable marker) may need to be included in the retroviral vector.

There are multiple types of retroviruses used in gene therapy research, including oncoviruses, lentiviruses, and spumaviruses (Table 40.3). To date, most retroviral vectors have been based on murine leukemia viruses. As described below, lentiviral vectors based on DNA sequences from human immunodeficiency virus (HIV) are better than oncoviruses at infecting nondividing cells. An alternative to murine leukemia viruses and HIV-1 vectors is the foamy virus vector (SFV-1). It is nonpathogenic and infects multiple cell types including hematopoietic cells (2). The basic cell biology of these viruses is not yet well defined, but preliminary studies showing infection of nondividing cells (3) suggest that this viral vector system should be pursued more thoroughly.

For safety reasons, all gene therapy vectors must be incapable of replication in the human host. By removal of the *pol* gene,

TABLE 40.3. COMMON VIRUSES USED AS VECTORS IN GENE THERAPY RESEARCH

Family	Maximum Insert Size	Examples	References
Retroviruses (single-stranded RNA)	Approx. 8 kb	—	(43)
Oncoviruses	—	Murine leukemia virus	(44)
—	—	Spleen necrosis virus	(45)
—	—	Rous sarcoma virus	(46)
—	—	Avian leukocytosis virus	(47)
Lentiviruses	—	HIV 1	(22,48)
—	—	HIV 2	(49)
Spumaviruses	—	Foamy virus	(50)
Adenovirus (double-stranded DNA)	Approx. 8 kb (1st generation) Up to 37 kb (new generation)	Adenovirus type 5	(51,52)
Adeno-associated virus (single-stranded DNA)	Approx. 5 kb	AAV 2	(53)

HIV, human immunodeficiency virus; AAV, adeno-associated virus.

replication-incompetent retroviruses (RIR) are produced. Because the removed *gag, pol,* and *env* genes are necessary for packaging the RNA genome into retrovirus particles, special "packaging" cells are required to produce retrovirus for use in gene therapy. These packaging cells permanently express the *gag, pol,* and *env* genes within their genomes. When an RIR vector containing the LTRs and the packaging signal is introduced into such packaging cell lines, its RNA is packaged into infectious particles by the gag, pol, and env proteins encoded by the cells. Importantly, these viral *gag, pol,* and *env* genes are not contained within the viral particles produced, so that even though these retroviruses are capable of infecting target cells they are not capable of replication. Prior to exposing target cells to the RIRs produced by the packaging cells, the presence of replication-competent retroviruses must be assessed and ruled out. Only then can that lot of RIRs be used to infect cells for clinical trials.

TABLE 40.4. VIRAL VECTORS AND THEIR RECEPTORS

Virus	Receptor or Coreceptor	Reference
Retrovirus		
Ecotropic murine leukemia virus	CAT-1	(54) (10) (11)
Amphotropic murine leukemia virus	Pit-2	
HIV	CD4, CXCR4	(55)
Adenovirus	CAR	(56)
—	Alpha Vbeta5 or Alpha Vbeta3 integrins	(57)
Adeno-associated virus		
Parvovirus B19	RBC-specific protein	(58)
AAV2	Heparin sulfate proteoglycans	(59)
—	Fibroblast growth factor receptor 1	(60)
—	Alpha Vbeta5	(61)

CAT-1, cationic amino acid transporter; Pit-2, sodium-dependent phosphate transporter; HIV, human immunodeficiency virus; CAR, coxsackie virus and anenovirus receptor; RBC, red blood cell; AAV, adeno-associated virus.

Some of the best target cells for in vitro retrovirus infection are hematopoietic cells. Highly proliferative hematopoietic progenitors, measured by in vitro colony-forming assays, have been successfully infected by retroviruses. The biggest obstacle to using retroviruses to infect hematopoietic stem cells is that retroviruses in general do not infect nondividing cells, and hematopoietic stem cells are very slow to cycle and are usually in G_0 phase of the cell cycle. The efficiency of infection of hematopoietic stem cells, which are best assayed by their ability to reconstitute the bone marrow after bone marrow transplantation, has been increased in recent years by addition of cytokines to the ex vivo culture medium prior to and during retroviral infection. Combinations of cytokines used vary. Unfortunately, most of the combinations of growth factors tested to date induce the cells to differentiate and thus to lose their long-term repopulating "stem cell" capacity.

Retroviral infection and modification of mouse hematopoietic stem cells has been demonstrated using mouse bone marrow transplantation (4,5), and efficiencies obtained have been very high with 80% to 100% of mouse stem cells being infected with retrovirus. Unfortunately, equally efficient infection of human hematopoietic stem cells has not yet been reported. Because there is no ideal experimental in vivo transplantation model for human hematopoietic stem cells, assays for human stem cells take advantage of the ability of human cells to engraft the bone marrow of immunocompromised animal hosts. These xenogeneic in vivo models have been quite useful as preclinical systems. One such model uses sublethally irradiated nonobese diabetic/severe combined immunodeficient (NOD/SCID) mice. The human cells that maintain multilineage engraftment long term in these mice are referred to as SCID repopulating cells (SRC) (6). In a related immunodeficient mouse system, human $CD34^+$ bone marrow

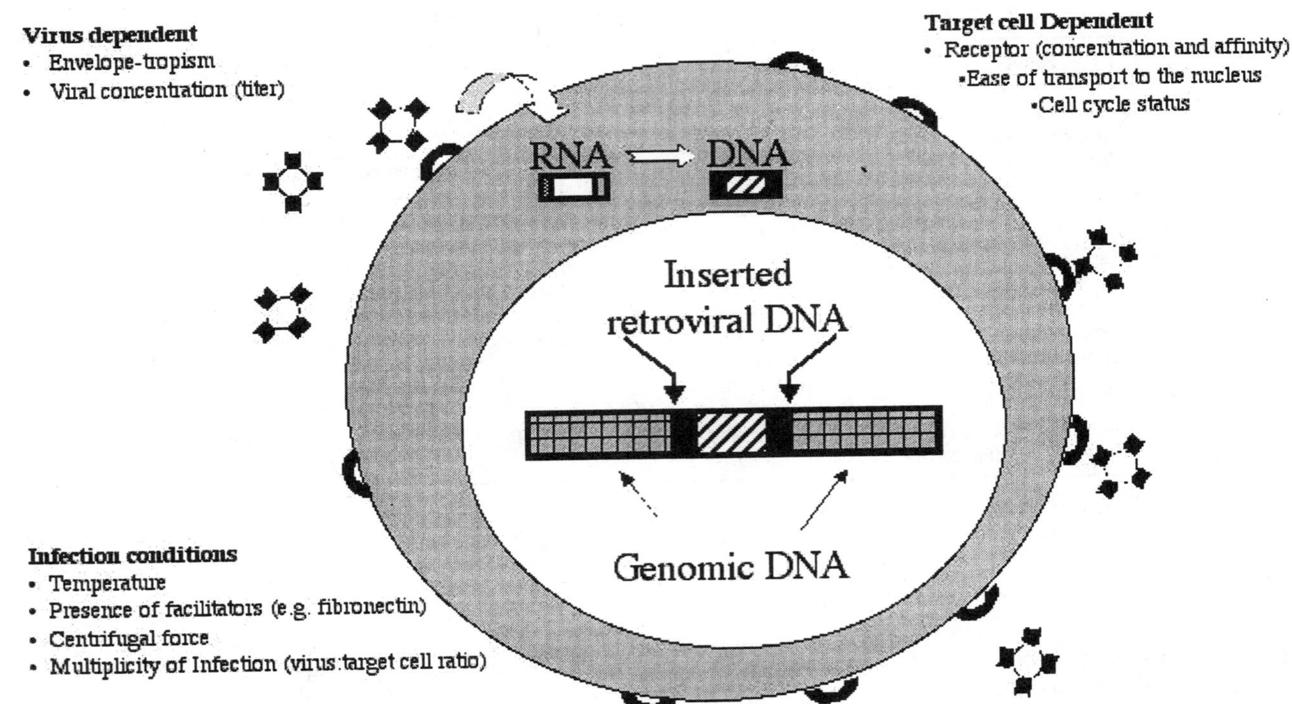

FIGURE 40.1. Factors that affect retroviral infection efficiency.

cells were infected with an efficiency of approximately 10% by retroviral vectors, and these cells survived in immunocompromised mouse hosts for at least 8 months (7).

The different degree of retroviral infection between mouse and human hematopoietic stem cells is due to multiple factors that must be optimized to obtain high levels of infection as shown in Figure 40.1. Much research has focused on two major differences between infection of mouse and human cells, a) the percentage of stem cells in mitosis and b) the surface expression of appropriate retroviral receptors. In mice, approximately 8% of hematopoietic stem cells enter the cell cycle per day, and about 75% are quiescent in G_0 phase at any time (8). It is estimated that human hematopoietic stem cells cycle less often than murine cells, and therefore a higher percentage of human hematopoietic stem cells is in G_0 phase than in murine cells (8, 9). The efficiency of retroviral infection is highly dependent upon whether the retrovirus can bind to and enter the cell. Different retroviruses have different receptors. For the murine retrovirus used most often to date, the receptor on the cell is CAT-1, an amino acid transporter (10). In contrast, the retroviruses that have been used to infect human cells, called amphotropic retroviruses, bind to Pit-2, which is a phosphate transporter (11). It is estimated that the CAT-1 retroviral receptor is expressed on a higher percentage of mouse hematopoietic stem cells than is Pit-2 on human hematopoietic stem cells (12,13). Preselection of a subpopulation of hematopoietic cells that expresses high levels of the retroviral receptor and stimulation of receptor expression are two strategies that have been attempted to increase retroviral infection efficiency of human hematopoietic stem cells (14,15). Higher levels of infection of human cells have also been achieved using "pseudotyped" retroviruses in which the envelope-encoding gene *env,* which encodes the ligand on the virus coat that binds to the target cells, has been replaced with a gene that is known to bind well to hematopoietic stem cells (16,17). One protein that has been studied extensively is the gibbon ape leukemia virus (GaLV) envelope protein, which binds to a receptor called Pit-1 (18). Retroviruses pseudotyped with GaLV infect more than twice as many hematopoietic progenitors than the standard amphotropic retrovirus (19,20).

Risks

The significant risks of retroviral vectors for gene therapy were elucidated when primate studies were initially performed prior to 1992. CD34-selected bone marrow cells of the monkeys were infected with RIRs from packaging cell lines. There were, however, some RIRs that formed by rearrangement that had not been detected by the existing assays for replication-competent viruses. Upon infusion, three of eight monkeys subsequently developed lymphomas containing the active rearranged retrovirus (21). Advances in retroviral vector production that decrease the chance of recombination with potential host virus have greatly decreased the risk of replication-competent virus being present. Currently, all clinical trials require very stringent testing to guarantee that the retroviral vector to be used in humans is entirely replication incompetent. Of hundreds of patients who have been treated with retroviral vectors, none has developed a lymphoma due to replication competent retrovirus. Clinical trials using retroviruses have given quite promising safety and efficacy results.

Challenges

One of the major problems with using the oncoviruses for gene therapy is their inability to infect nondividing cells. The retrovirus may be able to bind to and enter the cell, but it cannot enter the nucleus and become stably incorporated into the cell genome unless it can cross the nuclear membrane. It is able to enter the genomic DNA of dividing cells because there is breakdown of the nuclear membrane during mitosis. In contrast, lentiviruses such as HIV produce proteins that allow them to cross the nuclear membrane in nondividing cells. Several researchers have shown that lentivirus-based vectors are capable of incorporating stably into the genomic DNA of nondividing cells such as brain and liver. The HIV gene products that are responsible for this entry across the nuclear membrane are not yet fully characterized. At least three HIV genes appear to be involved, the matrix protein, the integrase protein, and the virion protein R. The matrix protein may function by interacting with importin-α and -β at the nuclear pore complex (22), optimizing retroviral infection of nondividing cells.

Because the majority of hematopoietic stem cells are in G_1 or G_0 phase of the cell cycle, lentiviral vectors have the potential to infect hematopoietic stem cells with higher efficiency (23) than the oncoretroviruses. The results with lentivirus-based vectors have been very promising; they have been shown to infect human progenitors cells as well as human SRC (24). Although based in part on the HIV genome, these vectors do not contain the genes in the virus that can cause AIDS.

Additional problems with long-term retroviral infection of hematopoietic stem cells currently being addressed include establishing techniques for concentrating retrovirus onto the cells (25, 26), improving retroviral survival in vivo (27,28), and optimizing infection into specific target cells (17).

Adeno-associated Virus

Adeno-associated virus (AAV) is a nonpathogenic, replication-defective human 4.68-kb single-stranded DNA virus, which requires external factors for infection. The name AAV was given because helper virus, usually adenovirus, is necessary for infection. Advantages to AAV vectors include the ability to infect nondividing cells and insertion as DNA rather than RNA. This is a potential advantage over retroviral vectors because some genes, most notably β-globin, require the presence of introns for optimal expression, and these introns are likely be spliced out when the retroviral RNA is reverse transcribed into DNA.

The inverted terminal repeats (ITRs) that are located at each end of the AAV genome are sufficient to package the single-stranded DNA into viral particles. When making a gene therapy vector from AAV, the therapeutic gene can be inserted in place of nearly the entire normal viral protein coding domain (4.5 kb) as long as the flanking ITRs remain intact. These vectors are packaged into virions by supplying the required rep and cap AAV proteins separately. This is usually achieved by inserting both a vector plasmid encoding the therapeutic gene and a packaging plasmid encoding the *rep* and *cap* genes into cells infected with adenovirus. Replication-incompetent AAV vectors are produced by lysing the cells to release virion, and destroying the "helper" adenovirus with heat. In the absence of helper virus, AAV does not replicate and remains integrated in the genomic DNA of the producer cell.

Adeno-associated viral vectors efficiently infect human marrow $CD34^+$ progenitor cells. From 80% to 90% of $CD34^+$ cells in suspension cultures and 50% to 95% of myeloid colonies differentiating in vitro from transduced $CD34^+$ cells demonstrate transgene expression. In murine transplantation models with AAV-infected hematopoietic cells, no cytotoxic response to AAV occurs. Mice transplanted with AAV-transduced bone marrow show evidence of long-term multilineage reconstitution (29). The transgene is still detectable after 6 months. In secondary mouse recipients (another "test" for stem cell infection), a small but significant percentage (1%) of bone marrow cells were still transduced. Results from a phase I clinical trial using AAV vectors to treat cystic fibrosis have achieved gene transfer with little or no cytopathic or host immune response (30). No clinical trials using AAV-infected hematopoietic cells have been reported.

Challenges

The major problem with using AAV vectors has been that the efficiency of infectivity with AAV varies highly from lab to lab. Unfortunately, one possible explanation for this variability is that different labs have different amounts of remaining intact adenovirus, which is coinfected with the AAV. This is problematic because adenoviral vectors are replication competent. Improved techniques to effectively remove contaminating helper virus are currently being developed. Also, because stable packing systems for AAV are not yet fully developed, it is difficult to obtain high titers of pure AAV. Recently, a "hybrid" between viral AAV vectors and liposomes has been proposed for gene therapy use in which the AAV ITRs are used to flank the gene of interest in order to facilitate its insertion into the host genomic DNA, but rather than a viral particle, the DNA is packaged simply in a liposome carrier.

Adenoviral Vectors

Adenoviral vectors have been tested extensively in models to treat cystic fibrosis, but it is not yet clear whether they will be of use in gene therapy protocols using hematopoietic cells. Adenoviruses are double-stranded DNA viruses that are approximately 36 kb. There are four early regions, which are expressed at the beginning of viral cycle and are required for DNA replication and viral propagation. The late genes, which encode structural proteins, are transcribed after DNA replication. Unlike retroviruses, they are quite stable in vitro and can be produced and concentrated to high titers. They can infect quiescent or postmitotic cells. Once the adenovirus enters a cell, its genome is released and can be maintained as an episome (circular DNA in the cytoplasm which is separate from the nuclear genomic DNA) in the cell. Because the adenoviral DNA does not incorporate stably into the genomic DNA of the cell, adenoviral gene expression is transient. The duration of expression of a gene on an adenoviral vector varies significantly based on the longevity and cell cycle status of the cell that is infected. Adenoviruses infect many different cell types, and there are over 50 different types of adenoviruses that are associated with disease in humans. The diseases caused by adenoviruses are transient and usually are not serious unless the patient is immunocompromised. The cell membrane receptor for adenovirus fiber protein is called CAR for coxsackievirus and adenovirus receptor. The normal cellular function of CAR is not yet known. Similar to other types of viruses, interaction with a second membrane coreceptor is necessary for internalization of bound adenovirus. For adenoviruses, this second interaction is between the penton base of the virus and integrins on the cell surface including $\alpha_v\beta_3$ and $\alpha_v\beta_5$.

Whether adenoviral vectors can infect hematopoietic stem and progenitor cells has been controversial. It appears that CAR is not expressed on most hematopoietic cells. When hematopoietic cells are exposed to adenovirus, there is only low-level transgene expression and primarily mature monocytes and macrophages are infected (31). This is accounted for by the relatively low abundance of $\alpha_v$integrin and CAR on most blood cells. Normal human monocytes in contrast have relatively high levels of $\alpha_v$integrin and CAR and are more easily infected by adenoviruses than are early hematopoietic stem and progenitor cells (32). In at least one report, adenovirus was used to transiently express genes in $CD34^+$ human hematopoietic cells after cytokine stimulation in vitro (33). Attempts are currently being made to target adenoviruses to hematopoietic cells by modifying both the target cells and the virus (34,35).

Challenges

Ongoing challenges with adenoviral vectors include the immune response mounted by the host, the transient nature of transgene expression due to lack of genomic insertion, and the inherent low affinity for hematopoietic cells. In clinical trials using adenoviral vectors to treat cystic fibrosis, problems arose due to an inflammatory response to the vectors. In addition to inflammatory reactions against the viral vector, another hindrance to using adenoviral vectors to treat cystic fibrosis may be a relatively low level of integrin expression on the airway epithelium (36). Inflammation against adenovirus was also to blame in September 2000, when an 18-year-old patient with ornithine transcarbamylase (OTC) deficiency, an inherited liver disease that causes life-threatening levels of ammonia to build up in the blood, became the first known death caused by gene therapy. This event demanded the attention of the public as well as that of regulatory agencies and committees that oversee and approve human gene therapy protocols. The patient, who had managed his disease with oral medication and a special diet, developed acute hepatitis after receiving an adenoviral gene therapy vector via the portal vein. Since that time, for example, the Food and Drug Administration (FDA) has investigated several laboratories across the country and has found one failure to comply with National Institutes of Health (NIH) and FDA procedures. These findings raise the ethical question of whether to stop or slow the progress of gene therapy by tightening all regulations or to move ahead because patients with rare and untreatable diseases and their families want the trials to continue.

NONVIRAL VECTORS

Nonviral vectors for gene therapy are also undergoing intensive investigation (37). Unlike viral vectors, nonviral vectors will not need to overcome the extensive immune mechanisms that destroy some viral vectors in vivo, and they do not have the risk of there being replication-competent forms of the vector. Among the technologies being developed are liposomes, and direct gene gun injection, injection of "naked" DNA, and complexing the DNA with polylysine residues or asialoglycoproteins.

CLINICAL PROTOCOLS

Ongoing Protocols

As of 1996, the worldwide enrollment in gene therapy trials included 1,537 patients on 232 different protocols. As of December 2000, a total of 409 human gene therapy clinical protocols had been submitted to the NIH for review. Of those, approximately 70% were designed to treat cancer, 7% HIV-related disease, 7% vascular disease, and 7% cystic fibrosis. Approximately 1% of the trials were designed to treat monogenic diseases including Gaucher disease, hemophilia, Canavan disease, chronic granulomatous disease, and Fanconi anemia. The remaining 3% were designed to treat other diseases including muscular dystrophy, Alzheimer disease, and α_1-antitrypsin deficiency. Internationally, (at that time) nearly 40 clinical gene therapy trials had begun or had been proposed (38). Approximately 60% of current protocols use retroviral vectors, 12% use adenoviral vectors, and 1% use adeno-associated virus.

Basic Design

In designing a clinical trial, different goals are defined for phases I–IV. In phase I trials, researchers test the treatment in a small group of people (usually 20 to 80) for the first time to evaluate its safety, determine a safe dosage range, and identify side effects. Phase I studies are thus primarily concerned with safety and secondarily with the feasibility of the work proposed. In phase II clinical trials, more people (100 to 300) are recruited in order to evaluate whether the therapy is effective and to further evaluate its safety. Most gene therapy protocols are currently in the phase I or phase II stages. In phase III studies, larger groups of people (1,000 to 3,000) are treated in order to confirm that the therapy is effective, monitor side effects, and to compare it with existing treatments. Factors involved in safety include production of sterile replication-incompetent vectors, prevention of adverse reactions, and minimization of patient immune responses against vector. Phase IV studies are premarket trials that provide additional confirmation of the efficacy and safety of the regimen. Regulatory considerations for all clinical trials are assessed by multiple reviewers with different levels of oversight, including an institutional scientific review committee, institutional human investigation committee, institutional biosafety committee, the NIH recombinant advisory committee, and the FDA.

Clinical Gene Therapy Successes

Two very promising clinical gene therapy trials have been reported for the treatment of SCID in children (39,40). In the first, retroviral vectors containing the missing gene ADA were used to transfect autologous cord blood cells, which were then returned to three newborns who had been diagnosed with ADA deficiency in utero. Using in vitro retroviral infection protocols that achieve levels of infection of 5% to 40% of hematopoietic stem and progenitor cells, the patients had low percentages (0.01 to 0.001%) of detectable circulating blood cells containing vector sequences after 1 year (39). In these human studies, no replication-competent retrovirus has been detected. After 5 years, the authors have reported, there are still some circulating cells that contain the transgene. Because these children are being treated with an oral form of pegylated-ADA, the standard of care for the disease, the potential therapeutic effect of the inserted transgene, cannot be assessed in these patients.

Early results were reported for a gene therapy trial to treat X-linked SCID-X1 disease, in which there is a complete lack of functional T and natural killer (NK) lymphocytes in affected boys due to mutation of the gene encoding the shared subunit of the receptors for interleukins 2, 4, 7, 9, and 15 (40). A murine retrovirus vector was used to introduce the complementary DNA (cDNA) for the missing receptor ex vivo into $CD34^+$ cells of two children with the disease, and the cells were then transplanted back into the patients. After 10 months, circulating T and NK cells that contained the therapeutic transgene were detected in the patients and the functional activity of the T and NK cells were the same as in normal unaffected children. This is the first report of gene therapy providing full correction of a disease phenotype.

DESIGNING A CLINICAL VECTOR LABORATORY

Gene therapy holds much promise for the treatment of malignant and nonmalignant diseases. But, just as there is the potential for benefit, there is also the potential to cause harm. Safety measures are being put into place at all levels from the basic science laboratories and centers where the work is being tested to the establishment of federal regulations designed to safeguard the patients, the people working with the transgenes, and the general public. The clinical stem cell laboratory where gene therapy vectors are applied to the cells ex vivo must be compliant with very stringent regulations designed to maintain safety and sterility. These complex and thorough regulations need to be followed in order to be within the limits of current Good Manufacturing Practices (cGMPs). By definition, "cGMPs are methods to be used in, and the facilities or controls to be used for, the manufacture, processing, packing, or holding of a drug to assure that such drug meets [safety] requirements . . . , and has the identity and strength and meets the quality and purity characteristics that it purports or is represented to possess" (41).

The cGMPs are put into place to ensure that all procedures are performed in as safe and controlled a manner as possible. All of the general principles of cGMP are outlined by the FDA in the Code of Federal Regulations (CFR) in 21 CFR 210 and 211, 21 CFR 600s, and 21 CFR 820. Some of the key elements of cGMP encompass raw materials, maintenance of equipment, complete standard operating protocols, validation, record keeping, and personnel training. Several professional organizations including the American Association of Blood Banks and the Foundation for the Accreditation of Cell Therapy have voluntarily established comprehensive standard setting, inspection, and accreditation programs that encompass all phases of cell collection, processing, and transplantation. Additional standards specifically for gene therapy are being developed by the United States Pharmacopoeia (USP), the USP Biotechnology and Gene Therapy Subcommittee, and its Advisory Panel on Gene and Cell Therapies (42).

SUMMARY

Gene therapy continues to offer much promise for the treatment of genetic and acquired diseases. Gene therapy has been used to treat patients with SCID, and applications to other diseases are currently being tested in clinical trials. The characteristics, advantages, and disadvantages of several gene therapy vectors are reviewed herein. Transfusion medicine laboratories are currently involved in clinical gene therapy trials and, in the future when these therapeutic modalities are FDA approved, will oversee the "routine" administration of gene therapy vectors and vector-infected cells. This oversight requires extensive knowledge of cGMP as well as risk prevention–infection control in gene therapy.

REFERENCES

1. Phillips K, Gentry T, McCowage G, et al. Cell-surface markers for assessing gene transfer into human hematopoietic cells. *Nat Med* 1996; 2:1154–1156.
2. Hirata RK, Miller AD, Andrews RG, et al. Transduction of hematopoietic cells by foamy virus vectors. *Blood* 1996;88:3654–3661.
3. Mergia A, Chari S, Kolson DL, et al. The efficiency of simian foamy virus vector type-1 (SFV-1) in nondividing cells and in human PBLs. *Virology* 2001;280:243–252.
4. Williams DA. Expression of introduced genetic sequences in hematopoietic cells following retroviral-mediated gene transfer. *Hum Gene Ther* 1990;1:229–239.
5. Karlsson S. Treatment of genetic defects in hematopoietic cell function by gene transfer. *Blood* 1991;78:2481–2492.
6. Larochelle A, Vormoor J, Haneberg H, et al. Identification of primitive human hematopoietic cells capable of repopulating NOD/SCID mouse bone marrow: implications for gene therapy. *Nat Med* 1996;2: 1329–1337.
7. Dao M, Hannum C, Kohn D, et al. FLT3 ligand preserves the ability of human $CD34^+$ progenitors to sustain long-term hematopoiesis in immune-deficient mice after ex vivo retroviral-mediated transduction. *Blood* 1997;89:446–456.
8. Cheshier SH, Morrison SJ, Liao X, et al. In vivo proliferation and cell cycle kinetics of long-term self-renewing hematopoietic stem cells. *Proc Natl Acad Sci U S A* 1999;96:3120–3125.
9. Gothot A, van der Loo JC, Clapp DW, et al. Cell cycle–related changes

in repopulating capacity of human mobilized peripheral blood CD34+ cells in non-obese diabetic/severe combined immune-deficient mice. *Blood* 1998;92:2641–2649.

10. Wang H, Kavanaugh MP, North RA, et al. Cell-surface receptor for ecotropic murine retroviruses is a basic amino-acid transporter. *Nature* 1991;352:729–731.
11. Kavanaugh MP, Miller DG, Zhang W, et al. Cell-surface receptors for gibbon ape leukemia virus and amphotropic murine retrovirus are inducible sodium-dependent phosphate symporters. *Proc Natl Acad Sci U S A* 1994;91:7071–7075.
12. Crooks GM, Kohn DB. Growth factors increase amphotropic retrovirus binding to human CD34+ bone marrow progenitor cells. *Blood* 1993;82:3290–3297.
13. Orlic D, Girard LJ, Anderson SM, et al. Transduction efficiency of cell lines and hematopoietic stem cells correlates with retrovirus receptor mRNA levels. *Stem Cells* 1997;15:23–29.
14. Orlic D, Girard LJ, Jordan CT, et al. The level of mRNA encoding the amphotropic retrovirus receptor in mouse and human hematopoietic stem cells is low and correlates with the efficiency of retrovirus transduction. *Proc Natl Acad Sci U S A* 1996;93:11097–11102.
15. Scott-Taylor TH, Gallardo HF, Gansbacher B, et al. Adenovirus facilitated infection of human cells with ecotropic retrovirus. *Gene Ther* 1998;5:621–629.
16. Miller N, Vile R. Targeted vectors for gene therapy. *FASEB J* 1995; 9:190–199.
17. Kasahara N, Dozy AM, Kan YW. Tissue-specific targeting of retroviral vectors through ligand-receptor interactions. *Science* 1994;266: 1373–1376.
18. Kavanaugh MP, Kabat D. Identification and characterization of a widely expressed phosphate transporter/retrovirus receptor family. *Kidney Int* 1996;49:959–963.
19. Dybing J, Lynch CM, Hara P, et al. GaLV pseudotyped vectors and cationic lipids transduce human CD34+ cells. *Hum Gene Ther* 1997; 8:1685–1694.
20. von Kalle C, Kiem HP, Goehle S, et al. Increased gene transfer into human hematopoietic progenitor cells by extended in vitro exposure to a pseudotyped retroviral vector. *Blood* 1994;84:2890–2897.
21. Donahue RE, Kessler SW, Bodine D, et al. Helper virus induced T cell lymphoma in nonhuman primates after retroviral mediated gene transfer. *J Exp Med* 1992;176:1125–1135.
22. Popov S, Rexach M, Ratner L, et. al. Viral protein R regulates docking of The HIV-I prointegration complex to the nuclear pore complex. *J Biol Chem* 1998;273:13347–13352.
23. Naldini L, Blomer U, Gallay P, et al. In vivo gene delivery and stable transduction of nondividing cells by a lentiviral vector. *Science* 1996; 272:263–267.
24. Miyoshi H, Smith KA, Mosier DE, et al. Transduction of human CD34+ cells that mediate long-term engraftment of NOD/SCID mice by HIV vectors. *Science* 1999;283:682–686.
25. Chuck AS, Palsson BO. Consistent and high rates of gene transfer can be obtained using flow-through transduction over a wide range of retroviral titers. *Hum Gene Ther* 1996;7:743–750.
26. Chuck A, Palsson B. Membrane adsorption characteristics determine the kinetics of flow-through transductions. *Biotechnol Bioeng* 1996;51: 260–270.
27. Takeuchi Y, Porter C, Strahan K, et al. Sensitization of cells and retroviruses to human serum by α(1-3)galactosyltransferase. *Nature* 1996; 379:85–88.
28. Rother R, Fodor W, Springhorn J, et al. A novel mechanism of retrovirus inactivation in human serum mediated by abti-α-galactosyl natural antibody. *J Exp Med* 1995;182:1345–1355.
29. Chatterjee S, Lu D, Podsakoff G, et al. Strategies for efficient gene transfer into hematopoietic cells: the use of adeno-associated virus vectors in gene therapy. *Ann N Y Acad Sci* 1995;770:79–90.
30. Wagner JA, Messner AH, Moran ML, et al. Safety and biological efficacy of an adeno-associated virus vector-cystic fibrosis transmembrane regulator (AAV-CFTR) in the cystic fibrosis maxillary sinus. *Laryngoscope* 1999;109:266–274.
31. Chen L, Pulsipher M, Chen D, et al. Selective transgene expression for detection and elimination of contaminating carcinoma cells in hematopoietic stem cell sources. *J Clin Invest* 1996;98:2539–2548.
32. Huang S, Kamata T, Takada Y, et al. Adenovirus interaction with distinct integrins mediates separate events in cell entry and gene delivery to hematopoietic cells. *J Virol* 1996;70:4502–4508.
33. Neering SJ, Hardy SF, Minamoto D, et al. Transduction of primitive human hematopoietic cells with recombinant adenovirus vectors. *Blood* 1996;88:1147–1155.
34. Leon RP, Hedlund T, Meech SJ, et al. Adenoviral-mediated gene transfer in lymphocytes. *Proc Natl Acad Sci U S A* 1998;95:13159–13164.
35. Gu DL, Gonzalez AM, Printz MA, et al. Fibroblast growth factor 2 retargeted adenovirus has redirected cellular tropism: evidence for reduced toxicity and enhanced antitumor activity in mice. *Cancer Res* 1999;59:2608–2614.
36. Goldman MJ, Wilson JM. Expression of $\alpha_v\beta_5$integrin is necessary for efficient adenovirus-mediated gene transfer in the human airway. *J Virol* 1995;69:5951–5958.
37. Ferry N, Heard JM. Liver-directed gene transfer vectors. *Hum Gene Ther* 1998;9:1975–1981.
38. Human gene marker/therapy clinical protocols (complete updated listings). *Hum Gene Ther* 2000;11:2543–2617.
39. Kohn DB. The current status of gene therapy using hematopoietic stem cells. *Curr Opin Pediatr* 1995;7:56–63.
40. Cavazzana-Calvo M, Hacein-Bey S, de Saint Basile G, et al. Gene therapy of human severe combined immunodeficiency (SCID)-X1 disease. *Science* 2000;288:669–672.
41. Burger SR. Design and operation of a current good manufacturing practices cell-engineering laboratory. *Cytotherapy* 2000;2:111–122.
42. States PU. Cell and gene therapy products. *Cytotherapy* 2000;2: 123–167.
43. Hu WS, Pathak VK. Design of retroviral vectors and helper cells for gene therapy. *Pharmacol Rev* 2000;52:493–512.
44. Mann R, Mulligan RC, Baltimore D. Construction of a retrovirus packaging mutant and its use to produce helper-free defective retrovirus. *Cell* 1983;33:153–159.
45. Dougherty JP, Wisniewski R, Yang SL, et al. New retrovirus helper cells with almost no nucleotide sequence homology to retrovirus vectors. *J Virol* 1989;63:3209–3212.
46. Petropoulos CJ, Hughes SH. Replication-competent retrovirus vectors for the transfer and expression of gene cassettes in avian cells. *J Virol* 1991;65:3728–3737.
47. Thacker EL, Fulton JE, Hunt HD. In vitro analysis of a primary, major histocompatibility complex (MHC)-restricted, cytotoxic T-lymphocyte response to avian leukosis virus (ALV), using target cells expressing MHC class I cDNA inserted into a recombinant ALV vector. *J Virol* 1995;69:6439–6444.
48. Naldini L, Blomer U, Gage FH, et al. Efficient transfer, integration, and sustained long-term expression of the transgene in adult rat brains injected with a lentiviral vector. *Proc Natl Acad Sci U S A* 1996;93: 11382–11388.
49. Poeschla E, Gilbert J, Li X, et al. Identification of a human immunodeficiency virus type 2 (HIV-2) encapsidation determinant and transduction of nondividing human cells by HIV-2-based lentivirus vectors. *J Virol* 1998;72:6527–6536.
50. Linial ML. Foamy viruses are unconventional retroviruses. *J Virol* 1999; 73:1747–1755.
51. Bett AJ, Prevec L, Graham FL. Packaging capacity and stability of human adenovirus type 5 vectors. *J Virol* 1993;67:5911–5921.
52. Parks RJ, Chen L, Anton M, et al. A helper-dependent adenovirus vector system: removal of helper virus by Cre-mediated excision of the viral packaging signal. *Proc Natl Acad Sci U S A* 1996;93: 13565–13570.
53. Monahan PE, Samulski RJ. AAV vectors: is clinical success on the horizon? *Gene Ther* 2000;7:24–30.
54. Palu G, Parolin C, Takeuchi Y, et al. Progress with retroviral gene vectors. *Rev Med Virol* 2000;10:185–202.
55. Feng Y, Broder CC, Kennedy PE, et al. HIV-1 entry cofactor: functional cDNA cloning of a seven-transmembrane, G protein-coupled receptor. *Science* 1996;272:872–877.

56. Nemerow GR, Stewart PL. Role of $\alpha_v$integrins in adenovirus cell entry and gene delivery. *Microbiol Mol Biol Rev* 1999;63:725–734.
57. Wickham TJ, Mathias P, Cheresh DA, et al. Integrins $\alpha_v\beta_3$ and $\alpha_v\beta_5$ promote adenovirus internalization but not virus attachment. *Cell* 1993;73:309–319.
58. Ponnazhagan S, Weigel KA, Raikwar SP, et al. Recombinant human parvovirus B19 vectors: erythroid cell-specific delivery and expression of transduced genes. *J Virol* 1998;72:5224–5230.
59. Summerford C, Samulski RJ. Membrane-associated heparan sulfate proteoglycan is a receptor for adeno-associated virus type 2 virions. *J Virol* 1998;72:1438–1445.
60. Qing K, Mah C, Hansen J, et al. Human fibroblast growth factor receptor 1 is a co-receptor for infection by adeno-associated virus 2. *Nat Med* 1999;5:71–77.
61. Summerford C, Bartlett JS, Samulski RJ. $\alpha_v\beta_5$integrin: a co-receptor for adeno-associated virus type 2 infection. *Nat Med* 1999;5:78–82.

Rossi's Principles of Transfusion Medicine, Third Edition, edited by Toby L. Simon, Walter H. Dzik, Edward L. Snyder, Christopher P. Stowell, and Ronald G. Strauss. Lippincott Williams & Wilkins, Philadelphia © 2002.

PART IV
Surgery Patients

41

RED BLOOD CELL SUPPORT IN THE PERIOPERATIVE SETTING

LAWRENCE T. GOODNOUGH

PHYSIOLOGIC BASIS OF BLOOD TRANSFUSION

The appropriate indication for transfusion of blood is to restore or maintain the blood's oxygen-carrying capacity. Friedman (1) looked at the epidemiologic aspects of blood usage and used the term "transfusion trigger" to identify the criteria used by clinicians for a blood transfusion. Their data suggested that the actual determination for blood administration is most often based on a single laboratory value, hemoglobin concentration. In a review of the basic principles of oxygen transport, Finch and Lenfant (2) described the oxygen transport system as "a corporate process involving several organs, each with its own regulatory system." The traditional determinants of oxygen transport are pulmonary gas exchange, blood flow, hemoglobin mass, and hemoglobin-oxygen affinity. Because the system is regulated so that an alteration in one component may be balanced by compensatory changes in other determinants to maintain oxygen equilibrium, a single laboratory value such as hemoglobin concentration may not be the only appropriate determinant of an individual patient's need. The oxygen transport process and its relevance in transfusion practice is therefore summarized.

L.T. Goodnough: Division of Laboratory Medicine, Washington University School of Medicine, St. Louis, Missouri.

Normal Oxygen Transport

Oxygen delivery (DO_2) is defined as the product of blood flow (cardiac output) and arterial oxygen content (CaO_2):

$$DO_2 = \text{cardiac output} \times CaO_2$$

The actual utilization of oxygen by the tissues is the oxygen consumption (VO_2), which is calculated from the cardiac output and arteriovenous oxygen content difference ($CaO_2 - CvO_2$) by using the Fick relationship:

$$VO_2 = \text{cardiac output} \times (CaO_2 - CvO_2)$$

The oxygen content of blood depends on the hemoglobin

concentration, the binding coefficient of hemoglobin (β equals 1.39 ml oxygen/g hemoglobin), the saturation of the hemoglobin (Sat), and the physically dissolved oxygen. The oxygen content is calculated as follows:

$$\text{Oxygen content} = (\text{hemoglobin concentration} \times \beta \times \text{Sat}) + (0.0031 \times PO_2)$$

Because the dissolved oxygen is minimal at ambient partial pressure of oxygen (PO_2) levels, it is usually omitted. Because β is constant, the oxygen content therefore depends primarily on hemoglobin concentration and saturation.

The saturation of the hemoglobin molecule depends on the PO_2 and the hemoglobin-oxygen affinity state, described by the sigmoidal hemoglobin-oxygen dissociation curve (Fig. 41.1). The *y axis* indicates the saturation of the hemoglobin molecule at each oxygen tension shown on the *x axis*. The oxyhemoglobin affinity state is characterized by the P_{50} of the dissociation curve, which is the oxygen tension at which the hemoglobin is 50% saturated. The normal P_{50} for human blood is 27 torr. As oxygen affinity increases (more tightly bound), the dissociation curve shifts to the left and the P_{50} falls. The saturation is independent of hemoglobin concentration and at any PO_2 is affected only by left or right changes in the oxygen affinity state. Because oxygen content reflects hemoglobin concentration and saturation, the oxygen content curve will have the same sigmoidal shape as the oxygen dissociation curve. Changes in hemoglobin concentration will determine the height of the curve, while P_{50} shifts move the curve to the left or the right.

The oxygen content curve provides a simple means of illustrating the unloading of oxygen or the (CaO_2 − CvO_2) (Fig. 41.2). The arterial PO_2 (PaO_2) is the oxygen tension at which oxygen is loaded onto the hemoglobin molecule in the lung. The arterial content can then be read from the content curve for a known hemoglobin concentration. Oxygen is consumed during the circulation throughout the body, and the mixed venous PO_2 (PvO_2) is the oxygen tension of pulmonary arterial blood at the completion of the oxygen unloading. By using the PvO_2, the venous oxygen content can merely be read from the curve. The CaO_2 − CvO_2 can then be calculated or can be read from the curve (Fig 41.2). The CaO_2 − CvO_2 and cardiac output are then multiplied to obtain oxygen consumption.

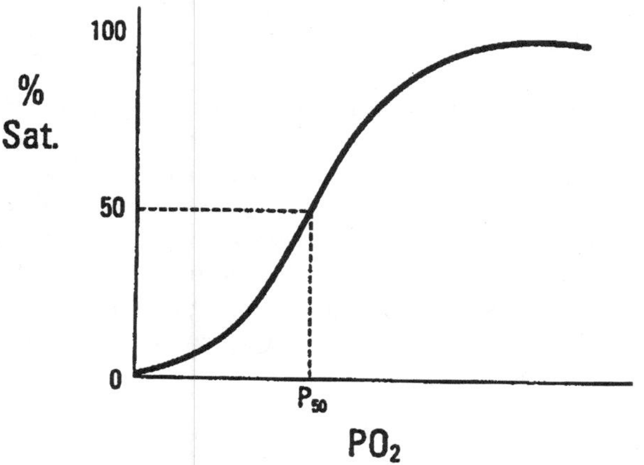

FIGURE 41.1. Hemoglobin-oxygen dissociation curve for whole blood.

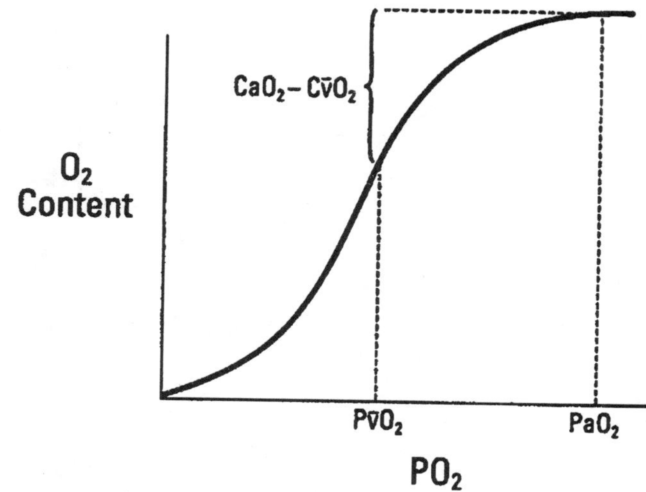

FIGURE 41.2. Oxygen content curve for whole blood, illustrating CaO_2 − CvO_2 and PvO_2.

The mathematics of these relationships indicates the enormous reserve that normally exists:

Normal oxygen consumption = cardiac output × (CaO_2 − CvO_2)
= 5 liters/min × 5 vol%
= 5 liters/min × 50 ml/liter
= 250 ml/min

Normal O_2 delivery = cardiac output × CaO_2
= 5 liters/min × 20 vol%
= 5 liters/min × 200 ml/liter
= 1,000 ml/min

The oxygen extraction ratio (oxygen consumed/oxygen delivered), or O_2ER, is 0.25; in other words, the available oxygen is four times the normally consumed oxygen.

$$O_2ER = VO_2/DO_2$$

Oxygen demand is the volume of oxygen that is needed by the tissue to function aerobically. If the demand for oxygen exceeds consumption, anaerobic metabolism must take over to supply the tissues with adequate energy. When the physiologic response to situations in which the usual relationship between oxygen delivery and oxygen utilization has been altered, a decision must be made concerning the merits of a blood transfusion.

Disorders of Oxygen Transport

A reduction in hemoglobin concentration during the natural hemodilution of surgical blood loss and crystalloid fluid replacement in a healthy normovolemic person is accompanied by an

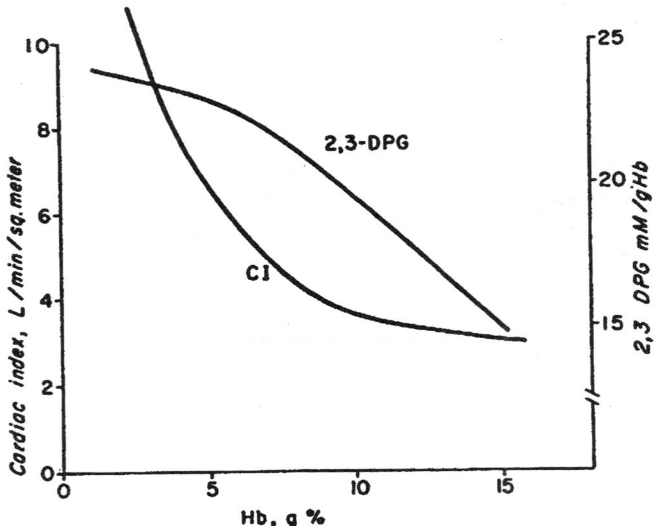

FIGURE 41.3. Effect of anemia on cardiac index and diphosphoglycerate (DPG). (From Finch CA, Lenfant C. Oxygen transport in man. *N Engl J Med* 1972;286:407–415, with permission.)

increased cardiac output to maintain oxygen delivery (Fig 41.3). This response has been observed during purposeful, acute normovolemic hemodilution in both normal subjects (3) and in patients (4), demonstrating the ability of the cardiovascular system to maintain oxygen equilibrium during anemia. Tissue oxygenation was maintained at hemoglobin concentration as low as 4.8 g/dl, with preservation of VO_2 down to DO_2 as low as 7.3 ml oxygen $\times$ kg^{-1} $\times$ min^{-1}; the critical DO_2, at least in healthy humans, appears to be less than this value (Fig 41.4). Such results suggest that hemoglobin concentration alone should not be used to assess the need for a blood transfusion. It may be more appropriate to assess the need for red blood cell therapy

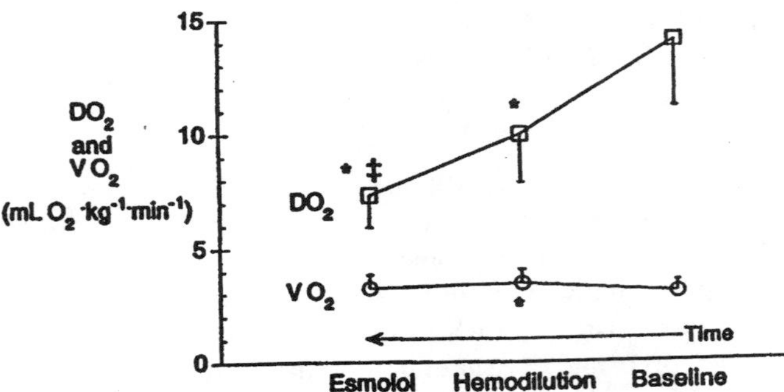

FIGURE 41.4. Oxygen delivery (DO_2) and oxygen consumption (VO_2) in eight healthy adults before (hemoglobin concentration, 12.5 ± 0.8 g/dl) and after (hemoglobin concentration, 4.8 ± 0.2 g/dl) isovolemic hemodilution and during intravenous infusion of a β-adrenergic antagonist, esmolol (with hemoglobin concentration of 4.7 ± 0.2 g/dl). *Indicates $P < 0.05$ versus baseline; indicates $P < 0.05$ versus hemodilution without esmolol. (From Lieberman JA, Weiskopf RB, Kelley SD, et al. Critical oxygen delivery in conscious humans is less than 7.3 ml O_2 $\times$ kg^{-1} $\times$ min^{-1}. *Anesthesiology* 2000;92:407–412, with permission.)

in terms of disorders of oxygen transport, including not only hemoglobin concentration but also blood flow, oxygen loading, hemoglobin–oxygen affinity, and tissue demands.

In the interrelationships between the determinants of oxygen transport and the reserve mechanisms, isolated changes are rare—a change in one factor is often balanced by one or more changes in the remainder to maintain oxygen equilibrium. It is not necessary to treat every clinical disorder in the oxygen transport system because the system itself has a large reserve capacity. Therapeutic interventions are required only when the reserve becomes inadequate. Because the PvO_2 is the best indicator of mean tissue oxygen tension, it becomes a key measurement in assessing the overall adequacy of oxygen transport in the critically ill patient. The normal value for PvO_2 in resting persons is 40 torr. Although a traditional concept has stated that a reduced PvO_2 indicates a low cardiac output, low PvO_2 and high cardiac output may occur simultaneously. It is more appropriate to consider a fall in PvO_2 as an indication of either a decrease in oxygen supply (delivery) or an increase in oxygen demand, serving as an important monitor of the oxygen transport system, including an indicator of oxygen reserve.

There are five etiologies of a decreased PvO_2:

1. Arterial oxygen saturation (Sat)
2. Cardiac output
3. Hemoglobin concentration
4. P_{50}
5. Oxygen consumption (VO_2)

The first four measurements constitute oxygen delivery, and the fifth constitutes oxygen demand. If the supply (delivery) is decreased and oxygen consumption is maintained, the reserve is depleted because of an increase in the oxygen extraction ratio (oxygen consumed/oxygen delivered). The actual utilization of oxygen remains constant except in a situation of an increased oxygen requirement and thus consumption. It is likely that in clinical situations with an altered PvO_2, a combination of changes exists, with more than one compensatory response. The above list provides a qualitative guide to the influence of the changes on PvO_2. A quantitative assessment of the importance of each determinant may be more helpful in the critically ill patient.

Data in primates have permitted quantitative assessment to facilitate diagnostic and therapeutic decisions. The influence of these variables on venous content, $CaO_2 - CvO_2$, and the oxygen extraction ratio also have been analyzed in an effort to identify other critical values that should be treated, regardless of the stability of the patient. As indicated earlier, a fall in PvO_2 indicates a lowered oxygen reserve. However, because venous oxygen content actually represents the volume of oxygen remaining after the oxygen exchange process in the periphery, it may be an even more accurate predictor of a marginal reserve. Animal data suggest that "critical" values that may indicate marginal reserve and warrant therapy are:

PvO_2 <25 torr
Extraction ratio >50%
VO_2 <50% of baseline

The above criteria formed the basis of a clinical trial to evaluate the efficacy of the perfluorocarbon Fluosol DA (Alpha Therapeutics, Los Angeles, CA), a synthetic oxygen carrier. Surgical patients with acute blood loss and religious objections to receiving blood transfusions (5) were studied. Fifteen moderately anemic patients with a mean hemoglobin level of 7.2 ±0.5 g/dl had no evidence of a physiologic need (discussed above) for increased arterial oxygen content and did not receive Fluosol DA. Fourteen of these 15 patients with moderate anemia survived. Eight severely anemic patients with a mean hemoglobin level of 3.0 ± 0.4 g/dl met these physiologic criteria of need and received the synthetic oxygen carrier. Six of these eight patients died, ascribed to the poor oxygen-loading ability of this early synthetic oxygen carrier. Nevertheless, this clinical trial confirmed the clinical relevance of the physiologic criteria of the need for blood transfusion.

Physiologic Benefit of Transfusion

The therapeutic goal of a blood transfusion is to increase oxygen delivery according to the physiologic need of the recipient. To achieve this outcome, the decision to transfuse each unit of blood should be based on the physiologic mechanisms that may be causing the deficit in oxygen delivery. If a physiologic need exists, a transfusion should be given on a unit-by-unit basis. If no physiologic need is identified, there is no role for transfusion. Understanding the complexities associated with the human body's ability to compensate for anemia (in both normal and abnormal settings) and the dynamic nature of perioperative blood loss is essential.

The usual response to an acute reduction in hemoglobin concentration in the normovolemic state is to increase cardiac output (6). This compensatory mechanism is an attempt to maintain adequate oxygen delivery. The heart is therefore the principal organ at risk in acute anemia. Myocardial anaerobic metabolism, indicating inadequate oxygen delivery, occurs when lactate metabolism in the heart converts from lactate uptake to lactate production. The normal whole-body oxygen extraction ratio—the ratio of oxygen consumption to oxygen delivery—is 20% to 25%. The oxygen extraction ratio approaches 50% when myocardial lactate production occurs, indicating anaerobic metabolism. In a normal heart, this lactate production and an oxygen extraction ratio of 50% occur at a hemoglobin concentration of approximately 3.5 to 4.0 g/dl (7). In a model of coronary stenosis, the anaerobic state occurs at a hemoglobin concentration of approximately 6.0 to 7.0 g/dl (8). These values also coincide with the onset of ventricular wall motion abnormalities.

The observations that the critical extraction ratio and anaerobic threshold occur at a different hemoglobin concentration in different physiologic states suggest that the oxygen extraction ratio represents a reasonable indicator of the adequacy of oxygen delivery and, therefore, need for transfusion. There is thus a spectrum of oxygen extraction ratios that ranges from 20% to 50%. No single number, either extraction ratio or hemoglobin concentration, can serve as an absolute indicator of transfusion need. However, the use of such a physiologic value in conjunction with clinical assessment of the patient status permits a rational decision regarding the appropriateness of transfusion prior to the onset of hypoxia or ischemia (9).

If a transfusion is appropriate, then a benefit should occur. The benefits of transfusion are difficult to define and measure with precision. When a change in clinical status occurs, it is often difficult to separate the effect of the transfusion from a change in the patient's underlying disease. In a literature assessment of the benefit of transfusion in terms of mortality, morbidity, and function, the data on mortality are the clearest. In a review of 16 reports of the surgical outcomes in Jehovah's Witnesses who underwent major surgery without blood transfusion, mortality associated with anemia occurred in 1.4% of the 1,404 operations (10). In one large study, the risk of death was found to be higher in patients with cardiovascular disease than in those without (11). These data suggest that in surgery-induced anemia, survival may be improved with blood transfusion. In a study of patients undergoing repair of hip fracture, 84 patients were randomly assigned to receive transfusions either at a predetermined threshold (a hemoglobin concentration level of 10.0 g/dl) or only if symptoms of anemia occurred (with the lower limit of hemoglobin concentration set a 8.0 g/dl); the respective mortality rates at 60 days were 4.8% and 11.9% (12). Because of the small numbers of patients in the study, one should be cautious about drawing definitive conclusions regarding mortality benefits ascribed to transfusion. In a large retrospective study of elderly patients who underwent surgical repair of hip fracture, the use of perioperative transfusion in patients with hemoglobin levels as low as 8.0 g/dl did not appear to influence 30- or 90-day mortality (13).

In a multicenter Canadian study by Hebert et al. (14), 418 critical care patients were randomized to receive red blood cell transfusions when the hemoglobin concentration dropped below 7.0 g/dl, with hemoglobin concentration maintenance in the range of 7.0 to 9.0 g/dl, and 420 patients were randomized to receive transfusions when the hemoglobin concentration dropped below 10.0 g/dl, with hemoglobin concentration levels maintained in the range of 10.0 to 12.0 g/dl. The 30-day mortality rates were not different in the two groups (18.7% versus 23.3%, $P = 0.11$), indicating that a transfusion threshold as low as 7.0 g/dl is as safe as a higher transfusion threshold of 10.0 g/dl in critical care patients. Clearly, more data are needed to determine when transfusion in this setting is beneficial.

Data on morbidity, on the other hand, are much less clear. Gore et al. (15) described the tendency for many clinicians to maintain a hematocrit near 30% in critically ill patients, especially those with hypoxia or sepsis, in an attempt to optimize oxygen delivery and minimize the frequency of ischemic events and other potential complications. Those authors hypothesized that a reduction in morbidity may be possible with transfusion. In their study, hemodynamic and oxygen transport measurements were examined in five severely burned male patients who did not receive blood transfusions for 36 to 48 hours after the operative incision. The hemoglobin concentration level was then raised 3.0 g/dl with multiple transfusions. Although transfusion raised the red blood cell mass significantly and increased oxygen delivery, the physiologic benefit seems marginal. The oxygen extraction ratio, in particular, was not markedly deranged before the transfusion, which indicates that the compensation for the

TABLE 41.1. HEMODYNAMIC MEASUREMENTS IN CRITICALLY ILL POSTOPERATIVE PATIENTS (N = 30)

Variable	Before Transfusion	After Transfusion
Hb (g/dl)	9.4	10.4[a]
Cardiac index (l/min/m^2)	3.2	3.2
Oxygen delivery (ml/min/m^2)	401	433[a]
Oxygen consumption (ml/min/m^2)	117	115
Oxygen extraction ratio (%)	31	29[a]

[a]$P < .01$
Hb, hemoglobin.
From Goodnough LT, Brecher ME, Kanter MH, et al. Medial progress: transfusion medicine, part II. Blood conservation. *N Engl J Med* 1999;340:525–533, with permission.

anemia was quite adequate. In addition, there was no change in oxygen consumption, which suggests that blood transfusion may not have benefited these critically ill patients.

In a report by Babineau et al. (16), the benefit of transfusion was examined in 30 surgical intensive care unit patients who were normovolemic and hemodynamically stable. The data are summarized in Table 41.1. Once again, transfusion increased the hemoglobin concentration level and total oxygen delivery but had a negligible effect on oxygen consumption. There were no important hemodynamic benefits in this group of patients. One can conclude from these data that the assumed benefit of an increase in the red blood cell mass does not always translate into a true benefit in terms of oxygen transport in critically ill patients.

Silent perioperative myocardial ischemia has been observed in patients undergoing noncardiac (17) as well as cardiac (18) surgery. Hemoglobin levels ranging from 6.0 to 10.0 g/dl—a range in which indicators other than hemoglobin concentration may identify patients who may benefit from blood transfusion—therefore need to be the most closely scrutinized (19, 20). A study of elderly patients who were undergoing elective noncardiac surgery found that intraoperative or postoperative myocardial ischemia was more likely to occur in patients with hematocrits below 28%, particularly in the presence of tachycardia (21). In the absence of a physiologic need in a stable nonbleeding patient, a rise in hemoglobin concentration level alone is not a good reason to give a transfusion (22).

Published data related to the benefit of transfusion on function are scant. Some investigators have studied possible benefits to the transfusion of autologous blood. Kim et al. (23) did not find a relationship between hemoglobin concentration and length of hospital stay for 332 patients who underwent total hip arthroplasty. Johnson et al. (24) did not identify any overall correlation between hematocrit value and exercise capacity in a randomized prospective trial of two transfusion strategies in 39 patients undergoing elective myocardial revascularization. No significant differences in postoperative exercise endurance were found between patients who received transfusions in order to maintain a hematocrit of 32% and patients who received transfusions only if the hematocrit dropped below 25%.

There are no documented effects on length of hospital stay, rehabilitation, return to work, or health care costs as a consequence of transfusion. Whether blood transfusion is associated with a clinically significant immunomodulatory effect (e.g., perioperative infections) is the object of debate (25,26), and is discussed in detail in Chapter 60.

TRANSFUSION PRACTICES

Utilization Review

Audits of a facility's transfusion practices can improve the efficiency and appropriateness of transfusion if they are performed in a timely manner and if the results are communicated to physicians who order transfusions for their patients (27). Audits of the use of plasma and platelet products are particularly amenable to this approach and can reduce the use of blood components by up to 50% (28). However, a recent multihospital study found that a retrospective utilization review did not reduce the use of red blood cell transfusions (29).

This lack of success may be a consequence of several factors. First, it is difficult to evaluate the appropriateness of transfusion in patients with hemorrhage who are seen in emergency rooms and trauma units, operating rooms, and intensive care units. Second, some studies have found that fewer than 5% of red blood cell transfusions are unjustified (30). One reason for this low rate may be that clinical indicators for transfusion appropriateness are too generous. It is difficult to improve transfusion practices if over 95% of transfusions are found to be justified. Third, there is often no clearly documented information in a medical chart that explains why a transfusion was administered. In only two-thirds of cases in which postoperative transfusions are administered on the day of surgery is blood loss or a change in vital signs noted in the medical record, and the rationale for transfusion is documented in fewer than a third of cases (31). This lack of success has raised questions regarding the overall value and effectiveness of retrospective utilization review (30). Point-of-care testing and transfusion algorithms show promise in improving transfusion appropriateness (32).

Surgery

The discharge hematocrit levels of patients who underwent orthopedic surgery ranged from 31% to 34% in the mid-1980s, suggesting that perisurgical anemia was being treated too aggressively with transfusion (33). Subsequently however, the overall rate of transfusions for patients undergoing hip and knee arthroplasty has declined by 15% to 35% (34). The patient's gender has been found to influence the outcome of transfusion in such patients (1,35) and has been attributed to physicians' use of the same hematocrit value as a threshold for transfusion for both women and men, without taking into account that women have lower hematocrit levels. Studies found substantial variability in the use of red blood cell transfusions for patients undergoing total hip and knee arthroplasty (34), and the variability was attributed to the lack of clearly defined criteria for transfusion and to hospital-specific differences.

There is also considerable variation in transfusion practices among institutions with respect to patients who undergo cardiac surgery. A multicenter audit of 18 institutions demonstrated a wide range in the outcomes of allogeneic transfusions among patients who underwent primary coronary artery bypass grafting (36). A subsequent study reported similar findings (37). The variability in transfusion outcomes in these patients has also been attributed to differences in training that are specific to hospitals and physicians, rather than to differences in patient populations (38).

Guidelines for Transfusion

Guidelines for blood transfusion have been issued by several organizations, including a National Institutes of Health consensus conference on perioperative transfusion of red blood cells (39), the American College of Physicians (40), the American Society of Anesthesiologists (20), and the Canadian Medical Association (41). These guidelines recommend that blood not be transfused prophylactically and suggest that, in patients who are not critically ill, the threshold for transfusion should be a hemoglobin level of 6.0 to 8.0 g/dl. Adherence to these guidelines has raised questions about whether transfusion is now underused (42). A hemoglobin concentration of 8.0 g/dl seems an appropriate threshold for transfusion in surgical patients with no risk factors for ischemia, whereas a threshold of 10.0 g/dl can be justified for patients who are considered at risk. However, prophylactic transfusion of blood (i.e., in anticipation of blood loss) cannot be endorsed, particularly because studies have found that overuse of transfusion in critically ill patients (14) may be associated with less favorable outcomes. It is unlikely that any level of hemoglobin can be used as a universal threshold for transfusion.

AUTOLOGOUS BLOOD TRANSFUSION

Interest in autologous blood procurement was stimulated in the 1980s by a renewed awareness that infectious diseases are transmissible by blood transfusion, including not only posttransfusion hepatitis but also human immunodeficiency virus (HIV). Preoperative autologous blood donation (PAD), acute normovolemic hemodilution (ANH), and intraoperative and postoperative autologous blood cell recovery and reinfusion were techniques identified and promoted (43) in the surgical arena in response to medical and legal pressures to minimize allogeneic blood exposure.

The role of autologous blood procurement in surgery remains in evolution, based on improved blood safety, increased blood costs, and emerging pharmacologic alternatives to blood transfusion (44). In certain elective surgical settings, such as total joint replacement surgery, PAD became accepted as a standard practice, so that over 6% of the blood transfused in the United States in 1992 was autologous (45). In contrast, ANH was rarely practiced and published data regarding its merits were scant. Subsequently, substantial improvements in blood safety have been accompanied by a decline in PAD (Table 41.2) as well as an interest in ANH as an alternative lower-cost autologous blood procurement strategy. Current applications of autologous blood procurement strategies and techniques in the surgical setting will be summarized.

Preoperative Autologous Blood Donation

Efficacy

Patients undergoing PAD may donate a unit (450 ± 45 ml, or up to 10.5 ml/kg body weight) of blood as often as twice weekly until 72 hours before surgery. Under routine conditions, patients usually donate once weekly. Oral iron supplements are routinely prescribed. This iatrogenic blood loss is accompanied by a response in endogenous erythropoietin levels that, while increased significantly over basal levels, remain within the range of normal. The erythropoietic response that occurs under these conditions is therefore modest (46). A summary of prospective controlled trials (47–52) of patients undergoing such blood loss via autologous phlebotomy is presented in Table 41.3, along with calculated estimates of red blood cell volume expansion (erythropoiesis in excess of basal rates). With routine PAD, 220 to 351 ml, representing 11% to 19% red blood cell expansion (47,48) or the equivalent of 1.0 to 1.75 blood units, are produced in excess of basal erythropoiesis, defining the efficacy of this blood conservation practice.

TABLE 41.2. COLLECTION AND TRANSFUSION OF AUTOLOGOUS BLOOD IN THE UNITED STATES

Source	1980	1986	1989	1992	1994	1997
Transfused	(Thousand of Units)					
Autologous	N/A	N/A	369	566	482	421
(% of total)	—	—	(3.1%)	(5.0%)	(4.3%)	(3.7%)
Total	9,934	12,159	12,059	11,307	11,107	11,476
Collected						
Autologous	28	206	655	1,117	1,013	611
(% of total)	(0.25%)	(1.5%)	(4.8%)	(8.5%)	(7.8%)	(4.9%)
Total	11,174	13,807	13,554	13,169	12,908	12,550

From Goodnough LT, Brecher ME, Kanter MH, et al. Medical progress: transfusion medicine, part I. Blood transfusion. *N Engl J Med* 1999;340:439–447, with permission.

TABLE 41.3. ERYTHROPOIESIS DURING AUTOLOGOUS BLOOD DONATION

Patients (n)	Blood Removed (Donated): Baseline RBC (ml)	Requested/ Donated Units		RBC (ml)	Blood Produced: RBC (ml)	Expansion (%)	Iron Therapy	Ref
Standard phlebotomy								
108	1,884	3	2.7	522	351	19%	PO	(47)
22	1,936	3	2.8	590	220	11%	None	(48)
45	1,881	3	2.9	621	331	17%	PO	(48)
41	1,918	3	2.9	603	315	16%	PO, IV	(48)
Aggressive phlebotomy								
30	2,075	≥3	3.0	540	397	19%	None	(49)
30	2,024	≥3	3.1	558	473	23%	PO	(49)
30	2,057	≥	2.9	522	436	21%	IV	(49)
24	2,157	6	4.1	683	568	26%	PO	(50,51)
23	2,257	6	4.6	757	440	19%	PO	(52)

Data expressed as means
PO, oral; IV, intravenous; RBC, red blood cell
From Goodnough et al. *Blood* 2000; 96:823–833, with permission.

For patients subjected to more aggressive (up to two units weekly) phlebotomy, the endogenous erythropoietin response is more substantial (49–52). In one clinical trial (50), a linear logarithmic relationship was demonstrated between change in hemoglobin level and the endogenous erythropoietin response (53). Erythropoietin-mediated erythropoiesis in this setting is 397 to 568 ml (19% to 26% red blood cell expansion) (49–52), or the equivalent of two to three blood units.

Patient Selection

Preoperative autologous collections are most beneficial for patients at risk for blood transfusion who are undergoing procedures associated with substantial blood loss, such as orthopedic joint replacement, vascular surgery, cardiac or thoracic surgery, and radical prostatectomy. Autologous blood is unnecessary for procedures that seldom require transfusion, such as transurethral resection of the prostate, cholecystectomy, herniorrhaphy, vaginal hysterectomy, and uncomplicated obstetric delivery (54). A hospital's maximal surgical blood order schedule (MSBOS) for blood crossmatch can provide estimates of transfusion needs for specific procedures; the generally accepted cut-off at which transfusion is "unlikely" and autologous blood procurement should not be recommended is 10% (55).

It is important to establish guidelines for the appropriate number of units to be collected, so that patient exposure to allogeneic blood in minimized. Collection of units should be scheduled as far in advance of surgery as possible for liquid blood storage (up to 42 days), in order to allow compensatory erythropoiesis (46) to correct the induced anemia. If the erythropoietic response to autologous blood phlebotomy is not able to maintain the patient's level of hematocrit during the donation interval, the predeposit of autologous blood may actually be harmful. A study of patients undergoing hysterectomy (56) demonstrated that preoperative autologous blood donation resulted in perioperative anemia and an increased likelihood of any blood transfusion. Table 41.4 summarizes the rates of allogeneic blood exposure in patients undergoing total joint replacement, with or without PAD, in the United States in 1996 and 1997 (57).

While the most important indicator for autologous blood procurement is the effectiveness in reduced allogeneic transfusions, the "wastage" rate of autologous units is an index of its efficiency and costs. Even for procedures such as total joint replacement surgery, discard rates of up to 50% of collected units are common (57). When autologous blood is collected for procedures that seldom require transfusion, such as vaginal hysterectomies, up to 90% of units collected for these procedures are wasted (56). The additional costs associated with the collection

TABLE 41.4. *ALLOGENEIC BLOOD TRANSFUSION OUTCOMES IN PATIENTS UNDERGOING TOTAL JOINT REPLACEMENT: USA 1996–1997*

Procedure	Autologous Blood Predonated: No (n = 3741)	Yes (n = 5741): Nonanemic	Yes (n = 5741): Anemic (hct < 39%)
Knee			
Unilateral	18	6	11
Revision	30	11	18
Bilateral	57	16	21
Hip			
Unilateral	32	9	14
Revision	59	21	33

Data shown represent (%) of patients receiving allogeneic blood.
Hct, hematocrit.
From Bierbaum BE, Callaghan JJ, Galante JO, et al. An analysis of blood management in patients having total hip or knee arthroplasty. *J Bone Joint Surg Am* 1999;81: 2–10, with permission.

of autologous units and the inherent "wastage" of these units, along with advances in the safety of allogeneic blood, now make the predonation of autologous blood poorly cost effective (58). Some suggestions that have been made to make autologous blood programs less costly include: abbreviate the donor interview for autologous collection, use only whole blood and discontinue component production, limit the use of frozen autologous blood, apply the same transfusion guidelines for autologous and allogeneic blood, and test only the first donated autologous blood unit for infectious disease markers. Attempts to stratify patients into groups at high and low risk for transfusion based on the baseline level of hemoglobin and on the type of procedure show some promise. In a study using a point score system, 80% of patients undergoing total joint replacement procedures were identified to be at low risk (less than 10%) for transfusion, so that autologous blood procurement for these patients would not be recommended (59).

Safety Considerations

Autologous blood donation and the transfusion of autologous blood are both associated with risks. One in 16,783 autologous donations is associated with an adverse reaction severe enough to require hospitalization, which is 12 times the risk associated with community donations by healthy individuals (60). Ischemic events have also been reported to occur in association with autologous blood donation (61). The transfusion of autologous blood has many of the same complications as transfusion of allogeneic units, including bacterial contamination, hemolysis due to errors in the administration of units, and volume overload. Advantages and disadvantages of PAD are summarized in Table 41.5. Because mortality from allogeneic blood transfusion is now more likely due to administrative error (62) rather than to blood-transmitted infection (45), the risks of banked autologous blood units are similar to banked allogeneic blood units.

Acute Normovolemic Hemodilution

Acute normovolemic hemodilution is a technique that comprises the removal of whole blood from a patient while restoring the circulating blood volume with acellular fluid shortly before an anticipated significant surgical blood loss. Blood is collected in standard blood bags containing anticoagulant on a tilt-rocker with automatic cutoff via volume sensors. The blood is then stored at room temperature and reinfused in the operating room after major blood loss has ceased, or sooner if indicated. Simultaneous infusions of crystalloid (3 ml crystalloids to 1 ml blood withdrawn) and colloid (dextrans, starches, gelatin, albumin, 1 ml to 1 ml) have been recommended. Subsequent intraoperative fluid management is based on the usual surgical requirements. Blood units are reinfused in the reverse order of collection. The first unit collected, and therefore the last unit transfused, has the highest hematocrit and concentration of coagulation factors and platelets.

Withdrawal of whole blood and replacement with crystalloid or colloid solution decreases arterial oxygen content, but compensatory hemodynamic mechanisms and the existence of surplus oxygen-delivery capacity make ANH safe. A sudden drop in red blood cell mass increases cardiac output and lowers blood viscosity, thereby decreasing peripheral resistance. If cardiac output can compensate effectively, oxygen delivery to the tissues at a hematocrit of 25% to 30% is as good as, but no better than, delivery at a hematocrit of 35% to 45% (3).

Because blood collected by ANH is stored at room temperature and is usually returned to the patient within 8 hours of collection, there is little deterioration of platelets or coagulation factors. The hemostatic value of blood collected by ANH is of questionable benefit for orthopedic or urologic surgery because plasma and platelets are rarely indicated in this setting. Its value in protecting plasma and platelets from the acquired coagulopathy of extracorporeal circulation in cardiac surgery (known as "blood pooling") is better established (63).

Efficacy

The chief benefit of hemodilution has been recognized to be the reduction of red blood cell losses when whole blood is shed perioperatively at lower hematocrit levels after ANH is complete. Mathematic modeling has suggested that severe hemodilution to preoperative hematocrit levels of less than 20%, accompanied by substantial blood losses, would be required before the red blood cell volume "saved" by hemodilution became clinically important (64). An analysis of patients who had undergone "minimal" ANH (representing 15% of patients' blood volumes) estimates that only 100 ml red blood cells (the equivalent of one-half unit of blood) is "saved" under these conditions (65). With moderate hemodilution (target hematocrit levels of 28%) the "savings" becomes more substantial, as illustrated in Figure 41.5. The removal of three blood units from a patient who subsequently undergoes a blood loss of 2,600 ml results in an estimated 732 ml of red blood cells lost, compared to 947 ml of red blood cells that would have been lost if hemodilution had not been performed. The surgical red blood cells losses "saved" in this instance by hemodilution are 215 ml, or the equivalent of one allogeneic blood unit. The safety and efficacy of more extensive hemodilution is controversial and may provide little additional blood conservation.

TABLE 41.5. AUTOLOGOUS BLOOD DONATION

Advantages	Disadvantages
1. Prevents transfusion-transmitted disease	1. Risk of bacterial contamination or volume overload remains
2. Prevents red cell alloimmunization	2. Does not eliminate risk of administrative error with ABO incompatibility
3. Supplements the blood supply	3. More costly than allogeneic blood
4. Provides compatible blood for patients with alloantibodies	4. Wastage of blood not transfused
5. Prevents some adverse transfusion reactions	5. Causes perioperative anemia and increased likelihood of transfusion

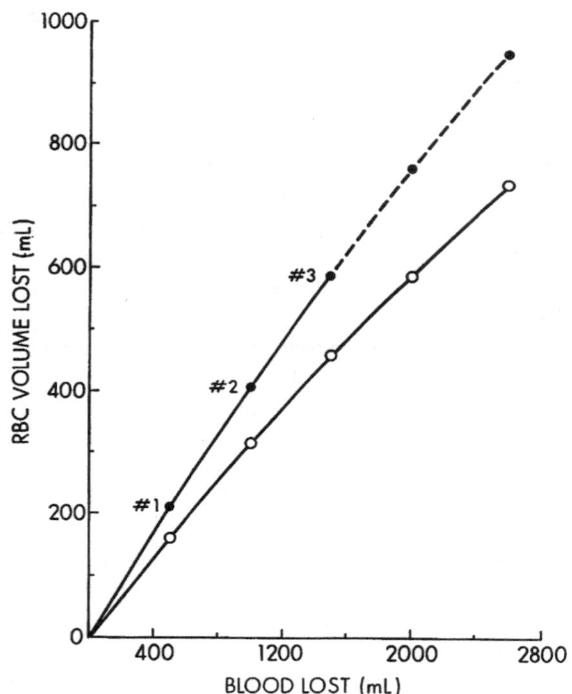

FIGURE 41.5. The relationship between whole blood volume (ml) lost *(abscissa)* and red blood cell (RBC) volume lost *(ordinate)* in a 100-kg patient undergoing hemodilution. Red blood cell volume lost with 2,800 ml whole blood lost intraoperatively after hemodilution of 1,500 ml whole blood *(o—o)*. Red blood cell volume lost with 2,800 ml whole blood lost during hemodilution at each of three 500-ml volumes *(—)*. Cumulative RBC volume lost intraoperatively, derived for 2,800 ml whole blood lost if hemodilution had not been performed *(- - -)*. A net 215-ml reduction in RBC volume lost with hemodilution is illustrated by the divergence of the two curves. (From Goodnough LT, Grishaber JE, Monk TG, et al. Acute preoperative hemodilution in patients undergoing radical prostatectomy: a case study analysis of efficacy. *Anesth Analg* 1994;78:932–937, with permission.)

Clinical Studies

It had been recommended previously that patients scheduled for radical prostatectomy predonate three units of autologous blood; this reduced the prevalence of allogeneic exposure from 66% to 70% in patients without autologous blood to 14% to 16% in patients who have predonated three units of autologous blood (66). A study of 250 patients in this setting reported that 21% of patients undergoing ANH alone received allogeneic blood (67). Two prospective randomized trials (68,69) and a case-controlled retrospective comparison (70) of ANH and PAD in patients undergoing radical prostatectomy demonstrated that subsequent allogeneic blood exposure (10% to 20%) was not different for patients undergoing either method of autologous blood procurement.

The benefit of ANH as determined in a mathematic model (71) is illustrated in Figure 41.6. An adult with an estimated 5-liter blood volume and an initial hematocrit of 40%, with surgical blood losses of up to 3,000 ml, would result in a level of hematocrit that would remain ≥25% postoperatively without an autologous blood intervention. This level of hematocrit is generally considered safe for patients with known risk factors (20). Note that in this model, the performance of ANH with initial hematocrit levels of 40% to 45% would allow up to 2,500- to 3,500-ml surgical blood losses, yet the nadir level of hematocrit could be maintained ≥28%. The benefit of ANH in this model is to protect patients who have substantial blood losses that cannot be predicted and maintain perioperative levels of hematocrit that minimize risks related to ischemia. Blood conservation strategies need to address both of these issues. The theoretic relationship between the number of red blood cell units saved via moderate ANH as a function of estimated surgical blood loss (72) is illustrated in Figure 41.7.

In a randomized trial in patients undergoing total hip arthroplasty, 23 patients were randomized to the ANH and 25 patients to the PAD group (73). No differences were noted between groups, including estimated intraoperative blood losses and calculated red blood cell losses for the surgical hospitalization. Four (17%) of 23 ANH patients received allogeneic blood, not different than none in the PAD group ($P = 0.30$).

Because ANH represents "point of care" autologous blood procurement, it is less costly than PAD. First, autologous blood units procured by ANH are retransfused before leaving the operating room and require no inventory or testing costs. The procedure therefore reduces the possibility of an administrative error that could lead to an ABO-incompatible blood transfusion and

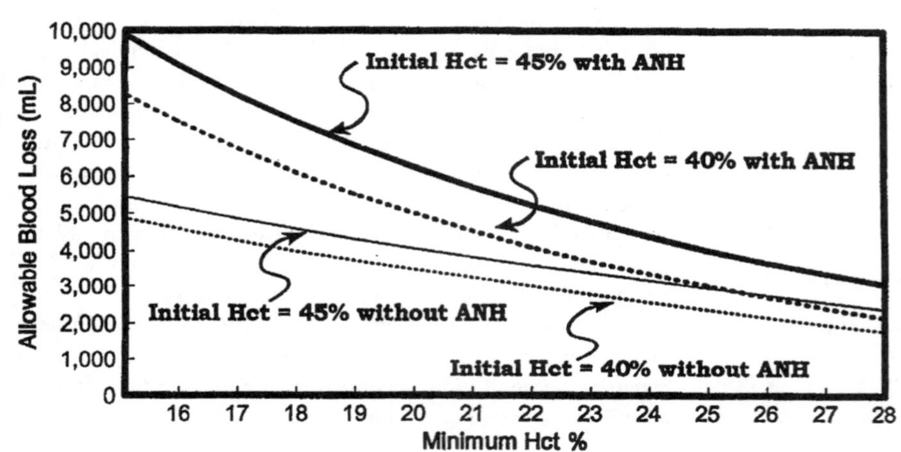

FIGURE 41.6. The maximal allowable blood loss in a patient with a blood volume of 5 liters and an initial hematocrit level of 45% *(the solid lines)* or 40% *(the dotted lines)*, with and without acute normovolemic hemodilution (ANH). (From Goodnough LT, Monk TG, Brecher ME. Acute normovolemic hemodilution in surgery. *Hematology* 1997; 2:413–420, with permission.)

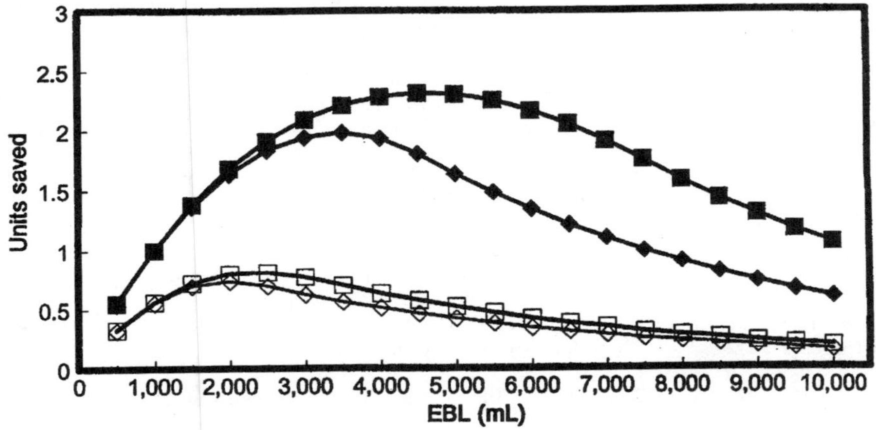

FIGURE 41.7. The theoretic relationship between the number of red blood cell units saved as a function of estimated blood loss (EBL) following acute isovolemic hemodilution to minimum hematocrit of 28% *(open symbols)* or a hematocrit of 18% *(shaded symbols)* for a patient with a blood volume of 5 liters and an initial hematocrit of 45%. Replacement strategies were either to infuse ml-for-ml of blood lost *(diamond symbols)* or to transfuse so as to maintain the hematocrit at the minimal hematocrit *(square symbols)*. (From Goodnough LT, Monk TG, Brecher, ME. A review of autologous blood procurement in the surgical setting: lessons learned in the last 10 years. *Vox Sang* 1996;71:13–21, with permission.)

death, while PAD does not eliminate this risk; the estimated risk of death from a hemolytic transfusion reaction (62) now approximates the risk of mortality from HIV or hepatitis infection from blood transfusion (45). Because ANH and reinfusion is accomplished in the operating room by on-site personnel, procurement and administration costs are minimized. In addition, blood obtained during ANH does not require the commitment of patient time, transportation, and loss of work associated with PAD. Finally, the wastage (54) of autologous blood units (approximately 50% of units collected) is eliminated with ANH. Hemodynamic monitoring and absence of adverse events in 250 consecutive patients undergoing ANH (74) indicate that moderate hemodilution can be performed safely. A pro and con debate on the merits of ANH has been published (75,76).

Intraoperative Autologous Blood Recovery and Reinfusion

Intraoperative recovery of blood involves the collection and reinfusion of autologous red blood cells lost by a patient during surgery. Cell-washing devices can provide the equivalent of up to ten units of banked blood per hour to a patient with massive bleeding. The survival of the red blood cells that are recovered appears to be similar to that of transfused allogeneic red blood cells (77). Relative contraindications include the potential for the aspiration of malignant cells, the presence of infection, and the presence of other contaminants such as amniotic or ascitic fluid in the operative field. Because washing does not completely remove bacteria from the recovered blood, intraoperative recovery should not be used if the operative field has gross bacterial contamination (78).

As with other strategies of autologous blood procurement, the relative benefits, safety, and costs of intraoperative recovery of autologous blood should be carefully scrutinized. A prospective randomized trial of patients who were undergoing repair of abdominal aortic aneurysms or aortofemoral artery bypass procedures found that intraoperative recovery and reinfusion of blood did not result in the need for fewer blood transfusions (79). Four deaths related to intraoperative blood recovery were reported to the New York Department of Health from 1990 through 1995, for an estimated rate of 1 per 35,000 procedures (80). With the use of automated cell-washing devices, the equivalent of at least two units of washed blood needs to be recovered in order for this method to be cost effective (81). Intraoperative recovery of blood may be of most value, not because it reduces the requirements for blood transfusion, but because it provides blood that is less costly to obtain and is more immediately available in the event of rapid blood loss.

Postoperative Autologous Blood Recovery and Reinfusion

Postoperative recovery of blood involves the collection of blood from surgical drains followed by reinfusion, with or without processing. The blood recovered is dilute, is partially hemolyzed and defibrinated, and may contain high concentrations of cytokines. For these reasons, programs establish an upper limit to the volume of unprocessed blood (1,400 ml at one of the author's hospitals) that may be reinfused.

The safety and the benefit of the use of unwashed blood obtained from surgical drains after orthopedic surgery remain in question (82). One center that initially found this approach to be beneficial subsequently reported that this costly practice is of no clinical benefit (83). Because the blood-cell volume of the fluid collected is low (hematocrit, 20%), the volume of red blood cells reinfused is often small. Selective use of the method in situations in which large postoperative blood losses are anticipated, such as in bilateral joint replacement surgery, would improve the efficacy for the procedure, but such blood losses are difficult to predict.

CONCLUSION

The use of blood transfusion has declined, probably as a result of more conservative transfusion practices during an era of concerns about the safety of the blood supply. It is unlikely that any level of hemoglobin can be used as a universal threshold for transfusion. Increased attention to the costs and safety of health care delivery has caused the relative benefits and costs of both blood transfusion and conservation to be scrutinized. The prospective identification of surgical candidates who will need transfusion and will therefore truly benefit from blood conservation must be based on patient-specific factors, such as the baseline hematocrit, cardiac performance, and the anticipated blood loss during surgery. The decision to conserve blood needs may no longer be based on the safety of the blood supply, but on evidence that blood conservation is safe and of value for individual patients.

REFERENCES

1. Friedman BA, Burns TL, Schork MA. An analysis of blood transfusion of surgical patients by sex: a quest for the transfusion trigger. *Transfusion* 1980;20:179–188.
2. Finch CA, Lenfant C. Oxygen transport in man. *N Engl J Med* 1972; 286:407–415.
3. Lieberman JA, Weiskopf RB, Kelley SD, et al. Critical oxygen delivery in conscious humans is less than 7.3 ml $0_2 \times kg^{-1} \times min^{-1}$. *Anesthesiology* 2000;92:407–412.
4. Messmer K, Sunder-Plassman L, Jesch F, et al. Oxygen supply to the tissues during limited normovolemic hemodilution. *Res Exp Med* 1973; 159:152–166.
5. Gould SA, Rosen AL, Sehgal LR, et al. Fluosol DA as a red-cell substitute in acute anemia. *N Engl J Med* 1986;314:1653–1656.
6. Woodson RD, Willis RE, Lenfant C. Effect of acute and established anemia on O_2 transport at rest, submaximal and maximal work. *J Appl Physiol* 1978;44:36–43.
7. Levy PS, Chavez RP, Crystal GJ, et al. Oxygen extraction ratio: a valid indicator of transfusion need in limited coronary reserve? *J Trauma* 1992;32:769–774.
8. Levy PS, Kim SJ, Eckel PK, et al. Limit to cardiac compensation during acute isovolemic hemodilution: influence of coronary stenosis. *Am J Physiol* 1993;265:H340–349.
9. Goodnough LT, Despotis GJ, Hogue CW. On the need for improved transfusion indicators in cardiac surgery. *Ann Thorac Surg* 1995;60: 473–480.
10. Kitchens CS. Are transfusions overrated? Surgical outcome of Jehovah's Witnesses [Editorial]. *Am J Med* 1993;94:117–119.
11. Carson JL, Duf A, Poses RM, et al. Effect of anaemia and cardiovascular disease on surgical mortality and morbidity. *Lancet* 1996;348:1055.
12. Carson JL, Terrin ML, Barton FB, et al. A pilot randomized trial comparing symptomatic vs hemoglobin-level driven red blood cell transfusions following hip fractures. *Transfusion* 1998;38:522–529.
13. Carson JL, Duff A, Berlin JA, et al. Perioperative blood transfusion and postoperative mortality. *JAMA* 1998;279:199–205.
14. Hebert PC, Wells G, Blajchman MA, et al. A multicenter, randomized, controlled clinical trial of transfusion requirements in critical care. *N Engl J Med* 1999;340:409–417.
15. Gore DC, DeMaria EJ, Reines HD. Elevations in red blood cell mass reduce cardiac index without altering the oxygen consumption in severely burned patients. *Surg Forum* 1992;43:721–723.
16. Babineau TJ, Dzik WH, Borlase BC, et al. Reevaluation of current transfusion practices in patients in surgical intensive care units. *Am J Surg* 1992;164:22–25.
17. Mangano DT, Browner WS, Hollenberg M, et al. Association of perioperative myocardial ischemia with cardiac morbidity and mortality in men undergoing noncardiac surgery. *N Engl J Med* 1990;323: 1781–1788.
18. Rao TLK, Montoya A. Cardiovascular, electrocardiographic and respiratory changes following acute anemia with volume replacement in patients with coronary artery disease. *Anesth Dev* 1985;12:49–54.
19. Goodnough LT, Despotis GJ, Hogue CW Jr, et al. On the need for improved transfusion indicators in cardiac surgery. *Ann Thorac Surg* 1995;60:473–480.
20. Practice guidelines for blood component therapy: a report by the American Society of Anesthesiologists Task Force on Blood Component Therapy. *Anesthesiology* 1996;84:732–747.
21. Hogue CW Jr, Goodnough LT, Monk TG. Perioperative myocardial ischemic episodes are related to hematocrit level in patients undergoing radical prostatectomy. *Transfusion* 1998;38:924–931.
22. Welch HG, Mehan KR, Goodnough LT. Prudent strategies for elective red blood cell transfusion. *Ann Int Med* 1992;116:393–402.
23. Kim DM, Brecher ME, Estes TJ, et al. Relationship of hemoglobin level and duration of hospitalization after total hip arthroplasty: implications for the transfusion target. *Mayo Clin Proc* 1993;68:37–41.
24. Johnson RG, Thurer RL, Kruskall MS, et al. Comparison of two transfusion strategies after elective operations for myocardial revascularization. *J Thorac Cardiovasc Surg* 1992;104:307–314.
25. Blajchman MA. Transfusion-associated immunomodulation and universal white cell reduction. Are we putting the cart before the horse? *Transfusion* 1999;39:667–670.
26. Goodnough LT. The case against universal leukoreduction (and for the practice of evidence-based medicine). *Transfusion* 2000;40: 1552–1557.
27. Toy PTCY. Effectiveness of transfusion audits and practice guidelines. *Arch Pathol Lab* 1994;118:435–437.
28. Barnette RD, Fish DJ, Eisenstaedt RS. Modification of fresh-frozen transfusion practices through educational intervention. *Transfusion* 1990;30:253–257.
29. Lam HTC, Schweitzer SO, Petz L, et al. Are retrospective peer-review transfusion monitoring systems effective in reducing red blood cell utilization? *Arch Pathol Lab* 1996;120:810–816.
30. Goodnough LT, Audet AM. Retrospective utilization review for blood transfusions. Are we just going through the motions? *Arch Pathol Lab Med* 1996;120:802.
31. Audet AM, Goodnough LT, Parvin CA. Evaluating the appropriateness of red blood cell transfusions: the limitations of retrospective medical record reviews. *Int J Qual Health Care* 1996;8:41–49.
32. Despotis GJ, Grishaber J, Goodnough LT. The effect of an intraoperative transfusion algorithm on physician transfusion behavior in cardiac surgery. *Transfusion* 1994;34:290–296.
33. Toy PTCY, Kaplan EB, McVay PA, et al. Blood loss and replacement in total hip arthroplasty: a multicenter study. *Transfusion* 1992;32: 63–67.
34. Churchill WH, McGurk S, Chapman RH, et al: The Collaborative Hospital Transfusion Study: variations in use of autologous blood account for differences in red cell use during primary hip and knee surgery. *Transfusion* 1998;38:530–539.
35. Goodnough LT, Verbrugge D, Vizmeg K, et al. Identification of elective orthopedic surgical patients transfused with blood volumes in excess of blood needs: the "transfusion trigger" revisited. *Transfusion* 1992;32:648–653.
36. Goodnough LT, Johnston MFM, Toy PTCY. The variability of transfusion practice in coronary artery bypass graft surgery. *JAMA* 1991; 265:86–90.
37. Stover EP, Siegel LC, Parks R, et al. Variability in transfusion practice for coronary artery bypass surgery persists despite national consensus guidelines. *Anesthesiology* 1998;88:327–333.
38. Surgenor DN, Churchill WH, Wallace EL, et al: The specific hospital significantly affects red cell and component transfusion practice in coronary artery bypass graft surgery: a study of five hospitals. *Transfusion* 1998;37:122–134.
39. Consensus Conference. Perioperative red cell transfusion. *JAMA* 1988; 260:2700–2703.
40. American College of Physicians. Practice strategies for elective red blood cell transfusion. *Ann Int Med* 1992;116:403–406.
41. Expert Working Group. Guidelines for red blood cell and plasma transfusions for adults and children. *CMAJ* 1997;156[Suppl 1]1:S1–S24.
42. Valeri CR, Crowley JP, Loscalzo J. The red cell transfusion trigger: has a sin of commission now become a sin of omission? *Transfusion* 1998;38:602–610.
43. NHLBI Expert Panel. Transfusion alert: use of autologous blood. *Transfusion* 1995;35:703–711.
44. Goodnough LT, Brecher ME, Kanter MH, et al. Medial progress: transfusion medicine, part II. Blood conservation. *N Engl J Med* 1999; 340:525–533.
45. Goodnough LT, Brecher ME, Kanter MH, et al. Medial progress:

transfusion medicine, part I. Blood transfusion. *N Engl J Med* 1999; 340:439–447.

46. Goodnough LT, Skikne B, Brugnara C. Erythropoietin, iron, and erythropoiesis. *Blood* 2000;96:823–833.
47. Kasper SM, Gerlich W, Buzello W. Preoperative red cell production in patients undergoing weekly autologous blood donation. *Transfusion* 1997;37:1058–1062.
48. Kasper SM, Lazansky H, Stark C, et al. Efficacy of oral iron supplementation is not enhanced by additional intravenous iron during autologous blood donation. *Transfusion* 1998;38:764–770.
49. Weisbach V, Skoda P, Rippel R, et al. Oral or intravenous iron as an adjunct to autologous blood donation in elective surgery: a randomized, controlled study. *Transfusion* 1999;39:465–472.
50. Goodnough LT, Rudnick S, Price TH, et al. Increased preoperative collection of autologous blood with recombinant human erythropoietin therapy. *N Engl J Med* 1989;321:1163–1167.
51. Goodnough LT, Price TH, Rudnick S, et al. Preoperative red blood cell production in patients undergoing aggressive autologous blood phlebotomy with and without erythropoietin therapy. *Transfusion* 1992;32:441–445.
52. Goodnough LT, Price TH, Friedman KD, et al. A phase III trial of recombinant human erythropoietin therapy in non-anemic orthopedic patients subjected to aggressive autologous blood phlebotomy: dose, response, toxicity, efficacy. *Transfusion* 1994;34:66–71.
53. Goodnough LT, Price TH, Parvin CA, et al. Erythropoietin response to anaemia is not altered by surgery or recombinant human erythropoietin therapy. *Br J Haematol* 1994;87:695–699.
54. Renner SW, Howanitz PJ, Bachner P. Preoperative autologous blood donation in 612 hospitals. *Arch Pathol Lab Med* 1992;116:613–619.
55. Mintz PD, Nordine RB, Henry JB, et al. Expected hemotherapy in elective surgery. *N Y State J Med* 1976;76:532.
56. Kanter MH, Van Maanen D, Anders KH, et al. Preoperative autologous blood donation before elective hysterectomy. *JAMA* 1996;276: 798–801.
57. Bierbaum BE, Callaghan JJ, Galante JO, et al. An analysis of blood management in patients having total hip or knee arthroplasty. *J Bone J Surg Am* 1999;81:2–10.
58. Etchason J, Petz L, Keeler E, et al. The cost-effectiveness of preoperative autologous blood donations. *N Engl J Med* 1995;332:7.
59. Larocque BJ, Gilbert K, Brien WF. Prospective validation of a point score system for predicting blood transfusion following hip or knee replacement. *Transfusion* 1998;38:932–937.
60. Popovsky MA, Whitaker B, Arnold NL. Severe outcomes of allogeneic and autologous blood donations: frequency and characterization. *Transfusion* 1995;35:734–737.
61. Goodnough LT, Monk TG. Evolving concepts in autologous blood procurement. Case reports of perisurgical anemia complicated by myocardial infarction. *Am J Med* 1996;101:33A–37S.
62. Linden JV, Wagner, K, Voytovich AE, et al. Transfusion errors in New York State: an analysis of 10 years' experience. *Transfusion* 2000;40: 1207–1213.
63. Petry AF, Jost T, Sievers H. Reduction of homologous blood requirements by blood pooling at the onset of cardiopulmonary bypass. *J Thorac Cardiovasc Surg* 1994;1097:1210.
64. Brecher ME, Rosenfeld M. Mathematical and computer modeling of acute normovolemic hemodilution. *Transfusion* 1994;34:176–179.
65. Goodnough LT, Grishaber JE, Monk TG, et al. Acute preoperative hemodilution in patients undergoing radical prostatectomy: a case study analysis of efficacy. *Anesth Analg* 1994;78:932–937.
66. Goodnough LT, Grishaber JE, Birkmeyer JD, et al. Efficacy and cost-effectiveness of autologous blood predeposit in patients undergoing radical prostatectomy procedures. *Urology* 1994;44:226–231.
67. Monk TG, Goodnough LT, Brecher ME. Acute normovolemic hemodilution can replace preoperative autologous donation as a method of autologous blood procurement in radical prostatectomy. *Anesth Analg* 1997;85:953–958.
68. Monk TG, Goodnough LT, Brecher ME, et al. A prospective randomized trial of three blood conservation strategies for radical prostatectomy. *Anesthesiology* 1999;91:24–33.
69. Ness PM, Bourke DL, Walsh PC. A randomized trial of perioperative hemodilution versus transfusion of preoperatively deposited autologous blood in elective surgery. *Transfusion* 1991;31:226–230.
70. Monk TG, Goodnough LT, Birkmeyer JD, et al. Acute normovolemic hemodilution is a cost-effective alternative to preoperative autologous blood donation by patients undergoing radical retropubic prostatectomy. *Transfusion* 1995;35:559–565.
71. Goodnough LT, Monk TG, Brecher ME. Acute normovolemic hemodilution in surgery. *Hematology* 1997;2:413–420.
72. Goodnough LT, Monk TG, Brecher, ME. A review of autologous blood procurement in the surgical setting: lessons learned in the last 10 years. *Vox Sang* 1996;71:13–21.
73. Goodnough LT, Despotis GJ, Merkel K, et al. A randomized trial of acute normovolemic hemodilution compared to preoperative autologous blood donation in total hip arthroplasty. *Transfusion* 2000;40: 1054–1057.
74. Bovill DF, Moulton CW, Jackson WS, et al. The efficacy of intraoperative autologous transfusion in major orthopaedic surgery: a regression analysis. *Orthopedics* 1986;9:1403–1407.
75. Goodnough LT, Monk TG, Brecher ME. Acute normovolemic hemodilution should replace preoperative autologous blood donation before elective surgery. *Transfusion* 1998;38:473–476.
76. Rottman G, Ness PM. Is acute normovolemic hemodilution a legitimate alternative to allogeneic blood transfusions? *Transfusion* 1998;38: 477–480.
77. Williamson KR, Taswell HF. Intraoperative blood salvage: a review. *Transfusion* 1991;31:662–675.
78. Napier JA, Bruce M, Chapman J, et al. Guidelines for autologous transfusion II. Perioperative haemodilution and cell salvage. *Br J Anaesth* 1997;78:768–771.
79. Clagett GP, Valentine RJ, Jackson MR, et al. A randomized trial of intraoperative transfusion during aortic surgery. *J Vasc Surg* 1999;29: 22–31.
80. Linden JV, Tourault MA, Scribner CL. Decrease in frequency of transfusion fatalities. *Transfusion* 1997;37:243–244.
81. Goodnough LT, Monk TG, Sicard G, et al. Intraoperative salvage in patients undergoing elective abdominal aortic aneurism repair. An analysis of costs and benefits. *J Vasc Surg* 1996;24:213–218.
82. Clements DH, Sculco TP, Burke SW, et al. Salvage and reinfusion of postoperative sanguineous wound drainage. *J Bone Joint Surg* 1993; 74A:646–651.
83. Ritter MA, Keating EM, Faris PM. Closed wound drainage in total hip or total knee replacement. *J Bone Joint Surg Am* 1994;76:35–38.

Rossi's Principles of Transfusion Medicine, Third Edition, edited by Toby L. Simon, Walter H. Dzik, Edward L. Snyder, Christopher P. Stowell, and Ronald G. Strauss. Lippincott Williams & Wilkins, Philadelphia © 2002.

42

COAGULATION SUPPORT IN THE PERIOPERATIVE SETTING

KENDALL P. CROOKSTON
BRUCE D. SPIESS

Surgery is the ultimate test of hemostasis. The physiologic sealing of interrupted blood vessels is fundamental to the success of any operation; the failure of this process can have disastrous results. Hemostasis is the arrest of blood flow from a vessel and comprises a number of interdependent physiologic processes (Table 42.1) (1,2). Hemostatic abnormalities are not rare. It is increasingly common for patients who need procedures to have underlying disease or to be undergoing medical treatments that alter hemostasis. The clinician must recognize clinically significant hemostatic abnormalities before performing an invasive procedure or taking a patient to surgery. Hemostatic competence should be carefully assessed for all patients undergoing procedures of any magnitude. Even a minor operation on a patient with an undiagnosed bleeding disorder can be a major undertaking with life-threatening consequences. Hemostatic failure also can have dire consequences among patients undergoing invasive diagnostic and therapeutic interventions, such as arteriography, arterial monitoring, or placement of extended-use infusion catheters. Assessment of hemostasis is as important for these persons as it is for patients undergoing surgery.

The consequences of an undetected hemorrhagic defect depend on the magnitude of the operation and on the severity of the defect. Uncontrolled, life-threatening hemorrhage is an occasional complication of major vascular trauma and ruptured abdominal aortic aneurysms but is rarely encountered in elective surgical settings. Profuse intraoperative or postoperative bleeding is most common among patients undergoing emergency surgery with uncompensated disseminated intravascular coagulation (DIC), severe liver disease, extensive trauma, massive transfusion of blood, or hyperfibrinolysis (3). Excessive bleeding is frequently due to surgical causes or uncorrected vascular lesions rather than defects in coagulation. In these settings, bleeding usually is anticipated and controlled accordingly. However, differentiating between postoperative bleeding due to coagulopathy and a lesion than can be corrected with surgical reexploration is not always straightforward.

The location and type of surgery are important determinants of the consequences of undetected hemorrhagic defects. Bleeding may be the principal indication for surgery, as in trauma or aneurysm rupture. Bleeding also can develop unexpectedly because of unrecognized preoperative conditions or as a result of the surgery and intraoperative events themselves. Even relatively

K.P. Crookston: Transfusion Medicine and Coagulation, University of New Mexico Health Sciences Center, United Blood Services of New Mexico, Department of Pathology, University of New Mexico School of Medicine, Albuquerque, New Mexico.

B.D. Spiess: Department of Anesthesiology, Virginia Commonwealth University/Medical College of Virginia, Richmond, Virginia.

TABLE 42.1. HEMOSTASIS OVERVIEW

The arrest of blood flow from a vessel involves five interdependent processes (2). The first two constitute *primary* hemostasis and the next two constitute *secondary* hemostasis:
- Interaction of blood vessels and supporting structures
- Interaction of circulating platelets
- Fibrin clot formation by means of the coagulation system
- Regulation of clot extension by coagulation inhibitors and the fibrinolytic system
- Remodeling and repair after arrest of bleeding

small amounts of blood collecting in tightly confined spaces and fascial planes, such as the cranial vault, orbit, spinal canal, epidural space, or axillary sheath, can jeopardize the success of an operation. Mild bleeding disorders can have a serious effect in this regard. These mild acquired and congenital disorders are much more commonly encountered than are the major forms of coagulopathy associated with severe liver disease, uncompensated DIC, and hyperfibrinolysis. Mild bleeding disorders can lead to severe neurologic impairment when blood collects in the tightly confined spaces of the cranial vault and spinal canal. Collections of blood in the tongue, oropharynx, epiglottis, and neck can produce life-threatening airway compression. In orthopedic operations, hematoma can complicate bone healing, cause compartment syndromes, and lead to wound infections that can compromise prostheses. Collections of blood in the deep body cavities are prone to infection and complicate gynecologic, urologic, thoracic, and general surgical operations. Intramural hematoma after gastrointestinal repairs and anastomoses can cause anastomotic leakage and dehiscence. Abdominal operations complicated by retroperitoneal hematoma and intramesenteric bleeding can cause prolonged postoperative ileus.

Some surgical procedures are inherently associated with a higher risk of perioperative bleeding, and mild hemostatic abnormalities can increase the risk. Continued oozing from the raw prostatic fossa bathed in urokinase presents a problem after open or closed prostatectomy. The use of thrombolytic therapy or antiplatelet drugs such as abciximab in the care of patients undergoing coronary angioplasty can lead to severe bleeding problems if emergency coronary artery bypass becomes necessary. In cardiac and vascular operations, the cumulative effects of intraoperative anticoagulation, cardiopulmonary bypass, and platelet-inhibitor therapy render patients vulnerable to continued blood loss.

This chapter addresses the diagnosis and management of bleeding disorders encountered before and during invasive bedside procedures or surgery. Some of these bleeding disorders develop acutely because of specific clinical circumstances. Others arise from predisposing conditions that can result in pathologic hemorrhage when hemostatic mechanisms are stressed. Most causes of abnormal bleeding among surgical patients can be readily identified with a careful review of the patient's clinical situation, bleeding history, and medication history and with the assistance of a few judiciously chosen laboratory tests.

CLINICAL ASSESSMENT OF PATIENTS WHO NEED AN INVASIVE PROCEDURE OR SURGERY

Most clinically significant bleeding disorders can be detected by means of clinical examination without a battery of expensive laboratory tests (4–6). A detailed medical history directed at uncovering abnormal bleeding is the mainstay of clinical assessment and is mandatory before surgery or invasive procedures. These tests must not be postponed until the day of surgery because this leaves inadequate time for appropriate laboratory testing when follow-up evaluation is warranted because of the history. A list of standard presurgical questions and topic areas is presented in Table 42.2. The history should focus on whether the patient bleeds easily in response to minor trauma or spontaneously in the absence of trauma. Responses about major and

TABLE 42.2. BLEEDING HISTORY

Hemostatic Response to Surgery and Trauma
1. What operations have you had, including minor ones, such as tonsillectomy, circumcision, or biopsies? Was bleeding after surgery hard to stop? Have you ever had unusual bruising in the skin around an area of surgery?
2. Have you ever needed a blood transfusion?
3. Have you ever bled for a long time or had a swollen tongue or mouth after cutting or biting your tongue, cheek, or lip? What was the longest time it took to stop bleeding from cuts or scrapes? Has bleeding from a cut or scrape ever restarted after stopping completely?
4. How many times have you had teeth pulled, and what was the longest time that you bled afterward? Has bleeding ever restarted the day after tooth extraction?
5. Have you ever borne children? Did you have any bleeding problems associated with delivery?

Spontaneous Bleeding
1. Do you have bruises larger than a silver dollar without remembering when or how you injured yourself? If so, how big was the largest of these bruises?
2. Do you ever have nosebleeds?
3. Do your gums bleed easily?
4. Do you ever have abnormally heavy menstrual periods or spotting between periods?
5. Do you have blood in your urine or stool? Do you ever have black, tarry stools?
6. Have you ever had bleeding into joints or muscles?
7. Have you ever been told you had anemia or iron deficiency?

Medication History
1. What medications, including aspirin or any other pills or powders for headaches, colds, menstrual cramps, arthritis, joint pains, back aches, or other pains, have you taken within the last 2 weeks? What other herbal remedies, vitamins, or medications have you taken recently?
2. Do you take medicine to thin the blood or to prevent blood clots?
3. Have you had a medical problem within the past 5 years requiring a doctor's care? If so, what is its nature?

Family History
1. Are there any bleeders in your family?
2. Has any blood relative had a problem with unusual bleeding or bruising after surgery? Were blood transfusions needed to control this bleeding?

minor surgery and dental extractions are particularly helpful. A patient who has recently undergone surgery without bleeding complications has been subjected to a test of hemostasis as good as any laboratory assay.

The manifestations of abnormal bleeding provide clues to the nature of the bleeding abnormality. It is useful for the clinician to differentiate lesions of primary and secondary hemostasis, because these have different causes (Table 42.1). A history of easy bruising, ecchymosis, petechial hemorrhage, and mucosal bleeding, such as nosebleed, gingival bleeding, or heavy menses, generally indicates a lesion of primary hemostasis such as thrombocytopenia, von Willebrand disease, or a qualitative platelet disorder. Joint hemorrhage, deep muscular hematoma, and retroperitoneal bleeding usually are signs of a lesion of secondary hemostasis (coagulation defect) such as a congenital factor deficiency or anticoagulant use. Lesions of either primary or secondary hemostasis can cause unexpected or excessive bleeding during surgery. Because any bleeding is disturbing to the typical patient, it is important to quantify the bleeding history whenever possible. For example, bleeding that necessitates blood transfusion usually is significant. Likewise, questions about the number of pads used by a patient with menorrhagia help to determine the magnitude of this symptom. Gathering a family history of bleeding and hemostatic challenges is essential. Classic hemophilia A (factor VIII deficiency) and hemophilia B (factor IX deficiency) are transmitted as X-linked traits with only male family members affected. Most other inherited deficiencies of coagulation factors affect both sexes. A careful medication history is important, though sometimes overlooked, during the history and physical examination. All patients should be asked specifically about ingestion of aspirin and other drugs that interfere with platelet function. In summary, a bleeding history, including recent medications and family history, provides clues to possible hemostatic defects. A truly informative history is one in which there have been substantial hemostatic challenges to the patient and there is a large extended family known to the patient. A physician can take a detailed bleeding history, but if, for example, the patient was adopted and has never had hemostatic challenges such as surgery, trauma, or childbirth, the history is not especially informative.

The physical examination also provides evidence of abnormal hemostasis. The skin should be examined for evidence of excessive bruising, petechiae, or subcutaneous hematoma. Hyperelasticity of the skin and joint hypermobility suggest hereditary connective tissue diseases such as Marfan or Ehlers-Danlos syndrome, both of which are associated with platelet-mediated bleeding tendency. Joints arthritic owing to old hemarthrosis can provide clues to congenital coagulation abnormalities. Vascular anomalies such as giant hemangioma can be associated with thrombocytopenia. Hepatomegaly and splenomegaly should alert the physician to the possibility of liver or myeloproliferative disease with thrombocytopenia or platelet dysfunction. Jaundice is indicative of severe liver dysfunction; the possibility of an associated coagulation defect should not be overlooked. A digital rectal examination with testing of the stool for the presence of occult blood is valuable. In addition to detecting gastrointestinal hemorrhage from mucosal lesions, this test can be an important clue to uncovering a hemostatic defect.

Despite the importance of an informative history in the detection of bleeding problems, several pitfalls must be avoided. False-positive and false-negative conclusions derived from the standard bleeding questionnaire are common. In a series of adult patients undergoing elective general surgery who responded to a bleeding history, 50% of all patients gave positive responses to the history, but only 8% had abnormal results of coagulation studies (7). Among the remaining 50% who gave negative responses, 5% had abnormalities in coagulation tests that influenced the course of surgery. It is common for patients to give histories of abnormal bleeding during past surgery or dental extractions, but it is uncommon to find hemostatic defects. It is often impossible to determine whether the complication was caused by mechanical factors or impaired hemostasis. Of the 20% of patients in this series who reported excessive bleeding with past surgery, none was found to have a hemostatic defect (7). Some patients who have withstood surgery without abnormal bleeding later acquire hemostatic defects, such as thrombocytopenia or drug-induced platelet dysfunction. A patient who has never undergone an operation or serious trauma also can have an unknown abnormality. In the face of these uncertainties, the following section evaluates whether there is a role for routine laboratory testing before surgery or invasive procedures.

SCREENING TESTS FOR HEMOSTASIS

Most coagulation tests are based on artificial initiation of complicated enzyme cascades that ultimately result in formation of a fibrin clot detected by the instrument. These tests are inherently much more variable and less precise than the typical chemistry test. Preanalytical variables can have profound effects on the test results (8). For example, a specimen can be drawn from a line that once contained the anticoagulant heparin, or a specimen drawn in the operating suite can be diluted owing to crystalloid infusion in the same arm. Platelets and coagulation factors may be partially activated owing to traumatic phlebotomy. In addition to preanalytical error, clotting times also vary greatly with the model of coagulation analyzer, the reagents used, and even with the individual lot numbers of the same reagent (this is why the normal references ranges at a given institution may vary slightly from year to year). To minimize these problems for the prothrombin time (PT) assay, the international normalized ratio (INR) was developed. In a strict sense, it was developed only for use in evaluating multiple factor deficiencies secondary to warfarin treatment. It has become convenient to use the INR as a surrogate for PT in other situations to lessen the reagent and instrument variation involved in comparisons between institutions or in the literature.

Table 42.3 summarizes the effects of common anticoagulants on laboratory parameters of hemostasis. Dilution studies (mixing studies) of the patient's plasma are theoretically useful in differentiating true factor deficiency from the effects of anticoagulants and acquired inhibitors. If a 1:1 mix of patient plasma with normal plasma corrects a prolonged PT or activated partial thromboplastin time (aPTT), a factor deficiency (congenital or acquired through warfarin or vitamin K deficiency) is responsible. Little correction of a prolonged clotting time suggests the

TABLE 42.3. LABORATORY EVALUATION OF HEMOSTATIC DISORDERS

	Representative Results of Basic Coagulation Testing[a]					
Potential Defect	**aPTT**	**PT**	**Platelet Count**	**Fibrinogen**	**Platelet Function Screen (PFA-100)**	**Ancillary Testing**
Factor VIII, IX, XI, or XII[b] deficiency	↑	nl	nl	nl	nl	↓ Factor level
Factor II, V, or X deficiency	↑	↑	nl	nl	nl	↓ Factor level
Factor VII deficiency	nl	↑	nl	nl	nl	↓ Factor VII level
Factor XIII deficiency	nl	nl	nl	nl	nl	Abnormal urea clot lysis
Dysfibrinogenemia (Factor I)	nl	nl	nl	↓ or nl	nl	Abnormal reptilase time with or without abnormal thrombin time
von Willebrand disease	↑ or nl	nl	nl	nl	Abnormal	↓ vWF activity; ↓ vWF antigen; ↓ or nl factor VIII
Lupus-like inhibitor[b] (lupus anticoagulant)	↑	nl or slt ↑	nl or ↓	nl	nl	Abnormal result of dilute Russell viper venom test; abnormal hexagonal phospholipid competition
Thrombocytopenia	nl	nl	↓	nl	Abnormal	Platelet antibody screen
Qualitative platelet defect (e.g., inherited lesion, drug effect)	nl	nl	nl	nl	Abnormal	Abnormal platelet aggregation studies
Severe liver disease	↑	↑	nl or ↓	nl or ↓	Abnormal	
Uremia	nl	nl	nl	nl	Abnormal	PFA-100 moves toward normal after administration of desmopressin
Fulminant DIC	↑	↑	↓	↓ or nl	Abnormal	↑ Fibrin D-dimer
Cardiopulmonary bypass	slt ↑	slt ↑	>75,000/μL	nl	Abnormal	
Drug effects						
Unfractionated heparin (therapy or line contamination)	↑	nl	nl	nl	nl	Heparin level
Low-molecular-weight heparin	nl	nl	nl	nl	nl	Heparin level
Aspirin	nl	nl	nl	nl	Abnormal	
Warfarin	nl or slt ↑	↑	nl	nl	nl	↓ Vitamin K–dependent factors[c]
Direct thrombin inhibitor (e.g., argatroban)	↑	↑	nl	nl or ↓	nl	
Thrombolytic therapy (e.g. tPA)	nl or ↑	nl or ↑	nl	nl or ↓	nl	↑ Fibrin D-dimer
Hyperfibrinolysis	nl or ↑	nl or ↑	nl	nl or ↓	nl	↑ Fibrin D-dimer

[a]The representative results shown may be quite variable in clinical practice. Results can be affected by active bleeding and clotting, acute phase reactants, and preanalytical variables.
[b]Not associated with a bleeding tendency.
[c]The vitamin K–dependent factors are II, VII, IX, and X.
aPTT, activated partial thromboplastin time; PT, prothrombin time; ↑, increased; nl, normal; ↓, decreased; vWf, von Willebrand factor; slt, slightly; DIC, disseminated intravascular coagulation; tPA, tissue plasminogen activator.

presence of heparin or another circulating anticoagulant, such as fibrin degradation products or lupus-like inhibitors). However, the results of this exercise often are more difficult to interpret than is suggested by the theory. Experienced coagulation technologists may prefer to perform the definitive testing suggested by the clinical situation, rather than performing a screening test with the 1:1 mix. Consultation with the laboratory is helpful in this situation.

There are occasional situations in which the history suggests the possibility of a bleeding diathesis, but the cause of a prolonged aPTT is difficult to determine in a timely manner or a strong lupus-like anticoagulant may be present, possibly masking a factor deficiency. The clinician may be nervous about taking such a patient to surgery. Normal activity levels of factors VIII, IX, and XI often are reassuring, because these are the most common congenital deficiency states that would lead to excess surgical bleeding in this situation.

The PT and aPTT entail testing of proteins in an artificial

environment of in vitro activation and inherently give an incomplete idea of the true biologic activity of the coagulation system. A contemporary view of coagulation reveals that the coagulation proteins function on the surface of activated platelets and bind to specific sites, such as glycoprotein (GP) IIb/IIIa (9). However, impaired interaction of coagulation proteins with platelet surfaces is not detected with the PT or aPTT test.

Bleeding time once was used as a screening test for platelet function. However, skin bleeding time does not necessarily correlate with bleeding at other anatomic sites. Bleeding time is not a particularly sensitive test for von Willebrand disease, and it is known to vary in patients with von Willebrand disease who undergo repeated studies. Lind (10) reviewed 13 studies in the medical literature regarding the use of bleeding time as a preoperative screening test. A prolonged bleeding time per se was not associated with increased perioperative bleeding or transfusion requirements in studies with patients who underwent cardiac and patients who underwent noncardiac surgical procedures. An analysis of 862 articles describing bleeding time showed that bleeding time was not related to any given risk of perioperative coagulopathic bleeding (11). In cardiopulmonary bypass, in which platelet dysfunction is extremely common, the bleeding time has never been shown to have predictive value either preoperatively or postoperatively. There are no data to suggest that any particular bleeding time is predictive of risk of bleeding deep in tissue. There also is no known increased risk with any particular bleeding time for either epidural or spinal anesthesia. Thus bleeding time is not useful in the perioperative setting. There is a trend among major medical centers to remove the bleeding time from the test menu or restrict its use.

Considerable progress has been made in the clinical assessment of platelet function. Harrison (12) reviewed the advantages of various methods, including whole-blood methods with turnaround times suited to the perioperative setting. A platelet function screen with an instrument known as the PFA-100 offers an attractive alternative to bleeding time (13, 14). Although not exactly equivalent, it can be thought of as an in vitro bleeding time. Many major medical centers have this test available for use as a screening test for platelet function. Because the test must be performed on a fresh specimen within 4 hours of draw, it usually is not available as a send-out test. Citrated whole blood is drawn by means of negative pressure through a capillary tube and across a membrane through a tiny laser-cut hole. The membrane is coated with collagen and either adenosine diphosphate (ADP) or epinephrine (platelet agonists). The time it takes the platelets to plug the hole and stop the flow of blood (closure time) is reported in seconds. The pattern of prolongation when the ADP cartridge is used helps discriminate between drug-induced and intrinsic platelet defects. A limitation of use of the PFA-100 and related instruments is that abnormal results can occur solely from thrombocytopenia or pronounced anemia.

Thromboelastography (TEG) has been used since 1947 as a whole-blood clotting test (15). It has gained popularity in the perioperative setting (16). Thromboelastography is used to test clot strength over time through examination of the elastic shear modulus. A small sample of blood is placed in a warmed cuvette that rotates back and forth through a 45-degree arc. Suspended within the cuvette is a piston with a torsion wire attached. As coagulation proceeds, fibrin-platelet interactions occur and the movement of the cuvette is transferred to the piston. As the turning motion continues, tension is placed on the fibrin platelet strands, and the shear modulus is tested. Thromboelastography is now understood to test the interaction between fibrin and GP IIb/IIIa. Work with abciximab has shown a direct dose-dependent relation between drug and maximum amplitude during TEG. Although TEG has been advertised as a bedside test, it requires considerable maintenance and quality assurance and should not be considered a typical point-of-care test. It has been misconstrued as an excellent test of platelet function, but in reality is a poor test of the effect of aspirin on platelets. Thromboelastography is an excellent test of clot strength, hypercoagulability, and fibrinolysis. It helps differentiate DIC from primary fibrinolysis. Thromboelastography was revitalized with the advent of liver transplantation, but since that time it has been widely applied to cardiac surgery and to a number of other surgical procedures. Several publications have shown it to be a useful predictor of abnormal postoperative bleeding after cardiac surgery (17) or bleeding after renal biopsy (18). Incorporation of TEG into transfusion decision trees has shown that it decreases blood use and outperforms decision trees based solely on PT, aPTT, and platelet count (19). Results of TEG, which have shown good correlation with postoperative bleeding in cardiac patients, show no correlation between results of preoperative testing and postoperative bleeding (16–19). Routine screening of patients with TEG before open-heart surgery does not help identify the patients most likely to bleed, nor does it help identify which patients could benefit the most from prophylactic aprotinin or lysine analogue therapy.

The Sonoclot analyzer is a whole-blood viscometer used to examine viscoelastic clot function in response to a vertically vibrating probe. The Sonoclot has been advertised as a platelet function analyzer, but few published data define what platelet or platelet-protein abnormalities are associated with a given degree of signature deviation. Data do show a relation between Sonoclot abnormalities and postoperative bleeding in cardiac surgery (20).

The Hemodyne instrument is used to examine platelet contractile force as well as viscoelastic modulus in a manner similar to TEG. The Hemodyne platelet contractile force measurement is used to examine both the platelet-fibrin interaction and the function of the cytoskeleton and pseudopod formation. Although some work with the Hemodyne has been described, there are few data on whether the results can affect transfusion practice or be predictive of bleeding outcome after cardiac surgery.

Hemostatus is another test of platelet function. Platelet-activating factor and a more typical activated clotting time assay are used to assess clot formation. When the results of stimulated and unstimulated assays are compared, overall platelet function can be estimated (reserve available for stimulation).

Assessment of platelet function and platelet-protein interactions remains imperfect. Thromboelastography facilitates assessment, but a dedicated person is needed who understands the test and is willing to become knowledgeable about the various applications. Much perioperative surgical bleeding is caused by platelet dysfunction, particularly by the interaction of platelet surface glycoproteins with coagulation proteins.

Useful coagulation screening tests and the disorders detected are shown in Table 42.3. The advantages and limitations of routine screening tests have been debated. When the aPTT was used as a screening test, 11% of results had prolongations in a study of more than 1,000 patients in a hospital (21). The most common reasons for an abnormal aPTTs included liver disease, anticoagulant therapy, vitamin K deficiency from starvation or malabsorption, and undiagnosed hereditary factor deficiencies. The authors concluded that the relatively inexpensive screening with aPTT was cost effective.

The arguments against routine preoperative hemostasis screening tests are based on issues of cost-effectiveness. Most abnormal test results have little clinical significance and may delay needed procedures unnecessarily. In a prospective study with 2,000 patients who underwent routine screening with a platelet count, aPTT, and PT, 77% of aPTT and PT tests and 90% of platelet counts were not indicated because of normal clinical histories (22). Abnormalities were detected in only 0.5% of these patients, and in no case was there postponement of surgery or a change in clinical treatment based on the abnormal test results. It was concluded that it is rare for a patient to have abnormal results of bleeding tests without clinical indications of hemostatic dysfunction and that even if test results are abnormal, it is unlikely that the results will influence anesthetic or surgical management. Eliminating such tests would save both time and money. In a similar study (6), preoperative coagulation tests (PT, aPTT, platelet count, and bleeding time) were performed on 282 patients before elective general and vascular surgery. Of the 1,119 tests performed, 605 were considered to be indicated on the basis of predefined clinical indications. Of the 514 tests performed without predefined clinical indications, results of 4.1% were abnormal, but none defined a clinically significant bleeding abnormality. In contrast, results of 7.4% of the indicated tests were abnormal, and all clinically significant cases of coagulopathy were found in this group. The authors concluded that screening tests for coagulopathy not suspected on a clinical basis are unnecessary and should not be performed.

The value of routine preoperative screening tests also has been evaluated in subpopulations with known tendencies toward acquired coagulopathy. Screening of 322 patients with gynecologic cancer was performed for coagulation abnormalities, particularly a compensated form of chronic DIC, with PT, aPTT, fibrinogen, and fibrin D-dimer tests (23). Abnormal results of coagulation tests were found in 188 patients, but none of these abnormalities was associated with significant perioperative bleeding complications. Similarly, routine preoperative testing for occult coagulopathy provided little clinically useful information about these patients. Routine preoperative screening tests in the care of patients in preparation for cardiopulmonary bypass procedures detected only one completely unsuspected abnormality (mild factor IX deficiency) among 5,000 consecutively screened patients (24).

The value of specific preoperative screening tests for coagulopathy has been examined. The importance of the aPTT and PT as preoperative screening tests was assessed in the care of 750 patients undergoing general and gynecologic surgical procedures (25). Among the 611 (82%) patients who had no indication of a bleeding abnormality at history or physical examination, only 2.7% had abnormal PT or aPTT test results. In many of these tests, factors unrelated to a hemostatic lesion were responsible for the abnormal result. In the remainder, the abnormal result was ignored, and the operations were performed as scheduled with no adverse clinical consequences. A more cost-conscious approach with laboratory tests to confirm suspicious findings of the history and physical examination was advocated. This approach was justified given the low prevalence of unsuspected bleeding disorders (1 in 1,000), compared with the variations in aPTT and PT test results, according to statistical differences from mean values (1 in 40).

Who, then, should undergo preoperative screening tests, and which ones should be performed? In general, a screening test should be based on the bleeding history and the magnitude of the planned operation. The following guidelines are adapted from Rappaport (4), who advocates assigning patients to levels of risk:

Level I. An informative bleeding history is normal, and the procedure is relatively minor. No screening tests are recommended.

Level II. The bleeding history is normal, but the proposed operation is major. A platelet count and an aPTT should be performed. These tests help detect acquired bleeding disorders such as thrombocytopenia, the presence of an anticoagulant, and occult DIC that have developed without symptoms owing to the absence of a hemostatic challenge in the form of recent trauma or surgery.

Level III. The bleeding history raises the possibility of bleeding disorders. The operations are of such magnitude that hemostasis will be severely challenged (e.g., cardiopulmonary bypass, major vascular surgery, or extensive general surgical procedures in which numerous transfusions are anticipated) or even minimal bleeding could be hazardous (e.g., intracranial and spinal surgery). For such patients, screening tests such as an aPTT, PT, platelet count, and possibly use of a PFA-100 are indicated (Table 42.3)

Level IV. The bleeding history strongly suggests the presence of a bleeding disorder. The procedure can be either major or minor. In addition to screening tests, specific testing to characterize the hemostatic lesion is prudent. Testing may include measuring specific factor levels or running multitest panels to identify lupus-like inhibitors or von Willebrand disease. The specific ancillary tests ordered are based on the suspected hemostatic lesion. Consultation with a hematologist or pathologist knowledgeable in coagulation is recommended.

PREPROCEDURE CONDITIONS THAT MAY IMPAIR HEMOSTASIS

A number of conditions may be present before invasive procedures or operations that can impair hemostasis. Those discussed in this section include platelet abnormalities, drugs affecting coagulation, renal and hepatic failure, hyperfibrinolysis, and unrecognized hemostatic defects. Disseminated intravascular coagulation is discussed later.

Qualitative and Quantitative Platelet Abnormalities

Acquired platelet dysfunction is one of the most commonly encountered hemostatic defects among patients undergoing surgical procedures (3). Although usually caused by ingestion of drugs that impair platelet function, platelet abnormalities occur in a variety of medical illnesses among patients who need surgery (26). Clinically significant platelet defects have been associated with myeloproliferative disorders. Patients with autoimmune disorders sometimes have immune-mediated thrombocytopenia coupled with severe platelet dysfunction from immunoglobulin coating of platelet membranes. Acute and chronic liver disease is associated with clinically significant platelet dysfunction caused by elevated levels of circulating fibrinogen degradation products, aggregation defects, and advanced platelet age (26). Surgical procedures on uremic patients sometimes are complicated by abnormal bleeding. The multifactorial pathogenesis seems related to anemia, acquired defects in specific receptors that impair platelet binding to fibrinogen and von Willebrand factor, and other ill-defined abnormalities in platelet aggregation (27,28).

Commonly used drugs can induce platelet dysfunction. However, in otherwise healthy patients, isolated drug-induced platelet dysfunction rarely causes clinically significant intraoperative hemorrhage. Drugs known to affect platelet function are listed in Table 42.4. When platelet dysfunction combines with another mild hemostatic abnormality, such as uremia, mild thrombocytopenia, or coagulation defects produced by malnutrition, liver disease, or anticoagulants, the effects can be additive, and serious bleeding can result (29). For example, low-dose heparin, commonly used in the care of patients undergoing surgery for prophylaxis of deep venous thrombosis, does not interfere sufficiently with hemostasis to cause major hemorrhage. However, the incidence of wound hematoma (5% to 8%) is significantly higher than it is among patients who do not receive heparin (30). When platelet function is impaired, low-dose heparin can cause hemorrhagic side effects.

Aspirin is the most commonly ingested drug that impairs platelet function. In one study, 50% of patients undergoing surgery had biochemical evidence of recent aspirin ingestion (31). Aspirin irreversibly inhibits platelet function by acetylation of the active site of the platelet enzyme cyclooxygenase and blocks platelet synthesis of thromboxane A_2. Because of its effects in reducing stroke, myocardial infarction, and cardiovascular mortality, aspirin is increasingly prescribed to middle-aged and elderly patients. Many cold remedies and pain relievers contain aspirin or aspirin-like components. Assessing every medication the patient has taken recently, including over-the-counter and alternative medicine compounds, is the only way to determine whether there will be a drug effect on hemostasis. Studies with very large series of patients have shown that aspirin does not influence postoperative bleeding. However, other historical literature shows that aspirin ingestion does increase bleeding. Other nonsteroidal antiinflammatory drugs inhibit platelet function, but the effects are typically transient, lasting only for as long as the drug is in the circulation. Alcohol in moderate doses has little effect on platelet function but can potentiate the effects of aspirin (32).

TABLE 42.4. DRUGS THAT CAN AFFECT PLATELET FUNCTION

Anesthetics
Cocaine
Halothane
Procaine
Xylocaine
Antiinflammatory agents
Aspirin
Other nonsteroidal antiinflammatory agents
Antibiotics (predominantly β-lactam)
Ampicillin
Carbenicillin
Cephalosporins
Nitrofurantoin
Penicillin G (high dose)
Piperacillin
Ticarcillin
Antiplatelet, antithrombotic drugs
Abciximab
Cilostazol
Clopidigrel
Dypyridamole
Eptifibatide
Ticlopidine
Tirofiban
Cardiovascular drugs
Isoproterenol
Nitroglycerin
Propranolol
Quinidine
Verapamil
Psychotropic drugs
Phenothiazines
Tricyclic antidepressants
Miscellaneous agents
Aminophylline
Antihistamines
Caffeine
Cyclosporine
Dextran
Ethanol
Furosemide
Glucocorticoids
Papaverine
Sulfinpyrazone

Antibiotics are associated with bleeding among patients undergoing surgery. The penicillins produce dose-dependent inhibition of platelet receptors for ADP and epinephrine. High doses in patients with hemostatic disorders can lead to serious intraoperative bleeding. Interestingly, cephalosporins can cause short-term and rather profound platelet dysfunction. Cephalosporins are often the antibiotics of choice for routine antimicrobial prophylaxis. Dextran is a plasma expander with mild antithrombotic effects (33). At sufficiently high concentrations, it inhibits platelet aggregation and adhesion, impairs fibrin polymerization, and promotes clot lysis. Another popular perioperative plasma expander is hydroxyethyl starch. At high doses, it can impair von Willebrand factor–dependent platelet function. However, platelet function is not affected at doses less than 1 L. Research in both renal dialysis and cardiac surgery, wherein the starches are used to prime perfusion systems, has never shown an increased bleeding tendency with these volume expanders. The effects of plasma expanders can persist for days, until they are cleared from the circulation. A variety of other drugs, including vasodilators and calcium channel blockers, inhibit platelet function, but the impairment of hemostasis does not appear to be clinically significant (34). Nitrates are profound platelet inhibitors (most patients with cardiac disease receive either nitroglycerin or nitroprusside). However, it is unclear how much these drugs effect the risk of bleeding because of the emphasis on aspirin.

Several classes of antiplatelet drugs are in use. These include agents that block membrane receptor sites (e.g. abciximab, clopidogrel) prostaglandin biosynthetic pathways (e.g. aspirin), or phosphodiesterase activity (e.g. cilostazol, dipyridamole) (26). Many novel platelet inhibitors have been introduced (35,36). Ticlopidine and clopidogrel, which act on the cyclic adenosine monophosphate pathway to irreversibly inhibit platelets, are increasingly popular substitutes for aspirin in the management of arterial thromboembolism. In the field of cardiovascular intervention, a number of antibodies and peptides have been developed that specifically block the platelet integrin GP IIb/IIIa. This is the principal receptor responsible for fibrinogen binding and platelet aggregation. These drugs can totally block platelet aggregation when administered in concentrations sufficient to saturate 80% of the receptors.

In addition to qualitative platelet defects, quantitative defects are important in the perioperative setting. Thrombocytopenia is common and easily detected with a platelet count. Drug-related thrombocytopenia is particularly noteworthy, because platelet transfusion rarely is necessary if the offending agent is removed (37). Drugs that inhibit platelet function should be avoided in the care of all such patients.

Some studies suggest that recent aspirin ingestion is associated with a greater risk of surgical blood loss, but this has not been borne out by others (10). The truth is probably that aspirin and most platelet inhibitors rarely cause a major bleeding tendency on their own. However, a major hemorrhagic diathesis can develop when the defects induced by other drugs, uremia, or open heart surgery are combined with drug-induced platelet dysfunction (38). A platelet function screen with a PFA-100, TEG, Hemodyne, or Sonoclot can be performed when impairment of platelet function by drugs is suspected; a normal result helps to rule out drug-induced platelet dysfunction. When hemorrhage is caused by impaired platelet hemostasis, platelet transfusion corrects the deficit, if the responsible drug is no longer in the circulation. Desmopressin can also be used to manage drug-induced platelet dysfunction (39).

Novel platelet inhibitors such as antibodies or peptides directed against integrin receptors (e.g. abciximab) can cause major hemorrhage, especially in association with invasive arterial procedures and the use of heparin. If a patient needs emergency cardiac surgery after cardiac catheterization, these inhibitors may still be present. In such cases, repeated platelet transfusion despite a normal platelet count is the only therapy for serious bleeding (40). Abciximab has a long half-life, and platelet transfusion may be of limited efficacy. The goal of therapy is to transfuse enough platelets to bind all of the drug and leave sufficient receptors to function in hemostasis.

Thrombocytopenia can be managed with administration of platelet concentrates. If bleeding is present and the platelet count decreases to less than 50×10^9/L, platelet transfusion may be indicated. A single apheresis unit or a pool of 4 to 6 units of whole blood–derived platelets is a typical adult dose. Inability to arrest bleeding suggests either an anatomic lesion (unrepaired bleeding site), ongoing coagulopathy unrelated to pure thrombocytopenia, or ineffective platelet transfusion.

Drugs That Affect Plasma Coagulation

Deficiencies in the vitamin K–dependent clotting factors may result from drug therapy, dietary insufficiency, or gastrointestinal dysfunction. The drug warfarin prevents activation of factors II, VII, IX, X, protein C, and protein S. The anticoagulant effect can persist as long as 1 week after discontinuation of the drug (41). Vitamin K deficiency is not uncommon among patients in hospitals, especially those referred for bleeding. Many patients with overt vitamin K deficiency manifest as bleeding, which often necessitates transfusion therapy. In addition to dietary sources, endogenous vitamin K supplied by intestinal flora is an important source for hepatic synthesis of coagulant factors. Systemic antibiotics and intestinal preparation may impair vitamin K–dependent factor synthesis by eliminating the intestinal flora. Alterations in gastrointestinal function and enterohepatic circulation potentiate this effect by decreasing absorption of fat-soluble vitamin K. Vitamin K–dependent factor deficiency most commonly causes major bleeding complications in the postoperative period.

Bleeding complications occur more frequently with the therapeutic use of heparin than with prophylactic use owing to the substantially higher doses needed in treatment (42). Bleeding is more likely to occur when heparin therapy causes excessive prolongation of the aPTT or when there is coexisting impairment of platelet function. After cardiovascular surgery, heparin is commonly neutralized with protamine, but excessive bleeding can result from incomplete neutralization. The heparin-protamine complex is detrimental to platelet function, and the complex can cause sudden thrombocytopenia with a rebound of the platelet count approximately 45 to 90 minutes after infusion. This explains how the surgical team can see a good clot form initially but see oozing approximately 10 minutes after protamine infusion. This oozing often triggers a reflex response of ordering blood products. This practice occurs most often where rapid coagulation monitoring capabilities are not available. Heparin rebound occurs most commonly after cardiopulmonary bypass when the heparin effect reappears hours after administration of protamine. This phenomenon may result from reequilibration between heparin bound to protamine and other plasma proteins (43). Though often studied, it is actually uncommon.

Although heparin is best known as an inhibitor of the plasma coagulation cascade, it also can interfere with platelet hemostasis. Heparin inhibits the hemostatic interactions between platelets and von Willebrand factor. This property of heparin may explain episodes of heparin-related hemorrhage that occur despite clotting times that are not excessive. Heparin can also induce a serious form of autoimmune thrombocytopenia that is accompanied by platelet activation and thromboembolism (44). This heparin-induced thrombocytopenia (HIT), which occurs among 1% to 3% of patients receiving heparin, is immune mediated and typically occurs 5 to 7 days after primary exposure to heparin. However, among patients who have been exposed to heparin within the previous 100 days, HIT may occur in less than 24 hours (45). Low-molecular-weight heparin also can precipitate this condition. As many as 20% to 50% of patients with HIT experience catastrophic thrombosis if all heparin is not withdrawn. Any heparin, including the small amounts used to flush lines or heparin used during surgery, can trigger severe clotting. Although mainly a clinical diagnosis, several laboratory tests have become available for assessing HIT; these include an enzyme-linked immunosorbent assay, a radioactive serotonin release assay, and modified platelet aggregation. All of these tests produce false-positive and false-negative results, and they usually are unavailable on an urgent basis, because they are performed by off-site reference laboratories. Therefore the diagnosis of HIT usually is clinical with laboratory tests serving a supporting role. Alternative anticoagulants such as hirudin and argatroban are available as substitutes for heparin in the care of patients with HIT (46).

Management of cardiopulmonary bypass for patients with active HIT is controversial. The direct thrombin inhibitors (e.g., argatroban and hirudin) are a new family of anticoagulant drugs being used more widely in situations in which heparin is contraindicated. At routine therapeutic doses these agents prolong the aPTT in a dose-dependent manner. However, in the large doses used for cardiopulmonary bypass, hirudin effects cannot be monitored with the aPTT or the activated clotting time. Ecarin clotting time has been used instead. Ecarin is a snake venom that converts prothrombin to mezzothrombin and activates clotting. Other agents for treating patients with HIT include danaparoid, a combination of chondroitin sulfate, dermatan sulfate, and heparan. Although this therapy has been reported successful, approximately 50% of patients have had massive postoperative bleeding. Ancrod is another snake venom that digests fibrinogen. When it is administered up to 24 hours before an operation, slow defibrinogenation can be accomplished. When the fibrinogen level is less than 50 mg/dl, cardiopulmonary bypass is possible. All current heparin alternatives share the disadvantage that they cannot be pharmacologically reversed at the end of the operation.

Approach to the Care of Patients Receiving Warfarin for Hypercoagulable States

Many patients are given warfarin after a thrombotic event for management of hypercoagulable states. Comprehensive recommendations for anticoagulation treatment of these patients in the perioperative period have been made by Kearon and Hirsh (47). These recommendations vary according to the type of thrombotic event, how recently the event occurred, and the risk of another event. The type of heparin used perioperatively (regular intravenous or low molecular weight) depends on the clotting risk. In general, if the event was not recent and the risk of an additional event is low, warfarin can be held 4 to 5 days before major surgical procedures. If the risk of a recurrent thrombotic event is high, intravenous heparin can be started when the INR decreases to less than 2.0 then held 6 hours before surgery. For all patients, administration of heparin is started as soon postoperatively as feasible to allow sufficient wound hemostasis. Administration of warfarin can be restarted before the heparin is discontinued. If emergency surgery is needed, transfusion of fresh-frozen plasma (FFP) is indicated. A typical dose is 15 ml/kg of FFP (4 to 5 units for adults) adjusted according to correction of the INR to approximately 1.5. It is not unusual for the INR to slowly increase after FFP correction owing to the short half-life of factor VII (7 hours) and reequilibration of small factors to the extravascular space.

Management of Bleeding Complications Caused by Drugs That Affect Plasma Coagulation

Acquired deficiency of vitamin K can develop insidiously in the postoperative period. The effects of parenterally administered vitamin K (2 to 10 mg) should be evident within 8 to 12 hours. If there is active hemorrhage, FFP transfusion provides more rapid correction of the deficiency. If there is profuse bleeding that appears to be responsive to plasma infusion, FFP infusion can be considered to keep the INR less than 1.5. Concomitant administration of vitamin K to bleeding patients is indicated, because the procoagulant effect of FFP can wane.

When hemorrhagic complications develop in patients receiving heparin, the heparin dose should be reduced or discontinued. In unusual circumstances, a heparin level can be useful, because the relation between aPTT and the true heparin level is somewhat unpredictable (48). If the heparin level is within the therapeutic range, other causes of bleeding should be considered. Individualization of heparin dosages, careful laboratory monitoring of anticoagulant effect, and correct neutralization with protamine when indicated can help prevent bleeding complications. Persistence of heparin effect after protamine neutralization usually can be corrected by means of administration of 25 to 50 mg of additional protamine guided by the activated clotting time or aPTT. Antithrombin drugs such as hirudin have no antidote but have a short duration of action. Hirudin is cleared through renal filtration, so in the care of patients with renal failure, argatroban may be a preferred direct thrombin inhibitor. Within several hours, the anticoagulant effects generally wane; this can be monitored with the aPTT or ecarin clotting time.

Renal and Hepatic Failure

Patients with uremia may have excessive surgical bleeding due to platelet dysfunction (49). The cause of the hemorrhagic diathesis in uremia is complex (27). The primary defect is caused by accumulation of substances in the plasma that are normally cleared by the kidney. Platelet calcium and prostaglandin metabolism and adhesion to von Willebrand factor may be impaired. Factor IX deficiency can be secondary to urinary loss of plasma protein in nephrotic syndrome. Anemia also contributes to bleeding because the decrease in erythrocytes diminishes the margination of platelets needed for effective vessel wall hemostasis.

Disseminated intravascular coagulation often develops in patients with liver disease because of release of thromboplastin into the circulation during hepatic necrosis, defective clearance of activated coagulation factors, and decreased levels of antithrombin III. The associated platelet consumption is worsened by qualitative platelet dysfunction. Portal hypertension leads to hypersplenism and increased platelet pooling. In addition to having these hemostatic abnormalities, patients with portal hypertension are at high risk of severe hemorrhage from injury to distended, friable veins during intraabdominal operations.

Hepatic synthesis of clotting factors can be impaired by liver resection, liver disease, hypotension, or sepsis. Compounded by the consumption and dilution of existing coagulation factors, massive transfusion, or the effects of acquired vitamin K deficiency, impaired hepatic synthesis can be an important contributor to bleeding diathesis in a surgical patient (49). Severe hepatic failure can cause generalized hemostatic failure that resembles DIC. Not only is the synthesis of clotting factors decreased but also dysfunctional forms of fibrinogen may be present. Advanced liver disease produces complex derangement of hemostasis that is difficult to manage. Parenchymal cell dysfunction is associated with impaired synthesis of fibrinogen and other coagulation factors, the extent of the synthetic defect reflecting the degree of liver dysfunction. Liver transplantation represents a unique form of this derangement (see Chapter 43). First, the preexisting hepatic dysfunction may manifest as low levels of clotting factors, a prolonged PT, elevated levels of fibrin degradation products, and thrombocytopenia. The hemostatic stress and trauma of surgery and the absence of the liver during the anhepatic phase can promote profound derangements of hemostasis. Before and during the operation, excessive fibrinolysis due to decreased clearance of tissue plasminogen activator (tPA) by the liver can cause prominent fibrinolytic derangement. After surgery, an excess of plasminogen activator inhibitor-1 combined with increased clearance of tPA by the new liver can induce a hypercoagulable state (50).

Results of platelet function studies, as with the PFA-100, TEG, and Hemodyne, typically are abnormal in patients with uremia. The defective platelet function of patients with uremia is partially corrected by renal dialysis, an important part of preoperative preparation. Red blood cell transfusion and correction of severe anemia to a hematocrit of approximately 30% also improve platelet function. Platelet transfusion is ineffective in the care of patients with uremia unless thrombocytopenia also is present. In emergencies, infusion of cryoprecipitate often improves the platelet defect in uremia, the effects lasting 24 hours. An alternative is to use desmopressin to improve intraoperative and postoperative hemostasis (39). This agent increases plasma levels of factor VIII and von Willebrand factor by stimulating release from endogenous stores. It also may decrease transfusion requirements in other surgical settings in which platelet dysfunction exists, such as cardiopulmonary bypass. The effects of desmopressin begin relatively quickly; the maximum effects occur in 4 hours. The time course makes it an ideal choice for temporary improvement of hemostasis in patients with uremia undergoing procedures or surgery without the risk associated with transfusion of a blood product. The effect of desmopressin on hemostasis diminishes with repeated administration, because the endogenous stores of factors must have time to be renewed.

In the bleeding patient with liver failure, the PT may be corrected to an INR of 1.5 or less by means of repletion of vitamin K stores and infusion of FFP. If fibrinogen is deficient or dysfunctional, cryoprecipitate infusion should be considered (FFP also contains fibrinogen, if volume is not an issue). In severe liver failure, even massive transfusion of FFP does not always decrease the INR to less than 1.5, possibly because unidentified substances present in these patients interfere with the in vitro coagulation assay. In these cases, the surgical team may be forced to settle for a more realistic target INR. The patient's condition should be evaluated clinically to assess the response to plasma administration. Thromboelastography can be used to assess overall clot function. Maximum amplitude within the normal range without evidence of early clot lysis should reassure the team that clinical bleeding is unlikely.

Hyperfibrinolysis and Fibrinolytic Drugs

Systemic hyperfibrinolysis has been reported with heat stroke, cardiac arrest, and cardiopulmonary bypass. It is a frequent manifestation of DIC, particularly in patients with severe hepatic decompensation. More common among preoperative patients, however, is systemic fibrinolysis induced by tPA, urokinase, or streptokinase. These agents are used increasingly to dissolve thrombi in the arterial and venous circulation. Even with so-called regional use (catheter-directed infusion of a single bed with low doses of fibrinolytic agents), systemic fibrinolysis frequently occurs with associated impairment of hemostasis (51). Procedures such as emergency coronary or vascular surgery sometimes are necessary in the care of such patients because of worsening of the ischemic process for which the fibrinolytic treatment was initiated.

Bleeding may ensue when fibrinolysis affects the hemostatic clots at catheterization sites or in fresh surgical wounds. Excessive fibrinolysis leads to systemic fibrinogenolysis, consumption of plasma fibrinogen, and generation of fibrinogen degradation products that can interfere with platelet function and the coagulation cascade. The effects of most fibrinolytic drugs usually are not long lasting, and most bleeding complications can be managed by simply stopping the drug. In cases of severe hemorrhage with hypofibrinogenemia (<100 mg/dl), cryoprecipitate should be administered. If heparin also is being administered, it should be stopped. The thrombotic risk of using antagonists such as protamine and ϵ-aminocaproic acid must be balanced against the need for rapid restoration of hemostasis.

Unrecognized Congenital Defects in Hemostasis

Unrecognized congenital disorders of coagulation are seldom the cause of surgical hemorrhage. However, routine hemostatic screening with the history and physical examination can miss some inherited bleeding diatheses. Mild deficiencies of factor VIII, factor IX, and von Willebrand factor as well as dysfibrinogenemia can exist despite normal results of preoperative screening tests and previously uneventful hemostatic stress. Mild deficiencies of factor VIII, factor IX, factor XI, and von Willebrand factor are associated with subclinical disease in which bleeding usually occurs only with significant trauma or surgery. In rare instances, acquired autoantibodies to factor VIII develop spontaneously in a person without hemophilia. This acquired hemophilia sometimes is associated with pregnancy or occurs in elderly persons with an autoimmune disorder, malignant disease, or infection. This disorder has even been identified in postoperative surgical patients (52).

Rare congenital platelet disorders include Glanzmann's thrombasthenia and Bernard-Soulier disease. Specific platelet membrane receptors or platelet granules are absent or defective. Most of these disorders are likely to be known preoperatively and may be confirmed with platelet aggregation studies. Platelet transfusion, administration of desmopressin, or both may be helpful, depending on the lesion (53).

PROPHYLACTIC COAGULATION SUPPORT OF PATIENTS UNDERGOING AN INVASIVE PROCEDURE OR SURGERY

The hemostatic challenge has been reduced for many surgical procedures owing to advances in laparoscopic technique and other minimally invasive procedures. At the same time, the invasiveness of procedures performed outside the operating suite ("bedside" procedures) has been increasing. It is not uncommon that a patient with mild to moderate laboratory anomalies of hemostasis needs an invasive procedure, such as a biopsy, catheter placement, or major conduction (regional) anesthesia. Clinicians sometimes order blood products "to prevent bleeding" in patients whose only bleeding risk may be a laboratory test. Although results of randomized, controlled trials are not yet available, a number of studies contain useful clinical information. For example, data are available on 202 central venous catheter insertions in liver transplant patients with severe hemostatic abnormalities typical of end-stage liver disease (mean aPTT, 92 seconds; mean platelet count, $<50 \times 10^9$/L) (54). No attempts were made to correct coagulation abnormalities, and no serious bleeding complications occurred. Another group studied internal jugular vein catheterization in the care of patients with significant hemostatic abnormalities and reported only 1 hematoma in 1,000 attempts (55). A report of the evaluation of 5,223 lumbar punctures in children with acute lymphoblastic leukemia described no serious complications regardless of platelet count. The authors concluded that prophylactic platelet transfusion is not necessary in the care of children with platelet counts greater than 10×10^9/L (56).

Do the results of studies such as those just described justify the use of blood products before invasive bedside procedures? An extensive review has been made of the predictive value of laboratory screening tests for bleeding in various invasive procedures (57). The conclusions vary by procedure. In central venous catheterization, prophylactic transfusion is not of any value, except perhaps to patients with extreme coagulopathy. In liver biopsy, the risk of bleeding is related more to the presence of vascular lesions than to preprocedure laboratory values. Bleeding complications of renal biopsy are far less common than those of liver biopsy, and these patients are at low risk. (A trial is needed to see whether desmopressin treatment improves this already favorable outcome.) Bleeding in paracentesis, thoracentesis, and gastrointestinal biopsy is not predicted by laboratory testing or aspirin use; no prophylaxis is warranted. There are insufficient data on epidural anesthesia and upper airway manipulation to evaluate whether prophylactic transfusion based on laboratory testing has an effect. Given the poor predictive value of current coagulation screening tests, the correction of mild laboratory abnormalities in most patients who need an invasive bedside procedure is not justified. In general, the decision to perform transfusion is most defensible in the management rather than the prevention of hemorrhage. Because any transfusion has inherent risks, the risk to benefit ratio supports selective transfusion. The cost to benefit ratio also strongly supports this approach.

COAGULATION SUPPORT OF BLEEDING SURGICAL PATIENTS

Clinical Assessment

The surgeon and anesthesiologist at the operative field often are the first to notice abnormal hemostasis, which is characterized by oozing from cut surfaces in the wound where hemostasis previously seemed adequate. Postoperatively, when the incision is closed, it may be more difficult to differentiate purely surgical hemorrhage (a missed bleeding vessel) and failure of hemostasis. Rapid localized blood loss would favor a surgical cause, whereas bleeding from nonoperative sites, such as line insertion sites and mucous membranes, suggests generalized impairment of hemostatic mechanisms. In the complex case of a surgical patient who has received numerous transfusions or heparin or undergone cardiopulmonary bypass, the cause of excessive bleeding may be more difficult to define precisely as surgical or nonsurgical because the hemostatic deficits frequently play a permissive role.

Table 42.5 outlines a general differential diagnosis of the causes of abnormal bleeding in the perioperative period. With the aid of a systematic approach to the care of a bleeding surgical

TABLE 42.5. DIFFERENTIAL DIAGNOSIS OF PERIOPERATIVE BLEEDING

- Preoperative conditions
  - Platelet abnormalities
  - Drug effects
  - Renal and hepatic failure
  - Hyperfibrinolysis
  - Unrecognized congenital disorders
- Intraoperative conditions
  - Massive transfusion
  - Disseminated intravascular coagulation
  - Cardiopulmonary bypass, liver transplantation
  - Local fibrinolytic syndromes
  - Inadequate surgical hemostasis

patient, therapy can be expedited, and increased risk of hemorrhagic complications can be identified preoperatively. Likely factors contributing to the hemorrhagic diathesis should be identified. Did the patient have a preoperative conditions or receive drugs that may now be influencing hemostasis? Has the patient received massive transfusions? Are conditions present that can lead to DIC? Is the surgery in question associated with specific known derangements of clotting? Is the patient cold? The answers will lead the clinician to the diagnostic laboratory tests appropriate and specific for the suspected problem.

Certain basic laboratory tests should be performed for all patients believed to have abnormal surgical bleeding. These include a hematocrit, platelet count, PT, aPTT, and fibrinogen level. The results of these simple tests are used to evaluate the contributions of thrombocytopenia and the effects of factor deficiencies and anticoagulants that may inhibit the intrinsic or extrinsic pathways of coagulation. When abnormalities are encountered or when specific diagnoses are needed, specialized laboratory testing may be indicated. These laboratory studies are summarized in Table 42.3 and discussed throughout this chapter according to diagnosis. The addition of TEG results sometimes is useful (15,17,19). The use of treatment algorithms based on PT, fibrinogen level, platelet count, and TEG findings significantly decreases the need for blood transfusion and incidence of postoperative bleeding (19). For these results to be realized, a member of the surgical-anesthesia team must take an interest in appropriate blood use and improved monitoring.

Treatment of the Bleeding Patient

Transfusion of blood products is best guided by timely laboratory testing during the surgical procedure, because the results can suggest which blood components are needed and prevent anticipation or "blind" use of blood products. Timely acquisition of laboratory results is a challenge at most institutions. This is partly because so many tests are run "stat" in most hospitals that "emergency" specimens from the operating room are delayed among less urgent test requests. Another contributing factor is that many test results submitted from the surgical suite are abnormal because of the nature of the procedures and the patient population. For each test, the laboratory has a protocol to verify an abnormal result before it is released. For example, for a low platelet count, the specimen may be tested again and a manual blood smear evaluated. For a prolonged result of coagulation test, heparin contamination should be ruled out. This means that the turnaround time for abnormal stat specimens may be 45 minutes or longer, even in efficient laboratories. An attractive solution is used by the department of laboratory medicine at the University of Washington. This laboratory offers an "emergency hemorrhage panel" that includes a platelet count, PT, and fibrinogen level with results reported less than 20 minutes after the specimen reaches the technologist (mean, 11 minutes). All unnecessary delays have been eliminated. The specimen is delivered directly to the hematology section of the laboratory, where previously printed "emergency" bar codes are attached. The ordering physician is aware that as long as the instruments are functioning properly and controls are within appropriate limits, abnormal results will not be investigated before the results are faxed or called directly to the operating room. To save time, the specimen need not be logged into the computer or results entered until after the results are reported to the surgery-anesthesia team.

In the absence of other causes of abnormal perioperative bleeding, inherited disorders of coagulation should be investigated (58). The evaluation and management of these disorders are discussed in Chapter 31. Clues to the diagnosis are indicated by isolated abnormalities in the intrinsic or extrinsic coagulation pathways as indicated by the aPTT or PT (factor deficiency) or by prolongation of the platelet function screen. Diagnosis of an inherited disorder is best made before surgery, because the specific testing needed usually cannot be completed on a stat basis. Consultation with a transfusion medicine expert is useful in guiding transfusion therapy before the specific disorder can be characterized. Consultation is helpful in differentiating the various subtypes of and appropriate therapies for von Willebrand disease (59). Specialized advice is particularly needed in the management of acquired antibodies to coagulation factors. In emergencies, cryoprecipitate is a concentrated source of von Willebrand factor, factor VIII, and fibrinogen, and FFP is a source of these and most other factors.

Congenital, heritable abnormalities of the vessel wall can be mistaken for bleeding disorders (Table 42.1). In type IV Ehlers-Danlos syndrome, there is a genetic defect in the synthesis of type III collagen in the vessel wall. These patients can bruise easily and are predisposed to spontaneous aneurysm formation and arterial rupture. Surgery should be avoided and limited to arterial ligation when needed. Other vascular causes of bleeding include amyloidosis, vitamin C deficiency, hemorrhagic purpura, and vasculitis.

Adjuncts to Hemostasis during Surgery

Topical Agents

Local bleeding in the absence of severe derangements of systemic coagulation is best managed with local hemostatic agents (60). Oxidized regenerated cellulose is an absorbable material that is applied directly to the bleeding tissues. It serves as a matrix for the formation and deposition of fibrin clot. Topical bovine thrombin (solution or powder) can be applied to bleeding sites and is especially helpful in the care of patients receiving heparin for anticoagulation. If thrombin does not induce blood clotting at the operative field, there may be a deficiency or abnormality of fibrinogen itself. Microcrystalline preparations of collagen are useful topical agents for hemostasis on large raw bleeding surfaces such as the liver and spleen. Collagen is a potent activator of platelets. Biologic surgical glues have grown increasingly popular for their efficacy in promoting hemostasis at localized sites of refractory bleeding. Bovine thrombin and a source of human fibrinogen (e.g., cryoprecipitate or a commercial fibrinogen preparation) can be rapidly mixed in situ on the bleeding area. These fibrin glues are clearly beneficial when the cumulative effects of technical and local factors combine with systemic hemostatic derangements to make hemostasis difficult, as at leaky suture lines or on the bleeding surface of solid organs. Viral inactivation steps are now applied to plasma-derived topical fibrin sealants.

Hemostatic Drugs

Desmopressin (DDAVP; 1-diamino-8-D-arginine vasopressin), a synthetic derivative of vasopressin, has been used successfully in the clinical management of bleeding associated with specific subtypes of von Willebrand disease, factor VIII deficiency, and uremia (39). Desmopressin infusion not only improves hemostatic competence when platelet–von Willebrand factor interaction is impaired but also seems to partially correct unrelated disorders of platelet function (39). Hyponatremia and paradoxic thrombosis are possible side effects. Early results of the use of desmopressin in cardiac surgery were impressive, but many studies could not reproduce early findings. However, when TEG was used to demonstrate platelet function defects, desmopressin was found effective.

Aprotinin is a naturally occurring serine protease inhibitor derived from bovine lung tissue. It blocks contact activation of the blood along kallikrein-dependent pathways. Aprotinin potently inhibits fibrinolysis by blocking the conversion of plasminogen to plasmin. This drug may have a role in controlling the excessive fibrinolysis associated with liver transplantation and cardiopulmonary bypass (61). Aprotinin has been shown repeatedly to be highly effective in decreasing bleeding after cardiac surgery. Reductions in bleeding and blood transfusion of 30% to 70% have been demonstrated. The exact mechanism of this effect continues to be debated. Because of the risk of allergic reactions, a test dose is recommended, and treatment with aprotinin should be repeated only with caution (62). The highest risk of anaphylaxis occurs within 1 to 3 months after initial exposure.

ε-Aminocaproic acid and tranexamic acid are older antifibrinolytic drugs with a narrower profile of activity. By binding the lysine binding sites of plasminogen for fibrin and fibrinogen, ε-aminocaproic acid interferes with localization of plasminogen and plasmin on the fibrin clot. ε-Aminocaproic acid can be useful as an antidote to drugs that activate plasminogen (such as tPA) in the management of bleeding associated with excessive fibrinolysis. As with desmopressin, there remains a theoretic concern about inducing a paradoxic hypercoagulable state through administration of aprotinin or ε-aminocaproic acid. For this reason, antifibrinolytic drugs are generally contraindicated in the care of patients with DIC. Debate continues as to whether the lysine analogues are as effective as aprotinin. It would seem from metaanalysis of published reports as well as from clinician belief that aprotinin is more effective, particularly in complex operations. The question of cost-effectiveness continues to be debated, because aprotinin is considerably more expensive than lysine analogues. Aprotinin appears to have marked antiinflammatory effects. These and other long-term benefits are being investigated.

MANAGEMENT OF INTRAOPERATIVE CONDITIONS THAT AFFECT HEMOSTASIS

Massive Transfusion

Transfusion is considered massive when the entire blood volume is replaced within minutes or hours. Patients undergoing massive transfusion are heterogeneous, but typically have life-threatening hemorrhage associated with shock, trauma, and organ system failure. The specific hemostatic deficits resulting from massive transfusion often are difficult to differentiate from the clotting abnormalities of the associated conditions. The lack of prospective, randomized, clinical trials also limits understanding of the ideal methods to prevent and control the bleeding diathesis associated with massive transfusion. Dilution, consumption, and decreased production of procoagulant factors and platelets can occur in injured patients who have undergone massive transfusion. One-third to more than one-half of these patients experience clinical coagulopathy that manifests as bleeding from nonoperative sites (e.g., mucous membranes, sites of intravenous cannulation, and epistaxis). Results of laboratory tests of hemostasis may be abnormal in as many as 90% of patients who receive massive transfusions (Table 42.3); however, neither results of laboratory studies nor total transfusion volume correlates well with the development of a clinical hemorrhagic diathesis (63).

Thrombocytopenia is the abnormality most frequently associated with massive transfusion. Although platelets are lost to hemorrhage and consumption, they are not replaced by means of red blood cell transfusions or administration of plasma or volume expanders. The decrease in platelet count associated with massive transfusion is less than would be predicted on the basis of dilution alone because of release of platelets from storage in the bone marrow and spleen (64). The platelet count may decrease initially as much as one-half for each blood volume transfused. Patients who undergo massive transfusion become reconstituted with a cohort of platelets sharing a single life span. The result is a predictable decline in platelet count during the first 2 or 3 postoperative days. In addition to the decrease in platelet number due to consumption and dilution, platelet function can be impaired by systemic acidosis, hypothermia, subtle changes in the function of platelet membrane receptors, subclinical dilution of von Willebrand factor, and the less effective hemostatic function of transfused platelets (65). Although a defect in platelet plug formation can occur at any platelet count less than 100×10^9/L, not all patients experience bleeding, even with counts close to 50×10^9/L. The clinical significance of thrombocytopenia depends in part on the degree of concomitant platelet dysfunction.

Comparison of coagulation profiles between groups of animals resuscitated from severe hemorrhagic shock with FFP or factor-free solutions shows equivalent dilution of the coagulation factors (66). Elective total plasma exchange to treat humans, a procedure uncomplicated by shock and hemorrhage, does not reduce the coagulation factor activities below a level necessary for effective hemostasis. However, a patient who has sustained trauma and hypotension often experiences hypothermia, acidosis, hepatic ischemia, and activation of thrombosis and fibrinolysis, all of which can diminish overall hemostatic function (66). Acid-base and electrolyte changes can be severe and correlate independently with survival (67). Thus the hemorrhagic diathesis in these complex cases is the sum of many challenges to normal hemostatic mechanisms, including dilution.

Disseminated intravascular coagulation can be superimposed on the other consequences of massive transfusion. In the rush of transfusing 10 or 20 units of blood components to a patient with rapid bleeding, a hemolytic transfusion reaction may be mistaken for a "generalized bleeding diathesis." Disseminated intravascular coagulation also can be induced by extensive brain injury or soft-tissue crush injuries and lead to the consumption of platelets and coagulation factors with activation of the fibrinolytic system. Most patients with severe head injury have some element of DIC that continues for up to 72 hours postoperatively.

Effects of Autotransfusion of Shed Blood

Systems designed to collect and reinfuse shed blood range from the very simple to the complex. During cardiopulmonary bypass, the patient is given systemic heparin, and shed blood is recirculated into an oxygenator. If the blood has not been excessively activated by means of frothing and contact with tissue thromboplastin, the red blood cells, platelets, and clotting factors are all returned to the circuit. Shed blood also can be suctioned from the operative field and rapidly washed to produce a suspension of viable red blood cells (absent platelets and clotting factors).

In the simplest methods of autotransfusion, shed blood is collected by means of suction or drainage from wounds or chest tubes and stored briefly in a sterile reservoir, which is used for reinfusion after filtration of macroscopic clots. Analysis shows that this reinfused blood contains red blood cells but few clotting factors or platelets. The blood is rich in thromboplastins, fibrin degradation products, and activated clotting factors. Reinfusion of large volumes (>800 ml) of this activated blood can contribute to a generalized bleeding diathesis in patients with compromised hemostatic reserve (68).

Treatment of a Bleeding Patient during Massive Transfusion

Transfusion support during massive transfusion can be guided with a series of basic laboratory tests (Table 42.3). The goal of this testing is to avoid extremes of hemodilution due to inadequate replacement of platelets and FFP. It is not to generate normal coagulation values intraoperatively. The platelet count most strongly correlates with development of abnormal bleeding after massive transfusions. Transfusion of less than two blood volumes without FFP replacement rarely reduces the levels of plasma clotting factors to less than the critical concentrations needed for hemostasis. The PT and aPTT frequently are prolonged slightly after massive transfusion, but the values may normalize without specific therapy. More profound abnormalities of PT and aPTT (more than two times control) can occur in patients who undergo massive transfusion who have additional risk factors for coagulopathy, such as hypotension, soft-tissue injury, drug effects, sepsis, liver disease, and organ failure. Fibrinogen levels may decrease with massive transfusion, and the abnormality often signals the uncommon case in which DIC or pathologic fibrinolysis is contributory. Laboratory testing during massive transfusion leads to improved use of blood products and patient outcome (69). Figure 42.1 is a sample algorithm for massive transfusion.

It is difficult to establish standard clinical guidelines for the prevention, management, and correction of a bleeding diathesis associated with massive transfusion (70). The patients are a heterogeneous group, and there have been few prospective, randomized studies of therapy. Loss of platelet function and number is the most common cause of coagulopathy, and correction of thrombocytopenia is the mainstay of therapy for bleeding associated with massive transfusion. There are two dominant philosophies in the management of massive transfusion—routine, prophylactic administration of component therapy before coagulopathy is evident and selective replacement of platelets and factors on the basis of laboratory abnormalities and clinical signs. The efficacy of the former has been compared with that of the latter. One study showed that routine empiric transfusion of platelets or FFP did not reduce the transfusion requirements or the incidence of bleeding among patients undergoing massive transfusion (63). Results of other studies suggest that platelet transfusion should be withheld until clinical bleeding is evident (71). Despite severe reductions in platelet number and function, no abnormal bleeding developed in the patients in the series undergoing massive transfusion. Nevertheless, the experiences of several trauma centers suggest that bleeding due to massive transfusion is a preventable complication caused primarily by consumption and dilution. They advocate routine administration of FFP and platelets before the onset of a clinical coagulopathy. Although some patients may be overtreated, the investigators justify this approach by citing the high mortality associated with the hemorrhagic diathesis of massive transfusion (72).

Treatment of patients undergoing massive transfusion should be individualized to the extent of the patient's injuries and associated conditions and the anticipated transfusion requirement. If the patient is in stable condition, the primary source of bleeding has been controlled, and the transfusion requirement appears finite, an expectant approach to platelet and FFP therapy is appropriate. There should be close monitoring of the PT, fibrinogen level, platelet count, and possibly TEG, but laboratory abnormalities need not be corrected unless there is clinical evidence of abnormal bleeding. Therapy is guided by the deficiencies identified with laboratory testing. If the patient is in unstable condition and bleeding is not controlled, the course is marked by extensive trauma, shock, or other complicating factors, and laboratory results are not immediately available, empiric administration of 2 to 4 units of FFP and 6 units of platelets 1 apheresis unit for every 10 to 12 units of packed red blood cells transfused is justified.

Disseminated Intravascular Coagulation

Disseminated intravascular coagulation is a disorder of inappropriate thrombin generation that results in a chaos of hypercoagulation and hyperfibrinolysis with activation and consumption of the factors and inhibitors of both systems (73). Equilibrium exists between the formation and dissolution of thrombus at the site of vascular injury. The same biochemical events that initiate thrombosis activate the process of fibrinolysis, which is regulated by its own system of activators and inhibitors (74). Fibrinolysis is enhanced by stress, trauma, surgery, and even exercise. During surgery, thrombosis occurs in response to vascular injury, and the fibrinolytic system helps confine the thrombosis to the area of injury and ultimately removes the thrombus once hemostasis

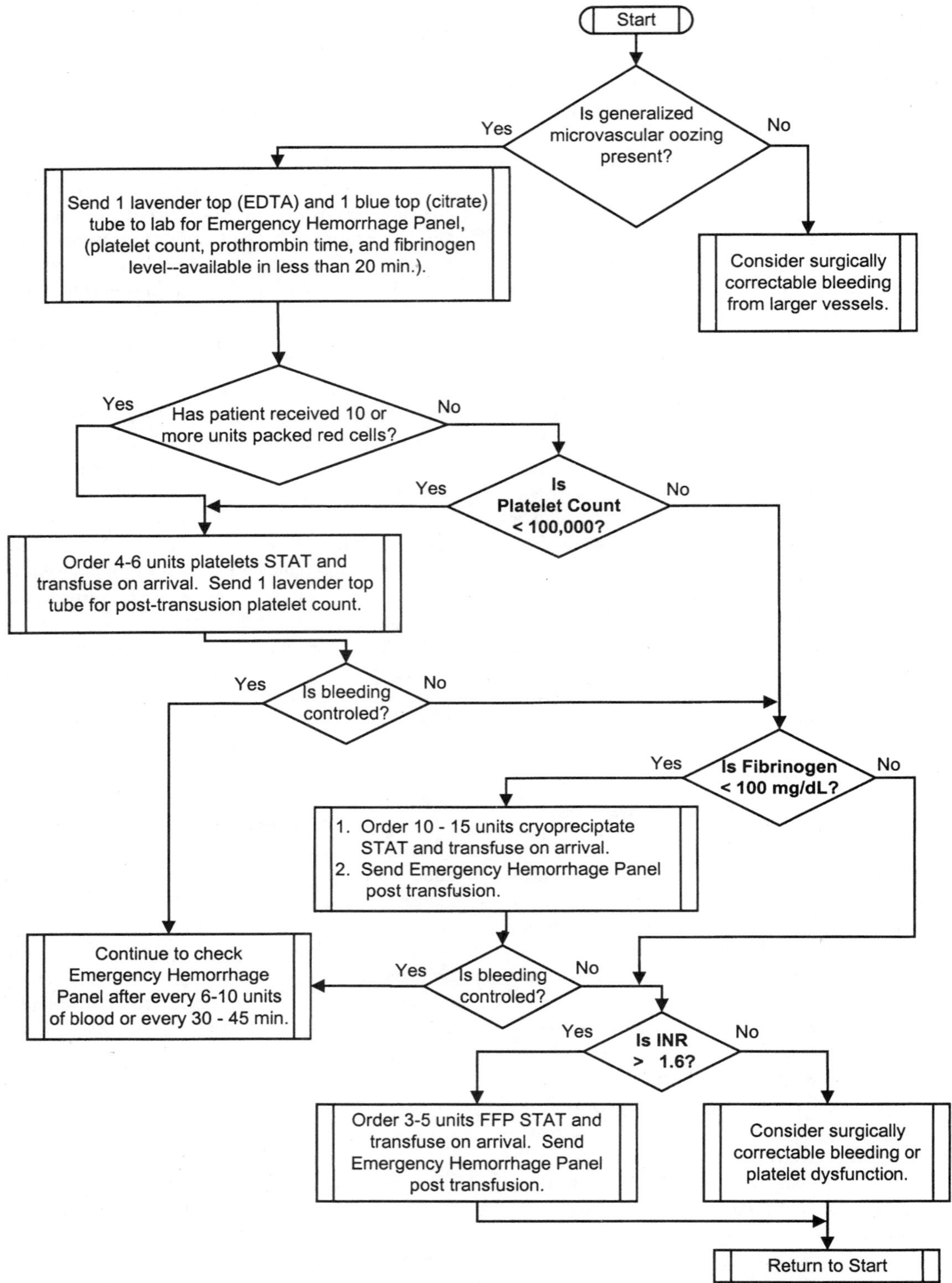

FIGURE 42.1. Sample protocol for management of bleeding during massive transfusion. (Adapted from a pathway courtesy of T. Gernsheimer, Puget Sound Blood Center, Seattle, Washington.)

TABLE 42.6. CAUSES OF DISSEMINATED INTRAVASCULAR COAGULATION IN THE PERIOPERATIVE PERIOD

Adult respiratory distress syndrome
Aortic aneurysm, dissection, balloon pumping
Cirrhosis, hepatic necrosis
Complications of pregnancy
Disseminated malignant disease
Extensive soft-tissue or brain injury
Fat embolism
Hemolytic transfusion reaction
Sepsis
Shock

has occurred. However, if the balance between thrombosis and thrombolysis is upset, pathologic clotting, consumptive coagulopathy, or hemorrhage can result.

Pathologic fibrinolysis most often accompanies DIC. The hemorrhagic diathesis of DIC results first from consumption and depletion of coagulation factors and platelets by the thrombotic process. Second, the induction of fibrinolysis results in accelerated digestion of fibrinogen and fibrin by plasmin. The resulting degradation products may act as circulating anticoagulants. These fragments of fibrin and fibrinogen interfere with coagulation, impair platelet function, and inhibit fibrin polymerization. The original clot is destabilized and digested, and bleeding occurs where once it was stopped. Because DIC can cause unexpected nonsurgical bleeding, this diagnosis should be considered in the evaluation of bleeding surgical patients when likely clinical factors are present. Unique stimuli in injured or critically ill surgical patients can promote pathologic activation of the coagulation system, resulting in DIC. These clinical conditions are summarized in Table 42.6. In surgical patients, the most commonly encountered conditions are sepsis, extensive soft-tissue trauma, tissue ischemia, and malignant disease. It is not uncommon for patients with advanced malignant disease to have biochemical or clinical evidence of activated clotting and chronic subclinical DIC.

There are numerous clinical settings for intraoperative coagulopathy in patients undergoing surgery, including hemolytic transfusion reactions, septicemia, malignant disease, viral infection, burns, crush injury, liver disease, and the presence of certain prosthetic devices (73). The surgeon should be alert to the possibility of underlying DIC, because surgery can augment the process and lead to severe hemorrhagic complications. For example, it has been estimated that 4% to 5% of patients with large aortic aneurysms have chronic partially compensated DIC (75). Aortic surgery on such patients can be associated with severe bleeding. Ecchymosis at the preoperative examination in the hospital is a cardinal feature of DIC and should prompt immediate laboratory investigation.

The diagnosis of DIC begins with identification of the clinical condition inciting pathologic thrombosis and fibrinolysis (Table 42.6). A typical laboratory profile shows low platelet and fibrinogen levels, prolonged PT and aPTT, and elevated levels of fibrin degradation products or fibrin D-dimers (Table 42.3). However, because fibrinogen is an acute-phase protein, the level may remain in the normal range even while fibrinogen is being consumed.

Control of DIC requires management of the underlying condition. Replacement of consumed platelets and coagulation proteins may only temporarily improve the hemorrhagic diathesis. Replacement therapy is appropriate while management of the underlying disorder producing DIC is in progress. In the surgical setting, platelets should be administered when the platelet count decreases to less than 50×10^9/L and when hemorrhage persists. Fresh-frozen plasma or cryoprecipitate can be used if levels of fibrinogen decrease to less than 100 mg/dl. Therapy should be guided by following the PT, aPTT, platelet count, and fibrinogen level. If the fibrinogen level decreases to much less than 100 mg/dl, results of the aPTT and PT are meaningless, because there is insufficient substrate to form the fibrin clot end points of the assays. Factor concentrates or drugs affecting hemostasis to augment standard blood component therapy for DIC should be used only in consultation with a physician highly experienced in the management of DIC. Early clinical results suggest that administration of antithrombin III in cases of DIC may help arrest the pathologic thrombotic process and possibly improve survival (76). Inhibitors of fibrinolysis, such as ϵ-aminocaproic acid, usually should be avoided, because inhibition of fibrinolysis can result in diffuse thrombosis. Heparin therapy for DIC is not recommended unless a life-threatening thrombotic process is evident.

Cardiopulmonary Bypass

Alterations of hemostatic mechanisms occur in almost all patients undergoing open heart surgery and extracorporeal circulation. The average transfusion requirement historically ranges from 1 to 3 units of packed red blood cells for uncomplicated operations or 3 to 5 units for more complex procedures (77). A growing number of programs suggest that "bloodless" cardiac surgery may be better for their patients (78). There is no "best" hematocrit for heart surgery. The science regarding the transfusion trigger in heart surgery is complex and under great debate. Data from the Multicenter Study of Perioperative Ischemia (McSPI), which involved 2,200 patients, show that patients undergoing coronary artery bypass graft surgery actually do better with lower hematocrits when they are admitted to the intensive care unit (79). Other database research, however, has shown an increased frequency of adverse events with very low hematocrits during bypass. These other databases may actually be finding low hematocrits as surrogates for transfusion use. It may well be that transfusion itself carries adverse outcome risks in cardiac surgery.

The definition of excessive bleeding differs from institution to institution but generally amounts to 100 to 200 ml/h. Approximately 2% to 3% of all open-heart procedures are followed by reexploration for bleeding (80). Patients who undergo cardiac surgical procedures frequently receive medications that can impair hemostatic mechanisms, including aspirin, warfarin, heparin, nitrates, calcium channel blockers, β-blockers, and antibiotics. Despite the use of heparin during cardiopulmonary bypass, interaction of blood with the foreign surfaces of the extracorporeal circuit results in stimulation and activation of coagulation proteins and platelets.

Platelet abnormalities account for most of the nonsurgical bleeding that occurs after cardiac surgery. Platelet dysfunction and thrombocytopenia are principally the result of dilution, sequestration, and contact with the extracorporeal circuits, pumps, and oxygenators as well as the partial activation caused by heparin. The coagulopathy after cardiopulmonary bypass is complex and highly variable. One article described 250-fold variability in fibrinolytic response to bypass. Dilution by the non-blood-priming solutions of the extracorporeal circuit reduces the platelet count to approximately 50% of baseline value, but the platelet count rarely decreases to less than 75 × 10^9/L. Platelet consumption by the pump and oxygenator as well as splenic and hepatic sequestration may contribute to this decrease. Normalization of the platelet count occurs within 3 to 5 days postoperatively. A defect in platelet function is important to the bleeding diathesis that occurs with cardiopulmonary bypass (81). Extracorporeal circulation depletes platelets of their stores of ADP, adenosine triphosphate, and other constituents, making them hemostatically less effective. Low levels of fibrin degradation products appear in the circulation of most patients undergoing cardiopulmonary bypass and contribute to platelet dysfunction. Formation of tPA and fibrin degradation products leads to dysfunction of platelet binding sites after cardiac surgery.

Although plasma coagulation factors are diluted by the non-blood-priming solutions to 50% of normal, the levels remain well above the minimum needed for normal hemostasis. Clotting factors are not depleted or consumed by the extracorporeal circuits or oxygenator, and the degree of postoperative bleeding correlates poorly with the occurrence of prolonged clotting times after the operation. If one looks at only PT and aPTT, these two tests can account for only 12% of cases of bleeding after cardiac surgery (82). Disseminated intravascular coagulation is rare after cardiopulmonary bypass, probably because of the protective effect of large doses of heparin used during the operation. However, excessive fibrinolysis and contact activation of the blood may be important contributors to bleeding, as exemplified by the salutary hemostatic effects of the protease inhibitor aprotinin (61).

A bleeding diathesis that develops intraoperatively is most apparent after the bypass is complete, when the patient approaches normothermia and attempts at controlling all surgical bleeding points are underway. At this juncture, heparin anticoagulation is reversed with intravenous protamine according to standard calculations. Circulating protamine-heparin complexes may activate complement pathways, induce systemic mediators of inflammation, and cause leukopenia and thrombocytopenia (83).

Bleeding after cardiopulmonary bypass is most frequently caused by platelet dysfunction induced by the extracorporeal circuit and oxygenator. Patients with valvular heart disease and those taking aspirin may have a preexisting defect in platelet function that is worsened by the bypass procedure. These conditions as well as long bypass times, intraaortic balloon pumping, and repeated operations are major risk factors for increased postoperative bleeding. Consumption and depletion of clotting factors rarely occur, except in the unusual case of insufficient heparin with thrombosis of the extracorporeal circuits.

When there is excessive bleeding after cardiopulmonary bypass, initial laboratory studies should include PT, aPTT, platelet count, fibrinogen level, and TEG where available. Clotting times frequently are mildly prolonged (Table 42.3), but these abnormalities bear little relation to the occurrence of clinically significant bleeding. The platelet count may decrease to as low as 75 × 10^9/L immediately after bypass. In the absence of excessive bleeding, isolated laboratory abnormalities should be observed, as they will often resolve within 4 to 6 hours after bypass. Greater prolongations of PT may result from subclinical vitamin K deficiency. When the aPTT is prolonged more than 10 to 15 seconds, heparin excess should be suspected. Assessment of platelet function is largely academic, because platelet dysfunction always accompanies cardiopulmonary bypass. However, TEG and possibly measurement with a Hemodyne device allow the clinician to estimate the degree of platelet dysfunction. With the use of heparinase, these tests can be performed on samples of blood just before bypass is discontinued. A treatment algorithm can be used as bypass is being discontinued or soon after protamine is administered (19). Treatment of patients with coagulation blood products should be reserved for patients who are bleeding. Although the incidence of viral transmission is low, the risk of mistransfusion, perioperative infection, and other adverse outcomes from blood transfusion is not.

If active bleeding continues after bypass is discontinued, platelet transfusion should be considered, even if the platelet count is more than 75 × 10^9/L. Platelet transfusions should usually be withheld until the conclusion of bypass. Heparin excess should be managed with small (25 to 50 mg) doses of protamine. Infusion of FFP does not neutralize the anticoagulant activity of remaining heparin. Therapy with FFP rarely is indicated except in unusual cases of isolated factor deficiency or truly massive transfusion. Because FFP can replenish antithrombin, the activated clotting time may rise when circulating heparin is present and may account for some instances of "heparin rebound."

The routine prophylactic use of desmopressin to improve platelet function after bypass has been questioned (84,85). Desmopressin can be useful to selected patients with impaired von Willebrand factor–dependent hemostasis, but a method to identify these patients (TEG or Hemodyne) is not available at all centers. Many protocols for aprotinin call for administration at the onset of bypass, ostensibly to block the initial contact activation of the blood and its fibrinolytic system. Dosage and the appropriate patient population remain areas of controversy. Data suggest that aprotinin treatment of patients who are bleeding after surgery is useful (85).

Local Fibrinolytic Syndromes

Hemorrhage can occur among patients with congenital or acquired bleeding disorders when fibrinolysis is not offset by continued formation and polymerization of fibrin. Bleeding in such patients usually manifests itself in the postoperative period and often is confined to the area of operative trauma. The development of a localized hyperfibrinolytic state in surgical patients probably is not recognized as often as it occurs. Specific conditions and procedures associated with enhanced fibrinolysis are as follows.

Bleeding during and after ureteral, bladder, and prostate surgery may be excessive because of fibrinolytic factors present in the tissues as well as the urokinase present in the urine. Bleeding usually is mild rather than life threatening and more likely to occur after open, rather than closed, procedures (86). Antifibrinolytic therapy for bleeding originating in the ureters or renal pelvis carries the danger of urinary obstruction by thrombus. Thrombosis in the bladder is not as dangerous.

Fibrinolytic factors are present in the eye, and the most serious complication of ocular trauma is recurrent, or secondary, bleeding into the eye. The abundant tPA present in the eye provides local fibrinolysis as a protective mechanism to clear blood from the anterior chamber. As many as 38% of patients with traumatic hyphema may have recurrent bleeding within 1 week of injury resulting in visual impairment or blindness (86). Efforts to prevent the natural fibrinolytic process can delay the clearance of thrombus from the chambers of the eye.

Brain tissue injury can induce local fibrinolysis with secondary bleeding into the area of injury. In rare instances, severe brain injuries cause DIC from the release of thromboplastic brain tissue into the circulation. Heightened fibrinolytic activity can be detected locally and systemically during pulmonary and mediastinal surgery and after the release of an arterial tourniquet during orthopedic operations. Such fibrinolysis rarely is pathologic or the cause of excessive postoperative bleeding. The routine use of inhibitors of fibrinolysis such as ε-aminocaproic acid and tranexamic acid is controversial and carries the risk of thrombotic complications. Inhibitors of fibrinolysis have been used to control postoperative bleeding in the lower urinary tract, but not all studies show a beneficial reduction in transfusion requirements (87). Pleural and pericardial tissues are rich in mesothelial cells able to release plasminogen activators. Excessive mediastinal tube or pleural chest tube bleeding can result from localized excessive clot lysis. This is best managed by means of clearing the retained blood or the use of antifibrinolytic agents (85).

Hypothermia

Hypothermia can result from deliberately hypothermic surgery, such as cardiac surgery, or from environmental exposure and multiple trauma. Hypothermia also can occur during lengthy procedures involving exposed body cavities or as the result of infusion of crystalloids and blood products at temperatures less than physiologic. Hypothermia appears to worsen existing coagulopathy, possibly because of decreased enzyme activity in platelets and clotting factors at the lower temperature (88). Personal observation with needle temperature probes has found the wound edge often to be 24°C or colder. Clot function is abnormal at this level of hypothermia, and it matters little what the systemic temperature is if the local vascular temperature does not support normal protein and platelet coagulation.

SUMMARY

A bleeding history is mandatory before surgery. It should disclose the hemostatic response to previous surgery or trauma, episodes of spontaneous bleeding, and medical, family, and medication history. Laboratory tests should be based on the magnitude of the planned operation and the history of bleeding. Particular attention should be given to the possible presence of other conditions that diminish hemostatic reserve, such as uremia, liver disease, anticoagulant administration, or chronic, low-grade DIC. Diminished hemostatic reserve is more easily managed when it is diagnosed.

Prophylactic transfusion treatment of patients scheduled for invasive bedside procedures cannot be justified solely on the basis of mildly to moderately abnormal results of laboratory screening tests. The patient's clinical condition must weigh heavily into the decision, because the predictive value of screening laboratory tests is poor when there is no history of bleeding. There is little correlation between actual surgical bleeding and mild prolongation of the aPTT and PT. Work with the PFA-100, TEG, and other tests of platelet function is encouraging, but these methods are not available at all centers. The coupling of reasonable algorithms with fast turnaround of coagulation tests has improved blood use.

The diagnosis and management of abnormal bleeding in surgical patients are most difficult when the hemorrhage is unanticipated. The evaluation must proceed in concert with therapy. This emphasizes the importance of the preoperative assessment to identify congenital bleeding disorders, drug ingestion, renal and hepatic dysfunction, and unique clinical conditions that may predispose to perioperative hemostatic defects. When there is serious, life-threatening hemorrhage, empiric treatment should begin even before the results of the more definitive laboratory tests are known. Close communication and cooperation between the surgical team, hematologist, blood bank, and clinical laboratories will expedite diagnosis and therapy and should improve patient outcome. Physicians who champion appropriate blood use and improved coagulation management are needed to create the systems that bring success.

REFERENCES

1. Triplett DA. Coagulation and bleeding disorders: review and update. *Clin Chem* 2000;46:1260–1269.
2. Goodnight SH, Hathaway WE. *Hemostasis and thrombosis: a clinical guide,* 2nd ed. New York: McGraw-Hill, 2001.
3. Edmunds LH. Hemostatic problems in surgical patients. In: Colman RW, Hirsh J, Marder VJ, et al., eds. *Hemostasis and thrombosis: basic principles and clinical practice,* 4th ed. Philadelphia: Lippincott, Williams & Wilkins, 2001:956–968.
4. Rapaport SI. Preoperative hemostatic evaluation: which tests, if any? *Blood* 1983;61:229–231.
5. Narr BJ, Hansen TR, Warner MA. Preoperative laboratory screening in healthy Mayo patients: cost- effective elimination of tests and unchanged outcomes. *Mayo Clin Proc* 1991;66:155–159.
6. Rohrer MJ, Michelotti MC, Nahrwold DL. A prospective evaluation of the efficacy of preoperative coagulation testing. *Ann Surg* 1988;208:554–557.
7. Borzotta AP, Keeling MM. Value of the preoperative history as an indicator of hemostatic disorders. *Ann Surg* 1984;200:648–652.
8. Narayanan S. The preanalytic phase: an important component of laboratory medicine. *Am J Clin Pathol* 2000;113:429–452.
9. Ereth MA. A contempory view of coagulation. In: Spiess BD, ed. *The relationship between coagulation, inflammation and endothelium: a pyramid towards outcome.* Philadelphia: Lippincott, Williams & Wilkins, 2000:129–146.

10. Lind SE. The bleeding time does not predict surgical bleeding. *Blood* 1991;77:2547–2552.
11. Rodgers RP, Levin J. A critical reappraisal of the bleeding time. *Semin Thromb Hemost* 1990;16:1–20.
12. Harrison P. Progress in the assessment of platelet function. *Br J Haematol* 2000;111:733–744.
13. Mammen EF, Comp PC, Gosselin R, et al. PFA-100 system: a new method for assessment of platelet dysfunction. *Semin Thromb Hemost* 1998;24:195–202.
14. Favaloro EJ. Utility of the PFA-100(R) for assessing bleeding disorders and monitoring therapy: a review of analytical variables, benefits and limitations. *Haemophilia* 2001;7:170–179.
15. Chandler WL. The thromboelastography and the thromboelastograph technique. *Semin Thromb Hemost* 1995;4:1–6.
16. Spiess BD, Tuman KJ, McCarthy RJ, et al. Thromboelastography as an indicator of post-cardiopulmonary bypass coagulopathies. *J Clin Monit* 1987;3:25–30.
17. Essell JH, Martin TJ, Salinas J, et al. Comparison of thromboelastography to bleeding time and standard coagulation tests in patients after cardiopulmonary bypass. *J Cardiothorac Vasc Anesth* 1993;7:410–415.
18. Davis CL, Chandler WL. Thromboelastography for the prediction of bleeding after transplant renal biopsy. *J Am Soc Nephrol* 1995;6: 1250–1255.
19. Shore-Lesserson L, Manspeizer HE, DePerio M, et al. Thromboelastography-guided transfusion algorithm reduces transfusions in complex cardiac surgery. *Anesth Analg* 1999;88:312–319.
20. Miyashita T, Kuro M. Evaluation of platelet function by Sonoclot analysis compared with other hemostatic variables in cardiac surgery. *Anesth Analg* 1998;87:1228–1233.
21. Robbins JA, Rose SD. Partial thromboplastin time as a screening test. *Ann Intern Med* 1979;90:796–797.
22. Kaplan EB, Sheiner LB, Boeckmann AJ, et al. The usefulness of preoperative laboratory screening. *JAMA* 1985;253:3576–3581.
23. Myers ER, Clarke-Pearson DL, Olt GJ, et al. Preoperative coagulation testing on a gynecologic oncology service. *Obstet Gynecol* 1994;83: 438–444.
24. Ellison N, Campbell FW, Jobes DR. Preoperative hemostasis. *Semin Thorac Cardiovasc Surg* 1990;3:33–38.
25. Eisenberg JM, Clarke JR, Sussman SA. Prothrombin and partial thromboplastin times as preoperative screening tests. *Arch Surg* 1982;117: 48–51.
26. Bick RL. Acquired platelet function defects. *Hematol Oncol Clin North Am* 1992;6:1203–1228.
27. Weigert AL, Schafer AI. Uremic bleeding: pathogenesis and therapy. *Am J Med Sci* 1998;316:94–104.
28. Noris M, Remuzzi G. Uremic bleeding: closing the circle after 30 years of controversies? *Blood* 1999;94:2569–2574.
29. Barbui T, Buelli M, Cortelazzo S, et al. Aspirin and risk of bleeding in patients with thrombocythemia. *Am J Med* 1987;83:265–268.
30. Geerts WH, Heit JA, Clagett GP, et al. Prevention of venous thromboembolism. *Chest* 2001;119:132S–175S.
31. Ferraris VA, Swanson E. Aspirin usage and perioperative blood loss in patients undergoing unexpected operations. *Surg Gynecol Obstet* 1983; 156:439–442.
32. Deykin D, Janson P, McMahon L. Ethanol potentiation of aspirin-induced prolongation of the bleeding time. *N Engl J Med* 1982;306: 852–854.
33. Fitzgerald GA, Meagher EA. Antiplatelet drugs. *Eur J Clin Invest* 1994; 24[Suppl 1]:46–49.
34. George JN, Shattil SJ. The clinical importance of acquired abnormalities of platelet function. *N Engl J Med* 1991;324:27–39.
35. Bennett JS. Novel platelet inhibitors. *Annu Rev Med* 2001;52: 161–184.
36. Patrono C, Coller B, Dalen JE, et al. Platelet-active drugs: the relationships among dose, effectiveness, and side effects. *Chest* 2001;119: 39S–63S.
37. Rizvi MA, Kojouri K, George JN. Drug-induced thrombocytopenia: an updated systematic review. *Ann Intern Med* 2001;134:346.
38. Levine MN, Raskob G, Landefeld S, et al. Hemorrhagic complications of anticoagulant treatment. *Chest* 2001;119:108S–121S.
39. Mannucci PM. Desmopressin (DDAVP) in the treatment of bleeding disorders: the first twenty years. *Haemophilia* 2000;6[Suppl 1]:60–67.
40. Lemmer JH Jr, Metzdorff MT, Krause AH Jr, et al. Emergency coronary artery bypass graft surgery in abciximab-treated patients. *Ann Thorac Surg* 2000;69:90–95.
41. Hirsh J, Dalen J, Anderson DR, et al. Oral anticoagulants: mechanism of action, clinical effectiveness, and optimal therapeutic range. *Chest* 2001;119:8S–21S.
42. Hirsh J, Warkentin TE, Shaughnessy SG, et al. Heparin and low-molecular-weight heparin: mechanisms of action, pharmacokinetics, dosing, monitoring, efficacy, and safety. *Chest* 2001;119:64S–94S.
43. Teoh KH, Young E, Bradley CA, et al. Heparin binding proteins: contribution to heparin rebound after cardiopulmonary bypass. *Circulation* 1993;88:420–425.
44. Baglin TP. Heparin induced thrombocytopenia thrombosis (HIT/T) syndrome: diagnosis and treatment. *J Clin Pathol* 2001;54:272–274.
45. Warkentin TE, Kelton JG. Temporal aspects of heparin-induced thrombocytopenia. *N Engl J Med* 2001;344:1286–1292.
46. Lewis BE, Wallis DE, Berkowitz SD, et al. Argatroban anticoagulant therapy in patients with heparin-induced thrombocytopenia. *Circulation* 2001;103:1838–1843.
47. Kearon C, Hirsh J. Management of anticoagulation before and after elective surgery. *N Engl J Med* 1997;336:1506–1511.
48. Levine MN, Hirsh J, Gent M, et al. A randomized trial comparing activated thromboplastin time with heparin assay in patients with acute venous thromboembolism requiring large daily doses of heparin. *Arch Intern Med* 1994;154:49–56.
49. DeLoughery TG. Management of bleeding with uremia and liver disease. *Curr Opin Hematol* 1999;6:329–333.
50. Crookston KP, Marsh CL, Chandler WL. A kinetic model of the circulatory regulation of tissue plasminogen activator during orthotopic liver transplantation. *Blood Coagul Fibrinolysis* 2000;11:79–88.
51. Smith CM, Yellin AE, Weaver FA, et al. Thrombolytic therapy for arterial occlusion: a mixed blessing. *Am Surg* 1994;60:371–375.
52. Rice L. Surreptitious bleeding in surgery: a major challenge in coagulation. *Clin Lab Haematol* 2000;22[Suppl 1]:17–20.
53. DiMichele DM, Hathaway WE. Use of DDAVP in inherited and acquired platelet dysfunction. *Am J Hematol* 1990;33:39–45.
54. Foster PF, Moore LR, Sankary HN, et al. Central venous catheterization in patients with coagulopathy. *Arch Surg* 1992;127:273–275.
55. Goldfarb G, Lebrec D. Percutaneous cannulation of the internal jugular vein in patients with coagulopathies: an experience based on 1,000 attempts. *Anesthesiology* 1982;56:321–323.
56. Howard SC, Gajjar A, Ribeiro RC, et al. Safety of lumbar puncture for children with acute lymphoblastic leukemia and thrombocytopenia. *JAMA* 2000;284:2222–2224.
57. Dzik S. The use of blood components prior to invasive bedside procedures: a critical appraisal. In: Mintz PD, ed. *Transfusion therapy: clinical principles and practice.* Bethesda, MD: American Association of Blood Banks, 1999:151–169.
58. Teitel JM. Unexpected bleeding disorders: algorithm for approach to therapy. *Clin Lab Haematol* 2000;22[Suppl 1]:26–29.
59. Mannucci PM. How I treat patients with von Willebrand disease. *Blood* 2001;97:1915–1919.
60. Tuthill DD, Bayer V, Gallagher AM, et al. Assessment of topical hemostats in a renal hemorrhage model in heparinized rats. *J Surg Res* 2001; 95:126–132.
61. Mojcik CF, Levy JH. Aprotinin and the systemic inflammatory response after cardiopulmonary bypass. *Ann Thorac Surg* 2001;71: 745–754.
62. Dietrich W, Spath P, Ebell A, et al. Prevalence of anaphylactic reactions to aprotinin: analysis of two hundred forty-eight reexposures to aprotinin in heart operations. *J Thorac Cardiovasc Surg* 1997;113:194–201.
63. Mannucci PM, Federici AB, Sirchia G. Hemostasis testing during massive blood replacement: a study of 172 cases. *Vox Sang* 1982;42: 113–123.
64. Reed RL, 2nd, Ciavarella D, Heimbach DM, et al. Prophylactic platelet administration during massive transfusion: a prospective, randomized, double-blind clinical study. *Ann Surg* 1986;203:40–48.
65. Ferrara A, MacArthur JD, Wright HK, et al. Hypothermia and acidosis

worsen coagulopathy in the patient requiring massive transfusion. *Am J Surg* 1990;160:515–518.
66. Martin DJ, Lucas CE, Ledgerwood AM, et al. Fresh frozen plasma supplement to massive red blood cell transfusion. *Ann Surg* 1985;202: 505–511.
67. Wilson RF, Binkley LE, Sabo FM Jr, et al. Electrolyte and acid-base changes with massive blood transfusions. *Am Surg* 1992;58:535–544.
68. Schonberger JP, van Oeveren W, Bredee JJ, et al. Systemic blood activation during and after autotransfusion. *Ann Thorac Surg* 1994;57: 1256–1262.
69. Reiss RF. Hemostatic defects in massive transfusion: rapid diagnosis and management. *Am J Crit Care* 2000;9:158–165.
70. Practice parameter for the use of fresh-frozen plasma, cryoprecipitate, and platelets. Fresh-Frozen Plasma, Cryoprecipitate, and Platelets Administration Practice Guidelines Development Task Force of the College of American Pathologists. *JAMA* 1994;271:777–781.
71. Harrigan C, Lucas CE, Ledgerwood AM, et al. Serial changes in primary hemostasis after massive transfusion. *Surgery* 1985;98:836–844.
72. Phillips TF, Soulier G, Wilson RF. Outcome of massive transfusion exceeding two blood volumes in trauma and emergency surgery. *J Trauma* 1987;27:903–910.
73. Levi M, Ten Cate H. Disseminated intravascular coagulation. *N Engl J Med* 1999;341:586–592.
74. Chandler WL. The human fibrinolytic system. *Crit Rev Oncol Hematol* 1996;24:27–45.
75. Fisher DF, Jr., Yawn DH, Crawford ES. Preoperative disseminated intravascular coagulation associated with aortic aneurysms: a prospective study of 76 cases. *Arch Surg* 1983;118:1252–1255.
76. Lee WL, Downey GP. Coagulation inhibitors in sepsis and disseminated intravascular coagulation. *Intensive Care Med* 2000;26: 1701–1706.
77. Hardy JF, Perrault J, Tremblay N, et al. The stratification of cardiac surgical procedures according to use of blood products: a retrospective analysis of 1480 cases. *Can J Anaesth* 1991;38:511–517.
78. Rosengart TK, Helm RE, DeBois WJ, et al. Open heart operations without transfusion using a multimodality blood conservation strategy in 50 Jehovah's Witness patients: implications for a "bloodless" surgical technique. *J Am Coll Surg* 1997;184:618–629.
79. Spiess BD, Ley C, Body SC, et al. Hematocrit value on intensive care unit entry influences the frequency of Q-wave myocardial infarction after coronary artery bypass grafting. The Institutions of the Multicenter Study of Perioperative Ischemia (McSPI) Research Group. *J Thorac Cardiovasc Surg* 1998;116:460–467.
80. Munoz JJ, Birkmeyer NJ, Dacey LJ, et al. Trends in rates of reexploration for hemorrhage after coronary artery bypass surgery. Northern New England Cardiovascular Disease Study Group. *Ann Thorac Surg* 1999;68:1321–1325.
81. Despotis GJ, Goodnough LT. Management approaches to platelet-related microvascular bleeding in cardiothoracic surgery. *Ann Thorac Surg* 2000;70:S20–32.
82. Gravlee GP, Arora S, Lavender SW, et al. Predictive value of blood clotting tests in cardiac surgical patients. *Ann Thorac Surg* 1994;58: 216–221.
83. Carr JA, Silverman N. The heparin-protamine interaction: a review. *J Cardiovasc Surg (Torino)* 1999;40:659–666.
84. Cattaneo M, Harris AS, Stromberg U, et al. The effect of desmopressin on reducing blood loss in cardiac surgery: a meta-analysis of double-blind, placebo-controlled trials. *Thromb Haemost* 1995;74:1064–1070.
85. Levi M, Cromheecke ME, de Jonge E, et al. Pharmacological strategies to decrease excessive blood loss in cardiac surgery: a meta-analysis of clinically relevant endpoints. *Lancet* 1999;354:1940–1947.
86. Verstraete M. Clinical application of inhibitors of fibrinolysis. *Drugs* 1985;29:236–261.
87. Risberg B. Current research review: surgery and fibrinolysis. *J Surg Res* 1979;26:698–715.
88. Watts DD, Trask A, Soeken K, et al. Hypothermic coagulopathy in trauma: effect of varying levels of hypothermia on enzyme speed, platelet function, and fibrinolytic activity. *J Trauma* 1998;44:846–854.

Rossi's Principles of Transfusion Medicine, Third Edition, edited by Toby L. Simon, Walter H. Dzik, Edward L. Snyder, Christopher P. Stowell, and Ronald G. Strauss. Lippincott Williams & Wilkins, Philadelphia

43

TRANSFUSION THERAPY IN SOLID-ORGAN TRANSPLANTATION

GLENN RAMSEY

ORGAN TRANSPLANTATION SCENE

Organ transplantation is at once a life-extending tour de force of modern medicine and a routine operation performed dozens of times a day (1). The blood bank has a vital place on the hospital-wide team that makes transplantation possible for severely ill patients. Approximately 1% of all red blood cell (RBC) and platelet transfusions and approximately 5% of all plasma and cryoprecipitate transfusions are used in organ transplantation surgery (2).

In the United States, 261 programs perform organ transplantation. Table 43.1 shows the number of transplants of each organ performed in the United States in 1999 (3). Also shown are the 3-year graft and patient survival percentages for transplantation procedures performed on adults in the United States in 1995–1996 with follow-up data through 1999. Pediatric results are similar.

ORGAN PROCUREMENT

In the United States, the federal government established the National Organ Procurement and Transplantation Network, which began in 1987 (1). The United Network for Organ Sharing, in Richmond, Virginia, holds the contract from the U.S. Department of Health and Human Services for managing the Organ Procurement and Transplantation Network. The United Network for Organ Sharing oversees all aspects of procurement, organ sharing, and waiting lists and compiles statistical information on donor and patient activity and outcome. Organ procurement is coordinated by 59 regional and local organ procurement organizations, which are approved and regulated by Health and Human Services. Organ donation is widely promoted, and hospitals are required by Medicare to evaluate all deaths for eligibility to donate organs. The organ procurement organization usually obtains the necessary consent from the next of kin in concert with the deceased person's physicians.

The circulation of a brain-dead donor is maintained until the organs are harvested by transplantation surgeons. Sometimes blood component transfusions are needed for oxygenation and hemostasis. After cadaveric organs are removed, the hearts and lungs must be used within 4 to 6 hours, liver within 12 hours, pancreas within 16 hours, and kidneys within 18 to 30 hours. Preservative solutions are used during cold ischemia until transplantation.

The systems for ranking the priorities of patients are specific for each organ and incorporate severity of illness and waiting time. For each organ within a region, the patient waiting lists are compiled according to ABO blood group, although patients

G. Ramsey: Department of Pathology, Northwestern University School of Medicine, Chicago, Illinois.

TABLE 43.1. U.S. ORGAN TRANSPLANTS, WAITING LISTS, AND ADULT 3-YEAR GRAFT AND PATIENT SURVIVAL RATES

Organ	1999 Transplants	2000 Waiting List	Graft Survival Rate (%)	Patient Survival Rate (%)
Kidney	12,483	47,770	79	91
Kidney and pancreas	946	2,466	83 Kidney 76 Pancreas	90
Liver	4,698	16,839	69	76
Heart	2,185	4,147	77	77
Lung	885	3,688	55	56
Heart-lung	49	207	55	55
Pancreas	363	1,025	51	88
Intestine	70	151	45	49

Some patients are listed for more than one organ or at more than one center. Waiting lists are as of December 30, 2000. Survival rates are for transplantation procedures performed in 1995–1996 with 3 years of follow-up evaluation (3).

who need urgent treatment may receive an ABO-unmatched transplant (e.g., O to A) if necessary.

Cadaveric kidney donations have a slightly longer timeframe than that of other organs. Patients can be maintained on dialysis, and the kidneys can be stored long enough for HLA matching, crossmatch compatibility, and shipping across regions if warranted. Patients who are six-antigen HLA-A, B, and DR matches receive the highest priority because of slightly better graft survival.

For each transplantation performed, two to four persons are on the waiting lists for each organ (Table 43.1). Organs and organ donors are still scarce. The need for organs has stimulated efforts to expand the supply by using organs from living donors and by splitting livers. Approximately one fourth of the kidney transplantation procedures performed in the United States are from living donors. The graft and patient survival rates are better than for renal transplantation from cadavers. A small but cautiously growing number of liver transplants are from living donors, from whom the right lobe is removed. Cadaveric livers sometimes are split. The right lobe is given to one patient and the rest of the liver to another patient. Both the graft split liver and the living donor's liver regenerate to normal size in a few weeks.

Like blood donors, organ donors, both cadaver and living, are screened and tested for transmissible diseases and infectious agents. Unlike blood, however, organs from donors who have antibody to hepatitis B core antigen are used by some programs in operations on patients with hepatitis B. Some programs accept donors with hepatitis C for patients with hepatitis C. The U.S. Food and Drug Administration (FDA) has issued rules for infectious disease testing of organ donors (4). If a cadaver donor has received voluminous transfusions and fluids before death, hemodilution of the plasma can lead to false-negative results of testing for viral markers. Therefore the FDA requires that a pretransfusion sample be tested whenever large infusions have been administered. The donor hospital transfusion service may be asked to provide the compatibility-testing specimen for this purpose, because it is available for at least 7 days.

IMMUNOSUPPRESSION

Much of the credit for the modern clinical success of transplantation is due to the immunosuppressive medications used to prevent and manage rejection (5). Cyclosporine (Sandimmune, Neoral, SangCyA) and tacrolimus (formerly FK-506; Prograf) suppress T-cell activation. These drugs block the activity of calcineurin, a crucial cytosolic protein in the major signaling pathway leading to interleukin-2 gene activation. Rapamycin (sirolimus, Rapamune) inhibits various effects of interleukin-2. Daclizumab (Zenapax) and basiliximab (Simulect) are monoclonal antibodies that bind to and block the interleukin-2a receptor on T cells. Prednisone suppresses cytokines in the inflammatory response and affects cell migration. Azathioprine (Imuran) and the newer, less toxic mycophenolate mofetil (CellCept) inhibit T-cell and B-cell proliferation by blocking nucleic acid synthesis. Antilymphocyte antibodies for managing rejection are formulated as polyclonal preparations from horses (Atgam) or rabbits (Thymoglobulin), or as a murine monoclonal antibody (Orthoclone; OKT3). More agents are under development to block other steps in the signaling pathways of the immune response.

IMMUNOHEMATOLOGY

ABO Transplantation Barrier

The fundamental test for organ donation and transplantation is the ABO group, because solid organs almost always must be ABO compatible. Anti-A and anti-B antibodies bind to endothelial cells, setting off a cycle of complement fixation, vascular damage, and thrombosis that leads to ischemia and rejection. ABO-incompatible liver transplants are less susceptible to hyperacute rejection than are other organs. The transplantation procedure occasionally is performed in extreme emergencies, but the risk of eventual rejection is still high. As group O RBCs are sometimes in shortest supply in relation to demand, so are group O organs. Group O patients often wait longer than other patients for nonemergency cadaveric transplantation.

In efforts to extend organ availability, there have been two approaches to surmounting the ABO barrier in renal transplantation. A few centers have investigated transplantation of ABO-incompatible kidneys (6,7). When intensive immunosuppression and plasmapheresis are used to temporarily lower antibody levels, respectable results are achieved.

The other strategy is to use A_2 kidneys for O or B patients or A_2B kidneys for B patients. Twenty percent of group A persons are A_2. Their RBCs have approximately one-fourth the content of A_1 persons, and the same is true of their endothelial cells and other organ group A antigens. The A_2 antigen also is qualitatively different, with fewer repeating A-epitopes, from the A_1 antigen (see Chapter 8). In the largest U.S. experience, prospective recipients of A_2 organs had their anti-A titers assessed

(8,9). Approximately 30% of group O patients and 75% of group B patients had anti-A levels considered low enough to receive an A_2 transplant. Standard immunosuppression is used, along with plasmapheresis if the anti-A level increases after transplantation. Results are comparable with those for ABO-matched transplantation.

Another use of intentional ABO-incompatible organ transplantation is care of neonates who need scarce cardiac grafts (10). Because these patients have not yet developed ABO antibodies, ABO-incompatible hearts have been successfully implanted without hyperacute rejection. In the initial experience, long-term survival was similar to that of ABO-compatible transplants, and the mortality of infants on the center's waiting list decreased from 58% to 7%. In many clinical studies of ABO-incompatible transplants, however, the titration methods for evaluating anti-A or anti-B levels are not well defined or are not standard techniques. Immunosuppressive agents that help block antibody responses, such as mycophenolate mofetil, may play an adjunctive role in breaching the ABO barrier.

Patient Alloantibodies

In the 1980s, 6% to 8% of adult recipients of kidney or liver transplants had clinically significant RBC alloantibodies. Another 8% of recipients of a liver developed antibodies after the large number of transfusions given during surgery (11,12). Both of these patient groups now are receiving fewer transfusions before and during surgery. Most patients with renal failure receive erythropoietin. Patients with cirrhosis often are treated to reduce variceal bleeding from portal hypertension with medications to reduce venous pressure (β-blockers, octreotide), sclerotherapy or band ligation of varices, and if necessary, transjugular intrahepatic portosystemic shunting. Consequently, pretransplantation RBC antibody problems are less frequent than they were in the past.

Advance screening for the presence of antibodies to non-ABO antigens is still advisable for candidates for liver transplantation. Some liver transplantation patients have a complex antibody problem, and the supply of antigen-negative units is limited. The following strategy has been successful in my program: (a) give at least the first blood volume of RBCs as compatible antigen negative, (b) after this degree of hemodilution of the antibodies, give antigen-positive units, (c) reserve additional antigen-negative units for after surgery, when transfusions return to small volumes and the antibodies may return anamnestically after immune stimulation (13).

When Rh-negative patients need large amounts of RBCs during liver or other organ transplantation, it may be necessary to give Rh-positive RBCs. Follow-up tests show that these patients usually do not make anti-D antibodies (14). Transplantation immunosuppression greatly reduces the expected high rate of Rh sensitization among patients with normal immune function. HLA alloantibodies against the donor can cause prompt rejection of renal and cardiac grafts. Candidates for this type of transplantation undergo periodic HLA antibody tests, and then HLA cross-matching against donor lymphocytes to confirm compatibility.

Antibodies from Passenger Lymphocytes

Like hematopoietic stem cell transplants, organ transplants contain lymphocytes that sometimes can make antibodies against antigens in the recipient (15). This is most common when group O organs are placed into non-O patients. In approximately 40% of liver transplant recipients and 10% of kidney recipients, the patient develops IgG antibodies from graft lymphocytes against his or her own A or B antigens. A few cases have been caused by A or B organs in group AB patients. The patient's direct antiglobulin test becomes reactive 1 to 2 weeks after transplantation, and some of these antibodies produce sudden marked hemolysis. The antibodies typically persist for a few weeks. Immunoglobulin allotyping has proved that these antibodies are of donor origin and are not patient autoantibodies. This phenomenon emerged after azathioprine for immunosuppression was replaced by cyclosporine, which is more permissive for secondary antibody responses, and it has occurred with tacrolimus as well.

Non-ABO RBC antibodies can develop in a similar manner when the organ donor is alloimmunized against an antigen in the recipient. Rh and other antibodies have been reported, and some have caused temporary hemolysis (15,16). Women donating kidneys to their children or their partner sometimes transmit pregnancy-induced antibodies. When an organ donor is found to have a large number of RBC alloantibodies, it may be prudent to notify the organ procurement agency or in the case of a living donor the recipient's physician. If a donor is known to have a clinically significant RBC alloantibody, patients in my program receive RBC transfusions that are negative for the target antigen whether the patient is antigen positive or antigen negative.

Anti-platelet antibodies have been transferred from organs of a donor who died of cerebral hemorrhage due to immune thrombocytopenic purpura (17). Perhaps any antibody in the organ donor can be temporarily transferred to the recipient.

Anti-α-Galactose in Xenotransplantation

Another possible method for increasing the supply of transplant organs is to use animals, particularly pigs (18). However, the presence of anti-α-galactose is a major antibody barrier resulting in hyperacute rejection of xenografts. Residues containing α-galactose are the immunodominant carbohydrate antigens in mammals other than humans and Old World monkeys. These residues are the target of rejection similar in pathogenesis to ABO incompatibility. All humans have naturally occurring antibodies to α-galactose. This antigen resembles the group B galactose antigen (Fig. 43.1). Because some of the naturally occurring anti-α-galactose cross-reacts in vitro with group B cells, a significant proportion of the anti-B antibody observed in routine blood bank testing is actually anti-α-galactose (19). However, group B and AB persons also have anti-α-galactose, and xenotransplants probably would not be more compatible in them than in group O or A persons.

Lewis Blood Group in Organ Transplantation

Lewis antigens are present in secretory tissues, including the renal tubules. Conflicting data were reported in the 1980s on

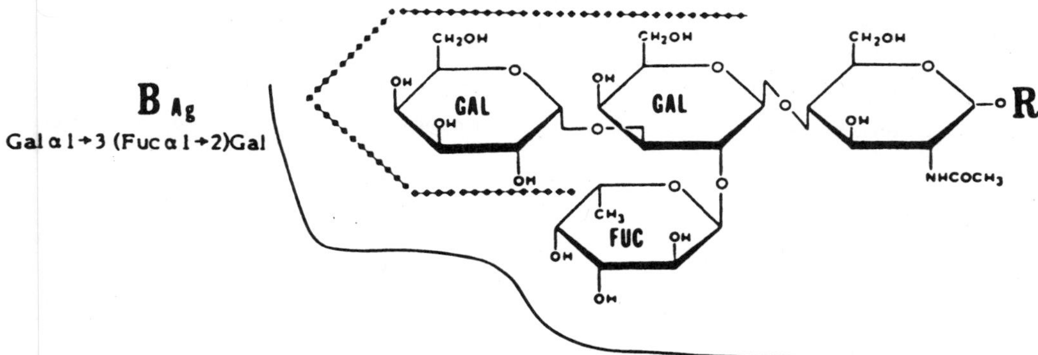

FIGURE 43.1. α-1,3-Galactose (α-galactose) is the major animal tissue antigen target in the hyperacute rejection of xenotransplants. α-Galactose is similar to the human group B antigen. *CPH,* ceramide pentahexose containing the α-galactose antigen. *Dark hatched line,* binding site of anti-α-galactose. *Dotted line,* anti-α-galactose in group A or group O sera binding to the group B antigen. *Solid line,* B antigen for anti-B. (From Galili U, Buehler J, Shohet SB, et al. The human natural anti-Gal IgG, III: the subtlety of immune tolerance in man as demonstrated by crossreactivity between natural anti-Gal and anti-B antibodies. *J Exp Med* 1987;165:693–704, with permission of the Rockefeller University Press.)

whether Lewis-antigen-positive kidneys in Lewis-antigen-negative recipients represented an independent risk factor for graft survival (20,21). However, Lewis antibodies in a recipient of a kidney transplant may be problematic. Terasaki et al. (22) in 1988 reported that repeat renal graft survival was sharply reduced when the recipient had Lewis antibodies against the Lewis antigens of the graft. Whether this is a factor with current immunosuppression has not been investigated.

Lewis antigens on RBCs are adsorbed from the plasma. The source of plasma Lewis antigens is uncertain, but the small intestine has been proposed (23). It has abundant amounts of Lewis antigens in configurations similar to those in the plasma. In my program, the laboratory has found that candidates for small-intestinal transplantation, most of whom have undergone complete resection of the small intestine for various problems, have the RBC phenotype Le(a − b −) (24). This supports the concept that RBC Lewis antigens originate in the small intestine. As experience with small-intestinal transplantation grows, it should be possible to assess whether the RBC Lewis antigens of a recipient of a small-intestinal transplant change to those of the donor, when they are different, and whether RBC Lewis expression could be clinically useful in monitoring graft function.

BLOOD TRANSFUSION NEEDS

Table 43.2 shows recent data for mean blood component usage in organ transplantation. Primary cardiac transplantation without previous cardiac surgery is similar to routine cardiac surgery, but use of components increases in operations on patients who have undergone previous sternotomy. The use of aprotinin in the care of patients undergoing second operations reduced overall blood component needs in a randomized study (25). Patients undergoing transplantation after use of a cardiac support device need large amounts of blood, even when treated with aprotinin, in part because of anticoagulation before transplantation (26). Double-lung transplantation uses more blood than does single-lung transplantation. Uncomplicated renal transplantation usually is a type-and-screen procedure. As shown in Figure 43.2, blood component transfusions for liver transplantation are quite variable. Although some patients need large amounts of blood, the median perioperative use for adults at my center is 7 units of RBCs, 8 units of plasma, and one platelet dose. Living donors of liver and kidney grafts usually do not need transfusions. However, advance autologous donation of 2 units of RBCs by liver donors may be prudent.

TABLE 43.2. MEAN BLOOD COMPONENT USAGE IN ORGAN TRANSPLANTATION

Organ	Red Blood Cells	Plasma	Platelets	Reference
Liver				
Adult	12	15	11	NMH
Pediatric ≥20 kg	9	13	8	CMH
Pediatric <20 kg	6	7	4	CMH
Cardiac				
Primary	1	1–3	1–4	25,26
Repeated sternotomy	1–2	1–6	1–8	25,26
After support device (with aprotinin)	8	13	12	26
Lung				
Single	2	1	2	27
Double	6	4	6	27
Pancreas	2	0	0	28
Kidney	1	0	0	29

Units are rounded to whole numbers. Platelets are expressed as platelet concentrates, with apheresis units counted as 6 units. The perioperative liver transplantation data shown here include use during the operation and through the first day after the operation. The cardiac transplantation range is from two centers. In one center, aprotinin reduced overall component transfusions in repeated sternotomy cases in a randomized study (25).
NMH and CMH, Northwestern Memorial Hospital (n = 106) and Children's Memorial Hospital (n = 58 <20 kg, 34 ≥20 kg), Northwestern University, Chicago, 1997–2000.

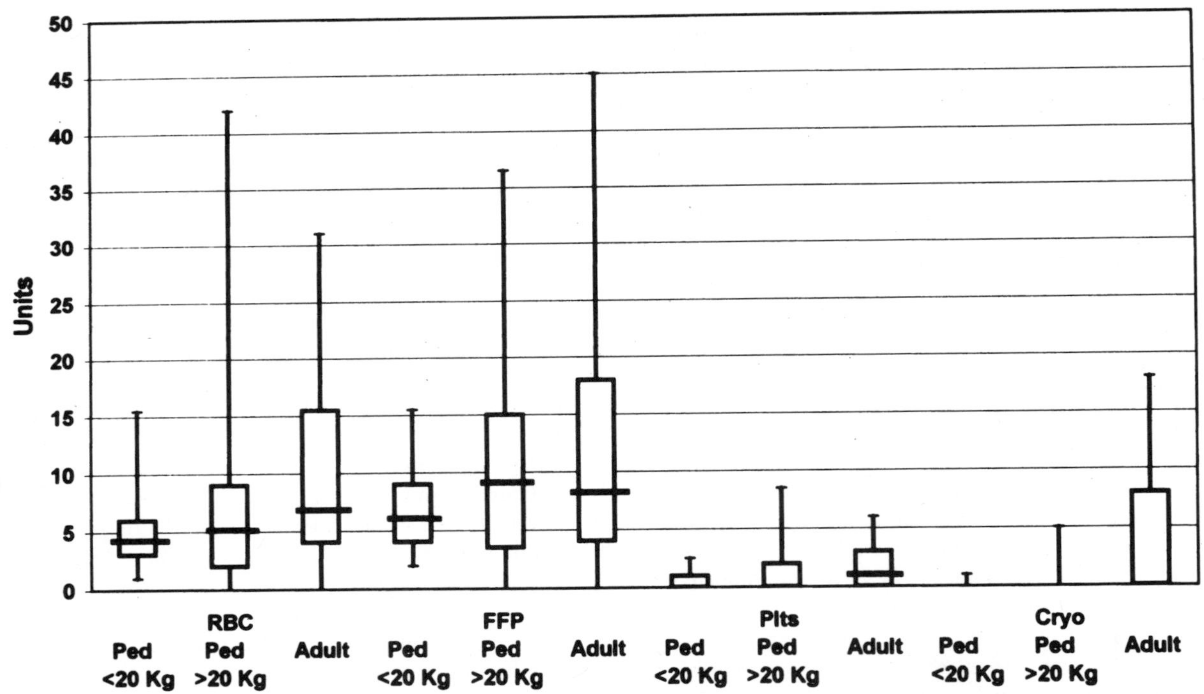

FIGURE 43.2. Perioperative blood use in adult and pediatric liver transplantation, Northwestern Memorial Hospital and Children's Memorial Hospital, Chicago, 1997–2000. Figures include the operation through the day after the operation. *Boxes,* 25th and 75th percentiles. *Whiskers,* 5th and 95th percentiles. *Lines,* medians. When *no line* is present, the median is zero. Platelets are expressed as plateletpheresis units.

LIVER TRANSPLANTATION

The various indications for liver transplantation have been reviewed elsewhere (1). Hepatitis C cirrhosis is the leading cause, and many of these infections are attributed to past blood transfusions from before the discovery of the virus.

The liver transplantation operation is simple in concept, but complex complications can develop at any time (30). In the preanhepatic first stage, the vascular and biliary connections of the liver are dissected and exposed—portal vein, bile duct, hepatic artery, and inferior vena cava. The liver is separated from the diaphragm and the retroperitoneum, often exposing a raw, bare surface prone to bleeding. In the typical procedure, the major vessels are clamped, the vascular and bile duct connections are transected, and the liver is removed. The first stage usually takes 4 to 8 hours. In the anhepatic second stage, the graft and recipient suprahepatic and infrahepatic vena cava and portal vein are anastomosed end to end. The liver is flushed to remove most of its preservative solution. This second stage usually takes 1 to 1.5 hours. At the beginning of the third stage, the post-anhepatic stage, the large vessels are unclamped to restore portal inflow, and the hepatic artery and bile duct are connected. If all goes well, the third stage is completed in 2 to 4 hours. The anastomoses are diagrammed in Figure 43.3.

Liver transplantation presents a unique set of challenges for transfusion and hemostasis needs. Patients with acute liver failure have low levels of clotting factors. Patients with cirrhosis also usually have thrombocytopenia due to splenomegaly and low levels of thrombopoietin, much of which is made by the liver. Platelet function may be reduced by liver failure, uremia in hepatorenal syndrome, or anemia. On the other hand, some patients may have a hypercoagulability syndrome due to high levels of factor VIII and decreased levels of fibrinolytic proteins.

During the operation, certain problems can arise in each stage. During dissection, portal hypertension can contribute to venous bleeding from the areas around the liver. Before and during the anhepatic stage, fibrinolysis sometimes develops from imbalance of its inhibitors and promoters. The graft is flushed, but when the new liver is unclamped, the patient often is partly anticoagulated by heparin present from the donor's anticoagulation and by heparin-like substances from injured endothelium released into the circulation.

To counteract all the possible problems, the liver transplantation, anesthesia, and laboratory team uses an array of tactics to meet the transfusion and hemostatic needs of the patient. Surgeons use an argon-beam laser to coagulate bleeding surfaces. Two surgical techniques are used in the care of selected patients to improve hemodynamics. If the anatomic features of the graft

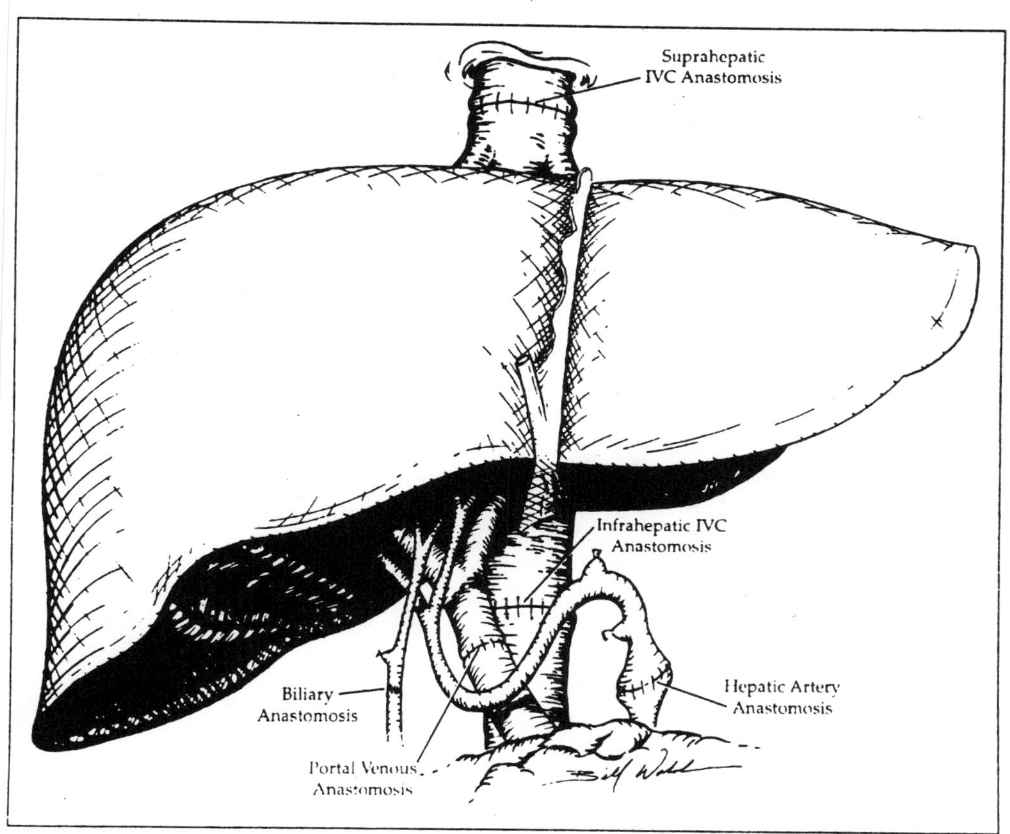

FIGURE 43.3. A conventional liver transplant has anastomoses to the suprahepatic and infrahepatic vena cava, the portal vein, the hepatic artery, and the common bile duct. (From Stuart FP, Abecassis MM, Kaufman DB, eds. *Organ transplantation.* Georgetown, TX: Landes Bioscience, 2000:186, with permission. Illustration by William E. Walsh, CMI.)

are favorable, the liver can be sewn on to the inferior vena cava in a so-called piggyback manner to maintain partial blood flow through the vena cava during the operation. Some surgeons use venovenous bypass during the anhepatic stage, either routinely or if interruption of vena caval flow causes too much hypotension. This perfusion technique shunts venous return from the inferior vena cava and the portal vein up to the subclavian vein and improves cardiac output if needed.

To monitor coagulation status and to anticipate transfusion needs, hemoglobin, platelet count, prothrombin time, activated partial thromboplastin time, and fibrinogen are measured regularly. Many programs use thromboelastography (TEG) to supplement routine clotting tests (31). The TEG instrument measures the initiation, rate, and strength of whole-blood clotting, displays the results in the operating room as they develop over 20 to 60 minutes, and has the following three functions not available in routine coagulation testing: (a) Fibrinolysis can be readily detected. (b) The patient's blood can be tested in vitro with protamine or ϵ-aminocaproic acid to assess whether these medications would help correct heparinization or fibrinolysis. (c) Hypercoagulability, although not as well clinically correlated as its opposite, is observed in some patients' TEG results.

To meet the patient's transfusion needs, intraoperative blood salvage is helpful. One-third or more of the patient's total RBC transfusions can be provided by recovering shed blood during the operation. The anesthesiologist can give large volumes of warmed blood and fluids through a rapid-infusion pump that delivers more than 1 L per minute if necessary.

Plasma usage usually closely parallels RBC use in operations with large transfusion needs, in effect reconstituting whole blood for the transfusions. If available, whole blood is suitable for the first blood volume or so, because these patients usually have normal levels of factor VIII. Solvent-detergent plasma has been used successfully, although it may be deficient in some antifibrinolytic proteins (32,33).

In my program, approximately 15% of adults need more than 40 units of RBCs. Although some of these patients have preoperative coagulopathy, this usually can be corrected with appropriate transfusions in the first stage of the transplantation procedure. The underlying factors in these large hemorrhages usually are intraoperative problems such as unusually severe portal hypertension, cardiopulmonary instability, and anatomic and technical complications causing surgical blood loss. These problems often are not predictable from the patient's transplantation evaluation, and large blood use frequently is unexpected.

Prophylactic intraoperative administration of antifibrinolytic agents was studied in two double-blind, randomized trials. Tranexamic acid (not available in the United States) reduced the number of transfusions compared with needs when ϵ-aminocaproic acid or placebo was used (34). Two dosage levels of aprotinin reduced blood use compared with the need when a placebo was used (35). No differences in the rates of thrombotic complications were seen in these studies, although this is still a concern for some investigators (36).

Even without medications, thrombosis, either systemic or localized to the hepatic artery, is an occasional complication during liver transplantation operations. In some patients, this complication is associated with hypercoagulability found during TEG, and moderate heparinization may be advisable. Aggressive correction of coagulopathy should be avoided when clotting would present special difficulties, as during venovenous bypass, or when the hepatic artery is small or not flowing well.

SPECIAL NEEDS

Prevention of Cytomegalovirus Infection

Cytomegalovirus (CMV) infection is a major infectious complication of organ transplantation because of the cellular immunosuppression needed. If a candidate for solid-organ transplantation is anti-CMV negative, cellular blood products should be CMV safe (37). When an anti-CMV-negative transplant recipient receives an anti-CMV-negative organ, CMV-safe transfusions are recommended when possible to prevent third-party CMV infection from the blood donor. The growing availability of leukoreduced products has increased the supply of CMV-safe products for liver transplantation operations.

For patients who are already anti-CMV-positive or who receive an anti-CMV-positive graft, CMV-safe transfusion generally is not necessary. The risk of CMV infection comes from the new organ or from reactivation of the original infection. There is no evidence to date of transfusion-transmitted CMV disease in a patient who already had CMV infection. A second strain of CMV from the organ donor has caused disease in anti-CMV-positive organ recipients, but second-strain infections from transfusion have not been documented (see Chapter 52).

Leukoreduction

The leukoreduction of blood components for organ transplantation presents a paradox. This is one clinical setting in which transfused white blood cells were historically beneficial (38). In the 1970s and early 1980s, transfusions were commonly given to candidates for renal transplantation to achieve better graft survival. Red blood cell transfusions leukoreduced by means of freezing and thawing did not render the same advantage. The effect was attributed to immunosuppression by transfused white blood cells. When immunosuppression improved, the transfusion advantage decreased. Opelz et al. (39), however, have found evidence that even in the cyclosporine era, there is still a slight advantage in renal graft survival when the patient has undergone transfusion before transplantation. Recipients of liver transplants who had undergone previous transfusions had fewer rejection episodes than did patients who had not undergone transfusion (40).

The other side of the paradox is that if the transplant recipient has previous HLA antibodies against the prospective graft kidney, transplantation is contraindicated because rejection of these organs may ensue. From this perspective, leukoreduction of pretransplant transfusions would be desirable to prevent difficulty in finding a compatible transplant. HLA alloimmunization also adversely affects survival of heart and lung grafts.

The balance of current opinion probably falls on the side of leukoreduction to avoid development of HLA antibodies in candidates for kidney, heart, and lung transplantation. Research continues on transfusion immunomodulation in transplantation (see Chapter 60).

Blood Irradiation

Graft versus host disease (GVHD) has occurred from passenger leukocytes in transplanted organs. However, GVHD from transfusions in these patients is rare (41). Solid-organ transplantation usually is not included in recommended indications for blood irradiation (see Chapter 59).

Microchimerism and Stem Cell Transplantation

Starzl and others have advanced the paradigm that in organ transplantation, the continuing presence of donor leukocytes in the body after transplantation helps induce immune tolerance against the graft, not unlike transfusion immunomodulation (42). In large-scale investigations, bone marrow cells from the same cadaveric donor as the organ have been given at the time of transplantation. Rejection episodes were reduced in some of these studies, compared with controls, but benefits in graft survival have been limited to date.

Applications of Therapeutic Apheresis

Therapeutic apheresis has several applications in organ transplantation for providing plasma, managing rejection, and controlling complications. In the care of patients with critically severe liver failure, plasma exchange sometimes is performed to assist with temporary metabolic and hemostatic support while a new liver is sought. Plasma exchange has been performed to reduce the level of HLA antibodies causing transplant rejection and the level of ABO antibodies in patients receiving ABO-incompatible organ transplants.

Photopheresis is under study as therapy for organ rejection (43,44). In this process, as in the management of T-cell lymphoma, the patient is given psoralen, which binds to circulating cellular DNA. Lymphocytopheresis is performed, and the harvested cells are exposed to ultraviolet light before they are reinfused. The ultraviolet light cross-links the DNA and suppresses the proliferative immune response of the cell to the graft. Initial results in heart and lung transplantation have been promising.

Posttransplantation immunosuppression sometimes is associated with the development of thrombotic thrombocytopenic purpura or hemolytic uremic syndrome. Plasma exchange has been used to manage these disorders.

ARTIFICIAL ORGANS

Numerous types of ventricular assist devices are in use or under development for the care of patients with severe cardiac failure (45). Some are for temporary use or use as a bridge to cardiac transplantation. Others are intended for permanent implantation. While using these devices, patients often have coagulopathy from platelet dysfunction or anticoagulation. Mechanical hemolysis may occur from shearing in the pump. Transfusions during these treatments can cause HLA alloimmunization, and leukoreduction should be performed if transplantation is planned.

Hepatic assist devices are perfused with the patient's blood or plasma to remove toxins (46). These systems are in clinical trials to support patients until their liver recovers, as in poisoning, or until a liver transplant is available. One category of these systems passes the blood through various absorbent materials such as charcoal, resins, or albumin. The other type metabolizes toxins in the blood with immobilized porcine or human hepatocytes in a perfused bioreactor.

XENOTRANSPLANTATION

Pigs are the most likely potential source of animal organs for human transplantation, because their size and anatomic features are somewhat similar to those of humans. Unlike primates, pigs are not endangered, and use of these animals for human consumption and other purposes is widely accepted (47). The heart and the liver would be the most useful organs. Early research protocols have aimed at temporary use of pig organs to treat severely ill patients until a human organ becomes available. In addition to in vivo transplantation of the pig heart and liver, the pig liver can be perfused in an ex vivo blood circuit to provide temporary metabolism of toxins without the need for surgical implantation. Reduction of levels of anti-α-galactose antibody may help such patients, either through regular plasmapheresis or through immunoadsorption of antibody from the patient's plasma. Plasma products needed for hemostatic support also have anti-α-galactose, of course, and immunoadsorption of the plasma's antibody before transfusion in such patients has been proposed.

To help ameliorate the barrier of hyperacute rejection by anti-α-galactose antibodies, transgenic pigs were produced with the human genes for the complement-inactivating proteins CD55 (decay-accelerating factor, DAF, which incidentally gives these pigs the human Cromer blood group) and CD59 (membrane inhibitor of reactive lysis, MIRL). The human *PIG-A* gene is needed for the RBC membrane attachment of these proteins (see Chapter 10). The presence of these human proteins on the endothelium of the transgenic animal inhibits activation of the patient's complement cascade and therefore reduces vascular injury and inflammation.

Pigs have been cloned, which further advances the prospects of genetic manipulations to promote graft tolerance (48). Cloning and gene transfer may make it possible to reduce α-galactose expression, or perhaps even replace α-galactose with the human H carbohydrate antigen, resulting in "humanized" group O pigs.

Concern about novel infections transmitted from animal organs has slowed clinical research in xenotransplantation. All pigs carry a porcine retrovirus, although no human infections or diseases have been recognized from exposures to porcine heart valves or porcine clotting factor concentrates. As a precaution, the FDA is considering prohibition of blood donation by recipients of xenotransplants and their contacts (49). The prospects for human xenotransplantation are long term at this time, but research is continuing.

SUMMARY

Since the early 1980s, organ transplantation has grown dramatically. With more experience, medications, and other therapies, the average transfusion needs for each patient have declined. Unfortunately, as the success rate increases, the field is limited by an insufficient supply of organs to treat all the patients whose lives could be extended by transplantation. In the next 20 years, we can look forward to additional means to replace the functions of failing body systems, including artificial organs, cellular transplants, tissue engineering to build new organs, the use of animal tissues and organs, and immune system modulation to prevent graft rejection. Transfusion medicine will continue to be a vital partner in the management of organ failure.

REFERENCES

1. Stuart FP, Abecassis MM, Kaufman DB, eds. *Organ transplantation.* Georgetown, TX: Landes Bioscience, 2000.
2. Ramsey G, Sherman LA. The new age of organic blood banking. *Transfusion* 1998;38:9–11.
3. UNOS Transplant Patient DataSource. United Network for Organ Sharing, Richmond, VA, January 2001. Available at: www.unos.org.
4. US Food and Drug Administration. Guidance for industry: screening and testing of donors of human tissue intended for transplantation. Bethesda, MD: US Food and Drug Administration, 1997.
5. Stuart FP. Immunosuppression. In: Stuart FP, Abecassis MM, Kaufman DB, eds. *Organ transplantation.* Georgetown, TX: Landes Bioscience, 2000:45–59.
6. Alexandre GPJ, Squifflet JP, De Bruyère M, et al. Present experience in a series of 26 ABO-incompatible living donor renal allografts. *Transplant Proc* 1987;19:4538–4542.
7. Tanabe K, Takahashi K, Sonda K, et al. Long-term results of ABO-incompatible living kidney transplantation: a single-center experience. *Transplantation* 1998;65:224–228.
8. Nelson PW, Landreneau MD, Luger AM, et al. Ten-year experience in transplantation of A_2 kidneys into B and O recipients. *Transplantation* 1998;65:256–260.
9. Nelson PW, Hughes TM, Beck ML, et al. Stratification and successful transplantation of patients awaiting ABO-incompatible (A_2 into B and O) transplantation by A-isoagglutinin-titer phenogroup. *Transplant Proc* 1996;28:221–223.
10. West LJ, Pollock-Barziv SM, Dipchand AI, et al. ABO-incompatible heart transplantation in infants. *N Engl J Med* 2001;344:793–800.
11. Brantley SG, Ramsey G. Red cell alloimmunization in multitransfused HLA-typed patients. *Transfusion* 1988;28:496–498.
12. Ramsey G, Cornell FW, Hahn LF, et al. Red cell antibody problems in 1000 liver transplants. *Transfusion* 1989;29:396–400.
13. Ramsey G, Cornell FW, Hahn LF, et al. Incompatible blood transfusions in liver transplant patients with significant red cell alloantibodies. *Transplant Proc* 1989;21:3531.
14. Ramsey G, Hahn LF, Cornell FW, et al. Low rate of Rhesus immunization from Rh-incompatible blood transfusions during liver and heart transplant surgery. *Transplantation* 1989;47:993–995.
15. Ramsey G. Red cell antibodies arising from solid organ transplants. *Transfusion* 1991;31:76–86.
16. Seltsam A, Hell A, Heymann G, et al. Donor-derived alloantibodies and passenger lymphocyte syndrome in two of four patients who received different organs from the same donor. *Transfusion* 2001;41:365–370.
17. Friend PJ, McCarthy LJ, Filo RS, et al. Transmission of idiopathic (autoimmune) thrombocytopenic purpura by liver transplantation. *N Engl J Med* 1990;323:807–811.
18. Morris PJ. Xenotransplantation. *Br Med Bull* 1999;55:446–459.
19. Galili U, Buehler J, Shohet SB, et al. The human natural anti-Gal IgG, III: the subtlety of immune tolerance in man as demonstrated by crossreactivity between natural anti-Gal and anti-B antibodies. *J Exp Med* 1987;165:693–704.
20. Spitalnik S, Pfaff W, Cowles J, et al. Correlation of humoral immunity to Lewis blood group antigens with renal transplant rejection. *Transplantation* 1984;37:265–268.
21. Smith WJ, Hopkins KA, Schaefer KL, et al. Failure of Lewis blood group antigens to influence renal allograft outcome. *Transplant Proc* 1987;19:4503–4506.
22. Terasaki PI, Chia D, Mickey MR. The second histocompatibility locus in humans. *Transplant Proc* 1988;20[Suppl 1]:21–25.
23. Henry S, Oriol R, Samuelsson B. Lewis histo-blood group system and associated secretory phenotypes. *Vox Sang* 1995;69:166–182.
24. Ramsey G, Fryer JP, Teruya J, et al. Lewis (a − b −) red blood cell phenotype in patients undergoing evaluation for small intestinal transplantation. *Transfusion* 2000;40[Suppl]:114S.
25. Prendergast TW, Furukawa S, Beyer III AJ, et al. Defining the role of aprotinin in heart transplantation. *Ann Thorac Surg* 1996;62:670–674.
26. Wegner JA, DiNardo JA, Arabia FA, et al. Blood loss and transfusion requirements in patients implanted with a mechanical circulatory support device undergoing cardiac transplantation. *J Heart Lung Transplant* 2000;19:504–506.
27. Triulzi DJ, Griffith BP. Blood usage in lung transplantation. *Transfusion* 1998;38:12–15.
28. Nyman T, Elmer DS, Shokouh-Amiri MH, et al. Improved outcome of patients with portal-enteric pancreas transplantation. *Transplant Proc* 1997;29:637–638.
29. Danielson CFM, Filo RS, O'Donnell JA, et al. Institutional variation in hemotherapy for solid organ transplantation. *Transfusion* 1996;36:263–267.
30. Abecassis M, Blei AT, Flamm S, et al. Liver transplantation. In: Stuart FP, Abecassis MM, Kaufman DB, eds. *Organ transplantation.* Georgetown, TX: Landes Bioscience, 2000:169–207.
31. Kang Y. Thromboelastography in liver transplantation. *Semin Thromb Hemost* 1995;21[Suppl 4]:34–44.
32. Williamson LM, Llewelyn CA, Fisher NC, et al. A randomized trial of solvent/detergent-treated and standard fresh-frozen plasma in the coagulopathy of liver disease and liver transplantation. *Transfusion* 1999;39:1227–1234.
33. Sarode R, Yomtovian R. Efficacy of SD-treated plasma during liver transplantation. *Transfusion* 2000;40:886–888.
34. Dalmau A, Sabaté, A, Acosta F, et al. Tranexamic acid reduces red cell transfusion better than ϵ-aminocaproic acid or placebo in liver transplantation. *Anesth Analg* 2000;91:29–34.
35. Porte RJ, Molenaar IQ, Begliomini B, et al. Aprotinin and transfusion requirements in orthotopic liver transplantation: a multicentre randomised double-blind study. *Lancet* 2000;355:1303–1309.
36. Segal H, Hunt BJ. Aprotinin: pharmacological reduction of perioperative bleeding. *Lancet* 2000;355:1289–1290.
37. Smith DM Jr, Lipton KS. Leukocyte reduction for the prevention of transfusion-transmitted cytomegalovirus (TT-CMV). Association bulletin 97-2. Bethesda, MD: American Association of Blood Banks, 1997.
38. Wilkinson SL, Lipton KS. Leukocyte reduction. Association bulletin 99-7. Bethesda, MD: American Association of Blood Banks, 1999.
39. Opelz G, Vanrenterghem Y, Kirste G, et al. Prospective evaluation of pretransplant blood transfusions in cadaver kidney recipients. *Transplantation* 1997;63:964–967.
40. Koneru B, Harrison D, Rizwan M, et al. Blood transfusions in liver recipients: a conundrum or a clear benefit in the cyclosporine/tacrolimus era? *Transplantation* 1997;63:1587–1590.
41. Triulzi DJ, Nalesnik MA. Microchimerism, GVHD, and tolerance in solid organ transplantation. *Transfusion* 2001;41:419–426.
42. Salgar SK, Shapiro R, Dodson F, et al. Infusion of donor leukocytes to induce tolerance in organ allograft recipients. *J Leukoc Biol* 1999;66:310–314.
43. Barr ML, Meiser BM, Eisen HJ, et al. Photopheresis for the prevention

of rejection in cardiac transplantation. *N Engl J Med* 1998;339: 1744–1751.
44. Salerno CT, Park SJ, Kreykes NS, et al. Adjuvant treatment of refractory lung transplant rejection with extracorporeal photopheresis. *J Thorac Cardiovasc Surg* 1999;117:1063–1069.
45. Clark RE, Zafirelis Z. Future devices and directions. *Prog Cardiovasc Dis* 2000;43:95–100.
46. McLaughlin BE, Tosone CM, Custer LM, et al. Overview of extracorporeal liver support systems and clinical results. *Ann N Y Acad Sci* 1999;875:310–325.
47. Soin B, Vial CM, Friend PJ. Xenotransplantation. *Br J Surg* 2000;87: 138–148.
48. Prather RS. Pigs is pigs. *Science* 2000;289:1886–1887.
49. Food and Drug Administration. Draft PHS guideline on infectious disease issues in xenotransplantation. Bethesda, MD: US Food and Drug Administration, 2000.

Rossi's Principles of Transfusion Medicine, Third Edition, edited by Toby L. Simon, Walter H. Dzik, Edward L. Snyder, Christopher P. Stowell, and Ronald G. Strauss. Lippincott Williams & Wilkins, Philadelphia

44

TRANSFUSION THERAPY IN THE CARE OF TRAUMA AND BURN PATIENTS

KIMBERLY A. DAVIS
RICHARD L. GAMELLI

HISTORY OF TRANSFUSION THERAPY FOR TRAUMA AND BURNS

Although the first described blood transfusion was performed in the early nineteenth century, widespread acceptance of transfusion therapy did not occur until Landsteiner described the ABO blood groups. Experience gained during World War I and the Spanish Civil War led to technologies to collect, store, and transfuse blood in emergencies. Bernard Fantus in 1937 opened the first blood bank in the United States at Cook County Hospital in Chicago. The use of the preservative acid-citrate-dextrose was practiced by the end of World War II, further expanding the ability to store blood (1). During this same period, the importance of resuscitation was recognized and the use of crystalloids began.

The ability to store blood in large quantities was a boon for trauma surgery. The liberal use of O-negative blood during the Vietnam War significantly reduced mortality (2). This coupled with rapid transport time, aggressive fluid resuscitation, and early operative intervention for patients not responding to resuscitation marked the beginning of modern trauma surgery. The lessons learned from the wartime experience with the resuscitation of injured patients were applied to the civilian injured, and by the late 1960s, organized prehospital emergency services were rapidly transporting patients to trauma centers.

The use of blood for the resuscitation and treatment of thermally injured patients was advocated as early as the 1920s and 1930s (3). Blood and blood products have been components of various treatment regimens and burn formulas for the initial resuscitation of burned patients. The ready availability of blood and blood products has improved survival among elderly patients and patients with associated medical problems who otherwise would not have tolerated a low hemoglobin level. Intraoperative transfusion has allowed wider, more aggressive débridement and decreased the number of surgical procedures needed by a patient.

The current indications for transfusion in trauma and burn care recognize the merits of this form of treatment but acknowledge the practical considerations regarding transfusion. The limitations of the blood supply are apparent, demand exceeding supply at times. In the United States, 12 million units of blood are transfused yearly into approximately 4 million recipients, most transfusions being administered in the perioperative period. Red blood cells have a limited shelf life and are discarded after 42 days. In addition, the incidence of transfusion reactions and of the transmission of hepatitis was well documented by the 1970s. The risk of transmission of human immunodeficiency virus is estimated to be 1 in approximately 1,000,000 units of blood; that of hepatitis C virus transmission is 1 in approximately 100,000 units. On a yearly basis, approximately 35 patients die per year of major transfusion reactions or bacterial contamination (4).

Beyond disease transmission, several studies have shown the immunosuppressive effect of blood transfusion. One such study with burn patients identified the number of transfusions received as an independent variable predictive of the increased incidence

K.A. Davis and Richard L. Gamelli: Department of Surgery, Loyola University Medical Center, Maywood, Illinois.

of infectious complications (5). In patients with colon cancer, only Dukes classification and administration of blood were predictive of recurrence (6).

Although a transfusion is still a life-saving treatment in the appropriate circumstances, the foregoing observations have led to a more judicious use of blood and blood products as the risk-to-benefit considerations are more fully understood. It is also known that 50% of severely injured patients who survive the immediately posttrauma phase have a clinical course complicated by inflammatory or infectious episodes. These patients are at markedly increased risk of development of the systemic inflammatory response syndrome with a dysregulated cytokine milieu. It is possible that transfusion may exacerbate this posttraumatic systemic inflammatory response syndrome by contributing cytokine precursors to an already disrupted environment. Current blood use in trauma and burns therefore must combine judgment and careful assessment of the risk-to-benefit ratio.

DEFINITION OF SHOCK

Shock is defined as inadequate organ perfusion and tissue oxygenation. After trauma, the most common type of shock is hemorrhagic. Neurogenic shock after high cervical spinal injuries and septic shock after penetrating trauma also are possible. After burns, hypovolemic shock is caused by fluid sequestration at the site of injury and in unburned injured tissue as a systemic response to injury and by evaporative loss due to loss of the dermal barrier.

THE TRAUMA PATIENT

Hemorrhagic Shock

Hemorrhage results in decreased cardiac output and total body ischemia, which cannot be corrected until circulating volume is restored. Acute loss of intravascular volume results in increased vascular tone and redistribution of blood flow to the heart and brain at the expense of cutaneous, splanchnic, and renal vascular beds. Acidosis develops as tissues switch from aerobic to anaerobic metabolism. This acidosis initially facilitates the unloading of oxygen at the tissues with a shift of the oxygen dissociation curve to the left. Urine output decreases as the kidneys work to retain water and sodium in response to decreased renal perfusion.

Without transfusion therapy, this correction requires the movement of fluid and protein from the interstitium to the plasma, or transcapillary plasma refill (7). Initially triggered by a decrease in capillary hydrostatic pressure, this results in movement of protein-free fluid from the interstitium to the plasma. A second phase involves movement of protein into the plasma space in support of plasma oncotic pressure. This results in restoration of plasma volume and protein concentration with reduced oxygen-carrying capacity owing to decreases in total red blood cell mass, that is, normovolemic anemia. Transcapillary refill is capable of sustaining a relatively fixed level of plasma volume, equal to approximately two thirds of the initial plasma volume, irrespective of the rate of bleeding. Laboratory studies have shown that plasma refill reaches 33% by 0.5 hours after hemorrhage, and 50% by 3 hours, allowing fairly rapid restoration of circulating blood volume (8,9). The amount of transcapillary refill is a function of the severity of pressure-driven hemorrhage but does not correlate with arterial pressure or cardiac output.

In evaluating an injured patient, it rapidly becomes apparent that trauma patients are an extremely heterogeneous population. Each patient's resuscitative needs are different and can be broadly anticipated on the basis of initial hemodynamic status and the response to resuscitative efforts. The American College of Surgeons committee on trauma (10), in an effort to guide and standardize the initial resuscitation of trauma patients, has defined four classes of shock (Table 44.1). Whereas crystalloid resuscitation alone is adequate for class I and II shock, early consideration should be given to administering blood to patients in class III and IV shock.

Initial Resuscitation of the Trauma Patient

The initial resuscitation fluid of choice after trauma is an isotonic crystalloid solution, usually Ringer lactate. The American College of Surgeons committee on trauma advanced trauma life support course (10) recommends insertion of two large-bore intravenous catheters and immediate infusion of 2,000 ml warmed crystalloid solution, 20 ml/kg for a child. Because shock after trauma most often is hypovolemic, the response to initial fluid resuscitation determines subsequent resuscitative measures. Hypothermia must be prevented during the resuscitation phase.

The response to fluid resuscitation determines which if any subsequent resuscitative measures are needed. A patient with minimal injury and normal vital signs with initial crystalloid resuscitation is called a *responder* to fluid resuscitation. The condition of these patients, by definition class I or II shock, remains hemodynamically normal without ongoing resuscitation. Such patients need evaluation and management of the injuries but rarely need transfusion during the initial evaluation.

A patient in compensated shock, defined as hypovolemia coexistent with normotension but with serious metabolic derangement, often is difficult to identify. The conventional end points of resuscitation—heart rate, blood pressure and urine output—are crude assessments of the adequacy of resuscitation. Early identification of compensated shock is facilitated by recognition of a transient response to fluid resuscitation. Patients in class III shock often have hypotension and tachycardia, but vital signs normalize in response to initial fluid resuscitation. During observation, such patients have physiologic signs of shock and need aggressive ongoing resuscitation to maintain relatively normal vital signs. Early identification of the site of hemorrhage and prompt surgical intervention minimize the period of hypoperfusion and the subsequent risk of multiple organ dysfunction. Transfusion with cross-matched or type-specific blood is indicated.

A patient in class IV, or uncompensated, shock has pallor, diaphoresis, apathy, and hyperventilation, clinical signs and symptoms that must be correctly interpreted. These patients also have tachycardia, hypotension, and tachypnea not responsive to aggressive fluid resuscitation with crystalloid and banked blood. Any injured or burned patient who is cool and tachycardic is

TABLE 44.1. ESTIMATED FLUID AND BLOOD LOSSES BASED ON PATIENT'S INITIAL PRESENTATION

	Class I	Class II	Class III	Class IV
Blood loss (ml)	Up to 750	750–1,500	1,500–2,000	>2,000
Blood loss (% blood volume)	Up to 15	15–30	30–40	>40
Pulse rate (beats/min)	<100	>100	>120	>140
Blood pressure	Normal	Normal	Decreased	Decreased
Pulse pressure (mm Hg)	Normal or increased	Normal	Normal	Normal
Respiratory rate (breath/min)	14–20	20–30	30–40	>35
Urine output (ml/h)	>30	20–30	5–15	Negligible
Mental status	Slighly anxious	Mildly anxious	Anxious, confused	Confused, obtunded
Fluid replacement (3:1 rule)	Crystalloid	Crystalloid	Crystalloid and blood	Crystalloid and blood

Patient is a 70-kg man.
These guidelines are based on the 3-for-1 rule. This rule derives from the empiric observation that most patients in hemorrhagic shock need as much as 300 ml of electrolyte solution for each 100 ml of blood loss. Applied blindly, these guidelines can result in excessive or inadequate fluid administration.
From American College of Surgeons Committee on Trauma Advanced Trauma Life Support Course. Chicago: American College of Surgeons, 1997, with permission.

in shock until proved otherwise. These patients are described as *nonresponders,* in that their vital signs do not improve with aggressive resuscitative techniques. In this population, early identification of the site of hemorrhage and surgical intervention are paramount to survival. Early transfusion with group O red blood cells is indicated.

The decision regarding early administration of blood, that is, in the trauma department, should be reserved for patients who have a transient response to initial resuscitation or those who have no response to resuscitation. These two groups have lost more than 30% of their blood volume or are still actively bleeding. Transfusion of blood in the trauma department must not delay definitive surgical intervention, and these patients should be transported to the operating room urgently.

In a retrospective study with 1,000 trauma patients, Knottenbelt (11) found an interesting correlation between initial low hemoglobin level and mortality. He found that patients who came to medical attention in shock and died had significantly lower hemoglobin levels than did patients who did not arrive for treatment in shock. The mean hemoglobin levels of patients who died of hemorrhagic causes were significantly lower regardless of initial blood pressure. In this study, 48% of patients received no prehospital resuscitation, indicating that hemodilution was not the cause of a low initial hemoglobin level. Knottenbelt hypothesized that patients with a low hemoglobin level may have suffered blood loss exceeding their compensatory mechanisms. He concluded that a low initial hemoglobin level indicated severe, ongoing blood loss.

Once the decision to perform a transfusion has been reached, there are several options for the type of blood used. Blood ideally should by typed and cross-matched before transfusion, although this can take as long as 1 hour in many blood banks. This is an unacceptably long delay for a patient in class III or IV shock. An alternative is to use type-specific blood, although this also is associated with a processing delay of 20 to 30 minutes, which often also is an unacceptable delay. In most trauma units, group O red blood cell is immediately available and is the blood of choice in the care of trauma patients in hemodynamically unstable condition not responding to crystalloid resuscitation. Numerous studies have shown that administration of group O red blood cell is a safe and rapid means by which to restore circulating red blood cell volume in a patient in severe shock.

Future Directions for Initial Resuscitation of Trauma Patients

Although crystalloid and blood are the standards in initial resuscitation of trauma patients, there is active investigational interest in developing alternative resuscitative materials. Although few would argue that blood is the ideal resuscitative fluid in that it rapidly expands circulatory volume and improves oxygen transportation, there are many disadvantages to blood. It must be cross-matched, has a short shelf life, and must be refrigerated. Massive transfusion can produce dilutional coagulopathy, hypocalcemia, and hypomagnesemia. Blood-borne viral pathogens can be transfused.

Hemoglobin-based red blood cell substitutes offer many of the advantages of red blood cell transfusion with theoretically fewer limitations. A number of blood substitutes are being evaluated in efficacy trials in North America and Europe (Table 44.2) (see Chapter 13). These solutions are attractive compared with banked blood in that they are potentially readily available, have a long shelf life, are free of bacterial and viral contamination,

TABLE 44.2. HEMOGLOBIN SUBSTITUTES

Manufacturer	Product	Type of Hemoglobin	Adverse Effect	Trial
Baxter (Deerfield, IL)	HemAssist	Human outdated blood, diaspirin cross-linked	Increase vasomotor tone, nitric oxide scavenger	Closed
Northfield Laboratories (Evanston, IL)	PolyHeme	Polymerized human	Mild hyperbilirubinemia	Phase III
Hemosol (Etobicoke, Ontario, Canada)	Hemolink	Human outdated blood, o-raffinose polymerized	Mild gastrointestinal discomfort	Phase II
Biopure/Pharmacia and Upjohn (Cambridge, MA)	Hemopure	Bovine, gluteraldehyde polymerized	Increased SVR and PVR, decreased cardiac output	Phase II

SVR, systemic vascular resistance; PVR, pulmonary vascular resistance.

and do not require typing and cross-matching. They also may lack the immunosuppressive activity of transfused blood. Most blood substitutes under development are based on either human or animal hemoglobin. The disadvantage of human hemoglobin relates to a limitation in the availability of outdated red blood cells; only 5% to 15% of the 14 million units of blood donated in the United States are being discarded. Animal hemoglobin, particularly bovine hemoglobin, is potentially inexpensive and is readily available, although uncertainty regarding the purification of animal pathogens remains a concern (12).

Several companies have hemoglobin-based blood substitutes in efficacy trials. One company, Baxter Healthcare (Deerfield, IL) terminated work with a diaspirin cross-linked hemoglobin when a multicenter trial with trauma patients with hypotension showed increased mortality during interim review (13). PolyHeme (Northfield Laboratories, Evanston, IL) is in phase III trials and appears to lack the vasopressive effects of diaspirin cross-linked hemoglobin. A randomized, clinical trial of PolyHeme versus red blood cells in the treatment of trauma patients showed a lower overall red blood cell transfusion requirement; there was no difference in circulating hemoglobin level, and there were no adverse events (14). Other blood substitutes, including Hemopure (Biopure Corporation, Cambridge MA), a bovine hemoglobin-based solution that appears to have some vasopressor effects, and Hemolink (Hemosol, Toronto, Ontario, Canada) are in phase II and phase III trials in the United States, Canada, and Europe.

Although blood substitutes remain in clinical trials, other solutions have been evaluated for use in immediate resuscitation of trauma patients. Colloid solutions are theoretically more efficient than crystalloid at restoring intravascular volume. The colloid-crystalloid debate is at least 50 years old. A potential indication for colloid administration is ongoing resuscitation of critically injured patients. The principle reason for the ongoing debate is a lack of quality data to support the choice of either solution for resuscitation. No adequate prospective, randomized, controlled trials have been performed with sufficient numbers of patients to generate a statistically significant difference in outcome. There is little doubt that smaller volumes of colloid than of crystalloid are needed to restore intravascular volume. It also is generally accepted that allergic reactions to colloid can occur. Beyond these two facts, there is little agreement. Current clinical practice appears to reflect dogma and local bias rather than evidence-based medicine.

To clarify the colloid versus crystalloid debate, several studies have examined outcome, including survival and generation of extravascular lung water. Investigators in favor of crystalloid resuscitation argue that after severe trauma, there is depletion of interstitial volume as well as intravascular volume, a deficit not adequately addressed with colloid resuscitation. Crystalloid has been proposed as the best resuscitation fluid, because it has been shown to restore the volume of both the intravascular and interstitial spaces without worsening pulmonary function (15). Pulmonary lymphatic vessels increase their flow at least severalfold in animals, and the increase likely occurs in humans, minimizing the development of pulmonary edema after crystalloid resuscitation. Proponents of colloid resuscitation, however, believe that resuscitation of the intravascular component alone is beneficial and that use of colloid may decrease the incidence of pulmonary edema (16). Although this debate has been subjected to several metaanalyses, the results are conflicting owing to highly heterogeneous patient populations and study designs.

Advocates of crystalloid use note the lower cost of crystalloids than of colloids, although larger volumes are needed to reach similar end points. Although colloids remain in the intravascular space, in states of increased vascular permeability, colloids can leak into the interstitium, increasing the colloid oncotic pressure of the extravascular space. This increased oncotic pressure can hamper mobilization of third-space fluids after the acute resuscitative phase has been completed. Velanovich (17) reviewed eight randomized, prospective trials comparing crystalloid to colloid resuscitation. He found a 5.7% relative decrease in mortality in the group receiving crystalloid resuscitation. When nontrauma trials were excluded, a 12.3% decrease in mortality favored crystalloid resuscitation.

Several studies have examined use of hypertonic saline solution in the resuscitation of animals and humans from shock. Hypertonic saline solution has the advantage of requiring smaller volumes to reach end points similar to those of standard crystalloid resuscitation. This makes hypertonic saline solution particularly attractive for use in the prehospital setting. Administration of hypertonic saline solution has been shown to elevate mean arterial pressure and cardiac output and to increase renal, mesenteric, total splanchnic, and coronary blood flow. Hypertonic saline solution also causes a small and transient increase in circulatory volume by means of transcapillary refill. These effects are well established after controlled hemorrhage. However, the utility of hypertonic saline solution in the management of uncontrolled hemorrhage has yet to be firmly established.

Gross et al. (18), using a model of uncontrolled hemorrhage in rats, found increased blood loss and mortality after administration of hypertonic saline solution. They concluded that hypertonic saline resuscitation must be delayed until after definitive control of hemorrhage (18). This study was criticized for its use of an anesthetic agent that may have exacerbated hypotension and affected the outcome. Coimbra et al. (19) compared hypertonic saline and shed blood resuscitation with crystalloid and shed blood resuscitation in a model of hemorrhage and cecal ligation and puncture in rats. They found improved survival among animals resuscitated with hypertonic saline solution and shed blood, improvement in pulmonary histologic features, and decreased local peritoneal sepsis. They hypothesized that resuscitation with hypertonic saline solution caused less impairment in cellular immune function, possibly contributing to the improvement in survival that they documented.

In a prospective, randomized trial with 105 patients in hypovolemic shock, Younes et al. (20) found that infusion of 250 ml of hypertonic saline solution was not associated with any complications and did not affect mortality. It did improve mean arterial blood pressure significantly, acutely expanded plasma volume 24%, and significantly reduced the volume of crystalloid and blood needed for resuscitation. A multicenter trial evaluated the use of hypertonic saline and dextran in the prehospital treatment of trauma patients with hypotension. The investigators found improved survival among patients undergoing surgery. The difference reached statistical significance, although there was no overall improvement in survival rate. Use of hypertonic saline solution and dextran, however, appeared to be associated with a lower incidence of adult respiratory distress syndrome, renal failure, and coagulopathy. The authors concluded that although hypertonic solutions appeared useful in the prehospital resuscitation of trauma patients, further studies are needed (21). Reports by others have similarly described a survival benefit among patients receiving hypertonic saline solution versus conventional resuscitative fluids in prehospital therapy for hypotension associated with trauma (22). It appears that judicious administration of hypertonic solution early in resuscitation may offer some benefit.

Ongoing Resuscitation of the Trauma Patient

It is of paramount importance to assess the adequacy of resuscitation. The search continues for valid markers of adequate resuscitation. Many believe that base deficit accurately reflects the hemodynamic and tissue perfusion changes associated with shock and resuscitation (23). Serum lactate is a reliable marker of hypoperfusion in hemorrhagic shock, because failure to clear lactate within 24 hours of injury has been associated with increased mortality (24). Although identification of serum markers is helpful for guiding the treatment of trauma patients, it is at best a global measure of perfusion. Organ-specific monitoring therefore may be useful in ensuring adequate end-organ perfusion. Ivatury et al. (25) have proposed gastric tonometry for such monitoring. They documented improved survival among patients whose gastric pH normalized within 24 hours.

Once a patient has survived the initial insult and resuscitation has begun, the patient enters a new phase of recovery based on the injuries and the need for surgical intervention. Because this is a very heterogeneous group of patients, it is perhaps best to consider three separate stages—the intraoperative stage, nonsurgical management of solid organ injuries, and recovery.

Intraoperative Phase

The initial surgical treatment of a trauma patient involves rapid control of bleeding. In the case of severe abdominal trauma, this may necessitate use of damage control techniques or rapid packing of the abdomen to achieve hemostasis and rapid control of injuries to hollow viscera (26). Damage control allows the anesthesia team to administer intravenous fluids and rapidly restore intravascular volume. The use of heated ventilator circuits and warmed intravenous fluids reduces the risk of hypothermia and the coagulopathy associated with reduced body temperature.

The decision to perform intraoperative transfusion can be somewhat complex and involves both the surgeon and the anesthesiologist. Despite a traditional hemoglobin-based transfusion trigger of 10 g/dl, numerous studies have documented the safety of a lower hemoglobin level (27,28). In a study of Jehovah's Witness patients with anemia undergoing elective surgery, Spence et al. (27) found that active bleeding was an independent predictor of survival only when hemoglobin level decreased to less than 4 g/dl. Low hemoglobin levels became an independent predictor of mortality only when they decreased to less than 3 g/dl. How these data are used relative to the care of a trauma patient must be tempered with the recognition that hemoglobin levels obtained during active hemorrhaging may be falsely elevated because the intravascular and interstitial spaces have not equilibrated. In addition, the compensatory mechanisms of chronic anemia require more time to develop than that afforded by acute hemorrhage. Although results of these studies support the concept that the use of an arbitrary hemoglobin transfusion trigger is probably inappropriate, the intraoperative decision to perform transfusion must be based on an assessment of the patient's overall physiologic condition and the severity of ongoing blood loss.

Autotransfusion of the patient's blood has become a widely accepted practice in elective surgery and can be used as an adjunct to transfusion in the care of trauma patients. The benefits of this practice include the conservation of the blood supply, avoidance of transfusion-related complications, and the absence of viral pathogens. Although intraoperative salvage has been successfully used in cases of thoracic trauma, intraoperative salvage of blood from abdominal injuries has not been universally accepted because of the risk of contamination from injuries to hollow viscera.

Nonoperative Management of Solid Organ Injuries

At the beginning of the 1900s, the mortality rate for nonoperative management of splenic injuries was 100%, thus splenectomy was readily accepted as the standard of care for splenic rupture. However, King and Schumaker reported on overwhelming postsplenectomy sepsis among children who had undergone splenectomy. Despite this report, the practice of splenectomy remained unchallenged through the first half of the twentieth century, until pediatric surgeons began to realize that children in hemodynamically stable condition with splenic injuries could be safely observed. With the advent of improved imaging techniques, including computed tomography (CT) of the abdomen and pelvis, splenic injuries can be identified in patients with normal hemodynamic values. The pediatric experience has been extended to the treatment of adults who have sustained trauma but are in hemodynamically stable condition. Benefits of splenic salvage include avoidance of overwhelming postsplenectomy sepsis and avoidance of unnecessary laparotomy. In the 1990s, these principles were extended to the nonoperative treatment of selected patients with liver trauma (29).

In determining whether a patient needs operative therapy for a splenic injury, the most important factor is hemodynamic stability. Patients in hemodynamically unstable condition (approximately 35% of patients with splenic injury) need exploration and splenectomy or splenorrhaphy depending on the decision of the operating surgeon. However, 65% of patients arrive for treatment in hemodynamically stable condition and are candidates for nonoperative treatment. When nonoperative management fails, hemodynamic instability necessitates exploration, or hemoglobin level decreases, necessitating transfusion. Feliciano, using decision analysis, found that the relative risk of blood transfusion was higher than the risk of overwhelming postsplenectomy sepsis and advocated early exploration for any patient with a blunt splenic injury necessitating transfusion (29). Most patients with splenic injury do not need transfusion. However, in the present environment, the relative risk of a 1- or 2-unit transfusion if the patient is in otherwise stable condition seems a reasonable alternative to splenectomy. Adjuncts to improve the success of nonoperative management of splenic injuries include the use of angiography. Schurr et al. (30) described a contrast blush on helical CT scans of the spleen. This finding corresponded to a traumatic pseudoaneurysm on an angiogram. In a follow-up article, Davis et al. (31) reported that aggressive identification and embolization of splenic artery pseudoaneurysms decreased the failure rate of nonoperative management to 6%.

In a landmark article in 1990, Knudson et al. (32) described 52 patients with blunt liver trauma who were observed carefully with serial CT. No failures of nonoperative management were reported. This was followed by a report from the group at the University of Tennessee, Memphis, documenting the safety of nonoperative management of even the most severe liver injuries. The authors found transfusion requirements were markedly lower than for patients who underwent surgery. Again the only criterion for initial nonoperative management was hemodynamic stability. The most common complication described in a large series of nonoperative management of blunt hepatic injury was the need for transfusion. As with splenic trauma, early identification of contrast extravasation on helical CT scans of the liver with subsequent angiographic embolization of the bleeding vessel has improved the success rate of nonoperative management (33).

Recovery Phase

The time between operative or nonoperative treatment of a patient who has sustained trauma until discharge from acute care may be the period in which transfusion can be decreased the most without compromising the patient's condition. During this period, there is no ongoing blood loss, and the intravascular volume has successfully equilibrated with the interstitial space, so dramatic changes in hematocrit are not expected. The decision to perform transfusion during this period should be based not on maintaining an arbitrary hematocrit but on results of assessment of the physiologic need for transfusion.

A critical goal in the care of trauma and burn patients is optimization of oxygen delivery and prevention of tissue hypoxia. Although it would be ideal for a simple laboratory value to identify the need for transfusion to optimize oxygen delivery, such a magic bullet does not exist. The decision to perform transfusion must be based on an understanding of the role of hemoglobin in the definition of oxygen delivery.

Oxygen delivery (DO_2) is the product of arterial oxygen content (CaO_2) and cardiac output (CO): $DO_2 = CaO_2 \times CO$. Arterial oxygen content is a measure of both hemoglobin-bound and free oxygen. It is calculated with the following equation:

$$CaO_2 = 1.34 \times SaO_2 \times Hb \times 10 + (0.003 \times PaO_2)$$

where 1.34 is an estimate of the mean volume of oxygen that can be bound to 1g of fully saturated normal hemoglobin, SaO_2 is oxygen saturation, and PaO_2 is the partial pressure of arterial oxygen. Ten is a correction factor converting grams per deciliter to grams per liter. From this equation, it is apparent that dissolved oxygen contributes little to total CaO_2 at atmospheric pressure. This contribution would be increased with the use of hyperbaric oxygen.

Oxygen consumption (VO_2) is a measure of total oxidative metabolism and is a product of the arterial-venous oxygen difference ($CaO_2 - CvO_2$) and the cardiac output. In most cases, oxygen consumption is independent of hemoglobin concentration over a wide range of oxygen delivery values; compensation occurs with increases in cardiac output and oxygen uptake by the tissues. The oxygen extraction ratio, the ratio between oxygen consumption and oxygen delivery, is approximately 25% to 30% under normal conditions. However, different tissues have a variable ability to increase oxygen extraction, further increasing tissue oxygen availability in those tissues. The heart is at maximal oxygen extraction under baseline conditions and depends on increased delivery to meet increasing oxygen demands.

It has been shown in experiments that in the normovolemic state, cardiac output progressively increases with decreases in hematocrit to a hematocrit between 6% and 8.6% (34). This occurs through reductions in blood viscosity (35), increases in vasomotor tone resulting in increased venous return (35), and

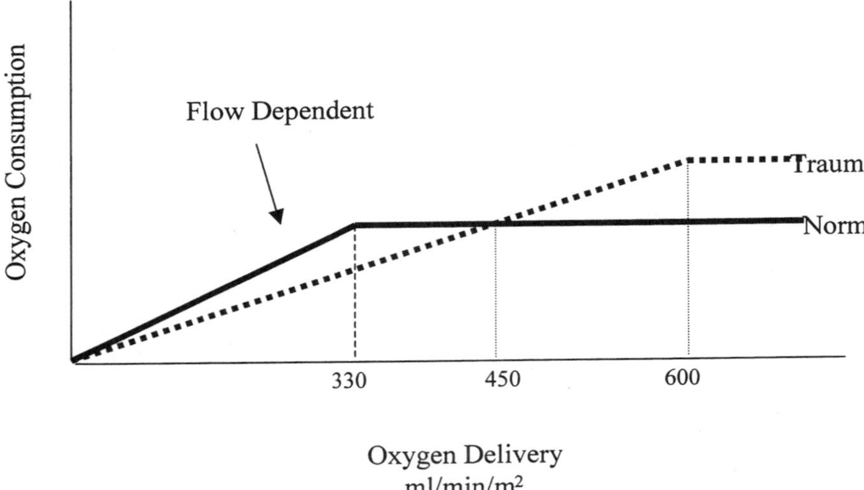

FIGURE 44.1. Unrecognized flow-dependent oxygen consumption (VO_2) under normal conditions and in a trauma state. Critical oxygen delivery (DO_2) in anesthetized adult is 330 ml/min per square meter. The normal oxygen delivery index is 450 ml/min per square meter. The survivor response after normal resuscitation is 600 ml/min per square meter. (From Moore FA, Moore EE, Sauaia A. Postinjury multiple-organ failure. In: Mattox KL, Feliciano DV, Moore EE, eds. *Trauma,* 4th ed. New York: McGraw-Hill, 2000:1439, with permission.)

increased sympathetic activity resulting in increased cardiac contractility (36,37). As the hematocrit decreases from normal value to 30%, oxygen delivery increases to approximately 110% of baseline level (35). These compensatory mechanisms allow maintenance of oxygen delivery until the hematocrit decreases to approximately 10%, after which there is a marked decline (36).

The relation between oxygen delivery and oxygen consumption is biphasic (Fig. 44.1). At less than a critical level of oxygen delivery, consumption is related to delivery in a linear manner. At greater than critical oxygen delivery, consumption is independent of delivery, the flow-independent portion of the curve (35). Analysis of patients under anesthesia showed that the critical value of oxygen delivery differentiating flow-dependent and flow-independent oxygen consumption is 333 ml/min per square meter (38). Shoemaker et al. (39) compared survivors with nonsurvivors of elective surgery. They found that nonsurvivors had lower myocardial performance indicators, higher pulmonary artery pressures and pulmonary vascular resistance, and lower oxygen delivery than did the survivors. A study by Boyd et al. (40) showed a reduced mortality rate and reduced incidence of postoperative complications if inotropic agents were used to increase cardiac output with a target oxygen delivery of 600 ml/min per square meter. After major trauma, several factors alter the DO_2/VO_2 relation. First, VO_2 increases to 150 ml/min per square meter to repay ongoing oxygen debts and to support the systemic inflammatory response syndrome. At the same time, peripheral oxygen extraction is impaired, which decreases the slope of the flow-dependent portion of this relation (Fig. 44.1). It is possible that a trauma patient with a normal DO_2 of 450 ml/min per square meter may be on the flow-dependent portion of the curve (41). In the care of critically ill patients in whom maximal increases in cardiac output have occurred without the necessary improvements in oxygen delivery needed to reach the flow-independent portion of the curve, transfusion is indicated to optimize oxygen delivery. However, this strategy may not be effective for patients in whom oxygen delivery is normal (42).

Traditional teaching that all patients should have a hematocrit of 30% (or a hemoglobin level of 10 g/dl) for optimal oxygen delivery has not been borne out in recent studies. Persons with normal blood volume and normal cardiopulmonary function tolerate hemoglobin levels as low as 5 g/dl (43). In the care of critically ill patients younger than 55 years with Acute Physiology and Chronic Health Evaluation II (APACHE II) scores less than 20, mortality may be reduced if a restrictive transfusion strategy is adopted and hemoglobin levels are maintained at 7 to 9 g/dl (44). Decisions to perform transfusion should be based on evidence of symptomatic anemia, including chest pain, dyspnea, fatigue, and significant tachycardia. In the absence of symptoms, transfusion is not warranted. A more liberal transfusion trigger is probably warranted in the care of older patients and those with underlying coronary disease.

Complications of Transfusion Therapy

Massive resuscitation with fluids and blood products after hemorrhagic shock is associated with complex metabolic derangements and high morbidity and mortality rates. The clinical hallmark of severe hemorrhagic shock is the lethal triad of acidosis, hypothermia, and coagulopathy. Massive transfusion has been defined as replacement of a patient's entire blood volume in 24 hours, transfusion of more than 20 units of red blood cells, or replacement of more than 50% of the circulating blood volume within 3 hours (45,46).

Banked blood undergoes a number of metabolic and structural changes (46). When it is transfused in large volumes, the blood can theoretically cause severe derangements in physiologic values. It appears, however, that the severity and duration of shock rather than the volume of transfused blood are the primary determinants of physiologic derangement and ultimately patient outcome (47,48). It is vital that patients receiving massive transfusion also receive adequate fluid resuscitation such that oxygen delivery and organ perfusion are maintained. Survival after massive transfusion is no longer uncommon. One patient received

186 units of blood and blood components within 12 hours and had a successful outcome (49,50).

Many debates in the literature surround transfusion of blood products. One problem associated with massive resuscitation is microvascular bleeding, or so-called medical bleeding. This is to be clearly differentiated from surgical bleeding. Medical bleeding is associated with mucous membrane bleeding, oozing from surgical wounds and raw tissue surfaces, oozing from catheter sites after application of direct pressure, and generalized petechiae and enlarging ecchymoses (51). It has been recommended that prophylactic transfusion of platelets and fresh-frozen plasma be administered according to the volume of red blood cells transfused (51–53). This practice pattern may not decrease the risk of microvascular bleeding and may markedly increase the patient's exposure to viruses such as hepatitis.

Several studies have evaluated changes in level of coagulation factors and platelet count and their role in microvascular bleeding after trauma and massive transfusion (52–54). These studies document a decrease in both coagulation factors and platelet counts. One explanation is the development of a washout phenomenon, or dilutional coagulopathy, resulting from the use of stored blood deficient in both platelets and coagulation factors (54). Although dilution appears to play a role in thrombocytopenia and coagulopathy after massive resuscitation, it does account for all changes after massive transfusion.

In a regression analysis of thrombocytopenia after massive transfusion, Reed et al. (51) found that only 35% of the decrease in platelet count could be attributed to dilution. They found further that 50% of patients with microvascular bleeding needed large volumes of platelet transfusions well after the period of massive resuscitation. This finding suggested that dilution did not play a role in persistent thrombocytopenia in these patients. In a related study (54), investigators hypothesized that platelet consumption accounted for this persistent thrombocytopenia, which was related to the pathophysiologic response accompanying lung, brain, massive tissue injury, sepsis, and endothelial damage.

Several authors have examined the concentration of coagulation factors to determine whether dilution plays a contributing role. Martin et al. (55) found that although levels of coagulation factors decreased significantly at the end of a shock insult, the levels remained much higher than those considered adequate for normal hemostasis. Reed et al. (51,52) evaluated coagulation studies in the treatment of patients who received massive transfusions. They found mild to moderate prolongation of prothrombin time (PT) and partial thromboplastin time (PTT) were common in this patient population but were not predictive of microvascular bleeding. Regression analysis showed that 15% to 35% of the elevation of the PT and PTT could not be attributed to coagulation factor deficiencies. This finding indicated that other, unidentifiable factors had a role in the elevation of the PT and PTT.

Although no one study alone can confirm which patients at risk of microvascular bleeding may benefit from transfusions of platelets and fresh-frozen plasma, certain tests are more useful than others. A PT less than 1.3 times control value has a 94% predictive value in indicating the absence of microvascular bleeding. Although the sensitivity of PT or PTT in identifying microvascular bleeding is only 50%, values greater than 1.8 times control value are 96% specific for microvascular bleeding. Bleeding time is of no value in determining which patients will have microvascular bleeding. The most sensitive laboratory predictors are a platelet count less than 50×10^9/L and a fibrinogen level less than 0.5 g/L, with a combined sensitivity of 87% and a negative predictive value of 96%. This has led to the following recommendations: platelet transfusion for patients with a platelet count less than 100×10^9/L and evidence of microvascular bleeding; prophylactic platelet transfusion for patients with a platelet count less than 50×10^9/L; and administration of supplemental fresh-frozen plasma or cryoprecipitate to patients with fibrinogen levels of 0.8 g/L or less (52).

Hypothermia is a contributing factor to platelet and coagulation factor dysfunction after massive transfusion. Villalobos et al. (56) studied the effects of hypothermia on platelets in dogs and found that thrombocytopenia was caused by sequestration by the liver, spleen, and other sites in the portal circulation rather than by platelet destruction. No change in platelet production was found during either cooling or rewarming.

Johnson and Reed et al. (57–59) reported on coagulation factor dysfunction secondary to hypothermia. Standard coagulation testing in the laboratory typically is performed at 37°C. This method detects clotting abnormalities only if the actual factor content is decreased. The function of the coagulation cascade, however, depends on enzymatic activity, which can be adversely affected by hypothermia. The result is prolongation of clotting times even in the face of normal factor concentrations (Fig. 44.2). Reed et al. found that PTT was prolonged at all temperatures less than 35°C and that PT was prolonged at temperatures less than 33°C (58). These authors concluded that if clinical oozing exists in a patient with hypothermia and results of coagulation studies performed at 37°C are within the normal range, rewarming the patient is more appropriate and more effective than empiric transfusion of fresh-frozen plasma.

Recognition of the contributions of hypothermia to the development of medical bleeding has revolutionized the field of trauma surgery. The concept of the damage-control laparotomy has been reborn. In this procedure all efforts are directed at control of surgical bleeding and containment of intraabdominal contamination. However, the operation is truncated to minimize the on-table time. The patient often is closed with laparotomy packs in place in a temporary abdominal wall closure (26). The patient is returned to the surgical intensive care unit, where aggressive rewarming and resuscitation continue. Only when acidosis, coagulopathy, and hypothermia have been corrected is the patient returned to the operating room for definitive management of injuries.

THE BURN PATIENT

Initial Resuscitation

The large number of resuscitation formulas available for use in the treatment of thermally injured patients is a tribute to the fact that no one formula is an accurate predictor of the fluid requirements of every patient. No formula replaces the role of the physician, who must continually assess the adequacy of resus-

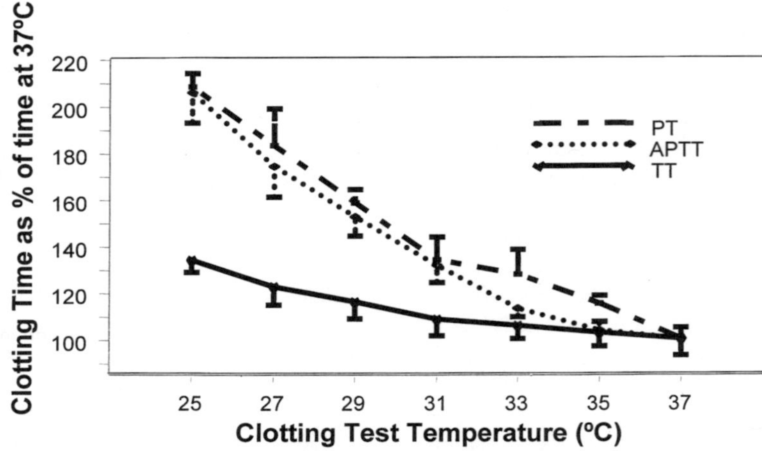

FIGURE 44.2. Clotting times relative to clotting test temperature—the effect of hypothermia. PT, prothrombin time; APTT, activated partial thromboplastin time; TT, thrombin time. (From Reed RL, Bracey AW, Hudson JD, et al. Hypothermia and blood coagulation: dissociation between enzyme activity and clotting factor levels. *Circ Shock* 1990;32:141–152, with permission.)

citation. Ongoing controversies about resuscitation involve the use of colloid, the differences between adults and children, and the influence of inhalation injury on fluid requirements.

In the first 24 hours of resuscitation, most patients need 2 to 4 ml/kg of fluid per percentage of total body surface area (TBSA) burned. This fluid is given as lactated Ringer solution. The first half of the calculated requirement is given over the first 8 hours, measured from time of injury not beginning of resuscitation. The rest is given over the next 16 hours (Parkland formula). Children also need maintenance fluids containing dextrose in addition to the resuscitative fluid. The presence of inhalation injury increases the volume of fluid needed to achieve adequate resuscitation. Whether colloid is used in the first 24 hours is determined on a case by case basis; administration of colloid should not be routine. Regardless of the volume of resuscitative fluid initially chosen, ongoing resuscitation should be dictated by the patient's response to resuscitation. Urinary output of 1 ml/kg per hour is an adequate measure of resuscitation.

Release of vasoactive mediators from injured tissue results in a diffuse capillary leak starting soon after injury. This loss of microvascular integrity results in extravasation of crystalloid and colloid solutions for the first 18 to 24 hours after thermal injury. This pathophysiologic process explains the enormous fluid requirements of burn patients for the first 24 hours. This is the reason that most burn resuscitation formulas incorporate the use of colloids after 24 hours—microvascular integrity apparently is restored at that time. After 24 hours, colloid remains largely intravascular. Colloid, generally 5% albumin in lactated Ringer solution, is infused at a dose based on burn size (generally 0.3 to 0.5 ml/kg per percentage of TBSA burned over 24 hours). During this period, crystalloid requirements decrease markedly.

Transfusion Therapy in the Care of Thermally Injured Patients

Like severely injured trauma patients, thermally injured patients often have anemia throughout the hospital course. The cause of this anemia is very different from that of the anemia of trauma (60–64). A thermally injured patient presents a different challenge during evaluation for transfusion therapy. The factors that predominate as the cause of anemia vary with respect to time from injury; they must be considered in evaluation for transfusion (61,62).

Soon after burn injury, anemia is caused by direct destruction of erythrocytes within the cutaneous circulation and by hemorrhage into the burn wound. As time progresses, the factors resulting in anemia include hemolysis of injured erythrocytes and blood loss during dressing changes. Further hemolysis also occurs as blood flows through injured tissue and burn eschar. Additional blood loss occurs during burn wound débridement, split-thickness skin grafting, and postoperative dressing changes. Because of the stress associated with thermal injury, blood loss can occur into the gastrointestinal tract as well as from unnecessary "routine" blood work.

The response of burn patients to anemia is different from that of trauma patients (61–64). Several but not all studies have documented an increase in erythropoietin level after thermal injury as well as a decrease in reticulocyte numbers (63,64). In a study with 27 patients, erythropoietin levels were inversely related to hemoglobin levels, and patients had persistent reticulocytopenia (64). The results of this study suggested a relative resistance to erythropoietin at the bone marrow level. An elevated level of circulating erythropoietin did not result in an expected increase in erythrocyte production. It does appear that the erythropoietic response to thermal injury is inversely proportional to the size of the burn (63). Results of studies of the use of recombinant erythropoietin in the management of postburn anemia have not been encouraging. A study with pediatric burn patients did not show a statistically significant increase in hematocrit for either burn patients or healthy volunteers, although increases in reticulocyte count occurred (60).

The relative resistance of the bone marrow of thermally injured patients to erythropoietin may be caused by an inhibitory factor in the serum. A study was performed in which serum from patients with more than 20% TBSA burned was cultured with mouse bone marrow. The authors found the number of erythroid colonies decreased when erythropoietin was added to the system. Granulocytosis was not affected. When erythropoietin activity was assayed in vivo, no decrease in activity was detected. This finding suggests the inhibition did not occur at the level of the erythropoietin (62). Another study showed that erythroid colony-forming cells appeared to return to normal as healing occurred. This study also showed that granulocytopoiesis and thrombocytopoiesis were unaffected and proceeded at an accelerated rate (61). These authors postulated redirection of the pluripotent stem cells away from the erythroid line to the granulocyte and monocyte cell lines may offer a survival advantage to burned patients because infection and sepsis are major sources of morbidity and mortality in this population.

As in the care of trauma patients, the safety of lower hemoglobin and hematocrit levels in the care of burn patients has been demonstrated (65,66). Mann et al. (66) retrospectively examined the transfusion requirements of patients with burns of more than 10% TBSA who needed at least one operation. They found a fivefold decrease from 1980 to 1990 in the volume of blood transfused per percentage TBSA without adverse cardiac complications or increased morbidity. Because of their findings, the authors recommended that healthy patients do not need transfusion unless the hematocrit decreases to less than 15% in patients who need one operation or 25% in patients who need more than one operative procedure. As with trauma patients, thermally injured patients with underlying cardiovascular disease should be treated with a more liberalized transfusion policy. Sittig and Deitch (65) confirmed the foregoing findings and found a greater than a threefold decrease in transfusion requirements when a more selective transfusion policy was implemented (Fig. 44.3) whereby 86% of blood transfused was given at the time of an operative procedure (Fig. 44.4).

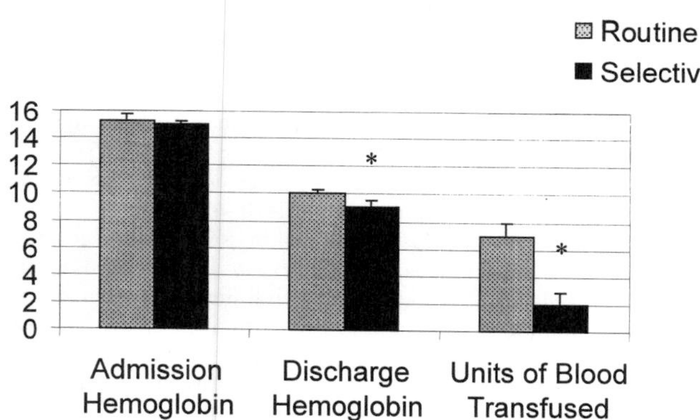

FIGURE 44.3. Comparison of admission and discharge hemoglobin levels (g/dl) between burn patients who received transfusions to maintain a hemoglobin of 10 g/dl (*Routine*) versus burn patients who received selective transfusions once the hemoglobin level decreased to less than 6 to 6. 5 g/dl (*Selective*) *$P < .01$. (From Sittig KM, Deitch EA. Blood transfusion: for the thermally injured or for the doctor? *J Trauma* 1994; 36:369–372, with permission.)

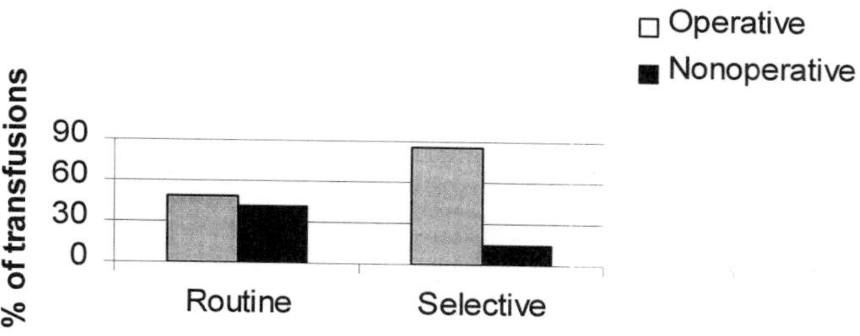

FIGURE 44.4. Timing of transfusion in the care of burn patients who received transfusions to maintain a hemoglobin level of 10g/dl (*Routine*) compared with that in the care of burn patients who received selective transfusions once the hemoglobin level decreased to less than 6.65 g/dl (*Selective*). (From Sittig KM, Deitch EA. Blood transfusion: for the thermally injured or for the doctor? *J Trauma* 1994;36:369–372, with permission.)

Intraoperative use of hemostatic agents can further decrease transfusion requirements. It is well known that intraoperative blood loss is the limiting factor of the extent of excision and grafting performed. Thrombin spray and laparotomy pads saturated with thrombin and epinephrine have been used extensively to limit intraoperative blood loss (65,67). The use of tourniquets for excision and grafting of extremities has further decreased blood loss (68). Fibrin sealants may prove effective. Results of preliminary studies of the use of intraoperative blood salvage techniques with cell savers are promising—recovery and reinfusion of approximately 40% of shed blood without adverse inflammatory or infectious complications (69). As in the care of trauma patients, the importance of normothermia in preventing coagulopathy is recognized, and patients are aggressively warmed at the time of surgery.

SUMMARY

Massive hemorrhage continues to be the leading cause of death during resuscitation of severely injured trauma patients. The early use of blood and blood products combined with aggressive crystalloid resuscitation and early surgical intervention has significantly decreased mortality. However, the risk of disease transmission has prompted reevaluation of the transfusion practices of both trauma and burn surgeons. Although it is recognized that these patients tolerate a lower hemoglobin level than was originally thought, the lower limit of safe hemoglobin level is not known. Although data from other surgical populations have helped to demonstrate that previously accepted transfusion triggers are not appropriate, the unique characteristics of injured patients do not allow universal application of these findings. It is possible to optimize transfusion practices once it is realized that injured patients experience distinct clinical phases based on time from injury. Although blood transfusion continues to be a life-saving therapy, judicious use of blood and blood products can provide maximal benefit and minimize unnecessary risk to the patient after injury.

REFERENCES

1. Bordley J III, Harvey AM. *Two centuries of American medicine.* Philadelphia: WB Saunders, 1976:303–314.
2. Whelan RJ Jr, Burkhalter WE, Gomez A. Management of war wounds. *Adv Surg* 1968;3:227–350.
3. Artz CP. Historical aspects of burn management. *Surg Clin North Am* 1970;50:1193–1200.
4. Goodnough LT, Brecher ME, Kanter MH, et al. Transfusion medicine, I: blood transfusion. *N Engl J Med* 1999;340:438–447.
5. Graves TA, Cioffi WG, Mason AD Jr, et al. Relationship of transfusion and infection in a burn population. *J Trauma* 1898;29:948–954.
6. Tartter PJ. The association of perioperative blood transfusion with colorectal cancer recurrance. *Ann Surg* 1992;216:633–638.
7. Drucker WR, Chadwick CDJ, Gann DS. Transcapillary refill in hemorrhage and shock. *Arch Surg* 1981;116:1344–1353.
8. Barrientos T, Hillman N, Peoples JB. The effects of dehydration on the dynamics of transcapillary refill. *Am Surg* 1982;48:412–416.
9. Prist R, Rocha-e-Silva M, Scalabrini A, et al. A quantitative analysis of transcapillary refill in severe hemorrhagic hypotension in dogs. *Shock* 1994;1:188–195.
10. American College of Surgeons Committee on Trauma. *ACS advanced trauma life support for doctors,* 6th ed. Chicago: American College of Surgeons, 1997.
11. Knottenbelt JD. Low initial hemoglobin levels in trauma patients: an important indicator of ongoing hemorrhage. *J Trauma* 1991;31: 1396–1399.
12. Cohn SM. Blood substitutes in surgery. *Surgery* 2000;127:599–602.
13. Sloan E, Koenigsberg M, Gens D, et al. Diaspirin cross-linked hemoglobin (DCLHb) in the treatment of severe traumatic hemorrhagic shock: a randomized controlled efficacy trial. *JAMA* 1999;282: 1857–1864.
14. Gould SA, Moore EE, Hoyt DB, et al. The first randomized trial of human polymerized hemoglobin as a blood substitute in acute trauma and emergent surgery. *J Am Coll Surg* 1998;187:113–122.
15. Shires GT, Barber AE, Illner HP. Current status of resuscitation: solutions including hypertonic saline. *Adv Surg* 1995;28:113–170.
16. Henry S, Scalea TM. Resuscitation in the new millennium. *Surg Clin North Am* 1999;79(6):1259–1267.
17. Velanovich V. Crystalloid versus colloid fluid resuscitation: a meta-analysis of mortality. *Surgery* 1989;105:65–71.
18. Gross D, Landau EH, Klin B, et al. Treatment of uncontrolled hemorrhagic shock with hypertonic saline solution. *Surg Gynecol Obstet* 1990; 170:106–112.
19. Coimbra R, Hoyt D, Junger W, et al. Hypertonic saline resuscitation decreases susceptibility to sepsis after hemorrhagic shock. *J Trauma* 1997;42:602–607.
20. Younes RN, Aun F, Accioly CQ, et al. Hypertonic solutions in the treatment of hypovolemic shock: a prospective, randomized study in patients admitted to the emergency room. *Surgery* 1992;111:380–385.
21. Mattox KL, Maningas PA, Moore EE, et al. Prehospital hypertonic saline/dextran infusion for post-traumatic hypotension. *Ann Surg* 1991; 213:482–491.
22. Vassar MJ, Perry CA, Holcroft JW. Prehospital resuscitation of hypotensive trauma patients with 7. 5% NaCl versus 7.5% NaCl with added dextran: a controlled trial. *J Trauma* 1993;34:622–632.
23. Davis J, Shackford S, Mackersie R, et al. Base deficit as a guide to volume resuscitation. *J Trauma* 1988;28:1464–1467.
24. Abramson D, Scalea T, Hirchcock R, et al. Lactate clearance and survival following trauma. *J Trauma* 1993;35:584–588.
25. Ivatury R, Simon R, Islam S, et al. A prospective randomized study of endpoints of resuscitation after major trauma: global oxygen transport indices versus organ-specific gastric mucosal pH. *J Am Coll Surg* 1996; 183:145–154.
26. Shapiro MB, Jenkins DH, Schwab CW, et al. Damage control: collective review. *J Trauma* 2000;49:969–978.
27. Spence RK, Costabile JP, Young GS, et al. Is hemoglobin level alone a reliable predictor of outcome in the severely anemic surgical patient? *Am Surg* 1992;58:92–95.
28. Czer LSC, Shoemaker WC. Optimal hematocrit value in critically ill postoperative patients. *Surg Gynecol Obstet* 1978;147:363–368.
29. Knudson MM, Maull KI. Nonoperative management of solid organ injuries: past, present and future. *Surg Clin North Am* 1999;79: 1357–1371.
30. Schurr MJ, Fabian TC, Gavant M, et al. Management of blunt splenic trauma: computed tomographic contrast blush predicts failure of nonoperative management. *J Trauma* 1995;39:507–513.
31. Davis KA, Fabian TC, Croce MA, et al. Improved success in nonoperative management of blunt splenic injuries: embolization of splenic artery pseudoaneurysms. *J Trauma* 1998;44:1008–1015.
32. Knudson MM, Lim RC Jr, Oakes DD, et al. Nonoperative management of blunt liver injuries in adults: the need for continued surveillance. *J Trauma* 1990;30:1494–500.
33. Carrillo EH, Spain DA, Wohltmann CD, et al. Interventional techniques are useful adjuncts in nonoperative management of hepatic injuries. *J Trauma* 1999;46:619–624.
34. Levy PS, Chavez RP, Crystal GJ, et al. Oxygen extraction ratio: a valid indicator of transfusion need in limited coronary vascular reserve? *J Trauma* 1992;32:769–774.
35. Tuman KJ. Tissue oxygen delivery: the physiology of anemia. *Anesthesiol Clin North Am* 1990;8:451–469.
36. Chapler CK, Cain SM. The physiologic reserve in oxygen carrying capacity: studies in experimental hemodilution. *Can J Physiol Pharmacol* 1986;64:7–12.
37. Glick G Jr, Plauth WH, Braunwald E. Role of the autonomic nervous system, I: the circulatory response to acutely induced anemia in unanesthetized dogs. *J Clin Invest* 1964;43:2112–2124.
38. Shibutani K, Komatsu T, Kubal K, et al. Critical level of oxygen delivery in anesthetized man. *Crit Care Med* 1983;11:640–643.
39. Shoemaker WC, Kram HB, Appel PL. Therapy of shock based on pathophysiology, monitoring, and outcome prediction. *Crit Care Med* 1990;18:S19–S25.
40. Boyd O, Grounds RM, Bennett ED. A randomized clinical trial of the effect of deliberate perioperative increase of oxygen delivery on mortality in high-risk surgical patients. *JAMA* 1993;270:2699–2707.
41. Shah DM, Newell JC, Saba TM. Defects in peripheral oxygen utilization following trauma and shock. *Arch Surg* 1981;116:1277–1281.
42. Gramm J, Smith S, Gamelli RL, et al. Effect of transfusion on oxygen transport in critically ill patients. *Shock* 1996;5:190–193.
43. Weiskopf RB, Viele MK, Feiner J, et al. Human cardiovascular and metabolic response to acute, isovolemic anemia. *JAMA* 1997;279: 217–221.
44. Hebert PC, Wells G, Blajchman MA, et al. A multicenter, randomized, controlled clinical trial of transfusion requirements in critical care. *N Engl J Med* 1999;340:409–417.
45. Rutledge R, Sheldon GF, Collins ML. Massive transfusion. *Crit Care Clin* 1986;2:791–805.
46. Lovric V. Alterations in blood components during storage and their clinical significance. *Anaesth Intensive Care* 1984;12:246–251.
47. Waxman K, Shoemaker WC. Physiologic responses to massive intraoperative hemorrhage. *Arch Surg* 1982;117:470–475.
48. Canizaro PC, Pessa ME. Management of massive hemorrhage associated with abdominal trauma. *Surg Clin North Am* 1990;70:621–634.
49. Kivioja A, Myllynen P, Rokkanen P. Survival after massive transfusions exceeding four blood volumes in patients with blunt injuries. *Am Surg* 1991;57:398–401.
50. Michelsen T, Salmela L, Tigerstedt I, et al. Massive blood transfusion: is there a limit? *Crit Care Med* 1989;17:699–700.
51. Reed RL, Ciavarella D, Heimback DM, et al. Prophylactic platelet administration during massive transfusion. *Ann Surg* 1986;230:40–48.
52. Ciavarella D, Reed RL, Counts RB, et al. Clotting factor levels and the risk of diffuse microvascular bleeding in the massively transfused patient. *Br J Haematol* 1987;67:365–368.
53. Lucas CE, Ledgerwood AM. Clinical significance of altered coagulation tests after massive transfusion for trauma. *Am Surg* 1981;47;125–130.

54. Counts RB, Haisch C, Simon TL, et al. Hemostasis in massively transfused trauma patients *Ann Surg* 1979;190:91–99.
55. Martin DJ, Lucas CE, Ledgerwood AM, et al. Fresh frozen plasma supplement to massive red blood cell transfusion. *Ann Surg* 1985;202: 505–511.
56. Villalobos TJ, Adelson E, Riley PA Jr. A cause of the thrombocytopenia and leukopenia that occur in dogs during deep hypothermia. *J Clin Invest* 1958;37:1–7.
57. Johnston TD, Chen Y, Reed RL. Functional equivalence of hypothermia to specific clotting factor deficiencies. *J Trauma* 1994;37:413–417.
58. Reed RL, Bracey AW, Hudson JD, et al. Hypothermia and blood coagulation: dissociation between enzyme activity and clotting factor levels. *Circ Shock* 1990;32:141–152.
59. Reed RL, Johnston TD, Hudson JD, et al. The disparity between hypothermic coagulopathy and clotting studies. *J Trauma* 1992;33: 465–470.
60. Fleming RYD, Herdon DN, Vaidya S, et al. The effect of erythropoietin in normal healthy volunteers and pediatric patients with burn injuries. *Surgery* 1992;112:424–432.
61. Wallner S, Vautrin R, Murphy J, et al. The haematopoietic response to burning: studies in an animal model. *Burns* 1984;10:236–251.
62. Wallner S, Vautrin R. The anemia of thermal injury: mechanism of inhibition of erythropoiesis. *Proc Soc Exp Biol Med* 1986;181:144–150.
63. Deitch EA, Sittig KM. A serial study of the erythropoietic response to thermal injury. *Ann Surg* 1993;217:293–299.
64. Vasko SD, Burdge JJ, Ruberg RL, et al. Evaluation of erythropoietin levels in the anemia of thermal injury. *J Burn Care Rehabil* 1991;12: 437–441.
65. Sittig KM, Deitch EA. Blood transfusions: for the thermally injured or for the doctor? *J Trauma* 1994;36:369–372.
66. Mann R, Heimback DM, Engrav LH, et al. Changes in transfusion practices in burn patients. *J Trauma* 1994;37:220–222.
67. Prasad JK, Taddonio TE, Thomson PD. Prospective comparison of a bovine collagen dressing to bovine spray thrombin for control of haemorrhage of skin graft donor sites. *Burns* 1991;17:70–71.
68. Housinger TA, Lang D, Warden GD. A prospective study of blood loss with excisional therapy in pediatric burn patients. *J Trauma* 1993; 34:262–263.
69. Jeng JC, Boyd TM, Jablonski KA, et al. Intraoperative blood salvage in excisional burn surgery: an analysis of yield, bacteriology and inflammatory mediators. *J Burn Care Rehabil* 1998;19:305–311.

Rossi's Principles of Transfusion Medicine, Third Edition, edited by Toby L. Simon, Walter H. Dzik, Edward L. Snyder, Christopher P. Stowell, and Ronald G. Strauss. Lippincott Williams & Wilkins, Philadelphia © 2002.

CASE 44A

EMERGENCY TRANSFUSION

CASE HISTORY

A 53-year-old man with a history of hepatitis C and end-stage liver disease was transferred from a small suburban hospital because of intractable gastrointestinal bleeding. The patient had arrived at the outlying hospital the previous day with nausea, vomiting, melena, and hematemesis. He received a transfusion of 2 units of red blood cells and underwent endoscopy, which revealed esophageal varices and a bleeding duodenal ulcer. The patient was treated with epinephrine injection. Arteriography did not show a bleeding artery. The night of the endoscopic procedure, the patient received 10 units of fresh-frozen plasma and an additional 12 units of red blood cells because of continued bleeding. The patient's condition became hemodynamically unstable with deteriorating blood gas values, and he was intubated. The next morning, he was transferred to a referral hospital. When the patient arrived in the intensive care unit, the blood pressure was 74/42 mm Hg and the heart rate was 122 beats/min. Blood was oozing blood from the patient's mouth, the nasogastric tube, and a rectal tube.

The medical history included numerous episodes of upper gastrointestinal bleeding over a period of 25 years and three major events in the past 10 years. The patient was presumed to have contracted hepatitis C caused by a transfusion in the 1970s. A biopsy confirmed that he had cirrhosis. The patient also had chronic renal failure (creatinine concentration, approximately 1.5 mg/dl), chronic thrombocytopenia (platelet count, 70 to 120×10^9/L), hypertension, depression, and benign prostatic hypertrophy. The patient had been taking hydrochlorothiazide, paroxetine, omeprazole, and lactulose before admission and had no known allergies to medications. The family and social history provided no relevant information, and the patient's family denied alcohol or intravenous drug abuse. The hematocrit was 18.9%, the platelet count was 115×10^9 per L, the PT was 15.7 seconds, the aPTT was 41.7 sec, the fibrinogen level was 148 mg/dl, the D-dimer level was borderline elevated at 0.5 to 2.0 μg/ml, and the result of a fibrin split product test was negative.

As the patient was being brought to the intensive care unit, one of the residents called the blood bank for the emergency release of blood. He identified the patient according to the provisional identification number assigned in the emergency department when the patient arrived. Four units of type O Rh-negative red blood cells that were not cross-matched were issued with a waiver form. Soon thereafter, a blood bank specimen was sent with a requisition for red blood cells and fresh-frozen plasma. The patient was found to be group O Rh-positive, but the technologists were horrified to discover that he had a positive result of the antibody screen—1+ at the antiglobulin phase with one of the screening cells (R_2R_2). They promptly called the resident covering the blood bank, who called the resident in the intensive care unit.

DISCUSSION

This case highlights a classic dilemma in blood banking—what to do about a bleeding patient who has an unidentified alloantibody. The situation calls for balancing the risk of severe anemia in a patient who is losing blood against the risk of a hemolytic reaction. The resident covering the blood bank had the right instincts, namely to call the physicians taking care of the patient to alert them of the situation and to assess the urgency of the patient's transfusion requirement. In this case, the patient's condition was hemodynamically unstable and he was bleeding actively, so the need for red blood cell transfusion was pressing.

The other part of the equation is the risk of hemolysis. Alloimmunization is not common among patients in hospitals. Most large series show rates of 1% to 1.5% (1). The rates are higher among patients with heavy transfusion requirements, such as this one. Issitt and Anstee (1) reviewed several published series and found rates averaging 18% among patients with sickle cell disease, 5% among patients with β thalassemia major and 8.7% in a mixed group of surgical and medical patients. Not all red blood cell alloantibodies are hemolytic. Some, such as room temperature–reactive immunoglobulin M (IgM) alloantibodies to M or P_1, for example, are routinely ignored. Even among the IgG alloantibodies generally regarded as clinically significant, few produce the catastrophic intravascular hemolysis one associates with the anti-A and anti-B isoagglutinins. With a few notable exceptions, such as the Jk alloantibodies, most IgG alloantibodies are responsible for accelerated extravascular clearance of allogeneic red blood cells. Clearance usually occurs over hours to days and is rarely associated with disseminated intravascular coagulation, renal failure, or hemodynamic instability. The three most common significant alloantibodies encountered in clinical practice are anti-D, anti-E, and anti-K (2). This patient had Rh-positive blood, so he was not at risk to make anti-D. Anti-E and anti-K are IgG alloantibodies, and although they usually consist of IgG1 and IgG3, most do not fix complement nor do they cause intravascular hemolysis. The complications of an extravascular hemolytic reaction are outweighed in this situation by the evidence of vascular collapse in this bleeding patient with hypotension.

In a situation such as this one, in which there is not enough time to identify the alloantibody or to find and crossmatch antigen-negative units, it may be necessary to issue group O or type-specific units of red blood cells. The degree of risk sometimes can be assessed. On the basis of the likelihood that the alloantibody is anti-E or anti-K, it is comforting to know that 90% of units are K-negative. The frequency of Rh-positive units that are E-negative is approximately 68%, whereas more than 95% of Rh-negative units are also E-negative. A moment's inspection of the phenotype of the screening cells would show which is E-positive—the second cell of a three-cell screen usually is R_2R_2—and which is K-positive. If inspection of the screening cell phenotypes indicates that anti-E rather than anti-K is a good possibility, issuing type O Rh-negative units is likely to avert a hemolytic reaction.

It is possible that the patient will be found to have another alloantibody that happens to react with the E-positive or K-positive cells, but once again, most clinically significant alloantibodies cause accelerated extravascular hemolysis, which is not too difficult to manage clinically. Nonetheless, a patient's unstable condition may necessitate basing a decision about transfusion on partial information from the blood bank. In that case, a solid understanding of the pathophysiologic mechanism of extravascular and intravascular hemolysis and a good grasp of serology are essential.

The other issue that such a case raises is the necessity of having a well-devised plan for emergency transfusion when serologic information is incomplete. Perhaps the most important aspect of such a plan is to have a means of identifying the patient so that specimens for the blood bank and other laboratories can be accurately related to the patient. Many hospitals have protocols for assigning temporary identification numbers to patients until identification is complete. If the patient already has a hospital identification number, the files can be merged when the dust settles. Identification systems with generic descriptors, such as "Caucasian male" have obvious problems. The use of an identification number similar to those in routine use is preferable. Some hospitals have kits containing identification bracelets, addressograph cards, and requisitions already made out with unique identification numbers that can be rapidly deployed in an emergency when other means of identification are not available or reliable.

The second part of such a plan is to set up a system for providing blood rapidly, including in situations in which serologic information is lacking. Most institutions have a tiered system for accelerating the process for providing blood, moving from group O units to type specific (electronically crossmatched) units to immediate spin crossmatched units to fully serologically crossmatched units, as the urgency of the situation decreases and the amount of serologic information increases. The standard operating procedure should spell out the circumstances in which the blood bank staff should move from one level to the next. When serologic testing is abbreviated, it is good practice and an American Association of Blood Banks standard to obtain documentation from the physician ordering the blood that the clinical circumstances dictate the need to abbreviate the usual serologic testing. It is also helpful to the technologists in the blood bank if the standard operating procedure indicates when they should contact their medical director to help assess the situation and to facilitate communication between the clinicians and the blood bank.

CODA

After a brief conversation with the rather preoccupied resident in the intensive care unit, it was apparent to the blood bank resident that the patient was in very unstable condition and would likely need a substantial amount of blood. He informed the intensive care unit resident about the alloantibody, gave him an idea of what the risks were likely to be, and told him that he would call back with an update as the serologic evaluation progressed in the blood bank. The patient eventually needed 12 units of red blood cells, 10 units of fresh-frozen plasma and 10 units of cryoprecipitate during the first 24 hours.

The technologists in the blood bank set up a panel that included another R_2R_2 cell, which was K-negative, and a cell that was E-negative but homozygous for K. The panel showed that the alloantibody was anti-E reactive at the antiglobulin phase. The panel was being read at approximately the time one of the technologists succeeded in contacting someone in the laboratory in the referring hospital, who confirmed the original hospital also had identified an anti-E. The technologist also learned the patient had received 2 noncrossmatched units at the first facility that had been found after emergency transfusion to be E-positive. By this point, 4 units of type O Rh-positive cells had been transfused in addition to the 4 units of type O Rh-negative cells. All 8 units were tested for the E antigen, and one of the Rh-positive units was found to be E-positive. The patient's red blood cells gave a mixed field reaction with anti-E, probably because of the E-positive units he had received at the other hospital.

The blood bank called the resident in the intensive care unit to see whether the E-positive unit could be retrieved (it had already been transfused), described the blood bank findings, and told the resident to be alert for signs of extravascular hemolysis. The waiver form was returned later that afternoon.

Endoscopic examination revealed grade 2 esophageal varices and a large ulcer in the second portion of the duodenum that was oozing bright red blood. The patient was not considered a good surgical candidate and was treated with octreotide, a somatostatin analogue. The bleeding abated, and the patient did well for 5 days. At this point, the direct antiglobulin test result was positive with anti-IgG reagent, and anti-E was eluted. The bilirubin level increased slightly over baseline, but soon thereafter, results of all liver function tests began to deteriorate rapidly. On the sixth hospital day, the bleeding recurred, and the patient needed 10 units of red blood cells and 10 units of fresh-frozen plasma. He had several more episodes of bleeding over the next 2 weeks, and these were managed with embolization and cauterization. Sepsis, acute hepatic decompensation, and acute renal failure developed. The patient was not considered a candidate for liver transplantation. The patient remained intubated and unconscious. The family decided to withdraw support, and the patient died on the twenty-fourth hospital day.

Case contributed by Christopher P. Stowell, M.D., Ph.D., Massachusetts General Hospital, Boston, MA.

REFERENCES

1. Issitt PD, Anstee DJ. *Applied blood group serology,* 4th ed. Durham, NC: Montgomery Scientific Publications, 1998:873–877.
2. Hoeltge GA, Domen RE, Rybicki LA, et al. Multiple red cell transfusions and alloimmunization: experience with 6996 antibodies detected in a total of 159,262 patients from 1985–1993. *Arch Pathol Lab Med* 1995; 119:42–45.

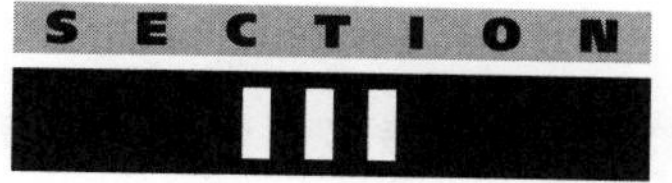

APHERESIS

45

APHERESIS: PRINCIPLES AND TECHNOLOGY OF HEMAPHERESIS

RONALD O. GILCHER

HISTORICAL BACKGROUND AND GENERAL INFORMATION

Apheresis, a word of Greek derivation, means "removal" in its broadest sense. In this chapter, it refers to any procedure performed on a donor or patient in which blood is withdrawn from the person and separated ex vivo into some or all of its components. Some of these components are retained for donation or therapeutic purposes. The others are returned to the person. The word *pheresis* once was used synonymously with the word *apheresis*; however, *apheresis* is the preferred word. *Hemapheresis* also is frequently used synonymously with *apheresis.*

The first experimental apheresis was performed in 1660 by Richard Lower of Oxford, England, who performed a manual procedure on dogs. Plasmapheresis (removal of plasma with return of red blood cells [RBCs]) was first performed in France in 1902 and in Russia in 1914 (1). In 1914 at Johns Hopkins University, Roundtree and Turner used plasmapheresis in artificial kidney research (1).

In 1960, Soloman and Fahey used manual plasmapheresis therapeutically to reduce elevated globulin levels in a patient with a hyperviscosity syndrome, and thus began the era of therapeutic apheresis (1,2). Apheresis became a practical reality with technologic developments, which included plastic bags, integrally connected tubing, and ex vivo centrifugation. It began with blood separation as an "off line" disconnected process in laboratories with freestanding component separation centrifuges. Now apheresis is routinely performed as an "on line" procedure with fully automated blood cell separators at the donor's or patient's bedside.

Manual donor plasmapheresis with paid plasma donors was the major method of collecting source plasma for fractionation into plasma derivatives (albumin, immunoglobulins, factor VIII, and factor IX) between 1950 and 1980. Because the process was off line, requiring separation of the donor from the unit of whole blood during plasma separation, the possibility of returning the RBCs to the wrong donor existed and occasionally was realized. The long time of 1.5 to 2 hours to generate 500 to 700 ml of plasma led to the use of paid donors and to the contamination of many plasma derivatives with hepatitis B and C viruses and human immunodeficiency virus (HIV). In the 1980s, automated on-line cell separation devices were developed by Haemonetics, Baxter Fenwal, and Organon Teknika for collection of source plasma in the United States and Europe. By 1985, an estimated 120,000 to 150,000 automated donor plasmapheresis procedures had been performed in the United States; however, 15 years later that number was more than 12 million a year.

Granulocytes, platelets, and fresh-frozen plasma were the original components collected by means of apheresis technology. In 2001, numerous products are collected from a single donor by means of apheresis technology. Donor products collected include platelets, plasma, RBCs and RBC plasma (RBCP), double RBCs (2RBC), platelets and RBCs, platelets and plasma, granulocytes stimulated with steroids or colony-stimulating factors, and peripheral blood progenitor cells (PBPC) stimulated with granulocyte colony-stimulating factor (G-CSF) or granulocyte-macrophage colony-stimulating factor (GM-CSF). From 1989 to 1990, a 42% increase in plateletpheresis procedures was reported within American Association of Blood Banks (AABB) member organizations (171,200 plateletpheresis procedures in

R.O. Gilcher: Oklahoma Blood Institute, Oklahoma City, Oklahoma.

1989 to 243,700 in 1990) (3,4). Red blood cell apheresis procedures, especially 2RBC, are rapidly increasing. Of the 149,763 collections of allogeneic RBCs at the Oklahoma Blood Institute in 2000, 13,944 (9.3%) were performed with RBC apheresis procedures.

By 1985, an estimated 60,000 to 80,000 therapeutic apheresis procedures (therapeutic plasma exchange and therapeutic cytapheresis) had been performed in the United States. On the basis of results of a survey conducted in 1998, the National Blood Data Resource Center estimated 92,000 therapeutic apheresis procedures were performed in 1997. The use of hemapheresis technology to remove RBCs provides a new approach to removal of RBCs (iron) from patients with hemochromatosis. The results of 2000 survey by the National Blood Data Resource Center indicated that in 1999 approximately 21,716 therapeutic phlebotomies had been performed at blood centers and 129,451 at U.S. hospitals. Apheresis for 2RBC can remove 360 ml of RBCs (350 mg iron) per donation. This would greatly increase the number of therapeutic apheresis procedures performed in the United States. The expanding role of photopheresis in managing conditions such as graft versus host disease and host versus graft disease also is increasing the use of therapeutic apheresis procedures.

CURRENT TECHNOLOGY OVERVIEW

E. J. Cohn, originator of plasma fractionation processes to produce plasma derivatives such as albumin and γ-globulin, developed a prototype machine for centrifugal separation of the cellular elements of blood from plasma. Allen "Jack" Latham, cofounder of Haemonetics, working with Cohn's prototype, developed a disposable polycarbonate plastic bowl with a rotary seal, which was first used to collect platelets in 1971. Concurrently, George Judson, an IBM engineer on loan to the National Cancer Institute, developed another machine to facilitate white blood cell (granulocyte) collection (1). Plasmapheresis and eventually therapeutic plasma exchange and therapeutic cytapheresis were natural developments in the use of these early apheresis devices to manage human diseases known or thought to be mediated by plasma or cellular factors.

The apheresis devices currently approved by the U.S. Food and Drug Administration (FDA) for donor and patient (therapeutic) use are outlined in Table 45.1. These devices are either discontinuous flow (Haemonetics) or modified continuous flow (Baxter/Fenwal, Fresenius, Gambro BCT) systems that can be used for one- or two-arm venous access for apheresis procedures. The spinning membrane technology used in the Autopheresis-C (Baxter/Fenwal) and the new flexible bowl technology of Transfusion Technologies (acquired by Haemonetics in 2000) are unique. The latter actually produces a potential-space bowl that I liken to the blood bottles of the 1940s and 1950s being developed into the plastic bags in use since the 1960s. This device has an expandable membrane over a flat disk. Fluid pressure controls the shape and volume of the collecting apheresis chamber and offers unique options for future blood component collection and separation. This unique flexible bowl is being developed into a chair-side whole-blood collection and separation device and is being used in an intraoperative autotransfusion device.

Baxter/Fenwal Technology

Fenwal uses continuous-flow technology and a seal-less system in the CS3000 blood cell separator originally introduced in the early 1980s. The device is fully automated and computer controlled. The CS3000 concentrates platelets during collection into a final volume of approximately 200 ml. An enhancement of the CS3000 with a platelet-collection chamber called the TNX-6 separation chamber has decreased the frequency of white blood cell (WBC) contamination of the platelet product. The CS3000 is now the CS3000 Plus. The CS3000 Plus can be used to collect granulocyte-platelet concentrates and PBPC.

TABLE 45.1. APHERESIS DEVICES USED IN THE UNITED STATES FOR DONOR COLLECTION AND PATIENT THERAPEUTICS

Manufacturer	Device	Type	Product	Venous Access	Intended Use
Baxter/Fenwal	CS-3000	C/CF	SP, AFFP	1 or 2	D/P
	Amicus	C/CF	PLAP, AFFP, PBPC	1 or 2	D/P
Fresenius	Autopheresis-C	SM/DF	PLAP, AFFP	1	D
Gambro BCT	104	C/CF	PLAP, AFFP, PBPC	1 or 2	D/P
	Spectra	C/CF	PLAP, PLAP + RBC, PLAP + 2RBC	1 or 2	D/P
Haemonetics	Trima	C/CF	PLAP, AFFP	1	D
	MCS + (LN9000)	C/DF	RBCP, 2RBC	1 or 2	D/P
	MCS + (8150)	C/DF	SP, AFFP	1	D
	PCS-2	C/DF	WBC-MR	1	D
Therakos/Johnson & Johnson	UVAR-XTS	C/DF	PC-WBC	1	P

C, centrifugal; CF, continuous flow; SP, source plasma; AFFP, apheresis fresh frozen plasma; D, donor; P, patient; SM, spinning membrane; DF, discontinuous flow; PLAP, platelets by apheresis; PBPC, peripheral blood progenitor cell; RBC, red blood cells; 2RBC, double red blood cells; RBCP, red blood cells plus plasma; WBC-MR, mononuclear enriched white blood cells; PCWBC, photochemically modified white blood cells.

Fenwal has developed a cell separator called the Amicus, which operates in a similar manner to the CS-3000, but has a smaller footprint and operates as a one-arm venous access device for platelet collection. The high extraction coefficient for platelets allows frequent collection of double products, such as two platelet apheresis products each 3.0×10^{11} platelets or more and leukocyte reduced to 1.0×10^{6} residual WBCs or less without use of a leukoreduction filter. In donors with platelet counts of 250×10^{9}/L or more before donation, double plateletpheresis products are obtained more than 75% of the time at the Oklahoma Blood Institute.

Fenwal also uses a device called the Autopheresis-C with a spinning membrane, thus incorporating both membrane and centrifugation technology to collect plasma. In the United States, this device is commonly used to collect source plasma as well as apheresis fresh-frozen plasma (AFFP). This is a discontinuous system in which only a single venipuncture is performed. Fenwal attempted to change the porosity of the membrane to collect platelet-rich plasma (5). This procedure has been abandoned.

Fresenius Technology

Fresenius of Germany introduced a cell separator into Europe in 1987 primarily for the collection of platelets. The Fresenius AS104 is currently licensed in the United States for the collection of single-donor platelets and is licensed for therapeutic plasma exchange and collection of PBPC. It is a continuous-flow, double-venipuncture system. Fresenius has introduced an upgraded version called the AS204 in Europe but not in the United States.

GAMBRO BCT (COBE) TECHNOLOGY

Gambro BCT (formerly COBE) acquired the IBM biomedical services technology (the IBM-2997 cell separator) and then developed the COBE Spectra as a seal-less system based on the original IBM-2997 rotating-channel belt. The Spectra is a continuous-flow system in which one- or two-arm venous access is used for platelet collection. Spectra uses a leukoreduction system to collect leukoreduced platelet units. The Spectra device indicates when units may contain excessive numbers of leukocytes and thus when counting is needed to document leukoreduction status. The Spectra device also is used to collect PBPC and to perform therapeutic apheresis procedures (6,7).

The newest cell separator added into the Gambro BCT Technology is the Trima. This device is fully automated; the technology is similar to that of the Spectra device. The Trima device is a single-venous-access device, has no rotating seal, and has a smaller footprint than does the Spectra. The Trima is capable of collecting double units ($\geq 6.0 \times 10^{11}$ platelets) that are leukoreduced to 1.0×10^{6} or fewer residual WBCs. The Trima device has been designed and is licensed to collect a single or double RBC unit along with the apheresis platelet product. To date it has not been used for therapeutic procedures. Collection of 1 or 2 RBC units with a platelet unit ($\geq 3.0 \times 10^{11}$ platelets) that is leukoreduced is a novel idea and has the advantage of increasing the RBC supply of a blood center. The disadvantage is the possibility deferring a donor on the next visit if the donor's hematocrit decreases to less than 38% (FDA/AABB minimum requirement). Because of the low extracorporeal RBC mass in the Trima device, a donor giving RBCs and a plateletpheresis product can return within 72 hours to donate another plateletpheresis product with the Trima device (8). For donors with a predonation platelet count of 250×10^{9}L or more double plateletpheresis products can be collected more than 75% of the time at the Oklahoma Blood Institute.

Gambro had developed a therapeutic plasma exchange membrane cell separator called the TPE, which was a continuous-flow device with a flat membrane for blood separation. This device is now obsolete in the United States and no longer used. The COBE/IBM 2997 also is obsolete.

Haemonetics Technology

The discontinuous-flow cell separators (MCS Plus-LN-9000; MCS Plus-8150; PCS-2) produced by the Haemonetics, operate with a fixed centrifuge speed and a variable centrifugal force to separate a donor's or patient's blood into components. A disposable rotating bowl separates the incoming blood in such a way that RBCs move to the periphery and plasma to the inside of the rotating bowl. The buffy coat, which contains the WBCs and platelets, forms a layer between the RBCs and plasma. Platelets or mononuclear cells are collected with the aid of optical detectors by means of a fluid-surge elutriation process. The remaining RBCs and plasma are returned to the donor, and the platelets are retained until the desired yield is obtained with multiple passes or cycles. This discontinuous technology is amenable to a one- or a two-arm protocol, although the one-arm venous access technique is used more often because of donor preference for a single needle stick (6).

The Haemonetics plasma collection system-2 (PCS-2) has a special disposable bowl specifically designed to collect plasma. This has become the most commonly used automated cell separator for collection of source plasma in the United States and the world. The PCS-2 also is used to collect transfusable plasma in clinically useful volumes of 500 to 600 ml; the product is designated AFFP. The mobile collection system plus (MCS Plus) cell separators are the newest of the Haemonetics discontinuous-flow technology. They are lightweight (60 to 70 pounds [27 to 31.5 kg]), extremely portable and mobile, fully automated, and flexible in terms of blood components collected. The MCS Plus LN-9000 is used strictly to collect platelets with or without concurrent plasma. Unlike the Fenwal Amicus and Gambro Trima or Spectra leukoreduction system, the initial platelet product is not leukoreduced to an acceptable level ($\leq 1.0 \times 10^{6}$ residual WBCs) and must undergo leukoreduction filtration, which is now accomplished with an on-line process that produces a final transfusable product that contains 1.0×10^{6} residual WBCs or fewer in 3.0×10^{11} platelets or more.

The MCS Plus 8150 has been developed for collection of either RBCP (red blood cell unit plus a plasma unit) or 2RBC (double red blood cell units) (9–11). This device is a fixed-RBC-mass collection machine. Each unit of RBCs contains approximately 180 to 200 ml of absolute RBC mass. Both MCS Plus devices (LN-9000 and 8150) have a functionally closed rotating seal to maximize product shelf life. The MCS Plus 8150 operates with an anticoagulant to anticoagulated whole blood (AC:WB) collection ratio of 1:16 with citrate–phosphate–double dextrose (CP2D), which further reduces the amount of citrate in the RBC units of RBCP or 2RBC but markedly reduces the citrate in the plasma collected. The plasma of the RBCP collection contains one-half the citrate of whole blood–derived fresh-frozen plasma (WBD-FFP). The RBCs from the 2RBC procedure can be filtered on line to yield two leukoreduced RBC units.

Therakos (Johnson & Johnson) Technology

The newest photopheresis device (UVAR-XTS system) essentially is a discontinuous-flow cell separator that collects buffy coat that contains mononuclear cells from patients with a variety of conditions such as cutaneous T-cell lymphoma, graft versus host disease due to bone marrow transplantation, or solid-organ host versus graft disease. These mononuclear cells are incubated with methoxsalen (Uvadex) and subjected to ultraviolet radiation and transfused back to the patient. Amelioration of the pathologic process is the desired outcome. The older and no longer supported Therakos photopheresis system was used with oral administration of methoxypsoralen.

Other Technology

Other devices, both centrifugal and membrane based, are used outside the United States. The Dideco Excel is an automated blood cell separator made in Italy for the collection of apheresis platelets. Organon Teknika developed a hollow-fiber membrane plasma collection system, which was previously used in Europe to collect source plasma. Immunoadsorption technologies continue to be tried for removal of pathologic antibodies and various lipid fractions from patients with homozygous type II hypercholesterolemia. These technologies (see Chapter 47) are expensive and for the most part remain research based (12–14).

DONOR APHERESIS

General Information

The key forces driving transfusion medicine into the twenty-first century are safety and quality, availability of blood, legal and regulatory issues, and cost. The issues of safety and quality of blood products are enhanced with the use of apheresis-derived products. Metered anticoagulation, automation during collection, reduced variables, fewer donor exposures enhance safety and quality. The issues of blood availability and cost have, as of 2000, become critical and major issues, respectively. Availability of blood products, especially RBCs, is an increasing and worsening problem, as is increasing cost, especially with a movement toward universal leukoreduction of blood products. Apheresis products that have been clearly more expensive to produce are now being produced as double- and triple-yield products or as multiple types of products (RBCP and RBCs plus platelets). This reduces costs while increasing availability. The advantages of use of apheresis-derived blood components are listed in Table 45.2. Blood components that can be obtained are presented in Table 45.3.

TABLE 45.2. ADVANTAGES OF USE OF APHERESIS DERIVED BLOOD COMPONENTS

Reduced donor exposure: full transfusion dose
Frequent repeat donor: "pedigreed" donors
Higher quality products: more quality control per product collected
Consistent and standardized products (yields)
Matching donors to patients
Reduced donor reactions
High donor acceptance
Double yield or multiple full-dose blood product collections

Donor Care

Donors who undergo automated apheresis procedures must go through routine screening and testing procedures. At minimum, component donors must meet all the requirements of a whole-blood donors. The main difference is that the "needle in to needle out" time for a 500-ml whole-blood donation is only 8 to 12 minutes, whereas the needle in to needle out time for plasmapheresis and RBC pheresis is 35 to 45 minutes and for plateletpheresis is 60 to 120 minutes. The total donation time therefore is much longer for apheresis donation and requires more precise scheduling and a more dedicated donor. When 2 units of RBCs are donated, the interval between donations is 112 days. The allowed frequency of donation is greater with non-RBC collection procedures, that is, plasma and platelet donation—up to 24 donations per year for a plateletpheresis donor versus six donations for whole-blood donors. Donors of transfusable plasma (AFFP) can make up to 13 donations per year (every

TABLE 45.3. APHERESIS-DERIVED BLOOD COMPONENTS FROM A SINGLE PROCEDURE

Procedure	Instrument
Primary	
PLAP	MCS+(LN9000), Spectra, Trima, CS-3000, Amicus, AS104
PLAP + plasma	MCS+(LN9000), Spectra, Trima, CS-3000, Amicus, AS104
PLAP + RBC	Trima
2RBC	MCS+(8150)
RBCP	MCS+(8150)
Plasma	PCS-2, Autopheresis-C
Granulocytes	MCS+(LN9000), Spectra, CS-3000
PBPC	Spectra, CS-3000, AS104
Secondary	
Cryoprecipitate	PCS-2, Autopheresis-C
Cryoreduced Plasma	PCS-2, Autopheresis-C

PLAP, plateletpheresis; RBC, red blood cells; 2RBC, double red blood cells; RBCP, red blood cells plus plasma; PBPC, perpheral blood progenitor cells.

TABLE 45.4. DONOR REACTIONS

Reaction	Whole Blood	AFFP	Plateletpheresis	2RBC, RBCP
Vasovagal	Occasional	Rare	Rare	Rare
Hypovolemia	Occasional	Rare	Rare	Rare
Allergic	Very rare	Very rare	Very rare	Very rare
Citrate				
effect	None	Rare	Frequent	Rare
toxicity	None	Very rare	Occasional	Very rare

AFFP, apheresis fresh frozen plasma; 2RBC, double red blood cells; RBCP, red blood cells plus plasma; Occasional, 0.5% to 2.5%; Rare, <0.5%; Very rare, <0.01%; Frequent, 5% to 20%.

4 weeks) by obtaining a variance from the FDA with relief from the obligation to meet the FDA regulations for source plasma donors.

In the United States, source plasma, that is, plasma obtained for fractionation into albumin, intravenous immune globulin, factor VIII, and factor IX, is almost totally obtained from paid donors who donate at commercially operated plasma donation centers. These donors may donate up to 800 ml of absolute plasma per donation as frequently as twice a week, depending on the donor's weight. The donor must be examined at defined intervals by a physician and must have total protein and serum protein electrophoresis determinations made at FDA-required intervals as specified in the *Code of Federal Regulations.*

Apheresis donors for platelets, plasma, and RBCs tend to have lower reaction rates than do donors of whole blood (Table 45.4). Vasovagal reactions are most common among first-time blood donors; apheresis donors usually are repeated donors (15). Hypovolemia is less common among apheresis donors than among whole-blood donors for two reasons. First, the total volume removed in plateletpheresis, RBC apheresis, and plasmapheresis for transfusion is less than that in whole-blood donation because the component has a lower volume, as in plateletpheresis, or volume is returned to the donor as crystalloid solution in the anticoagulant and saline solution. Second, the relatively long time at rest during apheresis donation allows transcapillary refilling of the intravascular compartment from the interstitial space. Allergic reactions to iodine skin preparations are very rare. However, a mild citrate effect (circumoral paresthesia, feelings of vibration or buzzing, tingling, or coldness) is not uncommon for most plateletpheresis donors. More severe citrate toxicity (muscle cramping, total body shivering, nausea, vomiting, and tetany) is uncommon but is potentially serious and necesitates slowing the rate of return of citrate-containing plasma (16,17). The intravenous administration of calcium-containing solutions is generally not recommended, unless the reactions are unusually severe or prolonged.

Hemolysis occurs rarely and when it does almost always has a mechanical cause, such as occlusion or partial occlusion of RBC-containing tubing. On rare occasions (1 in 3,000 to 5, 000 donations), hyperlipemic plasma in platelet donors causes elevated and visible free hemoglobin levels in the collected component. The mechanism of this hemolysis remains unclear.

Venous access is an important consideration in donor apheresis procedures because of the need for (a) long needle in to needle out time, (b) a prolonged high flow rate, (c) increased frequency of donation, and (d) the occasional need for two venipunctures with continuous-flow equipment. Possible venous access injuries include blood infiltration and bruising but rarely venous thrombosis. Cutaneous nerve injuries are rare, and deep nerve injuries (median, ulnar, and radial nerves) are almost nonexistent. The development of smaller-needle technology for venous access will help reduce these problems.

Extracorporeal blood volume (ECBV) in apheresis procedures—the total amount of blood out of the donor—is greatly reduced with use of newer apheresis devices, such as the Amicus and Trima. With the older devices, especially the discontinuous-flow devices, ECBV tends to be greater but generally is not a problem except in therapeutic apheresis involving pediatric patients. The supine position of donors and access to oral fluids during the procedure tend to eliminate problems. However, from a regulatory standpoint, loss of ECBV during malfunction of a machine can lead to a 56-day donor deferral when the older, higher ECBV devices are used. The low ECBV of the newer devices allows another plateletpheresis procedure within 3 days if necessary. If the ECBV of the apheresis device is 100 ml or less, plateletpheresis may be done less than 8 weeks after a whole-blood donation (18).

In the early years of donor apheresis, lymphocyte depletion with loss of immunologic memory was a concern because of high WBC levels in apheresis components, especially in plateletpheresis. This has proved not to be a problem, and with the current focus on WBC-reduced apheresis components, it is no longer a concern even for very frequent apheresis donors (19).

Specific Products and Procedures

Plateletpheresis donations are limited to 24 per year by the AABB and the FDA. Plateletpheresis donation can occur every 72 hours but not more than twice a week. If the interval between plateletpheresis donation is 4 weeks or more, a predonation platelet count is not required. If the interval is less than 4 weeks, a predonation platelet count must be obtained and must be ≥$150 $\times 10^9$/L for the procedure to be performed. If RBC loss during the procedure exceeds 200 ml, the waiting period is 8 weeks before the next donation. Donors with predonation platelet counts of 300 $\times 10^9$/L or more usually can donate a double-dose platelet product (≥6.0 $\times 10^{11}$ platelets). Almost all plateletpheresis products in the United States are produced as leukoreduced, that is, 1.0 $\times 10^6$ or fewer residual WBCs. Currently a leukoreduced product (platelet or RBC) in the United States must be 5.0 $\times 10^6$ or fewer residual WBCs. However, the European standard is 1.0 $\times 10^6$ or fewer residual WBCs per product. Prestorage leukoreduction, as is done after many plateletpheresis procedures, has clear advantages over filtration after storage or bedside leukoreduction filtration in reducing febrile reactions and other leukocyte-derived complications by preventing accumulation of cytokines and leukocyte fragments during storage (20–22).

The intravascular volume deficit during the procedure should not exceed 10.5 ml per kilogram of the donor's weight by AABB standards (18). Only rarely, when fluids are administered intravenously or orally to plateletpheresis donors, does the donor even come close to that value. Plateletpheresis units must contain 3.0×10^{11} or more platelets per unit in at least 75% of the units tested at maximal storage time. The physician in charge of the donor apheresis unit can make a medical decision to accept a donation from someone not eligible at the time if the benefits to the intended recipient outweigh the risks to the donor. This can occur when the donor is an HLA match or is HPA-1a (Pl^{A1}) negative and no other donor is available. Use of single venous access and high platelet extraction coefficients in the newer plateletapheresis devices (Amicus, Trima) allows shorter collection time or higher product yields in normal collection times.

Automated RBC collection with apheresis technology can be performed using the Haemonetics MCS Plus 8150, which can collect 2 units of RBCs (2RBC) or 1 unit of RBCs and one large volume plasma unit (RBCP), or the Gambro Trima which can collect one plateletpheresis product and 1 or 2 units of RBCs (10,11,23). The 2RBC procedure is becoming rapidly more popular in the United States to collect group O and Rh-negative RBCs with the intent of reducing RBC availability shortages, which are becoming increasingly more common in the United States. The advantages are (a) a standardized RBC mass collection (180 to 200 ml per unit of RBCs), (b) metered anticoagulation, which obviates mixing and reduces clot formation, (c) the ability to return fluids to the donor and reduce any risk of hypovolemia, (d) on-line separation of RBCs and plasma, 2RBCs, or RBCP, eliminating secondary separation procedures, and (e) the use of smaller needles. For the collection of 1 unit of RBCs along with another component (plasma or platelets) the standard hematocrit criteria apply. However, for 2RBC collection, the FDA has imposed specific donor hematocrit, height, and weight requirements (11). Table 45.5 outlines the current criteria for allogeneic 2RBC collection. Unless the FDA changes the criteria, the use of 2RBC collection from female donors will be limited. After 2RBC apheresis donation, donor deferral for any procedure (whole blood or apheresis) is 16 weeks. The RBCP criteria for collection of 1 unit of RBCs and 1 unit of jumbo plasma are outlined in Table 45.6. The anticoagulant used in RBCP and 2RBC procedures with the Haemonetics MCS Plus 8150 is CP2D at an AC:WB ratio of 1:16. This markedly reduces (50%) the citrate returned to the donor during these procedures as well as the citrate in the plasma collected. The absolute volume of plasma collected (~90%) is higher than that derived from a whole-blood collection (approximately 80% of which is absolute).

TABLE 45.5. CRITERIA FOR ALLOGENEIC DONATION OF DOUBLE RED BLOOD CELLS

Donor Weight (lb)	Donor Height (in)	Donor Hematocrit (%)	Maximum Absolute RBC Volume (ml)
Men			
130–149	≥61	≥40	180 × 2
150–174	≥61	≥40	200 × 2
≥175	≥61	≥40	210 × 2
Women			
150–174	≥65	≥40	180 × 2
≥175	≥65	≥40	200 × 2

TABLE 45.6. CRITERIA FOR ALLOGENEIC RED BLOOD CELL AND PLASMA DONATION

Donor Weight (lb)	Donor Hematocrit (%)	Maximum Red Blood Cell Volume (ml)	Absolute Maximum Plasma Volume (ml)
Men			
110–129	≥38	185	450
130–149	≥38	195	500
≥150	≥38	210	550
Women			
110–129	≥38	180	450
130–149	≥38	190	450
150–174	≥38	190	500
≥175	≥38	200	550

Automated collection of plasma (AFFP) can be done with all of the apheresis devices, either as a sole collection product (Fenwal Autopheresis-C and Haemonetics PCS-2) or as a concurrent product with apheresis platelets or as part of an RBC apheresis procedure (RBCP). Table 45.6 shows the volume of plasma that can be collected during the RBCP procedure according to donor weight and hematocrit. Plasma collected with the Autopheresis-C or PCS-2 is collected at a 1:16 AC:WB ratio, as is the plasma of the RBCP.

Apheresis fresh-frozen plasma is a unique component and differs substantially from WBD-FFP (Table 45.7). There is more absolute plasma per milliliter of anticoagulated plasma (90% in AFFP versus 80% in WBD-FFP), much less glucose, and only one half to two thirds of the citrate. A truly transfusable dose can be obtained that markedly affects the clotting factor status of an adult patient depending on patient size and the severity of the clotting deficiency. This component meets the criteria for a source of FFP espoused at the 1984 National Institutes of Health consensus conference on the use of plasma (24). The number of residual platelets and WBCs in AFFP also is less than in WBD-FFP. This may be important in reducing the recipient reactions to plasma transfusion caused by the release of cytokines or leukocyte fragments into the plasma by passenger leukocytes (20,21).

Apheresis cryoprecipitate is derived by means of cryoprecipitation of AFFP. At the Oklahoma Blood Institute, the apheresis cryoprecipitate (APH-CRYO) is prepared from a volume of absolute plasma equivalent to 3 units of WBD-FFP. Correspondingly the APH-CRYO has a volume of approximately 100 ml (wet cryo) and does not require pooling or dilution but can be simply thawed and infused. This is in contrast to WBD-CRYO, which is prepared as a dry CRYO (volume, 15 to 20 ml) and requires dilution and pooling before administration (11). The

TABLE 45.7. AUTOMATED PLASMA VERSUS WHOLE BLOOD–DERIVED PLASMA

	Collection Technique			
	MCS+8150	PCS-2/Auto-C	Concurrent	WBD-FFP
Total volume (ml)	450–550	500–800	250–450	200–250
Absolute plasma (%)	90	90	80–85	80
Anticoagulant (% citrate)	CP2D (3%)	Sodium citrate (4%)	ACD (3%)	CPDA-1, CPD, CP2D (3%)
Anticoagulant to whole blood ratio	1:16	1:16	1:8–1:12	1:8
Grams of citrate (100 ml plasma)	0.3	0.4	0.6–0.45	0.6

WBD-FFP, Whole blood–derived fresh frozen plasma; CP2D, citrate–phosphate–double dextrose; ACD, acid-citrate-dextrose; CPDA–1, citrate-phosphate-dextrose-adenine; CPD, citrate-phosphate-dextrose.

apheresis cryopoor plasma (APH-CPP) remaining has a volume of approximately 400 ml and is used as replacement fluid for plasma exchange in the care of patients with thrombotic thrombocytopenic purpura (TTP).

Granulocyte donations are relatively infrequent because of the development of better antibiotics to prevent and manage the infections associated with granulocytopenia and because of the availability of cytokines such as GM-CSF and G-CSF, which help reduce the duration of the granulocytopenic period in patients with bone marrow failure. When granulocytes are needed, as in the management of neutropenia with bacterial or fungal sepsis not responding to antibiotics, collection of granulocytes poses problems for the donor and the patient. To collect an adequate number of granulocytes (see Chapter 20), the donor must be stimulated before donation with steroids and G-CSF to increase the circulating pool of granulocytes. Then hydroxyethyl starch (HES), available in low- and high-molecular-weight forms, must be infused during collection to increase RBC sedimentation and to facilitate separation and collection of granulocytes (25,26). The use of G-CSF, steroids, and HES (pharmacomanipulation of the donor) can cause problems such as musculoskeletal pain, weight gain, fluid overload, allergic reaction to the starch, and reactivation of peptic ulcer disease by the steroids. However, only rarely are these problems severe.

Peripheral blood progenitor cells can be collected with a variety of cell separators, but the Spectra (Gambro BCT), the CS-3000 (Fenwal), and the AS-104 (Fresenius) are the most commonly used cell separators for PBPC collection in the United States (14,27–29). Peripheral blood progenitor cells are collected by means of harvesting the buffy coat–rich portion of the blood and specifically extracting the mononuclear cell–rich portion of the buffy coat, which contains the CD34-positive progenitor or stem cells (29). The number of CD34+ cells needed to repopulate the bone marrow varies from 4 to 10 $\times$ 10^6 per kilogram of body weight. The PBPC usually are cryopreserved in autologous plasma with a 5% final concentration of dimethyl sulfoxide and are frozen in a controlled-rate freezer and stored at less than −135°C.

Collection of autologous PBPC now is commonplace as a method for autologous bone marrow "rescue" of patients with certain malignant diseases undergoing extensive chemotherapy (see Chapter 37). Collection of allogeneic PBPC stimulated with G-CSF or GM-CSF as a replacement for classic allogeneic bone marrow transplantation (see Chapter 38) is slowly increasing in frequency (30).

Adverse Effects on Donors and Recipients

Donor apheresis procedures have not proved more hazardous than donation of whole blood and are generally proving to be as safe as or safer because of the ability to return fluids to donors and because the longer collection times of apheresis procedures allow better fluid equilibration and a lower risk of hypovolemia occurring. Hematoma with use of single venous access devices (MCS Plus, Amicus, Trima) are no more frequent than in donation of whole blood. The major "expected" adverse consequence is related to the effects of the citrate anticoagulant returned to the donor. Donors of lower body weight are more likely to experience citrate symptoms. Almost all plateletpheresis donors and 2RBC donors have some citrate effects (circumoral paresthesia, buzzing sensation, and nasal stuffiness). These effects are not worrisome but when they occur suggest slowing the procedure before more serious toxic effects occur, such as muscle tightening, chills, nausea, vomiting, or tetany. Administration of oral antacids, warming donors, and slowing flow rate reduce the citrate effects. Calcium gluconate (10 ml of 10% solution given slowly intravenously) rarely is needed (31,32). A single plateletpheresis procedure can remove 25% to 50% of circulating platelets, but the release of normally splenic sequestered platelets almost always prevents significant thrombocytopenia in the donor. In frequent plateletpheresis procedures, it is not uncommon for the donor's platelet count to decrease and then rebound after 1 to 2 weeks.

Adverse effects in recipients of plateletpheresis products are equal to or less than the reactions that occur with administration of WBD platelet products. The use of leukoreduction with almost all plateletpheresis products has markedly reduced but not eliminated transfusion-associated febrile reactions. The greatest transfusion-associated infectious disease risk today is bacterial contamination. Because plateletpheresis products are from a single donor and one collection event unlike WBD platelets, which are from several donors and collection events, the risk of bacterial contamination is less with plateletpheresis products than with WBD platelets.

THERAPEUTIC APHERESIS OVERVIEW

Therapeutic apheresis can be classified as therapeutic cytapheresis or therapeutic plasma exchange. Strictly speaking, therapeutic plasma exchange implies removal of the patient's plasma with replacement of a crystalloid or colloid solution to maintain a normovolemic state in the patient. Plasmapheresis generally implies removal of an aliquot of plasma without fluid replacement. Because these procedures are discussed completely in Chapter 46, only basic principles are mentioned here.

Critical factors involved in therapeutic apheresis procedures include (a) what is to be removed and how it is best removed, such as plasma, WBCs, or platelets, (b) how much is to be removed with each procedure, (c) how often the procedure should be performed, (d) how many procedures should be performed, (e) what the replacement solution should be, if any, (f) what special considerations involving the patient are present, such as presence of other disease or medications, (g) what equipment should be used, (h) what type of vascular access should be used, (i) what anticoagulant should be used and how much, (j) where the procedure should be performed, such as at the blood center or in the inpatient or outpatient areas of a hospital, (k) whether the presence of a physician is needed throughout each procedure, (l) whether the request complies with established therapeutic apheresis guidelines, (m) what complications or adverse reactions are to be expected, such as thrombocytopenia, bleeding, thrombosis, arrhythmia, plasma-induced immune reactions, (n) whether the patient needs testing for infectious diseases, as in routine donor screening, (o) whether special precautions must be taken by the apheresis staff, (p) who should perform the therapeutic apheresis procedure—physician, nurse, physician's assistant, or trained technician, and (q) how fast the removed substance will regenerate or redistribute into the bloodstream.

What is to be removed from the patient depends on the diagnosis. How it is to be removed depends on the equipment available to do it. For patients with disease mediated by a known plasma factor such as an autoantibody, immune complex, a drug or toxin that is protein bound, and a high cholesterol or triglyceride level, it is clear what must be removed. There are diseases, such as TTP, in which it is still not completely clear whether a plasma factor has to be removed, replaced, or both. For a patient with hemophilia A and an inhibitor to factor VIII, the inhibitor should be removed, and factor VIII should be replaced in the presence of life-threatening bleeding. For patients with hypercholesterolemia, the use of chromatographic columns that selectively remove cholesterol and allow return of cholesterol-depleted plasma would be preferable to therapeutic plasma exchange. In therapeutic cytapheresis, the cells to be removed can be platelets in a patient with severe thrombocytosis (generally more than $1{,}500 \times 10^9$ platelets per liter), blast cells in a patient with acute leukemia with a leukostasis syndrome (generally more than 100×10^9 blasts per liter), or RBCs in a patient with sickle cell disease in a life-threatening sickle cell crisis.

TABLE 45.8. PLASMA VOLUMES EXCHANGED: FRACTION REMOVED AND REMAINING

Plasma Volume Removed	Fraction Removed (%)	Fraction Remaining (%)
0.5	40	60
1.0	62	38
1.5	78	22
2.0	85	15
2.5	91	9
3.0	94	6

How much plasma is to be removed with each procedure and the frequency of procedures depends on the plasma factor involved. The removal of one calculated plasma volume results in a net overall exchange of only 62% because of progressive dilution by replacement solutions during the procedure (33). This is true whether plasma or RBCs are being removed (Table 45.8). The most effective therapeutic plasma exchanges remove 1.0 to 1.5 plasma volumes (62% to 78% overall exchange). If the plasma factor is an IgG antibody, the total IgG within the intravascular compartment is only approximately 45% to 50%; the rest is in the extravascular spaces. Because equilibration is rapid, it is difficult to reduce IgG antibodies with one therapeutic plasma exchange; daily therapeutic plasma exchanges are necessary. On the other hand, approximately 90% to 92% of IgM antibodies reside in the intravascular compartment and are more easily removed with one large volume therapeutic plasma exchange. I limit therapeutic plasma exchange to 1.0 to 1.5 calculated plasma volumes per procedure in most instances because of a lower rate of complications than with larger-volume plasma exchanges (2.0 volumes or greater).

A simple method for estimating the blood volume of adults is shown in Table 45.9. I developed this modified rule of fives to quickly estimate blood and plasma volumes. It agrees with results of recent blood volume studies within ±15% (34,35). Plasma volume is calculated by means of multiplying the obverse of the hematocrit (1.0 minus the decimal equivalent of the hematocrit) by the estimated blood volume. How often a therapeutic apheresis procedure should be performed depends on how ill the patient is and the rate of regeneration or redistribution of the substance being removed. Removal of IgG antibodies generally requires daily therapeutic plasma exchanges because of regenera-

TABLE 45.9. ESTIMATING BLOOD VOLUME: MODIFIED RULE OF FIVES, BODY MASS AND BUILD

Sex	Fat	Thin	Normal	Muscular
Men	60	65	70	75
Women	55	60	65	70

Values are in milliliters of whole blood per kilogram body weight.

tion and redistribution from the extravascular to the intravascular space. Therapeutic plasma exchange occasionally must be performed every 12 hours to save a patient with florid liver failure awaiting a liver transplant.

The end point of therapeutic apheresis (therapeutic plasma exchange or therapeutic cytapheresis) with regard to the number of procedures needed depends on the patient's clinical response and specific laboratory measurements. For example, in TTP the patient's clinical response is critical (e.g., resolution of altered sensorium) and generally parallels a decrease in lactate dehydrogenase level and an increase in platelet count. In disorders mediated by antibodies, because therapeutic plasma exchange is generally a treatment that buys time during the wait for other therapeutic measures, such as immunosuppression, to take effect, only a limited number of procedures usually are needed (5 to 10 therapeutic plasma exchanges). Recurrence or exacerbation of some diseases, such as TTP or inflammatory neuropathy, frequently necessitate extending the therapeutic apheresis time frame to achieve durable remissions.

Replacement solutions can be crystalloid or colloid (Table 45.10). Although they are less expensive, crystalloid solutions are less useful for large-volume daily plasma exchanges because of the rapid onset of hypoproteinemia and dilutional coagulopathy. In addition, the volume of crystalloid needed is at least two to three times the plasma removed because of the rapid movement of the crystalloid solution into the extravascular space. The most commonly used replacement solution in therapeutic plasma exchange is 5% albumin, a true natural colloid, which is slightly hyperoncotic. This form of albumin is stripped of its calcium and acts like a calcium sponge by binding calcium ions. It is a safe product, never having been associated with transmission of any known viral infection (hepatitis A, B, and C viruses or HIV). Because it is slightly hyperoncotic, albumin can be diluted with saline solution to 4.0% to 4.5% for plasma exchange. The other natural colloid is FFP. However, because of an increased incidence of allergic reactions and slightly increased risk of transmission of infectious disease, FFP is used only when clotting factors or other proteins must be replaced or in the management of TTP, in which studies have established it as the replacement fluid of choice (36). The issue of whether cryoprecipitate-poor plasma, solvent-detergent plasma, or unaltered FFP is best in the management of TTP is still not resolved. Artificial colloid solutions (HES or dextran) are used relatively infrequently in the United States and offer no medical advantage over 5% albumin.

TABLE 45.10. REPLACEMENT SOLUTIONS FOR TOTAL PLASMA EXCHANGE

Solution	Comment
Crystalloid Solutions	
Saline 0.9%	Least expensive, high sodium and chloride
Ringer solution	Inexpensive, less sodium and chloride
Lactated Ringer solution	Inexpensive, less sodium and chloride
Balanced electrolyte solution	Most physiologic and expensive
Colloids (Natural)	
Albumin 5%	Safe, hyperoncotic, and expensive
Plasma protein fraction 5%	No advantage over albumin
Fresh frozen plasma (FFP)	Potentially the least safe but is isooncotic, contains all clotting factors
Donor retested FFP	Safer than regular FFP and more expensive
Solvent-detergent treated plasma	Very expensive, risk of nonlipid enveloped viral transmission, pooled
Colloids (Artificial)	
Hydroxethyl starch (high MW)	450,000 average MW
Hydroxethyl starch (low MW)	150,000 average MW
Dextran	Infrequently used
Modified fluid gelatin	Not in United States, used in Europe

MW, molecular weight.

The development of pathogen-inactivated plasma will further reduce the risk of transmission of infectious agents. Solvent-detergent plasma is currently available but does not inactivate viruses that do not have a lipid envelope, such as hepatitis A or human Parvovirus B19. Solvent-detergent plasma is a pooled product that does not transmit HIV or hepatitis B or C viruses. Solvent-detergent plasma has normal amounts of clotting factors but is deficient in some of the anticlotting factors (protein C, protein S, and antithrombin III) and plasminogen. Another plasma product with reduced infectious disease risk is donor retested plasma. The donor is retested at least 110 days after the initial donation. The unit is not transfused until the retest has been performed and the results are negative for all viral markers tested.

The type of equipment used depends on the particular needs of the therapeutic apheresis service. Each of the different manufacturers' equipment has certain advantages. Most therapeutic plasma exchange procedures are performed with centrifuge-based machines. Add-on devices such as staphylococcal protein A immunoadsorption columns can be used ex vivo to remove IgG selectively and then to return the immunoadsorbed plasma to the patient (12,13,37). Another special type of therapeutic apheresis, called *photopheresis,* is used to manage a hematologic malignant lesion called *cutaneous T-cell lymphoma* or *Sezany syndrome.* Photopheresis is the use of extracorporeal photochemotherapy to modify circulating malignant T cells. The process involves giving a patient with diagnosed disease 8-methoxypsoralen, a drug that enters these cells and bonds to the DNA. These psoralen-containing T cells are harvested from the peripheral blood with a special cell separator, which exposes the harvested T cells to ultraviolet A radiation ex vivo. These ultraviolet irradiated and altered T cells in some way modulate an antitumor effect when reinfused (38,39). The new model of the Therakos photopheresis system (UVAR XTS) operates with a form of psoralen (methoxsalen) that is injected into the product collected with the device and reduces the risks of systemic exposure to psoralen in the patient.

Vascular access can be through peripheral veins, central veins, or both. If many therapeutic plasma exchanges are planned, central venous catheters usually are necessary. Double- or triple-lumen dialysis catheters are ideal for central venous access. Strict catheter care is critical to prevent clotting of the catheter and infections at the catheter site. Flushing the catheter with a heparinized solution immediately after exchange is critical to prevent clotting. If catheter clotting should occur, injection of plasminogen-activating drugs into the clotted lumen frequently lyses the clot and restores patency. Placement of central venous catheters is critical so that the catheter tip is not in the heart (right atrium) but in the superior vena cava. Cardiac irritability with premature ventricular beats can occur if the catheter is in the right atrium. The irritation is caused directly by the catheter or indirectly by return of fluids that are cold, hypocalcemic, hypokalemic, or high in citrate ion. A chest radiograph should be obtained after placement of a subclavian central venous catheter, not only to locate the tip of the catheter within the superior vena cava but also ensure that the catheter did not perforate the subclavian vein and cause hemothorax or pneumothorax. For some patients, surgical placement of an arteriovenous shunt, such as an expanded polytetrafluoroethylene (Gore-Tex) graft tunneled under the anterior thigh to connect the femoral artery and vein, may be necessary for long-term therapeutic plasma exchange.

The use of anticoagulants in therapeutic apheresis usually is limited to citrate anticoagulants (acid-citrate-dextrose A [ACD-A], ACD-B, and sodium citrate), heparin, or both. Acid-citrate-dextrose A is a 3% citrate anticoagulant and ACD-B a 2% citrate anticoagulant. Sodium citrate is available as a 4% citrate anticoagulant. The advantage of citrate as an anticoagulant is that any amount returned to the patient during the RBC return in a therapeutic plasma exchange procedure is rapidly metabolized. Citrate never produces systemic anticoagulation. This, however, can be a disadvantage when flow is low, because catheter clotting can occur. If the flow rate is low and heparin is not contraindicated, heparin can be used alone or in combination with citrate. Heparin may enhance systemic anticoagulation more than is expected because of the additional effect of dilution of clotting factors by the nonplasma replacement solutions. The half-life of heparin in the body is approximately 90 minutes. Citrate is not an issue because it has a short in vivo half-life and does not systemically anticoagulate. When heparin is used to anticoagulate blood in the draw line and is not used systemically, 17,500 U is added to 500 ml of saline solution (35 U of heparin per milliliter of saline solution). With an AC:WB ratio of 1:8, this formula delivers 5 U of heparin per milliliter of whole blood collected. At an AC:WB ratio of 1:10, it delivers 3.9 U of heparin per milliliter of whole blood collected (3.5 U of heparin per milliliter of anticoagulated blood collected).

Therapeutic apheresis procedures should be performed only when emergency care is readily available. If the procedure is performed at the blood center on an outpatient basis, the blood center must have a knowledgeable physician. The nursing staff performing the procedure must be trained in resuscitation care, and a crash cart with a cardiac monitor and defibrillator must be available. In the hospital, the same requirements apply for outpatient procedures. Critically ill patients, such as those with acute TTP, should be treated in an intensive care setting where emergency care is readily available. A physician must be available for each procedure, but the severity of the patient's illness determines whether a physician is needed at the bedside for each therapeutic apheresis procedure. At the Oklahoma Blood Institute, a patient services department handles all therapeutic apheresis procedures, and all procedures are performed by knowledgeable registered nurses.

Complications and adverse reactions can and do occur. Volume overload, venous access problems, bleeding, thrombosis, immunoglobulin depletion, citrate reactions, hypokalemia, hypocalcemia, hypotension, allergic reactions, infection, viral transmission from blood products, thrombocytopenia, anemia, and death can occur. The mortality has been estimated at 3 deaths per 10,000 procedures (16).

SUMMARY

Apheresis technology has rapidly advanced and eventually will replace some of the manual whole-blood collection techniques. Although more expensive and requiring personnel with greater skill levels to operate the equipment, the new techniques make it possible to collect two or more transfusion doses of blood components from a single donor, theoretically making safer and higher-quality blood components available from a smaller donor base. The ability to use smaller needles and to return fluids will make procedures safer for donors as well. Therapeutic apheresis will continue to advance as new agents such as immunoadsorbents are combined with cell and plasma separation devices, whether centrifugal or membrane. The development of PBPC for bone marrow repopulation, especially when allogeneic donors are routinely stimulated with cytokines (e.g., G-CSF), is signaling an even newer era of apheresis advancement. The new era of pathogen inactivation technology and its application to replacement fluids will improve safety in the use of FFP derivatives for therapeutic apheresis.

REFERENCES

1. Huestis DW, Bove JR, Busch S. *Practical blood transfusion,* 3rd ed. Boston: Little, Brown, 1981:315–372.
2. Barnes A. Hemapheresis perspectives. In: Kolins J. Jones JM, eds. *Therapeutic apheresis.* Bethesda, MD: American Association of Blood Banks, 1983:1–13.
3. Devine P, Postoway N, Hoffstadter L, et al. Blood donation and transfusion practices: the 1990 American Association of Blood Banks institutional membership questionnaire. *Transfusion* 1992;32:683–687.
4. Devine P, Linden JV, Hoffstadter LK, et al. D. Blood donor, apheresis, and transfusion- related activities: results of the 1991 American Association of Blood Banks institutional membership questionnaire. *Transfusion* 1993;33:779–782.
5. Simon T, Lee EJ, Heaton A, et al. Storage and transfusion of platelets collected by an automated two-stage apheresis procedure. *Transfusion* 1992;32:624–628.
6. Simon TL. The collection of platelets by apheresis procedures. *Transfus Med Rev* 1994;8:132–145.
7. Simon TL, Sierra ER, Ferdinando B, et al. Collection of platelets with a new cell separator and their storage in a citrate-plasticized container. *Transfusion* 1991;31:335–339.
8. Murphy MF, Seghatchian J, Krailadsiri P, et al. Evaluation of Cobe Trima for the collection of blood components with particular reference to the in vitro characteristics of the red cell and platelet concentrates and the clinical responses to transfusion. *Transfus Sci* 2000;22:39–43.
9. Klein HG. It seemed a pity to throw away the red cells: selective component collection [Editorial]. *Transfusion* 1993;33:788–790.
10. Meyer D, Bolgiano DC, Sayers M, et al. Red cell collection by apheresis technology. *Transfusion* 1993;33:819–824.
11. Smith JW and Gilcher RO. Red blood cells, plasma, and other new apheresis-derived blood products: improving product quality and donor utilization. *Transfus Med Rev* 1999;13:118–123.

12. Bosch T. State of the art of lipid apheresis. *Artif Organs* 1996;20: 292–295.
13. Bosch T. Lipid apheresis: from a heroic treatment to routine clinical practice. *Artif Organs* 1996;20:414–419.
14. Bandarenko N, Owen HG, Mair DC, et al. Apheresis: new opportunities. *Clin Lab Med* 1996;16:907–929.
15. Newman BH. Donor reactions and injuries from whole blood donation. *Transfus Med Rev* 1997;11:64–75.
16. Huestis DW. Adverse effects in donors and patients subjected to hemapheresis. *J Clin Apheresis* 1984;2:81–90.
17. Simon TL, Moore RC, Sierra ER, et al. Storage of platelets from a new cell separator in a citrate-plasticized container. In: Rock G, ed. *Apheresis.* New York: Wiley-Liss, 1990:11–14.
18. Gorlin JB, ed. *Standards for blood banks and transfusion services,* 20th ed. Bethesda, MD: American Association of Blood Banks, 2000.
19. Strauss RG. Effects on donors of repeated leukocyte losses during plateletpheresis. *J Clin Apheresis* 1994;9:130–134.
20. Heddle NM, Klama L, Singer J, et al. The role of the plasma from platelet concentrates in transfusion reactions. *N Engl J Med* 1994;331: 625–628.
21. Brand A. Passenger leukocytes, cytokines, and transfusion reactions [Editorial]. *N Engl J Med* 1994;331:670–671.
22. Dzik WH. Effects on recipients of exposure to allogeneic donor leukocytes. *J Clin Apheresis* 1994;9:135–138.
23. Shi PA, Ness PM. Two unit red cell apheresis and its potential advantages over traditional whole-blood donation. *Transfusion* 1999;39: 218–225.
24. National Institutes of Health Consensus Conference. Fresh-frozen plasma: indications and risks. *JAMA* 1985;253:551–553.
25. Herzig RH. Granulocyte transfusion therapy: past, present, and future. In: Garratty G, ed. *Concepts in transfusion therapy.* Bethesda, MD: American Association of Blood Banks, 1985:267–294.
26. Price TH. The current prospects for neutrophil transfusions for the treatment of granulocytopenic infected patients. *Transfus Med Rev* 2000;14:2–11.
27. Norol F, Scotto F, Duedari N, et al. Peripheral blood stem cell collection with a blood cell separator. *Transfusion* 1993;33:894–897.
28. Leibundgut K, Muff J, Hirt A, et al. Evaluation of the Fresenius cell separator AS 104 for harvesting peripheral blood stem cells in pediatric patients. *Transfus Sci* 1994;15:93–99.
29. Hester JP, Wallerstein RO. Peripheral blood stem cell transplantation for breast cancer patients with bone marrow metastases using GM-CSF priming. *Transfus Sci* 1993;14:65–69.
30. Heuft HG, Dubiel M, Kingreen D, et al. Automated collection of peripheral blood stem cells with the Cobe Spectra for autotransplantation. *Vox Sang* 2000;79:94–99.
31. Hester JP, McCullough J, Mishler JM, et al. Dosage requirements for citrate anticoagulants. *J Clin Apheresis* 1983;1:149–157.
32. Olson PR, Cox C, McCullough J. Laboratory and clinical effects of the infusion of ACD solution during plateletpheresis. *Vox Sang* 1987; 33:79–87.
33. Chopek M, McCullough J. Protein and biochemical changes during plasma exchange. In: Berkman EM, Umlas J, eds. *Therapeutic hemapheresis: a technical workshop.* Bethesda, MD: American Association of Blood Banks, 1980:13–52.
34. Heaton A, Holme S. Blood donation and red cell volume (RCV) regeneration in donors of different weights. *Vox Sang* 1994;67[Suppl]: 13(abst).
35. Holme S, Heaton A. Red cell volume (RCV) distribution in volunteers: implications for eligibility for two-unit red cell donation. *Transfusion* 1994;34[Suppl]:S58(abst).
36. Rock GA, Shumak KH, Buskard NA, et al. Comparison of plasma exchange with plasma infusion in the treatment of thrombotic thrombocytopenic purpura. *N Engl J Med* 1991;325:393–397.
37. Weinstein R, Sato PTS, Shelton K, et al. Successful management of paraprotein-associated peripheral polyneuropathies by immunoadsorption of plasma with staphylococcal protein A. *J Clin Apheresis* 1993; 8:72–77.
38. Rook AH, Wolfe JT. Role of extracorporeal photopheresis in the treatment of cutaneous T-cell lymphoma, autoimmune disease, and allograft rejection. *J Clin Apheresis* 1994;9:28–30.
39. Edelson RL. Photopheresis. *J Clin Apheresis* 1990;5:77–79.

Rossi's Principles of Transfusion Medicine, Third Edition, edited by Toby L. Simon, Walter H. Dzik, Edward L. Snyder, Christopher P. Stowell, and Ronald G. Strauss. Lippincott Williams & Wilkins, Philadelphia © 2002.

CASE 45A

A CALL ONE SATURDAY MORNING YEARS AGO . . .

CASE HISTORY

Early on a Saturday morning, a transfusion medicine specialist was called to initiate emergency plasmapheresis for a patient with alveolar hemorrhage and a clinical diagnosis of thrombotic thrombocytopenic purpura (TTP). The patient was in the intensive care unit and had anemia due to a microangiopathic process, thrombocytopenia, fever, and mild renal failure. This was the tenth day of the patient's hospital stay. After chart review and examination of the patient, the following history emerged.

A 55-year-old white woman, an elementary school principal, was transferred to a tertiary care hospital with respiratory failure. She had been well until approximately 2 months before admission, when she noticed the onset of exertional dyspnea. One week before admission, a dry, nonproductive cough developed. Outpatient treatment with clarithromycin (Biaxin) was started. Five days before admission to the tertiary care hospital, the patient had been admitted to a community hospital with anemia, diffuse lung infiltrates, and hypoxemia. An endotracheal tube was inserted. Bronchoscopy revealed bloody airway secretions without obvious pathogens on Gram stain. The transfer to the teaching hospital was arranged because of failing oxygenation despite 100% FiO_2. There was no history of fever, chills, purulent sputum, or chest pain.

The medical history included hypertension and depression but did not reveal cardiovascular or lung disease. The social history was unremarkable. Medication before admission to the community hospital included sertraline (Zoloft), atenolol, Biaxin, progestin, estrogen, and promethazine (Phenergan). On the transfer to the teaching hospital she was taking erythromycin, steroids, and several cardiac medicines.

The initial physical examination at the teaching hospital revealed a temperature of 99.8°F (37.7°C), heart rate of 128 beats/min, and blood pressure of 216/90 mm Hg. An endotracheal tube was inserted, and the patient was supported with a ventilator administering 100% oxygen. She was sedated yet slightly agitated. The physical examination showed diffuse, coarse breath sounds bilaterally. The skin was clear without rash. The examination of other systems produced no remarkable findings. There were no neurologic focal deficits. A Swan-Ganz catheter produced no evidence of left-sided cardiac failure. A chest radiograph revealed bilateral fluffy alveolar infiltrates. The electrocardiogram showed sinus tachycardia at a rate of 130 beats/min and evidence of left ventricular hypertrophy.

The laboratory data revealed normal electrolyte levels; blood urea nitrogen, 51 mg/dl; creatinine, 1.9 mg/dl; and glucose, 222 mg/dl. Initial arterial blood gas values were pH, 7.27; PO_2 56 mmHg; and PCO_2 53 mm Hg. The hemoglobin level was 9.6 g/dl with hematocrit of 28.7%. The platelet count was 129×10^9/L. The white blood cell count was 26×10^9/L. The calcium concentration was 7.9 mg/dl and magnesium 1.9 mEq/L. Urinalysis was remarkable for the absence of cellular casts.

The initial impression of the clinical team was alveolar hemorrhage syndrome of unknown causation (1). The differential diagnosis included Wegener's granulomatosis, systemic lupus erythematosus, anti-GBM (glomerular basement membrane) disease, rheumatic heart disease, and other immune complex–mediated diseases. Atypical pneumonitis progressing on to adult respiratory distress syndrome also was considered. The patient had negative results of tests for anti-GBM, antineutrophil cytoplasmic antibodies, and antinuclear antibodies. The only positive serologic finding was an elevated level of immunoglobulin G (IgG) anticardiolipin antibody of 226 IU/dl (normal value, <15 IU/dl). On the second hospital day, the patient underwent bronchoscopy, which revealed bloody lavage in essentially all lung segments. Gram stains of this lavage and cultures were negative for microbial forms. To further evaluate the cause of alveolar hemorrhage, the patient underwent open lung biopsy, which revealed acute pulmonary hemorrhage and changes of ongoing, diffuse, alveolar damage with capillaritis. There were rare, small arterial thrombi most likely due to in situ thrombosis. The potential causes of these histologic features included Wegener's granulomatosis, Goodpasture's disease, collagen vascular disorders, cryoglobulinemia, cardiolipin antibodies, and embolic disease superimposed on diffuse alveolar damage. Special stains for organisms were negative.

Mechanical ventilation could not be discontinued, and the alveolar hemorrhage was refractory to steroids. The hematology and nephrology services favored the diagnosis of TTP because of the thrombocytopenia and fever despite the absence of schistocytes on a peripheral blood smear.

On hospital day 10, the transfusion medicine specialist was asked to initiate plasma exchange for a presumed diagnosis of TTP. At this point, the patient had the following relevant laboratory results: platelet count, 113×10^9L; hematocrit, 29%; lactate dehydrogenase, 665 IU/L; alanine aminotransferase, 130 IU/L; aspartate aminotransferase, 26 IU/L; blood urea nitrogen, 101 mg/dl; and creatinine, 2 mg/dl. The review of a peripheral blood smear revealed few microcytes without schistocytes. The haptoglobin level was 166 mg/dl. Anticardiolipin antibody titers for IgG and IgM were 150 IU/dl and 15 IU/dl, respectively. The transfusion medicine consultant did not believe the findings supported the diagnosis of TTP.

After consultation with other services, the decision was made to institute pulse steroid therapy, administration of cyclophosphamide, and plasma exchange to manage catastrophic antiphospholipid antibody syndrome (APAS). On the fourteenth hospital day, mechanical ventilation was successfully discontinued, and the endotracheal tube was removed. The patient was transferred to a medical floor, where oxygenation continued to improve and the pulmonary infiltrates gradually regressed. The patient underwent a total of seven plasma exchanges.

The patient was discharged in good condition to a rehabilitation facility with prescriptions for steroids, lorazepam (Ativan), and diltiazem. Anticoagulation was not initiated at this point because of a perceived increased risk of recurrent pulmonary hemorrhage.

DISCUSSION

Thrombocytopenia, thrombosis, or recurrent fetal loss in the presence of antiphospholipid antibodies (e.g., anticardiolipin antibodies) found on two occasions separated by at least 6 weeks defines APAS. Pulmonary involvement can occur alone or simultaneously with other manifestations of APAS and can range from mild to severe. Pulmonary capillaritis and alveolar hemorrhage are infrequent complications of APAS (2–7). In catastrophic APAS, rapidly progressive disease leads to the multiple organ failure and not uncommonly to death. The treatment of choice is anticoagulation combined with immunosuppressive therapy.

Neither the American Society for Apheresis nor the American Association of Blood Banks lists APAS as an indication for apheresis in their consensus documents. In such a situation, it should be assumed that APAS is a category III indication if case reports are identified in the literature. Well-established therapies such as anticoagulation combined with immunosuppression render other therapies, including apheresis, unnecessary in the care of most patients. There is a theoretical rationale, however, for use of plasmapheresis in the care of patients with catastrophic APAS, such as the one in this case. This patient's signs and symptoms were complicated by diffuse alveolar hemorrhage, which is a rare complication of catastrophic APAS and hampers introduction of standard therapy with anticoagulation. Associating bleeding complications in APAS seems counterintuitive. A possible explanation of the pathogenesis of alveolar hemorrhage is that microvascular thrombosis causes an increase in vascular permeability, which facilitates perivascular IgG and complement deposition and leads to development of capillaritis. Whether the vascular disease is thrombosis or vasculitis or both is important in choosing the proper management strategy.

At this stage of the disease described in this case, the use of anticoagulation was contraindicated. Plasmapheresis combined with immunosuppression was chosen as the therapy with the highest chance of success, although the prognosis for this patient was guarded. Informed consent was obtained from the family and ex-husband of the patient after careful explanation of the experimental, although theoretically justifiable, nature of the treatment. Apheresis procedures are frequently performed on patients with a poor prognosis when other therapies have failed. Under such circumstances, it is important that the informed consent not only list potential expected complications of apheresis but also discuss the role of plasmapheresis in the particular clinical setting.

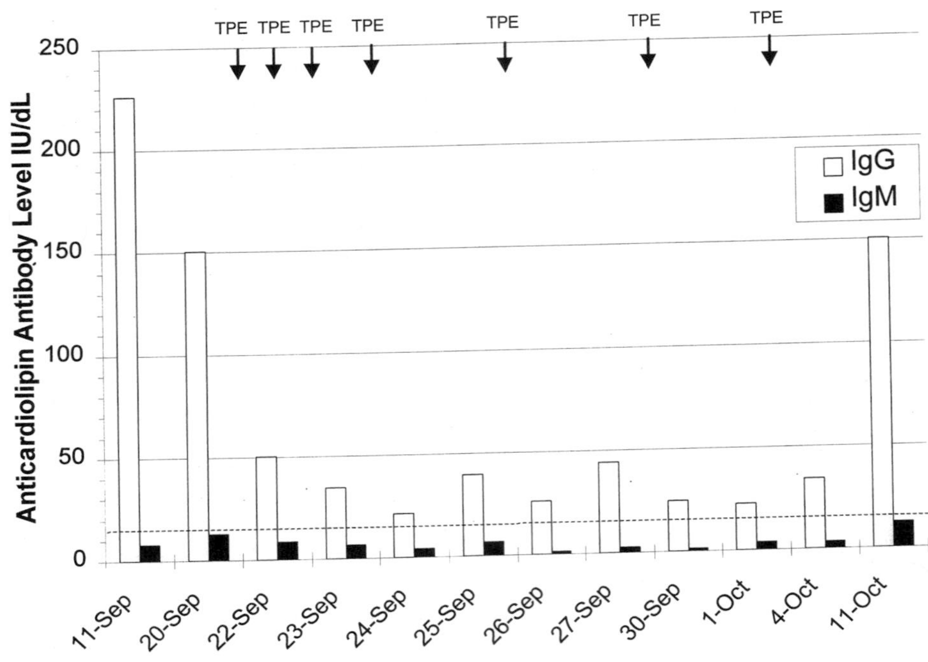

FIGURE 45A.1. Levels of IgG and IgM anticardiolipin antibodies in the serum during the first admission. There is significant decrease in IgG antibody titer after several plasmapheresis procedures with return to pre-apheresis levels within 1 week after discontinuation of the procedures. *Open bars,* IgG. *Closed bars,* IgM. *TPE,* therapeutic plasmapheresis.

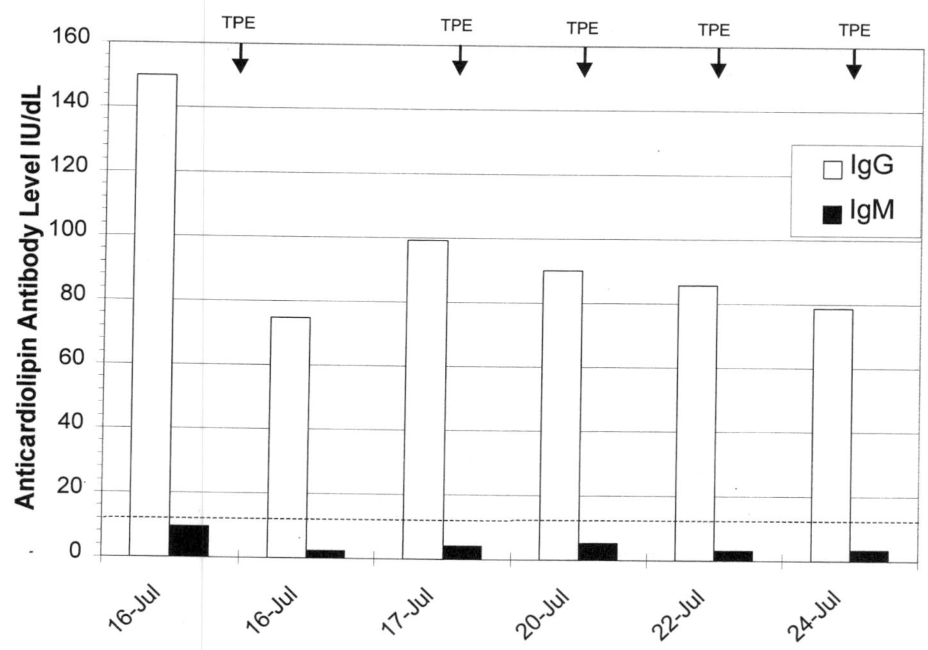

FIGURE 45A.2. Levels of IgG and IgM anticardiolipin antibodies in patient's serum during the second admission. There is much less effect of therapeutic plasmapheresis on the IgG anticardiolipin titer in comparison with the first admission. *Open bars,* IgG. *Closed bars,* IgM. *TPE,* therapeutic plasmapheresis.

Therapeutic plasmapheresis was initiated immediately with replacement fluid consisting of 5% albumin and fresh-frozen plasma. The use of fresh-frozen plasma minimized the risk of coagulopathy due to transient multiple factor deficiencies induced by apheresis. The effect of plasmapheresis on the titer of anticardiolipin antibodies is shown in Figure 45A.1.

This case illustrates two important aspects of consultation in transfusion medicine regarding apheresis. First, it emphasizes the importance of a critical review of the presumed diagnosis for which apheresis has been requested before the therapy is initiated. Second, it emphasizes the need for a transfusion medicine specialist as a consultant when the use of apheresis is considered.

A SECOND HOSPITALIZATION

After discharge from the hospital, the patient underwent a period of rehabilitation during which she developed deep venous thrombosis that necessitated anticoagulation. During the follow-up period, the titer of anticardiolipin antibodies increased to more than 200 IU/dl. Therapy with azathioprine (Imuran) was started on an outpatient basis. The patient continued to take warfarin (Coumadin) and Imuran for 18 months, after which the Imuran was discontinued because of symptoms suggestive of recurrent tracheobronchitis. Three years later, the patient returned to the hospital with shortness of breath on exertion, low-grade fever, and nosebleed.

The initial evaluation showed evidence of hypoxemia, bilateral pulmonary infiltrates, new anemia, normal platelet count, and an international normalized ratio of 1.8. Results of bronchoscopy performed soon after admission were consistent with alveolar hemorrhage. Cytologic examination of the bronchoalveolar lavage fluid revealed hemosiderin-laden macrophages. The IgG anticardiolipin antibody was greater than 150 IU/dl. The patient was treated with a series of five plasmapheresis procedures in addition to reinitiation of immunosuppression (Fig. 45A.2). Over the following week, the patient responded well to this treatment with complete resolution of symptoms and clearing of the bilateral alveolar infiltrates. There was no need for intubation during this admission because of the quick clinical response. The patient was discharged home with prescriptions for Imuran and Coumadin for the near future for the management of APAS. She has not needed hospital care for 3 years.

Case contributed by Zbigniew M. Szczepiorkowski, M.D., Ph.D., Massachusetts General Hospital, Boston, MA.

REFERENCES

1. Crausman RS, Achenbach GA, Pluss WT, et al. Pulmonary capillaritis and alveolar hemorrhage associated with the antiphospholipid antibody syndrome. *J Rheumatol* 1995;22:554–556.
2. Gertner E, Lie JT. Pulmonary capillaritis, alveolar hemorrhage, and recurrent microvascular thrombosis in primary antiphospholipid syndrome. *J Rheumatol* 1993;20:1224–1228.
3. Castellino G, La Corte R, Santilli D, et al. Wegener's granulomatosis associated with antiphospholipid syndrome. *Lupus* 2000;9:717–720.
4. Specs U. Diffuse alveolar hemorrhage syndromes. *Curr Opin Rheumatol* 2001;13:12–17.
5. Waterer GW, Latham B, Waring JA, et al. Pulmonary capillaritis associated with the antiphospholipid antibody syndrome and rapid response to plasmapheresis. *Respirology* 1999;4:405–408.
6. Gertner E. Diffuse alveolar hemorrhage in the antiphospholipid syndrome: spectrum of disease and treatment. *J Rheumatol* 1999;26:805–807.
7. Maggiorini M, Knoblauch A, Schneider J, et al. Diffuse microvascular pulmonary thrombosis associated with primary antiphospholipid antibody syndrome. *Eur Respir J* 1997;10:727–730.

46

THERAPEUTIC PLASMA EXCHANGE

BRUCE C. MCLEOD

Therapeutic plasma exchange (TPE) has been compared to the practice of bloodletting to remove evil humors. The notion of therapeutic removal has changed little since medieval times; however, the concept of an evil humor has been discarded in favor of an evidence-based understanding that some blood cells and plasma components can be harmful. Three subtypes that can be distinguished among plasma macromolecules that are candidates for therapeutic removal follow: a) antibodies that are troublesome because of their binding specificity—these are often autoantibodies; b) molecules that confer abnormal physical properties, such as hyperviscosity or cold insolubility, on plasma and hence on the blood—these, too, are usually antibodies, although they may be bound in immune complexes; and c) molecules such as low-density lipoproteins (LDL) that have nonimmune toxicity. From a theoretic point of view, it is easier to envision a significant therapeutic effect when the molecule to be removed is relatively large and has a relatively long half-life in the circulation, with a correspondingly low rate of synthesis. In practice the majority of successfully treated disorders are caused by pathogenic immunoglobulin G (IgG), which has these properties. It has been suggested from time to time that removal of complement or coagulation proteins, or inflammatory mediators derived from immunocytes, might contribute to a therapeutic effect. Such proposals have seemed unlikely to the author because the candidate molecules are rapidly synthesized and relatively short lived, and in fact no therapeutic effect involving such molecules has been proven to date.

Therapeutic plasma exchange can be employed in a fourth way, not foreseen by medieval barbers or eighteenth-century physicians, and that is to achieve relatively high levels of a normal plasma constituent that is deficient in patient plasma and is not available in a concentrated form for simple infusion.

B.C. McLeod: Department of Medicine and Pathology, Rush Medical College, Rush-Presbyterian-St. Luke's Medical Center, Chicago, Illinois.

GENERAL PRINCIPLES OF THERAPEUTIC PLASMA EXCHANGE

Mathematic Principles

Patients often compare TPE to an automobile oil change, and it is instructive to consider the factors that make this analogy inapt. A 100%-efficient 5-liter oil change can be accomplished in 10 minutes, because the engine need not operate during the procedure. In TPE, limitations are imposed on rate and efficiency by the need to keep the heart pumping and the bloodstream nearly full, so that only a small portion of the total blood volume can be outside the body at any time. Because TPE must proceed gradually, either continuously or in small increments, an ever-increasing proportion of the material being removed is not patient plasma but rather replacement fluid infused earlier in the procedure.

In this process, the level of an entirely intravascular substance that is absent in the replacement medium can be predicted by the formula:

$$y_x = y_0 e^{-x},$$

on which y_0 is the starting concentration of the substance, e is the base natural logarithm, and y_x is the concentration of the substance after x patient plasma volumes have been exchanged. If y_0 is assigned a nominal value of 1.0, the function yields the smooth asymptotic middle curve plotted in Figure 46.1 for a continuous exchange. The flanking curves, describing small incremental discontinuous exchanges, are similar. This formula accurately forecasts the outcome of an exchange for macromolecules such as LDL and IgG that have a substantial extravascular reservoir, provided that equilibration between the intra- and extravascular compartments is slow relative to the removal rate (1).

Because the molecule targeted for removal by TPE is often an IgG antibody, which is approximately 50% extravascular (1), and because removal of accessible (that is, intravascular) IgG becomes progressively less efficient during a TPE procedure, most practitioners limit an exchange to 1 to 1.5 times the patient's estimated plasma volume. An exchange of this magnitude will remove 60% to 75% of intravascular material while limiting side effects from depletion of normal plasma components. The intravascular IgG level will rise during the ensuing 1 to 2 days by equilibration with extravascular sources, and further removal by a subsequent exchange can then be undertaken more efficiently. The effects of a series of TPEs on extravascular, intravascular, and total IgG are shown schematically in Figure 46.2.

Human serum albumin is the most common replacement fluid in TPE, for reasons that are given below. In such exchanges, all plasma constituents are removed while only albumin is replaced; thus plasma component depletion in an individual exchange is almost completely nonselective (1). However, because most other plasma constituents are synthesized much more rapidly than IgG, a series of such exchanges will result in a reasonably selective depletion of IgG over the course of treatment. This is shown in Figure 46.3.

Regulation of IgG Metabolism

Because IgG removal is often the goal of TPE, it is worthwhile to consider certain aspects of IgG metabolism. The subclasses IgG1, IgG2, and IgG4 together constitute about 90% of total IgG. Their catabolic rates are proportional to total IgG level and

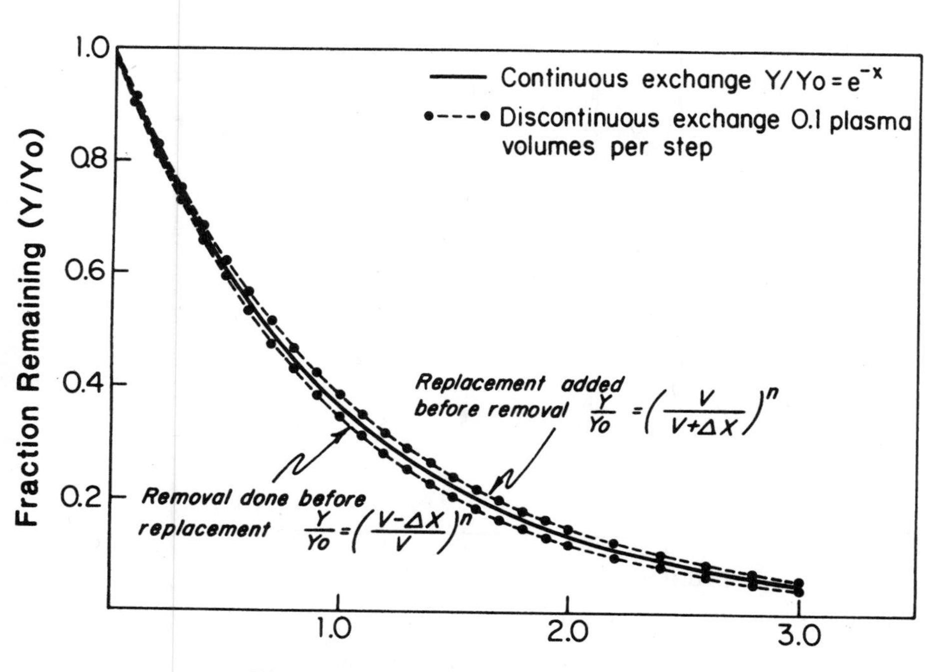

FIGURE 46.1. Calculated fraction of intravascular substance remaining during a plasma exchange, assuming no equilibration with extravascular material. (From Chopek M, McCullough J. Protein and biochemical changes during plasma exchange. In: Berkman EM, Umlas J, eds. *Therapeutic hemapheresis—a technical workshop.* Washington DC: American Association of Blood Banks, 1980: 17, with permission.)

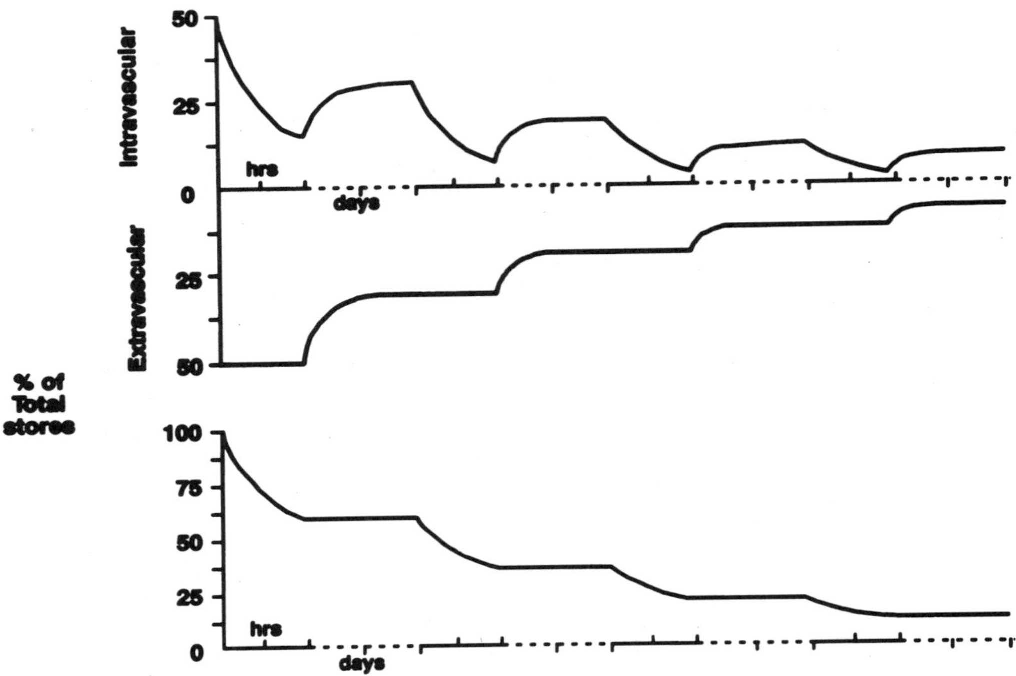

FIGURE 46.2. Computer-generated curve estimating amounts of intravascular and extravascular IgG *(upper curves),* and total IgG *(lower curve)* during a course of four one-plasma-volume therapeutic plasma exchanges with an IgG-free replacement medium. Published formulas were used for rates of removal during exchanges and reequilibration after exchanges. No correction was made for continuing synthesis.

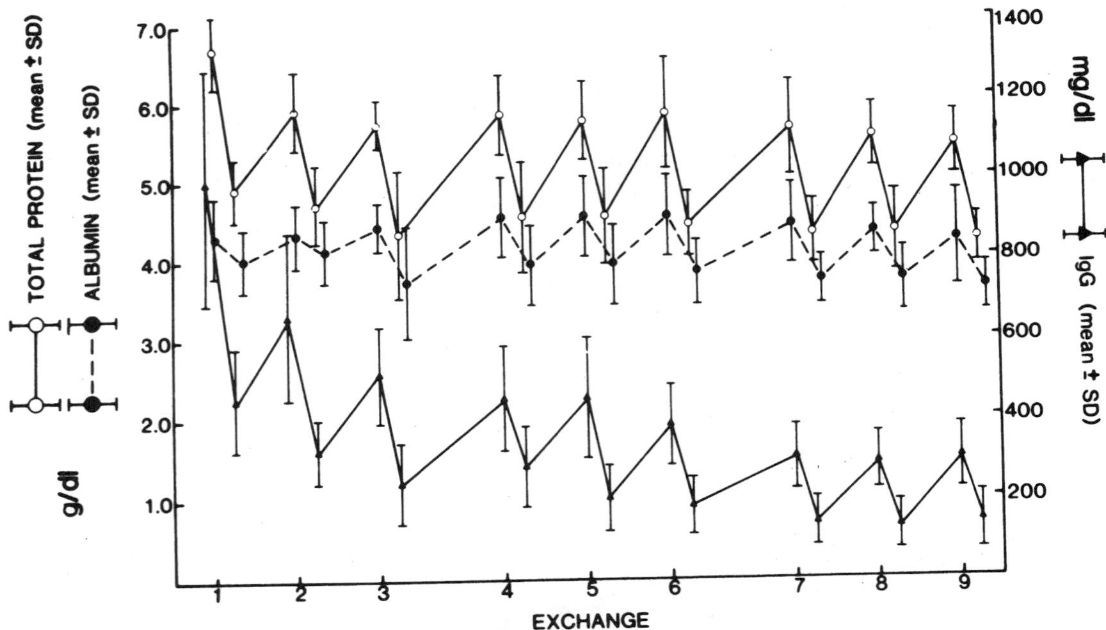

FIGURE 46.3. Total protein, albumin, and IgG levels before and after therapeutic plasma exchange with albumin/saline replacement. Exchanges were carried out three times per week for 3 weeks on seven patients. Points and ranges represent means and standard deviations. Note this disproportionate decrease in IgG levels. (From McLeod BC, Sassetti RJ, Stefoski D, et al. Partial plasma protein replacement in therapeutic plasma exchange. *J Clin Apheresis* 1983;1:117, with permission.)

their half-lives are therefore inversely proportional to concentration. This pattern has been taken to indicate the existence of a saturable receptor that protects IgG from catabolism. A receptor on endothelial cells having this property has recently been discovered and characterized; it appears to be identical to the FcRn receptor that transports intact maternal antibody in breast milk across the neonatal intestinal epithelium (2).

It is difficult to measure the IgG synthetic rate in humans. Previous animal studies concerning levels of specific antibody were interpreted to show that the synthetic rate for IgG exhibits negative feedback, increasing when IgG or specific antibody levels or both are lower (3). More recently, Junghans has shown that "knock-out" mice genetically deficient for the FcRn receptor catabolize IgG quite rapidly and maintain very low IgG levels, but they have the same IgG synthetic rate as normal mice (4). This argues against negative feedback regulation of IgG synthesis and suggests that a reduction in antibody levels induced by TPE would not produce a meaningful "rebound" increase in IgG synthesis.

Intravenous immune globulin (IVIG) has been reported to be effective in some of the same antibody-mediated diseases as TPE. Yu and Lennon (5) recently proposed that exogenous immune globulin competes with endogenous IgG for FcRn receptors and thereby promotes accelerated catabolism of the latter, including any pathogenic antibodies. In this view the beneficial effects of IVIG and TPE are essentially the same; both lead to lower levels of harmful antibodies. Therapeutic plasma exchange lowers levels quickly but may be followed by slower catabolism, whereas IVIG presumably has a slower onset of action but promotes rapid catabolism. This concept of the effect of IVIG could provide a compelling rationale for sequential treatment of autoantibody diseases with TPE followed by IVIG.

Replacement Fluids

Saline alone can suffice when only 500 to 1,000 ml of plasma is removed in a manual plasmapheresis, but colloid replacement must be given in a multiliter plasma exchange. Available colloid replacement fluids are listed in Table 46.1, which also summarizes their relative advantages and disadvantages. For the majority of indications the standard replacement medium is 5% human serum albumin in normal saline; however, substitution of 25% to 50% of the total with saline has been shown to be well tolerated in certain patient groups. Although it is a pooled product, 5% albumin is preferred over plasma as a source of replacement colloid because a) it can be pasteurized to inactivate all known blood-borne pathogens, b) it can be given without regard to blood type, and c) it does not require thawing or other preparation prior to use. Adverse reactions to albumin are rare (6). Exchanges of plasma for albumin produce temporary deficiencies of other plasma proteins, such as coagulation factors; however, these are usually subclinical and levels are rapidly restored by ongoing synthesis and reequilibration (1).

There are a few circumstances in which replacement of patient plasma with donor plasma seems prudent. Prominent among these is the treatment of thrombotic microangiopathies. Affected patients customarily receive exchanges with fresh-frozen plasma (FFP) in light of abundant evidence that patients with thrombotic thrombocytopenic purpura (TTP) respond better to plasma than to albumin. Cryoprecipitate-poor plasma is also effective for this purpose (7). Some plasma may also be given toward the end of an exchange to patients with preexisting thrombocytopenia or humoral coagulopathy, who are considered to be at increased risk for bleeding complications when the dilutional coagulopathy of an albumin exchange is superimposed. Plasma replacement carries a higher risk of urticarial and hypocalcemic reactions (8).

One group has tried infusing a solution of hydroxyethyl starch (HES), a less costly volume expander, in the early part of an exchange. They reason that recommended dosage limitations for HES will not actually be exceeded, because much of the infused HES will be removed in exchange for albumin infused later. This group has reported successes, albeit with a higher incidence of side effects (9).

TABLE 46.1. COLLOID REPLACEMENT FLUIDS FOR TPE

Fluid	Advantages	Disadvantages
5% Albumin	Viral inactivation Ease of use Reactions rare	High cost Most proteins not replaced
Single-donor plasma[a]	All proteins replaced	High cost Inconvenient[b] Citrate reactions Urticaria Viral infection risk
Solvent-detergent plasma	All proteins partially replaced[c] Lipid-coated viruses inactivated	Very high cost Inconvenient[b] Citrate reactions Urticaria Pooled product
6% Hetastarch	Low cost Viral safety Ease of use Slow catabolism	No proteins replaced Hypotensive reactions Dosage limit

TPE, therapeutic plasma exchange.
[a]Fresh-frozen plasma or cryoprecipitate-poor plasma.
[b]Must be thawed prior to use; must match patient ABO type.
[c]Coagulation factors ≥80% of normal levels.

Selective Extraction of Plasma Components

Practitioners of TPE have long recognized the inherent wastefulness in removing and discarding all plasma components in order to deplete just one. Selective extraction of a pathogenic component from separated plasma, with recovery and reinfusion of normal constituents, has been considered an attractive goal. Several applications and methods for on-line separation have been explored (10), but commercial availability and widespread acceptance have only recently begun to be realized.

Obstacles to commercially practical devices include the high cost and limited capacity of truly selective, biocompatible sorbents and the high extracorporeal volume associated with sorbent modules having a depletion capacity equivalent to TPE. In the past decade, two systems that use pairs of small, low-capacity sorbent modules have become available. In both, flow cycles are alternated, with one module absorbing material from patient plasma while the absorbent capacity of the other is restored by elution of bound material. This approach to selective extraction lowers the volume and cost of sorbent modules but requires an additional instrument to manage the cycling-elution-regeneration process. A semiselective device of this kind in which a staphylococcal protein A sorbent used to deplete IgG is approved in Europe, while a Japanese device for selective extraction of LDL from patients with familial hypercholesterolemia (FH) has also been approved in the United States (10).

Indication and Treatment Intensity Categories

The remainder of this chapter will describe use of TPE in specific diseases. To assist practitioners in assessing the value of apheresis in specific circumstances, the American Society for Apheresis (ASFA) (11) has described indication categories for therapeutic apheresis. The definitions can be summarized as follows. Category I denotes diseases for which apheresis therapy is a standard first-line therapy, although it may not always be necessary. Category II denotes diseases in which apheresis is a valuable second-line therapy when first line measures fail or are poorly tolerated. Category III may indicate uncertainty due to inadequate data or controversy due to conflicting reports. Category IV is reserved for diseases in which there is negative data from controlled trials or anecdotal reports. The indication categories assigned by ASFA are provided in tabular form for the diseases in each of the following sections.

In addition, these tables include the author's perceptions of the customary intensity (frequency and duration) of TPE therapy for most of the diseases. The four categories used are: aggressive (A), which implies daily TPE until remission or improvement; routine (R), which implies five to seven treatments every other day (or three times per week); prolonged (P), which implies one to three treatments per week for 3 to 8 weeks; and chronic (C), which implies one treatment every 1 to 4 weeks, continuing indefinitely. These intensity categories, which need not be mutually exclusive, are summarized in Table 46.2. Note that more than one category may be applicable to a given disease, or even a given patient, depending on extant clinical circumstances.

The number of references cited in the following discussions is limited by editorial policy. For that reason, controlled trials of TPE have been emphasized. Readers seeking a more extensive bibliography may consult the chapters on TPE in a recent text devoted to apheresis (1,10,12–14) and articles in a recent journal issue devoted to therapeutic apheresis (11,15–18).

TABLE 46.2. INTENSITY OF TREATMENT CATEGORIES FOR TPE

Level	Schedule	Duration
Aggressive (A)	q day	3–indefinite
Routine (R)	3 ×/week	5–7 treatments
Prolonged (P)	1–2 ×/week	3–8 weeks
Chronic (C)	q 1–4 weeks	Indefinite

TPE, therapeutic plasma exchange.

THERAPEUTIC PLASMA EXCHANGE IN NEUROLOGIC DISORDERS

Immune processes, especially formation of circulating antibody to structures in the nervous system, have been implicated in several neurologic diseases, and TPE has become an important therapy for some of them. The diseases to be considered in this section appear in Table 46.3 along with their respective indication and intensity categories.

Guillain-Barré Syndrome

Guillain-Barré syndrome (GBS) affects the peripheral nervous system. It is the most common cause of acute paralysis with areflexia in the Western world, with an incidence of 1 to 2 cases per 100,000 population per year. A typical clinical course begins with symmetric distal paresthesias, which are followed by leg and arm weakness. Symptoms spread proximally and reach a peak of severity by 14 to 30 days after onset. About one-fourth of patients with GBS have mild illness and remain ambulatory throughout. The remainder are disabled by paralysis and may have oropharyngeal and respiratory weakness as well. One-fourth will require assisted ventilation at some point, and the worst cases are marked by quadriplegia, ophthalmoplegia, and prolonged ventilator dependence. Unusual variants with predominating arm weakness or with symptoms limited to ophthalmoplegia, ataxia, and areflexia (Fisher's syndrome) are also possible. The spinal fluid usually contains few cells and only a moderately elevated concentration of protein. A conduction block indicating demyelination is the usual finding in electrophysiologic studies, although inexcitability may be seen in the axonal form of GBS (19).

Demyelination is believed to be caused by circulating antineuronal antibodies. Early experiments showed that sera from patients with GBS produced demyelination in animals. Later studies have found antimyelin antibodies in the serum of many patients. Guillain-Barré syndrome is often associated with a history of recent infection, especially with *Campylobacter jejuni*. It has been postulated that antibodies are formed in response to a strain-specific lipopolysaccharide that is antigenically similar to the myelin ganglioside GM-1 (20). Epidemic Chinese acute motor neuropathy is an illness of rural Chinese children that has epidemiologic characteristics of an infectious disease. It is clinically similar to GBS and is also associated with evidence of *C. jejuni* infection and anti-GM-1 antibodies.

Spontaneous recovery is the usual outcome of GBS and may be associated with the decline in antibody levels expected after recovery from infection. Patients with mild illness require no treatment, but more severely affected patients need careful observation so that appropriate supportive therapies, such as mechanical ventilation, can be implemented when needed. Neither oral

TABLE 46.3. INDICATION AND INTENSITY OF TREATMENT CATEGORIES FOR TPE IN NEUROLOGIC DISORDERS

Disorder	Antibody Specificities	ASFA Indication Category[a]	Intensity Category[b]
Guillain-Barré syndrome	Peripheral nerve myelin	I	R
Chronic inflammatory demyelinating polyneuropathy	Peripheral nerve myelin	I	P
Peripheral neuropathy with monoclonal gammopathy	Myelin-associated glycoprotein	I,II	P
Myasthenia gravis	AChR	I	A,R,P,C
Lambert-Eaton myasthenic syndrome	Voltage-gated calcium channel	II	R
Paraneoplastic neurologic syndromes	Various	III	R
Rasmussen's encephalitis	Glu R3	III	R
Sydenham's chorea	Unknown	II	R
PANDAS	Unknown	III	R
Multiple sclerosis	Unknown	III	R

TPE, therapeutic plasma exchange; ASFA, American Society for Apheresis; AChR, acetylcholine receptor molecule; Glu R3, glutamate receptor; PANDAS, pediatric autoimmune neuropsychiatric disorders associated with streptococcal (infection).
[a]I, standard first-line therapy; II, second-line therapy; III, controversial; IV, no efficacy.
[b]A, aggressive; R, routine; P, prolonged; C, chronic (see Table 46.2).

nor pulse intravenous steroids are helpful in GBS; however, large randomized controlled trials have documented that TPE can shorten recovery time and reduce disability (21–24).

The North American trial enrolled 245 disabled patients, 142 of whom received TPE (24). At 4 weeks, 59% of treated patients versus 39% of controls had improved by one grade in a clinical grading scale devised for the study. Mean improvements were 1.1 and 0.4 grades, respectively. The median time to improve one grade was 19 days in treated patients versus 40 days in controls, while median times to walk unassisted were 53 and 85 days, respectively. In the subgroup of ventilated patients, the median times to weaning were 24 and 48 days, respectively, and the median times to walk unassisted were 97 versus 169 days. A similar shortening of recovery time in severely affected patients was shown in the French Cooperative Group trial involving 220 patients (22). In another study of 556 patients, this group showed benefit from TPE in mildly affected patients as well (23). A typical treatment schedule in these trials consisted of five to six exchanges of 1 to 1.5 plasma volumes over 7 to 14 days. Patients with GBS may need careful monitoring, perhaps in an intensive care unit, because they may have autonomic neuropathy and are more prone to hemodynamic instability during TPE.

Later studies have shown that IVIG is also beneficial in GBS. A large multicenter trial compared IVIG, TPE, and TPE followed by IVIG, with 121 to 130 patients in each treatment group (25). Mean disability grades at 4 weeks improved by 0.8, 0.9, and 1.1 respectively, while the median times to walk unassisted were 51, 49, and 40 days. The trends favored TPE plus IVIG, although none of the differences was statistically significant.

Chronic Inflammatory Demyelinating Polyneuropathy

Chronic inflammatory demyelinating polyneuropathy (CIDP) is an acquired neuropathy that may follow either a continuously progressive or an intermittent, relapsing course. Both weakness and sensory loss are usually present, and both distal and proximal sites may be affected. Proximal weakness can help to differentiate CIDP from other chronic neuropathies, while progression for more than 2 months helps to distinguish it from GBS. Nerve conduction studies should suggest demyelination, which should be apparent in nerve biopsy tissue if this is done. Patchy inflammatory infiltrates may be seen in nerve root biopsies. The cerebrospinal fluid usually has a moderately elevated protein concentration and a cell count less than 10/μl. If certain exclusionary criteria are met, the diagnosis of CIDP is deemed "possible" if made on the basis of clinical findings and nerve conduction studies, "probable" if compatible cerebrospinal fluid findings are also documented, and "definite" if appropriate nerve pathology is also demonstrated. Treatment is recommended for all groups, and the results of treatment are similar in all three. Although it may be idiopathic, CIDP may also occur in an associated condition, such as inflammatory bowel disease, chronic active hepatitis, connective tissue disease, Hodgkin's disease, human immunodeficiency virus (HIV) infection, or monoclonal gammopathy (26).

The precise cause of CIDP remains unknown; however, the disease associations, the clinical similarities to GBS, and the histopathology suggest an immune process. The presence of a monoclonal protein in some cases points to an antibody-mediated disorder, as does the finding that an animal model of

CIDP (experimental allergic neuritis) can be passively transferred with serum. Recent studies have demonstrated antibody-to-myelin components such as GM-1, P_0 and P_2 proteins, and β-tubulin in the sera of patients with CIDP, although a definite cause-and-effect relationship has not been established (12).

Most patients with CIDP will respond to moderately high doses of glucocorticoids. Standard initial therapy consists of prednisone at perhaps 100 mg/d for an adult, followed by tapering to alternate-day dosing when a functional plateau is reached (26). Early trials of TPE were conducted in patients with CIDP who had failed to improve with steroids or were unable to tolerate them. A double-blind, sham-controlled crossover trial reported by Dyck et al. in 1986 showed improvement in 5 of 15 patients treated with TPE for 3 weeks; after crossover a similar proportion responded in the sham group (27). However, many patients worsened after TPE was stopped. A similar study in 18 previously untreated patients was reported in 1996 by Hahn et al. (28). Of the 15 patients who completed the trial, 12 improved during the TPE portion. These patients were put on prednisone for 6 months after completing TPE and, following recovery from a brief relapse when TPE was stopped, many maintained good function.

Intravenous immune globulin therapy has also been investigated in CIDP. Hahn et al. published a double-blind, placebo-controlled crossover trial in 30 patients (29). Study patients were permitted to take prednisone at stable low doses. Overall 63% (19 patients) responded to IVIG, while 17% (five patients) improved on placebo. Two studies have compared IVIG to TPE. In a retrospective study by Choudhary and Hughes, 21 of 33 patients (64%) improved after TPE treatment, while a response to IVIG was seen in 14 of 21 patients (67%) treated at the same institution (30). A prospective observer-blinded crossover study of 20 patients at the Mayo Clinic suggested that both therapies were able to produce rapid, statistically significant improvement; the authors concluded that either was appropriate as a primary treatment (31). The TPE protocols used in CIDP have tended to specify relatively prolonged treatment. A proposed schedule is three one-plasma-volume exchanges each week for 2 weeks, followed by two exchanges each week for another 4 weeks (26).

Peripheral Neuropathy and Monoclonal Gammopathy

The background incidence of a circulating monoclonal immunoglobulin is only 1% in adults over 50 (3% in adults over 70), while about 10% of patients with polyneuropathy have such a protein (32). Thus principles of epidemiology suggest a causal relationship in at least some cases. This idea is supported by studies showing that antimyelin antibody activity is expressed by the monoclonal proteins of many patients with neuropathy. Specificity for a carbohydrate epitope on myelin-associated glycoprotein (MAG) can be identified in a majority of IgM-associated neuropathies. The same epitope is found on myelin glycoprotein P_0 and on other gangliosides in nerve cell membranes. Injection of anti-MAG into experimental animals is known to produce demyelination. Additional patients have antibody activity against myelin sheath sulfatides, membrane-associated chondroitin sulfate C moieties, or the GM-1 ganglioside (18).

Most clinical features of neuropathies associated with a monoclonal gammopathy are similar to CIDP (26); however, sensory abnormalities tend to be more prominent and, while progression may be slower overall, it is also more relentless, so that instances of spontaneous improvement are uncommon. The prevalence of neuropathy is higher in patients with IgM paraproteins than in those with IgG or IgA except in osteosclerotic myeloma, where the prevalence of neuropathy with IgG or IgA proteins is quite high, sometimes as a part of the POEMS syndrome (polyneuropathy, organomegaly, endocrinopathy, monoclonal protein, skin changes). Nerve biopsies show demyelination, axonal degeneration and fiber loss, and immunofluorescence may demonstrate IgM and complement in IgM-associated cases (32).

Patients with multiple myeloma or Waldenström's macroglobulinemia should be treated with appropriate chemotherapy and may experience improvement in the neuropathy as a result. However, many patients have neuropathy in addition to a monoclonal gammopathy of undetermined significance (MGUS) and are usually treated with immunosuppressive regimens similar to those used in CIDP (32).

Therapeutic plasma exchange can be helpful in MGUS-associated neuropathy. In a sham-controlled trial in 39 patients, twice-weekly exchange led to improvement in disability scores, weakness scores, and electrodiagnostic parameters in the blinded portion of the trial. Scores also improved in sham-treated patients who received true TPE in an open follow-up (33). In this and other studies a response was noted more frequently in patients with IgG and IgA paraproteins than in those with IgM (12).

Myasthenia Gravis

Myasthenia gravis is a disease of the neuromuscular junction that is characterized clinically by fatigability, with or without weakness in skeletal muscle. Ocular myasthenia, with diplopia and ptosis, may be the initial symptoms, but other muscles are eventually affected in most patients. Involvement of muscles enervated by lower cranial nerves leads to the most serious symptoms, including dysphagia and respiratory insufficiency.

Most patients with myasthenia have circulating antibody to a portion of the α-subunit of the acetylcholine (ACh) receptor molecule (AChR) on the motor end plate of muscle cells (34). Such antibodies can cause weakness by at least three mechanisms. a) They can occupy receptors, so that ACh released from the nerve ending cannot gain access. b) They can cross-link receptors, increasing turnover in a manner that leads to a decrease in the number of receptors available to receive signals. c) They can mediate damage to muscle cells by complement or inflammatory cell attack or both.

There are two kinds of drug therapy for myasthenia. Acetylcholinesterase inhibitors, such as neostigmine and pyridostigmine, slow the degradation of ACh at the neuromuscular junction, enhancing its action on remaining receptors. Immunosuppressive drugs, such as prednisone and azathioprine, are also useful. These agents reduce damage to receptors through general antiinflammatory properties or decreased antibody synthesis or both (35).

Surgical treatment is also employed. Malignant thymoma is sometimes associated with myasthenia. Strength sometimes improves in such patients after surgical resection of the thymus. This observation led to trials of thymectomy in patients without tumors, who may also experience disease remission (35).

Because of the relationships between circulating antibody, pathology, and symptoms, TPE has seemed a very reasonable approach to treatment for myasthenia. Although a controlled trial has never been published, numerous open trials have shown that TPE can lead to rapid symptomatic improvement in concert with lower levels of circulating anti-AChR antibody. Therapeutic plasma exchange has also been effective in patients who test negative for antibody, perhaps suggesting that not all pathogenic antibodies are detected by current assays (18,35).

As a result of favorable experience, TPE is a widely accepted therapy for myasthenia; however, it is not recommended for all patients. It is instead reserved for those with severe disease and those who are intolerant of, or unresponsive to, other therapies. Patients whose breathing, swallowing, or walking is inadequate are good candidates for the rapid improvement brought by TPE, even as on initial treatment (35). Therapeutic plasma exchange can also be useful to optimize muscle function prior to thymectomy or other surgery. An occasional patient will need regular TPE at 2- to 4-week intervals in addition to maintenance drug therapy for optimal function. Semiselective adsorption of IgG with protein A-sepharose has also been effective in myasthenia (18).

Myasthenia may respond to IVIG. No randomized trials have been done to prove efficacy; however, in a controlled study comparing IVIG to TPE in 87 patients, either three or five infusions of 0.4 g/kg IVIG were equivalent to three TPE treatments. The median time to response was shorter for TPE-treated patients (9 days versus 15 days), but not significantly so ($P = 0.14$) (36). A multicenter retrospective chart review found that ventilatory status at 2 weeks and functional status at 1 month were significantly better in patients treated with TPE (37).

Lambert-Eaton Myasthenic Syndrome

Lambert-Eaton myasthenic syndrome (LEMS) is also characterized by weakness and fatigue. Neither bulbar nor oculomotor symptoms are likely to be prominent in LEMS, but signs of dysautonomia, such as dry mucous membranes and orthostatic hypotension, are common. The syndrome is most often seen in patients with cancer, with about 60% of cases being in patients with small cell lung cancer. Neuromuscular symptoms may precede any other sign of tumor.

The pathophysiology of LEMS also involves the neuromuscular junction, but the defect is in the nerve cell ending instead of the muscle cell. Symptoms are due to circulating antibody against "active zones" in the nerve terminus, which house the voltage-gated calcium channels that mediate electrical events in neuromuscular impulse transmission. These antibodies reduce the amount of ACh released during depolarization events, causing weakness in affected skeletal muscles as well as dysfunction in autonomic nerves (38).

Curiously, cholinesterase inhibitors are not as effective in LEMS as they are in myasthenia gravis (39). More useful are agents that prolong nerve action potentials by blocking voltage-gated potassium channels. These drugs may improve muscle strength in patients with LEMS, presumably by enhancing ACh release; 3,4-diaminopyridine is a promising agent of this type (40). Immunosuppressive drugs such as prednisone and azathioprine may also be beneficial in LEMS, and paraneoplastic cases may respond to specific antitumor therapy.

Therapeutic plasma exchange has been helpful in LEMS. Responses are usually less dramatic than those seen in myasthenia gravis, perhaps suggesting that a damaged nerve ending needs more time to heal than a motor end plate (39). In recent trials IVIG has also been reported to be active in both the short and long term (41).

Other Paraneoplastic Neurologic Syndromes

Several other neurologic syndromes associated with malignant tumors are characterized by circulating antibody to structures in the nervous system. Paraneoplastic encephalomyelitis includes seizures, mental changes, and cerebellar and autonomic dysfunction. It is often associated with anti-Hu (also called ANNA-1), an antibody to a 38- to 40-kd antigen in the nuclei of neurons and of small cell lung cancer cells. Paraneoplastic cerebellar degeneration is characterized by ataxia, dysarthria, and down-beating nystagmus. It may be associated with ovarian, breast, and small cell lung cancers, as well as with Hodgkin's disease. About 40% of these patients have an antibody to 34- and 62-kd antigens in Purkinje cells (anti-Yo). Paraneoplastic opsoclonus-myoclonus syndrome produces both vertical and horizontal dysrhythmic conjugated eye movements. It may occur in children with neuroblastoma and in adults with lung, breast, or other tumors. Cases seen with breast or gynecologic cancers may have circulating anti-Ri (also called ANNA-2), an antibody to 55- and 80-kd antigens in neuronal nuclei. Paraneoplastic stiff-man syndrome is characterized by stiffness and spasm in axial muscles. It is associated with antibody to amphiphysin, a 128-kd synaptic vesicle protein. Cancer-associated retinopathy produces photosensitivity and gradual vision loss. It is associated with anti-CAR, an antibody to antigens shared by retinal neurons and small cell lung cancer cells (42).

Treatment of these syndromes is uniformly difficult. They seldom respond well to immunosuppressive drugs or to antitumor measures, even when these are otherwise effective. Therapeutic plasma exchange has been tried in these syndromes, usually with disappointing results (42).

Nonneoplastic Disorders with Anti–Central Nervous System Antibodies

Rasmussen's encephalitis is a rare, acquired disorder that begins in childhood, often following a viral infection. Seizures are prominent but, unlike patients with idiopathic epilepsy, those with Rasmussen's encephalitis develop progressive, predominantly unilateral neurologic deficits including hemiparesis and mental retardation. The histopathology includes inflammation and atrophy of brain tissue, usually confined to one hemisphere (43). Recent studies have revealed circulating IgG antibody to the Glu R3 receptor for the central nervous system (CNS) neurotransmitter glutamate, which may arise in response to a cross-reactive microbial antigen. Treatment with either TPE or IVIG has been followed by temporary improvement (18). Sydenham's chorea is a movement disorder that may follow a group A streptococcal infection in children. Patients with Sydenham's may also exhibit obsessive-compulsive symptoms, while children who develop obsessive-compulsive behaviors, tics, and other neurologic symptoms in the absence of chorea may also have evidence of streptococcal infection (pediatric autoimmune neuropsychiatric disorders associated with streptococcal infection; PANDAS) (44). A cross-reactive antibody response to streptococcal antigens could mediate symptoms in some of these patients, and small controlled trials have indicated that both TPE and IVIG can be beneficial in either Sydenham's chorea or PANDAS (18).

Multiple Sclerosis

Multiple sclerosis (MS) is a disease characterized by localized neurologic dysfunction that is due to demyelinated "plaques" in the CNS. Two clinical patterns are observed. About 70% of patients will have acute attacks that resolve fully or partially (relapsing-remitting). The other 30% have slow, continual progression of disease (chronic progressive). The frequency of attacks in relapsing-remitting MS tends to decrease with disease duration, and some patients evolve to a chronic progressive pattern (45).

Discrete areas or plaques of demyelination in white matter, which are easily visualized with magnetic resonance imaging (MRI), are the hallmarks of MS. Histopathologically these areas are initially inflammatory but progress to fibrosis (45). The mechanism of their appearance remains unexplained, but most authorities in the field suspect involvement of the immune system. Experimental allergic encephalomyelitis, an animal model of MS, can be induced by immunization with myelin basic protein or other myelin proteins. Experimental allergic encephalomyelitis is mediated by T cells and can be passively transferred with T cells from immunized animals. Most evidence suggests a misdirected cellular immune response in MS as well, and it has been difficult to assign a primary pathogenic role to circulating antibody.

The study of treatments for MS is complicated by the natural history of the disease, particularly the tendencies for acute attacks to subside and for attack frequency to decline, but also by other spontaneous fluctuations in disease activity. Clinical measurement tools such as the Expanded Disability Status Scale are used to quantify improvement or progression of disability. Although these bring some degree of objectivity to clinical studies, they are subject to interrater variability (46).

Immunosuppressive and immunomodulatory agents have been the mainstays of drug therapy in MS. Resolution of acute attacks is thought to be hastened by brief courses of either glucocorticoids or adrenocorticotrophic hormone, both of which may promote faster restoration of normal nerve conduction by decreasing edema and inflammation in and around new plaques. The relentless progression of disability is probably not halted by these measures, although aggressive treatment of optic neuritis with intravenous steroids may delay the onset of frank MS that often follows. Cyclosporin, total lymphoid irradiation, and cytotoxic immunosuppressants such as azathioprine and cyclophosphamide have only modest benefits that may not warrant the risks such drugs entail. Mitoxantrone has also been tried. Interferon-β has shown promise in more recent studies, as has glatiramer acetate, a mixture of synthetic polypeptides that may modulate immune responses to myelin-basic protein. These agents reduce the frequency of acute attacks and the appearance of new lesions seen with MRI (12,18,45).

Prophylactic administration of IVIG to patients with MS in open trials was reported to reduce the frequency of attacks. In three later controlled trials there was also an apparent decrease in the frequency of attacks; however, MRI monitoring was not done in one study, while in another fewer gadolinium-enhancing lesions were found in IVIG-treated patients. In the third study the number of lesions seen without enhancement was the same after 2 years in both treatment and control groups. A recent review concludes that IVIG should still be regarded as experimental (47).

The rationale for TPE in MS is uncertain, given the paucity of evidence that any circulating factor has a role in the etiology of acute attacks or chronic progression. Therapeutic plasma exchange has nevertheless been used, and encouraging results have been reported from uncontrolled studies. In controlled trials, however, it has been difficult to discern benefit, even with vigorous TPE regimens (12). The first randomized, double-blind, sham-controlled study in chronic progressive MS was reported to show significant benefit for patients receiving TPE in addition to cyclophosphamide and prednisone (48). The study was subsequently questioned because of anomalies in statistical analysis, and because dramatic recoveries in several of the TPE patients, not seen in subsequent trials, suggested that some relapsing-remitting patients were misclassified and entered into the trial during attacks that would have improved spontaneously (46). Two later sham-controlled trials have not shown convincing benefit (49,50). A recent trial suggested that TPE may be useful in a subset of patients with MS with prolonged severe demyelination (51); however, this study will require confirmation (45). The American Academy of Neurology recently classified TPE as "possibly useful" in MS (52).

THERAPEUTIC PLASMA EXCHANGE IN HEMATOLOGIC AND ONCOLOGIC DISORDERS

Therapeutic plasma exchange has been tried in a variety of hematologic and oncologic conditions. These are listed in Table 46.4 along with their respective indication and intensity categories.

Monoclonal Proteins

In addition to peripheral neuropathy (discussed above), four other syndromes associated with monoclonal immunoglobulins are regarded as clinical indications for TPE. Hyperviscosity, coagulopathy, and renal failure, which almost always occur in the setting of a malignant B-cell disorder, are discussed here while cryoglobulinemia is covered in a later section.

Hyperviscosity was the first condition to be treated successfully with manual plasmapheresis, the precursor to TPE. The

TABLE 46.4. INDICATION AND INTENSITY OF TREATMENT CATEGORIES FOR TPE IN HEMATOLOGIC AND ONCOLOGIC DISORDERS

Disorder	Antibody Specificities	ASFA Indication Category[a]	Intensity Category[b]
Hyperviscosity syndrome	Not applicable	I	P,C
Hemolytic disease of the newborn	Rh(D) or other	III	R
ABO-incompatible marrow transplant	A or B	II	A
Platelet alloimmunization and refractoriness	HLA antigens	III	R
Thrombotic thrombocytopenia purpura	vWF-cleaving enzyme	I	A
Hemolytic uremic syndrome	Unknown	III	A
Posttransfusion purpura	HPA-1a or other	I	A
Idiopathic thrombocytopenic purpura	Unknown	III	R
Autoimmune hemolytic anemia	Unknown	III	R
Aplastic anemia	Unknown	III	R
Pure red blood cell aplasia	Unknown	III	R
Coagulation factor inhibitors	Factor VIII or other	II	A

TPE, therapeutic plasma exchange; ASFA, American Society for Apheresis; HLA, human leukocyte antigen; vWF, von Willebrand factor; HPA, human platelet antigen.
[a]I, standard first-line therapy; II, second-line therapy; III, controversial; IV, no efficacy.
[b]A, aggressive; R, routine; P, prolonged; C, chronic; see Table 46.2.

full-blown syndrome consists of neurologic symptoms, a bleeding diathesis, a peculiar retinopathy marked by alternating dilated and constricted segments in retinal veins, and hypervolemia due to expansion of plasma volume. Symptoms are uncommon if the relative serum viscosity is below 4 and become more likely when it exceeds 6. The hyperviscosity syndrome is most often seen in patients with Waldenström's macroglobulinemia, who have IgM paraproteins, but it may also occur in multiple myeloma.

At higher paraprotein levels a relatively large change in viscosity may follow a relatively small change in concentration. It is this nonlinear relationship that allowed the two-unit manual plasmapheresis technique available in the 1950s to lower viscosity enough to relieve symptoms. Because most IgM paraproteins are roughly 80% intravascular, the same relationship also predicts that a one-plasma-volume automated exchange will provide a wide margin of safety and can therefore be repeated less frequently for hyperviscosity than is necessary for many other conditions. Viscosity measurements should guide therapy, of course, but treatment every 1 to 2 weeks may be adequate.

Paraproteins may interfere in platelet and clotting factor interactions in the absence of hyperviscosity. Such coagulopathies are found in 60% of patients with macroglobulinemia, 40% of patients with IgA myeloma, and 15% of patients with IgG myeloma (53). In instances that are clinically significant, TPE therapy can help restore adequate hemostasis.

Renal failure develops in 3% to 9% of patients with myeloma and confers a poor prognosis. In many cases, renal biopsy demonstrates accumulation of free light chains in renal tubules. Urinary excretion of light chains will greatly exceed the amount that could be removed by TPE if renal function is normal, but the reverse may be true in renal failure. Two controlled studies have shown higher rates of recovery of renal function in patients who received TPE therapy. In one study, three of seven dialysis-dependent patients who received TPE recovered renal function while none of five control patients did (54). In the other, 13 of 15 patients in the treatment group recovered renal function compared with only 2 of 14 controls (55).

Alloantibodies to Blood Cells

Alloantibodies to red blood cells and platelets may be problematic in a number of disease processes. Treatment by antibody removal has been tried in several of these.

Hemolytic disease of the newborn was one of the first problems to be approached with automated apheresis instruments. In the hope of slowing fetal hemolysis, sensitized D-negative mothers carrying D-positive fetuses underwent TPE to lower anti-D titers. Since the original reports, the number of sensitized mothers has declined as prophylaxis with Rh immune globulin has become more widespread. Furthermore, intrauterine transfusion with D-negative red blood cells has proven to be a better treatment for affected fetuses. For these reasons, TPE is seldom called for now, but it may still be useful in an occasional pregnancy when there is very early evidence of fetal involvement, because intrauterine transfusion is not feasible prior to about 18 weeks of gestation (56). Prompt, early institution of TPE was followed by successful delivery after multiple prior abortions in compelling case reports involving mothers with anti-M and anti-P (16).

Therapeutic plasma exchange has also been used to remove isoagglutinins in the setting of hematopoietic stem cell transplantation. Allogeneic transplantation across a major ABO barrier (e.g., group A donor into group O recipient) is feasible if a hemolytic transfusion reaction to red blood cells in the transplant can be avoided. This was first accomplished in bone marrow transplants by exhaustive pretransplant TPE of the recipient; however, most centers have preferred to simply remove most of the red blood cells (e.g., <20 ml remaining) from an incompatible bone marrow graft prior to transplantation (57). Peripheral blood stem cell collections include far fewer red blood cells (usually <10 ml). Such grafts can be infused safely without any manipulation. Red blood cell engraftment may be delayed in this situation. Therapeutic plasma exchange has been used, both prior to transplant to avoid delayed engraftment and after transplant to correct it, with uncertain results in both cases (58). Transplantation of a solid organ, such as a liver or kidney, across a major ABO barrier can result in hyperacute rejection and is usually avoided for this reason. When organ availability is limited, however, desperate circumstances have sometimes led to transplantation of an ABO-incompatible liver after extensive TPE of the recipient, often with a satisfactory outcome (17).

Organ transplantation across a minor ABO barrier (e.g., group O donor into group A recipient) does not carry an increased risk of rejection. Some patients, however, develop hemolytic anemia caused by isoagglutinins derived from B lymphocytes in the transplant. Red blood cell destruction mediated by these "passenger lymphocytes" is most often seen in heart and lung or liver transplantation, in which the volume of lymphoid tissue transplanted is relatively high, and is usually evident by 1 to 3 weeks after transplantation (59). Severe hemolysis may improve after TPE and compatible (e.g., group O) red blood cell transfusion (60).

Alloimmunization to human lymphocyte antigens (HLAs) or platelet antigens can cause refractoriness to platelet transfusions. To restore responsiveness, antibody removal by means of TPE or a protein A–silica column has been attempted. Intravenous immune globulin has also been tried (16). However, the results have been inconclusive and the best option for alloimmunized patients is transfusion of compatible platelets.

Thrombotic Thrombocytopenia Purpura and Hemolytic Uremic Syndrome

Thrombotic Thrombocytopenic Purpura

Thrombotic thrombocytopenic purpura is characterized by microangiopathic hemolytic anemia and thrombocytopenia, often severe. Central nervous system changes, fever, and renal abnormalities may be seen in advanced cases, although frank renal failure is unusual. A rare relapsing form begins in childhood, but the majority of cases in adults are sporadic, with women accounting for 70%. Thrombotic thrombocytopenic purpura is most often idiopathic but may be seen in association with other illnesses, such as systemic lupus erythematosus (SLE) and HIV infection. Idiopathic TTP formerly carried a mortality rate of 95%, but empiric studies in the 1970s and 1980s demonstrated much improved survival in patients treated with TPE and plasma replacement. Some patients, including children with the relapsing form of the disease, will respond to simple plasma infusion (61).

A convincing account of the pathogenesis of TTP has recently been offered. It involves a plasma enzyme (a metalloproteinase) that cleaves ultralarge von Willebrand factor (ULvWF) multimers secreted by endothelial cells, yielding the smaller vWF polymers found in normal plasma. Children with relapsing TTP have an inherited deficiency of this enzyme (62), while in idiopathic adult cases an "acquired deficiency" arises due to the formation of an autoantibody inhibitor to the enzyme (63,64). In either case, persistence of ULvWF in the circulation promotes inappropriate adherence of platelets to endothelial cells and to each other, leading to consumptive thrombocytopenia and to microvascular obstructions that cause mechanical trauma to red blood cells and varying degrees of end-organ ischemia. Periodic plasma infusion may abort or prevent attacks in congenitally deficient patients by supplying active enzyme (62). Idiopathic cases respond better to TPE (78% response rate versus 63% for plasma infusion in the Canadian study) (65), presumably because exchanges remove inhibitory antibody as well as replacing the deficient enzyme. Exchanges are usually carried out daily until the platelet count and LDH (as a marker of hemolysis) have normalized.

Various immunosuppressive maneuvers, including glucocorticoid therapy, vincristine, and splenectomy have been advocated as adjunctive treatments. Discovery of a causative autoantibody provides support for their use in idiopathic, but not in congenital, cases. Further work may clarify whether SLE- and HIV-associated cases are due to a similar autoantibody (16).

A syndrome resembling TTP has been identified in some patients taking the antiplatelet drugs ticlopidine (66) and clopidogrel (67). Antibody to the metalloproteinase enzyme has been detected in such cases (68), and TPE has been reported to improve outcome (76% survival versus 50% for unexchanged patients in a retrospective study of ticlopidine recipients) (66).

Hemolytic Uremic Syndrome

The hemolytic uremic syndrome (HUS) usually involves microangiopathic hemolysis, renal insufficiency, and mild-to-moderate thrombocytopenia. It occurs in children in a self-limited form that follows infection with a verotoxin-producing *Escherichia coli* (diarrhea positive or D positive); however, not all pediatric cases have this association (D negative). Both a familial and a nonfamilial form may be seen in adults. Some nonfamilial cases are associated with prior chemotherapy or stem cell transplantation.

Because of the striking overlap in clinical manifestations, it has long been supposed that the pathogenesis of HUS was the same as, or similar to, that of TTP. Largely on this basis, TPE and protein A-column therapy have been recommended for D− childhood HUS and for adult HUS. Responses have generally been less favorable than in TTP, especially in HUS associated with chemotherapy or hematopoietic stem cell transplantation (69,70).

Studies of the vWF-cleaving metalloproteinase in adult patients with familial and nonfamilial forms of HUS have revealed neither severe deficiency nor inhibitory activity (63). Thus the hypothesis that HUS has the same pathogenic mechanism as

TTP would seem to be in error. Deficiency of complement factor H has been identified in some patients with familial HUS (71). This might provide some rationale for plasma replacement therapy; however, for most cases of HUS the role of TPE is unclear at this time. This is also true for the role of TPE in the HELLP syndrome of hemolysis, elevated liver enzymes, and low platelets in pregnant women (72), which shares clinical features with TTP, HUS, and preeclampsia.

Posttransfusion Purpura

Posttransfusion purpura (PTP) is a rare syndrome in which the platelet count falls to dangerously low levels about 1 week after an allogeneic transfusion. Patients who develop the syndrome lack the common allele for one of the platelet-specific glycoprotein antigens, most often the HPA-1a antigen on glycoprotein IIIa. Most patients have had multiple prior transfusions or pregnancies, and have been immunized thereby to the platelet-specific antigen coded by the prevalent allele. The transfusion that precedes the illness appears to stimulate an anamnestic increase in the titer of IgG antiplatelet-specific alloantibody, most often anti-HPA-1a. Posttransfusion purpura is self-limited and should resolve without treatment after a few weeks; however, bleeding complications, including fatal CNS hemorrhage, may occur in the interim.

Although it is somehow linked to a platelet-specific alloantibody response, the mechanism of extensive destruction of antigen-negative autologous platelets in PTP remains uncertain. The following four possibilities have been proposed: a) immune complexes consisting of platelet antigen and antiplatelet antibody bind to autologous platelets and mediate their destruction, b) soluble platelet-specific alloantigen derived from the transfusion is adsorbed by autologous platelets, c) a simultaneous platelet autoantibody response occurs, or d) a broad polyclonal alloimmune response produces some antibodies that cross-react with autologous platelets.

Treatment of PTP is recommended, because many patients will have bleeding complications. High-dose glucocorticoids are usually given empirically and pulse methylprednisolone at 1g/d has been reported effective. Platelet transfusions, even those from antigen-negative donors, seldom raise the platelet count but are likely to cause severe reactions. Daily TPE usually promotes a rise in platelet count within several days and is thought to be an effective treatment for this reason, even though no controlled trials have been done (73). Exchanges usually include FFP replacement to avoid a superimposed humoral coagulopathy. Intravenous immune globulin produces a similarly rapid increase in platelet count and has become the favored treatment modality for this group of patients (74).

Idiopathic Thrombocytopenic Purpura

Idiopathic thrombocytopenic purpura (ITP) is an autoimmune illness affecting platelets. Most patients have an autoantibody of the IgG class directed against a platelet-membrane glycoprotein antigen. Idiopathic thrombocytopenic purpura is sometimes accompanied by warm autoimmune hemolytic anemia (WAHA; Evans syndrome). In pediatric patients, ITP is acute and self-limited; recovery is the rule regardless of treatment. Adults with ITP, most of whom are women, seldom recover without treatment and their disease often progresses to a chronic form. An ITP syndrome may also be seen in patients with SLE or HIV (75).

The goal of treatment in ITP is to prevent bleeding. Fortunately most of the circulating platelets in patients with ITP are relatively young and have above-average hemostatic activity, so that a normal platelet count is not needed to avoid hemorrhage. Glucocorticoids, splenectomy, and IVIG are the mainstays of therapy (75). A few favorable anecdotal reports of TPE in ITP appeared in the 1970s, and one small trial suggested a lower rate of splenectomy in exchanged patients (76). In the absence of confirmatory controlled trials, however, enthusiasm for this approach has waned.

Favorable responses to protein A–silica column treatment have been reported in ITP associated with HIV infection (77), as well as in patients with chronic ITP without HIV (78). The mechanism of action of protein A in this effect is unknown. A purely subtractive mechanism (i.e., removal of antiplatelet antibody) seems unlikely, because responses have been reported when as little as 250 ml plasma per week was treated. Bearing this uncertainty in mind, the protein A–silica column remains an option for chronic ITP refractory to more standard therapies.

Autoimmune Hemolytic Anemia

Autoimmune hemolytic anemia (AHA) is caused by autoantibodies to red blood cells. Such antibodies are classified as either "cold" or "warm" agglutinins, depending on the temperature of maximal activity. Cold agglutinins are usually IgM antibodies directed against the I/i antigens; they bind most strongly at low temperatures and may produce a syndrome of complement-mediated intravascular hemolysis (cold agglutinin disease; CAD). Warm agglutinins are usually IgG and are often directed against an antigen that does not appear on Rh_{null} cells; they bind better at body temperature and produce a predominantly extravascular hemolytic syndrome, WAHA. Autoimmune hemolytic anemia can be idiopathic but can also be associated with infections, lymphoproliferative disorders, or other autoimmune diseases.

Most patients need treatment. Standard therapy is aimed at lowering antibody production and inhibiting destruction of sensitized cells. Glucocorticoids, IVIG, and splenectomy are often effective in WAHA, and other immunosuppressive drugs may be tried if these measures fail. All of these approaches are less successful in CAD.

Therapeutic plasma exchange to deplete circulating antibody has been tried in both WAHA and CAD when conventional treatments have failed. Because the IgM antibodies in CAD are predominantly intravascular and only loosely bound to cells, their removal by TPE should be relatively efficient. Such therapy, when added to conventional drug treatment, has been reported to lower antibody titers and transfusion requirements, albeit only temporarily. In WAHA much of the circulating antibody is bound to red blood cells; TPE has been tried in this disorder also, but it is less likely to be helpful (76).

Aplastic Anemia and Pure Red Blood Cell Aplasia

Pure red blood cell aplasia and aplastic anemia are bone marrow disorders. In the former there is reticulocytopenic anemia, while the latter leads to pancytopenia. At least some cases of both conditions likely have an immunologic basis. Allogeneic bone marrow transplantation is the preferred treatment for severe aplastic anemia if a suitable donor is available, but immunosuppressive therapies, such as glucocorticoids, cytotoxic drugs, cyclosporin, and antithymocyte globulin may be effective, especially in milder cases.

In the serum of a minority of patients it is possible to demonstrate a factor, probably antibody, that inhibits the growth of marrow-derived precursor cells in culture (79). This provides a rationale for TPE, which has been reported in both disorders in a few cases. Results in aplastic anemia have been mixed; responses appear to be more likely in patients with serum inhibitory activity. All reported instances of TPE treatment for pure red blood cell aplasia have led to improvement, which is sometimes quite dramatic in patients with serum inhibitory activity. Thus, although TPE is not a primary therapy for either disorder, it can be offered to patients who have failed to improve after receiving conventional treatment, especially those found to have serum inhibitory factors (76).

Coagulation Factor Inhibitors

Coagulation factor inhibitors are IgG antibodies to components of the clotting cascade. They interfere with clotting by inactivating the targeted factor. Inhibitors may be autoantibodies that arise in individuals with no prior bleeding history. Alternatively they may be alloantibodies that form in genetically deficient patients after exposure to "foreign protein" in the course of factor replacement therapy. Factor VIII is the clotting protein most often affected by antibodies of either type, and most of the following concerns factor VIII inhibitors.

The two goals of treatment for patients with inhibitor are control of individual bleeding episodes and suppression of inhibitor synthesis. Depending on inhibitor titer, the first goal can usually be achieved by infusion of high doses of human factor VIII, porcine factor VIII (which cross-reacts only partially with anti–human factor VIII antibodies) or, for patients with the highest titers, factor VIII-bypassing products, including recombinant factor VIIa. Therapeutic plasma exchange during a bleeding episode may reduce inhibitor titers enough to allow infused human or porcine factor VIII to bring about hemostasis. Suppression of inhibitor synthesis is approached with immunosuppressive measures, including high-dose glucocorticoids, cytotoxic agents, cyclosporine, and IVIG. Tolerance-inducing protocols that include regular infusion of exogenous factor VIII have been devised for patients with alloimmune inhibitors (13). In the so-called Malmö protocol, extensive TPE or IgG depletion with protein A–sepharose column procedures is used to reduce the inhibitor level at the onset of treatment so that infused "tolerizing" factor can circulate (80). Frequent, large (two to three plasma volumes) exchanges with FFP replacement are recommended for patients with inhibitor. Central venous access is often required; placement of a catheter in a patient with a refractory bleeding diathesis is a challenge for all concerned and often mandates infusion of a factor VIII-bypassing product for wound hemostasis (81).

Therapeutic plasma exchange has also been reported for treatment of patients with antiphospholipid antibodies (82), which may interfere with in vitro assays of coagulation, such as the partial thromboplastin time. In contrast to the inhibitory antibodies described above, however, they usually promote inappropriate coagulation in vivo and cause thrombotic events.

THERAPEUTIC PLASMA EXCHANGE IN OTHER IMMUNOLOGIC DISORDERS

Therapeutic plasma exchange has been tried in a number of rheumatic diseases and other diseases that are considered to have an immune or autoimmune etiology. These are listed in Table 46.5 along with the author's intensity guidelines and the indication categories assigned by ASFA.

Cryoglobulinemia

Cryoglobulins are abnormal serum proteins that precipitate reversibly at 4°C; some will precipitate at higher temperatures. Such precipitates always contain immunoglobulin, and immunoelectrophoretic or immunofixation analysis allows distinction of three types. Type I cryoglobulins consist of a single species of monoclonal immunoglobulin. These are usually found in B-cell lymphoproliferative disorders such as myeloma or Waldenström's macroglobulinemia. Cryoglobulin levels are often quite high (>500 mg/dl) and may cause Raynaud phenomenon or acral necrosis due to microvascular obstruction, as well as other symptoms. Type II cryoglobulins contain both monoclonal and polyclonal immunoglobulins. The former is usually an IgMκ with anti-IgG activity while the latter is polyclonal IgG bound to the IgMκ in an immune complex. Many cases occur in association with chronic hepatitis C infection (83). They typically manifest a cutaneous vasculitis on the lower extremities and may have visceral manifestations of immune complex disease as well. Type III cryoglobulins are mixed polyclonal, often with IgM anti-IgG that binds IgG in immune complexes. These may arise in acute infections, such as hepatitis B, or in chronic inflammatory states such as severe rheumatoid arthritis. Clinical manifestations resemble serum sickness.

If there is an underlying condition, cryoglobulin levels and related symptoms may decrease with treatment of this primary disorder, for example, chemotherapy for myeloma or interferon for hepatitis C virus infection. For idiopathic and secondary cases of mixed cryoglobulinemia, prednisone therapy often relieves symptoms, while alkylating agents may be useful in patients with severe symptoms resistant to prednisone.

Therapeutic plasma exchange will reduce cryoglobulin levels and control symptoms, even in the absence of other treatments (84,85), but inconvenience and expense mitigate against such use. It should be started promptly for patients who seek treatment for severe acral ischemia or visceral manifestations of vascu-

TABLE 46.5. INDICATION AND INTENSITY OF TREATMENT CATEGORIES FOR TPE IN RHEUMATIC AND OTHER IMMUNE DISORDERS

Disorder	Antibody Specificity	ASFA Indication Category[a]	Intensity Category[b]
Cryoglobulinemia	IgG	II	A,R,P,C
Rheumatoid arthritis	IgG	III, (II for IA)	R ?
Systemic lupus erythematosus	dsDNA and others	IV	R,P
Systemic vasculitis	ANCAs	III	R ?
Polymyositis and dermatomyositis	Unknown	IV	R ?
Goodpasture syndrome	Type IV collagen	I	A
Rapidly progressive glomerulonephritis	Unknown	II	R
Renal transplantation	—	—	—
Rejection	HLA antigen	IV	NA
Presensitization	HLA antigen	III	Unknown
Recurrent focal glomerulosclerosis	Unknown	III	R
Heart transplant rejection	HLA antigen	III	R

[a]I, standard first-line therapy; II, second-line therapy; III, controversial; IV, no efficacy; IA, protein A-silica immunoadsorption.
[b]A, aggressive; R, routine; P, prolonged; C, chronic; see Table 46.2.
TPE, therapeutic plasma exchange; ASFA, American Society for Apheresis; IgG, immunoglobulin G; dsDNA, double-stranded DNA; ANCAs, antineutrophil cytoplasmic antibodies; HLA, human lymphocyte antigen.

litis, in whom it can help achieve control of symptoms until aggressive drug therapy takes hold (86). Patients with chronic vasculitic skin ulcers may also benefit (87). In all cases replacement fluids should be warmed to body temperature prior to infusion.

Rheumatoid Arthritis

Rheumatoid arthritis (RA) is a disease of unknown cause that is more prevalent in women. It is the most common chronic inflammatory joint disease and a leading cause of disability. Most patients have rheumatoid factor, an IgM autoantibody to IgG; however, because this antibody is absent in many clinically typical cases, and because it is also found in patients who do not have arthritis, it is not likely to be directly involved in pathogenesis.

Conservative treatment includes nonsteroidal antiinflammatory agents, oral glucocorticoids in low doses, and intraarticular steroids. More severely affected patients eventually receive slow-acting "disease-modifying antirheumatic drugs" that are probably immunomodulatory, such as antimalarials, gold compounds, and methotrexate. Tumor necrosis factor inhibitors are also approved for treatment of RA.

Therapeutic plasma exchange was tried for RA in the 1970s and 1980s, but controlled trials did not show benefit. There were subsequent reports of lymphapheresis, with or without accompanying TPE. Some controlled trials investigating this approach showed significant but short-lived benefit, while others did not. In practice, the prospect of only a modest chance of modest benefit from a costly, inconvenient therapy has discouraged treatment with therapeutic apheresis (15).

A recent sham-controlled trial of 12 weekly protein A–silica column treatments produced improvement in 33% of 48 treated patients versus only 9% of 43 controls. Benefit persisted for about 8 months on average, and a subsequent course was again beneficial in 7 of 9 initial responders (88). Although its mechanism of action is unclear, this device has gained Food and Drug Administration approval for use in RA.

Systemic Lupus Erythematosus

Systemic lupus erythematosus has long been regarded as the prototypic autoimmune disease. The most important diagnostic criterion, circulating antibodies to DNA, especially double-stranded DNA (anti-dsDNA), identifies patients who may have a variety of other autoantibodies and a disparate array of clinical syndromes in which skin disease, joint disease, cytopenias, or nephritis may be the sole or dominant problem.

Immunosuppressive measures are the cornerstone of therapy for SLE. Most patients are given prednisone in varying doses, and those with severe disease may also receive azathioprine or cyclophosphamide. The plethora of autoantibodies that seem relevant to clinical signs made SLE an obvious target for TPE. It was one of the first illnesses to be treated with automated TPE in the early 1970s, and early case reports and uncontrolled series suggested a favorable effect (15).

Lupus nephritis is a particularly devastating manifestation in which glomerular deposition of immune complexes and anti-dsDNA is believed to have a prominent role in pathogenesis. Thus it seemed an attractive setting for randomized trials of TPE. A controlled trial with only eight patients suggested benefit (89). However, in a multicenter randomized controlled trial comparing oral cyclophosphamide plus TPE to oral cyclophosphamide alone, there was no advantage for the patients receiving TPE (90). A later international trial, which enrolled patients with a variety of severe manifestations, was structured to exploit enhanced sensitivity to a properly timed pulse dose of intravenous cyclophosphamide that was believed to follow pathogenic antibody removal by TPE (91). As mentioned above, subsequent work with knock-out mice deficient for the FcRn receptor suggests that enhanced susceptibility would not occur (4). In any case, this trial also failed to show any advantage for all patients treated with TPE (92) or for a subgroup with nephritis (93). Thus large controlled studies have failed to confirm any worthwhile effect of TPE in SLE.

Systemic Vasculitis

The term *systemic vasculitis* encompasses a group of disorders that cause inflammation in blood vessel walls and ischemic tissue damage. Vasculitis syndromes are conveniently classified on the basis of the size of vessels typically involved, but most are of unknown etiology. Immune complexes are found in patients with some syndromes, and autoantibodies such as antineutrophil cytoplasmic antibodies (ANCA) in Wegener's granulomatosis (c-ANCA) and polyarteritis (p-ANCA), can be demonstrated in others. This has lent credence to the notion that humoral immune factors are somehow involved.

Prednisone is the first-line therapy for most vasculitic syndromes and cyclophosphamide is often added in more severe cases. Randomized controlled trials in renal vasculitis (94), as well as in a group of patients with polyarteritis or Churg-Strauss angiitis (95), have shown little evidence that addition of TPE to drug therapy confers long-term benefit. Nevertheless, it may be requested for patients who are not responding to maximal drug therapy.

Polymyositis and Dermatomyositis

Polymyositis and dermatomyositis are inflammatory diseases affecting skeletal muscle. A characteristic dermatitis involving the eyelids, knuckles, neck, and shoulders is also part of the latter condition. The usual clinical picture includes proximal weakness with biochemical evidence of muscle cell enzyme leakage; the diagnosis is confirmed by muscle biopsy. The natural history is progressive fiber loss, eventually leading to profound, irreversible weakness. An autoimmune etiology is suspected, but circulating antibody specific for skeletal muscle has not been implicated. Initial treatment is high-dose prednisone, which can often be tapered to maintenance levels. Resistant disease is treated with azathioprine, methotrexate, an alkylating agent, or a combination. Controlled trials have also shown that IVIG infusion reduces muscle enzyme levels and improves strength temporarily (18).

Several uncontrolled series were interpreted to show that TPE was beneficial, but they were unfortunately confounded by concurrent escalations in immunosuppressive drug therapy (18). A randomized controlled trial in which 12 patients received TPE, 12 received lymphapheresis, and 12 received sham apheresis, with no changes in drug therapy, showed no difference in the response rate among the three groups (96). Thus despite the successes with IVIG there appears to be no role for TPE in the treatment of polymyositis.

Goodpasture Syndrome

Goodpasture syndrome (GPS) is characterized clinically by pulmonary hemorrhage and rapidly progressive glomerulonephritis. Light microscopy of renal biopsies shows crescent formation in many glomeruli, while immunofluorescent and electron microscopy reveal linear subendothelial immune deposits that may also be evident in a lung biopsy. In 95% of cases there is a circulating antibody that binds to glomerular basement membrane (anti-GBM). Such antibodies are specific for a noncollagenous sequence near the carboxy terminus of the $\alpha3$ chain of type IV collagen, which is found in appreciable quantities only in renal and pulmonary basement membranes. Untreated GPS progresses quickly and relentlessly, and most patients die of uremia or complications of lung hemorrhage (97). The preferred treatment for GPS is high-dose prednisone and cyclophosphamide, combined with aggressive TPE, to quickly reduce anti-GBM levels and minimize progression of tissue damage (17). Exchanges are usually carried out daily and may be continued for up to 2 weeks. It is prudent to give some FFP replacement in the latter part of each exchange to avoid a dilutional coagulopathy that might cause exacerbation of lung bleeding.

A single controlled trial failed to show an advantage for GPS patients who received TPE; however, this study has been largely discounted because the TPE schedule (every 3 days) was not sufficiently aggressive and because the extent of renal damage at entry was worse in the TPE than in the control group (98). Early treatment is recommended because patients who are already dialysis-dependent at the onset of TPE are unlikely to recover renal function (99). It follows that the subset of patients whose renal biopsies show irreversible lesions are not likely to benefit from TPE unless they also have pulmonary hemorrhage.

Other Rapidly Progressive Glomerulonephritis

In addition to GPS, there are two other categories of rapidly progressive glomerulonephritis (RPGN)—those with an immune complex disease, who have granular subendothelial immune deposits, and those with pauci-immune RPGN, who have scant immune deposits, if any. Light microscopic findings in both are similar to those found in GPS, with severe glomerular inflammation and crescent formation. Some cases also have associated lung hemorrhage. Patients in either group may have isolated renal disease or may have accompanying features that suggest a diagnosis of systemic vasculitis, mixed cryoglobulinemia, or Henoch-Schönlein purpura for granular–immune complex RPGN and microscopic polyangiitis, or Wegener's granulomatosis for pauci-immune RPGN patients, many of whom test positive for ANCA (17).

Therapies are similar for these two categories of RPGN, and some trials and series have included patients with both types. Virtually all patients receive prednisone and most receive either oral or intravenous cyclophosphamide. Therapeutic plasma exchange has been used extensively in patients with both types of disease. Two controlled trials, one published in 1988 (100) and the other in 1992 (101), showed no advantage for patients who received TPE in addition to immunosuppressive drugs. However, a subgroup analysis in the second study suggested that patients who have dialysis-dependent renal failure are more likely to recover renal function if they receive TPE. No such trend was noticed in the more recent trial conducted by Guillevin and colleagues (102). A prospective, randomized trial by Stegmayr et al. compared TPE with immunoadsorption. Among 38 patients with non-GPS RPGN, 87% of whom had ANCA, 70% avoided long-term dialysis (99). Therapeutic plasma exchange and immunoadsorption were equally effective. Thus TPE continues to be controversial in non-GPS RPGN. It is probably not justified as a first-line therapy, except (paradoxically) in patients who are dialysis dependent (103), but it may be offered to patients whose disease progresses despite immunosuppressive drug therapy.

Solid Organ Transplantation

In organ transplant recipients TPE has been used both to treat and to prevent rejection, as well as for recurrence of certain diseases in a transplanted organ. Photopheresis, which has also been tried for the same purposes, primarily in heart transplantation, is covered in Chapter 47.

Rejection

Cellular immune mechanisms mediate rejection of most organ allografts; however, antibody-mediated rejection may occur rapidly in patients who have preexisting antibodies to ABO or HLA antigens expressed by the graft. Such "hyperacute" rejection is characterized histologically by neutrophil infiltration, fibrin deposition, and endothelial damage in small blood vessels; failure of the graft is mainly due to ischemic damage. All treatments have been futile in hyperacute rejection, including TPE. Vascular changes, which may be seen microscopically in later rejection episodes, are sometimes taken to indicate antibody-mediated rejection, even when immunofluorescence microscopy and tests for circulating antibody are negative (104).

Standard posttransplant management for kidney and liver transplantation consists of prophylactic immunosuppression with glucocorticoids and either cyclosporin or tacrolimus. Heart recipients may also receive azathioprine or mycophenolate mofetil. Rejection episodes that occur in spite of these measures are treated with pulse steroids or anti-T cell antibody preparations or both.

Case reports and uncontrolled series published in the late 1970s and early 1980s suggested TPE was beneficial in renal transplant rejection. Then five controlled trials (17) were reported in the mid- and late 1980s. Four showed no significant benefit for patients receiving TPE in addition to standard drug therapy, even in the subgroups whose transplant biopsies showed vascular histologic changes. In the one study suggesting benefit, the mean treatment time was 10 to 11 months after transplant, when antibody-mediated rejection is unlikely. The last and largest study concluded that TPE therapy for renal transplant rejection could no longer be recommended (105). Nevertheless, use of TPE for this purpose continues to be reported (17).

Its apparent ineffectiveness in renal transplantation notwithstanding, TPE has also been employed in cases of cardiac allograft rejection. Favorable outcomes have been reported in individual patients who were also receiving other therapies, but no controlled trials have been done. It is more difficult to detect or exclude vascular rejection in the endomyocardial biopsies done to monitor cardiac allografts because sizable vessels are seldom found in this part of the heart muscle. Detection of specific deposits of IgG by immunofluorescence is the usual criterion for humoral rejection, although one group has suggested that this diagnosis be made, and TPE performed, in patients who have relatively normal biopsies in the face of deteriorating cardiac function (106). Controlled data to support this assertion are lacking.

More recently pretransplant TPE has been tried in patients previously sensitized to HLA antigens. Transplant candidates whose sera react with lymphocytes from a large fraction of the population are less likely to have a compatible crossmatch with a cadaveric donor and hence have a lower likelihood of receiving a transplant. Prospective immunosuppression, combined with antibody removal by TPE or protein A-sepharose immunoadsorption, has been explored as a means to achieve a compatible crossmatch prior to transplantation and thereby prevent hyperacute rejection. Several centers have reported groups of patients who received kidney transplants after being prepared in this way and achieved quite respectable graft survival rates. Such protocols have also facilitated transplantation of ABO-incompatible kidneys and livers (17).

In summary, evidence from controlled trials suggests that TPE is ineffective in reversing established rejection of renal allografts. However, pretransplant antibody removal can allow transplantation of otherwise ineligible candidates, especially those with high-titer antibodies to one or two HLA antigens whose titer-sensitive cross-reactions can be suppressed.

Recurrence of Disease

Focal glomerulosclerosis (FGS) is a disease that causes nephrosis and renal failure, predominantly in children. It recurs in about 30% of allografted patients, which suggests that a humoral factor may have a role in its pathogenesis. A 50-kd plasma factor that binds to protein A has been implicated but has not been further characterized (107). Reduced proteinuria and improved renal function have been reported when recurrence in an allograft is treated with stepped-up immunosuppression and TPE (17).

Goodpasture syndrome may occasionally recur in a transplanted kidney; however, this can usually be avoided by delaying transplantation until the anti-GBM response has subsided spontaneously. Should the syndrome recur in spite of this precaution it should be treated promptly with TPE and cyclophosphamide.

Allograft vasculopathy, a diffuse coronary artery disease that sometimes develops in transplanted hearts, is the leading cause of morbidity and mortality in heart transplant recipients who survive beyond 1 year. It may be related either to continuing hyperlipidemia or to chronic rejection. Selective depletion of LDLs, which is discussed in greater detail in the section on hypercholesterolemia, has been reported helpful in a few such patients with persistent lipoprotein abnormalities (108).

TABLE 46.6. INDICATION AND INTENSITY OF TREATMENT CATEGORIES FOR TPE IN METABOLIC DISORDERS

Disease	ASFA Indication Category[a]	Intensity Category[b]
Homozygous familial hypercholesterolemia	II, (I for LDL-P)	C
Refsum's disease	I	A,R,P
Overdose or poisoning	III	A
Acute hepatic failure	III	A

[a]I, standard first-line therapy; II, second-line therapy; III, controversial; IV, no efficacy; LDL-P, LDL-apheresis; i.e., selective depletion of LDL.
[b]A, aggressive; R, routine; P, prolonged; C, chronic; see Table 46.2.
TPE, therapeutic plasma exchange; ASFA, American Society for Apheresis.

THERAPEUTIC PLASMA EXCHANGE IN TOXIC AND METABOLIC DISORDERS

This section covers conditions in which removal of plasma constituents other than immunoglobulin is potentially beneficial. These are listed in Table 46.6 along with indication and intensity categories.

Hypercholesterolemia

Familial hypercholesterolemia is a genetically determined deficiency of cell surface LDL receptors that interferes with cholesterol off-loading from LDL into cells and with the normal negative-feedback regulation of LDL synthesis, leading to highly elevated levels of circulating LDL, cholesterol (650 to 1,000 mg/dl), and lipoprotein(a) (Lp[a]). Skin xanthomas and coronary atheromas develop in the first decade of life in homozygotes, and death from myocardial infarction prior to age 20 is common. Heterozygotes also have elevated LDL, cholesterol (350 to 500 mg/dl), and Lp(a) levels; they may develop xanthomas by age 20 and coronary atherosclerosis by age 30 (109).

Milder forms of hypercholesterolemia can be influenced by dietary modifications and are amenable to drug treatment with agents such as HMG-CoA reductase inhibitors, bile acid–binding resins, and nicotinic acid. However, FH homozygotes and some FH heterozygotes respond only modestly to these measures and remain at risk for premature death. Drastic surgical measures, such as ileal bypass, portacaval shunt, and liver transplantation may be recommended for such patients if they have evidence of coronary artery disease (109). Alternatively, removal of LDL and its associated cholesterol from the blood can be accomplished repeatedly by various modalities of therapeutic apheresis.

A standard TPE will lower LDL and cholesterol levels by 50% or more, and long-term treatment every 1 to 2 weeks can lead to shrinkage of cutaneous xanthomas and regression of coronary artery deposits (17). Although TPE removes both LDL and Lp(a), it also depletes high-density lipoproteins (HDL), which are believed to have an antiatherogenic action. This disadvantage has stimulated efforts to deplete LDL semiselectively and on-line from patient plasma separated by an apheresis device, and then return the LDL-depleted plasma to the patient.

Several systems have been designed to accomplish this goal (10). Filtration systems employ a plasma filter with the pore size chosen such that the very large LDL molecules are retained while smaller ones such as albumin are sieved; these systems are only partially selective and typically remove about half of plasma HDL. In heparin extracorporeal LDL precipitation (HELP) systems, LDLs are precipitated by heparin at acid pH and separated from patient plasma by filtration; LDL-depleted plasma is then dialyzed on-line to restore a physiologic pH. Lipoprotein(a) is efficiently depleted by HELP systems, and HDL levels fall by only 15%. Low-density lipoprotein immunoadsorption columns utilize an LDL-specific antibody linked to sepharose particles. A pair of reusable columns must be assigned to each patient to hold costs within realistic limits. A final system, the Kaneka Liposorber, uses a pair of regenerable dextran sulfate columns that absorb LDL efficiently, but not HDL or Lp(a). Although all the above systems remove LDL effectively, only the dextran sulfate system has received Food and Drug Administration approval for marketing in the United States. For a given decrement in LDL, this system lowers HDL less than TPE; however, because it has no application other than treatment of hypercholesterolemia, a facility acquiring it must use it regularly on multiple patients to make it economically feasible.

Refsum's Disease

Refsum's disease results from deficiency of the peroxisomal enzyme phytanoyl-CoA hydroxylase, which participates in degradation of phytanic acid by α-oxidation. Accumulation of diet-derived phytanic acid in plasma lipoproteins and in tissue lipid stores leads to symptoms, which may include peripheral neuropathy, cerebellar ataxia, retinitis pigmentosa, anosmia, deafness, ichthyosis, renal failure, and arrhythmias. Slow progression is the usual course, but rapid deterioration and even sudden death may follow a marked increase in plasma phytanic acid.

Restriction of dietary intake of phytanic acid via dairy products, meats, and ruminant fats is the mainstay of treatment. It leads to gradual clearing of phytanate stores by slow ω-oxidation and gradual symptomatic improvement in most patients. Nutrition must be maintained, however, because mobilization of calories from endogenous fat can increase plasma phytanic acid levels acutely and cause clinical exacerbations. Therapeutic plasma exchange will remove large quantities of phytanic acid incorporated into plasma lipids (110). Selective lipoprotein depletion is also effective (111). Apheresis therapy is most appropriate for patients who have very high plasma phytanate levels and an associated exacerbation of symptoms. Skin disease, neuropathic symptoms, and ataxia usually improve as plasma levels drop. Cranial nerve defects usually do not.

Drug Overdose and Poisoning

Toxic effects may occur after exposure to excessive doses of pharmacologic agents or to harmful agents in the environment. Management techniques for both types of event are similar and may include removal of toxin still in the gastrointestinal tract, enhancement of renal elimination, and direct removal from blood by hemodialysis, hemoperfusion (e.g., over charcoal columns), or TPE (112). Specific antidotes may also be given if available. Serious events are usually treated with multiple measures.

Therapeutic plasma exchange has been reported to be beneficial, when combined with other therapies, in cases involving substances that bind tightly to plasma proteins such as methyl parathion, vincristine, and cisplatin. It has also been reported for severe hyperthyroidism, either endogenous or exogenous, in which its effectiveness may be limited by extensive binding of L-thyroxine to tissue proteins. Therapeutic plasma exchange has been reported in poisonings due to ingestion of the *Amanita phalloides* mushroom; however, diuresis clears more Amanita toxin (17).

Unfortunately the literature on this topic is older and entirely anecdotal. Furthermore, TPE has always been used in combination with other therapies that are presumably effective. This complicates formulation of firm, rational guidelines. Nevertheless it seems reasonable to offer TPE to a severely affected patient with an overdose or poisoning who has a high blood level of an agent that binds to plasma proteins. It should also be noted that TPE has shown minimal or no beneficial effect in overdosage of drugs known to bind to tissue proteins and lipids, including barbiturates, chlordecone, aluminum, tricyclic antidepressants, benzodiazepines, quinine, phenytoin, digoxin, digitoxin, prednisone, prednisolone, tobramycin, and propranolol (17).

Acute Hepatic Failure

Acute hepatic failure may develop after a severe liver insult, such as overwhelming hepatitis B infection or acetaminophen overdosage. Cases may also be due to drug reactions, Wilson's disease, vascular anomalies, acute fatty liver of pregnancy, and a variety of toxins. Acute hepatic failure results in many metabolic imbalances and synthetic defects. Clinical symptoms include jaundice, coagulopathy, encephalopathy, and renal failure. The treatment of choice is liver transplantation, which leads to 60% to 80% long-term survival versus >60% mortality for untransplanted patients. Cerebral edema accounts for fatal outcomes (113).

Conservative treatment is basically supportive. Fluid, electrolyte, and nutritional supplements are adjusted in response to metabolic abnormalities. Bowel sterilization with enteral antibiotics minimizes production of ammonia by intestinal bacteria. Pressors are infused if needed for hemodynamic support. Osmotic diuretics, sedatives, hyperventilation, and proper positioning are all employed to reduce intracranial pressure. Platelets and plasma products are infused to improve coagulation (113).

Therapeutic plasma exchange with plasma replacement has seemed appealing as a means to restore metabolic homeostasis, remove toxic metabolites that may cause cerebral edema, and supply coagulation factors and other deficient plasma proteins in quantity without causing volume overload. Practical evaluations of this approach have produced mixed results (113). Some investigators have found TPE helpful in stabilizing and maintaining patients until an organ for transplant becomes available. Improvements in blood pressure, cerebral blood flow, and neurologic status were attributed to TPE in one study (114), however intracranial pressure, a key prognostic indicator, did not fall. Hemoperfusion over activated charcoal, which will lower plasma ammonia levels, has also shown no advantage over intensive supportive care alone.

Potential problems with extensive TPE arise from the diminished ability of patients with acute hepatic failure to metabolize the citrate in infused plasma. Accumulation of citrate leads to ionized hypocalcemia and to alterations in arterial ketone body ratios that may interfere with regeneration of hepatocytes (115). Thus, although TPE can partially reverse coagulopathy and other synthetic deficits in these patients, a favorable net impact on outcome has been difficult to demonstrate.

The bioartificial liver being tested by Circe Biomedical is an interesting new development. It contains a suspension of pig liver cells in the exterior space surrounding the hollow fibers in a filter cartridge. Patient plasma, having been separated by an apheresis device and passed through a charcoal column to remove ammonia, is brought into "metabolic contact" with the porcine hepatocytes by flowing through the hollow fibers before being returned to the patient. A nonrandomized study showed decreases in both ammonia levels and intracranial pressure readings in patients treated for 6 to 8 hours per day with the device, which is intended primarily as a bridge to liver transplantation (116).

CONCLUSION

Therapeutic plasma exchange is an effective therapy for a number of diseases, especially those mediated by paraproteins or autoreactive antibodies. Improvements in apheresis instruments that are outside the scope of this chapter have made it a very safe treatment as well. Thus it should continue to have an important role in the management of selected diseases.

REFERENCES

1. Weinstein R. Principles of blood exchange. In: McLeod BC, Price TH, Drew MJ, eds. *Apheresis: principles and practice.* Bethesda, MD: American Association of Blood Banks, 1997:263–286.
2. Junghans RP, Anderson CL. The protection receptor for IgG catabolism is the β_2-microglobulin-containing neonatal intestinal transport receptor. *Proc Natl Acad Sci U S A* 1996;93:5512–5516.
3. Dau PC. Immunologic rebound. *J Clin Apheresis* 1995;10:210–217.
4. Junghans RP. IgG Biosynthesis. No "immunoregulatory feedback." *Blood* 1997;90:3815–3818.
5. Yu Z, Lennon VA. Mechanism of intravenous immune globulin therapy in antibody-mediated autoimmune diseases. *N Engl J Med* 1999; 340:227–228.
6. Pool M, McLeod BC. Pyrogen reactions to human serum albumin in plasma exchange. *J Clin Apheresis* 1995;10:81–84.
7. Owens MR, Sweeney JD, Tahhan RH, et al. Influence of type of exchange fluid on survival in therapeutic apheresis for thrombotic thrombocytopenic purpura. *J Clin Apheresis* 1995;10:178–182.
8. McLeod BC, Price TH, Owen H, et al. Frequency of immediate adverse effects associated with therapeutic apheresis. *Transfusion* 1999; 39:282–288.
9. Owen HG, Brecher ME. Partial colloid replacement for therapeutic plasma exchange. *J Clin Apheresis* 1997;12:146–153.
10. Vamvakas EC, Pineda AA. Selective extraction of plasma constituents. In: McLeod BC, Price TH, Drew MJ, eds. *Apheresis: principles and*

practice. Bethesda, MD: American Association of Blood Banks, 1997: 378–407.
11. McLeod BC. Introduction to the 3rd special issue on clinical applications of therapeutic apheresis. *J Clin Apheresis* 2000;15:1–5.
12. McLeod BC. Therapeutic plasma exchange in neurological disorders. In: McLeod BC, Price TH, Drew MJ, eds. *Apheresis: principles and practice.* Bethesda, MD: American Association of Blood Banks, 1997: 287–306.
13. Drew MJ. Therapeutic plasma exchange in hematologic diseases and dysproteinemia. In: McLeod BC, Price TH, Drew MJ, eds. *Apheresis: principles and practice.* Bethesda, MD: American Association of Blood Banks, 1997:307–333.
14. Trainor LD, Hillyer CD. Therapeutic plasma exchange in renal, rheumatic and miscellaneous disorders. In: McLeod BC, Price TH, Drew MJ, eds. *Apheresis: principles and practice.* Bethesda, MD: American Association of Blood Banks, 1997:335–354.
15. Koo AP. Therapeutic apheresis in autoimmune and rheumatic disorders. *J Clin Apheresis* 2000;15:18–27.
16. Grima KM. Therapeutic apheresis in hematological and oncological disorders. *J Clin Apheresis* 2000;15:28–52.
17. Wilkins JL, Pineda AA, McLeod BC, et al. Therapeutic apheresis in renal and metabolic disorders. *J Clin Apheresis* 2000;15:53–73.
18. Weinstein R. Therapeutic apheresis in neurological disorders. *J Clin Apheresis* 2000;15:74–128.
19. Hughes RA, Rees JH. Guillain-Barré syndrome. *Curr Opin Neurol* 1994;7:386–392.
20. Rees JH, Soudain SE, Gregson NA, et al. *Campylobacter jejuni* infection and Guillain-Barré syndrome. *N Engl J Med* 1995;333: 1374–1379.
21. The Guillain-Barré Syndrome Study Group. Plasmapheresis and acute Guillain-Barré syndrome. *Neurology* 1985;35:1096–1104.
22. French Cooperative Group on Plasma Exchange and Guillain-Barré Syndrome. Efficiency of plasma exchange in Guillain-Barré syndrome: role of replacement fluids. *Ann Neurol* 1987;22:753–761.
23. French Cooperative Group on Plasma Exchange in Guillain-Barré Syndrome. Plasma exchange in Guillain-Barré syndrome: one-year follow-up. *Ann Neurol* 1992;32:94–97.
24. Jansen PW, Perkin RM, Ashwal S. The Guillain-Barré syndrome in childhood: natural course and efficacy of plasmapheresis. *Pediatr Neurol* 1993;9:16–20.
25. Plasma Exchange/Sandoglobulin Guillain-Barré Syndrome Trial Group. Randomised trial of plasma exchange, intravenous immunoglobulin, and combined treatments in Guillain-Barré syndrome. *Lancet* 1997;349:225–230.
26. Mendell JR, Chronic inflammatory demyelinating polyradiculopathy. *Annu Rev Med* 1993;44:211–219.
27. Dyck PJ, Daube J, O'Brien P, et al. Plasma exchange in chronic inflammatory demyelinating polyradiculoneuropathy. *N Engl J Med* 1986;314:461–465.
28. Hahn AF, Bolton CF, Pillay N, et al. Plasma-exchange therapy in chronic inflammatory demyelinating polyneuropathy. A double-blind, sham-controlled, cross-over study. *Brain* 1996;119: 1055–1066.
29. Hahn AF, Bolton CF, Zochodne D, et al. Intravenous immunoglobulin treatment in chronic inflammatory demyelinating polyneuropathy. A double-blind, placebo-controlled, cross-over study. *Brain* 1996; 119:1067–1077.
30. Choudhary PP, Hughes RAC. Long-term treatment of chronic inflammatory demyelinating polyradiculoneuropathy with plasma exchange or intravenous immunoglobulin. *Q J Med* 1995;88:493–502.
31. Dyck PJ, Litchy WJ, Kratz KM, et al. A plasma exchange versus immune globulin infusion trial in chronic inflammatory demyelinating polyradiculoneuropathy. *Ann Neurol* 1994;36:838–845.
32. Bosch EP, Smith BE. Peripheral neuropathies associated with monoclonal proteins. *Med Clin North Am* 1993;77:125–139.
33. Dyck PJ, Low PA, Windebank AJ, et al. Plasma exchange in polyneuropathy associated with monoclonal gammopathy of undetermined significance. *N Engl J Med* 1991;325:1482–1486.
34. Masselli, RA. Pathophysiology of myasthenia gravis and Lambert-Eaton syndrome. *Neurol Clin* 1994;12:285–303.
35. Sanders DB, Scoppetta C. The treatment of patients with myasthenia gravis. *Neurol Clin* 1994;12:343–368.
36. Gajdos P, Chevret S, Clair B, et al. Clinical trial of plasma exchange and high-dose intravenous immunoglobulin in myasthenia gravis. *Ann Neurol* 1997;41:789–796.
37. Qureshi AI, Choudhry MA, Akbar MS, et al. Plasma exchange vs. intravenous immunoglobulin treatment in myasthenic crisis. *Neurology* 1999;52:629–632.
38. Hewett SJ, Atchison WD. Specificity of Lambert-Eaton myasthenic syndrome immunoglobulin for nerve terminal calcium channels. *Brain Res* 1992;599:324–332.
39. Dau PC, Denys EH. Plasmapheresis and immunosuppressive drug therapy in the Eaton-Lambert syndrome. *Ann Neurol* 1982;11: 570–575.
40. Cooke JD, Hefter H, Brown SH, et al. Lambert-Eaton syndrome: evaluation of movement performance following drug therapy. *Clin Neurophysiol* 1994;34:87–93.
41. Takano H, Tanaka M, Koike R, et al. Effect of intravenous immunoglobulin in Lambert-Eaton myasthenic syndrome with small-cell lung cancer: correlation with the titer of anti-voltage-gated calcium channel antibody. *Muscle Nerve* 1994;17:1073–1075.
42. Moll JWB, Vecht CJ. Immune diagnoses of paraneoplastic neurological disease. *Clin Neurol Neurosurg* 1995;97:71–81.
43. Oguni H, Andermann F, Rasmussen TB. The natural history of the syndrome of chronic encephalitis and epilepsy: a study of the MNI series of forty-eight cases. In: Andermann F, ed. *Chronic encephalitis and epilepsy: Rasmussen's syndrome.* Boston: Butterworth-Heinemann, 1991:7–36.
44. Swedo SE, Leonard HL, Garvey M, et al. Pediatric autoimmune neuropsychiatric disorders associated with streptococcal infections: clinical description of the first 50 cases. *Am J Psychiatry* 1998;155: 264–271.
45. Noseworthy JH, Lucchinetti C, Rodriguez M, et al. Multiple sclerosis. *N Engl J Med* 2000;343:938–952.
46. Noseworthy JH, Ebers GC, Vandervoort MK, et al. The impact of blinding on the results of a randomized, placebo-controlled multiple sclerosis clinical trial. *Neurology* 1994;44:16–20.
47. Arnason BGW. Immunologic therapy of multiple sclerosis. *Annu Rev Med* 1999;50:291–302.
48. Khatri BO, McQuillen MP, Harrington GJ, et al. Chronic progressive multiple sclerosis: double-blind controlled study of plasmapheresis in patients taking immunosuppressive drugs. *Neurology* 1985;35: 312–319.
49. Weiner HL, Dau P, Khatri BO, et al. Double-blind study of true versus sham plasma exchange in patients being treated with immunosuppression for acute attacks of multiple sclerosis. *Neurology* 1989; 39:1143–1149.
50. The Canadian Cooperative Multiple Sclerosis Study Group. The Canadian cooperative trial of cyclophosphamide and plasma exchange in progressive multiple sclerosis. *Lancet* 1991;337:441–446.
51. Weinshenker BG, O'Brien PC, Petterson TM, et al. A randomized trial of plasma exchange in acute central nervous system inflammatory demyelinating disease. *Ann Neurol* 1999;46:878–886.
52. Assessment of plasmapheresis. Report of the Therapeutics and Technology Assessment Subcommittee of the American Academy of Neurology. *Neurology* 1996;47:840–843.
53. Glaspy JA. Hemostatic abnormalities in multiple myeloma and related disorders. *Hematol Oncol Clin North Am* 1992;6:1301–1314.
54. Johnson WJ, Kyle RA, Pineda AA, et al. Treatment of renal failure associated with multiple myeloma. Plasmapheresis, hemodialysis, and chemotherapy. *Arch Int Med* 1990;150:863–869.
55. Zucchelli P, Pasquali S, Cagnoli L, et al. Controlled plasma exchange trial in acute renal failure due to multiple myeloma. *Kidney Int* 1988; 33:1175–1180.
56. Watson WJ, Katz VL, Bowes WA. Plasmapheresis during pregnancy. *Obstet Gynecol* 1990;76:451–457.
57. Braine HG, Sensenbrenner LL, Wright SK, et al. Bone marrow transplantation with major ABO incompatibility using erythrocyte depletion of marrow prior to infusion. *Blood* 1982;60:420–425.
58. Gmur JP, Burger J, Schaffner A, et al. Pure red cell aplasia of long

duration complicating major ABO incompatible bone marrow transplantation. *Blood* 1990;75:290–295.
59. Ramsey G. Red cell antibodies arising from solid organ transplants. *Transfusion* 1991;31:76–86.
60. Lundgren G, Asaba H, Bergstrom J, et al. Fulminating anti-A autoimmune hemolysis with anuria in a renal transplant recipient: a therapeutic role of plasma exchange. *Clin Nephrol* 1981;16:211–214.
61. Moake JL. Thrombotic thrombocytopenic purpura. *Thromb Haemost* 1995;74:240–245.
62. Furlan M, Robles R, Solenthaler M, et al. Deficient activity of von Willebrand factor–cleaving protease in chronic relapsing thrombotic thrombocytopenic purpura. *Blood* 1997;89:3097–3103.
63. Furlan M, Robles R, Galbusera M, et al. Von Willebrand factor–cleaving protease in thrombotic thrombocytopenic purpura and the hemolytic-uremic syndrome. *N Engl J Med* 1998;339:1578–1584.
64. Tsai H-M, Lian EC-Y. Antibodies to von Willebrand factor–cleaving protease in acute thrombotic thrombocytopenic purpura. *N Engl J Med* 1998;339:1585–1594.
65. Rock GA, Shumak KH, Buskard NA, et al. The Canadian Apheresis Study Group. Comparison of plasma exchange with plasma infusion in the treatment of thrombotic thrombocytopenic purpura. *N Engl J Med* 1991;325:393–397.
66. Bennett CL, Weinberg PD, Rozenberg-Ben-Dor K et al. Thrombotic thrombocytopenic purpura associated with ticlopidine. A review of 60 cases. *Ann Intern Med* 1998;128:541–544.
67. Bennett CL, Connors JM, Carwile JM, et al. Thrombotic thrombocytopenic purpura associated with clopidogrel. *N Engl J Med* 2000;342: 1773–1777.
68. Tsai H-M, Rice L, Sarode R, et al. Antibody inhibitors to von Willebrand factor metalloproteinase and increased binding of von Willebrand factor to platelets in ticlopidine-associated thrombotic thrombocytopenic purpura. *Ann Intern Med* 2000;132:794–799.
69. Snyder HW, Mittelman A, Oral A, et al. Treatment of cancer chemotherapy–associated thrombotic thrombocytopenic purpura/hemolytic uremic syndrome by protein A immunoadsorption of plasma. *Cancer* 1993;71:1882–1892.
70. Sarode R, McFarland JG, Flomenberg N, et al. Therapeutic plasma exchange does not appear to be effective in the management of thrombotic thrombocytopenic purpura/hemolytic uremic syndrome following bone marrow transplantation. *Bone Marrow Transplant* 1995;16: 271–275.
71. Zipfel PF, Hellwage J, Friese MA, et al. Factor H and disease: a complement regulator affects vital bodily functions. *Mol Immunol* 1999;36:241–248.
72. Martin JN, Files JC, Blake PG, et al. Plasma exchange for preeclampsia. I. Postpartum use for persistently severe preeclampsia-eclampsia with HELLP syndrome. *Am J Obstet Gynecol* 1990;162:126–137.
73. Laursen B, Morling N, Resenkvist J, et al. Post-transfusion purpura treated with plasma exchange by Haemonetics cell separator. *Acta Med Scand* 1978;203:539–543.
74. Mueller-Eckhardt C, Kiefel V. High dose IgG for post-transfusion purpura—revisited. *Blut* 1988;57:163–167.
75. George JN, Rizvi MA. Thrombocytopenia. In: Beutler E, Lichtman MA, Coller BS, et al., eds. *Williams hematology,* 6th ed. New York: McGraw-Hill, 2000:1495–1539.
76. McLeod BC, Strauss RG, Ciavarella D, et al. Clinical applications of therapeutic apheresis: management of hematological disorders and cancer. *J Clin Apheresis* 1993;8:211–230.
77. Mittelman A, Bertram J, Henry DH, et al. Treatment of patients with HIV thrombocytopenia and hemolytic uremic syndrome with protein A (Prosorba column) immunoadsorption. *Semin Hematol* 1989;26[Suppl 11]:15–18.
78. Snyder HW Jr, Cochran SK, Balint JP, et al. Experience with protein A-immunoadsorption in treatment resistant immune thrombocytopenic purpura. *Blood* 1992;79:2237–2245.
79. Fitchen JJ, Cline MJ, Saxon A, et al. Serum inhibitors of hematopoiesis in a patient with aplastic anemia and systemic lupus erythematosus. *Am J Med* 1979;6:537–542.
80. Nilsson IM, Berntorp E, Zettervoll O. Induction of immune tolerance in patients with hemophilia and antibodies to factor VIII by combined treatment with intravenous IgG, cyclophosphamide, and factor VIII. *N Engl J Med* 1988;318:947–950.
81. Smith OP, Hann IM. rVIIa Therapy to secure haemostasis during central line insertion in children with high-responding FVIII inhibitors. *Br J Haematol* 1996;92:1002–1004.
82. Nakamura Y, Yoshida K, Itoh S, et al. Immunoadsorption plasmapheresis as a treatment for pregnancy complicated by systemic lupus erythematosus with positive antiphospholipid antibodies. *Am J Reprod Immunol* 1999;41:307–311.
83. Bloch KJ. Cryoglobulinemia and hepatic C Virus. *N Engl J Med* 1992; 327:1521–1522.
84. Berkman EM, Orlin JB. Use of plasmapheresis and partial plasma exchange in the management of patients with cryoglobulinemia. *Transfusion* 1980;20:171–178.
85. McLeod B, Sassetti R. Plasmapheresis with return of cryoglobulin depleted autologous plasma (cryoglobulinpheresis) in cryoglobulinemia. *Blood* 1980;55:866–870.
86. Bombardieri S, Maggiore Q, L'Abbate A, et al. Plasma exchange in essential mixed cryoglobulinemia. *Plasma Ther Transfus Technol* 1981; 2:101–109.
87. McGovern TW, Enzenauer RJ, Fitzpatrick JE. Treatment of recalcitrant leg ulcers in cryoglobulinemia types I and II with plasmapheresis. *Arch Dermatol* 1996;132:498–500.
88. Felson DT, La Valley MP, Baldassare AR, et al. The Prosorba column for the treatment of refractory rheumatoid arthritis: a randomized, double-blind, sham controlled trial. *Arthritis Rheum* 1999;42: 2153–2159.
89. Huston DP, White MJ, Maltiolo C, et al. A controlled trial of plasmapheresis and cyclophosphamide therapy of lupus nephritis. *Arthritis Rheum* 1983;26[Suppl]:S33.
90. Lewis EJ, Hunsicker LG, Lan SP, et al. A controlled trial of plasmapheresis therapy in severe lupus nephritis. *N Engl J Med* 1992;326: 1371–1379.
91. Euler HH, Schwab UM, Schroeder JO, et al. The lupus plasmapheresis study group: rationale and updated interim report. *Artif Organs* 1996;20:356–359.
92. Schroeder JO, Schwab U, Zennet R, et al. Plasmapheresis and subsequent pulse cyclophosphamide in severe systemic lupus erythematosus. Preliminary results of the LPSG Trial. *Arthritis Rheum* 1997;40: S325.
93. Wallace DJ, Goldfinger D, Pepkowitz S, et al. Randomized control of pulse/synchronization cyclophosphamide/apheresis for proliferative lupus nephritis. *J Clin Apheresis* 1998,13:163–166.
94. Pusey CD, Rees AJ, Evans DJ, et al. Plasma exchange in focal necrotizing glomerulonephritis without anti-GBM antibodies. *Kidney Int* 1991;40:757–763.
95. Guillevin L, Fain O, Lhote F, et al. Lack of superiority of steroids plus plasma exchange to steroids alone in the treatment of polyarteritis nodosa and Churg-Strauss syndrome. A prospective, randomized trial in 78 patients. *Arthritis Rheum* 1992;35:208–215.
96. Miller FW, Leitman SF, Cronin ME, et al. Controlled trial of plasma exchange and leukapheresis in polymyositis and dermatomyositis. *N Engl J Med* 1992;326:1380–1384.
97. Wiseman KC. New insights on Goodpasture's syndrome. *ANNA J* 1993;20:17–24.
98. Johnson JP, Moore J, Austin HA, et al. Therapy of anti-glomerular basement membrane antibody disease: analysis on the prognostic significance of clinical, pathologic, and treatment factors. *Medicine (Baltimore)* 1985;64:219–227.
99. Stegmayr BG, Almroth G, Berlin G, et al. Plasma exchange or immunoadsorption in patients with rapidly progressive glomerulonephritis. a Swedish multicenter study. *Int J Artif Organs* 1999;22:81–87.
100. Glöckner WM, Sieberth HG, Wichmann HE, et al. Plasma exchange and immunosuppression in rapidly progressive glomerulonephritis: a controlled, multi-center study. *Clin Nephrol* 1988;29:1–8.
101. Cole E, Cattran D, Magil A, et al. A prospective randomized trial of plasma exchange as additive therapy in idiopathic crescentic glomerulonephritis. *Am J Kidney Dis* 1992;20:261–269.
102. Guillevin L, Fain O, Lhote F, et al. Lack of superiority of steroids plus plasma exchange to steroids alone in the treatment of polyarteritis

nodosa and Churg-Strauss syndrome. A prospective, randomized trial in 78 patients. *Arthritis Rheum* 1992;35:208–215.
103. Levy JB, Pusey CD. Still a role for plasma exchange in rapidly progressive glomerulonephritis? *J Nephrol* 1997;10:7–13.
104. Croker BP, Ramos EL. Pathology of the renal allograft. In: Tishler CC, Brenner BM, eds. *Renal pathology: with clinical and functional correlations.* Philadelphia: JB Lippincott Co, 1994:1591–1640.
105. Blake P, Sutton D, Cardella C. Plasma exchange in acute renal transplant rejection. *Prog Clin Biol Res* 1990;337:249–252.
106. Costanzo-Nordin MR, Heroux AL, et al. Role of humoral immunity in acute cardiac allograft rejection. *J Heart Lung Transplant* 1993;12: S143–S146.
107. Savin VJ, Sharma R, Sharma M, et al. Circulating factor associated with increased glomerular permeability to albumin in recurrent focal segment of glomerulosclerosis. *N Engl J Med* 1996;334:878–883.
108. Thiery J, Meiser B, Wenke K, et al. Heparin-induced extracorporeal low-density-lipoprotein plasmapheresis (HELP) and its use in heart transplant patients with severe hypercholesterolemia. *Transplant Proc* 1995;27:1950–1953.
109. Goldstein JL, Hobbs HH, Brown MS. Familial hypercholesterolemia. In: Scriver CR, Beuadet AL, Sly WS, et al., eds. *The metabolic and molecular basis of inherited disease.* New York: McGraw-Hill, 1995: 1981–2030.
110. Gibberd FB. Plasma exchange for Refsum's disease. *Transfus Sci* 1993; 14:23–26.
111. Gutsche H-U, Siegmund JB, Hoppmann I. Lipapheresis: an immunoglobulin-sparing treatment for Refsum's disease. *Acta Neurol Scand* 1996;94:190–193.
112. Giorgi DF, Jagoda A. Poisoning and overdose. *Mt Sinai J Med* 1997; 64:283–291.
113. Lee WM. Acute liver failure. *New Engl J Med* 1993;329:1862–1872.
114. Larsen FS, Hansen BA, Ejlersen E, et al. Cerebral blood flow, oxygen metabolism and transcranial Doppler sonography during high-volume plasmapheresis in fulminant hepatic failure. *Eur J Gastroenterol Hepatol* 1995;8:261–265.
115. Saibara T, Maeda T, Onishi S, et al. Plasma exchange and the arterial blood ketone body ratio in patients with acute hepatic failure. *J Hepatol* 1994;20:617–622.
116. Chen SC, Hewitt WR, Watanabe FD, et al. Clinical experience with a porcine hepatocyte-based liver support system. *Int J Artif Organs* 1996;19:664–669.
117. Chopek M, McCullough J. Protein and biochemical changes during plasma exchange. In: Berkman EM, Umlas J, eds. *Therapeutic hemapheresis—a technical workshop.* Washington DC: American Association of Blood Banks, 1980:17.
118. McLeod BC, Sassetti RJ, Stefoski D, et al. Partial plasma protein replacement in therapeutic plasma exchange. *J Clin Apheresis* 1983; 1:117.

Rossi's Principles of Transfusion Medicine, Third Edition, edited by Toby L. Simon, Walter H. Dzik, Edward L. Snyder, Christopher P. Stowell, and Ronald G. Strauss. Lippincott Williams & Wilkins, Philadelphia © 2002.

CASE 46A

WHAT'S YOUR DIAGNOSIS?

CASE HISTORY

A 76-year-old man who was transferred to our facility for plasma exchange. He had been admitted 2 weeks earlier to another hospital with urinary problems. At that hospital he was found to have daily fevers to 102°F (38.9°C). A urine culture was positive for coagulase-negative staphylococci. The white blood cell (WBC) count was 11×10^9/L, and the platelet count was 189×10^9/L. Urine output was markedly low, and the diagnosis of acute renal failure was soon made. Evaluation showed no evidence of obstruction. Several blood tests were done to investigate the possibility of rapidly progressive glomerulonephritis, but no diagnosis could be made. A catheter was placed for possible hemodialysis, but dialysis was not needed before transfer to our hospital. The patient was treated with ciprofloxacin and metronidazole. A gallium scan showed no evidence of infection or tumor.

During the week before transfer, other problems surfaced. The patient had a known history of hypertension, but at the end of the first week, marked hypotension developed, and the patient was transferred to the intensive care unit. A pulmonary arterial catheter was placed, and an echocardiogram showed no evidence of endocarditis or pericardial effusion. At this time, the creatinine concentration had increased to 5.5 mg/dl. The WBC count was 21×10^9/L, and the lactate dehydrogenase (LDH) level was 1,100 IU/ml. The platelet count had decreased to 38×10^9/L. The prothrombin time (PT) increased to 24.6 seconds with an international normalized ratio of 4.3. The patient was given a transfusion of 10 units of platelet concentrates. Serum protein electrophoresis showed no evidence of multiple myeloma. Bone marrow examination showed all three marrow lineages present, and there was no evidence for tumor. Schistocytes were seen in the peripheral blood smear, and the diagnosis of thrombotic thrombocytopenic purpura (TTP) or hemolytic uremic syndrome was made. The patient was transferred to our hospital for plasma exchange.

The medical history included gout. Medications at home included ibuprofen, colchicine, allopurinol, and atenolol. On transfer to our intensive care unit, the patient was receiving dopamine, imipenem, and cilastatin. On arrival, the blood pressure was 90/50 mm Hg (with dopamine); heart rate, 95 beats/min; and temperature, 103°F (39.5°C). A faint systolic murmur was heard in the chest. The abdomen was diffusely tender with normal bowel sounds. There were no focal neurologic defects, but the patient responded only to painful stimuli.

On transfer, the laboratory results were as follows: hematocrit, 22%; WBC count, 15.6×10^9/L; platelets, 50×10^9/L; creatinine, 3.4 mg/dl; LDH, 935 IU/ml; total bilirubin, 1.9 mg/dl; alkaline phosphatase, 62 U/L; aspartate aminotransferase, 28 IU/ml; fibrinogen, 410 mg/dl; PT, 17.4 seconds; and D-dimer, positive 1:8. A peripheral blood smear showed anisocytosis and poikilocytosis of the red blood cells but very few schistocytes.

The attending staff believed the patient had TTP and needed immediate plasma exchange. However, there was discussion regarding features that did not fit the diagnosis of TTP, including the prolonged PT, positive D-dimer, elevated WBC count, and absence of significant schistocytes. Most important, it was noted that the patient first arrived at the referring hospital with a normal platelet count and that the decline in platelets was precipitous and associated with the development of hypotension necessitating pressors. The transfusion medicine consultants believed the onset of TTP 1 week after admission to the referring hospital was distinctly unlikely. An alternative diagnosis was sepsis characterized by hypotension, high fever, decline in consciousness, and disseminated intravascular coagulation. To evaluate a possible source of sepsis, the patient underwent chest radiography, computed tomography (CT) of the abdomen and pelvis, CT scan of the thorax, CT of the head, and several blood cultures—all of which provided no diagnosis. Oliguria persisted. Metabolic acidosis worsened, and the patient began to have periods of ventricular tachycardia. A gingival biopsy was performed in an attempt to find TTP, but the result was negative. Several blood smears showed minimal (if any) evidence of microangiopathic hemolysis.

The patient remained unconscious. In discussion with the patient's family, it was agreed that aggressive treatment, including plasma exchange, would not be pursued. Four days after transfer, the patient died. An autopsy was performed.

DISCUSSION

The diagnosis in this case was a matter of considerable debate in the intensive care unit. Some members of the health care team believed the patient had "classic TTP" because he had a fever, renal insufficiency, neurologic impairment, thrombocytopenia, and although not obvious microangiopathic hemolysis, a high LDH level. Others equally strongly believed he did not

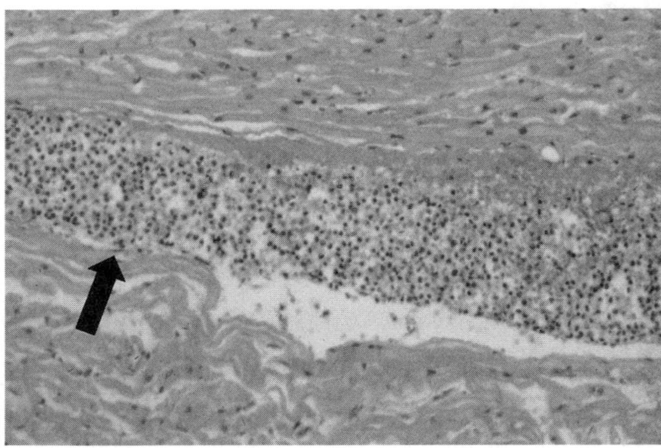

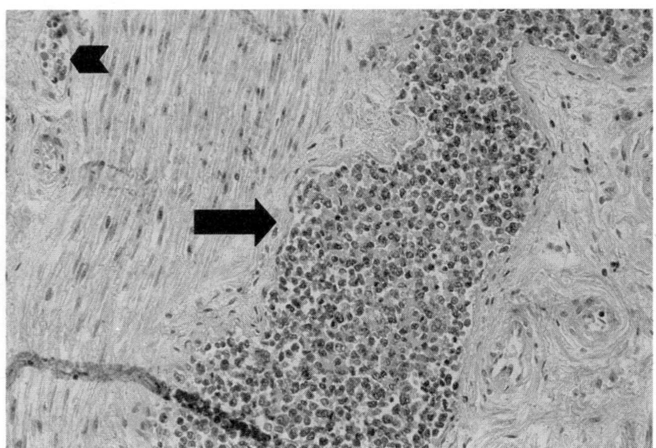

FIGURE 46A.1. A: Section through the heart. The striated muscle fibers of the heart run horizontally. A large vessel (*arrow*) runs diagonally and is filled with lymphomatous cells. **B:** Section through the prostate. A prominent vessel packed with lymphomatous cells is evident (*arrow*). *Arrowhead,* small venule also containing lymphoma cells. (Original magnification, ×40; photomicrographs courtesy of Zoe Tang, M.D.)

have TTP and pointed out that nearly all extremely sick patients in the medical intensive care have most of the features of TTP.

Physicians on both sides of the diagnostic debate wanted the best care for the patient. Those in favor of plasma exchange as a "diagnostic" effort believed there was little real toxicity to daily plasma exchange. Others believed that once exchange was begun, blood exchanges would mask other diagnostic results and that the source of sepsis would be neither identified nor controlled.

The patient had been examined with numerous scans and many diagnostic laboratory tests, including a bone marrow examination, without a unifying diagnosis. Gingival biopsy was performed in an attempt to identify thrombotic microangiopathic changes, but the result was negative. However, the sensitivity of this test is poor, and a negative result cannot be used to exclude the diagnosis of TTP.

CODA

The results of the autopsy were a surprise to everyone. The patient had diffuse intravascular large B-cell lymphoma (Fig. 46A.1). Lymphomatous cells were found packed within the lumens of blood vessels of the heart, lungs, liver, spleen, kidneys, adrenal glands, thyroid, pancreas, prostate, bladder, and lymph nodes. Despite extensive lymphoma within the lumens of vessels, circulating lymphoma cells were not seen in the peripheral blood smear. This is characteristic of intravascular lymphoma. Of note, there was no thrombotic microangiopathic process in any organ. Diffuse intravascular large B-cell lymphoma is an unusual condition, and the diagnosis rarely is made during life. The lesion often masquerades as another multisystem condition.

Case contributed by Walter H Dzik, M.D., and Zoe Tang, M.D., Massachusetts General Hospital, Boston, MA.

47

SPECIALIZED THERAPEUTIC HEMAPHERESIS PROCEDURES

ELEFTHERIOS C. VAMVAKAS
ALVARO A. PINEDA

The word apheresis is derived from the Greek word *aphaeresis* that means removal. Hemapheresis is the process of removing normal or abnormal blood constituents from circulating blood. It can be divided into cytapheresis and plasmapheresis which refer, respectively, to the removal of the cellular components or the plasma fraction of blood. Donor hemapheresis procedures are used to collect red blood cells, platelets, leukocytes, or plasma for transfusion, and they are discussed in Chapter 45. Therapeutic hemapheresis procedures are used to remove cellular components of blood or plasma constituents known or presumed to cause disease. Therapeutic cytapheresis procedures are selective, removing red blood cells (erythrocytapheresis), platelets (plateletpheresis), or leukocytes (leukapheresis). Therapeutic plasmapheresis is, by definition, nonselective, and refers to the removal of all plasma constituents, with simultaneous replacement of the removed plasma with an equal volume of plasma or plasma substitute. Thus, the term therapeutic plasma exchange (TPE) better describes the two processes that take place in the course of a therapeutic plasmapheresis procedure (1). Therapeutic plasma exchange is discussed in Chapter 46. Selective removal of specific plasma constituents is achieved through plasma perfusion. In this case, plasma collected by plasmapheresis is perfused through columns that selectively remove a substance of interest, while the modified plasma is returned to the patient (2).

This chapter reviews the therapeutic apheresis procedures used to remove leukocytes, platelets, or red blood cells from circulating blood, and the procedures used to selectively extract plasma constituents from circulating plasma. Table 47.1 lists these specialized hemapheresis procedures and the diseases for which each procedure is indicated. Therapeutic cytapheresis procedures are performed using the same equipment, and protocols similar to those used for the respective donor cytapheresis procedures. Accordingly, the rationale, side effects, and technical aspects of therapeutic cytapheresis procedures are not discussed in this chapter. The rationale, side effects, and technical aspects of photopheresis, staphylococcal protein A immunoadsorption,

E.C. Vamvakas: New York University Medical Center, Associate Professor of Pathology, New York University School of Medicine, New York, New York.
A.A. Pineda: Division of Transfusion Medicine, Mayo Clinic, Professor of Laboratory Medicine, Mayo Medical School, Rochester, Minnesota.

TABLE 47.1. INDICATIONS FOR SPECIALIZED THERAPEUTIC HEMAPHERESIS PROCEDURES[a]

Procedure/Indication	Indication Category[b]
Therapeutic Leukapheresis	
Hyperleukocytosis in patients with acute myelogenous leukemia	I
Therapeutic Plateletpheresis	
Thrombocytosis in patients with a chronic myeloproliferative disease	I
Therapeutic Erythropheresis	
Sickle cell disease	I
Polycythemia vera	II
Secondary erythrocytosis	II
Malaria and babesiosis	III
Photopheresis	
Cutaneous T-cell lymphoma	I
Cardiac allograft rejection	III
Graft versus host disease	NL[c]
Autoimmune diseases	NL[c]
Immunoadsorption with Staphylococcal Protein A/Agarose Column	
Preparation of hyperimmunized patients for renal transplantation	NL[c]
Acute humoral rejection of renal allograft	NL[c]
Rapidly progressing glomerulonephritis	NL[c]
Factor VIII or IX inhibitors	NL[c]
Autoimmune diseases	NL[c]
Immunoadsorption with Staphylococcal Protein A/Silica Column	
Rheumatoid arthritis	II
Idiopathic thrombocytopenic purpura (ITP)	II
Platelet alloimmunization and refractoriness	III
Paraneoplastic syndromes with central nervous system manifestations	III
Paraproteinemic polyneuropathies	III
Cancer chemotherapy–associated TTP/HUS syndrome	NL[c]
Malignant disease failing conventional chemotherapy	NL[c]
Selective Extraction of Low-Density Lipoproteins	
Familial hypercholesterolemia	I
Selective Extraction of Bile Acids	
Intractable pruritus secondary to cholestasis	NL[c]

TTP/HUS, thrombotic thrombocytopenic purpura hemolytic uremic syndrome.
[a]From McLeod, BC. Clinical applications of therapeutic apheresis. *J Clin Apheresis* 2000;15:1–159.
[b]Therapeutic apheresis is standard treatment for category I indications and adjunctive treatment for category II indications. Category III indications include diseases for which the available evidence is insufficient to establish or refute the benefit from therapeutic apheresis. For these diseases, therapeutic apheresis is indicated when other conventional therapies have failed, or as part of a research protocol with Institutional Review Board approval.
[c]Indication discussed in the text, but not listed in the table of Indications of clinical applications of therapeutic apheresis *J Clin Apheresis* 2000;15:2–3.

and the procedures used to selectively extract low-density lipoproteins (LDLs) or bile acids are described, because these latter procedures have not been discussed in Chapters 45 and 46.

THERAPEUTIC LEUKAPHERESIS

Acute myelogenous leukemia (AML), especially the M4 and M5 types, can cause extreme leukocytosis (i.e., a white blood cell count exceeding 100,000/μl). When such hyperleukocytosis develops, the large circulating myeloblasts can cause both a hyperviscosity syndrome and obstruction of the microcirculation, especially in the lungs and brain. The clinical syndrome associated with hyperleukocytosis is highly and rapidly fatal, requiring emergency leukapheresis for the removal of the circulating myeloblasts. Although leukapheresis is standard therapy for hyperleukocytosis and potentially life saving, its efficacy is debated.

Leukapheresis may also be indicated with white blood cell counts between 50,000/μl and 100,000/μl and a diagnosis of AML if there are symptoms of leukostasis, such as dizziness, fainting, headache, altered sensorium, visual disturbances, priapism, dyspnea, tachypnea, rales, hypoxemia without hypercapnia, and diffuse pulmonary infiltrates without evidence of pneumonia. Cerebral leukostasis may also produce similar symptoms in patients with the accelerated or blast-crisis phase of chronic myelogenous leukemia (CML). However, before the blast-crisis phase, CML does not ordinarily produce a hyperleukocytosis syndrome even when the white blood cell count exceeds 300,000/μl.

When a patient is experiencing a hyperleukocytosis syndrome, leukapheresis is performed to decrease the white blood cell count and to relieve the patient's symptoms. There is no defined goal, however, in terms of the magnitude of the desired reduction in white blood cell count, because no correlation has been observed between the degree of cytoreduction and the subsequent duration of survival (3). Usually, two blood volumes are processed in a leukapheresis procedure, and this results in a 50% to 85% reduction in white blood cell count (4). An erythrocyte-sedimenting agent (6% hydroxyethyl starch) is added to the patient's blood to achieve more efficient extraction of mature and immature myeloid cells.

Leukapheresis has also been used to control the symptoms of cutaneous T-cell lymphoma, a disease for which leukapheresis may be an effective palliative therapy. As shown in Table 47.1, however, the hemapheresis treatment of choice for cutaneous T-cell lymphoma is photopheresis. Finally, randomized double-blind trials of lymphocytapheresis or lymphoplasmapheresis were performed in the early 1980s in patients with rheumatoid arthritis, and they produced mixed results. At the present time, and as discussed later in this chapter, the hemapheresis treatment of choice for rheumatoid arthritis is protein A immunoadsorption (Table 47.1).

THERAPEUTIC PLATELETPHERESIS

Chronic myeloproliferative diseases are often associated with extreme thrombocytosis when platelet counts exceed 1,000,000/μl. Such primary thrombocytosis may lead to thrombotic or hemorrhagic complications in some patients, and findings can range from severe headache to stroke. Plateletpheresis is standard therapy for symptomatic thrombocytosis in patients with a chronic myeloproliferative disease, and the procedure should be performed as soon as possible. Platelet counts show only a very weak correlation with the occurrence of symptoms, however, and patients with primary thrombocytoses who are at risk for thrombosis or hemorrhage cannot be identified prior to the appearance of symptoms. A consensus has thus not been reached as to whether a) plateletpheresis should be performed only in the presence of signs or symptoms of thrombosis or hemorrhage, or b) the procedure is indicated prophylactically in patients with a myeloproliferative disease and platelet counts exceeding 1,000,000/μl. In the latter case, the procedure may be indicated prophylactically only in patients who have additional risk factors for thrombosis or hemorrhage, including elderly patients and patients with underlying cardiovascular disease, pregnant women, or patients scheduled to undergo general anesthesia or an invasive procedure or both.

Plateletpheresis is not indicated in patients with secondary thrombocytoses (5). Secondary thrombocytosis may appear in association with malignancy (especially lung cancer or mucin-producing tumors), chronic inflammatory disease (such as rheumatoid arthritis, sarcoidosis, or ulcerative colitis), bone marrow recovery after therapy with myelosuppressive drugs, or following splenectomy or acute hemorrhage. Platelet counts may exceed 1,000,000/μl in some secondary thrombocytoses, but these patients are not at risk for thrombosis or hemorrhage.

In primary thrombocytosis, plateletpheresis is performed to decrease the platelet count and relieve the patient's symptoms. There is no defined target, however, in terms of the magnitude of the desired reduction in platelet count. Usually, 1.0 to 1.5 blood volumes are processed (6), or the procedure is continued for a specific length of time, such as 3 hours (4).

THERAPEUTIC ERYTHROCYTAPHERESIS

Therapeutic erythrocytapheresis differs from donor erythrocytapheresis (described in Chapter 45), in that the removed patient red blood cells are isovolemically replaced by donor red blood cells. Thus, another term for therapeutic erythrocytapheresis is therapeutic red blood cell exchange. Erythrocytapheresis has been helpful in treating patients with cerebral malaria or patients with extreme parasitemia of malaria or babesiosis (7). As discussed in Chapter 11, erythrocytapheresis has also been used in lieu of simple phlebotomy in patients with polycythemia vera or secondary erythrocytosis, in order to lower red blood cell mass more rapidly than can be achieved with phlebotomy. The usual indication for erythrocytapheresis, however, is the management of a severe infarctive crisis in a patient with sickle cell disease.

Stroke, acute chest syndrome, intrahepatic cholestasis and hemolysis, acute splenic sequestration, retinal infarction, or priapism are well-accepted indications for erythrocytapheresis in patients with sickle cell disease, although no controlled studies have been conducted to demonstrate clinical benefit from erythrocytapheresis in these patients. Prophylactic erythrocytapheresis is universally recommended for patients with sickle cell disease who have had a stroke, and it is also used, at some centers, for patients who have had disabling pain crises in the past. There also seems to be general agreement that prophylactic erythrocytapheresis is indicated for patients with sickle cell disease who are scheduled to undergo general anesthesia, but the use of erythrocytapheresis during pregnancy is controversial (8).

Therapeutic Erythrocytapheresis Procedure

A procedure undertaken to relieve a sickle cell crisis may aim at a) reducing the hemoglobin S (HbS) concentration to below 30% and b) increasing the hematocrit to approximately 30%. A prophylactic procedure usually aims at maintaining the HbS concentration below 50%. For patients who have not been recently transfused, a preprocedure HbS level of 100% can generally be assumed. The procedure removes the patient's HbS-containing red blood cells, replacing them with donor red blood cells that contain hemoglobin A. The fraction of the patient's own red blood cells remaining in the blood stream after the procedure, as a percentage of the total number of red blood cells circulating in the patient after the procedure (FCR%), is calculated as:

$$\text{Desired FCR\%} = 100 \times (\text{desired HbS concentration/preprocedure HbS concentration})$$

For example, if the desired HbS concentration is 30%, and the preprocedure HbS concentration is 100%, the desired FCR% = 30% ÷ 100% = 30%. In addition, the procedure may aim at increasing the patient's hematocrit, as follows:

Adjusted FCR% = Desired FCR% × (current hematocrit/ desired hematocrit) × 100

For example, if the desired hematocrit is 30% and the current hematocrit is 25%, the desired FCR% should be multiplied by 25% ÷ 30% = 0.83 to obtain the adjusted FCR%. In such a case, the adjusted FCR% would equal 30% × 0.83 = 25%. Thus, the patient's own red blood cells will represent 25% of circulating red blood cells after the procedure.

Based on a) the adjusted FCR%, b) the patient's hematocrit and estimated blood volume, and c) an average hematocrit for the donor red blood cell units, one can calculate the number of donor red blood cell units that must be used for the procedure. Usually, the FCR% and the information about the patient are entered into the hemapheresis instrument, which determines the volume of donor red blood cells necessary to achieve the specified targets of HbS concentration and hematocrit.

A syndrome consisting of association of sickle cell disease, priapism, exchange transfusion, and neurologic events (ASPEN syndrome) has been reported to occur in some patients with sickle cell disease and priapism treated with erythrocytapheresis. The syndrome consists of neurologic events, ranging from headache and seizures to obtundation that requires mechanical ventilation. The syndrome is thought to arise from decreased cerebral blood flow, perhaps secondary to the abrupt elevation in hematocrit after an erythrocytapheresis procedure, and from the release of vasoactive substances as a result of the penile detumescence (9). Many, although not all, of the reported cases had a postprocedure hematocrit above 36%, or above 150% of baseline. Thus, maintenance of the preprocedure hematocrit throughout the procedure, or an increase of no more than 120% of baseline, would seem prudent and may help avoid this complication (10).

In patients with sickle cell disease, either red blood cell transfusion or erythrocytapheresis can achieve the HbS concentration and hematocrit targets, and a choice must be made between simple transfusion and erythrocytapheresis for each treatment episode (8). At tertiary-care medical centers where erythrocytapheresis is readily available, erythrocytapheresis is usually preferred to simple transfusion, because it can achieve the desired HbS concentration faster and without causing an increase in blood viscosity. Also, by removing red blood cells, erythrocytapheresis contributes less to iron overload than does simple transfusion.

Donor red blood cell units used for erythrocytapheresis should be screened for the sickle cell trait, with the positive units excluded. Selected units should be crossmatch compatible with the patient's serum, and the patient should be watched during the procedure for signs and symptoms of a hemolytic transfusion reaction. Antigenic disparity between the donor population and patients with sickle cell disease makes these individuals especially likely to form red blood cell alloantibodies, and thus these subjects are at increased risk for immediate (or delayed) hemolytic transfusion reactions. In addition, these multitransfused patients are at increased risk for nonhemolytic transfusion reactions and may also present difficulties in obtaining vascular access.

PHOTOPHERESIS

Photopheresis is currently standard therapy for cutaneous T-cell lymphoma. In this procedure, buffy coat separated from whole blood and chemically treated with 8-methoxypsoralen (either ingested orally or instilled into the collection bag) is exposed to light (ultraviolet A irradiation) and returned to the patient. 8-Methoxypsoralen is a drug that irreversibly binds covalently to one or both strands of the DNA of nucleated cells following photoactivation. The photochemically damaged alloreactive T-cell clones returned to the patient appear to induce suppressor or cytotoxic T cell formation, which might be responsible for the "antitumor" effect attributed to the procedure.

It is theorized that the patient's own T cells mount an immune response to the treated neoplastic T cells, but the mechanism of such an immune-mediated "antitumor" effect is poorly understood (11). The beneficial effects of the procedure cannot be traced to direct cytotoxicity of 8-methoxypsoralen and ultraviolet A irradiation (UVA) on T cells or tumor cells, because only 10% to 15% of the lymphocyte pool is harvested by the leukapheresis procedure, and fewer than 5% of the cutaneous T-cell lymphoma cells are exposed to UVA (12). Photopheresis is known to induce a $CD8^+$ T-cell response against pathologic T-cell clones (13). Thus, patients with cutaneous T-cell lymphoma who are treated early after diagnosis—when they are still immunologically competent and have nearly normal counts of $CD8^+$ lymphocytes—respond best to photopheresis.

The photopheresis procedure is performed using the UVAR II or the newer UVAR XTS (Therakos, Inc., Exton, PA). Six cycles of whole blood collection are performed intermittently, and in each cycle the whole blood is separated into components in a pediatric Latham centrifuge bowl; the buffy coat is retained in a collection bag and the remaining blood components are returned to the patient. The buffy coat is pumped through a photoactivation chamber, which consists of transparent acrylic plates between which is sandwiched a tortuous channel. Adjacent to the plates is a UVA light source that irradiates the 8-methoxypsoralen-containing buffy coat. Because photopheresis relies on both UVA and 8-methoxypsoralen, it is also known as extracorporeal photochemotherapy. A typical course of photopheresis consists of two treatments on consecutive days every 4 weeks. Following improvement in disease symptoms, the interval between procedures may be prolonged, or the patient may be weaned from photopheresis (12).

Patients undergoing photopheresis may experience side effects of 8-methoxypsoralen, such as nausea, vomiting, vertigo, cutaneous erythema, or facial edema. In addition, patients receiving 8-methoxypsoralen are sensitive to sunlight and must avoid sun exposure (12). There also exists a theoretic risk of mutagenesis, because of the DNA damage that the procedure causes in the leukocytes that are returned to the patient. These cells could conceivably give rise to hematologic malignancies if they were still capable of cell division following the photopheresis treatment. Although evidence of secondary malignancies has not been reported, mutagenesis remains a theoretic risk of photopheresis, because there has not yet been sufficient follow-up of patients treated with this procedure (11).

Cutaneous T-cell Lymphoma

In the study of Edelson et al., photopheresis was performed on 2 consecutive days every 4 weeks to treat cutaneous T-cell lymphoma, with clinical evaluation of the patients at 6 months after the beginning of therapy. A skin scoring system that ranged from 0 (entirely uninvolved skin) to 400 (universal involvement, with maximal erythroderma and induration) was used for clinical evaluation. Patients who demonstrated significant clinical improvement were maintained on this treatment schedule until they achieved maximal clearing of their skin lesions. An additional 6 months of therapy was then administered to ensure the stability of the response. Patients were weaned off photopheresis by gradually increasing the interval between treatments (14).

Twenty-seven of 37 (73%) patients were judged to respond, based on a greater than 25% improvement in skin score. Nine (24%) patients achieved a complete response with clearing of skin lesions. Patients with generalized exfoliative erythroderma responded better than those with skin plaques or tumors; the recorded response rates were 83% and 38%, respectively. Responses were observed after an average of five to six cycles of photopheresis treatments (mean ± SD duration of therapy, 22.4 ± 9.6 weeks) (14).

Continued follow-up of the patients enrolled in the trial of Edelson et al. demonstrated that photopheresis can achieve better long-term results than conventional therapy. Four of nine complete responders remained disease free for 6 to 10 years after their photopheresis treatment without further therapy. These patients did not have malignant lymphoma cells, either in their skin biopsies or in their blood (15).

Zic et al. pooled the data from seven North American trials of the use of photopheresis in cutaneous T-cell lymphoma. They demonstrated an objective response to treatment in 54% of patients, with 19% of subjects achieving a complete remission. The median time until clearing of skin lesions in responding patients was 11 months. Patients who showed early response to treatment (i.e., clearing of skin lesions within 6 to 8 months) were less likely to experience relapse of their disease (16).

Other Indications for Photopheresis

Photopheresis has also been used in various other diseases (Table 47.2). Several teams have described patients with cardiac, pulmonary, or renal allograft rejection who appeared to improve after photopheresis (17). Controlled studies have been conducted in patients having cardiac allograft rejection. In a study reported by Meiser et al., five cardiac allograft recipients receiving standard immunosuppression had more histologic rejection episodes, compared with ten patients who received either 10 or 20 photopheresis treatments (18). Barr et al. randomized 60 patients to receive standard immunosuppressive therapy with or without photopheresis. Neither the probability of survival nor the frequency of allograft rejection associated with hemodynamic compromise differed between the treatment and control arms.

TABLE 47.2. DISEASES FOR WHICH PHOTOPHERESIS HAS BEEN REPORTED AS EFFECTIVE

Graft Versus Host Disease
Solid Organ Allograft Rejection
Cardiac
Renal
Pulmonary
Autoimmune Diseases
Systemic lupus erythematosus
Rheumatoid arthritis
Psoriatic arthritis
Progressive systemic sclerosis
Juvenile dermatomyositis
Pemphigus vulgaris
Epidermolysis bullosa acquisita
Infectious Diseases
Chronic Lyme Arthritis
AIDS-related complex
Other Diseases
Severe atopic dermatitis
Psoriasis

From van Iperen HP, Beijersbergen van Henegouwen GM. Clinical and mechanistic aspects of photopheresis. *J Photochem Photobiol B* 1997;39:99–109, with permission.
From Zic JA, Miller JL, Stricklin JP, et al. The North American experience with photopheresis. *Ther Apher* 1999;3:50–62, with permission.

However, there were fewer histologic rejection episodes in the treatment arm (mean ± SD of 0.91 ± 1.0), compared with the control arm (1.44 ± 1.0; P = 0.04) (19). This finding is hard to evaluate, because Barr et al. did not report the histologic grade of rejection in either arm. Histologic evidence of mild rejection in endomyocardial biopsies often resolves without a change in the immunosuppressive regimen (20) and may thus not affect a patient's clinical outcome.

In graft versus host disease (GVHD), photopheresis has produced improvement in cutaneous manifestations, as well as in mucosal manifestations (17). Greinix et al. reported on 21 patients who developed steroid-refractory acute GVHD grade II to IV after allogeneic stem cell grafting. Three months after initiation of photopheresis, 60% of patients achieved a complete resolution of all GVHD manifestations. Complete responses were obtained in 100% of patients with grade II, 67% of patients with grade III, and 12% of patients with grade IV disease. Thirteen of 21 patients had hepatic manifestations of GVHD, and 67% of them responded to treatment. Four patients had gastrointestinal manifestations, and none of them responded to photopheresis (21).

Finally, photopheresis has also been used in various autoimmune diseases (Table 47.2) and is presently undergoing evaluation in patients with ulcerative colitis. Rook et al. examined the efficacy of photopheresis in treating patients with progressive systemic sclerosis (PSS) (22). Patients were randomized to receive either monthly photopheresis treatments on 2 consecutive days or treatment with D-penicillamine at a maximum dose of 750 mg per day. After 6 months of treatment, significant improvement in skin severity score occurred in 21 (68%) of 31 patients receiving photopheresis, compared with 8 (32%) of 25 patients receiving D-penicillamine treatment. In addition, 3 (10%) of 31 patients receiving photopheresis, as compared with 8 (32%) of 25 patients receiving D-penicillamine treatment, manifested significant worsening in skin severity score. At 10 months, however, there were no significant differences in skin severity score between the photopheresis and D-penicillamine arms of this trial, and subsequent studies have not demonstrated any significant benefit from photopheresis in patients with PSS (23). Moreover, the trial of Rook et al. (22) was criticized for its methodology and for the optimistic conclusion that photopheresis is an effective intervention for the treatment of PSS (24). Further studies are needed to define the role of photopheresis in the treatment of this disease.

IMMUNOADSORPTION WITH THE STAPHYLOCOCCAL PROTEIN A–AGAROSE COLUMN

Therapeutic plasma exchange is usually performed to remove paraproteins, autoantibodies, lipids, toxins or drugs, or circulating immune complexes that mediate (or are believed to mediate) a particular disease process. The pathogenic substance (e.g., a specific autoantibody) is usually present at very low levels in the circulation, and a typical plasmapheresis removes 150 g of healthy plasma protein in order to eliminate 1 to 2 g of the culprit substance (2). To preserve the various healthy plasma proteins that are essential to homeostasis, selective extraction of pathologic plasma constituents has been proposed as a more physiologic, and at least as efficacious, approach to the management of patients with specific diseases as therapeutic plasmapheresis (25,26).

Immunoadsorption systems make use of the principle of affinity chromatography and are highly specific for the removal of a particular pathogenic substance. The plasma constituents are extracted by perfusion of plasma over affinity columns containing immobilized sorbents or ligands. Ligands have binding affinity for a specific antigen, antibody, immune complex, or other immune reactant in the patient's circulation. Examples include staphylococcal protein A or sheep anti-human immunoglobulin (IgG) antibody for extraction of IgG and immune complexes from the circulation, sheep anti-human LDL or apolipoprotein B antibody for extraction of LDL, synthetic blood group substances for removal of ABO isoagglutinins, and DNA for removal of anti-DNA antibody. Two immunoadsorption systems that have received approval from the U.S. Food and Drug Administration (FDA) and are currently commercially available are discussed in this chapter. These are the staphylococcal protein A–agarose column (Immunosorba), and the staphylococcal protein A–silica column (Prosorba).

Protein A is a cell-wall constituent of the Cowan I strain of *Staphylococcus aureus.* It carries five homologous regions at its N-terminus which bind IgG from mammalian species, and its interaction with other plasma proteins is insignificant. Binding of IgG is nonimmunologic but of high affinity. Protein A interacts strongly with IgG1, IgG2, and IgG4, but only to a variable extent with IgG3, IgM, and IgA. Moreover, the affinity of protein A is higher for complexed IgG than for free IgG. Gjörstrup and Watt reported that treatment of 2.5 plasma volumes with a protein A–agarose column resulted in a 97% reduction in IgG1, a 98% reduction in IgG2, a 40% reduction in IgG3, a 77% reduction in IgG4, a 56% reduction in IgM, and a 55% reduction in IgA. Plasma levels of albumin, fibrinogen, and antithrombin III were reduced by less than 20% (27).

Thus, the protein A–agarose column permits more vigorous removal of IgG from the circulation than TPE. More intense treatment is possible with the protein A–agarose column because of its selectivity, which permits larger amounts of plasma to be processed without lowering the concentration of essential plasma proteins below acceptable levels. More vigorous treatment can have a major impact in situations where pathogenic antibodies rapidly produce irreversible tissue damage (e.g., in Goodpasture's syndrome [GPS] or in rapidly progressing glomerulonephritis [RPGN]).

Use of the Protein A–agarose Column

The protein A–agarose column is marketed by Excorim AB (Lund, Sweden) as part of an immunoadsorption system that combines two protein A columns and an elution monitor. Protein A is covalently linked to beaded agarose (Sepharose), and the columns have a shelf life of 18 months when stored in the refrigerator. Patient plasma is pumped into the elution monitor, which directs the flow of plasma through one of the protein A–agarose columns. After one column is perfused to the point of saturation, the plasma is directed to the other column, and while this column is adsorbing IgG, the saturated column is eluted (with regard to the adsorbed IgG), using an elution fluid. The previously saturated column is thus regenerated and ready for a new adsorption cycle. Treated plasma leaving the column is combined with the cellular components of blood in the plasmapheresis device and is returned to the patient. Every 10 minutes the plasma flow is automatically switched to the other column, and the two-column arrangement gives the adsorption system almost unlimited capacity to remove immunoglobulins. The procedure can thus continue until a desired amount of IgG has been removed. Processing of three plasma volumes takes 3 to 5 hours and involves 20 to 30 adsorption cycles. One pair of columns is assigned to each patient to be used throughout the treatment period (27).

The protein A–agarose column has been used in European countries for the removal of alloantibodies or autoantibodies from the serum of hyperimmunized patients awaiting renal transplantation, renal allograft recipients having acute humoral rejection, patients with GPS or RPGN, and patients with congenital or acquired hemophilia and antoantibodies to factors VIII or IX. The column has also been used in the treatment of patients with other diseases that are thought to be autoimmune in origin. These have included myasthenia gravis and the Eaton-Lambert myasthenic syndrome, the acute Guillain-Barré syndrome, microscopic polyarteritis and Wegener's granulomatosis (mostly in the context of RPGN), pemphigus vulgaris, systemic lupus erythematosus, and idiopathic thrombocytopenic purpura (ITP). In the United States, the protein A–agarose column is approved by the FDA for the extraction of autoantibodies to factors VIII or IX. The results of studies of the efficacy of the protein A–agarose column for the treatment of various diseases have been reported as case reports or case series, and no controlled studies are available (2).

Preparation of Hyperimmunized Patients for Renal Transplantation

Patients awaiting renal transplantation who have developed HLA class I antibodies reacting with more than 75% of lymphocytes from random donors have been successfully transplanted following an intensive course of treatment with the protein A–agarose column (28–30). In most reports, such patients underwent an initial intensive course of four to six immunoadsorptions combined with immunosuppressive therapy (e.g., cyclophosphamide and prednisolone), and then received additional immunoadsorptions if the initial course did not result in a negative crossmatch between the patient's serum and the lymphocytes of renal allograft donors. Successfully transplanted patients usually received renal allografts within 2 months of the start of treatment. If patients were not transplanted soon after treatment, they experienced rapid resynthesis of HLA class I antibodies within a few weeks after receiving immunoadsorption.

Based on the available data, it would appear that treatment with the protein A–agarose column is effective in reducing the alloreactivity of sera of prospective renal allograft recipients. Patients transplanted with a current negative and historic positive crossmatch can manifest long-term graft survival as high as 60%. Some grafts are lost because of acute humoral rejection, but a substantial percentage are lost for other reasons (e.g., recurrence of disease, chronic rejection, technical failures). Variability in response to treatment is substantial, and criteria for selecting patients likely to benefit from this procedure need to be better defined.

Acute Humoral Rejection of Renal Allograft

Protein A–agarose column treatments have also been used in renal allograft recipients having acute humoral rejection (31–33). Persson et al. reported on 12 patients with deteriorating graft function who received one to seven immunoadsorption treatments each (mean, 3.6 treatments). Five (42%) patients had good graft function after 8 to 77 months of follow-up (32). Pretagostini et al. reported on 23 patients in whom acute humoral rejection developed within 1 to 3 weeks of transplantation. These subjects received from 4 to 23 immunoadsorption treatments each (mean, 7.3 treatments) over 3 to 44 days (mean, 12.3 days). Immediately after treatment, a negative crossmatch was obtained in 22 (96%) of 23 patients. Graft function was recovered in 16 (70%) of 23 patients (33).

Rapidly Progressing Glomerulonephritis

Palmer et al. concluded that treatment with the protein A–agarose column produces better results than therapeutic plasmapheresis in patients with RPGN. They treated ten patients with RPGN and acute renal failure who were dialysis dependent at the start of the treatment. Nine patients rapidly regained renal function within 2 weeks of commencing immunoadsorption (34). In contrast, Esnault et al. observed improvement in only three of five patients with RPGN treated with protein A immunoadsorption (35).

Inhibitors to Factor VIII or IX

Several reports have described the use of immunoadsorption to manage patients with inhibitors to factors VIII or IX. Gjörstrup and Watt (27) presented the experience with 32 patients with congenital (20 cases) or acquired (12 cases) hemophilia reported prior to 1990. Further case reports also appeared (36), and Gjörstrup et al. presented a more recent series of ten patients in 1991 (37). In addition, Uehlinger et al. reported the successful treatment of a patient with acquired von Willebrand factor antibody (38). In the report of Gjörstrup et al., ten patients underwent a combined total of 17 treatments with the protein A–agarose column. From 1.3 to 15.3 plasma volumes were processed per treatment over one to six sessions. Seven treatments involved only one session and six treatments entailed two daily procedures; in the remaining four treatments, three to six daily sessions were needed. The seven patients with congenital hemophilia responded better than the three patients with acquired hemophilia. In the former group, antibody titers were reduced to less than 10 Bethesda units (BU) in six of seven patients. In contrast, antibody titers were reduced to less than 10 BU in only one of three patients with acquired hemophilia (37).

Autoimmune Diseases

The Canadian Apheresis Group assessed the efficacy of the protein A–agarose column in patients with myasthenia gravis. Ten of 12 patients included in this case series experienced an improvement in their neurologic function, as measured by a 20-point scoring system. These subjects received an average of 2.2 procedures over a 3- to 5-day treatment period, and a total 6.0 plasma volumes was processed per patient. The mean ± SD percent decrease in acetylcholine receptor antibody titers was 68.1 ± 21.7%. The authors concluded that, in patients with myasthenia gravis, treatment with the protein A–agarose column may achieve a clinical response similar to that obtained with standard therapeutic plasmapheresis, but following a smaller number of procedures. More specifically, an average of 2.2 immunoadsorption procedures per patient were used in this study, compared with the historic therapeutic plasmapheresis experience of 4.3 procedures per patient. However, the authors acknowledged that their observations need to be corroborated by a study randomizing myasthenic subjects to receive treatment with the protein A–agarose column or therapeutic plasmapheresis. They also cautioned readers that treatment with the protein A–agarose column is more expensive than therapeutic plasmapheresis, despite the smaller number of procedures needed to achieve a clinical response, because of the added cost of the protein A column (39).

IMMUNOADSORPTION WITH THE STAPHYLOCOCCAL PROTEIN A–SILICA COLUMN

The Prosorba column is currently marketed in the United States by Fresenius Hemocare, Inc. (Redmond, WA). It received approval from the FDA initially for the treatment of ITP and recently for the treatment of moderate-to-severe rheumatoid arthritis. Perfusion of patient plasma over the Prosorba column can be done off-line, with perfusion of as little as 250 ml of plasma, or on-line, typically with perfusion of 1 to 2 liters of plasma. In the off-line mode, one unit of whole blood is collected from the patient, the plasma is separated from the cellular components by centrifugation, and the cellular components of blood are returned to the patient. The collected plasma is then perfused through the Prosorba column, and the treated plasma is reinfused to the patient. In the on-line mode, the patient is connected to an apheresis instrument, the Prosorba column is attached to the plasma return line, and plasma is perfused through the column. Treated plasma is then reunited with the cellular components and returned to the patient. The Prosorba column contains 200 mg of staphylococcal protein A, immobilized on 125 mg of a silica matrix. The column is saturated with as little as 1 g of IgG and is incapable of either regeneration or reuse. Thus, the mechanism of action of the Prosorba column is not based on the removal of pathogenic IgG.

It is believed that the treated plasma exercises an obscure immunomodulatory effect when it is returned to patients, perhaps causing a long-lasting change in a patient's immune system. The Prosorba column is reported to facilitate the clearance of circulating immune complexes—which consist of disease-associated antigen and antibody or idiotypic autoantibody and regulatory antiidiotypic antibody—and to unblock the production of protective antibody which targets either disease-associated antigen or idiotypic autoantibody. Thus, in promoting the formation of antiidiotypic antibody, the Prosorba column is believed to exercise an effect similar to that of intravenous immune globulin (IVIG) (40,41).

Circulating immune complexes can be present in patients with autoimmune diseases, cancer, and persistent viral infections. Snyder et al. presented evidence that circulating immune complexes in ITP contain autoantibody to a platelet-associated antigen (such as GP IIb/IIIa) and a corresponding antiidiotypic antibody directed against the idiotope of the autoantibody (42). Circulating immune complexes in patients with breast adenocarcinoma contain tumor-associated glycosphingolipid antigens ("Le^x glycolipids") (43). Circulating immune complexes in patients with cancer chemotherapy–associated thrombotic thrombocytopenic purpura/hemolytic uremic syndrome (CCATTP/HUS) contain platelet-associated antigens (GP IIb/IIIa) with or without tumor-associated antigens (Le^x glycolipids), with or without antiplatelet autoantibody complexed with antiidiotypic antibody (44).

Moreover, the Prosorba column causes complement activation (45) and has a mitogenic effect on T and B lymphocytes (46). Complement activation by the Prosorba column may explain some of its therapeutic effects as well as some of its toxicity. Activated complement components bind to circulating immune complexes and stimulate their clearance by the reticuloendothelial system. The mitogenic effect of the column results in an increased T helper to suppressor cell ratio, as well as in increased natural killer cell activity. These effects, singly or in combination, may account for the immunologic changes observed in patients with autoimmune or malignant disease receiving Prosorba treatment (24).

Immunoadsorption with the Prosorba column has been used in the treatment of HIV (human immunodeficiency virus)-associated ITP (47), non-HIV-associated ITP (48), CCATTP/HUS (44), refractory TTP (49), and malignant disease failing conventional chemotherapy (50). If the mechanism of action of the column is similar to that of IVIG, this treatment could be used in a variety of autoimmune diseases, including myasthenia gravis, acute Guillain-Barré syndrome, systemic lupus erythematosus, hemophilia with inhibitors, autoimmune cytopenias other than ITP, rheumatoid arthritis, allograft rejection, paraneoplastic syndromes with central nervous system (CNS) manifestations, paraproteinemic polyneuropathies, and others. The last two conditions have been included as potential indications for Prosorba column treatment in the third Consensus Statement of the American Society for Apheresis (Table 47.1), and rheumatoid arthritis is currently the most common indication for the use of the Prosorba column in the United States.

Rheumatoid Arthritis

Felson et al. conducted a randomized, double-blind, sham-controlled trial to assess the efficacy and safety of the Prosorba column for the treatment of patients with active rheumatoid arthritis that is refractory to conventional therapy. Ninety-one patients who had failed to respond to methotrexate or at least two other second-line drugs were enrolled in this study. Forty-seven subjects were randomized to receive 12 weekly Prosorba on-line treatments, and 44 patients were randomized to receive 12 weekly sham apheresis procedures. The efficacy of the treatment was evaluated 7 to 8 weeks after treatment ended.

Included patients had had rheumatoid arthritis for an average of 15.5 years (range, 1.7 to 50.6), and they had failed to respond to an average of 4.2 second-line drug therapies prior to entry into the study. Patients also had high tender-joint counts and high swollen-joint counts. Fifteen of 47 (31.9%) patients treated with the Prosorba column, compared with 5 of 44 (11.4%) subjects receiving sham apheresis, experienced improvement ($P = 0.019$). The number of respondents in the Prosorba arm increased from five at 5 weeks of treatment, to seven at week 9, to 13 at week 13, to 14 at week 16, and to 15 at weeks 19 and 20. Among patients receiving sham apheresis, the number of responders ranged from four to six over the 20 weeks of the study period.

Tender- and swollen-joint counts were used to assess response to treatment. At 20 weeks, the tender-joint count was 62% of baseline in patients treated with immunoadsorption, compared with 85% in control subjects; the swollen-joint count was, respectively, 74% or 93%. Other outcome measures included a physician's global assessment, the patient's own global assessment, the patient's pain score, the level of C-reactive protein, and a score obtained from a Health Assessment Questionnaire.

The benefit from the use of the Prosorba column persisted (P = 0.03) after the authors adjusted statistically for baseline differences between the treatment and control arms in disease duration, physician global assessment score, and Health Assessment Questionnaire score.

Side effects of treatment were common, but their frequency did not differ between the treatment and control arms. For example, 78% and 88% of patients from the control and treatment arms, respectively, reported joint pain as a side effect of treatment. Felson et al. concluded that the Prosorba column is an efficacious treatment for patients with refractory rheumatoid arthritis but could not explain the mechanism of action of this treatment (51).

Idiopathic Thrombocytopenic Purpura

The Prosorba column is presently considered to be appropriate adjunctive therapy for patients with chronic ITP who are refractory to steroids and splenectomy (52). In the case series of Snyder et al., immunoadsorption produced a response, in terms of an increased platelet count, in 33 of 72 (46%) refractory ITP patients who had failed at least two other treatments (including steroids and splenectomy) (48). Seven of these 33 responders experienced only a transient increase in platelet count for a period of less than 1 month. The majority of the responding patients (79%) did not experience a relapse of thrombocytopenia over a mean follow-up period of 8 months. However, 29 of 72 patients continued receiving other ITP treatments during the trial of the Prosorba column. Also, there was no control group of untreated patients with chronic ITP, making it difficult to conclude that the observed improvements could be attributed specifically to treatment with the Prosorba column.

Platelet Alloimmunization and Refractoriness

Christie et al. reported on ten thrombocytopenic patients who received Prosorba treatment to overcome refractoriness to random-donor platelet transfusions. Nine of these subjects were also refractory to HLA-matched platelets, and nine had been previously treated with steroids, IVIG, with or without other forms of immunosuppressive therapy. Antibodies to HLA class I antigens, ABO antigens, or platelet-specific antigens could be demonstrated in the serum of eight of ten patients. Included subjects received from 1 to 14 off-line or on-line treatments, and six of ten patients responded to therapy (53). Two other teams reported similar results, suggesting that there are some platelet-refractory patients who respond to immunoadsorption with improvement in the corrected count increment following transfusion of non-HLA-matched platelets (54,55). However, one group that reported on three refractory patients concluded that immunoadsorption is not beneficial in this situation (56).

Paraneoplastic Syndromes with CNS Manifestations

Paraneoplastic syndromes with CNS manifestations affect approximately 1% of cancer patients. These syndromes include paraneoplastic cerebellar degeneration (PCD) associated with anti-Yo (anti-Purkinje cell) antibodies; paraneoplastic encephalomyelitis (PEM) associated with anti-Hu (antineuronal nuclear) antibodies; paraneoplastic opsoclonus-myoclonus (POM) associated with anti-Ri (antineuronal nuclear 2) antibodies; paraneoplastic stiff-man syndrome associated with antiamphiphysin antibodies; and cancer-associated retinopathy associated with antirecoverin antibodies (57). Cher et al. treated six patients with such paraneoplastic syndromes with the Prosorba column. Three patients with POM, treated six times over a 2-week period, experienced complete remission of their CNS signs and symptoms. One patient with PEM received 14 treatments over 7 weeks with substantial improvement. Another patient with PEM received four treatments and had only a partial, transient response. One patient with PCD did not respond, but this patient did not complete the Prosorba column treatment because he developed cutaneous vasculitis after the second procedure (58).

Paraproteinemic Polyneuropathies

Immunoadsorption has been used to treat demyelinating polyneuropathy with IgG/IgA as well as polyneuropathy with IgM (with or without Waldenström's). Responses to therapy have been reported from uncontrolled case series (59–61), and it appears that treatment with the Prosorba column may be helpful in predominantly sensory demyelinating polyneuropathies associated with M components of all major immunoglobulin classes.

Cancer Chemotherapy-associated TTP/HUS

Cancer chemotherapy-associated TTP/HUS is a syndrome that mimics classic TTP/HUS, but it probably has an immunologic origin. It occurs in 2% to 10% of patients with cancer and a history of mitomycin C, bleomycin, or cisplatin therapy. The syndrome arises most frequently 2 to 9 months after cessation of chemotherapy and even when the tumor—usually an adenocarcinoma—is in remission. Immunosuppressive drugs with or without plasmapheresis are ineffective in CCATTP/HUS, and immunoadsorption with the Prosorba column possibly offers a critical therapeutic option for these patients who would otherwise have an abysmal prognosis.

Synder et al. reported on 55 patients with CCATTP/HUS who were treated with the Prosorba column. Twenty-five (45%) of these 55 patients achieved a clinical response, according to criteria specified by the authors. Most responses to treatment were evident by the time six treatments had been administered (i.e., within 2 to 3 weeks). All responses were evident by the time 12 procedures had been performed. Of the included patients, 14 had a tumor that was in remission, whereas 35 subjects had stable or progressing tumors. Patients who entered the study with their tumor in remission experienced a survival benefit from the treatment, whereas patients with stable or progressing tumors did not (44). No series corroborating these findings has been reported, in part because of the rarity of CCATTP/HUS.

Malignant Disease Failing Conventional Chemotherapy

Messerschmidt et al. reported on 142 patients treated with immunoadsorption for malignant disease unresponsive to conventional chemotherapy. These subjects received a total of 12 treatments, usually administered three times a week. Patients with stable or regressing disease were permitted to continue treatment beyond the twelfth procedure. Partial remission (PR) was defined as a 50% decrease in the size of the tumor, providing that no new lesions had appeared. A less-than-PR was defined as a greater than 25%, but less than 50%, decrease in tumor size. Twenty-two of 101 (21.8%) evaluable subjects exhibited a PR or a less-than-PR in response to treatment. Subjects with breast adenocarcinoma or Kaposi's sarcoma responded best to this therapy. Patients who received on-line (compared with off-line) therapy had better responses, and the difference between the two treatment modes was statistically significant (50). However, based on the available data, immunoadsorption may be offered to patients with advanced cancer only as experimental treatment. Despite a favorable response in 20% to 25% of subjects, the findings cited here remain controversial, because controls were not included in the study of Messerschmidt et al. and the duration of the observed responses was brief. Moreover, occasional patients experienced severe reactions to the Prosorba column treatment, as discussed in the next section.

TOXICITY OF THE STAPHYLOCOCCAL PROTEIN A COLUMNS

Early human trials of staphylococcal protein A in the treatment of malignant disease reported frequent and severe reactions to the procedure (62). These reactions included severe cardiovascular and respiratory toxicity, as well as severe neutropenia and thrombocytopenia; two deaths from respiratory failure were attributed to the procedure. However, the more recent evaluation of the Prosorba column in patients with ITP (47,48), CCATTP/HUS (44), and malignant disease failing conventional chemotherapy (50) uncovered a much lower frequency and severity of complications than had been reported previously (62). The reasons for the sharp contrast between the early and the more recent experience are not well understood but may be related to the purity of the currently available protein A preparations.

Huestis and Morrison presented a comprehensive review of the adverse effects of immunoadsorption with protein A columns (63). These authors separated the reactions caused by the withdrawal of blood and the apheresis circuit (e.g., vasovagal reactions and citrate toxicity, respectively) from the side effects that can be ascribed directly to the perfusion of plasma through the column. They concluded that protein A immunoadsorption is associated with a significant incidence of adverse effects, and that most patients undergoing a series of treatments will experience one or more untoward effects, although most procedures will be completed without an adverse reaction.

Huestis and Morrison also noted the lower frequency of reactions reported with the protein A–agarose column than with the Prosorba column. They emphasized that reported reaction rates cannot be directly compared, because the two protein A preparations have been used in different clinical settings and in different countries, employing different reporting criteria for recording adverse effects. The nature of the reactions associated with each type of column has also differed, and there have been differences in the complications attributed to the Prosorba column when patients with ITP versus CCATTP/HUS versus cancer were treated.

Among 444 patients undergoing 3,253 treatments with the Prosorba column, 34% of the procedures were complicated by a reaction and 70% of the patients experienced a complication. The most frequent side effects were fever and chills (8.5% of procedures), nausea and vomiting (7.0%), pain (6.0%), hypotension (4.5%), dyspnea (4.0%), allergic manifestations (4.0%), headache (2.5%), hypertension (2.0%), and tachycardia (2.0%). Among 134 and 54 patients, respectively, undergoing 891 and 300 treatments with the protein A–agarose column in Europe and the United States, 26% and 30% of the procedures were complicated by a reaction, and 60% and 37% of the patients experienced a complication. Pain was the most frequently reported side effect in Europe (9.5%), while nausea and vomiting (8.5%) and hypotension (8.5%) were the most frequently reported adverse reactions in the United States (63). The most frequent side effects (fever, chills, nausea, pain, and perhaps also dyspnea) are probably the result of complement activation. Enterotoxin contamination of the staphylococcal protein A and leaching of protein A may also contribute to the observed side effects.

A fatal pulmonary reaction attributed to the Prosorba column occurred in a patient with pure red blood cell aplasia. The patient was severely anemic and had refused red blood cell transfusion due to religious convictions. He received four on-line daily perfusions and reacted during the first procedure with rigors and bronchospasm. For procedures 2, 3, and 4 the patient was heavily premedicated. However, 40 minutes after the fourth procedure was completed the patient developed dyspnea and bronchospasm, which progressed to full respiratory arrest and death (64).

Despite the possibility of such serious reactions to the procedure, however, most reactions to the Prosorba column can be regarded as mild or moderate, and immunoadsorption using protein A columns can be performed on an outpatient basis. Similar to TPE and all other procedures entailing extracorporeal manipulation of blood, protein A immunoadsorption is contraindicated in patients who are currently receiving angiotensin-converting enzyme (ACE) inhibitor medications. The Prosorba manufacturer's instructions recommend that such medications be withheld for at least 72 hours prior to the administration of a protein A immunoadsorption treatment.

SELECTIVE EXTRACTION OF LOW-DENSITY LIPOPROTEINS

Familial hypercholesterolemia (FH) is a dominantly inherited disorder that causes accelerated atherosclerosis, predisposing to premature death from coronary heart disease (CHD). Homozygotes occur with a frequency of one per million population. They are usually unresponsive to diet and drugs and require other treatments to reduce LDL concentrations. These include portocaval shunt, liver transplantation, and long-term TPE. Therapeutic plasma exchange slows the rate of progression of aortic and coronary atherosclerosis, but—in addition to LDL—it removes high-density lipoproteins (HDL) that reduce the risk of developing atherosclerosis. Various approaches have been used to selectively remove LDL from the plasma of patients with homozygous FH. These approaches are collectively referred to as "LDL apheresis" and include a) secondary filtration (65), b) heparin-induced extracorporeal LDL precipitation (HELP) (66), c) dextran sulfate adsorption (67), and d) immunoadsorption (68). Low-density lipoprotein apheresis is both appropriate and life-saving therapy for patients with homozygous FH. In these patients, LDL apheresis should be initiated at as early an age as technically feasible (although generally not before the age of 15) (69).

Patients with heterozygous FH occur with a frequency of 1 per 500 population. LDL apheresis is used infrequently in these patients. Among FH heterozygotes, LDL apheresis is generally reserved for patients who are refractory to LDL-lowering drugs. The Liposorber LA-15 system (Kaneka Pharma America Corp., New York, NY) and the HELP-LDL Apheresis system (Braun-Melsungen, Melsungen, FRG) received FDA approval for use in the following patients: a) functional hypercholesterolemic homozygotes with LDL cholesterol exceeding 500 mg/dl, b) functional hypercholesterolemic heterozygotes with LDL cholesterol exceeding 300 mg/dl, and c) functional hypercholesterolemic heterozygotes with LDL cholesterol exceeding 200 mg/dl and documented CHD (Table 47.3).

The dextran sulfate–cellulose column (Liposorber LA-15) was evaluated by Mabuchi et al. who compared the efficacy of two aggressive LDL-lowering strategies between 87 patients receiving LDL-lowering drugs and 43 patients receiving LDL apheresis along with LDL-lowering drugs. Total serum cholesterol, serum LDL cholesterol, and clinical outcomes were compared after approximately 6 years of therapy. LDL-lowering drugs reduced LDL cholesterol levels by 28%, and LDL apheresis combined with drugs reduced LDL cholesterol levels by 58%. Moreover, the rate of coronary events (including nonfatal myocardial infarction, percutaneous transluminal coronary angioplasty, coronary artery bypass grafting, and death from CHD) was 72% lower in the LDL-apheresis group, compared with the drug therapy group (10% versus 36%, respectively; P = 0.0088). Patients included in this study had CHD secondary to heterozygous FH, and the authors concluded that LDL apheresis is an effective treatment for CHD in FH heterozygotes (70).

Low-density lipoprotein apheresis has also been used in cardiac transplant-associated CHD, because accelerated CHD is seen frequently in cardiac transplant recipients. Furthermore, subjects with steroid-resistant nephrotic syndrome have been treated with LDL apheresis, because hyperlipidemia in these patients is sometimes associated with the progression of glomerulosclerosis.

TABLE 47.3. CHARACTERISTICS AND TREATMENT OF HOMOZYGOUS AND HETEROZYGOUS FAMILIAL HYPERCHOLESTEROLEMIA

	Homozygous Disease	Heterozygous Disease
Usual total cholesterol level	≥600 mg/dl (15.5 mmol/l)	≥300 mg/dl (7.6 mmol/l)
Usual LDL cholesterol level	≥500 mg/dl (14.2 mmol/l)	≥250 mg/dl (6.5 mmol/l)
Onset of atherosclerosis	In adolescence	Between the ages of 30 and 50
Indication(s) for LDL apheresis	LDL cholesterol ≥500 mg/dl (12.9 mmol/l)[a]	LDL cholesterol ≥300 mg/dl[a] (7.6 mmol/l), or LDL cholesterol ≥200 mg/dl[a] (5.2 mmol/l), along with: Documented coronary heart disease, and Failure of treatment with diet and LDL lowering drugs

LDL, low-density lipoprotein.
[a]Following at least a 6-month trial of the American Heart Association Step II diet, along with maximally tolerated combination therapy with LDL-lowering drugs.

Low-density Lipoprotein Apheresis Systems

The Liposorber LA-15 system uses dextran sulfate as the ligand and cellulose as the carrier to selectively extract LDL cholesterol from plasma. In this system, plasma is initially separated from the cellular components of blood by filtration, and the separated plasma is perfused over adsorption columns. The system has two columns connected in parallel, each capable of binding 7.1 g of LDL. One column is perfused with 500 ml of plasma, and then the plasma is diverted to the second column, allowing for the desorption of the first column to its original adsorption capacity. The two columns thus alternate in a manner similar to that described for the protein A–agarose system.

In the HELP system, plasma is also separated from the cellular components by a plasma filter. Heparin in an acidic acetate solution is added to cell-free plasma to precipitate LDL, and the precipitate is removed by filtration. Excess heparin and acetate solution are then removed from the filtered plasma by heparin adsorption and bicarbonate dialysis. Treated plasma is finally recombined with the cellular components of blood and returned to the patient. This system takes advantage of heparin's ability to precipitate LDL at acidic pH by forming complexes with apolipoprotein B complexes.

Comparisons of the four available systems for the selective extraction of LDL (68–71) have shown similar reductions in LDL cholesterol with all systems (71). Table 47.4 shows the efficacy of the immunoadsorption system used in the study of Stoffel et al. (72) in extracting LDL and cholesterol from plasma. Only the dextran sulfate adsorption and HELP systems, however, are currently FDA approved for use in the United States. Both of these systems require heparinization to prevent blood coagulation within the extracorporeal circuit. Patients in whom adequate anticoagulation cannot be achieved safely, as well as patients with known hypersensitivity to heparin or ethylene oxide (which is present in the dextran sulfate columns), cannot undergo LDL apheresis with these systems and, as already discussed, it is prudent to withhold ACE medications prior to any procedure that entails extracorporeal manipulation of blood.

TABLE 47.4. EFFICACY OF IMMUNOADSORPTION IN REDUCING CHOLESTEROL LEVELS IN A PATIENT WITH FAMILIAL HYPERCHOLESTEROLEMIA

Total Plasma Cholesterol (mg/dl)				Lipids Removed From Circulation[a]		
Before Treatment	After Treatment	Between Treatments	Interval Between Treatments (weeks)	LDL (g)	Total Cholesterol (g)	Total Cholesterol (%)
448	171	—	—	11	5.3	62
—	—	228	0.5	—	—	—
285	88	—	—	8	3.9	69
—	—	183	2	—	—	—
278	103	—	—	10	4.9	63
—	—	150	0.5	—	—	—
196	53	—	—	6	3.0	74

LDL, low-density lipoprotein.
[a]Lipids recovered from the immunoadsorption columns used in this LDL apheresis system.
From Stoffel W, Borberg H, Greve V. Application of specific extracorporeal removal of low density lipoprotein in familial hypercholesterolemia. *Lancet* 1981;2:1005–1007, with permission.

Low-density lipoprotein apheresis procedures are generally well tolerated. Four percent (142 of 3,902) of the LDL apheresis procedures performed by Mabuchi et al. were associated with adverse reactions. Hypotension was the most common adverse event, occurring in 0.9% of procedures. Other adverse events included nausea and vomiting (0.7%), flushing (0.5%), chest pain (0.3%), fainting (0.2%), and lightheadedness (0.2%) (70). Plasma volumes of 2 to 5 liters are processed in LDL apheresis procedures. Procedures are usually performed every other week, because studies have demonstrated equivalent results with weekly versus biweekly therapy (73).

SELECTIVE REMOVAL OF BILE ACIDS

Approximately 20% of patients with cholestasis may suffer from severe pruritus that is refractory to conventional modes of treatment (i.e., surgery and medications such as phenobarbital, cholestyramine, or activated charcoal capsules). This symptom may be caused by accumulation in the skin of either bile acids or some other pruritogenic agent that possibly travels in the company of bile acids. Plasma perfusion through charcoal-coated glass beads has been used for the treatment of intractable pruritus in cholestatic patients who are refractory to other modes of treatment, based on the affinity of *U.S. Pharmacopeia* charcoal for bile acids. Pineda et al. treated 34 patients with severe cholestasis and intractable pruritus with plasma perfusion, and 29 (85%) of these patients reported subjective benefit from the treatment (74).

CONCLUSION

Therapeutic leukapheresis, therapeutic plateletpheresis, or therapeutic erythropheresis is standard treatment for patients with AML and a hyperleukocytosis syndrome, chronic myeloproliferative disease and thrombocytosis, or sickle cell disease and a severe infarctive crisis, respectively. Similarly, photopheresis is standard treatment for patients with cutaneous T-cell lymphoma; and LDL apheresis is standard treatment for patients with homozygous FH, as well as selected patients with heterozygous FH. Immunoadsorption with the protein A–silica (Prosorba) column is an important adjunctive therapy for patients with moderate to severe rheumatoid arthritis, as well as some other conditions for which the mechanism of action of this treatment is poorly understood (Table 47.1).

Immunoadsorption with the protein A–agarose column shows great promise for the future, and it is unfortunate that no controlled studies of this therapeutic modality have been reported. For diseases whose pathogenesis is well established, selective extraction of plasma constituents (by such means as immunoadsorption with the protein A–agarose column) is preferable to the wholesale removal of plasma proteins that takes place with therapeutic plasmapheresis. For example, columns that selectively remove IgG (or, better yet, specifically extract glomerular basement membrane or acetylcholine receptor antibodies) could be used in lieu of plasmapheresis in patients with GPS or myasthenia gravis in the future, provided that their superiority is demonstrated by randomized controlled trials.

Selective extraction of plasma constituents cannot be expected, however, to replace plasmapheresis in the majority of diseases for which plasmapheresis is currently used. Such a change could occur only if knowledge of the pathophysiology of each disease advanced to a point that would permit the targeting of a specific injurious agent for removal. Until that happens, wholesale removal of plasma proteins, which include various mediators of inflammation (e.g., cytokines, complement components, kinins, and others), will likely be preferred to selective extraction. Even in diseases for which the therapeutic benefit from plasmapheresis is well established (e.g., in CIDP), the specific injurious agent that is targeted for removal remains unknown. Thus, the development of new materials for selective extraction of plasma constituents (e.g., for the specific removal of antibodies to peripheral nerve myelin in patients with CIDP) may contribute to a better understanding of disease pathogenesis. Clinical success of a column designed to selectively extract antibodies to peripheral nerve myelin may establish the importance of these antibodies in the causation of CIDP (2,25,26).

Various selective extraction systems developed in other countries are not commercially available or in clinical use in the United States. In addition to the protein A–agarose column discussed in this chapter, these include cryofiltration, columns for the removal of anti-B isoagglutinins or DNA antibodies, and columns using amino acids such as tryptophan as ligands. In all likelihood, the next several years will see a wider application of existing technologies for selective extraction of plasma constituents, possibly with an increasing variety of sorbents and carriers. The manufacture of new monoclonal antibodies and the recombinant synthesis of biomaterials may create new opportunities to selectively extract undesirable elements from human plasma and to provide specific treatment for diseases with established pathogenesis.

REFERENCES

1. Winters JL, Pineda AA. Hemapheresis. In: Henry JB, ed. *Clinical diagnosis and management by laboratory methods,* 20th ed. Philadelphia: WB Saunders, 2001.
2. Vamvakas EC, Pineda AA. Selective extraction of plasma constituents. In: McLeod BC, Price TH, Drew MJ, eds. *Apheresis: principles and practice.* Bethesda, MD: American Association of Blood Banks, 1997: 375–407.
3. Porcu P, Danielson CF, Orazi A, et al. Therapeutic leukapheresis in hyperleukocytic leukemias: Lack of correlation between degree of cytoreduction and early mortality rate. *Br J Haematol* 1997; 98:433–436.
4. Burgstaler EA, Pineda AA. Therapeutic cytapheresis: continuous flow versus intermittent flow apheresis systems. *J Clin Apheresis* 1994;9: 205–209.
5. Schafer AI. Management of thrombocythemia. *Curr Opin Hematol* 1996;3:341–346.
6. Baron BW, Mick R, Baron JM. Combined plateletpheresis and cytotoxic chemotherapy for symptomatic thrombocytosis in myeloproliferative disorders. *Cancer* 1993;72:1209–1218.
7. Lercari G, Paganinin G, Malfanti L, et al. Apheresis for severe malaria complicated by cerebral malaria, acute respiratory distress syndrome, acute renal failure, and disseminated intravascular coagulation. *J Clin Apheresis* 1991;7:93–96.
8. Wayne AS, Kevy SV, Nathan DG. Transfusion management of sickle cell disease. *Blood* 1993; 81:1109–1123.
9. Siegel JF, Rich MA, Brock WA. Association of sickle cell disease, priapism, exchange transfusion, and neurologic events: ASPEN syndrome. *J Urol* 1993; 150:1480–1482.
10. Pepkowitz S. Red cell exchange and other therapeutic alterations of red cell mass. In: McLeod BC, Price TH, Drew MT, eds. *Apheresis: principles and practice.* Bethesda, MD: American Association of Blood Banks, 1997:355–374.
11. van Iperen HP, Beijersbergen van Henegouwen GM. Clinical and mechanistic aspects of photopheresis. *J Photochem Photobiol B* 1997; 39:99–109.
12. Christensen I, Heald P. Photopheresis in the 1990s. *J Clin Apheresis* 1991;6:216–220.
13. Stevens SR, Bowen GM, Duvic M, et al. Effectiveness of photopheresis in Sézary syndrome. *Arch Dermatol* 1999;135:995–997.
14. Edelson RL, Berger C, Gasparro F, et al. Treatment of cutaneous T-cell lymphoma by extracorporeal photochemotherapy. *N Engl J Med* 1987;316:297–303.
15. Heald P, Rook A, Perez M, et al. Treatment of erythrodermic cutaneous T-cell lymphoma with extracorporeal photochemotherapy. *J Am Acad Dermatol* 1992;27:427–433.
16. Zic JA, Miller JL, Stricklin JP, et al. The North American experience with photopheresis. *Ther Apher* 1999;3:50–62.
17. Sniecinski I. Photopheresis. In: McLeod BC, Price TH, Drew MJ, eds. *Apheresis: principles and practice.* Bethesda, MD: American Association of Blood Banks, 1997:521–535.
18. Meiser BM, Kur F, Reichensparner H, et al. Reduction of the incidence of rejection by adjunct immunosuppression with photochemotherapy after heart transplantation. *Transplantation* 1994;57:563–564.
19. Barr ML, Meiser BM, Eisen HJ, et al. Photopheresis for the prevention of rejection in cardiac transplantation. *N Engl J Med* 1998;339: 1744–1751.
20. Lloveras JJ, Escourrou G, Delisle MB, et al. Evolution of untreated mild rejection in heart transplant recipients. *J Heart Lung Transplant* 1992;1:751–756.
21. Greinix HT, Volc-Platzer B, Kalhs P, et al. Extracorporeal photochemotherapy in the treatment of severe steroid-refractory acute graft-versus-host disease: a pilot study. *Blood* 2000; 96:2426–2431.
22. Rook AH, Freundlich B, Jegasorthy BV, et al. Treatment of systemic sclerosis with extracorporeal photochemotherapy. Results of a multicenter trial. *Arch Dermatol* 1992;128:337–346.
23. Zachariae H, Bjerring P, Heickendorff L, et al. Photopheresis and systemic sclerosis. *Arch Dermatol* 1992;128:1651–1653.
24. Fries JF, Seibold JR, Medsger TA. Photopheresis for scleroderma? No! *J Rheumatol* 1992;19:1011–1013.
25. Pineda AA. *Selective plasma component removal.* Mount Kisco, NY: Futura Publishing, 1984.
26. Pineda AA. Immunoaffinity apheresis columns: clinical applications and therapeutic mechanisms of action. In: Sacher RA, Brubaker DB, Kaspisin DO, et al., eds. *Cellular and humoral immunotherapy and apheresis.* Arlington, VA: American Association of Blood Banks, 1991: 31–45.
27. Gjörstrup P, Watt RM. Therapeutic protein A immunoadsorption: a review. *Transfus Sci* 1990;11:281–302.
28. Hiesse C, Kriaa F, Rousseau P, et al. Immunoadsorption of anti-HLA antibodies for highly sensitized patients awaiting renal transplantation. *Nephrol Dial Transplant* 1992;7:944–951.
29. Ross CN, Gaskin G, Gregor-MacGregor S, et al. Renal transplantation following immunoadsorption in highly sensitized patients. *Transplantation* 1993;55:785–789.
30. Higgins RM, Bevan DJ, Vaughan RW, et al. Five-year follow-up of patients successfully transplanted after immunoadsorption to remove anti-HLA antibodies. *Nephron* 1996;74:53–57.
31. Mastrangelo F, Pretagostini R, Berloco P, et al. Immunoadsorption with protein A in humoral acute rejection of kidney transplants: multicenter experience. *Transplant Proc* 1995;27:892–895.
32. Persson NH, Bucin D, Ekberg H, et al. Immunoadsorption in acute vascular rejection after renal transplantation. *Transplant Proc* 1995;27: 3466.
33. Pretagostini R, Berloco P, Poli L, et al. Immunoadsorption with protein A in humoral rejection of kidney transplants. *ASAIO J* 1996;42: M645–648.
34. Palmer A, Cairns T, Gluck G, et al. Treatment of rapidly progressive glomerulonephritis by extracorporeal immunoadsorption, prednisolone and cyclophosphamide. *Nephrol Dial Transplant* 1991;6: 536–542.
35. Esnault VLM, Testa A, Jayne DRW, et al. Influence of immunoadsorption on the removal of immunoglobulin G autoantibodies in crescentic glomerulonephritis. *Nephron* 1993;65:180–184.
36. Negrier C, Dechavanne M, Alfonsi F, et al. Successful treatment of acquired factor VIII antibody by extracorporeal immunoadsorption. *Acta Haematol* 1991;85:107–110.
37. Gjörstrup P, Berntorp E, Larsson L, et al. Kinetic aspects of the removal of IgG and inhibitors in hemophiliacs using protein A immunoadsorption. *Vox Sang* 1991;61:244–250.
38. Uehlinger J, Rose E, Aledort LM, et al. Successful treatment of an acquired von Willebrand factor antibody by extracorporeal immunoadsorption. *N Engl J Med* 1989;320:254–255.
39. Benny WB, Sutton DM, Oger J, et al. Clinical evaluation of a staphylococcal protein A immunoadsorption system treatment of myasthenia gravis patients. *Transfusion* 1999;39:682–687.

40. Jones FR, Balint JP, Snyder HW Jr. Selective extracorporeal removal of immunoglobulin G and circulating immune complexes: a review. *Plasma Ther Transfus Technol* 1986;7:333–349.
41. Snyder HW Jr, Balint JP, Jones FR. Modulation of immunity in patients with autoimmune disease and cancer treated by extracorporeal immunoadsorption with PROSORBA column. *Semin Hematol* 1989; 26[Suppl. 1]:31–41.
42. Snyder HW Jr, Seawell BW, Cochran SK, et al. Specificity of antibody responses affected by extracorporeal immunoadsorption of plasma over columns of protein A silica. *J Clin Apheresis* 1992;7:110–118.
43. Singhal AK, Singhal MC, Nudelmen E, et al. Presence of fucolipid antigens with mono and dimeric X determinant (Le^x) in the circulating immune complexes of patients with adenocarcinoma. *Cancer Res* 1987; 47:5566–5571.
44. Snyder HW, Mittleman A, Oral A, et al. Treatment of cancer chemotherapy-associated thrombotic thrombocytopenic purpura/hemolytic-uremic syndrome by protein A immunoadsorption of plasma. *Cancer* 1993;71:1882–1892.
45. Langone JJ, Boyle MDP, Borsos T. Studies on the interaction between protein A and immunoglobulin G. II. Composition and activity of complexes formed between protein A and IgG. *J Immunol* 1978;121: 333–338.
46. Bertram JH, Hengst JCD, Mitchell MS. Staphylococcal protein A immunoadsorptive column induces mitogenicity in perfused plasma. *J Biol Response Mod* 1984;3:235–240.
47. Snyder HW Jr, Bertram JH, Henry DH, et al. Use of protein A immunoadsorption as a treatment for thrombocytopenia in HIV-infected homosexual men: a retrospective evaluation of 37 cases. *AIDS* 1991; 5:1257–1260.
48. Snyder HW Jr, Cochran SK, Balint JP, et al. Experience with protein A-immunoadsorption in treatment-resistant adult immune thrombocytopenic purpura. *Blood* 1992;79:2237–2245.
49. Drew MJ. Resolution of refractory, classic thrombotic thrombocytopenic purpura after staphylococcal protein A immunoadsorption. *Transfusion* 1994;34:536–538.
50. Messerschmidt GL, Henry DH, Snyder HW Jr, et al. Protein A immunoadsorption in the treatment of malignant disease. *J Clin Oncol* 1988; 6:203–212.
51. Felson DT, LaValley MP, Baldassare AR, et al. The Prosorba column for treatment of refractory rheumatoid arthritis: A randomized, double-blind, sham-controlled trial. *Arthritis Rheum* 1999;42:2153–2159.
52. George JN, Woolf SH, Raskob GE, et al. Idiopathic thrombocytopenic purpura: a practice guideline developed by explicit methods for the American Society of Hematology. *Blood* 1996;88:3–40.
53. Christie DJ, Howe RB, Lennon SS, et al. Treatment of refractoriness to platelet transfusion by protein A column therapy. *Transfusion* 1993; 33:234–242.
54. Kim HC, Dugan NP, Snyder HW, et al. Protein A immunoadsorption treatment in children with refractoriness to platelet transfusion. *Blood* 1992;80:222a(abst).
55. Hussein MA, Long T, Bolwell B, et al. Response to Prosorba A column in alloimmunized platelet refractory patients. *Transfusion* 1994;34: 66S(abst).
56. Lopez-Plaza I, Miller K, Leitman SF. Ineffectiveness of protein A adsorption in the treatment of platelet refractoriness. *J Clin Apheresis* 1992;7:33(abst).
57. Weinstein R. Therapeutic apheresis in neurological disorders. *J Clin Apheresis* 2000;15:74–128.
58. Cher LM, Hochberg FH, Teruya J, et al. Therapy for paraneoplastic neurologic syndromes in six patient with Protein A column immunoadsorption. *Cancer* 1995;75:1678–1683.
59. Siciliano G, Moriconi L, Gianni G, et al. Selective techniques of apheresis in polyneuropathy associated with monoclonal gammopathy of undetermined significance. *Acta Neurol Scand* 1994;89:117–122.
60. Weinstein R, Sato PTS, Shelton K, et al. Successful management of paraprotein-associated peripheral polyneuropathies by immunoadsorption of plasma with staphylococcal protein A. *J Clin Apheresis* 1993; 8:72–77.
61. Niemierko E, Weinstein R. Response of patients with IgM- and IgA-associated peripheral polyneuropathies to "off line" immunoadsorption treatment using the Prosorba protein A column. *J Clin Apheresis* 1999; 14:159–162.
62. Young JB, Ayus JC, Miller LK, et al. Cardiopulmonary toxicity in patients with breast carcinoma during plasma perfusion over immobilized protein A: pathophysiology of reaction and attenuating methods. *Am J Med* 1983;75:278–288.
63. Huestis DW, Morrison FS. Adverse effects of immune adsorption with staphylococcal protein A columns. *Transfus Med Rev* 1996;10:62–70.
64. Garey DC, Perry E, Jackson B. Fatal pulmonary reaction with staph protein A immune adsorption for pure red cell aplasia. *Transfusion* 1988;28:245(abst).
65. Leitman SF, Smith JW, Gregg RE. Homozygous familial hypercholesterolemia: selective removal of low-density lipoproteins by secondary membrane filtration. *Transfusion* 1989;29:341–346.
66. Lane DM, McConathy WJ, Laughlin LO, et al. Weekly treatment of diet/drug-resistant hypercholesterolemia with the heparin-induced extracorporeal low-density lipoprotein precipitation (HELP) system by selective plasma low-density lipoprotein removal. *Am J Cardiol* 1993; 71:816–822.
67. Schulzeck P, Olbricht CJ, Koch KM. Long-term experience with extracorporeal low-density lipoprotein cholesterol removal by dextran sulfate cellulose adsorption. *Clin Invest* 1992;70:99–104.
68. Richter WO, Jacob BG, Ritter MM et al. Three-year treatment of familial heterozygous hypercholesterolemia by extracorporeal low-density lipoprotein immunoadsorption with polyclonal apolipoprotein B antibodies. *Metabolism* 1993;42:888–894.
69. Gordon BR, Stein E, Jones P, et al. Indications for low-density lipoprotein apheresis. *Am J Cardiol* 1994;74:1109–1112.
70. Mabuchi H, Koizumi J, Shimizu M, et al. Long-term efficacy of low-density lipoprotein apheresis on coronary heart disease in familial hypercholesterolemia. *Am J Cardiol* 1998;82:1489–1495.
71. Jovin IS, Taborski U, Muller-Berghaus G. Comparing low-density lipoprotein apheresis procedures: difficulties and remedies. *J Clin Apheresis* 1996;11:168–170.
72. Stoffel W, Borberg H, Greve V. Application of specific extracorporeal removal of low density lipoprotein in familial hypercholesterolemia. *Lancet* 1981;2:1005–1007.
73. Lane DM, McConathy WJ, Laughlin LO, et al. Selective removal of plasma low density lipoprotein with the HELP system: biweekly vs weekly therapy. *Atherosclerosis* 1995;114:203–211.
74. Pineda AA, Burgstaler EA, Dickson R, et al. Treatment of intractable pruritus of cholestasis by plasma perfusion through USP charcoal-coated glass beads. In: Atsumi, Kazuhiko, Maekawa, et al., eds. *Progress in artificial organs,* vol 2. Cleveland, OH: ISAO Press, 1984:750–753.

Rossi's Principles of Transfusion Medicine, Third Edition, edited by Toby L. Simon, Walter H. Dzik, Edward L. Snyder, Christopher P. Stowell, and Ronald G. Strauss. Lippincott Williams & Wilkins, Philadelphia © 2002.

CASE 47A

TOO MUCH DUST IN THE BLOOD

CASE HISTORY

A 43-year-old woman was transferred from another hospital for diagnosis and management of the acute onset of quadriplegia and bulbar weakness. She had a complex history of neurologic problems beginning 16 years earlier when she had an episode of lower extremity hypesthesia accompanied by bowel and bladder dysfunction. Results of the evaluation did not suggest multiple sclerosis or Guillain-Barré syndrome, but the symptoms resolved spontaneously. Ten years previously, the patient had had brain stem encephalitis with magnetic resonance imaging evidence of infarction in the pons, midbrain, and diencephalon. At that time, she came to medical attention with headache and fever followed by rapid onset of quadriparesis (right more than left) and bulbar paresis. The patient was treated with steroids and had some improvement but was left with significant right hemiparesis and had to stay in bed or use a wheelchair. Since that time, the medical history included only numerous headaches associated with a visual aura, for which she took ibuprofen.

The patient presented at the admitting hospital with a several-month history of intermittent abdominal pain and several days of malaise, anorexia, and headache, which became much worse on the day of admission and was accompanied by frequent vomiting. Lumbar puncture revealed a white blood cell count of 420/μl (90% polymorphonuclear leukocytes [PMNs]); red blood cell count, 210/μl; protein, 110 mg/dl; and glucose, 57 mg/dl. Magnetic resonance images showed changes consistent with the previous neurologic events. The patient was treated for several days with analgesics and antiemetics for aseptic meningitis. Her condition improved initially, but then over 24 hours quadriparesis and diplopia developed, as did so much difficulty clearing secretions that intubation was necessary. Intravenous steroids were administered, and the patient was transferred to the neurologic intensive care unit at a referred hospital.

At the time she was admitted to the neurologic intensive care unit, the patient had a blood pressure of 135/80 mm Hg; heart rate, 120 beats/min; temperature, 102.7°F (39.3°C); and adequate oxygenation with a ventilator. The neurologic examination showed a lack of spontaneous movement except for the ability to blink and move the eyes on command. The patient had flaccid quadriplegia with posturing in the upper extremities and triple flexion in the legs. There also was extensive bulbar paresis. The laboratory results were a WBC count of 32 × 10^9/L with 91% PMNs; hematocrit, 39.4%; and platelet count, 631 × 10^9/L, which was initially believed to be reactive thrombocytosis associated with an inflammatory or infectious disorder. Magnetic resonance images revealed areas of acute and subacute infarction in the pons, medulla and midbrain most consistent with small-vessel vasculitis or an infectious process producing small vessel ischemia, although thromboembolism was a consideration. Over the next several days, an extensive investigation for vasculitis and infection was performed but did not yield a diagnosis. Two days after admission, brain biopsy was performed and showed no evidence of vasculitis but did reveal multiple foci of parenchymal hemorrhage and an area of acute infarction in the midcortex with intraluminal fibrin thrombi.

Meanwhile, the platelet count continued to climb to 939 × 10^9/L. The hematology and transfusion medicine services were consulted. The clinical impression at this time was essential thrombocythemia complicated by cerebral infarction. Despite initiation of therapy with hydroxyurea, the platelet count increased from 794 × 10^9/L to 1,657 × 10^9/L over the next 3 days. The decision was made to perform therapeutic plateletpheresis in light of the marked increase in platelet count despite hydroxyurea treatment and because of the acute nature of the neurologic changes. A single plateletpheresis procedure was performed that processed close to two blood volumes. The next day the platelet count was 344 × 10^9/L. Thereafter the platelet count decreased to as low as 122 × 10^9/L and was maintained between 300 and 700 × 10^9/L by means of titration with hydroxyurea. There was little change in neurologic status, however, and the patient was discharged to a rehabilitation facility for respirator-dependent patients.

DISCUSSION

This patient had what at first looked like a recurrence of the same type of neurologic insult she had sustained 10 years previously and which had been diagnosed as brain stem encephalitis. The normal results of the evaluation for vasculitis and infection were frustrating until the brain biopsy results and the sudden escalation in platelet count pointed the way to a diagnosis. The diagnosis of essential thrombocythemia is largely one of exclusion. Other causes of secondary thrombocytosis were not evident in this patient, including malignant disease, chronic inflammatory disorders, acute infection, and iron deficiency.

When platelets were first found at microscopic examination, they were considered a form of blood "dust." Patients with essential thrombocythemia often have no symptoms, even with platelet counts exceeding 1,000 × 10^9/L. Thrombotic complications are major causes of morbidity and mortality among these

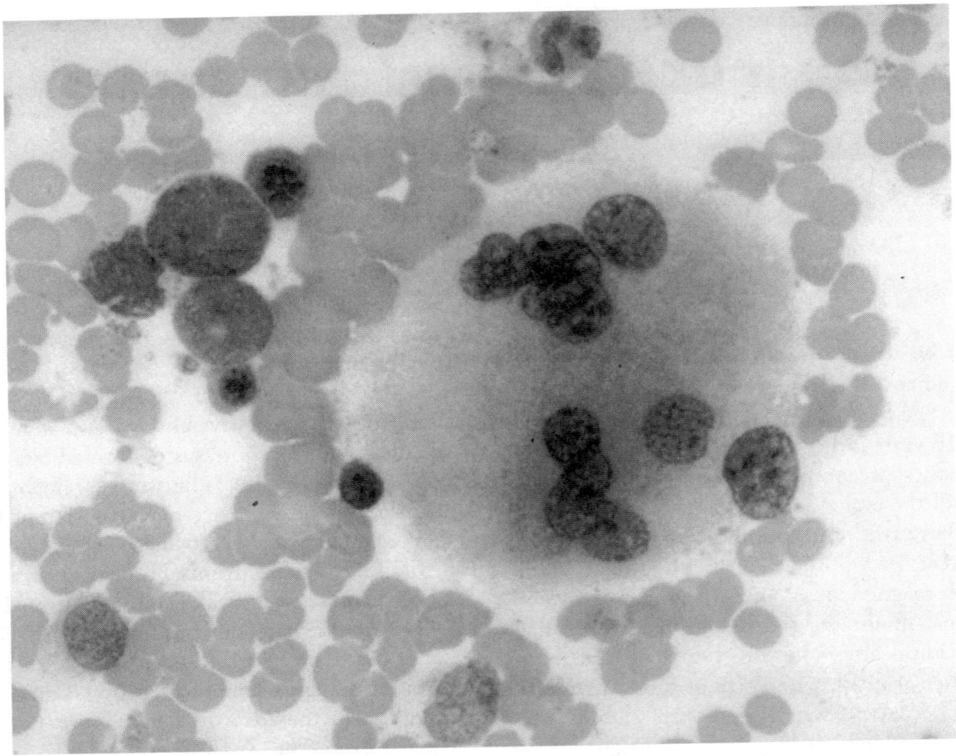

FIGURE 47A.1. Photograph of bone marrow biopsy specimen shows megakaryocyte.

patients; hemorrhagic complications are less common. Bleeding complications, which are attributed to defects in platelet function, can occur independently or in association with thrombosis. Arterial thrombosis is more common than venous thrombosis and occurs in large vessels and in the microvasculature. Patients with essential thrombocythemia are particularly predisposed to cerebrovascular events and digital microvascular ischemia, which produces intense pain in the extremities (erythromelalgia). Central nervous system involvement can manifest as nonspecific symptoms, such as headache, impaired mentation, or migraine-like symptoms, or with focal neurologic signs, including peripheral paresthesia, hemiparesis, and seizures.

The pivotal therapeutic decision in the care of patients with essential thrombocythemia is whether to reduce the platelet count. No data suggest that reduction in the platelet count of patients who do not have symptoms alters the prognosis or even the occurrence of thrombotic events. There is a consensus, however, that cytoreduction in the care of patients with active or recurrent bleeding or thrombosis may relieve symptoms, especially for patients with microvascular digital or cerebrovascular ischemia. Patients with a history of thrombotic events or who are older than 60 years are at risk of additional thrombotic events and need treatment to decrease the platelet count. In this setting, cytoreduction therapy was shown to prevent additional thrombotic events in a randomized clinical trial (1).

Cytoreduction is commonly accomplished with hydroxyurea; alkylating agents have been largely abandoned because of leukemogenic potential. Anagrelide and interferon-alfa also have been used. The use of antiplatelet drugs in the treatment of patients with thrombotic complications is controversial. These agents are contraindicated in the presence of hemorrhage but are useful in the care of patients with digital microvascular ischemia. Plateletpheresis usually is reserved for patients with platelet counts exceeding $1,000 \times 10^9/L$ and serious bleeding or thrombotic complications when rapid cytoreduction is desirable (2). Both the American Society of Apheresis (3) and the American Association of Blood Banks (4) consider this situation a category I indication (standard, acceptable therapy).

CODA

Results of bone marrow biopsy confirmed the clinical impression of essential thrombocythemia. The specimen exhibited moderate hypercellularity with megakaryocytic hyperplasia and clusters of giant megakaryocytes (Fig. 47A.1). The number and maturation of myeloid elements were normal. Iron stores were adequate, and there was no evidence of fibrosis. Mechanical ventilation was successfully discontinued at the rehabilitation center, but the patient recovered little function otherwise and remained quadriplegic. She was transferred to an extended care facility.

Case contributed by Christopher P. Stowell, M.D., Ph.D., Massachusetts General Hospital, Boston, MA.

REFERENCES

1. Cortelazzo S, Finazzi G, Ruggeri M, et al. Hydroxyurea for patients with essential thrombocythemia and a high risk of thrombosis. *N Engl J Med* 1995;332:1132–1136.
2. Baron BW, Mick R, Baron JM. Combined plateletpheresis and cytotoxic chemotherapy for symptomatic thrombocytosis in myeloproliferative disorders. *Cancer* 1993;72:1209–1218.
3. McLeod B. Introduction to the third special issue: clinical applications of therapeutic apheresis. *J Clin Apheresis* 2000;15:1–5.
4. American Association of Blood Banks Hemapheresis Committee. *Guidelines for therapeutic hemapheresis.* Bethesda, MD: American Association of Blood Banks, 1995.

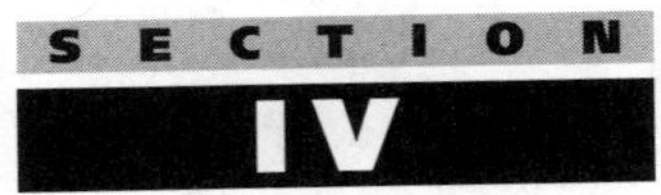

ADVERSE SEQUELAE

PART I
Disease Transmission

48

TRANSFUSION-TRANSMITTED INFECTION RISK FROM BLOOD COMPONENTS AND PLASMA DERIVATIVES

STEVEN KLEINMAN

GENERAL CONSIDERATIONS

Accurate estimates of the risks of transfusion-transmitted infection are important in order to provide an informed basis for patients and physicians to decide on allogeneic transfusion versus

S. Kleinman: Department of Pathology, University of British Columbia, Vancouver, British Columbia, Canada.

other therapeutic options, and to enable policy makers to evaluate the expected benefits and costs of proposed interventions to further reduce such risk. In addition, such estimates may reassure the public about the safety of transfusion, provided that the information can be communicated in a manner that is clearly understood and overcomes fears that have arisen subsequent to the association of blood transfusion with human immunodeficiency virus (HIV) transmission.

Risk estimates have limitations. In addition to yielding a single best estimate of risk (known as the point estimate), these estimates will usually include wide ranges or confidence limits. Unfortunately, confidence intervals often confuse physicians, patients, and the media, all of whom want to quote a single best number; therefore, ranges and confidence limits are usually forgotten, even if they have been initially communicated. Transfusion-transmitted risk estimates obtained in previous years may become obsolete when newer, more sensitive donor screening protocols are adopted, and estimates obtained in particular geographic areas may not be applicable to other locations. However, because the data needed to make risk estimates are difficult to gather, estimates that appear in the literature are often quoted for many years despite their limitations.

Early studies expressed infection risk on a per-recipient basis, making it difficult to compare the risk for patients receiving different numbers of transfused units. More recently, it has become standard practice to express the risk of infection on a per-unit or per–blood component basis when possible; the risk per unit is a given percentage (i.e., 0.001%) or 1 in a given number (i.e., 1 in 100,000). This per-unit risk needs to be adjusted for the number of units (or more precisely, the number of donor exposures) received by a particular patient. In practice, the per-patient risk can be obtained by multiplying the per-unit risk by the number of units transfused. More precisely, the mathematically correct way to determine per-patient risk is as follows: if p represents the probability of infection from a given unit of blood and n represents the number of units transfused, then the probability that a single unit is free of infection is $(1-p)$, the probability that all n units are infection free is $(1-p)^n$, and therefore, the probability that a recipient would get infected would be 1 minus the probability that he would not get infected or $1 - (1-p)^n$. Because transfusion risks are small, this formula simply reduces to $p \times n$.

HISTORIC FRAMEWORK OF RISKS

The transfusion-transmitted risk of three viral agents that cause significant morbidity and mortality are shown in a timeline in Figure 48.1 (1). It is apparent that the risk of transfusion-transmitted hepatitis has diminished steadily since the early 1980s; not shown in the figure are the even higher rates from the 1960s and early 1970s. Transfusion-transmitted HIV infection peaked in the early to mid-1980s (ranging up to 1 per 100 units in San Francisco, the location with the highest incidence) and diminished significantly with the implementation of HIV antibody

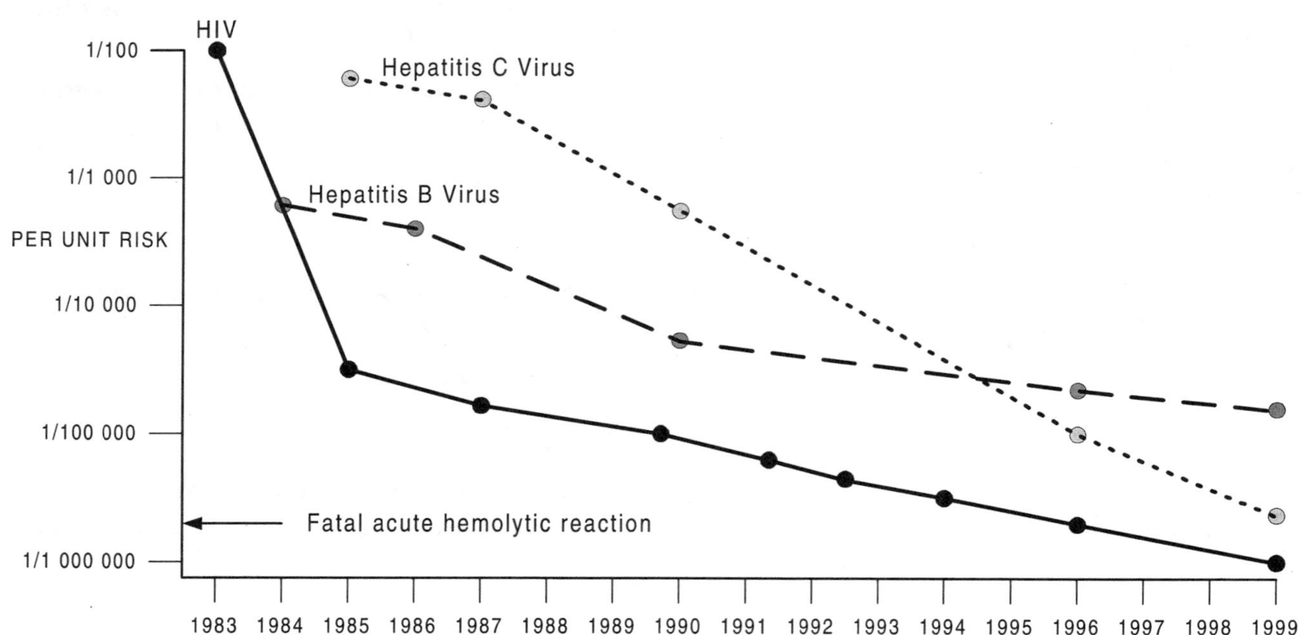

FIGURE 48.1. Declining risk of transfusion-transmitted HIV, HBV, and HCV infection in the United States. Risk is expressed per transfusable unit and plotted on a logarithmic scale. HIV, *solid line;* HBV, *dashed line;* HCV, *dotted line.* Per-unit risk estimates for 2001 are HIV, 1:971,000; HBV, 1:81,000; HCV, 1:813,000. The *arrow* shows an estimate for fatal acute hemolytic reaction for comparison. (From AuBuchon JP, Birkmeyer JD, Busch MP. Safety of the blood supply in the United States: opportunities and controversies. *Ann Intern Med* 1997;127:904–909, with permission.)

testing in 1985. The risk has continued to diminish as new laboratory tests have been added.

The large number of cases of transfusion-transmitted HIV in 1983 through 1985 led to a paradigm shift in the way the public viewed the safety of blood transfusion (2). Prior to the emergence of acquired immunodeficiency syndrome (AIDS), the general public and the medical profession regarded blood transfusion as a life-saving measure, despite the historically high risk of transmitting hepatitis. Transfusion came to be viewed as high risk because of AIDS, with the very real possibility of severe complications or death. In the 1990s, many countries retrospectively undertook inquiries reviewing the policies they had adopted in the 1980s to reduce the risk of transfusion-transmitted AIDS. These investigations contributed to a paradigm shift among national blood safety policy–making and regulatory agencies toward the principle that recipient safety was paramount at any cost. This paradigm has subsequently been applied to decisions concerning other potential transfusion-transmitted agents with low risks or risks that are theoretic but unproved (3,4).

Risk can be termed theoretic when adequate data to quantify risk do not exist. Many transfusion medicine specialists misunderstand the concept of theoretic risk. They assume that theoretic risk is equivalent to a risk that is extremely negligible or only slightly above zero. This assumption is true for agents for which there is a large amount of data documenting lack of transfusion transmission; risk is termed theoretic because despite such data, it is virtually impossible to prove that transfusion transmission can never occur. Examples are classic Creutzfeldt-Jakob disease (CJD) and hepatitis G virus (HGV). However, for other agents with theoretic risk, the data are insufficient for evaluation, and biologic mechanisms for transfusion transmission with resulting disease are plausible. In such cases, if the risk subsequently turns out to prove real, it is possible that the degree of risk may be shown to be high. This was the case when it was first hypothesized that AIDS might be transmitted by transfusion and is currently the case for variant CJD. In summary, theoretic risk should not be equated with zero risk or negligible risk in all circumstances.

RISK-REDUCTION GOALS

In establishing policies for decreasing the risk of infectious disease transmission by blood transfusion, it is important to define the target goal. The three possibilities are: zero risk, minimal risk, and minimal risk at an acceptable cost. Events related to HIV in the mid-1980s resulted in subsequent adoption of a zero-risk goal (2,5). Soon after this goal was adopted, it was postulated that zero risk would not be attainable due to certain theoretic limitations (6). These are:

- In a biologic system (e.g., blood transfusion) it is unlikely that any single method could be 100% effective. Therefore, approaching zero risk would require the use of multiple overlapping methods.
- When multiple methods are used, procedures become administratively more complex and the potential for error increases.
- Successive risk reductions achieve less but cost more.
- If the risk is already low, it will be extremely difficult to measure the effect of adding additional procedures that are designed to provide further safeguards.

Evaluations of blood safety policy interventions in the past decade have shown that these theoretic concerns have proven to be true.

More recently, with the diminished risk of transfusion-transmitted infections, two competing decision-making principles have emerged. Decisions regarding agents other than HIV may attempt to assess the efficacy and cost impact of an intervention prior to its implementation (1). On the other hand, certain decisions have been guided by the precautionary principle, which originated in the environmental protection field in the mid-1970s. This principle has been adapted to blood safety decision making and articulated in the report of the Krever Commission of Inquiry on the Blood System in Canada as follows: "... preventative action should be taken when there is evidence that a potentially disease-causing agent is or may be blood borne, even when there is no evidence that recipients have been affected. If harm can occur, it should be assumed that it will occur" (7). Applications of the precautionary principle in transfusion medicine have been based on the following (4):

- The amount of evidence needed to implement an intervention decreases as the potential adverse outcome of a given threat to safety increases.
- Worst-case scenarios in transfusion recipients have been used to consider the potential benefits of interventions.
- Actions should be taken quickly even when scientific data do not conclusively establish that harm to recipients will occur.
- A partial solution to a particular problem should be introduced as long as it causes no harm.

Although the precautionary principle provides a decision-making framework, problems arise when deciding how to apply the principle in specific situations. A recent set of guidelines urging consistent application of this principle across various decisions with careful evaluation of existing scientific data has been published (8). However, the precautionary principle has not been applied consistently in transfusion medicine; its application has been influenced by subjective and emotional concern from the general public and policy makers with regard to certain infectious agents and not others (9).

RISK-REDUCTION METHODS

Multiple methodologies have been used to reduce the risk of transfusion transmission of infectious agents. More than one method may be employed to reduce the risk of transmission of all infectious agents or of a specific agent. Methods applicable to all agents include (1,6):

- Minimizing unnecessary transfusion (e.g., establishing autologous donation and blood conservation programs and establishing audit criteria and clinical best-practice parameters for blood product transfusion);

- Minimizing exposures to multiple donors (e.g., using apheresis platelets rather than whole blood–derived platelets, collecting multiple directed donations from the same donor for pediatric recipients).

Methods applicable to multiple agents concurrently include:

- Inactivation of infectious agents (e.g., solvent-detergent treatment of plasma; research initiatives aimed at pathogen inactivation of cellular blood components);
- Removal of infectious cells (e.g., leukodepletion for cell-associated viruses).

Methods applicable to individual agents (which may also result in improved safety for other agents that may be carried by a coinfected donor) include:

- Donor selection and screening procedures (e.g., donor interview, confidential unit exclusion, donor deferral registries, elimination of cash payment to donors);
- Laboratory testing;
- Consignee notification and removal of potentially infectious units from inventory based on postdonation donor information or improper laboratory testing.

METHODS TO ASSESS TRANSFUSION RISK

The most basic method of establishing that a disease is transmitted by transfusion is through posttransfusion clinical case reporting. Clinical case reporting has several limitations, including physicians' awareness of the need to report such cases and proper recognition of a transfusion association if there is a prolonged incubation period prior to the development of clinical disease. A variation on case reporting is a look-back investigation which assesses whether disease has developed in a recipient when a donor to that recipient is subsequently documented to have evidence of a potentially transfusion-transmissible infection. Despite their limitations, clinical case reporting and look-back case investigations are the methods currently used to estimate the risk of transmitting bacteria, parasites, malaria, and viruses for which donated blood is not routinely screened. Recently, some European countries have established active hemovigilance or surveillance programs (10,11). Although these programs may have some success in detecting an acute infectious complication such as bacterial sepsis, they are subject to the same limitations as clinical case reporting for detection of transfusion-transmissible agents with long incubation periods.

The most scientifically accurate method of establishing transfusion-transmitted infection risk is a prospective controlled study of transfusion recipients in which blood specimens from recipients are obtained prior to transfusion and at periodic intervals posttransfusion. Transfusion transmission is presumptively proven by establishing that a recipient a) who tests positive for an agent posttransfusion was negative for that agent pretransfusion and b) received blood from a donor who was positive for the same agent. The use of a group of nontransfused patients or recipients of units that test negative as controls helps to rule out a confounding nontransfusion etiology. Such studies are further strengthened when serum samples from recipients and donors are frozen in a repository so that they may be reevaluated when more sensitive blood screening assays become available. More detailed reviews of the repository-based studies discussed below can be found elsewhere (12,13).

Over the past three decades, the U.S. National Heart, Lung, and Blood Institute (NHLBI) has funded several prospective recipient follow-up studies: the Transfusion-transmitted Virus Study (recipients transfused from 1974 through 1979), the Frequency of Agents Communicated by Transfusion Study (recipients transfused from 1985 to 1991) and ongoing studies of posttransfusion hepatitis at the National Institutes of Health Clinical Center (14–16). These studies have used their repository samples to measure the transfusion-transmitted risk of non-A, non-B hepatitis, hepatitis C virus (HCV), HIV, human T-cell lymphotropic viruses 1 and 2 (HTLV-1 and -2), HGV, and TT virus (TTV) (14–18).

An alternative approach to direct risk estimation involves retention of very large repositories of donor specimens, followed by testing for infectious agents and selective recipient follow-up. Human immunodeficiency virus and HTLV antibody testing of the Transfusion Safety Study repository of over 200,000 representative blood donor samples collected in 1984 and 1985 identified seropositive donor units, and the components were traced to the transfusing hospitals and subsequently to the transfusion recipients. These studies established the rate of HIV and HTLV-1 and -2 transmission from known seropositive units (19,20).

From 1991 to 1995, the Retrovirus Epidemiology Donor Study (REDS) established large donor repositories of over 600,000 donor samples, and subsequently used a selective approach for testing these donor specimens to evaluate a) *T. cruzi* seroprevalence (and transmission via look-back studies), b) the rate of HBV viremia in anti-HBc positive units, and c) to establish donor prevalence for human herpesvirus 8 (HHV-8) antibody, TTV viremia, and cytomegalovirus (CMV) viremia (21, 22).

Because transfusion-transmitted risks are currently so low in developed countries, it is exceedingly difficult to directly measure these risks with accuracy. Furthermore, it is unlikely that many future prospective studies of transfusion recipients will be conducted due to the requirement for very large sample sizes and the associated expense. It is therefore necessary to rely on mathematic approaches that evaluate a limited data set, and using reasonable assumptions, model the data to generate an estimate of risk. Mathematic modeling has been used to generate estimates of HIV, HTLV, HCV, and hepatitis B virus (HBV) risk.

TRANSFUSION-TRANSMITTED INFECTION RISK FROM BLOOD COMPONENTS

Agents for Which Laboratory Testing Is Routinely Performed (HIV, HTLV, HCV, HBV)

Although each unit of donated blood is tested for evidence of HIV, HTLV, HBV, and HCV infection, transmission of these viral agents can still occur (23). The primary contributor to such risk is from donations collected during the window period, defined as the time during the early stage of infection when the donor is infected with a virus but has negative results in blood donor screening assays; hence, REDS investigators developed the incidence-window period model to estimate per-unit risk. A more thorough discussion of this model and its assumptions can be found elsewhere (24,25). Briefly, this approach estimates risk by measuring the incidence of new infection (seroconversion) in a blood donor population over a specific time interval and then multiplying this incidence by the average time interval that a seroconverting donor would be expected to be capable of transmitting infection (i.e., the length of the window period) (24).

Incidence data are obtained from direct observation of blood donor populations and are measured as the number of newly infected (seroconverting) donors divided by the observed person-years at risk. Incidence is calculated using data obtained from donors who gave more than one donation during the study period. Determination of the window period requires data from specialized studies of the early events following viral infection (24,25). The infectious window period is defined as the interval between the time a donor is infectious (by the route of blood transfusion) and the time that a particular laboratory test becomes positive. This infectious window period may be shorter than that predicted from the time of exposure to the agent, due to a sequestering of the agent in tissue such as lymph nodes, introducing a lag time before the donor can transmit infection (26).

In 1996, Schreiber et al. published the results of the incidence-window period model using data collected from 1991 to 1993 to establish the per-unit risks of HIV, HTLV, HCV, and HBV (27). Recently, minipool nucleic acid testing (NAT) has shortened the window period for HCV, from 70 days using the most sensitive antibody assays to an estimated 12 days. For HIV, minipool NAT (in addition to p24 antigen testing) has shortened the 22-day window period to an estimated 13 to 15 days (28). These newer window periods can be combined with more contemporary and geographically representative HCV and HIV incidence estimates (HCV: 2.2 per 100,000 person-years; HIV: 1.7 per 100,000 person-years; American Red Cross data from 1998 and 1999) and an estimate from HCV NAT programs that the incidence of infection is 4.5-fold higher in first-time than in repeat donors to recalculate the estimated risk of HIV and HCV transmission (28,29). Using the newer hepatitis B surface antigen (HbsAg) incidence data, the same 59-day HBsAg window period, and the 4.5-fold adjustment for first-time donor incidence leads to a new risk estimate for HBV of 1 per 81,000 units.

Thus, the contemporary point estimates for risk are:

- HCV: 1 per 813,000 units
- HIV: 1 per 971,000 units
- HBV:1 per 81,000 units
- HTLV: 1 per 641,000 units

The HBV risk estimate is the most controversial aspect of the incidence-window period model. Because HBsAg is a transient marker, detection of HBsAg incident cases will underestimate new HBV infections in blood donors, some of whom may have acquired HBV infection and cleared HBsAg prior to their next donation. Investigators for REDS adjusted for this by calculating an incidence adjustment factor of 2.38 based on the average interdonation interval for donors who became HBsAg positive (30).

In the window period model, the per-unit risk must be multiplied by the likelihood that such a potentially infectious blood component will transmit the agent to the recipient. For HIV, HCV, and HBV the per-unit risk is the same for each type of blood component transfused (e.g., red blood cells, platelets, fresh-frozen plasma [FFP], cryoprecipitate). Recipients of HIV or HCV seropositive components have an 80% to 90% likelihood of acquiring the infection; it is assumed that the risk from an HCV- or HIV NAT-negative, seronegative window-period unit is similar (19,31). Alternatively, it is possible that units collected during the very early phase of viremia may not contain enough viral particles to transmit an infectious dose; data are currently insufficient to evaluate this possibility (32).

Given the high HBV transmission rate from needlestick injury, it is likely that the transfusion-transmission rate for HBV is at least as high as that for HIV (33). The situation is different for HTLV, for which there is no risk of transmission from acellular components (such as FFP or cryoprecipitate) due to the exclusive cell-associated nature of the virus (34). Furthermore, transmission rates of HTLV from cellular products obtained from infected donors vary with the length of storage of the blood components; although overall transmission rates in the United States are 35% from red blood cells or platelets, there has been no transmission documented from red blood cell units stored longer than 14 days (20).

Three factors other than window-period donation might contribute to the risk of transfusion transmission of these viruses. These factors are a) the existence of a chronic carrier state in which a clinically asymptomatic donor will persistently test negative on an antibody screening assay, b) viral variation such that screening assays fail to identify some infectious donors who harbor a particular atypical genetic variant, and c) laboratory error. Minipool NAT testing for HIV and HCV should detect these types of infectious units (with the possible exception of rare genetic variants), thereby confining the current risk only to those units that are in the NAT-negative window. It has been documented that errors in blood donor laboratory screening occur at low frequency (0.05%; 95% CI, zero to 1.5%); to result in risk, a testing error would need to occur in a seropositive unit that is screened by a single assay method (35). However, because HIV screening currently includes three independent laboratory assays, and HCV and HBV screening use two assays each, it is extremely unlikely that testing error contributes to risk.

Agents for Which Laboratory Testing Is not Routinely Performed

The risk of many rare transfusion-transmitted agents cannot be estimated using the incidence-window period model and therefore such estimates rely on clinical case reporting to establish a minimum transfusion risk. Factors such as the prevalence of donors infected with the agent, the survival of the agent in stored blood components, the rate of transmission when a potentially infectious unit is transfused, and the susceptibility or immunity of the transfused recipient population are important parameters that need to be considered when evaluating whether the true risk of the agent exceeds that predicted from clinical case reporting.

Hepatitis A Virus

Because HAV does not induce a chronic carrier state, it can be transmitted only by transfusion if a person donates during the several-week interval of viremia prior to development of acute clinical symptoms (36). As a result of this biologic property, only rare cases of transfusion-transmitted hepatitis A from blood components have been reported, with approximately 25 case reports in the literature through 1989 (37). One author used these data to estimate that transmission-transmitted HAV risk was 1 per 1 million units (37); however, the case reporting data, if accurate, would suggest an even lower risk, in the order of 1 per 10 million transfused units.

Non-A-E Hepatitis

Clinical and laboratory evidence in the 1970s and 1980s suggested that a viral agent other than HCV causes some cases of transfusion-transmitted non-A, non-B hepatitis. Prior to the discovery of HCV, such cases constituted approximately 5% to 10% of non-A, non-B cases. Although the current transfusion-transmission risk of the non-A-E agent is unknown, it is probably less than it was previously. It is likely that the non-A-E virus primarily affects many donors who also have exposure to HCV; hence many of these donors will be deferred by HCV screening assays.

Two recently discovered viruses, HGV and TTV, were both thought to represent the agent of non-A-E hepatitis soon after their initial discovery; however, subsequent intensive study has shown that neither of these agents is the non-A-E virus (13,17, 18,38). Recently, variants of a new class of viral agents termed SEN-V, which are related to the expanding class of TTVs, have been hypothesized to be this causative agent. Studies are currently underway to prove or disprove this hypothesis.

Cytomegalovirus

Cytomegalovirus-reduced-risk blood products are routinely used for immunocompromised recipients. Traditionally, these products have been supplied from CMV-seronegative donors. Fresh-frozen plasma and cryoprecipitate have not been implicated in CMV transmission. CMV is transmitted by infected leukocytes. Leukodepletion of cellular blood components to $< 5 \times 10^6$ leukocytes has been demonstrated to provide the same level of safety as CMV-seronegative cellular products, and leukodepletion has been accepted by most experts as another method of supplying CMV-reduced-risk blood (39).

Despite these preventive measures, primary CMV infection has been demonstrated in recipients of CMV-reduced-risk blood products. It has not been proven whether these apparent breakthrough infections were transfusion transmitted or whether they resulted from other nosocomial sources; if transfusion related, limited data from one study would indicate that the transfusion risk was about 1 in 100 recipients or 1 in 7,500 CMV-reduced-risk units (40). However, this 1% per-recipient risk estimate from CMV-reduced-risk blood components (which has also been found in several other studies of CMV-seronegative transfusions) has wide 95% confidence limits, and several small studies with leukodepleted blood showed no evidence of CMV transmission (39). Given these limited and incomplete data, most experts have tended to assume that the risk of transfusion-transmitted CMV from CMV-reduced-risk blood products is virtually zero. The risk of clinically important transfusion-transmitted disease is much lower than is the risk of CMV transmission, but an accurate figure is not available.

Human Herpesvirus 8

Human herpesvirus 8 (HHV-8) is a leukocyte-associated herpes virus discovered in the mid-1990s that has been implicated as the causative agent of Kaposi's sarcoma (41,42). Sexual transmission of HHV-8 has been proven, whereas data on parenteral transmission are less clear. A recent report provides some epidemiologic evidence that such transmission may occur (42a). Transmission during renal transplantation has been documented. There is a single case report of HHV-8 cultured from an asymptomatic blood donor infecting allogeneic lymphocytes in the in vitro culture system (43). Preliminary studies have indicated no risk of transfusion transmission. Human herpesvirus 8 was not detected in small numbers of recipients of blood from HHV-8 antibody-positive blood donors, and the rate of HHV-8 seropositivity in hemophiliacs transfused with clotting factor concentrates prior to viral inactivation has been shown to be low (41,42).

Parvovirus B19

Parvovirus B19 viremia rates in blood donor populations (as detected by NAT) have been reported to range from 0.03% to 0.1% (44). Nevertheless, only three cases of clinical disease (anemia) associated with Parvovirus B19 transmission by blood component transfusion have been reported in North America and Europe during the past 5 years (45).

Malaria

Transfusion-transmitted malaria is common in some parts of the world but is rare in the United States. The Centers for Disease Control and Prevention conducts annual surveillance of clinical malarial cases; 103 transfusion-transmitted cases have been reported during the 40-year period from 1958 through 1998, for an average of two to three cases per year (46–48). The estimated rate of occurrence is 1 per 4 million red blood cells transfused.

Babesia

Babesia microti is a small protozoan parasite that infects red blood cells. It is the second most commonly reported cause of transfusion-transmitted parasitic infection in the United States, with over 25 cases reported in the literature during the last two decades (48). Most cases involved transfusion of red blood cells, but at least four cases have been attributed to the transfusion of platelets, most likely contaminated with red blood cells. This clinical case–reporting data would suggest an incidence of approximately 1 per 9.6 million red blood cell units. Multiple cases have been reported in each of the last 3 years, suggesting that the transfusion-transmission rate may be increasing. Recently, Babesia-like organisms with increased virulence, termed WA-1 and MO-1, have been documented to be transmitted by transfusion (49). Most transfusion-transmitted Babesia cases have occurred in immunocompromised or asplenic patients.

Chagas Disease

Chagas disease is caused by a protozoan parasite, *Trypanosome cruzi*. This parasite is endemic to Mexico and Central and South America, where large numbers of transfusion-transmitted cases have been documented. Since the mid-1980s, only five cases of acute transfusion-transmitted Chagas disease have been reported in the United States and Canada, all involving immunocompromised recipients (48). Platelets have been the implicated blood component in cases in which data were available. Most recently, an additional case of asymptomatic transfusion-transmitted *T. cruzi* infection has been documented in a recipient transfused with a *T. cruzi*-seropositive platelet unit (50). This latter case supports the assertion that due to lack of acute symptoms, other cases of asymptomatic transfusion-transmitted *T. cruzi* infection may have occurred, particularly in immunocompetent patients. Several studies in the United States have documented rates of *T. cruzi* seropositivity in blood donors ranging from none to 0.48% (with the higher rates in geographic regions with more Hispanic donors), suggesting that a greater number of cases may be transmitted by transfusion but go undetected (48,51).

Bacteria

Recently, the 1998 and 1999 results of a national voluntary surveillance study of transfusion-transmitted bacterial sepsis (BaCon study) have been reported (52). Cases were detected by investigation of transfusion reactions that met a set of predetermined clinical criteria and these cases were confirmed by strict bacteriologic culture criteria. Bacterial infection from transfused platelet concentrates was documented to occur at a higher rate than from red blood cell transfusions. The rate of clinically detectable sepsis by component type was: 1 per 116,00 platelet apheresis units, 1 per 557,000 platelet concentrates (or 1 in 93,000 platelet transfusion episodes, estimated as six whole blood–derived platelet concentrates per transfusion episode), and 1 per 3.9 million red blood cell units. The rate of fatal septic reaction was 1 per 263,000 platelet apheresis units, 1 per 740,000 whole blood–derived platelet transfusion episodes, and 1 per 5.2 million red blood cell units (52). There were a total of 21 symptomatic cases with eight fatalities in the 2-year reporting period; five of the fatalities were from platelet transfusion and three from red blood cell transfusion. These BaCon study results are consistent with but somewhat lower than transfusion-sepsis fatalities reported to the Food and Drug Administration (FDA); these have averaged about five cases per year since the mid-1970s but rose to seven cases per year between 1996 and 1998 (53).

Many experts believe that data from voluntary national surveillance and FDA reporting underestimate the true incidence of morbidity and mortality from platelet-induced sepsis. For example, an ongoing study over a 12-year period at a major hospital found that septic transfusion reactions ranged from 1 per 4,000 platelet transfusion episodes (pools of six whole blood–derived platelets) to 1 per 15,000 platelet apheresis units transfused; a rate that is 8- to 25-fold higher than that reported in the BaCon study (54). A similar frequency has been reported by the French Hemovigilance system (55). Multiple studies that have performed automated culturing of platelet units have shown bacterial contamination rates in the range of 1 in 2,000 to 1 in 3,000 per platelet concentrate or platelet apheresis unit (56). Very few similar studies have been performed for red blood cells; the results suggest a positive culture rate of about 1 per 38,000.

Variant Creutzfeldt-Jakob Disease

Variant CJD (vCJD) is a newly discovered degenerative and fatal neurologic disease. To date, no cases of transfusion-transmitted vCJD have been reported anywhere in the world (57). However, because vCJD is a new disease and other transmissible spongiform encephalopathies are known to have long incubation periods, the 5-year observation period since the discovery of the disease is too short to draw any firm conclusions about transfusion transmission. Furthermore, the spread of the vCJD agent (probably a prion) from cattle to man, and the detection of the vCJD prion in lymphoid tissue, have raised concern that there is a biologic basis for vCJD to be transmitted by peripheral routes, including blood transfusion (57).

Variant CJD is an example of a transfusion-transmitted agent with a risk that is theoretic and not documented. The rationale for implementing policies that might decrease this theoretic risk has been based upon the precautionary principle that action should be taken in the absence of firm data when the potential consequences of inaction could be catastrophic (e.g., transmission of an untreatable, fatal disease) (4).

EVALUATING THE SIGNIFICANCE OF TRANSFUSION-TRANSMITTED INFECTIONS

Data from look-back studies indicate that there is a greater than 50% probability that a specific blood component will have been transfused to an individual who will die within 1 year from the underlying disease that necessitated the transfusion (58). (This should not be misinterpreted to indicate that 50% of blood recipients die within 1 year, but rather that large-volume users with poor prognoses receive a high percentage of transfused blood components.) Because some transfusion-transmitted infections produce clinical disease only after many years (e.g., HIV, HCV), it is obvious that the deleterious effects of these agents will occur in fewer patients than would be predicted from per-unit risk estimates.

Concern about long-term chronic sequelae due to infectious

agents is greatest for those recipients transfused at a young age who have a good disease prognosis. For surviving recipients, follow-up studies have documented the progression to AIDS in a significant number of HIV-infected recipients (59). In the case of HCV, significant liver disease develops in only approximately 20% of recipients 2 to 3 decades posttransfusion (60). Most transfusion recipients who acquire HBV resolve the initial infection and develop immunity, whereas those who develop chronic infection are unlikely to experience severe outcomes. A long-term follow-up study of patients who acquired HBV in adulthood from exposure to contaminated yellow fever vaccine demonstrated lack of serious sequelae and no progression to liver cancer (61). Most HTLV-infected recipients remain asymptomatic, but a very small percentage develop a neurologic disease (HTLV-associated myelopathy) after incubation periods as short as 1 to 2 years (62).

In contrast to these agents, other transfusion-transmissible agents produce acute morbidity and mortality. The effects of bacterial sepsis are immediate and can be lethal. In immunocompromised patients, Chagas disease, babesiosis, and CMV disease have relatively rapid onset and can cause death. Transfusion-associated malaria also causes acute morbidity and mortality.

TRANSFUSION-TRANSMITTED INFECTION RISK FROM PLASMA DERIVATIVES

Plasma derivatives (fractionated plasma products) are preparations of purified plasma proteins prepared commonly by a process known as Cohn alcohol fractionation. Plasma derivatives include antihemophilic factor (factor VIII concentrate), factor IX concentrate, albumin, plasma protein fraction (PPF), intravenous immune globulin (IVIG), and intramuscular immune globulin (IMIG). Because the preparation of plasma derivatives by commercial manufacturers involves the pooling of plasma from tens of thousands of donors, there is a significant likelihood that the pool includes plasma from at least one infectious donor, even if the prevalence of the infectious agent in the donor population is low. Furthermore, plasma for fractionation is often collected from donor populations with higher rates of infectious disease and from very-frequent donors (up to twice per week), thereby increasing the likelihood of donation during a presymptomatic, high-titer viremic phase of infection (63).

Coagulation Factor Preparations

Prior to the application of viral inactivation procedures during the early to mid-1980s, factor VIII and IX preparations prepared from human plasma transmitted HIV and HCV at high rates. Since 1987, coagulation factor products prepared by solvent-detergent treatment or wet heating (pasteurization) methods have not transmitted any cases of HIV, HBV, or HCV to recipients (64).

Solvent-detergent treatment is only partially effective against non-lipid-enveloped viruses such as HAV and Parvovirus B19 (45,65). In an attempt to reduce the risk of these viral infections, plasma derivative manufacturers have recently introduced minipool NAT for these agents (65). Prior to introduction of minipool NAT, six documented outbreaks of HAV from coagulation factor concentrates occurred worldwide from 1987 to 1997. These involved approximately 100 recipients of particular batches of factor VIII concentrate treated only by the solvent-detergent procedure; one of these outbreaks was also associated with factor IX concentrate (66). Parvovirus B19 has been more frequently transmitted by coagulation factor concentrates than has HAV. Recipients of clotting factor concentrates treated by multiple viral inactivation methods have high rates of infection (estimated at 40%) with Parvovirus B19. Despite this high transmission rate, very few clinical sequelae have been observed; as of 1999, only one case of hypoplastic anemia and three cases of erythema infectiosum had been reported in hemophilia patients (45).

Because the agents of classic CJD and variant CJD are thought to be prions (which are highly resistant to any viral inactivation procedures), there is a theoretic risk that plasma derivatives might transmit these agents. Experimental evidence suggests that if prions are present in input plasma, they are more likely to partition to the coagulation factor fraction rather than to other fractions. Recent epidemiologic evidence in patients with hemophilia and laboratory evidence in experimental animal models provides evidence against classic CJD transmission by plasma derivatives and therefore strongly suggests that classic CJD is not transmitted (or very rarely transmitted) by plasma derivatives (67). Similar data are not yet available for vCJD, which remains a theoretic, but unproven, risk.

In the last few years, recombinant factor VIII and IX preparations have replaced human-derived products. Initially, these factor concentrates were stabilized with human albumin, thereby raising the theoretic concern that the concentrates might pose an infectious risk due to the presence of the albumin. Recently, recombinant factor VIII and IX concentrates which do not use albumin as a stabilizer have been introduced; these factor concentrates should be considered to be risk free with respect to transfusion-transmitted agents.

Immune Globulin Preparations

There are two theoretic reasons why immune globulin preparations have historically been of very low risk for infectious disease transmission: a) the plasma derivative manufacturing process has been shown to result in partitioning of viruses into plasma products other than the immunoglobulin fraction, and b) the immunoglobulin fraction contains antibodies from thousands of donors that may serve to neutralize any viruses that partition into this fraction (64). In the past, several IVIG preparations used in Europe and a single manufacturer's product in the United States was documented to transmit non-A, non-B hepatitis or HCV (64). Subsequent to the U.S. episode in 1994, IVIG products have been subjected to viral inactivation procedures, and more recently input plasma has been screened by minipool NAT for HCV, HIV, and HBV (64,65). The current risk of IVIG transmitting any known viral agents is virtually zero. Human immunodeficiency virus has never been transmitted by IMIG, and the only outbreak of IMIG-associated HBV transmission occurred prior to HBsAg screening of blood donors in the 1970s. Although HCV has never been transmitted by IMIG in North

America, Rh immune globulin manufactured by different methods than those used in North America has transmitted HCV in separate outbreaks in Ireland and Eastern Europe (64). Currently, IMIG products manufactured in North America are either subjected to virus inactivation and removal procedures or undergo final product testing for HCV RNA. The current risk of transmitting any known viral agents is virtually zero.

Albumin and Plasma Protein Fraction

Two theoretic reasons why albumin and PPF have been virtually risk free follow: a) the plasma derivative manufacturing process has been shown to result in partitioning of viruses into different plasma products (other than albumin and PPF) and b) albumin and PPF have long been subjected to pasteurization procedures. There have been no documented transmissions of HBV, HIV, or HCV by albumin in its 50 years of clinical use and only one instance of HBV transmission by PPF, which occurred prior to the use of pasteurization procedures (64).

Solvent-detergent–treated Plasma

Solvent-detergent–treated (SD) plasma is a pooled plasma product manufactured by pooling approximately 2,000 to 2,500 units of ABO-identical FFP prior to solvent-detergent treatment. Extensive experience in Europe has established that SD plasma does not transmit HIV, HBV, or HCV (68). In the United States, some lots of SD plasma have transmitted Parvovirus B19 infection and theoretically may transmit HAV or other non-lipid-enveloped viruses. Subsequent to the Parvovirus B19 transmissions, the manufacturer of this product has initiated mini-pool high-titer Parvovirus B19 NAT of input plasma (44).

TRANSFUSION-TRANSMITTED INFECTION RISKS IN PERSPECTIVE

Based on data from the early 1990s, Schreiber et al. concluded that the cumulative risk of a unit being donated during the window period for the four viruses they considered (HIV, HTLV, HBV, and HCV) was 1 in 34,000 (27). In 1994, Dodd concluded that when data for all transfusion-transmitted agents were taken into account, approximately 2.6 per 10,000 blood components caused transfusion-transmitted infection (37). He further calculated that only about 10% of these transmissions (3.1 to 4.2 per 100,000 transfused components) resulted in fatal transfusion-transmitted disease; the range depended on projections of how may patients would survive their underlying disease long enough to develop transfusion-transmitted disease complications. He attributed 50% of transfusion-infection–related mortality to bacterial sepsis. Linden recently reported a 10-year experience in New York State. She used error reports submitted to the state to estimate that the risk of transfusing an ABO-incompatible unit due to human error was 1 per 38,000 red blood cell units, and the risk of a resulting fatality was 1 per 1.8 million recipients. She concluded that these risks were of comparable magnitude to those associated with transfusion-transmitted infectious agents (69). The estimate, however, represents a gross underestimation of the true frequency of ABO fatalities, because many episodes are thought to go unrecognized and unreported.

In 1997, the U.S. Government Accounting Office (GAO) issued a report on infectious and noninfectious risks of blood transfusion (63). The GAO authors calculated that 5 in 10,000 transfused units carried an infectious risk to the recipient. In reviewing their estimates, it is apparent that 60% of their estimated risk was due to their extremely high estimates for transmission of HCV and non-A-E hepatitis. Adjusting their calculations to reflect current, more realistic risk estimates for these two agents results in one that is very similar to Dodd's 2.6 per 10,000 components. By factoring in the average number of blood components per transfusion episode (estimated as five) and recipient mortality from underlying disease (estimated as 30%), the GAO authors further calculated that approximately 3.2 per 10,000 patients would develop chronic disease or die from transfusion-transmitted infection (and an additional 0.8 would die from noninfectious complications of transfusion). As with their per-unit risk calculations, this is probably a substantial overestimate of such risk.

The risk estimate in the United States for various transfusion-transmitted agents as of early 2001 is presented in Table 48.1. Estimates for aggregate risk of transfusion-transmitted infections from red blood cell and from FFP or cryoprecipitate units range from 1 in 60,000 to 1 in 69,000 per unit and are not sensitive to the estimate chosen for the risk of bacterial infection. In contrast, the risk from platelet concentrate transfusion may be as high as 1 per 17,000 if the higher estimate for bacterial infection is considered, or 1 per 55,000 if the lower estimate is used. It is estimated that 282 to 434 transfusion-transmitted infections occur annually in the United States, leading to an overall risk estimate of infectious agent transmission of 1:40,000 to 1:62,000 for all components transfused.

These current risk estimates are substantially lower than those published previously. The reasons for this are two-fold, a) the availability of better data which enable more accurate risk estimates to be calculated and b) improvements in blood safety due to implementation of effective interventions.

As is evident, it is difficult to accurately calculate projected rates of adverse outcomes in recipients due to uncertainties inherent in the data. It is noteworthy that in their 1997 analysis, the GAO authors deliberately selected the highest-available estimates for transfusion risks and compared this worst-case transfusion outcome scenario against other medical and nonmedical risks (63). Their comparative analysis is presented in Tables 48.2 and 48.3. In brief, the risks of chronic disease or death from transfusion-transmitted infections was 15-fold lower than the risk that a hospital stay would result in death or chronic disability due to factors other than the underlying disease, 33-fold lower than the risk of dying from a direct result of surgery, 162-fold lower than the risk of suffering an injury from hospital drug therapy, and 187-fold lower than the risk of developing an infection of unknown cause in the intensive care unit. Furthermore, the annual risk to the average person of dying from transfusion without an anticipated surgical operation was shown to be comparable to that of dying from electrocution or drowning. Current

TABLE 48.1. ESTIMATED RISK OF TRANSFUSION-TRANSMITTED INFECTION BY BLOOD COMPONENT TYPE IN THE UNITED STATES IN EARLY 2001

	Risk Per Component[a]			Infected Components Transfused Annually[b,c]		
Agent	RBC	Platelet Concentrate[a]	FFP or Cryoprecipitate	RBC	Platelet Concentrate	FFP or Cryoprecipitate
HIV[d]	1:971,000	1:971,000	1:971,000	11	4	3
HCV[d]	1:813,000	1:813,000	1:813,000	13	4	4
HBV[d]	1:81,000	1:81,000	1:81,000	131	44	41
HTLV	1:1,923,000[e]	1:641,000	0	6	6	0
HAV[f]	1:10,000,000	1:10,000,000	1:10,000,000	1	0.4[c]	0.3
Non A-E[g]	rare	rare	rare	NC[h]	NC	NC
CMV[i]	rare	rare	0	NC	NC	0
Parvovirus B19[j]	rare	rare	rare	NC	NC	NC
Malaria	1:4,000,000	rare[k]	0	3	NC	0
Babesia	1:9,000,000	rare[k]	0	1	NC	0
Chagas	rare	1:9,000,000	0	NC	0.4[c]	0
Bacteria[l]	—	—	—	—	—	—
High	1:1,000,000	1:24,000	rare	11	150	NC
Low	1:3,900,000	1:557,000	rare	3	6	NC
Total[m]	—	—	—	—	—	—
High	1:60,000	1:17,000	1:69,000	177	209	48
Low	1:63,000	1:55,000	1:69,000	169	65	48

HHV-8, human herpes virus-8; vCJD, variant Creutzfeldt-Jakob disease.
RBC, red blood cells; FFP, fresh-frozen plasma; HIV, human immunodeficiency virus; HCV, hepatitis C virus; HBV, hepatitis B virus; HTLV, human T cell lymphocyte virus; HAV, hepatitis A virus; CMV, cytomegatovirus.
HHV-8 and vCJD have been excluded because transfusion-transmission has not been documented (42,57).
[a]Risk calculated per individual component transfused. Platelet transfusion episodes often consist of six platelet concentrates (risk factor is multiplied by six) or one platelet apheresis unit. Risk per component rounded to the nearest thousand.
[b]Annual number of transfused components is from published 1994 data. RBC, 10.6 million units; platelets, 3.6 million platelet concentrates; FFP/cryo, 3.3 million units combined.
Published 1992 annual usage for each component type is similar as is published 1997 RBC usage (75–77).
[c]Annual risk estimates have been rounded to the nearest whole number, except when this number is less than one case per year.
[d]Newer estimates for HIV, HCV, HBV using 1998–1999 data; these differ from previously published estimates.
[e]HTLV RBC risk estimated from look-back studies indicating that 35% of potentially infectious RBCs resulted in HTLV transmission (20).
[f]HAV risk estimate has been stated as 1:1,000,000 in previous reports (37,63).
[g]Non A-E hepatitis risk cannot be quantitated due to insufficient data.
[h]NC, not calculable due to insufficient data, but should be close to zero.
[i]CMV risk cannot be accurately quantitated. One study suggests it may be as high as 1:7500 units, even with the use of CMV-safe blood components in CMV at-risk recipients; however, this high estimate has not been verified (39,40).
[j]Parvovirus B19 risk appears to be extremely low but studies of asymptomatic transfusion-transmitted infection have not been conducted.
[k]Malaria and babesia are intraerythrocytic infections; very rare transmissions by platelets may occur due to residual red blood cells in platelet concentrates (48).
[l]Bacterial transmission rates are very difficult to estimate. The higher risk estimates are from older data; the lower risk estimates are from the BaCon study (52–54).
[m]Total risk is given as both a high and low estimate; these differ based upon the estimate chosen for bacterial infection risk.

TABLE 48.2. A COMPARISON OF ADVERSE EFFECTS FROM TRANSFUSION-TRANSMITTED INFECTIONS WITH OTHER MEDICAL PROCEDURES/CONDITIONS

Outcome	Per 10^5 Patients Or Hospitalizations
Chronic disease or death from blood if:	
General surgery patient	5
Received blood transfusion	40
Hospital stay ends in death or disability	600
Death as direct result of surgery	1333
Injury related to drug therapy during hospitalization	6500
Infection of unknown cause in intensive care	7500

From United States General Accounting Office. Blood supply: transfusion-associated risks. GAO/PEMD-97-2, Washington DC, 1997:16, with permission.

risk estimates for transfusion-transmitted infection are 20- to 30-fold lower than those in the GAO report (Table 48.1), which further illustrates the marked safety of transfusion when compared to other health outcomes.

RISK COMMUNICATION

A challenge for transfusion medicine professionals is to communicate these rather dry risk estimates and comparisons to the general public in a way that will be readily understood. It is particularly difficult for the general public to comprehend low-probability events and their relative frequency. One approach to making quantifiable risk estimates more understandable to the public has been the development of graphic tools. One such tool is the Paling perspective scale, which is a graphic representation of comparative risks on a log scale (70). The scale uses the

TABLE 48.3. ANNUAL RATES OF VARIOUS HEALTH OUTCOMES

Outcome	Condition	Per 100,000 Population
Chronic disease or death by transfusion without surgery plans	—	0.5
Hospitalization for	Septicemia	105
	Accidental poisoning by drugs/medicines	128
	Adverse effects of therapeutic drugs	142
	Infections or parasitic diseases	311
	Cerebrovascular disease	328
	Pneumonia	462
	Malignant tumor	578
	Injury and poisoning	1060
	Heart disease	1541
Death from	Electrocution	0.5
	Tuberculosis	0.8
	Drowning	2.8
	Arteriosclerosis	9
	Motor vehicle crash	15
	Pneumonia or influenza	32
	Stroke	59
	Cancer	206
	Heart Disease	296

From United States General Accounting Office. Blood supply: transfusion-associated risks. GAO/PEMD-97-2, Washington DC, 1997:17, with permission.

risk of 1 per million (10^{-6}) as effective zero, under the assumption that this is an acceptable level of risk for most people in their daily activities. Originally used to communicate risks of environmental hazards, the Paling scale has recently incorporated transfusion risk; Figure 48.2, reproduced from a recently published article, uses the Paling scale to compare the risk of death from transfusion to death associated with violent crime.

RISK PERCEPTION

Public fear about HIV infection from transfusion was heightened in the mid-1980s by the lack of scientific knowledge about the actual risk. At that time, medical experts quoted risks that reflected the number of known transfusion-associated AIDS cases detected. When it was later discovered that actual risks were far greater than had been stated, the public lost faith in the credibility of the estimates provided by the experts. Many people have remained suspicious and distrustful of subsequent statements about risk made by transfusion medicine specialists (5,71).

Patients and their families tend to be influenced by psychologic and emotional factors when they assess risk. Consequently, perceived risk may differ substantially from actual risk, and presentation of quantitative estimates of risk may do little to change the perception of individual patients or the lay public. One approach to understanding factors involved in the public's risk perception is a cognitive model derived from psychometric research (72). This model plots risks on a grid consisting of two axes that divide the plotted risks into four quadrants: the *x-axis* plots increasing amount of dread and the *y-axis* plots the degree to which the true risk is unknown or unclear (Fig. 48.3). Studies have concluded that events scoring high on the dread scale and low on the "clear" knowledge scale (events which locate in the upper right quadrant of the grid in Figure 48.3) will be perceived as riskier than predicted by quantitative estimates. As a consequence, the public will make a greater effort to avoid these situations and will expect government or industry regulators to adopt policies to decrease these risks. Elements that contribute to increased dread include the assessment that the event is uncontrollable, involuntary, unjust, or unfair and that the outcome of the event is catastrophic or fatal. Using this model, it is easy to see why transfusion risk is of such concern to the public; some transfusion-transmitted diseases have dreaded outcomes (e.g., HIV infection), the source of the donated units is beyond the recipient's control, the decision to be transfused may not have been perceived by the patient as entirely voluntary (because the alternative might be worsening of a medical condition or even death), and the certainty of the risk estimate, as communicated by the experts, is not believed by the public.

These predictions of the model with regard to attitudes toward transfusion safety are borne out by a recent study (73). A telephone survey conducted in late 1997 of over 1,200 respondents showed that 33% to 47% gave answers to each of three questions about blood transfusion safety that indicated substantial concerns. Respondents' perception of transfusion risk was related to their attitudes about retaining control over hazardous activities and to their level of trust in experts.

Although virtually all experts now make the statement (and the data support) that blood transfusion is safer than ever, a segment of the general public does not feel this way (73,74). Is there any way to change this perception? The best suggestions

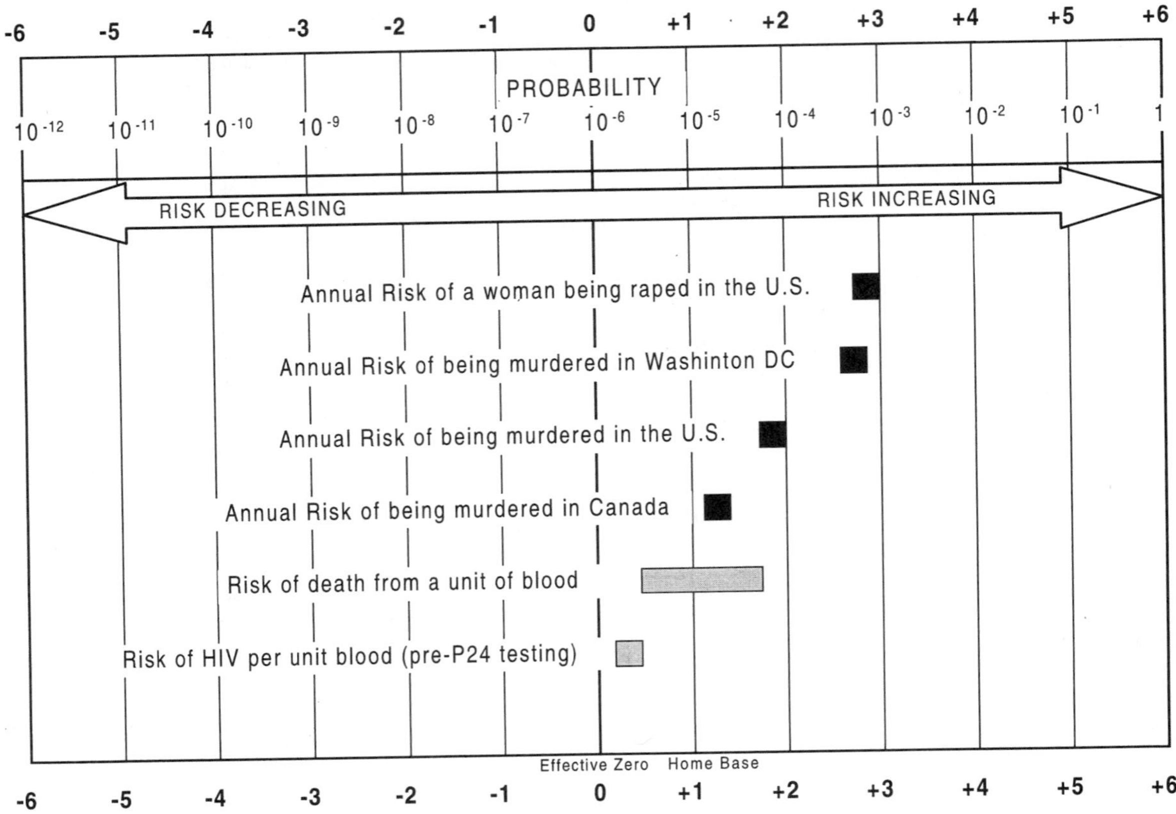

FIGURE 48.2. Risk of violent crime versus infectious risks of blood transfusion. Data plotted using the Paling Perspective Scale. Effective zero is equivalent to a risk of 10 to 6. Home base refers to 0 to 2 on the Paling scale. (From Lee DH, Paling JE, Blajchman MA. A new tool for communicating transfusion risk information. *Transfusion* 1998;38:184–188, with permission.)

of how to do so are to a) highlight the life-saving benefits of transfusion, thereby making the risk an acceptable tradeoff and b) compare transfusion risks with other medical and nonmedical formats in a manner that is easily understood.

EVALUATING THE RISK OF NEW AGENTS

As molecular biology techniques improve, newly identified infectious agents will continue to be discovered (42). Concerns that these agents will cause severe disease in transfusion recipients will likely arise; these may originate from the media, advocacy organizations for plasma product recipients, research scientists, epidemiologists, and transfusion medicine specialists. It is not unusual for the media to compare a newly identified pathogen to HIV and its spread by transfusion in the early 1980s. The media often amplifies this comparison and the fear that it engenders (13).

Although the initial discovery of a transfusion-transmitted agent often leads to the assumption that it is an etiologic agent of disease, it is very possible that such a newly discovered agent will be benign. Thus, the question of whether to screen the blood supply for an infectious agent that is transfusion transmitted but not proven to cause disease is likely to arise frequently, as it has recently for agents such as HGV (38). Logically, before blood screening is implemented, one needs to show that an infectious agent is transfusion transmitted, that acquiring this agent has adverse consequences, that a blood screening test can detect some infectious donors, and that the anticipated deferral of donors does not have an overly adverse impact on blood availability (38,42). A reflex reaction to advocate screening of the blood supply for all such newly discovered agents should be avoided.

The usual process to initiate medical and scientific research often requires years to plan, fund, and implement, and is not suited to quickly evaluating the possibility of transfusion transmission of new infectious agents. A solution to this problem is to establish an infrastructure for transfusion-related research and surveillance studies in advance of a specific problem (13). A recently begun collection of a new contemporary linked donor-recipient repository termed the REDS Allogeneic Donor and Recipient Repository (RADAR) is intended to accrue samples from at least 10,000 recipients through 2003. This repository has been designed as a resource that can be accessed rapidly to determine whether a newly discovered agent is likely to be transmitted by transfusion. Frozen repository samples are retained from donors whose units are transfused into enrolled

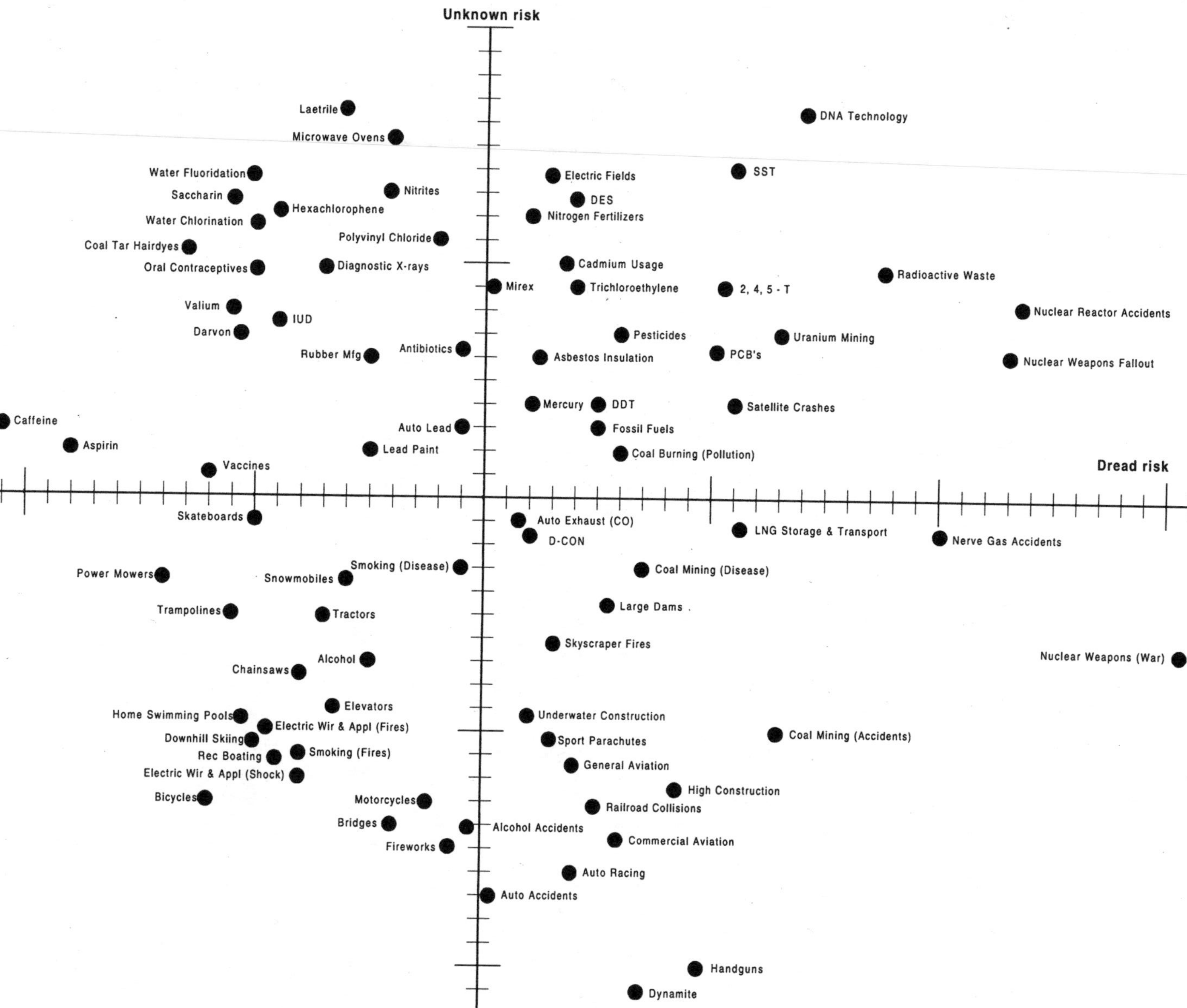

FIGURE 48.3. The public's rating of risk for many hazards. The *x-axis* shows public "dread risk" defined at its high end by a combination of perceived lack of control, dread, the potential for catastrophic consequences, and the inequitable distribution of risks and consequences. The *y-axis* shows public "unknown risk" which is defined at its high end by a combination of risks that are unobservable, unknown, new, and have delayed manifestations. Using these two axes, the public rating of risk for many hazards is shown. (From Slovic P. Perception of risk. *Science* 1987;236:280–285, with permission.)

recipients, as well as from the recipients at the time of study enrollment and 6 months posttransfusion. The major purpose of RADAR is to document, with a reasonable level of certainty (i.e., 95%), whether or not a given agent is transmissible by transfusion. More precisely, the repository has been designed so that if negative test results are obtained in recipients who receive positive donor units, the data will provide a high degree of statistical confidence that the transmission rate of a given agent is less than a given low number (i.e., the transmission rate approaches zero). These data should be important in assuring the public that policy makers have mechanisms in place that can accurately establish risk or lack of risk from newly discovered infectious agents.

REFERENCES

1. AuBuchon JP, Birkmeyer JD, Busch MP. Safety of the blood supply in the United States: opportunities and controversies. *Ann Intern Med* 1997;127:904–909.
2. Blachjman MA, Klein HG. Looking back in anger: retrospection in the face of a paradigm shift. *Transfus Med Rev* 1997;11:1–5.
3. Kleinman S. Transfusion safety decisions in the 1990s: reactions to the past. In: Smit Sibinga C, Alter H, eds. *Risk management in blood transfusion: the virtue of reality.* Kluwer Academic Publishers, 1999: 81–94.
4. Kleinman S. New variant Creutzfeldt-Jakob disease and white cell reduction: risk assessment and decision making in the absence of data [Editorial]. *Transfusion* 1999;39:920–924.
5. Perkins HA. Safety of the blood supply: making decisions in transfusion medicine. In: Nance SJ, ed. *Blood safety: current challenges.* Bethesda, MD: American Association of Blood Banks, 1992:125–150.
6. Kleinman S. Donor screening procedures and their role in enhancing transfusion safety. In: Smith D, Dodd RY, eds. *Transfusion transmitted infection.* Chicago: American Society of Clinical Pathologists, 1991: 207–242.
7. Krever, H. *Commission of inquiry on the blood system in Canada. Final report.* Ottawa: Canadian Government Publishing, 1997:994–1049.
8. Foster KR, Vecchia P, Repacholi MH. Science and the precautionary principle. *Science* 2000;2888:979–980.
9. Aubuchon JP, Kruskall MS. Transfusion safety: realigning efforts with risks. *Transfusion* 1997;37:1211–1216.
10. Debeir J, Noel L, Aullen JP, et al. The French Haemovigilance system. *Vox Sang* 1999;77:77–81.
11. Williamson LM. Systems contributing to the assurance of transfusion safety in the United Kingdom. *Vox Sang* 1999;77:82–87.
12. Busch M, Chamberland M, Epstein J, et al. Oversight and monitoring of blood safety in the United States. *Vox Sang* 1999;77:67–76.
13. Kleinman S. Transfusion safety when you don't know what you are looking for: issues related to emerging pathogens. In: Stramer S, ed. *Blood safety in the new millennium.* Bethesda, MD: American Association of Blood Banks, 2000.
14. Aach RD, Szmuness W, Mosley JW, et al. Serum alanine aminotransferase of donors in relation to the risk of non-A, non-B hepatitis in recipients. The transfusion-transmitted viruses study. *New Engl J Med* 1981;304:989–994.
15. Nelson KE, Donahue JG, Muñoz A, et al. Transmission of retroviruses from seronegative donors by transfusion during cardiac surgery. A multicenter study of HIV-1 and HTLV-I/II infections. *Ann Intern Med* 1992;117:554–559.
16. Alter HJ, Purcell RH, Holland PV, et al. Donor transaminase and recipient hepatitis. Impact on blood transfusion services. *JAMA* 1981; 246:630–634.
17. Alter HJ, Nakatsuji Y, Melpolder J, et al. The incidence of transfusion-associated hepatitis G virus infection and its relation to liver disease. *New Engl J Med* 1997;336:747–754.
18. Matsumoto A, Yeo AET, Shih JWK, et al. Transfusion-associated TT virus infection and its relationship to liver disease. *Hepatology* 1999; 30:283–288.
19. Donegan E, Stuart M, Niland JC, et al. Infection with human immunodeficiency virus type 1 (HIV-1) among recipients of antibody-positive blood donations. *Ann Intern Med* 1990;113:733–739.
20. Donegan E, Lee H, Operskalski EA, et al. Transfusion transmission of retroviruses: human T-lymphotropic viruses types I and II compared with human immunodeficiency virus type 1. *Transfusion* 1994;34: 478–483.
21. Zuck TF, Thomson RA, Schreiber GB, et al. The Retrovirus Epidemiology Donor Study (REDS): rationale and methods. *Transfusion* 1995;35:944–951.
22. Handa A, Dickstein B, Young NS, et al. Prevalence of the newly described human circovirus, TTV, in United States blood donors. *Transfusion* 2000;40:245–251.
23. Busch MP, Stramer SL, Kleinman SH. Evolving applications of nucleic acid amplification assays for prevention of virus transmission by blood components and derivatives. In: Garraty G, ed. *Applications of molecular biology in blood transfusion.* Bethesda, MD: American Association of Blood Banks, 1997:123–176.
24. Kleinman SH, Busch MP, Korelitz JJ, et al. The incidence/window period model and its use to assess the risk of transfusion-transmitted HIV and HCV infection. *Transfus Med Rev* 1997;11:155–172.
25. Kleinman S. Residual risk of transfusion transmitted viral infections in seronegative blood donors: application of the incidence/window period model. In: Brown F, Vyas G, eds. *Advances in transfusion safety.* Basel: S Karger 2000:61–66.
26. Busch MP, Satten GA. Time course of viremia and antibody seroconversion following primary HIV infection: implications for management of exposed health care workers. *Am J Med* 1997;102[Suppl 5B]: 117–124.
27. Schreiber GB, Busch MP, Kleinman SH, et al. The risk of transfusion-transmitted viral infections. *New Engl J Med* 1996;334:1685–1690.
28. Kleinman SH, Stramer SL, Mimms L, et al. Comparison of preliminary observed yield of HCV and HIV minipool nucleic acid testing with predictions from the incidence/window period model. *Transfusion* 2000;[Suppl S]:40(abst).
29. Aberle-Grasse JM, Dodd RY, Stramer SL. Recent trends in seroprevalence and incidence of HIV1/2, HCV, and HBV in US allogeneic blood donors *Transfusion* 2000;[Supplement:3S]:40(abst).
30. Korelitz JJ, Busch MP, Kleinman SH, et al. A method for estimating hepatitis B virus incidence rates in volunteer blood donors. *Transfusion* 1997;37:634.
31. Alter HJ, Purcell RH, Shih JW, et al: Detection of antibody to hepatitis C virus in prospectively followed transfusion recipients with acute and chronic non-A, non-B hepatitis. *New Engl J Med* 1989;321: 1494–1500.
32. Ling AE, Robbins KE, Brown TM, et al. Failure of routine HIV-1 tests in a case involving transmission with preseroconversion blood components during the infectious window period. *JAMA* 2000;284: 210–214.
33. Masuko K, Mitsui T, Iwano K, et al: Factors influencing postexposure immuno-prophylaxis of hepatitis B virus infection with hepatitis B immune globulin. High deoxyribonucleic acid polymerase activity in the inocula of unsuccessful cases. *Gastroenterology* 1982;82:502.
34. Okochi K, Satao H, Hinuma Y. A retrospective study on transmission of adult T cell leukemia virus by blood transfusion: seroconversion in recipients. *Vox Sang* 1984;46:245.
35. Busch MP, Watanabe KK, Smith JW, et al. for the Retrovirus Epidemiology Donor Study. False-negative testing errors in routine viral marker screening of blood donors. *Transfusion* 2000;40:585–589.
36. Brower WA, Nainan OV, Han X, et al. Duration of viremia in hepatitis A virus infection. *J Infect Dis* 2000;182:12–17.
37. Dodd RY. Adverse consequences of blood transfusion: quantitative risk estimates. In: Nance ST, ed. *Blood supply risks, perceptions and prospects for the future.* Bethesda, MD: American Association of Blood Banks, 1994:1–24.
38. Alter HJ. G-pers creepers, where'd you get those papers? A reassessment of the literature on the hepatitis G virus. *Transfusion* 1997;37:569–572.
39. Preiksaitas JK. The cytomegalovirus "safe" blood product: is leukore-

duction equivalent to antibody screening? *Transfus Med Rev* 2000;14: 112–136.
40. Bowden RA, Slichter SJ, Sayers M, et al. A comparison of filtered leukocyte-reduced and cytomegalovirus (CMV) seronegative blood products for the prevention of transplant-associated CMV infection after marrow transplant. *Blood* 1995;86:3598–3603.
41. Kedes DH, Operskalsi E, Busch P, et al. The seroepidemiology of human herpesvirus 8 (Kaposi's sarcoma associated herpesvirus): distribution of infection in KS risk groups and evidence for sexual transmission. *Nat Med* 1996;2:918–924.
42. Allain JP. Emerging viruses in blood transfusion. *Vox Sang* 1998; 74[Suppl 2]:125–129.
42a. Cannon MJ, Dollard SC, Smith DK, et al. Blood-borne and sexual transmission of human herpesvirus 8 in women with or at risk for human immunodeficiency virus infection. *N Engl J Med* 2001;344: 637–643.
43. Blackbourne DJ, Ambroziak J, Lennette E, et al. Infectious human herpesvirus 8 in a healthy North American blood donor. *Lancet* 1997; 349:609–611.
44. Koeningbauer UF, Eastland T, Day JW. Clinical illness due to parvovirus B19 infection after infusion of solvent/detergent-treated pooled plasma. *Transfusion* 2000;40:1203–1206.
45. Azzi A, Morfini M, Manucci M. The transfusion-associated transmission of Parvovirus B19. *Transfus Med Rev* 1999;13:194–204.
46. Guerrero IC, Weniger BC, Schultz MG. Transfusion malaria in the United States, 1972–1981. *Ann Intern Med* 1983;99:221.
47. Centers for Disease Control and Prevention. Transfusion-transmitted malaria—Missouri and Pennsylvania. *MMWR* 1999;48:253.
48. Leiby DA. Parasites and other emergent infectious agents. In Stramer S, ed. *Blood safety in the new millennium.* Bethesda, MD: American Association of Blood Banks, 2000.
49. Herwaldt BL, Kjememtrup AM, Conrad AM, et al. Transfusion transmitted babesiosis in northern Washington state: first reported case by a WA-1 type parasite. *J Infect Dis* 1997;175:1259–1262.
50. Leiby DA, Lenes BA, Tibbals MA, et al. Prospective evaluation of a patient with *Trypanosoma cruzi* infection transmitted by transfusion. *N Engl J Med* 1999;341:1237–1239.
51. Leiby DA, Read EJ, Lenes BA, et al. Seroepidemiology of *Trypanosoma cruzi,* etiologic agent of Chagas' disease, in US blood donors. *J Infect Dis* 1997;176:1047–1052.
52. Kuehnert MJ. Bacterial contamination of blood components: what is the problem, what is the solution? BaCon study update [Corporate evening]. Presented at the 53rd Annual Meeting of the American Association of Blood Banks, November 4–8, 2000, Washington, DC.
53. Lee JH. FDA's surveillance for bacterial safety of blood. Bacterial Contamination of Platelets Workshop, FDA/CBER. Sept 1999.
54. Ness P. Long-term review of septic outcome among platelet recipients. Bacterial contamination of blood components: what is the problem, what is the solution? BaCon study update [Corporate evening]. Presented at the 53rd Annual Meeting of the American Association of Blood Banks, November 4–8, 2000, Washington, DC.
55. Morel P. The French experience in the prevention of transfusion incidents due to bacterial contamination. Bacterial Contamination of Platelets Workshop, FDA/CBER. Sept 1999.
56. Blachjman MA. Overview of the magnitude and mechanisms of transfusion-associated bacterial sepsis. Bacterial Contamination of Platelets Workshop, FDA/CBER. Sept 1999.
57. Turner ML, Ludlum CA. Variant Creutzfeldt-Jakob disease. *Transfus Med Rev* 2000;14:216–224.
58. Goldman M, Juodvalkis S, Gill P, et al. Hepatitis C look-back. *Transfus Med Rev* 1998;12:84–93.
59. Operskalski EA, Stram DO, Lee H, et al. Human immunodeficiency virus type 1 infection: relationship of risk group and age to rate of progression to AIDS. *J Infect Dis* 1995;172:648–655.
60. Seeff LB. Why is there such difficulty in defining the natural history of hepatitis C? *Transfusion* 2000;40:1161–1164.
61. Seeff LB, Beebe GW, Hoofnagle JH, et al. A serologic follow-up of the 1942 epidemic of post-vaccination hepatitis in the United States Army. *New Engl J Med* 1991;316:965–970.
62. Murphy EL, Fridey J, Smith JW, et al. HTLV-associated myelopathy in a cohort of HTLV-I and HTLV-II-infected blood donors. *Neurology* 1997;48:315–320.
63. United States General Accounting Office. Blood supply: transfusion-associated risks. GAO/PEMD-97-2, Washington, DC, 1997.
64. Tabor E. The epidemiology of virus transmission by plasma derivatives: clinical studies verifying the lack of transmission of hepatitis B and C viruses and HIV-1. *Transfusion* 1999;39:1160–1168.
65. Tabor E, Yu MW, Hewlitt I, et al. Summary of a workshop on the implementation of NAT to screen donors of blood and plasma for viruses. *Transfusion* 2000;40:1273–1275.
66. Richardson LS, Evatt BL. Risk of hepatitis A virus infection in persons with hemophilia receiving plasma derived products. *Transfus Med Rev* 2000;14:64–73.
67. Drohan WN, Cervenekova L. Safety of blood products: are transmissible spongiform encephalopathies (prion diseases) a risk? *Thromb Haemost* 1999;82:486–493.
68. Klein HG, Dodd RY, Dzik WH, et al. Current status of solvent/detergent-treated detergent plasma. *Transfusion* 1998;38:102–107.
69. Linden JV, Wagner K, Voytovich AE, et al. Transfusion errors in New York state: an analysis of 10 years' experience. *Transfusion* 2000;40: 1207–1213.
70. Lee DH, Paling JE, Blajchman MA. A new tool for communicating transfusion risk information. *Transfusion* 1998;38:184–188.
71. Menitove JE. Perception of risk. In: Nance ST, ed. *Blood supply risks, perceptions and prospects for the future.* Bethesda, MD: American Association of Blood Banks, 1994:45–59.
72. Slovic P. Perception of risk. *Science* 1987;236:280.
73. Finucane ML, Slovic P, Mertz CK. Public perception of the risk of blood transfusion. *Transfusion* 2000;40:1017–1022.
74. Klein HG. Will blood transfusion ever be safe enough? [Editorial] *JAMA* 2000;284:238–240.
75. Wallace EL, Churchill WH, Surgenor DM, et al. Collection and transfusion of blood and blood components in the United States, 1994. *Transfusion* 1998;38:625–636.
76. Wallace EL, Churchill WH, Surgenor DM, et al. Collection and transfusion of blood and blood components in the United States, 1992. *Transfusion* 1995;35:802–812.
77. Goodnugh LT, Brecher ME, Kanter MH, et al. Transfusion medicine. *New Engl J Med* 1999;340:438–447.

Rossi's Principles of Transfusion Medicine, Third Edition, edited by Toby L. Simon, Walter H. Dzik, Edward L. Snyder, Christopher P. Stowell, and Ronald G. Strauss. Lippincott Williams & Wilkins, Philadelphia © 2002.

49

TRANSFUSION-TRANSMITTED HEPATITIS C AND NON-A, NON-B, NON-C VIRUS INFECTIONS

HARVEY J. ALTER

After more than a decade of virologic and serologic frustration, the nature of the non-A, non-B hepatitis virus (NANBV) yielded to the sophisticated approaches of molecular biology. Although it has still not been definitively visualized, the primary agent of NANB hepatitis has been cloned, its molecular sequence has been unraveled, and expressed epitopes now serve as the basis for highly specific serologic assays routinely used for blood donor screening. This agent has been designated the *hepatitis C virus* (HCV) and is responsible for at least 90% of cases of transfusion-associated hepatitis (TAH). A marked reduction in the incidence of TAH has been observed since the introduction of screening assays to detect antibody to HCV. This virus-specific antibody assay combined with existing sensitive assays for the detection of the hepatitis B virus (HBV), the recent addition of routine nucleic acid testing (NAT) for HCV RNA, the routine use of viral inactivation procedures for pooled plasma products, and the possible use of viral inactivation for cellular products presages the final days of TAH.

H.J. Alter: Department of Transfusion Medicine, National Institutes of Health, Bethesda, Maryland.

DEFINITIONS

In the mid 1970s, it was recognized that the major cause of TAH was neither the hepatitis A virus (HAV) nor HBV, and the term *non-A, non-B hepatitis* was coined and persisted much longer than anticipated. Non-A, non-B hepatitis was defined according to biochemical evidence of hepatic inflammation and the clinical and serologic exclusion of other viral and nonviral causes of hepatocellular injury. Reproducible elevations in transaminase levels, associated or not associated with clinical disease, served as the foundation for the diagnosis if there was no discernible nonviral etiologic factor and if serologic tests for HAV, HBV, cytomegalovirus (CMV), and Epstein-Barr virus (EBV) showed no evidence of recent seroconversion. The diagnosis was imprecise, and undoubtedly a proportion of the cases classified as NANB hepatitis represented other unrecognized viral or nonviral etiologic factors. Despite this inaccuracy, there was an unequivocal form of viral hepatitis unrelated to the four viruses (HAV, HBV, CMV, EBV) generally associated with hepatitis among humans. Studies with the chimpanzee model proved that NANB hepatitis was caused by a transmissible agent (1,2). Before HCV was cloned, NANB hepatitis was characterized by several distinct clinical and pathologic features, particularly progression to chronic liver disease and induction of characteristic ultrastructural tubules in the livers of infected chimpanzees (3). The NANB hepatitis agent was biophysically characterized as small (<60 mm) and lipid encapsulated (4,5). The agent with these physical characteristics was subsequently cloned and shown to be an RNA virus of approximately 9,500 bases (6) coding for approximately 3,000 amino acids. This small lipid-enveloped RNA virus has been designated *hepatitis C virus* (HCV) and classified in the family Flaviviridae.

A problem in nomenclature exists because there are cases that have been clinically defined as NANB hepatitis that are negative for HCV serologic markers and lack HCV RNA in the polymerase chain reaction (PCR). These instances might be attributed to a different NANB virus (non-A, non-B, non-C), be due to a known hepatitis agent the presence of which is below the detection limit of current assays, or be nonviral in origin. In this chapter, the term *non-A, non-B virus* (NANBV) designates the agent described in studies conducted before the cloning of HCV. *Hepatitis C virus* (HCV) denotes the serologically and molecularly defined agent. *NANBV/HCV* is used to discuss this class of hepatitis agents generically, with the understanding that 80% to 90% of NANBV-related hepatitis is caused by HCV. *Hepatitis C* denotes the disease specifically caused by HCV, and *non-A, non-B, non-C hepatitis* (or *non-A–E*) relates to hepatitis of presumed viral causation in which no established hepatitis virus can be serologically or molecularly implicated.

SPECTRUM OF NON-A, NON-B HEPATITIS

In the absence of a specific serologic marker, NANB hepatitis became a catchall for a variety of hepatocellular, inflammatory processes that lacked serologic evidence of HAV or HBV infection. The entity NANB hepatitis evolved from prospective studies of TAH and the observation that a relatively high percentage of patients had elevations in transaminase levels after transfusion that were not attributable to underlying disease, medication, or other forms of viral hepatitis (7). Until the development of the HCV assay, transfusion was the primary arena of diagnosis of NANB hepatitis. Subsequently, cases fulfilling the exclusion criteria for NANB hepatitis were observed in other settings, including community-acquired NANB hepatitis and epidemic or enterically transmitted NANB hepatitis. Community-acquired (sporadic) NANB hepatitis has been investigated extensively in prospective studies conducted in four selected (sentinel) counties in the United States (8). The sentinel counties studies initially revealed that among patients with clinically overt NANB hepatitis, only 15% gave a history of previous blood transfusion, 25% used intravenous drugs, fewer than 10% were in health-related fields or had a presumed sexual or household contact, and more than 50% had no known route of exposure to this agent. More recent evaluations (9) have shown that fewer than 1% of cases of community-acquired hepatitis are related to transfusion. Hepatitis C virus is the principal agent of community-acquired NANB hepatitis, as it is for TAH. The clinical course of acute hepatitis C and its progression to chronic hepatitis appear to be independent of the presumed source of exposure. The precise routes of nonparenteral transmission of NANBV/HCV remain an enigma even in the face of sensitive serologic assays for HCV.

There is evidence that HCV, like HBV and the acquired human immunodeficiency virus (HIV), has a sexual and perinatal, as well as parenteral, route of transmission. However, HCV is much less efficiently spread by these nonparenteral routes than are HBV and HIV.

An epidemic form of NANB hepatitis has resulted in massive outbreaks, most prominently in India, other parts of the Asian subcontinent, and South America (10,11). These explosive outbreaks are waterborne and epidemiologically resemble HAV infection, but they are serologically and to some degree clinically distinct. Particles ranging from 27 to 38 nm have been associated with the epidemic form of NANBH, and a specific serologic assay has been developed (12). The patients do not have antibodies to HCV, and the hepatitis is now known to be caused by a distinct RNA virus designated *hepatitis E virus* (HEV). The characterized human hepatitis viruses thus range from A to E, including HAV (infectious), HBV (serum), HCV (former NANBV), HDV (δ agent), and HEV (enterically transmitted NANBH).

It has been suggested that some cases of NANB hepatitis represent a seronegative variant or cryptic form of HBV infection (13). Previous evidence indicating the absence of immunologic cross-protection between HBV and NANBV, along with more recent evidence that HCV is an RNA rather than a DNA virus, rules out a virologic relation between HCV and HBV. It is possible, however, that some cases of NANB hepatitis that are negative for HCV markers actually represent HBV infection in which the usual HBV markers are not expressed. At most, this would account for a small proportion of cases of NANB hepatitis.

HEPATITIS C VIRUS

Historical Perspective

Before HCV was cloned, a considerable amount was learned about this agent from experiments with chimpanzees. In 1978, it was found that serum from patients with acute or chronic NANB hepatitis and that from asymptomatic carriers could transmit NANBV infection to chimpanzees (1,2). Although they did not have clinical illness, the chimpanzees had small elevations in transaminase levels and had liver biopsy evidence of hepatitis after an appropriate incubation period. Animals inoculated with serum from patients with NANB hepatitis did not develop HBV markers. This finding emphasized the clear distinction between HBV and the agent of NANB hepatitis. In addition to elevations in transaminase levels, infected chimpanzees generally had characteristic tubular ultrastructures in hepatocyte cytoplasm (3). These tubular structures, consisting of an electron-dense center and a double-unit membrane, represent proliferation of the rough endoplasmic reticulum, a change now shown to be induced by interferon. The tubules are an epiphenomenon of NANBV/HCV infection and in chimpanzees are useful indicators of such infection because of their relative specificity. They are not induced during the course of HAV or HBV infection and are not seen in human NANBV/HCV infection.

The findings of elevation of transaminase levels, light microscopic changes of hepatocellular damage, and electron microscopic evidence of cytoplasmic tubules made it possible to define NANB hepatitis in chimpanzees, even in the absence of a specific serologic marker. These findings led to the finding that the cytoplasmic tubule-inducing agent was sensitive to chloroform and other lipid solvents and that it contained essential lipid, presumably in its surface membrane (5,14). Filtration studies subsequently showed that the NANB agent was 30 to 60 nm in diameter (4). Among known viruses, only the flaviviruses (formerly called *togaviruses*), the hepadnaviruses (HBV, woodchuck hepatitis virus, duck hepatitis virus), and the δ agent are lipid encapsulated and fall into this size range. It was predicted that the NANB agent was a flavivirus. The subsequent cloning and characterization of HCV (6) proved this prediction correct.

Flaviviruses are a large and diverse family, formerly known as arboviruses (arthropod-borne viruses) and togaviruses. They include the dengue and yellow fever viruses, the Rubivirus (rubella), and the pestiviruses (bovine diarrheal virus, hog cholera virus, and other mucosal disease viruses of animals). It is now considered that HCV represents a new genus in the family Flaviviridae and that it is most closely related to pestiviruses. Although there is only limited homology with the pestiviruses, the genomic structure and hydrophobicity patterns are similar. The pestiviruses, like HCV, are characterized by blood-borne transmission and by lifelong viremia. Unlike dengue and yellow fever viruses, they do not have a mosquito vector.

Cloning and Molecular Characterization

In 1988, a long series of experiments conducted by Houghton et al. at the Chiron Corporation, in collaboration with Bradley at the Centers for Disease Control, culminated in the cloning and serologic characterization of HCV (6). Using large volumes of plasma derived from a chimpanzee with chronic NANB hepatitis, these investigators extracted whole nucleic acid and made complementary DNA (cDNA) from RNA and single-stranded DNA templates. The cDNA then was inserted into a gt11-phage expression vector and used to infect *Escherichia coli.* Expressed proteins were blotted and overlaid with serum from patients with NANB hepatitis. A single clone was identified that expressed an antigen reactive with chronic- and convalescent-phase serum from persons with NANB hepatitis but not with serum from control subjects without infection or from patients with type A or type B hepatitis (6). Cloned nucleic acid was used to generate probes that were shown hybridized with RNA derived from the starting plasma, thus closing the loop between the cloned agent and the infectious plasma. Once the cloned agent of NANB hepatitis was molecularly characterized, it was designated *hepatitis C virus.* Amplification of the reactive clones and later expression of the genome in large cultures of yeast produced sufficient antigen to formulate radioimmune and enzyme-linked assays for the detection of antibody to HCV.

Characterization of HCV indicated that the viral genome consists of single-stranded, linear RNA of 9.6 kb that is positively stranded and hence can serve directly as message for the synthesis of viral proteins (6,15). The viral proteins are encoded from a single, large open reading frame that produces a polyprotein that is posttranslationally cleaved (15). The genome is characterized by a highly conserved, untranslated region at the 5′ terminus (5′UTR) that is now used as the primary target for molecular amplification assays to detect HCV RNA and for viral genotyping. The 5′UTR contains an internal ribosomal entry site that is essential for viral protein synthesis and that initiates translation at the start codon of the large open reading frame (15). Downstream of the 5′UTR are the coding regions for envelope proteins designated E1 and E2, followed by the coding region for the viral core (nucleocapsid). In the terminal portion of the E1 region is a hypervariable segment (HVR1), which is the most highly mutable region of the genome, presumably because its position in the viral envelope places it under a high degree of immune pressure. It is presumed that this region is the target for neutralizing antibody responses, but such antibodies have been difficult to measure. Downstream from the structural genomic regions are a series of nonstructural coding regions designated NS2, NS3, NS4, and NS5. The full function of these regions is not known, but they have been shown to code for critical enzymes, including an NS3 protease, an NS3 helicase, and an NS5 polymerase.

Evidence of Multiple Non-A, Non-B Hepatitis Agents

Evidence for the existence of more than one NANB hepatitis agent initially derived from clinical observation of more than one episode of HBV- and HAV-negative hepatitis occurring in the same patient (16) and the observation that some episodes of NANB hepatitis among persons with hemophilia occurred after an unusually short incubation period (17). Results of initial chimpanzee cross-challenge studies further supported the existence of two NANB agents (18). One of these agents proved to be HCV, and the other is still undefined (see later). Further confounding the issue of whether there are NANB agents in addition to HCV is the observation in chimpanzees that animals can sustain more than one episode of HCV infection (19). Thus what appeared to be two episodes of NANB hepatitis caused by two distinct agents may instead have been two distinct episodes of hepatitis C. Nonetheless, 10% to 30% of cases of chronic NANB hepatitis cannot be accounted for by HCV infection, and most cases of fulminant hepatitis and hepatitis-associated aplastic anemia appear to be unrelated to hepatitis viruses A, B, or C. This finding suggests the existence of an additional, as yet undefined, agent of hepatitis among humans.

Encouraged by the blind cloning of HCV, investigators have used sophisticated molecular approaches to search for the agent or agents of non-A, non-B, non-C hepatitis. The findings have led to the sequential discovery of the GB virus (GBV), the hepatitis G virus (HGV), the TT virus, and the SEN virus. None of these agents has yet been proved a hepatitis virus, but each has been shown to be transmitted by transfusion and to result in persistent infection in some recipients of blood. The GB agent derives from the blood of a surgeon (G.B.) who in the 1950s contracted acute icteric hepatitis. Inoculation of GB serum into marmosets reproducibly caused hepatitis, but controversy arose about whether this represented transmission of a human hepatitis agent or activation of a latent marmoset hepatitis virus. The controversy was never resolved. Decades later, investigators at Abbott Laboratories analyzed frozen samples that had been collected during serial passages in the marmoset model. Using representational difference analysis to compare preinoculation and postinoculation marmoset serum (20), the investigators identified unique nucleic acid sequences in the postinoculation specimens (21). Sequencing of the full genome identified three distinct GB agents that were designated *GBV-A, GBV-B,* and *GBV-C* (21). The genomic structure identified these agents as in the Flaviviridae family, but the agents showed little homology to HCV or other members of that family. Extensive population studies, studies involving patients with and without liver disease and studies of marmosets established that GBV-A was a primary marmoset agent, that GBV-C was a human virus, and that GBV-B might be able to infect both species.

In independent investigations, Gene Labs, in collaboration with investigators at the National Institutes of Health and the Centers for Disease Control and Prevention, used sequence-independent single primer amplification to identify what was considered a novel hepatitis agent and called the agent *hepatitis G virus* (22). Subsequent sequence comparisons revealed that GBV-C and HGV were essentially the same agent and represented strain variants of this new member of the Flaviviridae family. Although GBV-C/HGV was found unequivocally transfusion-transmitted, extensive clinical studies did not show a causal relation between the presence of the virus and the development of hepatitis (23). The designation HGV now appears a misnomer. It would be better to refer to this agent as the *GB virus* because that designation does not infer causality.

In 1997, Nishizawa et al. (24) in Japan used representational difference analysis to compare prehepatitis and posthepatitis serum from 5 patients with TAH. A unique viral clone was found in 3 of the 5 cases of TAH studied, and viral titers generally correlated with the level of alanine aminotransferase (ALT). The presumed virus was designated *TT virus* after the initials of the person with the index case. Biophysical characterization (25) suggested that TT virus was a novel, 3,700 bp, nonenveloped, circular, single-stranded human DNA virus most closely related to Circoviridae, a family of plant and animal viruses not previously associated with human disease (26). The TT virus family is highly divergent; at least 16 genotypes have been identified.

The TT virus has been reported to replicate in the liver, according to results of PCR detection and in situ hybridization studies (27). There were no morphologic changes in the liver cells that showed hybridization signals, and there was no correlation between the percentage of TT virus–infected hepatocytes and the histologic activity index or its composite scores. Although the TT virus can infect liver cells, it may not cause hepatitis.

Epidemiologic studies have shown that TT virus is transmitted by both parenteral and enteral routes. The original studies of TT virus suggested a relation to acute and chronic liver disease (24), but subsequent studies with inclusive primers that targeted conserved sequences showed an exceedingly high background prevalence (93%) and thus established that most persons with TT virus infection did not have hepatitis (28).

Matsumoto et al. (29) studied TT virus infection in the transfusion setting using the more restrictive primers used in the original publications. The background prevalence in the volunteer U.S. donor population was 7.5%. The key finding of this NIH study was that the frequency of transfusion-associated TT virus infection was identical among patients with non-A–E hepatitis (23%) and control patients who did not have hepatitis (22%). Overall, fewer than 4% of cases of TT virus infection were associated with hepatitis, and there was poor correlation between TT virus DNA levels and ALT levels. Hence, as had occurred in investigations with HGV, the NIH prospective series did not support a causal association between TT virus infection and posttransfusion hepatitis. However, there are caveats to the interpretation that the TT virus lacks pathogenicity in that the agent may cause disease in only a small number of persons with infection who have particular host susceptibility factors or that there may be particular TT virus variants that are pathogenic while the wild-type virus is not.

Many other isolates subsequently were identified in the TT virus family, including agents designated *SANBAN, YONBAN,* and *TLMV* (30). Each of these agents is phylogenetically distant from the prototype TT virus agent and shows only 50% to 60% sequence homology. Unlike in HCV, variants of which primarily represent strain differences of 1% to 2% (quasispecies) or genotypes diverging by approximately 15%, in the TT virus family, sequence differences between variants frequently exceed 30% and sometimes exceed 50%. These differences are so great that the agents, although linked by common biophysical characteristics, may have totally different clinical spectrums and disease associations.

A virus detection program conducted by the Diasorin Corporation uncovered what was at the time considered a novel infectious agent. It was designated *SEN virus* for the initials of the patient in whom it was initially found. Like TT virus, SEN virus proved to be a small, nonenveloped, circular, single-stranded DNA virus (31). The SEN virus represented a subfamily of very heterogeneous agents differing in nucleotide sequences by 15% to 50% from each other and by 40% to 60% from the prototype TT virus sequence. The SEN virus is now considered a member of the TT virus family Circoviridae.

The clinical significance of SEN virus is uncertain. At the NIH, two SEN virus variants, designated *SENV-D* and *SENV-H,* have been studied. SENV-D and H were found in 1.5% to 2% of volunteer donors and were shown to be transfusion transmitted. They were present in 40% of 155 subjects who underwent transfusion but in only 3% of 97 control subjects who did not undergo transfusion ($P < .0001$) (32). A significant relation of infection to transfusion volume was observed, and donor-recipient linkage was established by means of sequencing. It is noteworthy that new SEN virus infections occurred in 3% of patients who did not receive transfusions. This finding suggested that, as with TT virus, there was nosocomial transmission or reactivation of latent virus.

In the NIH prospective study of transfusion-associated hepatitis (32), 13 cases of non-A–E hepatitis were found. One of these patients was infected with SEN virus before transfusion. Among the remaining 12 susceptible recipients, 11 (92%) became SENV-D or SENV-H positive after transfusion. There was a good, though imperfect, temporal association between the level of virus and the level of elevation of ALT value. In contrast, acute SEN virus infection was found in 24% of patients who underwent transfusion who did not have hepatitis ($P < .0001$).

Despite the strong statistical link to cases of transfusion-associated non-A–E hepatitis, it was projected that no more than 5% of cases of SEN virus infection were accompanied by biochemical evidence of hepatitis. If SEN virus is a hepatitis agent, it causes disease in only a small number of persons with infection, the difference perhaps depending on host susceptibility, viral load, or immune responsiveness. A parallel can be drawn to viruses such as CMV or EBV that also cause disease in only a small number of persons with infection.

Long-term follow-up study of a subset of 31 patients with either SEN virus infection alone or SEN virus/HCV coinfection showed that the virus was cleared within 1 year in 61% and within 5 years in 87% of cases. The infection persisted more than 10 years in 6% of cases (32). Two of the 11 patients (18%) with acute SEN virus–associated hepatitis had persistent infection with biochemical evidence of chronic hepatitis. In separate studies, there has been no significant association between SEN virus infection and acute liver failure or cryptogenic cases of chronic hepatitis, cirrhosis, or hepatocellular carcinoma (HCC). It is important to emphasize that the statistical association between SEN virus infection and transfusion-associated hepatitis does not establish causality. There is currently no proof that either GB virus, TT virus, or SEN virus represents the elusive agent of non-A, non-B, non-C (non-A–E) hepatitis.

INCIDENCE OF TRANSFUSION-ASSOCIATED NON-A, NON-B HEPATITIS

The incidence of TAH in the United States was formerly based on data from prospective studies, but as the incidence decreased to rates less than 1%, it became logistically and economically unfeasible to conduct prospective studies with sufficiently large numbers of subjects to achieve a statistically valid incidence. The incidence of TAH is now derived from mathematical modeling based on the incidence of HBV and HCV infection among donors who repeatedly give blood and estimates of the window period between exposure to these agents and the first detectable marker of infection in recipients. The switch to mathematical models is a reflection of the success of blood bank programs at interdicting donors with high-risk behavior or those with serologic or molecular markers of hepatitis virus infection.

Before mathematical modeling was used, determination of the incidence of TAH required performance of prospective studies to find biochemical evidence of liver disease because 75% of cases of TAH are clinically inapparent and because fewer than 10% of overt cases are reported to blood banks. Before 1970, a prospective study at the NIH with patients undergoing open-heart surgery (33) showed that the incidence of TAH exceeded 30%. The introduction of an all-volunteer donor system and first-generation assays for hepatitis B surface antigen (HBsAg) dramatically reduced the incidence of TAH to the range of 10% to 12%. That incidence persisted through the 1970s despite increasingly sensitive tests for HBsAg but declined to the 6% to 10% range through the mid 1980s (33). By 1988, the cumulative effect of more stringent donor questioning regarding high-risk behaviors, the introduction of HIV testing and surrogate marker testing for NANBH, the routine viral inactivation of plasma products, and the more judicious use of blood in wake of the epidemic of acquired immunodeficiency syndrome (AIDS) served to decrease the incidence of TAH to approximately 4% (33). The introduction of specific anti-HCV assays in 1990 led to a further marked decline in the incidence of TAH to approximately 1%. Testing of stored donor and recipient serum revealed that first-generation anti-HCV assays could have prevented 80% of cases of TAH that occurred before 1990 and that second-generation assays, introduced in 1992, could have prevented 90% of cases of TAH (34). On the basis of the prevalence of HCV in the donor population in 1990, it is estimated that the introduction of anti-HCV testing prevented 40,500 cases of hepatitis per year (111 cases per day) in the United States alone.

The results of the NIH prospective study indicated that the incidence of TAH had decreased to less than 1% by 1995 and that the incidence of transfusion-associated hepatitis C approached zero by 1997 (33), a remarkable decline from rates that exceeded 30% in the 1960s. It also is apparent that clotting factor concentrates have been rendered almost hepatitis virus free by the combination of donor screening and a spectrum of inactivation procedures, including heat and solvent-detergent treatment.

Mathematical modeling conducted before the implementation of routine NAT of donor blood estimated the risk of HCV transmission to be 1 case per 100,000 transfusions and the risk of HBV transmission to range from 1 in 65,000 to 1 in 150,000 transfusions. After the implementation of minipool NAT testing, the calculated risk of HCV infection was 1 in 300,000 to 1 in 625,000. Individual unit NAT testing will decrease that risk further but will not have a dramatic effect on HCV transmission. Nucleic acid testing for HBV has not been implemented as of this writing, but individual NAT for HBV should decrease the current seronegative window by 25 days and bring the risk of HBV infection into the same range as the risk of HCV infection.

CLINICAL SPECTRUM OF HEPATITIS C VIRUS INFECTION

Acute Manifestations

As is apparent from results of prospective studies, only 25% of cases of NANB/HCV hepatitis manifest as jaundice or substantial clinical symptoms; the remaining cases are detected only through biochemical abnormalities, primarily elevations of ALT level. Long-term observation has revealed that these mild cases have the same propensity to evolve into chronic liver disease, including cirrhosis, as do the more overt cases. Thus silent TAH may have major clinical significance. Although patients with HCV rarely have sufficient symptoms to seek medical care, some have chronic fatigue syndrome or other low-grade morbidity that deleteriously alters their lifestyle. In addition, individual cases can be acutely severe and even fulminant. Although fulminant hepatitis is an exceedingly rare complication of hepatitis C, many cases of fulminant hepatitis are thought to be etiologically related to a non-A, non-B, non-C hepatitis agent.

Three major patterns of elevation of ALT level have been observed in NANB/HCV hepatitis—monophasic, polyphasic (fluctuating), and plateau (35). The monophasic pattern involves a single acute phase peak followed by complete normalization of ALT level. The polyphasic pattern is the most characteristic and includes dramatic fluctuations of ALT level over brief intervals. Over time, the amplitude of the fluctuation diminishes, but the periodicity persists into chronicity. In the plateau pattern, a relatively constant and generally low-level ALT abnormality is observed in the acute and chronic phases of the disease. Such patients often have biopsy evidence of chronic liver disease early in the posttransfusion course. These patterns have prognostic implications. In one study (35), 42% of patients with a monophasic peak contracted chronic hepatitis, compared with 87% of patients with the fluctuating pattern and 95% of patients with the plateau pattern. Levels of ALT occasionally normalize for prolonged intervals that suggest recovery but are followed months to years later by secondary elevations that indicate the presence of chronic liver disease. This prolonged normalization of ALT level followed by recrudescence makes it difficult to ascertain when, or if, recovery from NANB/HCV infection truly has occurred. The best current assessment of recovery from HCV infection is serial measurement of HCV RNA. Three negative determinations of HCV RNA over the course of 3 to 6 months generally connote sustained clearance of the virus and full recovery from the infection.

Chronic Sequelae

The most important component of HCV infection is its ability to evolve into chronic hepatitis, cirrhosis, and more rarely, HCC. Long-term follow-up evaluation of transfusion-associated cases indicates that at least 50% of patients contract chronic hepatitis evidenced by elevations in ALT level that persist longer than 1 year. More recent data indicate that chronic hepatitis may occur in nearly 70% of cases. Similar frequencies of chronic hepatitis have been documented among community-acquired cases of hepatitis C.

In eight early studies, 339 patients with transfusion-associated NANBH underwent prospective observation (36); 47% had biochemical evidence of chronic hepatitis. Of 102 patients who underwent biopsy, 41% had chronic active hepatitis and 20% had cirrhosis; 5 of the 20 patients with cirrhosis died of liver disease. Subsequent studies in which serial liver biopsies were performed provided unequivocal documentation of the progression of histologic abnormalities from acute to chronic hepatitis to cirrhosis (37–40). In summary, numerous studies in which the subjects were transfusion recipients have revealed the following: (a) at least 50% of patients with acute hepatitis C eventually have biochemical evidence of chronic hepatitis; (b) approximately 20% of patients with chronic hepatitis C have biopsy evidence of cirrhosis; and (c) progression from acute hepatitis to cirrhosis can be documented histologically and generally evolves slowly over the course of decades but sometimes can occur in only a few years, the mean time to the development of cirrhosis being approximately 20 years; (d) the progression to cirrhosis is enhanced in patients with HCV infection who abuse alcohol—the cumulative effect of alcohol and HCV infection is more than additive, and the risk of cirrhosis may be 15-fold higher among persons who abuse alcohol than among persons with HCV infection alone (41); (e) when HCC occurs, it is almost always in patients with established cirrhosis—the risk of development of HCC among patients with cirrhosis has been estimated to be 1.7% per year (42).

Untoward occurrences among recipients of standard blood transfusion are exaggerated in recipients of clotting factor concentrates. Before recent inactivation procedures were developed, such concentrates, derived from massive pools of paid blood donors, were invariably contaminated with HBV and HCV. Overall, more than 50% of patients with hemophilia have ALT elevations and serologic results that suggest chronic hepatitis C (43). That proportion increases to 80% among severe patients with hemophilia who receive clotting factor concentrates before viral inactivation (44). In a landmark multicenter study (44), liver biopsy specimens from 155 patients with hemophilia and chronic elevations in ALT level had cirrhosis in 15% and severe chronic active hepatitis, likely to progress to cirrhosis, in an additional 7%. Similar severe outcomes were found in a subsequent prospective study in England (45) wherein 71% of 79 patients with hemophilia had persistent abnormalities in ALT level, 25% of the 34 patients who underwent biopsy had cirrhosis, and 12% had radiographic evidence of esophageal varices. One patient died of complications of portal hypertension. Before AIDS, chronic liver disease accounted for 5% to 11% of deaths of patients with hemophilia. The advent of AIDS has further complicated the course of hepatitis C in this population. It is now evident that HIV infection accelerates the course and increases the severity of coexistent HCV infection (46). Now that patients with HIV infection have long survival periods because of highly active anti-retroviral therapy, severe liver disease is emerging as a major cause of morbidity and mortality among patients with HCV and HIV infection.

In Japan, where hepatitis C is common and where a similar progression from acute to chronic hepatitis has been well documented, it has been possible to examine the role of blood transfusion in the development of chronic liver disease. Kiyosawa et al. (47) found that among patients with chronic hepatitis and cirrhosis, presumably related to NANBH, 44% and 38% of patients, respectively, had a history of previous transfusion. In NANBV-related chronic liver disease, a history of previous transfusion was 6 to 12 times more frequent than in HBV-related disease. This finding suggested a causal relation in the former, but less so in the latter, whereby the virus tends to be transmitted more readily by sexual and maternal-fetal routes. Another important observation in the study by Kiyosawa et al. was the long interval between transfusion and the first clinical manifestations of chronic liver disease. The mean interval from transfusion to the clinical recognition of chronic hepatitis was 11.3 years; to the development of overt cirrhosis, 21.2 years; and to the development of clinically apparent HCC, 29.0 years (47). These long intervals may account for the apparent disparity between the number of expected cases of transfusion-associated cirrhosis and the number of cases actually detected. Because patients who undergo transfusion tend to be elderly, many die of underlying illness before chronic liver disease becomes clinically evident. Such intercurrent deaths obscure the course of this slowly evolving disease and mask the possible effect of NANB/HCV-related chronic hepatitis and cirrhosis on younger blood recipients.

Infection with HCV can unequivocally lead to HCC (48).

In a composite of prospective studies, it appears that the incidence of HCV-associated HCC is 1% to 5%. The rate of HCC is relatively low in Western nations and relatively high in Japan. Okuda et al. (49) conducted a study with 113 patients with nonalcoholic HCC. They found that 69% of the cases of HCC were HBsAg negative and presumably related to NANB/HCV infection. This finding was subsequently supported by results of serology testing for HCV that showed anti-HCV antibody in as many as 70% of patients with HBsAg-negative HCC (50).

The long-term consequences of transfusion-associated hepatitis were comprehensively studied by Seeff et al. (51). Patients who had TAH in five major prospective studies conducted in the 1970s were traced after a mean interval of 18 years and prospectively evaluated for evidence of chronic hepatitis. Over this interval, there was no increase in overall mortality among patients who sustained an episode of TAH compared with controls who underwent transfusion who did not have an episode of TAH. Although the mortality was not different, 35% of patients with previous episodes of hepatitis had biochemical and histologic evidence of chronic hepatitis; 1% of controls did so. The results of this study have now been updated to a mean follow-up period of 23 years (52). Overall mortality was similar among patients with hepatitis cases and control subjects without hepatitis, but patients with hepatitis had a small but significant increase in liver-related mortality (4.1% versus 1.3%; $P = .05$). Among 103 patients with positive results for anti-HCV in 1974, 76% were still anti-HCV positive and HCV RNA–positive approximately 20 years later. An additional 17% had specific anti-HCV antibody but no longer had viremia. This finding suggested they had spontaneously cleared the infection. A surprising finding was that 7% of patients had no residual markers of HCV infection. This finding suggested these patients not only had cleared the virus but also had lost anti-HCV antibodies. Hence prevalence estimations based on serologic status may be slight underestimates of the extent of HCV infection in the population. More important, this study showed that the spontaneous clearance rate of HCV infection may exceed the commonly accepted estimate of 15% and actually be between 20% and 25%. In a separate study of longer duration, Seeff et al. (53) found that only 1 of 17 persons with HCV infection died of liver disease in the nearly 50 years after their HCV infection had first been documented.

Milder outcomes of HCV infection have been observed in studies of blood donors who did not have symptoms. In an NIH study (54), it was found that 15% of donors appeared to have spontaneously cleared HCV infection on the basis of the presence of recombinant immunoblot assay (RIBA)–confirmed anti-HCV and repeatedly negative determinations for HCV RNA. Among those with persistent HCV infection, the peak ALT level exceeded two times the upper limit of normal in only 16%, and clinical symptoms were minimal. Liver biopsy was performed on 94 patients. No patients had severe inflammatory changes, 13% had stage 3 of 4 fibrosis, and only 2% had cirrhosis after an average duration of infection of 19 years on the basis of a defined parenteral exposure. Repeated liver biopsies were performed 5 years later on 60 of these patients. Fibrosis progression over that interval was minimal; no new cases of cirrhosis were found even when the follow-up was extended to a mean of 24 years (55).

Three additional long-term outcome studies are of importance. Kenny-Walsh et al. (56) performed a 17 year follow-up study with 376 women with HCV infection from a contaminated lot of Rh immune globulin. Liver biopsies were performed on 363 patients a mean of 17 years after exposure. Only 4% had moderate to severe grades of inflammation (histologic activity index, 9 to 18). Periportal fibrosis (stage 1) was found in 34% of patients; bridging fibrosis (stage 3), a potential precirrhotic lesion, was found in 15%; cirrhosis in only 2%; and no fibrosis in 49%. Two of seven patients with cirrhosis also had a history of alcohol abuse. A similar study in Germany with 152 women with infection from Rh immune globulin (57) showed that none had cirrhosis or severe degrees of inflammation or fibrosis after a mean follow-up period of 15 years. Last, a 20-year follow-up study (58) of children with HCV infection showed a surprisingly high rate of spontaneous recovery from HCV infection. Forty-five percent of the children were found to be anti-HCV positive, but persistently HCV RNA negative, the serologic and molecular profile of recovery. Among the children with viremia who underwent biopsy, only 2 of 17 had portal fibrosis and only 1 had cirrhosis 20 years after exposure. The one patient with cirrhosis also had chronic HBV infection.

There is a paradox in the course of HCV infection. If one examines the relation of infection to disease outcome by examining patients who already have evidence of severe liver disease, one finds that HCV causes many of these cases. From this perspective, HCV projects as a frequent cause of cirrhosis, end-stage liver disease, and HCC. On the other hand, if one prospectively evaluates entire cohorts of persons with HCV infection, a more balanced picture emerges. First, it is now apparent that at least 15% and possibly as many as 25% of adults spontaneously recover from HCV infection, usually within the first year of infection. The rate of recovery among children with infection may be even higher. In one study (58), it was 45%. It is now also apparent that in the absence of alcohol abuse or coexistent HIV infection, chronic hepatitis C is generally an indolent process in which severe outcomes may never occur or may take decades to evolve. Most adults who undergo transfusion die of the disease for which the transfusion was necessary or of an intercurrent illness before the potentially fatal complications of chronic hepatitis C become manifest. Nonetheless, over the span of 20 or more years, 20% to 30% of patients with HCV infection may have histologic evidence of cirrhosis that can ultimately lead to liver failure and the need for liver transplantation. That perhaps 70% of patients with HCV infection spontaneously recover or have a nonprogressive form of chronic liver disease gives hope to the individual patient; however, it does not diminish the global impact of HCV infection engendered by the sheer magnitude of the population with infection. On a global scale, the absolute number who face life-threatening events related to HCV is staggering even if the proportion that encounters these events is encouragingly small.

MECHANISMS OF VIRAL PERSISTENCE

Quasispecies

The most striking feature of HCV is its ability to persist in the host. Measurements of HCV RNA in serum and liver suggest that the prevalence of persistent infection is higher than the prevalence of chronic hepatitis and may be in the range of 75% to 85%. The mechanism of persistence appears to involve the ability of the virus to mutate rapidly under immune pressure and to exist simultaneously as a series of related but immunologically distinct variants, any one of which can become the predominant strain when a coexistent strain comes under immune pressure. This coexistence of multiple genetic variants has been termed *quasispecies.* It provides an efficient and rapid mechanism for the virus to escape the host immune response. Although mutations occur throughout the HCV genome, most occur in a relatively short hypervariable segment of the envelope domain. This finding suggests that this region contains important target epitopes that are under intense immune attack. Among HCV isolates, the average mutation rate for HCV is 10^{-3} to 10^{-4} base substitutions per genome site per year (59). This high rate of mutation, reflected in the quasispecies nature of the virus and in the ability of HCV to rapidly evolve escape mutants, appears to be the primary mechanism underlying the absence of effective neutralization and the development of persistent infection. A 2000 study by Farci et al. (60) showed that early in HCV infection patients who ultimately recover have a decreased degree of viral diversity after the appearance of anti-HCV antibody. In these persons, antibody or coexistent cell-mediated immune responses seem to contain viral replication and quasispecies formation such that the virus becomes increasingly homogeneous and is eventually cleared. In contrast, in most patients, the development of antibody appears to drive viral diversity until the population becomes so heterogeneous that it cannot be fully contained by the immune system.

Hepatitis C virus has evolved to become an efficient machine for survival. In this survival scheme, a master strain is accompanied by a series of subservient strains that under immune pressure can themselves become the master. Defective particles are formed that can protect replicative particles, and a low level of replication can allow the virus to both hide from the host and protect its environment by inducing disease so indolent that the cells that nurture the virus are well maintained or only incrementally destroyed. These efficient mechanisms of self-survival have allowed HCV to chronically infect approximately 1% of the world's population.

Neutralizing Antibody and Cell-mediated Immunity

There is little evidence that HCV is directly cytopathic. It is generally believed that liver damage is the result of the host's immune response, including cytotoxic T cells (CTLs), cytokines, and apoptotic factors. The immune response to HCV infection is brisk and yet generally ineffective in viral clearance. High titers of antibody coexist with high levels of virus. Antibodies broadly directed across the entire genome rarely have neutralizing potential. Those directed at the critical neutralizing epitopes in the viral envelope more often tend to drive viral diversity than to eradicate the agent. Nonetheless, neutralizing antibodies to HCV have been found in mixing experiments in which chimpanzee infectivity was used as the end point. These neutralizing responses, however, have been shown to be transient and highly strain specific (61). Because HCV has not been grown in culture, there are no reliable and reproducible in vitro neutralizing antibody assays.

It has been difficult to measure cell-mediated immunity to HCV. In recent years, however, an increasing array of assays have been used to measure in vitro lymphoproliferative and cytotoxic responses to HCV. With conventional lymphoproliferative and CTL assays, enzyme-linked immunospot assays, and more recently tetramer assays, the cellular immune responses to HCV infection are gradually being dissected (62). It has been found that cell-mediated immune responses occur soon (1 to 2 weeks) after the onset of infection. The initial responses to viral infection generally involve innate immunity primarily effected by $CD56^+$ natural killer cells. Interesting is that the liver is particularly rich in natural killer cells, but it has been suggested that HCV may have mechanisms to bypass innate immunity. Results suggest that the class II major histocompatibility complex restricted helper T-cell (T_H) response is particularly important in determining the outcome of acute HCV infection (63). Patients with acute, self-limited hepatitis C have been shown to mount an early, vigorous, and multispecific T_H response that can be measured in the peripheral blood. In contrast, if this T_H response is weak or poorly sustained, persistent infection and chronic hepatitis ensue. It appears that in most patients with HCV infection, the T_H response is blunted. With the immune escape potential provided by the quasispecies nature of HCV, persistent viremia is perpetuated.

In addition to the early stimulation of T_H responses, there is a corresponding HCV-specific $CD8^+$ CTL response. This is probably driven by cytokines (interferon, interleukin-2) released by T_H1 lymphocytes. Early, vigorous, and multispecific CTL responses have been associated with viral clearance and recovery from HCV infection. Conversely, in patients with persistent HCV infection, CTL responses are weak and targeted against fewer HCV epitopes (63). Of interest is that although patients with chronic HCV infection have blunted CTL responses to HCV, they have normal CTL responses to other viruses such as influenza and EBV. Hence there is no generalized immunodeficiency but rather a specific tolerance to HCV.

It appears that several mechanisms are at play in the development of persistent HCV infection. First, because HCV has a rapid rate of replication and a polymerase with poor proof-reading capability, many mutations occur during normal replication so that the virus always exists as a swarm of closely related but immunologically distinct variants called the *quasispecies.* This genetic diversity occurs even in the absence of immune pressure. For unknown reasons, this swarm of infecting virus is able to enter the liver without generating significant innate immunity (natural killer cells). Avoidance of innate immunity is probably facilitated by the fact that HCV almost always enters the body by means of direct passage into the blood stream. Early in infection, replication occurs without accompanying liver damage or clinical symptoms. Although the total number of virions produced is large, the number of viruses per cell is small. This small intracellular viral burden may decrease the display of viral antigens on the cell surface, blunt the lymphoid immune response, and protect the cell from immune destruction. Nonetheless, HCV epitopes are expressed on liver cells in linkage to HLA class I and class II molecules, and these induce CTL and T_H responses within the first weeks of infection. If these cell-mediated responses are brisk, the virus appears to be contained and is eventually cleared through the combined action of CTLs and specific antibody. If the cell-mediated immune responses are weak, some viral variants may be contained, but other members of the quasispecies circumvent the initial cellular immune attack. When antibodies appear 6 to 12 weeks after infection, the immune system has a second chance to clear the virus, but more commonly the targeted immune attack on the hypervariable region of the viral envelope drives additional mutations, and the quasispecies rapidly expands to the point at which the swarm cannot be eradicated, and persistent infection ensues. From that point forward, host immunity can contain the rate of viral replication but cannot achieve viral clearance. There is little evidence that HCV is directly cytopathic, so it is probable that CTL and other immune responses while attempting to contain the virus also cause liver cell damage through a variety of mechanisms, including Fas-ligand apoptosis, cytokine injury including tumor necrosis factor α injury, and perforin-induced injury (62). It has been shown that Fas is up-regulated on HCV infected hepatocytes and on uninfected bystander cells and that Fas ligand is expressed on activated liver-infiltrating T cells (62). Such apoptotic cell death may account for liver cell destruction that is sometimes out of proportion to the number of cells actually infected. The T cell–mediated attack on the HCV-infected liver may lead to sufficient inflammation and fibrotic repair that cirrhosis develops. However, in most patients with HCV infection, an equilibrium seems to develop in which ongoing viral replication and T cell– and cytokine-mediated cell destruction are balanced by controlled hepatic regeneration such that chronic hepatitis develops without progressive fibrosis and without impairment of liver function.

DETECTION SYSTEMS

Surrogate Tests

Mounting evidence of the role of blood transfusion in the induction of chronic liver disease and continuing frustration in the development of a specific assay for the agent of NANB hepatitis prompted the adoption of surrogate (nonspecific) tests for the detection of NANB hepatitis virus carriers. These surrogate tests, ALT and antibody to hepatitis B core antigen (anti-HBc), were implemented for routine donor screening early in 1987. Use of these tests evolved from retrospective analyses of prospective studies of TAH conducted by the Transfusion Transmitted Virus Study Group (64,65) and by the department of transfusion medicine at the NIH (66,67). These two groups found a threefold to fourfold increase in hepatitis risk among recipients of ALT-elevated or anti-HBc–positive blood compared with the rate among recipients of blood negative for these two indices. It was predicted from these studies that the adoption of ALT or anti-HBc tests for donor screening may produce a 30% to 40% reduction in NANB hepatitis and that the combined use of these tests may reduce the incidence of NANB hepatitis 50%. The value of surrogate assays as an interim measure in the prevention of hepatitis C has been validated with the specific anti-HCV assay. Approximately one third of donors with confirmed anti-HCV also had positive results for either or both of these surrogate markers (68). A controlled prospective study conducted in Canada validated the use of surrogate assays for the prevention of TAH (69).

Unresolved is whether the specific assay for HCV negates the use of the surrogate tests or whether these tests must be maintained to exclude the possibility that some carriers of HCV are not found with existing screening assays. The introduction of donor screening assays for HCV RNA has so dramatically decreased the window for HCV infection that it is unlikely that donors will be infectious in the window before nucleic acid detection and even more unlikely that such donors would be recognized with surrogate markers such as anti-HBc or ALT. There is little current justification for maintaining surrogate testing for the prevention of hepatitis C. One can still argue that these assays may be useful in the prevention of hepatitis B or non-A, non-B, non-C hepatitis, but the data supporting this argument are weak.

Specific Hepatitis C Virus Assays

Humoral responses to HCV are vigorous and are directed to a multiplicity of antigenic sites (15,70). As shown in Figure 49.1, the original clone produced a protein designated 5-1-1, which was then expanded and fused to form the c100-3 antigen that served as the basis of first-generation anti-HCV assays. This early assay was highly effective in interdicting HCV carrier blood donors. The problem with the anti-c100-3 assay was that antibody often did not appear for a protracted period after exposure, creating a window of infectivity that ranged from 12 to more than 26 weeks. Some patients with HCV infection never developed antibody reactive in the first-generation assay. The second-generation assays added two critical epitopes to both the screening enzyme immunoassay (EIA) and the confirmatory RIBA. These were a core protein, designated *c22-3,* and an NS3 protein, designated *c33c.* Antibodies to these new epitopes generally appear much earlier than do anti-c100-3, and the window period in which a donor might be seronegative has considerably narrowed. In the NIH prospective study, 41% of persons with HCV infection had specific antibody detected with second-generation assays within 10 weeks of exposure, 80% had antibody within 15 weeks, and all patients had antibody within 6 months. Third-generation EIA tests added an HCV antigen from the NS-5 region and have shown a marginal increase in sensitivity with a further reduction of the window period of approximately 1 week compared with second-generation assays. Because this increment in sensitivity would have minimal benefit in disease prevention, the use of third-generation anti-HCV assays has not been mandated by the U.S. Food and Drug Administration.

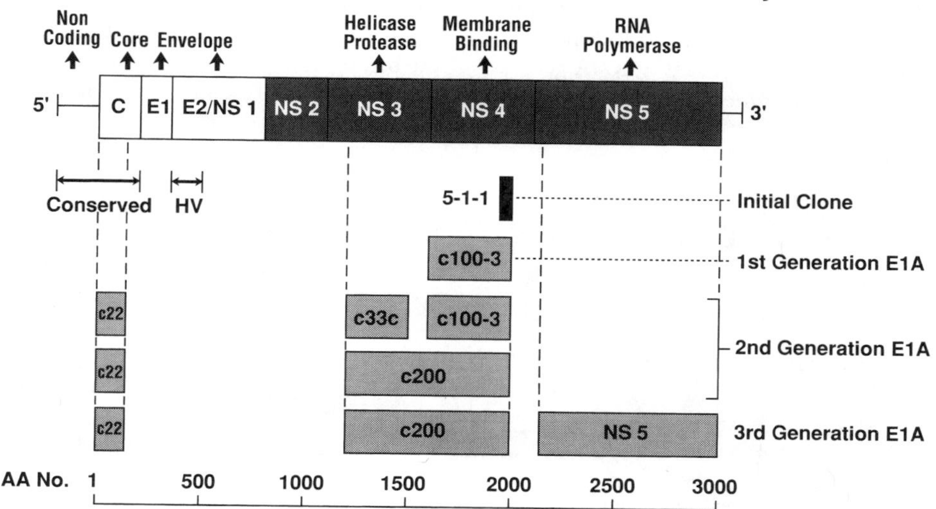

FIGURE 49.1. Proposed genome of hepatitis C virus (HCV). Functional equivalents and major antigens used in antibody detection assays. The structural organization of the HCV genome has been deduced from genomic sequencing and from parallels with other flaviviruses. The entire genome contains approximately 9,500 bases coding for approximately 3,000 amino acids. The 5′ end has a highly conserved noncoding region, the one generally used for polymerase chain reaction amplification and presumed to have important regulatory functions. Downstream to the noncoding region are the regions coding for the structural elements, including the core or nucleocapsid (*C*) and the envelope (*E1, E2/NS1*). It is unclear whether NS1 is part of the envelope region or the first nonstructural gene. The 5′ end of E2/NS1 contains a hypervariable region (*HV*) that mutates rapidly and probably plays a key role in the ability of the virus to escape neutralization. There follow a series of nonstructural genes (*NS2–NS5*) with enzymatic or membrane-binding functions. The initial clone discovered was from the NS4 region; the derived protein was designated *5-1-1*. This was expanded to form the c100-3 antigen, the basis of the first-generation anti-HCV assay. Second-generation assays added the c22 core antigen and the c33c antigen from the NS3 region. These antigens increased the sensitivity of the second-generation assay approximately 20% over the first-generation test. The third-generation assay (pending licensure in the United States) adds an NS5 protein and reconfigures some of the earlier antigens. (From Alter HJ. To C or not to C: these are the questions. *Blood* 1995;85:1681–1695, with permission.)

Antibodies, particularly to 5-1-1, c100-3, and E1, may disappear spontaneously, during immunosuppression, or after successful antiviral therapy. Antibodies to c22-3 and c33c rarely disappear from persons with chronic infection and only infrequently disappear even from those persons with apparent recovery. In most persons, anti-HCV antibodies persist for long periods, perhaps for a lifetime. The prevalence of anti-HCV antibody, found with second-generation EIAs and confirmed with RIBA, among U.S. blood donors ranges from 0.2% to 0.4%. Similar rates have been observed in Europe and higher rates in Japan and other Eastern nations. These rates among highly selected blood donors are underestimates of the prevalence in the general population.

Because of the problem of nonspecificity, it is important to confirm EIA reactivity with a supplemental assay. The only licensed supplemental test is an RIBA that displays the key epitopes in a linear format on a nitrocellulose strip. With second-generation assays, approximately 40% of EIA-reactive samples are confirmed by means of RIBA in a low-risk blood donor setting. Among high-risk populations or EIA-reactive donors who have elevated ALT levels, the confirmation rate is much higher (60% to 80%). In the initially licensed supplemental assay, approximately 30% of EIA-positive samples were classified as indeterminate because only one band appeared on the strip. A third-generation RIBA replaces the recombinant proteins c22-3 and c100-3 with synthetic peptides representing only a portion of the respective coding regions and replaces 5-1-1 antigen with recombinant NS5. This new format resolves many RIBA-2-indeterminate patterns. Approximately 60% of RIBA-2 indeterminates are negative with RIBA-3, whereas 20% are RIBA-3 positive and 20% remain indeterminate even in the RIBA-3 assay. Thus RIBA-3 resolves approximately 80% of RIBA-2 indeterminate results. There is good, but not absolute, correlation between a positive RIBA result and PCR documentation of HCV RNA. Patients who have resolved HCV infection are RIBA positive but PCR negative. In contrast, almost all anti-HCV-positive persons who are PCR positive also are RIBA positive.

The most sensitive way to detect HCV is measurement of HCV RNA by means of PCR or another gene amplification technique. Tests with the PCR have shown that HCV RNA is almost universally detected in the early phase of HCV infection. Most patients have HCV RNA in the serum within 2 to 3 weeks of exposure. Thus HCV RNA detection precedes the increase in serum ALT level, sometimes by as much as 10 to 12 weeks.

It also has been shown by means of quantitative PCR or branched DNA assay that the highest levels of HCV RNA appear early in the course of infection, generally preceding or coinciding with the first significant elevation in ALT level (71). In persons who appear to recover from HCV infection, HCV RNA generally declines or disappears near the time of the peak of ALT elevation. However, in at least 75% of persons, HCV RNA persists, generally with associated fluctuating ALT elevations but sometimes even in the absence of biochemical abnormalities. These temporal relations imply that infectiousness must be greatest before signs or symptoms of acute hepatitis develop, that chronic HCV infection is more frequent than is indicated by

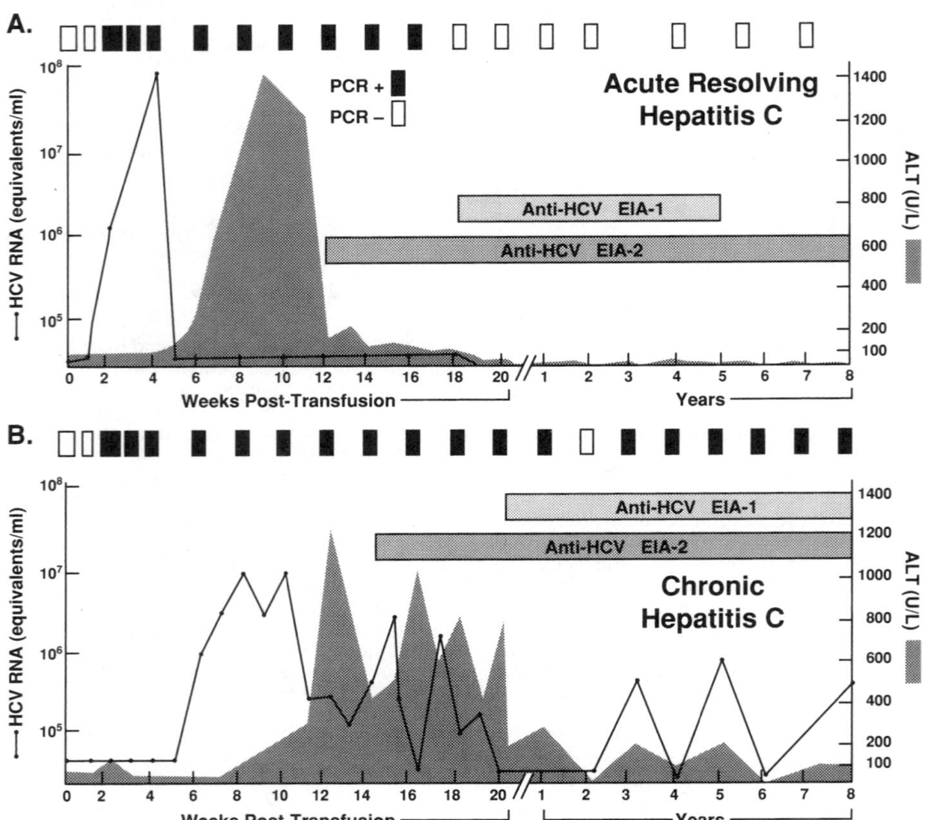

FIGURE 49.2. Biochemical, serologic, and molecular biologic profile of acute and chronic transfusion-associated hepatitis C virus (HCV) infection. Acute, resolving hepatitis C is shown in **A** and chronic hepatitis C in **B.** Resolving disease cannot be differentiated from progressive disease by the time of onset of detectable HCV RNA by means of polymerase chain reaction (*PCR*), the magnitude of HCV RNA elevation as measured by means of branched DNA assay, the interval to the first elevation in the level of alanine aminotransferase (*ALT*), the magnitude of ALT elevation in the acute phase, or the interval between exposure and the first appearance of antibody. Progression to chronic disease cannot be predicted in the acute phase, and the only distinguishing features in these patterns are the persistence of ALT elevation and the persistence of HCV RNA in persons with chronic hepatitis C. The acute, resolving pattern **(A)** occurs in 10% to 15% of patients with transfusion-associated hepatitis C and the chronic pattern **(B)** in 85% to 90%. Note: (a) HCV RNA is detectable soon after exposure. Here the PCR results was positive 2 weeks after exposure, but it can become positive even sooner. (b) HCV RNA may be detected by means of branched DNA assay coincident with PCR reactivity, but the reaction may be delayed, as shown here. (c) The major peak of viral replication (assessed with HCV RNA level) occurs before the first increase in ALT level and before any clinical or biochemical evidence of hepatitis; it is presumed that persons might be most infectious in this interval before the acute phase. (d) In acute resolving infection, HCV RNA levels increase rapidly before the decline in serum ALT level. (e) In chronic infection, HCV RNA level diminishes and can remain low, fluctuate, or become undetectable; HCV RNA levels sometimes show a periodicity that parallels the fluctuations in ALT level; in **B,** the level of HCV RNA increases a short time before ALT level does and decreases before the decline in ALT. (f) Second-generation anti-HCV assays shorten the seronegative window in HCV infection much more than do first-generation assays; nonetheless, anti-HCV was not detectable for 12 to 15 weeks after exposure and for 6 to 7 weeks after the first significant rise in ALT level. Antibody to HCV (detected with second-generation assays) almost always persists in chronic cases and generally persists in acute resolving cases. Antibodies detected with the first-generation assay (anti-C100, anti-5-1-1) generally disappear in resolving cases. (From Alter HJ. To C or not to C: these are the questions. *Blood* 1995;85:1681–1695, with permission.)

ALT elevations alone, and that a small number of persons with infection may be true asymptomatic carriers with normal serum ALT levels and minimal histologic abnormalities in the liver.

The extreme sensitivity of nucleic acid amplification techniques and the long seronegative window between the first detection of virus and the first detection of anti-HCV has prompted the introduction of NAT into routine donor screening. NAT assays are now licensed and they have been universally implemented in U.S. blood establishments and in most blood centers in developed nations. Nucleic acid testing is being performed by two primary methods—standard reverse-transcription PCR and transcription-mediated amplification. Transcription-mediated amplification offers two advantages to the blood bank setting in that extraction and amplification take place in the same tube under isothermal conditions and that the test lends itself to a duplex configuration whereby HIV and HCV RNA can be measured simultaneously. Under development is a triplex assay that would incorporate detection of HBV DNA. As indicated earlier, the routine use of NAT has generated a better understanding of the dynamics of HCV and HBV viremia. With serial collections from commercial plasma donors who suddenly have positive NAT results, it has been shown that HCV RNA usually is undetectable until the level increases precipitously to reach peak levels in a brief period. This phase of rapid acceleration has been termed the *ramp-up phase,* and it usually occurs 2 to 4 weeks after exposure. During ramp-up, the doubling time of the virus has been calculated to be 17 hours (72). There is now evidence from these commercial panels that the ramp-up may be preceded by transient, very low elevations of HCV RNA. It is unknown at this time whether a donor may be infectious during the NAT-negative phase before ramp-up or during the very low, transient elevations (blips). The pattern of HBV viremia differs in that the ramp-up is more delayed and not as steep and in that the ramp-up is preceded by a persistent low-level of viremia (72). During the period of low-level HBV viremia before the ramp-up phase, possibly infectious donations can be missed at minipool testing but detected with individual unit testing. The doubling time for HBV during the ramp-up phase is calculated to be 2.8 days.

Another distinction between HBV testing and HCV testing is that minipool NAT testing dramatically decreases the infectious window for HCV (60-day [85%] reduction) compared with detection of antibody to HCV. In contrast, minipool NAT testing for hepatitis B reduce the window by only 6 days (13%) compared with detection of HBsAg; individual donor NAT for HBV would decrease the window 25 days (55%) compared with that for HBsAg testing (72). In essence, to have a significant effect on HBV transmission compared with current practice, one would have to implement individual-unit NAT testing. For HCV, minipool testing seems sufficient in most instances. A serologic test for HCV core antigen has been developed (73) and has shown sensitivity similar to that of minipool HCV NAT testing. This test may be an option for blood establishments that have not committed to NAT technology.

The foregoing considerations allow a schematic depicting the typical course of acute resolving and chronic hepatitis C (Fig. 49.2). The essential features of viral replication, humoral immune responses, hepatocellular inflammation, and clinical outcome are described earlier and in the legend to Figure 49.2. These are representative diagrams of classic cases— there is considerable variability in these patterns from case to case. The most consistent features are that viral replication can be detected soon after exposure, that peak viremia occurs in the acute or preacute phase in patients who recover and in those who have chronic hepatitis, and that progression to chronic hepatitis cannot be predicted with the time of onset or the peak level of viremia.

MECHANISMS OF VIRAL INACTIVATION

Heat Inactivation

Pasteurization (wet heat at 60°C for 10 hours) has been the staple of plasma inactivation and has rendered albumin a hepatitis-free blood product. Throughout its long history, albumin has not been implicated in hepatitis transmission unless there has been an error in manufacturing. It was thought initially that heating could not be used to inactivate clotting factor concentrates because of the lability of the individual components, particularly the antihemophiliac factor (factor VIII). However, it was found subsequently that lyophilization stabilized the clotting components against heat injury and provided approximately 70% recovery of clotting factor activity. Unfortunately, hepatitis breakthroughs occurred from products that had been inactivated in the lyophilized state. This encouraged a return to pasteurization, various stabilizers being added to protect the labile clotting factors. These wet-heated products do not appear to transmit hepatitis and provide adequate clotting factor activity (74). Subsequent approaches entailed affinity chromatography with monoclonal antibodies to factor VIII to purify the coagulation factor before heating (75). Production of factor VIII by means of recombinant technology ultimately removed the need for pasteurization steps.

Lipid Solvents

The membranes of HCV, HBV, and the AIDS virus (HIV-1) all contain essential lipid, and disruption of the lipid coat should theoretically inactivate these viruses. This premise led to the investigation of a variety of lipid solvents and detergents. The most thoroughly studied, and seemingly the safest and most efficacious, appears to be the combination of an organic solvent, tri(n-butyl)phosphate (TNBP), and a detergent, sodium cholate (CA). In chimpanzee experiments, this mixture inactivated 10^4 50% chimpanzee infective doses per milliliter (CID_{50}/ml) of HBV and NANBV. In tissue culture experiments, it inactivated 10^4 tissue culture infectious doses of HIV-1 (76). The first lipid-disrupting agent licensed for plasma decontamination in the United States, TNBP/CA is an alternative to wet heat and actualizes safe and effective plasma components. Unfortunately, the cellular elements of blood also contain essential lipids and are destroyed by lipid solvents. Solvent-detergent inactivation has become the method of choice for pooled plasma derivatives such as clotting factor concentrates. However, the method has not been widely adopted for fresh-frozen plasma because it requires pooling and introduces the theoretic risk that an emerging non-enveloped pathogen may be widely disseminated by the pooling process. High cost also has limited use of this method for generally low-risk fresh-frozen plasma.

Chemical Pathogen Reduction

See Chapter 56 for a discussion of this topic.

SUMMARY

A marked decline in the incidence of transfusion-associated hepatitis was observed in the early 1970s as commercial blood supplies were phased out and the United States adopted an all-volunteer donor system. No subsequent interdictive measure has had such dramatic effect, although additional contributions were made by the development of more sensitive assays for HBsAg and by the introduction of surrogate tests for NANBV. Ironically, AIDS had the next most profound effect on the incidence of hepatitis. The development of a highly sensitive test for antibody to HIV and the intensified donor screening initiated to exclude high-risk AIDS groups served to exclude the primary source of donors transmitting viral hepatitis. The overlap between groups at risk of AIDS and groups at risk of viral hepatitis is so marked that a single exclusionary process diminishes both occurrences. The effect of these AIDS-related measures on the incidence of TAH has not been documented experimentally, but it appears that the incidence of TAH had declined significantly even before the introduction of anti-HCV testing. In sequential prospective studies at the NIH, the incidence of TAH had decreased from more than 8% to less than 5% just before routine anti-HCV donor screening.

Implementation of anti-HCV testing has had a remarkable effect on the incidence of TAH. A prospective study conducted in Barcelona (77) showed that immediately before the introduction of anti-HCV screening, the incidence of TAH was 9.6%. One year after the exclusion of anti-HCV-positive donors, the incidence had decreased to 1.9%, an 80% reduction attributed solely to first-generation anti-HCV testing. In a large study of anti-HCV seroconversion among transfusion recipients, Donahue et al. (78) showed that the HCV seroconversion rate per transfusion recipient decreased from 4.4% before anti-HCV screening to 1.1% after testing, a 76% reduction. The per unit risk of anti-HCV seroconversion after second-generation donor screening was calculated to be 0.07%.

It can be calculated from the prevalence of the HCV carrier state (0.3%), the number of units of blood products transfused (15 million annually), and the infectivity of anti-HCV-positive, RIBA-positive blood (90%) that the introduction of first-generation assays initially prevented 111 transfusion-associated HCV infections per day in the Untied States alone, or approximately 40,000 infections per year. A subsequent analysis showed that second-generation assays would find 1 additional true positive donor in every 1,000 tested (68) and thus could have prevented an additional 15,000 HCV transmissions per year. A prospective study at the NIH (33) in which the second-generation anti-HCV assay was used for donor screening showed that the risk of transfusion-transmitted hepatitis C is now exceedingly low and indeed approaches zero—a remarkable achievement given that the incidence of hepatitis at the NIH was 33% in the 1960s and 10% to 12% in the early 1980s.

The risk of transfusion-associated hepatitis C after minipool NAT testing is calculated to be 1:300,000 to 1:600,000. When NAT is performed for HBV and HCV on individual units, the risk of transmission of either agent is predicted to be less than 1:500,00 and possibly less than 1 in 1 million. Although anti-HCV screening has been a critical determinant in risk reduction, it has been only one of many interventions since 1985 that have increased blood safety. Other measures include the more judicious use of blood components and derivatives by physicians and a concerned recipient population, the increasing use of autologous blood by predeposit or intraoperative salvage, intensive donor questioning and interdiction based on high-risk behavior, the shift to use of single donor-platelets, the introduction of surrogate assays, HIV and human T-lymphotrophic virus testing, and viral inactivation of clotting factor concentrates. Under development are chemical pathogen reduction procedures for plasma, platelets, and red blood cells. These combined sociologic, serologic, molecular, and viral inactivation measures increase the realistic potential that transfusion-associated viral hepatitis will be totally eradicated and soon will become a historical footnote in the practice of transfusion medicine.

REFERENCES

1. Alter HJ, Purcell RH, Holland PV, et al. Transmissible agent in non-A, non-B hepatitis. *Lancet* 1978;1:459–463.
2. Tabor E, Gerety RJ, Drucker JA, et al. Transmission of non-A, non-B hepatitis from man to chimpanzee. *Lancet* 1978;1:463–466.
3. Shimizu YK, Feinstone SM, Purcell RH, et al. Non-A, non-B hepatitis: ultrastructural evidence for two agents in experimentally infected chimpanzees. *Science* 1979;205:197–200.
4. Li-Fang HE, Alling DW, Popkin TJ, et al. Non-A, non-B hepatitis virus: determination of size by filtration. *J Infect Dis* 1987;156: 636–640.
5. Feinstone JM, Mihalik KB, Kamimura J, et al. Inactivation of hepatitis B virus and non-A, non-B virus by chloroform. *Infect Immun* 1983; 4:816–821.
6. Choo Q-L, Kuo G, Weiner AJ, et al. Isolation of cDNA clone derived from blood-borne non-A, non-B viral hepatitis genome. *Science* 1989; 244:359–362.
7. Dienstag JL, Feinstone SM, Purcell RH, et al. Non-A, non-B post-transfusion hepatitis. *Lancet* 1977;1:560–562.
8. Alter MJ, Gerety RJ, Smallwood LA, et al. Sporadic non-A, non-B hepatitis: frequency and epidemiology in an urban U.S. population. *J Infect Dis* 1982;145:886–893.
9. Alter MJ, Kruszon-Moran D, Nainan OV, et al. The prevalence of hepatitis C virus infection in the United States, 1988 through 1994. *N Engl J Med* 1999;341:556–562.
10. Khuroo MS. Study of an epidemic of non-A, non-B hepatitis: possibility of another human hepatitis virus distinct from post-transfusion non-A, non-B type. *Am J Med* 1980;68:818–824.
11. Kane MA, Bradley DW, Shrestha JM, et al. Epidemic non-A, non-B in Nepal: recovery of a possible etiologic agent and transmission studies in marmosets. *JAMA* 1984;252:3140–3145.
12. Tsarev SA, Tsareva TS, Emerson SU, et al. ELISA for antibody to hepatitis E virus (HEV) based on complete open-reading-frame 2 protein expressed in insect cells: identification of HEV infection on primates. *J Infect Dis* 1993;168:369–378.

13. Muller R, Stephan B, Helmstedt D. Occurrence of viral hepatitis type B and type non-B in three patients. *J Infect Dis* 1975;132:195–199.
14. Bradley DW, McCaustland KA, Cook EH, et al. Posttransfusion non-A, non-B hepatitis in chimpanzees: physicochemical evidence the tubule-forming agent is a small, enveloped virus. *Gastroenterology* 1985; 88:773–779.
15. Branch AD. Hepatitis C virus RNA codes for proteins and replicates: does it also trigger the interferon response? *Semin Liver Dis* 2000;20: 57–68.
16. Mosley JW, Redeker AG, Feinstone SM, et al. Multiple hepatitis viruses in multiple attacks of acute viral hepatitis. *N Engl J Med* 1977;296: 75–78.
17. Craske J, Dilling N, Stern D. An outbreak of hepatitis associated with intravenous injection of factor VIII concentrate. *Lancet* 1975;2: 221–223.
18. Yoshizawa H, Itoh Y, Iwakiri S, et al. Demonstration of two different types of non-A, non-B hepatitis by reinjection and cross-challenge studies in chimpanzees. *Gastroenterology* 1981;81:107–113.
19. Lai ME, Mazzoleni AP, Argiolu F, et al. Hepatitis C virus in multiple episodes of acute hepatitis in polytransfused thalassaemic children. *Lancet* 1994;343:388–390.
20. Simons JN, Leary TP, Dawson GJ, et al. Isolation of novel virus-like sequences associated with human hepatitis. *Nat Med* 1995;6:564–569.
21. Leary TP, Muerhoff AS, Simons JM, et al. Sequence and genomic organization of GBV-C: a novel member of the Flaviviridae associated with human non-A-E hepatitis. *J Med Virol* 1996;48:60–67.
22. Linnen J, Wages J Jr, Zhang-Keck ZY, et al. Molecular cloning and disease association of Hepatitis G virus: a transfusion-transmissable agent. *Science* 1996;271:505–508.
23. Alter HJ, Nakatsuji Y, Melpolder J, et al. The incidence of transfusion-associated HGV infection and its relation to liver disease. *N Engl J Med* 1997;336:747–754.
24. Nishizawa T, Okamoto H, Konisi K, et al. A novel DNA virus (TTV) associated with elevated transaminase levels in posttransfusion hepatitis of unknown etiology. *Biochem Biophys Res Commun* 1997;241:92–97.
25. Okamoto H, Nishizawa T, Kato N, et al. Molecular cloning and characterization of a novel DNA virus (TTV) associated with posttransfusion hepatitis of unknown etiology. *Hepatol Res* 1998;10:1–16.
26. Mushahwar IK, Erker JC, Muerhoff AS, et al. Molecular and biophysical characterization of TT virus: evidence for a new virus family infecting humans. *Proc Natl Acad Sci U S A* 1999;96:3177–3182.
27. Rodriguez-Inigo E, Casqueiro M, Bartolome J, et al. Detection of TT virus DNA liver biopsies by in situ hybridization. *Am J Pathol* 2000; 156:1227–1234.
28. Okamato H, Takahashi M, Nishizawa T, et al. Marked genomic heterogeneity and frequent mixed infection of TT virus demonstrated by PCR with primers from coding and noncoding regions. *Virology* 1999; 259:428–436.
29. Matsumoto A, Yeo AE, Shih JW, et al. Transfusion-associated TT Virus infection and its relationship to liver disease. *Hepatology* 1999; 30:283–288.
30. Hijikata M, Takahashi K, Mishiro S. Complete circular DNA genome of a TT virus variant (isolate name SANBAN) and 44 partial ORF2 sequences implicating a great degree of diversity beyond genotypes. *Virology* 1999;260:17–22.
31. Tanaka Y, Primi D, Wang RY, et al. Genomic and molecular evolutionary analysis of a newly identified infectious agent (SEN virus) and its relationship to the TT virus family. *J Infect Dis* 2001;183:359–367.
32. Umemura T, Yeo AET, Sottini A, et al. SEN virus infection and its relationship to transfusion-associated hepatitis. *Hepatology* 2001;33: 1303–1311.
33. Alter HJ. Hepatitis C virus and eliminating post-transfusion hepatitis. *Nat Med* 2000;6:12–14.
34. Alter HJ, Purcell RH, Shih JN, et al. Detection of antibody to hepatitis C virus in prospectively followed transfusion recipients with acute and chronic non-A and non-B hepatitis. *N Engl J Med* 1989;321: 1494–1500.
35. Pastore G, Monno L, Santantonio T, et al. Monophasic and polyphasic pattern of alanine aminotransferase in acute non-A, non-B hepatitis: clinical and prognostic implications. *Hepatogastroenterology* 1985;32: 155–158.
36. Dienstag JL. Non-A, non-B hepatitis, I: recognition, epidemiology, and clinical features. *Gastroenterology* 1983;85:439–462.
37. Alter HJ, Hoofnagle JH. Non-A, non-B: observations on the first decade. In: Vyas GN, Dienstag JL, Hoofnagle JH, eds. *Viral hepatitis and liver disease.* Orlando, FL: Grune & Stratton, 1984:345–354.
38. Realdi G, Alberti A, Rugge M, et al. Long-term follow-up of acute and chronic non-A, non-B post-transfusion hepatitis: evidence of progression to liver cirrhosis. *Gut* 1982;23:270–275.
39. Omata M, Iwama S, Sumida M, et al. Clinico-pathological study of acute non-A, non-B post-transfusion hepatitis: histological features of liver biopsies in acute phase. *Liver* 1981;1:201–208.
40. Iwarson S, Lindberg J, Lundin P. Progression of hepatitis non-A, non-B to chronic active hepatitis: a histologic follow-up of two cases. *J Clin Pathol* 1979;32:351–355.
41. Corrao G, Arico S. Independent and combined action of hepatitis C virus infection and alcohol consumption on the risk of symptomatic cirrhosis. *Hepatology* 1998;27:914–919.
42. Kato Y, Nakata K, Omagari K, et al. Risk of hepatocellular carcinoma in patients with cirrhosis in Japan: analysis of infectious hepatitis viruses. *Cancer* 1994;74:2234–2238.
43. Seeff LB. Hepatitis in hemophilia: a brief review. In: Burk PB, Chalmers C, eds. *Frontiers in liver disease.* New York: Thieme-Stratton, 1981:231–241.
44. Aledort LM, Levine PH, Hilgartner M, et al. A study of liver biopsies and liver disease among hemophiliacs. *Blood* 1985;66:367–372.
45. Hay CRM, Preston FE, Triger DR, et al. Progressive liver disease in haemophilia: an understated problem? *Lancet* 1985;1:1495–1497.
46. Tefler P, Sabin C, Devereux H, et al. The progression of HCC-associated liver disease in a cohort of hemophiliac patients. *Br J Haemotol* 1994;87:555–561.
47. Kiyosawa K, Akahane Y, Nagata A, et al. Significance of blood transfusion in non-A, non-B chronic liver disease in Japan. *Vox Sang* 1982; 43:45–52.
48. Kiyosawa K, Akahane Y, Nagata A, et al. Hepatocellular carcinoma after non-A, non-B posttransfusion hepatitis. *Am J Gastroenterol* 1984; 79:777–781.
49. Okuda H, Obata H, Motoike Y, et al. Clinicopathological features of hepatocellular carcinoma: comparison of hepatitis B seropositive and seronegative patients. *Hepatogastroenterology* 1984;31:64–68.
50. Bruix J, Calvet X, Costa J, et al. Prevalence of antibodies to hepatitis C virus in Spanish patients with hepatocellular carcinoma. *Lancet* 1989; 2:1004–1006.
51. Seeff LB, Buskell-Bales Z, Wright EC, et al. Long-term mortality after transfusion-associated non-A, non-B hepatitis. *N Engl J Med* 1992; 327:1906–1911.
52. Seeff LB, Hollinger FB, Alter HJ, et al. Long-term mortality and morbidity of transfusion-associated non-A, non-B and type C hepatitis—a National Heart, Lung and Blood Institute collaborative study. *Hepatology* 2001;33:455–463.
53. Seeff LB, Miller RN, Rabkin CS, et al. 45-Year follow-up of hepatitis C virus infection in healthy young adults. *Ann Intern Med* 2000;132: 105–111.
54. Conry-Cantilena C, VanRaden M, Gibble J, et al. Routes of infection, viremia, and liver disease in blood donors found to have hepatitis C virus infection. *N Engl J Med* 1996;334:1691–1696.
55. Shakil AO, Conry-Cantilena C, Alter HJ, et al. Volunteer blood donors with antibody to hepatitis C virus: clinical, biochemical, virologic and histologic features. *Ann Intern Med* 1995;123:330–337.
56. Kenny-Walsh E, Irish Hepatology Research Group. Clinical outcomes after hepatitis infection from contaminated anti-globulin. *N Engl J Med* 1999;340:1228–1233.
57. Muller R. The natural history of hepatitis C: clinical experiences. *J Hepatol* 1996;24[Suppl]:52–54.
58. Vogt M, Lang T, Frosner G, et al. Prevalence and clinical outcome of hepatitis C infection in children who underwent cardiac surgery before the implementation of donor screening. *N Engl J Med* 1999;341: 866–870.
59. Ogata NR, Alter HJ, Miller RH, et al. Nucleotide sequence and muta-

tion rate of the H strain of hepatitis C virus. *Proc Natl Acad Sci U S A* 1991;88:3392.
60. Farci P, Shimoda A, Coiana A, et al. The outcome of acute hepatitis C predicted by the evolution of the viral quasispecies. *Science* 2000; 288:339–344.
61. Farci P, Alter HJ, Govindarajan S, et al. Lack of protective immunity against reinfection with hepatitis C virus. *Science* 1992;258:135–140.
62. Rehermann B. Interaction between the hepatitis C virus and the immune system. *Semin Liver Dis* 2000;20:127–141.
63. Ferrari C, Valli A, Galati L, et al. T-cell response to structural and non-structural hepatitis C virus antigens in persistent and self-limited hepatitis C virus infections. *Hepatology* 1994;19:286–295.
64. Aach RD, Szmuness W, Mosley JW, et al. Serum alanine aminotransferase of donors in relation to the risk of non-A, non-B hepatitis in recipients: the transfusion-transmitted viruses study. *N Engl J Med* 1981;304:989–994.
65. Stevens CE, Aach RD, Hollinger FB, et al. Hepatitis B virus antibody in blood donors and the occurrence of non-A, non-B hepatitis in transfusion recipients: an analysis of the transfusion-transmitted viruses study. *Ann Intern Med* 1984;101:733–738.
66. Alter HJ, Purcell RH, Holland PV, et al. The relationship of donor transaminase (ALT) to recipient hepatitis: impact on blood transfusion services. *JAMA* 1981;246:630–634.
67. Koziol DE, Holland PV, Alling DW, et al. Antibody to hepatitis B core antigen as a paradoxical marker for non-A, non-B hepatitis agents in donated blood. *Ann Intern Med* 1986;104:488–495.
68. Kleinman S, Alter HJ, Busch M, et al. Increased detection of hepatitis C virus (HCV)-infected blood donors by multiple-antigen HCV enzyme immunoassay. *Transfusion* 1992;32:805–813.
69. Blajchman MA, Bull SB, Feinman SV. Post-transfusion hepatitis: impact of non-A, non-B hepatitis surrogate tests. Canadian Post-Transfusion Hepatitis Prevention Study Group. *Lancet* 1995;345:21–25.
70. Kuo G, Choo OL, Alter HJ, et al. An assay for circulating antibodies to a major etiologic virus of non-A, non-B hepatitis. *Science* 1989;244: 362–364.
71. Alter HJ. To C or not to C: these are the questions. *Blood* 1995;85: 1681–1695.
72. Busch MP. Closing the windows on viral transmission by blood transfusion. In: Stramer SL, ed. *Blood safety in the new millennium.* Bethesda, MD: American Association of Blood Banks, 2001:33–54.
73. Tanaka E, Ohue C, Aoyagi K, et al. Evaluation of a new enzyme immunoassay for hepatitis C virus (HCV) core antigen with clinical sensitivity approximating that of genomic amplification of HCV RNA. *Hepatology* 2000;32:388–393.
74. Schimpf K, Mannuci PM, Kreutz W, et al. Absence of hepatitis after treatment with a pasteurized factor VIII concentrate in patients with hemophilia and no previous transfusion. *N Engl J Med* 1987;316: 918–922.
75. Bretler D, Fosberg A, Levine P, et al. Factor VIII-C purified from plasma via monoclonal antibodies. *Thromb Haemost* 1987;58:307.
76. Horowitz B, Wiebe ME, Lippin A, et al. Inactivation of viruses in labile blood derivatives: disruption of lipid enveloped viruses by tri(n-butyl)phosphate detergent combinations. *Transfusion* 1985;25: 516–522.
77. Esteban JI, Gonzalez A, Hernandez JM, et al. Open prospective efficacy trial of anti-HCV screening of blood donors to prevent post-transfusion hepatitis. In: Hollinger FB, Lemon SM, Margolis HS, eds. *Viral hepatitis and liver disease.* Baltimore: Williams & Wilkins, 1991:431–433.
78. Donahue JG, Munoz A, Ness PM, et al. The declining risk of post-transfusion hepatitis C virus infection. *N Engl J Med* 1992;1327: 369–373.

Rossi's Principles of Transfusion Medicine, Third Edition, edited by Toby L. Simon, Walter H. Dzik, Edward L. Snyder, Christopher P. Stowell, and Ronald G. Strauss. Lippincott Williams & Wilkins, Philadelphia © 2002.

50

TRANSFUSION-TRANSMITTED HEPATITIS B, A, AND D

JULES L. DIENSTAG

HISTORIC BACKGROUND

Epidemic hepatitis, presumed to be caused by hepatitis A virus (HAV) infection but possibly also by hepatitis E virus (HEV), is believed to date back to Biblical times (1). In contrast, percutaneously transmitted hepatitis was not recognized until contemporary times, the first reported outbreak having been described little more than a century ago, in 1885. In that year, jaundice occurred in 15% of dockyard workers in Bremen, Germany, who had been vaccinated earlier against smallpox with glycerinated lymph derived from persons convalescent from the disease (2). Although, in retrospect, hepatitis C virus (HCV) cannot be excluded, in all probability, the responsible agent was hepatitis B virus (HBV) (3). Of course, HBV infection has afflicted humankind since ancient times, judging by the extraordinary prevalence of the virus on the Asian and African continents, where it has been perpetuated by percutaneous and maternal-neonatal transmission.

Percutaneous spread of viral hepatitis gained notoriety once again in the early part of the twentieth century, when medical clinics began to routinely obtain blood samples and inject medications. Reports followed describing jaundice affecting persons attending diabetic (4), venereal disease (5,6), and arthritis (7) clinics. Because the disease seemed to be associated with the communal use of inadequately sterilized needles, the term "postinoculation jaundice" was introduced, although the initial consideration was that the jaundice reflected toxic responses to such drugs as salvarsan, arsenic, bismuth, and gold. Further support for a link between needle exposure and viral infection came from reports of severe hepatitis among children and British troops who had been inoculated prophylactically with convalescent measles and mumps sera (8,9); similar outbreaks were noted, as well, among recipients of yellow fever vaccine (10,11,12). Of course, the specific virus responsible for these instances of jaundice could not then, and cannot now, be pinpointed.

During World War II, viral hepatitis research increased dramatically. Not only was "epidemic" hepatitis once again found to be a common disease of war (affecting military troops and civilian populations alike), but also the growth of blood transfusion as a vital part of war-related health care introduced the serious complication of blood-transmitted hepatitis. The first reports of transfusion-transmitted hepatitis appeared in 1943 (13,14), prompting intensive investigations that included experimental human transmission studies. These studies all pointed to the existence of two, and only two, separate viruses, distinguished by differences in modes of transmission, incubation periods, and severity and outcome (15–17). Hepatitis B virus was held responsible for all cases of hepatitis following transfusion, and the terms "serum hepatitis" and "homologous serum jaundice" were used interchangeably for "posttransfusion hepatitis." The current terminology, *hepatitis B,* was proposed in the late 1940s and was adopted by the World Health Organization in the mid-1970s.

Proof that HBsAg (then referred to as the Australia Antigen) was associated with a transmissible infectious agent came from the earliest studies, even though the diagnostic assay employed was an insensitive immunodiffusion test (18). Approximately 75% of recipients of HBsAg-positive donor blood were found to have either hepatitis or serologic markers of HBV infection,

J.L. Dienstag: Gastrointestinal Unit (Medical Services), Massachusetts General Hospital and Department of Medicine, Harvard Medical School, Boston, Massachusetts.

although hepatitis also was noted in recipients of HBsAg-negative donor blood. Investigators concluded that fewer than 25% of the cases of transfusion-transmitted hepatitis could be attributed to HBV, suggesting that either the test was not sufficiently sensitive or the HBsAg-negative cases were caused by another hepatitis virus (18). Both suspicions proved to be correct. Following the introduction of more sensitive assays for HBsAg and the recognition that most occurrences of transfusion-transmitted hepatitis were not caused by HBV, the facile assumption was that these cases must have been caused by HAV infection. Initially, this view was challenged by the observations that transfusion-associated hepatitis occurred after incubation periods incompatibly long for HAV (19). The development of a specific assay for HAV (following identification of the virus in 1973) (20) provided the means to exclude HAV definitively as an agent of transfusion-associated hepatitis. Examinations of stored sera from earlier prospective screening studies failed to implicate HAV in any of these instances (21). Therefore, the cases identified were recognized as not being attributable to either HBV or HAV, introducing a new concept—non-A, non-B (NANB) hepatitis. The years that followed were devoted not only to confirming these original observations but also to developing a simpler and more sensitive test for HBsAg, which would facilitate mass screening of blood donations. Voluntary at first, the test was made mandatory by federal regulation in July 1972. After 1975, federal regulation required that all blood donors be tested for HBsAg by a third-generation test.

HEPATITIS B

Hepatitis B virus is a 42-nm DNA virus (Table 50.1) composed of an outer shell (7 nm in width) and an inner core (27 nm in diameter). It belongs to a novel class called hepadnaviruses; HBV is designated hepadnavirus type 1. The outer coat material (or envelope), referred to as hepatitis B surface antigen (HBsAg), is synthesized by infected host hepatocytes, contains lipid and three major polypeptides, is DNA free and, therefore, is noninfectious. It can be detected in serum not only as a part of the intact virus but also as separate 22-nm spheric or tubular particles. These particles circulate in amounts that far exceed the number of complete HBV particles. Highly immunogenic but noninfectious, nonvirion HBsAg constituted the source for the first generation of plasma-derived HBV vaccines. Current HBV vaccines rely upon recombinant yeast-produced HBsAg as the immunogen. Clinically, HBsAg is detected in serum by serologic assays, can be visualized in the cytoplasm of hepatocytes by electron microscopy, and can be identified in liver biopsy material of infected persons with non-virus-specific special stains (e.g., orcein, aldehyde fuchsin, Victoria blue) or by virus-antigen–specific immunohistochemical staining.

The inner icosahedral nucleocapsid core of HBV contains partially double-stranded DNA, endogenous DNA polymerase with reverse transcriptase activity, and protein kinases. Hepatitis B core antigen (HBcAg), is a particulate antigen expressed on the surface of the nucleocapsid. The genomic information of the virus is present on the long strand of the DNA (3,200 nucleotides), which comprises four overlapping open reading frames (referred to as *S, C, P,* and *X* genes), each encoding different polypeptides. The viral polymerase has reverse transcriptase activity that effects the transcription from a pregenomic RNA template of negative-strand DNA; in turn, the DNA polymerase activity of the polymerase results in transcription of the positive DNA strand, which tends to be incomplete and to account for the partially double-stranded, partially single-stranded genomic structure of HBV. The HBcAg, which cannot be detected in serum unless the lipid envelope of the intact virus is first disrupted by detergent, can be visualized by immune electron microscopy in hepatocyte nuclei and, occasionally, in cytoplasm; it also can be identified immunochemically in liver biopsy specimens. Within the core particle is a nonparticulate soluble antigen, called hepatitis B e antigen (HBeAg). This antigen is associated intimately with, and believed to be a cleavage product of, HBcAg, requiring translation of the precore region of the *C* gene for its expression. Its presence in serum reflects active viral replication and, hence, a state of high infectivity. A replicating HBeAg-negative, HBV DNA-positive mutant has been described; it is concentrated in Mediterranean countries, broadly distributed in Asia, but uncommon in the United States. Each of the HBV antigens induces production of its own antibody; anti-HBs, anti-HBc, and anti-HBe. A variety of long-recognized HBV serologic subtypes exist; HBV subtypes vary geographically and have little impact on the clinical expression of viral infection.

TABLE 50.1. CHARACTERISTICS OF HEPATITIS B, A, AND D VIRUSES

	Hepatitis B	Hepatitis A	Hepatitis D
Classification	Hepadnavirus	Picornavirus	? Satellite
Size	42 nm	27 nm	36 nm
Genome (length)	DNA (3.2 kb)	RNA (7.5 kb)	RNA (1.7 kb)
Envelope	HBsAg	None	None
Carrier state	Yes	No	Yes
Chronic hepatitis	Yes	No	Yes
Predominant mode of transmission	Sexual Percutaneous Maternal-neonatal	Fecal-oral	Percutaneous Sexual

HBsAg, hepatitis B surface antigen.

Recently, at least six distinct viral genotypes, A through F, have been identified. Like the serologic subtypes, they vary in their geographic distribution; however, emerging data suggest that pathogenicity, outcome (22), and even response to antiviral therapy is influenced by viral genotype. In the United States, genotype A is the most common, while genotypes B and C are most common in Asian countries.

A complex pattern of serologic manifestations marks the development of acute and chronic HBV infection (23). Acute infection is characterized by the appearance of HBsAg (generally 2 to 6 weeks after exposure but occasionally as early as 1 week), HBeAg, and HBV DNA, followed soon thereafter by anti-HBc (initially of the immunoglobulin M [IgM] and then the IgG class). Hepatitis is defined by the observed onset of increased aminotransferase activity, 25% or fewer of the cases being associated with jaundice. Usually, markers of viral replication (HBeAg, HBV DNA detectable with insensitive hybridization assays that have a sensitivity of 10^5 to 10^6 particles per ml) disappear early, and HBsAg titers decline as the illness peaks. Soon thereafter, the enzyme values begin to decline. What remains is IgM anti-HBc which, after 6 months or longer, is replaced by IgG anti-HBc, which persists for life, although in decreasing titers. The period between loss of HBsAg and development of anti-HBe and anti-HBs, which also can extend for weeks or months, generally is referred to as the *window period.* In the past, the window period was identified in approximately 10% of acute cases and represented a potential low-level carrier state; however, as the sensitivity of immunoassays for HBsAg and anti-HBs has increased, the frequency of identification of patients with acute hepatitis B infection in the window period has declined to negligible levels. The appearance of anti-HBs defines recovery from the acute disease and immunity to reinfection.

The usual recovery sequence begins with the loss of replicative markers, the disappearance of HBsAg, the return of aminotransferase levels to normal and, finally, the appearance of anti-HBs. Persistence of HBsAg and (usually) of HBeAg beyond 6 months defines chronic infection and the likelihood of progression to chronic liver disease. The worst of the sequelae is the development of primary hepatocellular carcinoma (HCC).

Epidemiologically, HBV is a percutaneously transmitted agent, but the presence of HBV (albeit at lower levels than in blood) in physiologic (e.g., semen, cervicovaginal fluid, and saliva, but not urine or stool) and pathologic body fluids (e.g., ascites, pleural effusions) establishes HBV as an infection also readily transmitted by transfer of secretions (transmucosally as well as percutaneously). Two patterns of infection exist. In Asia and sub-Saharan Africa, the disease is transmitted predominantly during the perinatal period by carrier mothers, and the infected newborn almost invariably becomes a carrier with a high likelihood of progression to cirrhosis and, ultimately, HCC. A striking inverse relationship has been noted between age at infection and the occurrence of chronic infection and hepatitis (24,25). In Western countries, the disease affects mainly adolescents and young adults through sexual behavior (heterosexual and homosexual) or percutaneous exposure (injection drug use, tattoos, multiple transfusions, accidental needlestick exposure, etc.). It much less commonly culminates in chronicity. Hepatocellular carcinoma almost never occurs unless the infected host is immunologically compromised as a consequence of intrinsic disease or immunosuppressive drug therapy.

HEPATITIS B AND TRANSFUSION

Clinical Features

Data from several prospective studies conducted during the early 1970s indicate that transfusion-transmitted HBV infection begins after an average incubation period of 11 to 12 weeks (26). In general, the clinical symptoms of the different types of viral hepatitis are indistinguishable from one another, although symptoms are more frequently absent among persons with HCV than among those with HBV infections. The accompanying biochemical dysfunction also tends to be more severe with HBV disease than with HCV transfusion-transmitted disease, as evidenced by higher mean alanine aminotransferase (ALT) values (705 versus 471 U/liter) and the higher frequency of jaundice (60% versus 25%) (26). It is difficult to assess the disease course after transfusion because of the sparsity of well-defined cases studied prospectively. The widely held early view, based on analyses of cases of HBV infection of diverse origin, was that 5% to 10% of acutely infected adults progressed to chronic infection. More recent studies suggest that evolution to chronic infection is far less common (27). Too few large-scale, prospective, long-duration studies have been conducted to establish whether a very low frequency of chronicity applies to transfusion-related cases as well. A single small-volume percutaneous exposure in healthy young adults does not seem to carry this high risk of persistence; fewer than 1% of the 350,000 army personnel infected in 1942 through yellow fever vaccine injections (whether or not the illness was accompanied by jaundice) could be identified as carriers 40 years later (12). Limited observations suggest that high levels of HBV markers (HBsAg, HBeAg, and HBV DNA) during the early course of acute hepatitis B may predict progression to chronic HBV infection (28). The prognostic value of viral replication during acute hepatitis has not been confirmed in other studies, but the persistence of high-level HBV replication beyond the third month of acute illness does appear to portend chronicity of infection.

Demographic and Epidemiologic Features

Donors

Demographic characteristics of HBV-positive donors were established in several studies undertaken soon after the identification of HBsAg as a marker for HBV infection. These studies showed that HBsAg was more common in males than in females, in blacks and Asian Americans than in whites, and in paid than in volunteer donors. In addition, the prevalence of detectable HBsAg was found to be more common among certain at-risk population groups (including injection drug abusers and sexually promiscuous homosexual men). Further, paid donors were more likely than volunteer donors to be HBsAg positive as well as HBeAg positive (29). This was consistent with the evidence that had accrued during the late 1950s and afterward, especially in several large prospective studies conducted during the 1970s

(30–32), that paid donors represented a particularly serious health threat to blood recipients. Collectively, these prospective studies established that in comparison to receipt of volunteer-donor blood, receipt of paid-donor blood was associated with a two- to six-fold increase in the frequency of hepatitis B and non-A, non-B hepatitis (hepatitis C). In 1978, labeling of donor blood (paid versus volunteer) became required, with the aim of reducing reliance on nonvolunteer blood donors. Voluntary nonpaid donations are considered a key requirement for the safety of the blood supply. Nevertheless, donor screening questions used to identify persons potentially at high risk for blood-borne infections may not identify all such donors (33), and the pursuit of additional refinements in the donor screening process will need to continue. With regard to HBsAg-positive donors, several retrospective analyses have shown that they have a higher than normal risk of dying from liver-related diseases, such as cirrhosis and HCC (34,35). A recent study of the risk of transfusion-transmissible viral infections at five blood donor centers from 1991 to 1996 and involving 1.9 million donors showed no reduction in the frequency (0.2%, of HBsAg in first-time blood donors during this recent 6-year period). This stability contrasts with a reduction in both the frequency of HCV and HIV infections among first-time blood donors in this longitudinally monitored population (36).

Recipients

During the 1970s, extensive prospective monitoring studies were undertaken to gather data on the frequency of hepatitis and to evaluate the efficacy of immune globulin prophylaxis. These studies coincided with the appearance of serologic assays for HBV and for HAV. Data generated in these studies documented the impact of screening tests with greater assay sensitivity. For example, in a study performed at the blood bank of the National Institutes of Health, the frequency of transfusion-related hepatitis was 4.8% when the gel diffusion test was used. The rate decreased to 3.7% when counterelectrophoresis (CEP) screening was introduced and fell to 0.6% after screening by radioimmunoassay (RIA) became available (31). Similar findings were noted in other studies.

No additional prospective monitoring studies were performed in the United States during the 1980s or 1990s and, therefore, accurate data on the current frequency of transfusion-transmitted hepatitis B do not exist. Table 50.2 shows data on cases of suspected posttransfusion hepatitis reported to the American Red Cross. However, such data are retrospective, subject to reporting bias, and cannot be used to estimate true frequency. Numerous prospective studies have been reported for this period from other countries, including the Far East, the Middle East, Europe, Canada, and Australia (37–47). These investigations revealed that transfusion-related hepatitis is global, the frequency ranging from 3% to 19%, and as in studies of a decade earlier, few of the cases can be attributed to hepatitis B (Table 50.3). In over 50% of the studies, no cases of hepatitis B were identified (38,40,42,43,45,47), and hepatitis B accounted for 7% or fewer of total cases in three of the remaining five studies (37,41,46) and 18% to 26% of the cases in the last two studies (39,44). The unusually high rate of hepatitis B in the last two studies was attributed to the relatively low sensitivity of the donor screening test used for HBsAg. Only 1 of these 11 studies (the one conducted in Toronto, Canada) has geographic proximity to the United States and furnishes data directly relevant to the United States (47). During the 3 years in which that study was conducted (1983 through 1985), the frequency of transfusion-related hepatitis was 9.2%; none of the cases could be attributed to hepatitis B. In view of the similarity in population traits of Toronto and most large cities in the United States, we can assume that the frequency and characteristics of transfusion-related hepatitis in the two countries are similar.

Testing for anti-HBc was originally introduced in 1986 and 1987 as a surrogate marker for the presence of non-A, non-B infection. With the advent of specific testing for HCV, anti-HBc testing was retained because of its potential value for the detection of early HBV infection. The effectiveness of screening

TABLE 50.2. TRANSFUSION-ASSOCIATED HEPATITIS REPORTED TO THE AMERICAN RED CROSS, 1981–1994

	Number of Cases			
Year	Hepatitis B	Non-A, Non-B	Other	Total
1981–1982	222	434	318	974
1985–1986	166	401	276	843
1986–1987	141	353	190	684
1987–1988	108	194	113	415
1988–1989	68	163	139	370
1989–1990	126	208	152	486
1990–1991	135	112	147	394
1991–1992	83	75	153	311
1992–1993	64	89	96	249
1993–1994	87	100	74	261

Personal communication, Roger Dodd.
[a] Reporting categories changed to hepatitis B; hepatitis C; hepatitis other viral; hepatitis non-A, non-B, non-C; and hepatitis unspecified.

TABLE 50.3. WORLDWIDE FREQUENCY OF TRANSFUSION-TRANSMITTED HEPATITIS DURING THE 1980S

Author (Reference)	Country	Patients (N)	Hepatitis Frequency (%)	Percentage of Total Cases Caused by Hepatitis B
Tateda (37)	Japan	676	11.6	7
Katchaki (38)	Netherlands	380	3.4	0
Cossart (39)	Australia	842	2.0	18
Grillner (40)	Sweden	74	18.9	0
Tremolada (41)	Italy	297	18.5	4
Collins (42)	England	248	2.4	0
Tur-Kaspa (43)	Israel	50	8.0	0
Hernandez (44)	Spain	230	16.9	26
Aymard (45)	France	64	6.3	0
Colombo (46)	Italy	676	14.0	3
Feinman (47)	Canada	576	9.2	0

of blood donors for anti-HBc as a means to reduce HBV transmission is questionable. Although occasional case reports have described hepatitis B infection in recipients of HBsAg-negative, anti-HBc-positive blood, a considerable body of data suggests that anti-HBc screening is of little value in low-prevalence populations (48). In contrast to studies from high-prevalence regions, where HBV DNA has been identified by polymerase chain reaction (PCR) in nearly 5% of HBsAg-negative, anti-HBc-positive donors (49), in low-prevalence populations such as the blood donor pool in the United States and western Europe, HBV DNA has not been detected. These observations are consistent with the notion that a considerable proportion of the anti-HBc reactivity identified in low-prevalence populations represents false-positive test results.

The most recent study of anti-HBc-reactive blood donors and recipients was conducted in the United Kingdom (50). Among 103,869 blood donations screened, 586 (0.56%) were anti-HBc-reactive, but none contained HBV DNA by PCR amplification. Moreover, among 171 blood recipients who had been transfused with blood products obtained from these anti-HBc-reactive blood donors, only 12 had any markers of HBV infection, one-half of whom had other risk factors for infection. Of the other six recipients, in whom an association with transfusion was deemed probable in two and possible in four, the blood donors from whom their transfusions were derived did not have detectable HBV DNA 6 to 40 months after the potentially implicated transfusion. These investigators estimated that the risk of acquiring HBV infection from HBsAg-negative HBV carriers was 1 in 52,000 donations and concluded that nucleic acid amplification screening of blood donors would be unlikely to reduce the minuscule frequency of transfusion-associated hepatitis B (50). Additional studies to assess the value of such nucleic acid testing of donated blood are continuing (51).

A recent analysis of HBV risk after transfusion was derived from data between 1991 and 1993 on 587,507 blood donors at five blood centers, representing more than 2 million blood donations. Standard serologic screening tests were negative in all these blood donors, and the risk of transfusion-transmitted hepatitis B among recipients of these blood products was estimated to be 1 in 63,000, quite low but higher than the estimated frequency of transfusion-acquired HCV infection (1 in 103,000) or HIV infection (1 in 641,000) (52).

Simultaneous transfusion-associated infection with HBV and HCV or other non-A, non-B, non-C hepatitis viruses appears to be a very rare event (53). Dual infections appear to result in delayed onset of circulating HBsAg, lower levels of HBsAg, a shorter duration of HBsAg detectability, and lower serum ALT levels than are seen in transfusion-associated HBV infection alone (54). Coinfected patients may show a biphasic pattern of ALT elevations. These observations suggest that HCV may reduce the replication of HBV when coinfection occurs. Hepatitis B virus did not influence the high risk of chronicity following HCV infection.

Plasma Derivatives

Among the manufactured plasma derivatives, three—albumin, plasma protein fraction, and immune globulin—are considered low risk for transmission of HBV (55). The first two are rendered safe by heating to 60°C for 10 hours; the safety of the third comes, in part, from the neutralizing effect of anti-HBs. In early reports, immune globulin produced by the Cohn fractionation method was shown not to transmit HBV, even if derived from apparent infectious material (56). Presumably this is because the Cohn fractionation process causes HBV markers to bypass fraction II (the immune globulin component) with migration to later fractions (fraction III in particular) (57,58). This accounts for the few, no more than a handful, reported cases of apparent (not documented) transmission of hepatitis B by immune globulins, despite the administration of millions of doses of the product over the past 40 years.

In contrast to these three products, several untreated plasma derivatives were previously known to carry a high risk of hepatitis transmission: factors VIII (antihemophilic factor) and IX, antithrombin III, fibronectin, α_1-antitrypsin, C-1 inactivator, and factor XIII (59). As noted, HBsAg is distributed to the very fractions that are the sources of these plasma products. Even though factors VIII and IX were derived from plasma pools (generally containing 1,000 or more donor units) that were prescreened for HBsAg, HBV infection among hemophiliacs was extraordinarily high. To address this, plasma fractionation programs introduced several treatment steps designed to reduce the infectivity of plasma-derived protein concentrates. These included vapor-heat treatment, chemical treatment, and solvent-detergent treatment of the source plasma. Plasma products derived from treated pooled plasma have proved extraordinarily safe with respect to HBV transmission. For many concentrates, such as factor VIII and factor IX, the development of recombinant proteins has virtually eliminated any residual risk of infectious disease transmission.

HEPATITIS A

Hepatitis A virus is a 27-nm, nonenveloped picornavirus, within the genus Hepatovirus, with a 7,500-nucleotide single-stranded RNA genome and four virion polypeptides (60,61) (Table 50.1). Unusually stable to environmental exposure, HAV can withstand heat and cold; its hardiness contributes to its efficient transmission through contaminated food and water. Infection occurs after an incubation period of about 4 (but rarely, as long as 6) weeks. The virus can be detected in the liver and stool during the late incubation period and early phase of acute illness. For practical clinical purposes, almost all viral shedding, which essentially is completed by the time jaundice appears, is limited to fecal excretion; fecal shedding of virus and infectivity decline rapidly thereafter. Viremia is limited and lasts only a few days during the acute illness. Prolonged viremia, lasting a few months, detected by PCR, has been described, but neither liver injury nor infectivity have been associated with such late, barely quantifiable, circulating viral RNA. Thus, no chronic viremic or fecal carrier state or chronic HAV infection has been recognized clinically although, rarely, infectivity may be somewhat more prolonged under unusual circumstances (such as among premature babies infected in a neonatal intensive care unit). A diagnosis can be made by detection of antibody to HAV of the IgM class

(IgM anti-HAV) in acute-phase serum. Following recovery and becoming the predominant class of antibody approximately 3 months after acute infection, IgG antibody to HAV (IgG anti-HAV) persists indefinitely after HAV infection and correlates with protection from reinfection.

In nature, HAV is transmitted almost exclusively by the fecal-oral, or enteric, route. The vehicles for transmission of common-source outbreaks, therefore, are fecally contaminated food or water. Transmission readily occurs within families, institutions, day-care centers, and persons traveling to endemic areas. In developing countries, exposure to HAV is almost uniform in early childhood; in developed countries, improvements in environmental and personal hygiene limit the spread of HAV infection and the prevalence of anti-HAV. As a result, the frequency of HAV infection has been declining in modern developed countries.

Hepatitis A causes an acute illness, and symptoms and signs can be indistinguishable from those of acute hepatitis B; the former, however, tends to be milder and is much less likely to cause fulminant hepatitis. Hepatitis A does not cause chronic hepatitis. Prevention is accomplished by avoiding potentially contaminated food and water and, in situations promoting exposure, by timely administration of immune globulin, all lots of which contain substantial levels of protective anti-HAV or, more recently, by active immunization with HAV vaccines. Inactivated hepatitis A vaccines have been shown to provide extraordinarily high protective efficacy rates in field trials when administered prior to exposure (62). Modeling studies have suggested that the rate of decay of protective levels of anti-HAV is such that protection may persist for at least 10 years (63) and more likely up to 20 years after primary immunization.

Hepatitis A and Transfusion

As already noted, before HAV was recognized and tests were developed to identify HAV infection, hepatitis A was blamed for cases of transfusion-associated non-B hepatitis. During the 1970s, application of anti-HAV testing to the seroepidemiologic analysis of patient groups with transfusion-associated hepatitis failed to implicate HAV in any of these cases (21). In fact, instances of transfusion-transmitted HAV infection were considered unlikely because of the absence of an asymptomatic HAV carrier state and the very limited (brief duration and low concentration) viremia associated with acute infection. For transfusion-associated hepatitis to occur, an unusual set of rare circumstances must coincide. A person with asymptomatic acute hepatitis A, presymptomatic late–incubation period acute hepatitis A, very early acute symptomatic HAV infection, or relapsing hepatitis A must donate blood during the limited time (a few days) in which sufficient-level viremia occurs. In cases of clinical hepatitis A, nonspecific symptoms of malaise and fatigue occur during the late-incubation preicteric period—symptoms that normally would discourage a person from donating blood. Considering how rare these circumstances are and how low the frequency of hepatitis A is in the general population, the singular rarity of transfusion-associated HAV infection is not unexpected. The infrequency with which blood is contaminated by HAV is reflected as well in the absence of cases of transfusion-associated hepatitis A in reports of sporadic hepatitis (64,65) and in the absence, until 1992 (see below), of an association between HAV infection and exposure to blood products among hemophiliacs and other multiply transfused patients, hemodialysis patients, health workers, and comparable populations exposed to blood-borne HBV and HCV (66,67).

As unlikely as it might seem, the short-lived viremia of HAV infection occasionally does coincide with blood donation. Serologically bona fide cases of transfusion-associated hepatitis A are so rare that they tend to be reported. Only a few documented cases have been described (68–78), but in nearly all of these patients, the report documents or relies on the assumption that a blood donor gave blood during the late incubation period of hepatitis A. Several of these reports involved transfusion-transmitted hepatitis in premature babies, whose resulting asymptomatic hepatitis A led to amplification of enteric transmission of HAV to staff in the nursery (68,73–75). Contamination of blood products with HAV remains rare, but recent outbreaks have attracted attention to the need for vigilance. In 1992, the transmission of HAV by processed plasma derivatives was reported from Italy in patients with hemophilia receiving factor VIII concentrates in which ion-exchange chromatography and solvent-detergent treatment had been used for virus inactivation (79). Similar reports quickly followed from Germany, Ireland, and Belgium (80–82). Hepatitis A virus nucleotide sequences in implicated factor VIII concentrate and recipients were shown to be identical (83).

To study the removal or neutralization of HAV during processing, investigators spiked human plasma and factor VIII intermediates with HAV (84). The combination of antibody-mediated neutralization, partitioning during cryoprecipitation, anion-exchange chromatography, and lyophilization resulted in a minimum of a 5.5 to 8.85 $\log_{10}$ reduction in the infectious titer of HAV in a contaminated plasma pool. These data suggest that ion-exchange chromatography–treated, solvent-detergent–inactivated factor VIII concentrates are unlikely to transmit HAV, assuming that plasma pools used for their preparation contain low HAV levels. This experience strongly suggests that solvent-detergent inactivation, although very effective in the inactivation of enveloped blood-borne viruses, will not eliminate the risk of HAV transmission if the nonenveloped HAV contaminates plasma pools or factor VIII lots. Virus inactivation by manufacturing processes that rely upon pasteurization may be preferable to those that rely on ion-exchange chromatography and solvent-detergent methods. In the United States, transmission of HAV by plasma-derived factor VIII preparations has not been recognized.

Despite these caveats, most physicians and blood bank workers probably will never see a case of transfusion-associated hepatitis A. For all practical purposes, HAV infection is not, and should not be, categorized as a blood-borne disease. Even though highly sensitive PCR techniques capable of detecting as few as four HAV particles have been described (85), donor screening for viremia by PCR for HAV RNA does not seem justifiable. However, it has been proposed and studied by some manufactures for an in-process control test for pooled plasma products.

HEPATITIS D

Hepatitis D virus, also known as hepatitis delta virus, is a 35- to 37-nm defective RNA virus that can infect only a host harboring HBV infection (Table 50.1). Hepatitis D virus relies on HBV for its surface coat, which consists of HBsAg, and requires concurrent infection with HBV to support its replication and clinical expression (86). A hybrid virus, HDV has an outer coat of host-contributed HBsAg and a nucleocapsid core that expresses HDV antigen, and it contains a 1,700-nucleotide RNA genome similar to that of plant satellite viruses and viroids. Hepatitis B virus and HDV infections can occur simultaneously, or a patient with chronic HBV infection can become superinfected with HDV. Ultimately, the duration of HDV infection is determined by the duration of HBV infection; because HDV relies on HBV for its expression, HDV cannot outlast HBV infection. A diagnosis of infection with HDV can be made by demonstrating antibody to HDV (anti-HDV); both IgG and IgM antibodies circulate. Detection of HDV antigen (HDAg) is difficult; HDAg is, therefore, not a practical diagnostic marker. A diagnosis of hepatitis D and ongoing HDV replication can be made by identifying HDAg in liver nuclei by immunohistochemical staining or by detecting HDV RNA in serum or liver by cDNA hybridization.

Hepatitis D tends to segregate into two different epidemiologic patterns. In endemic areas, such as Mediterranean countries, HDV infection appears to be transmitted from person to person. In contrast, in nonendemic areas, such as northern Europe and North America, transmission of HDV infection appears to be confined to certain populations, such as drug users and hemophiliacs, who have frequent exposure to blood, blood products, and blood-contaminated needles. Occasionally, even in nonendemic areas, protracted outbreaks of hepatitis D do occur; examples of such outbreaks of simultaneous acute coinfection with HBV and HDV have been described. Sizable outbreaks of superinfection with HDV in patients chronically infected with HBV also have been noted in the literature. In nonendemic areas, such outbreaks have a tendency to amplify HDV infection in the community and to blur the epidemiologic distinction between endemic and nonendemic areas. The frequency of HDV infection, even in endemic areas of the world, has been declining.

The clinical features of hepatitis D are similar to those of hepatitis B, and most of the more severe outcomes of hepatitis B also can be associated with hepatitis D. Although simultaneous acute coinfection with HDV and HBV can cause clinical features indistinguishable from those of acute hepatitis B alone, superinfection with HDV of a chronically HBV-infected person often leads to more serious, rapidly progressive liver disease. Hepatitis D virus superinfection can resemble an acute hepatitis-like exacerbation in a patient with chronic hepatitis B. Commonly, such HDV superinfection transforms asymptomatic or mild chronic hepatitis B into severe chronic hepatitis and cirrhosis. Fulminant hepatitis can follow coinfection or superinfection. In short, hepatitis D tends to exacerbate and accelerate liver injury in patients with chronic (rarely acute) hepatitis B (87).

Because HDV infection cannot occur in a patient immune to HBV, prevention of HDV infection is accomplished readily by HBV vaccination in persons susceptible to hepatitis B. For those already infected by HBV, prevention of superinfection is limited to mechanical efforts to avoid intimate contact with HDV-infected persons.

Hepatitis D and Transfusion

Because blood is routinely screened for HBsAg as well as for antibody to hepatitis B core antigen (anti-HBc), the likelihood of receiving a unit of blood containing HBV is extraordinarily low. Because, under ordinary circumstances, HDV infection cannot occur in the absence of HBV infection, the chance that a blood donor screened and found to be negative for HBsAg and anti-HBc could harbor HDV is exceedingly small. Prior to the advent of current screening techniques, transmission of HDV undoubtedly occurred and contributed to the previously identified high frequency of HDV infection in multiply transfused persons (such as hemophiliacs and thalassemics) (88). In a study of American patients with hemophilia A, 75% had a serologic marker of previous HBV infection, and 13% of them had antibodies to HDV (89).

Although HDV is a blood-borne viral agent, contemporary, highly sensitive screening methods used in blood banks should be effective in reducing the frequency of transfusion-associated HDV hepatitis to a negligible level, at least in HBsAg-negative blood recipients. Such complacency might not be warranted in HBsAg-positive recipients of blood products, especially recipients of pooled blood derivatives.

SUMMARY

Hepatitis B virus, a hepadnavirus, causes an acute infection characterized by the appearance of HBsAg 2 to 6 weeks after exposure. It is transmitted by blood and secretions and was a major cause of posttransfusion hepatitis until the risk was reduced by elimination of paid donors and by screening donors for HBsAg. Hepatitis B vaccine is widely available in the developed world. Hepatitis A is very rarely a blood-borne disease, and screening for HBV has kept HDV infection at negligible levels. The near elimination of the risk of HBV transmission by transfusion has been a major part of the success of contemporary transfusion medicine.

REFERENCES

1. Zuckerman AJ. *Hepatitis-associated antigen and viruses,* 1st ed. New York: Elsevier Science, 1972:1.
2. Lurman A. Eine Icterusepidemie. *Klin Wochenschr* 1885;22:20–23.
3. Koff RS. *Viral hepatitis,* 1st ed. New York: John Wiley and Sons, 1978: 39.
4. Flaum A, Malmros H, Perrson E. Eine Nosocomiale Ikterus Epidemic. *Acta Med Scand* 1926;16[Suppl]:544–553.
5. MacCallum FO. Transmission of arsenotherapy jaundice by blood: failure with faeces and nasopharyngeal washings. *Lancet* 1945;1:1342.
6. Bigger JW. Jaundice in syphilitics under treatment: possible transmission of virus. *Lancet* 1943;1:457–458.
7. Hartfall SJ, Garland HG, Goldie W. Gold treatment of arthritis: a review of 900 cases. *Lancet* 1937;2:784–788.

8. Propert SA. Hepatitis after prophylactic serum. *BMJ* 1938;2:677–678.
9. Beeson PB, Chesney G, McFarlane AM. Hepatitis following injection of mumps convalescent serum. 1. Use of plasma in the mumps epidemic. *Lancet* 1944;1:814–815.
10. Findlay GM, MacCallum FO. Note on acute hepatitis and yellow fever immunization. *Trans Soc Trop Med Hyg* 1937;31:297–308.
11. Fox JP, Manso C, Penna HA, et al. Observations on occurrence of icterus in Brazil following vaccination against yellow fever. *Am J Hyg* 1942;36:63–116.
12. Seeff LB, Beebe GB, Hoofnagle JH, et al. A serologic follow-up of the 1942 epidemic of post-vaccination hepatitis in the United States Army. *N Engl J Med* 1987;316:965–970.
13. Beeson PB. Jaundice occurring one to four months after transfusion of blood or plasma: report of seven cases. *JAMA* 1943;121:1332–1334.
14. Morgan HW, Williamson DA. Jaundice following administration of human blood products. *BMJ* 1943;1:750–753.
15. Paul JR, Havens WP, Sabin AB, et al. Transmission experiments in serum jaundice and infectious hepatitis. *JAMA* 1945;128:911–915.
16. Neefe JR, Gellis SS, Stokes J Jr. Homologous serum hepatitis and infectious (epidemic) hepatitis. Studies in volunteers bearing on immunologic and other characteristics of the etiologic agents. *Am J Med* 1946;1:3–22.
17. Krugman S, Giles JP, Hammond J. Infectious hepatitis: evidence for two distinctive clinical, epidemiological, and immunological types of infection. *JAMA* 1967;200:365–373.
18. Gocke DJ. A prospective study of posttransfusion hepatitis: the role of the Australia antigen. *JAMA* 1972;219:1165–1170.
19. Prince AM, Grady GF, Hazzi C, et al. Long-incubation post-transfusion hepatitis without serologic evidence of exposure to hepatitis-B virus. *Lancet* 1974;2:241–246.
20. Feinstone SM, Kapikian AZ, Purcell RH. Hepatitis A detection by immune electron microscopy of a virus-like antigen associated with acute illness. *Science* 1973;182:1026–1028.
21. Dienstag JL, Feinstone SM, Purcell RH, et al. Non-A, non-B post-transfusion hepatitis. *Lancet* 1977;1:560–562.
22. Kao JH, Chen PJ, Lai MY, et al. Hepatitis B genotypes correlate with clinical outcomes in patients with chronic hepatitis B. *Gastroenterology* 2000;118:554–559.
23. Hoofnagle JH, Seeff LB, Bales ZB, et al. Serologic responses in HB. In: Vyas GN, Cohen SN, Schmid R, eds. *Viral hepatitis.* Philadelphia: Franklin Institute Press, 1978:219–242.
24. Beasley RP, Hwang LY, Lin CC, et al. Hepatitis B immune globulin (HBIG) efficacy in the interruption of perinatal transmission of hepatitis B virus carrier state. *Lancet* 1981;2:388–393.
25. McMahon BJ, Alward WLM, Hall DB, et al. Acute hepatitis B virus infection: relation of age to the clinical expression of disease and subsequent development of the carrier state. *J Infect Dis* 1985;151:599–603.
26. Dienstag JL. Non-A, non-B hepatitis. I. Recognition, epidemiology, and clinical features. *Gastroenterology* 1983;85:439–462.
27. Koff RS. Natural history of acute hepatitis B in adults re-examined. *Gastroenterology* 1987;92:2035–2037.
28. Fong TL, Di Bisceglie AM, Biswas R, et al. High levels of viral replication during acute hepatitis B infection predict progression to chronicity. *J Med Virol* 1994;43:155–158.
29. Tabor E, Goldfield M, Black HC, et al. Hepatitis Be antigen in volunteer and paid donors. *Transfusion* 1980;20:192–198.
30. Goldfield M, Black HC, Bill J, et al. The consequences of administering blood pretested for HBsAg by third generation techniques: a progress report. *Am J Med Sci* 1975;270:335–342.
31. Alter HJ, Holland PV, Purcell RH, et al. Transfusion hepatitis after exclusion of commercial and hepatitis-B antigen-positive donors. *Ann Intern Med* 1972;77:691–699.
32. Aach RD, Lander JJ, Sherman LA, et al. Transfusion-transmitted viruses: interim analysis of hepatitis among transfused and non-transfused patients. In: Vyas GN, Cohen SN, Schmid R, eds. *Viral hepatitis.* Philadelphia: Franklin Institute Press, 1978:383–396.
33. Williams AE, Thomson RA, Schreiber GB, et al. Estimates of infectious disease risk factors in US blood donors. *JAMA* 1997;277:867–972.
34. Hall AJ, Winter PD, Wright R. Mortality of hepatitis B positive blood donors in England and Wales. *Lancet* 1985;1:91–93.
35. Dodd RY, Nath N. Increased risk for lethal forms of liver disease among HBsAg-positive blood donors in the United States. *J Virol Methods* 1987;17:81–94.
36. Glynn SA, Kleinman SH, Schreiber GB, et al. Trends in incidence and prevalence of major transfusion-transmissible viral infections in US blood donors, 1991 to 1996. *JAMA* 2000;284:229–235.
37. Tateda A, Kikuchi K, Numazaki Y, et al. Non-B hepatitis in Japanese recipients of blood transfusion: laboratory screening of donor blood for hepatitis B surface antigen. *J Infect Dis* 1979;139:511–518.
38. Katchaki JM, Siem TH, Brouwer R, et al. Posttransfusion non-A, non-B hepatitis in the Netherlands. *BMJ* 1981;282:197–198.
39. Cossart YE, Kirsch S, Ismay SL. Post-transfusion hepatitis in Australia: report of the Australian Red Cross Study. *Lancet* 1982;1:208–213.
40. Grillner L, Bergdahl S, Jyrala A. Non-A, non-B hepatitis after open-heart surgery in Sweden. Scand *J Infect Dis* 1982;14:171–175.
41. Tremolada F, Chiapetta F, Noventa F, et al. Prospective study of post-transfusion hepatitis in cardiac surgery patients receiving only blood or also blood products. *Vox Sang* 1983;44:25–30.
42. Collins JD, Bassendine MF, Codd AH, et al. Prospective study of post-transfusion hepatitis after cardiac surgery in a British center. *BMJ* 1983;287:1422–1424.
43. Tur-Kaspa R, Shimon DV, Shalit M, et al. Posttransfusion non-A, non-B hepatitis after cardiac surgery: a prospective study. *Vox Sang* 1983;45:312–315.
44. Hernandez JM, Pigueras J, Carrera A, et al. Posttransfusion hepatitis in Spain: a prospective study. *Vox Sang* 1983;44:231–237.
45. Aymard JP, Janot C, Gayet S, et al. Post-transfusion non-A, non-B hepatitis after cardiac surgery: prospective analysis of donor blood anti-HBc activity as a predictor of the occurrence of non-A, non-B hepatitis in recipients. *Vox Sang* 1986;51:236–238.
46. Colombo M, Oldani S, Donato MF, et al. A multicenter, prospective study of posttransfusion hepatitis in Milan. *Hepatology* 1987;7:709–712.
47. Feinman SV, Berris B, Bojarski S. Post-infusion hepatitis in Toronto, Canada. *Gastroenterology* 1988;95:464–469.
48. Douglas DD, Taswell HF, Rakela J, et al. Absence of hepatitis B virus DNA detected by polymerase chain reaction in blood donors who are hepatitis B surface antigen negative and antibody to hepatitis B core antigen positive from a United States population with a low prevalence of hepatitis B serologic markers. *Transfusion* 1993;33:212–216.
49. Wang JT, Wang TH, Sheu JC, et al. Detection of hepatitis B virus DNA by polymerase chain reaction in plasma of volunteer blood donors negative for hepatitis B surface antigen. *J Infect Dis* 1991;163;397–399.
50. Allain JP, Hewitt PE, Tedder R, et al. Evidence that anti-HBc but not HBV DNA testing may prevent some HBV transmission by transfusion. *Br J Haematol* 1999;107:186–195.
51. Sacher RA, Schreiber GB, Kleinman SH. Prevention of transfusion-transmitted hepatitis. *Lancet* 2000;355:331–332.
52. Schreiber GB, Busch MP, Kleinman SH, et al. The risk of transfusion-transmitted viral infections: the retrovirus epidemiology donor study. *N Engl J Med* 1996;334:1685–1690.
53. Baginski I, Chemin I, Hantz O, et al. Transmission of serologically silent hepatitis B virus along with hepatitis C virus in two cases of post-transfusion hepatitis. *Transfusion* 1992;32:215–220.
54. Mimms LT, Mosley JW, Hollinger FB, et al. Effect of concurrent acute infection with hepatitis C virus on acute hepatitis B virus infection. *BMJ* 1993;307:1095–1097.
55. Hoofnagle JH, Gerety RY, Thiel J, et al. The prevalence of hepatitis B surface antigen in commercially prepared plasma products. *J Lab Clin Med* 1976;88:102–113.
56. Murray R, Ratner F. Safety of immune serum globulin with respect to homologous serum hepatitis. *Proc Soc Exp Biol Med* 1953;83:554–555.
57. Schroeder DD, Mozen MM. Australia antigen: distribution during Cohn ethanol fractionation of human plasma. *Science* 1970;168:1462–1464.
58. Trepo C, Hantz O, Jacquier MF, et al. Different fates of hepatitis B markers during plasma fractionation: a clue to the infectivity of blood derivatives. *Vox Sang* 1978;35:143–148.
59. Gerety RJ, Aronson DL. Plasma derivatives and viral hepatitis. *Transfusion* 1982;22:347–351.

60. Lemon SM. Type A viral hepatitis. New developments in an old disease. *N Engl J Med* 1985;313:1059–1067.
61. Cohen JI. Hepatitis A virus: insights from molecular biology. *Hepatology* 1989;9:889–895.
62. Innis BL, Snitbhan R, Kunasol P, et al. Protection against hepatitis A by an inactivated vaccine. *JAMA* 1994;271:1328–1334.
63. Wiedermann G, Ambrosch F, Andre FE, et al. Persistence of vaccine-induced antibody to hepatitis A virus. *Vaccine* 1992;10[Suppl 1]: S129–S131.
64. Dienstag JL, Alaama A, Mosley JW, et al. Etiology of sporadic hepatitis B surface antigen-negative hepatitis. *Ann Intern Med* 1977;87:1–6.
65. Francis DP, Hadler SC, Prendergast TJ, et al. Occurrence of hepatitis A, B, and non-A/non-B in the United States: CDC sentinel hepatitis study I. *Am J Med* 1984;76:69–74.
66. Mayor GH, Klein AM, Kelly TJ, et al. Antibody to hepatitis A and hemodialysis. *Am J Epidemiol* 1982;116:821–827.
67. Stevens CE, Silbert JA, Miller DR, et al. Serologic evidence of hepatitis A and B virus infections in thalassemia patients: a retrospective study. *Transfusion* 1978;18:856–860.
68. Seeberg S, Brandberg A, Hermodsson S, et al. Hospital outbreak of hepatitis A secondary to blood exchange in a baby. *Lancet* 1981;1: 1155–1156.
69. Hollinger FB, Khan NC, Oefinger PE, et al. Posttransfusion hepatitis type A. *JAMA* 1983;250:2313–2317.
70. Barbara JAJ, Howell DR, Briggs M, et al. Post-transfusion hepatitis A [Letter]. *Lancet* 1982;1:738.
71. Skidmore SJ, Boxall EH, Ala F. A case of post-transfusion hepatitis A. *J Med Virol* 1982;10:223.
72. Sheretz RJ, Russell BA, Reuman PD. Transmission of hepatitis A by transfusion of blood products. *Arch Intern Med* 1984;144:1579–1580.
73. Noble RC, Kane MA, Reeves SA, et al. Posttransfusion hepatitis A in a neonatal intensive care unit. *JAMA* 1984;252:2711–2715.
74. Azimi PH, Roberto PR, Guralnik J, et al. Transfusion-acquired hepatitis A in a premature infant with secondary nosocomial spread in an intensive care nursery. *Am J Dis Child* 1986;140:23–27.
75. Klein BS, Michaels JA, Rytel MW, et al. Nosocomial hepatitis A: a multinursery outbreak in Wisconsin. *JAMA* 1984;252:2716–2721.
76. Ishikawa K, Sato S, Sugai S, et al. A case of post-transfusion hepatitis A. *Gastroenterol Jpn* 1984;19:247–250.
77. Giacoia GP, Kasprisin DO. Transfusion-acquired hepatitis A. *South Med J* 1989;82:1357–1360.
78. Nigro G, Del Grosso B. Transfusion acquired hepatitis A in a patient with β-thalassemia major. *J Infect* 1990;20:175–176.
79. Mannucci PM. Outbreak of hepatitis A among Italian patients with haemophilia. *Lancet* 1992;339:819.
80. Gerritzen A, Schneweis KE, Brackmann HH, et al. Acute hepatitis A in haemophiliacs. *Lancet* 1992;340:1231–1232.
81. Temperley JJ, Cotter KP, Walsh TJ, et al. Clotting factors and hepatitis A. *Lancet* 1992;340:1466.
82. Peerlinch K, Vermylen J. Acute hepatitis A in patients with haemophilia A. *Lancet* 1993;341:179.
83. Mannucci PM, Gdovin S, Gringeri A, et al. Transmission of hepatitis A to patients with hemophilia by factor VIII concentrates treated with organic solvent and detergent to inactivate viruses. *Ann Intern Med* 1993;120:1–7.
84. Lemon SM, Murphy PC, Smith A, et al. Removal/neutralization of hepatitis A virus during manufacture of high purity, solvent/detergent factor VIII concentrate. *J Med Virol* 1994;43:44–49.
85. Deng MY, Day SP, Cliver DO. Detection of hepatitis A virus in environmental samples by antigen-capture PCR. *Appl Environ Microbiol* 1994;60:1927–1933.
86. Rizzetto M. The delta agent. *Hepatology* 1983;3:729–737.
87. Smedile A, Farci P, Verme G, et al. Influence of delta infection on severity of hepatitis B. *Lancet* 1982;2:945–947.
88. Jacobson IM, Dienstag JL, Werner BG, et al. Epidemiology and clinical impact of hepatitis D virus (delta) infection. *Hepatology* 1985;5: 188–191.
89. Kumar A, Kulkarni R, Murray DL, et al. Serologic markers of viral hepatitis A, B, C, and D in patients with hemophilia. *J Med Virol* 1993;41:205–209.

Rossi's Principles of Transfusion Medicine, Third Edition, edited by Toby L. Simon, Walter H. Dzik, Edward L. Snyder, Christopher P. Stowell, and Ronald G. Strauss. Lippincott Williams & Wilkins, Philadelphia © 2002.

51

RETROVIRAL INFECTIONS

EBERHARD FIEBIG
MICHAEL P. BUSCH

Retroviruses owe their name to reverse transcriptase, an essential enzyme in the viral life cycle, which allows transcription of viral RNA to DNA after infection of a host cell (Fig. 51.1). This sizable family of RNA viruses had long been known as a relatively obscure cause of malignant lesions in animals, but they were not considered significant human pathogens or a threat to transfusion recipients. The discovery of human immunodeficiency virus (HIV) (Fig. 51.2), a transfusion-transmissible retrovirus in the lentivirus group and the etiologic agent of acquired immunodeficiency syndrome (AIDS), changed all this almost overnight and made retroviruses one of the most feared and studied pathogens ever. It is difficult to overstate the effect of the HIV/AIDS pandemic on almost all aspects of blood banking and transfusion medicine since the mid 1980s. Although the HIV crisis had profound negative repercussions in the field when it first emerged, the reaction to the threat posed by the virus has vastly improved blood and transfusion safety in general, which is now at a higher level than ever before in history (1). This chapter focuses on the remarkable role of human retroviruses HIV-1 and HIV-2 and human T-lymphotrophic virus types 1 and 2 (HTLV-1, HTLV-2) in transfusion medicine. The emphasis is on blood safety issues, donor testing and counseling, and recipient infection. Details on the virologic aspects, clinical diagnosis, and management of retroviral infections are contained in textbooks (2–5), reviews (6–10), and Internet resources (http://hivinsite.ucsf.edu).

E. Fiebig: Department of Laboratory Medicine, University of California, San Francisco, Transfusion Service and Hematology Divisions, Clinical Laboratories, San Francisco General Hospital, San Francisco, California.

M.P. Busch: Department of Laboratory Medicine, University of California, San Francisco, Blood Centers of the Pacific and Blood Systems, Inc., San Francisco, California, and Scottsdale, Arizona.

HISTORICAL SUMMARY AND OVERVIEW

Retroviruses were among the first viruses described at the beginning of the twentieth century. They are a major class of membrane-coated, diploid, single-stranded RNA viruses with wide distribution in genera ranging from insects to reptiles to almost all mammals. The first definitive report of human retrovirus infection appeared in 1980. The patient had a rare type of leukemia, now known as adult T-cell leukemia (ATL) (11). In recognition of its role in pathogenesis, the virus was called *human T-cell lymphoma virus type I* (HTLV-1). Subsequently, HTLV-1 also was identified as cause of a rare neurologic condition called *HTLV-associated myelopathy–tropical spastic paraparesis* (HAM-TSP) (12). A second, closely related human retrovirus (HTLV-2) was isolated in 1982. For more than a decade, HTLV-2 could not be clearly associated with pathogenesis in humans, although recent studies have shown it to cause HAM-TSP and possibly other diseases (12). A third human retrovirus, initially called HTLV-3, was isolated from patients with lymphadenopathy and immune deficiencies in 1983 and was recognized as cause of AIDS the following year (4). In light of substantial genomic differences from HTLV-1 and HTLV-2, the virus was later renamed *human immunodeficiency virus.*

The full pathogenic potential of HIV was not realized until 1984. By then, it became increasingly clear that this virus was the cause of one of the worst pandemics in the century. More than 20 million deaths from AIDS had occurred since the beginning of the pandemic, and an estimated 36 million persons were

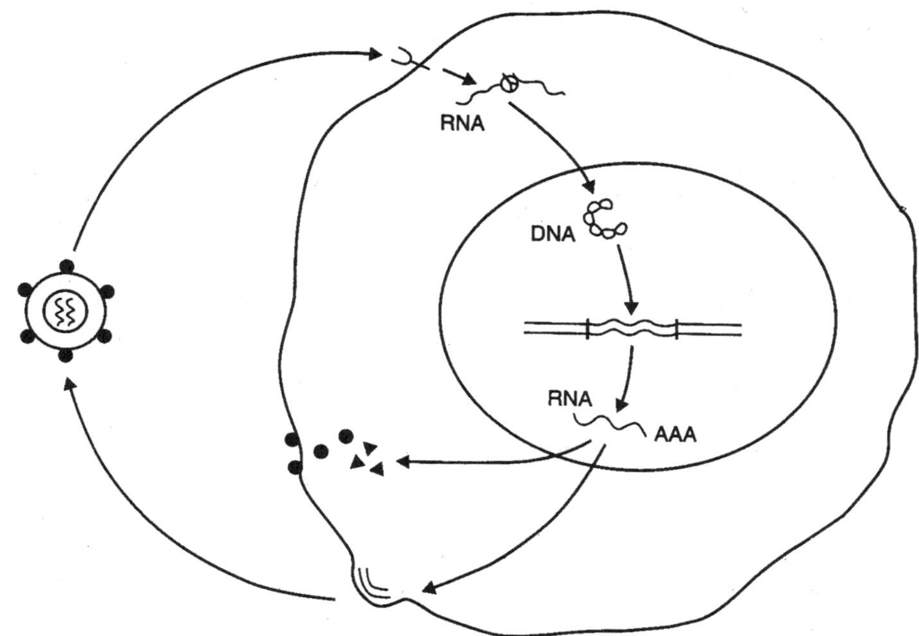

FIGURE 51.1. Simplified replication cycle of a retrovirus. The virion containing two RNA genome copies enters the cell via a specific cell surface receptor. The single-stranded RNA genome is converted into a double-stranded RNA provirus by the virion enzyme reverse transcriptase. The provirus inserts into host chromosomal DNA in the same orientation as the original virion RNA. Transcription of RNA from the integrated DNA provirus is mediated by cellular RNA polymerases, and this RNA serves both as messenger RNA for the synthesis of viral antigens and as genomic RNA, which becomes packaged into progeny virion budding from the cell surface. (From Weiss RA, Dalgleish AG, Loveday C. Human immunodeficiency viruses. In: Zuckerman AJ, Banatvala JE, Pattison JR, eds. *Clinical virology,* 4th ed. Chichester, UK: J Wiley & Sons, 2000:660, with permission.)

living with the infection in 2000 (13). Human immunodeficiency virus is a member of the lentivirus group of retroviruses, which includes other animal immunodeficiency viruses (4). Closely related to HIV-1 is a second human immunodeficiency virus, HIV-2, which causes similar, although usually milder disease than does HIV-1. Numerous genetic variants of HIV-1 have been identified and designated group M (main) with at least 11 subtypes A through K, an outlier group O, and a new group N. It appears that HIV^{S} originated in chimpanzee species and were introduced to native peoples of the central African rain forest through zoonotic exposure (14). There probably have been multiple introductions of the virus into humans over the past 50 years. Although so far the earliest documented proof of HIV infection in humans comes from a blood sample collected in 1959 (15), analysis of genetic variation of HIV-1 strains suggests the virus appeared in humans in approximately 1930 (16) with very limited spread within Africa over the subsequent two to three decades. Human immunodeficiency virus type 1 initially

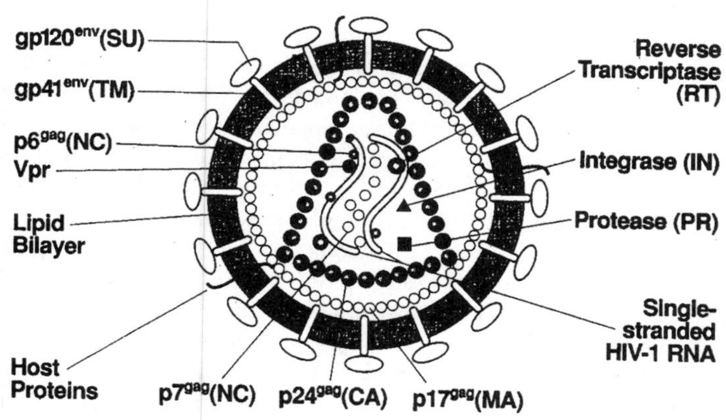

FIGURE 51.2. Schematic of the human immunodeficiency virus type 1 (HIV-1) virion. Each of the virion proteins making up the envelope (*gp120env* and *gp41env*) and inner core (*p24gag, p17gag, p7gag,* and *p6gag*) is identified. The diploid RNA genome is shown associated with reverse transcriptase (*RT*), an RNA- and DNA-dependent DNA polymerase. Integrase (*IN*) and protease (*PR*) also are present in the mature HIV-1 virion. The auxiliary protein Vpr is incorporated into the HIV-1 virion through interaction with the p6gag protein, which composes the carboxyl terminus of the p55gag precursor protein. *CA,* capsid protein; *MA,* matrix protein; *NC,* nucleocapsid protein; *SU,* surface protein; *TM,* transmembrane protein. (From Geleziunas R, Greene WC. Molecular insights into HIV-1 infection and pathogenesis. In: Sande MA, Volberding PA, eds. *The medical management of AIDS,* 6th ed. Philadelphia: WB Saunders, 1999:25, with permission.)

emerged in the male gay community in the United States in the late 1970s to early 1980s. From there it spread to the heterosexual population. By late 1982, reports of AIDS-like illnesses among persons with hemophilia (17) and recipients of blood components (18) suggested blood-borne transmission of HIV in addition to spread through sexual contact.

Deferral of high-risk blood donors (and in some regions surrogate testing for HIV), as well as heat-treatment of factor VIII concentrates for hemophilia treatment, began in 1983. These practices effectively reversed the trend toward increased transmission of the virus in blood and blood products. By the time the first HIV test was introduced in 1985, the incidence of transfusion-transmitted HIV infection in the San Francisco Bay area, one of the worst hit geographic regions in the United States, had already declined precipitously (19). Still, in the United States alone, more than 12,000 transfusion recipients and approximately one half of 16,000 persons with hemophilia contracted infection in the early period of the epidemic, before viral inactivation of clotting factor concentrates and blood and plasma donor screening for HIV antibodies became available (20). From the mid 1980s on, new cases of transfusion-transmitted AIDS became rare in the United States. Through continuation of strict screening of blood donors by means of interview of prospective donors, focused physical examinations, and periodically upgraded laboratory testing, the risk of HIV infection from blood transfusion decreased to an estimated 1 case per 725,000 units transfused by 2000 (21). For plasma products such as coagulation factor concentrates, which are submitted to effective virus inactivation procedures, the risk of HIV transmission is considered remote. Table 51.1 lists major milestones on the way from emergence of retroviral infections toward near elimination of these infections from the blood supply.

Once HIV was identified as a threat to blood safety, attention also turned to HTLV as a risk for transfusion recipients. Human T-lymphotrophic virus, a member of the oncovirus subfamily of retroviruses, is thought to be derived from related viruses in nonhuman primates, as is HIV (22). Unlike the situation for HIV, however, evidence of human infection with HTLV goes back to prehistoric times (23). Results of studies in the early 1980s suggested HTLV, which is endemic around the globe, can be transmitted by means of blood transfusion. Fortunately, HTLV is highly cell associated and does not survive blood storage for more than 2 weeks (24,25). Consequently, transmission of HTLV in fresh frozen plasma and older blood units is unlikely, and plasma-derived products have never been associated with HTLV transmission. The association with disease and pathogenicity of HTLV, although not trivial, are not as immediate and severe as those of HIV. There is less concern over HTLV in regard to blood safety. Nevertheless, testing for HTLV was implemented in blood donor screening in the United States in 1988 and a combination test for HTLV-1 and HTLV-2 was introduced in 1998. In Japan, screening for HTLV-1 began in 1986. In Europe, screening of blood donors for HTLV is performed in some but not all countries (26), in part a reflection of variable prevalence of HTLV infection in different geographic areas of the continent (27).

Globally, the issue of retrovirus transmission by transfusion is split along geographic and economic lines. Although the risk approaches zero in developed nations, the outlook is rather bleak in the poorest countries in sub-Saharan Africa and southeast Asia, where incidence rates of HIV infection are soaring and the prevalence in some communities reaches 20% to 30% (13). Heterosexual transmission drives the epidemic in these areas and makes effective deferral of donors at high risk difficult. Blood safety also is compromised because there are insufficient funds and infrastructure to establish and maintain effective blood donor screening programs (28).

TABLE 51.1. MAJOR EVENTS RELATED TO HUMAN RETROVIRUSES AND THE U.S. BLOOD SUPPLY

1980	First conclusive report of human retrovirus infection with HTLV-I (11)
1981	First report of AIDS in homosexuals
1982	AIDS reported in three persons with hemophilia (17) Case of TA-AIDS reported in San Francisco infant (18)
1983	Joint statement by collection agencies (165) U.S. Public Health Service recommends high-risk-donor deferral FDA licensure of first heat-treated factor VIII concentrate
1984	Report on 20 cases of TA-AIDS (166) HTLV-III (HIV-1) virus recognition (167) Report of HTLV-I transmission by means of blood transfusion in Japan (85)
1985	First commercial kit for HIV-1 antibody screening licensed; all blood tested; alternative test site network established; revised definition of high-risk groups
1986	Look-back programs initiated; confidential unit exclusion programs recommended
1988	HTLV-I antibody EIA implemented for blood donor screening
1992	HIV-1/HIV-2 combination antibody EIA tests implemented
1995	HIV-1 antigen (p24) EIA test implemented
1998	HTLV-I,II combination test implemented
1999	Minipool NAT for HIV (and HCV) begun under IND application to FDA

HTLV, human T-cell lymphotropic virus; TA, transfusion-associated; FDA, Food and Drug Administration; HIV, human immunodeficiency virus; EIA, enzyme immunoassay; NAT, nucleic acid testing; IND, investigational new drug.
Numbers in parentheses are references.

INCIDENCE AND PREVALENCE AMONG BLOOD DONORS

From a blood safety perspective, the number of new cases of HIV infection (incidence) among blood donors is the most important epidemiologic variable, because blood donated by newly infected persons may not be recognized as being infectious and may enter the blood supply if the donation fell into the window period of the screening tests used in the blood donor setting (29). The incidence of HIV infection among U.S. blood donors who gave more than once held steady at a low rate of approximately 2.9 cases per 100,000 person-years, according to a cross-sectional survey of 1.9 million nonautologous donors in 1991 through 1996, the latest period for which such data have been published (30). This figure reflects observed seroconversion among donors who gave blood at least twice during a 2-year period at five U.S. blood centers joined in the Retrovirus Epidemiology Donor Study (REDS). Unpublished REDS data covering the period from 1996 through 1998 suggest a further decrease in incidence among repeated donors to approximately 1.9 per 100,000 person-years (P. Glynn, personal communication, 2001). The incidence among first-time donors cannot be calculated directly but can be estimated with a recently developed sensitive–less sensitive HIV-1 enzyme immunoassay (EIA) testing strategy (31). According to this approach, the overall incidence of HIV infection among more than 2.7 million first-time donors who gave blood in 32 American Red Cross regions from 1993 through 1996 was approximately 7.2 cases per 100,000 person-years, more than twice the observed rate among repeated donors (31). The number of existing cases of HIV infection (prevalence) among first-time donors approximately halved from 0.03% to 0.015% from 1991 through 1996 (30) while the prevalence in the general U.S. population was 10 times higher and remained stable (32), demonstrating the effectiveness of behavioral risk factor screening of prospective blood donors.

Available data from other high-income nations show similar low incidence and prevalence of HIV infection among local blood donors (33–35). In contrast, epidemiologic data from many low-income nations, particularly those in sub-Saharan Africa, India, and southeast Asia, project staggering rates of HIV infection in the general population—for example, 8.8% of the entire adult population in sub-Saharan Africa, according to the latest figures from the Joint United Nations Programme on HIV/AIDS (13)—with equally disturbing prevalence and incidence among blood donors (28,36).

For HTLV, the overall incidence among repeat U.S. blood donors in 1991 through 1996 was approximately 1.6 cases per 100,000 person-years, according to REDS data, and the seroprevalence among first-time donors averaged approximately 0.04% (30). Infection with HTLV-2 is approximately two to three times more prevalent than is HTLV-1 infection among first-time donors. This in part reflects the epidemic of HTLV-2 infection transmitted by injection drug use and secondary sexual transmission that began in the late 1960s (37).

DONOR TESTING AND COUNSELING

Testing of all allogeneic blood donations for HIV-1, HIV-2, HTLV-1, and HTLV-2 is mandated by federal regulations and standards of the American Association of Blood Banks (38). The primary goal of testing is prevention of virus transmission to blood recipients, but consideration also is given to accurate notification of blood donors of test results that suggest or show infection. The first objective is achieved with screening assays designed to have maximum sensitivity both to immunovariant viruses and to low-titer antibody during seroconversion to intercept any potentially infectious donations. The obligation of blood-collecting facilities to inform blood donors of possible infection is addressed with so-called confirmatory or supplemental testing, which is performed to clarify whether the donor has infection. Tests for both purposes can be divided into indirect assays used to detect antibodies to viral antigens and direct viral

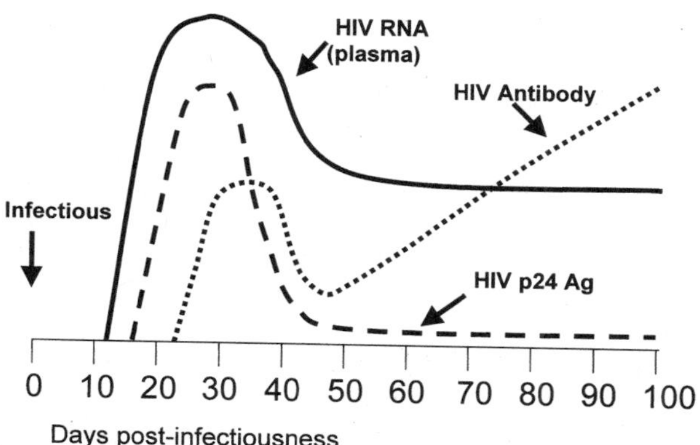

FIGURE 51.3. Virologic events during primary human immunodeficiency virus (HIV) infection. After initial infection and propagation of HIV in lymph nodes, a blood donor becomes infectious (defined as day 0), point estimates of HIV RNA becoming detectable in plasma on days 10 through 12, HIV-1 antigen (p24) on day 17, and HIV antibody on day 22. Subsequently, HIV p24 antigen often becomes undetectable, and HIV antibody level may decrease temporarily owing to complexing with HIV-1 antigen. After temporal decline, HIV antibody levels continue to increase during the initial 3 to 6 months of infection and persist indefinitely but may be lost in the preterminal stage of the disease, paralleled by a surge in viral burden that heralds collapse of the immune system. Plasma levels of HIV RNA generally remain detectable throughout the course of infection but may decrease to undetectable levels with highly active antiretroviral therapy. (Adapted from Busch MP. HIV and blood transfusions: focus on seroconversion. *Vox Sang* 1994;67:[Suppl 3]:13–18, with permission.)

assays used to detect viral antigens or viral genomic sequences in the form of nucleic acids (Fig. 51.3). Screening tests are performed on serum or plasma from pilot tubes collected at donation. If this initial test result is reactive, testing is repeated on both the originally tested serum or plasma and either a second pilot tube or an aliquot of plasma obtained from segmented tubing attached to the blood components. This element of the algorithm is designed as an additional safeguard to identify and resolve possible specimen-labeling errors. If the results of one or both repeated tests are reactive, the unit is designated *repeat reactive* and discarded. A look-back process is initiated to identify and quarantine all in-date components from any previous donations from that donor and to notify facilities and recipients who received blood components from previous donations (39).

SCREENING TESTS

Current routine blood center screening assays for antibodies to HIV and HTLV are based on an EIA format in which carefully selected recombinant and synthetic peptide antigens are the target of donor antibodies. Earlier versions of EIAs, in which crude HIV-1 and HTLV-I viral lysates were used, have been periodically updated to improve window-phase sensitivity and ensure detection of both predominant and variant viral strains (HIV-2, group O HIV-1, and HTLV-2). A recombinant "antigen sandwich" EIA format used in anti-HIV-1 and HIV-2 assays has allowed use of lower dilutions of donor serum and detection of immunoglobulin M (40,41). The advances led to marked narrowing of the seroconversion window with a concomitant reduction in the risk of use of screened blood (see later). Concerns that HIV group O strains may not be reliably detected with EIAs commonly used in the United States and Europe (42) led the U.S. Food and Drug Administration to mandate deferral of blood donors with close links to West Africa, the geographic region where HIV group O is most common. In the United States, group O infections have been rare (43), but an increase, apparently due to immigration from Africa, has been noticed in Europe (44).

With regard to HTLV screening, earlier versions of the HTLV-1 EIA were made more sensitive for HTLV-2 by means of addition of a recombinant HTLV-1 envelope glycoprotein 21 that has cross-reactivity for both viral types. True HTLV-1–HTLV-2 combination tests with viral lysates and recombinant peptides from both HTLV-1 and HTLV-2 subsequently were introduced. The resultant combination HTLV-1–HTLV-2 assay has good sensitivity for both viruses; it was licensed and introduced to blood donor screening in 1998 (45).

Testing for HIV-1 antigens (in practice, p24 antigen) became mandatory in the United States in 1996 because of the premise that HIV-1 antigens can be detected approximately 1 week earlier than can antibodies. Mathematical models constructed with findings from geographic areas with a very high incidence of HIV infection suggested that routine antigen testing would help detect 8 antigen-positive–antibody-negative donations per year, or 1 per 1.5 million screened units (29). In reality this projection was not achieved, and only 8 donations from infected window-phase (p24 antigen positive–anti-HIV negative) volunteer donors were intercepted solely on the basis of results of p24 antigen testing in the first 5 years of screening. This is an observed yield of approximately 1 in 8 million donations (21). A possible explanation for the underperformance of HIV-1 antigen testing in the detection of HIV-1 antibody–negative window-period infection is that blood donors in the HIV-1-antigen-only early phase of HIV-1 infection may be experiencing symptoms of acute retroviral infection that deter them from donation or result in rejection during the predonation history interview and physical examination (21).

Nucleic acid testing for HIV (HIV NAT), usually performed for HIV-1 as well as hepatitis C virus (HCV), relies on the polymerase chain reaction (PCR) or an alternative nucleic acid amplification method, most commonly transcription-mediated amplification (46). Testing was begun in several European countries in 1998 and in the United States in 1999 (47). On the basis of model projections similar to those for HIV-1 antigen, it was predicted that HIV NAT would help detect infected blood donors approximately 7 to 9 days before the antibody test with a projected incremental yield of approximately 1 per 1.2 to 1.5 million units screened, an almost ten times lower yield than projected for HCV NAT (21). In the United States volunteer donor setting, NAT is currently performed on plasma pooled for 16 to 24 donations under an investigational new drug exemption from the FDA. A positive test result on the pool is resolved by means of testing intermediate pools or individual pool members. Units that are NAT reactive are discarded, and the donor is notified and counseled (see later). Units that have a negative test result can be released for transfusion. Because the test has not been licensed, testing is not mandatory, and blood units are not labeled as to whether they have been subjected to NAT. Nevertheless, by mid 1999 almost all blood donations collected in the United States were screened before release by means of HIV-HCV NAT in addition to tests for HIV and HCV antibodies and HIV-1 antigen. Licensure of HIV-HCV NAT occured in 2002. Although controversial, it is likely that NAT performed on individual donations will replace testing of plasma donor pools once the necessary instrumentation is in place to handle the additional workload and to ensure completion of testing for timely release of cellular blood components. There is also active consideration of introduction of NAT for additional agents, including hepatitis B virus, hepatitis A virus, Parvovirus B19, and cytomegalovirus.

SUPPLEMENTAL TESTING AND DONOR COUNSELING

Because of the exquisite sensitivity of EIAs in blood donor screening and the low pretest probability of HIV or HTLV infection among blood donors, most positive screening results are falsely positive, despite excellent specificity of the tests. Supplemental assays therefore are essential for confirmation of positive screening results and for donor counseling (48). Supplemental assays for HIV must be performed with FDA-licensed reagents and must rule out both HIV-1 and HIV-2 infection (49). Although combination HIV-1 and HIV-2 supplemental assays with recombinant DNA-derived or synthetic peptide antigens have been developed that appear accurate in detecting and discriminating anti-HIV-1 and anti-HIV-2 (50), these are not yet approved by the FDA. Therefore current confirmatory algorithms in U.S. blood banks include HIV-1 viral lysate-based Western blots or immunofluorescence assays in combination with a licensed anti-HIV-2 EIA and unlicensed HIV-2 supplemental assays (49). Interpretive criteria for Western blots have evolved as tests have improved and understanding of the meaning of various banding patterns has increased. For currently licensed assays, a positive interpretation requires antibody reactivity to two of the following three HIV antigens: p24 (the major gag protein), gp41 (transmembrane env protein) or gp120/160 (external env protein/env precursor protein). Although these criteria are generally accurate, it is clear that some donors who show antibody reactivity only to the envelope glycoproteins or to env and p24 gag antigens are not infected with HIV-1 (51). It is important, therefore, that all initial positive Western blot results be confirmed with a separate follow-up sample, both to rule out specimen mix-up or testing errors and to discriminate nonspecific patterns from early seroconversion. A negative test result on Western blot is, by definition, the absence of any bands. Any other pattern of reactivity is classified as indeterminate. Only a small proportion of donors with indeterminate results of Western blot testing are infected with HIV-1 (51).

Repeatedly reactive donors with negative or persistent indeterminate Western blot patterns are deferred from further blood donations and notified that their screening and supplemental test results represent false positivity. Donors with confirmed positive results are appropriately counseled, and recipients of previous donations are traced in a process called *look-back* (39). Donors whose supplemental test results are completely negative are eligible for possible reentry into the donor pool according to an FDA-specified protocol (49), although in practice, logistical and legal considerations have generally prevented reinstatement of these donors.

Supplemental testing of HIV-1 antigen results relies on neutralization assays. When the EIA screening test for HIV-1 antigen is repeatedly reactive, the confirmatory neutralization test is performed to aid in counseling the donor and to determine the need for product quarantine, look-back, and deferral (52). Although donors whose serum shows neutralization are classified as having confirmed positive results for HIV-1 antigen and must be permanently deferred, studies involving reverse transcriptase PCR and follow-up evaluation of such donors have established that only a small proportion actually have HIV infection; that is, most have false-positive neutralizations (53). Donors whose serum cannot be neutralized are currently considered not confirmed but must be reported as HIV-1 antigen indeterminate. They should be temporarily deferred from donation for a minimum of 8 weeks. Donors can be reentered into the supply if they have been retested after this period and are found to be nonreactive in the HIV-1 antigen screening test and in the HIV antibody test. Unfortunately, approximately 70% of donors with indeterminate results remain p24 antigen indeterminate at follow-up testing and must be indefinitely deferred. As with antibody-reactive units, units from HIV-1 antigen repeatedly reactive donations cannot be used for transfusion or for further manufacturing into injectable products and must be quarantined and destroyed.

Supplemental testing for HTLV-1 and HTLV-2 has continued to be more difficult than for HIV-1 and HIV-2 because of the limited diagnostic market for HTLV test reagents. The earliest and most commonly used test is the Western blot. However, because of a deficiency in viral envelope protein, Western blots containing only HTLV-1 native viral proteins are relatively nonspecific and may be insensitive to HTLV-2 antibodies. Western blots supplemented with recombinant HTLV-1 transmembrane glycoprotein (rgp21e) are available and have increased sensitivity to HTLV-2 because of greater antibody cross-reactivity. However, false-positive reactions to rgp21 in combination with nonspecific reactivity with gag p19 or p24 bands, has occasionally led to false-positive Western blot interpretations (54). Radioimmunoprecipitation has been used in research and reference laboratories for many years to determine more specifically the presence of antibodies to envelope proteins of HTLV-1 and HTLV-2 (55). However, the radioimmunoprecipitation assay necessitates handling of radioactive substances and is labor intensive and therefore not suitable for routine supplemental testing in blood banks.

Second-generation Western blots have been developed that contain native HTLV-1 proteins supplemented with a refined version of the rgp21e to decrease nonspecific reactions in addition to two synthetic peptides specific to HTLV-1 (rgp46-1) and HTLV-2 (rgp46-2) (56,57). In the research setting, these assays have proved highly sensitive and specific for the diagnosis of HTLV-1 and HTLV-2 infection. Because of the presence of the type-specific peptide epitopes, they allow differentiation of HTLV-1 from HTLV-2 infection in most cases (56,57). This is important because counseling of a donor who has infection should be specific to the disease outcomes expected with either HTLV-I or HTLV-2 infection (58).

Unfortunately, no HTLV supplemental tests have been licensed by the FDA. For purposes of decision making about blood product quarantine, donor deferral and look-back, FDA allows "supplemental testing" with a second licensed screening EIA from a different manufacturer, so that only samples with repeatedly reactive results of two screening tests are considered reactive (45). This leaves many nonspecific reactions unresolved. Although unlicensed supplemental tests have been performed on donor samples under provisions for research, the counseling of infected donors on the basis of results of these unlicensed assays has carried regulatory risk. Because of the complexity of some of these supplemental assays, proficiency of laboratories depended on the local expertise and the volume of supplemental tests performed. This led the FDA to ban the use of unlicensed supplemental assays in the diagnosis of HTLV infection among blood donors. This is a concern because only 10% to 25% of EIA-reactive blood donors are in fact seropositive for HTLV-1 or HTLV-2, and seroindeterminate results are unlikely to indicate HTLV infection in the absence of definite risk factors (59). The lack of a licensed supplemental test thus results in a large number of EIA-reactive donors' being falsely informed that they may have HTLV infection. The effect of such a message is not trivial. Many donors have evidence of considerable psychosocial stress after being notified of such test results (60). Development of supplemental assays for HTLV-1 and HTLV-2 that meet criteria for licensing is urgently needed.

Nucleic acid testing for blood donor screening has not yet been licensed in the United States. Therefore official algorithms for supplemental testing have not been developed. Proposals have been made, however, to use an independent donor sample in a second NAT assay as a confirmatory test based on different primers, detection probes, and technology (47). Although the counseling message to donors with NAT-positive and HIV antigen and antibody–negative results will have to emphasize that infection is possible, most such results are caused by cross-contamination. Follow-up testing to document persistent NAT positivity and seroconversion is essential for definitive confirmation.

WINDOW PERIOD AND RISK OF TRANSFUSION-TRANSMITTED RETROVIRAL INFECTION

The window period of acute viral infection usually is defined as the lag time between exposure to the virus or onset of infectiousness in the host and the appearance of a diagnostic marker of the infection in the bloodstream. In blood donation, the time between onset of infectiousness through secondary blood transfusion and detectability of infection with the screening test is the critical period during which blood donated by an infected donor, who typically has no symptoms at this early stage of infection, would not be rejected and could enter the blood supply and infect the blood recipient. Blood donation during the pre-seroconversion window period of HIV or HTLV infection is by far the most common reason screened blood units still carry a small risk of transmission of human retrovirus (61). This became evident in the late 1980s when well-documented cases of HIV-1 transmission from screened blood transfusions were reported (62). It was therefore clear that a small number of transmissions continued, despite screening with antibody tests. On the basis of investigations of HIV infection among patients who received transfusions from 1986 through 1991, investigators at the U.S. Centers for Disease Control and Prevention (CDC) estimated that approximately five cases of transfusion-associated AIDS had occurred per year during that period owing to infection from anti-HIV–negative window-phase blood transfusions (63). Reports of isolated cases of HIV transmission from screened blood have continued. They include a case involving transfusion of HIV antibody– and antigen (p24)–negative blood that had been donated during the window period of HIV infection and would have escaped detection even with minipool NAT because of the low viral copy number (64).

In the United States, two prospective studies conducted between 1985 and 1991 estimated the risk of HIV transmission from antibody-screened donations at approximately 1 case in 60,000 units (65,66). These studies were discontinued in 1992 because of high cost and the realization that prospective monitoring of donors and recipients represents an insensitive and inadequate approach for assessing the small residual risk of HIV transmission from screened transfusions. Since then an alternative approach has been developed for estimating the risk of HIV infection from transfusions, now known as the *incidence–window period model* (29). It is based on the premise that the risk of virus transmission by means of blood transfusion in a given geographic area is primarily a function of the incidence (number of newly infected blood donors per person-time of observation) and the length of the window period (time from infectiousness to seroconversion according to results of screening tests). The risk of HIV-1 transmission from repeated donors and, with some adjustments, from first-time donors can be calculated. Window-period estimates for HIV-1 infection in the United States decreased from a median of 45 days (95% confidence interval, 34–55 days) for the overall period from 1985 to 1990 to approximately 22 to 25 days with routine introduction in 1992 of new format for anti-HIV-1–HIV-2 combination tests to detect HIV-specific immunoglobulin M antibody 10 to 15 days earlier than with previously available assays (40). By combining the 25-day window-period estimate with data on the frequency of HIV seroconversion in large U.S. donor populations, two independent studies derived point estimates for the risk of HIV transmission during the 1992 through 1995 period of 1:450,000 (67) and 1:495,000 (68) (Table 51.2). Introduction of HIV-1 antigen screening in 1995 is likely to have further reduced the risk, but because fewer than expected HIV-1 antigen–positive HIV-1 and HIV-2 antibody–negative units were intercepted since the test was introduced, it is thought that its contribution to risk reduction has been minimal (21). On the other hand, incorporation of NAT of pooled samples into routine blood donor screening, which began on a research basis in 1999, decreased the risk to an estimated 1 per 725,000 to 835,000 screened donations (Table 51.2). By multiplying the per-unit risk estimates by 18 million transfused components per year in the United States, it can be expected that a maximum 22 to 25 recipients per year receive transfusions with blood infected with HIV-1. Fewer than 5 of these infected recipients would be expected to contract AIDS-related diseases before dying of other causes (63). The risk of transmission of HIV-2 has been estimated at less than 1 in 15 million (69), other rare subtypes (e.g., HIV-1 subtype O) (70) being of even lesser concern. It is impressive to recognize that these combined risks are nearly 7,000-fold lower than the risk that existed at the peak of the transfusion AIDS epidemic between 1982 and 1984 (19).

With regard to HTLV infection, a study of U.S. transfusion recipients estimated the risk of HTLV infection at 12 per 100,000 units before and 1.4 per 100,000 units after the institution of HTLV screening in 1988 (65). More recent projections based on the incidence–window period model are a residual risk of HTLV-1–HTLV-2 infection of 1.6 per 1 million screened donations, which is comparable to the risk of HIV infection (Table 51.2) (68). Although the risk of transmission of HTLV-1 and HTLV-2 in cell-free plasma is undoubtedly small, the issue of whether it is possible is controversial. Studies in Jamaica and the United States showed no episodes of transfusion transmission among persons receiving only plasma transfusions (71). Laboratory studies have shown that cell-free transmission of HTLV-1 is difficult. It also appears that transfusion of blood products containing residual leukocytes carries a higher risk of HTLV transmission than does transfusion free of leukocytes (65).

TABLE 51.2. ESTIMATED RISK OF VIRAL INFECTION

	Window Period	Viral Variants	Chronic Antibody-Negative Carriers	Testing Error	Total
HIV *before* p24, MP NAT	24	<0.6	<0.1	0.4	25
HIV *after* p24, MP NAT	12–13	<0.6	0	0	13–14
HTLV	15	<1	<1	0.8	16

In the United States per 10 million donations by source of risk before and after implementation of HIV-1 p24 antigen and minipool HIV NAT.
HIV, human immunodeficiency virus; MP NAT, minipool nucleic acid testing; HTLV, human T-cell lymphotropic virus.
Adapted from Kleinman SH, Busch MP. The risks of transfusion-transmitted infection: direct estimation and mathematical modelling. *Baillieres Best Pract Res Clin Haematol* 2000;13:631–649, with permission.

RECIPIENT INFECTION

Human immunodeficiency virus is not inactivated by blood refrigeration and survives freezing of plasma. The virus is therefore readily passed by means of transfusion of cellular and frozen plasma components. Clinical, virologic, and immunologic studies of exposed transfusion recipients and persons with hemophilia have yielded important insights into the significance of factors that might influence transmission of HIV-1 infection and disease course. The Transfusion Safety Study (TSS), which is unique in being the only U.S. study that traced and enrolled recipients of known seropositive units (72,73), offers some of the clearest data addressing these issues. In the TSS, 111 (89.5%) of 124 enrolled recipients of transfusions of anti-HIV-1–positive blood components experienced seroconversion to anti-HIV-1 positivity (73). Neither characteristics of the infection of the donor nor inherent recipient susceptibility factors significantly influenced transmission of HIV-1 by means of transfusion (74). Variables identified as correlating with the likelihood of HIV-1 transmission are type of blood component transfused and duration of storage (75). Washed red blood cell units and red blood cell units stored more than 26 days had lower transmission rates than did other components. This observation and experimental evidence (76) suggest that component manipulations that reduce the number of viable leukocytes or free virus in plasma may reduce but not eliminate infectiousness.

With regard to recipients of clotting factor concentrates, an average of approximately 50% of persons with hemophilia treated with factor VIII in the early 1980s experienced seroconversion (77,78). However, persons with hemophilia treated with very high doses of factor VIII (>500,000 units) experienced seroconversion to anti-HIV-l positivity at a rate approaching 100% (78). This indicates that perhaps with the rare exception of persons lacking HIV-1 coreceptors required for infection (see later), no one is resistant to HIV-1 infection given a large enough inoculum and repeated exposures. There was early hope that a proportion of persons with hemophilia and seropositive results might have experienced seroconversion as a result of exposure to denatured HIV-1 proteins rather than infectious virus. Several large studies, however, performed with sensitive viral culture and PCR techniques have confirmed the presence of persistent HIV-1 infection in 100% of persons with hemophilia and positive serologic results (79,80). On the other hand, although several early studies with PCR showed detection of HIV-1 DNA in a subset of exposed persons with hemophilia and seronegative results (81), subsequent studies refuted these reports (82,83) as well as the general concept of seronegative (so-called immunosilent) HIV-1 infection (84).

Human T-cell lymphoma virus type 1 was shown in Japan to be transmitted by means of blood transfusion with an efficiency of at least 50% (85,86). In contrast, a cohort study in Jamaica in the late 1980s showed a 25% to 30% risk of HTLV-1 infection after transfusion of 1 unit of blood infected with HTLV-1. There was a 50-day mean latency period between the implicated transfusion and the development of de novo anti-HTLV antibodies (71). The TSS, undertaken in the mid 1980s, showed an even lower rate of transmission of only 10% to 20% for HTLV-1 and HTLV-2 (87). Differences between these transmission rates may be due to the requirement that HTLV-infected viable lymphocytes must be present in the unit transfused. In agreement with this hypothesis, the TSS investigators found a significant inverse correlation between the duration of refrigerated storage (presumably related to lymphocyte viability) and the risk of HTLV transmission. Although such data were not reported, it is probable that the storage time of blood units studied in Japan and Jamaica was shorter than in the U.S. study.

CLINICAL COURSE

The clinical courses of HIV and HTLV infection are quite different. Human immunodeficiency virus is more infectious, and in most instances it causes a relentlessly progressive, generalized immunodeficiency, and most patients, if left untreated, eventually die of AIDS. Human T-lymphotrophic virus, however, causes lifelong asymptomatic infection, and only in a small number of persons with the infection does autoimmune-like myelopathy or an unusual type of T-cell leukemia or lymphoma develop.

The course of HIV infection begins with an asymptomatic incubation period of approximately 2 to 3 weeks that culminates in an acute flulike illness in approximately 40% to 90% of patients (88). Signs and symptoms of acute HIV-1 infection include fever, enlarged lymph nodes, sore throat, rash, joint and muscle pain, headache, diarrhea, and vomiting. This syndrome usually lasts less than 2 weeks but may continue for several months. Because of the nonspecific nature of the symptoms and negative results of HIV antibody tests at this early stage of infection, the correct diagnosis often is not made until later in the disease. The infection enters a clinically latent stage, but viral replication and dissemination continue unabated (89). The virus can be transmitted in blood or genital secretions during this asymptomatic carrier phase.

Persistent asymptomatic infection lasts a median of approximately 10 years in the absence of treatment (90). After years of lack of clinical progression, however, both plasma viremia and the percentage of infected T lymphocytes increase, immune functions served by helper T cells decline resulting in impaired immune reactivity, and there are inappropriate immune activation and cytokine secretion. Eventually a sharp decline in the number of $CD4^+$T lymphocytes leads to profound immunosuppression, and persons with the infection die of opportunistic illnesses.

Enumeration of viral load and $CD4^+$ cells is used to guide the treatment of patients with HIV infection. The AIDS classification system devised by the CDC is based on the number of $CD4^+$ T cells ($\leq$200/μl defines AIDS), the presence or absence of systemic symptoms, and the existence of any of numerous conditions considered to be AIDS-defining illnesses (91). Among these conditions are otherwise unusual malignant tumors, such as Kaposi sarcoma and central nervous system lymphoma, and an array of devastating, potentially lethal opportunistic infections with fungi and parasites, such as *Pneumocystis carinii* pneumonia. Advances in management of HIV and opportunistic infections coupled with new tools for measuring HIV replication have dramatically enhanced survival (92). Unfortunately, worldwide the disease is spreading rapidly and for most persons with HIV infection in developing countries, effective therapy is either not available or not affordable (93).

Investigating the course of HIV-1 infection in transfusion recipients provides data for counseling and treatment of patients with infection and those at risk. It also is of medical scientific interest because the date of infection and transfusion is precisely known and because recipients lack many cofactors (e.g., other sexually transmitted diseases or intravenous drug use) that can influence the course of disease in other infected cohorts. The transfusion setting is unique in that the course of disease in a recipient can be compared with that in a linked donor to allow study of whether a relation exists between disease progression in a donor and his or her recipients (74,94,95). Of the 112 recipients with infection enrolled in the TSS, 37 had AIDS (CDC 1987 revised definition) after 7 years of posttransfusion follow-up study (96). According to Kaplan-Meyer analysis, the actuarial risk of AlDS at 7 years was 51%. This rate was faster than the rate of progression observed for donors with infection and persons with hemophilia whose cases were followed in parallel in that study (96,97). As observed by others (98), an effect of age on rate of disease progression was found in all three TSS groups, older patients having symptoms of AIDS earlier than did younger persons. Once age and underlying disease were controlled for, progression rates to clinical AIDS were almost identical for TSS recipients and persons with hemophilia, whereas the rate of diagnosis of AIDS was slightly higher for enrolled donors (most of whom were homosexual men) (96). This suggests that factors such as route of infection, inoculum size, and proposed cofactors, such as other viral infections (e.g., with cytomegalovirus or hepatitis B virus), are not highly significant in determining the course of HIV disease.

Further analyses of TSS data illustrate the importance of the level of viremia to HIV transmission in cases of transfusion-acquired infection (99) and in heterosexual transmission from persons infected through transfusion to their sexual partners (100). With regard to factors influencing disease progression, data from the study point to host factors rather than differences in viral strains within B-type HIV-1 as determinants of disease progression (101). Archived samples from the TSS also were used to investigate the role of the β-chemokine CCR5, a more recently discovered coreceptor for non-syncytium-inducing strains of HIV-1, in parenteral transmission of virus. Recipients of HIV-seropositive blood units and coagulation factor concentrates who had a 32-bp deletion in the CCR5 gene were less susceptible to infection, although in those with infection disease progressed at the same rate as in recipients with a normal CCR5 gene (102). Finally, the significance of a virulence gene, *nef,* was demonstrated in an Australian cohort of a blood donor and eight transfusion recipients infected with an HIV-1 viral strain lacking a functioning *nef* gene. The cohort members had a milder than usual course of disease and prolonged disease-free survival without therapy (103).

Transfusion provides a mode of transmission of HIV, and there is evidence that transfusion affects the course of disease in patients with AIDS. Observations from retrospective and small prospective studies suggested that allogeneic transfusion may accelerate disease progression and shorten survival among patients with HIV infection (104). In vitro experiments provided evidence that allogeneic leukocytes, presumably through immunologic activation of lymphocytes and macrophages, increase replication of HIV, whereas autologous leukocytes and allogeneic red blood cells, platelets, and plasma do not have this effect (105). However, the results of the Viral Activation by Transfusion Study, a large, multicenter U.S. clinical trial of provision of leukoreduced blood to patients with late-stage HIV infection, showed no evidence that leukoreduction benefits this patient group (106).

Infection with HTLV in general rarely causes insignificant clinical disease, although HTLV-1 infection is clearly associated with the $CD4^+$ T-lymphocytic lymphoma known as *adult T-cell leukemia or lymphoma* (107,108). This lymphoma, which has a leukemic phase in one fourth to one third of persons with HTLV-1 infection, also is associated with hypercalcemia, skin lesions, and hepatosplenomegaly (109). Atypical malignant lymphocytes with convoluted nuclei called *flower cells* are present in a large number of patients with leukemic-phase ATL and may be present in low numbers in persons with asymptomatic, seropositive HTLV-1 infection (110,111). The prognostic significance of flower cells is not well defined, although it appears that persons with relatively high numbers of circulating flower cells may be predisposed to increased risk of ATL (112). A person with HTLV-1 infection at birth has an estimated 4% lifetime risk of development of ATL, the risk presumably being lower among those infected sexually as adults (113). There are two case reports of ATL occurring after apparent transfusion-related HTLV-1 infection (114). Chemotherapy often is less effective than for other forms of lymphoma and leukemia, and a high mortality is associated with this hematologic malignant disease (115,116).

Although both HTLV-1 and HTLV-2 are known to cause spontaneous lymphocytic proliferation in vitro (12), HTLV-2 does not appear to cause hematologic malignant disease. Although HTLV-2 was initially isolated in two cases of atypical T-lymphocytic hairy cell leukemia, subsequent epidemiologic studies of hairy cell leukemia have not revealed an association with HTLV-2 infection (117–120). Further studies also have ruled out an association between HTLV-2 infection and mycosis fungoides or large granular cell leukemia (121–123).

The other major disease association of both HTLV-1 and HTLV-2 is HTLV-associated HAM-TSP. Initially described by Gessain et al. in Martinique (124), the association with HAM-TSP was soon confirmed by investigators in Japan and elsewhere (125–128). This disorder is a slowly progressive form of myelopathy characterized by spastic paraparesis of the lower extremity, hyperreflexia, bowel and bladder symptoms, and relative sparing of upper extremity strength and cognitive function (129). The course is slow but progressive, 10 years often elapsing between the first signs and severe paraplegia necessitating use of a wheelchair. Despite considerable disability, this disease does not appear to be associated with increased mortality. There is no definitive therapy for HAM-TSP, although use of systemic steroids, immunosuppression with azathioprine, and the use of the androgenic agent danazol have had transient success (129).

In a cohort study, the risk of HAM-TSP was estimated to be approximately 2% among persons with positive results for HTLV-1 (130). Sexual acquisition of HTLV-1 may be a risk factor for HAM-TSP (131); however, the incubation period may be shortest after transfusion-acquired infection (132–134). Persons with positive results for HTLV-2 have been less well studied, but the risk of HAM-TSP appears to be slightly less than or equal to that associated with HTLV-1 infection (130). In contrast to some initial reports, there is no association of either HTLV-1 or HTLV-2 infection with classic multiple sclerosis (135–137). Likewise, implication of HTLV-1 and HTLV-2 infection in other neurologic syndromes is controversial because persons with HTLV-2 infection may have confounding genetic or environmental factors that predispose to neurologic disease (138).

Other immunologic diseases and phenomena have been reported in association with HTLV-1 and HTLV-2 infection. Infection with HTLV-1 has been associated with lymphocytic pneumonitis and uveitis (139,140). Cases of HTLV-1 polymyositis have been reported, and both HTLV-1 and HTLV-2 may be associated with an increased incidence of arthritis (141,142). Of particular interest, a cohort study showed that HTLV-2 and to a lesser extent HTLV-1 are associated with an increased incidence of other infections, including pneumonia, acute bronchitis, and urinary tract infection (143). This finding is consistent with the HTLV-1 association with infective dermatitis among children (144). Although the mechanism of immunologic dysfunction has not been described, these results do indicate a mild degree of virus-induced immunosuppression. It is not clear whether either HTLV-1 or HTLV-2 contributes to an increased incidence of other types of malignant disease. A study in Japan showed an increased risk of "virus-associated" malignant tumors such as hepatoma (145). However, a study in the United States showed no increased association between any nonhematologic malignant disease and HTLV-1 or HTLV-2 infection (143).

TREATMENT

Antiretroviral therapy plays a central role in the management of HIV infection. Prophylaxis and management of opportunistic infections, therapy for HIV-associated malignant lesions, and support with hematopoietic stimulating factors are essential adjuncts in the overall management of the disease (3). Antiviral regimens have evolved from monotherapy, typically with a nucleoside analogue, to combination treatment with a variety of antiviral agents that target different viral structures. The result is much more effective and longer-lasting virus suppression (146). This treatment strategy, often called *highly active antiretroviral therapy* (HAART), has achieved remarkable success in decreasing mortality from AIDS and in causing durable remissions among patients with HIV infection (92). Highly active antiretroviral therapy is effective in suppressing HIV to often undetectable levels but cannot eradicate the virus, which predictably has a resurgence when treatment is interrupted. An important controversy is the optimal time point at which treatment should begin. Proponents of early treatment initially argued that patients have less damage to the immune system and have a better prognosis if aggressive antiretroviral therapy is started before signs of immune deficiency develop and therapy is continued indefinitely (147). In light of serious drug toxicities and risk of selection of multi-drug-resistant viral strains with this regimen, more recent recommendations are to begin HAART later in the disease (148,149). The principles of antiretroviral therapy for established HIV infection are likely to evolve as experience with these agents increases.

A special situation is chemoprophylaxis to prevent HIV infection after high-risk exposure to the virus, such as through injury with contaminated needles, unprotected sexual relations with an infected partner, or receipt of blood transfusion from an HIV-positive donor. Although definitive proof of effectiveness has not been established, case reports suggest that combination antiretroviral therapy provided within hours of exposure may prevent infection. Most data reflect experience with needle-stick injuries in the health care setting, which has led to recommendations for administering prophylactic treatment under certain conditions (150). An extremely rare situation is transfusion of blood from a donor with known HIV infection. A case from Denmark suggested that antiretroviral therapy begun 50 hours after transfusion of an HIV-infected red blood cell unit may have prevented transmission to the recipient (151).

Despite the success of HAART, its medical limitations and high cost have spawned a search for additional and alternative treatment modalities. Gene therapy (152) and immune-based strategies of HIV control (153) are novel treatment strategies under active research. Perhaps most important, development of an HIV vaccine is making slow but steady progress (154). Unlike many traditional vaccines, a realistic goal for an HIV vaccine may not be conferring sterilizing immunity but may be control of viral replication. In conjunction with intermittent antiviral therapy, control of replication could allow persons with infection to stay healthy and reduce the likelihood of secondary transmission of the virus to others. Given the almost insurmountable problems in managing HIV infection in developing countries with currently available therapies, even such a partially effective vaccine would offer the best hope to cope with the pandemic (155).

Unlike that of HIV infection, management of asymptomatic infection with HTLV has not been considered, given the low likelihood of development of clinical disease. Patients with HAM-TSP have been given immunosuppressive therapy, but treatment responses are limited, variable, and often transient (129). Better responses to glucocorticoid treatment have been reported among patients who acquired HTLV-1 infection from blood transfusion (156). More aggressive intervention is required in the management of ATL, in which the median survival time is less than 1 year. Conventional combination chemotherapy, experimental regimens including combinations of antiretroviral agents, interferon, and etretinate, and allogeneic bone marrow transplantation have been used with limited success.

SURVEILLANCE FOR ADDITIONAL RETROVIRUSES AMONG BLOOD DONORS AND RECIPIENTS

The discovery of HIV and HTLV, and the appreciation that they are important transfusion-transmissible agents, has raised concerns that other human retroviruses have not been discovered. It is also well established that retroviruses from other species can be transmitted to humans and pose a risk to the blood supply (157,158). There is a critical need for active surveillance for new or emerging retroviruses of potential relevance to transfusion safety.

It is known that 5% to 10% of the genome of humans and many other species comprises endogenous retroviral sequences. The origin and function of human endogenous retroviral sequences remain unclear, although it is generally believed that these sequences represent relics of ancestral retroviral infections that have been conserved through evolution for functional properties, including protection from exogenous retroviral infection. There is no convincing evidence that human endogenous retroviral sequences are associated with any disease or that they can be transmitted horizontally by means of blood transfusion or other routes. There is concern, however, that endogenous retroviruses in the genomes of other species can be activated into exogenous retroviruses and be transmitted to humans (159–161). This concern has been highlighted by demonstration of in vitro transmission of porcine endogenous retrovirus sequences to human cells (159). There is particular concern with regard to use of animal-derived blood constituents (e.g., porcine-derived clotting factors, bovine albumin, equine immunoglobulins) or organs in xenotransplantation protocols. Studies with sensitive serologic and molecular assays conducted to examine whether endogenous retroviruses from other species infect humans exposed to blood products or organs from these species have not documented any cases of infection (160,161).

There is concern regarding cross-species transmission of exogenous retroviruses with the potential that such transmission can result in accelerated transmission patterns and increased pathogenicity among humans similar to what likely happened with simian immunodeficiency virus and HIV. For example, a clinical syndrome called *idiopathic (HIV-negative) CD4 lymphocytopenia,* described in the early 1990s, was speculated to result from a novel retrovirus infection. However, subsequent studies with both high risk and blood donor populations did not confirm a retroviral or other infectious etiologic factor, with the exception of a subset of cases caused by group O HIV-1 (162). There has been speculation over the years that donors with indeterminate seroreactivity for HIV or HTLV may harbor cross-reactive primate or ungulate retroviruses (163). However, most studies that have probed samples from donors with indeterminate test results have not identified evidence of infection based on type-specific serologic or PCR analyses (163).

Over the past several years, novel assays have been developed that allow for probing of donor and other specimens for evidence of unknown retroviruses. These include amplified reverse transcriptase assays, also called product-enhanced reverse transcriptase assays, and generic PCR assays that target conserved regions of polymerase and *gag* genes that are common among highly divergent retrovirus families (164). Continued application of these tools to samples from blood donor-recipient repositories in both developed and developing countries will be important to reassure the public that additional retroviral agents do not pose a risk to blood safety.

REFERENCES

1. Blood supply: transfusion-associated risks. Washington, DC: U.S. General Accounting Office, 1997.
2. Fields BN, Knipe DM, Howley PM. *Fields virology.* New York: Lippincott– Raven, 1996.
3. Cohen P, Sande M, Volberding P. *The AIDS knowledge base.* Philadelphia: Lippincott Williams & Wilkins, 1999.
4. Levy J. *HIV and the pathogenesis of AIDS,* 2nd ed. Washington, DC: ASM Press, 1998.
5. Sande M, Volberding P. *The medical management of AIDS.* Philadelphia: WB Saunders, 1999.
6. Fauci AS. Host factors and the pathogenesis of HIV-induced disease. *Nature* 1996;384:529.
7. Gallo RC. Human retroviruses in the second decade:a personal perspective. *Nat Med* 1995;1 (8):753.
8. Greene WC. The molecular biology of human immunodeficiency virus type 1 infection. *N Engl J Med* 1991;324:308.
9. Manns A, Hisada M, La Grenade L. Human T-lymphotropic virus type I infection. *Lancet* 1999;353:1951.
10. Hahn BH, Shaw GM, De Cock KM, et al. AIDS as a zoonosis: scientific and public health implications. *Science* 2000;287:607.
11. Poiesz BJ, Ruscetti FW, Gazdar AF, et al. Detection and isolation of type C retrovirus particles from fresh and cultured lymphocytes of a patient with cutaneous T-cell lymphoma. *Proc Natl Acad Sci U S A* 1980;77:7415.
12. Blattner W. *Human retrovirology: HTLV.* New York: Raven Press, 1990.
13. Joint United Nations Programme on HIV/AIDS. AIDS epidemic update: December 2000. Geneva, Switzerland: UNAIDS, 2000.
14. Gao F, Bailes E, Robertson DL, et al. Origin of HIV-1 in the chimpanzee Pan troglodytes troglodytes. *Nature* 1999;397:436.
15. Zhu T, Korber BT, Nahmias AJ, et al. An African HIV-1 sequence from 1959 and implications for the origin of the epidemic. *Nature* 1998;391:594.
16. Korber B, Muldoon M, Theiler J, et al. Timing the ancestor of the HIV-1 pandemic strains. *Science* 2000;288:1789.
17. Centers for Disease Control. Update on acquired immune deficiency syndrome (AIDS) among patients with hemophilia A. *MMWR Morb Mortal Wkly Rep* 1982;31:644.
18. Centers for Disease Control. Possible transfusion-associated acquired immune deficiency syndrome (AIDS): California. *MMWR Morb Mortal Wkly Rep* 1982;31:652.
19. Busch MP, Young MJ, Samson SM, et al. Risk of human immunodeficiency virus (HIV) transmission by blood transfusions before the implementation of HIV-1 antibody screening. The Transfusion Safety Study Group. *Transfusion* 1991;31:4.
20. Leveton L, Sox H, Stoto M. *HIV and the blood supply: an analysis of crisis decisionmaking.* Washington, DC: National Academy Press, 1995.
21. Kleinman SH, Busch MP. The risks of transfusion-transmitted infection: direct estimation and mathematical modelling. *Baillieres Best Pract Res Clin Haematol* 2000;13:631–649.
22. Slattery JP, Franchini G, Gessain A. Genomic evolution, patterns of global dissemination, and interspecies transmission of human and simian T-cell leukemia/lymphotropic viruses. *Genome Res* 1999;9:525.
23. Li HC, Fujiyoshi T, Lou H, et al. The presence of ancient human T-cell lymphotropic virus type I provirus DNA in an Andean mummy. *Nat Med* 1999;5:1428.
24. Kleinman S, Swanson P, Allain JP, et al. Transfusion transmission of human T-lymphotropic virus types I and II: serologic and polymerase chain reaction results in recipients identified through look-back investigations. *Transfusion* 1993;33:14.
25. Sullivan MT, Williams AE, Fang CT, et al. Transmission of human T-lymphotropic virus types I and II by blood transfusion: a retrospective study of recipients of blood components (1983 through 1988). The American Red Cross HTLV-I/II Collaborative Study Group. *Arch Intern Med* 1991;151:2043.

26. Vrielink H, Reesink HW. Transfusion-transmissible infections. *Curr Opin Hematol* 1998;5:396.
27. Taylor GP. The epidemiology of HTLV-I in Europe. *J Acquir Immune Defic Syndr Hum Retrovirol* 1996;13[Suppl 1]:S8.
28. Lackritz EM. Prevention of HIV transmission by blood transfusion in the developing world:achievements and continuing challenges. *AIDS* 1998;12[Suppl A]:S81.
29. Kleinman S, Busch MP, Korelitz JJ, et al. The incidence/window period model and its use to assess the risk of transfusion-transmitted human immunodeficiency virus and hepatitis C virus infection. *Transfus Med Rev* 1997;11:155.
30. Glynn SA, Kleinman SH, Schreiber GB, et al. Trends in incidence and prevalence of major transfusion-transmissible viral infections in US blood donors, 1991 to 1996. Retrovirus Epidemiology Donor Study (REDS). *JAMA* 2000;284:229.
31. McFarland W, Busch MP, Kellogg TA, et al. Detection of early HIV infection and estimation of incidence using a sensitive/less-sensitive enzyme immunoassay testing strategy at anonymous counseling and testing sites in San Francisco. *J Acquir Immune Defic Syndr* 1999;22: 484.
32. Trends in the HIV epidemic. Atlanta: Centers for Disease Control and Prevention, 1998.
33. Remis RS, Delage G, Palmer RW. Risk of HIV infection from blood transfusion in Montreal. *CMAJ* 1997;157:375.
34. Schwartz DW, Simson G, Baumgarten K, et al. Risk of human immunodeficiency virus (HIV) transmission by anti-HIV-negative blood components in Germany and Austria. *Ann Hematol* 1995;70:209.
35. Whyte GS, Savoia HF. The risk of transmitting HCV, HBV or HIV by blood transfusion in Victoria. *Med J Aust* 1997;166:584.
36. Fleming AF. HIV and blood transfusion in sub-Saharan Africa. *Transfus Sci* 1997;18:167.
37. Murphy EL, Watanabe K, Nass CC, et al. Evidence among blood donors for a 30-year-old epidemic of human T lymphotropic virus type II infection in the United States. *J Infect Dis* 1999;180:1777.
38. *Standards for blood banks and transfusion services.* Bethesda, MD: American Association of Blood Banks, 2000.
39. Food and Drug Administration. Current good manufacturing practices for blood and blood components: notification of consignees receiving blood and blood components at increased risk for transmitting HIV infection. *Federal Register* 1996:61:47413.
40. Busch MP, Lee LL, Satten GA, et al. Time course of detection of viral and serologic markers preceding human immunodeficiency virus type 1 seroconversion: implications for screening of blood and tissue donors. *Transfusion* 1995;35:91.
41. Gallarda JL, Henrard DR, Liu D, et al. Early detection of antibody to human immunodeficiency virus type 1 by using an antigen conjugate immunoassay correlates with the presence of immunoglobulin M antibody. *J Clin Microbiol* 1992;30:2379.
42. Apetrei C, Loussert-Ajaka I, Descamps D, et al. Lack of screening test sensitivity during HIV-1 non-subtype B seroconversions. *AIDS* 1996;10:F57.
43. Sullivan PS, Do AN, Ellenberger D, et al. Human immunodeficiency virus (HIV) subtype surveillance of African-born persons at risk for group O and group N HIV infections in the United States. *J Infect Dis* 2000;181:463.
44. Couturier E, Damond F, Roques P, et al. HIV-1 diversity in France, 1996-1998. The AC 11 laboratory network. *AIDS* 2000;14:289.
45. *Guidance for industry: donor screening for antibodies to HTLV-2.* Rockville, MD: U.S. Food and Drug Administration, 1998.
46. Busch M, Stramer S, Kleinman S. Evolving applications of nucleic acid amplification assays for prevention of virus transmission by blood components and derivatives. In: Garratty G, ed. *Applications of molecular biology to blood transfusion medicine.* Bethesda, MD: American Associations of Blood Banks, 1997:123.
47. Busch MP, Kleinman SH, Jackson B, et al. Nucleic acid amplification testing of blood donors for transfusion-transmitted infectious diseases: report of the Interorganizational Task Force on Nucleic Acid Amplification Testing of Blood Donors. *Transfusion* 2000;40:143.
48. Dodd RY, Stramer SL. Indeterminate results in blood donor testing: what you don't know can hurt you. *Transfus Med Rev* 2000;14:151.
49. U.S. Food and Drug Administration. *Revised recommendations for the prevention of human immunodeficiency (HIV) transmission by blood and blood products.* Rockville, MD: Center for Biologics Evaluation and Research, 1992.
50. Tobler LH, Kaufman E, Gefter N, et al. Use of human immunodeficiency virus (HIV) type 1 and 2 recombinant strip immunoblot assay to resolve enzyme immunoassay anti-HIV-2- repeatably reactive samples after anti-HIV-1/2 combination enzyme immunoassay screening. *Transfusion* 1997;37:921.
51. Kleinman S, Busch MP, Hall L, et al. False-positive HIV-1 test results in a low-risk screening setting of voluntary blood donation. Retrovirus Epidemiology Donor Study. *JAMA* 1998;280:1080.
52. Recommendation for donor screening with a licensed test for HIV-1 antigen [memorandum]. Rockville, MD: U.S. Food and Drug Administration Congressional and Consumer Affairs, 1995.
53. Stramer S, Aberle-Grasse J, Brodsky J, et al. United States blood donor screening with p24 antigen: one year experience. *Transfusion* 1997; 37:1S.
54. Kleinman SH, Kaplan JE, Khabbaz RF, et al. Evaluation of a p21e-spiked western blot (immunoblot) in confirming human T-cell lymphotropic virus type I or II infection in volunteer blood donors. The Retrovirus Epidemiology Donor Study Group. *J Clin Microbiol* 1994;32:603.
55. Gallo D, Penning LM, Diggs JL, et al. Sensitivities of radioimmunoprecipitation assay and PCR for detection of human T-lymphotropic type II infection. *J Clin Microbiol* 1994;32:2464.
56. Lal RB, Brodine S, Kazura J, et al. Sensitivity and specificity of a recombinant transmembrane glycoprotein (rgp21)-spiked western immunoblot for serological confirmation of human T-cell lymphotropic virus type I and type II infections. *J Clin Microbiol* 1992;30:296.
57. Brodine SK, Kaime EM, Roberts C, et al. Simultaneous confirmation and differentiation of human T-lymphotropic virus types I and II infection by modified western blot containing recombinant envelope glycoproteins. *Transfusion* 1993;33:925.
58. Guidelines for counseling persons infected with human T-lymphotropic virus type I (HTLV-I) and type II (HTLV-2). Centers for Disease Control and Prevention and the USPHS Working Group. *Ann Intern Med* 1993;118:448.
59. Busch MP, Laycock M, Kleinman SH, et al. Accuracy of supplementary serologic testing for human T-lymphotropic virus types I and II in US blood donors. Retrovirus Epidemiology Donor Study. *Blood* 1994;83:1143.
60. Guiltinan AM, Murphy EL, Horton JA, et al. Psychological distress in blood donors notified of HTLV-I/II infection. Retrovirus Epidemiology Donor Study. *Transfusion* 1998;38:1056.
61. Busch MP, Watanabe KK, Smith JW, et al. False-negative testing errors in routine viral marker screening of blood donors. *Transfusion* 2000;40:585.
62. Ward JW, Holmberg SD, Allen JR, et al. Transmission of human immunodeficiency virus (HIV) by blood transfusions screened as negative for HIV antibody. *N Engl J Med* 1988;318:473.
63. Selik RM, Ward JW, Buehler JW. Trends in transfusion-associated acquired immune deficiency syndrome in the United States, 1982 through 1991. *Transfusion* 1993;33:890.
64. Ling AE, Robbins KE, Brown TM, et al. Failure of routine HIV-1 tests in a case involving transmission with preseroconversion blood components during the infectious window period. *JAMA* 2000;284: 210.
65. Nelson KE, Donahue JG, Munoz A, et al. Transmission of retroviruses from seronegative donors by transfusion during cardiac surgery: a multicenter study of HIV-1 and HTLV-I/II infections. *Ann Intern Med* 1992;117:554.
66. Busch MP, Eble BE, Khayam-Bashi H, et al. Evaluation of screened blood donations for human immunodeficiency virus type 1 infection by culture and DNA amplification of pooled cells. *N Engl J Med* 1991;325:1.
67. Lackritz EM, Satten GA, Aberle-Grasse J, et al. Estimated risk of transmission of the human immunodeficiency virus by screened blood in the United States. *N Engl J Med* 1995;333:1721.
68. Schreiber GB, Busch MP, Kleinman SH, et al. The risk of transfusion-

transmitted viral infections. The Retrovirus Epidemiology Donor Study. *N Engl J Med* 1996;334:1685.

69. Sullivan MT, Guido EA, Metler RP, et al. Identification and characterization of an HIV-2 antibody-positive blood donor in the United States. *Transfusion* 1998;38:189.
70. Loussert-Ajaka I, Ly TD, Chaix ML, et al. HIV-1/HIV-2 seronegativity in HIV-1 subtype O infected patients. *Lancet* 1994;343:1393.
71. Manns A, Wilks RJ, Murphy EL, et al. A prospective study of transmission by transfusion of HTLV-I and risk factors associated with seroconversion. *Int J Cancer* 1992;51:886.
72. Kleinman SH, Niland JC, Azen SP, et al. Prevalence of antibodies to human immunodeficiency virus type 1 among blood donors prior to screening. The Transfusion Safety Study/NHLBI Donor Repository. *Transfusion* 1989;29:572.
73. Donegan E, Stuart M, Niland JC, et al. Infection with human immunodeficiency virus type 1 (HIV-1) among recipients of antibody-positive blood donations. *Ann Intern Med* 1990;113:733.
74. Busch MP, Donegan E, Stuart M, et al. Donor HIV-1 p24 antigenaemia and course of infection in recipients Transfusion Safety Study Group [letter]. *Lancet* 1990;335:1342.
75. Donegan E, Lenes BA, Tomasulo PA, et al. Transmission of HIV-1 by component type and duration of shelf storage before transfusion [letter] [published erratum appears in *Transfusion* 1991;31:287]. *Transfusion* 1990;30:851.
76. Rawal BD, Busch MP, Endow R, et al. Reduction of human immunodeficiency virus-infected cells from donor blood by leukocyte filtration. *Transfusion* 1989;29:460.
77. Kroner BL, Rosenberg PS, Aledort LM, et al. HIV-1 infection incidence among persons with hemophilia in the United States and western Europe, 1978-1990. Multicenter Hemophilia Cohort Study. *J Acquir Immune Defic Syndr* 1994;7:279.
78. Kim HC, Nahum K, Raska K Jr, et al. Natural history of acquired immunodeficiency syndrome in hemophilic patients. *Am J Hematol* 1987;24:169.
79. Jackson JB, Sannerud KJ, Hopsicker JS, et al. Hemophiliacs with HIV antibody are actively infected. *JAMA* 1988;260:2236.
80. Jackson JB, Kwok SY, Sninsky JJ, et al. Human immunodeficiency virus type 1 detected in all seropositive symptomatic and asymptomatic individuals. *J Clin Microbiol* 1990;28:16.
81. Hewlett IK, Laurian Y, Epstein J, et al. Assessment by gene amplification and serological markers of transmission of HIV-1 from hemophiliacs to their sexual partners and secondarily to their children. *J Acquir Immune Defic Syndr* 1990;3:714.
82. Jason J, Ou CY, Moore JL, et al. Prevalence of human immunodeficiency virus type 1 DNA in hemophilic men and their sex partners. Hemophilia-AIDS Collaborative Study Group. *J Infect Dis* 1989;160: 789.
83. Gibbons J, Cory JM, Hewlett IK, et al. Silent infections with human immunodeficiency virus type 1 are highly unlikely in multitransfused seronegative hemophiliacs. *Blood* 1990;76:1924.
84. Sheppard HW, Busch MP, Louie PH, et al. HIV-1 PCR and isolation in seroconverting and seronegative homosexual men: absence of long-term immunosilent infection. *J Acquir Immune Defic Syndr* 1993;6: 1339.
85. Okochi K, Sato H, Hinuma Y. A retrospective study on transmission of adult T cell leukemia virus by blood transfusion: seroconversion in recipients. *Vox Sang* 1984;46:245.
86. Kamihira S, Nakasima S, Oyakawa Y, et al. Transmission of human T cell lymphotropic virus type I by blood transfusion before and after mass screening of sera from seropositive donors. *Vox Sang* 1987;52: 43.
87. Donegan E, Lee H, Operskalski EA, et al. Transfusion transmission of retroviruses: human T-lymphotropic virus types I and II compared with human immunodeficiency virus type 1. *Transfusion* 1994;34: 478.
88. Kahn JO, Walker BD. Acute human immunodeficiency virus type 1 infection. *N Engl J Med* 1998;339:33.
89. Pantaleo G, Graziosi C, Demarest JF, et al. HIV infection is active and progressive in lymphoid tissue during the clinically latent stage of disease. *Nature* 1993;362:355.
90. Cohen P. Natural History, Clinical Spectrum, and General Management of HIV Disease. In: Cohen P, Sande M, Volberding P, eds. *The AIDS knowledge base.* Lippincott, Williams & Wilkins, 1999.
91. Centers for Disease Control and Prevention. From the Centers for Disease Control and Prevention. 1993 revised classification system for HIV infection and expanded surveillance case definition for AIDS among adolescents and adults. *JAMA* 1993;269:729.
92. Palella FJ, Jr, Delaney KM, Moorman AC, et al. Declining morbidity and mortality among patients with advanced human immunodeficiency virus infection. HIV Outpatient Study Investigators. *N Engl J Med* 1998;338:853.
93. Essex M. Human immunodeficiency viruses in the developing world. *Adv Virus Res* 1999;53:71.
94. Ward JW, Bush TJ, Perkins HA, et al. The natural history of transfusion-associated infection with human immunodeficiency virus: factors influencing the rate of progression to disease. *N Engl J Med* 1989; 321:947.
95. Ashton LJ, Learmont J, Luo K, et al. HIV infection in recipients of blood products from donors with known duration of infection. *Lancet* 1994;344:718.
96. Operskalski EA, Stram DO, Lee H, et al. Human immunodeficiency virus type 1 infection:relationship of risk group and age to rate of progression to AIDS. Transfusion Safety Study Group. *J Infect Dis* 1995;172:648.
97. Busch MP, Operskalski EA, Mosley JW, et al. Epidemiologic background and long-term course of disease in human immunodeficiency virus type 1-infected blood donors identified before routine laboratory screening. Transfusion Safety Study Group. *Transfusion* 1994;34:858.
98. Blaxhult A, Granath F, Lidman K, et al. The influence of age on the latency period to AIDS in people infected by HIV through blood transfusion. *AIDS* 1990;4:125.
99. Busch MP, Operskalski EA, Mosley JW, et al. Factors influencing human immunodeficiency virus type 1 transmission by blood transfusion. Transfusion Safety Study Group. *J Infect Dis* 1996;174:26.
100. Operskalski EA, Stram DO, Busch MP, et al. Role of viral load in heterosexual transmission of human immunodeficiency virus type 1 by blood transfusion recipients. Transfusion Safety Study Group. *Am J Epidemiol* 1997;146:655.
101. Operskalski EA, Busch MP, Mosley JW, et al. Comparative rates of disease progression among persons infected with the same or different HIV-1 strains. The Transfusion Safety Study Group. *J Acquir Immune Defic Syndr Hum Retrovirol* 1997;15:145.
102. Wilkinson DA, Operskalski EA, Busch MP, et al. A 32-bp deletion within the CCR5 locus protects against transmission of parenterally acquired human immunodeficiency virus but does not affect progression to AIDS-defining illness. *J Infect Dis* 1998;178:1163.
103. Learmont JC, Geczy AF, Mills J, et al. Immunologic and virologic status after 14 to 18 years of infection with an attenuated strain of HIV-1. A report from the Sydney Blood Bank Cohort. *N Engl J Med* 1999;340:1715.
104. Busch MP, Collier A, Gernsheimer T, et al. The Viral Activation Transfusion Study VATS: rationale, objectives, and design overview. *Transfusion* 1996;36:854.
105. Busch MP, Lee TH, Heitman J. Allogeneic leukocytes but not therapeutic blood elements induce reactivation and dissemination of latent human immunodeficiency virus type 1 infection: implications for transfusion support of infected patients. *Blood* 1992;80:2128.
106. Collier A, Kalish L, Busch M, et al. Double-blind, randomized study of leukocyte-reduced red blood cell transfusions in patients with anemia and human immunodeficiency virus infection: results of the Viral Activation Transfusion Study. *JAMA* 2001;285:1592–1601.
107. Hinuma Y, Gotoh Y, Sugamura K, et al. A retrovirus associated with human adult T-cell leukemia: in vitro activation. *Gann* 1982;73:341.
108. Hinuma Y, Nagata K, Hanaoka M, et al. Adult T-cell leukemia: antigen in an ATL cell line and detection of antibodies to the antigen in human sera. *Proc Natl Acad Sci U S A* 1981;78:6476.
109. Bunn PA Jr, Schechter GP, Jaffe E, et al. Clinical course of retrovirus-associated adult T-cell lymphoma in the United States. *N Engl J Med* 1983;309:257.
110. Kinoshita K, Amagasaki T, Ikeda S, et al. Preleukemic state of adult

T cell leukemia:abnormal T lymphocytosis induced by human adult T cell leukemia-lymphoma virus. *Blood* 1985;66:120.
111. Seiki M, Eddy R, Shows TB, et al. Nonspecific integration of the HTLV provirus genome into adult T-cell leukaemia cells. *Nature* 1984;309:640.
112. Tachibana N, Okayama A, Ishihara S, et al. High HTLV-I proviral DNA level associated with abnormal lymphocytes in peripheral blood from asymptomatic carriers. *Int J Cancer* 1992;51:593.
113. Murphy EL, Hanchard B, Figueroa JP, et al. Modelling the risk of adult T-cell leukemia/lymphoma in persons infected with human T-lymphotropic virus type I. *Int J Cancer* 1989;43:250.
114. Chen YC, Wang CH, Su IJ, et al. Infection of human T-cell leukemia virus type I and development of human T-cell leukemia lymphoma in patients with hematologic neoplasms: a possible linkage to blood transfusion. *Blood* 1989;74:388.
115. Prince H, Kleinman S, Doyle M, et al. Spontaneous lymphocyte proliferation in vitro characterizes both HTLV-I and HTLV-2 infection [letter]. *J Acquir Immune Defic Syndr* 1990;3:1199.
116. Wiktor SZ, Jacobson S, Weiss SH, et al. Spontaneous lymphocyte proliferation in HTLV-2 infection. *Lancet* 1991;337:327.
117. Katayama I, Maruyama K, Fukushima T, et al. Cross-reacting antibodies to human T cell leukemia virus-I and -II in Japanese patients with hairy cell leukemia. *Leukemia* 1987;1:401.
118. Lion T, Razvi N, Golomb HM, et al. B-lymphocytic hairy cells contain no HTLV-2 DNA sequences. *Blood* 1988;72:1428.
119. Rosenblatt JD, Gasson JC, Glaspy J, et al. Relationship between human T cell leukemia virus-II and atypical hairy cell leukemia: a serologic study of hairy cell leukemia patients. *Leukemia* 1987;1:397.
120. Rosenblatt JD, Giorgi JV, Golde DW, et al. Integrated human T-cell leukemia virus II genome in CD8 + T cells from a patient with "atypical" hairy cell leukemia: evidence for distinct T and B cell lymphoproliferative disorders. *Blood* 1988;71:363.
121. Busch MP, Murphy E, Nemo G. More on HTLV tax and mycosis fungoides [letter]. *N Engl J Med* 1993;329:2035.
122. Loughran TP Jr, Coyle T, Sherman MP, et al. Detection of human T-cell leukemia/lymphoma virus, type II, in a patient with large granular lymphocyte leukemia. *Blood* 1992;80:1116.
123. Zucker-Franklin D, Coutavas EE, Rush MG, et al. Detection of human T-lymphotropic virus-like particles in cultures of peripheral blood lymphocytes from patients with mycosis fungoides. *Proc Natl Acad Sci U S A* 1991;88:7630.
124. Gessain A, Barin F, Vernant JC, et al. Antibodies to human T-lymphotropic virus type-I in patients with tropical spastic paraparesis. *Lancet* 1985;2:407.
125. Bhagavati S, Ehrlich G, Kula RW, et al. Detection of human T-cell lymphoma/leukemia virus type I DNA and antigen in spinal fluid and blood of patients with chronic progressive myelopathy. *N Engl J Med* 1988;318:1141.
126. Jacobson S, Raine CS, Mingioli ES, et al. Isolation of an HTLV-1-like retrovirus from patients with tropical spastic paraparesis. *Nature* 1988;331:540.
127. Maloney EM, Cleghorn FR, Morgan OS, et al. Incidence of HTLV-I-associated myelopathy/tropical spastic paraparesis (HAM/TSP) in Jamaica and Trinidad. *J Acquir Immune Defic Syndr Hum Retrovirol* 1998;17:167.
128. Osame M, Usuku K, Izumo S, et al. HTLV-I associated myelopathy, a new clinical entity [letter]. *Lancet* 1986;1:1031.
129. Gessain A, Gout O. Chronic myelopathy associated with human T-lymphotropic virus type I (HTLV-I). *Ann Intern Med* 1992;117:933.
130. Murphy EL, Fridey J, Smith JW, et al. HTLV-associated myelopathy in a cohort of HTLV-I and HTLV-2-infected blood donors. The REDS investigators. *Neurology* 1997;48:315.
131. Kramer A, Maloney EM, Morgan OS, et al. Risk factors and cofactors for human T-cell lymphotropic virus type I (HTLV-I)-associated myelopathy/tropical spastic paraparesis (HAM/TSP) in Jamaica. *Am J Epidemiol* 1995;142:1212.
132. Gout O, Baulac M, Gessain A, et al. Rapid development of myelopathy after HTLV-I infection acquired by transfusion during cardiac transplantation. *N Engl J Med* 1990;322:383.
133. Kurosawa M, Machii T, Kitani T, et al. HTLV-I associated myelopathy (HAM) after blood transfusion in a patient with CD2+ hairy cell leukemia. *Am J Clin Pathol* 1991;95:72.
134. Osame M, Janssen R, Kubota H, et al. Nationwide survey of HTLV-I-associated myelopathy in Japan: association with blood transfusion. *Ann Neurol* 1990;28:50.
135. Madden DL, Mundon FK, Tzan NR, et al. Serologic studies of MS patients, controls, and patients with other neurologic diseases: antibodies to HTLV-I, II, III. *Neurology* 1988;38:81.
136. Reddy EP, Sandberg-Wollheim M, Mettus RV, et al. Amplification and molecular cloning of HTLV-I sequences from DNA of multiple sclerosis patients [published erratum appears in *Science* 1989;246: 246]. *Science* 1989;243:529.
137. Richardson J, Wucherpfennig K, Endo N. PCR analysis of DNA from multiple sclerosis patients for the presence of HTLV-I. *Science* 1989;246:821.
138. Hjelle B, Appenzeller O, Mills R, et al. Chronic neurodegenerative disease associated with HTLV-2 infection. *Lancet* 1992;339:645.
139. Mochizuki M, Watanabe T, Yamaguchi K, et al. HTLV-I uveitis: a distinct clinical entity caused by HTLV-I. *Jpn J Cancer Res* 1992;83: 236.
140. Sugimoto M, Nakashima H, Watanabe S, et al. T-lymphocyte alveolitis in HTLV-I-associated myelopathy [letter]. *Lancet* 1987;2:1220.
141. Morgan OS, Rodgers-Johnson P, Mora C, et al. HTLV-1 and polymyositis in Jamaica. *Lancet* 1989;2:1184.
142. Kitajima I, Maruyama I, Maruyama Y, et al. Polyarthritis in human T lymphotropic virus type I-associated myelopathy [letter]. *Arthritis Rheum* 1989;32:1342.
143. Murphy EL, Glynn SA, Fridey J, et al. Increased incidence of infectious diseases during prospective follow-up of human T-lymphotropic virus type II- and I-infected blood donors. Retrovirus Epidemiology Donor Study. *Arch Intern Med* 1999;159:1485.
144. LaGrenade L, Hanchard B, Fletcher V, et al. Infective dermatitis of Jamaican children: a marker for HTLV-I infection. *Lancet* 1990;336: 1345.
145. Stuver SO, Okayama A, Tachibana N, et al. HCV infection and liver cancer mortality in a Japanese population with HTLV-I. *Int J Cancer* 1996;67:35.
146. Volberding PA. Advances in the medical management of patients with HIV-1 infection: an overview. *AIDS* 1999;13[Suppl 1]:S1.
147. Ho DD. Time to hit HIV, early and hard [editorial]. *N Engl J Med* 1995;333:450.
148. Henry K. The case for more cautious, patient-focused antiretroviral therapy. *Ann Intern Med* 2000;132:306.
149. Harrington M, Carpenter CC. Hit HIV-1 hard, but only when necessary. *Lancet* 2000;355:2147.
150. Henderson DK. Postexposure chemoprophylaxis for occupational exposures to the human immunodeficiency virus. *JAMA* 1999;281:931.
151. Katzenstein TL, Dickmeiss E, Aladdin H, et al. Failure to develop HIV infection after receipt of HIV-contaminated blood and postexposure prophylaxis. *Ann Intern Med* 2000;133:31.
152. Bauer G, Selander D, Engel B, et al. Gene therapy for pediatric AIDS. *Ann N Y Acad Sci* 2000;918:318.
153. Pinto LA, Shearer GM, Blazevic V. Immune-based approaches for control of HIV infection and viral-induced immunopathogenesis. *Clin Immunol* 2000;97:1.
154. Gotch F, Rutebemberwa A, Jones G, et al. Vaccines for the control of HIV/AIDS. *Trop Med Int Health* 2000;5:A16.
155. Gray CM, Puren AJ. Rethinking globally relevant vaccine strategies to human immunodeficiency virus type-1. *Arch Immunol Ther Exp* 2000;48:235.
156. Hollsberg P, Hafler DA. Seminars in medicine of the Beth Israel Hospital, Boston. Pathogenesis of diseases induced by human lymphotropic virus type I infection. *N Engl J Med* 1993;328:1173.
157. Busch M, Chamberland M, Epstein J, et al. Oversight and monitoring of blood safety in the United States. *Vox Sang* 1999;77:67.
158. Chamberland M, Khabbaz RF. Emerging issues in blood safety. *Infect Dis Clin North Am* 1998;12:217.
159. Patience C, Takeuchi Y, Weiss RA. Infection of human cells by an endogenous retrovirus of pigs. *Nat Med* 1997;3:282.
160. Heneine W, Tibell A, Switzer WM, et al. No evidence of infection

with porcine endogenous retrovirus in recipients of porcine islet-cell xenografts. *Lancet* 1998;352:695.
161. Heneine W, Switzer WM, Soucie JM, et al. Evidence of porcine endogenous retroviruses in porcine factor VIII and evaluation of transmission to recipients with hemophilia. *J Infect Dis* 2001;183:648.
162. Busch MP, Holland PV. Idiopathic CD4+ T-lymphocytopenia (ICL) and the safety of blood transfusions: what do we know and what should we do? *Transfusion* 1992;32:800.
163. Busch MP, Switzer WM, Murphy EL, et al. Absence of evidence of infection with divergent primate T-lymphotropic viruses in United States blood donors who have seroindeterminate HTLV test results. *Transfusion* 2000;40:443.
164. Busch M, Stramer S, Garcia-Lerma J. Use of a PCR-amplified reverse transcriptase assay (Amp-RT) to rule out occult retrovirus infection in donors with positive HIV p24 antigen neutralization results. In preparation.
165. Joint statement on acquired immune deficiency syndrome (AIDS) related to transfusion. *Transfusion* 1983;23:87–88.
166. Curran JW, Lawrence DN, Jaffe H, et al. Acquired immunodeficiency syndrome (AIDS) associated with transfusions. *N Engl J Med* 1984; 310:69.
167. Gallo RC, Salahuddin SZ, Popovic M, et al. Frequent detection and isolation of cytopathic retroviruses (HTLV-2I) from patients with AIDS and at risk for AIDS. *Science* 1984;224:500.

Rossi's Principles of Transfusion Medicine, Third Edition, edited by Toby L. Simon, Walter H. Dzik, Edward L. Snyder, Christopher P. Stowell, and Ronald G. Strauss. Lippincott Williams & Wilkins, Philadelphia © 2002.

52

CYTOMEGALOVIRUS AND PARVOVIRUS TRANSMISSION BY TRANSFUSION

EDWARD C.C. WONG
NAOMI L.C. LUBAN

CYTOMEGALOVIRUS

Cytomegalovirus (CMV) belongs to the β-herpesvirinae subfamily of the human Herpesviridae family (Table 52.1). Among hosts with competent immune systems, CMV, like many other herpesviruses, produces self-limited disease. However, among immunosuppressed persons, these viruses can produce considerable morbidity and mortality. Herpesviruses share the ability to remain latent in tissues after acute infection. Unlike some herpesviruses, such as herpes simplex virus and varicella virus, which have restricted tissue expression, CMV can be isolated from many different organs, excretions, and secretions as well as from both fresh and anticoagulated stored blood components. As organ transplantation has expanded and therapy for malignant disease has become more immunosuppressive, CMV infection has become a major problem, the epidemiologic features of which are just now being elucidated.

Molecular Biology

The CMV genome is a linear double-stranded DNA molecule, approximately 229 kb long. The genome is helically associated with protein and forms a viral core particle encapsulated in an envelope composed of both viral envelope proteins and portions of the phospholipid bilayer (derived from the internal nuclear membrane and the endoplasmic reticulum of the infected cell). The total virion is 180 nm long (1).

The CMV genome is divided into two regions. The unique short (U_S) region is 35 kb long and is bounded by two 2.5-kb repeats designated IR_S and TR_S. The unique long (U_L) region is approximately 170 kb long and is flanked by two 11-kb repeats (the IR_L and the TR_L regions). The U_S and U_L segments can be oriented in either direction with respect to each other. The result is four distinct isomeric forms of the virion DNA, which are generally present in equimolar amounts in CMV-infected cells. Studies with restriction fragment length polymorphism have shown that clinical isolates of CMV are distinct in that they contain different-sized fragments when digested with restriction endonucleases. Most of this genetic heterogeneity is located in the U_S and U_L segments. The entire CMV genome is rich in guanine and cytosine residues, which account for cross-hybridization with human genomic DNA, even under stringent hybridization conditions (2). Between the U_L and the U_S sequences is an area called the *L-S junction.* The hypervariability in the repeat elements within this junction represents strain differences. This area, also called *seq* (α sequence), has homology with herpes simplex virus types 1 and 2. Zaia et al. (3) used a polymerase chain reaction (PCR) targeted at *seq* to catalog viral strains obtained from clinical isolates.

When CMV infects a host cell, the viral genome is released from the capsid and immediately circularizes. After infection, the genes of CMV are expressed in three distinct phases, designated immediate early (*IE*), early (*E*), and late (*L*) genes (2). For clinical diagnosis, the most important antibodies are made to these antigens. Immediate early antigens (IEAs) are produced independently of DNA synthesis within 1 to 4 hours after infection (1,

E.C.C. Wong and N.L.C. Luban: Departments of Laboratory Medicine, Pediatrics, and Pathology, The George Washington University School of Medicine, Washington, D.C.

TABLE 52.1. COMMON VIRUSES IN THE HUMAN HERPESVIRUS FAMILY

Common Name	Subfamily
Herpes simplex virus type 1 and type 2	α
Varicella-zoster virus	α
Cytomegalovirus	β
Human herpesvirus (HHV) 6	β
HHV-7	β
Epstein-Barr virus	γ
Kaposi sacrcoma–associated virus (HHV-8)	γ

2). The IE region contains four major transcription units—IE-1, IE-2, IE-3, and IE-4—that function as transactivators for the promoters of both viral and cellular genes and hence are necessary for progression of viral infection (1,4).

Expression of E genes depends on IE gene products. Early antigens (EAs) are produced after IEAs and have been mapped to all regions of the CMV genome. These gene products include the virus-encoded DNA polymerase that allows viral replication as well as other DNA binding proteins (5). The L genes encode the late structural antigens (LAs), which are needed for production of an infective viral particle and include matrix and tegument proteins as well as the envelope glycoproteins.

An estimated 35 to 40 structural proteins are present in the infectious CMV viral particle (5). With restriction endonuclease mapping, some of these proteins have been assigned to particular regions of the genome. Four of nine known phosphoproteins (pp150, pp71, pp65, and pp28) are located in the matrix region of the viral particle and are among the proteins most consistently recognized by antibodies in human serum (5).

The viral envelope consists of at least three glycoprotein complexes. Glycoprotein B (gB; gp58 or gel) is the carboxy terminus of a 160-kd glycosylated protein precursor that is proteolytically cleaved to a 58-kd mature product. It shows considerable homology to the major membrane glycoproteins of the other herpesviruses. In both human and murine systems, the gB region appears critical to host humoral and cellular immune responses (6). This led to the initial development of gB-based vaccines to induce both classes of immune response (7). However, more recent work has suggested that the cellular response to gB protein is of minor importance compared with cellular responses to pp65 and certain E proteins (see later). Glycoprotein H (gH; gp86 or gcII) is expressed on the viral envelope and the plasma membrane of CMV-infected cells and shows less homology between species than does gB. Both gB and gH have been localized to the U_L55 region. Glycoprotein gcII is a complex of two envelope glycoproteins, gp47 and gp52 (2,4).

Many other proteins have been mapped to particular regions of the genome, but their functions are unclear. Many of these regions of DNA are conserved, which indicates their importance in the viral life cycle. Further characterization of the CMV genome may help explain many of the paradoxes of CMV infection, including different antibody neutralization to different strains, infectivity, and the discrepancy observed between in vitro immune response and in vivo immune protection.

Patterns of Infection

The distinction between *CMV infection* identified by means of seroconversion or viral isolation and *CMV disease* is important in interpretation of the vast amount of literature on posttransfusion CMV infection. *Cytomegalovirus disease* is defined as laboratory evidence of infection coupled with specific symptoms attributable to the virus in the absence of other culpable pathogens or the patient's primary disease. The clinical manifestations of posttransfusion CMV range from a heterophile-negative mononucleosis syndrome to disseminated disease. Lymphadenopathy, lymphocytosis, fever, and pharyngitis with hepatitis constitute the mononucleosis-like syndrome. Interstitial pneumonitis, thrombocytopenia, hemolytic anemia, meningoencephalitis, and polyneuropathy are other associated findings. Immunosuppressed persons have a wide range of associated symptoms and signs. These include the aforementioned findings as well as retinitis, colitis, gastritis, nephritis, and rash. Rejection of renal allografts (8) and atherosclerosis of transplanted hearts (9) have been associated with primary CMV infection.

Primary Infection

Primary infection can occur in a seronegative recipient of blood or an organ transplant from a donor who has active or latent infection. Primary infection also results from community-acquired natural infection among children and adolescents who do not have symptoms. In primary infection, viremia, viruria, and immunoglobulin M (IgM)–specific antibody response and later an immunoglobulin G (IgG)–specific antibody response occur. Zanghellini et al. (10), studying asymptomatic primary CMV infection among adolescents found CMV PCR positivity in isolated white blood cells in 75% to 80% of adolescents within 16 weeks of infection. This number declined to zero to 25% after 48 weeks. After 6 to 8 weeks, IgG antibody to CMV, gB, and neutralizing antibody were seen. Peak lymphocyte proliferation responses to CMV (24 weeks after infection) and gB (48 weeks after infection) were threefold to fourfold lower than those of healthy adults with seropositive results. Viral shedding in urine was approximately 90% to 100% in all specimens in the first 36 weeks after infection. After 48 weeks, viruria was present in 40% to 50% of urine samples from adolescents. Despite relatively vigorous and rapid antibody responses, viruria and viremia did not clear until several months after seroconversion.

Transfusion-associated primary CMV infection has been the subject of numerous reviews (11–14). In many studies, the rate of seroconversion alone has been used to calculate the risk of primary infection from seropositive donor units. This calculated incidence has varied widely according to patient group and year of study. The reported incidence of primary posttransfusion CMV infection ranges from 10% to 50% (12,14), although figures of only 1.2% (15) and 0.9% (16) were reported in a large population of patients admitted to the hospital for burns, major surgery, pregnancy and delivery, neonatal complications, and oncologic treatment. The latter studies (15,16), however, had a relatively high number of patients with normal immune function. In contrast, studies with immunosuppressed patients such as low-birth-weight neonates have shown an incidence of

CMV infection ranging from 2% to 32% and associated with significant morbidity and mortality (17–22). The variation in incidence was attributed to donor seropositivity, number of donor exposures, amount of blood transfused, and age of the blood. Of particular importance was implementation of donor self-referral guidelines in March 1983. In addition to the reducing risk of transmission of human immunodeficiency virus (HIV), adherence to these guideline also likely reduced the risk of CMV infection in the more recent studies.

Determination of the actual risk of posttransfusion CMV infection among transplant recipients has been complicated by the high prevalence of infection among both donors and recipients. In studies in which seronegative recipients of transplants from seronegative donors were given blood products either seronegative or seropositive for CMV, the incidence of CMV infection and the morbidity and mortality were significantly higher when the blood donors were seropositive. The incidence of CMV infection among seronegative recipients of bone marrow transplants who received a seronegative transplant has ranged from 25% to 65% after transfusion of CMV-seropositive blood products (23,24) versus zero to 18% after transfusion of seronegative blood products (23–26). In one small study of transfusion-associated CMV infection among seronegative recipients of seronegative-donor heart transplants, 1 of 5 transplant recipients receiving unscreened blood contracted CMV infection; none of 8 recipients contracted CMV infection after receiving only screened blood (27). Although most authorities have considered blood transfusion not to represent a serious CMV risk factor for the recipients of renal transplants, primary infection secondary to transfusion has been reported (8) and has led to the frequent use of CMV-reduced-risk blood in the care of seronegative renal transplant recipients.

A prospective, randomized, controlled study of transfusion-associated CMV infection among children with malignant disease randomized to receive either unscreened blood products or CMV-seronegative blood components was performed (28). There were no cases of transfusion-acquired CMV infection among 62 patients in the study, but there was a low rate of nosocomial CMV infection. These findings are in contrast to those of previous studies (15,24,29–31) in which the median rate of CMV infection was 22.5% (range, zero to 37%). A number of factors have likely contributed to the lower rate of CMV infection than in previous studies. These include lower transfusion requirements, use of CMV-seronegative blood before randomization, low seroprevalence of CMV antibody in the donor population, use of older blood, and use of leukoreduction filters for reasons other than prevention of CMV infection. Recipient factors contributing to a lower incidence of posttransfusion CMV include the use of acyclovir and intravenous immunoglobulin for the management of non-CMV herpesvirus infections and the milder immunosuppression used in the oncologic treatment than in bone marrow transplantation. Overall, no significant transfusion-related CMV morbidity or mortality was found.

Early reports described increased rates of CMV infection among CMV-seronegative immunosuppressed patients receiving CMV-seropositive granulocyte transfusions. For example, patients receiving prophylactic leukocyte transfusions contracted more cases of CMV infection or symptomatic disease (19 of 31 patients [61%]) than did a control group receiving no leukocyte transfusions (7 of 27 patients [26%]; $P = .01$) (32). However, when the patients were stratified by serologic status, only seronegative patients and not seropositive patients had significantly higher rates of CMV infection. Hersman et al. (33), however, evaluating recipients of allogeneic bone marrow transplants, found no effect of seropositive granulocyte transfusions on the incidence of CMV pneumonitis. In a retrospective study, Kaufman et al. (34) examined the effect of ABO-compatible, HLA-matched prophylactic granulocyte transfusions on the development of CMV viremia and disease among recipients of peripheral blood stem cells. The authors concluded that CMV-seropositive granulocyte transfusion did not increase the overall risk of CMV viremia or mortality among CMV at-risk recipients of peripheral blood stem cells (donor or recipient or both CMV seropositive). Because CMV-seropositive granulocytes often are given in life-threatening situations, it is difficult to document CMV-related morbidity or mortality among seronegative immunosuppressed patients with a high predicted mortality. At present, most investigators would agree that use of CMV-seropositive granulocytes should be avoided in the treatment of seronegative patients.

Secondary Infection

Secondary infection can occur as either reactivation or coinfection. Reactivation of latent virus occurs in a previous CMV-seropositive recipient of either seropositive or seronegative donor blood or organ. Reactivation infections are accompanied by a fourfold or greater increase in the titer of CMV IgG and shedding of the virus. An IgM response occasionally is elicited. Viral shedding also can occur without an increase in IgG or IgM antibody response. Reinfection, which is better called *coinfection,* occurs in a seropositive patient who is exposed to a strain of CMV different from that which caused the original infection. In this case, an IgM antibody response, viral shedding, and an IgG CMV antibody response occur. In reactivation, as in primary infection, the primary IgG response is directed against gp150, appears later in infection, and remains elevated longer than the antibody response to other epitopes (35).

The frequency of reactivation and coinfection has not been determined in different patient groups because of the difficulty in differentiating these two types of infections with antibody quantification or immunoblotting assays. Molecular epidemiologic techniques, however, allow identification of strain differences. Tolpin et al. (36) were the first to identify two different strains of CMV by means of restriction endonuclease DNA patterns in a neonate who received blood from a seropositive donor. Since that report, similar molecular epidemiologic studies have been performed for infant-donor transfusion pairs (37), for transplant recipients (38,39), and in day-care centers (40). Such techniques have not been applied to large enough populations of persons with normal immune function to allow calculations of frequency of reactivation or coinfection.

Donor and Recipient Factors Predisposing to Infection

Not all seropositive donor units are capable of causing infection. Both recipient and donor factors predispose certain recipients to posttransfusion CMV infection and certain donors to transmit this cell-associated virus. In seroepidemiologic studies, posttransfusion CMV infection has been attributed to transfusion of all cellular blood components but has not been associated with transfusion of plasma products (41,42). High-titer antibody to CMV, in the form of either CMV hyperimmune globulin (27) or intravenous immune globulin (IVIG) (43) protects against CMV and has been used prophylactically in the care of transplant recipients with variable results. It is unknown whether platelets transmit CMV more readily than do red blood cells. Leukoreduction through washing of blood (44) reduces and deglycerolization (45–47) eliminates the risk of CMV transmission, even when the red blood cell units are seropositive for CMV. Third-generation leukoreduction filters appear effective (48–51).

The seroepidemiologic features of the virus coupled with attenuation or prevention of posttransfusion CMV by means of leukoreduction imply that CMV is harbored in white blood cells. In 1985, Schrier et al. (52) detected CMV RNA in circulating mononuclear cells using a hybridization probe unique to the IE proteins. These probes were selected because they were likely to be heavily transcribed in early infection. Furthermore, this group established through flow cytometry that 24% of CMV-hybridizing cells are $CD4^+$, whereas 0.8% are $CD8^+$, suggesting that the lymphocyte is the major source of CMV (52).

The PCR has been used to study CMV in both transplant patients and healthy blood donors. Several groups of investigators have optimized techniques for peripheral blood leukocytes. In one study, PCR did not help detect CMV in seropositive and seronegative controls without symptoms and became negative after acute viremia in patient samples. In serial samples obtained from 13 recipients of kidney or bone marrow transplants, the PCR estimate of infection levels was more than 60 genomes per sample of 10^5 leukocytes (38). Latent infection with CMV was not detected, however, implying that healthy seropositive persons have fewer CMV genome–bearing cells.

A dissociation between antigenemia and presence of CMV DNA has been reported (53). In the study, DNA dot blot hybridization was used in place of PCR, and DNA was quantitated in mononuclear and polymorphonuclear populations of blood and saliva from transplant recipients by means of an optical scanning system. Cytomegalovirus DNA was recovered from 16 of 17 (94%) polymorphonuclear cell specimens and from 7 of 15 (47%) mononuclear cell specimens obtained from EDTA specimens of patients with viremia. The number of cells required for detection was 1.6×10^5 for polymorphonuclear cells (range, 5.5×10^3 to 1.3×10^6) and 2.3×10^5 for mononuclear cells (range, 8.6×10^3 to 1×10^6). More viral DNA was present in polymorphonuclear cells (13.1 viral genome equivalents per 100 cells) than in mononuclear cells (9.1 viral genome equivalents per 100 cells). In patients without positive viral cultures, less viral DNA was obtained (4 viral genome equivalents per 100 cells), with no difference in cell type. No CMV DNA was detected in the leukocytes of 25 IgG CMV seropositive blood donors.

The disparity between culture and molecular hybridization techniques for identifying virus in mononuclear cells is not completely explained. One can speculate that CMV exists within the granulocyte in a mature infectious form. As a result, studies with patients who have infection are more likely to identify CMV in granulocytes. In contrast, results of studies with blood donors who do not have symptoms suggest that CMV may remain latent in mononuclear cells. Understanding the cellular tropism for infectious versus latent viral infection has implications for the screening of donors and for processes designed to reduce the infectivity of blood.

Immunology

The interaction of CMV with both the humoral and cellular immune systems is complex. Cytomegalovirus can both suppress and enhance the host response to specific viral and nonviral antigens. Antibody response to CMV may develop but does not result in protective immunity. Therapeutic immunosuppression activates viral expression and replication. Patients with congenital immunodeficiency who lack the ability to mount antibody responses are at risk of fulminant CMV disease.

Humoral Immune Response

The humoral immune response to CMV, initially with IgM and later with IgG anti-CMV antibody production, provides a means of classifying the type of CMV infection. In the presence of preexisting antibody, there may be moderation of pathogenicity but not prevention of disease. For example, mothers with preexisting antibody are less likely to contract CMV disease, as are their fetuses (54). In renal transplantation, CMV-seropositive recipients of CMV-seropositive renal allografts have less morbidity from CMV than do CMV-seronegative recipients of CMV-seropositive living-related donor allografts (55). Cytomegalovirus serologically discordant heart, heart-lung, liver, and bone marrow donor-recipient pairs have been described who have had similar results. Among premature infants, however, CMV-seropositive premature infants receiving seropositive blood have been reported to have severe morbidity (56,57). Although not mentioned or specifically investigated in these studies, other sexually transmitted diseases in the mother, particularly gonorrhea (58), might have compounded the clinical course among the infants. Gradual loss of protective immunity from the mother also might have resulted in more severe CMV disease.

Supportive evidence of humoral attenuation of CMV infection and disease comes from the literature on bone marrow transplantation. Studies have been conducted to evaluate the efficacy of CMV hyperimmune plasma (59), IVIG (43), and CMV-specific intravenous immune globulin (23,59–61). Results have been conflicting, some studies showing a decrease in the incidence of CMV pneumonia (43,59,60,62) and others not (42, 62). Reasons for the discrepancies include variability in the titers of antibody to CMV in the product, total dose and schedule of administration, and discordance in kind of blood product used or serologic status of donor-recipient pairs. Bowden et al. (63) used a CMV IgG product prepared from donors selected for a high concentration of "naturally" occurring CMV antibody, in a randomized placebo-controlled study of 123 seronegative recipients of seropositive bone marrow. The product was administered at 200 mg/kg on days 8 and 6 before transplantation, on the day of marrow infusion, and weekly for 7 weeks for a total of 10 doses. There was less CMV infection and viremia in the treated group. However, similar numbers of patients (14 in the treatment group, 17 in the control group) had CMV syndrome with CMV disease documented as tissue invasion. There was also no difference in the median number of days after transplantation until onset of infection, viremia, or tissue-invasive CMV disease. The results of this study differed from those of others (43,59, 60). The difference might have been caused in part by the failure of CMV IVIG to affect the incidence of acute graft versus host disease (GVHD). The authors speculated that the decrease in the incidence of CMV disease in previous studies might have been caused by a reduction in the incidence of GVHD by IVIG, although the mechanism by which IVIG attenuates GVHD is not understood (64).

Neutralizing antibodies are responsible for inactivating extracellular virions by binding to the virus. Purified gB envelope protein induces neutralizing antibodies in both human and murine models. In one study, 40% to 70% of neutralizing antibodies were directed toward gB (65). In recombinant vaccinia-gB vaccine studies, 50% to 88% of total virus-neutralizing activity was directed toward gB protein (66). Evaluation with a radioimmunoprecipitation assay and specific absorption experiments of 20 CMV-seropositive subjects who had normal immune function for neutralizing antibody to gB protein showed that 48% of specimens had neutralizing activity to gB (67). Intracellular viral proliferation and reactivation are under the control of helper and cytotoxic T cells. Cytotoxic T cells respond to gB protein by increasing cytolysis (68). In one study (69), the gB-specific cytotoxic response was isolated to the N-terminal 513 amino acids of gB. Exposing helper-T-cell clones derived from CMV-seropositive and CMV-seronegative donors to whole virus and immunoaffinity-purified segments of the gB glycoprotein complex showed variability in the response of different clones to the different epitopes. The results of this study implied that helper-T-cell precursors recognize a variety of immunodominant epitopes on gB. The results showed that only in some subjects were neutralizing antibody, helper T cells, and cytotoxic T cells detected.

Data from a study by Chou and Dennison (70) support future development of monoclonal antibodies of high purity and specificity. The investigators found peptide homology ranging from 91% to 98% in the gB gene of more than 28 clinical strains and suggested that the number of gB variants among clinical strains is limited. They speculated that sequence differences may determine tissue tropism, as occurs in herpes simplex virus, in which gB sequence differences correlate with neurovirulence. Results of further studies suggested that gB genotype differences may be associated with increased virulence in recipients of bone marrow transplants (71–73) but not of renal transplants (74) and not with neurodevelopmental outcome of intrauterine infection (75). The role of strain-specific neutralizing antibody in attenuating CMV infection remains incompletely understood and may be related to the degree of immunosuppression and GVHD.

Vaccination is yet another mechanism that can be used to study humoral response. In a study evaluating the efficacy of the Towne vaccine, a live attenuated CMV vaccine, 237 renal transplant recipients were entered into a double-blind, randomized, placebo-controlled trial. The vaccine was ineffective in protecting against CMV disease in seropositive recipients. Seronegative recipients of seropositive kidneys had less severe CMV disease and improved graft survival, although the infection rate was the same in both the placebo and vaccination groups. Restriction fragment length polymorphism analysis showed that the virus excreted after transplantation differed from the live vaccine virus. This finding confirmed that Towne virus does not become latent in vaccine recipients. Antibody response did not correlate with outcome. These findings were confirmed in a larger multicenter trial (76). Because of the speculation that the cellular immune response to the vaccine may provide more information about protection against CMV and that the antibody response was poor in some patients who received vaccinations (76), several additional approaches to improving antibody response have been attempted. These include use of a canarypox vector expressing CMV gB to prime for antibody response to the Towne vaccine (77), naked DNA vaccines (78), and the use of canarypox vector expressing CMV pp65. Use of a canarypox vector expressing pp65 has been implemented in a phase I trial and has been shown to elicit both antibody response and long-lasting CMV pp65 $CD8^+$ cytotoxic T lymphocytes (CTLs) (79).

Cell-mediated Immunity

The importance of cell-mediated immunity in CMV infection is supported by the direct correlation between the degree of cellular immunosuppression and the severity of CMV disease. Patients with severe immunodeficiency or those with HIV infection have the most severe forms of CMV infection. In several early studies, investigators evaluated cell-mediated immunity by measuring lymphocyte transformation and blastogenesis to different mitogens and antigens. Persons immune to CMV were found to have proliferative responses to both mitogens and viral antigens, the latter occurring within 1 to 2 months after primary infection. In contrast, infants with congenital infection and their mothers were found to have a decreased proliferative response to CMV antigens as well as mitogen-specific responses. Recipients of cardiac, renal, or bone marrow transplants were found to have similar depressed in vitro responses (80,81).

Using murine CMV (MCMV) as an animal model of human CMV, researchers have evaluated many different cellular immune responses. During acute MCMV infection, there is depression of the humoral response to other antigens, T-cell response to mitogens, and monocyte release of interleukin-1. The cytotoxic T-lymphocyte response to MCMV has been extensively investigated and appears to be restricted by the major histocompatibility locus, H2. The process in mice may be due to recognition of an H2 complex modified by viral antigens or to simultaneous recognition of independent viral and histocompatibility antigens. In mice, CTLs respond to the immunogenic protein encoded by the IEA or the structural gB protein. In several studies, $CD8^+$ T cells were found to confer resistance to MCMV. In the presence of selective deficiency of $CD8^+$ cells, $CD4^+$ T cells facilitate production of CMV-specific antibodies that neutralize virus (82). An alternative explanation is that selective deficiency of $CD4^+$ cells in mice with normal immune function resulted in persistent viral latency. Remaining $CD8^+$ T cells functioned independently of $CD4^+$ T cells to restrict virus to acinar glandular epithelial cells of the salivary gland (83). In adoptive transfer experiments, immune $CD8^+$ T cells protected immunosuppressed mice from primary MCMV and attenuated disease in mice with established MCMV infection. Other investigators have evaluated antibody-dependent cell-mediated cytotoxicity and natural killer (NK) cell function in MCMV. A lack of H2 restriction for NK cells appears early in infection, whereas antibody-dependent cell-mediated cytotoxicity is more likely to be found in chronic and latent phases of murine infection and is likely to be H2 restricted (1).

Virus-specific CTLs are responsible for at least some of the cytopathic effects of CMV. Murine lymphocytic choriomeningitis virus, for example, injected into immunosuppressed mice produces neither encephalitis nor hepatitis. However, when immune spleen cells also are injected, encephalitis develops. If $CD8^+$ T cells ($Ly2^+$) are adoptively transferred, hepatic necrosis and periportal infiltrates form. These findings suggest that CTLs may protect in early infection through lysis of small numbers of infected cells and elaboration of cytokine responses. In late infection, however, cytolysis of infected tissues and the subsequent inflammatory response produce pathologic changes. Pasternack et al. (84) reviewed some of the factors that may be involved in the balance between protective immunity and cytopathologic changes in the mouse model. The size and route of the inoculum, temporal relation between infection and development of T cell–mediated immunity or adoptive transfer, strain of virus, characteristics of host, and nature of immunosuppressive regimen used may be critical to the development of CMV-mediated disease. Many parallels can be drawn to human CMV infection in immunosuppressed persons.

Analyzing Cellular Immune Response with Flow Cytometry

In a study with 112 healthy volunteer blood donors stratified according to CMV IgG and IgM antibody status, flow cytometric analysis, including human natural killer (HNK) fluorescent intensity, and morphologic evaluations were performed (85). Cytomegalovirus-seropositive subjects had larger numbers of $HNK1^+$ ($Leu7^+$) lymphocytes than did CMV-seronegative subjects. Lymphocytes with strong HNK1 fluorescence had greater granularity. This finding suggested that these cells with HNK1 epitopes may serve as adhesion or interaction sites between cytotoxic lymphocytes and their targets (85). Work has centered on the characterization of the $CD8^+$ CTL population in vivo. Studies have shown a high frequency of $CD8^+$ memory CTLs in healthy carriers of CMV. DNA analysis of the T-cell receptor use of these $CD8^+$ memory CTLs has revealed extensive oligoclonal expansion of $CD8^+$ CTLs from a $CD57^+CD28^-$population (86,87). These findings are similar to clonal expansion of CMV-specific $CD8^+$ CTLs from a $CD57^+$ population in recipients of bone marrow transplants (88).

The development of the major histocompatibility complex (MHC) tetramer assay has allowed rapid, real-time, flow cytometric monitoring of the CMV-specific $CD8^+$ CTL response. Engstrand et al. (89), using an MHC tetramer consisting of HLA-A2 and NLVPMVATV, an immunodominant peptide of pp65, characterized the pp65 $CD8^+$ CTL percentages in healthy HLA-A2 CMV-seropositive carriers and in immunosuppressed recipients of renal transplants who had latent infection. The percentages of pp65 $CD8^+$ CTLs in healthy carriers (seropositive and seronegative) and immunosuppressed recipients of renal transplants who had latent CMV infection were less than 3% and 0.2% to 9%, respectively. With CMV reactivation, however, pp65 $CD8^+$ CTL percentages increased to 9% to 15%. In one healthy patient with primary infection who was not immunosuppressed, levels cell activation markers (CD45RO, CD38, and HLA-DR) were found increased on tetramer identified cells.

Tetramer analysis has shown that antigen-specific cells for human CMV peptides may exceed 4% of the $CD8^+$ T cells (90). In combination with antibodies to cell surface markers and intracellular cytokines, functional heterogeneity within the CMV-specific population was identified. In two of three subjects, most CMV-specific cells were cytotoxic T cells. This finding correlated with the ability of these cells to lyse peptide-pulsed targets in "fresh killing" assays. Gillespie et al. (90) found much higher CMV-specific $CD8^+$ T-cell frequencies in healthy seropositive donors when they used tetramer analysis rather than limiting dilution analysis. It is likely that limiting dilution analysis underestimates the number of circulating CTLs because the assay requires that T lymphocytes retain the ability to proliferate in vitro. However, effector T cells often have poor proliferative potential and are likely to be excluded or underestimated in this type of analysis (91–93). One of the most promising features of tetramer analysis is the potential to study specific cellular responses in real time. Coupled with other flow cytometric techniques, such as sorting, tremendous advances in understanding of the CMV cellular responses will undoubtedly occur.

Mechanisms by Which Cytomegalovirus Escapes Immune Clearance

Cytomegalovirus has developed many biologic mechanisms to evade the host immune system. The simplest way that CMV has accomplished this is by not expressing viral proteins. This is established by a latency state in a variety of cell types, including circulating monocytes, macrophages, bone marrow progenitor cells, and possibly endothelial cells (94–99). This concept is supported by observations in which a substantial number of seronegative, healthy persons have positive PCR results for CMV (99) and the finding that 30% to 40% of bone marrow progenitor cells of healthy persons have evidence of CMV latency (96). Another means of evading the immune system is not presenting IE protein to the cell surface by means of phosphorylation of IE proteins by phosphoprotein pp65 (100). A third means of avoiding immune detection is blockade of class I and II MHC antigen expression on CMV-infected cells. This is believed to occur by means of inhibition of cytokine-induced class II MHC expression and inhibition of class I MHC expression. Class I MHC expression is inhibited by CMV proteins such as US2, US3, US6, and US11, which disrupt peptide translocation on the MHC molecule, destabilize class I MHC heavy chains, and dissociate class I heavy chains from the endoplasmic reticulum (101–105).

A fourth means of evading the immune system is chemokine sequestration. Chemokines such as RANTES, monocyte chemoattractant protein 1 (MCP-1), MCP-3, macrophage inflammatory protein 1α (MIP-1), and MIP-β affect lymphocyte and monocyte effector mechanisms (106). Evidence of this mechanism comes from studies of expression of US27 and US28 that show homology to chemokine receptors and bind RANTES and MCP-1 (107). US28 binds MCP-3, MIP-1α and MIP-β as well as the CX3C chemokine, fractalkine (107,108). US28 also is involved in cell to cell fusion, which may allow intercellular passage of the virus without exposure to neutralizing antibodies (109). In vitro studies have shown that monocyte chemoattraction is significantly attenuated by wild-type CMV virus but not by CMV viruses lacking US28 or US27 genes (110).

A fifth means by which CMV can evade the immune system is absorption of neutralizing antibodies. Infection by CMV typically leads to a 100-fold increase in Fc receptor expression on infected fibroblasts and leads to increased expression on endothelial cells (111,112). These Fc receptors bind all four IgG isotypes with highest affinity to IgG1, which incidentally composes most (approximately 96%) of the anti-CMV response (113,114). Cytomegalovirus may inhibit interferon-α antiviral activity. Evidence in CMV-infected fibroblasts and endothelial cells from humans has shown that CMV inhibits Janus kinase 1 and p48, two essential components of the IFN-α signal transduction pathway leading to down-regulation of these antiviral effectors (115, 116). Last, CMV encodes its own unique interleukin-10 homologue, which may be involved in down-regulation of inflammatory responses and antigen presentation of foreign CMV epitopes (117). Future research is needed to identify the extent to which each of these mechanisms of immune evasion contributes to CMV disease and whether different CMV strains use different mechanisms of immune evasion.

Blood Product Variables Influencing Infectivity

Several variables are important in the transmissibility of CMV in a blood product. These include the number of white blood cells containing CMV virions capable of proliferation in the recipient; the cellular and humoral immune status of the recipient, the presence of neutralizing antibody in the product or the recipient, and associated clinical conditions in the recipient, such as GVHD, that promote viral activation. Blood products vary widely in the quantity of leukocytes present, owing at least in part to the method of collection (see Chapter 21). Products with the greatest number of leukocytes would be expected to transmit CMV infection most efficiently. This has been substantiated by studies with persons receiving granulocyte transfusions (32,33). With increase in storage time, fewer lymphocytes can be isolated from either red blood cell concentrates (118) or whole-blood platelet concentrates (119).

Fluorescence activated cell sorter analysis and mixed lymphocyte culture have shown a progressive decline in class II HLA antigen expression on residual leukocytes in platelet concentrates stored at room temperature (119). Class I HLA antigens, however, were consistently expressed throughout storage in 95% of the platelet concentrates analyzed. These findings may have implications for CMV transmission. As the total white blood cell count decreased, presumably because of cytolysis, the percentage of cells remaining as lymphocytes increased (119). If polymorphonuclear cells or mononuclear cells harbor CMV, then the infectivity of aged products might be less than that of recently obtained products.

Data from four studies addressing the age of stored blood provide conflicting information at least in part owing to differences in study design. Two studies showed higher rates of seroconversion to CMV in recipient of fresh red blood cells (15, 120), and in two the higher seroconversion rate was correlated with greater number and volume of transfusions (16,121). Red blood cell storage of 3 to 8 days versus 20 to 42 days was specifically assessed for a group of 84 seropositive patients undergoing surgery. There was no statistically significant increase in antibody titer as a consequence of reactivation between the two groups (121). Despite variable rates of seroconversion in different studies (15,16,120,121) and viral excretion found in one study (120), no mortality or morbidity was attributable to CMV infection. Reactivation of latent CMV remains subclinical for patients not severely immunosuppressed.

There are few data on class II expression by residual lymphocytes in stored red blood cells. At least one study with recipients of renal transplants showed that those receiving stored refrigerated red blood had less HLA sensitization than did those receiving fresh red blood cells (122). Diminished class II–dependent allogeneic stimulation from older red blood cell products may contribute to the lower rate of reactivation of CMV in recipients of both CMV-seropositive and CMV-seronegative aged blood units. Human CMV-specific CTLs expressing class I antigenicity have been identified in the lymphocytes of persons with symptomatic, persistent CMV infection. These cells may be the T cells responsible for reestablishing latent infection in the nonimmune host and for further immune perturbations in the immune host, and they may be selectively depleted under certain storage conditions.

Recipient Groups at Risk of Transfusion-transmitted Cytomegalovirus Infection

Numerous investigators (11–14,21) have attempted to classify patients to streamline provision of blood products that may be difficult to obtain. Recipients can switch between classification groups as chemotherapy, adoptive immunotherapy, and treatment protocols increase in immunosuppressive intensity. Table 52.2 details the classification system used by Sayers et al. (123).

Methods to Prevent Transfusion-transmitted Cytomegalovirus Infection

Blood obtained from seronegative donors is considered by many authorities to be the standard of care of patients who need CMV-reduced-risk blood products. Seronegativity can be defined with one of several methods. The commercial assays entail measurement of either IgG-specific or total anti-CMV antibody with

TABLE 52.2. INDICATIONS FOR THE USE OF CYTOMEGALOVIRUS-REDUCED-RISK CELLULAR BLOOD PRODUCTS

High risk of serious infection and disease. Controlled trials show less morbidity and a lower incidence of infection.
- Low-birth-weight infants born to seronegative mothers
- Seronegative recipients of seronegative donor bone marrow (allogeneic) or peripheral blood stem cell transplants
- Seronegative recipients of autologous bone marrow transplants

High risk of serious morbidity as the result of transfusion-acquired CMV infection, but the incidence of transfusion-acquired CMV infection in these populations has not been clearly documented or the benefit of using CMV-reduced-risk cellular blood products has not been proved.
- Seronegative pregnant women who need antepartum transfusion and seropositive women who need antepartum transfusion
- Low-birth-weight infants born to seronegative or seropositive mothers; seronegative immunosuppressed patients who need granulocyte transfusions
- Recipients of fetal transfusions
- Infants and children with suspected or confirmed congenital immunodeficiencies
- Seronegative recipients of seronegative donor lungs and livers and possibly other organs, excluding heart and kidney recipients
- Seronegative patients with human immunodeficiency virus (HIV) infection or acquired immunodeficiency syndrome (AIDS)

Populations who may be at higher risk of trasfusion-acquired CMV infection or its morbidity but in whom the incidence or morbidity of transfusion-acquired CMV infection is low or poorly documented.
- Low-birth-weight infants born to seropositive mothers
- Infants with birth-weights >1,500 g born to seronegative mothers
- Neonates receiving extracorporeal membrane oxygenation and other neonates who need extensive transfusion support (e.g., exchange transfusion, cardiovascular surgery)
- Seronegative recipients of seronegative donor kidneys and hearts
- Seronegative patients with malignant disease receiving chemotherapy
- Seronegative patients with hematologic or genetic disorders who need repetitive transfusions for whom bone marrow transplantation may be a future therapeutic option
- Seronegative patients experiencing major trauma or undergoing splenectomy

Populations in which the incidence and morbidity associated with transfusion-acquired CMV infection is low. The use of CMV-"safe" cellular blood products is not indicated.
- Infants with birthweights >1,500 g born to seropositive mothers
- Other seronegative patients with normal immune function
- Seropositive transfusion recipients (excluding neonates)
- Seropositive patients with HIV infection or AIDS.

Modified from Preiksaitis JK. The cytomegalovirus "safe" blood product: is leukoreduction equivalent to antibody screening? *Transfusion Med Rev* 2000;14:112–136.

indirect hemagglutination, latex agglutination, enzyme-lined immunosorbent assay, or solid-phase immunofluorescence techniques. A review of methods commonly available in clinical laboratories has shown differences in sensitivity and specificity that may account for the few anecdotal cases of posttransfusion CMV in seronegative recipients of seronegative blood and blood products (149).

Immunoglobulin M testing of donors is a serologic technique not widely used, predominantly because assay systems for IgM CMV are not well established. The theory is that IgM-seropositive donors would be more likely to harbor infectious virus that could transmit infection. In one study, 7 of 22 seronegative infants who had seroconversion and shed virus had received at least one IgM-seropositive donor transfusion. In the second phase of the study, 1 of 141 seronegative infants receiving IgM-seronegative blood showed seroconversion. The donor was later found seropositive according to another assay system (124). The serologic prevalence of IgM in donor populations ranges from less than 1% to 6% (21,44,124), far lower than the reported 70% serologic prevalence of IgG. Owing to the paucity of clinical trials conducted with IgM-seronegative, IgG seropositive blood, other methods of prevention have received more attention.

Because CMV is probably harbored in the white blood cells, leukoreduction of blood products has been advocated as a method to abrogate CMV transmission. This is supported by clinical studies showing no or reduced seroconversion with either untested or seropositive frozen deglycerolized and washed red blood and fresh-frozen plasma. Filtration, particularly with leukodepletion filters capable of greater than 3 log removal of white blood cells, has become a common method used to avoid CMV transmission (Table 52.3) (see Chapter 21).

Although the minimum number of infected white blood cells and the specific subtype of white blood cell (monocyte, granulocyte, lymphocyte) harboring sufficient virus to cause CMV disease remain unknown, results of early clinical studies conducted with filtration or double spinning of platelet concentrate pools or pheresis platelets were promising for patients with leukemia

TABLE 52.3. CYTOMEGALOVIRUS (CMV) INFECTION IN CMV-SERONEGATIVE TRANSFUSION RECIPIENTS RECEIVING PRODUCTS PROCESSED WITH LEUKOREDUCTION

Population	Author	Year	Leukocyte Reduction		Number of Patients Infected/Number Studied	
			Red Blood Cells	Platelets		Standard
Low-birth-weight Neonates	Gilbert	1989	Filter	N/A	0/30	9/42
	Eisenfeld	1992	Spincool, filter	No treatment	0/48[a]	None
	Ohto	1999	Filter	N/A	3/33[b]	1/19
Leukemia, lymphoma	Murphy	1988	Filter	Centrifuge	0/11[c]	6/42
	DeGraan	1989	Filter	Centrifuge	0/59[c]	10/86
	Pamphilon	1999	Filter	Single needle	0/62	None
Bone marrow transplantation	Verdonk	1987	Single needle	Filter	0/29	None
	DeWitte	1990	Filter	Centrifuge	0/37[c]	None
	Bowden	1991	Filter	Centrifuge	0/17	7/30
	Van Prooijien	1994	Filter	Filter	0/60	None
	Bowden	1995	Filter	Filter	3/247	2/249
	Narvious	1998	Filter	Filter	1/45	None
Cardiac surgery	Lang	1977	Centrifuge	N/A	2/8[d]	4/6

[a] Spincool filtration for some of study units.
[b] Infants breast-fed with milk not tested for CMV.
[c] Centrifugation plus filtration.
[d] Centrifugation, fresh whole blood.
N/A, not applicable.

(125), recipients of bone marrow transplants (94), and neonates (48). Each of these studies was performed with filters no longer used in the United States. Bowden et al. (31) compared use of CMV-seronegative red blood cells and double-spun platelets with use of unscreened blood and blood products in a randomized study of seronegative recipients of either autologous or CMV-seronegative bone marrow allografts. The investigators found no cases of CMV infection in 17 patients who could be evaluated until day 100 after transplantation. Seven cases of infections occurred among the 30 patients who served as controls. The investigators estimated a 1.5- to 2-log reduction in white blood cells in the platelets used. The number of donor exposures was substantial— a mean of 164 platelet concentrates and 25 units of red blood cells in the leukodepletion group and 165 platelet concentrates and 20 units of red blood cells in the control group (31).

Bowden et al. (126) subsequently undertook a prospective, randomized trial with CMV-seronegative marrow recipients to determine whether filtered, 3-log leukoreduced red blood cells and platelets were as effective as CMV-seronegative blood products for the prevention of transfusion-transmitted CMV infections after bone marrow transplantation. Five hundred two patients were randomized to receive either type of product and were observed for the development of CMV infection or disease 21 and 100 days after transplantation. Cytomegalovirus infection was defined as identification of CMV (antigen based or culture positive) in weekly urine, throat, and blood cultures. Cytomegalovirus disease was defined as the presence of CMV in tissue specimens or bronchoalveolar lavage fluid and associated clinical symptoms. There was no significant difference between the randomized groups as far as the number of products received. In a primary analysis of the data (end point at day 100 after transplantation), there were a total of 5 cases of CMV infection in the two population groups—2 cases among the 249 recipients receiving seronegative products and 3 cases among the 247 recipients receiving filtered blood products. This difference was not statistically significant. In a secondary analysis, 5 additional patients were found to have contracted early CMV infection between randomization and day 21 after transplantation—2 in the seronegative group and 3 in the group who underwent leukoreduction. The investigators concluded that the rates of infection from leukoreduced and seronegative products were comparable (2.4% versus 1.4%) but that the probability of development of CMV disease was higher among persons receiving the leukoreduced products (2.4% versus 0%, $P = .03$). The authors concluded that filtration was an effective alternative to use of seronegative blood products.

A European prospective study compared the rates of CMV infection among 60 seronegative recipients of bone marrow transplants. Recipients of allogeneic (n = 23) and autologous (n = 37) bone marrow transplants were given filtered (leukoreduced) blood products; none had positive serologic results for CMV (127). Another study (128) was performed to evaluate use of leukoreduced versus seronegative blood in 45 recipients of CMV-seronegative allogeneic marrow transplants. Cytomegalovirus pneumonitis developed in 1 patient (2.7%). The investigators claimed equivalency between seronegative and leukoreduced blood and blood products. However, the study was not powered sufficiently to make this claim.

A subsequent study with pediatric patients was performed to examine the practice of using CMV-reduced-risk (seronegative or leukoreduced blood products) in the care of patients with newly diagnosed malignant disease that might ultimately be managed by means of transplantation (28). The investigators attempted to determine the rate of CMV infection among persons receiving seronegative and untested products. Seventy-six CMV-seronegative children with hematopoietic or solid malignant lesions were randomized to receive CMV-untested or CMV-seronegative red blood cells and platelets. The patients were examined monthly for 1 year after diagnosis or 6 months after the last transfusion. Serologic tests for CMV-specific IgG and IgM were performed, as were throat swabbing and urine collection for culture. Additional specimens were obtained from various sources when there was a clinical suspicion of CMV disease. There were no significant differences in the number or type of blood products received by the two groups. Children in the CMV-seronegative group were observed a median of 19 months and those in the untested group a mean of 234 months. No case of transfusion-acquired CMV was documented. One factor that may have contributed to this observation was a relatively low number of donor exposures (median, 11 platelet products for the untested group and 14 for the seronegative group). Donor characteristics may have been important in determining the infectivity of the blood product. In this population, there was relatively low frequency of CMV IgM among the donors (0.9%), indicating a low incidence of acute or subacute infection among these children.

Another study (129) was performed to examine CMV-seropositive products for the presence of free infectious virus particles in the plasma. This study showed that the plasma of seropositive red blood cell and platelet concentrates contained CMV DNA according to PCR results, but it also contained virus particles able to infect tissue culture cells in vitro. The presence of these infective virus particles was associated with an increased length of storage and was attributed to the release of infective agents with the progressive breakdown of the white blood cells.

Recommendations from the American Association of Blood Banks augmented by other reviews (130) summarize the indications for use of CMV-reduced-risk (seronegative or leukoreduced) blood. The use of CMV-reduced-risk products is not indicated for general hospital patients, persons receiving non-neutropenia-promoting chemotherapy, persons receiving glucocorticoids, and term infants, regardless of CMV status. Persons who are CMV seropositive and undergoing chemotherapy that may promote neutropenia, who are pregnant, or who have HIV infection do not need CMV-seronegative products (131). Similar CMV-seronegative patients should receive CMV-reduced-risk products.

Cytomegalovirus-seronegative recipients of CMV-seronegative solid organ allografts should receive CMV-reduced-risk products. Cytomegalovirus-seropositive transplant recipients or persons receiving allografts from CMV-positive donors do not need CMV-reduced-risk products. For persons undergoing bone marrow or hematopoietic stem cell transplantation, the CMV status of the donor is not considered, and use of CMV-reduced-risk blood is indicated except when the allograft recipient is CMV seropositive. Some institutions give CMV-seropositive recipients undergoing bone marrow transplantation leukoreduced products, and formal evaluation of this practice is underway. All low-birth-weight or premature infants (<1,200 g), seronegative pregnant women, and fetuses receiving intrauterine transfusion need CMV-reduced-risk blood products.

Some seronegative patient populations may require a compromise between acquisition of CMV and induction of tolerance. In renal transplantation, for example, transfusion of cells with a common HLA haplotype or shared HLA-B and HLA-DR antigens induces tolerance to donor antigens. In one study of 23 renal allograft recipients who received buffy-coat-depleted red blood cells up to 36 hours after donation, CTLs were quantitated over time. The T-cell response against donor alloantigens disappeared 4 to 16 weeks after transfusion and was long lasting (132). The investigators theorized that under certain conditions, donor lymphocytes may travel to certain sites and induce low-grade mixed chimerism. The result is T-cell inactivation and improvement in graft survival. Another theory is that peripheral blood stem cells present in blood units produce permanent chimerism, but this is probably less likely in the case of buffy-coat-poor transfusion. If either transient or permanent chimerism were the cause of transplant tolerance, viable leukocytes with adequate HLA antigen presentation would be needed. Leukoreduction of blood units would not promote such an effect.

PARVOVIRUS B19

Biology and Pathology

Parvovirus B19 is a single-stranded nonenveloped DNA virus of 5,500 nucleotides. It encodes one major nonstructural protein, two capsid proteins (VP1 and VP2), and several small peptides of unknown function and is encased in an icosahedral structure. In productive infection, the major (VP2) and minor (VP1) capsid proteins are synthesized. VP1 and VP2 are identical except for the additional 226 amino acids at the amino terminus end of VP1. Most of the capsid protein is VP2, which is critical to the development of the immune response. VP1 and VP2 together lead to self-assembly of viral particles; VP1 does not self-assemble to form capsids. The presence of the nonstructural proteins is cytotoxic to cells in which viral capsid proteins are not produced (133).

The cellular receptor for Parvovirus B19 is a globoside, also known as *blood group P antigen.* Persons lacking the P blood group are not susceptible to infection with Parvovirus B19 (134). Globoside is found on a wide range of cell types, perhaps accounting for the pathologic changes of fetal disease and the clinical manifestations of Parvovirus B19 infection in children and adults. These cells include erythroid precursors and megakaryocytes in bone marrow, fetal myocardium, placenta, liver, kidney, and thyroid cells.

Parvovirus B19 tropism for erythroid progenitors is caused by high expression of globoside on erythroid progenitors. Productive infection in this cell line occurs because Parvovirus B19 depends on mitotically active cells for replication. Erythroid progenitors infected with Parvovirus B19 are characterized by giant pronormoblasts with cytoplasmic vacuolization, immature chromatin, and eosinophilic nuclear inclusion bodies, which represent actual Parvovirus capsids. Concentration of globoside on nonhematopoietic tissue and lack of active proliferation result in less active infection.

The development of neutralizing antibody to VP1 is critical to an adequate immune response. Persons susceptible to recurrent or prolonged Parvovirus B19 infection are missing anti-VP1, according to results of assays with erythroid progenitors (135). Vaccine development has concentrated on the use of VP1-enhanced capsids with adjuvants, and commercial development has begun. The cellular immune response to the virus is not as well studied, and whether Parvovirus B19 resides latently in cellular reservoirs is not known.

Diagnostic Methods

The diagnosis of Parvovirus B19 infection can be made with serologic assays, nucleic acid testing, histopathologic examination, in situ hybridization, or erythroid culture assays. The classic serologic tests include IgM and IgG antibody assays, which are most often performed with enzyme linked immunoassays and capture antibody assays. Use of the capture antibody format with whole-virus antigen increases the sensitivity and specificity of the IgM assays, whereas indirect IgM assays are more sensitive (136). Nucleic acid testing for viral DNA is more routinely available and preferred in selected clinical circumstances. Nucleic acid testing is particularly useful in the care of patients who do not yet have IgM or IgG responses or the care of immunosuppressed patients with blunted or absent IgM or IgG responses. Nucleic acid testing can be used with fetal blood or tissue to diagnose congenital infection and may be helpful in monitoring response to therapy when treatment with immunoglobulin makes results of monitoring with antibody levels difficult to interpret. Parvovirus B19 variants have been described that are not identified if PCR is used alone. Direct hybridization assays may be necessary to fully identify variants and to interpret pathologic ramifications (137).

Epidemiology

Infection with Parvovirus B19 is common, especially in late winter, spring, and summer. Episodic epidemics recur at 3- or 4-year intervals. Parvovirus B19 is spread in nasopharyngeal secretions during the viremic phase of the host. This respiratory droplet route makes Parvovirus B19 infection common in schools, day-care centers, and other closed environments. The infection occurs in two phases. The initial viremic period can result in bone marrow suppression. In persons with shortened red blood cell survival periods or those with profound immunodeficiency, severe aplastic anemia can occur. The second phase occurs when a specific antibody response neutralizes the viremia. Formation of immune complexes in skin, joints, or organs can cause specific symptoms, such as rash (erythema infectiosum, fifth disease), rheumatologic manifestations, hepatitis, and nephropathy. The clinical manifestations include erythema infectiosum, polyarthropathy, transient aplastic crisis, chronic bone marrow failure, and in rare instances myocardiopathy, vasculitis, and neurologic disease. Among pregnant women, infection can lead to fetal death, severe hydrops fetalis, myocardiopathy, and other congenital malformations. In utero fetal transfusion has proved successful in saving fetuses with infection and bringing them to term (138). Patients with cellular and humoral immune deficiency may have chronic Parvovirus B19 infection in the absence of systemic symptoms.

Groups of patients at risk of nosocomial or epidemic Parvovirus B19 infection include those with congenital or acquired hemolytic anemia who have a high turnover of erythroid precursors, those with acquired or congenital immunodeficiency who have immune paresis, others who are serologically naive because of age (fetus, infants, children), and serologically naive pregnant women. Intravenous immune globulin with variable titers of VP1 and VP2 has been used therapeutically to treat selected patients, especially those with immune paresis and immunodeficiency from HIV. Intravenous immune globulin neutralizes the virus and leads to viral clearance and erythroid recovery.

Parvovirus B19 and Blood Transfusion

Blood and plasma donors have been tested for evidence of Parvovirus B19 in several studies conducted with a variety of PCR-based methods. Variability in donor virus titer has been found to range from 10^3 to 10^{10} genome copies per milliliter (139–141). Copy number increases when the virus is epidemic in the community. The number of genome copies per milliliter to transmit viremia in blood products is unknown. According to data derived from solvent-detergent plasma, at least 10^3 genome copies per milliliter are needed to transmit viremia.

Plasma-derived products, especially plasma-derived coagulation products, can transmit Parvovirus B19. Persons with hemophilia have a high serologic prevalence of Parvovirus B19 infection, and they have participated in extensive studies (142,143). Transmissibility in coagulation products has occurred among patients who received heat-treated, pasteurized, monoclonally purified, and solvent-detergent–treated concentrates. Minor clinical symptoms, including fatigue, arthralgia, transient hypoplasia, and rash, have occurred among a small number of patients. Only one severe case of pancytopenia has been reported. The patient had hemophilia and ankylosing spondylitis (144). In the large Multicenter Hemophilia Cohort Study of persons with hemophilia and HIV infection, no reactivation of Parvovirus B19 infection or persistent viremia was identified. This finding supported the concept that Parvovirus B19 antibodies were protective in this population (145). Nucleic acid testing for Parvovirus B19 of plasma pools is being instituted by plasma providers to reduce the risk of Parvovirus B19 transmission in pooled products.

Infection with Parvovirus B19 as a result of transfusion with cellular blood products has been reported twice with red blood cells and once with platelets (140,146,147). In 2 of the 3 cases, the donor was putatively infected with Parvovirus B19, as evidenced by either IgM-positive or Parvovirus B19 DNA in donor blood. No reports of transmission from polyethylene glycol or alkylated IVIG or albumin have surfaced. Transmission has been reported among recipients of solvent-detergent plasma (148) and prompted institution of nucleic acid testing of plasma pools to ensure less than 10^4 genome copies per milliliter. Universal testing for Parvovirus B19, particularly for cellular products, is unlikely in the future unless more substantial clinical adverse effects can be documented (136).

REFERENCES

1. Landini MP, Michelson S. Human cytomegalovirus proteins. *Prog Med Virol* 1988;35:152–185.
2. Emery VC, Griffiths PD. Molecular biology of cytomegalovirus. *Int J Exp Pathol* 1990;71:905–908.
3. Zaia J, Gallez-Hawkins G, Churchill MA. Comparative analysis of human cytomegalovirus sequence in multiple clinical isolates by using polymerase chain reaction and restriction length polymorphism assays. *J Clin Microbiol* 1990;28:2602–2607.
4. Lehner R, Stamminger J, Mach M. Comparative sequence analysis of human cytomegalovirus strains. *J Clin Microbiol* 1991;29: 2494–2502.
5. Mach M, Stamminger R, Jahn G. Human cytomegalovirus: recent aspects from molecular biology. *J Gen Virol* 1989;70:3117–3146.
6. Gerna G, Revello MC, Pervivalle E, et al. Quantification of human cytomegalovirus viremia by using monoclonal antibodies to viral different proteins. *J Clin Microbiol* 1990;28:2681–2688.
7. Adler SP. Current prospects for immunization against cytomegalovirus disease. *Infect Agents Dis* 1996;5:29–35.
8. Rubin RH, Tolkoff-Rubin NE, Oliver D, et al. Multicenter seroepidemiologic study of the impact of cytomegalovirus infection on renal transplantation. *Transplantation* 1985; 40:243–249.
9. Grattan MT, Moreno-Cabral E, Starnes VA, et al. Cytomegalovirus infection is associated with cardiac allograft rejection and atherosclerosis. *JAMA* 1989; 261:3561–3566.
10. Zanghellini F, Boppana SB, Emery VC, et al. Asymptomatic primary cytomegalovirus infection: virologic and immunologic features. *J Infect Dis* 1999;180:702–707.
11. Hillyer CD, Snydman DR, Berkman EM. The risk of cytomegalovirus infection in solid organ and bone marrow transplant recipients: transfusion of blood products. *Transfusion* 1990;30:659–666.
12. Tegtmeier GE. Posttransfusion cytomegalovirus infections. *Arch Pathol Lab Med* 1989;113:236–245.
13. Blajchman MA, Goldman M, Freedman J, et al. Proceedings of a consensus conference: prevention of post transfusion CMV with era of universal leukoreduction. *Transfusion Med Rev* 2001;15:1–20.
14. Preiksaitis JK. The cytomegalovirus "safe" blood product: is leukoreduction equivalent to antibody screening? *Transfusion Med Rev* 2000; 14:112–136.
15. Wilhelm JA, Matter L, Schopfer K. The risk of transmitting cytomegalovirus to patients receiving blood transfusion. *J Infect Dis* 1986;154; 169–171.
16. Preiksaitis JK, Brown L, McKenzie M. The risk of cytomegalovirus infection in seronegative transfusion recipients not receiving exogenous immunosuppression. *J Infect Dis* 1988;157:523–529
17. Yeager AS, Grumet FC, Hafleigh EB, et al. Prevention of transfusion acquired cytomegalovirus infections in newborn infants. *J Pediatr* 1981;98:281–287.
18. Adler SP, Chandrika T, Lawrence L, et al. Cytomegalovirus infections in neonates acquired by blood transfusions. *Pediatr Infect Dis J* 1983; 2:114–118.
19. Smith D Jr, Wright P, Estes W, et al. Posttransfusion cytomegalovirus infection in neonates weighing less than 1250 grams. *Transfusion* 1988;23:420.
20. Ohto H, Ujiie N, Hirai H. Lack of difference in cytomegalovirus transmissions via the transfusion of filtered-irradiated and nonfiltered-irradiated blood to newborn infants in an endemic area. *Transfusion* 2000; 39: 201–205
21. Lamberson HV, McMillan JA, Weiner LB, et al. Prevention of transfusion associated cytomegalovirus (CMV) infection in neonates by screening blood donors for IgM to CMV. *J Infect Dis* 1988;157: 820–823.
22. Preiksaitis JK, Brown L, McKenzie M, et al. Transfusion acquired cytomegalovirus infection in neonates: a prospective study. *Transfusion* 1988;28:205–209.
23. Bowden RA, Sayers M, Flounoy N, et al. Cytomegalovirus immune globulin and seronegative blood products to prevent primary cytomegalovirus infection after marrow transplantation. *N Engl J Med* 1986;314:1006–1010.
24. Miller WJ, McCollough J, Balfour HH Jr, et al. Prevention of cytomegalovirus infection following bone marrow transplantation: a randomized trial of blood product screening. *Bone Marrow Transplant* 1991;7:227–234.
25. MacKinnon S, Burnett AK, Crawford RJ, et al. Seronegative blood products prevent primary cytomegalovirus infection after bone marrow transplantation. *J Clin Pathol* 1988;41:948–950.
26. Rubie H, Altal M, Compardou AM, et al. Risk factors for cytomegalovirus infection in BMT recipients transfused exclusively with seronegative blood products. *Bone Marrow Transplant* 1993;11:209–214.
27. Preiksaitis JK, Rosno S, Grumet C, et al. Infections due to herpes viruses in cardiac transplant recipients: role of the donor heart and immunosuppressive therapy. *J Infect Dis* 1983;147:974–981.
28. Preiksaitis JK, Desai S, Vaudry W, et al. Transfusion and community-acquired cytomegalovirus infection in children with malignant disease: a prospective study. *Transfusion* 1997;37:941–946.
29. Cox F, Hughes WT. The value of isolation procedures for cytomegalovirus infections in children with leukemia. *Cancer* 1975;36: 1158–1161.
30. Murphy MF, Grint PC, Hardiman AE, et al. Use of leucocyte poor blood components to prevent primary cytomegalovirus (CMV) infection in patients with acute leukaemia [letter]. *Br J Haematol* 1988; 70:253–254.
31. Bowden RA, Slichter SJ, Sayers MH, et al. Use of leukocyte depleted platelets and cytomegalovirus-seronegative red blood cells for prevention of primary cytomegalovirus infection after marrow transplant. *Blood* 1991;78:246–250.
32. Winston DJ, Ho WG, Howell CL, et al. Cytomegalovirus infections associated with leukocyte transfusions. *Ann Intern Med* 1980;93: 671–675.
33. Hersman J, Meyers JD, Thomas ED, et al. The effect of granulocyte transfusions on the incidence of cytomegalovirus infection after allogeneic marrow transplantation. *Ann Intern Med* 1982;96:149–152.
34. Kaufman RM, Goodnough LT, Dynis M, et al. Selection of donors for granulocyte transfusion: is donor CMV serologic status important? *Transfusion* 2000;40[Suppl]:21S.
35. Landini MP, Rossier E, Schmitz H. Antibodies to human cytomegalovirus structural polypeptides during primary infection. *J Virol Methods* 1988;22:309–317.
36. Tolpin MD, Stewart JA, Warren D, et al. Transfusion transmission of cytomegalovirus confirmed by restriction endonuclease analysis. *J Pediatr* 1985;107:953–956.
37. Adler SP, Baggett J, Wilson M, et al. Molecular epidemiology of cytomegalovirus in a nursery: lack of evidence for nosocomial transmission. *J Pediatr* 1986;108:117–123.
38. Jiwa NM, Van Gemert GW, Raap AK, et al. Rapid detection of human cytomegalovirus DNA in peripheral blood leukocytes of viremic transplant patients by the polymerase chain reaction. *Transplantation* 1989;48:72–76.
39. Chou S. Differentiation of cytomegalovirus strains by restriction analysis of DNA sequences amplified from clinical specimens. *J Infect Dis* 1990;162:738–742.
40. Adler SP. Cytomegalovirus and child day care. *N Engl J Med* 1989; 321:1290–1296.
41. Adler SP. Data that suggests that FFP does not transmit CMV [letter]. *Transfusion* 1988;28:604.
42. Bowden RA, Sayers M. The risk of transmitting cytomegalovirus by fresh frozen plasma. *Transfusion* 1990;30: 762–763.
43. Winston DJ, Ho WG, Lin C et al. Intravenous immune globulin for prevention of cytomegalovirus infection and interstitial pneumonia after bone marrow transplantation. *Ann Intern Med* 1987;106:12–18.

44. Luban NLC, Williams AE, MacDonald MG, et al. Low incidence of acquired cytomegalovirus infections transfused with washed red blood cells. *Am J Dis Child* 1987;141:146–149.
45. Brady MT, Milam JD, Anderson DC, et al. Use of deglycerolized red blood cells to prevent posttransfusion infection with cytomegalovirus in neonates. *J Infect Dis* 1984;150:334–339.
46. Taylor BJ, Jacobs RF, Baker RL, et al. Frozen deglycerolized red blood cells prevents transfusion acquired cytomegalovirus transmission in neonates. *Pediatr Infect Dis J* 1986;5:188–191.
47. Simon T, Johnson J, Koffler H, et al. Impact of previously frozen deglycerolized red blood cells in cytomegalovirus transmission to newborn infants. *Plasma Ther Transfus Technol* 1987;8:51–56.
48. Gilbert GL, Hayes K, Hudson IL, et al. Prevention of transfusion-acquired cytomegalovirus infection in infants by blood filtration to remove leukocytes. Neonatal Cytomegalovirus Infection Study Group. *Lancet* 1989;1:1228–1231.
49. De Graan-Hentzen YCE, Gratama JW, et al. Prevention of primary cytomegalovirus infection in patients with hematologic malignancy by intensive white cell depletion of blood products. *Transfusion* 1989: 29:757–760.
50. DeWitte T, Schattenberg A, Van Dijk BA, et al. Prevention of primary cytomegalovirus infection after allogeneic bone marrow transplantation by using leukocyte-poor random blood products from cytomegalovirus unscreened blood bank donors. *Transplantation* 1990;50: 964–968.
51. Preiksaitis JK. Indications for the use of cytomegalovirus-seronegative blood products. *Transfus Med Rev* 1991;5:1–17.
52. Schrier RD, Nelson JA, Oldstone MB. Detection of human cytomegalovirus in peripheral blood lymphocytes in a natural infection. *Science* 1985; 230:1048–1051.
53. Saltzman RL, Quirk MR, Jordan MC. Disseminated cytomegalovirus infection: molecular analysis of virus and leukocyte interaction in viremia. *J Clin Invest* 1988;81:75–81.
54. Stagno S, Cloud GA. Changes in the epidemiology of cytomegalovirus infection: molecular analysis of virus. *Adv Exp Med Biol* 1990;278: 93–104.
55. Weir MR, Henry ML, Blackmore M, et al. Incidence and morbidity of cytomegalovirus disease associated with a seronegative recipient receiving seropositive donor-specific transfusion and living-related donor transplantation. *Transplantation* 1988;45:111–116.
56. de Cates CR, Robertson NR, Walker JR. Fatal acquired cytomegalovirus infection in a neonate with maternal antibody. *J Infect* 1988;17; 235–239.
57. Griffin MP, O'Shea M, Brazy JE, et al. Cytomegalovirus infection in a neonatal intensive care unit: subsequent morbidity and mortality of seropositive infants. *J Perinatol* 1990;10:43–45.
58. Fowler KB, Pass RF. Sexually transmitted diseases in mothers of neonates with congenital cytomegalovirus infection. *J Infect Dis* 1991; 164;259–264.
59. Winston DJ, Pollard RB, Ho WG, et al. Cytomegalovirus immune plasma in bone marrow transplant recipients. *Ann Intern Med* 1982; 97:11–18.
60. Condie RM, O'Reilly RJ. Prevention of cytomegalovirus infection by prophylaxis with an intravenous, hyperimmune mature, unmodified cytomegalovirus globulin. *Am J Med* 1984;76:134–141.
61. Kubanek B, Ernest P, Ostendorf P, et al. Preliminary data of a controlled trial of intravenous hyperimmune globulin in the prevention of cytomegalovirus in bone marrow transplant recipients. *Transplant Proc* 1985;17:468.
62. Meyers JD, Leszczynski J, Zaia JA, et al. Prevention of cytomegalovirus infection by cytomegalovirus immune globulin after marrow transplantation. *Ann Intern Med* 1983;98:442–446.
63. Bowden RA, Fisher LD, Rogers K, et al. Cytomegalovirus (CMV)–specific intravenous immunoglobulin for the prevention of primary CMV infection and disease after marrow transplant. *J Infect Dis* 1991;164:483–487.
64. Sullivan KM, Kopecky KJ, Jocom J, et al. Immunomodulatory and antimicrobial efficacy of intravenous immunoglobulin in bone marrow transplantation. *N Engl J Med* 1990;323;705–712.
65. Britt WJ, Vugler L, Butfiloski EJ, et al. Cell surface expression of human cytomegalovirus (HCMV) gp 55-116 (gB): use of HCMV recombinant vaccinia virus-infected cells in analysis of the human neutralizing antibody response. *J Virol* 1990;64:1079–1085.
66. Gonczol E, de Taisene C, Hirka G, et al. High expression of human cytomegalovirus (HCMV) gB protein in cells infected with a vaccinia gB recombinant-derived glycoprotein B after natural human cytomegalovirus infection correlate with neutralizing activity. *Vaccine* 1991; 9:631–837.
67. Marshall GS, Rabalais GP, Stout GG, et al. Antibodies to recombinant-derived glycoprotein B after natural human cytomegalovirus infection correlate with neutralizing activity. *J Infect Dis* 1992;165; 381–384.
68. Borysiewicz LK, Hickling JK, Graham S, et al. Human cytomegalovirus-specific cytotoxic T cells: relative frequency of stage-specific CTL recognizing the 72-kD immediate early protein and glycoprotein expressed by recombinant vaccinia viruses. *J Exp Med* 1988;168; 919–931.
69. Liu Y-N, Klaus A, Kari B, et al. The N-terminal 513 amino acids of the envelope glycoprotein gB of human cytomegalovirus stimulates both B and T cell immune responses in humans. *J Virol* 1991;65; 1644–168.
70. Chou S, Dennison KM. Analysis of interstrain variation in cytomegalovirus glycoprotein B sequences encoding neutralization-related epitopes. *J Infect Dis* 1991;163:1229–1234.
71. Fries BC, Chou S, Boeckh M, et al. Frequency distribution of cytomegalovirus envelope glycoprotein genotypes in bone marrow transplant recipients. *J Infect Dis* 1994;169:769–774.
72. Torok-Storb B, Boeckh M, Hoy C, et al. Association of specific cytomegalovirus genotypes with death from myelosuppression after marrow transplantation. *Blood* 1997;90:2097–2102.
73. Hebart H, Greif M, Krause H, et al. Interstrain variation of immediate early DNA sequences and glycoprotein B genotypes in cytomegalovirus clinical isolates. *Med Microbiol Immunol (Berl)* 1997;186: 135–138.
74. Vogelberg C, Meyer-Konig U, Hufert FT, et al. Human cytomegalovirus glycoprotein B genotypes in renal transplant recipients. *J Med Virol* 1996;50:31–34.
75. Bale JF Jr, Morph JR, Demmler GJ, et al. Intrauterine cytomegalovirus infection and glycoprotein B genotypes. *J Infect Dis* 2000;182: 933–936.
76. Plotkin SA, Starr SE, Friedman HM, et al. Effect of Towne live virus vaccine on cytomegalovirus disease after renal transplant: a controlled trial. *Ann Intern Med* 1991;114;525–531.
77. Adler SP, Plotkin SA, Gonczol E, et al. A carnarypox vector expressing cytomegalovirus (CMV) glycoprotein primes for antibody responses to a live attenuated CMV vaccine (Towne). *J Infect Dis* 1999;180: 843–846.
78. Endresz V, Kari L, Berensci K, et al. Induction of human cytomegalovirus (HCMV) glycoprotein B (gB)–specific neutralizing antibody and phosphoprotein 65 (pp65)–specific cytotoxic lymphocyte responses by naked DNA immunization. *Vaccine* 1999;17:50–58.
79. Berensci K, Gyulai Z, Gonczol E, et al. A canarypox vector-expressing cytomegalovirus (CMV) phosphoprotein 65 induces long-lasting cytotoxic T cell responses in human CMV-negative subjects. *J Infect Dis* 2001;183:1171–1179.
80. Quinnan GV, Ennis FA. Cell-mediated immunity in cytomegalovirus: a review. *Comp Immunol Microbiol Infect Dis* 1980:3:283–290.
81. Quinnan GV, Kirmani N, Rook AN, et al. Cytotoxic T cells in cytomegalovirus infection: HLA-restricted T-lymphocyte and non-T lymphocyte cytotoxic responses correlate with recovery from cytomegalovirus infection in bone marrow transplant recipients. *N Engl J Med* 1982;307:7–13.
82. Koszinowski UH. Molecular aspects of immune recognition of cytomegalovirus. *Transplant Proc* 1991;23:70–73.
83. Jonjic S, Mutter W, Weiland F, et al. Site-restricted persistent cytomegalovirus infection after selective long-term depletion of CD4+ T lymphocytes. *J Exp Med* 1989;169:1199–1212.
84. Pasternack MS, Medearis DN, Rubin RH. Cell-mediated immunity in experimental cytomegalovirus infections: a perspective. *Rev Infect Dis* 1990;12:S720–S726.

85. Gratama JW, Kluin-Nelemans HC, Langelaar RA, et al. Flow cytometric and morphologic studies of HNK1+ (Leuk 7+) lymphocytes in relation to cytomegalovirus carrier status. *Clin Exp Immunol* 1988; 74:190–195.
86. Weekes MP, Wills MR, Mynard K, et al. The memory cytotoxic T lymphocyte (CTL) response to human cytomegalovirus infection contains individual peptide-specific CTL cones that have undergone extensive expansion in vivo. *J Virol* 1999;73:2099–2108.
87. Weekes MP, Wills MR, Mynard K, et al. Large clonal expansions of human virus-specific memory cytotoxic T lymphocytes within the CD57+CD28-CD8+ T-cell population. *Immunology* 1999;98: 443–449.
88. Dolstra H, Van de Wiel–van Kemenade E, De Witte T, et al. Clonal predominance of cytomegalovirus-specific CD8+ cytotoxic T lymphocytes in bone marrow recipients. *Bone Marrow Transplant* 1996; 18:339–345.
89. Engstrand M, Tournay C, Peyrat MA, et al. Characterization of CMV pp65-specific CD8+ T lymphocytes using MHC tetramers in kidney transplant patients and healthy participants. *Transplantation* 2000; 69:2243–2250.
90. Gillespie GMA, Wills MR, Appay V, et al. Functional heterogeneity and high frequencies of cytomegalovirus-specific CD8+ T lymphocytes in healthy seropositive donors. *J Virol* 2000;74:8140–8150.
91. Lewis DC, Tang DS, Adu-Oppong A, et al. Anergy and apoptosis in CD8+ T cells from HIV-infected persons. *J Immunol* 1994;153: 412–420.
92. Lloyd TE, Yang L, Tang DN, et al. Regulation of CD28 costimulation in human CD8+ T cells *J Immunol* 1997; 158:1551–1558.
93. Monteiro J, Batliwalla F, Ostrer H, et al. Shortened telomeres in clonally expanded CD28-CD8+ T cells imply a replicative history that is distinct from their CD28+CD8+ counterparts. *J Immunol* 1996;156:3587–3590.
94. Taylor-Wideman J, Sissons JG, Borysievicz LK, et al. Monocytes are the major site of persistence of human cytomegalovirus in peripheral blood mononuclear cells. *J Gen Virol* 1991;72:2059–2064.
95. Kondo K, Kaneshima H, Mocarski ES, et al. Human cytomegalovirus latent infection of granulocyte-macrophage progenitors. *Proc Natl Acad Sci U S A* 1994;91:11879–11883.
96. Kondo K, Mocarski ES. Cytomegalovirus latency and latency-specific transcription in hematopoietic progenitors. *Scand J Infect Dis* 1995: 63–67.
97. Hahn G, Jores R, Mocarski ES. Cytomegalovirus remains latent in a common precursor of dendritic and myeloid cells. *Proc Natl Acad Sci U S A* 1998;95:3937–3942.
98. Mendelson M, Monard S, Sissons P, et al. Detection of endogenous human cytomegalovirus in CD34(+) bone marrow progenitors. *J Gen Virol* 1996;77:3099–3102.
99. Hendrix RMB, Wagenaar M, Slobbe RL, et al. Widespread presence of cytomegalovirus DNA in tissues of healthy trauma victims. *J Clin Pathol* 1997;59–63.
100. Gilbert MJ, Riddell SR, Plachter B, et al. Cytomegalovirus selectively blocks antigen processing and presentation of its immediate-early gene product. *Nature* 1996;383:720–722.
101. Jones, TR, Sun L. Human cytomegalovirus US2 destabilizes major histocompatibility complex class I heavy chains. *J Virol* 1997;71: 2970–2979.
102. Jones, TR, Wiertz E, Sun L, et al. Human cytomegalovirus US3 impairs transport and maturation of major histocompatibility complex class I heavy chains. *Proc Natl Acad Sci U S A* 1996;93: 11327–11333.
103. Wiertz E, Totorella D, Bogyo M, et al. Sec61-mediated transfer of a membrane protein from the endoplasmic reticulum to the proteasome for destruction. *Nature* 1996;384:432–438.
104. Wiertz EJ, Jones TR, Sun L, et al. The human cytomegalovirus US11 gene product dislocates MHC class I heavy chains from the endoplasmic reticulum to the cytosol. *Cell* 1996;84:769–779.
105. Ahn K, Gruhler A, Galocha B, et al. The ER-luminal domain of the HCMV glycoprotein US6 inhibits peptide translocation by TAP. *Immunity* 1997;6:613–621.
106. Baggiolini M, Dewald B, Moser B. Human chemokines: an update. *Ann Rev Immunol* 1997;15:675–705.
107. Bodaghi B, Jones TR, Zipeto D, et al. Chemokine sequestration by viral chemoreceptors as a novel viral escape strategy: withdrawal of chemokines from the environment of cytomegalovirus-infected cells. *J Exp Med* 1998;188:855–866.
108. Kledal TN, Rosenkilde MM, Schwartz TW. Selective recognition of the membrane-bound CX3C chemokine, fractalkine, by the human cytomegalovirus-encoded broad-spectrum receptor US28. *FEBS Lett* 1998;441:209–214.
109. Pleskoff O, Treboute C, Alizon M. The cytomegalovirus-encoded chemokine receptor US28 can enhance cell-cell fusion mediated by different viral proteins. *J Virol* 1998;72:6389–6397.
110. Randolph-Habecker J. The HCMV beta chemokine receptor homolog, US28, acts as "chemokine sink" by binding endogenously and exogenously produced beta chemokines. *J Clin Virol* 1999;12:138.
111. Mackowiak PA, Marling-Cason M. Immunoreactivity of cytomegalovirus-induced Fc receptors. *Microbiol Immunol* 1987;31:427–434.
112. Murayama T, Natsume-Sakai S, Shimokawa K, et al. Fc receptors(s) induced by human cytomegalovirus bind differentially with human immunoglobulin G subclasses. *J Gen Virol* 1986;67:1475–1478.
113. Gilljam G, Wahren B. Properties of IgG subclasses to human cytomegalovirus. *J Virol Methods* 1989;25:139–151.
114. Gupta CK, Leszczynski J, Gupta RK, et al. IgG subclass antibodies to human cytomegalovirus (CMV) in normal human plasma samples and immune globulins and their neutralizing activities. *Biologicals* 1996;24:117–124.
115. Darnell JE, Kerr IM, Stark GR. Jak-Stat pathways and transcriptional activation in response to IFNs and other extracellular signaling proteins. *Science* 1994;264:1415–1421.
116. Miller DM, Zhang Y, Rahill BM, et al. Human cytomegalovirus inhibits IFN-α stimulated antiviral and immunoregulatory responses by blocking multiple levels of IFN-α signal transduction. *J Immunol* 1999;162:6107–6113.
117. Kotenko SV, Saccani S, Izotova LS, et al. Human cytomegalovirus harbors its own unique IL-10 homolog (cmvIL-10). *Proc Natl Acad Sci U S A* 2000;97:1695–1700.
118. McCullough J, Yunis EJ, Benson SJ, et al. Effect of blood bank storage on leukocyte function. *Lancet* 1969;1:1333.
119. Sherman ME, Dzik WH. Stability of antigens in leukocytes in banked platelet concentrates: decline in HLA-DR antigen expression and mixed lymphocyte culture stimulating capacity following storage. *Blood* 1988;72:867–872.
120. Paloheimo JA, von Essen R, Klemola JE, et al. Subclinical cytomegalovirus infections and cytomegalovirus mononucleosis after open heart surgery. *Am J Cardiol* 1968;22:624–630.
121. Adler SP, McVoy MM. Cytomegalovirus infections in seropositive patients after transfusion. *Transfusion* 1989;29:667–671.
122. Light JA, Metz S, Oddenino K, et al. Donor-specific transfusion with diminished sensitization. *Transplantation* 1982;34:322.
123. Sayers MH, Anderson KC, Goodnough LT, et al. Reducing the risk for transfusion-transmitted cytomegalovirus. *Ann Intern Med* 1992; 116:55–62.
124. De Graan-Hentzen YCE, Gratama JW, Mudde GL, et al. Prevention of primary cytomegalovirus infection during induction treatment of acute leukemia using at random leukocyte poor blood products. *Br J Haematol* 1987;66:421.
125. Verdonck LF, De Graan-Hentzen YC, Dekker AW, et al. Cytomegalovirus seronegative platelets and leukocyte poor red blood cells can prevent primary cytomegalovirus infection after bone marrow transplantation. *Bone Marrow Transplant* 1987;2:73–78.
126. Bowden RA, Slichter SJ, Sayers MH, et al. A comparison of filtered leukocyte reduced and cytomegalovirus (CMV) seronegative blood products for the prevention of transfusion-associated CMV infection after marrow transplant. *Blood* 1995;86:3598–3603.
127. Van Prooijen HC, Visser JJ, van Oostendorp WR, et al. Prevention of primary transfusion-associated CMV infection after marrow transplant recipients by the removal of white cells from blood components with high affinity filters. *Br J Haematol* 1994; 87:144–147.
128. Narvious AB, Przepiorka D, Tarrand J, et al. Transfusion support

using filtered unscreened blood products for cytomegalovirus-negative allogeneic marrow transplant recipients. *Bone Marrow Transplant* 1998;22:575–577.
129. James DJ, Sikotra S, Sivakumaran M, et al. The presence of free infectious cytomegalovirus (CMV) in the plasma of donated CMV-seropositive blood and platelets. *Transfusion Med* 1997;7:123–126.
130. American Association of Blood Banks. Leukocyte reduction for the prevention of transfusion-transmitted cytomegalovirus (TT-CMV). Association Bulletin 97-2. Bethesda, MD: American Association of Blood Banks, 1997;2:1–15.
131. Collier AC, Kahshla, Busch MP, et al. Leukocyte-reduced red blood cell transfusions in patients with anemia and human immunodeficiency virus infection. *JAMA* 2001;285:1592–1601.
132. Van Twuyver E, Mooijarart RJD, ten Berge IJM, et al. Pretransplantation blood transfusion revisited. *N Engl J Med* 1991;325:1210–1213.
133. Brown KE, Young NS, Liu JM. Molecular, cellular and clinical aspects of parvovirus B19 infection. *Crit Rev Oncol Hematol* 1994;16:1–31.
134. Brown KE, Hibbs JR, Gallinella G, et al. Resistance to Parvovirus B19 infection due to lack of virus receptor (erythrocyte P antigen). *N Engl J Med* 1994;330:1192–1196.
135. Kurtzman GJ, Ozawa K, Cohen B, et al. Chronic bone marrow failure due to persistent B19 Parvovirus infection. *N Engl J Med* 1987;317: 287–294.
136. Brown KE, Young NS, Barbosa LH. Parvovirus B19: implications for transfusion medicine: summary of a workshop. *Transfusion* 2001; 41:130–135.
137. Nguyen QT, Sifer C, Schneider V, et al. Novel human erythrovirus associated with transient aplastic anemia. *J Clin Microbiol* 1999;37: 2483–2487.
138. Rogers BB. Parvovirus B19: twenty-five years in perspective. *Pediatr Dev Pathol* 1999;2:296–315.
139. Wakamatsu C, Takakura F, Kojima E, et al. Screening of blood donors for human parvovirus B19 and characterization of the results. *Vox Sang* 1999;76:14–21.
140. Jordan J, Tiangco B, Kiss J, et al. Human parvovirus B19: prevalence of viral DNA in volunteer blood donors and clinical outcomes of transfusion recipients. *Vox Sang* 1998;75:97–102.
141. McComish F, Yap PL, Jordan A, et al. Detection of Parvovirus B19 in donated blood: a model system for screening by polymerase chain reaction. *J Clin Microbiol* 1993;31:323–328.
142. Azzi A, Morfini M, Mannucci PM. The transfusion-associated transmission of parvovirus B19. *Transfus Med Rev* 1999;13:194–204.
143. Luban NLC. Human parvoviruses: implications for transfusion medicine. *Transfusion* 1994;34:821–827.
144. Yee TT, Cohen BJ, Pasi KS, et al. Transmission of symptomatic parvovirus B19 infection by clotting factor concentrate. *Br J Haematol* 1996;93:457–459.
145. Goedert JJ, Erdman DD, Konkle BA, et al. Parvovirus B19 quiescence during the course of human immunodeficiency virus infection in persons with hemophilia. *Am J Hematol* 1997;56:248–251.
146. Cohen BJ, Beard S, Knowles WA, et al. Chronic anemia due to Parvovirus B19 infection in a bone marrow transplant patient after platelet transfusion. *Transfusion* 1997;37:947–952.
147. Zanella A, Rossi F, Cesana C, et. al. Transfusion-transmitted human Parvovirus B19 infection in a thalassemic patient. *Transfusion* 1995; 35:769–772.
148. Koenighauer UF, Eastland T, Day JW. Clinical illness due to Parvovirus B19 infection after infusion of solvent-detergent treated pooled plasma. *Transfusion* 2000;10:1203–1206.
149. Kraat YJ, Hendrix RN, Landini MP, et al. Comparison of four techniques for detection of antibodies to cytomegalovirus. *J Clin Microbiol* 1992;30:522–524.

Rossi's Principles of Transfusion Medicine, Third Edition, edited by Toby L. Simon, Walter H. Dzik, Edward L. Snyder, Christopher P. Stowell, and Ronald G. Strauss. Lippincott Williams & Wilkins, Philadelphia © 2002.

CASE 52A

CYTOMEGALOVIRUS INFECTION IN AN IMMUNOSUPPRESSED INFANT

CASE HISTORY

As an infant, J.L. had cholestatic liver disease caused by biliary atresia. This led to progressive hepatic fibrosis, and liver function deteriorated progressively during the first 10 months of life. At 9 months of age, worsening hepatic function resulted in a coagulopathy, and transfusion of fresh frozen plasma (FFP) was administered. Liver transplantation was being planned at this time, and serum was obtained prior to the infusion of FFP. Testing of this serum showed negative results for all viruses tested, including cytomegalovirus (CMV).

At 10 months of age, J.L. received a segmental liver transplant from his father. The father was chosen because he was healthy, had the same blood group as J.L., and had a large enough liver. The father had positive serologic results for CMV, but this does not exclude potential organ donors. During the operation, J.L. needed transfusion of red blood cells and FFP. The surgery had no complications, and J.L. recovered uneventfully. The transplanted liver segment functioned normally. Prophylactic drugs for liver rejection included prednisone, cyclosporine, and azathioprine.

Approximately 1 month after the operation, J.L. had fever, malaise, intermittent abdominal cramps, loss of appetite, nausea, vomiting, and diarrhea. There was blood in the stool and the vomitus. Results of liver function tests were normal. The prednisone dose was slowly decreased, but the symptoms did not resolve. Liver biopsy showed no evidence of rejection.

The gastrointestinal problems persisted. Endoscopic examination revealed moderate ulcers in the stomach and small intestine. A biopsy of the stomach revealed cytoplasmic and nuclear inclusions typically present in CMV infection (Fig. 52A.1). Similar findings were seen in biopsy specimens from the small intestine (not shown). Cytomegalovirus early antigens (pp65) were detected in the blood, confirming the diagnosis of active CMV infection. J.L. was treated with intravenous ganciclovir for 2 weeks, after which he was given oral ganciclovir. The symptoms resolved.

DISCUSSION

Like most children, J.L. did not have CMV infection before liver transplantation. Although many persons acquire CMV at some point in their lives, few become ill. The immunosuppressive drugs used after liver transplantation made J.L. susceptible to symptomatic CMV disease.

There were several possible sources of CMV infection in this case, including the donated liver segment, the FFP, and the red blood cell transfusion. The FFP is unlikely to have been the source of the CMV because FFP is practically acellular and is not associated with transmission of CMV. Although the CMV could have been community acquired, this mode is not as likely as the other two possible modes of transmission. That the red blood cells were the source of the CMV is theoretically possible, but this mode of transmission usually does not cause symptomatic CMV disease. The donor liver segment is the most likely

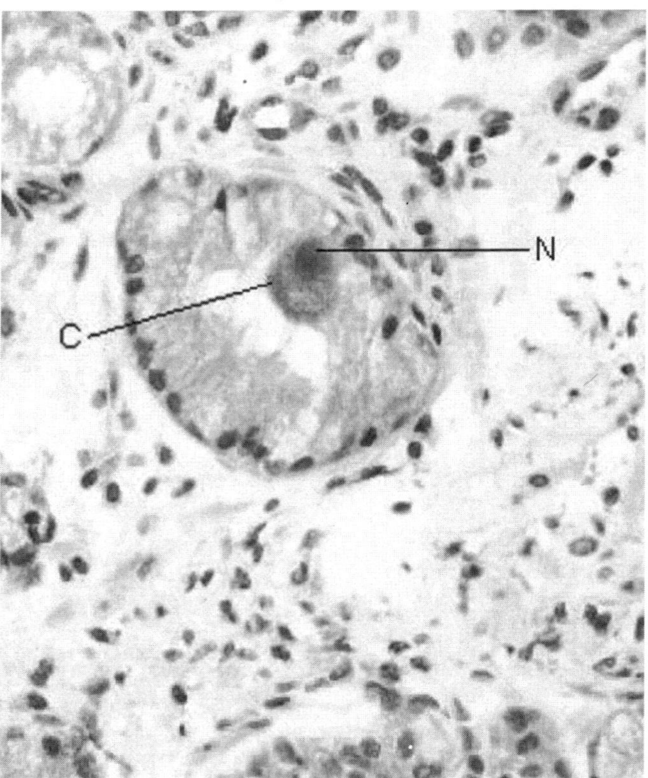

FIGURE 52A.1. Specimen from gastric biopsy shows an intranuclear inclusion (*N*) and a cytoplasmic inclusion (*C*). These are typical finding of cytomegalovirus infection. (Courtesy of Sara O. Vargas, M.D.)

source. Studies of risk factors associated with symptomatic CMV infection among liver transplant recipients have shown that CMV is most likely to arise in a CMV-seronegative patient who receives a liver from a CMV-seropositive donor (1,2). This risk associated with CMV transmission by the donor liver is caused at least in part by the fact that the donor liver contains a large number of "fresh" lymphocytes that can harbor CMV.

Transfused blood components are not often associated with CMV transmission in this patient population, probably because blood components contain fewer leukocytes than do donor livers. Results of studies that show leukoreduction of blood products decreases the risk of CMV transmission suggest that the risk of CMV transmission is proportional to the dose of leukocytes administered. The leukocytes present in blood components usually have been stored at 4°C for some time and are less likely to proliferate and release CMV than are leukocytes present in a fresh donor liver.

There is no method to ascertain with complete accuracy which patients are at risk of CMV disease. Patients who are CMV seropositive before transplantation can still acquire symptomatic CMV disease. In some patients, the disease is caused by reactivation of latent infection; in others, is caused by infection with a different strain of CMV. There is no way to be certain that a blood product is free of CMV. Some infected donors do not mount a sufficient antibody response to allow detection in the serologic screening assay. Recently infected donors may not have positive test results for CMV antibody. Process-controlled leukoreduction provides an alternative method for reducing the risk of CMV transmission, but there also have been cases of CMV transmission despite the use of leukoreduced blood components. For these reasons, the preferred term is *CMV-reduced-risk* rather than "CMV-negative" or "CMV-safe" blood.

Case contributed by Steven R. Sloan, M.D., Children's Hospital, Boston, MA.

REFERENCES

1. Gorensek MJ, Carey WD, Vogt D, et al. A multivariate analysis of risk factors for cytomegalovirus infection in liver-transplant recipients. *Gastroenterology* 1990;98:1326–1332.
2. Paya CV, Wiesner RH, Hermands PE, et al. Risk factors for cytomegalovirus and severe bacterial infections following liver transplantation: a prospective multivariate time-dependent analysis. *J Hepatol* 1993;18: 185–195.

53

TRANSMISSION OF PARASITIC INFECTIONS BY BLOOD TRANSFUSION

IRA A. SHULMAN
MARCIA D. HAIMOWITZ

The possibility the transfusion of blood in the United States will result in transmission of a parasitic infection is currently less than 1 in 1 million. This small risk is greatest for components such as red blood cells and platelets currently not subjected to pathogen reduction processes. International travel, immigration, and wars provide a reservoir of potential blood donors within the United States who have asymptomatic parasitemia. This chapter discusses the parasitic infections of most concern to the safety of the U.S. blood supply as well as steps that can be taken to minimize the likelihood of transfusing parasite-containing blood.

MALARIA

Malaria is caused by the intraerythrocytic protozoan parasites *Plasmodium vivax, P. falciparum, P. ovale,* and *P. malariae.* Malaria is a serious global problem, an estimated 300 to 500 million cases occurring annually (1). The usual mode of transmission is the bite of an infected anopheles mosquito, although transfusion of infected blood also transmits malaria. According to reports to the Centers for Disease Control and Prevention (CDC), 103 transfusion-associated cases of malaria occurred in the United States from 1958 through 1998, for an average of 2 or 3 cases per year or 0.25 cases per 1 million units of blood collected (2). Although transfusion-transmitted malaria is rare in comparison with transmission of other parasites, malaria is currently the most common reported parasitic infection to complicate blood transfusion therapy in the United States.

Malaria usually is characterized by fever, which can be episodic, tachycardia, rigors, and sweating. Other manifestations include anemia, hepatosplenomegaly, cerebral involvement, renal failure, and shock (3). Transfusion-transmitted malaria often manifests with nonspecific clinical signs and symptoms, and the severity and speed of onset depend on the species (4). The infection can be fatal (2). The incubation period tends to be shortest for *P. falciparum* and longest for *P. malariae* (4).

Infection in blood donors can escape detection at the time of donor screening because asymptomatic parasitemia can occur, especially among residents of malaria-endemic areas. Transfusion-transmitted malaria is possible if a person with asymptomatic malaria arrives to give blood in the United States, but the infection is not recognized. There are different periods of asymptomatic infection for each malaria species. *Plasmodium falciparum* infection usually resolves within 1 to 2 years, although longer periods (up to 13 years) have been described (2,4). Infections with *P. vivax* and *P. ovale* can last as long as 5 years and 7 years, respectively; *P. malariae* infectivity can last a lifetime (4). Asymptomatic persistence of *P. malariae* at low blood levels has occurred for as long as 40 years (2). Donation of malaria-infected blood can cause infection in the recipient because malaria parasites survive for at least 1 week in blood stored at 4°C. Cases of *P. falciparum* malaria have been transmitted by blood stored longer than 10 days (4). The parasites can survive cryopreservation (4).

Because no blood donor screening tests for malaria have been approved for use in the United States, careful questioning is the only way to identify prospective donors at risk of transmitting

I.A. Shulman: Departments of Pathology, Keck School of Medicine, University of Southern California, and Los Angeles County/University of Southern California Medical Center, Los Angeles, California.

M.D. Haimowitz: Department of Pathology, Keck School of Medicine, University of Southern California, and American Red Cross Blood Services, Los Angeles, California.

malaria. Recommendations have been established to defer persons at risk of malaria from donating blood. The deferral criteria are based on donors' having been in endemic areas. These areas are defined in the CDC *Health Information for International Travelers,* known as the *CDC yellow book,* which is revised periodically by the CDC and can be found on the CDC website http://www.cdc.gov/. Standard operating procedures and deferral practices for blood establishment should keep pace with such revisions. The last guidance implemented by the Food and Drug Administration (FDA) for deferring donors in the United States at risk of malaria was published in July 1994 (5). As of this writing, a new guide is in draft form (6).

According to the current recommendations of the FDA (5) and of the American Association of Blood Banks (7), the following guidelines should be followed to decrease the risk of transfusion-transmitted malaria:

1. Permanent residents of nonendemic countries who travel to an area considered endemic for malaria by the malaria branch of the CDC should not be accepted as donors of whole blood or blood components within 1 year of departure from the endemic area. One year after departure, such otherwise suitable prospective donors may be accepted whether or not they have received antimalarial chemoprophylaxis, provided they have been free of unexplained symptoms suggestive of malaria.
2. Prospective donors who have had malaria should be deferred for 3 years after symptoms are no longer present. Immigrants, refugees, citizens, or residents of endemic countries should not be accepted as donors of whole blood or blood components within 3 years of departure from the area. After the 3-year period, otherwise suitable prospective donors may be accepted if they have remained free of unexplained symptoms suggestive of malaria.

When more than one of these deferral periods apply to a prospective donor, the longest period of deferral must be observed. These recommendations apply only to donations containing intact red blood cells. Donations for preparing plasma, plasma components, or derivatives devoid of intact red blood cells are excluded (5). Donations from which only the plasma is to be used are exempt from current American Association of Blood Banks standards (7). These deferral criteria are based on unpublished data from the CDC that show 97% of reported cases of malaria among U.S. and foreign civilians are diagnosed within 1 year and 99% within 3 years of the person's having been present in an area considered endemic for malaria (2).

The following is the proposed FDA guideline. When finalized, it will replace the foregoing guideline (6):

1. Permanent residents of non-endemic countries who travel to an area considered endemic for malaria by the Malaria Epidemiology Section, CDC, should not be accepted as donors of Whole Blood and blood components, including platelets, prior to one year after departure from the endemic area. After one year has passed since departure from the malarious area, such otherwise suitable prospective donors may be accepted provided that they have been free of unexplained symptoms suggestive of malaria and regardless of whether or not they have received antimalarial chemoprophylaxis.
2. Prospective donors who have had malaria and received an appropriate treatment should be deferred for three years after becoming asymptomatic.
3. Persons that have previously resided in endemic countries and now reside in the US, such as immigrants, refugees, citizens, or residents (for at least five years) of endemic countries, should not be accepted as donors of Whole Blood or blood components, including platelets, prior to three years after departure from the area. After the three year period, otherwise suitable prospective donors may be accepted if they have remained free of unexplained symptoms suggestive of malaria.
4. Persons that may possess a partial acquired immunity to malaria, such as those that have previously resided in a malarious region for at least five years (immigrants, refugees, citizens, persons who have been or who are residents of endemic countries), should not be accepted as donors of Whole Blood or blood components, including platelets, for a period of three years since their last visit to a malarious region.
5. The following questions should be added to the donor questionnaire:

a) "Were you born in the US?"

If the answer is yes, the donor should be asked,

b) "Have you traveled outside the US in the last three years?"

If so, determine if the area visited was a malarious area that should result in donor deferral.

If the answer to the question "Were you born in the US?" is no, the donor should be asked,

i) "When did you arrive in the US?" and

ii) "Since your arrival, have you traveled outside the US?"

If the answer to the question in "5a" (above) is yes, or if in question "ii" (above) it is determined that the prospective donor has traveled out of the US, follow-up questions should be asked to determine the country or geographical regions that have been visited.

When more than one of the deferral periods apply to a prospective donor, the longest period of deferral must be observed. These recommendations apply only to donations containing intact red blood cells or platelets. Donations used for preparing plasma, plasma components, or derivatives devoid of intact red blood cells or platelets are excluded (6).

A variety of laboratory methods have been developed to establish a diagnosis of malaria. These tests include: (a) microscopic examination of thick and thin blood smears, (b) flow cytometric analysis, (c) immunodiagnostic testing, including enzyme immunoassay methods, (d) fluorescent microscopy, (e) centrifugal diagnosis, and (f) nucleic acid probe methods, including polymerase chain reaction (8,9). Studies have been done in endemic countries to consider how best to screen and test donors (10). Investigation in countries other than the United States has attempted to show that use of additional testing may help recover units from donors being deferred because of travel to endemic areas (11,12). However, at the time of this writing, none of the aforementioned test strategies is being used routinely in the United States for mass screening of blood donors.

When a case of transfusion-transmitted malaria occurs, the patient can be treated with therapy that kills the erythrocytic parasites, because the transfusion-transmitted form of malaria in humans is limited to red blood cells (4). In severe cases, exchange transfusion may be indicated (4,13). The donor responsible for the transfusion-transmitted malaria should be determined, so that the donor can be treated and other recipients traced. There is hope for development of a malaria vaccine (14).

BABESIOSIS

Babesiosis occurs among animals and humans and is caused by several species of intracellular protozoan parasites of the genus *Babesia* (15). The usual mode of transmission of babesiosis is the bite of an infected tick, although transfusion of infected blood also can transmit the infection. Most cases in the United States are acquired in the northeastern states and the midwest (15,16). Several species of *Babesia* can infect humans, *B. microti* causing most infections in the United States. European cases usually have been caused by *B. divergens* (17). In the United States, newly recognized *Babesia* species include MO1-type and WA1-type *Babesia* (15,16).

Symptoms of babesiosis vary widely (17–19). The disease can range from silent infection to a fulminant, malaria-like disease with severe hemolysis and a fatal outcome (17). One report (20) described 139 patients hospitalized with babesiosis in the state of New York. Nine patients (6.5%) died, 35 (25.2%) were admitted to the intensive care unit, and 35 (25.2%) needed hospitalization for more than 14 days. The most common symptoms were fatigue, malaise, weakness, fever, shaking chills, and diaphoresis (20). Severe *B. divergens* infection usually has been characterized by severe intravascular hemolysis with hemoglobinuria. The clinical manifestations of *B. microti* infection vary widely, from asymptomatic infection to a severe, rapidly fatal disease (19). Infection with *B. microti* often remains subclinical or asymptomatic, detected only through serologic testing, the frequency of parasitemia ranging from less than 1% to 85% (19). In general, the most seriously affected patients are those who do not have a spleen, are elderly, have human immunodeficiency virus infection, or are immunosuppressed (18,19).

Babesiosis is the most common tick-borne disease related to transfusion reported in the United States (15). More than 25 cases of babesiosis transmitted by red blood cell transfusion and at least 4 cases attributed to platelet administration have been documented (15,21–25). One case of infection with WA1-type *Babesia* transmitted in a red blood cell transfusion has been reported (15). With the frequent recent reporting of cases of transfusion-transmitted babesiosis, babesiosis may soon surpass malaria as the most commonly reported transfusion-transmitted parasitic infection in the United States.

Few studies have been done to determine the exact risk of transfusion-transmitted babesiosis. Seroprevalence among blood donors has been investigated (24). One study in which blood donors from endemic areas were compared with those from non-endemic areas showed that a significantly larger number of seropositive donors came from endemic areas. Of the seropositive donors who underwent subsequent polymerase chain reaction testing, 4 of 19 (21%) had positive results, suggesting they may be at risk of transmitting *B. microti* (24). Risk also was assessed in an endemic area in an investigation involving 155 transfusion recipients; 149 received 601 total units of packed red blood cells, and 48 received 371 total units of platelets (25).

Because infection with *Babesia* is intraerythrocytic, red blood cells and platelets, which can contain some red blood cells, are the components most likely to contain these parasites (15). *Babesia microti* organisms remain viable in blood stored at room temperature for 3 days (26) and in refrigerated blood for at least 17 to 21 days (15,22,26). At least one case of babesiosis has occurred after transfusion of refrigerated blood that was stored for 35 days (15). Babesiosis has been reported to occur after transfusion of frozen-thawed blood. (27).

As with malaria, persons with asymptomatic babesiosis may arrive to donate blood. Current blood safety control measures call for indefinite deferral of those with a history of babesiosis because of the possibility of ongoing asymptomatic parasitemia (7,18,28). Prospective donors currently are not deferred because of residence in an endemic area or if they report a recent tick bite. This approach can be supported by the observation that seropositive donors with antibodies to tick-borne pathogens reportedly are no more likely to remember tick bites than are those who are seronegative, nor is someone who remembers a tick bite at greater risk of infection than is someone who does not remember a bite (15,18). Although there is risk of transfusion transmission of babesiosis, this risk must be balanced with the effect of stricter donor criteria on the availability of blood (15). Deferring donors because they have lived in an endemic area or have had a recent tick bite would exclude a large number of healthy donors. Therefore changes in current donor questioning would not likely be useful (15). There also is no test in routine use for mass blood donor screening of carriers of asymptomatic *B. microti* infection. The development of such a test could be useful, especially in some regions of the United States (15). On the other hand, if an infected donor or recipient is identified, retrieval of involved blood components should be initiated immediately (18). Donors should be encouraged to provide postdonation information to the blood collection center if symptoms suggestive of babesiosis are encountered (15).

Persons with babesiosis can be treated with quinine and clindamycin (18,29), which typically shorten the illness. However, infection can persist, and recrudescence and side effects have been commonly reported (28). Atovaquone and azithromycin have been shown as effective as clindamycin and quinine with fewer adverse reactions (30). In cases of severe babesiosis, red blood cell or whole-blood exchange transfusion in combination with appropriate antimicrobial therapy is beneficial (16,31–33).

TRYPANOSOMAL INFECTION

Trypanosoma cruzi is the protozoan hemoflagellate that causes Chagas disease, which is endemic in parts of South America, Central America, and Mexico but is extremely rare in the United States. Chagas disease is a major public health problem in endemic countries, where an estimated 16 to 18 million persons are infected (34–36). The usual mode of disease transmission is contact with triatomid (reduviid) bugs that have *T. cruzi* infection of the digestive system. The parasite can be transmitted to human or other mammalian hosts after a bug bite and blood meal, soon after which the bug excretes feces containing *T. cruzi.* The parasite can pass from the feces directly through the site of the bite or be transferred to a mucous membrane when the host scratches or rubs the bite and then touches the eyes or mouth with the infected feces (36). The natural habitat of triatomid bugs is woodlands; however, the bugs can come in close contact with humans who live in houses constructed with thatched roofs, mud walls, stick walls, and tiled roofs.

Vigorous efforts, through the Southern Cone Initiative (http://www.who.int/ctd/chagas/epidemio.htm), are underway to eliminate the chief regional vector of Chagas disease to interrupt disease transmission in some endemic countries (35). It remains a possibility, however, that in areas endemic for *T. cruzi,* donors may have parasitemia with *T. cruzi* at the time of blood collection, so transfusion of most blood components except plasma derivatives carries risk of disease transmission (36). Transfusion is the second most common mechanism of spread of *T. cruzi* disease in Latin America (34,37). In the United States, the emigration of persons with *T. cruzi* infection from Mexico, Central America, and South America has increased the risk of blood donation by persons who have no symptoms but may have parasitemia (36,38). Other modes of infection, such as congenital transmission (39) and infection after transplantation, including kidney (40) and bone marrow (41) transplantation, have been described. There is also a concern regarding Chagas disease as a complication of hematopoietic progenitor stem cell therapy (42). Bugs and mammals infected with *T. cruzi* have been found in some regions of the United States, but only a small number of cases of Chagas disease (autochthonous transmission) have been attributed to this vector contact (43,44).

More than 90% of cases of acute Chagas disease are mild and self-limiting, although in rare situations acute Chagas disease can cause serious morbidity, including cardiac complications (myocarditis, congestive heart failure), meningoencephalitis, and death (36). Infection with *T. cruzi* can be a severe problem among immunosuppressed patients (45). Acute cases can progress to chronic asymptomatic infection. After years to decades of chronic infection, Chagas disease causes serious sequelae in 20% to 30% of persons, including cardiac arrhythmia, cardiomegaly, cardiac failure, megaesophagus, or megacolon (35,36). In one study of patients undergoing cardiac surgery in the United States who received more than one transfusion (46), 6 postoperative patients (0.05%) had confirmed positive results for *T. cruzi* at serologic testing or histologic examination of excised heart tissue or both. The investigators stated that although several of the 6 patients had histories and clinical findings suggestive of Chagas disease, none of the cases was diagnosed and no patient underwent tests for *T. cruzi* before the discovery of the infection at surgery. Five of the patients with infection were Hispanic, and overall, 2.7% of the Hispanic patients in the study had positive results. No evidence in this study linked *T. cruzi* infection with transfusion. Because the diagnosis of Chagas disease was not known or even considered for any of these patients, there is concern that Chagas disease is an underdiagnosed cause of cardiac disease in the United States, particularly among patients born in countries endemic for *T. cruzi* (46).

Chagas disease has been gaining attention in the United States because *T. cruzi* infection has been transmitted in the United States and in Canada after blood transfusions (47–51). In a study of ten Central and South American countries conducted with data collected in 1993, the probability of administering a unit infected with *T. cruzi* was determined to be 219/10,000 in Bolivia, 24/10,000 in Colombia, 17/10,000 in El Salvador, and approximately 2 to 12/10,000 in the other countries. The assumed infectivity risk of *T. cruzi,* that is, the likelihood of contracting infection when receiving an infected unit, was 20% (37). In the United States, information from look-back investigations does not reflect a similar level of infectivity (39,52). In a case of transfusion transmission of *T. cruzi* reported in 1999 (51), a platelet recipient received a unit that was subsequently confirmed to contain *T. cruzi* antibodies. The risk in some endemic areas is decreasing. Screening procedures in Venezuela appear to have been effective in decreasing the risk of disease transmission through transfusion (53).

Infection with *T. cruzi* can be transmitted by means of transfusion because the parasite is viable for at least 18 to 21 days in refrigerated blood and may survive cryopreservation and thawing (36). However, in most transfusion-associated cases of *T. cruzi* infection reported in the United States and Canada, platelets were the implicated component (54). Therefore platelets appear to be the most likely blood component to transmit *T. cruzi* infection in the United States (54).

The risk of collecting a donor unit infected with *T. cruzi* is highest in areas of the United States where the greatest numbers of Latin American immigrants have settled (34,36,38,44, 55–57). Data indicate the distribution of *T. cruzi*–seropositive donors varies within the United States from none to nearly 200 per 100,000 donors (39,44,52,55–58). Results of polymerase chain reaction studies indicated that more than one half of *T. cruzi*–seropositive donors who underwent testing (10 of 16 donors) had evidence of parasitemia (59). Although the likelihood of collecting blood from a *T. cruzi*–seropositive donor appears regionally dependent, a unit infected with *T. cruzi* could be distributed to an area where the collection of seropositive blood would be unlikely to occur, because blood components are frequently shipped between geographic regions of the United States.

At present, a history of Chagas disease is cause for indefinite deferral of a prospective donor (7). Establishing further donor history criteria on which to base deferral decisions, such as a history of birth, extended stay, or transfusion in an endemic area, has been investigated. Questions regarding these factors have been shown effective in determining whether a prospective donor has serologic evidence of *T. cruzi* infection or has parasitemia (52,57,58). Although they may help determine whether someone is at high risk of infection, questions before donation may not be as sensitive as other policies, such as serologic testing, in the prevention of transfusion-transmitted Chagas disease (54). Some *T. cruzi*–seropositive donations can be missed if a questionnaire regarding risk factors for *T. cruzi* infection is the only screening tool used (52). There also is concern that an excessive number of healthy persons would be unnecessarily deferred (54).

A policy to test donors for evidence of *T. cruzi* infection is not currently used in the United States, because there is no available FDA-approved serologic test for screening blood donors. A confirmatory test also would be necessary (60). Once a *T. cruzi* screening test is approved and in use, an important advantage would be identification of donors who do not admit or realize that they have a risk factor (39).

Leukoreduced blood products for all transfusions is another potential means to reduce transmission of *T. cruzi.* Results of a study by Moraes-Souza et al. (61) suggested that leukoreduction filters are effective in decreasing the number of parasites in blood artificially spiked with low concentrations of *T. cruzi.* It is not known, however, whether leukoreduction by means of a nonfiltration method effectively decreases the number of *T. cruzi* parasites in plateletpheresis units or reduces the risk of transmission of *T. cruzi.* organisms. Plateletpheresis units are more likely to be leukoreduced by means of differential centrifugation than by leukocyte filtration. Whether the risk of transfusion-transmitted Chagas disease is reduced with routine use of leukoreduced blood components, regardless of the method of leukoreduction, is not known and requires further study (54).

TRANSFUSION-TRANSMITTED LEISHMANIASIS

Many species of *Leishmania* can cause disease (leishmaniasis) in humans. The usual mode of disease transmission is the bite of infected sandflies (62). Several clinical forms of leishmaniasis exist, including visceral (also known as *kala azar*), cutaneous, and mucosal (63). If infection is clinically evident but the person is not treated, cutaneous leishmaniasis can cause chronic skin sores, mucosal leishmaniasis can lead to facial disfigurement, and visceral leishmaniasis can be a life-threatening systemic infection (63). Kala azar is the most severe manifestation of leishmanial infection; however, leishmanial infection can manifest as an asymptomatic syndrome, an acute febrile illness, or a prolonged, nonspecific systemic illness that does not progress to kala azar (64). Visceral leishmaniasis is characterized by fever, hepatosplenomegaly, weight loss, and emaciation and can be deadly if the person is not treated (62). It has also become an acquired immunodeficiency syndrome (AIDS)–associated opportunistic infection (63). Kala azar was nearly eradicated but has reemerged with an annual worldwide estimated incidence of 0.5 million cases and a prevalence of 2.5 million cases; 90% of the confirmed cases were found in India, Nepal, Bangladesh, and Sudan (65). Visceral leishmaniasis was thought to be all but absent from the United States but has recently been discovered in hunting dogs in 21 states in the United States and in Ontario, Canada (66).

The *Leishmania* parasite is found in reticuloendothelial cells and leukocytes (38). Because the parasite infects leukocytes, the disease can be transmitted to recipients of blood transfusions. A few cases of transfusion-transmitted disease have been reported in the literature, affecting mainly newborns and immunosuppressed patients (38,67–69). Transfusion-transmitted leishmaniasis has never been reported in the United States.

A concern about the safety of the U.S. blood supply and leishmaniasis arose in the 1990s during the Persian Gulf conflict. In November 1991, the U.S. Department of Defense recommended that persons participating in Operation Desert Storm be deferred as blood donors after leishmaniasis was diagnosed among some members of the armed forces (64,70). A study of the survivability and infectivity of *Leishmania* in human blood donors (64) conducted soon thereafter supported the concern of the Department of Defense. The investigators concluded that the parasite can survive 30 days in refrigerated whole blood, 25 days in refrigerated red blood cells, at least 5 days in platelet concentrates at 24°C, and at least 35 days in frozen red blood cells at −70°C. All results of fresh-frozen plasma cultures were negative. Infected blood administered to mice was infective to most of the animal recipients (64).

Two years after initiating its deferral policy, the Department of Defense in December 1993 stopped asking leishmaniasis-related questions of blood donors. The rare number of cases of infection identified and follow-up screening that showed an extremely small number of donors with symptoms of possible leishmaniasis led to the change (71). Although leishmaniasis did not pose a significant threat to blood safety in the United States, this episode draws attention to our need to be constantly vigilant for diseases that could affect our blood supply. The concern about transfusion-transmitted leishmaniasis continues in endemic areas, where studies have been conducted to investigate the occurrence of asymptomatic infection among blood donors (69,72,73).

As of the August 2000 edition of the *Circular of Information for the Use of Human Blood and Blood Components* (74), there were no routinely available tests to predict or prevent disease transmission of *Leishmania* oragnisms. However, stringent screening procedures are in place to reduce to a minimum the risk of transmitting infectious agents. The use of leukoreduced blood products has been suggested as a means to prevent the transmission of leishmaniasis through blood transfusion (72).

TOXOPLASMOSIS

The ubiquitous *Toxoplasma gondii* is an obligate intracellular protozoan parasite that causes toxoplasmosis (38). The usual mode of transmission is zoonotic, and members of the cat family are the definitive host (38). A human can be infected with *T. gondii* in the following ways: (a) accidental ingestion of *T. gondii* oocysts after handling infected cat feces in cat litter or soil; (b) eating undercooked infected meat (pork, goat, lamb, or beef) (75,76); (c) direct contamination through contact with open wounds; (d) blood transfusion (the parasite can infect white blood cells present in cellular blood products (77); (e) organ transplantation; and (f) congenital transmission from infected mother to child (38,76). Most *T. gondii* infections probably go unnoticed clinically. *Toxoplasma gondii* is a rare cause of mononucleosis (78,79) and occasionally causes lymphadenopathy, malaise, fever, headache, and sore throat (38). Splenomegaly, hepatomegaly (78), and rash (38) may be present. Although healthy persons usually have a relatively mild disease course, immunosuppressed patients, including those with AIDS and recipients of organ, bone marrow, or hematopoietic stem cell transplants, may experience serious disease that includes encephalitis, chorioretinitis, myocarditis, and pneumonitis (38,80–82).

Although the organism can be recovered from blood donors who do not have symptoms or from persons with infection for 14 months to 4 years after the onset of infection (83) and can survive for as long as 50 days at 4°C in citrated whole blood (84,85), reported cases of transfusion-transmitted *T. gondii* infection are rare. Such cases have occurred among patients with acute leukemia receiving chemotherapy and leukocyte transfusions—from donors with chronic myelogenous leukemia (86), who would not meet current acceptance criteria for allogenic donors (7)—and in one case, a platelet transfusion (87). Most cases of toxoplasmosis have been attributed to reactivation of latent infection after bone marrow and hematopoietic stem cell transplantation, because many recipients had positive serologic results before the procedure (88). Among several recipients of cardiac transplants, however, disease transmission was attributed to the donor organ (80).

Because of the low risk, there is no reason to perform serologic testing of donors to determine whether they are carriers of asymptomatic *T. gondii* infection (38). Use of leukoreduced blood may be considered when immunosuppressed patients undergo transfusion because these patients are at greater risk of symptomatic transfusion-transmitted toxoplasmosis (38).

MICROFILARIASIS

Eight filarial worms can affect the lymphatic, subcutaneous, or cutaneous tissue of humans: *Wuchereria bancrofti,* which is widely distributed in tropical and subtropical areas; *Brugia malayi,* found in Asia and the Indian subcontinent; *Onchocerca volvulus,* in Central Africa, Latin American, and the Middle East; *Loa Loa* and *Mansonella streptocerca,* found in Africa; *Mansonella perstans,* in tropical Africa and South America; *Mansonella ozzardi,* which is restricted to the western hemisphere; and *Brugia timori,* limited to some Indonesian islands (89). These worms share the characteristic that the adult female worm produces a microfilaria, a primitive larva (89). Except for those of *O. volvulus* and *M. streptocerca,* which usually are found in the skin, the microfilariae of most of the species circulate in the peripheral blood (89). This creates the possibility of transfusion-transmitted infection. Microfilariae that circulate in the bloodstream have been observed to be transmitted in blood, except for *B. timori* (83).

The microfilariae of *W. bancrofti* have been reported to survive in blood stored at 4°C to 6°C for at least 12 days. When blood was examined 21 days after collection, the microfilariae were inactive on wet smear but were revived when the slide was warmed to 37°C (90). In a study of *Loa Loa,* the concentration of microfilariae in banked blood steadily decreased to 66% of the initial concentration during the first 18 days of storage. Counts decreased sharply thereafter. Filtration of stored blood removed a large proportion of *Loa Loa* microfilariae (91).

Serious infection of humans can be caused by filarial worms, including lymphatic filariasis (elephantiasis), typically caused by *W. bancrofti,* but 10% of cases are caused by *B. malayi* and *B. timori* (92). The disease is endemic in 73 countries, yet the World Health Organization is hopeful that because of available and effective treatment and diagnostic tools, this disease can be eliminated as a global public health problem by 2020 (92).

Filarial infection is transmitted by arthropod vectors. Of clinical importance is that transfusion of microfilariae in blood does not transmit filariasis (90). Transfusion-acquired microfilaremia is self-limited because transfused microfilariae do not develop into adult filarial worms (85). Microfilaria develop to the infective stage only in the arthropod vector and then must be passed back to a person for an adult worm to develop (85,89).

There have been isolated reports of transfusion of blood containing microfilariae to humans (85), but none of the reports is recent. In one report, microfilariae of *W. bancrofti* transfused into a healthy person survived 14 days. In other transfusion experiments with human subjects, however, there usually has been an immediate disappearance of most of the transfused microfilariae, without any evidence of anaphylaxis (85). In another study, Gönnert injected himself with blood containing microfilariae of both *Loa Loa* and *M. perstans; Loa Loa* disappeared by the fourth day, but *M. perstans* persisted for 3 years (85). Transfusion experiments with human subjects have shown that *M. ozzardi* microfilariae can persist for more than 2 years (93).

Acute inflammatory reactions to destroyed microfilariae that often occur in true filarial infection have not been seen in transfusion recipients (85), although there is a concern that allergic reactions to breakdown products of the dead microfilariae can occur (94). Fever, headache, and rash have occurred among persons intentionally given transfusions of blood containing microfilariae, but these reactions may have been caused by other factors (85). Only one blood donor in the United States has been found to have microfilaremia (in this case, with *M. ozzardi*); however, transfusion-transmitted microfilariasis has not been proved to occur in any of the recipients of that donor's blood (93). Because the clinical consequences of transfusion of microfilariae appear limited, routine testing of donors does not appear warranted. It seems prudent, however, not to transfuse blood known to contain microfilariae because an allergic reaction is a theoretic possibility (85).

SUMMARY

Transfusion-transmitted parasitic infections will continue to occur at a very low rate in the United States because donor screening and testing methods are less than 100% effective in stopping all persons with parasitemia from donating blood. As demographic characteristics change, an increased incidence of parasitic infection in the United States may increase the number of cases of posttransfusion parasitic infection. The organisms that pose an increasing threat to the U.S. blood supply are *B. microti* and *T. cruzi.* It is anticipated that serologic tests will become available for testing donors for evidence of possible infection with *T. cruzi* or *B. microti.* This testing may become routine on a national, regional, or local level.

REFERENCES

1. Malaria surveillance—United States, 1995. *MMWR Morb Mortal Wkly Rep* 1999;48(SS-1):1–21.
2. Transfusion-transmitted malaria—Missouri and Pennsylvania, 1996–1998. *MMWR Morb Mortal Wkly Rep* 1999;48:253–256.
3. Croft A. Malaria: prevention in travellers. *BMJ* 2000;321:154–160.
4. Turc JM. Malaria and blood transfusion. In: Westphal RG, Carlson KB, Turc JM, eds. *Emerging global patterns in transfusion-transmitted infections.* Arlington, VA: American Association of Blood Banks, 1990.
5. Zoon K. Recommendations for deferral of donors for malaria risk: memorandum to all registered blood establishments. Washington, DC: Department of Health and Human Services, Food and Drug Administration, July 26, 1994.
6. Guidance for industry: recommendations for donor questioning regarding possible exposure to malaria. *Federal Register* 2000;65: 36452–36453.

7. Gorlin JB, ed. *Standards for blood banks and transfusion services,* 20th ed. Bethesda, MD: American Association of Blood Banks, 2000.
8. Makler MT, Gibbins B. Laboratory diagnosis of malaria. *Clin Lab Med* 1991;11:941–956.
9. Makler MT, Palmer CJ, Ager AL. A review of practical techniques for the diagnosis of malaria. *Ann Trop Med Parasitol* 1998;92:419–433.
10. Contreras CE, Pance A, Marcano N, et al. Detection of specific antibodies to *Plasmodium falciparum* in blood bank donors from malaria-endemic and non-endemic areas of Venezuela. *Am J Trop Med Hyg* 1999;60:948–953.
11. Davidson N, Woodfield G, Henry S. Malarial antibodies in Auckland blood donors. *N Z Med J* 1999;112:181–183.
12. Chiodini PL, Hartley S, Hewitt PE, et al. Evaluation of a malaria antibody ELISA and its value in reducing potential wastage of red cell donations from blood donors exposed to malaria, with a note on a case of transfusion-transmitted malaria. *Vox Sang* 1997;73:143–148.
13. Tejura B, Sass DA, Fischer RA, et al. Transfusion-associated falciparum malaria successfully treated with red blood cell exchange transfusion. *Am J Med Sci* 2000;320:337–341.
14. Plebanski M, Hill AV. The immunology of malaria infection. *Curr Opin Immunol* 2000;12:437–441.
15. McQuiston JH, Childs JE, Chamberland ME, et al. Transmission of tick-borne agents of disease by blood transfusion: a review of known and potential risks in the United States. *Transfusion* 2000;40:274–284.
16. Herwaldt BL, Springs FE, Roberts PP, et al. Babesiosis in Wisconsin: a potentially fatal disease. *Am J Trop Med Hyg* 1995;53:146–151.
17. Homer MJ, Aguilar-Delfin I, Telford SR 3rd, et al. Babesiosis. *Clin Microbiol Rev* 2000;13:451–469.
18. Popovsky MA. Transfusion-transmitted babesiosis. *Transfusion* 1991; 31:296–297.
19. Gorenflot A, Moubri K, Precigout E, et al. Human babesiosis. *Ann Trop Med Parasitol* 1998;92:489–501.
20. White DJ, Talarico J, Chang HG, et al. Human babesiosis in New York State: review of 139 hospitalized cases and analysis of prognostic factors. *Arch Intern Med* 1998;158:2149–2154.
21. Gorlin JB, Jensen KA, Perry EH, et al. Transmission of *Babesia microti* through multiple donations from the same blood donor. *Transfusion* 2000;40[Suppl).:42S(abst).
22. Linden JV, Kolakoski MH, Wong SJ, et al. Transfusion-associated babesiosis in two recipients. *Transfusion* 2000;40[Suppl).:96S(abst).
23. Linden JV, Kolakoski MH, Wong SJ, et al. Transfusion-associated babesiosis in an elderly patient. *Transfusion* 2000;40[Suppl).:96S(abst).
24. Leiby DA, Chung AP, Triano LR, et al. Serologic and nucleic acid evidence for *Babesia microti* in Connecticut blood donors. *Transfusion* 2000;40[Suppl).:2S(abst).
25. Gerber MA, Shapiro ED, Krause PJ, et al. The risk of acquiring Lyme disease or babesiosis from a blood transfusion. *J Infect Dis* 1994;170: 231–234.
26. Eberhard ML, Walker EM, Steurer FJ. Survival and infectivity of Babesia in blood maintained at 25C and 2-4C. *J Parasitol* 1995;81: 790–792.
27. Grabowski EF, Giardina PJV, Goldbery D, et al. Babesiosis transmitted by a transfusion of frozen-thawed blood. *Ann Intern Med* 1982;96: 466–467.
28. Krause PJ, Spielman A, Telford SR 3rd,et al. Persistent parasitemia after acute babesiosis. *N Engl J Med* 1998;339:160–165.
29. Clindamycin and quinine treatment for *Babesia microti* infections. *MMWR Morb Mortal Wkly Rep* 1983;32:65–66,72.
30. Krause PJ, Lepore T, Sikand VK, et al. Atovaquone and azithromycin for the treatment of babesiosis. *N Engl J Med* 2000;343:1454–1458.
31. Jacoby GA, Hunt JV, Kosinski KS, et al. Treatment of transfusion-transmitted babesiosis by exchange transfusion. *N Engl J Med* 1980; 303:1098–1100.
32. Dorman SE, Cannon ME, Telford SR 3rd, et al. Fulminant babesiosis treated with clindamycin, quinine, and whole-blood exchange transfusion. *Transfusion* 2000;40:375–380.
33. Machtinger L, Telford SR 3d, Inducil C, et al. Treatment of babesiosis by red blood cell exchange in an HIV-positive, splenectomized patient. *J Clin Apheresis* 1993;8:78–81.
34. Schmunis GA. *Trypanosoma cruzi,* the etiologic agent of Chagas' disease: status in the blood supply in endemic and nonendemic countries. *Transfusion* 1991;31:547–557.
35. Annex A: fact sheets for candidate diseases for elimination or eradication. *MMWR Morb Mortal Wkly Rep* 1999;48:154–203.
36. Gudino MD, Linares J. Chagas' disease and blood transfusion. In: Westphal RG, Carlson KB, Turc JM, eds. *Emerging global patterns in transfusion-transmitted infections.* Arlington, VA: American Association of Blood Banks, 1990.
37. Schmunis GA. Prevention of transfusional *Trypanosoma cruzi* infection in Latin America. *Mem Inst Oswaldo Cruz* 1999;94[Suppl 1).:93–101.
38. Wendel S. Current concepts on transmission of bacteria and parasites by blood components. *Vox Sang* 1994;67[Suppl 3).:161–174.
39. Leiby DA, Fucci MH, Stumpf RJ. *Trypanosoma cruzi* in a low to moderate risk blood donor population: seroprevalence and possible congenital transmission. *Transfusion* 1999;39:310–315.
40. Ferraz AS, Figueiredo JF. Transmission of Chagas' disease through transplanted kidney: occurrence of the acute form of the disease in two recipients from the same donor. *Rev Inst Med Trop Sao Paulo* 1993; 35:461–463.
41. Altclas J, Jaimovich G, Milovic V, et al. Chagas' disease after bone marrow transplantation. *Bone Marrow Transplant* 1996;18:447–448.
42. Guidelines for preventing opportunistic infections among hematopoietic stem cell transplant recipients: recommendations of CDC, the Infectious Disease Society of America, and the American Society of Blood and Marrow Transplantation. *MMWR Morb Mortal Wkly Rep* 2000;49:1–125.
43. Navin TR, Roberto RR, Juranek DD, et al. Human and sylvatic *Trypanosoma cruzi* infection in California. *Am J Public Health* 1985;75: 366–369.
44. Barrett VJ, Leiby DA, Odom JL, et al. Negligible prevalence of antibodies against Trypanosoma cruzi among blood donors in the southeastern United States. *Am J Clin Pathol* 1997;108:499–503.
45. Kirchhoff LV. Chagas disease: American trypanosomiasis. *Infect Dis Clin North Am* 1993;7:487–502.
46. Leiby DA, Rentas FJ, Nelson KE, et al. Evidence of *Trypanosoma cruzi* infection (Chagas' disease) among patients undergoing cardiac surgery. *Circulation* 2000;102:2978–2982.
47. Geiseler PJ, Ito JI, Tegtmeier BR, et al. Fulminant Chagas disease (CD) in bone marrow transplantation (BMT). In: *Abstracts of the 1987 Interscience Conference on Antimicrobial Agents and Chemotherapy.* 1987; 169(abst).
48. Grant IH, Gold JWM, Wittner M, et al. Transfusion–associated acute Chagas disease acquired in the United States. *Ann Intern Med* 1989; 111:849–851.
49. Cimo PL, Luper WE, Scouros MA. Transfusion-associated Chagas' disease in Texas: report of a case. *Texas Med* 1993;89:48–50.
50. Nickerson P, Orr P, Schroeder M, Sekla L, et al. Transfusion-associated *Trypanosoma cruzi* infection in a non-endemic area. *Ann Intern Med* 1989;111:851–853.
51. Leiby DA, Lenes BA, Tibbals MA, et al. Prospective evaluation of a patient with *Trypanosoma cruzi* infection transmitted by transfusion. *N Engl J Med* 1999;341:1237–1239.
52. Leiby DA, Read EJ, Lenes BA, et al. Seroepidemiology of *Trypanosoma cruzi,* etiologic agent of Chagas' disease, in US blood donors. *J Infect Dis* 1997;176:1047–1052.
53. Schmunis GA, Zicker F, Segura EL, et al. Transfusion-transmitted infectious diseases in Argentina, 1995 through 1997. *Transfusion* 2000; 40:1048–1053.
54. Shulman IA. Intervention strategies to reduce the risk of transfusion-transmitted *Trypanosoma cruzi* infection in the United States. *Transfus Med Rev* 1999;13:227–234.
55. Kerndt P, Waskin HA, Kirchhoff LV, et al. Prevalence of antibody to *Trypanosoma cruzi* among blood donors in Los Angeles, California. *Transfusion* 1991;31:814–818.
56. Brashear RJ, Winkler MA, Schur JD, et al. Detection of antibodies to *Trypanosoma cruzi* among blood donors in the southwestern and western United States, I: evaluation of the sensitivity and specificity of an enzyme immunoassay for detecting antibodies to *T. cruzi. Transfusion* 1995;35:213–218.
57. Shulman IA, Appleman MD, Saxena S, et al. Specific antibodies to

Trypanosoma cruzi among blood donors in Los Angeles, California. *Transfusion* 1997;37:727–731.
58. Appleman MD, Shulman IA, Saxena S, et al. Use of a questionnaire to identify potential blood donors at risk for infection with *Trypanosoma cruzi. Transfusion* 1993;33:61–64.
59. Tibbals MA, Leiby DA, Herwaldt BL, et al. Evidence of circulating parasites in *Trypanosoma cruzi* seropositive blood donors. *Transfusion* 1998;38:103S.
60. Leiby DA, Wendel S, Takaoka DT, et al. Serologic testing for *Trypanosoma cruzi:* comparison of radioimmunoprecipitation assay with commercially available indirect immunofluorescence assay, indirect hemagglutination assay, and enzyme-linked immunosorbent assay kits. *J Clin Microbiol* 2000;38:639–642.
61. Moraes-Souza H, Bordin JO, Bardossy L et al. Prevention of transfusion-associated Chagas disease: efficacy of white cell-reduction filters in removing *Trypanosoma cruzi* from infected blood. *Transfusion* 1995; 35:723–726.
62. Tropical Disease Research: progress 1995–96. In: *Thirteenth Programme Report of the UNDP/World Bank/WHO Special Programme for Research & Training in Tropical Diseases.* Available at: http://www.who.int/tdr/publications/publications/PR13.htm.
63. Herwaldt BL. Leishmaniasis. *Lancet* 1999;354:1191–1199.
64. Grogl M, Daugirda JL, Hoover DL, et al. Survivability and infectivity of viscerotropic *Leishmania tropica* from Operation Desert Storm participants in human blood products maintained under blood bank conditions. *Am J Trop Med Hyg* 1993;49:308–315.
65. Bora D. Epidemiology of visceral leishmaniasis in India. *Natl Med J India* 1999;12:62–68.
66. Enserink M. Has leishmaniasis become endemic in the U.S.? *Science* 2000;290:1881–1882.
67. Cohen C, Corazza F, De Mol P, et al. Leishmaniasis acquired in Belgium. *Lancet* 1991;338:128.
68. Cummins D, Amin S, Halil O, et al. Visceral leishmaniasis after cardiac surgery. *Arch Dis Child* 1995;72:235–236.
69. Otero AC, da Silva VO, Luz KG, et al. Short report: occurrence of *Leishmania donovani* DNA in donated blood from seroreactive Brazilian blood donors. *Am J Trop Med Hyg* 2000;62:128–131.
70. Viscerotropic leishmaniasis in persons returning from Operation Desert Storm: 1990–1991. *MMWR Morb Mortal Wkly Rep* 1992;41: 131–134.
71. Rutherford BD. In: Proceedings of the Department of Health and Human Services, Public Health Service, Food and Drug Administration, Transmissible Spongiform Encephalopathies Advisory Committee meeting June 2, 1999, Gaithersburg, Maryland. Available at: http://www.fda.gov/ohrms/dockets/ac/99/transcpt/3518t1.rtf.
72. le Fichoux Y, Quaranta JF, Aufeuvre JP, et al. Occurrence of *Leishmania infantum* parasitemia in asymptomatic blood donors living in an area of endemicity in southern France. *J Clin Microbiol* 1999;37:1953–1957.
73. Luz KG, da Silva VO, Gomes EM, et al. Prevalence of anti–*Leishmania donovani* antibody among Brazilian blood donors and multiply transfused hemodialysis patients. *Am J Trop Med Hyg* 1997;57:168–171.
74. Circular of information for the use of human blood and blood components. Bethesda, MD: American Association of Blood Banks, America's Blood Centers, and the American Red Cross, 2000. Available at: http://www. aabb. org/all about blood/coi/coiv2.pdf..
75. Cook AJ, Gilbert RE, Buffolano W, et al. Sources of toxoplasma infection in pregnant women: European multicentre case-control study. European Research Network on Congenital Toxoplasmosis. *BMJ* 2000; 321:142–147.
76. Tenter AM, Heckeroth AR, Weiss LM. *Toxoplasma gondii:* from animals to humans. *Int J Parasitol* 2000;30:1217–1258.
77. Channon JY, Seguin RM, Kasper LH. Differential infectivity and division of *Toxoplasma gondii* in human peripheral blood leukocytes. *Infect Immun* 2000;68:4822–4826.
78. Kanegane H, Shintani N, Miyamori C, et al. Peripheral blood lymphocyte subpopulations in three infants with hepatosplenomegaly caused by cytomegalovirus infection. *Acta Paediatr Jpn* 1995;37:370–373.
79. Evans AS. Infectious mononucleosis and related syndromes. *Am J Med Sci* 1978;276:325–339.
80. Michaels MG, Wald ER, Fricker FJ, et al. Toxoplasmosis in pediatric recipients of heart transplants. *Clin Infect Dis* 1992;14:847–851.
81. Saad R, Vincent JF, Cimon B, et al. Pulmonary toxoplasmosis after allogeneic bone marrow transplantation: case report and review. *Bone Marrow Transplant* 1996;18:211–212.
82. Rose I. Morphology and diagnostics of human toxoplasmosis. *Gen Diagn Pathol* 1997;142:257–270.
83. Tabor E. *Infectious complications of blood transfusion.* New York: Academic Press, 1982.
84. Raisanen S. Toxoplasmosis transmitted by blood transfusions. *Transfusion* 1978;18:329–332.
85. Wolfe MS. Parasites, other than malaria, transmissible by blood transfusion. In: Greenwalt TJ, Jamieson GA, eds. *Transmissible disease and blood transfusion.* New York: Grune & Stratton, 1975:267–277.
86. Siegel SE, Lunde MN, Gelderman AH, et al. Transmission of toxoplasmosis by leukocyte transfusion. *Blood* 1971;37:388–394.
87. Nelson JC, Kauffmann JH, Ciavarella D, et al. Acquired toxoplasmic retinochoroiditis after platelet transfusions. *Ann Ophthalmol* 1989;21: 253–254.
88. Martino R, Maertens J, Bretagne S, et al. Toxoplasmosis after hematopoietic stem cell transplantation. *Clin Infect Dis* 2000;31:1188–1195.
89. Orihel TC, Ash LR. Tissue helminths. In: Murray PM, ed. *Manual of clinical microbiology,* 6th ed. Washington DC: ASM Press, 1995.
90. Bird GWG, Menon KK. Survival of *Microfilaria bancrofti* in stored blood. *Lancet* 1961:2;721.
91. AuBuchon JP, Dzik WH. Survival of Loa loa in banked blood. *Lancet* 1983;1:647–648.
92. Candidate parasitic diseases. *MMWR Morb Mortal Wkly Rep* 1999;48: 80–85.
93. Weller PF, Simon HB, Parkhurst BH, et al. Tourism-acquired *Mansonella ozzardi* microfilaremia in a regular blood donor. *JAMA* 1978; 240:858–859.
94. Hira PR, Husein SF. Some transfusion-induced parasitic infections in Zambia. *J Hyg Epidemiol Microbiol Immunol* 1979;23:436–444.

Rossi's Principles of Transfusion Medicine, Third Edition, edited by Toby L. Simon, Walter H. Dzik, Edward L. Snyder, Christopher P. Stowell, and Ronald G. Strauss. Lippincott Williams & Wilkins, Philadelphia © 2002.

CASE 53A

FEVER AFTER BLOOD TRANSFUSION

CASE HISTORY

An 85-year-old man was admitted to the hospital because of acute gastrointestinal bleeding. He received a transfusion of 5 units of red blood cells. He was discharged only to be readmitted soon thereafter because of another episode of acute gastrointestinal bleeding and a fever to 104°F (40.0°C). The peripheral blood smear contained intraerythrocytic parasites resembling those in Figure 53A.1. The patient was treated with oral quinine and doxycycline; however, his mental status deteriorated the next day and treatment was changed to intravenous quinidine gluconate and doxycycline. A computed tomographic scan showed evidence of a cerebral vascular accident. The patient died 18 days after the second admission (1,2).

DISCUSSION

Figure 53A.1 shows *Plasmodium falciparum* rings. The microscopic diagnosis in this case is malaria. One or more of four species of *Plasmodium* (*P. falciparum, P. vivax, P. ovale,* and *P. malariae*) causes malaria among humans. Signs and symptoms of malaria can be vague, although most patients have fever (1). Other symptoms include headache, back pain, myalgia, chills, increased sweating, nausea, vomiting, diarrhea, and cough (1). Malaria should be considered in the differential diagnosis of fever of unknown origin. A comprehensive travel history should be obtained, although a diagnosis of malaria should be considered regardless of travel history (1).

As in this case, treatment should be started immediately after the diagnosis is confirmed with a positive result of a blood smear. Malaria not caused by *Falciparum* rarely causes complications; however, patients with *P. falciparum* infection are at risk of coma, renal failure, pulmonary edema, and death (1).

The source of malaria in this case must be ascertained. All cases of malaria in the United States are thoroughly investigated by state or local health departments and the Centers for Disease Control and Prevention (CDC) (1,3). Most cases of malaria in the United States have been imported from malaria-endemic regions throughout the world. In rare instances, local mosquito-borne transmission is identified in the United States. Every year congenital infections and those from blood exposure (induced malaria, that is, malaria acquired through artificial means such as blood transfusion or use of shared syringes) also are reported (1). This was one of two cases of induced malaria reported in the United States in 1997. The other case involved a nurse who contracted malaria after a needle-stick injury from an infected patient (1). Because transfusion-transmitted malaria usually occurs in recipients with other underlying illnesses or those who have undergone surgery, the proper diagnosis may be delayed because the fever is attributed to the underlying disease, postoperative infection, or tissue reaction to surgical trauma (2).

Reports of transfusion-transmitted malaria in the United States from 1963 through 1999 (3) revealed that of 93 cases reported, 35% were caused by *P. falciparum,* 27% were caused by *P. vivax,* 27% were caused by *P. malariae,* 5% were caused by *P. ovale,* 3% were mixed infections, and 2% were caused by unidentified species. Ten (11%) recipients died; 6 had *P. falciparum* infection, 2 had *P. vivax,* and 2 had *P. malariae.* The CDC considers a donor the source of transfusion-transmitted malaria if at least one of three criteria are met—the donor has a positive blood smear result, the donor has a positive serologic test result, or the patient has received blood from no other donor (3). In cases in which complete information on donors is available, it was found that 62% of implicated donors were not acceptable according to guidelines in place at the time of donation. This shows that obtaining accurate travel and immigration histories from donors can be difficult (3). Careful donor screening with recommended exclusion guidelines is considered the best way to prevent transfusion-transmitted malaria (3).

If investigation of the source suggests posttransfusion infection, the blood center should carefully investigate the implicated donor's history and determine the pertinent time frames and risk behavior for malaria. Previous involved donations should be retrieved and the recipients evaluated. The donor must also receive appropriate treatment.

CODA

This patient was a World War II veteran, but he had no recent history of international travel (1). The serum was tested by means of immunofluorescent assay from all five of the donors whose blood this patient received during the first admission (1). One donor was a military training base recruit who had immigrated to the United States from West Africa in 1995 and donated at a civilian blood center (2). The results of his serologic tests for malaria were positive (titers were as follows: *P. falciparum,* 1:16,384; *P. malariae,* 1:4,096; *P. ovale,* 1:1,024; and *P. vivax,* 1:64) (2). Malaria parasites were not seen in a blood smear obtained after his donation, but polymerase chain reaction

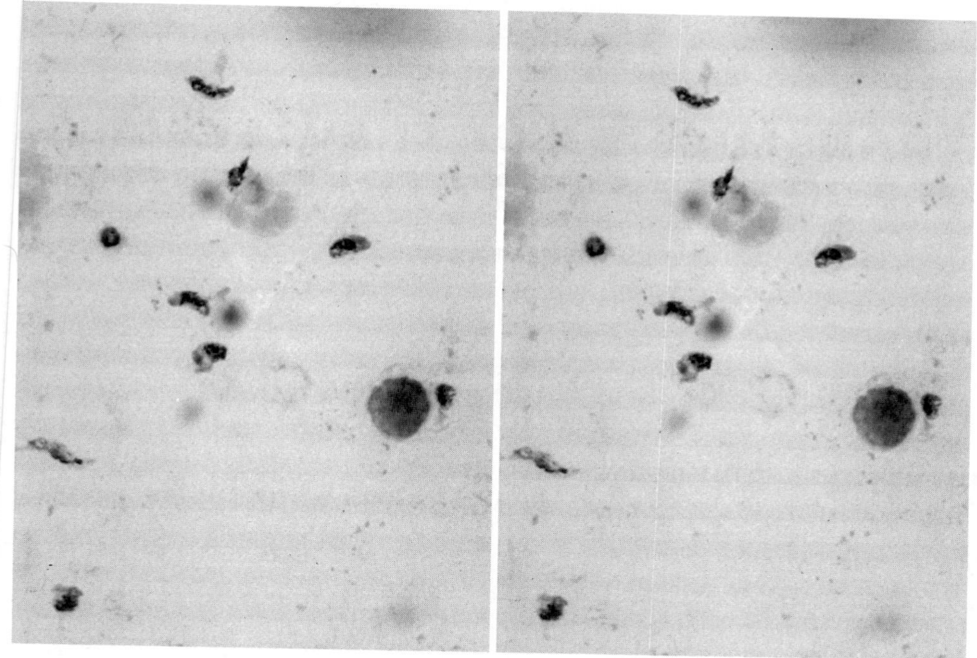

FIGURE 53A.1. Blood smear shows *Plasmodium falciparum* rings. (Courtesy of M. Crossey, M.D. and C. Steven, M.D., Tricore Reference Laboratories.)

tests showed *P. falciparum* DNA, and this donor was treated with quinine and doxycycline (2).

The donation screening questions did not furnish accurate information in this case. Current malaria screening criteria should have prevented this case of transfusion-transmitted malaria (2). This case demonstrates the reality of transfusion-transmitted malaria in the United States, its life-threatening consequences, and the importance of the donor screening process. The case is based on a real event reported by the CDC (1,2).

Case abstracted from references 1 and 2 by Ira Shulman, M.D., Los Angeles County Medical Center, and Marcia Haimowitz, M.D., American Red Cross Blood Services, Southern California Region, Los Angeles, CA.

REFERENCES

1. Malaria surveillance—United States, 1997. *MMWR Morb Mortal Wkly Rep* 2001;50;25–44.
2. Transfusion-transmitted malaria—Missouri and Pennsylvania, 1996–1998. *MMWR Morb Mortal Wkly Rep*1999;48;253–256.
3. Mungai M, Tegtmeier G, Chamberland M, et al. Transfusion-transmitted malaria in the United States from 1963–1999. *N Engl J Med* 2001; 344:1973–1978.

54

TRANSMISSION OF CREUTZFELDT-JAKOB DISEASE BY TRANSFUSION

PAUL BROWN

CHARACTERISTICS AND CAUSES OF CREUTZFELDT-JAKOB DISEASE

Creutzfeldt-Jakob disease (CJD) is a neurodegenerative disorder in which dementia and a variety of physical abnormalities including incoordination, visual deterioration, and involuntary movements usually progress to a fatal termination within a year of onset. The great majority of cases occur at random, without any evident cause, typically affecting individuals between the ages of 50 and 75 years, at an annual incidence of about one per million population (i.e., about 300 cases per year in the United States). Approximately 10% of cases have a genetic basis as a result of mutations in a gene on chromosome 20 that encodes the so-called *prion* protein, a normal glycoprotein that is vulnerable to a variety of mutation-induced transformations into β-sheeted amyloid. Most of the remaining cases result from iatrogenically acquired infections, such as neurosurgical cross-contaminations, or contamination of pools of dura mater grafts or pituitary extracts from cadavers with unsuspected disease (Table 54.1). Recently, another source of acquired infection has been found to result from oral exposure to bovine spongiform encephalopathy (BSE, or "mad cow" disease), causing a variant form of CJD (vCJD).

BLOOD INFECTIVITY IN HUMANS AND IN EXPERIMENTAL MODELS

The infectious agent (perhaps the prion protein itself) is concentrated in the central nervous system but may also be present at much lower levels in many other organs and tissues. The question of iatrogenic transmission as a result of therapy with blood, blood components, or plasma protein concentrates is still hypothetical. Blood has transmitted disease to experimental animals but is not known to have done so to humans, and this discordance between positive laboratory results and negative epidemiologic observations underlies all of the uncertainties that surround the issue of risk.

The numerous studies of experimentally and naturally infected animals, and of humans with CJD, can be very simply summarized by the statement that only in experimentally infected animals has disease transmission unequivocally been shown to occur (Table 54.2) (1,2). In experiments done on rodents, whole blood and plasma have been found to contain extremely low levels of infectivity, in the range of 2 to 20 infectious units per ml, and buffy coat may contain up to 100 infectious units per ml (Table 54.3) (3–6). Furthermore, even when whole blood, buffy coat, or plasma can be shown to contain infectivity when inoculated intracerebrally, substantially larger volumes are needed to transmit disease by the intravenous route. Levels of infectivity during the presymptomatic incubation phase

TABLE 54.1. SUMMARY OF IATROGENIC CASES CREUTZFELDT-JAKOB DISEASE (2000)

Mode of Infection	Number of Patients	Median Incubation Period (Range)
Corneal transplant	3	16, 18, 320 mos
Stereotactic EEG	2	16, 20 mos
Neurosurgery	5	17 mos (12–28)
Dura mater graft	114	6 yrs (1.5–18)
Growth hormone	139	12 yrs (5–30)
Gonadotrophin	4	13 yrs (12–16)

P. Brown: Laboratory of Central Nervous System Studies, National Institute of Neurological Disorders and Stroke, National Institutes of Health, Bethesda, Maryland.

TABLE 54.2. SUMMARY OF ATTEMPTS TO DEMONSTRATE INFECTIVITY IN THE BLOOD OF HUMANS AND ANIMALS WITH TRANSMISSIBLE SPONGIFORM ENCEPHALOPATHY

Host	Type of Infection	Infectivity in Blood
Animal	Experimental	Yes
Animal	Natural	No
Human	Natural	Unknown

TABLE 54.3. INFECTIVITY LEVELS IN THE BLOOD OF RODENTS EXPERIMENTALLY INFECTED WITH DIFFERENT STRAINS OF TRANSMISSIBLE SPONGIFORM ENCEPHALOPATHY

		Infectious Units (IU) Per ml		
Host	Agent	Whole Blood	Plasma	Buffy Coat
Mouse	CJD	NT	10–20	50–100
Hamster	Scrapie	10	2	30
Mouse	BSE	NT	4–5	NT

CJD, Creutzfeldt-Jakob disease; NT, not tested; BSE, bovine spongiform encephalopathy.

of disease are even lower than during the symptomatic phase and are often undetectable in plasma (Table 54.4) (4). By way of comparison, brain tissue from the same animals contains up to 10^6 infectious units per gram (ml).

BLOOD DONOR POLICIES AND RATIONALE

Any level of infectivity in blood, however low, would be sufficient cause to prohibit its therapeutic use, and it would be imprudent to dismiss results in experimentally infected rodents as irrelevant to human transfusion medicine. It is for this reason, and because of the few published reports of experimentally transmissible infectivity in the blood of humans with CJD (1), that the U.S. Food and Drug Administration in 1996 issued a guidance to the blood banking and plasma derivatives industries to destroy or quarantine any product tainted by a contribution from an individual who was discovered to have later died from CJD.

This guidance was countermanded in 1998, and although it was still considered inadvisable to transfuse whole blood or administer labile blood components from an individual with CJD, the use of plasma or plasma derivatives was permitted unless the patient had, or was suspected to have, vCJD. A number of considerations went into this policy reversal. They include potential and in some cases real shortages of certain plasma products, such as factor VIII and immune globulin, as a result of product batches being removed from distribution; evidence that significant reductions of infectivity occur during the fractionation and purification of plasma into therapeutic protein concentrates; calculations showing that, even if not recognized, most large plasma pools would probably contain at least one contribution by a person incubating CJD; and perhaps most importantly, epidemiologic evidence that despite intensive searching, CJD has never been identified as having resulted from blood or blood product administration, and probably does not occur.

Donor Pool Size

Calculations about the probability of a plasma pool being contaminated by a contribution from a donor who subsequently died of CJD were based upon the size of the donor pool, the prevalence of CJD in the donor population, and estimates of the preclinical period of blood infectivity (7). Reasoning from infectivity data obtained from experimental rodent models, and from incubation periods following peripheral-route iatrogenic infections in humans suggesting a preclinical infectivity period of 10 years, the frequency of potentially contaminated pools was calculated to range from 13% (for a pool of 10,000 donors) to 75% (for a pool of 100,000 donors). This rather surprising result

TABLE 54.4. INFECTIVITY LEVELS IN THE BUFFY COAT AND PLASMA OF MICE DURING THE INCUBATION PERIOD FOLLOWING INOCULATION WITH A HUMAN STRAIN OF TRANSMISSIBLE SPONGIFORM ENCEPHALOPATHY (FUKUOKA-1). MICE WERE ASYMPTOMATIC AT 5, 9, AND 13 WEEKS, AND SHOWED EARLY SIGNS OF DISEASE AT 18 WEEKS

Time After Inoculation	Specimen	Number of Infectious Units Per ml (CI)
5 weeks	Buffy coat	11.8 (3–29)
	Plasma	1.7 (0.1–8)
9 weeks	Buffy coat	6.8 (0.4–30)
	Plasma	0.0 (0–11)
13 weeks	Buffy coat	6.4 (0.4–28)
	Plasma	0.0 (0–11)
18 weeks	Buffy coat	106.0 (55–184)
	Plasma	21.9 (8–47)

CI, 95% confidence interval.

TABLE 54.5. INFECTIVITY LEVELS IN PLASMA AND PLASMA FRACTIONS OF MICE INFECTED WITH A HUMAN STRAIN OF TRANSMISSIBLE SPONGIFORM ENCEPHALPATHY (FUKUOKA-1)

	Number of Infectious Units (IU) Per ml	
Specimen	Experiment No 1	Experiment No 2
Plasma	11.7	19.4
Cryoprecipitate	1.1	13.6
Fraction I, II, III	0.9	NT
Fraction II	NT	1.5
Fraction I, III	NT	0.3
Fraction IV	0.0	0.3
Fraction V	0.0	0.0

NT, not tested.

TABLE 54.7. SUMMARY OF INFECTIVITY CLEARANCE DURING THE PURIFICATION OF CRYOPRECIPITATE INTO FACTOR VIII, USING SPECIMENS THAT HAD BEEN 'SPIKED' WITH A HAMSTER-ADAPTED STRAIN OF SHEEP TRANSMISSIBLE SPONGIFORM ENCEPHALOPATHY (SCRAPIE STRAIN 263K)

Purification Step	Log_{10} Reduction
Monoclonal antibody column	4.4
Sepharose (QSFF) column	6.3

Assuming 2,500 ($10^{3.4}$) infective units per batch of cryoprecipitate, the processing steps yield a safety margin of 7.3 logs (10.7 − 3.4 = 7.3). Data presented by Dr. Robert Rohwer at Cambridge HealthTech Institute meeting in February 2000.

not only reoriented thinking about restricting the use of plasma pools to which a donor incubating CJD had contributed, but also led to a voluntary agreement by the plasma industry to reduce the size of individual processing pools to 60,000 or fewer donations.

Blood Processing

The low levels of infectivity that might be present in plasma from patients in the preclinical phase of CJD are further reduced during the processing of plasma into therapeutic end products. In experimentally infected mice, plasma infectivity diminishes with each sequential fractionation step such that no infectivity remains in the final two fractions, which are the sources of α-1 proteinase inhibitor and albumin (Table 54.5) (3,4). In experiments conducted on "spiked" plasma or plasma fractions, purification steps involving precipitations, depth filtration, or chromatography result in reductions of between one and six orders of magnitude, with most showing 3- to 4-log reductions (Tables 54.6 and 54.7) (8–11). Given a maximum endogenous infectivity input of about 1 log per milliliter of plasma, these processing reductions guarantee a very large margin of safety in the end products.

TABLE 54.6. CLEARANCE OF INFECTIVITY DURING SUCCESSIVE PLASMA FRACTIONATION STEPS USING SPECIMENS THAT HAD BEEN "SPIKED" WITH A HAMSTER-ADAPTED STRAIN OF SHEEP-TRANSMISSIBLE SPONGIFORM ENCEPHALOPATHY (SCRAPIE STRAIN 263K)

Fractionation Step	Infectivity Clearance (Logs)
Cryoprecipitation	1.0
Fraction II, III	2.2
Fraction III	5.3
Fraction IV-1	3.7
Fraction IV-4	4.6

Epidemiology

The epidemiology of CJD confirms this high degree of safety. Many studies have been conducted during the past 15 years in an effort to define risk factors for the disease, and several have addressed the question of an association with prior blood transfusion (12–17). Five of these included sufficient information to permit systematic evaluation and metaanalysis; whether considered individually or together, the statistical evidence for any association was uniformly negative (18,19).

In addition to these statistical studies, surveillance has been carried out on individuals who received blood from patients later dying of CJD, and on the occurrence of CJD in high-risk groups such as hemophiliacs. In one report, among 35 of 55 identified recipients, 21 had died from non-CJD illnesses up to 22 years after having received transfusions, and 14 recipients were still alive without evidence of neurologic disease after an average survival of 12 years (20). Unpublished studies of other incidents have been carried out by the American Red Cross and European CJD surveillance teams, with similarly negative results. With respect to high-risk groups, no cases have been identified in hemophiliacs receiving either crude or purified factor VIII (21) or in patients with congenital immune deficiency who were receiving immune globulin (unpublished data, 2001).

VARIANT CREUTZFELDT-JAKOB DISEASE

The risk to recipients of blood from patients with vCJD is unknown. Assuming the most plausible explanation for its occurrence in the United Kingdom to be the consumption of beef products contaminated by central nervous system tissue from cattle affected with BSE, it may be supposed that virtually the entire nonvegetarian British population was exposed to the infectious agent during the period from 1980 to 1996. Today, the number of cases of vCJD is approaching 100, with 5 to 20 new cases each year since 1994, and the future upper and lower limits of the outbreak have been estimated by mathematic modeling to span a range from 100 to 100,000 cases (22,23). There is some reason to believe that blood from patients with vCJD might pose more of a risk than blood from patients with other forms of CJD, because their lymphoreticular tissues (e.g., spleen, tonsils, appendix) contain the proteinase-resistant isoform of prion protein (PrP), which in most circumstances is inseparable from infectivity (24). Also, the strain of BSE responsible for vCJD has been transmitted by the transfusion of blood from an experimentally infected sheep to a healthy sheep (25), and brain tissue from BSE-infected monkeys apparently transmits disease by the intravenous route almost as easily as by the intracerebral route (26).

The British government has therefore taken the precautionary measure of leukoreduction of all blood donated by U.K. residents before use as whole blood or labile components, and of importing all plasma and plasma derivatives. Several other governments have adopted donor deferral policies for individuals who visited the United Kingdom for cumulative periods of 6 months or more during the period from 1980 to 1996. Even more restrictive measures have been recommended, which would defer donors who spent 3 months or more in the United Kingdom from 1980 to 1996, cumulative travel or residence of 5 years or more in Europe, 6 months or more on a U.S. Department of Defense base 1980–1996 (before 1990 for Northern Europe), or receipt of blood in the United Kingdom from 1980 to the present (33). The need for such precautions will be clarified as we gain a better understanding of how the vCJD outbreak will evolve, as surveillance of people who have already received blood or blood products from patients incubating vCJD continues, and as information becomes available from studies of vCJD in experimental models (including primates) that are currently in progress.

SCREENING TESTS FOR PRECLINICAL INFECTION

A simple, accurate, and inexpensive screening test for preclinical infection would eliminate all of the uncertainty surrounding the possible iatrogenic human-to-human transmission of CJD via blood or blood products, and several tests are presently under development for the detection of PrP in the blood of preclinical cases of CJD (2). If the distribution of infectivity in human blood parallels that in rodents, the highest concentrations of PrP would be found in buffy coat, and although the purified white blood cell component of buffy coat has not yet been assayed, differential measurements of infectivity in purified platelets and whole buffy coat of infected hamsters indicates that white blood cells are the major infectious component (RG Rohwer, personal communication).

Substantial species differences in the amount of PrP precursor protein in different blood cell components have been reported, including the observation that the precursor protein is not detectable in hamster platelets, whereas it is abundant in human platelets (27). Measurements of the precursor in normal human blood indicate that leukocytes contain a higher concentration (per ml) than either platelets or plasma, although these two components contribute over 90% of the total quantity of the precursor in blood (28,29). Moreover, the ability of cells to express the normal precursor does not parallel the tissue distribution of either PrP or infectivity—muscle cells, for example, contain large amounts of the precursor (30) but no PrP and no infectivity. An interesting recent observation that both fibrinogen and plasminogen show a high in vitro binding affinity to PrP (but not its precursor) has both diagnostic and perhaps therapeutic implications, but is irrelevant to the question of endogenous PrP in the plasma of infected patients (31).

Taken together, these observations suggest that unpurified buffy coat would be the most appropriate material to detect the presence of PrP, but they do not imply that buffy coat in the blood of humans in either the preclinical or clinical stages of CJD contains enough PrP to be detectable. In any case, none of the tests under development has achieved a level of sensitivity sufficient to detect even the maximal amount of PrP that might be expected to be present in buffy coat, which is estimated to be in the range of picograms per ml (2). With continued refinement, it is still possible that at least one test method may reach this level. The application of an immuno-PCR assay, which could detect fewer than 1,000 molecules of some purified proteins (32), and the selective use of a successful screening test for CJD in "high-risk" blood donors would virtually eliminate any hazard of disease transmission through blood or blood products.

REFERENCES

1. Brown P. Can Creutzfeldt-Jakob disease be transmitted by transfusion? *Curr Opin Hematol* 1995;2:472–477.
2. Brown P, Cervenáková L, Diringer H. Blood infectivity and the prospects for a diagnostic screening test in Creutzfeldt-Jakob disease. *J Lab Clin Med* 2001;137:5–13.
3. Brown P, Rowher RG, Dunstan BS, et al. The distribution of infectivity in blood components and plasma derivatives in experimental models of transmissible spongiform encephalopathy. *Transfusion* 1998;38: 810–816.
4. Brown P, Cervenáková L, McShane LM, et al. Further studies of blood infectivity in an experimental model of transmissible spongiform encephalopathy, with an explanation of why blood components do not transmit Creutzfeldt-Jakob disease in humans. *Transfusion* 1999;39: 1169–1178.
5. Rohwer RG. Titer, distribution, and transmissibility of blood-borne TSE infectivity. Presented at Cambridge Healthtech Institute 6th Annual Meeting: blood product safety: TSE, perception versus reality, Feb 13–15, 2000, MacLean, VA.
6. Taylor DM, Fernie K, Reichl HE, et al. Infectivity in the blood of mice with a BSE-derived agent. *J Hosp Infect* 2000;46:78–79.
7. Brown, P. Donor pool size and the risk of blood-borne Creutzfeldt-Jakob disease. *Transfusion* 1998;38:312–315.
8. Foster PR. Assessment of the potential of plasma fractionation processes to remove causative agents of transmissible spongiform encephalopathy. *Transfus Med* 1999;9:3–14.
9. Lee DC, Stenland CJ, Hartwell RC, et al. Monitoring plasma processing steps with a sensitive Western blot assay for the detection of the prion protein. *J Virol Methods* 2000;84:77–89.
10. Foster PR, Welch AG, McLean C, et al. Studies on the removal of abnormal prion protein by processes used in the manufacture of human plasma products. *Vox Sang* 2000;78:86–95.
11. Lee DC, Stenland CJ, Miller JLC, et al. A direct relationship between partitioning of the pathogenic prion protein and transmissible spongiform encephalopathy infectivity during the purification of plasma proteins. *Transfusion* 2001;41:449–455.
12. Kondo K, Kuroiwa Y. A case-control study of Creutzfeldt-Jakob disease: association with physical injuries. *Ann Neurol* 1982;11:377–381.
13. Harries-Jones R, Knight R, Will RG, et al. Creutzfeldt-Jakob disease in England and Wales 1980–1984: a case-control study of potential risk factors. *J Neurol Neurosurg Psychiatry* 1988;51:1113–1119.
14. Esmonde TFG, Will RG, Slattery JM, et al. Creutzfeldt-Jakob disease and blood transfusion. *Lancet* 1993;341:205–207.

15. Van Dujin CM, Delasnerie-Laupretre N, Masullo C, et al. Case-control study of risk factors of Creutzfeldt-Jakob disease in Europe during 1993–1995. *Lancet* 1998;351:1081–1105.
16. Collins S, Law MG, Fletcher A, et al. Surgical treatment and risk of sporadic Creutzfeldt-Jakob disease: a case-control study. *Lancet* 1999; 353:693–697.
17. Zerr I, Brandel JP, Masullo C, et al. European surveillance on Creutzfeldt-Jakob disease: a case-control study for medical risk factors. *J Clin Epidemiol* 2000;53:747–754.
18. Wientjens DPWM, Davanipour Z, Hofman A, et al. Risk factors for Creutzfeldt-Jakob disease: a reanalysis of case-control studies. *Neurology* 1996;46:1287–1291.
19. Wilson K, Code C, Ricketts MN. Risk of acquiring Creutzfeldt-Jakob disease from blood transfusions: systematic review of case-control studies. *BMJ* 2000;321:17–19.
20. Heye N, Hensen S, Müller N. Creutzfeldt-Jakob disease and blood transfusion. *Lancet* 1994;343:298–299.
21. Evatt B, Austin E, Barnhart L, et al. Surveillance for Creutzfeldt-Jakob disease among persons with hemophilia. *Transfusion* 1998;38: 817–820.
22. Cousens SN, Vynnycky E, Zeidler M, et al. Predicting the CJD epidemic in humans. *Nature* 1997;385:197–198.
23. Ghani AC, Ferguson NM, Donnelly CA, et al. Predicted vCJD mortality in Great Britain. *Nature* 2000;406:583–584.
24. Hill AF, Butterworth RJ, Joiner S, et al. Investigation of variant Creutzfeldt-Jakob disease and other human prion diseases with tonsil biopsy samples. *Lancet* 1999;353:183–189.
25. Houston F, Foster JD, Chong A, et al. Transmission of BSE by blood transfusion in sheep. *Lancet* 2000;356:999–1000.
26. Lasmézas CI, Fournier JG, Nouvel V, et al. Adaptation of the bovine spongiform encephalopathy agent to primates and comparison with Creutzfeldt-Jakob disease: implications for human health. *Proc Natl Acad Sci U S A* 2000;98:4142–4147.
27. Holada K, Simák, Vostal JG. Letter to the editor. *Lancet* 2000;356: 1772.
28. MacGregor I, Hope J, Barnard G, et al. Application of a time-resolved fluoroimmunoassay for the analysis of normal prion protein in human blood and its components. *Vox Sang* 1999;77:88–96.
29. Völkel D, Zimmermann K, Zerr I, et al. Immunochemical determination of cellular prion protein in plasma from healthy subjects and patients with sporadic Creutzfeldt-Jakob disease or other neurological diseases. *Transfusion* 2001;41:441–448.
30. Bendheim PE, Brown HR, Rudelli RD, et al. Nearly ubiquitous tissue distribution of the scrapie agent precursor protein. *Neurology* 1992;42: 149–156.
31. Fischer MB, Roeckl C, Parizek P, et al. Binding of disease-associated prion protein to plasminogen. *Nature* 2000;408:479–483.
32. Sano T, Smith CL, Cantor CR. Immuno-PCR: very sensitive antigen detection by means of specific antibody-DNA conjugates. *Science* 1992; 258:120–122.
33. CBER, Guidance for Industry. Revised preventive measures to reduce the possible risk of transmission of Creutz-Feldt-Jakob disease (CFJ) and variant Creutzfeldt-Jakob disease (vCJD) by blood and blood products, US Food and Drug Administration, Rockville, MD, January 2002.

Rossi's Principles of Transfusion Medicine, Third Edition, edited by Toby L. Simon, Walter H. Dzik, Edward L. Snyder, Christopher P. Stowell, and Ronald G. Strauss. Lippincott Williams & Wilkins, Philadelphia © 2002.

55

BACTERIAL CONTAMINATION OF BLOOD PRODUCTS

MARK E. BRECHER

Bacterial contamination of blood products is a persistent but often overlooked problem in transfusion medicine. The incidence of platelet bacterial contamination is approximately 1 in 1,000, and the number of instances of severe morbidity or death may be as high or higher than 150 cases per year in the United States (1). Although recent public attention has focused on transfusion-transmitted viral infection, improved methods of screening through donor questioning and testing have greatly reduced the transmission of hepatitis viruses and retroviruses. Bacterial contamination, therefore, poses the greatest infectious threat in transfusion medicine. The risks of receiving bacterially contaminated platelets may be 50- to 250-fold higher than the combined risk of transfusion-related infection per unit associated with human immunodeficiency virus (HIV-1), hepatitis C virus (HCV), hepatitis B virus (HBV), and human T-lymphotropic virus (HTLV)-1 and -2 (1).)

TRANSFUSION-TRANSMITTED BACTERIAL INFECTION OF RED BLOOD CELLS

Sepsis associated with the transfusion of bacterially contaminated red blood cell products is generally regarded as a very rare event. From 1976 through September 1998, 26 fatalities thought to be secondary to contamination of whole blood or red blood cells were reported to the U.S. Food and Drug Administration (FDA) (Fig. 55.1) (2). During this period approximately 10 to 12 million units of whole blood or packed red blood cells were transfused per year in the United States, resulting in an approximate risk of less than one death per every 10 million units transfused (3,4). Unrecognized cases, under-reporting, and regional variation may account for observed differences in this incidence. For example, reports from New Zealand indicate a *Yersinia enterocolitica* transfusion-transmitted incidence rate of 1 in 65,000, with a fatality rate of 1 in 104,000 red blood cell units transfused (5).

The most commonly implicated organism in bacterial contamination of red blood cells is *Y. enterocolitica,* usually serotype O3, followed by *Serratia* spp. *(liquifaciens* or *marcescens)* and *Pseudomonas* spp. (6–24). These organisms are all capable of growth at 1° to 6°C. Sepsis associated with the transfusion of gram-negative bacterially contaminated red blood cells are typically severe and rapid in onset. Patients frequently develop high fever (temperatures as high as 109°F have been observed) and chills during or immediately following transfusion. From 1987 to 1996, 20 cases of *Yersinia*-infected red blood cells in 14 states were reported to the Centers for Disease Control (CDC) (14). Twelve of the 20 recipients died in 37 days or less following transfusion. The median time from transfusion to death was 25 hours. Of the seven who developed disseminated intravascular

M.E. Brecher: Department of Pathology and Laboratory Medicine, and Transplantation and Transfusion Services, University of North Carolina Hospitals, Chapel Hill, North Carolina.

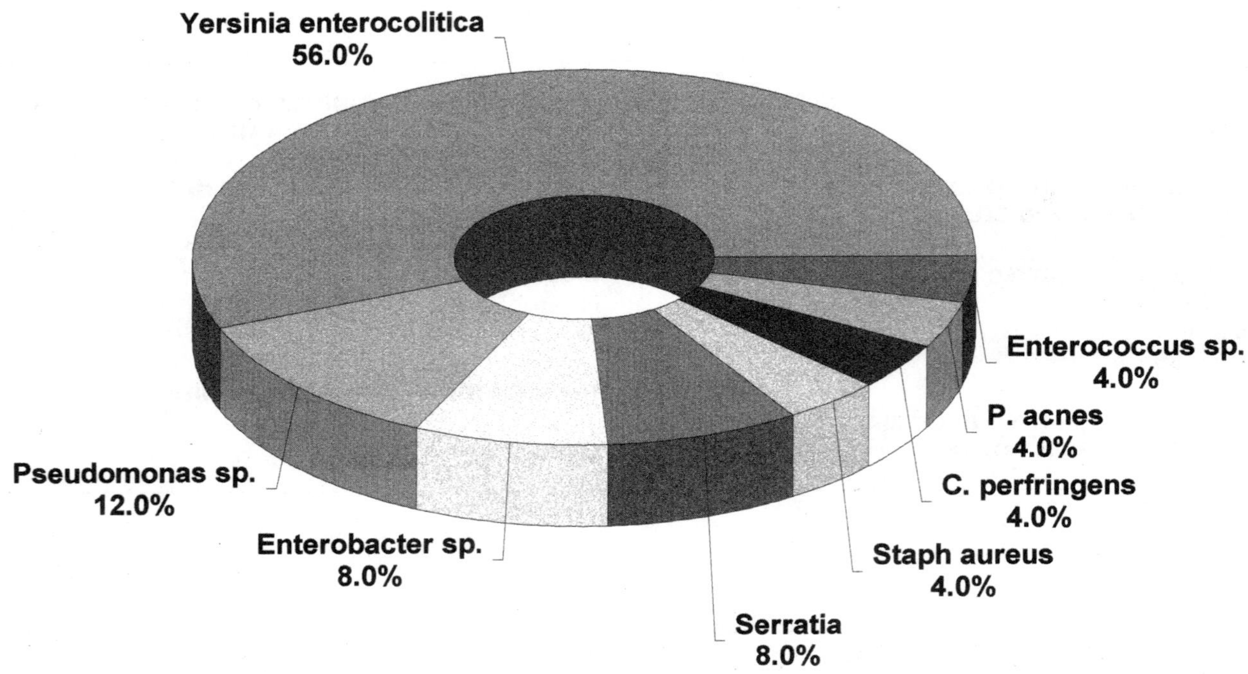

FIGURE 55.1. Transfusion fatalities, by organism, in red blood cell units or whole blood as reported to the United States Food and Drug Administration from 1976 to 1998. (From Lee J. United States Food and Drug Administration. Presented at the FDA/CBER Bacterial Contamination of Platelets Workshop; September 1999, Bethesda, MD, with permission.)

coagulation, six died. Signs, symptoms, and complications are summarized in Table 55.1.

Asymptomatic donors with transient *Yersinia* bacteremia are presumed to be responsible for contamination. Implicated donors typically are found to have elevated antibody titers (immunoglobulin M [IgM] or IgG) to *Y. enterocolitica,* implying a recent infection (6–8). The possibility of contamination of red blood cell products is directly related to its storage time; most cases of *Yersinia* contamination of red blood cell products occur in blood bags older than 25 days (23).

Serratia marcescens has been linked to an outbreak caused by red blood cell contamination in Denmark and Sweden (20,21). This outbreak was thought to involve the manufacturing process, because the sterile bag sets were autoclaved and put in a clean but not sterile outer plastic package. It was thought that *S. marcescens* present in the dust in the factory contaminated the outside of the containers, and in the presence of moisture and a nutrient (the plasticizer diethyl hexyl phthalate) the bacteria proliferated and somehow gained entry into the bag (22).

TABLE 55.1. MORBIDITY AND MORTALITY ASSOCIATED WITH 20 CASES OF *YERSINIA ENTEROCOLITICA*-CONTAMINATED RED BLOOD CELLS

Signs, Symptoms, and Mortality	Number	Percentage
Chills	16	80%
Fever	14	70%
Hypotension	13	65%
DIC	7	35%
Death	12	60%

Prospective bacterial culture of whole blood or packed red blood cells have shown a much higher incidence of bacterial contamination (Table 55.2); however, the organisms commonly cultured are *Staphylococcus species,* or *Propionibacterium species* which do not proliferate during storage at 1° to 6°C.
DIC, disseminated intravascular coagulation.
From (14).

TABLE 55.2. SELECTED CULTURE STUDIES OF RED BLOOD CELL CONCENTRATES AND WHOLE BLOOD

Country	Product	Sample Volume	Method	Day of Sampling	No of Samples	Initial Positive	Confirmed Positive	Rate Per 1,000 Units	Ref
Brazil	RCC	2 ml	Bact-Alert	0	20,206	108 (0.53%)	55 (0.27%)	2.7	15
New Zealand	RCC	1 drop	Plate	7–9 and 15–17	46,500	1–3%	1 (0.002%)	0.021	16
Canada	RCC	10 ml	Broth	NS	26,576	88 (0.33%)	NS	3.3	12,16,18
Netherlands	WB	NS	Bact-Alert	1	18,263	NS	71 (0.39%)	3.9	19
					7,115[a]		15 (0.21%)	2.1	

RCC, red cell concentrates; NS, not stated; WB, whole blood.
[a]After diversion of the first 10 ml of the blood withdrawal.

TRANSFUSION-TRANSMITTED BACTERIAL INFECTION OF AUTOLOGOUS RED BLOOD CELL UNITS

Although autologous blood is generally considered a "safer" blood product, there have been at least five reported cases of bacterial contamination of autologous red blood cell units, four due to *Y. enterocolitica* and one due to *S. liquifaciens* (24–28). Fortunately, all recipients survived, possibly due to preformed immunity. Upon retrospective questioning, all patients infected by *Yersinia* recalled gastrointestinal symptoms in days prior to donation. In the case of *Serratia* contamination, the patient's infected toe ulcer was presumed to be the source.

TRANSFUSION-TRANSMITTED BACTERIAL INFECTION OF PLATELETS

Sepsis due to transfusion of bacterially contaminated platelets is the most common transfusion-transmitted disease, because platelets are stored for up to 5 days at 20° to 24°C. From 1976 through 1998, 51 fatalities thought to be secondary to contaminated platelets were reported to the FDA (Fig. 55.2) (2). However, it is widely suspected that platelet bacterial sepsis is frequently unrecognized and, thus, under-reported. Single-unit contamination is similar for both platelet concentrates made from whole blood and single-donor apheresis concentrates (approximately 1 in 2,000 units; Table 55.3), but the ultimate risk

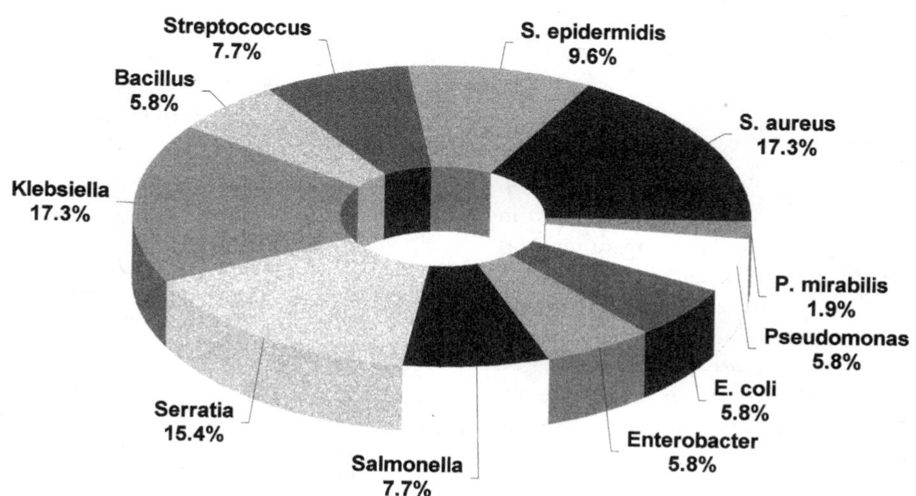

FIGURE 55.2. Transfusion fatalities, by organism, in platelets as reported to the United States Food and Drug Administration from 1976 to 1998. (From Lee J. United States Food and Drug Administration. Presented at the FDA/CBER Bacterial Contamination of Platelets Workshop; September 1999, Bethesda, MD, with permission.)

TABLE 55.3. SELECTED CULTURE STUDIES OF PLATELET CONCENTRATES AND SINGLE-DONOR APHERESIS

Country	Product	Sample Volume	Method	Day of Sampling	No of Samples	Initial Positive	Confirmed Positive	Rate Per 1,000 Units	Ref
Belgium	PC	NS	BacT/Alert	NS	17,675	294 (1.7%)	143 (0.81%)	8.1	31
	Aph				6,885	98 (1.4%)	12 (0.17%)[a]	1.7	
Belgium	PC	2.5–5.0	BacT/Alert	0	7,644	140 (1.8%)[b]	NS	18	32
	Aph				1,949	34 (1.8%)[b]		18	
Brazil	PC	2	BacT/Alert	0	13,454	35 (0.26%)	21 (0.16%)	1.6	14
	Aph				3,553	21 (0.59%)	16 (0.45%)	4.5	
US	PC	5	Broth	6–12	4,995	NS	4 (0.08)	0.8	33
US	PC	NS	Plate	4–5	23,390	NS	12 (0.05%)	0.5	34
	Aph				5,147	NS	3 (0.06%)	0.6	
Canada	PC	2	Bac Tec	1	16,290	NS	4 (0.02%)	0.2	35
				3	10,065	NS	7 (0.07%)	0.7	

PC, platelet concentrates; Aph, apheresis; Ns, not stated; US, United States.
[a]Extrapolated from units available for retesting (125 PCs and 27 Aph).
[b]Based on the successful subculture of the culture bottle (originally 144, 1.9% and 38, 2.0%, respectively).

of sepsis is likely to be 6 to 10 times greater with pooled units, because there is a 6- to 10-fold increased donor exposure (28–35). It has been estimated that as many as 150 people per year in the United States suffer severe morbidity or mortality as a consequence of a platelet transfusion (1).

In a study of symptomatic bacteremia following platelet transfusion in 161 bone marrow transplant recipients in Hong Kong, it was found that 1 in 2,000 units of platelet concentrates were bacterially contaminated (36). This translated to 1 in 350 pooled platelet units being contaminated. Of those patients who were febrile (a rise in temperature of >1°C) following platelet transfusion, 1 in 4 (27%) were found to have received a bacterially contaminated unit. Of those found to have a >2°C-rise in temperature following a platelet transfusion, 50% were found to have received a bacterially contaminated unit. In this multiply transfused patient population, the chance of receiving a bacterially contaminated platelet was 1 in 16. Of the ten patients who are known to have received a bacterially contaminated unit, four suffered from septic shock.

Organisms and Sources

Skin commensal organisms such as *Staphylococcus epidermidis* and *Bacillus cereus* are the organisms most often implicated in platelet bacterial contamination (11,30). These organisms typically do not grow at 0° to 6°C but survive and multiply readily at 20° to 24°C, the storage temperature of platelets. However, fatalities due to platelet contamination tend to be equally divided between gram-positive and gram-negative organisms (Fig. 55.2). Potential sources of organisms include contamination of the collection bag, tubing, or anticoagulant, and donor-related factors such as transient bacteremia. In some cases retrograde flow from vacuum tubes used in the collection or retrograde flow from the recipient have been implicated as a source of contamination (37, 38). However, contamination of platelets is principally thought to occur during phlebotomy due to inadequate disinfection or skin core removal by the collection needle.

Clinical Presentation

The clinical sequelae due to transfusion of bacterially contaminated platelets may range from asymptomatic to mild fever (which may be indistinguishable from a nonhemolytic transfusion reaction) to acute sepsis, hypotension, and death. The clinical picture is much more varied and often less severe than that of patients infected by transfusion of bacterially contaminated red blood cells (39). In fact, it is felt that sepsis due to transfusion of contaminated platelets is vastly under-recognized and under-reported. Ironically, those patients who receive the greatest number of platelets (patients being treated with chemotherapy who are both thrombocytopenic and immunosuppressed) are those most at risk of sepsis (Table 55.4). In such patients fever can be readily attributed to other infectious causes. In one well-documented outbreak of *Salmonella choleraseus* sepsis in seven patients linked to one common repeat platelet donor with an occult chronic osteomyelitis, the time to the onset of illness ranged from 5 to 12 days (mean 8.6 days) (41). One patient died, and two had long-term recurrences. The overall mortality rate of platelet-associated sepsis reported in the literature is 26% (12). Broad-spectrum antibiotics should be considered for any patient who develops fever within 6 hours of platelet infusion (36,40).

TABLE 55.4. FACTORS AFFECTING OUTCOME OF TRANSFUSION OF BACTERIALLY CONTAMINATED BLOOD PRODUCTS

V	Virulence of the organism
I	Immune status and general condition of the recipient
C	Concentration and bolus dose of bacteria transfused
T	Timely recognition and therapeutic intervention
I	Intensity of patient monitoring—i.e, inpatient vs. outpatient
M	Medicines the patient is receiving—i.e., antibiotics

From Krishnan LS, Brecher ME. Transfusion transmitted bacterial infection. *Hematol Oncol Clin North Am* 1995;9:167–185, with permission.

TRANSFUSION-TRANSMITTED BACTERIAL INFECTION OF PLASMA AND CRYOPRECIPITATE

Cell-free products, such as plasma and cryoprecipitate, are stored in the frozen state and thus are rarely associated with contamination. However, in some cases *Pseudomonas cepacia* and *Pseudomonas aeruginosa* have been cultured from cryoprecipitate and plasma thawed in contaminated water baths (42,43).

TRANSFUSION-TRANSMITTED BACTERIAL INFECTION OF PLASMA PROTEIN CONCENTRATES

Human serum albumin is a good culture medium and preserves viability of contaminants. The heating step (60°C for 10 hours) in the manufacturing of albumin is performed to inactivate certain viruses, not to assure bacterial sterility (44,45). This would require autoclaving (super-heated steam under pressure), which would cause albumin to denature. On occasion, specific lots of albumin product have been found to be contaminated with bacteria, typically *Pseudomonas* spp. (46). These lots have produced endotoxic shock, transient bacteremias, and febrile reactions in recipients. Most recently, two patients in different hospitals developed *Enterobacter cloacae* septicemia after receiving albumin (46,47). This resulted in a worldwide recall of 5%, 20%, 25% albumin, Monoclate-P (antihemophilic factor), and plasma protein fraction. It is suspected that cracks in the glass were responsible for the contamination. Manufacturing problems, therefore, are a source of bacterial risk from these derivatives.

STRATEGIES FOR THE REDUCTION OF THE RISK OF POSTTRANSFUSION SEPSIS

There are a variety of approaches to the reduction of risk of posttransfusion sepsis, which can be grouped into four major categories: bacterial avoidance, growth inhibition, detection, and elimination.

Bacterial Avoidance

Donor History

Upon retrospective questioning, approximately one-half of donors implicated in *Yersinia* red blood cell sepsis have had gastrointestinal symptoms in the 30 days preceding donation (6–8). Unfortunately, routine questioning of donors has shown that up to 13% of donors have had gastrointestinal symptoms in the 30 days prior to donation (48). Thus, donor questioning about gastrointestinal symptoms appears not to be a specific predictor of *Yersinia* bacteremia. In addition, this method lacks sensitivity, because only 13 of 20 donors associated with *Y. enterocolitica*–contaminated red blood cells recalled a history of gastrointestinal symptoms (14). Histories of recent dental procedures, gastrointestinal or genitourinary manipulation, and breast-feeding (which can be associated with skin cracks) may all be associated with bacteremia and are cause to defer a potential donor.

Skin Preparation and Phlebotomy

Despite excellent technique, one cannot assure a sterile venipuncture, because organisms harbored in sebaceous glands and hair follicles cannot be completely removed or killed, and skin fragments drawn up into the collection bag during the initial phase of donation can provide a source of infectious organisms (49,50).

Scarring or dimpling of the venipuncture site due to prior donations has also been recognized as a risk factor for bacterial contamination, because these areas frequently contain recessed pits that are difficult to disinfect (51). In one case, three episodes of platelet contamination with gram-positive organisms resulted in four cases of sepsis in recipients of those platelets, all of which were obtained from a dimpled site of a single donor.

Iodine solutions have been shown to be the most effective in reducing the donor skin bacterial burden (Table 55.5). Skin of donors who are allergic to iodine is often cleansed with a chlorhexidine solution. Alternatively, "green soap" has been used to disinfect the skin of iodine-sensitive donors. However, green soap, sometimes used for operative scrubs, has been shown to be a relatively ineffective method of skin disinfection (Table 55.5) in blood donors (52). In one study, 13 of 30 subjects had more bacteria colonies present after skin disinfection with green

TABLE 55.5. PERCENTAGE OF DONORS WITH BACTERIA GROWTH AFTER SKIN DISINFECTION

Bacterial Colonies Per Plate	Povidone Iodine	Isopropyl Iodine Alcohol and Tincture	Chlorhexidine Gluconate	Green Soap and Isopropyl Alcohol
0	34–49%	63%	60%	0%
1–100	35–43%	34%	25%	17%
11–100	10–14%	2%	12%	47%
>100	0–13%	1%	3%	36%
P value compared to povidone iodine		<0.001	>0.3	<0.001

From Goldman M, Roy G, Frechette, et al. Evaluation of donor skin disinfection methods. *Transfusion* 1997;37:309–312, with permission.

soap and isopropyl alcohol than before disinfection. Thus, the use of green soap is not recommended. Given the decreased reduction in skin bacterial load with some alternatives to iodine, it may be prudent either not to prepare platelets from iodine-sensitive donors or to use chlorhexidine to disinfect their skin.

Diversion of the Initial Collection

Diversion from the primary container of the first few milliliters of whole blood collected has been studied as a means of reducing the bacterial contamination arising from the skin. A study performed on 22,000 blood donations by the Red Cross in the Netherlands, in which the first 10 ml of donor blood were diverted from the primary bag, showed that 16 of the first 5-ml aliquots were bacterially contaminated, while only two of the second 5-ml aliquots were positive after culture (53). A second study from the Netherlands showed that removal of the first 10 ml of donor blood was associated with a significant decrease in bacterial contamination (n = 18,263 collections with 0.39% contamination, compared with n = 7,115 collections with a contamination rate of 0.21%, $P < 0.05$) (19). Similarly, an in vitro model with a medication site that was deliberately contaminated with *Staphylococcus aureus* and allowed to dry showed that diversion of the first 21 to 42 ml of whole blood reduces the downstream bioburden by approximately 1 log (54). These data suggest that diversion of the initial 10 to 40 ml of blood collection (which can be used for testing) would decrease, but not eliminate, the risk of bacterial contamination. Collection systems that accomplish this are now being evaluated.

Single-donor Apheresis Versus Pooled Platelets

As noted above, single-unit contamination is similar for platelet concentrates made from both whole blood and single-donor apheresis concentrates (approximately 1 in 2,000 units), but the ultimate risk of sepsis is likely to be 6 to 10 times greater with pooled units, because there is a 6- to 10-fold increase in donor exposure (29,39). Because of the increased risk associated with pooling of platelets, some institutions have elected to use single-donor platelets whenever possible. In one recent study from Johns Hopkins Hospital, the use of single-donor platelets was increased from 51.7% to 99.4% of all platelet transfusions over a 12-year period (1986 to 1998) (55). During this time, the incidence of reported septic reactions to platelet transfusion decreased from 1 in 4,818 transfusions to 1 in 15,098 transfusions, an approximate three-fold reduction. The three-fold reduction was compatible with their baseline rate of single-donor platelet transfusions of 50%.

Growth Inhibition

Optimizing Storage Time

In 1991, the Blood Product Advisory Committee (BPAC) of the FDA reviewed all cases of *Yersinia* sepsis from red blood cell units reported to either the FDA or the CDC during the late 1980s. At that time all reported cases of red blood cell–associated *Yersinia* sepsis in the United States had occurred in units older than 25 days. As a result of timing necessary for the bacteria to attain a lethal concentration, the BPAC proposed reducing the storage time of red blood cells from 42 to 25 days. This recommendation was subsequently rejected for the following reasons. a) A questionnaire distributed at the time revealed that 20% of red blood cell units in stock at over 1,500 blood banks and transfusion services were more than 28 days old (56,57). Discarding such units would have severely compromised the nation's blood supply. b) A shorter outdate would then require recruitment of new donors. It was estimated that the addition of a quarter of a million donations per year would be required to replace the loss due to outdates. This would involve additional risk, because first-time donors are known to be at a greater risk of carrying disease because their blood has not been repeatedly tested, as has the blood of veteran donors. c) Units less than 25 days old can also cause sepsis, so that decreasing the allowable storage time would lessen the problem but would not eliminate it (23,58,59). d) Older units are less likely to transmit viruses such as HIV and HTLV-1 and -2 (60,61).

Longer platelet storage time has also been associated with increased probability of contamination. In 1983, in the United States platelet storage was transiently approved for 7 days. This 7-day storage was based on acceptable in vitro function and in vivo recovery and survival data. However, due to the increasing risk of bacterial proliferation over time, the outdate was reduced in 1986 to the current 5 days. Unfortunately, merely decreasing the shelf life did not eliminate the problem of bacterial contamination. It has been shown that even a moderate inoculate (10 to 50 colony-forming units (CFU)/ml) of certain bacteria such as *B. cereus* and *P. aeruginosa* in platelets have a minimal lag phase with a doubling time of 1 to 2 hours (62). This can lead to a bacterial load of 10^8 CFU/ml in just 1 to 2 days.

Only by severely reducing the storage time of platelets to 1 to 2 days would one significantly impact the risk of bacterial overgrowth. However, operational changes affect the storage age of available platelets. With increased complexity of disease-marker testing, the availability of 1-day-old platelets has decreased. For example, in the United States in 1982 the mean age of distributed platelets was 1.6 days, in 1983 (after extension of the dating period to 5 days) it was 2.0 days, and in 1992 (after addition of increased laboratory testing) it was 2.5 days. In 1983, only 5% of issued platelets were older than 3 days. In 1992, just 10% were older than 3 days. But with the introduction of centralized testing by the American Red Cross, the mean age of issued platelets increased to 2.7 days with 20% older than 3 days (63). With the recent addition of nucleic acid testing for HIV and HCV, additional delays are likely. Not only can this decrease the available shelf life of an already precariously limited supply of platelets, it can also decrease the availability of fresh platelets, which are the most hemostatic and the least likely to be bacterially contaminated.

Optimizing Storage Temperature

Bacterial proliferation in red blood cells or whole blood is generally limited to a few gram-negative organisms capable of proliferation at 1° to 6°C (so-called *psychrophilic* organisms, most notably *Y. enterocolitica*, *Serratia* spp., and *Pseudomonas fluorescens*).

Freezing red blood cells with glycerol would prevent the proliferation of bacteria but would be associated with significant decreased availability and increased cost.

Platelets are stored for a limit of 5 days at 20° to 24°C, due principally to a potential concern of bacterial contamination (see above) and progressive decline in platelet function (storage lesion) if stored for longer periods at these temperatures. Although storage of platelets at 4°C results in a significantly lower rate of bacterial contamination, it also causes a temperature-induced activation of platelets and a rapid decline in functional ability and in vitro viability. Recent studies of cold-storage platelets with the addition of specific second-messenger stimulators have reported that platelets stored at 4°C were bacteriostatic and retained partial functional ability and viability compared with control platelets (64,65). If a practical method for storing platelets at 4°C or in a frozen state were perfected, it would have the potential to reduce the risk of bacterial contamination of this blood product.

Bacterial Detection

A simple low-cost method to detect bacterial overgrowth would be a valuable tool for screening units prior to release from the blood bank. A variety of systems for bacterial detection are under active investigation. Bacterial detection systems include simple inspection, microscopic examination, detection of metabolic changes in stored products, endotoxin assays, nucleotide-based assays, and bacterial culture. Unlike viral contamination of blood products, which is detected from a sample obtained at the time of donation, bacterial contamination of blood products frequently requires time for the organisms to proliferate prior to being detectable. Therefore, knowledge of the growth characteristics of bacteria in blood products must be considered for successful implementation of a detection strategy.

Blajchman et al. with the Canadian Red Cross, using an automated detection system (Bactec, Becton Dickinson, Cockeysville, MD) cultured whole blood platelet concentrates on days 1 ($n = 16{,}290$ platelet concentrates) and 3 ($n = 10{,}065$ platelet concentrates) following preparation (35). Of the 16,290 platelet concentrates cultured on the day of collection, four units were found to be culture positive; however, an additional three which were culture negative on the day of collection were culture positive after an additional 2 days of storage. Based on these results the authors concluded that cultures from the day of collection may be inadequate to detect all contaminated platelet concentrate units.

Bacterial growth characteristics were reported for 165 platelet units, each inoculated on the day of collection with one of the following organisms: *B. cereus, P. aeruginosa, Klebsiella pneumoniae, S. marcescens, S. aureus,* and *S. epidermidis* (66). All examples of *B. cereus, P. aeruginosa, K. pneumoniae, S. marcescens,* and *S. aureus* had concentrations $\geq 10^2$ CFU/ml by day 3 following inoculation. By day 4 all units with these organisms contained $\geq 10^5$ CFU/ml. Units contaminated with *S. epidermidis* showed slower and more varied growth. This study concluded that an assay capable of detecting 10^2 CFU/ml on day 3 of storage would detect the vast majority of bacterially contaminated platelet units.

In the case of red blood cell contamination, inoculation experiments of whole blood with *Y. enterocolitica* have demonstrated an initial rapid decline in the number of viable organisms followed by a resumption of growth after a lag phase of approximately 3 to 14 days (23,67–71). During this lag phase, *Yersinia* typically cannot be recovered from samples obtained from the bag.

Visual Inspection of Red Blood Cells to Detect Color Change

It is known that in cases of bacterially contaminated red blood cells, the attached tubing segments almost invariably remain sterile even when the organism is cultured from the blood bag (6, 7). An observation first noted by Kim et al. and subsequently confirmed by several authors is a darkening of the color of the unit compared to the attached segments in additive solution red blood cells (71–74). Compared with sterile units, the contaminated units became noticeably darker in color 1.5 to 2 weeks after the organism was detected by culture. This color change was very apparent when the contaminated units were compared with the attached segments of tubing, which did not darken. The sensitivity of visual identification of bacterial contamination in this manner is approximately 10^8 CFU/ml. A recent study found bacterial concentrations in the range of 1.8×10^4 to 1.6×10^9 CFU/ml at the time that whole blood units were first identified by visual inspection as potentially contaminated (74).

Microscopic Examination with Gram Stain and Acridine Orange

Microscopic examination has been used to detect bacterial contamination in both red blood cell products and platelets. Several authors have reported the use of the Gram stain for microscopic examination of blood products (29,75). One institution implemented a surveillance program that included pretransfusion Gram stains of platelet pools and apheresis units (75). In platelets aged 1 to 5 days, the sensitivity and specificity of this method were 80% and 99% to 96%, respectively. In 4- to 5-day-old platelets, the sensitivity was increased to 100%, with a specificity of 99.93%. The true-positive results were associated with bacterial concentrations $>10^6$ CFU/ml. Based on their analysis, these authors concluded that the use of pretransfusion Gram stain, combined with culture of 4- and 5-day-old units was more cost effective than discarding whole blood platelets stored for 5 days. However, Barrett et al. reported a higher rate of false positives. In their study, 8 of 5,334 platelet units yielded positive Gram stain results, six of which were negative by culture (29). Other investigators have reported on the use of acridine orange as a stain for bacteria (67,76).

Metabolic Measurements

Brecher et al. described a decrease in PO_2 and an increase in PCO_2 (with an associated decrease in pH) in platelets that supported the growth of *S. epidermidis.* The units, which had initial PO_2 levels of 79 to 137 mm Hg, often showed PO_2 levels below

20 mm Hg by the time the organisms reached a plateau concentration of 10^7 to 10^8 CFU/ml (77). Other groups have explored this method (78–81). Although this technique has the added advantage of being noninvasive, it detects contamination only at high levels. Because platelets (and white blood cells) also produce carbon dioxide, this complicates attempts to detect bacterial contamination by measurements of this analyte. Because proliferating bacteria consume glucose and generate acid, several investigators have explored the use of dipsticks to indicate metabolic changes consistent with bacterial proliferation (82,83). Prospective surveillance of 3,000 platelet concentrates at the M.D. Anderson Cancer Center in Houston using reagent strips found 12 platelets concentrates with a glucose concentration or pH outside of their reference range (84). Two of the twelve platelets were found to be culture positive for *B. cereus.* The remaining ten platelet concentrates did not demonstrate bacterial proliferation upon culture.

Endotoxin Assay

Investigators have used the Limulus amebocyte lysate assay for detection of endotoxin in blood components (23,67). This method is limited to detection of endotoxin-producing organisms such as *Y. enterocolitica.*

DNA/RNA Techniques

A variety of molecular biologic approaches have been applied to the detection of bacterial contamination of blood products. Feng et al. investigated the use of the polymerase chain reaction (PCR) in detection of *Y. enterocolitica* in whole blood (85). Recently, Sen developed a 5′ nuclease TaqMan PCR assay probe based on the nucleotide sequence of the 16S rRNA gene from *Y. enterocolitica* (86). The TaqMan PCR assay detected as few as six bacteria spiked in 200 microliters (30 CFU/ml) within 2 hours. Brecher et al. described the use of a nonamplified chemiluminescence-linked universal bacterial rRNA probe (62,77). This method uses an acridinium ester-labeled single-stranded DNA probe complementary to highly conserved bacterial rRNA regions. Although a multicenter trial confirmed the effectiveness of this technique in detecting platelet samples contaminated with one of four bacterial species, the company developing this assay has chosen not to pursue further assay development. Recently, Mosaic Technologies (Waltham, MA) has been developing a somewhat similar approach with the use of a nonamplified probe directed to a conserved region of bacterial 4.5S RNA (87). This approach employs a solid-phase capture gel, a brief electrophoresis followed by probe detection with a chemiluminescent probe.

Culture

Several investigators have explored the effectiveness of currently available automated liquid media culture systems (Bactec, Becton Dickinson and BacT/Alert, Organon Teknika). In one study, isolates of 15 organisms thought to be clinically significant platelet contaminants were inoculated into day-2 apheresis platelet units in order to obtain a final concentration of approximately 10 and 100 CFU/ml (two units per organism) and cultured in replicate (Fig. 55.3) (88). With the exception of *Propionibacterium acnes,* all of the contaminants were detected in 9.2 to 25.6 hours. *Propionibacterium acnes,* which can occasionally be isolated from platelets, grows poorly in the aerobic environment of platelet storage, is of questionable clinical significance, and takes considerably longer to detect (in either aerobic or anaerobic bottles). Using spiking experiments, Wagner and Robinette found that if samples were taken 24 hours after inoculation, on average an additional 24 hours was required for the BacT/Alert to detect the organisms in all units that ultimately resulted in positive cultures (89).

Balance of Sensitivity and Rapid Detection

Each of the different technologies for detection of bacterial overgrowth in blood components presents advantages and disadvantages. As a general rule, the more rapid a bacterial detection assay is, the lower is its sensitivity (Fig. 55.4). Decisions regarding the implementation of bacterial testing must balance the need for rapid detection versus sensitivity. The principal objectives in regard to detection of bacterially contaminated platelets are a) the prevention of posttransfusion-related sepsis and b) the extension of the platelet shelf life. The level and timing of detection to achieve these two interrelated objectives may differ. For example, a rapid test with limited sensitivity (e.g., $>10^2$ CFU/ml) performed late in storage, such as on day 4, may be sufficient to justify the extension of the platelet shelf life but would not be effective in preventing platelet transfusion–related sepsis caused by contaminated units that were transfused before they were 4 days old. Similarly, a very sensitive technique, such as culture performed on the day of collection, may require days to detect a positive unit and would likely miss many bacterially contaminated units due to initial sampling error. To achieve both objectives, a combination of detection strategies may be required (e.g., at the time of collection and after 2 to 3 days of storage) (90).

Bacterial Elimination

Filtration

Leukocyte reduction of blood products is widely used in North America, Europe, Asia, and Australia. Several countries, including Canada, England, Portugal, France, Ireland, and Norway, have announced plans to switch to a completely leukocyte-reduced blood supply (so-called "universal leukocyte reduction" or ULR) (91,92). Similarly, the FDA is currently encouraging voluntary implementation of ULR whenever feasible and plans to either create a regulatory requirement for ULR or enforce ULR as a product standard under current Good Manufacturing Practices regulations (93).

Due to concern regarding the accumulation of cytokines, leukocyte and platelet breakdown products, and possibly immunogenic white blood cell fragments in stored blood, emphasis has been placed on prestorage versus poststorage leukoreduction (94–96). A theoretic risk of prestorage filtration would be that early removal of the phagocytic leukocytes, which would nor-

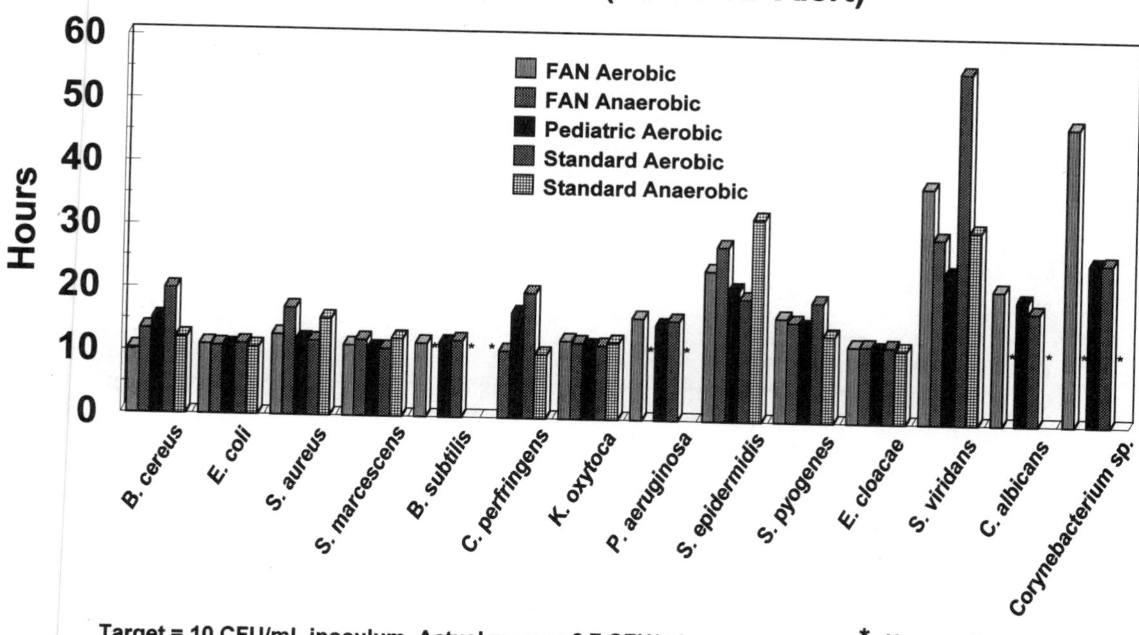

FIGURE 55.3. Mean time to detection for 14 microbial organisms inoculated at 10 CFU/ml displayed by bottle type. Mean detection times for 10 CFU/ml for these 14 organisms ranged from 10.2 to 23 hours. (From Brecher ME, Means N, Jere CS, et al. Evaluation of the BacT/ALERT 3D microbial detection system for platelet bacterial contamination: an analysis of 15 contaminating organisms. *Transfusion* 2001;41:477–482, with permission.)

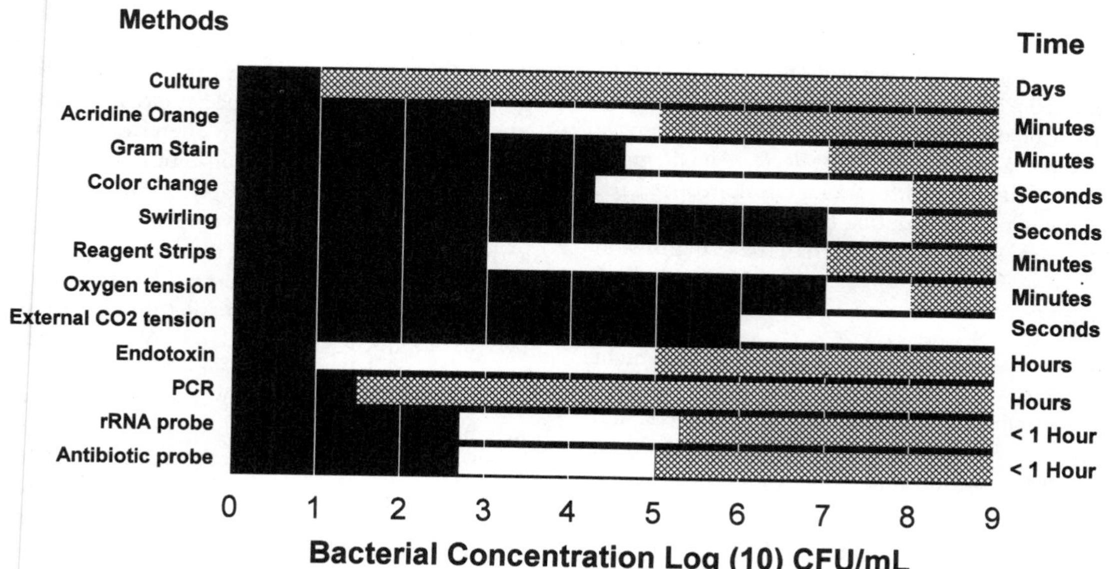

FIGURE 55.4. Methods of detection of bacterial contamination of blood products—approximate limits of detection as reflected in the current literature. *Areas of clear shading* represent concentrations (CFU/ml) at which some, but not all, bacteria are detected by each method. *Cross-hatched areas* represent ranges over which each method is considered reliable. The approximate time from beginning to end of the assay is reported (immunochromatographic assay is not included because clinical trials have not been published to date). (From Mitchell KT, Brecher ME. Approaches to the detection of bacterial contamination in cellular blood products. *Trans Med Rev* 1999;13:132–144, with permission.)

TABLE 55.6. SELECTED STUDIES OF *YERSINIA ENTEROCOLITICA* GROWTH AND PRESTORAGE LEUKOCYTE REDUCTION BY FILTRATION

Inoculating Concentration CFU/ml	Filtered Growth/ Total (%)	Control Growth/ Total (%)	Filter Type	P Value[a]	Reference
100	0/10 (0)	10/10 (100)	Sepacell PL-5N	<0.001	99
65	2/10 (20)	8/8 (100)	Leukotrap and Leukotrap RC (Pall RC300)	0.002	67
10/150	3/8 (37)	8/8 (100)	Pall BPF4	0.03	97
0.3–132	3/24 (12)	16/24 (67)	Sepacell R-500	<0.001	68
20–30,000	6/30 (20)	22/30 (70)	Cellselect, NPBI	<0.001	100
1.5	2/6 (33)	6/6 (100)	Leukotrap RC (Pall RC300)	0.06	98
Total	16/88 (18)	70/86 (81)		<0.001	

[a]Two-sided Fisher's exact test.
CFU, colony-forming unit.

mally remove low levels of bacteria present in these products, might lead to an increase in bacterial contamination of blood products and septic complications. In the case of *Y. enterocolitica* (the organism which has been most extensively studied), prestorage leukoreduction by filtration actually is associated with a decrease in bacterial growth in inoculated red blood cells (Table 55.6) (5,67,68,97–99).

The mechanism by which leukoreduction removes bacteria is multifactorial. Bacteria which have been phagocytized but not killed are removed with the white blood cells. Alternatively, organisms may be adsorbed to leukocytes or activated complement, to then be bound indirectly to the charged filter fibers, or the bacteria may directly adhere to the filter fibers. AuBuchon and Pickard showed with a panel of bacterial organisms differences in the affinity for bacteria by direct adherence of red blood cell leukoreduction filters and platelet leukoreduction (101). In general, red blood cell reduction filters are more efficient, removing 88% to 100% of organisms, while platelet filters remove only 67% to 97% of organisms. Unlike the decrease in *Y. enterocolitica* growth seen with filtered, prestorage leukoreduced red blood cells, leukoreduction by filtration failed to decrease bacterial growth in platelets spiked with bacteria (102–104).

Antibiotics

Although the use of antibiotics to assure a sterile product might be effective, it is not an acceptable solution. Fears of the selection and development of antibiotic-resistant strains of bacteria and of merely trading one rare event (idiosyncratic drug reaction) for another (bacterial sepsis) preclude their use (11,105).

Prolonged Room Temperature Hold of Red Blood Cells

When whole blood is placed immediately at 4°C, growth occurs more rapidly than if held at 10°C for 24 hours prior to 4°C storage (106). Bacterial growth of most pathogens is inhibited by cold temperatures, but host defense mechanisms present in fresh whole blood are also inhibited at 4°C. *Yersinia* with plasmid-encoded complement resistance can become complement sensitive when blood is transiently stored at 20°C (69). Because phagocytosis and complement activation are impaired at 4°C, it may be advantageous to allow red blood cells to remain in contact with plasma for several hours prior to separation and storage of components.

Chemical Pathogen Reduction

Several techniques to reduce pathogens in blood components using chemicals are under active investigation (see Chapter 56).

TRANSFUSION-TRANSMITTED SYPHILIS

Treponema pallidum is a thin-walled, motile, spiral gram-negative rod or spirochete, which cannot be visualized with Gram stain and does not grow on bacteriologic media or cell culture. Although it is a bacterium, it is often treated as a distinct entity, different from other transfusion-transmitted bacterial organisms and is thus addressed separately. Only 25% of patients with primary syphilis have a reactive serologic test for syphilis (STS), and the test does not become routinely positive until the fourth week after the onset of symptoms; therefore donors infected with *T. pallidum* may be asymptomatic with negative serology during periods of spirochetemia (107,108). Although the organism does not survive prolonged storage at 4°C, it may live for 1 to 5 days at these cold temperatures (109,110). Therefore, a rare infection may be associated with transfusion of a fresh unit of red blood cells from a donor who was in the seronegative phase at the time of donation. Platelets are stored at 20° to 24°C, however, provide a more hospitable environment for this organism. Since 1969, only three cases of transfusion-transmitted syphilis have been reported in the literature (111–113). The extremely low rate of transfusion-transmitted syphilis infection likely results from a) donor questioning targeting high-risk behavior; b) the cardiolipin-based assay, although an insensitive test in the acute postinfectious setting, which does pick up a number of infected donors; c) refrigerator storage, which results in the death of spirochetes;

d) antibiotics given to many patients at the time of platelet transfusion, which would be bactericidal for any viable organisms; and e) donors excluded for a positive test for HIV or hepatitis B or C, because of the high correlation between infection with *T. pallidum* and viruses such as these, even though the donors may have been in the seronegative phase of syphilis at the time of donation (114–119). Because syphilis testing plays only a minor role in protecting the blood supply and is associated with a high degree of false-positive reactions, elimination of syphilis testing has been advocated. Despite the shortcomings of syphilis testing, it has been argued that such testing provides a surrogate marker for individuals at risk of other sexually transmitted diseases and therefore should be retained.

CONCLUSION

At present, bacterial contamination of blood products is the most frequent cause of transfusion-transmitted infectious disease. The contamination rate of 1 in 2,000 for platelet units is orders of magnitude greater than that found for HIV, HBV, HCV, or HTLV-1 and -2. In addition, the fear of bacterial overgrowth of platelets currently is the limiting factor in many countries for the shelf life of platelets. Although no existing strategy can completely eliminate the risk of bacterial contamination of blood products, it is inevitable that additional partial solutions will be widely implemented in the near future. The first strategies will likely be diversion of the initial blood collection and bacterial detection by culture. In the case of platelets, bacterial detection will entail testing on day 2 or 3 of storage and possibly on the day of collection. However, detection by culture may be replaced by nucleic acid–based testing (which may allow testing closer to the time of issue). Already, recent reports from Denmark, Yugoslavia, the Netherlands, and the United Kingdom have advocated the use of bacterial culturing of platelets on days 2 or 3 of storage in order to extend the shelf life of platelets to 7 days, thereby reducing the waste and preserving a limited medical resource (100,120–122). Such a strategy is considered cost effective (120,123). If chemical pathogen reduction becomes available, this technology would be expected to largely eliminate the risk of bacterial contamination of blood products, except possibly for spore-forming organisms (e.g., *B. cereus*) (124).

REFERENCES

1. Bacterial contamination of blood components. Bulletin 96-6. AABB Faxnet 294. Bethesda, MD: American Association of Blood Banks, 1996.
2. Lee J. United States Food and Drug Administration. Presented at the FDA/CBER Bacterial Contamination of Platelets Workshop; September 1999, Bethesda, MD.
3. Wallace EL, Churchill WH, Surgenor DM, et al. Collection and transfusion of blood and blood components in the United States, 1994. *Transfusion* 1998;38:625–636.
4. Goodnough LT, Brecher ME, Kanter MH, et al. Medical progress: transfusion medicine, part I. Blood transfusion. *New Engl J Med* 1999; 340:438–447.
5. Theakston EP, Morris AJ, Streat SJ, et al. Transfusion transmitted *Yersinia enterocolitica* infection in New Zealand. *Aust N Z J Med* 1997; 27:62–67.
6. Tipple MA, Bland LA, Murphy JJ, et al. Sepsis associated with transfusion of red cells contaminated with *Yersinia enterocolitica. Transfusion* 1990;30:207–213.
7. Update. *Yersinia enterocolitica* bacteremia and endotoxin shock associated with red blood cell transfusion—United States, 1991. *MMWR* 1991;40:176–178.
8. Red blood cell transfusions contaminated with *Yersinia enterocolitica*—United States, 1991–1996, and initiation of a national study to detect bacteria-associated transfusion reactions. *MMWR* 1997;20; 46:553–555.
9. Roth VR, Arduino MJ, Nobiletti J, et al. Transfusion-related sepsis due to *Serratia liquefaciens* in the United States. *Transfusion* 2000; 40:931–935.
10. Wagner SJ, Friedman LI, Dodd RY. Transfusion-associated bacterial sepsis. *Clin Microbiol Rev* 1994;7:290–302.
11. Klein HG, Dodd RY, Ness PM, et al. Current status of microbial contamination of blood components: summary of a conference. *Transfusion* 1997;37:95–101.
12. Goldman M, Blajchman MA. Blood product–associated bacterial sepsis. *Transfus Med Rev* 1991;5:73–83.
13. Sazama K. Bacteria in blood for transfusion. A review. *Arch Pathol Lab Med* 1994;118:350–365.
14. Cookson ST, Arduino MJ, Aguero SM, et al. *Yersinia enterocolitica*–contaminated red blood cells (RBCs): an emerging threat to blood safety. In: Program and abstracts of the 36th Interscience Conference on Antimicrobial Agents and Chemotherapy, September 15–18, 1996, New Orleans. Washington, DC: American Society for Microbiology, 1996:237(abst).
15. Wendel S, Fontao-Wew Orleansendel R, Germano S, et al. Screening of bacterial for blood components production in a Brazilian blood bank. *Vox Sang* 2000:78[Suppl 1]:P376(abst).
16. Faed JM. A simple method for screening red cell and platelet units for bacteria. *Vox Sang* 2000;78[Suppl 1]:P381(abst).
17. Blajchman MA, Ali AM. Bacteria in the blood supply: an overlooked issue in transfusion medicine. In: Nance SJ, ed. Blood safety: current challenges. Bethesda, MD: American Association of Blood Banks, 1992:213–220.
18. Blajchman MA. Personal communication. January 2001.
19. de Korte D, Vlaar R, Marcelis J, et al. Reduction of the degree of bacterial contamination for whole blood collections. *Transfusion* 2000;40[Suppl]:36S(abst).
20. Hogman CF, Fritz H, Sandberg L. Post-transfusion *Serratia marcescens* septicemia [Editorial]. *Transfusion* 1993;33:189–191.
21. Heltberg O, Show F, Gerner-Smidt P, et al. Nosocomial epidemic of *Serratia marcescens* septicemia ascribed to contaminated blood transfusion bags. *Transfusion* 1993;33:221–227.
22. Szewzyk U, Szewzyk R, Stenstrom TA. Growth and survival of *Serratia marcescens* under aerobic and anaerobic conditions in the presence of materials from blood bags. *J Clin Microbiol* 1993;31: 1826–1830.
23. Arduino MJ, Bland LA, Tipple MA, et al. Growth and endotoxin production of *Yersinia enterocolitica* and *Enterobacter agglomerans* in packed erythrocytes. *J Clin Microbiol* 1989;27:1483–1485.
24. Richards C, Kolins J, Trindale CD. Autologous transfusion-transmitted *Yersinia enterocolitica* [Letter]. *JAMA* 1992;268:1541–1542.
25. Sire JM, Michelet C, Mesnard R, et al. Septic shock due to *Yersinia enterocolitica* after autologous transfusion [Letter]. *Clin Infect Dis* 1993;17:954–955.
26. Duncan KL, Ransley J, Elterman M. Transfusion-transmitted *Serratia liquefaciens* from an autologous blood unit [Letter]. *Transfusion* 1994; 34:738–739.
27. Haditsch M, Binder L, Gabriel C, et al. *Yersinia enterocolitica* septicemia in autologous blood transfusion. *Transfusion* 1994;34:907–909.
28. Cookson S. Personal communication—Centers for Disease Control. September 23, 1996.
29. Barrett BB, Andersen JW, Anderson KC. Strategies for the avoidance of bacterial contamination of blood components. *Transfusion* 1993; 33:228–233.
30. Halpin TJ, Kilker S, Epstein J, et al. Bacterial contamination of platelet pools. Ohio, 1991. *MMWR* 1992;41:36–37.
31. Claeys H, Verhaegle B. Bacterial screening of platelets. *Vox Sang* 2000; 78[Suppl 1]:P374(abst).
32. Schelstaete B, Bijnens B, Wuyts G. Prevalence of bacteria in leucode-

pleted pooled platelet concentrates and apheresis platelets: a 3 years experience. *Vox Sang* 2000;78[Suppl 1]:P373(abst).

33. Leiby DA, Kerr KL, Campos JM, et al. A retrospective analysis of microbial contaminants in outdated random-donor platelets from multiple sites. *Transfusion* 1997;37:259–263.
34. Dykstra A, Jacobs M, Yomtovian R. Prospective microbiologic surveillance (PMS) of random donor (RDP) and single donor apheresis platelets (SDP). *Transfusion* 1998;38[Suppl]:104S.
35. Blajchman MA, Ali A, Lyn P, et al. Bacterial surveillance of platelet concentrates: quantitation of bacterial load. *Transfusion* 1997; 37[Suppl]:74S.
36. Chiu EKW, Yuien KY, Lie AKW, et al. A prosective study of symptomatic bacteremia following platelet transfusion and its managment. *Transfusion* 1994;34:950–954.
37. Blajchman MA, Thornley JH, Richardson H, et al. Platelet transfusion-induced *Serratia marcescens* sepsis due to vacuum tube contamination. *Transfusion* 1979;19:39–44.
38. Engstrand M, Engstrand L, Hogman CF, et al. Retrograde transmission of *Proteus mirabilis* during platelet transfusion and the use of arbitrarily primed polymerase chain reaction for bacteria typing in suspected cases of transfusion transmission of infection. *Transfusion* 1995;35:871–873.
39. Morro JF, Braine HG, Kickler TS, et al. Septic reactions to platelet transfusions. A persistent problem. *JAMA* 1991;266:555–558.
40. Krishnan LS, Brecher ME. Transfusion transmitted bacterial infection. *Hematol Oncol Clin North Am* 1995;9:167–185.
41. Rhame FS, Root RK, MacLowry JD, et al. Salmonella septicemia from platelet transfusions. *Ann Intern Med* 1973;78:633–641.
42. Rhame FS, McCullough JJ, Cameron S, et al. *Pseudomonas cepacia* infections caused by thawing cryoprecipitate in a contaminated water bath. *Transfusion* 1979;19:653(abst).
43. Casewell MW, Slater NGP, Cooper JE. Operating theatre water-baths as a cause of *Pseudomonas* septicemia. *J Hosp Infect* 1981;2:237–240.
44. McClelland DB. Safety of human albumin as a constituent of biologic therapeutic products. *Transfusion* 1998;38:690–699.
45. Albumin recall. *Lancet* 1996;348:1026.
46. Steere AC, Tenney JH, Mackel DC, et al. *Pseudomonas* species bacteremia caused by contaminated normal human serum albumin. *J Infect Dis* 1977;135:729–733.
47. Wang SA, Tokars JI, Bianchine PJ, et al. *Enterobacter cloacae* bloodstream infections traced to contaminated human albumin. *Clin Infect Dis* 2000;30:35–40.
48. Grossman BJ, Kollins P, Lau PM, et al. Screening blood donors for gastrointestinal illness: a strategy to eliminate carriers of *Yersinia enterocolitica*. *Transfusion* 1991;31:500–501.
49. Gibson T, Norris W. Skin fragments removed by injection needles. *Lancet* 1958;2:983–985.
50. Lilly HA, Lowbury EJL, Wilkins MD. Limits to progressive reduction of resident skin bacteria by disinfecion. *J Clin Pathol* 1979;32: 382–385.
51. Anderson KC, Lew MA, Gorgone BC, et al. Transfusion-related sepsis after prolonged platelet storage. *Am J Med* 1986;81:405–411.
52. Goldman M, Roy G, Frechette, et al. Evaluation of donor skin disinfection methods. *Transfusion* 1997;37:309–312.
53. Olthuis H, Putlaert C, Verhagen C, et al. A simple method to remove contaminating bacteria during venipuncture. *Vox Sang* 1996; 70[Suppl 2]:113(abst).
54. Wagner SJ, Robinette D, Friedman LI, et al. Diversion of initial blood flow to prevent whole-blood contamination by skin surface bacteria: an in vitro model. *Transfusion* 2000;40:335–338.
55. Ness PM, Braine HG, Barrasso C, et al. Single donor platelets reduce the risk of septic transfusion reactions [Suppl]. *Transfusion* 1999;39: 89S(abst).
56. FDA committee endorses education and research to combat rare bacterial reaction: rejects operational changes for now. *Council of Community Blood Centers Newsletter* May 10, 1991:1–4.
57. FDA Blood Products Advisory Committee supports educational efforts on *Yersinia enterocolitica.Blood Bank Week* 1991;20:1–3.
58. Jensenius M, Hoel T, Heier HE. *Yersinia enterocolitica* septicemia after blood transfusion. *Tidsskr Nor Laegeforen* 1995;115:940–942.
59. Jacobs J, Jamaer D, Vandeven J, et al. *Yersinia enterocolitica* in donor blood: a case report and review. *J Clin Microbiol* 1989;27:1119–1121.
60. Donegan E, Lenes BA, Tomasulo PA, et al. Transmission of HIV-1 by component type and duration of shelf storage before transfusion [Letter]. *Transfusion* 1991;30:851–852.
61. Donegan E, Lee H, Operskalski EA, et al. Transfusion transmission of retroviruses: human T-lymphotropic virus types I and II compared with human immunodeficiency virus type 1. *Transfusion* 1994;34: 478–483.
62. Brecher ME, Hogan JJ, Boothe G, et al. The use of a chemiluminescence-linked universal bacterial ribosomal RNA gene probe and blood gas analysis for the rapid detection of bacterial contamination in white cell reduced and nonreduced platelets. *Transfusion* 1993;33:450–457.
63. Bacterial detection device. *Blood Bank Week* September 29, 1995:2.
64. Connor J, Currie LM, Allan H, et al. Recovery of in vitro functional activity of platelet concentrates stored at 4°C and treated with second-messenger effectors. *Transfusion* 1996;36:691–698.
65. Currie LM, Harper JR, Allan H, et al. Inhibition of cytokine accumulation and bacterial growth during storage of platelet concentrates at 4 degrees C with retention of in vitro functional activity. *Transfusion* 1997;37:18–24.
66. Brecher ME, Holland PV, Pineda A, et al. Bacterial growth in inoculated platelets: implications for bacterial detection and the extension of platelet storage. *Transfusion* 2000;40:1308–1312.
67. Kim DM, Brecher ME, Bland LA, et al. Prestorage removal of *Yersinia enterocolitica* from red cells with white cell-reduction filters. *Transfusion* 1992;32:658–662.
68. Buchholz DH, AuBuchon JP, Snyder EL, et al. Removal of *Yersinia enterocolitica* from AS-1 red cells. *Transfusion* 1992;32:667–672.
69. Gibb AP, Martin KM, Davidson GA, et al. Modeling the growth of *Yersinia enterocolitica* in donated blood. *Transfusion* 1994;34: 304–310.
70. Pietersz RNI, Reesink HW, Pauw W, et al. Prevention of *Yersinia enterocolitica* growth in red blood cell concentrates. *Lancet* 1992;340: 755–756.
71. Kim DM, Brecher ME, Bland LA, et al. Visual identification of bacterially contaminated red cells. *Transfusion* 1992;32:221–225.
72. Franzin L, Gioannini P. Growth of *Yersinia* species in artificially contaminated blood bags. *Transfusion* 1992;32:673–676.
73. Bradley RM, Gander RM, Patel SK, et al. Inhibitory effect of 0°C storage on the proliferation of *Yersinia enterocolitica* in donated blood. *Transfusion* 1992;37:691–695.
74. Pickard C, Herschel L, Seery P, et al. Visual identification of bacterially contaminated red blood cells. *Transfusion* 1998;38[Suppl]:12S.
75. Yomtovian R, Lazarus HM, Goodnough LT, et al. A prospective microbiologic surveillance program to detect and prevent the transfusion of bacterially contaminated platelets. *Transfusion* 1993;33: 902–909.
76. Chongokolwatana V, Morgan M, Feagin JC, et al. Comparison of microscopy and a bacterial DNA probe for detecting bacterially contaminated platelets. *Transfusion* 1993;33[Suppl]:50S.
77. Brecher ME, Boothe G, Kerr A. The use of chemiluminescence-linked universal bacterial ribosomal RNA gene probe and blood gas analysis for the rapid detection of bacterial contamination in white cell-reduced and nonreduced platelets. *Transfusion* 1993;33:450–457.
78. Arpi M, Bremmelgaard A, Abel Y, et al. A novel screening method for the detection of microbial contamination of platelet concentrates. An experimental pilot study. *Vox Sang* 1993;65:335–336.
79. Hogman CF, Gong J. Studies of one invasive and two noninvasive methods for detection of bacterial contamination of platelet concentrates. *Vox Sang* 1994;67:351–355.
80. Cortus M, Chong, Carmen R, et al. A new system to detect bacterial contamination in platelet concentrates. *Transfusion* 2000;440[Suppl]: 36S(abst).
81. Wenz B, Delgiacco G, Cortus MA, et al. A system designed to detect bacterial contamination in platelet concentrates. *Vox Sang* 2000; 78[Suppl 1]:65(abst).
82. Wagner SJ, Robinette D. Evaluation of swirling, pH, and glucose tests for the detection of bacterial contamination in platelet concentrates. *Transfusion* 1996;36:989–993.

83. Burstain JM, Brecher ME, Workman K, et al. Rapid identification of bacterially contaminated platelets using reagent strips: glucose and pH analysis as markers of bacterial metabolism. *Transfusion* 1997;37: 255–258.
84. Mhawech PY, Werch J, Stager C, et al. Detecting bacterial contamination in platelet concentrates using reagent strips—application in a major cancer center blood bank. *Transfusion* 1999;39[Suppl]: 36S–37S(abst).
85. Feng P, Keasler SP, Hill WE. Direct identification of *Yersinia enterocolitica* in blood by polymerase chain reaction amplification. *Transfusion* 1992;32:850–854.
86. Sen K. Rapid identification of *Yersinia enterocolitica* in blood by the 5′ nuclease PCR assay. *J Clin Microbiol* 2000;38:1953–1958.
87. Adams CP, Stone BB, Yan L, et al. Rapid detection of bacteria in platelets using a non-amplified nucleic acid probe assay. *Vox Sang* 2000;78[Suppl 1]:66.
88. Brecher ME, Means N, Jere CS, et al. Evaluation of the BacT/ALERT 3D microbial detection system for platelet bacterial contamination: an analysis of 15 contaminating organisms. *Transfusion* 2001;41: 477–482.
89. Wagner SJ, Robinette D. Evaluation of an automated microbiologic blood culture device for detection of bacteria in platelet components. *Transfusion* 1998;38:674–679.
90. Mitchell KT, Brecher ME. Approaches to the detection of bacterial contamination in cellular blood products. *Trans Med Rev* 1999;13: 132–144.
91. Dzik S, Aubuchon J, Jeffries L, et al. Leukocyte reduction of blood components: public policy and new technology. *Transfus Med Rev* 2000;14:34–52.
92. Wilkinson SL. Association Bulletin 99-7. American Association of Blood Banks.
93. Transcript of the Food and Drug Administration Blood Product Advisory Committee meeting, June 16, 2000. Available at http://www.fda-.gov/ohrms/dockets/ac/00/transcripts/3620t2.pdf.
94. Blajchman MA. The effect of leukodepletion on allogenic donor platelet survival and refractoriness in an animal model. *Semin Hematol* 1991;28[Suppl]:14–17.
95. Brecher ME, Pineda AA, Torloni AS, et al. Prestorage leukocyte depletion: effect on leukocyte and platelet metabolites, erythrocyte lysis, metabolism and in vivo survival. *Semin Hematol* 1991;28[Suppl]:3–9.
96. Heddle NM, Klama L, Singer J, et al. The role of the plasma from platelet concentrates in transfusion reactions. *New Engl J Med* 1994; 331:625–628.
97. Wenz B, Burns ER, Freundlich LF. Prevention of growth of *Yersinia enterocolitica* in blood by polyester fiber filtration. *Transfusion* 1992; 32:663–666.
98. Kim DM, Estes TJ, Brecher ME, et al. WBC filtration, blood gas analysis and plasma hemoglobin in *Yersinia enterocolitica* contaminated red cells. *Transfusion* 1992;32:41S.
99. Hogman CF, Gong J, Hambraeus A, et al. The role of white cells in the transmission of *Yersinia enterocolitica* in blood products. *Transfusion* 1992;32:654–657.
100. Vuetic D, Taseki J, Balint B, et al. The use of BacTAlert system for bacterial screening in platelet concentrates. *Vox Sang* 2000;[Suppl 1]: P371.
101. AuBuchon JP, Pickard C. White cell reduction and bacterial proliferation [Letter]. *Transfusion* 1993;33:533–534.
102. Buchholz DH, AuBuchon JP, Snyder EL, et al. Effects of white cell reduction on the resistance of blood components to bacterial multiplication. *Transfusion* 1994;34:852–857.
103. Sherburne B, McCullough A, Dzik WH, et al. Bacterial proliferation in platelet concentrates is unaffected by pre-storage leukocyte depletion. *Blood* 1991;78[Suppl]:350a.
104. Wenz B, Ciavarella D, Freundlich L. Effect of prestorage white cell reduction on bacterial growth in platelet concentrates. *Transfusion* 1993;33:520–523.
105. Food and Drug Administration. Proceedings of the 36th Meeting of the Blood Products Advisory Committee, Center for Biologist Evaluation and Research. Publication No. 92-026824, Rockville, MD: US Food and Drug Administration, May 29, 1992:440–445.
106. Pietersz RNI, Reesink HW, Dekker MA, et al. Elimination of *Yersinia enterocolitica* by a 20h hold of whole blood and removal of leukocytes by filtration. *Transfusion* 1992;32[Suppl]:253S(abst).
107. Seidl S. Syphilis screening in the 1990s. *Transfusion* 1990;30: 773–774.
108. Spangler AS, Jackson JH, Fiumara NJ, et al. Syphilis with a negative blood test reaction. *JAMA* 1964;189:87–90.
109. Van der Sluis JJ, Onvlee PC, Kothe FCHA, et al. Transfusion syphilis, survival of *Treponema pallidum* in donor blood I. Report of an orientating study. *Vox Sang* 1984;47:197–204.
110. Van der Sluis JJ, ten Kate FJW, Vuzevski VD, et al. Transfusion syphilis, survival of *Treponema pallidum* in donor blood II. Dose dependence of experimentally determined survival times. *Vox Sang* 1985;49:390–399.
111. Soendjojo A, Boedisantoso M, Ilias MI, et al. Syphilis *d'emblee* due to a blood transfusion. *Br J Venereal Dis* 1982;58:149–150.
112. Risseeuw-Appel IM, Kothe FC. Transfusion syphilis: a case report. *Sex Transm Dis* 1983;10:200–201.
113. Chambers RW, Foley HT, Schmidt PJ. Transfusion of syphilis by fresh blood components. *Transfusion* 1969;9:32–34.
114. Quinn TC, Cannon RO, Glasser D, et al. The association of syphilis with risk of human immunodeficiency virus infection in patients attending sexually transmitted disease clinics. *Arch Intern Med* 1990; 150:1297–1302.
115. Nelson KE, Vlahov D, Cohn S, et al. Sexually transmitted diseases in a population of intravenous drug users: association with seropositivity to the human immunodeficiency virus (HIV). *J Infect Dis* 1991; 164:457–463.
116. Potterat JJ. Does syphilis facilitate sexual acquisition of HIV? [Letter]. *JAMA* 1987;258:473.
117. Otten MW Jr, Zaidi AA, Peterman TA, et al. High rate of HIV seroconversion among patients attending urban sexually transmitted disease clinics. *AIDS* 1994;8:549–553.
118. Rosenblum L, Darrow W, Witte J, et al. Sexual practices in the transmission of hepatitis B virus and prevalence of hepatitis δ virus infection in female prostitutes in the United States. *JAMA* 1992;267: 2477–2481.
119. Thomas DL, Cannon RO, Shapiro CN, et al. Hepatitis C, hepatitis B, and human immunodeficiency virus infections among non-intravenous drug-using patients attending clinics for sexually transmitted diseases. *J Infect Dis* 1994;169:990–995.
120. Ollgaard M, Albjerg I, Georgen J. Monitoring of bacterial growth in platelet concentrates—one year's experience with the BactAlert System. *Vox Sang* 1998;74[Suppl 1]:1126(abst).
121. Laan E, Tros C. Improved safety and extended shelf-life of leucodepleted platelet concentrates by automated bacterial screening. *Transfusion* 1999;39[Suppl]:5S.
122. McDonald CP, Roy A, Lowe P, et al. The first experience in the United Kingdom of the bacteriological screening of platelets to increase shelf life to 7 days. *Vox Sang* 2000;[Suppl 1]:P375.
123. Cooper L, Leach MF, Tracy JE, et al. Application of a universal culturing approach to reduce the risk of bacterial contamination of apheresis platelet units. *Transfusion* 1999;39[Suppl]:119S–120S.
124. Knutson F, Alfonso R, Dupuis K, et al. Photochemical inactivation of bacteria and HIV in buffy-coat–derived platelet concentrates under conditions that preserve in vitro platelet function. *Vox Sang* 2000; 78:209–216.

Rossi's Principles of Transfusion Medicine, Third Edition, edited by Toby L. Simon, Walter H. Dzik, Edward L. Snyder, Christopher P. Stowell, and Ronald G. Strauss. Lippincott Williams & Wilkins, Philadelphia © 2002.

CASE 55A

IT AIN'T OVER 'TIL IT'S OVER

CASE HISTORY

A 36-year-old white male with a diagnosis of non-Hodgkin lymphoma, status post bone marrow transplantation and chemotherapy, came to the oncology clinic with severe thrombocytopenia. At the time of arrival, he had a white blood cell count of 3,100/μL with 50% polymorphonuclear cells and bands, and a platelet count of 8,000/μL. The patient's oncologist requested a five-unit pool of platelet concentrates be given.

Five units of 4-day-old cytomegalovirus-seronegative platelet concentrates were pooled and irradiated at 10:55 AM and signed out by the blood bank technologist at 11:33 AM.

The pooled platelet concentrates were administered at 12:00 noon through a leukoreduction filter. One and one-half hours into the transfusion and after 75 ml had been infused, the patient complained of chills, burning chest pain, and a headache. The transfusion was stopped immediately, and the transfusion service was notified. The platelet bag was returned to the blood bank, along with a posttransfusion blood sample from the patient. Shortly after, the patient spiked a temperature to 37.8°C and developed mild rigors. His blood pressure and pulse remained stable.

Vital signs before transfusion were temperature, 36.9°C; blood pressure, 120/70 mm Hg; heart rate, 78 beats/min; respiratory rate, 18 breaths/min. Two hours after the transfusion, the vital signs were temperature, 37.8°C; blood pressure, 126/75; heart rate, 75; respiratory rate, 20.

The patient was treated with 650 mg acetaminophen and 25 mg intramuscular meperidine hydrochloride; his symptoms resolved and he felt better by 2:20 PM. At that time, the posttransfusion reaction work-up from the blood bank was reported to be negative, including a negative direct antiglobulin test (DAT), no visible hemolysis, and no clerical errors found. The patient was evaluated by a transfusion medicine physician and was diagnosed with a probable febrile nonhemolytic transfusion reaction. His vital signs at 2:25 PM were stable, temperature, 36.7°C; blood pressure 115/78; heart rate, 75; respiratory rate 18.

DISCUSSION

An increase in temperature and chills after a blood transfusion could be the initial sign and symptom of several types of transfusion reactions, ranging from a benign febrile nonhemolytic transfusion reaction to a life-threatening hemolytic transfusion reaction, or a septic transfusion reaction. When a transfusion reaction such as this occurs, the infusion should be stopped immediately and the suspected transfusion reaction reported to the blood bank. The remainder of the implicated blood component(s) with tubing and attached fluids, the transfusion tag, and a blood sample from the patient should be sent to the blood bank. A posttransfusion platelet reaction work-up includes a clerical check to ensure that all identifying names and numbers are correct, and ABO/Rh retyping, DAT, and observation and evaluation of the sample for hemolysis or icterus are carried out.

In this case, the posttransfusion work-up was negative. In line with the findings that the patient had stable vital signs, mild chills, and a temperature elevation of less than 2°F (or 1°C), it seemed that the patient probably had a febrile nonhemolytic transfusion reaction (Fig. 55A.1).

Febrile nonhemolytic transfusion reactions are the most common type of transfusion reaction and often begin with fever, an increased temperature (often more than 1°C above baseline) and chills. They are mediated by cytokines produced during the storage of platelets or other blood products, or by cytokines generated when donor antigens react with antibodies present in the recipient. As a result of generalized use of prestorage leukoreduction filters, the incidence of febrile nonhemolytic transfusion reactions has decreased significantly (1).

CASE HISTORY, CONTINUED

At 3:30 PM, 3 hours after the transfusion, while sitting in the clinic awaiting discharge, the patient had a transient hypotensive episode (blood pressure dropped to 80/40) and a temperature rise to 40°C. Shortly after, he also developed severe rigors. He was immediately admitted to the emergency room and a working diagnosis of sepsis was made. The blood bank was quickly notified about the patient's new clinical symptoms. Blood cultures were drawn from the patient, and the blood bank sent the platelet bag to the laboratory to be evaluated for Gram stain and culture.

Subsequently, the patient remained febrile with a temperature of 40°C, and while in the emergency room his blood pressure dropped further to 63/21, with a pulse of 130 and a respiratory rate of 22. The patient was treated empirically with gentamicin and vancomycin and was admitted to the medical intensive care unit.

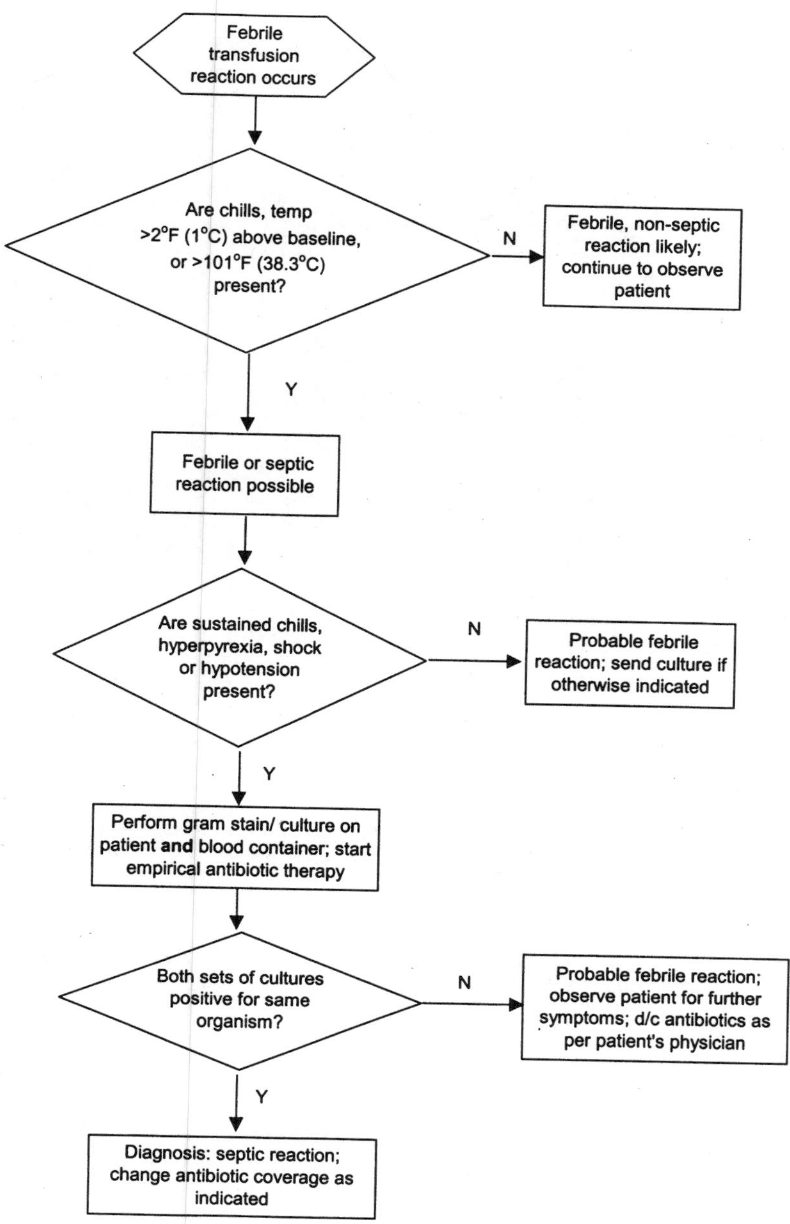

FIGURE 55A.1. Flow chart for work-up of febrile transfusion reaction.

DISCUSSION, CONTINUED

About 3 hours posttransfusion the patient's condition changed drastically, with a temperature elevation of more than 2°F (1°C) above baseline and over 101°F (38°C), along with rigors and hypotension. The diagnosis of a febrile nonhemolytic transfusion reaction had become less likely, based on the patient's worsening condition with an increased temperature and decreased blood pressure; a septic transfusion reaction thus had become more probable. In the case of a possible septic transfusion reaction, to trace the source of infection and to guide therapy, it is critical that specimens for Gram stain and culture of both the patient and the blood container be sent (Fig. 55A.1). While the results are pending, if clinically indicated, the patient should be treated empirically with antibiotics.

As exemplified here, all patients have their vital signs monitored closely posttransfusion, because transfusion reactions could become apparent up to several hours posttransfusion.

CASE HISTORY, CONTINUED

At 4:30 PM, gram-positive cocci were found in the bag of platelets that had been sent to the microbiology laboratory. At 4:40 PM, the local blood center that supplied the blood to the blood bank was notified of this finding.

On Day 2 at 9:00 AM the patient was stable with blood pressure, 102/65; heart rate, 100; respiratory rate, 23; and temperature, 37.8°C. All six of the patient's blood culture bottles (three aerobic and three anerobic) were reported as positive for growth, showing gram-positive cocci on Gram stain.

In response to questioning, the blood bank technologist stated that the platelets looked normal before pooling. Review of blood bank records showed that the platelet storage temperatures were all within required range (20° to 24°C).

At 2:00 PM, the microbiology laboratory reported that the organisms both in the patient's blood cultures and in the pooling bag were *Staphylococcus aureus,* based on colony morphology and biochemical profile. Both of the organisms were later found to be sensitive to cephalothin, chloramphenicol, clindamycin, gentamicin, oxacillin, tetracycline, trimethoprim and sulfamethoxazole, and vancomycin, but resistant to penicillin.

At 2:15 PM, the blood bank director notified the director of the local blood center of the positive culture reports.

At 5:00 PM, the patient was clinically stable with blood pressure, 90/60; pulse, 80; respiratory rate, 18; temperature 37.5°C; and was still maintained on gentamicin and vancomycin. Subsequently, by pulsed-field gel electrophoresis (Fig 55A.2), all bacteria were confirmed to be from identical strains.

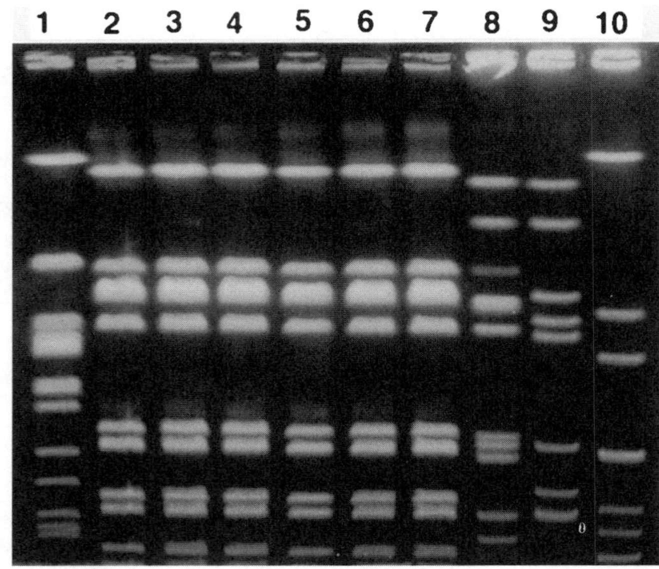

FIGURE 55A.2. Pulsed-field gel electrophoresis of whole cell DNA. Whole bacterial cell DNA was digested with restriction enzyme Sma I overnight, then incubated for 1 hour in TE (Tris-EDTA) buffer. The polarity of the electric field was switched every 5 to 35 seconds. The electrophoresis was run at 5°C for 23 hours at 198 volts. Note that the band patterns in lanes 2 through 7 are identical, showing that all of the bacteria in the samples were from the same strain. The patterns for lanes 8 to 10 are all different. These latter bacterial samples were of three different isolates of *S. aureus* obtained from three different patients.
Lane 1, molecular weight markers; *Lane 2,* patient's double lumen catheter, red port; *Lane 3,* patient's double lumen catheter, blue port; *Lane 4,* platelet pooling bag; *Lane 5,* first blood culture bottle drawn from patient; *Lane 6,* second blood culture bottle drawn from patient; *Lane 7,* blood culture from the corresponding red blood cell unit donated by the donor and quarantined by the blood supplier; *Lane 8,* sample of *Staphylococcus* isolate obtained from a different patient A; *Lane 9,* sample of *Staphylococcus* isolate obtained from a different patient B; *Lane 10,* sample of *Staphylococcus* isolate obtained from a different patient C.

DISCUSSION, CONTINUED

In the event of a positive culture result from any blood product, it is important to notify the patient's attending physician promptly so that appropriate therapy can be initiated (Fig. 55A.1). It is also crucial to notify the blood supplier so that other components (if any) from the same blood donation can be traced and quarantined pending further investigation. The blood supplier should also review donation records and interview the phlebotomist to assure that all procedures designed to prevent contamination of the collected blood were followed.

Pulsed-field gel electrophoresis has now become an important and reliable tool for bacterial identification and is being applied more and more for various epidemiologic studies (2). Basically, it is a fingerprinting technique. It can differentiate organisms based on heterogeneity of their DNA sequences. In principle, bacteria cells are placed into agarose plugs and lysed. Bacterial DNA is then digested with restriction enzymes, which cleave only at sites with a specific DNA sequence. Digested DNA fragments are then resolved by pulsed-field gel electrophoresis. As the name implies, during electrophoresis the polarity of the electric field is periodically reversed instead of remaining constant. As a result, relatively large DNA fragments can be separated cleanly. Restriction fragment length polymorphism (RFLP) patterns can be reliably generated. Based on whether organisms have the same or different RFLP, or fingerprints, it can be determined if they are derived from the same or different strains.

In this case, based on the identification of the same organism in the blood bag and in the patient by pulsed-field electrophoresis gel (Fig 55A.2), it is almost certain that the patient's bacteremia was due to contamination of a unit of platelets pooled for the implicated transfusion.

CASE HISTORY, CONTINUED

On Day 3 the director of the local blood center notified the director of the blood bank that all five units of red blood cells and fresh-frozen plasma (FFP) from the implicated donor units which made up the pool had been retrieved by the blood center, and that the implicated blood components and the corresponding blood donors would be evaluated.

Five days later, the local blood center reported that the culture of one red blood cell unit of the five implicated units was found to be positive for *Staphylococcus aureus.* Bacteria in that one red blood cell unit were subsequently found to have the identical sensitivity as the strain identified by the microbiology laboratory at the patient's hospital. The culture of the corresponding unit of the plasma was negative, as were those of the red blood cells and plasma of the other four implicated units.

Fourteen days later, after a full course of antibiotic treatment, the patient was discharged home with a referral to his primary care physician and a telephone number to call for follow-up. A sample of blood from the quarantined red blood cell unit was sent for pulsed-field gel electrophoresis and it, too, was found to contain a bacterial strain identical to the other samples from the patient and the platelet bag.

Review of the blood donor record disclosed that the donor had been afebrile and was acceptable by all health history criteria at the time of donation. The donor was contacted and gave a negative history for any signs or symptoms related to localized or systemic infection either before or after the donation. Prior to phlebotomy, the donor's antecubital areas had been inspected for scars, skin dimpling (pits), or evidence of intravenous drug use and were found to be negative.

The nurse who collected the unit was observed and found to be using proper preparation and phlebotomy technique. The blood center records did not show any evidence of product contamination or storage compromise.

DISCUSSION, CONTINUED

A culture of red blood cells from the implicated unit grew *S. aureus,* and this organism had the same antibiotic sensitivity as the *S. aureus* grown in the patient's blood culture and blood bag. This strongly suggests that bacterial contamination occurred at the time of donation. The contamination could be attributed to an asymptomatic donor infection, improper donor skin site preparation at the time of collection, improper handling of the blood units during processing, or another source. In this case, no clear source was ever identified.

Because platelets are stored at room temperature, the likelihood of contamination is much higher than other blood products (3–6). Indeed, the reported likelihood of platelet contamination has been reported as being several-fold higher than that of red blood cells. Fresh-frozen plasma cultures are almost always negative, such as was seen in this case, because these units are frozen within 8 hours of collection. Although the incidence of bacterial contamination of platelets is reported as 1:1,000 to 1:2,000, the incidence of a septic reaction after platelet transfusion is closer to 1:12,000 to 1:14,000. Septic transfusion reactions related to platelet infusion could develop as long as several hours after infusion, as was demonstrated in this case. Therefore, medical and nursing staff, as well as patients, should be warned about the signs and symptoms of a possible transfusion reaction. Optimally, arrangements should be made for a follow-up visit or for the patient to receive care in the emergency department in the event of a transfusion reaction which occurs after the patient has left the hospital outpatient or clinic area.

Case contributed by Yanyun Wu, M.D., and Edward L. Snyder, M.D., Yale-New Haven Hospital, New Haven, CT.

REFERENCES

1. Patterson BJ, Freedman J, Blanchette V, et al. Effect of premedication guidelines and leukoreduction on the rate of febrile nonhaemolytic platelet transfusion reactions. *Transfus Med* 2000;10:199–206.
2. Baribier N, Saulnier P, Chachaty E, et al. Random amplified polymorphic DNA typing versus pulsed-field gel electrophoresis for epidemiologic typing of vancomycin-resistant enterococci. *J Clin Microbiol* 1996; 34:953–958.
3. Illert WE, Sanger W, Weise W. Bacterial contamination of single-donor blood components. *Transfus Med* 1995;5:57–61.
4. Goldman M, Blajchman MA. Blood product–associated bacterial sepsis [Review]. *Transfus Med Rev* 1991;5:73–83.
5. Roth VR, Arduino MJ, Nobiletti J, et al. Transfusion-related sepsis due to *Serratia liquefaciens* in the United States. *Transfusion* 2000;8: 931–935.
6. Centers for Disease Control. Assessment of the frequency of blood component bacterial contamination association with transfusion reaction. (BaCon Study). Available at http://www.cdc.gov/ncidod/hip/bacon/index.htm.

56

PATHOGEN INACTIVATION IN BLOOD COMPONENTS

STEPHEN J. WAGNER

Careful donor selection and extensive laboratory testing have greatly improved the safety of the blood supply. Despite these measures, a small risk of virus transmission by transfusion still exists. Most transmission is thought to occur during the "window" period, prior to the development of antigen, antibody, or nucleic acid detectable by current test methods. The risk of viral transmission per unit has been estimated to be 1 in 1,000,000 for hepatitis A virus (HAV), 1 in 30,000 to 250,00 for hepatitis B virus (HBV), 1 in 223,000 for hepatitis C virus (HCV), 1 in 1,576,000 for human immunodeficiency virus (HIV), 1 in 250,000 to 2,000,000 for human T-cell lymphotropic viruses (HTLV) types 1 and 2, and 1 in 10,000 for human parvovirus B19 (1–3). Although these risks are generally considered to be low, more than one unit is typically transfused to patients, and their risk per transfusion is greater in proportion to the number of units transfused. In addition, the recent demonstration of transmission of HCV from a nucleic acid test (NAT)-negative unit, that was tested as a pool as well as a single unit, has emphasized that some residual risk will remain despite use of the most sensitive technology (4).

Second, a variety of viruses, bacteria, and parasites known to be capable of transmission by transfusion are currently not included in donor test screening. These pathogens may become more prevalent as donor demographics change.

Finally, there may be unrecognized or uncharacterized bloodborne agents which may become more prevalent. Because donor screening and testing are likely to be of limited use for reducing the risk of these agents, and improvements in screening and testing may not be able to substantially reduce the residual risk of known agents, appropriate pathogen reduction or inactivation methods represent an important additional safety measure in transfusion medicine.

S.J. Wagner: Product Development Department, American Red Cross Biomedical Services, Holland Laboratory for the Biomedical Sciences, Rockville, Maryland.

INACTIVATION

Plasma

Solvent-detergent Plasma

The solvent-detergent process for virus inactivation in fresh-frozen plasma (FFP) has been implemented after extensive in vitro and clinical studies. It uses thawed, group-specific, pooled plasma that is incubated at 30°C with 1% tri(n-butyl)phosphate and 1% of the nonionic detergent, Triton X-100, for 4 hours. Following incubation, the additives are removed via hydrophobic chromatography, and the plasma is sterile filtered and refrozen. Protein recovery and activity is generally more than 80% and coagulation factors are not activated. The 200-ml final product has a shelf life of more than 2 years when stored at −30°C. All tested enveloped viruses, including HIV, HBV, HCV, Sindbis, and vesicular stomatitis virus (VSV) are inactivated to the limit of detection (Table 56.1) (5). Extensive clinical studies support the general safety and efficacy of solvent-detergent plasma (6–8).

One disadvantage of the solvent-detergent process is the inability to inactivate nonenveloped viruses, such as HAV and human Parvovirus B19, in a pooled product (9). A phase IV clinical trial documented the seroconversion of 17 Parvovirus B19–seronegative individuals who were transfused with solvent-

TABLE 56.1. RANGE OF PATHOGENS AND TARGETS MODIFIED BY PATHOGEN INACTIVATION AGENTS

Inactivation Agent	Susceptible Pathogens	Target/Modification
Solvent-detergent	Enveloped viruses	Lipid envelope solubilization
S-59 + UVA	Intracellular viruses Enveloped viruses Intracellular viruses Some nonenveloped viruses Bacteria not including spores	Pyrimidine adducts and cross-links
Riboflavin plus light	Enveloped viruses Intracellular viruses Some nonenveloped viruses Bacteria (spores unknown)	Guanine oxidation and potential adducts to thymine or adenine
Methylene blue plus light	Enveloped viruses Some nonenveloped viruses	Guanine oxidation
S-303	Enveloped viruses Intracellular viruses Some nonenveloped viruses Bacteria (spores unknown)	Nucleic acid adducts and cross-links
PEN 110	Enveloped viruses Intracellular viruses Nonenveloped viruses Bacteria (spores unknown)	Guanine adducts
Pc 4 plus light	Enveloped viruses Intracellular viruses	Lipid envelope oxidation
DMMB plus light	Enveloped viruses Intracellular viruses Some nonenveloped viruses	Nucleic acid oxidation

UVA, ultraviolet A; DMMB, 1, 3-dimethoxy-5-methylbenzene.

detergent FFP units with $>10^7$ genome equivalents of Parvovirus B19 (10). No seroconversion was observed from individuals transfused with solvent-detergent units containing $<10^4$ genome equivalents of Parvovirus B19 (10). These results provided the rationale for Parvovirus B19 NAT testing of plasma minipools and final solvent-detergent plasma production of only those lots with $<10^4$-genome equivalents per milliliter. Finally, a cluster of fatal thrombotic events or excessive bleeding in liver transplant patients infused with solvent-detergent–treated plasma and other blood components was observed at a single institution (11). Complications from liver transplants are common, and no evidence has yet been identified that causally links the adverse events with the solvent-detergent product.

An improved version of the solvent-detergent process that would eliminate the need for group-specific plasma is being investigated. The process uses ligands to remove anti-A and anti-B group-specific antibodies from plasma, rendering it universal. Clinical trials of the universal solvent-detergent process are ongoing.

S-59 and Ultraviolet A Light

The structure of the synthetic psoralen, 4′-(4-amino-2-oxa)butyl-4,5′,8′-trimethylpsoralen, S-59 (Fig. 56.1), has been disclosed. S-59 and 3 J/cm^2 of long-wavelength ultraviolet (UVA) light has been used to inactivate viruses in single units of fresh human plasma containing 150 μmol/L of the drug. The method is based on light-activated adduct formation between the psoralen and pyrimidine residues in nucleic acid, resulting in DNA or RNA adduct formation and intrastrand cross-links (Table 56.1). In vitro studies have demonstrated inactivation of extracellular and cell-associated HIV (>5.9 and 6.4 $\log_{10}$, respectively), bovine viral diarrhea virus (BVDV) (5.4 $\log_{10}$), and duck hepatitis B virus (DHBV) (6.7 $\log_{10}$) in plasma (12). In addition, S-59 phototreatment has been shown to inactivate >4.5 $\log_{10}$ HCV and HBV in a chimpanzee infectivity model (13). Following photoinactivation, levels of unbound S-59 were reduced by using an affinity adsorption device and the treated plasma was frozen. Thawed phototreated units had satisfactory factor activities for fibrinogen (87%) and factors V (98%), VII (86%), VIII (73%), IX (95%), X (98%), and XI (91%) (12). No neoantigenicity against S-59 and UVA–treated plasma was observed in Ouchterlony assays (15).

In the Ames bacterial mutagenicity test using the *Salmonella* tester strain, TA1537, S-59 was positive at 44 and 103 μg per ml when samples were incubated in the absence or presence of metabolic activation (14). Use of the S-59 affinity removal device improves the genotoxicity profile of the compound.

Several clinical studies have been conducted with S-59 and UVA–treated plasma. A phase I stepwise ascending-dose clinical trial showed no adverse clinical reactions in 15 healthy subjects transfused with 1 liter of S-59 phototreated or control plasma. Subjects had similar factor activities prior to and following transfusion (16). Another clinical study in healthy subjects showed that the clearance, half-life, and mean residence time of factor VII was similar in subjects receiving control or S-59 and

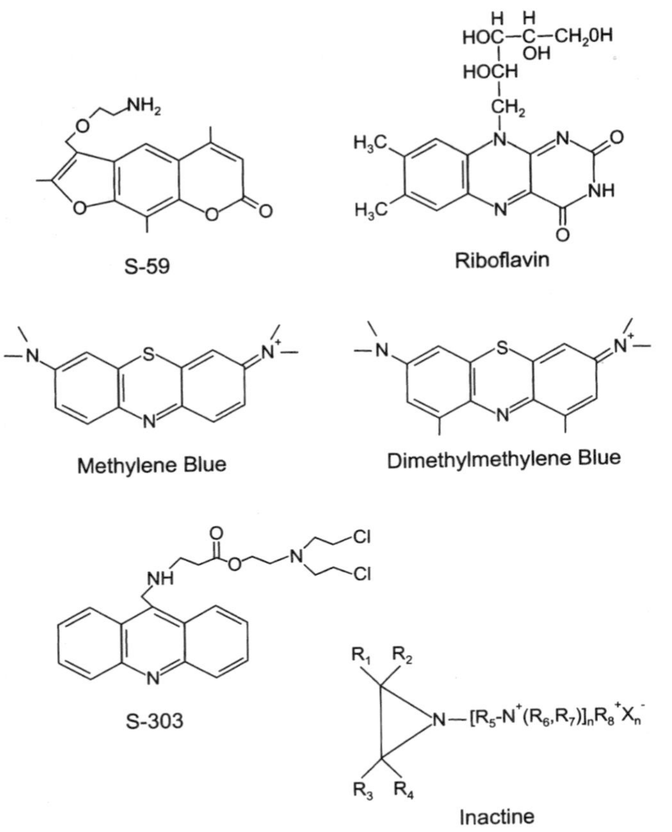

FIGURE 56.1. Structures and general formula for pathogen inactivation agents.

UVA–treated plasma to reverse a deliberate warfarin decrement in vitamin K–dependent clotting activities. Comparable vitamin K–dependent factor II, VII, IX, and X activities were also observed in subjects receiving phototreated and control plasma (17). In yet another clinical trial, investigators evaluated the ability of control or S-59 and UVA–treated plasma to reverse acquired coagulopathy due to liver disease in 13 patients. The prothrombin time (PT) and partial thromboplastin time (PTT) were found to be equivalent in patients receiving control FFP or those receiving S-59 phototreated plasma after data were normalized for FFP dose and patient weight (18). Finally, an open-label trial for reversal of congenital coagulation factor deficiencies has been initiated using S-59 and UVA–treated plasma. Preliminary data indicate all transfusions were well tolerated and achieved adequate homeostasis. For nine patients, mean initial recovery factor activities were: factor 1 (0.94 mg/dl)/(mg/kg), (n = 2); factor II (1.24 IU/dl)/(IU/kg); factor V (1.56 IU/dl)/(IU/kg), (n = 3); factor VII (1.19 IU/dl)/(IU/kg), and factor XI (1.67 IU/dl)/(IU/kg), (n = 2) (19).

Riboflavin and Light

Preliminary investigations have been conducted with vitamin B_2, or riboflavin, and light for pathogen inactivation in plasma. In the presence of light, riboflavin has been shown to generate oxidative damage to guanine and may form adducts with thymine or adenine (Table 56.1) (20,21). Riboflavin has a favorable toxicology profile; its primary photoproduct in neutral pH, lumichrome, is routinely produced in infants treated for hyperbilirubinemia with no adverse effects. Use of 10 mmol/L riboflavin and the quencher, ascorbic acid (10 mmol/L), with 250 J/cm^2 light from a halogen source resulted in ≥80% retention of factor VIII, IX, X, and fibrinogen activities. Factor V was more sensitive to riboflavin-mediated damage, with only 65% activity recovered following phototreatment. No virus inactivation data in plasma have been published, although similar conditions in platelets suspended in 90% plasma and 10% synthetic media resulted in >4 to 5 $\log_{10}$ inactivation of intracellular and extracellular HIV, BVDV, pseudorabies virus, HSV-1 and -2, and vaccinia virus (22).

Methylene Blue and Light

The virucidal action of illuminated phenothiazines, such as methylene blue, has been recognized for 70 years (23). These planar compounds appear to interact with nucleic acids through intercalative binding and produce singlet oxygen-mediated damage, primarily to nucleic acid guanosine residues (Table 56.1), upon illumination with red light (24,25). Seminal studies by Hiatt et al. in the 1950s demonstrated photoinactivation of a number of viruses in plasma by phenothiazines, with retention of electrophoretic properties of albumin and fibrinogen (26). Later work by Mohr in FFP documented inactivation of >6 $\log_{10}$ extracellular HIV-1 and Semliki Forest virus, and approximately 5 or more $\log_{10}$ inactivation of HSV and VSV with 1 μmol/L of methylene blue and 60 minutes of illumination with a 75-W halogen bulb (50,000 lux). Factor activities, including factors II, V, VII, VIII, IX, X, XI, XII, and antithrombin III, were reported to be >80% following phototreatment; however, factor 1 and C1 inactivator were more susceptible to photoinduced damage with 79.6% and 76.8% activity remaining, respectively, after phototreatment. Thrombin times of phototreated units were prolonged by approximately 25% (27). Methylene blue has routinely been used intravenously for the treatment of methemoglobinemia at >1,000-fold the levels used for virus inactivation (28). Genotoxicity studies suggest the compound is mildly positive in the mouse lymphoma–forward mutation assay in the presence of metabolic activation using concentrations three-fold greater than those used to photoinactivate viruses in plasma. However, a positive response was not elicited at any dose in the in vivo mouse micronucleus assay (29).

One problematic feature of methylene blue is that the dye does not effectively inactivate intracellular virus, such as cell-associated forms of HIV (30). The hydrophilicity of the dye has been postulated to inhibit permeation of the compound through plasma membranes and thus prevent inactivation of intracellular virus (31). Mohr et al. originally included a freeze-thaw step in their protocol that was designed to inactivate lymphocytes; however, later studies by Wieding documented substantial levels of viable leukocytes remaining after the freeze-thaw process (32). Residual leukocytes in the photoinactivation system have been eliminated by the development of a 0.2- to 1.0-μm–pore size plasma membrane filter (33); use of these types of filters reduced the infectivity of an HIV-infected Molt-4 line to the limits of detection (34). Other filters have been developed that simultaneously remove leukocytes and methylene blue by a filter element coupled to activated charcoal adsorbent (35).

A large number of units of methylene blue–phototreated plasma have been reported to be infused in Germany and other European countries, with adverse reactions similar in frequency, type, and severity to those associated with untreated plasma (36). Despite being included in the Guidelines for Blood Transfusion Services in the United Kingdom, leukocyte-depleted methylene blue–treated plasma has not gained acceptance from other European regulatory authorities.

Red Blood Cell Components

Alkylating Agents

FRALE Compounds

Frangible anchor linker effector compounds, or FRALE compounds, are alkylating agents which specifically inactivate virus via covalent adducts to viral nucleic acid (Table 56.1). The compounds consist of a nucleic acid–binding ligand that serves as an anchor and promotes nucleic acid specificity, an alkylating agent that functions as an effector, and an alkyl chain that joins the two moieties (37). The inventors designed the alkyl chain to be cleaved upon contact with blood to yield a negatively charged anchor at a rate slower than the rate of alkylation to nucleic acid. This would not inhibit pathogen inactivation, yet would help break down residual unreacted compound to negatively charged products that do not further interact with nucleic acid. Examples of anchors include intercalators such as psoralens, phenothiazines, and acridines; minor groove binders such as mitomycin and certain Hoerst dyes; major groove binders such as aflatoxins, electrostatic binders (phosphate backbone binders) such as spermidine; or nucleic acids themselves, which promote triple helix formation. The structure of the FRALE compound β-alanine, N-(acridin-9-yl), 2-(bis[2-chloroethyl]amino)ethyl ester, or S-303, has been disclosed in a patent application and appears in Figure 56.1 (38).

Investigators have used 150-μmol/L S-303 to inactivate >6 $\log_{10}$ of intracellular and extracellular HIV, DHBV, BVDV, VSV, HSV, and >4 $\log_{10}$ of the bacteria *Y. enterocolitica, S. marcescens,* and various species of *Salmonella, Pseudomonas,* and *Staphylococcus* in packed red blood cells at 60% hematocrit (39, 40). Under these conditions, levels of red blood cell hemolysis, adenosine triphosphate (ATP), 2,3-diphosphoglycerate (2,3-DPG, also known as 2,3-bisphosphoglycerate), glucose, and lactate were similar in treated and control units after 42 days of storage at 1° to 6°C (39). The 24-hour recovery of human red blood cells treated with 150 μmol/L S-303, stored for 35 days, and autologously infused resulted in 78.7 ± 5.69% 24-hour recovery, compared with 83.9 ± 6.05% recovery for untreated red blood cells (40). In a second clinical study, control and S-303-transfused subjects that were enrolled from the first trial received five infusions of S-303-treated red blood cells over a 35-day period, and the final infusion contained a radiolabel substance for 24-hour recovery measurements. The control group that later received five S-303 infusions had a 24 hour recovery of 84.2 ± 6.4%, and the S-303 group in the first clinical trial that received five additional S-303 infusions had a 24-hour recovery of 78.1 ± 6.1% (41).

Genotoxicity testing has been reported with one of the anchor linker effector compounds. The compound, quinacrine mustard, has structural similarities to S-303 and is highly mutagenic (thousands of histidine revertants per plate) in the Ames test system (TA 1537 indicator strain) using nanomolar concentrations of the compound in water or in red blood cells (37). Other quinacrine mustard studies have demonstrated positive results in the mouse lymphoma–forward mutation assay and sister chromatid exchanges in human chromosomes (42,43). Quinacrine mustard is degraded by prolonged incubation with red blood cell suspensions, and incubation with adsorbents such as Amberlite XAD-16 or activated charcoal can reduce its concentration. Breakdown and depletion of quinacrine mustard can reduce the number of colonies observed in the Ames test system to levels similar to an untreated control (37). However, use of highly genotoxic alkylating compounds necessitates that the concentration of the agent be carefully measured after the removal and breakdown steps, using highly sensitive and validated analytic chemistry assays capable of measuring to the picomolar level, in order to be convinced that levels of residual compound are well below those concentrations that cause mutagenesis in model systems. Finally, use of highly genotoxic compounds in the workplace may necessitate increased regulation in order to ensure occupational safety.

Aziridine Compounds

Aziridine compounds, such as ethyleneimine and its N-acetyl derivative, have been used in sera to produce vaccines for the past 30 years. The method inactivates both enveloped and nonenveloped viruses, including members of the difficult-to-inactivate Parvoviridae family (44). Inactivation of canine parvovirus suggests that ethyleneimine is small enough to permeate virus capsid pores. Although its mechanism of inactivation is not well characterized, virucidal treatment inhibits the ability to amplify viral and cell sequences following polymerase chain reaction (45), presumably by alkylation of nucleic acid via nucleophilic attack of guanine residues (Table 56.1). Virucidal concentrations of ethyleneimine (mmol/L range) (46) do not affect antigenicity or immunogenicity of viral proteins (47), do not impair the growth-promoting capacity of bovine serum in cell culture, and do not affect the antibody activity of guinea pig hyperimmune serum (46). Nevertheless, some amino acids in proteins such as lysozyme react with ethyleneimine (48), indicating that the compound does not react exclusively with nucleic acid.

The selectivity of aziridines for nucleic acids was improved by forming oligomers of ethyleneimine (49). Presumably, this was achieved by creating regularly spaced positive charges in the alkyl chain oligomer that would be electrostatically attracted to a polyanion such as nucleic acid. Approaches along these lines have been taken by a group of investigators to develop compounds for pathogen inactivation of red blood cells. The generic structure of these compounds, called inactines, has been disclosed in a patent application and appears in Figure 56.1 (50). Studies suggest that use of the inactine compound, PEN110, results in >5 $\log_{10}$ inactivation of porcine parvovirus, BVDV, extracellular HIV-1, and VSV in red blood cell concentrates (51). Other studies demonstrate >5 log_{10} inactivation of cell-associated HIV (52). In a phase I clinical trial, red blood cells were treated with 0.1% PEN110 for 6 hours at room temperature, radiolabeled, extensively washed, and subsequently treated with sodium thiosulfate to quench residual PEN110 prior to 28-day refrigerated storage and autologous infusion. These treatment conditions resulted in undetectable levels of the agent (<50 ng/ml), ≈250% increase in day-28 hemolysis (0.48 ± 0.15 versus 0.19 ± 0.1%), 59% reduced glucose consumption, 43% reduced lactate production, and 53% reduced ATP levels relative to untreated controls. Nevertheless, radiolabeled studies of treated and control red blood cell suspensions stored for 28 days demonstrated similar 24-hour recovery and survival (53).

There are no published studies of the genotoxicity of PEN110. Testing of other aziridine alkylating agents demonstrates the potential for mutagenesis, sister chromitid exchanges, and induction of micronuclei (54–56). If PEN110 has significant genotoxicity, additional safeguards and increased regulation of the workplace may be required to ensure staff safety.

Photosensitizers

Phthalocyanines

The silicon phthalocyanine dye, Pc4, has a planar structure which, like porphyrin, has a central chelating metal: $HOSiPc\text{-}OSi(CH_3)_2\text{-}(CH_2)_3N(CH_3)_2$. A hydrophobic compound, Pc4 cannot easily be formulated in water and tends to localize in membranes. In order to protect red blood cells from Pc4-mediated oxidative damage, various quenchers must be added to red blood cells and Pc4 must be added separately in a liposome formulation. Fifty milliliters of red blood cell concentrates containing 0.8 mmol/L tocopherol succinate, 4 mmol/L cysteine, 0.4 mmol/L carnitine, and 5μmol/L Pc4 were treated with 18 J/cm^2 of 670-nm red light, and resulted in reductions of >5.5 log_{10} HIV-1, >6.3 log_{10} VSV, >5.0 log_{10} PRV, and >5.0 log_{10} BVDV. Phototreatment of 350-ml volumes of red blood cell concentrates required 40 J/cm^2 light to achieve the same levels of virus inactivation as 50-ml samples with 18 J/cm^2 light. Under conditions used to treat 350-ml red blood cell concentrates, significantly more hemolysis (0.6%) is observed following 28 days of refrigerated storage compared with untreated controls (0.2%). In baboon red blood cell recovery and life span studies, Pc4-phototreated cells had a 15.9% reduction of 24-hour recovery and 26.7% reduction in 24-hour recovery relative to control values. Genotoxicity studies of Pc4 and photoproducts were negative on the Ames test, mouse lymphoma–forward mutation assay, and micronucleus test (57).

Dimethylmethylene Blue and Light

The structure of the photoactive phenothiazine, dimethylmethylene blue (DMMB), is given in Figure 56.1. Based on results from equilibrium dialysis experiments, DMMB strongly binds to nucleic acid (58). Deoxyribonucleic acid intercalation of DMMB has been demonstrated by diminution of fluorescence, red shift in the absorption maximum, and induced circular dichroism when DMMB is incubated with DNA (59). In the presence of oxygen, DMMB monomers absorb red light and inactivate virus by damaging viral nucleic acid (58,60).

Treatment of 30%-hematocrit red blood cell suspensions using 4-micromolar DMMB and 13.5-J/cm^2 cool white light resulted in >4.4-log_{10} inactivation of VSV, >5-log_{10} inactivation of pseudorabies virus, >4.7-log_{10} inactivation of bovine virus diarrhea virus, 5.8-log_{10} inactivation of bacteriophage $\phi6$, and 7.3-log_{10} inactivation of bacteriophage R17. Unlike methylene blue, DMMB can photoinactivate intracellular virus. Using an infectious center assay, >3 log_{10} of cell-associated VSV and >4.8 log_{10} cell-associated pseudorabies viruses were inactivated using 4-μmol/L DMMB and 13.5 J/cm^2 cool white light. The increased hydrophobicity of the compound compared to methylene blue has been attributed to improved plasma membrane permeation and inactivation of intracellular virus (61). In additional studies using higher-hematocrit red blood cells, DHBV was shown to be considerably more sensitive to photoinactivation than VSV (62). Another useful target for photoinactivation of cellular blood components are T lymphocytes, which play a crucial role in the development of transfusion-associated graft versus host disease. Based on studies using limiting dilution assays, virucidal treatment of red blood cell suspensions with DMMB and light has been shown to inactivate T lymphocytes by >5 log_{10} (63).

Treatment of red blood cells with DMMB under virucidal conditions resulted in no detectable immunoglobulin G (IgG) binding in 11 of 13 samples, unchanged red blood cell morphology, normal banding patterns of red blood cell membrane proteins on sodium dodecyl sulphate–polyacrylamide gel electrophoresis (SDS-PAGE), and unaltered characteristics of 12 of 13 red blood cell antigens during storage as measured by antibody titration (61). In addition, minimal changes were observed in red blood cell osmotic fragility, hemolysis, potassium efflux, ATP, and 2,3-DPG levels, and the strength of one Duffy system red blood cell antigen, Fy^a, during storage of phototreated samples compared to controls (61).

No genotoxicity studies of DMMB have been reported. Phenothiazines of similar structure, such as methylene blue, have been shown to be modestly positive on the mouse lymphoma–mutation assay, but negative on in vivo mouse micronucleus tests (29).

Platelet Components

Riboflavin and Light

Inactivation of viruses in platelet concentrates by the vitamin, riboflavin, and light has been studied. Treatment of apheresis platelets suspended in 20% plasma and 80% synthetic media with 10 μmol/L of riboflavin and 40, 80, and 120 J/cm^2 of 419-nm light resulted in 3.1, ≈4, and 6.6 log_{10} inactivation of BVDV, respectively (64). Bovine viral diarrhea virus is reported to be the enveloped virus most resistant to riboflavin photoinactivation. Platelet suspensions containing 20% plasma were treated with 10 μmol/L of riboflavin and 80 J/cm^2 419-nm light and resulted in similar extracellular pH and morphology following 5-day storage. However, these treatment conditions caused a 32.2% decrease in hypotonic shock response, 27.8%

TABLE 56.2. 24-HOUR SURVIVAL AND RECOVERY OF AUTOLOGOUS CYNOMOLGUS MONKEY PLATELETS TREATED WITH RIBOFLAVIN AND LIGHT

Plasma Concentration[a] (%)	Light Dose[b] (J/cm²)	24-Hour Recovery (% Decline)	Survival (% Decline)
90	40	3.4	16.0
90	80	No decline	23.3
30	40	No decline	36
30	80	65.6	33.1

Platelet suspensions were not stored prior to infusion.
[a] Riboflavin concentration: 10 Mmol.
[b] Light (360–460 nm).
J, joules.

increase in lactate concentration, and a 65% increase in P selectin levels compared to untreated controls at day 5 of storage (64). Additional studies were conducted in cynomolgus monkeys to determine the posttransfusion recovery and survival of radiolabeled platelets suspended in 30% or 90% plasma and treated with 10 μmol/L of riboflavin and 360- to 460-nm light (65). Results are given in Table 56.2. Although all treatment conditions reduced platelet life span by 16% to 36%, conditions using 90% plasma resulted in greater platelet survival than those using 30% plasma. Platelet 24-hour recoveries were similar to controls for all conditions tested except for the marked 64% reduction in survival observed in platelets suspended in 30% plasma and treated with 80 J/cm^2 of light. The extent of BVDV inactivation has not been reported for conditions used in the cynomolgus monkey study.

Psoralens and Ultraviolet A Light

The synthetic psoralen, S-59, has been used in the photochemical inactivation of pathogens in platelet components suspended in 30% plasma and a synthetic medium. Investigators have used 150 μmol/L of S-59 and 3 J/cm^2 of UVA to inactivate >6.6 $\log_{10}$ of intracellular and extracellular HIV, inhibition of expression of integrated HIV, >6.8 $\log_{10}$ inactivation of DHBV, >6.5 $\log_{10}$ inactivation of BVDV, >5.5 $\log_{10}$ inactivation of HBV, >4.5 $\log_{10}$ inactivation of HCV, as well as >5 $\log_{10}$ inactivation of *S. epidermidis* and *K. pneumoniae* (66,67). Other bacteria are also sensitive to S-59 and UVA. Bacterial spores, however, are resistant to photoinactivation (68).

As previously discussed, S-59 is mutagenic in the Ames test. An adsorption device reduces levels of unbound S-59 to approximately 25 μg in a 300-ml apheresis unit (69). In a trial investigating S-59 pharmacokinetics following infusion of residual S-59 from 300 ml of UVA-exposed and S-59-depleted apheresis platelets, recipients attained peak plasma levels of 988 pg/ml; levels declined to 293 pg/ml 1 hour after transfusion.

Leukocytes have been implicated in several adverse outcomes of transfusion ranging from transfusion-associated graft versus host disease (TAGVHD) to febrile reactions. Because psoralen phototreatment produces nucleic acid adducts that inhibit replication, S-59 phototreatment should inhibit leukocyte proliferation and thus prevent TAGVHD. Results from laboratory studies indicate that S-59 and UVA treatment inactivates >5.5$\log_{10}$ T cells (70). In a murine bone marrow transplant model of GVHD, Grass et al. demonstrated that S-59 phototreatment of 10^8 donor leukocytes prevented GVHD in a γ-irradiated heterozygous recipient (71). When recipient mice were infused with untreated leukocytes in this system, they developed severe TAGVHD, as measured by spleen weight, thymocyte count, percentage of lysis of target host cells, and white blood cell count. Unlike mice receiving phototreated leukocytes, recipients infused with untreated leukocytes eventually died. Further investigation will be required to determine if S-59 phototreatment can replace γ-irradiation for prevention of TAGVHD. In addition to inhibiting DNA replication and leukocyte proliferation, S-59 phototreatment should inhibit RNA transcription and thus prevent the induction of cytokine synthesis in leukocytes during platelet storage. Studies by Hei et al. have confirmed this hypothesis (72). Some investigators believe that cytokines play an important role in transfusion-associated febrile reactions (73).

Platelet in vitro properties have been studied after treatment with 150-μmol/L S-59 and UVA light during 5 days of storage. Photochemically treated platelets maintained pH, pCO_2, HCO_3-, platelet count, morphology, plasma glucose, plasma lactate, percentage of aggregation, secretory ATP, platelet shape change, and hypotonic shock response similar to untreated controls. Levels of P selectin expression and PO_2 were 13% and 20% greater, respectively, than untreated controls (67). In a rhesus monkey autologous transfusion model using four animals, the posttransfusion recovery and survival of S-59 and UVA–treated and control platelets were comparable to those of untreated platelets (66). Treatment of human platelets with S-59 and UVA did not result in the production of neoantigens in rabbits, as measured by crossed immunoelectrophoresis or flow cytometry assays (74).

Platelet recovery and survival of S-59 and UVA–treated platelets were measured in a clinical trial using healthy, normal subjects. Photochemically treated platelets stored for 5 days had a 15.5% reduced survival and 20.9% reduced life span compared to untreated platelets stored for 5 days. Despite the reduction in platelet survival and life span, results from S-59 and UVA–treated platelets were within the lower ranges of published values (75). In a further study, investigators combined S-59 phototreatment with γ-irradiation (2,500 cGy) and evaluated in vivo platelet viability following 5 days of storage. Platelets subjected to photochemical treatment and γ-irradiation had no additional reduction of in vivo platelet viability compared to photochemically treated platelets (76). The therapeutic efficacy of S-59 and UVA–treated platelets versus control platelets was investigated in profoundly thrombocytopenic patients in another clinical trial. Infusion of photochemically treated or control platelets in 13 of the patients resulted in a similar reduction (ranging from 38% to 71%) of patient bleeding time relative to bleeding times prior to transfusion. Comparison of responses to control and phototreated platelets in five additional patients revealed that those receiving phototreated platelets had 23.7% reduction of 1-hour count increment, 20.3% reduction of 24-hour count increment, 31.5% reduction of 1-hour corrected count increment, and 29.5% reduction of 24-hour corrected count increment compared to recipients infused with control platelets (77). A European phase III trial using S-59 and UVA–treated buffy-coat platelets for support of 100 thrombocytopenic patients has been completed. Results suggest that a similar number of patients had major hemorrhage, transfusion reactions, or refractory transfusions in control and photochemically treated arms. Recipients in the photochemically treated platelet group required 33.9% more platelet transfusions with 9.3% fewer platelets per transfusion than that of the control group. However, the total number of platelets used per patient in the control and treated arms was equivalent. Finally, the 24-hour corrected count increment of patients receiving photochemically treated platelets was 31% less than patients receiving untreated platelets, while the 1-hour corrected count increment was similar in control and photochemically treated groups (78). A similar but larger trial involving 600 thrombocytopenic patients is currently being conducted in the United States.

SUMMARY

An inactivation method to eradicate enveloped pathogens in pooled units of FFP has been implemented. Alternative photochemical methods for pathogen inactivation of single units of FFP are in clinical or preclinical development. For red blood cells, investigators have studied the use of alkylating agents or photochemicals for pathogen inactivation. Two methods employing alkylating agents have reached clinical trials; however, use of genotoxic agents may require changes in the current workplace to ensure worker safety. The use of a synthetic psoralen and UVA to eradicate pathogens in platelet components has been studied extensively in preclinical trials and is currently being evaluated in a large pivotal study. An alternative photoinactivation method using vitamin B_2, or riboflavin, is in preclinical development. In summary, pathogen inactivation methods for all blood components are being investigated extensively. Current inactivation methods can potentially prevent the transmission of known and unknown infectious agents from blood, yet may also introduce some less desirable outcomes of the technology, such as small reductions of cellular circulatory life span or functionality, increased complexity and regulation of component processing, the need for additional safety measures to protect blood center staff, environmental issues regarding genotoxic waste disposal, and infusion of residual drugs and breakdown products to recipients.

ACKNOWLEDGMENTS

The author gratefully acknowledges the continued support from the American Red Cross Biomedical Services and from the National Heart Lung and Blood Institute (1 RO1 HL53418 and 1 RO1 HL66779).

REFERENCES

1. Schreiber GB, Busch MP, Kleinman SH, et al. The risk of transfusion-transmitted viral infections. *N Engl J Med* 1996;334:1685–1689.
2. In vitro inactivation of viruses in blood components, RFA HL-00-010, National Heart, Blood and Lung Insititute, January 18, 2000.
3. Stramer SL. Nucleic acid testing for transfusion-transmissible agents. *Curr Opin Hematol* 2000;7:387–391.
4. Schuttler CG, Caspari G, Jursch CA, et. al. Hepatitis C virus transmission by a blood donation negative in nucleic acid amplification tests for viral RNA. *Lancet* 2000;355:41–42.
5. Horowitz B, Lazo A, Grossberg H, et al. Virus inactivation by solvent/detergent treatment and the manufacture of SD-plasma. *Vox Sang* 1998;74[Suppl]:203–206.
6. Beck KH, Mortelsman Y, Kretschmer V, et al. Comparison of solvent/detergent–inactivated plasma and fresh frozen plasma under routine clinical conditions. *Infus Ther Transfus Med* 2000;27:144–148.
7. Baudoux E, Margraff U, Coenen A, et al. Hemovigilance: clinical tolerance of solvent-detergent treated plasma. *Vox Sang* 1998;74[Suppl 1]: 237–239.
8. Horowitz MS, Pehta JC. SD plasma in TTP and coagulation factor deficiencies for which no concentrates are available. *Vox Sang* 1998; 74[Suppl 1]:231–235.
9. Koenigbauer UF, Eastlund T, Day JW. Clinical illness due to parvovirus B19 infection after infusion of solvent/detergent-treated pooled plasma. *Transfusion* 2000;40:1203–1206.
10. Davenport R, Geohas G, Cohen S, et al. Phase IV study of PLAS + SD: hepatitis A (HAV) and parvovirus B19 (B19) safety results. *Blood* 2000; 96:(abst).
11. Available at: www.fda.gov/medwatch/safety/2000/safety00.htm# plassd.
12. Alfonso R, Lin C, Dupuis K, et al. Inactivation of viruses with preservation of coagulation function in fresh frozen plasma. *Blood* 1996;88: 526a(abst).
13. Corten L, Wiesehahn G, Smyers JM, et al. Photochemical inactivation of hepatitis B (HBV) and hepatitis C (HCV) viruses in human plasma as assessed in a chimpanzee infectivity model. *Blood* 2000;96[Suppl 1]: 60a(abst).
14. Ciaravino V. Preclinical safety of a nucleic acid-targeted helix compound: A clinical prospective. *Semin Hemotol* 2001;38(4 Supp II): 12–19.
15. Damonte B, Behrman D, Hei G, et al. A comparative analysis of the antigen composition of native plasma to photochemically treated (PCT) plasma using the Ouchterlony assay. *Blood* 1997;90[Suppl 1]: 129b(abst).
16. Wages D, Smith D, Walsh J, et al. Transfusion of therapeutic doses of virally inactivated fresh frozen plasma in healthy subjects. *Blood* 1997;90[Suppl 1]:409a(abst).
17. Wages D, Radu-Radurescu L, Adams M, et al. Quantitative analysis of coagulation factors in response to transfusion of S-59 photochemically treated fresh frozen plasma. *Blood* 1998;92[Suppl 1]:503a(abst).
18. Wages D, Bass N, Keefe E, et al. Treatment of acquired coagulopathy by transfusion of fresh frozen plasma (FFP) prepared using a novel,

single unit photochemical pathogen inactivation (P.I.) process. *Blood* 1999;94[Suppl 1]:247a(abst).

19. DeAlercon P, Benjamin R, Shopnick R, et al. An open-label trial of fresh frozen plasma (FFP) treated by the Helinx single-unit photochemical pathogen inactivation system in patients with congenital coagulation factor deficiencies. *Blood* 2000;96[Suppl 1]:61a(abst).
20. Mori, T, Tano K, Takimoto K, et al. Formation of 8-hydroxyguanine and 2,6-diamino-4-hydroxy-5-formamidopyrimidine in DNA by riboflavin mediated photosensitization. *Biochem Biophys Res Commun* 1998;242:98–101.
21. Ennever JF, Speck WT. Short communication. Photochemical reactions of riboflavin: covalent binding to DNA and to poly (dA). poly (dT). *Pediatr Res* 1983;17:234–236.
22. Goodrich RP. The use of riboflavin for the inactivation of pathogens in blood products. *Vox Sang* 2000;78[Suppl 2]:211–215.
23. Clifton CE. Photodynamic action of certain dyes on the inactivation of staphylococcus bacteriophage. *Proc Soc Exp Biol Med* 1931;28: 745–746.
24. Hagmar P, Pierrou S, Nielsen P, et al. Ionic strength dependence of the binding of methylene blue to chromatin and calf thymus DNA. *J Biomolec Struct Dyn* 1992;9:667–679.
25. Buchko GW, Wagner JR, Cadet J, et al. Methylene blue–mediated photooxidation of 7,8-dihydro-8-oxo-2′-deoxyguanosine. *Biochim Biophys Acta* 1995;1263:17–24.
26. Heimets F, Kingston JR, Hiatt CW. Inactivation of viruses in plasma by photosensitized oxidation. Walter Reed Army Inst Res Report Number 1955;53–55.
27. Lambrecht B, Mohr H, Knuver-Hopf J, et al. Photoinactivation of viruses in human fresh plasma by phenothiazine dyes in combination with visible light. *Vox Sang* 1991;60:207–213.
28. Bodansky O. Methemoglobinemia and methemoglobin-producing compounds. *Pharmacol Rev* 1951;3:144–196.
29. Wagner SJ, Cifone MA, Murli H, et al. Mammalian genotoxicity assessment of methylene blue in plasma: implications for virus inactivation. *Transfusion* 1995;35:407–413.
30. Wagner SJ, Robinette D, Storry J, et al. Differential sensitivities of viruses in red cell suspensions to methylene blue photosensitization. *Transfusion* 1994;34:521–526.
31. Skripchenko A, Robinette D, Wagner SJ. Comparison of methylene blue and methylene violet for photoinactivation of intracellular and extracellular virus in red cell suspensions. *Photochem Photobiol* 1997; 65:451–455.
32. Wieding JU, Vehmeyer K, Dittman J, et al. Contamination of fresh-frozen plasma with viable white cells and proliferable stem cells. *Transfusion* 1994;34:185–186.
33. Walker WH, inventor. Blood bag system for the inactivation of pathogens in blood, blood components and plasma. European patent application EP 0933090 A1, January 21, 1999.
34. Abe H, Yamada-Ohnishi Y, Hirayama J, et al. Elimination of both cell-free and cell-associated HIV infectivity in plasma by a filtration/methylene blue photoinactivation system. *Transfusion* 2000;40: 1081–1087.
35. AuBuchon JP, Pickard C, Herschel L, et al. Removal of methylene blue from plasma via an adsorbent filter. *Vox Sang* 1998;74:1–6.
36. Mohr H, Pohl U, Lambrecht B, et al. Methylene blue/light treatment of virus inactivated plasma: production and clinical experience. *Infus Ther Transfus Med* 1993;20[Suppl 2]:19–24.
37. Cook D, Wollowitz D, inventors. Method for inactivating pathogens in red cell compositions using quinacrine mustard. US patent 5691132, November 25, 1997.
38. Greenman WM, Grass JA, Talib S, et al., inventors. Method of treating leukocytes, leukocyte compositions and methods of use thereof. European patent application WO 9903976, July 21, 1998.
39. Cook, D, Stassinopoulos A, Merritt J, et al. Inactivation of pathogens in packed red blood cells (PRBC) concentrates using S-303. *Blood* 1997;90S:409a(abst).
40. Cook D, Stassinopoulos A, Wollowitz S, et al. In vivo analysis of packed red blood cells treated with S-303 to inactivate pathogens. *Blood* 1998; 92[Suppl 1]:503a(abst).
41. Hambleton J, Greenwalt T, Viele M, et al. Post transfusion recovery after multiple exposures to red blood cell concentrates (RBCS) treated with a novel pathogen inactivation (P.I.) process. *Blood* 1999;94[Suppl 1]:376a(abst).
42. Rogers AM, Back KC. Comparative mutagenicity of 4 DNA-intercalating agents in L5178Y mouse lymphoma cells. *Mutat Res* 1982;102: 447–455.
43. Haglund U, Zech L. Simultaneous staining of sister chromatid exchanges and Q-bands in human chromosomes after treatment with methyl methane sulphonate, quinacrine mustard and quinacrine. *Hum Genet* 1979;49:307–317.
44. Press T, Kamstrup S, Kyvsgaard NC, et al. Comparison of two different methods for inactivation of viruses in serum. *Clin Diagn Lab Immunol* 1997;4:504–508.
45. Groseil C, Guerin P, Adamowicz P. Evaluaton by polymerase chain reaction on the effect of β-propiolactone and binary ethyleneimine on DNA. *Biologicals* 1995;23:213–220.
46. Bahnemann HG. Inactivation of viruses in serum with binary ethyleneimine. *J Clin Microbiol* 1976;3:209–210.
47. Hulskotte EG, Ding ME, Norley SG, et al. Chemical inactivation of recombinant vaccinia viruses and the effects on antigenicity and immunogenicity of recombinant simian immunodeficiency virus envelope glycoproteins. *Vaccine* 1997;15:1839–1845.
48. Yamada H, Imoto T, Noshita S. Modification of catalytic groups in lysozyme with ethylenimine. *Biochemistry* 1982;21:2187–2192.
49. Budowsky EI, Zalesskaya MA, Nepomnyashchaya M, et al. Principles of selective inactivation of the viral genome: dependence of the rate of viral RNA modification on the number of protonizable groups in ethyleneimine oligimers. *Vaccine Res* 1996;5:29–39.
50. Budowsky EL, Ackerman SK, Purmal AA, et al., inventors. Methods and compositions for the selective modification of nucleic acids. US patent 6093564, 2000.
51. Purmal A, Zhang QX, Edson C. INACTINE—A method to inactivate non-enveloped and enveloped viruses in red blood cell concentrates. *Blood* 1998;92[Suppl 2]:136b(abst).
52. Lazo A, Tassello J. Viral inactivation of U1 cell-associated HIV in red blood cell concentrates treated with the INACTINE technology. *Transfusion* 2000;40[Suppl]:38S(abst).
53. AuBuchon JP, Pickard CA, Herschel LH, et al. In vivo recovery of red blood cells virally inactivated by INACTINE and stored for 28 days. *Blood* 2000;96[Suppl 1]:818a–819a(abst).
54. Valencia R, Mason JM, Woodruff RC, et al. Chemical mutagenesis testing in *Drosophila*. III. Results of 48 coded compounds tested for the National Toxicology Program. *Environ Mutagen* 1985;7:325–348.
55. Nishi Y, Hasegawa MM, Taketomi M, et al. Comparison of 6-thioguanine-resistant mutation and sister chromatid exchanges in Chinese hamster V79 cells with forty chemical and physical agents. *Cancer Res* 1984;44:3270–3279.
56. Siboulet R, Grinfeld S, Deparis, et al. Micronuclei in red blood cells of the newt *Pleurodeles waltl Michah:* induction with X-rays and chemicals. *Mutat Res* 1984;125:275–281.
57. Ben-Hur E, Chan WS, Yim CZ, et al. Photochemical decontamination of red blood cell concentrates with the silicon phthalocyanine Pc4 and red light. In: Brown F, Vyas, eds. *Advances in transfusion safety, developments in biologicals,* vol 102. Basel: S Karger, 1999:149–156.
58. Wagner SJ, Skripchenko, A, Robinette D, et al. Factors affecting virus photoinactivation by a series of phenothiazine dyes. *Photochem Photobiol* 1998;67:343–349.
59. Mohammad T, Morrison H. Photonuclease activity of Taylor's blue. *Bioorg Med Chem Lett* 1999;9:2249–2254.
60. Skripchenko A, Wagner SJ. Identification of the target responsible for M13 virus inactivation by dimethylmethylene blue and light treatment. *Transfusion* 2000;40[Suppl]:37S(abst).
61. Wagner SJ, Skripchenko A, Robinette D, et al. Preservation of red cell properties after virucidal phototreatment with dimethylmethylene blue. *Transfusion* 1998;38:729–737.
62. Wagner SJ, Skripchenko A, Pugh JC, et al. Comparison of the sensitivity of duck hepatitis B and vesicular stomatitis virus to photoinactivation by dimethylmethylene blue. *Transfusion* 2000;40[Suppl]: 99S(abst).
63. Skripchenko A, Wagner SJ: Photoinactivation of leukocytes in erythro-

cyte suspensions: comparison of methylene blue and dimethylmethylene blue. *Transfusion* 2000;40:968–975.
64. McBurney LL, Goodrich TB, Hansen ET. The use of riboflavin for the viral inactivation of platelets. *Transfusion* 2000;40[Suppl]:37S(abst).
65. Tay-Goodrich BH, Schuyler RJ, Goodrich RP, et al. Evaluation of in-vivo survival of photochemically treated platelet concentrates in non-human primates. *Transfusion* 2000;40[Suppl]:38S(abst).
66. Lin L, Cook DN, Wiesehahn GP, et al. Photochemical inactivation of viruses and bacteria in platelet concentrates by use of a novel psoralen and long-wavelength ultraviolet light. *Transfusion* 1997;37:423–435.
67. Lin L, Corten L, Murthy KK, et al. Photochemical inactivation of hepatitis B (HBV) and hepatitis C (HCV) virus in human platelet concentrates as assessed by a chimpanzee infectivity model. *Blood* 1998; 92[Suppl 1]:502a(abst).
68. Knutson F, Alfonso R, Dupuis K, et al. Photochemical inactivation of bacteria and HIV in buffy-coat–derived platelet concentrates under conditions that preserve in vitro platelet function. *Vox Sang* 2000;78: 209–216.
69. Corash LM, Paton V, Wages D, et al. S-59 clearance and kinetics after transfusion of platelets treated with HELINX technology. *Transfusion* 2000;40[Suppl]:37S(abst).
70. Grass JA, Hei DJ, Metchette K, et al. Inactivation of leukocytes in platelet concentrates by photochemical treatment with psoralen plus UVA. *Blood* 1998;91:2180–2188.
71. Grass J, Wafa T, Reames A, et al. Prevention of transfusion-associated graft versus host disease (TA-GVHD) by photochemical treatment (PCT). *Blood* 1996;88[Suppl 1]:627a(abst).
72. Hei DJ, Grass J, Lin L, et al. Elimination of cytokine production in stored platelet concentrate aliquots by photochemical treatment with psoralen plus ultraviolet A light. *Transfusion* 1999;39:239–248.
73. Heddle NM, Klama L, Meyer R, et al. A randomized controlled trial comparing plasma removal with white cell reduction to prevent reactions to platelets. *Transfusion* 1999;39:231–238.
74. Behrman B, Damonte P, Metchette K, et al. Lack of neoantigenicity of human platelet concentrates treated with a novel psoralen and UVA. *Blood* 1996;88[Suppl 1]:335a(abst).
75. Corash L, Behrman B, Rheinschmidt M, et al. Post-transfusion viability and tolerability of photochemically treated platelet concentrates. *Blood* 1997;90[Suppl 1]:267a(abst).
76. Corash L. Inactivation of infectious pathogens and leukocytes in platelet concentrates, In: Seghatchian J, Snyder EL, Krailadsiri P, eds. *Platelet therapy: current status and future trends.* New York: Elsevier Science, 2000:439–466.
77. Slichler SJ, Corash L, Grabowski M, et al. Viability and hemostatic function of photochemically treated (PCT) platelets (PLTS) in thrombocytopenic patients. *Blood* 1999;94[Suppl 1]:376a(abst).
78. Van Rhenen D, Gulliksson H, Pamphilon D, et al. S-59 (HELINX) photochemically treated platelets (plt) are safe and effective for support of thrombocytopenia: results of the EUROSPRITE phase 3 trial. *Blood* 2000;96[Suppl 1]:819a(abst).

Rossi's Principles of Transfusion Medicine, Third Edition, edited by Toby L. Simon, Walter H. Dzik, Edward L. Snyder, Christopher P. Stowell, and Ronald G. Strauss. Lippincott Williams & Wilkins, Philadelphia © 2002.

PART II
Transfusion Reactions

57

HEMOLYTIC TRANSFUSION REACTIONS

ROBERTSON D. DAVENPORT

CLINICAL SPECTRUM

A hemolytic transfusion reaction (HTR) is the accelerated clearance or lysis of transfused red blood cells due to immunologic incompatibility. It is distinguished from other causes of shortened survival of transfused red blood cells that may be due to autoimmune hemolysis or nonimmune causes. Hemolytic transfusion reaction may occur when antigen-positive red blood cells are transfused to a patient with a preexisting alloantibody, or when a recently transfused patient makes a new alloantibody.

The great majority of HTRs are due to red blood cell transfusions. However, HTRs may also result from transfusion of plasma containing blood components, which contain red blood cell antibodies but very few, if any, red blood cells, such as fresh frozen plasma or platelet concentrates (1,2). Occasionally, an HTR may be due to incompatibility between red blood cells from one donor and antibody-containing plasma from a different donor transfused to the same recipient (3).

R.D. Davenport: Department of Pathology, University of Michigan and Blood Bank and Transfusion Service, University of Michigan Health Center, Ann Arbor, Michigan.

INCIDENCE

The actual incidence of HTRs is difficult to determine. In some cases the correct diagnosis is not made or is not reported. Delayed HTRs may be particularly hard to distinguish from more common conditions such as infection. Concomitant liver disease or bleeding may also make a definite diagnosis difficult.

The reported incidence of HTRs depends to some degree on the recipient patient population and is likely to be higher in academic medical centers with heavily transfused patient populations. Reports from blood centers have largely relied on surveys of transfusion services, which may result in underestimation. Improvement in antibody identification techniques over time, as well as increased knowledge of immunohematology, has undoubtedly resulted in a progressive decrease in HTRs.

Estimates of the incidence of HTR derived from both blood centers and transfusion services are summarized in Table 57.1. Some reports do not differentiate between acute and delayed reactions or between intravascular and extravascular hemolysis. Serologic and hemolytic transfusion reactions have not necessarily been differentiated, particularly in early reports. Overall, there has been an apparent increase in the incidence of delayed HTRs

TABLE 57.1. ESTIMATED INCIDENCE OF HEMOLYTIC TRANSFUSION REACTIONS

Study Setting	Time Period	HTR Risk Estimate Per Unit Transfused
Overall HTR (Acute and Delayed Reactions Not Differentiated)		
Blood center (77)	1981–1987	1:15,605
Oncology patients (78)	1974–1981	1:35,739
Acute HTR		
Tertiary care medical center (18)	1964–1973	1:12,100
Tertiary care medical center (25)	1974–1977	1:21,222
Reported transfusion errors[a] (23)	1990–1999	1:77,000
Delayed HTR		
Tertiary care medical center (79)	1964–1973	1:11,652
Tertiary care medical center[b] (25)	1974–1977	1:4,015
Tertiary care medical center (6)	1980–1992	1:5,405
Blood center (80)	1980–1981	1:6,875
Tertiary care medical center (5)	1986–1987	1:9,094
Tertiary care medical center (81)	1974–1978	1:2,339

HTR, hemolytic transfusion reaction.
[a] Clinical reactions in ABO transfusion errors.
[b] Same institution as previous, improved serologic detection.

and a decrease in acute HTRs with time. A higher rate of delayed reactions may be a reflection of improved serologic detection. Because most patients receive more than one unit of red blood cells, estimates of the incidence of HTR per transfused patient range from 1:854 to 1:524, which is higher than the incidence per unit transfused (4–6). The population incidence rate of delayed HTR has been estimated at 1.69 events per 100,000 population per year (4).

Hemolytic transfusion reactions are classified as acute or delayed reactions, based on whether they occur within or after 24 hours of the implicated transfusion. A more important distinction is between intravascular and extravascular hemolytic reactions. Intravascular hemolysis is characterized by hemoglobinemia and hemoglobinuria. In contrast, extravascular hemolysis lacks these dramatic signs but is characterized by shortened survival of transfused red blood cells along with the accumulation of hemoglobin breakdown products. Generally, intravascular hemolysis is seen with acute HTRs, while extravascular hemolysis is usually seen in delayed reactions. This distinction is not absolute, however. Occasional acute reactions result in extravascular hemolysis while some intravascular hemolytic reactions are delayed.

Accelerated clearance of incompatible red blood cells is an essential feature of HTRs. Transfusion may also stimulate the production of alloantibody without hemolysis. This phenomenon has been termed delayed serologic transfusion reaction (DSTR) and needs to be differentiated from delayed HTR (5, 6). Delayed serologic transfusion reaction is clinically benign. Earlier reports of hemolytic reactions have not necessarily differentiated clearly between serologic and true hemolytic reactions.

SIGNS AND SYMPTOMS

There is a broad range of initial clinical symptoms of HTR. The typical progression of intravascular and extravascular hemolysis is shown in Figures 57.1 and 57.2. In all cases, there is an unexpected degree of anemia due to the loss of transfused red blood cells. In some cases, particularly with extravascular hemolysis, this may be the only clue to HTR. Some reactions, both immediate and delayed, are asymptomatic. In intravascular hemolysis, however, most symptomatic patients experience fever and sometimes chills. Nausea or vomiting, pain, dyspnea, and hypotension or tachycardia are also common initial symptoms. The reported pain may be localized to the infusion site, back, flanks, chest, groin, or head. A subjective feeling of distress is sometimes reported. The cause of pain in HTR is unclear, but is most likely due to direct stimulation of nociceptive nerves in perivascular tissue by bradykinin generated from activation of the complement system (7).

In extravascular hemolysis, fever and sometimes chills are the most commonly reported initial symptoms. Jaundice also may be an initial sign, because elevation of serum bilirubin occurs with both intravascular and extravascular hemolysis. The degree of hyperbilirubinemia depends upon the patient's liver function and rate of red blood cell destruction. Conjugated and unconjugated bilirubin fractions tend to follow a parallel course, peaking at the same time (8). δ-Bilirubin, a minor albumin-bound fraction, persists past the peak of total bilirubin and may be a useful clue to previous hemolysis.

An acute HTR usually occurs during or shortly after the offending transfusion. The time from transfusion to symptoms of delayed HTR is quite variable. Although most delayed reactions become apparent within 2 weeks after transfusion, initial symptoms may occur more than 6 weeks later, due to the time required for antibody production.

COMPLICATIONS

In addition to loss of transfused cells, there may be evidence of complement deposition on autologous red blood cells, with a

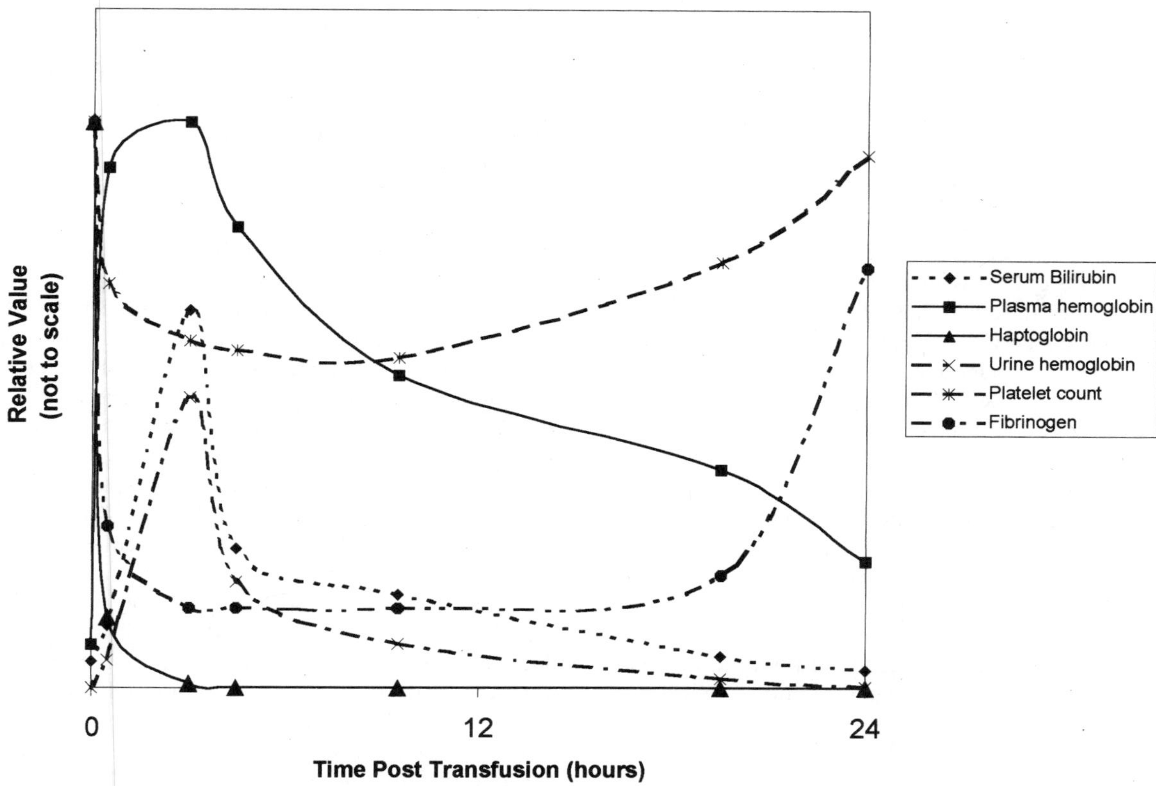

FIGURE 57.1. Time course of hemolytic and coagulation parameters in intravascular HTR. (From Duvall CP, Alter HJ, Rath CE. Hemoglobin catabolism following a hemolytic transfusion reaction in a patient with sickle cell anemia. *Transfusion* 1974;14:382–387, with permission.)

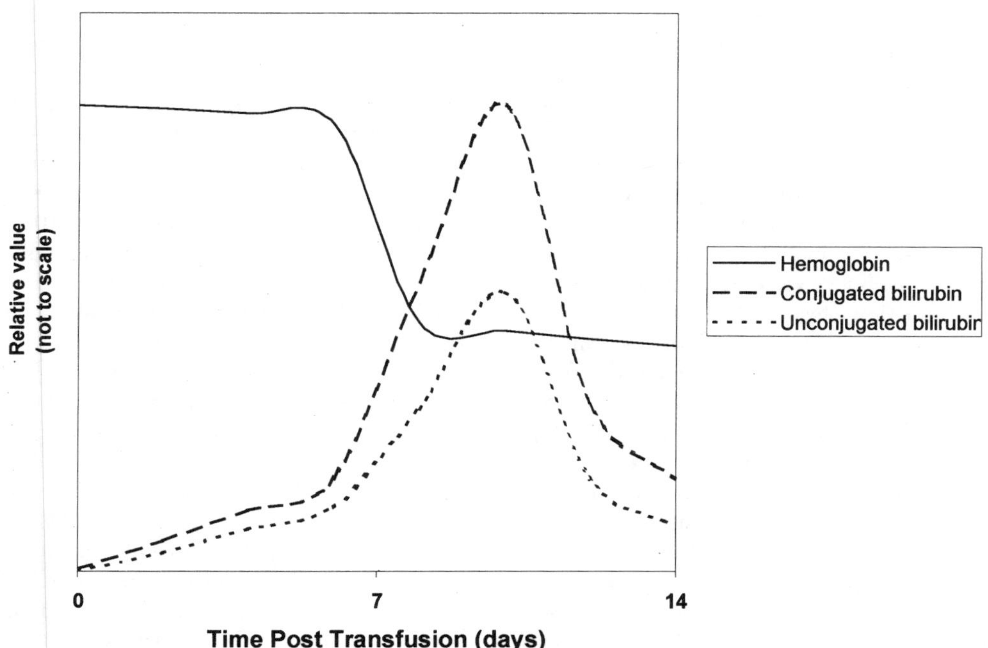

FIGURE 57.2. Time course of hemolytic parameters in extravascular hemolysis. (From Cummins D, Ferrier A, Murphy F. Bilirubinuria, conjugated hyperbilirubinaemia and δ-bilirubinaemia following acute haemolysis. *Ann Clin Biochem* 1997;24:109–110, with permission.)

positive direct antiglobulin test (DAT) due to C3 persisting for up to 100 days (9). This phenomenon has been called "bystander hemolysis." The absence of antiimmunoglobulin G (anti-IgG) reactivity in the DAT and the lack of autoantibody in the eluate often differentiate bystander hemolysis from autoimmune hemolytic anemia (AIHA).

Although in most cases the loss of autologous red blood cells is slight, a sickle cell crisis can be precipitated by an HTR in patients with sickle cell disease. Factors that contribute to the occurrence of sickle cell crisis include increased oxygen consumption due to fever, the relative loss of circulating hemoglobin A compared to hemoglobin S, and the release of vasoactive mediators causing reduction of local blood flow. Hemolytic transfusion reactions may be particularly severe in patients with sickle cell disease. In such reactions the degree of anemia may actually be greater than before transfusion, probably because of bystander hemolysis of autologous red blood cells. This phenomenon has been termed the sickle cell–hemolytic transfusion reaction syndrome (10). This diagnosis may be obscured, however, by suppression of erythropoiesis from hypertransfusion. The complete loss of transfused red blood cells several weeks after exchange transfusion may result in a more severe anemia than before transfusion. Thus, one explanation of this syndrome has been that the apparent loss of autologous red blood cells is not due to hemolysis but rather to underproduction. However, recent studies have shown that the corrected reticulocyte count actually increases during delayed HTR, and the absolute number of hemoglobin S–containing red blood cells similarly may increase (10,11). Pain crisis in a patient with sickle cell disease following transfusion should suggest the occurrence of sickle cell–hemolytic transfusion reaction syndrome. Further transfusion in this setting may exacerbate the anemia and even prove fatal. Serologic studies may not provide an explanation for HTR in these patients. In addition, the presence of multiple alloantibodies may make the serologic diagnosis difficult.

Hypotension occurs in some cases of intravascular HTR but is rare in extravascular reactions. Complement activation is likely to be the most important determining factor. The anaphylatoxins C3a, C4a, C5a, and C5a-des-arg are released during immune hemolysis. Additionally, the kinin pathway is activated, leading to generation of bradykinin. The proinflammatory cytokines, tumor necrosis factor and interleukin-1, produced by phagocytes during HTR, also may contribute to hypotension and shock.

Impairment of renal function may occur in both intravascular and extravascular HTRs, although it is more common in the former. The degree of renal function abnormality varies from an asymptomatic elevation of serum blood urea nitrogen (BUN) and creatinine to complete anuria. Renal failure is mostly due to acute tubular necrosis. Both hypotension and intravascular coagulation contribute to renal impairment. Thrombus formation in renal arterioles due to disseminated intravascular coagulation (DIC) may cause cortical infarcts. Free hemoglobin has been thought to be a major cause of renal failure. However, experience with purified hemoglobin-based oxygen-carrying solutions, which do not damage the kidneys, calls this assumption into question (12). On the other hand, hemoglobin binds bacterial endotoxin and increases the toxicity of lipopolysaccharide (LPS). Hemoglobin in the glomerular filtrate may deliver endotoxin to renal tubules in a septic patient, contributing to tubular cell damage.

Intravascular hemolysis may also cause labile blood pressure through alterations in the metabolism of the potent physiologic vasodilator nitric oxide (NO). Nitric oxide can combine with heme and thiol groups of hemoglobin (13). In oxyhemoglobin, nitric oxide causes reduction of ferrous iron (Fe^{2+}) to form ferric methemoglobin (Hb[Fe^{3+}]). Nitric oxide combines with deoxyhemoglobin to form Hb(Fe^{2+})NO but does not cause reduction. Scavenging of nitric oxide by free hemoglobin through these pathways results in vasoconstriction and hypertension. Nitric oxide can also combine with cysteine on the β-globin chain to form S-nitrosohemoglobin (SNO-Hb). This process is reversible, so SNO-Hb can act as an nitric oxide donor with resultant vasodilation. Free hemoglobin reacts with nitric oxide much more rapidly than do red blood cells (14). The effects of intravascular hemolysis may be very similar to that caused by the infusion of stroma-free hemoglobin. Indeed, prominent hypertensive effects limited early trials of hemoglobin solutions as a blood substitute (15).

Disseminated intravascular coagulation occurs in intravascular HTR but is relatively rare. Rarer still is the occurrence of DIC in extravascular HTR. The production of proinflammatory cytokines is likely to be a major factor in DIC. It can be difficult to distinguish DIC from other causes of coagulopathy, particularly in massive transfusion or liver disease. Uncontrolled bleeding due to DIC may be the initial manifestation of an acute HTR, particularly in the intraoperative setting. Unfortunately, if HTR is not recognized early in this situation, more incompatible blood may be transfused in an attempt to keep up with blood loss. In one report, out of 35 patients experiencing HTR while under anesthesia, nine received four to six additional units due to excessive bleeding (16).

Fatality due to HTR is usually associated with intravascular hemolysis, but severe extravascular reactions may also cause death (17,18). It is difficult to estimate the actual rate of mortality. The best available estimates are derived from reports to regulatory agencies. A review of transfusion-associated deaths reported to the Food and Drug Administration (FDA) from 1976 to 1985 attributed 158 fatalities to acute hemolysis and 26 to delayed hemolysis (19). Assuming that 100 million units of red blood cells were transfused in this time, the mortality rate for acute HTR would be 1:630,000 and that for delayed HTR would be 1:3,850,000 per unit transfused. Similarly, assuming that 30 million patients were transfused during this time, the per-patient mortality rate for acute HTR would be 1:190,00 and for delayed HTR would be 1:1,150,000. An earlier review of transfusion fatalities reported to the FDA covering 1976 to 1978 estimated the death rate from HTR to be 1:587,000 per unit transfused (20). A recent update has extended the analysis of FDA fatality reports through 1995 (21). Since 1990 the number of deaths reported to the FDA annually has increased, probably due to increased vigilance in reporting. The total number of deaths due to acute and delayed hemolysis reported from 1986 to 1995 (21) was essentially unchanged from the prior 10 years. However, acute hemolysis accounted for a higher proportion of deaths (62%) during the first decade than during the second decade (50%). The total number and proportion of deaths due to delayed HTRs was unchanged between the two reporting periods (26 or 10% versus 29 or 10%).

An analysis of blood transfusion errors reported to the New York State Department of Health from January 1990 to October 1991 reported a death rate of 1:600,000 per unit transfused (22). When these data were extended to cover the period from 1990 to 1999, the fatality rate from erroneous administration of red blood cells was 1:1,800,000 (23). It is not surprising that different studies result in discrepant estimates of mortality rate, because these figures are based on small numbers of events.

Mortality is dependent on the volume of incompatible red blood cells transfused. A review of 41 HTRs causing acute renal failure indicated that no deaths occurred among patients receiving less than 500 ml of incompatible blood, while there was 25% mortality in the group receiving 500 to 1,000 ml, and 44% mortality among those receiving greater than 1,000 ml of incompatible blood (24). However, transfusion of even small amounts of incompatible blood may not necessarily be safe. At least 12 deaths have been reported to the FDA involving transfusion of less than one unit of blood; in fact some volumes were as small as 30 ml (19).

CAUSES OF HEMOLYTIC TRANSFUSION REACTIONS

Hemolytic transfusion reactions usually result from inadvertent administration of incompatible blood components or the failure to detect a potential incompatibility. Rarely, incompatible blood components are deliberately transfused prior to ABO-incompatible bone marrow infusion or when compatible blood cannot be obtained, with an expectation of possible HTR. Among transfusion-related fatalities due to acute hemolysis reported to the FDA from 1976 to 1985, 86% were the result of process errors (19). Among these errors, 10% occurred in phlebotomy and ordering, 33% occurred within the blood bank, and 57% occurred during transfusion administration.

These frequencies are similar to reported transfusion errors in New York State, where 22% occurred in phlebotomy and ordering, 32% within the blood bank, and 46% during transfusion administration (22). More recent figures indicate that non–blood bank errors alone account for 56%, blood bank errors alone account for 29%, and compound errors account for the remaining 15% of transfusion errors (23). In part, differences between the FDA and New York figures may be accounted for by the inclusion of nonfatal errors in the latter. Serendipitously, a transfusion error may result in administration of compatible blood components, as occurred in one-third of the reported events in New York state.

Data on the failure of pretransfusion tests to detect potential incompatibility are scant. This is more likely to be a factor in delayed HTR than in acute HTR. A Mayo Clinic study suggested that at least 5 of 37 cases (14%) of delayed HTR could have been prevented by improving the sensitivity of red blood cell antibody screening procedures (25).

The deliberate, but physician guided, administration of incompatible blood components may occur in platelet transfusion, urgent transfusion required in patients with multiple alloantibodies or antibodies to high-incidence antigens, or in bone marrow transplantation. ABO-incompatible red blood cells have been successfully administered to patients prior to major ABO-incompatible bone marrow transplants in an effort to reduce the titer of isoagglutinins (26). These patients have predictable, but manageable, reactions. Some patients who have received incompatible transfusions due to antibodies outside of the ABO system and high-dose intravenous immune globulin (IVIG) have not experienced HTRs (27).

High levels of anti-A or anti-B in platelet concentrates, particularly apheresis products, can cause acute hemolysis (28,29,30). There is considerable variability in the strength of the implicated antibody, but a high-titer isoagglutinin is usually present in donor plasma when hemolysis occurs. There is no clear consensus as to what constitutes a critical anti-A or anti-B titer. At variance with reports of acute hemolysis, apheresis platelet concentrates can often be transfused across ABO types without adverse consequences. In a recent study, 16 patients who received both ABO-compatible and -incompatible platelet concentrates were evaluated for evidence of hemolysis (31). There was no difference between pre- and posttransfusion hemoglobin levels in 24 paired-transfusion episodes. Isoagglutinin titration studies were not performed.

DIAGNOSIS

Diagnosis of HTR requires clinical suspicion, especially when the transfusion may have occurred days to weeks previously. The initial laboratory evaluation includes a test for free hemoglobin and a DAT performed on a postreaction blood specimen (Table 57.2). Visual inspection of the postreaction plasma can detect hemoglobin in the range of 20 to 50 mg/dl, equivalent to the lysis of approximately 10 ml of red blood cells in an adult (32). It should be remembered that free serum hemoglobin also may be present in nonimmune hemolysis, red blood cell fragility syndromes, hemoglobinopathies, severe burns, polyagglutination, or infusion of hemoglobin-based oxygen-carrying solutions. A common cause of a false-positive test for free hemoglobin is drawing a sample through an indwelling catheter using inappropriate technique. A false-negative test for free hemoglobin may occur if too much time has been allowed to elapse before obtaining the postreaction specimen. A low level of free hemoglobin may be difficult to detect in an icteric specimen.

The DAT may be positive due to the effects of drugs, autoimmune disease, or autoantibodies. If the postreaction DAT is positive, then a test should be performed on a stored prereaction sample. If the prereaction sample is also positive, then the test is not valid for the purpose of detecting or excluding the presence of alloantibody-coated transfused cells, and further testing is required. The DAT can be negative if transfused antigen-positive cells have been cleared from circulation. In addition, when small numbers of antibody-coated allogeneic red blood cells are present, a DAT performed by routine methods may not be sufficiently sensitive. A recent study has compared the relative sensitivity of DATs performed with monospecific IgG antiglobulin technique, flow cytometry, and antibody elution performed by the chloroform-trichloroethylene method (33). In the authors'

TABLE 57.2. LABORATORY INVESTIGATION OF HEMOLYTIC TRANSFUSION REACTIONS

First-tier investigation
Posttransfusion serum hemoglobin (qualitative)
Posttransfusion direct antiglobulin test
Second-tier investigation
Repeat pretransfusion ABO-Rh
Posttransfusion ABO-Rh
Repeat antibody screen
Repeat special antigen typing
Crossmatch with pre- and postreaction specimens
Third-tier investigation
Antibody identification panels on pre- and postreaction samples
Enhanced antibody screening method: PEG, extended incubation, gel, enzymes
Red blood cell eluate on pre- and postreaction samples
Investigation of transfusion technique and blood storage conditions
Check of the blood bag, tubing, and segments for hemolysis
Enhanced crossmatches: PEG, enzymes
Minor crossmatches of implicated units
Antibody detection tests on donor units
Tests for polyagglutination
Hemoglobin electrophoresis
Quantitative serum hemoglobin
Serum bilirubin (conjugated and unconjugated)
Urine hemoglobin and hemosiderin
Bacterial culture and Gram stain of blood bags
Serum BUN and creatinine
Peripheral blood smear
Serial hemoglobin, hematocrit, and platelet count
Blood coagulation studies (PT, aPII, fibrinogen, FDP)
DAT on donor units

PEG, polyethylene glycol; BUN, blood urea nitrogen; PT, prothrombin time; FDP, fibrin degradation products; DAT, direct antiglobulin test, aPII, activated partial thromboplastin time.

hands, the DAT could detect 10% antibody-coated cells. Antibody could be detected in the eluate of the samples with as little as 1% antibody-coated red blood cells present, although in some cases it was not nearly as sensitive. Flow cytometry, however, was consistently the most sensitive method, with a detection limit of approximately 1%.

The hemoglobin and antiglobulin tests are useful for screening purposes. However, if either of these is positive, or if there is a strong clinical suspicion, then further testing must be performed. At this point, the implicated blood bags, with their attached administration sets, should be returned to the blood bank, and all units dispensed to the patient should be returned and quarantined. Units which were transfused within the past 24 hours should also be identified. The ABO and Rh typing of both pre- and postreaction blood specimens should be repeated. Care should be taken to look for mixed field agglutination. The antibody screen should be repeated on both specimens, and any special antigen typing of donor units should be repeated.

Blood from saved segments or recovered bags and tubing of units transfused within 24 hours should be crossmatched against both the pre- and postreaction specimens. This testing should include a 37°C reading and an indirect antiglobulin test. If a large number of units have been transfused during the last 24 hours, the blood bank medical director may elect to substitute reconfirmation of ABO typing of donor units. Negative results in these investigations usually rules out HTR, except in unusual circumstances.

Other causes of hemolysis or shortened red blood cell survival that should be considered in the differential diagnosis of HTR are listed in Table 57.3. Nonimmune hemolysis can have a similar clinical picture to HTR. Lysis of red blood cells can be caused by overheating in a blood warmer or by freezing. Hemolysis can also be caused by inadequate removal of glycerol from frozen red blood cells or by attempting to force blood through a filter or small-bore needle. The transfusion of outdated blood has been reported to cause hemoglobinuria and transient hemodynamic, pulmonary, and renal changes (34). Transfusion administered with hypotonic solutions or some drugs may also cause hemolysis (35). Reaction to intravenous dimethylsulfoxide infusion has been reported to mimic HTR (36). In general, patients tolerate the infusion of hemolyzed blood remarkably well. Often the only sign of an adverse event is hemoglobinuria. However, deaths have been reported due to the transfusion of hemolyzed blood (19).

Some hematologic abnormalities, particularly AIHA, can cause symptoms similar to those of HTR. Patients with congenital hemolytic anemias, such as glucose-6-phosphate dehydrogen-

TABLE 57.3. DIFFERENTIAL DIAGNOSIS OF HEMOLYTIC TRANSFUSION REACTIONS

Alloantibody-induced hemolysis
Delayed serologic transfusion reaction
Autoimmune hemolytic anemia
Cold hemagglutinin disease
Nonimmune hemolysis
- Incompatible fluids
- Improper storage
- Malfunctioning blood warmer
- Small needles, high hematocrit
- Improper deglycerolization
- Infusion pumps
- Bacterial contamination

Hemolytic anemia
- G6PD deficiency
- Congenital spherocytic anemia

Hemoglobinopathies
- Sickle cell disease
- Sickle cell transfusion reaction syndrome

Drug-induced hemolysis
Microangiopathic hemolytic anemias
- TTP
- HUS
- HELLP syndrome

Bleeding
Artificial heart valve dysfunction
Paroxysmal nocturnal hemoglobinuria
Polyaggultination
Infections
- Clostridium perfringens
- Malaria
- Babesiosis

G6PD, glucose-6-phosphate dehydrogenase; TTP, thrombotic thrombocytopenic purpura; HUS, hemolytic uremic syndrome; HELLP, hemolysis, elevated liver enzymes, low platelet count.

TABLE 57.4. GENERAL CLINICAL SIGNIFICANCE OF RED BLOOD CELL ANTIBODIES

Blood Group System	Generally Clinically Significant[a] Specificities	Generally Clinically Insignificant Specificities
ABO, H	All	−A1 not reactive at 37°C
Lewis	−Le^a, −Le^a + Le^b	−Le^b
P	−P, −P + P1 + Pk (Tj^a)	−P1, −P^k
I/i	−I, −i	−IH, −IA, −IB, −iH, −IP1 not reactive at 37°C
Rh	All	
Duffy	All	Possibly −Fy6
MNSs	All	−M not reactive at 37°C
Lutheran	−Lu^b	−Lu^a
Kell	All	—
Kidd	All	—
Cartwright	−Yt^a, −Yt^b	—
Diego	−Di^a, −Di^b, −Wr^a	—
Colton	−Co^a, −Co3	−Co^b
Dombrock	−Do^a, −Do^b	—
Cromer	−Cr^a, −Tc^a	—
Augustine	−At^a	—
Vel	−Vel	—
Lan	−Lan	—
Sid	—	−Sd^a
LW	—	All
Gerbich	—	All
Xg	—	All
Scianna	—	All
Chido/Rogers	—	All
Indian	−In^b	−In^a
Cost/York	—	−Cs^a, −Yk^a, −Yk^b
Knops/McCoy	—	−Kn^a, −Kn^b
JMH	—	−JMH
Holly/Gregory (Dombrock)	—	−Gy^a, −Hy
Bg (HLA)	—	All

[a]Resulting in hemolytic transfusion reaction or decrease red blood cell survival.

ase deficiency, may manifest hemolysis after blood transfusion (37). Conversely, blood donated by individuals with glucose-6-phosphate dehydrogenase deficiency can cause hemoglobinemia and hyperbilirubinemia in transfusion recipients (38).

Establishing the diagnosis of HTR may be particularly difficult in patients with liver disease, AIHA, or active bleeding. In chronic liver disease there is often a positive DAT, hyperbilirubinemia, and elevated lactate dehydrogenase (LDH). The clinical and laboratory features of AIHA may be identical to those of HTR. Concern has been raised that transfusion may aggravate hemolysis in AIHA, although one published study has suggested that this is not usually the case even in the face of serologic incompatibility (39). Characteristically, in both bleeding and AIHA there is proportionate loss of autologous and transfused red blood cells. One indication of HTR in these instances is the persistence of transfused red blood cells that lack the implicated antigen but the absence of transfused cells bearing the antigen.

Resorption of a hematoma can have manifestations very similar to those seen in extravascular HTR. In both disorders patients may have unconjugated hyperbilirubinemia, and elevated LDH and depressed haptoglobin levels. In addition, the presence in the serum of fibrin degradation products from the hematoma may cause one to suspect DIC. These patients, as do bleeding patients, show evidence of persistent circulating antigen-positive red blood cells and a negative posttransfusion DAT, which precludes the diagnosis of HTR.

The serologic specificity of a red blood cell antibody is an indication of its clinical significance. However, there is not an absolute correlation between specificity and presence or absence of red blood cell destruction. The general clinical significance of many red blood cell antibody specificities is summarized in Table 57.4.

PATHOPHYSIOLOGY

The pathophysiologic mechanisms involved in HTR are not well understood. There are essentially three phases: antibody-antigen interaction, phagocytosis and inflammatory cell activation, and systemic response. Initially, there is a binding of antibody to red blood cell antigens, which can result in complement activation. Subsequently, immunoglobulin and complement-coated cells interact with phagocytes, resulting in clearance and activation. Finally, the inflammatory mediators produced in the first two phases act on a variety of cell types, causing clinical manifestations of HTR.

The course of immune hemolysis is determined by antigen site density, immunoglobulin class of the alloantibody, and activation of complement. ABO antigens are present in high numbers on a red blood cell surface, approximately 5×10^5 per cell (32). In contrast, there are 10^3 to 10^4 antigens per cell in the Rh, Kell, Kidd, and Duffy systems. Complement fixation is facilitated by close proximity of antigens that allows bridging of IgG molecules by C1q. However, IgM antibodies can fix complement without a requirement for bridging between molecules. Immunoglobulin M antibodies are common in the ABO system but relatively unusual as alloantibodies to other antigens. Activation of the classical pathway of complement proceeds from C1q binding through C3 activation. Cleavage of C3 results in C3a liberation into circulation and C3b deposition on the red blood cell membrane. Activated C3 may then cleave C5 with release of C5a. Assembly of the membrane attack complex then may proceed with resultant intravascular hemolysis. Factor I is the major regulator of C3b activity. Cleavage of membrane-bound C3b by factor I results in the generation of iC3b and release of the small peptide fragment C3c. This terminates the complement cascade because iC3b is enzymatically inactive. iC3b is further degraded into C3dg and C3d by factor I and trypsin-like proteinases. Red blood cell–bound C3d is responsible for complement reactivity in the indirect antiglobulin test (Coombs test).

Erythrophagocytosis results from interaction of immunoglobulin or complement-coated red blood cells with phagocyte receptors or both. Cell-bound antibodies promote red blood cell clearance primarily through interaction of the Fc portion of IgG with specific receptors. Among the IgG receptors, FcγRI principally mediates red blood cell phagocytosis by monocytes (40). However, this receptor has a high affinity for monomeric IgG and is blocked by normal serum concentrations of IgG (41). FcγRIII appears to be the most important IgG receptor on splenic macrophages in alloimmune and autoimmune red blood cell clearance, as well as in autoimmune thrombocytopenia (42, 43,44). The principal complement receptor expressed by macrophages and monocytes, CR3, primarily recognizes iC3b. Receptors for C3a and C5a are present on a wide variety of cells including monocytes, macrophages, neutrophils, platelets, endothelium, and smooth muscle. The physiologic effects of C3a and C5a include oxygen radical production, granule enzyme release, leukotriene production, nitric oxide production, and cytokine production. These low-molecular-weight peptides can also produce vasodilation and bronchoconstriction.

Ligation of phagocyte receptors results in cellular activation and production of inflammatory response factors. An experimental model of ABO incompatibility has suggested that monocytes are the leukocyte subpopulation most directly involved in acute HTR (45). Incompatible red blood cells induce a reduction in CD14 (LPS receptor) expression on monocytes in whole blood. In addition, CD44 (hyaluronic acid receptor) expression is increased. After 24 hours of incubation with incompatible red blood cells, monocytes showed particularly high levels of CD44. These data demonstrate that monocyte activation is critical in the development of intravascular HTR.

Immune hemolysis stimulates the production of a variety of cytokines that are crucial to the initiation, maintenance, and ultimate resolution of HTR (Table 57.5). ABO incompatibility strongly stimulates production of tumor necrosis factor-α (TNF-

TABLE 57.5. CYTOKINES INVOLVED IN IMMUNE HEMOLYSIS

Terminology	Biologic Activities
Proinflammatory cytokines: Interleukin 1 (IL-1β) Tumor necrosis factor (TNF-α)	Fever Hypotension, shock, death (synergy) Mobilization of leukocytes from bone marrow Activation of T and B cells Induction of cytokines (IL-1β, IL-6, IL-8, TNF-α, MCP-1) Induction of adhesion molecules Induction of procoagulants
Interleukin 6 (IL-6)	Fever Acute phase protein response B-cell antibody production T-cell activation
Chemokines: Interleukin 8 (IL-8)	Chemotaxis of neutrophils Chemotaxis of lymphocytes Neutrophil activation Basophil histamine release
Monocyte chemoattractant protein-1 (MCP-1)	Chemotaxis of monocytes Induction of respiratory burst Induction of adhesion molecules Induction of IL-1β
Antiinflammatory Cytokines: Interleukin 1 Receptor Antagonist (IL-1ra, IRAP)	Competitive inhibition of IL-1 type I and II receptors

α) and the chemokines interleukin-8 (IL-8) and monocyte chemoattractant protein-1 (MCP-1) (46–49). Tumor necrosis factor-α indicates an early response, appearing in plasma within 2 hours, and has potent proinflammatory effects including pyrogenic activity, leukocyte activation, stimulation of procoagulant activity, and expression of a large number of gene products related to the inflammatory response. Tumor necrosis factor-α produced in blood during ABO incompatibility will stimulate endothelial cells to express leukocyte adhesion molecules, chemotactic cytokines, and procoagulant activity (50). The chemokines IL-8 and MCP-1 produced in blood during ABO incompatibility appear later than TNF-α and reach very high levels. Interleukin -8 primarily activates neutrophils to undergo the respiratory burst, release granule contents, and alter surface adhesion molecules (51). Monocyte chemoattractant protein-1 is primarily a chemotactic and activating factor for monocytes (52).

There is also evidence for the production of cytokines in IgG-mediated extravascular hemolysis (53,54). There appear to be two categories of cytokine responses in this disorder, those produced at levels greater than 1 ng/ml by 24 hours and others produced at lower levels in the range of 100 pg/ml (53). Low-level cytokine responses include IL-1β, IL-6, and TNF-α. Interleukin-8 production is a high-level response with a time course similar to that of ABO incompatibility. In contrast to the response associated with ABO incompatibility, TNF-α is produced in a delayed fashion in response to IgG-coated red blood cells, achieving a level of less than 100 pg/ml. However, cell-associated TNF-α can be demonstrated by immunocytochemical staining in monocytes engaged in erythrophagocytosis.

While the in vitro models employed in these studies are not directly comparable, these findings do suggest a possible reason for the clinical differences between intravascular and extravascular HTRs. In the former case, TNF-α is released into systemic circulation where it can have diverse effects on many cell types; whereas, in the latter case TNF-α effects may be confined to local effects at the site of erythrophagocytosis, primarily the spleen. Both IL-1β and IL-6 produced by monocytes in response to IgG-coated red blood cells increase progressively over 24 hours to levels approximating 100 pg/ml. Because IL-1β and IL-6 are B-cell growth and differentiation factors, the production of these two cytokines may promote the production of red blood cell allo- and autoantibodies that are often associated with delayed HTRs.

Immunoglobulin G–mediated hemolysis also results in the production of the IL-1β inhibitor IL-1ra (55). Significant levels of IL-1ra appear in a parallel fashion to IL-1β. Immunocytochemical staining has demonstrated strong reactivity for IL-1ra in monocytes engaged in erythrophagocytosis. Northern blot analysis of mononuclear cell RNA shows that IL-1β gene expression precedes that of IL-1ra in response to IgG-coated red blood cells. However, neutralizing antibodies to IL-1β do not suppress either IL-1ra or IL-1β gene expression in this setting. Therefore, it appears that IL-1ra production is a primary response to the IgG-coated red blood cell stimulus, rather than an autocrine phenomenon induced by initial IL-1β production. Treatment of mononuclear cells with the steroid dexamethasone inhibits IL-1ra production in response to IgG-coated red blood cells. These data suggest the possibility that the clinical variability of delayed HTR, and some of the clinical differences from intravascular HTR, may be accounted for, in part, by the relative balance of IL-1β and IL-1ra production.

Labile blood pressure is a feature of severe HTR, particularly with intravascular hemolysis. Both complement activation products (such as C5a) and cytokines (such as IL-1β and TNF-α) can contribute to hypotension. The common pathway of these mediators is the production of nitric oxide by endothelial cells. Nitric oxide, in turn, causes relaxation of vascular smooth muscle. Hypotension and deposition of thrombi in arterioles, which impair cortical blood flow, are the major factors that contribute to renal failure. In addition, there may be direct effects of inflammatory mediators on the kidneys.

There are several mechanisms by which HTR may result in intravascular coagulation. Tumor necrosis factor-α produced during immune hemolysis can induce tissue factor expression by endothelial cells (50). Tissue factor is an initiator of the extrinsic pathway that functions as a cofactor for factors VII and VIIa to accelerate the activation of factors IX and X. Tumor necrosis factor -α and IL-1β, acting on endothelial cells, will also decrease the cell surface expression of thrombomodulin. Thrombomodulin is normally present on endothelial cells and binds thrombin to activate the coagulation inhibitor protein C. Intravascular hemolysis, as in ABO incompatibility, will also induce procoagulant activity in blood leukocytes, largely due to tissue factor expression (55). This cellular procoagulant is partly inhibited by blocking antibodies to tissue factor and partly dependent of the multifunctional adhesion protein CD11b.

THERAPY

Patients who have minimal symptoms are best managed by careful observation. However, early and vigorous intervention in severe reactions saves lives. Therapeutic options in HTR are summarized in Table 57.6. The severity of HTR is directly related to volume and rate of infusion of incompatible blood. Thus, early recognition, stopping transfusion, and preventing the transfusion of additional incompatible units are the first essential steps of treatment. Immediate attention must be paid to cardiovascular support. If hypotension is present, fluid resuscitation and pressor support should be considered. Care should be taken to avoid fluid overload, however, especially in patients with impaired cardiac or renal function. Pulmonary artery catheterization is useful in selected patients to guide resuscitation.

Because intravascular hemolysis is an expected consequence of the infusion of ABO-incompatible bone marrow, some guidance can be obtained from published reports. Isoagglutinin titer clearly influences the clinical response to ABO-incompatible bone marrow infusion. In general, antibody titers below 1:64 are associated with mild or no reactions, while high titers such as 1:1,024 are associated with significant clinical reactions. The volume of incompatible red blood cells infused with the marrow also determines the magnitude of the response. One protocol reported to be successful in patients receiving major ABO-incompatible transplants involved preparatory hydration with 5% dextrose in one-half normal saline with 30 to 40 mEq/L sodium bicarbonate and 15 mEq/L potassium chloride at a rate of 3,000

TABLE 57.6. THERAPEUTIC OPTIONS IN HEMOLYTIC TRANSFUSION REACTION

Therapeutic Intervention	Indication	Typical Dose
Hydration	Prevention of renal impairment Maintain urine output >100 ml/hr	Normal saline and/or 5% dextrose 200 ml/m²/hr
Alkalinization of urine	Prevention of renal impairment Maintain urine pH >7.5	Bicarbonate 40–70 mEq in 1 liter 5% dextrose
Diuresis	Prevention of renal impairment	Mannitol 20% 100 ml/m²[a] Furosemide 40–80 mg
Vasodilation	Increase renal blood flow	Dopamine 1–5 μg/kg/min
Anticoagulation	Treatment of intravascular coagulation	Heparin 5–10 units/kg/hour
Red blood cell exchange transfusion	Decrease load of incompatible red cells	Exchange of one estimated red blood cell mass
Plasma or platelet transfusion	Treatment of hemorrhagic complications of DIC	Platelets: 1 unit platelets/10 kg (max/6 units) or 1 unit apheresis platelets Plasma: 10 ml/kg fresh-frozen plasma
Intravenous immunoglobulin	Prevention of extravascular hemolysis[b]	400 mg/kg

DIC, disseminated intravascular coagulation.
[a] Ensure adequate renal function to prevent fluid overload from increased intravascular volume.
[b] Investigational. Not standard therapy.

ml/m² per day, and 100 ml/m² mannitol 20% was given one hour prior to marrow infusion (56). During marrow infusion, the infusion rate of fluids was increased to 4,500 to 6,000 ml/m² per day, and additional mannitol was given at a rate of 30 ml/m² per hour for 12 hours. The rationale for this protocol was to maintain a high rate of urine output and prevent precipitation of hemoglobin in the renal tubules. All these patients had a preinfusion antibody titer no greater than 1:32. None experienced a clinical reaction to the infusion of approximately 120 to 160 ml of incompatible red blood cells.

The deliberate transfusion of ABO-incompatible red blood cells before transplantation has been employed to reduce isoagglutinin titers. In one such protocol, one unit of incompatible red blood cells was given over 8 hours on each of 2 days immediately before transplant (26). These patients were monitored in an intensive care unit and hydrated with normal saline and 5% dextrose (1:1 ratio) at a rate of 3,000 ml/m² per day. Sodium bicarbonate was administered to maintain the urine pH above 7.0. Of the 12 patients reported in this series, isoagglutinin titers before transfusion ranged from 1:32 to 1:1,024. One patient developed renal failure requiring hemodialysis for 17 days, but this resolved.

Because the severity and course of HTR is dictated by the load of incompatible red blood cells in circulation, exchange transfusion with antigen-negative blood may be considered. Although it is not appropriate to expose a patient to added risk of transfusion-related infectious disease if the hemolytic process is well tolerated, with a severe reaction to ABO incompatibility exchange transfusion might greatly reduce the chance of morbidity or death.

Early treatment of hypotension and DIC are the most important interventions to limit the extent of possible renal impairment. Maintenance of urine output with intravenous fluids and diuretics, such as mannitol or furosemide, early in the course of the reaction has been used successfully. However, if oliguria in the face of normovolemia is present, fluid loading may be contraindicated. The use of vasopressor agents with direct vasodilatory effects on the renal vascular bed, such as low-dose dopamine (1 to 5 μg/kg per minute) may also be considered.

The prevention and treatment of DIC is a controversial subject. Heparin has been advocated by some authors as a treatment of DIC (57). In addition, heparin may have a direct anticomplement effect, which limits intravascular hemolysis and the sequelae of complement activation (58). An obvious drawback of heparin therapy, especially in the intraoperative or postoperative patient, is the potential for hemorrhage. Therefore, heparin should be reserved for patients with clear evidence of intravascular coagulation (thrombocytopenia, hypofibrinogenemia, presence of fibrin degradation products and D-dimers). The use of fresh-frozen plasma or platelet concentrates in DIC is somewhat controversial, and transfusion of these components should be limited to those patients with active hemorrhage.

Most extravascular HTRs are not life-threatening and require no acute treatment; however, some patients with extravascular HTRs may benefit from IVIG infusion. A single dose of IVIG, 400 mg/kg infused within 24 hours of transfusion, has been used successfully to prevent transfusion reactions in alloimmunized patients for whom compatible blood was not obtainable (27). Five patients so treated did not experience transfusion reactions and had sustained increases in hematocrit. Such treatment, however, is generally not considered standard therapy.

The selection of blood components for a hemorrhaging patient undergoing HTR is a critical decision. The first consideration is that no patient should be allowed to suffer a fatal hemorrhage while a search for serologically compatible blood is undertaken. Second, red blood cells lacking known clinically significant antigens to which the patient currently has an antibody should be obtained, if at all possible. For instance, one should not reflexively issue O-negative red blood cells to a patient known to have anti-e. When the specificity of the antibody causing the reaction is not known, the results of serologic tests performed up to that point must be considered and clinical judgment exercised. Although the focus of attention in most HTRs is on red blood cells, care should be taken to avoid transfusion of type-incompatible plasma or platelets that may aggravate hemolysis, especially when ABO incompatibility is a possible cause. Undue haste in both serologic evaluation and decision making must be avoided, because human errors are often committed under pressure.

PREVENTION

Much of the activities of blood banking are directed toward the prevention of HTRs. Proper performance of donor unit typing, pretransfusion testing, antibody identification, and management of a transfusion service are critical but are beyond the scope of this chapter.

Proper identification of the transfusion recipient and pretransfusion blood specimen is the single most important aspect of the prevention of HTRs, because this is the single most common cause of HTRs. Every transfusion service must establish and enforce the procedures to be followed in its institution. At a minimum, these procedures should include meticulous identification of each patient using a permanent identification method, such as a wrist band, and confirmation of the proper labeling of blood specimens by comparison to the wrist band prior to starting the transfusion. Deviation from institutional policies on patient and specimen identification should be taken very seriously.

Because proper identification of the transfusion recipient is crucial to preventing HTR, barrier systems that are intended to physically prevent the transfusion of blood without correct identification of the patient have been devised. One such system uses a plastic lock that is preset to a three letter code at the time of blood component issuance by the blood bank. Before the unit can be administered, the identical code must be entered to unlock the system. Use of this system in one hospital over the course of 1 year detected two misidentified pretransfusion blood samples and prevented one attempt to transfuse blood to the wrong patient (59). Although systems such as this are promising for the prevention of mistransfusion, there is at present insufficient evidence of their effectiveness to warrant recommending them. In addition, sole reliance on such a device to prevent incorrect administration of blood may undermine other more important steps in proper patient identification.

In situations in which patient identification error has led to HTR, immediate consideration should be given to the possibility that another patient has been involved in the misidentification, and may, too, be at risk of receiving incompatible blood. This is especially likely if there are two patients with similar names, or if two blood samples for compatibility testing are received simultaneously from the same patient care location. Identification of such errors can prevent a second hemolytic reaction.

The optimal red blood cell antibody detection procedure would identify correctly all clinically significant antibodies while not detecting clinically insignificant reactions. No such perfect system exists, because all available methods have varying propensity for either false-positive or false-negative results, the latter resulting in failure to identify alloantibodies. The addition of reagents to the antibody screen test to enhance sensitivity is associated with an increased rate of false-positive results. One study showed that a procedure involving low-ionic-strength saline (LISS) with room temperature reading, 37°C reading, and polyspecific antihuman globulin detected all unexpected antibodies tested, but the rate of false-positive results was 1.41% (60). At the opposite end of the spectrum, the same study found that the use of albumin with 37°C reading and anti-IgG had a false-positive rate of only 0.1% but failed to detect ten antibodies present.

Performance of a serologic crossmatch may increase the rate of detection of incompatibility. In a study of crossmatch results by indirect antiglobulin technique (IAT) involving 81,444 blood samples in which the antibody screen was negative (2 cell, R_1R_1 and R_2R_2, LISS-37°C-IAT), 17 potentially significant alloantibodies were detected (61). However, 114 unwanted false-positive results were also encountered. In another study of 9,128 patients who received a total of 10,899 red blood cell units, there were 27 transfusion episodes in which the antiglobulin crossmatch on blood transfused was positive due to an IgG antibody, although the antibody screen was negative (62). Even though the transfused red blood cells were incompatible by the antiglobulin crossmatch, none of these patients had clinical or serologic evidence of hemolysis.

In rare instances, it is not possible to determine the clinical significance of a red blood cell antibody, or HTR occurs when serologic investigations have produced negative results. In such cases, a red blood cell survival study or "in vivo crossmatch" is useful (see Chapter 61). Red blood cell survival studies are based on the administration of a small aliquot of radiolabeled red blood cells and calculation of the fraction of transfused cells surviving in circulation over time.

Short of performing a red blood cell survival study, the monocyte monolayer assay (MMA) also provides clues to the clinical significance of red blood cell antibodies. This test is based on the ability of an antibody to mediate the binding of sensitized red blood cells to peripheral blood monocytes in vitro (63). A number of factors influence the reliability of the MMA to predict clinical significance, however. The conditions of in vitro sensitization of red blood cells may not reflect in vivo conditions, especially if any enhancement techniques are used. The addition of a source of fresh normal complement may be necessary for positive reactivity in the MMA but may also dilute the antibody during incubation with red blood cells. The source of red blood cells is critical if there is any variability in antigen expression. Ideally, the MMA should be carried out with a sample of the actual donor unit to be transfused. The source of monocytes used in the assay may also affect the results. Donors differ in the expression of IgG Fc receptors on their monocytes. It has been suggested that using the recipient's monocytes may give the most reliable results (64).

The published experience with the MMA in predicting clinical responses to serologically incompatible red blood cells suggests that this may be an alternative to in vivo red blood cell survival testing. One study on 18 examples of antibodies of little clinical significance demonstrated low MMA indices that correlated well with chromium 51 survival studies (65). Another study correlating MMA with red blood cell survival studies found positive MMA tests with three antibodies that also caused reduced red blood cell survival, and negative results with three other antibodies (anti-Ge, anti-Vel, and anti-Jk^b) that did not cause shortened red blood cell survival. In an extensive study of MMA activity in antibodies to high-frequency antigens, 11 examples of clinically significant antibodies gave positive MMA results, while one (anti-Yt^b) gave borderline MMA results and an abnormal red blood cell survival curve (66).

The chemiluminescent test (CLT) is another measure of the biologic response of monocytes in the presence of antibody-coated red blood cells, similar to the monocyte monolayer assay. In the CLT, monocytes are labeled with a fluorescent compound that indicates metabolic activity. Erythrophagocytosis or binding of IgG to Fc receptors results in increased metabolic activity of labeled monocytes and a measurable signal. The CLT has been compared to the MMA for predicting the clinical significance of red blood cell antibodies (67). In general, these two tests give similar results, although they may be discordant even for antibodies of known clinical significance. The amount of antibody bound to red blood cells as determined by flow cytometry does not correlate with CLT reactivity. Interestingly, both the MMA and the CLT may be positive in the presence of anti-Kn^a. This antibody specificity is not of clinical significance with respect to shortening red blood cell survival. However, Kn^a is part of the complement receptor CR1 that is present on monocytes. Cross-linking of this receptor by serum antibody is probably responsible for the false-positive assays.

The selection of donor units lacking antigens corresponding to alloantibodies is essential for prevention of HTR, but whether phenotype matching of donors and recipients is an appropriate strategy for the prevention of alloimmunization and HTR in the nonimmunized patient is controversial. Arguments in favor of this practice have been put forth for sickle cell disease in which, due to ethnic gene pool diversity, there is often a mismatch between the donor pool and recipient phenotypes. Examination of alloimmunization rates among children in one urban area indicated that children with non-American ethnic origins had a 42.9% incidence of alloimmunization compared to 17.6% in American patients (68). This was not due simply to variation in transfusion rates, because the American patients received more transfusions than the others. In another study that compared sickle cell patients to those with other forms of chronic anemia, 30% of the patients with sickle cell anemia were alloimmunized, in contrast to 5% in the group of patients with other forms of anemia (69). Of the 32 alloimmunized patients with sickle cell anemia, 17 had multiple antibodies and 14 had delayed transfusion reactions. These studies suggest that phenotype matching is beneficial for selected patients, but they do not provide sufficient evidence to recommend it as a routine practice.

Hemolytic transfusion reactions could be avoided entirely if the responsible antigens on the red blood cell surface could be removed or camouflaged. Recently, experimental work has suggested that treating red blood cells with polyethylene glycol (PEG) may be an effective means of camouflaging antigens (70). Polyethylene glycol modification appears to work by creating a sphere of hydration around the red blood cell that effectively excludes IgG or IgM from coming into contact with antigenic structures on the membrane surface. Polyethylene glycol–treated red blood cells have properties of size, shape, intracellular ion content, and oxygen binding that are identical to untreated red blood cells. However, PEG-treated red blood cells have a low shear viscosity compared to normal red blood cells. This also may be advantageous in sickle cell disease in which increased blood viscosity within capillaries can result in occlusive crises.

The effectiveness of PEG modification is dependent on the molecular weight and branching characteristics of PEG molecules and the chemistry of covalent attachment (71). Use of a dichlorotriazine derivative of 5-kd PEG results in complete inhibition of direct agglutination by anti-D. However, such cells are still agglutinated by anti-D in the indirect antiglobulin test. A and B epitopes are partially, but not completely, masked. In contrast, red blood cells coated with branched-chain 10-kd PEG after treatment with succinimidyl propionate–modified 20-kd PEG are not agglutinated by anti-A, anti-B, and anti-D.

Group A and group B red blood cells can be converted to group O by enzymatic cleavage of terminal determinant saccharides with α-N-acetylgalactosaminidase or α-D-galactosidase (72–74). The use of such technology for large-scale conversion of red blood cells raises the possibility that acute HTR due to ABO incompatibility may be completely avoidable in the future. However, there are issues with regard to completeness of antigen removal and the possibility of exposure of neoantigens by enzymatic treatment. Treatment of red blood cells with α-N-acetylgalactosaminidase results in rapid loss of A epitopes binding *Dolichos biflorus* lectin (72). Inhibition of complement-mediated hemolysis is somewhat slower. However, the epitopes of A antigen that react with human source anti-A are relatively resistant to enzymatic degradation. Additionally, there are differences in the enzymatic sensitivity of A epitopes on the red blood cell membrane. Glycosphingolipids with short oligosaccharide chains display the greatest resistance to enzymatic treatment.

Work on enzyme-converted group O (ECO) red blood cells from group B red blood cells has advanced to the stage of the clinical trials (75,76). An initial trial of a two-unit transfusion of ECO red blood cells to group O subjects demonstrated good 24-hour posttransfusion survival, 95%, with a half-life of 29.5 days (75). There was no clinical or laboratory evidence of hemolysis. A subsequent study with larger-volume transfusions had similar results. Subjects who received a second transfusion did not show evidence of alloimmunization or increase in anti-B titer (76).

SUMMARY

Although the prevention of HTRs continues to be a major focus in transfusion medicine, advances in serology and transfusion service practices have significantly reduced their incidence. Simultaneously, advances in the understanding of the pathophysiology of HTRs have given us insights to help guide the management of patients undergoing reactions. It is conceivable that technologic advances in red blood cell modification and oxygen-carrying solutions will significantly change red blood cell transfusion practice in the future and virtually eliminate the occurrence of HTRs. Until such time, however, HTRs will remain a major adverse consequence of blood transfusion.

REFERENCES

1. Murphy MF, Hook S, Waters AH, et al. Acute haemolysis after ABO-incompatible platelet transfusions [Letter]. *Lancet* 1990;335:974–975.
2. Reis MD, Coovadia AS. Transfusion of ABO-incompatible platelets causing severe haemolytic reaction. *Clin Lab Haematol* 1989;113: 237–240.
3. Abbott D, Hussain S. Intravascular coagulation due to inter-donor incompatibility. *CMAJ* 1970;103:752–753.
4. Vamvakas EC, Pineda AA, Moore SB. Incidence of delayed hemolytic transfusion reactions. *Vox Sang* 1995;69:86.
5. Ness PM, Shirey RS, Thoman SK, et al. The differentiation of delayed serologic and delayed hemolytic transfusion reactions: incidence, long-term serologic findings, and clinical significance. *Transfusion* 1990;30: 688–693.
6. Vamvakas EC, Pineda AA, Reisner R, et al. The differentiation of delayed hemolytic and delayed serologic transfusion reactions: incidence and predictors of hemolysis. *Transfusion* 1995;35:26–32.
7. Kindgen-Milles D, Klement W, Arndt JO. The nociceptive systems of skin, paravascular tissue and hand veins of humans and their sensitivity to bradykinin. *Neurosci Lett* 1994;181:39–42.
8. Cummins D, Ferrier A, Murphy F. Bilirubinuria, conjugated hyperbilirubinaemia and δ-bilirubinaemia following acute haemolysis. *Ann Clin Biochem* 1997;24:109–110.
9. Salama A, Mueller-Eckhardt C. Delayed hemolytic transfusion reactions. Evidence for complement activation involving allogeneic and autologous red cells. *Transfusion* 1984;24:188–193.
10. Petz LD, Calhoun L, Shulman IA, et al. The sickle cell hemolytic transfusion reaction syndrome. *Transfusion* 1997;37:382–392.
11. King KE, Shirey RS, Lankiewicz MW, et al. Delayed hemolytic transfusion reactions in sickle cell disease: simultaneous destruction of recipients' red cells. *Transfusion* 1997;37:376–381.
12. Whicher JT, Parry ES. Effects on renal tubular protein reabsorption of the infusion of free haemoglobin. *Eur J Clin Invest* 1984;14:116–121.
13. Patel RP. Biochemical aspects of the reaction of hemoglobin and NO: implications for Hb-based blood substitutes. *Free Radic Biol Med* 2000; 28:1518–1525.
14. Vaughn MW, Huang KT, Kuo L, et al. Erythrocytes possess an intrinsic barrier to nitric oxide consumption. *J Biol Chem* 2000;275: 2342–2348.
15. Gould SA, Moss GS. Clinical development of human polymerized hemoglobin as a blood substitute. *World J Surg* 1996;20:1200–1207.
16. Bluemle LW Jr. Hemolytic transfusion reactions causing acute renal failure. Serologic and clinical considerations. *Postgrad Med* 1965;38: 484–489.
17. Schorn TF, Knospe WH. Fatal delayed hemolytic transfusion reaction without previous blood transfusion. *Ann Int Med* 1989;110:241–242.
18. Pineda AA, Brzica SM Jr, Taswell HF. Hemolytic transfusion reaction. Recent experience in a large blood bank. *Mayo Clin Proc* 1978;53: 378–390.
19. Sazama K. Reports of 355 transfusion-associated deaths: 1976 through 1985. *Transfusion* 1990;30:583–590.
20. Honig CL, Bove JR. Transfusion-associated fatalities: review of Bureau of Biologics reports 1976–1978. *Transfusion* 1980;20:653–661.
21. Sazama K. Death from transfusion: a 20-year review (personal communication, 2001).
22. Linden JV, Paul B, Dressler KP. A report of 104 transfusion errors in New York state. *Transfusion* 1992;32:601–606.
23. Linden JV, Wagner K, Voytovich AE, et al. Transfusion errors in New York state: an analysis of 10 years' experience. *Transfusion* 2000;40: 1207–1213.
24. Bluemle LW Jr. Hemolytic transfusion reactions causing acute renal failure. Serologic and clinical considerations. *Postgrad Med* 1965;38: 484–489.
25. Moore SB, Taswell HF, Pineda AA, et al. Delayed hemolytic transfusion reactions. Evidence of the need for an improved pretransfusion compatibility test. *Am J Clin Pathol* 1980;74:94–97.
26. Nussbaumer W, Schwaighofer H, Gratwohl A, et al. Transfusion of donor-type red cells as a single preparative treatment for bone marrow transplants with major ABO incompatibility. *Transfusion* 1995;35: 592–595.
27. Kohan AI, Niborski RC, Rey JA, et al. High-dose intravenous immunoglobulin in non-ABO transfusion incompatibility. *Vox Sang* 1994;67: 195–198.
28. McManigal S, Sins KL. Intravascular hemolysis secondary to ABO incompatible platelet produces. *Am J Clin Pathol* 1999;111:202–206.
29. Conway LT, Scott EP. Acute hemolytic transfusion reaction due to ABO incompatible plasma in a platelet apheresis concentrate [Letter]. *Transfusion* 1984;24:413.
30. Larsson LG, Welsh VJ, Ladd DJ. Acute intravascular hemolysis secondary to out-of-group platelet transfusion. *Transfusion* 2000;40:902–906.
31. Mair B, Benson K. Evaluation of changes in hemoglobin levels associated with ABO incompatible plasma in apheresis platelets. *Transfusion* 1998;38:51–55.
32. Mollison PL, Engelfriet CP, Contreras PM. *Blood transfusion in clinical medicine,* 9th ed. Oxford: Blackwell Science, 1993.
33. Alvarez A, Rives S, Montoto S, et al. Relative sensitivity of direct antiglobulin test, antibody's elution and flow cytometry in the serologic diagnosis of immune hemolytic transfusion reactions. *Haematologica* 2000;85:186–188.
34. Gossinger H, Laggner A, Druml W, et al. Hemodynamic, pulmonary, and renal reactions to inadvertent transfusion of outdated blood. *Crit Care Med* 1986;14:70–71.
35. Whitelaw JP. Hemolysis caused by half-physiologic-strength saline [Letter]. *Transfusion* 1990;30:78.
36. Samoszuk M, Reid ME, Toy PT. Intravenous dimethylsulfoxide therapy causes severe hemolysis mimicking a hemolytic transfusion reaction [Letter]. *Transfusion* 1983;23:405.
37. Mimouni F, Shohat S, Reisner SH. G6PD-deficient donor blood as a cause of hemolysis in two preterm infants. *Isr J Med Sci* 1986;22: 120–122.
38. Shalev O, Manny N, Sharon R. Posttransfusional hemolysis in recipients of glucose-6-phosphate dehydrogenase-deficient erythrocytes. *Vox Sang* 1993;64:94–98.
39. Salama A, Berghofer H, Mueller-Eckhardt C. Red blood cell transfusion in warm-type autoimmune haemolytic anaemia. *Lancet* 1992;340: 1515–1517.
40. Ruegg SJ, Jungi TW. Antibody-mediated erythrolysis and erythrophagocytosis by human monocytes, macrophages and activated macrophages. Evidence for distinction between involvement of high-affinity and low-affinity receptors for IgG by using different erythroid target cells. *Immunology* 1988;63:513–520.
41. Leslie RGQ. Immunoglobulin and soluble immune complex binding to phagocyte Fc receptors. *Biochem Soc Trans* 1984;12:743–746.
42. Davenport RD, Kunkel SL. IgG receptor roles in red cell binding to monocytes and macrophages. *Transfusion* 1994;34:79S.
43. Unkeless JC. Function and heterogeneity of human Fc receptors for immunoglobulin G. *J Clin Invest* 1989;83:355–361.
44. Clarkson SB, Kimberly RP, Valinsky JE, et al. Blockade of clearence of immune complexes by anti-Fc γ-receptor monoclonal antibody. *J Exp Med* 1986;164:474–489.
45. Udani M, Rao N, Telen MJ. Leukocyte phenotypic changes in an in vitro model of ABO hemolytic transfusion reaction. *Transfusion* 1997; 37:904–909.
46. Butler J, Parker D, Pillai R, et al. Systemic release of neutrophil elastase

and tumour necrosis factor α following ABO incompatible blood transfusion. *Br J Haematol* 1991;79:525–526.
47. Davenport RD, Strieter RM, Kunkel SL. Red cell ABO incompatibility and production of tumour necrosis factor-α. *Br J Haematol* 1991;78: 540–554.
48. Davenport RD, Strieter RM, Standiford TJ, et al. Interleukin-8 production in red blood cell incompatibility. *Blood* 1990;76:2439–2442.
49. Davenport RD, Burdick MD, Strieter RM, et al. Monocyte chemoattractant protein production in red cell incompatibility. *Transfusion* 1994;34:16–19.
50. Davenport RD, Burdick M, Kunkel SL. Endothelial cell activation in hemolytic transfusion reactions. *Transfusion* 1992;32:53S.
51. Matsushima K, Oppenheim JJ. Interleukin 8 and MCAF: novel inflammatory cytokines inducible by IL-1 and TNF. *Cytokine* 1989;1:2–13.
52. Jiang Y, Beller DI, Frendl G, et al. Monocyte chemoattractant protein-1 regulates adhesion molecule expression and cytokine production in human monocytes. *J Immunol* 1992;148:2423–2428.
53. Davenport RD, Burdick M, Moore SA, et al. Cytokine production in IgG mediated red cell incompatibility. *Transfusion* 1993;33:19–24.
54. Hoffman M. Antibody-coated erythrocytes induce secretion of tumor necrosis factor by human monocytes: a mechanism for the production of fever by incompatible transfusions. *Vox Sang* 1991;60:184–187.
55. Davenport RD, Burdick MD, Strieter RM, et al. In vitro production of interleukin-1 receptor antagonist in IgG mediated red cell incompatibility. *Transfusion* 1994;34:297–303.
56. Slavc I, Urban Ch, Schwinger W, et al. ABO-incompatible bone marrow transplantation: prevention of hemolysis by alkaline hydration with mannitol diuresis in conjunction with red cell reduced buffy coat bone marrow. *Wien Klin Wochenschr* 1992;104:93–96.
57. Rock RC, Bove JR, Nemerson Y. Heparin treatment of intravascular coagulation accompanying hemolytic transfusion reactions. *Transfusion* 1969;9:57–61.
58. Gray JM, Oberman HA, Beck ML. Delay in the onset of immune hemolysis in vivo apparently due to heparinization. *Transfusion* 1973; 13:422–424.
59. Mercurilali F, Inghilleri F, Colotti MT, et al. One-year use of the Bloodloc system in an orthopedic institute. *Tranfus Clin Biol* 1994;1: 227–230.
60. Garratty G. The significance of complement in immunohematology. *CRC Crit Rev Clin Lab Sci* 1985;20:25–56.
61. Oberman HA, Judd WJ. Cost-containment in transfusion practice: a view from the United States. In: Cash JD, ed. *Progress in transfusion medicine.* Edinburgh: Churchill Livingstone, 1988.
62. Heddle NM, O'Hoski P, Singer J, et al. A prospective study to determine the safety of omitting the antiglobulin crossmatch from pretransfusion testing. *Br J Haematol* 1992;81:579–584.
63. Judd WJ. *Methods in immunohematology,* 2nd ed. Durham, NC: Montgomery Scientific Publications, 1994.
64. Garratty G. Predicting the clinical significance of red cell antibodies with in vitro cellular assays. *Transfus Med Rev* 1990;4:297–312.
65. Schanfield MS, Stevens JO, Bauman D. The detection of clinically significant erythrocyte allantibodies using a human mononuclear phagocyte assay. *Transfusion* 1981;21:571–576.
66. Nance SJ, Arndt P, Garratty G. Predicting the clinical significance of red cell alloantibodies using a monocyte monolayer assay. *Transfusion* 1987;27:449–452.
67. Hadley A, Wilkes A, Poole J, et al. A chemiluminescence test for predicting the outcome of transfusing incompatible blood. *Transfus Med* 1999;9:337–342.
68. Luban NL. Variability in rates of alloimmunization in different groups of children with sickle cell disease: effect of ethnic background. *Am J Pediatr Hematol Oncol* 1989;11:314–319.
69. Vichinsky EP, Earles A, Johnson RA, et al. Alloimmunization in sickle cell anemia and transfusion of racially unmatched blood. *N Engl J Med* 1990;322:1617–1621.
70. Scott MD, Bradley AJ, Murad KL. Camouflaged blood cells: low-technology bioengineering for transfusion medicine? *Transfus Med Rev* 2000;14:53–63.
71. Fisher TC, Armstrong JK, Meiselman HJ, et al. Second generation poly(ethylene glycol) surface coatings for red blood cells. *Transfusion* 2000;40:119S.
72. Hoskins LC, Larson G, Naff GB. Blood group A immunodeterminants on human red cells differ in biologic activity and sensitivity to α-N-acetylgalactosaminidase. *Transfusion* 1995;35:813–821.
73. Hobbs L, Mitra M, Phillips R, et al. Deantigenation of human type B erythrocytes with glycine max α-D-galactosidase. *Biomed Pharmacother* 1995;49:244–250.
74. Zhu A, Leng L, Monahan C, et al. Characterization of recombinant α-galactosidase for use in seroconversion from blood group B to O of human erythrocytes. *Arch Biochem Biophys* 1996;327:324–329.
75. Lenny LL, Hurst R, Goldstein J, et al. Transfusions to group O subjects of 2 units of red cells enzymatically converted from group B to group O. *Transfusion* 1994;34:209–214.
76. Lenny LL, Hurst R, Zhu A, et al. Multiple-unit and second transfusions of red cells enzymatically converted from group B to group O: report on the end of phase I trials. *Transfusion* 1995;35:899–902.
77. Henderson RA. Acute transfusion reactions. *N Z Med J* 1990;103: 509–511.
78. Lichtiger B, Perry-Thornton E. Hemolytic transfusion reactions in oncology patients: experience in a large cancer center. *J Clin Oncol* 1984; 25:438–442.
79. Pineda AA, Taswell HF, Brzica SM Jr. Transfusion reaction. An immunologic hazard of blood transfusion. *Transfusion* 1978;18:1–7.
80. Davis KG, Richard LA. Delayed haemolytic transfusion reactions. Review of three cases. *Med J Aust* 1982;1:335–337.
81. Croucher BEE. Differential diagnosis of delayed transfusion reactions. In: Bell CA, ed. *A seminar on laboratory management of hemolysis.* Washington: American Association of Blood Banks, 1979:151–160.
82. Duvall CP, Alter HJ, Rath CE. Hemoglobin catabolism following a hemolytic transfusion reaction in a patient with sickle cell anemia. *Transfusion* 1974;14:382–387.

Rossi's Principles of Transfusion Medicine, Third Edition, edited by Toby L. Simon, Walter H. Dzik, Edward L. Snyder, Christopher P. Stowell, and Ronald G. Strauss. Lippincott Williams & Wilkins, Philadelphia © 2002.

CASE 57A

A HEMOLYTIC TRANSFUSION REACTION: DOING IT THE HARD WAY

CASE HISTORY

Mrs. E. was a 37-year-old woman with diffuse, large cell non-Hodgkin lymphoma who was admitted for an allogeneic bone marrow transplantation from a human leukocyte antigen (HLA)-matched sibling. The patient had been well until 2 years prior to admission, when she began to experience intermittent substernal chest pressure which was noncardiac in origin. She subsequently developed a nonproductive cough, dyspnea on exertion, and right axillary pain. A chest radiographic examination showed a large mediastinal mass, and a biopsy of this mass led to the diagnosis. She was treated with two cycles of cyclophosphamide, doxorubicin, vincristine and prednislone (CHOP) and one of etoposide, methylprednisolone, cytosine arabinoside, and cisplatin (ESHAP), which resulted in only partial diminution of the mediastinal mass. She underwent peripheral blood progenitor cell collection after mobilization with granulocyte colony–stimulating factor, followed by high-dose chemotherapy with cyclophosphamide, V carinustine, and etoposide (VP16) and an autologous transplant. Three months after the peripheral blood progenitor cell transplant, she complained of pain on the right side of her neck and was found to have a new hilar mass. She received radiation therapy with little improvement.

At the time of admission, the patient's blood pressure was 116/70, the pulse was 72 and regular, and the temperature was 98.8°F. Her physical examination was unremarkable; there was no cervical or supraclavicular adenopathy, the lungs were clear to auscultation, and there was no tenderness in the neck, along the spine, or in the costovertebral angle. After receiving cyclophosphamide for 3 days and one dose of antithymocyte globulin, she was given bone marrow from her brother, who not only was a six-antigen match but was also group A RhD positive. In addition to the antithymocyte globulin, her immunosuppression consisted of cyclosporine and dexamethasone (Decadron). Her recovery was complicated by hypertension and elevation of liver function tests attributed to the immunosuppressive medications. She also developed a nonocclusive axillary vein thrombosis, which was treated with warfarin (Coumadin), and a bacteremia (coagulase-negative *Staphylococcus*) treated with intravenous vancomycin.

Engraftment was successful, with restoration of the absolute neutrophil count to 500/μL by posttransplant day 12 and a platelet count more than 50,000/μL by day 14. On the sixth posttransplant day, the patient's platelet count had fallen to 17,000/μL and a platelet transfusion was ordered. After receiving approximately 100 ml of a process-leukoreduced and irradiated plateletpheresis unit from a group O RhD-positive donor, she complained of severe, shaking chills and low back pain. Her blood pressure was noted to have increased from 110/70 to 140/96, her pulse increased from 82 to 100, and her temperature increased from 99.3°F to 101.1°F. The transfusion was stopped, and specimens were drawn and sent for a transfusion reaction work-up, including testing of the partially transfused plateletpheresis unit. She was given 25 mg diphenhydramine intravenously, 650 mg acetaminophen orally, and 2 mg morphine sulfate intravenously and her symptoms resolved.

In the laboratory, the technologists reviewed the clerical work, which was found to be in order. The plasma from the posttransfusion specimen showed no change compared with the pretransfusion specimen, and blood grouping agreed with the records, group A RhD positive. The direct antiglobulin test was weakly positive with polyspecific reagent and anti-C3 reagent but negative with antiimmunoglobulin G (anti-IgG). The pretransfusion specimen gave the same results. Being very efficient, the resident and attending physicians on the transfusion medicine service reviewed the blood bank work-up and went immediately to the patient care unit to check the patient's chart and to talk to the team in charge of the patient's care. They concluded that the reaction was a febrile nonhemolytic transfusion reaction (FNHTR).

The following day, however, the resident physician read the patient's record. Because of a transient rise in her liver function tests caused by the antithymocyte globulin given earlier in the hospitalization, she was being monitored periodically. The morning after the transfusion reaction, the patient's lactate dehydrogenase (LDH) had jumped from 291 to 953 U/L, the total bilirubin had increased from 1.0 to 1.2 mg/dl and the direct bilirubin from 0.7 to 1.2 mg/dl. A second blood bank specimen was obtained, and an eluate was prepared using a freeze-thaw technique (1). The eluate was tested against a three-cell screening panel, a group A_1 red blood cell, and a group B red blood cell and reacted with only the group A_1 red blood cell (Table 57A.1). The plasma from the plateletpheresis unit was titered against group A_1 red blood cells and had a titre of 1024 and an agglutination score of 119. The donor was female, but her pregnancy history was not known.

The resident and attending physicians wrote an amended transfusion reaction report, indicating that the patient had expe-

TABLE 57A.1. PATIENT ELUATE AND DONOR PLASMA TITRES

Test Cell	Patient Eluate	Donor Plasma Dilution 1	2	4	8	16	32	64	128	256	512	1024	2048
O R_1R_1	0	0	—	—	—	—	—	—	—	—	—	—	—
O R_2R_2	0	0	—	—	—	—	—	—	—	—	—	—	—
O rr	0	0	—	—	—	—	—	—	—	—	—	—	—
B	0	0	—	—	—	—	—	—	—	—	—	—	—
A_1	2+	4+	4+	4+	4+	4+	4+	4+	4+	3+	2+	1+	0
Score	—	12	12	12	12	12	12	12	12	10	8	5	119

rienced a hemolytic transfusion reaction due to the high-titre anti-A present in the plasma of the group O plateletpheresis unit. The patient's hemoglobin level decreased from 9.2 g/dl to 8.1 g/dl over the next 2 days, but she otherwise appeared to suffer no ill effects from the hemolytic episode.

DISCUSSION

This patient had the classic signs of a severe febrile reaction to an out-of-group plateletpheresis unit. Because we expect common events to occur commonly, and febrile reactions, along with urticarial reactions, are the most common complications of transfusion, it is not at all surprising that the initial impression was of an FNHTR. The patient did complain of low back pain, which always catches the attention of transfusion medicine specialists, but which is as common a complaint as it is nonspecific. In fact, the most common initial symptom of hemolytic transfusion reactions is fever, and not back pain or any of the other highly suggestive signs such as pain along the vein used for infusion or hemoglobinuria (2). In this instance, the weakly positive direct antiglobulin test performed on the pretransfusion specimen which might have been due to a medication or simply prolonged storage in the cold, may have lulled everyone into a false sense of security and made it easy to discount the results of the posttransfusion direct antiglobulin test, which appeared not to have changed. Had our heroes not leaped into the fray so quickly but waited to review the patient's chart the following morning, they might have had a chance to score a diagnostic coup. It was, however, appropriate for them to have reviewed the blood bank work-up and the chart when they did, even if it meant filing an amended report.

In this case of hemolysis, the tables were turned and it was the donor's anti-A which produced hemolysis of the recipient's red blood cells. It is not unusual to give pools of out-of-group platelet concentrates containing plasma that is incompatible with the transfusion recipient's red blood cells. Hemolysis is rarely a problem, because the plasma volumes are modest and the isoagglutinins are diluted. Even if one of the donors has high-titre anti-A or anti-B, the plasma volume of a platelet concentrate is only 45 to 65 ml and would be diluted out first in the pool and second in the recipient's plasma volume. If the product is a plateletpheresis unit and the isoagglutinin titre is high, however, it may be possible to deliver enough incompatible isoagglutinin to produce hemolysis in the recipient (3,4). In this case, the patient received approximately 100 ml of incompatible plasma with an anti-A titre of 1024, which was diluted into a plasma volume of approximately 3.5 liters. The resulting anti-A titre would have been expected to be on the order of 30, a respectable titre for a group O individual. Not all of the infused anti-A would be in the plasma, of course; most of it would presumably be bound to the recipient's red blood cells. A similar situation could occur transfusing platelet concentrates to an infant in which it is likely that a component from a single donor is used. For this reason, it is common to use ABO group-specific platelets for infants.

Isoagglutinin titres are not usually as high as in this donor unless the individual has been exposed to incompatible red blood cells by transfusion, or much more commonly, by the birth of an ABO-incompatible infant. It is worth noting that the donor of this unit of platelets was a group O female who may have given birth to group A infants. This donor should probably not be recruited for plateletpheresis donation in the future but encouraged to donate whole blood, particularly because she is group O. Red blood cell components prepared with additive solutions have so little residual plasma that there would be no danger of hemolysis should they be given to group A recipients. Platelet concentrates and plasma should probably not be made from this donor or should be used only as source plasma.

Case contributed by Christopher Stowell, M.D., Ph.D. Massachusetts General Hospital, Boston, MA.

REFERENCES

1. Feng CS, Kirkley KC, Eicher CA, et al. The Lui elution technique: a simple and efficient method for eluting ABO antibodies. *Transfusion* 1985;25:433–434.
2. Davenport RD. Hemolytic transfusion reactions (second edition). In Popovsky MA, ed. *Transfusion reactions.* Bethesda, MD: American Association of Blood Banks, 1996:1–44.
3. Larsson LG, Welsh VJ, Ladd DJ. Acute intravascular hemolysis secondary to out-of-group platelet transfusions. *Transfusion* 2000;40:902–906.
4. McManigal S, Sims KL. Intravascular hemolysis secondary to ABO-incompatible platelet products: an under-recognized transfusion reaction. *Am J Clin Path* 1999;111:202–206.

58

FEBRILE, ALLERGIC, AND NONIMMUNE TRANSFUSION REACTIONS

GARY STACK
GREGORY J. POMPER

The chapter reviews a variety of acute, nonhemolytic, and noninfectious transfusion reactions, the most common of which are febrile, nonhemolytic transfusion reactions (FNHTRs) and allergic reactions. Other acute, nonhemolytic reactions are reported less frequently and include transfusion-related acute lung injury (TRALI) and anaphylactic or anaphylactoid reactions. Additional acute adverse effects can occur in massive transfusion owing to the large volume of blood components transfused over a short period. The complications of massive transfusion include citrate toxicity, hypothermia, and electrolyte disturbances. Some patients cannot tolerate the acute increase in intravascular blood volume caused by transfusion and experience the complications of circulatory overload. Acute reactions can be caused by the toxicity of chemicals that leach into blood components from blood storage containers or filters or by chemicals added to improve storage conditions, such as dimethyl sulfoxide (DMSO). Other reactions are caused by endogenous mediators generated in the blood during filtration, processing, or storage, such as bradykinin-mediated hypotensive reactions. It is important that these complications of transfusion be recognized by patient care

G. Stack: Pathology and Laboratory Medicine Service, Veterans Affairs Connecticut Healthcare System, and Department of Laboratory Medicine, Yale University School of Medicine, New Haven, Connecticut.

G.J. Pomper: Department of Laboratory Medicine, Yale University School of Medicine, New Haven, Connecticut.

teams and blood bank staffs and that appropriate treatments and preventive measures be instituted for patient safety and well-being.

FEBRILE NONHEMOLYTIC TRANSFUSION REACTIONS

Description

An FNHTR is commonly defined as an increase in body temperature of 1°C or more unrelated to hemolysis, sepsis, or other known causes of fever that occurs during or within several hours of transfusion. The use of a 1°C increase in body temperature as a threshold for defining an FNHTR avoids undue concern over small fluctuations in body temperature unrelated to transfusion that do not justify discontinuation of transfusion and follow-up investigation. Many FNHTRs begin with the patient feeling uneasy and experiencing chills. In mild reactions, the signs and symptoms do not progress. Chills with or without an increase in body temperature can be classified as mild FNHTR if other possible causes of chills are unlikely and the time course of the reaction correlates with the transfusion. In the most severe reactions, patients may experience severe shaking chills (rigors) or a fever 2°C or more over baseline. Although signs and symptoms usually are limited to chills and fever, patients also can have headache and occasionally nausea and vomiting.

The fever of FNHTR usually persists no more than 8 to 12 hours after the start of transfusion. If fever persists 18 to 24 hours or longer, it is unlikely to be transfusion-related. Generally, FNHTRs are self-limited and have no sequelae. However, elderly patients, patients with compromised cardiovascular status, or critically ill patients are at risk of cardiorespiratory complications associated with FNHTR. Because fever increases oxygen demand and consumption an estimated 13% for every 1°C over 37°C and shivering increases oxygen demand approximately 300%, FNHTRs can aggravate preexisting cardiac, pulmonary, and cerebrovascular insufficiency. For that reason, prompt recognition and antipyretic management of FNHTRs is indicated.

An FNHTR almost always is associated with transfusion of cellular blood components, such as red blood cells (RBCs), platelets, and granulocyte preparations and rarely with noncellular components, such as plasma and cryoprecipitate. The incidence of FNHTR is commonly estimated at 0.5% per unit of nonleukoreduced RBCs (1,2). The reaction risk of blood components, however, varies according to numerous factors, such as method of preparation of the blood component, storage time of the blood component, and whether the patient population has a high rate of previous transfusion or pregnancy. These factors can vary among different geographic regions and medical centers. In addition, reaction rates based on reactions reported to blood banks are lower than those based on systematic surveillance of responses to all transfusions.

Published reaction rates to nonleukoreduced platelet concentrates, generally ranging from 2% to 30% per transfusion, vary more widely than do those to RBCs. Pools of random-donor platelet concentrates have been reported to cause a higher rate of FNHTR than single-donor apheresis platelets (3,4). Platelet concentrates prepared from platelet-rich plasma, which are commonly used in the United States, are reported to cause a higher rate of FNHTR than are platelet concentrates prepared with the buffy coat technique. Longer storage times of platelet concentrates also are associated with higher rates of FNHTR (5–7). Reactions also are more frequent among certain recipients, such as patients who undergo numerous transfusions or multiparous women who have had previous exposures to allogeneic leukocytes and platelets and are at risk of induction of leukocyte or platelet alloantibodies.

Etiology

An FNHTR appears to be part of the systemic inflammatory response syndrome provoked in transfusion recipients by the immune challenge of transfusing foreign cells or infusing soluble inflammatory mediators present in stored blood components. The term *systemic inflammatory response syndrome* was coined to describe the constellation of observed body responses to various insults, such as infection, trauma, burns, and ischemia. It is defined as the presence of two or more of the following: body temperature more than 38°C or less than 36°C; heart rate more than 90 beats/min; tachypnea (respiratory rate >20 breaths/min or $PaCO_2$ less than 32 mm Hg); white blood cell count more than 12×10^9/L or less than 4×10^9/L, or more than 10% immature neutrophils (band forms). Although a mild FNHTR may not completely fulfill these criteria, FNHTR is nevertheless an inflammatory response.

An FNHTR appears to have three possible underlying causes (Fig. 58.1): (a) infusion of passenger leukocytes into recipients alloimmunized to leukocytes or platelets, (b) infusion of pyrogenic cytokines or other inflammatory mediators (e.g., activated complement proteins or neutrophil-priming lipids) that accumulate in the plasma portion of cellular blood components during storage, and (c) infusion of blood components contaminated with bacteria or bacterial products (8,9). Each of these mechanisms is described in detail later. The common pathway by which these different stimuli induce posttransfusion fever is presumably an increase in circulating pyrogenic cytokines in the recipient, such as interleukin-6 (IL-6), IL-1β, and tumor necrosis factor α (TNF-α). Pyrogenic cytokines induce fever by mediating up-regulation of the thermostatic set point for body temperature in the thermoregulatory center of the hypothalamus (10).

The change in thermostatic set point initiates a series of responses that elevate the body temperature. These responses include rapid muscle contractions that cause shivering, rigors, and an increase in heat generation. Heat conservation is achieved through cutaneous vasoconstriction, which also contributes to the sensation of a chill. Perceived chills lead to behavioral changes that can further increase body temperature. For example, the patient may cover up, and the result is inhibition of heat dissipation.

Anecdotal reports suggest that patients with preexisting fever (Fig. 58.1, *middle left*) may be predisposed to FNHTRs (1). Although this phenomenon is unproved, the cytokine model provides a theoretic basis for how it could occur. Patients with preexisting fever sometimes have elevated levels of circulating cytokines because of recent or current fever, or their central nervous system pathways for fever may be primed by previous

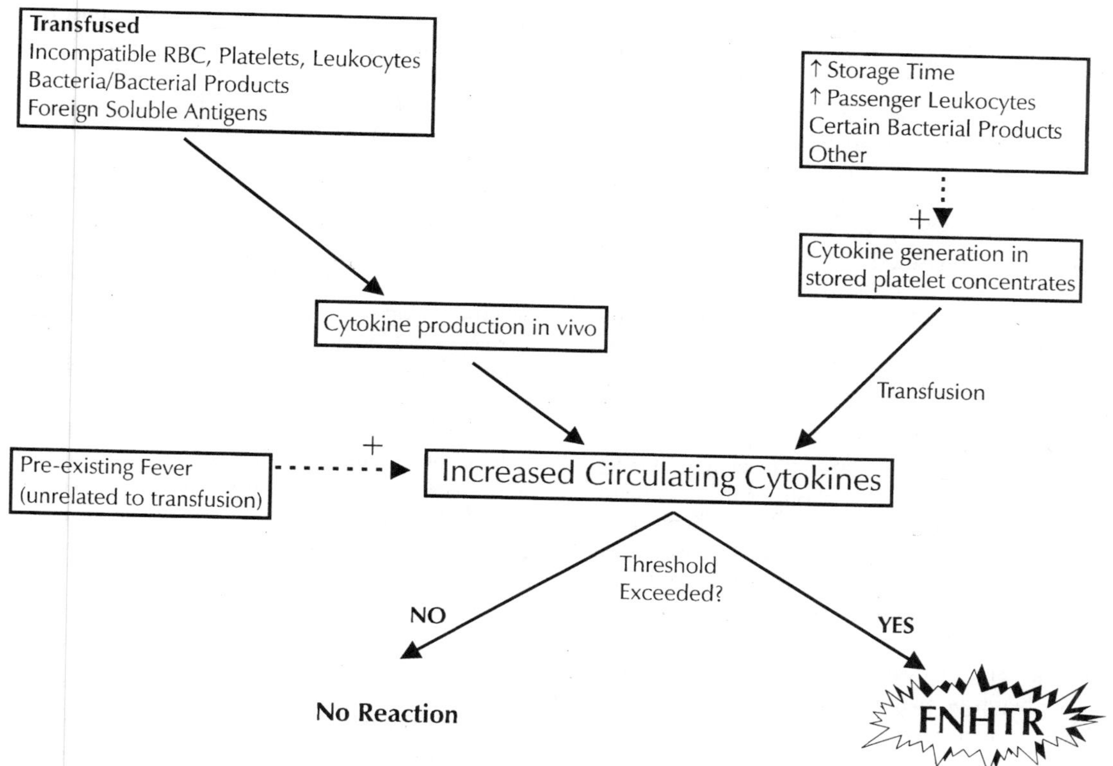

FIGURE 58.1. Cytokine model of febrile nonhemolytic transfusion reaction. Two potential sources of intravascular, pyrogenic cytokines in transfusion recipients are (1) endogenous production resulting from various transfusion-related immune stimuli or incompatibilities, and (2) infusion of cytokines generated in blood components during storage. Preexisting fever at the time of transfusion may prime the cytokine response and predispose transfusion recipients to a further febrile response. (From Stack G, Berkowitz D. Cytokines production during blood component storage. In: Davenport RD, Snyder EL, eds. *Cytokines in transfusion medicine: a primer.* Bethesda, MD: American Association of Blood Banks, 1997:46, with permission.)

pyrogenic stimuli. The transfusion provides a second stimulus for generation of cytokines and fever that acts in an additive or synergistic manner with the previous stimulus, causing an FNHTR to be induced more readily. Evidence for priming effects or synergism of multiple pyrogenic stimuli has been obtained in areas other than transfusion (8).

Alloimmunization to Leukocytes or Platelets

Transfusion recipients at greatest risk of an FNHTR are those with antileukocyte or antiplatelet antibodies who receive transfusions with blood components containing large numbers of passenger leukocytes or platelets (11,12). Less frequently, donor antibodies to leukocytes present in the plasma portion of blood components are associated with FNHTRs. The implicated antibodies most often have specificity for human leukocyte antigens (HLA), although they also may be platelet- or granulocyte-specific. A minimum of approximately 5×10^8 leukocytes per unit of RBCs appears necessary to cause an FNHTR, although this number varies among individuals (13,14). The role of donor leukocytes in FNHTR is supported by the finding that decreasing the leukocyte content of blood components below this threshold reduces the incidence of FNHTRs.

A variety of mechanisms are possible by which antibody-leukocyte or antibody-platelet interactions cause fever. For example, donor monocytes may be activated and secrete pyrogenic cytokines when recipient antibodies bind to them. An alternative explanation is that immune complex formation between recipient antibodies and donor leukocytes or platelets leads to generation of activated complement components, which stimulate the release of pyrogenic cytokines from recipient or donor monocytes.

Storage-generated Cytokines

Antibodies to leukocytes or platelets do not appear to account for all FNHTRs, particularly those caused by platelet transfusions. For example, some patients with no history of transfusion or pregnancy have an FNHTR to their first transfusion of platelets (3). It is unlikely that these reactions are mediated by recipient leukocyte or platelet antibodies because these recipients have no previous exposure to foreign cells. In addition, the rate of FNHTRs to platelet transfusion increases with increasing blood bank storage time of the transfused platelet concentrate (5–7). This indicates that time-dependent change occurs in the platelet concentrate during storage that has a role in stimulating an FNHTR in some patients. Furthermore, febrile reactions still occur with the use of bedside leukoreduction filters that are capable of 3-$\log_{10}$ (99.9%) or more leukocyte reduction (4,15). In some cases, this is the result of inappropriate filter use or filter failure. However, this observation also supports the possibility that a substance or substances in the plasma portion of blood components not removed by filtration may be responsible for mediating at least some FNHTRs. The discovery that proinflammatory cytokines accumulate in the plasma portion of platelet concentrates may account for many of these findings.

A variety of leukocyte-derived, proinflammatory cytokines, including IL-1β, IL- 6, IL-8, TNF-α, macrophage inflammatory protein 1α (MIP-1α), and growth-related oncogene α (GRO-α), are generated and accumulate in the plasma portion of platelet concentrates during storage (8,9,16–18). Extracellular levels of these cytokines generally increase with increasing component storage time and are roughly proportional to the passenger leukocyte content of the blood component bag. Prestorage or early-storage leukoreduction (within 1 to 2 days of collection) by means of filtration prevents or greatly reduces generation of these cytokines. Because they have pyrogenic activity, many of these cytokines if present in high enough concentration can induce febrile responses in transfusion recipients. Levels of IL-6, IL-1β, and TNF-α in the plasma portion of platelet concentrates correlate positively with the occurrence of an FNHTR (17,18). Some studies have shown that IL-6 levels in the plasma portion of platelet concentrates correlate best with the occurrence of FNHTR. In one study, chills, fever, or both occurred more frequently after infusion of the plasma portion of the platelet concentrates than after infusion the cellular portion containing platelets and leukocytes (18). The plasma portions that caused an FNHTR contained higher levels of IL-6 and IL-1β than did those that did not cause chills or fever. These data support the role of the plasma portion of platelet concentrate as a source of inflammatory mediators and as a possible stimulus of FNHTR in some transfusion recipients. Although levels of a variety of proinflammatory cytokines in the plasma portion of platelet concentrate correlate with the occurrence of FNHTRs, it is unknown which, if any, of these actually mediate FNHTRs. Other inflammatory mediators, such as activated complement fragments (19) and biologically active lipids (20) accumulate in platelet concentrates during storage and also may be implicated.

Platelet-derived cytokines, such as RANTES and transforming growth factor β1 (TGF-β1), are present in the plasma portion of platelet concentrates and apheresis platelets (8). These cytokines are not known to be directly pyrogenic, but they do have stimulatory effects on monocytes. For example, TGF-β1 stimulates monocytes to secrete IL-1β and TNF-α, which are pyrogenic. Because RANTES can activate basophils and mast cells and stimulate histamine release, it may play a role in mediating some allergic reactions (see later, Allergic Reactions).

Some proinflammatory cytokines, such as IL-1β and IL-8 have been detected in the supernatant portion of stored RBCs, although at much lower levels than in platelet concentrates (21). Because the cold storage temperature of RBC units (1°C to 6°C) has an inhibitory effect on cellular metabolism, the capacity of passenger leukocytes in RBC units to synthesize and secrete cytokines is less than those in platelet concentrates. As a result, the levels of cytokines in RBC units appear to be too low to mediate significant physiologic reactions.

The stimulus for cytokine generation during storage of blood components remains unknown. Measurements of cytokine messenger RNA levels and total cytokine levels (intracellular plus extracellular) in platelet concentrates indicates that accumulation of leukocyte-derived cytokines is due in part to new synthesis and secretion. The stimulus for synthesis and secretion of leukocyte-derived cytokines may be, for example, contact activation of monocytes after these cells interact with the plastic of the storage containers or tubing (22). Other possibilities include the stimulatory effects of activated complement components on monocytes or other leukocytes in the blood component bag. The presence of platelet-derived cytokines, such as RANTES and TGF-β1, in the plasma portion of platelet concentrates is likely due to their release from preexisting stores, because the biosynthetic activity of platelets is limited.

Bacterial Contamination of Blood Components

An FNHTR may result from infusion of a blood component contaminated with bacteria or bacterial products. Unless Gram stain and bacterial cultures are performed, mild septic transfusion reactions characterized by only fever and chills are likely to be classified clinically as FNHTR (23) (see Chapter 55).

Transfusion reactions caused by contaminating bacteria, whether mild or severe, are manifestations of the systemic inflammatory response syndrome (SIRS), described earlier. Proinflammatory cytokines, such as IL-1β, IL-6, IL-8, and TNF-α are implicated in the pathogenesis of SIRS associated with sepsis (24–27). The greatest source of cytokines if bacterial contamination of blood components has occurred is likely the transfusion recipients' cells stimulated by the infused bacteria or bacterial products. However, cytokine production by leukocytes in the component bag during storage stimulated by bacteria or bacterial products also may contribute to the reaction.

Diagnosis

As a routine part of the transfusion procedure, the vital signs of transfusion recipients (pulse, temperature, and respiratory rate) should be measured immediately before transfusion and at intervals during and soon after transfusion. The patient should be watched closely, particularly in the first 30 to 60 minutes of transfusion, for the onset of chills, shivering, or rigors, which often precede a fever.

A transfusion reaction is a possibility if chills, fever (1°C or more over pretransfusion temperature), or both develop any time during transfusion or up to several hours after the transfusion has ended. A febrile response to transfusion, however, is not specific for an FNHTR. For example, a fever may be the early manifestation of a more serious acute hemolytic or septic transfusion reaction. When a patient has a febrile reaction to transfusion, an evaluation to rule out hemolysis and possibly bacterial contamination should be undertaken promptly. Nursing staff should stop the transfusion immediately and notify the physician caring for the patient. They should verify that the identity of the transfusion recipient, based on the patient's identification bracelet and verbal confirmation with the recipient, if possible, matches that of the intended recipient, as indicated on the blood component tag. All containers and transfusion sets should be sent to the laboratory along with a posttransfusion blood specimen and a report that summarizes the clinical reaction. The clinical team should also have verbal communication with the blood bank staff to assure that the postreaction blood specimen, component bag, and infusion set are received by the blood bank as soon as possible.

Investigation of a febrile reaction in the blood bank generally begins with a recheck of the records for clerical errors. The posttransfusion serum must be visually evaluated for hemolysis and should be compared with the pretransfusion serum. A direct antiglobulin test, also called a direct Coombs test, must be performed on the posttransfusion blood specimen and ideally also on a pretransfusion specimen for comparison. The ABO typing of the patient and the donor unit should be repeated, and the crossmatch should be repeated for RBC transfusions to confirm patient-donor compatibility. The results of these tests confirm or exclude a hemolytic transfusion reaction as the basis for the fever. When a septic reaction is highly suspected, for example if the patient arrives with a high fever (2°C or more) or accompanying hypotension, the bag contents should be examined by means of Gram stain and culture for bacterial contamination. Blood cultures also should be obtained from a posttransfusion blood specimen from the transfusion recipient to look for bacteremia with the same organism that may be detected in the blood component bag. Most blood banks do not test for HLA-specific, platelet-specific, or granulocyte-specific antibodies in the recipient's serum as possible causes of an FNHTR. Identification of these antibodies and pyrogenic cytokinesis is reserved for specialized laboratories and does not play a role in the immediate evaluation of most reactions.

The patient is examined by the patient care team and the blood bank physician to determine whether associated symptoms or circumstances can explain the fever, such as drug reactions, sepsis, or other inflammatory conditions unrelated to transfusion. The time course of the development and resolution of fever should be examined in relation to the transfusion. In cases in which the transfusion recipient has a fever at the start of transfusion or is experiencing intermittent spiking fevers, a posttransfusion increase in body temperature can be difficult to interpret. In such cases *possible FNHTR* may be the most definitive diagnosis that can be made. An FNHTR is a diagnosis of exclusion, arrived at by means of eliminating the possibility of immune hemolysis, bacterial contamination of the blood component, or other causes of fever unrelated to transfusion.

Treatment

The transfusion should be stopped immediately. The intravenous line should be kept open with normal saline solution to provide ready access for the possible infusion of crystalloid and intravenous medication in case the fever is a sign of a more serious hemolytic or septic reaction. Most patients, however, should be reassured that febrile transfusion reactions usually are harmless and that the fever typically responds to antipyretic therapy. The antipyretic agent of choice is acetaminophen (adults, 325 to 650 mg orally; children, 10 to 15 mg/kg orally or rectally). Aspirin and nonsteroidal antiinflammatory drugs are contraindicated in the treatment of many transfusion recipients. Unless the patient has signs of an allergic reaction, such as urticaria, erythema, or pruritus, antihistamines are not indicated in the management of FNHTR.

Patients with severe shaking chills can be treated with meperidine (adults, 25 to 50 mg intravenously) (28). Because shivering can increase oxygen demand severalfold, it is important to control the shaking chills, particularly for patients with cardiac or respiratory insufficiency. Meperidine is effective in rapidly stopping shaking chills through mechanisms not clearly understood. Use of meperidine is generally contraindicated in the care of patients with renal failure owing to accumulation of the proconvulsant metabolite normeperidine. Use of meperidine also is contraindicated in the care of patients who have taken monoamine oxidase inhibitors within the previous 14 days because of the risk of serotonin syndrome (excess serotonin activity).

Any unused portion of the blood component should be returned to the blood bank and not subsequently transfused, even if blood bank testing rapidly rules out hemolysis. This is because no quick test is currently available that is sensitive enough to also rule out with confidence bacterial contamination of the blood component. Gram staining helps detect heavily contaminated units, but lower levels of contamination may be missed. If the febrile reaction is caused by bacterial contamination of the component bag, restarting transfusion of the same component can cause a severe and even fatal septic transfusion reaction as more bacteria or bacterial products are infused. For this reason, a new blood component unit should be used if transfusion is still needed after the patient's condition has been stabilized.

Restarting transfusion with the same platelet preparation that caused an FNHTR may be considered as a last resort in the treatment of patients who repeatedly have mild and uncomplicated febrile responses to platelet transfusions despite prophylactic measures (see later) (29). In this situation, it may be necessary to cautiously complete the transfusion with the same component, because the patient is likely also to react to other platelet preparations. The patient should have no other symptoms and the fever should be less than 1.5°C over the pretransfusion baseline. A septic reaction due to bacterial contamination of a unit is generally the major concern in this setting. Hemolysis of either donor or recipient RBCs usually is not significant owing to the small amount of RBCs and plasma in platelet preparations. The transfusion should generally not be restarted for at least 30 minutes as a precaution to allow other possible signs or symptoms of a serious reaction to develop. High transfusion-related fevers, such as a 2°C increment or more, are more likely to be associated with septic reactions and should preclude restarting the transfusion. However, lesser fevers do not rule out bacterial contamination of the blood component. If the transfusion is restarted, the patient should be made as comfortable as possible with appropriate antipyretic therapy, as described earlier. The transfusion should proceed slowly and the patient observed closely for further signs of a reaction or further temperature elevation throughout the transfusion, which should be stopped if symptoms reoccur. Restarting transfusion of a blood component that has caused an FNHTR should not be routine.

Prevention

Premedication

Premedication with acetaminophen but not diphenhydramine should be considered for patients with a history of FNHTR. Patients who have no history of FNHTR do not need premedication. Premedication with the glucocorticoid hydrocortisone sodium succinate (adults, 100 mg intravenously) may be useful in the care of reaction-prone patients when an antipyretic agent alone is ineffective. Glucocorticoids have antiinflammatory effects that may help prevent or reduce the severity of FNHTRs. For example, they inhibit the enzyme phospholipase A_2, thereby blocking production of arachidonic acid and its metabolites such as prostaglandin E_2, a key mediator of fever. Glucocorticoids also inhibit synthesis of pyrogenic cytokines, such as IL-1 and IL-6. A variety of glucocorticoids are available other than hydrocortisone. However, hydrocortisone has the advantage of being a short-acting glucocorticoid (biologic half-life, 8 to 12 hours), and it induces a shorter period of immunosuppression than do many other glucocorticoid preparations. Because glucocorticoids generally act through changes in gene expression, hydrocortisone should be administered at least 4 to 6 hours before transfusion so that its antiinflammatory action has time to take effect.

Rate of Infusion

Slowing the speed of infusion of a blood component can possibly prevent or decrease the severity of FNHTR. The rate of increase in body temperature in FNHTR due to leukocyte alloimmunization appears to be directly related to the rate of infusion of leukocytes in the blood components (13). A slower rate of infusion is of theoretic advantage in decreasing the severity of reactions due to bacterial contamination or storage-generated cytokines. Slower infusion avoids a sudden bolus of bacterial toxins or cytokines that may provoke an immediate and possibly massive inflammatory response.

Leukoreduction

The prophylactic transfusion of leukoreduced components in the treatment of patients receiving repeated transfusions is effective in avoiding alloimmunization to leukocytes, which is one of the major causes of FNHTR. Leukoreduced blood components ideally should be transfused into such patients beginning with the first transfusion. Leukoreduction is effective in the care of patients already alloimmunized to leukocytes, because FNHTRs in these patients are directly related to the number of and rate of infusion of passenger leukocytes. The threshold number of white blood cells associated with the development of an FNHTR generally ranges from 0.25×10^9 to 2.5×10^9 (13). The removal of approximately 90% of leukocytes (1 log10) which usually leaves less than 5×10^8 white blood cells per unit of RBCs, is sufficient to prevent most FNHTRs (14,30). For that reason, leukoreduction for the purpose of preventing FNHTRs often is defined as decreasing the passenger leukocytes to less than 5×10^8 per transfusion. Leukoreduction of blood components can be done either at the time of component preparation (prestorage leukoreduction) or immediately before transfusion (poststorage leukoreduction). Poststorage leukoreduction by means of filtration can be done in the blood bank before distribution of the component for transfusion or during administration of blood components. The latter often is called *bedside leukoreduction.*

Leukoreduced RBC units have in the past been prepared by means of a variety of poststorage techniques, including simple centrifugation with buffy-coat removal, saline washing, and deglycerolization of frozen RBCs (31,32). Saline-washed and frozen deglycerolized RBCs are rendered leukoreduced because approximately 1 to 2 $\log_{10}$ leukocytes are removed by means of repeated centrifugation and washing steps on automated cell washers. Filtration of RBCs through microaggregate filters designed to remove microaggregate debris more than 40 μm in diameter after an extra centrifugation step or after centrifugation and cooling (spin, cool, filter) also has been shown to leukoreduce RBC units sufficiently to reduce the incidence of FNHTRs (33–36).

High-efficiency leukoreduction filters have been developed for units of RBCs and platelets that are capable of removing both microaggregate debris and nonaggregated leukocytes (37). These leukoreduction filters can remove 3 or more log (99.9% or more) leukocytes, thereby decreasing the leukocyte content to approximately 1×10^6/unit or less. Despite their efficacy in leukoreduction, use of these filters at the bedside has had variable and sometimes disappointing results in reducing the incidence of FNHTRs to platelet concentrates (4,15). This may the result of causes of FNHTR other than leukocyte antibodies in the transfusion recipient (see earlier, Etiology). For example, storage-generated, extracellular cytokines in the component bag that either are not removed or are inadequately removed by means of poststorage filtration are now believed to mediate some reactions (see earlier, Etiology). As a result, the practice of prestorage leukoreduction is increasingly replacing poststorage leukoreduction. Prestorage leukoreduction not only removes leukocytes but also removes leukocytes before they have a chance to release cytokines that can accumulate extracellularly in blood component bags during storage.

Prestorage leukoreduction of platelet concentrates or RBC units is achieved by use of blood component containers with in-line leukoreduction filters in a closed system between the primary collection bag and satellite containers. Prestorage leukoreduced platelets also can be prepared with some automated apheresis instruments equipped with centrifugation chambers designed to minimize leukocyte collection (so-called *process leukoreduction*) (see Chapter 21). Because some data indicate that on average only approximately 15% of patients who experience an FNHTR will have a similar reaction to the next transfusion, some blood banks still provide a leukoreduced product (either prestorage or bedside leukoreduced) only when a patient has had two or more documented febrile reactions (2,38). This practice is cost-effective but has the disadvantage of subjecting some patients to two uncomfortable reactions before a preventive measure is taken. The U.S. Food and Drug Administration is considering making universal leukoreduction a national policy. Poststorage plasma removal from platelet preparations by saline washing techniques is an alternative to prestorage leukoreduction for eliminating extracellular cytokines (39–41). Prestorage leukoreduction by means of filtration is a more efficient and cost-effective way to eliminate extracellular leukocyte-derived cytokines while reducing passenger leukocytes. Moreover, in evaluations of plasma removal from platelet concentrates to reduce the risk of FNHTR, this technique still is associated with FNHTR in a relatively large percentage of recipients (42). Neither leukoreduction nor poststorage plasma removal has been effective in eliminating all FNHTRs to platelet transfusions.

ALLERGIC REACTIONS

Description

An allergic reaction is a type I immediate hypersensitivity response consisting of transient localized or generalized urticaria, erythema, and pruritus. More serious allergic reactions can be complicated by hypotension and angioedema of the face and larynx. In our classification, allergic reactions have only cutaneous manifestations and usually are mild, resolving soon after administration of antihistamines. If other organ systems—cardiovascular, respiratory, or gastrointestinal—are involved beyond mild hypotension, particularly if the reaction is serious enough to necessitate treatment beyond antihistamines, we refer to the reaction as *anaphylactic* or *anaphylactoid* (see later). Allergic and anaphylactic reactions, however, are part of a continuum. Allergic reactions occur during or soon after transfusion of plasma-containing blood components. Atopic individuals—those with other known allergies—appear at greater risk of allergic reactions.

Etiology

Allergic reactions are mediated by recipient immunoglobulin E (IgE) or non-IgE antibodies to proteins or other allergenic soluble substances in the donor plasma. The result of the hypersensitivity reaction is secretion of histamine from mast cells and basophils, which mediates cutaneous reactions by increasing vascular permeability.

Although the source of histamine in allergic reactions is believed in many cases to be the transfusion recipient's mast cells and basophils, it has been hypothesized that histamine generated by leukocytes in stored cellular blood components may play a role. Several studies have shown that histamine accumulates in the plasma portion of platelet concentrates and RBC units with increasing storage time (43,44). These data are consistent with the observation that allergic transfusion reactions also are more common with increasing storage time of blood components (5, 6,43). Several of the chemokines that accumulate in the plasma portion of platelet concentrates during blood bank storage, such as IL-8, RANTES, and MIP-1α, can recruit and activate basophils and stimulate histamine release. Therefore it is theoretically possible that the infusion of storage-generated donor cytokines during transfusion may contribute to the onset of allergic reactions among transfusion recipients. Consistent with this hypothesis, the platelet-derived cytokine, RANTES, is present at higher levels in platelet concentrates that cause allergic reactions (45).

Allergic (and anaphylactic) reactions have been reported after infusion of antibodies in donor plasma, such as antipenicillin antibody infused into recipients receiving penicillin or related antibiotics, and after infusion of drugs in donor plasma, such as penicillin infused into recipients already sensitized to penicillin.

Diagnosis

Urticaria is readily diagnosed clinically by the presence of the cutaneous wheal-and-flare reaction. Because allergic symptoms usually are mild and are not characteristic of hemolytic transfusion reactions, serologic blood bank investigations to rule out hemolysis usually are unrevealing. Isolated, mild urticarial reactions not accompanied by other signs and symptoms necessitate minimal diagnostic evaluation. If the reaction is severe, has atypical manifestations, or is accompanied by fever, which is uncharacteristic of allergic reactions, a more elaborate laboratory evaluation to rule-out a hemolytic or septic transfusion reaction is indicated. In the diagnosis of an allergic reaction as transfusion-related, it is important to rule out, if possible, urticarial drug reactions that may be circumstantially attributed to transfusions. Careful attention to the timing of onset of urticaria relative to the transfusion may help avoid this confusion. Administration of medication should generally be discouraged in the peritransfusion period to avoid such confusion.

Even mild allergic reactions should be reported to the blood bank. Monitoring allergic reactions and correlating reactions with any newly implemented changes in blood component collection, processing, storage, or filtration are important in detecting new and unexpected causes of reactions. In the care of patients with repeated allergic reactions, notification of the blood bank allows the blood bank medical director to consult on measures to manage or prevent such reactions in the future.

Treatment

The patient can be treated with a first-generation, H_1-blocking antihistamine (adults, 25 to 50 mg diphenhydramine intravenously or 25 mg hydroxyzine intramuscularly). If the sedating side effects of first-generation antihistamines must be avoided, newer, less-sedating antihistamines are available for oral administration (adults, cetirizine 10 mg orally, loratadine 10 mg orally, or fexofenadine 60 mg orally); however, parenteral antihistamines are preferred in the management of acute reactions because of their more rapid bioavailability. An H_2 blocker, such as cimetidine (adults, 300 mg intravenously) or ranitidine (adults, 50 mg intravenously) may be added to the H_1 blocker to speed resolution of the reaction. Combining H_1 and H_2 antagonists has given better results in treating patients with allergic reactions in nontransfusion settings than has use of an H_1 antagonist alone (46,47). For reactions characterized by only localized urticaria, such as a few hives, the transfusion can be temporarily discontinued while an antihistamine is administered. The transfusion can be resumed in approximately 30 minutes if the urticaria has cleared and if no further symptoms occur. For patients with generalized urticaria or a more serious allergic reaction accompanied by facial or laryngeal edema or hypotension, the transfusion should be discontinued and the infusion set with any untransfused blood returned to the blood bank. If laryngeal edema causes breathing difficulties or if hypotension is severe, epinephrine (adult dose, 0.2 to 0.5 ml of 1:1,000 solution [0.2 to 0.5 mg] subcutaneously) can be administered.

Prevention

Transfusion recipients often are given routine premedication with an antihistamine such as diphenhydramine in an effort to prevent or reduce the severity of allergic transfusion reactions, even when they have had no previous reactions. The value of this approach is uncertain, because few patients have allergic reactions. When premedication is restricted to patients who have had two or more previous allergic reactions, overall reaction rates do not increase. Accordingly, premedication with an antihistamine should probably be reserved for recipients who have had a previous allergic reaction. For patients with repeated reactions not eliminated by premedication with an H_1 blocker alone, a combination of H_1 and H_2 blockers has been shown more effective (46,47).

Should premedication not prevent repeated allergic transfusion reactions, another option is to reduce the plasma content of transfused blood components. This can be achieved in RBC and platelet preparations with automated saline "washing" (32, 39–41). However, washing or plasma removal steps generally should be reserved for patients with two or more serious allergic reactions (e.g., those that include angioedema or hypotension) that are not prevented with premedication with both H_1 and H_2 blockers, because cell washing is time-consuming and can delay transfusion. Patients with two or more allergic reactions can undergo testing for IgA deficiency, because this is a reported cause of both allergic and anaphylactic reactions.

ANAPHYLACTIC AND ANAPHYLACTOID REACTIONS

Description

Anaphylactic reactions are serious and potentially life-threatening type I immediate hypersensitivity reactions to allergens in the plasma of transfused blood components (48). These reactions can have a rapid onset beginning as early as seconds to minutes after the start of the transfusion and can occur with small transfused volumes. Anaphylactic reactions are differentiated from other allergic (urticarial) transfusion reactions by their systemic nature and severity. These reactions generally affect multiple organ systems, as evidenced by cutaneous, respiratory, cardiovascular, and gastrointestinal effects. The symptom complex often includes the rapid onset of laryngeal edema and bronchospasm with stridor, wheezing, coughing, and respiratory distress. Other symptoms include generalized urticaria, erythema, tachycardia, hypotension, nausea, vomiting, diarrhea, cramping abdominal pain, and pelvic pain (in women). Severe reactions can proceed rapidly to shock, syncope, respiratory failure, and death. Fatal anaphylactic reactions are less common than are fatal hemolytic or septic reactions.

Etiology

Anaphylactic reactions occur when an allergen present in plasma is transfused into a patient who through previous sensitization has a preexisting IgE directed against that allergen. Immunoglobulin E is bound by means of Fc receptors to mast cells and basophils. The binding of allergen to cell-bound IgE results in cross-linking of IgE and Fc receptors. This cross-linking activates the mast cells and basophils to secrete preformed mediators, such as histamine, as well as newly synthesized mediators, such as leukotrienes, prostaglandins, and cytokines (Fig. 58.2).

Anaphylactoid reactions are clinically identical to anaphylactic reactions but occur by mechanisms that do not involve IgE. For example, immune complexes involving antibodies other than IgE may result in complement fixation and generation of the anaphylatoxins C3a, C4a, and C5a, which activate basophils and mast cells. Some cytokines secreted by monocytes as part of the inflammatory cascade initiated by non-IgE immune complex formation also can directly activate basophils and mast cells and initiate anaphylactoid reactions. Moreover, IgG4 subclass antibodies can bind to Fc receptors of mast cells and basophils and, in a manner analogous to that of IgE, mediate cellular activation and degranulation after binding of allergen. The term *anaphylactoid* is sometimes mistakenly used to describe mild or a clinically atypical anaphylactic reactions. However, *anaphylactoid* is properly used to differentiate the mechanism of the reaction, not its clinical severity or presentation.

The best-documented anaphylactoid reactions have resulted from the infusion of donor plasma containing IgA into IgA-deficient recipients who have produced a class-specific IgG anti-IgA that reacts with all IgA subclasses. Less commonly, patients with normal total IgA levels have a subclass-specific IgA deficiency and may make an anti-IgA of restricted specificity. Although IgA deficiency is relatively common (approximately 1 case among 700 persons), anaphylactoid reactions occur only among some IgA-deficient transfusion recipients, because not all make anti-IgA. Anaphylactic or anaphylactoid reactions have been documented among patients with deficiencies of other plasma proteins, such as complement, von Willebrand factor, and haptoglobin (49–51). In an analogous manner, these patients produce an antibody to the missing factor that reacts with transfused, plasma-containing blood components. In most anaphylactic or anaphylactoid reactions, however, the allergen is never identified, nor is evidence obtained to differentiate anaphylactic from anaphylactoid mechanisms.

Diagnosis

Anaphylactic and anaphylactoid reactions are diagnosed from clinical signs and symptoms (see earlier, Description). The cutaneous signs and symptoms and the often rapid onset of the reaction help differentiate anaphylactic reactions from acute hemolytic and septic transfusion reactions. Serum β-tryptase levels may be measured to confirm an anaphylactic reaction, because it is a marker for mast cell degranulation. However, no laboratory measurement is available in time to meaningfully affect recognition and management of an anaphylactic reaction.

Recipient IgA levels should be measured in a pretransfusion

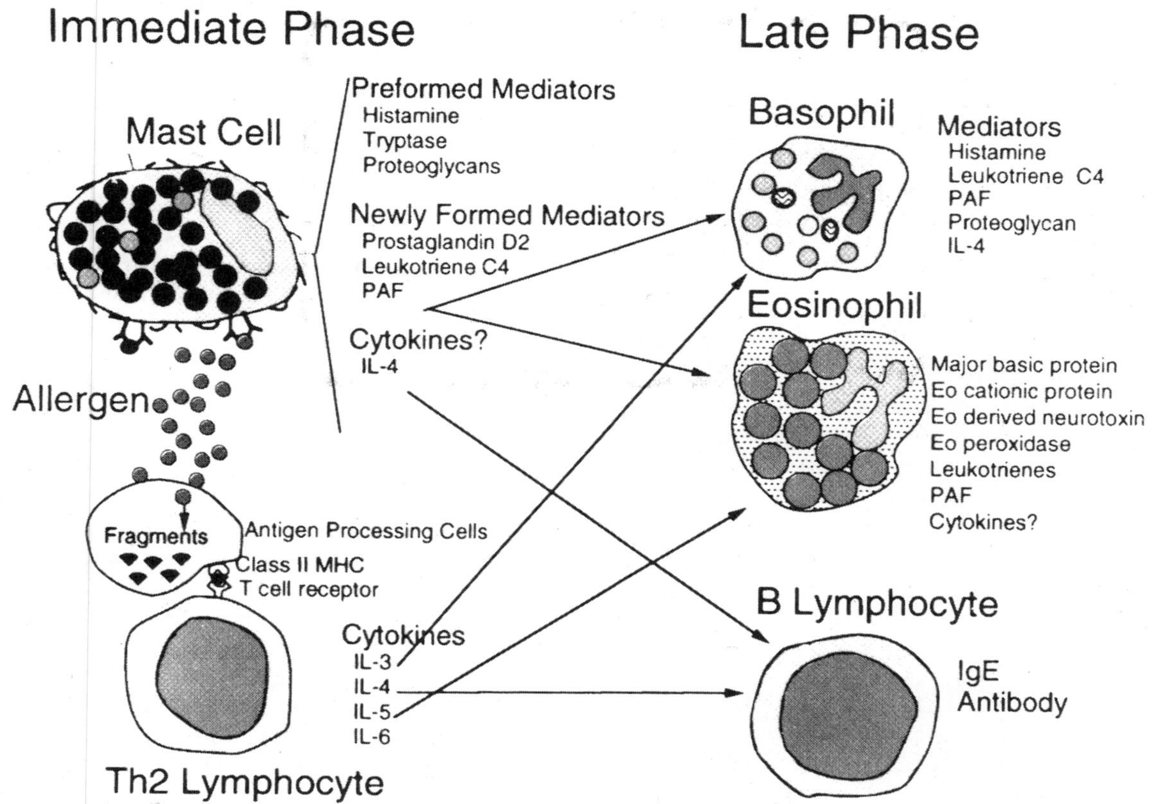

FIGURE 58.2. Mediators of immediate- and late-phase responses in allergic and anaphylactic reactions. The immediate phase is characterized by allergen-mediated activation of mast cells due to cross-linking of immunoglobulin E molecules on the mast cell surface. Activated mast cells release the indicated mediators of allergic responses. Lymphocytes also are activated to secrete cytokines. Mediators of the immediate-phase response can induce a secondary wave of late-occurring responses (late phase) through the activation basophils, eosinophils, and B lymphocytes. *PAF,* platelet activating factor; *Eo,* eosinophil; *IL,* interleukin. (From Norman PS. Current status of immunotherapy for allergies and anaphylactic reactions. *Adv Intern Med* 1996;41:682, with permission.)

blood specimen to determine whether the recipient is IgA-deficient. Although the results of tests for IgA deficiency do not affect diagnosis or management of the reaction at hand, it is important for avoiding future reactions. Testing should be done on a specimen drawn before transfusion, because IgA deficiency can be masked by any IgA provided by the transfusion. Recipient anti-IgA also can be measured, especially for rare cases in which the anti-IgA is subtype-specific and total IgA levels are within the reference range. Although IgA is the most commonly known allergen in anaphylactoid reactions, in most anaphylactic and anaphylactoid reactions, the offending allergen is not IgA and is never identified.

Treatment

Anaphylactic and anaphylactoid reactions are managed identically (52,53). Severe reactions are a true medical emergency and should be managed by experienced critical care staff, if possible. The patient should be placed in an intensive care unit as soon as it is practical without jeopardizing emergency care. Once anaphylaxis is evident clinically, 1:1000 epinephrine solution (1 mg/ml) should be administered subcutaneously in a dose of 0.2 to 0.5 ml for adults (0.01 ml/kg of body weight for children). The dose may be repeated every 15 to 30 minutes as needed. Intravenous crystalloid or colloid solution should be administered as needed to support the patient's blood pressure. For example, 500 ml to 1 L of normal saline solution can be administered in the first 15 to 30 minutes. Further infusion should be titrated to blood pressure. If the systolic blood pressure is less than 60 mm Hg, intravenous epinephrine in a dose of 1 to 5 ml of a 1:10,000 solution (0.1 mg/ml) for adults and 0.1 ml/kg for children, is administered over 2 to 5 minutes by means of intravenous push. An epinephrine drip (1 to 4 μg/min) may be started, and administration of other pressors, such as dopamine, can be considered. Blood pressure, pulse, and urine output should be monitored. It may be necessary to monitor the effectiveness of fluid replacement and pressor infusion through measurement of central venous pressure.

Respiratory distress is managed with supplemental oxygen. The patient's upper airway may have to be secured with endotracheal intubation if obstruction due to laryngeal edema is imminent. Stridor is a sign of laryngeal edema. Endotracheal intubation and mechanical assistance with ventilation are indicated if the $PaCO_2$ increases to more than 65 mm Hg. When intubation is difficult or impossible because of laryngeal obstruction, cricothyrotomy or tracheostomy is an option. Wheezing due to obstruction of small bronchi and bronchioles by increased mucus production and smooth muscle contraction can be managed with nebulized albuterol or metaproterenol and intravenous aminophylline.

Urticaria, angioedema, or gastrointestinal distress is managed with an antihistamine (adults, 50 mg diphenhydramine intravenously; children, 1 to 2 mg/kg intravenously). H_2-blocking antihistamines may be added as an adjunct to H_1 blockers. Glucocorticoids, such as hydrocortisone, 200 mg intravenously every 6 hours, usually are also administered because they reduce late-phase inflammatory responses. Glucocorticoids, however, are not expected to be of benefit in the initial management of anaphylaxis owing to their delayed onset of action.

Prevention

Patients with IgA deficiency who have already had an anaphylactic reaction or who are known to have anti-IgA should be treated by means of transfusion of RBC and platelet preparations that have been saline-washed with an automated cell washer (32, 39–41). If plasma transfusion is necessary, only IgA-deficient donors should be used. Patients who have anaphylactic reactions to any other known plasma allergen also should be treated with transfusion of saline-washed RBCs or platelet preparations. Because anaphylactic reactions can be induced by very small amounts of allergen, washing must be extensive. Washing and saline replacement by means of automated cell washers have been shown generally successful in removing IgA sufficiently to prevent recurrences of anaphylactoid reactions.

If a patient has had one anaphylactic reaction of unknown causation, the next transfusion need not necessarily be performed with washed RBCs or platelets, because the reaction might have been donor-specific. The next transfusion may be administered slowly with vigilance after premedication with both H_1 and H_2 blockers and a glucocorticoid. The following premedication regimen proposed for use as prophylaxis of anaphylactoid reactions to radiographic contrast media is suggested: 50 mg oral prednisone or 200 mg intravenous hydrocortisone 13 hours, 7 hours, and 1 hour before transfusion plus 50 mg oral or intravenous diphenhydramine and 25 mg ephedrine 1 hour before transfusion (54). The patient care team should be prepared to respond to an anaphylactic reaction. The patient ideally should be in a critical care unit with monitoring at the time of transfusion and with a critical care physician and nurses in attendance. Some blood banks with the capability of automated cell washing, nevertheless, may choose to provide saline-washed RBCs and platelet concentrates for future transfusions after a single anaphylactic reaction as a precautionary measure, particularly if the patient is not expected to receive many more transfusions.

TRANSFUSION-RELATED ACUTE LUNG INJURY

Description

Transfusion-related acute lung injury (TRALI), also known as *noncardiogenic pulmonary edema* or *pulmonary allergic or hypersensitivity reaction,* is a serious pulmonary complication that has an estimated incidence of 1 case in 5,000 to 10,000 transfusions with a fatality rate of 5% to 10%. Classic TRALI has an onset within 6 hours of transfusion, but an atypical form has been described as occurring as late as 2 days after transfusion. Noncardiogenic pulmonary edema following transfusion was first reported in the 1950s. The syndrome was later named *transfusion-related acute lung injury* and more clearly defined as a clinical entity by Popovsky in 1985 (55). Every commonly used blood component that contains plasma has been implicated in causing TRALI, including random-donor platelets, which is the most common, whole blood, RBCs, apheresis platelets, fresh-frozen plasma, cryoprecipitate, and granulocytes. Transfusion-related acute lung injury also has been reported as a complication of infusion of the plasma derivative intravenous immune globulin.

Transfusion-related acute lung injury manifests as adult respiratory distress syndrome with accelerating dyspnea, tachypnea, hypoxemia, fever, chills, cough, and occasionally hypotension (20,56,57). Physical examination reveals signs of pulmonary edema with crackles and decreased breath sounds in dependent lung areas. Chest radiographs show a normal cardiac silhouette with bilateral fluffy infiltrates that can progress to complete white-out of the lung fields. Copious amounts of frothy edema fluid may be found in the endotracheal tube. Although respiratory distress with a similar production of copious amounts of pulmonary edema fluid is characteristic of hypervolemia, other signs of hypervolemia, such as jugular venous distention, murmurs, or gallops are absent. Moreover, TRALI can follow infusion of blood volumes too small to produce fluid overload. Pulmonary wedge pressure and central venous pressure usually are normal during central monitoring. Surviving patients usually recover within 96 hours after the onset of symptoms (56).

Etiology

Two models for the mechanism of TRALI have been described (20,56). In both models, infusion of donor plasma results in activation of recipient neutrophils, which mediate pulmonary injury. One model implicates donor antineutrophil antibodies (55,56). The other implicates biologically active lipids or cytokines (20) (Fig.58.3).

One model of the mechanism for TRALI is based on the finding that approximately 90% of cases are associated with leukoagglutinating antibodies (HLA- or granulocyte-specific antibodies) in the donor plasma (55,56). In a smaller percentage of cases, leukoagglutinating antibodies are present in the recipient's plasma. According to this model, complement is activated after formation of immune complexes (antibody-leukocyte), and C5a-induced leukocyte aggregation results in pulmonary leukostasis (58). A role of immune complexes in TRALI is supported by the observation that in more than 50% of clinical cases, there is correspondence between the specificity of HLA-A or B antibodies of the donor with one or more HLA epitopes of

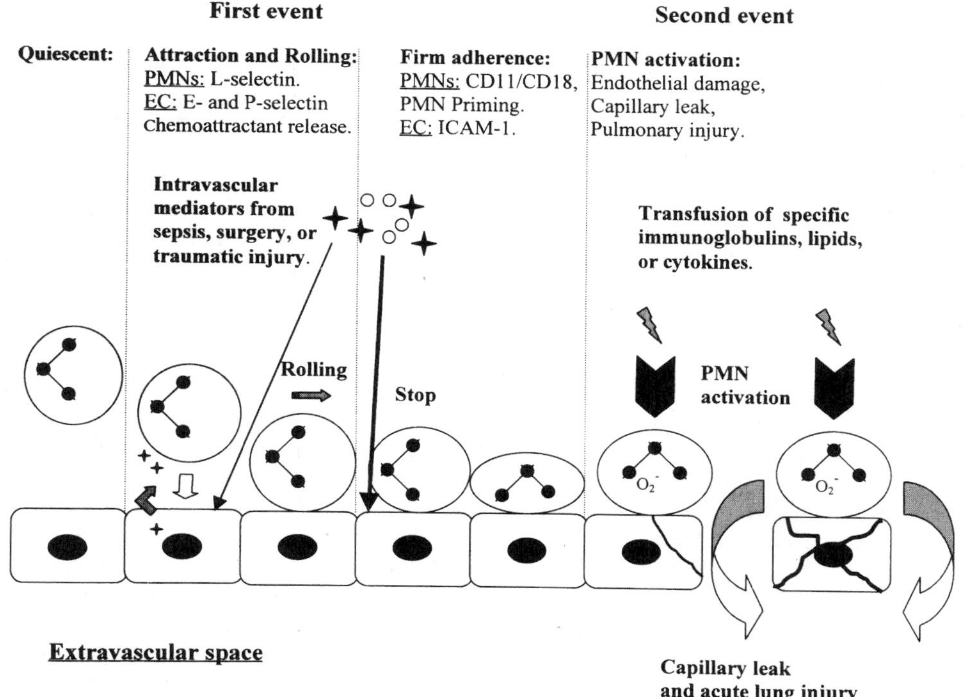

FIGURE 58.3. Two-event model of neutrophil activation in transfusion-associated acute lung injury. In the first event, proinflammatory, intravascular mediators, either endogenous or infused, activate vascular endothelial cells (*EC*). Activation of EC leads to loose attachment, rolling, and firm attachment of polymorphonuclear cells (*PMNs*). In the second event, activation of firmly attached, primed PMNs by means of infusion of biologically active lipids, leukocyte antibodies, or cytokines causes degranulation and oxidative burst. Resulting damage to EC leads to capillary leak and acute lung injury. (From Silliman CG. Transfusion-related acute lung injury. *Transfus Med Rev* 1999;13:181, with permission.)

the recipient. Pulmonary edema presumably occurs because of microvascular occlusion, endothelial damage, and capillary leakage. Leukocytes activated through generation of adhesion molecules are able to firmly attach to pulmonary endothelial cells. Degranulation of neutrophils and release of destructive lysosomal enzymes cause capillary leak syndrome. Complement-activated granulocytes produce oxygen radicals, which also may contribute to the pulmonary endothelial cell damage. Pathologic evidence of this model of TRALI has been reported (59).

In a more recently described model, TRALI is proposed to occur when biologically active lipid compounds or cytokines in the plasma fraction of stored blood are infused and activate the patient's neutrophils in the pulmonary vasculature (20). According to a two-event model, the patient's neutrophils must first be primed by lipopolysaccharide or other agents in the patient's blood as a result of clinical conditions such as sepsis or trauma (event 1) for them to respond to transfusion (event 2) (20). When neutrophils in the pulmonary vasculature are activated by lipid mediators in donor plasma after transfusion, they undergo a respiratory burst and release proteases. This leads to capillary leak, endothelial damage, and pulmonary injury. In support of this mechanism, Silliman (20) found that either stored plasma or a lipid extract of stored plasma but not fresh plasma caused acute lung injury in a rat model with lipopolysaccharide-pretreated lungs. This model may explain cases of TRALI that occur in the absence of identifiable leukoagglutinins.

Some studies have shown an association between TRALI and predisposing clinical conditions. A two-event model of TRALI involving priming due to a predisposing clinical condition and then activation of neutrophils by transfusion is consistent with mechanisms involving either antileukocyte antibodies or lipid activators. A requirement for coordination of two events under appropriate clinical conditions may explain the rare occurrence of TRALI.

Diagnosis and Treatment

The diagnosis of TRALI remains principally a clinical one based on the temporal association of noncardiogenic pulmonary edema with transfusion. In many cases, the patients are very ill with numerous complications, and it may be impossible to clearly distinguish the differential diagnoses, which include hypervolemia, pneumonia, and adult respiratory distress syndrome. Central venous monitoring helps to differentiate cardiogenic from noncardiogenic causes of pulmonary edema, but it often is unavailable. Identification of lymphocytotoxic, leukoagglutinating, or neutrophil antibodies in the donor or patient can be useful in supporting a clinical suspicion of TRALI, but results of these tests are generally not available in time to affect diagnosis and management.

When a patient has signs of noncardiogenic pulmonary edema, the transfusion should be stopped immediately. Treatment is then focused on supportive care. Fluid support to maintain blood pressure and cardiac output and ventilatory support are the mainstays of therapy. Hypervolemia and cardiac dysfunction are not components of TRALI; therefore diuretics are not useful and may even exacerbate the clinical symptoms in some patients (57).

Prevention

Transfusion-related acute lung injury is considered a donor-specific reaction and may never recur in a given patient. If, however, testing reveals that the recipient has circulating antileukocyte antibodies, the use of leukoreduced blood components for future transfusions in the care of that recipient is appropriate. Removing donor leukocytes, however, is not expected to benefit most patients because many cases of TRALI appear to be mediated by antileukocyte antibodies in donor plasma that act on recipient leukocytes. Because TRALI appears to be donor-specific, it is also unclear whether washing RBCs or platelets to remove the donor plasma provides any benefit for future transfusions of components from other donors. However, in the absence of data, some institutions routinely supply washed RBCs and platelets for subsequent transfusions as a theoretical precaution.

When possible, it is important to identify implicated donors and remove them from the donor pool to eliminate the possibility of episodes of TRALI in other recipients. Some blood centers routinely do not prepare plasma-containing blood components, such as fresh-frozen plasma or platelets, from donors with HLA antibodies or from donors who are at high risk of development of HLA antibodies. Because HLA antibodies or leukoagglutinins contained in donor plasma also can cause an FNHTR, removal of the plasma from blood donated by such persons has an additional benefit. In addition, plasma transfusion from multiparous women donors has been associated with impaired pulmonary function among patients in intensive care units (60).

No data exist regarding the role of recipient premedication in preventing recurrence of TRALI. Premedication is not expected to be useful, because TRALI appears to be an idiosyncratic, donor-specific reaction. Glucocorticoids are of theoretic but unproven benefit because of their immunosuppressive and antiinflammatory properties, including their ability to inhibit leukocyte chemotaxis.

In conclusion, TRALI is a highly morbid and possibly fatal reaction caused by the transfusion of leukoagglutinins, lipid mediators, or other agents into a clinically susceptible patient. The diagnosis relies on recognition of a constellation of clinical symptoms shared by other forms of pulmonary edema, and treatment is supportive. The correct diagnosis is critical for identifying implicated donors and preventing reactions among future recipients.

COMPLICATIONS OF MASSIVE AND RAPID TRANSFUSION

Massive transfusion is defined as the replacement of one blood volume within a 24-hour period. For adults of average size, this is roughly equivalent to 10 units of RBCs with any accompanying crystalloid, colloid, platelet, or plasma infusions. The possible complications include citrate toxicity, electrolyte imbalance (hypokalemia due to citrate toxicity, hyperkalemia due to transfusion of older RBCs), circulatory overload, and hypothermia. Recipients of massive transfusions are at increased risk of hemolytic transfusion reactions (including ABO incompatibility), FNHTR, and allergic reactions owing to the number of units they receive. Reactions can be more severe with massive transfusion because rapid infusion means the implicated unit often has been completely administered before the onset of symptoms. The large number of units transfused in a short time period complicates the investigation of transfusion reactions, because each transfused product must be investigated.

Rapid transfusion can occur during therapeutic apheresis and RBC exchange apheresis (erythrocytapheresis). During apheresis procedures, as many as 10 to 20 units of fresh-frozen plasma or 4 to 8 units of RBCs can be transfused over 1.5 to 2 hours. Although any acute transfusion reaction can occur during apheresis-associated transfusion, citrate toxicity in particular is a common but usually mild complication.

Citrate Toxicity

Rapid blood transfusion can cause a transient decrease in the level of ionized calcium because of the calcium-chelating properties of the citrate anticoagulant in stored blood components (61, 62). Citrate toxicity can occur whenever large volumes of plasma that contain citrate are transfused, such as during massive transfusion, plasma exchange, or apheresis procedures (63). Citrate toxicity is a recognized complication of liver transplantation, in which large amounts of plasma are transfused (64).

Citrate ordinarily is rapidly metabolized to bicarbonate in mitochondria-rich tissue, such as liver, skeletal muscle, and kidney (61). In routine transfusion of blood components, patients with normal liver function usually tolerate the citrate infusion without significant complications. However, patients with liver or renal failure or parathyroid dysfunction are at greater risk of citrate toxicity when they receive rapid transfusions of plasma or plasma-containing blood components.

Citrate anticoagulates by binding calcium, thus hypocalcemia is a primary symptom. During apheresis, citrate is administered as acid citrate dextrose formula A in constant proportion to the whole-blood flow rate. Healthy plateletpheresis donors receive relatively large doses of citrate, and many experience mild symptoms of the citrate effect, but the symptoms usually do not progress because of the short duration of the procedure. Donors of peripheral blood stem cells (PBSCs), however, receive smaller doses of citrate per unit of time but usually experience more severe citrate toxicity because of the longer duration of the procedure. Paresthesia due to transient hypocalcemia is common in apheresis. It typically occurs after the initial infusion of the priming solution (if citrate is used) or later as apheresis progresses. Apheresis practitioners should be aware that peripheral paresthesia due to hypocalcemia can be masked in patients with a preexisting neuropathy due to chemotherapy (vincristine) or as part of a neurologic condition.

Citrate toxicity is recognized clinically because of the signs and symptoms of hypocalcemia. It can be confirmed with measurement of plasma ionized calcium in the transfusion recipient. Symptoms of hypocalcemia include peripheral and perioral paresthesia (Chvostek and Trousseau signs can occasionally be elucidated), muscle spasm, cramping, nausea, vomiting, cardiac arrhythmia, bradycardia, hypotension, and if severe, tetany. An electrocardiogram (ECG) can show prolongation of the QT interval with hypocalcemia, but the relation is not linear with the ionized calcium level, and ECG findings are an unreliable guide to calcium therapy (see later). Citrate also binds other metallic divalent cations, such as magnesium and zinc. Accordingly, citrate toxicity can manifest clinically as hypomagnesemia (65).

Mild citrate toxicity during transfusion or apheresis is managed or prevented in part by means of slowing the rate of transfusion or reinfusion. When slowing the infusion rate is impossible or ineffective and the patient has signs and symptoms of hypocalcemia, calcium supplementation is indicated. The best guide to determining a need for calcium supplementation is measurement of the patient's ionized calcium levels, if results can be obtained rapidly. Calcium replacement during apheresis should generally be given when a patient has symptoms, when the patient's clinical condition may exacerbate citrate effects, or when prolonged large-volume leukapheresis is expected to cause citrate toxicity. Infusion of calcium itself, however, is associated with development of ventricular arrhythmia and even cardiac arrest. Therefore intravenous calcium replacement for the management or prophylaxis of apheresis-induced citrate toxicity should be administered only by experienced apheresis staff. Under no circumstances should calcium be added directly to a unit of blood, because it causes clots to form in the bag.

Citrate toxicity during apheresis is related to the citrate concentration of the reinfused blood or colloid solution, the infusion rate, the blood volume of the patient, and the total time over which the citrate is infused (66,67). It is difficult to establish a definitive safe rate of citrate infusion because of the large number of variables involved. However, citrate dosages of up to 1 mg/kg per minute given during platelet pheresis usually are well tolerated (68). The recommended safe rate of calcium replacement for controlling citrate toxicity during PBSC apheresis is 0.5 mg of calcium ion for every 1.0 ml of infused acid citrate dextrose formula A (69). This dosage has been successful for prophylaxis against citrate toxicity during large-volume leukapheresis. To avoid excessive volume during PBSC apheresis, administration of concentrated calcium solution (calcium chloride or calcium gluconate) appropriate. Care must be taken to coordinate the calcium infusion with whole blood flow during the apheresis procedure to avoid catheter thrombosis. Calcium administration should be halted soon after interruptions in whole blood flow.

Electrolyte Disorders

Because of inhibition of sodium–potassium–adenosine triphosphatase in RBC membranes by the cold storage temperature of RBC units, extracellular potassium accumulates with increasing blood bank storage times. Extracellular potassium increases at the rate of approximately 1 mEq/d during the first 3 weeks of RBC storage in citrate-phosphate-dextrose-adenine-1 (CPDA-1) (70). Potassium levels in additive solution (Adsol) units are markedly higher on day 7 of storage (17 mmol/L) than on day 0 (1.6 mmol/L). The increase is even greater by day 42 (46 mmol/L) (71).

Hyperkalemia resulting from massive transfusion of older units of RBCs with an elevated amount of extracellular potassium can cause significant cardiac complications in some patients, although these appear to be rare (71). Patients at greatest risk of hyperkalemic complications are neonates and those with renal failure. The diagnosis of hyperkalemia is made by means of measurement of potassium in the serum and observation of ECG changes, which include peaked T waves, prolongation of the PR interval, and ventricular arrhythmia.

In neonatal transfusions, hyperkalemia can be avoided by use of fresh units of RBCs (less than 7 days old) or older units that have been saline-washed to remove the extracellular fraction containing the potassium. However, transfusion of older RBC units does not place neonates at risk of hyperkalemia if small-volume transfusions (10 to 15 ml/kg) are given slowly (72) (see Chapter 33). Hypokalemia can be a problem during massive transfusion. As the anticoagulant citrate in blood components is metabolized to bicarbonate, the blood can become alkalotic, producing hypokalemia. The degree of hypokalemia may be sufficient to necessitate infusion of potassium if symptoms develop. However, the use of newer RBC additive solutions such as Adsol has helped to decrease the effect of hypokalemia. Red blood cell units are plasma-reduced before the addition of additive solution, which itself contains no additional citrate. Therefore most of the citrated plasma is removed from additive solution RBC units during production. Animal studies have shown fewer physiologic aberrations during massive transfusion with Adsol RBCs than with CPDA-1 units (73). The complications of hypokalemia therefore are more likely when large numbers of units of plasma rather than RBC units are transfused.

Hyperammonemia may be of concern in massive transfusions owing to increased levels of ammonia detected in an older generation of stored blood products (74). Elevated ammonia levels from transfusion can be a concern in the care of patients with liver failure or of premature newborns who receive large amounts of blood products. For such patients, washed products can be considered but are likely impractical in massive transfusion. Despite theoretic concerns, adverse reactions to transfused ammonia are not well documented.

Hypothermia

Hypothermia, defined as a core body temperature of less than 35°C, may be caused by rapid infusion of large quantities of cold (1°C to 10°C) blood or RBC units. Hypothermia during massive transfusion has been shown to induce cardiac arrhythmia and arrest (75). Even smaller quantities of cold blood can be cardiotoxic if transfused into central venous lines, because the newly infused cold blood can reach the heart before sufficient warming has occurred. Data published in the early 1960s showed that massive transfusion at a rate of approximately 1 unit every 5 to 10 minutes was sufficient to lower the temperature of an esophageal probe behind the right atrium to nearly 30°C (75). The resulting decrease in sinoatrial node temperature was associated with the development of ventricular fibrillation.

For most routine transfusions given at a standard rate of administration, blood does not have to be warmed (76). The patient may experience minor chills, but this is easily remedied by warming the patient, as with extra blankets. Transfusion of cold units of RBCs through central venous lines, however, should be avoided. Indications for warming blood include rapid transfusion, which are generally considered to be more than 50 ml/kg per hour for an adult and more than 15 ml/kg per hour for a child, and exchange transfusion for infants. Because blood warming during certain massive transfusions sometimes delays infusion and impedes resuscitation, it is not always practical. Warming blood for transfusion in the treatment of patients with cold agglutinin disease has a theoretic basis but is debatable because supportive outcome data are lacking.

If blood has to be warmed, an approved warming device should be used and the temperature must be kept below 42°C (76). Over-warming can produce hemolysis, and infusion of thermally injured cells can induce disseminated intravascular coagulation and shock. Heating blood with a device other than an approved blood-warming device, such as a commercial microwave oven, is unacceptable. Blood that has been warmed but not used should not be reissued for another patient because of the increased risk of bacterial proliferation at warmer temperatures.

The maximum flow rate that can be achieved with commercially available blood warmers is 850 ml/min; however, most can only provide a rate of 150 ml/min. An alternative to using mechanical blood warmers that circumvents such flow limitations is rapid admixture with warm (77) or hot saline solution (76) immediately before transfusion. This technique immediately warms a unit of RBCs, yet does not cause significant hemolysis. However, it necessitates that warmed saline solution be available at all times in trauma care and requires attention to technique to avoid the direct infusion of hot saline solution into the patient.

Reactions Attributed to Microaggregate Debris

Microaggregate debris ranges in diameter from 20 to 120 μm and consists of nonviable platelets, white blood cells, and strands of fibrin that form in blood during storage (33,78). Because of their size, microaggregates are not removed from transfused blood with the standard 170- to 260-μm screen filters. A variety of adverse events have been attributed to the presence of microaggregate debris after large-volume and massive transfusion.

Studies in the 1960s showed that patients undergoing open-heart surgery with cardiopulmonary bypass experienced postperfusion syndrome during the postoperative period. This symptom complex consisted of cerebral and renal dysfunction attributed in part to occlusion of end-organ capillaries with microaggregate debris. Cotton wool (Swank) microaggregate blood filters capable of retaining particles or debris with a size of 40 μm or more appeared to eliminate many of these reactions. During the Vietnam war, some soldiers who underwent massive transfusion experienced respiratory distress syndrome (shock lung), the cause of which was presumed to be the periodic acid–Schiff (PAS)–positive material found in soldiers' lungs at autopsy. Because microaggregate debris stains PAS-positive, this was taken at the time as evidence of the pathologic nature of microaggregate debris.

During the 1970s and 1980s, studies were undertaken to determine whether removal of microaggregate debris from blood was clinically significant (33,78). Several studies showed that microaggregate filtration of up to 6 units of blood during either hip or cardiac surgery provided no benefit. Collins et al. (79) concluded that the underlying clinical condition rather than the infusion of the microaggregate debris in blood led to the development of the respiratory distress syndrome reported earlier among patients undergoing massive transfusions. Microaggregate blood filters today are used mostly in conjunction with cardiopulmonary bypass pumps and only rarely otherwise.

CIRCULATORY OVERLOAD

Hypervolemia is a possible consequence of transfusion in the care of patients with cardiac insufficiency, renal impairment, or already expanded blood volumes, such as patients with chronic anemia. Moreover, patients with restricted blood volumes, such as infants and small children are at risk of circulatory overload if transfused blood is not reduced to an amount proportional to body mass and intravascular blood volume. Risk of hypervolemia increases with rapid infusion. Circulatory overload increases central venous pressure, causes congestion of the pulmonary vasculature, and decreases lung compliance, manifesting as dyspnea, tachycardia, acute hypertension, and in the extreme, pulmonary edema and left- or right-sided heart failure. Other signs and symptoms of circulatory overload include tachypnea, dry cough, chest or throat tightness, jugular venous distention, and pulmonary rales.

If symptoms of overload appear, the transfusion should be stopped, and intravascular volume reduction through diuresis should be instituted (e.g., administration of 40 mg furosemide intravenously). The patient should be placed in an upright (reverse Trendelenburg) position, if possible, with supplemental oxygen as necessary. Phlebotomy may be considered for severe volume overload, although this is not usually prudent in the setting of anemia or hypoxemia.

Rapid transfusion of any blood component into a patient who is not actively hemorrhaging produces no benefit and can cause harm. As a general guide, infusion should be at a rate not to exceed 2 to 4 ml/kg per hour, and the rate should be lower (~1 ml/kg per hour) for patients at high risk of circulatory overload (80). In neonates, a slower blood infusion rate increases the hematocrit and decreases cardiac demand without affecting pulmonary artery pressure. More rapid infusion rates are associated with decreased lung compliance and increased pulmonary airflow resistance (81,82).

For patients with volume overload due to medical reasons before transfusion, furosemide can be given prophylactically, and transfusion should proceed slowly (see earlier). The rate of transfusion can be even further slowed, if necessary, by dividing a unit of RBCs or anther component into smaller aliquots and transfusing a portion at a time over as much as 4 hours, the maximum allowable time a blood component should be kept outside blood-bank-monitored storage. The unused portion should be stored in the blood bank at 1°C to 6°C for up to 24 hours for RBCs and thawed fresh-frozen plasma while the initial aliquot is administered. It is important that transfusion of all or part of a blood component be completed within 4 hours and that any unused portion be stored under regulated blood bank conditions because of concerns about increased risk of bacterial contamination during improper storage. Red blood cell units, single-donor platelets, and random-donor platelet pools can be further concentrated by means of centrifugation and plasma removal, if other measures to prevent volume overload are inadequate.

TOXIC REACTIONS RESULTING FROM BLOOD MANUFACTURE OR PROCESSING

Hypotensive Reactions

Hypotension has been reported among patients receiving bedside, leukoreduced platelets who are also medicated with angiotensin-converting enzyme (ACE) inhibitors (83,84). These reactions appear to be caused by generation of bradykinin in transfused blood just as it is being passed through negatively charged leukoreduction filters. The mechanism is believed to involve the formation of activated factor XIIa when factor XII, a contact factor, is exposed to the negatively charged filter surface. The filter surface can mimic exposed, negatively charged subendothelium, which is the natural activating stimulus for the contact factors of the intrinsic coagulation pathway after blood vessel damage in vivo. Factor XIIa converts prekallikrein to kallikrein, which cleaves high-molecular-weight kininogen to form bradykinin. The biologic activity of the infused bradykinin is prolonged in transfusion recipients who are also receiving ACE inhibitors (e.g., captopril, enalapril), which inhibit kininase II, the enzyme that breaks down bradykinin. The combination of bradykinin generation just as the blood is being infused with inhibition of the transfusion recipient's ability to break down bradykinin produces prolonged bradykinin activity conducive to hypotensive reactions.

These reactions are less likely with use of prestorage leukoreduced blood components, because the bradykinin is broken down rapidly in the component bag during storage before transfusion. Although hypotensive reactions have been reported more frequently with negatively charged bedside leukoreduction filters, they also have been rarely reported with positively charged filters. This can be explained in part by the possibility that patients taking ACE inhibitors may be more prone to hypotensive reactions in general owing to their relative inability to rapidly break down bradykinin generated in vivo by any allergic mechanism. Hypotensive reactions to bedside leukoreduction among patients taking ACE inhibitors can be prevented by use of prestorage leukoreduced blood components or by means of temporary discontinuation of ACE inhibitor treatment.

Ocular Reaction to Leukoreduced Blood Components: Red Eye Syndrome

Some patients receiving transfusions of RBCs prestorage leukoreduced with a specific filtration system (LeukoNet Prestorage Leukoreduction Filtration System; HemaSure, Marlborough, MA) sustained bilateral conjunctival erythema (red eye syndrome) (85). The conjunctival erythema occurred within 24 hours of transfusion. Resolution occurred spontaneously within 2 to 21 days with a median duration of 5 days. The implicated prestorage leukoreduction system has been discontinued, and red eye syndrome has not been reported with other leukoreduction filters. The red eye symptoms are hypothesized to be an allergic or toxic reaction to an extractable chemical leached from the filtration set, although an exact cause has not been established.

Plasticizer Toxicity

Plasticizers are chemicals used to make rigid polyvinyl chloride plastics more malleable. The traditional plasticizer for blood storage bags is di-2-ethyl hexyl phthalate (DEHP), which leaches over time from the plastic into the blood and blood components with increasing exposure. The DEHP metabolite, mono-2-ethyl hexyl-phthalate (MEHP), also accumulates during storage (86). Infusion of blood that contains DEHP results in deposition of DEHP in various tissues; the greatest accumulation is in body fat. Results of some studies with animals have suggested that DEHP is toxic and may even be carcinogenic in large quantities (87). Other studies with animals have shown that MEHP is associated with formation of peroxisomes, indicating tissue alteration and toxicity. Although there have been no reports of transfusion-related plasticizer toxicity among humans, results of some in vitro experiments suggest that high concentrations of MEHP have a negative inotropic effect and can cause irregular contractions in isolated human myocardial cells. Some clinical data have described the production of antiplasticizer IgE in transfusion recipients and the incorporation of plasticizer into RBCs during storage (88,89). Despite the possible adverse effects of DEHP plasticizers, other data indicate that these substances stabilize RBC membranes (90) and improve the morphologic features of platelets during storage (91). No good evidence exists, however, of actual improvement in posttransfusion outcomes as the result of these effects.

Formulations for plastic blood bags are being developed with plasticizers other than DEHP that have a decreased capacity to leach into plasma. For example, one polyvinyl chloride–based material is made with plasticizer butyryl tri-n-hexyl citrate (BTHC). Although BTHC also leaches into blood components, it does so at a significantly slower rate than does DEHP. It also provides an antihemolytic effect similar to that of DEHP (92). Studies have shown this citrate-based plasticizer suitable for storage of both RBCs and platelets (93). Given the concerns over the risk of DEHP toxicity, other plasticizers and storage materials continue to be sought in an attempt to replace traditional storage materials (94,95). The possible human toxicity of DEHP continues to be evaluated (96,97).

Dimethyl Sulfoxide Toxicity during Infusion of Cryopreserved Progenitor Cells

Dimethyl sulfoxide is a versatile solvent that has been used as the principal cryopreservative for mononuclear cells since the 1950s. It is widely used as a cryopreservative for bone marrow and PBSCs used in human hematopoietic progenitor cell transplantation. Despite this, DMSO is not a Food and Drug Administration–approved pharmacologic agent for intravenous administration, and guidelines for intravenous administration are obscure. Toxicologic studies, however, have established the general safety of intravenous DMSO infusion (98–100). The metabolism of DMSO yields a characteristic harmless odor, described as a malodorous garlic or sulfur-like smell. Because of the exceptional solvent properties of the compound, DMSO is distributed throughout all tissues after administration. The two metabolites of DMSO are dimethyl sulfdioxide ($DMSO_2$) and dimethyl sulfide (DMS). Dimethyl sulfdioxide is an odorless compound excreted by the kidney, and DMS is excreted through the lungs and through other tissues and contributes to the characteristic odor.

The clinical toxicity of DMSO in bone marrow transplantation has been studied. Anaphylactoid symptoms attributable to the release of histamine and other mediators are common. Other toxic clinical signs and symptoms include hemolysis with hemoglobinuria, hyperosmolality, increased serum transaminase values, nausea, vomiting, abdominal cramping, fever, chills, tachypnea, cough, diarrhea, flushing, and headache (101,102). Patients who have been conditioned with chemotherapy or who have smaller body mass (<70 kg), seem more likely to experience nausea and vomiting after infusion of DMSO-preserved cells. Cardiovascular toxicities include decreased heart rate and bradycardia, occasionally increased heart rate and tachycardia, ectopic heartbeat, heart block, hypotension, hypertension, and other lesser blood pressure changes (101–105). Some studies, however, raise the question whether there is any significant cardiovascular toxicity of DMSO (105). It is possible that some adverse effects attributed to DMSO may be caused by the cellular infusion itself.

The mechanism of the clinical toxicities associated with DMSO infusion has not been well established. Histamine receptor binding of DMSO, histamine release, direct vagal tonic effects, cold thermal vagal responses (106), and renal failure secondary to hemolysis (101) explain many of the symptoms observed during cryopreserved cellular infusion. Increases in thrombin-antithrombin complex, β-thromboglobulin, platelet factor 4, and von Willebrand factor caused by DMSO have been described.

Several measures can be taken to prevent or reduce DMSO toxicity. Antihistamine prophylaxis is recommended routinely before any administration of DMSO. Intravenous DMSO should be given as a 10% to 40% solution to avoid local irritation. The recommended maximum daily dose of DMSO is 1 g/kg a day. Slowing an infusion containing DMSO or increasing the time between infusions of multiple aliquots greatly diminishes DMSO-related toxicity, which appears to be a dose-dependent but short-lived response. However, because DMSO is toxic to thawed mononuclear cells, hematopoietic progenitor cells can tolerate exposure to 10% DMSO for only as long as 1 hour (107). This limits how much the infusion rate can be slowed. Antiemetics and sedatives can help to ameliorate symptoms, and cellular products can be carefully washed before infusion to remove DMSO and other substances.

REACTIONS IN SPECIAL TRANSFUSION SETTINGS

Granulocyte Transfusion Reactions

Granulocyte transfusions are reemerging as a treatment option for neutropenic patients because of improved granulocyte collection yields after donor treatment with granulocyte colony-stimulating factor (G-CSF) (see Chapter 20). Febrile nonhemolytic transfusion reactions after granulocyte transfusion are common. Severe reactions can be accompanied by pulmonary complications (e.g., dyspnea, pulmonary infiltrates, and hypoxia), hypotension, and even cardiovascular collapse (108). In a recent study of dexamethasone- and G-CSF–stimulated granulocyte transfusions, 37% of patients (7% of transfusions) experienced chills, 32% of patients (7% of transfusions) experienced a fever, and 11% of patients (2% of transfusions) experienced hives or itching during a course of therapy (109). Oxygen desaturation of greater than 3% occurred in 7% of transfusions, and severe desaturation of greater than 6% occurred in 3 of 11 patients experiencing oxygen desaturation.

Concurrent administration of amphotericin B and granulocytes has been linked to severe pulmonary reactions, although the association has not been confirmed and remains in doubt. Nevertheless, it is prudent to separate amphotericin B administration and granulocyte therapy by at least 6 hours to avoid confusion about the cause of a severe reaction, which can occur with either of these reaction-prone treatments. Because of the relatively high rate and severity of febrile, pulmonary, and allergic reactions, it is prudent to give premedication with acetaminophen and diphenhydramine to recipients of granulocyte transfusions. Hydrocortisone may be added as premedication in the treatment of patients with severe reactions who otherwise cannot tolerate granulocyte transfusion, although the immunosuppressive effects of this agent are unwelcome among patients who need granulocyte transfusions to fight serious and life-threatening infections. Granulocyte concentrates should be transfused slowly.

Autologous Transfusion Reactions

A variety of reactions to autologous blood occur despite the complete compatibility. In a study involving 596 hospitals, the rate of reported FNHTRs to autologous blood was 0.12% and the rate of allergic reactions was 0.01% per transfused unit (110). Such rates are approximately fivefold to tenfold lower than those reported for allogeneic units. The cause of autologous transfusion reactions has not been clearly established. Mechanisms in many cases presumably are the same as for allogeneic transfusions. For example, autologous units can be contaminated with bacteria as can allogeneic units, and contamination leads to febrile or septic transfusion reactions. Because autologous donors

TABLE 58.1. TRANSFUSION REACTION SUMMARY

Type	Cause	Signs and Symptoms	Treatment	Prevention
Febrile, nonhemolytic	Recipient antibodies against leukocytes or platelets in donor blood components; cytokines in plasma or supernatant portion of stored components; undetected bacterial contamination of blood component	Chills, fever (>1°C increase in body temperature); rigors in severe reactions	Stop transfusion, notify physician and blood bank, maintain IV line, monitor vital signs. Physician may order acetaminophen.	Premedicate with acetaminophen (or glucocorticoid for refractory cases); give leukocyte-reduced RBCs.
Allergic	Allergen is a soluble substance in donor plasma	Localized or generalized urticaria, erythema and pruritus; if severe, may have laryngeal or facial angioedema, and hypotension	Hold transfusion, notify physician, monitor vital signs. Physician may order antihistamines. Physician may order restart of transfusion if mild urticaria clears and no other symptoms in 30 min.	Premedicate with H1 blocking antihistamine; add H2 blocker or glucocorticoid for refractory cases. Consider washed RBCs and platelets for repeated or severe reactions.
Anaphylactic or anaphylactoid	Recipient antibodies to a soluble substance in donor plasma; infusion of plasma with IgA into IgA-deficient recipient with anti-IgA	Uticaria, flushing, angioedema, stridor, wheezing, tachycardia, hypotension, shock, abdominal pain, diarrhea, pelvic pain	Stop transfusion; maintain IV line; notify physician and blood bank, monitor vital signs. Physician may order antihistamines, epinephrine, oxygen, IV crystalloid, or glucocorticoids.	Premedicate with antihistamines and glucocorticoid; transfuse washed RBCs and platelets for recurrent reactions; use IgA-deficient donors or washed RBCs and platelets for sensitized patients with IgA deficiency.
Transfusion-related acute lung injury	Donor (or recipient) leukoagglutinating antibodies (anti-HLA, anti-neutrophil) or lipid activators in a susceptible patient (two-event hypothesis)	Dyspnea, tachypnea, hypoxemia, cough, crackles, frothy edema fluid from endotracheal tube	Stop transfusion; supportive care—give oxygen, ventilatory and cardiac support; avoid unnecessary transfusions; report to blood bank for evaluation of donors for leukoagglutinating antibodies.	May be idiosyncratic reaction; identify donors or recipients with leukoagglutinating antibodies; transfuse slowly; consider washed products, but recall that plasma cannot be washed.
Circulatory overload	Blood volume too large or infusion too fast for compromised cardiovascular system	Dyspnea, orthopnea, systolic hypertension, headache, peripheral edema, coughing, cyanosis	Slow or stop transfusion; keep IV line open. Notify physician, monitor vital signs and input and output. Physician may order diuretics and oxygen.	Transfuse slowly; use split units; consider premedication with diuretics; carefully monitor aged, debilitated, or cardiac patients.
Hypothermia	Core body temperature <35°C caused by rapid infusion of cold blood products, such as RBCs, FFP, cryoprecipitate	Decreased body temperature, chills, cardiac arrhythmia (ventricular fibrillation)	Slow or stop transfusion; use an approved blood warmer, blankets, and other patient warming techniques (warm lavages, lamps).	Transfuse slowly, use an approved blood warmer.
Citrate toxicity	Excessive infusion of citrate during apheresis procedure or massive or rapid transfusion. Patients with liver failure are at increased risk	Perioral or peripheral paresthesia, tingling, buzzing, teeth chattering, bed or chair moving, cramps, nausea, vomiting, arrhythmia, bradycardia, hypotension, prolongation of QT interval, tetany	Slow or stop transfusion; slow or stop apheresis procedure; give IV calcium chloride or gluconate (for PBSC apheresis: 0.5 mg Ca^{2+}/1.0 ml ACD-A), or check ionized Ca^{2+} and dose per results; monitor relief of symptoms; consider hypomagnesemia.	More likely in lightweight patients (<70 kg) and patients with liver dysfunction, renal failure, or less skeletal muscle; observe patients closely for any symptoms, give IV calcium (for PBSC apheresis: 0.5 mg Ca^{2+}/1.0 ml ACD-A).

(*continued*)

TABLE 58.1. (CONTINUED)

Type	Cause	Signs and Symptoms	Treatment	Prevention
Electrolyte disorder	Hyperkalemia: transfusion of older blood products	Hyperkalemia: cardiac arrhythmia, ECG changes—peaked T waves, prolongation of PR interval (if severe, flat or lost P wave), widened QRS, ventricular arrhythmia	Hyperkalemia: give calcium to protect against cardiac effect, alkalinize blood, D50 plus insulin, sodium polystrene sulfonate; dialysis.	Hyperkalemia: give fresh products (<7 days old), or washed products).
	Hypokalemia: massive or rapid transfusion of citrate and metabolic alkalosis	Hypokalemia: cardiac arrhythmia, ECG changes—ST depression, U waves	Hypokalemia: give potassium.	Hypokalemia: give Adsol-1 preserved RBCs (not AS-3).
Hypotensive	Bradykinin generation with use of negatively charged bedside leukoreduction filters in patients taking angiotension-converting enzyme (ACE) inhibitors	Hypotension; sometimes also flushing, respiratory distress, nausea, abdominal pain, and loss of consciousness	Stop transfusion, notify physician and blood bank. Support blood pressure.	Avoid use of bedside leukoreduction filters in patients taking ACE inhibitors; use prestorage leukoreduced components or discontinue ACE inhibitor before transfusion.
DMSO toxicity	Cryopreservative for bone marrow, PBSCs, donor lymphocyte infusions, or any frozen cellular component; toxicity with >1.0 g DMSO per kg per day	Flushing, nausea, vomiting, abdominal cramping, throat tightness and cough, hypotension, hypertension, arrhythmia, fever, chills, headache, hemoglobinuria, hyperosmolality, increased liver enzymes	Antihistamines; antiemetics; slow or stop the infusion; supportive care. Wait between infusions for symptoms to clear.	Antihistamines; washed or plasma or volume depleted cellular infusions; antiemetics.

RBCs, red blood cells; FFP, fresh-frozen plasma; PBSC, peripheral blood stem cell; ACD, acid-citrate-dextrose; D50, dextrose 50% in water; DMSO, dimethyl sulfoxide.

are patients, not healthy volunteers, they may have various medical problems that put them at increased risk of bacteremia.

Accumulation of inflammatory mediators in blood component bags during storage, released from passenger leukocytes or platelets, may result in infusion of pyrogenic substances. That the mediators are derived from autologous leukocytes rather than allogeneic leukocytes should not make a difference. Allergic reactions may be provoked by histamine generation during storage of blood components or by chemicals leached from blood storage containers or filters. Moreover, autologous transfusions may contribute to volume overload and hypervolemic reactions in certain clinical settings just as allogeneic units do.

SUMMARY

A variety of acute, nonhemolytic and noninfectious reactions are reported after transfusion (Table 58.1). Many of these reactions have an immune basis and represent inflammatory or allergic responses to infused cells (e.g., many FNHTRs) or plasma (e.g., some FNHTRs, TRALI, and allergic and anaphylactic reactions). Although urgent transfusion can be lifesaving, it is important to recognize that a large volume of blood components given too quickly can itself have adverse chemical or physical effects, such as hypothermia, hyperkalemia, hypokalemia, hypocalcemia, and circulatory overload. Some reactions also are caused by unintended consequences of blood storage conditions or processing, such as generation of bradykinin by the contact of blood with some filter surfaces, leaching of toxic chemicals from filters or containers, and use of the chemical DMSO during hematopoietic progenitor cell preservation. It is important that these reactions and toxicities be recognized rapidly by the patient care team and blood bank personnel so that appropriate treatment and preventive measures can be instituted quickly. Care providers who administer transfusions must recognize that some symptoms of transfusion reactions, such as fever, are nonspecific and may be early manifestations of potentially life-threatening reactions, such as hemolysis or sepsis (Table 58.2). For that reason, the guiding rule regarding most transfusion reactions is to err on the side of conservatism and stop the transfusion immediately. Transfusion of a blood component that causes a reaction before complete infusion should not be restarted, with the possible exception of mild urticarial reactions. Several strategies are available to prevent repeated reactions among patients who are reaction-prone. These include leukoreduction for the prevention of FNHTR, cell washing for the prevention of allergic and anaphylactic reactions and possibly some FNHTRs and TRALI, and various premedication regimens.

TABLE 58.2. OVERLAPPING SIGNS AND SYMPTOMS OF TRANSFUSION REACTIONS

Sign or Symptom	Possible Reaction
Fever, chills	Febrile nonhemolytic
	Acute hemolytic
	Septic
	Transfusion-related acute lung injury
Urticaria, pruritus	Allergic
	Anaphylactic
Dyspnea	Hypervolemia
	Transfusion-related acute lung injury
	Anaphylactic
Hypotension	Septic
	Anaphylactic
	Acute hemolytic
	Hypotensive

Septic reactions are caused by the infusion of blood components contaminated with bacteria or bacterial products.
Hypotensive reactions are characterized by hypotension occurring in patients taking angiotensin-converting enzyme inhibitors, particularly in association with the use of bedside leukoreduction filters with a negatively charged filter surface.

REFERENCES

1. Walker RH. Special report: transfusion risks. *Am J Clin Pathol* 1987; 88:374–378.
2. Menitove JE, McElligott MC, Aster RH. Febrile transfusion reaction: what blood component should be given next? *Vox Sang* 1982;42: 318–321.
3. Chambers LA, Kruskall MS, Pacini DG, et al. Febrile reactions after platelet transfusion: the effect of single versus multiple donors. *Transfusion* 1990; 30:219–221.
4. Mangano MM, Chambers LA, Kruskall MS. Limited efficiency of leukopoor platelets for prevention of febrile transfusion reactions. *Am J Clin Pathol* 1991;95:733–738.
5. Muylle L, Wouters E, De Bock R, et al. Transfusion reactions to platelet concentrates: the effect of the storage time of the concentrate. *Transfus Med* 1992; 2:289–293.
6. Heddle NM, Klama LN, Griffith L, et al. A prospective study to identify the risk factors associated with acute reactions to platelet and red cell transfusions. *Transfusion* 1993;33:794–797.
7. Kelley DL, Mangini J, Lopez-Plaza I, et al. The utility of ≤3-day-old whole-blood platelets in reducing the incidence of febrile nonhemolytic transfusion reactions. *Transfusion* 2000;40:439–442.
8. Stack G, Berkowicz D. Cytokine production during blood component storage. In: Davenport R, Snyder E, eds. *Cytokines in transfusion medicine: a primer.* Bethesda, MD: American Association of Blood Banks, 1997:21–59.
9. Heddle NM. Pathophysiology of febrile nonhemolytic transfusion reactions. *Curr Opin Hematol* 1999;6:420–426.
10. Saper CB. Neurobiological basis of fever. *Ann N Y Acad Sci* 1998; 856:90–94.
11. de Rie MA, van der Plas–van Dalen CM, Engelfriet CP, et al. The serology of febrile transfusion reactions. *Vox Sang* 1985;49:126–134.
12. Brubaker DB. Clinical significance of white cell antibodies in febrile nonhemolytic transfusion reactions. *Transfusion* 1990;30:733–737.
13. Perkins HA, Payne R, Ferguson J, et al. Nonhemolytic febrile transfusion reactions: quantitative effects of blood components with emphasis on isoantigenic incompatibility of leukocytes. *Vox Sang* 1966;11: 578–600.
14. Lane TA, Anderson KC, Goodnough LT, et al. Leukocyte reduction in blood component therapy. *Ann Intern Med* 1992;117:151–162.
15. Trial to Reduce Alloimmunization to Platelets Study Group. Leukocyte reduction and ultraviolet B irradiation of platelets to prevent alloimmunization and refractoriness to platelet transfusions. *N Engl J Med* 1997;337:1861–1869.
16. Stack G, Snyder EL. Cytokine generation in stored platelet concentrates. *Transfusion* 1994;34:20–25.
17. Muylle L, Joos M. Wouters E, et al. Increased tumor necrosis factor

(TNFα), interleukin 1, and interleukin 6 (IL-6) levels in the plasma of stored platelet concentrates: relationship between TNFα and IL-6 levels and febrile transfusion reactions. *Transfusion* 1993; 33: 195–199.
18. Heddle NM, Klama L, Singer J, et al. The role of plasma from platelet concentrates in transfusion reactions. *N Engl J Med* 1994; 331: 625–628.
19. Miletic VD, Popovic O. Complement activation in stored platelet concentrates. *Transfusion* 1993;33:150–154.
20. Silliman CC. Transfusion-related acute lung injury. *Transfus Med Rev* 1999;13:177–186.
21. Stack G, Baril L, Napychank P, et al. Cytokine generation in stored, white cell-reduced, and bacterially-contaminated units of red blood cells. *Transfusion* 1995;35:199–203.
22. Elkattan I, Anderson J, Yun JK, et al. Correlation of cytokine elaboration with mononuclear cell adhesion to platelet storage bag plastic polymers: a pilot study. *Clin Diagn Lab Immunol* 1999;5:505–513.
23. Sharma AD, Grocott HP. Platelet transfusion reactions: febrile nonhemolytic reaction or bacterial contamination? Diagnosis, detection, and current preventive modalities. *J Cardiothorac Vasc Anesth* 2000;14: 460–466.
24. Elkattan I, Anderson J, Yun JK, et al. Correlation of cytokine elaboration with mononuclear cell adhesion to platelet storage bag plastic polymers: a pilot study. *Clin Diagn Lab Immunol* 1999;5:505–513.
25. Braine HG, Kickler TS, Charache P, et al. Bacterial sepsis secondary to platelet transfusion: an adverse effect of extended storage at room temperature. *Transfusion* 1986;26:391–393.
26. Goldman M, Blajchman M. Blood product associated bacterial sepsis. *Transfus Med Rev* 1991; 5:73–83.
27. Casey LC, Bolk RA, Bone RC. Plasma cytokine and endotoxin levels correlate with survival in patients with the sepsis syndrome. *Ann Intern Med* 1993;118:771–778.
28. Burks LC, Aisner J, Fortner CL, et al. Meperidine for the treatment of shaking chills and fever. *Arch Intern Med* 1980;140:483–484.
29. Oberman HA. Controversies in transfusion medicine: should a febrile transfusion response occasion the return of the blood component to the blood bank? *Con Transfusion* 1994;34:353–355.
30. Bordin JO, Heddle NM, Blajchman MA. Biologic effects of leukocytes present in transfused cellular blood products. *Blood* 1994;84: 1703–1721.
31. Hughes A, Mijovic V, Brozovic B, et al. Leukocyte-depleted blood: a comparison of cell-washing techniques. *Vox Sang* 1982;42:145–150.
32. Goldfinger D, Lowe C. Prevention of adverse reactions to blood transfusion by the administration of saline-washed red blood cells. *Transfusion* 1981;21:277–280.
33. Swank RL, Seaman GVF. Microfiltration and microemboli: a history. *Transfusion* 2000;40:114–119.
34. Schned AR, Silver H. The use of microaggregate filtration in the prevention of febrile transfusion reactions. *Transfusion* 1981;21: 675–681.
35. Wenz B. Microaggregate blood filtration and the febrile transfusion reaction. *Transfusion* 1983;23:95–98.
36. Parravicini A, Rebulla P, Apuzzo J, et al. The preparation of leukocyte-poor red cells for transfusion by a simple cost-effective technique. *Transfusion* 1984;24:508–509.
37. Dzik S. Leukodepletion blood filters: filter design and mechanisms of leukocyte removal. *Transfus Med Rev* 1993;7:65–77.
38. Kevy SV, Schmidt PJ, McGinniss MH, et al. Febrile, nonhemolytic transfusion reactions and the limited role of leukoagglutinins in their etiology. *Transfusion* 1962;2:7–16.
39. Silvergleid AJ, Hafleigh EB, Harabin MA, et al. Clinical value of washed-platelet concentrates in patients with non-hemolytic transfusion reactions. *Transfusion* 1977;17:33–37.
40. Kalmin ND, Brown DJ. Platelet washing with a blood cell processor. *Transfusion* 1982;22:125–127.
41. Buck SA, Kickler TS, McGuire M, et al. The utility of platelet washing using an automated procedure for severe platelet allergic reactions. *Transfusion* 1987;27:391–393.
42. Heddle NM, Klama L, Meyer R, et al. A randomized controlled trial comparing plasma removal with white cell reduction to prevent reactions to platelets. *Transfusion* 1999;39:231–238.
43. Frewin, DB, Jonsson JR, Frewin CF, et al. Influence of blood storage time and plasma histamine levels on the pattern of transfusion reactions. *Vox Sang* 1989;56:243–246.
44. Muylle L, Beert JF, Mertens G, et al. Histamine synthesis by white cells during storage of platelet concentrates. *Vox Sang* 1998;74: 193–197.
45. Kluter H, Bubel S, Kirchner H, et al. Febrile and allergic transfusion reactions after the transfusion of white cell–poor platelet preparations. *Transfusion* 1999;39:1179–1184.
46. Lin RY, Curry A, Pesola GR, et al. Improved outcomes in patients with acute allergic syndromes who are treated with combined H1 and H2 antagonists. *Ann Emerg Med* 2000;36:462–468.
47. Ring J, Behrendt H. H1- and H2-antagonists in allergic and pseudoallergic disease. *Clin Exp Allergy* 1990;20:43–49.
48. Sandler SG, Mallory D, Malamut D, et al. IgA anaphylactic transfusion reactions. *Transfus Med Rev* 1995;9:1–8.
49. Morishita K, Shimada E, Watanabe Y, et al. Anaphylactic transfusion reactions associated with anti-haptoglobin in a patient with ahaptoglobinemia. *Transfusion* 2000;40:120–121.
50. Westhoff CM, Sipherd BD, Wylie De, et al. Severe anaphylactic reactions following transfusions of platelets to a patient with anti–Ch. *Transfusion* 1992;32:576–579.
51. Bergamaschini L, Mannucci PM, Federici AB, et al. Posttransfusion anaphylactic reactions in a patient with severe von Willebrand disease: role of complement and alloantibodies to von Willebrand factor. *J Lab Clin Med* 1995;125:348–355.
52. Wyatt R. Anaphylaxis. How to recognize, treat and prevent potentially fatal attacks. *Postgrad Med* 1996;100:87–90,96–99.
53. Marino PL. *The ICU book,* 2nd ed. Baltimore: Williams & Wilkins. 1998:511–513.
54. Greenberger PA, Patterson R. Adverse reactions to radiocontrast media. *Prog Cardiovasc Dis* 1988;31:239–248.
55. Popovsky MA, Moore SB. Diagnostic and pathogenetic considerations in transfusion-related acute lung injury. *Transfusion* 1985;25: 573–577.
56. Popovsky MA. Transfusion-related acute lung injury. *Curr Opin Hematol* 2000;7:402–407.
57. Kopko PM, Holland PV. Transfusion-related acute lung injury. *Br J Haematol* 1999;105:322–329.
58. Jacob HS, Craddock PR, Hammerschmidt DE, et al. Complement-induced granulocyte aggregation: an unsuspected mechanism of disease. *N Engl J Med* 1980;302:789–794.
59. Dry SM, Bechard KM, Milford EL, et al. The pathology of transfusion-related acute lung injury. *Am J Clin Pathol* 1999;112:216–221.
60. Palfi M, Berg S, Ernerudh J, et al. A randomized controlled trial of transfusion-related acute lung injury: is plasma from multiparous blood donors dangerous? *Transfusion* 2001;41:317–322.
61. Dzik WH, Kirkley SA. Citrate toxicity during massive blood transfusion. *Transfus Med Rev* 1988;2:76–94.
62. Mollison PL. The introduction of citrate as an anticoagulant for transfusion and of glucose as a red cell preservative. *Br J Haematol* 2000; 108:13–18.
63. Weinstein R. Prevention of citrate reactions during therapeutic plasma exchange by constant infusion of calcium gluconate with the return fluid. *J Clin Apheresis* 1996;11:204–210.
64. Diaz J, Acosta F, Parrilla P, et al. Citrate intoxication and blood concentration of ionized calcium in liver transplantation. *Transplant Proc* 1994;26:3669–3670.
65. McLellan BA, Reid SR, Lane PL. Massive blood transfusion causing hypomagnesemia. *Crit Care Med* 1984;12:146–147.
66. Hester JP, Ayyar R. Anticoagulation and electrolytes. *J Clin Apheresis* 1984;2:41–51.
67. Hester JP, McCullough J, Mishler JM, et al. Dosage regimens for citrate anticoagulants. *J Clin Apheresis* 1983;1:149–157.
68. Olson PR, Cox C, McCullough J. Laboratory and clinical effects of the infusion of ACD solution during plateletpheresis. *Vox Sang* 1977; 33:79–87.
69. Korbling M, Huh YO, Durett A, et al. Allogeneic blood stem cell

transplantation: peripheralization and yield of donor-derived primitive hematopoietic progenitor cells (CD34+ Thy-1dim) and lymphoid subsets, and possible predictors of engraftment and graft-versus-host disease. *Blood* 1995;86:2842–2848.
70. Latham JT, Bove JR, Weirich FL. Chemical and hematologic changes in stored CPDA-1 blood. *Transfusion* 1982;22:158–159.
71. Carvalho B, Quiney NF. "Near-miss" hyperkalaemic cardiac arrest associated with rapid blood transfusion. *Anaesthesia* 1999;54: 1094–1096.
72. Liu EA, Mannino FL, Lane TA. Prospective, randomized trial of the safety and efficacy of a limited donor exposure transfusion program for premature neonates. *J Pediatr* 1994;125:92–96.
73. Buchholz DH, Borgia JF, Ward M, et al. Comparison of Adsol and CPDA-1 blood preservatives during simulated massive resuscitation after hemorrhage in swine. *Transfusion* 1999;39:998–1004.
74. Spear PW, Sass M, Cincotti JJ. Ammonia levels in transfused blood. *J Lab Clin Med* 1956;48:702–707.
75. Boyan C, Howland WS. Blood temperature: a critical factor in massive transfusion. *Anesthesiology* 1961;22:559–563.
76. Iserson KV, Muestis DW. Blood warming: current applications and techniques. *Transfusion* 1991;31:558–571.
77. Cohn SM, Stack G. In vivo comparison of heated saline-blood admixture to a heat exchanger for rapid warming of red blood cells. *J Trauma* 1993;35:688–691.
78. Snyder EL, Bookbinder M. Role of microaggregate blood filtration in clinical medicine. *Transfusion* 1983;23:460–470.
79. Collins JA, James PM, Bredenberg CE, et al. The relationship between transfusion and hypoxemia in combat casualties. *Ann Surg* 1978;188: 513–520.
80. Marriott HL KA. Volume and rate in blood transfusion for the relief of anemia. *Br Med J* 1940;1:1043–1046.
81. Sasidharan P, Heimler R. Alterations in pulmonary mechanics after transfusion in anemic preterm infants. *Crit Care Med* 1990;18: 1360–1362
82. Nelle M, Hoecker C, Linderkamp O. Effects of red cell transfusion on pulmonary blood flow and right ventricular systolic time intervals in neonates. *Eur J Pediatr* 1997;156:553–556.
83. Hume HA, Popovsky MA, Benson K, et al. Hypotensive reactions: a previously uncharacterized complication of platelet transfusion? *Transfusion* 1996;36:904–909.
84. Cyr M, Eastlund T, Blais Jr. C, et al. Bradykinin metabolism and hypotensive transfusion reactions. *Transfusion* 2001;41:136–150.
85. Adverse ocular reactions following transfusions—United States, 1997–1998. *MMWR Morb Mortal Wkly Rep* 1998;47:49–50.
86. Rock G, Secours VE, Franklin CA, et al. The accumulation of mono-2-ethylhexylphthalate (MEHP) during storage of whole blood and plasma. *Transfusion* 1978;18:553–558.
87. Kluwe WM, Haseman JK, Huff JE. The carcinogenicity of di(2-ethylhexyl) phthalate (DEHP) in perspective. *J Toxicol Environ Health* 1983; 12:159–169.
88. Barry YA, Labow RS, Keon WJ, et al. Perioperative exposure to plasticizers in patients undergoing cardiopulmonary bypass. *J Thorac Cardiovasc Surg* 1989; 97:900–905.
89. Salkie ML, Hannon JL. Anti-plasticizer specific IgE is present in the serum of transfused patients. *Clin Invest Med* 1995; 18:419–423.
90. Rock G, Tocchi M, Ganz PR, Tackaberry ES. Incorporation of plasticizer into red cells during storage. *Transfusion* 1984; 24:493–488.
91. Labow RS, Tocchi M, Rock G. Platelet storage: effects of leachable materials on morphology and function. *Transfusion* 1986; 26: 351–357.
92. Jaeger RJ, Rubin RJ. Plasticizers from plastic devices extraction, metabolism, and accumulation by biological systems. *Science* 1970; 170: 460–462.
93. Snyder EL, Hedberg SL, Napychank PA, et al. Stability of red cell antigens and plasma coagulation factors stored in a non-diethylhexyl phthalate-plasticized container. *Transfusion* 1993; 33:515–519.
94. Lee JH, Kim KO, Ju YM. Polyethylene oxide additive-entrapped polyvinyl chloride as a new blood bag material. *J Biomed Mater Res* 1999; 48:328–334.
95. Boomgaard MN, Gouwerok CW, de Korte D, et al. Platelets stored for 6 days in a polyolefin container in a synthetic medium with minimal plasma carry-over. *Vox Sang* 1994; 66:18–24.
96. Leadbitter J. Materials comment: PVC, why all the fuss? *Med Device Technol* 2000;11:30–32.
97. Doull J, Cattley R, Elcombe C, et al. A cancer risk assessment of di(2-ethylhexyl)phthalate: application of the new U.S. EPA risk assessment guidelines. *Regul Toxicol Pharmacol* 1999;29:327–357.
98. Jacob SW, Wood DC, Dimethyl sulfoxide (DMSO). Toxicology, pharmacology, and clinical experience. *Am J Surg* 1967;114:414–426.
99. Brobyn RD. The human toxicology of dimethyl sulfoxide. *Ann N Y Acad Sci* 1975;243:497–506.
100. Yellowlees P, Greenfield C, McIntyre N. Dimethylsulphoxide-induced toxicity. *Lancet* 1980;2:1004–1006.
101. Davis JM. Clinical toxicity of cryopreserved bone marrow graft infusion. *Blood* 1990;75:781–786.
102. Kessinger A, Schmit-Pokorny K, Smith D, et al. Cryopreservation and infusion of autologous peripheral blood stem cells. *Bone Marrow Transplant* 1990; 5 Suppl 1:25–27.
103. Keung YK. Cardiac arrhythmia after infusion of cryopreserved stem cells. *Bone Marrow Transplant* 1994; 14:363–367.
104. Zambelli A. Clinical toxicity of cryopreserved circulating progenitor cells infusion. *Anticancer Res* 1998;18:4705–4708.
105. Lopez-Jimenez J. Cardiovascular toxicities related to the infusion of cryopreserved grafts: results of a controlled study. *Bone Marrow Transplant* 1994;13:789–793.
106. Keung YK, Cobos E, Morgan D, et al. Higher cellular concentration of peripheral blood progenitor cells during cryopreservation adversely affects CFU-GM but not hematopoietic recovery. *J Hematother* 1996; 5:73–77.
107. Rowley SD. Effect of DMSO exposure without cryopreservative on hematopoietic progenitor cells. *Bone Marrow Transplant* 1993;11: 389–393.
108. Klein HG, Strauss RG, Schiffer CA. Granulocyte transfusion therapy. *Semin Hematol* 1996;33:359–368.
109. Price TH, Bowden RA, Boeckh M, et al. Phase I/II trial of neutrophil transfusions from donors stimulated with G-CSF and dexamethasone for treatment of patients with infections in hematopoietic stem cell transplantation. *Blood* 2000;95:3302–9.
110. Domen RE. Adverse reactions associated with autologous blood transfusion: evaluation and incidence at a large academic hospital. *Transfusion* 1998;38:296–300.

Rossi's Principles of Transfusion Medicine, Third Edition, edited by Toby L. Simon, Walter H. Dzik, Edward L. Snyder, Christopher P. Stowell, and Ronald G. Strauss. Lippincott Williams & Wilkins, Philadelphia © 2002.

59

TRANSFUSION-ASSOCIATED GRAFT VERSUS HOST DISEASE

PATRICIA M. CAREY
RONALD A. SACHER

Prior to the mid-1980s, graft versus host disease (GVHD) was considered a relatively rare adverse reaction to blood transfusion in some immunocompromised recipients. However, this complication has acquired greater significance, not only for immunocompromised patients, but also for apparently immunocompetent recipients. This change has been brought about by a number of new developments in blood transfusion and surgical practice, including the expanded use of hematopoietic and solid organ transplantation as a treatment modality, the institution of new chemotherapeutic regimens which induce additional immunocompromise in patients with hematologic and solid tumor malignancies, the prolonged survival of more very-low-birth-weight premature infants, use of new cardiac support devices which alter immune function similar to that seen with cardiopulmonary bypass, and use of directed donations from family members. This chapter defines the risk factors for transfusion-associated GVHD (TAGVHD) and its pathogenesis and outlines preventive measures against this unusual, but frequently fatal, complication of transfusion.

P.M. Carey and R.A. Sacher: Hoxworth Blood Center, University of Cincinnati Medical Center, Cincinnati, Ohio.

HISTORIC BACKGROUND

Graft versus host disease was probably first noted by Murphy in 1916, when he observed the development of disseminated nodules and splenic enlargement in chick embryos inoculated with cells from adult chicken spleens and bone marrows (1). Although Murphy was not explicit as to what these nodules meant, Simonsen subsequently interpreted the data as being consistent with GVHD (2) and showed that similar changes could be elicited not only in chick embryos but also in newborn and fetal mice (3). According to Simonsen, mouse GVHD could be elicited if the exposure to donor tissue occurred prenatally rather than postnatally. He also defined the basic requirements for a graft versus host reaction (GVHR), which include the following: a) the graft must contain immunologically competent cells, b) the host must be sufficiently different from the graft to be recognized as antigenically disparate, and c) the host must be immunologically incapable of mobilizing an effective rejection of the graft (3).

In experimental animals allowed to run the natural course of GVHD, two distinct clinical syndromes could be recognized, a) an acute fulminant form and b) a more chronic disease resulting in a "runting syndrome." Billingham and Brent (4) defined runting disease as an immunologic attack of the grafted cells against the host, resulting in weight loss, splenomegaly, diarrhea, anemia, leukopenia, lymphoid atrophy, and focal hepatic necrosis. This condition was ultimately fatal in the newborn mice challenged with allogeneic adult splenic lymphoid cells. A similar syndrome, produced in irradiated adult mice, is called *secondary disease.*

In 1959, the first instances of human GVHD were reported by Mathé, who described a condition similar to the runting syndrome in some patients after hematopoietic stem cell transplantation (HSCT) for acute leukemia (5). The susceptibility of human fetuses and newborns to TAGVHD was demonstrated in the 1950s and 1960s (6,7).

PATHOGENESIS OF GVHD

Graft versus host disease arises through transfer of viable cytotoxic allogeneic lymphocytes to a recipient unable to reject them. The nature of these cells was first demonstrated by Terasaki in 1959 (8). That blood could also cause GVHD was shown by Simonsen experimentally by the intravenous injection of adult allogeneic blood into 17-day-old embryos, which then developed splenomegaly in only 7 days (9). It is now known that the transfusion of immunocompetent blood cells into immunoincompetent hosts can evoke GVHD. This phenomenon has been observed in persons with primary and secondary immunodeficiency syndromes, and even in apparently immunocompetent recipients. The precipitating elements include:

1. Histocompatibility factors
2. Underlying medical conditions
3. Significant immunosuppression, regardless of etiology
4. Efficiency and maturity of host immune surveillance
5. Function and source of immunocompetent cells
6. Microbial factors

Controlling the incidence and severity of GVHD is the presence of recognizable antigenic disparity between host and donor (10). The ability to recognize differences resides in the human leukocyte locus antigens (HLA), both major and minor, which are also the triggers that initiate an immune response (10,11). Recipients of HSCT in animal and human models have increased the understanding of the pathophysiology of GVHD. The clinical picture of acute GVHD is most reminiscent of TAGVHD. The pathophysiology of chronic GVHD will also be discussed.

Pathophysiology of Acute GVHD

In HSCT, presentation of donor cells often occurs in an environment of damage, whether it is from the underlying disease, infection, or the conditioning regimen for transplantation. The donor cells are surrounded by foreign antigens, activated cytokines, expressed adhesion molecules, and cell surface recognition molecules. The cells involved in the immune process are T cells, natural killer (NK) cells, and monocytes.

The T-cell activity is of primary importance initially. Robert and Kupper (11) reviewed T cells and their immune function in the context of inflammatory skin disease. This model seems appropriate when discussing GVHD because skin is a principal target organ.

T-cell antigen receptors (TCRs) recognize fragments of macromolecules bound to antigen-presenting proteins on the surface of antigen-presenting cells (APCs) (Fig. 59.1). These proteins include class I and II major histocompatibility complex (MHC) molecules, which bind peptide antigens to present to $CD4^+$ or $CD8^+$ cells, and CD1 molecules, which bind nonpeptides for a different T-cell subgroup.

T cells that have never been activated by antigen (naive T cells) migrate from blood into lymph nodes and return to blood through lymphatics. This movement of T cells to lymph nodes involves adhesion molecules and chemokines on special postcapillary venules (high endothelial venules), L selectin and other adhesion molecules, and chemokine receptors on the T cells.

The presentation of antigen to T cells, in order to be activated, requires binding of antigen-HLA or antigen-CD1 complex to TCR and other costimulatory molecules provided by the APC. When the T cell is activated they proliferate, express activation molecules, and change into memory T cells. Cutaneous lymphocyte antigen (CLA) is the new cell marker that identifies T memory cells associated with skin. Additional cell surface molecules and their ligands facilitate the movement of the T cells to extranodal tissues.

Ferrara et al. (12) described the resulting pathology as occurring in the following three phases (Fig. 59.2): a) the conditioning regimen, b) donor T-cell activation, and c) inflammatory cell effectors. The pretransplant conditioning regimen, consisting of irradiation or chemotherapy or both, can cause host tissue damage and activate host cells to secrete inflammatory cytokines (i.e., tumor necrosis factor-α [TNF-α] and interleukin-1 [IL-1]). Such inflammatory substances can increase the expression of adhesion molecules and MHC antigens, creating a primed environment for donor cells to recognize major and minor host differences. This reaction of donor cells to host tissues can be reduced if the donor lymphocytes are presented after the tissue injury has resolved.

The second phase of acute GVHD includes presentation of antigen and activation of donor T cells, resulting in their differentiation and proliferation. Donor $CD4^+$ cells interact with MHC class II molecules of the APC. Donor $CD8^+$ cells interact with MHC class I molecules. Major HLA class disparity is one mechanism for T-cell activation. If donor and host are MHC identical, the T cell and its antigen receptor (TCR) may recognize foreign peptides, referred to as minor histocompatibility antigens bound to the MHC. The TCR responds to subtle variations in the peptide configuration presented by the MHC. The first signal for T-cell activation is provided by the TCR-peptide-MHC approximation. The second signal is referred to as a costimulatory signal, which determines the outcome of the activation sequence. Stimulation of T helper type 1 (T_H1) cell clones through the TCR without a costimulatory signal results in no IL-2 secretion and proliferation, and induction of a state of nonresponsiveness called anergy (13). The costimulatory signal is mediated by the CD28/B7 family and adhesion molecules such as lymphocyte function–associated antigen (LFA)-1, LFA-3, intercellular adhesion molecule (ICAM)-1, OX40 (CD134),

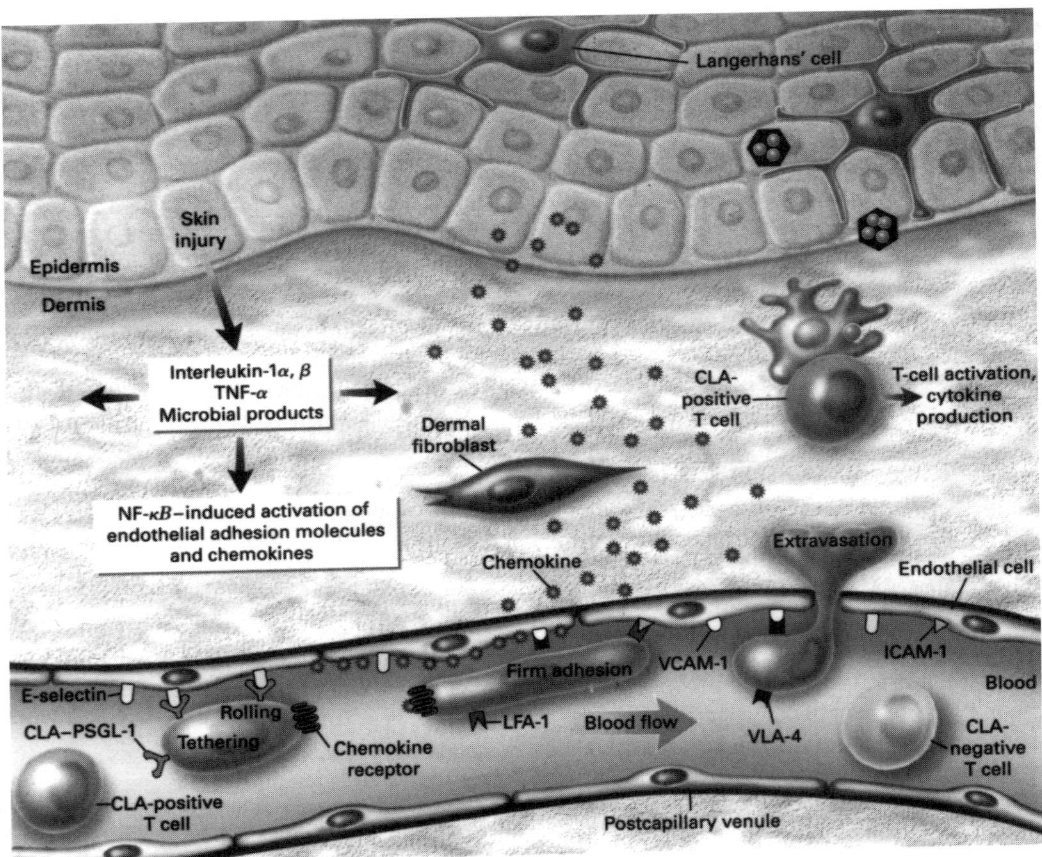

FIGURE 59.1. Extravasation of a cutaneous lymphocyte antigen (CLA)–positive memory T cell into inflamed skin. Skin injury or infection results in the activation of the nuclear factor-κB (NF-κB) pathway through cytokine receptors (interleukin-1 or tumor necrosis factor-α [TNF-α]) or toll-like receptors. Microbial products may directly activate this pathway. The result is the transcription of many genes that contain κB sites in their promoters in a variety of skin cells. In endothelial cells, these include the adhesion molecules E selectin, intercellular adhesion molecule 1 (ICAM-1), and vascular-cell adhesion molecule 1 (VCAM-1). To extravasate into skin, T cells must slow their velocity in the circulation. To do so, they use CLA–P selectin glycoprotein ligand 1 (CLA-PSGL-1) cell-surface molecules, located on the tips of microvilli, to bind to E selectin and P selectin on the luminal surface of the cutaneous postcapillary venules, a process called *tethering*. Once tethered, the T cells on the endothelial surface of the endothelium, where chemokines that have been produced on the abluminal side of the vessel by resident skin cells and transported to the luminal surface of the endothelial cells, can be displayed. The binding of chemokines to specific receptors on T cells results in a modification of the structure of the $\alpha_1\beta_2$ integrin (lymphocyte function–associated antigen 1 (LFA-1) and the $\alpha_1\beta_2$ integrin (very late antigen 4 [ULA-4]) so that they can bind to ICAM-1 and VCAM-1, respectively. Not only is the integrin binding of sufficiently high affinity to arrest the CLA-positive T cells, but it also favors the flattening of the lymphocytes in preparation for their extravasation through the endothelial layer. Once extravasated on the abluminal side of the vessel, the T cells are no longer subjected to shear forces from blood flow, and they can respond to chemotactic gradients emanating from the site of injury or infection. If these T cells encounter antigen in tissue, they will become activated. The subsequent release of T-cell cytokines will modify and expand the inflammatory infiltrate.

and 4-1BB (CD137). See Table 59.1 for a summary of costimulatory molecules and their roles. The complete activation of the T cell induces secretion of IL-2 and interferon-γ (INF-γ), type 1 cytokines. Both are potent mediators of GVHD (13).

The third phase involves inflammatory effectors. Most tissue damage in GVHD is not caused by direct cytotoxic T-cell activity. The cytokines produced by activated T cells recruit NK cells and mononuclear phagocytes as effector cells. Monocytes are secondarily stimulated to secrete TNF-α and IL-1. Lipopolysaccharide (LPS) (endotoxin) from damaged gut epithelium can be the stimulus. The LPS can also stimulate keratinocytes and dermal fibroblasts to release the same cytokines. Tumor necrosis factor-α can cause direct tissue damage by inducing necrosis of cells or it may induce apoptosis. Apoptosis is induced after activation of the TNF-α-Fas antigen pathway.

Cytokines, although important in systemic GVHD, play a limited role in specific target organ damage. This damage is mediated via cytolytic effectors. Two mouse models better describe the role this arm of immune damage plays in GVHD (14). Perforin-granzyme and Fas-FasL (Fas ligand) systems are

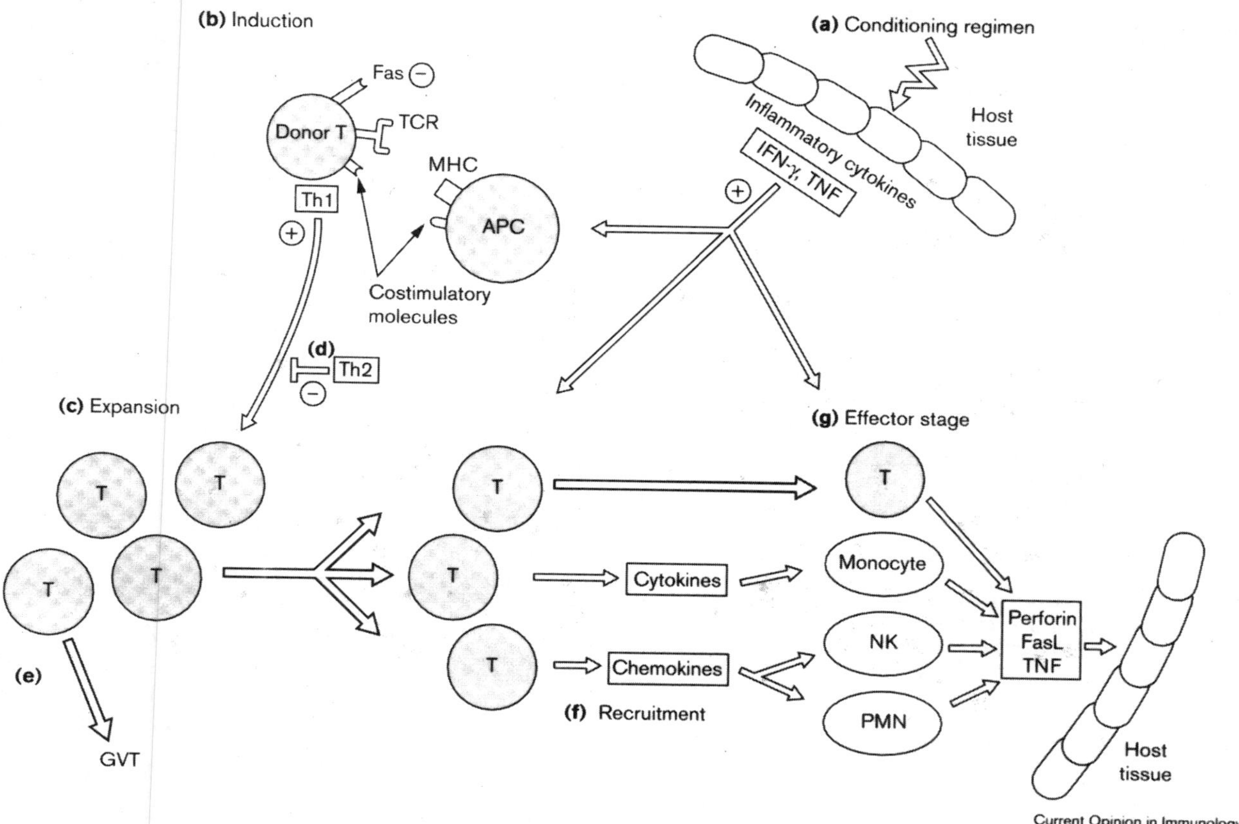

FIGURE 59.2. Various phases in acute GVHD. Circles containing + or − indicate positive or negative effects on GVHD, respectively. **A:** During the conditioning of the recipient, cytokines are released that can augment all phases of GVHD. **B:** During the induction phase the alloreactive donor T cells are sensitized to the host. **C:** During the expansion phase, they are driven by T_H1-type cytokines (e.g., IL-2). **D:** T_H2-type cytokines can inhibit GVHD. The expanded donor T cells can **(E)** mediate GVT effects or **(F)** release cytokines and chemokines, which recruit other host cell types (e.g., monocytes, natural killer cells, and polymorphonuclear leukocytes); these ultimately mediate the pathology of GVHD. **G:** The effector stage employs all the classical effector molecules (FasL, perforin, and tumor necrosis factor) to attack the host tissue.

important in class I– and class II–dependent GVHD, respectively. Looking at murine models, the number of cells necessary to induce GVHD is on the order of 1×10^7 lymphocytes per kilogram (2,15).

The presence of granulocyte colony–stimulating factor (G-CSF) has been shown to promote natural suppressor T lymphocytes (T_H2) which down-regulate mixed lymphocyte reactions and might suppress GVHD (16). This type-2 profile of cells may predispose to chronic GVHD as has been reported in the peripheral blood stem cell transplantation literature.

Pathophysiology of Chronic GVHD

Chronic GVHD is very different in its features and is frequently compared to autoimmune disorders. The skin is the primary organ of involvement. Next in frequency is the liver. Additional tissues cited are the eyes, salivary glands, oral mucosa, muscle, and possibly lung. Once again, T cells are the main protagonists with $CD8^+$ cells predominant. Alloreactive and autoreactive clones of antibodies are frequently present. These may develop secondary to thymic damage. The presence of INF-γ suggests that the cellular infiltrate is made up of T_H1 cells. Tumor necrosis factor-α and IL-1α are produced by the keratinocyte and are thought responsible for the inflammatory reaction with fibrosis seen in chronic GVHD. The fibroblasts are stimulated, by an unclear mechanism, to produce collagen. This is responsible for the variable degree of fibrosis noted in all chronic GVHD (17).

Syngeneic GVHD

The syngeneic or autologous GVHD (18) poses a challenging dilemma for immunologists in that it clearly violates one of the Simonsen and Billingham postulates (3,19), namely, that there must be HLA differences between graft and host for GVHD to occur. However, Glazier et al. (20) observed syngeneic GVHD (syn-GVHD) after HSCT to irradiated syngeneic hosts that were also treated with cyclosporine, which has been shown to cause ablation of the thymic medulla in rats and mice (21). It has

TABLE 59.1. T-CELL COSIGNALLING[a]

APC	—	T Cell
—	**First Signal**	—
MHC Class I	Recognition	CD8
MHC Class II	Recognition	CD4
Ag-Peptide	Recognition	CD3/TCR
—	**Cosignal**	—
CD11a/CD18(LFA-1)	Adhesion	CD54(ICAM-1)
CD54(ICAM-1)	Adhesion	CD11a/CD18(LFA-1)
CD58(LFA-3)	Adhesion	CD2
CD106(VCAM-1)	Adhesion	CD49d/CD29(VLA-4)
CD80(B7-1)	Costimulation	CD28
CD86(B7-2)	Costimulation	CD28
OX40L	Th2 differentiation	CD134(OX40)
4-1BBL	Th1 differentiation	CD137(4-1BB)
CD80(B7-1)	Inhibition	CD152(CTLA4)
CD86(B7-2)	Inhibition	CD152(CTLA4)
CD40	Up-regulation of B7 molecules Th1 Differentiation	CD154(CD40L)
CD95(Fas)	Apoptosis	CD95L(FasL) CD95(Fas)

[a] From Tanaka J, Asaka M, Imamura M. T-cell co-signalling molecules in graft-versus-host disease. *Ann Hematol* 2000;79:283–290, with permission.

been observed also that pathogen-free animals are less likely to develop syn-GVHD (22). Hess and Thoburn (23) reviewed syngeneic-autologous GVHD and characterized it as a two-phase process requiring active inhibition of thymic-dependent clonal deletion and the elimination of mature T cells with an immunoregulatory effect. The elimination occurs during the preparative regimen for HSCT. The autoreactive T cells recognize MHC class II determinants. This specificity seems related to peptide derived from the MHC class II invariant chain.

Role of Microbial Pathogens

Cytomegalovirus (CMV) is a major risk factor for mortality in allogeneic HSCT. It has considerable sequence homology and immunologic cross-reactivity with the human HLA-DRB chain, and CMV-infected cells are able to produce a glycoprotein homologous to class I MHC antigens (24). Herpes simplex virus and possibly human herpes virus-6 may be significant factors in GVHD in HSCT recipients. A viral illness may cause initiation or progression of GVHD (12).

CLINICAL FEATURES OF TAGVHD

Prevalence of TAGVHD

The actual prevalence of TAGVHD following blood transfusion is unknown, although the disease is common in patients with severe deficiency of cell-mediated immunity, either congenital or acquired. The recognition that immunocompetent individuals may also develop TAGVHD if they have received nonirradiated cellular products from relatives or other donors homozygous for one of the recipient's HLA haplotypes (25–27) resulted, for a time, in increased case reporting of TAGVHD. Based on this understanding of the association between probable mechanisms of TAGVHD and similarities of HLA haplotypes, it has been calculated that the risk of TAGVHD for nondirected transfusions in U.S. whites is 1 in 17,700 to 39,000, in Germans 1 in 6,900 to 48,500, and in Japanese 1 in 1,600 to 7,900. The risk in directed donations between children and parents is increased 21-fold for U.S. whites, 18-fold for Germans, and 11-fold for Japanese (28).

Clinical Risk Factors for Developing TAGVHD

The risk factors for developing TAGVHD are well recognized and reflect the inability of a transfused host to successfully reject graft tissue. The mechanisms are the same as those outlined for HSCT GVHD. Table 59.2 lists clinical diagnoses in which TAGVHD has been reported.

It is of particular interest that patients with acquired immune deficiency syndrome (AIDS) have never been reported to develop TAGVHD, in spite of the thousands of units of cellular blood products with which they have been transfused since the beginning of the epidemic. Why patients with AIDS should be immune to this risk is unclear, but it could be related to the HIV-induced inability of their macrophages to process antigen and the consequent failure to activate $CD45RA^{+}CD4^{+}$ T cells to $CD45RO^{+}CD4^{+}$ T cells (29). It has also been suggested that donor $CD4^{+}$ cells become infected by HIV and consequently are rendered immunologically incompetent (30).

TABLE 59.2. PATIENTS AT RISK FOR GVHD

Neonates
Intrauterine transfusion (IUT)
Postnatal transfusion in recipients of IUT
Very–low-birth-weight premature neonates
Neonatal alloimmune thrombocytopenia
Genetically Immunodeficient
Severe combined immunodeficiency
Wiskott-Aldrich syndrome
DiGeorge's syndrome
Other T-cell defects
Immunosuppression by Chemotherapy or Irradiation
Leukemia and Lymphoma
Acute lymphocytic leukemia
Acute nonlymphocytic leukemia
Hodgkin's disease
Non-Hodgkin's lymphoma
Fludarabine-treated lymphoma or lymphoid leukemia
Hematopoietic Stem Cell Transplantation
Allogeneic
Autologous
Syngeneic
Other Organ Transplant
Lung
Liver
Heart
Solid Tumors
Neuroblastoma
Glioblastoma
Other syndromes

Conditions Associated with TAGVHD

Fetuses and Newborns

The risk of TAGVHD in fetuses receiving intrauterine transfusion (IUT) and perinatal transfusion is theoretically high, although only a very few cases have been reported (31,32). These cases and those of newborn infants with TAGVHD have been reported (31–36). It is also conceivable that graft-host tolerance in fetuses may occur because of:

1. Lack of host immune surveillance due to immaturity
2. Inadequate expression of target antigens in fetal tissue
3. Maternal lymphocytes that may confer protection against GVHD (37,38).

Newborn GVHD from maternal-fetal transfer of lymphocytes occurs only infrequently (33). This suggests that the fetus has natural protective mechanisms against this condition, because although small-volume maternal-fetal hemorrhage reportedly occurs in approximately 25% of fetuses with severe combined immune deficiency syndrome (SCIDS), only a proportion of them develop TAGVHD (39). These infants are particularly vulnerable to TAGVHD, with at least 26 cases reported. Because these infants have thymic dysplasia, they are not protected against engraftment by donor immune response cells (IRCs), including those of maternal origin. However, the pathologic changes in the thymus of SCIDS patients with TAGVHD are virtually identical to those seen in GVHD not associated with SCIDS, raising the possibility that the latter condition may be secondary to TAGVHD induced by in utero maternal-fetal transfusion (40). It is possible that there is a dose-dependent relationship, because neonates have developed GVHD following transfusion of nonirradiated maternal platelets for neonatal alloimmune thrombocytopenia (34), and some cases of TAGVHD have occurred in neonates who were treated by IUT for erythroblastosis fetalis (EF) (6,31,32).

Although the occurrence of TAGVHD in neonates transfused postnatally appears to be extremely rare, this could be due to lack of recognition of the clinical syndrome in the complicated clinical picture of sick premature infants. Ohto and Anderson (41) reviewed TAGVHD in Japanese newborns reported from 1985 to 1994. Of the 27 cases reported, 20 were in premature and seven in full-term neonates. Twenty-three received whole blood less than 72 hours old (most from relatives), one received a platelet concentrate, three received cells reconstituted with plasma, and one received packed red blood cells. The interval from transfusion to clinical signs and symptoms of TAGVHD was a median of 28 days for development of fever, a median of 30 days for an erythematous rash, a median of 43 days for leukopenia, and a median of 51 days until death. The proposed mechanisms for latency in the appearance of TAGVHD follow: a) decreased frequency of donor-derived cytotoxic T-cell precursor (T_Cp) in blood transfusion recipients who share one HLA haplotype with the donor, b) a low frequency of host-specific T_Cp in donors associated with absent or mild GVHD in HSCT patients, and c) evidence that neonates may be tolerant of noninherited maternal human leukocyte antigens (41,42). Neonatal T cells simply might not be able to generate a host versus graft response regardless of tolerance (42).

In the cases of GVHD following IUT for EF, lymphoid and thymic atrophy were evident at autopsy, reflecting tissue atrophy induced by GVHD rather than primary immunologic deficiency (6). Nevertheless, the question why only a very few cases of TAGVHD have been reported in thousands of IUTs given to fetuses with EF remains unanswered.

Primary Immunodeficiency Syndromes

Transfusion-associated GVHD has been documented in more than 30 children with primary immunodeficiency syndromes (8,37–40,43–47). The majority of these patients had SCIDS (27 cases); other diagnostic groups were Wiskott-Aldrich syndrome (a condition associated with cellular immune dysfunction, humoral abnormalities, and thrombocytopenia), thymic dysplasia or hypoplasia, and purine nucleoside phosphorylase deficiency.

Secondary Immunodeficiencies

Secondary immunodeficiency is diagnosed when previously normal patients begin to manifest unusually increased susceptibility to infections. Such secondary deficiencies arise in a number of well-characterized situations, including lymphoreticular disease, malignancy, and immune system–altering chemotherapy or radiotherapy.

Malignancies

It is unclear if malignancy by itself is a risk factor for TAGVHD (48–63). Because the majority of reported cancer patients were treated with chemotherapy or irradiation or both, it has been difficult to separate the effect of malignancy from that due to treatment. However, there has been no correlation between the extent or duration of the therapies and the time taken to develop TAGVHD. Diagnostic groups include acute lymphocytic leukemia, acute nonlymphoid leukemia, Hodgkin disease, non-Hodgkin lymphoma, neuroblastoma, rhabdomyosarcoma, glioblastoma, and fludarabine (purine analogue)-treated lymphoreticular disease (primarily B cell–chronic lymphocytic leukemia) (64–65). Fludarabine is known to deplete the patient of $CD4^+$ T cells.

In a review of the Japanese experience with TAGVHD in immunocompetent recipients between 1985 and 1993 (66), patients with tumors involving the gastrointestinal system, biliary tract, urogenital system, lung, thyroid, and central nervous system were reported. This is most likely a reflection of the transfusion practices and HLA homology of residents in that country rather than immunosuppression related to therapy.

As in other clinical settings, the prevalence of TAGVHD in malignancy is unknown. It is likely that the reported cases represent only a small proportion of those recognized and that many instances go unrecognized. It could be that TAGVHD manifests an evolving clinical or laboratory syndrome that is aborted once normal hematopoiesis is reconstituted as cytotoxic therapy is reduced. Symptoms identical to GVHD occur in patients undergoing ablative chemotherapy, at a time when even skin biopsies may be equivocal. One way of proving engraftment of transfused donor cells is to demonstrate HLA class I and II antigen differences between host cells and donor cells.

Transfusion-associated GVHD in Immunocompetent Individuals

The observation that TAGVHD occurs in apparently immunocompetent individuals who receive cellular blood products from genetically related family members, or random donors from a genetically restricted community, are well described. Most of the reported TAGVHD occurring in immunocompetent hosts has arisen in genetically homogenous Japan (26,27).

The basis for developing TAGVHD in immunocompetent hosts lies in major HLA haplotype similarities between donor and recipient (26,27); specifically, the donor is homozygous for a class I haplotype for which the recipient is heterozygous. Transfusion-associated GVHD occurs in this setting because recipient immune surveillance recognizes class I antigen donor-recipient pairs as similar. This allows donor lymphocytes to go unrecognized as foreign and then be stimulated by, and do damage to, the dissimilar host tissues. In a heterogeneous society like North America, this type of TAGVHD is most likely to occur after transfusion between first- and even second-degree blood relatives (26). In Japan where random, as well as closely related, donors may share HLA class I and II haplotypes with recipients, the condition occurs more frequently (27,67).

Transfusion-associated GVHD in Surgery

Posttransfusion GVHD has frequently been recognized in patients who have had cardiac surgery (66). It is typically characterized by postoperative erythroderma, fever, rash, agranulocytosis, and marrow aplasia, usually within 10 days of surgery (63). It has been most commonly seen in Japan, where the most recent figures indicate a prevalence of 1:212 (0.47%) (68). It usually occurs in a patient who has received fresh (less than 7-day-old) cellular blood products from blood relatives or from an apparently unrelated donor in a community with HLA homology.

The reason cardiac surgery patients are at such a high risk for developing TAGVHD is unknown. It has been observed that surgery per se provokes immune suppression manifested by lymphopenia and depressed cell-mediated immunity within the first postoperative week (69,70). In addition, the old practice of transfusing fresh blood to patients undergoing cardiac surgery may have exposed them to viral pathogens, including leukocyte-borne CMV, which has been implicated in the postperfusion pump syndrome. Cytomegalovirus's close sequence homology to HLA antigens is believed to underlie its ability to enhance the severity of GVHD in bone marrow transplant recipients (24). However, the most remarkable factor was the presence, in the donors, of homozygosity of an HLA haplotype for which the recipient was heterozygous, namely a one-way HLA match. In many cases, the donor-recipient pairs were blood relatives. In more than one-half of the patients, however, there was no blood relationship between the donor and recipient, although the HLA haplotype conditions still prevailed, both in Japanese and non-Japanese patients.

Thus, the combination of circumstances most likely to lead to TAGVHD in immunocompetent hosts includes a) a one-way HLA match, b) use of fresh blood, c) cardiac surgery, d) a donor who is a blood relative. Of note is that TAGVHD in patients receiving nonirradiated blood components did not occur if the red blood cells were more than 7 days old (66). Fiebig et al. (71) reported continued T-cell activation after 8.1 days of cold storage and no activation at 21 days.

Risk is clearly not restricted to first-degree relatives, because the probability of one-way HLA match is still present at lower degrees of relatedness (26). Petz et al. (25) described TAGVHD in a 73-year-old man who, after a radical prostatectomy, had received a unit of red blood cells freshly donated by his grandson. Kanter (72) calculates the risk of TAGVHD among various degrees of blood relatedness and noted that in some situations, second-degree relatives are more likely than first-degree, to be homozygous for an HLA haplotype for which a recipient might be heterozygous.

Transfusion-associated GVHD in Solid Organ Transplantation

Most cases of GVHD in this patient population are from donor lymphocytes transported to the host with the transplanted organ. Transfusion-associated GVHD has been reported in orthotopic liver transplant recipients, a heart transplant recipient, and a recipient of a pancreas-spleen transplant (62,63,73,74). Two patients received transfusions at times of maximal immunosuppression. In one of the liver transplant cases and in the heart transplant report, the diagnosis was confirmed by HLA typing. It showed the presence of nonhost or organ-donor HLA types in the peripheral blood of the host (73,74).

Blood Components and Dosage of Immunocompetent Cells in TAGVHD

Transfusion-associated GVHD has been reported following transfusion of all cellular blood components and fresh plasma that contain viable lymphocytes (75). Graft versus host disease has not been reported following infusions with fresh-frozen plasma, cryoprecipitate, or coagulation factor concentrates devoid of viable cells. Cellular components with markedly reduced lymphocyte concentrations, such as deglycerolized red blood cells or washed red blood cells, also have not been associated with TAGVHD, despite the demonstration of viable lymphocytes in frozen washed blood (75,76). This is consistent with a dosage effect in the pathogenesis of TAGVHD. The number of immunocompetent cells transfused per unit of time during maximal immune suppression could also be important (77,78). The lymphocyte content of the various blood products is listed in Table 59.3; the ranges, in the implicated products, are from 1.5×10^5 cells per unit of fresh (nonfrozen) plasma to 5×10^9 lymphocytes in granulocyte concentrates (75). However, TAGVHD has been reported to occur following the infusion of as few as 8×10^4 lymphocytes per kilogram of body weight (79). Although transfusions of frozen deglycerolized red blood cells have not been associated with GVHD, 5×10^7 white blood cells can be present per transfused unit, representing 6% of the original

TABLE 59.3. LYMPHOCYTE CONTENT IN BLOOD COMPONENTS

Component	Lymphocytes per unit
Whole blood	$1.0–2.0 \times 10^9$
Washed red blood cells	$1.0–2.0 \times 10^8$
Frozen, degycerolyzed red blood cells	5.0×10^7
Single unit platelet pack	4.0×10^7
Plateletpheresis pack	3.0×10^8
Granulocyte concentrate	1.0×10^{10}
Single-donor plasma	1.5×10^5
Fresh-frozen plasma	0
Cryoprecipitate	0

From National Institutes of Health (Department of Transfusion Medicine) and Leitman SF. Post transfusion graft versus host disease. In: Smith DN, Silvergleid AJ, eds. *Special considerations in transfusing the immunocompromised patient.* Arlington, VA: American Association of Blood Banks, 1985:15–37.

unprocessed mononuclear cell total. These cells, moreover, can manifest mitotic activity and blast transformation in vitro (76).

Granulocyte concentrates were the component most associated with TAGVHD, before the clinical syndrome was well described, when granulocytes from patients with chronic myeloid leukemia (CML) were transfused (80). Transfusion of CML granulocytes in malignant disease has reportedly resulted in engraftment in as many as 50% of cases; however, death appears to occur less frequently than in other forms of TAGVHD. Eight of nine bone marrow transplant recipients who received these transfusions and who later developed TAGVHD suffered graft rejection without therapy.

Clinicopathologic Features of TAGVHD

Following HSCT, either acute or chronic GVHD syndromes can develop. The graft attacks all other susceptible tissues apart from itself. The transplanted bone marrow is not affected because it is of donor origin. By contrast, in TAGVHD all host tissues, including bone marrow, are targeted. Symptoms include dermatosis, diarrhea, liver enzyme elevation, and pancytopenia consequent to marrow hypoplasia. Two cases of chronic TAGVHD have been reported (51,81). The most recent case (81) occurred after an episode of unrecognized acute GVHD in an 84-year-old woman with non-Hodgkin lymphoma who had received recent nodal irradiation and chemotherapy for recurrent disease. Two units of leukoreduced red blood cells were transfused during that time. Symptoms of acute TAGVHD were an exfoliative erythroderma, massive edema of lower extremities with cutaneous ulceration, profuse watery diarrhea, fever, leukopenia, and elevated alkaline phosphatase levels. The diarrhea and fever resolved. Lichenoid skin changes developed after 4 months. These were diagnosed as chronic TAGVHD. Human leukocyte antigen typing demonstrated nonhost phenotypes. The dose of lymphocytes present must have been as few as 5×10^4 or 5×10^5 cells.

Pathology of TAGVHD

Cells expressing HLA antigens are targets for GVHD. Histologically, changes in GVHD have been classified according to two responses, a) the response seen in lymph nodes, splenic white pulp and intestinal lymph nodules, which show marked lymphoid stimulation and immunoblast transformation; and b) an aggressive lesion present on the epithelial surfaces of various tissues including the skin, associated with a lymphatic infiltration of the portal tracts of the liver, with focal hepatic cell necrosis (46). In TAGVHD, the bone marrow is hypoplastic (Table 59.4).

Diagnosis of GVHD

The diagnosis of GVHD is based on clinical features in the situations that are known to lead to the condition. The presence of skin lesions, diarrhea, elevated liver enzymes, and pancytopenia are sufficient clinical indicators for the diagnosis. When necessary, the diagnosis is usually confirmed histologically by skin biopsy. The skin biopsy in acute GVHD demonstrates vacuolar degeneration of basal cells, focal spongiosis in the epidermis, degenerated keratinocytes with pyknotic nuclei and eosinophilic cytoplasm throughout the epidermis, exocytosis of lymphoid cells, and mild infiltration of lymphocytes in the upper dermis. These findings are not pathognomonic for GVHD. The same findings have been described with skin changes in drug toxicity. Immunohistochemical analysis shows $CD8^+$ lymphocytes predominate in the epidermis. $CD4^+$ lymphocytes are mainly present around the blood vessels. Intercellular adhesion molecule 1 (CD54) expression in the epidermis is predominantly in the basal cells and the deepest layers of the stratum spinosum (82). Vascular endothelial cells also stained intensely with ICAM-1. Vascular cell adhesion molecule 1 was strongly expressed in the endothelial cells in almost all of the superficial vessels. Endothelial leucocyte adhesion molecule (ELAM-1) was only weakly expressed. Most infiltrating cells were positive for CD3, CD11a, CD18, and HLA-DR. Human leukocyte antigen-DR was also expressed in the epidermis on the surface of keratinocytes and in endothelial cells of superficial dermal vessels.

Chronic GVHD is characterized by a substantial increase in collagen deposition in the target organs and some T-cell infiltra-

TABLE 59.4. CLINICAL AND PATHOLOGIC COMPARISON OF GVHD ASSOCIATED WITH HEMATOPOIETIC STEM CELL TRANSPLANTATION AND TRANSFUSIONS

Manifestation	HSCTA-GVHD	TA-GVHD
Time sequence	35–70 d	2–30 d
Skin rash	+	+
Constitutional symptoms	Marked	Mild/moderate
Liver enzyme elevation	+	+
Pancytopenia	Rare/minimal	Marked
Bone marrow hypoplasia or aplasia	+/–	++
Occurrence of GVHD	70%	?0.1–1%
Response to therapy	80–90%	None
Mortality	10–15%	80–100%

GVHD, graft versus host disease; HSCTA-GVHD, hematopoietic stem cell transplantation–associated graft versus host disease.
From Brubaker DB. Transfusion associated graft versus host disease. *Hum Pathol* 1986;17:1085–1088, with permission.

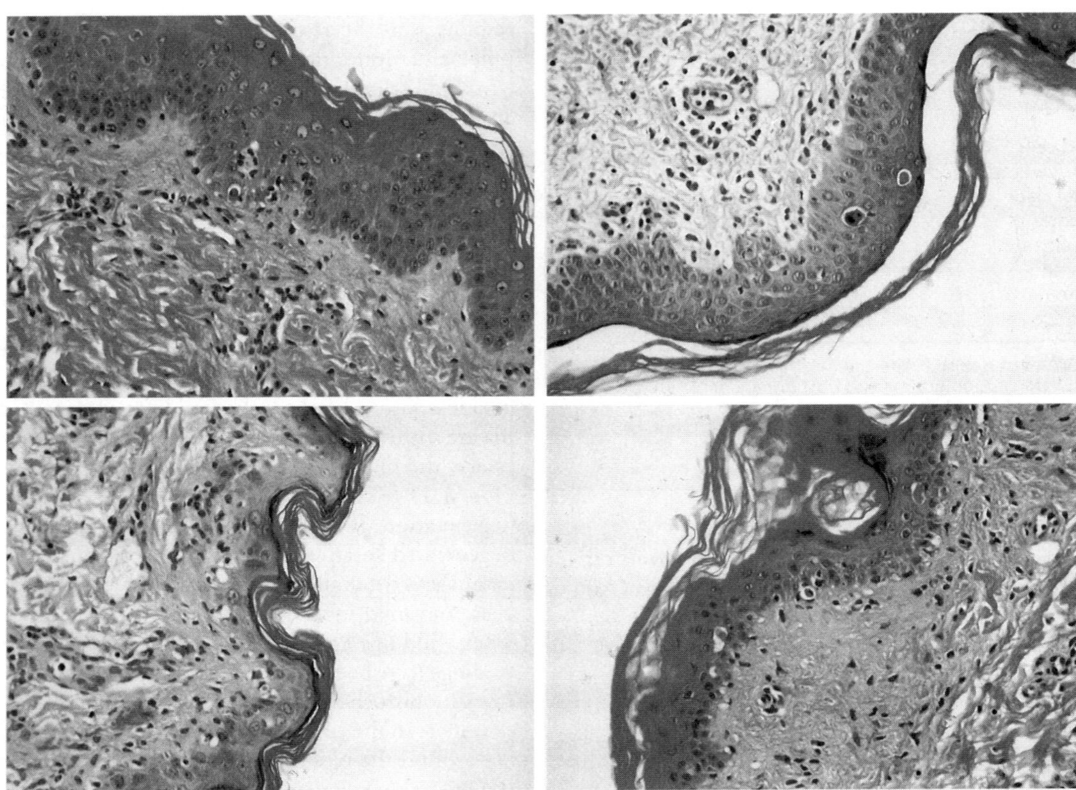

FIGURE 59.3. Hematoxylin and eosin stain. Chronic GVHD of skin. The lesions exhibit a superficial dermal infiltrate of lymphocytes, epidermal thickening with acanthosis, parakeratotic hyperkeratosis, and keratinocyte necrosis. (Photograph courtesy of Dr. Edgar Ballard, Children's Hospital Medical Center, Cincinnati, Ohio.)

tion. The lichenoid lesions in early chronic GVHD have the appearance of acute GVHD, a lymphocytic infiltrate of the superficial dermis with moderate exocytosis (Fig. 59.3). The epidermis is thickened with acanthosis, parakeratotic hyperkeratosis, hypergranulosis, and variable keratinocyte necrosis. The late chronic GVHD lesion is a sclerodermatous lesion. Present is a marked dermal atrophy with destruction of appendageal structures, linearization of dermal-epidermal junction, and superficial collagen fibrosis. Keratinocytes are small, flat, and full of melanin. The dermis contains discrete pericapillary infiltrates. Granular IgM deposits are at the dermal-epidermal junction in more than 80% of biopsied tissue.

Cell clones identified in TAGVHD (83–85) may contain $CD8^+$ cytotoxic T lymphocytes (T_C's), $CD4^+$ T_C's, or noncytotoxic $CD4^+$ cells. Each clone has its own target antigen, a class I or II MHC antigen. The TCR vβ gene populations are skewed to limited types, unlike normal controls (86).

Confirmation that an event of GVHD is the result of a blood transfusion can be obtained by demonstrating the presence of donor lymphocytes in the recipient's circulating blood. Current techniques for laboratory confirmation of TAGVHD include:

1. Histocompatibility testing, both by classic serology and by DNA typing of HLA *DR* and *DQ* using PCR amplification of relevant exons with allele-specific primers (48).
2. Cytogenetic analysis of graft cell and host cell chromosomes (87).
3. DNA analysis of graft and host tissue DNA microsatellite polymorphisms or variable normal tandem repeats (VNTRs) (88,89).

Tissues used for pretransfusion characterization of host cells are frequently fingernails or fibroblasts from skin biopsies. Host peripheral blood is the source of material for posttransfusion analysis of the mixed cell populations (host and blood donor) (85).

Cytogenetics are relatively simple but require the presence of recognizable distinguishing markers in the donor or recipient or both, of which sex chromosome difference is the most obvious (87). Wang et al. (89) have demonstrated the usefulness of polymorphic microsatellite markers in the diagnosis of TAGVHD.

Human leukocyte antigen class I and class II typing of circulating lymphocytes by classic serology may be difficult when the recipient is severely leukopenic. Deoxyribonucleic acid analysis of microsatellite polymorphisms or restriction fragment length polymorphisms is a suitable tool (25,85,89).

Treatment of TAGVHD

The treatment of HSCT-associated GVHD, using modalities such as antithymocyte globulin (ATG), cyclosporine, and high-dose corticosteroids is potentially more successful than the treatment for TAGVHD, which carries a mortality rate of 84% (90) to more than 90% (91). Additional current and experimental therapies for HSCT-associated GVHD are many. Interventions for acute GVHD include glatiramer acetate (Copaxone), nucleoside analogues (92), sirolimus (Rapamycin) (93), and serine protease inhibitors such as nafamostat mesylate (94). Therapies for chronic GVHD include monoclonal antibodies against various cellular antigens or receptors (95,96), thalidomide (97), photochemotherapy, extracorporeal photochemotherapy (98), tacrolimus, total lymphoid irradiation, mycophenolate mofetil, etretinate, ursodeoxycholic acid, penicillamine, cyclofenil halofuginone, nedocromil sodium (99), and UVB irradiation (100).

This multitude of interventions is aimed at prevention in addition to treatment of HSCT-related GVHD. Although TAGVHD has been difficult to treat, there may be benefit in trying some of the new modalities.

Spontaneous (101) and long-term survival (102) after TAGVHD have been reported. Therapeutic responses in TAGVHD have been reported using combination therapy that may involve anti-CD3 monoclonal antibodies, cyclosporine, methylprednisolone, G-CSF (103), or 15-deoxyspergualin (88) (not currently available in the United States).

Saigo and Ryo (104) outlined a strategy of treatment for TAGVHD dependent on vigilance, early diagnosis, and initiation of treatment before confirmation of the diagnosis is completed. The protocol involved a) suppression of T_C activity using nafamostat mesylate (serine protease inhibitor that acts on granzymes) and chloroquine (inhibits antigen processing and presentation), b) suppression of TNF-α using anti-TNF-α antibody or TNF-α receptor Fc-contained protein and pentoxifylline (inhibits TNF-α synthesis), c) immunomodulation using intravenous immune globulin (IVIG) to improve prognosis by reducing infections and G-CSF to increase the number of T_H2 lymphocytes, decreasing the release of INF-γ and IL-2, d) elimination of donor lymphocytes using corticosteroids, cyclophosphamide, methotrexate, and a strong adenosine deaminase inhibitor or purine analogue (reduces lymphocyte population) such as fludarabine, cladribine, pentostatin, or pegademase.

Nishimura (105) has also suggested that extracorporeal phototherapy using 8-methoxypsoralen (8-MOP) and UVA irradiation may be useful based on in vitro experiments using models of activated donor cells and resting patient cells. Low doses of 8-MOP and UVA irradiation were effective in inhibiting growth and cytotoxic activity of stimulated cells.

Prevention of TAGVHD

Because many of the risk factors for TAGVHD are known, we are theoretically positioned to eliminate the disease. At the recommended levels of exposure, γ-irradiation of cellular blood components destined for susceptible recipients eliminates the risk of GVHD. However, questions remain regarding other groups at risk, the potential role of leukodepletion filters (see Chapters 21 and 34), and other preventive measures.

Radiation Sources

γ-Irradiation is a high-energy form of radiation generated from several sources, including cesium 137, cobalt 60, and a linear accelerator (106). In general, cesium 137 is the more practical source because of its long half-life and high energy level. Although cobalt 60 can be substituted, it has a lower energy level and shorter half-life, so that it must be replaced more frequently; it also requires a longer exposure time.

Self-contained blood irradiators are available in blood banks and transfusion services. Despite their small size, they are extremely heavy because of the lead shielding (625 pounds per square foot) used to protect against leakage. Blood irradiators are easy to operate and are safe using cesium 137 or cobalt 60 as source materials. Operation costs vary according to the intensity of the source (in curies); the higher the source intensity, the shorter the time required to administer a set dose to a blood component. For example, a large cesium source (2,400 curies) delivers a dose of 20 Gy in 1.3 minutes, whereas a source of 600 curies takes nearly 4.5 minutes to achieve the same treatment. The cost of a 2,000-curie source is two to three times higher than a 600-curie source.

Radiation Practice

The most appropriate dose for blood component irradiation is 25 Gy at midplane (106–108). The Food and Drug Administration (FDA) has also recommended that a dose of 25 Gy be delivered to the internal midplane, with minimum of 15 Gy to any other point irradiated.

Effects of Irradiation on Nonlymphoid Cells

In vivo viability of irradiated red blood cells, when evaluated with 24-hour recovery, is reduced compared to nonirradiated red blood cells (106). Adenosine triphosphate (ATP) levels and in vitro hemolysis are not much changed. Potassium leakage is enhanced by irradiation. These observations have led to the FDA guideline that red blood cells must be limited to 28 days storage after irradiation.

Platelet properties are not significantly altered and they do not require any special handling. Slightly better function in single-donor apheresis leukoreduced platelets is noted if irradiation takes place before storage (109).

Polymorphonuclear leukocytes do not seem to exhibit significant functional changes following exposure to radiation doses below 40 Gy (110) and are relatively radioresistant, even at substantially higher doses (75). However, nitroblue tetrazolium reduction has been shown to be variably deficient in granulocytes receiving irradiation doses as low as 25 Gy, suggesting that defective oxidative metabolism may occur at therapeutic doses (75). In spite of this, granulocyte concentrates, because they are heavily contaminated with lymphocytes, must be irradiated prior to transfusion in order to reduce the likelihood of transfusing viable lymphocytes. In vitro human monocyte survival and function may also be impaired at doses designed to prevent TAGVHD (111).

A theoretic side effect of irradiation is the possibility that sublethal doses given to lymphocytes will impair DNA repair and induce oncogenic potential. Because irradiation can alter DNA structure or repair processes (112,113), there has been an effort to prevent the widespread use of irradiated blood components in other than the immunosuppressed patients. The fear of altered DNA structure remains hypothetical, however, and to date no evidence exists to restrict irradiated blood components for this reason.

Alternatives to γ-Irradiation

Irradiation of blood components is the proven modality for the prevention of TAGVHD. The process, easy to perform, is safe and does no harm to the transfusion component within the guidelines already mentioned. Irradiation of blood components should be standard practice for recognized high-risk recipients. Use of leukocyte depletion filters is a logical alternative, but efficiency is questionable: a patient receiving filtered blood developed TAGVHD (114). The postleukoreduction cell count in one case of chronic GVHD was estimated to be 5×10^4 to 5×10^5 cells (81). Thus, until leukocyte depletion filters become more efficient, they should not be used as an alternative to γ-irradiation.

A different strategy is to irradiate cellular blood products by ultraviolet light, a modality that has been shown to prevent TAGVHD in dogs (115) and reduces alloimmunization in humans (116). This approach needs further evaluation. Others have looked at the effect of photochemical treatment using a combination of 8-MOP and UVA irradiation (71) or dimethylmethylene blue and white light (117) for inactivation of white blood cells. Both have shown significant reduction in the activation of lymphocytes, similar to that demonstrated with 25 Gy of γ-irradiation.

SUMMARY

Transfusion-associated GVHD results from T lymphocytes being transfused in sufficient numbers to susceptible patients. Classically, these patients are immunodeficient either naturally or secondary to disease or therapy. Malignancy and transfusion of HLA haploidentical cells to immunocompetent patients are also recognized as risk factors for GVHD. Diagnosis of GVHD is based on the underlying disease, a transfusion within 4 to 30 days (median of 15 days), a fulminant illness (with rash, liver dysfunction, and diarrhea), and the presence of severe pancytopenia and bone marrow hypoplasia. Positive confirmation of GVHD is based on the demonstration of chimerism in the patient, either by HLA, sex chromatin, or DNA analysis. Irradiation of blood components, using a minimum dose of greater than 25 Gy, is the strategy of choice for preventing this dangerous condition.

REFERENCES

1. Murphy JB. The effect of adult chicken organ graft on the chick embryo. *J Exp Med* 1916;24:1.
2. Simonsen M. Graft-versus-host reactions. The natural history and applicability as tools of research. *Prog Allergy* 1962;6:349–467.
3. Simonsen M. The impact on the developing embryo and newborn animal of adult homologous cells. *Acta Pathol Microbiol Scand* 1957; 40:480.
4. Billingham RE, Brent LA. A simple method for inducing tolerance of skin homografts in mice. *Transplant Bull* 1957;4:67–71.
5. Mathé G, Bernard J, Schwarzenberg L, et al. Essai de traitment de sujets, atteints de, leuce mie aigue en rémission par irradiation totale suivie de transfusion de moelle osseuse homologue. *Rev Fr Études Clin Biol* 1959;4:675.
6. Naiman JL, Punnett H, Lischner HW, et al. Possible graft-versus-host reaction after intrauterine transfusion for erythroblastosis fetalis. *N Engl J Med* 1969;281:697–701.
7. Hathaway WE, Githens JH, Blackburn WR, et al. Aplastic anemia, histiocytosis and erythroderma in immunologically deficient children. *N Engl J Med* 1965;273:953.
8. Terasaki P. Identification of the type of blood cells responsible for the graft-versus-host reaction in chicks. *J Embryol Exp Morphol* 1959; 7:394.
9. Simonsen M. Graft-versus-host reactions. The history that never was, and the way things happened to happen. *Immunol Rev* 1985;88:5–23.
10. Klingebiel T, Schlegel PG. GVHD: overview on pathophysiology, incidence, clinical and biological features. *Bone Marrow Transplant* 1998;21[Suppl 2]:S45–S49.
11. Robert C, Kupper TS. Inflammatory skin diseases, T cells and immune surveillance. *N Engl J Med* 1999;341:1817–1828.
12. Ferrara JL, Levy R, Chao NJ. Pathophysiologic mechanisms of acute graft-vs.-host disease. *Biol Blood Marrow Transplant* 1999;5:347–356.
13. Tanaka J, Asaka M, Imamura M. T-cell signalling molecules in graft-versus-host disease. *Ann Hematol* 2000;79:283–290.
14. Pham CTN, Ley TJ. The role of granzyme B cluster proteases in cell-mediated cytotoxicity. *Semin Immunol* 1997;9:127–133.
15. Brubaker DB. Immunopathogenic mechanisms of posttransfusion graft vs host disease. *Proc Soc Exp Biol Med.* 1993;202:122–147.
16. Rutella S, Rumi C, Sica S, et al. Recombinant human granulocyte colony-stimulating factor (rHuG-CSF): effects on lymphocyte phenotype and function. *J Interferon Cytokine Res* 1999;19:989–994.
17. Aractingi S, Chosidow O. Cutaneous graft-versus-host disease. *Arch Dermatol* 1998;134:602–612.
18. Rappeport JM, Mihm M, Reinherz EL, et al. Acute graft-vs-host disease in recipients of bone marrow transplants from identical twin donors. *Lancet* 1979;2:717–720.
19. Billingham RE. The biology of graft-vs-host reactions. *Harvey Lecture* 1966–1967;62:21–78.
20. Glazier A, Totschka P, Farmer ER, et al. Graft-versus-host disease in cyclosporin-A treated rats after syngeneic and autologous bone marrow reconstitution. *J Exp Med* 1983;158:1–8.
21. Beschorner WE, Namnoum JD, Hess AD, et al. Cyclosporine and the thymus: immunopathology. *Am J Pathol* 1987;126:487–496.
22. Fischer AC, Berschorner WE, Hess AD. Age related factors in the induction of syngeneic GVHD. *Transplant Proc* 1989;21: 3033–3035.
23. Hess AD, Thoburn CJ. Immunobiology and immunotherapeutic implications of syngeneic/autologous graft-versus-host disease. *Immunol Rev* 1997;157:111–123.
24. Rubin RH, Tolkoff-Rubin NE. The impact of infection on the outcome of transplantation. *Transplant Proc* 1991;23:2068–2074.
25. Petz LD, Calhoun LP, Yam PM, et al. Transfusion-associated graft-versus-host disease in immunocompetent patients: report of a fatal case associated with transfusion of blood from a second-degree relative, and a survey of predisposing factors. *Transfusion* 1993;33: 742–750.
26. McMilin KD, Johnson RL. HLA homozygosity and the risk of related-donor transfusion-associated graft-versus-host disease. *Transfus Med Rev* 1993;7:37–41.
27. Ohto H, Yasuda H, Noguchi M, et al. Risk of transfusion-associated graft-versus-host disease as a result of directed donations from relatives [Letter]. *Transfusion* 1992;32:691–693.
28. Wagner FF, Flegel WA. Transfusion-associated graft-versus-host disease: risk due to homozygous HLA haplotypes. *Transfusion* 1995;35: 284–291.
29. Herbert MR, L'age-Stehr J, Mitchinson NA. Antigen presentation, loss of immunological memory and AIDS. *Immunology Today* 1993; 14:340–344.
30. Amman AJ. Hypothesis: absence of graft-versus-host disease in AIDS is a consequence of HIV-1 infection of $CD4^+$ T cells. *J Acquir Immune Defic Syndr* 1993;6:1224–1227.

31. Bohm N, Kleine W, Enzel U. Graft-versus-host disease in two newborns after repeated blood transfusions because of rhesus incompatibility. *Beitr Pathol* 1977;160:381–400.
32. Parkman R, Mosier D, Umansky, et al. Graft versus host disease after intrauterine exchange transfusions for hemolytic disease of the newborn. *N Engl J Med* 1974;290:359–363.
33. Tinaztepe K, Berkel AI. Thymic dysplasia-graft-versus-host disease due to maternofetal bleed. *Pediatr Res* 1979;13:953(abst).
34. Thompson JE, Stockman JA, Davey FR, et al. Development of apparent graft versus host (GVH) reaction following a maternal platelet transfusion in an immunocompetent infant. *Pediatr Res* 1981;15:604(abst).
35. Seemayer TA, Boland ERP. Thymic evolution mimicking thymic dysplasia. A consequence of transfusion induced graft versus host disease in a premature infant. *Arch Pathol Lab Med* 1980;104:141–144.
36. Hatley RM, Reynolds M, Paller AS, et al. Graft-versus-host following ECMO. *J Pediatr Surg* 1991;26:317–319.
37. Vaidya S, Mamlok R, Daeschner CW III, et al. Suppression of GVHD reaction in severe combined immunodeficiency with maternal-fetal T cell engraftment. *Am J Pediatr Hematol Oncol* 1991;13:172–175.
38. Fowler RJ, Schubert WK, West CD. Acquired partial tolerance to homologous skin grafts in the human infant at birth. *Ann N Y Acad Sci* 1960;87:403–428.
39. Goldmann SF, Niethammer D, Flad HD, et al. Hematopoietic and lymphopoietic split chimerism in SCID. *Transplant Proc* 1979;11:225–229.
40. Alain G, Carrier C, Beaumier L, et al. In utero acute graft-versus-host disease in a neonate with severe combined immunodeficiency. *J Am Acad Dermatol* 1993;29:862–865.
41. Ohto H, Anderson KC. Posttransfusion graft-versus-host disease in Japanese newborns. *Transfusion* 1996;36:117–123.
42. Luban NLC, DePalma L. Transfusion-associated graft-versus-host disease in the neonate-expanding the spectrum of disease [Editorial]. *Transfusion* 1996;36:101–103.
43. Park BH, Good RA, Gate J, et al. Fatal graft-vs.-host reaction following transfusion of allogeneic blood and plasma in infants with combined immunodeficiency disease. *Transplant Proc* 1974;6:385.
44. Niethammer D, Goldmann SF, Flad HD, et al. Graft-versus-host reaction after blood transfusion in a patient with cellular immunodeficiency: the role of histocompatibility testing. *Eur J Pediatr* 1979;132:43–48.
45. Frappat P, Coudere P, Marchal A, et al. Graft-versus-host reactions during primary combined immune deficiencise in children. *Ann Pediatr* 1974;21:1401–1409.
46. Brubaker DB. Transfusion associated graft versus host disease. *Hum Pathol* 1986;17:1085–1088.
47. Strobel S, Morgan G, Simmonds AH, et al. Fatal graft versus host disease after platelet transfusion in a child with purine nucleoside phosphorylase deficiency. *Eur J Pediatr* 1989;148:312–314.
48. Ford JM, Cullen MH, Lucey JJ, et al. Fatal graft-versus-host-disease following transfusion of granulocytes from normal donors. *Lancet* 1976;2:1167–1169.
49. Lowenthal RM, Menon C, Challis DR. Graft-versus-host disease in consecutive patients with acute myeloid leukemia treated with blood cells from normal donors. *Aust N Z J Med* 1981;11:179–183.
50. Szaley F, Buki B, Kalouics I, et al. Post transfusion GVHR in an adult with acute leukemia and aplastic anemia. *Orv Hetil* 1972;113:1275–1280.
51. Siimes MA, Koskimies S. Chronic graft versus host disease after blood transfusions by incompatible HLA antigens in bone marrow [Letter]. *Lancet* 1982;1:42–43.
52. Burgess MA, Garson OM. Homologous leukocyte transfusions in acute leukemia with cytogenetic evidence of myeloid graft. *Med J Aust* 1969;1:1243–1246.
53. Schmidmeier W, Feil W, Gebhart W, et al. Fatal graft-versus-host reaction following granulocyte transfusions. *Blut* 1982;45:115–119.
54. Kessinger A, Armitage JO, Klassen LW, et al. Graft vs host disease following transfusion of normal blood products to patients with malignancies. *J Surg Oncol* 1987;36:206–209.
55. Schaerer R, Schaerer L, Sotto JJ, et al. La réaction du greffon contre l'hote (GVHD) comme complication létale des transfusions de sang us cours dé là maladie de Hodgkin: a propos de deux observations. Premier Congress Français d' Hematologie, 1975(abst), Vittel, France.
56. Woods WG, Lubin BH. Fatal graft-versus-host disease following a blood transfusion in a child with neuroblastoma. *Pediatrics* 1981;67:217–221.
57. Kennedy JS, Rickets RR. Fatal graft-versus-host disease in a child with neuroblastoma following a blood transfusion. *J Pediatr Surg* 1986;21:1108–1109.
58. Remlinger K, Buckner CD, Clift RA, et al. Fatal graft versus host disease and probable graft versus host reaction due to an unradiated granulocyte transfusion after allogeneic bone marrow transplant. *Transplant Proc* 1983;15:1725–1728.
59. Murphy ML, Helson L. Chemotherapy of metastatic neuroblastoma stage IV. *Proc Am Soc Clin Oncol* 1977;18:338(abst).
60. Labotka RJ, Radvany R. Graft vs host disease in rhabdomyosarcoma following transfusion with nonirradiated blood products. *Med Pediatr Oncol* 1985;13:101–104.
61. Greenbaum B. Transfusion-associated graft-versus-host disease: historical perspectives, incidence, and current use of irradiated blood products. *J Clin Oncol* 1991;9:1889–1902.
62. Deierhol MH, Sollinger HW, Bozdech MJ, et al. Lethal graft-versus-host disease in a recipient of pancreas-spleen transplant. *Transplantation* 1986;41:544–546.
63. Burdick JF, Vogelsang GB, Smith WJH, et al. Severe graft-versus-host disease in a liver-transplant recipient. *N Engl J Med* 1988;318:689–691.
64. Williamson LM, Wimperis JZ, Wood ME, et al. Fludarabine treatment and transfusion-associated graft-versus-host disease [Letter]. *Lancet* 1996;348:472–473.
65. Deane M, Gor D, MacMahon ME, et al. Quantification of CMV viraemia in a case of transfusion-related graft-versus-host disease associated with purine analogue treatment. *Br J Haematol* 1997;99:162–164.
66. Ohto H, Anderson KC. Survey of transfusion-associated graft-versus-host disease in immunocompetent recipients. *Transfus Med Rev* 1996;10:31–43.
67. Takahashi K, Juji T, Miyazaki H. Post-transfusion graft-versus-host disease occurring in non-immunocompromised patients in Japan. *Transfus Sci* 1991;12:281–289.
68. Yasuura K, Okamoto H, Matsuura A. Transfusion-associated graft-versus-host disease with transfusion practice in cardiac surgery. *J Cardiovasc Surg* 2000;41:377–380.
69. Roth JA, Golub SH, Cuckingnam RA, et al. Cell-mediated immunity is depressed following cardiopulmonary bypass. *Ann Thorac Surg* 1981;31:350–356.
70. Marcus JN, Anderson C, DiMarzo L, et al. Selective depletion of T4+4B4+ ("helper-inducer") subset in lymphopenia associated with cardiopulmonary bypass. *J Histochem Cytochem* 1987;35:1023–1028(abst).
71. Fiebig E, Hirschkorn DF, Maino VC, et al. Assessment of donor T-cell function in cellular blood components by the CD69 induction assay: effects of storage, γ-radiation, and photochemical treatment. *Transfusion* 2000;40:761–770.
72. Kanter MH. Transfusion-associated-graft-versus host disease: do transfusions from second-degree relatives pose a greater risk than those from first-degree relatives? *Transfusion* 1992;32:323–327.
73. Wisecarver JL, Cattral MS, Langnas AN, et al. Transfusion-induced graft-versus-host disease after liver transplantation. *Transplantation* 1994;58:269–271.
74. Sola MA, Espana A, Redondo P, et al. Transfusion-associated acute graft-versus-host disease in a heart transplant recipient. *Br J Dermatol* 1995;132:626–630.
75. Leitman SF. Post transfusion graft versus host disease. In: Smith DN, Silvergleid AJ, eds. *Special considerations in transfusing the immunocompromised patient.* Arlington, VA: American Association of Blood Banks, 1985:15–37.
76. Crowley JP, Skrabut EM, Valeri CR. Immunocompetent lymphocytes in previously frozen washed red cells. *Vox Sang* 1974;26:513–517.

77. Brubaker DB. Human post transfusion graft versus host disease. *Vox Sang* 1983;45:401–420.
78. Luban NLC, Ness PM. Irradiation of blood products: invited comment. *Transfusion* 1985;25:301–303.
79. Ciccone E, Pende D, Viale O, et al. Specific recognition of human CD3⁻CD16⁺ natural killer cells requires the expression of an autosomic recessive gene on target cells. *J Exp Med* 1990;172:47–52.
80. Perkins HA. Granulocyte concentrates: should they be routinely irradiated. In: *Apheresis: development, applications and collection procedures.* New York: Alan R. Liss, 1981:49–57.
81. Hull RJ, Bray RA, Hillyer C, et al. Transfusion-associated chronic cutaneous graft-versus-host disease. *J Am Acad Dermatol* 1995;33: 327–332.
82. Arico M, Noto G, Pravata G, et al. Transfusion-associated graft-versus-host disease—report of two further cases with an immunohistochemical analysis. *Clin Exp Dermatol* 1994;19:36–42.
83. Nishimura M, Uchida S, Mitsunaga S, et al. Characterization of T-cell clones derived from peripheral blood lymphocytes of a patient with transfusion-associated graft-versus-host disease: Fas-mediated killing by CD4⁺ and CD8⁺ cytotoxic T-cell clones and tumor necrosis factor-β production by CD4⁺ T-cell clones. *Blood* 1997;89: 1440–1445.
84. Nishimura M, Uchida S, Mitsunaga S, et al. Identification of the target molecule of cytotoxic T cells presumably responsible for development of transfusion-associated graft-versus-host disease [Letter]. *Transfusion* 1996;36:846–847.
85. Nishimura M, Uchida S, Mitsunaga S, et al. Establishment of a T-cell line from lymphocytes presumably implicated in posttransfusion graft-versus-host disease. *Vox Sang* 1995;68:164–168.
86. Wang L, Tadokoro K, Uchida S, et al. Restricted use of T-cell receptor Vβ genes in posttransfusion graft-versus-host disease. *Transfusion* 1997;37:1184–1191.
87. Matsushita M, Shibata Y, Fuse K, et al. Sex chromatin analysis of lymphocytes invading host organs in transfusion-associated graft versus host disease. *Virch Arch* 1988;55:237–239.
88. Sakurai M, Moizumi Y, Uchida S, et al. Transfusion-associated graft-versus-host disease in immunocompetent patient: early diagnosis and therapy. *Am J Hematol* 1998;58:84–86.
89. Wang L, Juji T, Tokunaga K, et al. Brief report: polymorphic microsatellite markers for the diagnosis of GVHD. *N Engl J Med* 1994;330: 398–401.
90. Anderson KC, Weinstein HJ. Transfusion associated graft versus host disease. *N Engl J Med* 1990;323:315–321.
91. Leitman SF, Holland PV. Irradiation of blood products. *Transfusion* 1985;25:293–300.
92. Vogelsang GB. Advances in the treatment of graft-versus-host disease. *Leukemia* 2000;14:509–510.
93. Murphy WJ, Blazar BR. New strategies for preventing graft-versus-host disease. *Curr Opin Immunol* 1999;11:509–515.
94. Ryo R, Saigo K, Hashimoto M, et al. Treatment of post-transfusion graft-versus-host disease with nafamostat mesylate, a serine protease inhibitor. *Vox Sang* 1999;76:241–246.
95. Przepiorka D, Kernan NA, Ippoliti C, et al. Daclizumab, a humanized anti-interleukin-2 receptor α-chain antibody for treatment of acute graft-versus-host disease. *Blood* 2000;95:83–89.
96. Tse, JC, Moore TB. Monoclonal antibodies in the treatment of steroid-resistant acute graft-versus-host disease. *Pharmacotherapy* 1998; 18:988–1000.
97. Calabrese L, Fleischer AB. Thalidomide: current and potential clinical applications. *Am J Med* 2000;108:487–495.
98. Girardi M, McNiff JM, Heald PW. Extracorporeal photochemotherapy in human and murine graft-versus-host disease. *J Dermatol Sci* 1999;19:106–113.
99. Gaziev D, Galimberti M, Lucarelli G, et al. Chronic graft-versus-host disease: is there an alternative to the conventional treatment? *Bone Marrow Transplant* 2000;25:689–696.
100. Elad S, Garfunkel AA, Enk CD, et al. Ultraviolet B irradiation: a new therapeutic concept for the management of oral manifestations of graft-versus-host disease. *Oral Surg Oral Med Oral Pathol Oral Radiol Endod* 1999;88:444–450.
101. Mori S, Matsushita H, Ozaki K, et al. Spontaneous resolution of transfusion-associated graft-versus-host disease. *Transfusion* 1995;35: 431–435.
102. Klein C, Fraitag S, Foulon E, et al. Moderate and transient transfusion-associated cutaneous graft-versus-host disease in a child infected by human immunodeficiency virus. *Am J Med* 1996;101:445–446.
103. Yasukawa M, Shinozaki F, Hato T, et al. Successful treatment of transfusion-associated graft-versus-host disease. *Br J Haematol* 1994; 86:831–836.
104. Saigo K, Ryo R. Therapeutic strategy for post-transfusion graft-vs.-host disease. *Int J Hematol* 1999;69:147–151.
105. Nishimura M. Potential usefulness of photochemotherapy using 8-methoxypsoralen in the treatment of posttransfusion graft-versus-host disease [Letter]. *Vox Sang* 1998;75:306–307.
106. Moroff G, Luban NLC. The irradiation of blood and blood components to prevent graft-versus-host disease: technical issues and guidelines. *Trans Med Rev* 1997;11:15–26.
107. Pelszynski MM, Moroff G, Luban NLC, et al. Effect of γ-irradiation of red blood cell units on T-cell inactivation as assessed by limiting dilution analysis: implications for preventing transfusion-associated graft-versus-host disease. *Blood* 1994;83:1683–1689.
108. Luban NLC, Drothler D, Moroff G, et al. Irradiation of platelet components: inhibition of lymphocyte proliferation assessed by limiting-dilution analysis. *Transfusion* 2000;40:348–352.
109. Zimmermann R, Schmidt S, Zingsem J, et al. Effect of γ-radiation on the in vitro aggregability of WBC-reduced apheresis platelets. *Transfusion* 2001;41:236–242.
110. Valerius NH, Johansen KS, Nielsen OS, et al. Effect of in vitro X-irradiation on lymphocyte and granulocyte function. *Scand J Haematol* 1981;27:9–18.
111. Buescher ES, Gallin JI. Radiation effects on cultured human monocytes and on monocyte-derived macrophages. *Blood* 1984;63: 1402–1407.
112. Conrad RA. Quantitative study of irradiation effects in phytohaemagglutinin-stimulated leukocyte cultures. *Int J Radiat Biol* 1969;16: 157–165.
113. Klimov NA, Vaschenko VI, Kolyubaeva SN, et al. Changes in the supercoil structure of nuclear DNA in rat and human peripheral blood lymphocytes after γ-irradiation. *Int J Radiat Biol* 1982;41:221–225.
114. Hayashi H, Nishiuchi T, Tamura H, et al. Transfusion-associated graft-versus-host disease caused by leukocyte filtered stored blood. *Anesthesiology* 1993;79:1419–1421.
115. Deeg HJ, Graham TC, Gerhard-Miller L, et al. Prevention of transfusion-induced graft-versus-host disease in dogs by ultraviolet irradiation. *Blood* 1989;74:2592–2595.
116. Deeg HJ, Erickson K, Storb R, et al. Photoinactivation of lymphohemopoietic cells: studies in transfusion medicine and bone marrow transplantation. *Blood Cells* 1992;18:151–161.
117. Skripchenko AA, Wagner SJ. Inactivation of WBCs in RBC suspensions by photoactive phenothiazine dyes: comparison of dimethylmethylene blue and MB. *Transfusion* 2000;40:968–975.

CASE 59A

'O'H, IT'S BACK 'A'-GAIN

CASE HISTORY

Ms. K.I. was a 35-year-old woman with newly diagnosed acute myelocytic leukemia in January. She came to our hospital, after induction chemotherapy and an initial remission, for allogeneic bone marrow transplant. She was group A and received a transplant from her human leukocyte antigen (HLA)-matched brother who was group O. She received irradiated blood components during her transplant. Engraftment occurred on schedule and she was discharged to home in February.

One month later, in March, she had gradual onset of increasing diarrhea and fevers. In clinic her hematocrit was 32%, white blood cell count was 2,300/μL, and platelet count was 65,000/μL. She had a moderate elevation of her aspartate aminotransferase (AST) and alanine aminotransferase (ALT). There was no rash. Her clinicians suspected a graft versus host reaction. She was admitted for a 4-day hospitalization, was treated with higher doses of prednisone and cyclosporine, and her diarrhea and liver function test results improved. She was discharged and did well for the next year.

In February of one year after transplant she was seen in follow-up. She had few complaints other than vague weakness. Her complete blood count showed a hematocrit of 30%, white blood cell count of 4,600/μL, and platelet count of 175,000/μL. A review of Ms. K.I.'s blood grouping (recipient group A and donor group O) is shown in Table 59A.1.

What accounts for the weak expression of A antigen on her typing 1 year after transplant? A review of her blood transfusion record revealed that prior to the transplant Ms. K.I. had received seven units of A-positive red blood cells, during the transplant period she had received nine units of O-positive red blood cells, and since March of last year (posttransplant period) she had received no red blood cell transfusions. Thus, the weak group A antigen, found 1 year after transplant, could not be due to detection of previously transfused cells.

DISCUSSION

Bone marrow transplantation across ABO groups requires careful attention regarding blood support. In our hospital, we have a simple chart that we use as a guideline for blood support for each ABO combination (Table 59A.2). In this case, because the recipient was group A and the donor was group O, we supported the patient during the transplant with group O red blood cells. Using group O red blood cells decreases the risk of ABO hemolysis resulting from donor antibodies (anti-A and anti-B) that may develop as the new bone marrow engrafts. During the peritransplant period, we also used group A platelets and fresh-frozen plasma rather than group O in order to eliminate the risk of passive hemolysis of the patient's residual group A cells. The seemingly subtle finding of weak reactivity with anti-A 1 year after transplant raised concern for the technologist that the patient was developing a relapse and return of her original native group A bone marrow.

FOLLOW-UP

Because of the weak anti-A reactivity and concern for relapse of the original marrow, the patient underwent a bone marrow examination that showed no evidence of malignant relapse. Cytogenetics on the marrow showed that 20 of 20 metaphase cells demonstrated a normal male (XY) karyotype consistent with donor bone marrow. This information suggested that the weak A expression on her cells resulted from another cause. Because marrow sampling could miss relapse, further testing was done. We reasoned that the weak A antigen could have occurred either due to a small population of cells with normal A antigen expression (as might occur in an early relapse) or the weak expression of A antigen on all cells. The gel card system applied to ABO is a simple way to distinguish these two possibilities (Figure

TABLE 59A.1. BLOOD GROUPING RESULTS AFTER BONE MARROW TRANSPLANTATION

Date	Anti-A	Anti-B	Anti-D	A_1 Cells	B Cells
January: pretransplant	4+	neg	2+	neg	3+
March: 1 month posttransplant	1+	neg	3+	neg	3+
April: 2 months posttransplant	neg	neg	3+	neg	3+
Feb: 1 year posttransplant	weak+	neg	3+	neg	3+

TABLE 59A.2. TRANSFUSION SUPPORT GUIDELINES FOR ABO-MISMATCHED ALLOGENEIC BONE MARROW TRANSPLANTATION USED AT MASSACHUSETTS GENERAL HOSPITAL

				Platelets			
Recipient	Donor	Pretransplant	RBC	1st Choice	Next Choice	FFP	Posttransplant
O	A	Recipient type	O	A	AB, B, O	A, AB	Donor type
O	B	Recipient type	O	B	AB, A, O	B, AB	Donor type
O	AB	Recipient type	O	AB	A, B, O	AB	Donor type
A	O	Recipient type	O	A	AB, B, O	A, AB	Donor type
A	B	Recipient type	O	AB	A, B, O	AB	Donor type
A	AB	Recipient type	A	AB	A, B, O	AB	Donor type
B	O	Recipient type	O	B	AB, A, O	B, AB	Donor type
B	A	Recipient type	O	AB	B, A, O	AB	Donor type
B	AB	Recipient type	B	AB	B, A, O	AB	Donor type
AB	O	Recipient type	O	AB	A, B, O	AB	Donor type
AB	A	Recipient type	A	AB	A, B, O	AB	Donor type
AB	B	Recipient type	B	AB	B, A, O	AB	Donor type

59A.1). In Ms. K.I.'s case, the results were most consistent with a single population of cells that all expressed the A antigen weakly.

Where did the A antigen come from? A review of her blood grouping showed that the patient was originally typed as Le(a − b +) and that her donor was Le(a + b −). Thus, the recipient was a secretor and the donor was a nonsecretor. We wondered if the weak A antigen expression on the cells was due to adsorbed A substance, because the patient was still a genetic group A secretor. Secretors make type I ABH glycoproteins and glycolipids that express ABH antigens. A low concentration of these plasma glycoconjugates passively adhere to red blood cells, which accounts for routine Lewis typings. In support of this explanation for her blood grouping results was the finding that a new specimen (posttransplant) typed as Le(a − b +). The proposed adsorption of ABO antigens in this situation is unusual but has been reported by Garratty (1). It may be that the phenomenon is observed in only some recipients who are strong secretors and express large amounts of type I glycoconjugates.

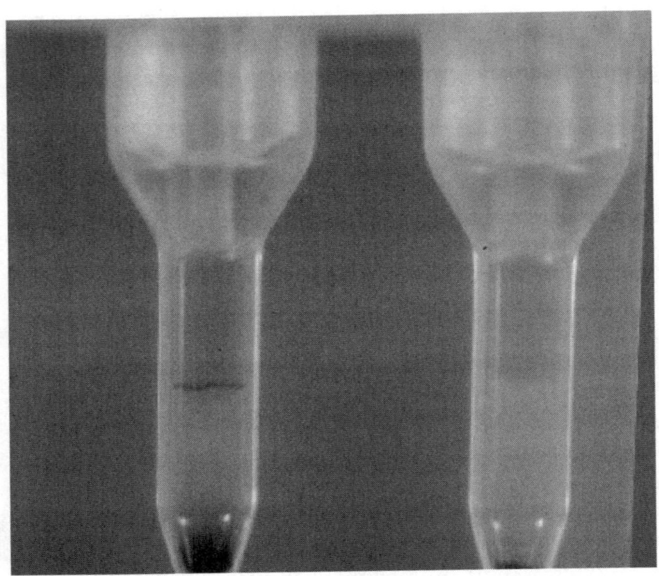

FIGURE 59A.1. ABO testing using gel technology. Reagent anti-A and the unknown cells are added to the top of the column and centrifuged. Cells reacting with anti-A form aggregates that fail to pass through the column during centrifugation and remain at the top. Nonreactive cells appear at the bottom. The gel column on the left shows findings typical of a small population of normal group A cells in a background of group O cells. This result would have occurred had the patient undergone relapse and return of her original group A cells. The column on the right shows the findings in our patient.

CODA

The patient and her physicians were very relieved to learn that there was an explanation for her findings other than bone marrow relapse. She has continued to do well with her transplant without recurrence of GVHD and without relapse for the last 3 years.

Case contributed by Kent D. Eliason, MT (ASCP) SBB, and Walter H. Dzik, M.D., Massachusetts General Hospital, Boston, MA.

REFERENCES

1. Arndt PA, Leger RM, Garratty G, et al. Use of flow cytometry for detecting uptake of A/B blood group substances on transfused/transplanted O RBCs. *Transfusion* 1999;[Suppl]:186P(abst).

60

TRANSFUSION-ASSOCIATED IMMUNOMODULATION

JOSÉ O. BORDIN
MORRIS A. BLAJCHMAN

Despite careful donor screening and blood donor selection as well as extensive pretransfusion laboratory testing, transfusion of allogeneic blood products can be associated with adverse effects on recipients (Table 60.1). These include alloimmunization, graft versus host disease, transmission of infectious agents, and immunosuppression (1). Over the past three decades, considerable data have accumulated indicating that allogeneic blood transfusion may be associated with the down-regulation of the recipient's immune response. This phenomenon has been called *transfusion-associated immunomodulation* (TRIM) (1,2). Such observations raised concern that allogeneic blood transfusion may adversely affect prognosis in the care of patients undergoing curative surgery for a malignant tumor by means of down-regulating the recipient's immune system and enhancing tumor growth and formation of metastatic lesions (3–5). Results of a large number of observational studies with human subjects appeared to implicate allogeneic blood transfusion as associated with increased risk of postoperative bacterial infection after abdominal, open-heart, and orthopedic surgery (6–9). Paradoxically, this allogeneic blood transfusion-associated immunosuppressive effect has been shown beneficial to selected patient groups. For example, allogeneic blood transfusion has been shown clinically beneficial in increasing allograft survival time in recipients of renal transplants (10), possibly reducing the relapse rate among patients with inflammatory bowel disease (11), and decreasing the incidence of recurrent spontaneous abortion (12). This chapter summarizes the data associating TRIM with allogeneic blood transfusion. Possible strategies to prevent some of these effects are discussed.

J.O. Bordin: Division of Hematology and Transfusion Medicine, Universidade Federal de Sao Paulo, Brazil.
M.A. Blajchman: Departments of Pathology and Medicine, McMaster University, and Canadian Blood Services, Hamilton, Ontario, Canada.

ALLOGENEIC BLOOD TRANSFUSION AND IMMUNE FUNCTION

Normal Immune Response

To initiate a normal immune response, T lymphocytes must be able to recognize alloantigens (peptides) associated with major histocompatibility complex (MHC) molecules. In humans, the latter are the HLA antigens. These peptide-MHC complexes are presented to the T-cell receptor by dendritic leukocytes that participate in the immune response process as antigen-presenting cells (13). Recipient T cells respond to alloantigens associated with allogeneic MHC molecules using one of two distinct pathways. The first involves direct presentation to recipient T cells of intact MHC molecules associated with the donor antigen-presenting cells. The second is an indirect pathway that involves presentation of processed MHC peptides on recipient antigen-presenting cells (14). Either pathway can induce production of various cytokines, particularly interleukin-2 (IL-2) and IL-4. These substances are produced by both antigen-presenting cells and recipient T cells and cause rapid cell expansion and differentiation of alloantigen-specific T lymphocytes. In addition to MHC antigen presentation to recipient T cells, costimulatory signals, derived from non-MHC molecules, present on the anti-

TABLE 60.1. ADVERSE AND BENEFICIAL RECIPIENT EFFECTS REPORTED TO BE ASSOCIATED WITH TRANSFUSION OF ALLOGENEIC BLOOD PRODUCTS

Adverse effects
Hemolytic and nonhemolytic transfusion reactions
Alloimmunization to donor alloantigens
Refractoriness to allogeneic platelet transfusions
Graft versus host disease
Transmission of infectious agents (viruses, bacteria, protozoa, and possibly prions)
TRIM causing susceptibility to infection
TRIM causing accelerated malignant cell growth
Beneficial effects
Improvement of renal allograft survival
Reduction in the prevalence of spontaneous recurrent abortion
Decrease in the relapse rate of Crohn's disease
Apoptive immunotherapy for chronic myelogenous leukemia preventing relapse after bone marrow transplantation

TRIM, transfusion-associated immunomodulation.

gen-presenting cells are required to enable generation and amplification of alloantigen-specific T cell responses that affect function (15,16). In this context, B7:CD28 interaction represents a critical pathway in determining immune reactivity (16). The B7-1 protein delivers a costimulatory signal mediated through the CD-28 and cytotoxic T lymphocyte A-4 T-cell receptors to regulate IL-2 secretion. The B7-2 protein provides a critical early costimulatory signal that results in T-cell clonal proliferation (16). Antigen-presenting cells thus present peptide-MHC complexes to T lymphocytes to deliver activation signals that initiate the T-cell-dependent immune response (13,16). These costimulatory signals increase production of IL-2, mainly by activated helper T (T_H) cells to stimulate their proliferation.

Interleukin-2 also directs the differentiation of naive T cells toward the T_H1 subset of cells, which are related to cell-mediated immunity. Similarly, IL-4 drives T cells to become T_H2 cells, which control antibody production by B lymphocytes (2,13). Helper T cells provide at least two signals to B cells during their interaction. B cells express CD40, and activated T_H cells express the complementary ligand, known as CD40L. B-cell proliferation is initiated by the interaction of CD40 with its ligand and is further stimulated by the presence of both IL-2 and IL-5. Interleukin-6 participates in B-cell maturation (17). Signals from T_H cells cause immunoglobulin class switching and the differentiation of B cells into antibody-producing plasma cells.

Cytokines produced during the immune response by antigen-presenting cells contribute to recruitment of host defense cells. Overproduction of some cytokines during this process can harm host tissues by producing fever, chills, rigors, and increased capillary permeability in the host (18). These cytokines also may cause cellular damage directly, such as damage of capillary endothelial cells by tumor necrosis factor α (18). Thus the immunogenicity of soluble, particulate, or cellular MHC antigens associated with transfused allogeneic blood products depends on the ability of either donor or host antigen-presenting cells to present such antigens to recipient T cells. The integrity of all relevant signals is crucial and the impairment of one, or more, of the costimulatory signals may result in T-cell unresponsiveness (15, 19).

Effects of Allogeneic Transfusion on Immune Function

Allogeneic transfusion of blood products appears to cause a variety of alterations of immune function in recipients, particularly function associated with cell-mediated immunity. These are summarized in Table 60.2. The most commonly observed effect is quantitative alteration in T-cell subset number, usually represented by a low CD4 count or an altered lymphocyte helper to suppressor (CD4/CD8) ratio. Such abnormalities have been reported to occur among patients with hemophilia after exposure to factor VIII concentrate (20). The use of very-high-purity factor VIII concentrates, either recombinant or produced from plasma by means of immunoaffinity chromatography, has been reported to retard the decline in CD4 count among patients with hemophilia and human immunodeficiency virus (HIV) infection compared with that among patients receiving factor VIII products of intermediate purity (21–24). It has not been established whether the retarded decline in CD4 count implies slower progression to symptomatic acquired immunodeficiency syndrome (AIDS) and improved survival. It has been reported that the use of high-purity products neither retards the development of AIDS nor decreases the risk of death among patients with hemophilia and HIV infection (25). Moreover, the prevalence of inhibitors (factor VIII alloantibodies) among patients treated with high-purity concentrates does not appear to be different from that among patients treated exclusively with intermediate-purity concentrates (26,27).

In addition to quantitative abnormalities of T-cell subsets, functional impairment of lymphocytes has been described among patients with hemophilia. These include a decrease in the extent of the proliferative responses to mitogens such as phytohemagglutinin and concanavalin A, decreased natural killer (NK) cell activity, diminished cell-mediated immunity, hypergammaglobulinemia associated with polyclonal B-cell activation, T-cell activation, and defective monocyte function (20, 28). The use of very-high-purity clotting factor concentrates has

TABLE 60.2. DOCUMENTED IMMUNE FUNCTION ALTERATIONS ASSOCIATED WITH TRANSFUSION OF ALLOGENEIC BLOOD PRODUCTS

Decreased helper T-cell (CD4) count
Decreased helper to suppressor (CD4/CD8) T-lymphocyte ratio
Decreased lymphocyte response to mitogens
Reduction in delayed-type hypersensitivity
Decreased natural killer cell function
B-cell activation
T-cell activation
Hypergammaglobulinemia
Decreased cytokine (IL-2; interferon-γ) production
Suppression of lymphocyte blastogenesis
Decreased monocyte-macrophage phagocytic function
Increased production of antiidiotypic antibodies
Increased production of anticlonotypic antibodies

been reported to prevent some of these immunologic alterations (29). Other alterations in immune function found in recipients of allogeneic cellular blood products include a decrease in NK cell function, a decrease in antigen presentation, suppression of lymphocyte blastogenesis, and a reduction in delayed-type hypersensitivity (7,8,11,30,31).

CLINICAL STUDIES

Allogeneic Blood Transfusion and Renal Allograft Survival

Since the first description of the beneficial effect of allogeneic blood transfusion in renal allograft transplantation in 1973, it has been widely accepted that allogeneic blood transfusion can improve renal allograft survival after transplantation (10,32,33). Patients given transfusions of allogeneic blood have been shown to have a significantly better renal allograft survival rate than do patients who do not undergo transfusion, regardless of the number of HLA-A, HLA-B, and HLA-DR locus mismatches between recipient and donor (10,34). This is true even when there is a common HLA haplotype, or shared HLA-B and HLA-DR antigens, between donors and recipients (35). This immunomodulatory effect has been reported also with allografts between HLA-identical siblings (36).

The beneficial effect of allogeneic transfusion on renal allograft survival was believed to have declined as a result of improved management of rejection and the availability of the newer, highly active immunosuppressive agents. However, results of a multicenter observational study of 58,036 renal transplants from cadaver donors since the advent of the use of cyclosporine suggested that patients receiving allogeneic blood transfusion were still more likely to have a successful renal allograft than were those who did not (10,37). This collaborative study showed that the 1-year renal allograft survival rate among patients receiving pretransplantation allogeneic blood transfusion was 3% to 5% better than that among patients who did not receive such transfusions (10). Similar results were reported for patients who received kidney transplants from living related donors (38).

The beneficial effect of pretransplantation allogeneic transfusion on the outcome of cadaveric kidney transplantation was confirmed in a prospective randomized clinical trial involving 14 transplant centers that included potential recipients of cadaveric renal grafts (39). The subjects enrolled in the study were randomly assigned to receive either three pretransplantation allogeneic unmodified red blood cell (RBC) transfusions or no RBC transfusions. The renal allograft survival rate was found to be significantly higher among the 205 patients who underwent transfusion than among the 218 patients who did not receive RBC transfusions (90% versus 82% at 1 year, $P = .02$; 79% versus 70% at 5 years, $P = .025$). The beneficial effect of allogeneic transfusion was found to be independent of age, sex, underlying disease, prophylaxis with lymphocyte antibodies, and the presence of preformed lymphocytotoxins (39).

The mechanism of allogeneic transfusion-associated improved renal allograft survival remains to be elucidated. Many questions about the optimal use of allogeneic blood transfusion in the care of such patients remain to be answered. The latter include the optimal number of allogeneic blood component transfusions needed to produce the TRIM effect, the volume of blood required with each transfusion, the timing of transfusions to produce the optimal TRIM effect, the concurrent hazards of the TRIM effect, and whether transfusions are still clinically necessary. Patients who receive more than 10 RBC units have been reported to have a better 1-year allograft survival rates than do patients who receive only one or two allogeneic RBC transfusions. However, patients who receive more than ten transfusions appear to have a poorer overall renal allograft survival rate than do those receiving fewer than ten transfusions (40). Such data suggest that patients who undergo more than one transfusion often develop cytotoxic antibodies and thus are at greater risk of earlier and more severe allograft rejection episodes (38). Allogeneic blood transfusions administered during surgical procedures have not been shown to affect subsequent renal allograft survival (33). Recipients of unmodified whole blood or RBC concentrates have been shown to have better 1-year cadaveric allograft survival rates than have patients given leukocyte-poor blood components, such as washed concentrates of frozen-deglycerolized RBCs. Such data indicate that allogeneic donor leukocytes are involved in eliciting the beneficial allogeneic TRIM effect (41).

It has been suggested by data from an animal model of experimental transplantation that the beneficial effect of donor-specific allogeneic blood transfusion may be related to the type of transplanted organ. Whereas allogeneic blood transfusions appear to lead to permanent acceptance of all renal allografts, this was not observed for pancreas, skin, or heart allografts (42). Although additional data are needed to understand how allogeneic blood transfusion induces a beneficial effect in renal transplantation, the use of pretransplantation allogeneic transfusion remains a possibly useful intervention in the treatment of selected patients scheduled for renal transplantation.

Allogeneic Blood Transfusion and Tumor Growth

The possible association between allogeneic blood transfusion and cancer recurrence was first suggested by Gantt (43) in 1981, who raised concern that patients undergoing curative surgery for malignant disease may be affected adversely by the immunosuppressive effects of allogeneic blood transfusions administered perioperatively. Since then, more than 100 observational reports and three randomized clinical trials have shown the effect of perioperative allogeneic blood transfusion on tumor recurrence or overall prognosis among patients with a malignant tumor undergoing curative cancer surgery, and the results are equivocal. Definitive clinical data proving that an allogeneic TRIM effect occurs in patients with cancer have not yet been provided (44).

The results of the observational studies involving patients with various forms of cancer have been subjected to three meta-analyses (3–5). There is general agreement among the three about the magnitude and statistical significance of the risk of cancer recurrence, death due to cancer recurrence, or overall mortality among patients who do undergo transfusion compared with those who do not for seven cancer sites for the 80 observational studies in which adjustments were not made for possible confounding factors (unadjusted studies). When the unadjusted study results were integrated into a metaanalysis, a statistically significant adverse clinical outcome was found among patients who underwent allogeneic transfusion compared with those who did not undergo transfusion for all cancer sites evaluated, except for the cervix (3). A statistically significant transfusion-associated adverse effect in the observational studies adjusted for the effects of confounding factors was found in 24 observational studies. These included 11 studies of colorectal cancer, 4 studies of head and neck cancer, 1 study of breast cancer, 2 studies of gastric cancer, 4 studies of lung cancer, and 2 studies of prostate cancer (3).

Three randomized, controlled studies (45–47) were performed to compare the incidence of cancer recurrence between patients with colorectal carcinoma who received buffy-coat-reduced allogeneic RBC units and patients who received autologous whole blood, unmodified RBCs, or leukoreduced and buffy-coat-reduced allogeneic RBCs (Table 60.3). The first (45) was a well-designed prospective trial conducted in the Netherlands with patients with colorectal cancer. The subjects were randomized to receive either allogeneic or autologous blood components perioperatively. The data from this study indicate that the risk of cancer recurrence was higher among patients who received transfusions with either allogeneic or autologous blood components than among patients who did not undergo transfusion. Although not stated in the article, blood centers throughout the Netherlands have routinely produced buffy-coat-depleted cellular blood products for a number of years. The investigators thus actually compared outcomes for patients receiving autologous blood with outcomes for patients receiving buffy-coat-depleted allogeneic blood. It is possible that the degree of leukoreduction in the buffy-coat-depleted allogeneic recipients may have sufficed to reduce the allogeneic TRIM effect that would have been observed had unmodified blood products been used. In the second study (46), also from the Netherlands, investigators compared allogeneic leukodepleted blood transfusion with buffy-coat-depleted allogeneic blood transfusion in the care of patients undergoing surgery for colorectal cancer. This study showed a similar association between blood transfusion and poor overall patient survival. However, all patients who received blood (allogeneic or autologous) had a significantly poorer 3-year survival rate than did patients who did not undergo transfusion (69% versus 81%, $P < .001$). Colorectal cancer recurrence rates were not influenced by the blood transfusion (30% versus 26%, $P = .22$). In the third prospective randomized study (47), conducted in Germany, investigators concluded that the transfusion of allogeneic blood components in the care of patients with colorectal carcinoma was an independent predictor of tumor recurrence. The results of these three randomized controlled trials do not prove a causal relation between allogeneic blood transfusion and cancer recurrence according to the tenets of evidence-based medicine. We believe that whether allogeneic blood transfusion influences prognosis in the care of patients with colorectal carcinoma is still unresolved.

Transfusion history and cancer risk were evaluated for more than 37,000 women between 55 and 69 years of age. The available data indicate that relative risk among the subjects who underwent allogeneic transfusion was 2.20 (95% confidence interval [CI], 1.35–3.58) for non-Hodgkin's lymphoma and 2.53 (95% CI, 1.34—4.78) for renal carcinoma (48).

Allogeneic Blood Transfusion and Bacterial Infection

The association between perioperative allogeneic blood transfusion and the increased incidence of bacterial infection after surgery has been explored in several clinical studies (6–9,49–54). The available data from observational studies indicated the existence of an adverse effect that related perioperative allogeneic blood transfusion as an independent risk factor for postoperative infection (2,55). However, the results from seven randomized clinical trials in which investigators compared the incidence of postoperative infection between patients given transfusions of buffy-coat-reduced or standard allogeneic RBCs or whole blood and recipients of autologous or leukoreduced, buffy-coat-reduced allogeneic RBCs or whole blood are statistically heterogeneous (7,8,46,56–59). Two studies showed a significant ($P <$

TABLE 60.3. RESULTS OF THREE PROSPECTIVE RANDOMIZED TRIALS OF THE EFFECT OF BLOOD TRANSFUSION ON CLINICAL OUTCOME OF COLORECTAL CARCINOMA

Variable	Busch et al., 1993 (45)	Houbiers et al., 1994 (46)	Heiss et al., 1994 (47)
Total number of patients	475	697	120
Type of blood transfusion per group	1. Autologous BC-PRBCs	1. LR-BC-PRBCs or allogeneic BC-PRBCs	1. Autologous BC-PRBCs
	2. Allogeneic BC-PRBCs	2. No transfusion	2. Allogeneic BC-PRBCs
Number of patients per group	1. 133 2. 112	1. 337 2. 360	1. 48 2. 52
Relative risk of tumor recurrence among patients who underwent transfusion compared with those who did not	1. 1.8; $P = .04$ 2. 2.1; $P = .01$	1. 0.91; $P = .53$	1. 0.96; $P = .96$ 2. 7.01; $P = .006$
Cancer-specific survival rate	1. 68% 2. 64% $P = .60$	1. 69% 2. 81% $P < .001$	1. Versus 2; $P = .20$

BC-PRBCs, buffy-coat-reduced packed red blood cells; LR-BC-PRBCs, leukoreduced BC-PRBCs.

.05) adverse allogeneic transfusion effect (7,57). Two studies showed a marginally significant ($P < .10$) transfusion effect (8, 59). Three studies did not show a deleterious transfusion effect (46,56,58).

The role of allogeneic leukocytes in the development of postoperative infection has been investigated. A prospective, randomized trial involving patients who underwent colorectal surgery showed that patients given transfusions of nonleukoreduced allogeneic whole blood had a significantly higher frequency of postoperative infection than did those who received 99.98% leukoreduced allogeneic blood (7). In another clinical trial, patients undergoing surgery for colorectal cancer were randomly assigned to receive leukoreduced RBCs or buffy-coat-depleted RBCs. Although cancer recurrence was not influenced by allogeneic blood transfusion, recipients of allogeneic or autologous blood had a significantly higher postoperative infection rate than did patients who did not received transfusions (47).

It has been suggested that the risk of bacterial infection may increase with the number of allogeneic blood units transfused. In a retrospective study of patients who underwent surgery for penetrating colonic injury, the risk of an infection was 7.5% for patients who did not undergo transfusion, 25% for patients who received 1 to 5 units, 37% for those who received 6 to 9 units, and 57% for those who received 10 or more allogeneic blood units (60). A retrospective analysis of patients who underwent surgery for gastric carcinoma similarly showed that patients who contracted postoperative infection had received transfusions of a significantly larger number of allogeneic blood component units than did those who did not receive transfusions (61). The randomized clinical trial by van de Watering et al. (59) showed that the number of RBC units transfused was an important predictor of both the incidence of postoperative infection and mortality (2,55).

The available clinical data suggest that the bacterial infection rate among patients who undergo allogeneic transfusion ranges from 20% to 30% compared with 5% to 10% among either patients who did not undergo transfusion or those receiving autologous blood. Despite such data, the relation between allogeneic blood transfusion and increased risk of bacterial infection is still unproved. This is partially because of the problem of defining the term *bacterial infection* in such patients. Limiting the definition of bacterial infection to patients who had positive results of bacterial cultures leads to underestimation of prevalence, but extending the definition to include fever leads to overestimation of prevalence. The presence of comorbid conditions (diabetes mellitus or heart, lung, liver, or kidney failure) and the number of days with an indwelling urinary catheter or endotracheal tube may be important determinants, as well as confounders, of postoperative infection. It has been estimated that a rather large ($n > 20{,}000$ patients) randomized clinical trial is needed to validate definitively the association between allogeneic blood transfusion and increased risk of infection (2). Nonetheless, five randomized clinical trials have been conducted in which leukoreduced rather than autologous RBCs were transfused into control subjects. These five studies cannot be evaluated together for a metaanalysis because there is a high degree of heterogeneity among the five studies. Nonetheless, four of five of these randomized clinical trials investigating the relation between transfusion of leukocyte-containing versus leukoreduced allogeneic blood and postoperative infection showed a trend toward an increased incidence of postoperative infection in association with transfusion of allogeneic leukocytes (62).

Allogeneic Blood Transfusion and Recurrent Spontaneous Abortion

The fetus represents a semi-allogeneic graft to its mother, thus maintenance of pregnancy depends on immunologic equilibrium between the implanted fetus and the maternal immune response to the fetus. When the genetic parents share HLA antigens, this balance can be altered if maternal blocking antibodies do not form, and the pregnant woman becomes predisposed to recurrent pregnancy loss. According to such a hypothesis, the use of allogeneic leukocyte transfusions has been proposed as a form of immunotherapy to treat women with a history of recurrent spontaneous abortion (62). Different allogeneic leukocyte transfusion protocols have been used with leukocytes obtained from either sexual partner or third-party donors. Allogeneic leukocytes have been transfused to women with recurrent spontaneous abortion as pooled buffy coats, as single-donor buffy coats, or as RBC suspensions containing leukocytes. These have been administered intravenously, intracutaneously, or as intradermal injections of mononuclear cells obtained by means of gradient separation. The number of allogeneic cells inoculated may influence outcome. It has been postulated that infusion of fewer than 60 million mononuclear cells may result in a suboptimal effect and that inoculation of more than 400 million cells either has no benefit or has only a slightly reduced success rate (63,64).

The efficacy of allogeneic leukocyte transfusion in the treatment of patients with recurrent spontaneous abortion remains to be established by appropriately sized, prospective, randomized clinical studies. Nonetheless, nonrandomized studies have shown a success rate of approximately 75% with transfusion of either paternal or third-party leukocytes. The success rate has been approximately 50% when maternal cells have been given (65–67).

On the basis of results of analyses by two separate expert teams, the American Society for Reproductive Immunology (ASRI) conducted a worldwide collaborative individual patient data metaanalysis to examine the efficacy of allogeneic leukocyte immunotherapy in the care of patients defined as having recurrent spontaneous abortions (12). Agreement was reached in the ASRI study that leukocyte immunotherapy is an effective therapy for recurrent spontaneous abortion. The effect was small, because only 8% to 10% of affected women appeared to benefit from such treatment (12). Nonetheless, the ASRI data appear to indicate that approximately 11 patients have to be treated with immunotherapy to achieve 1 additional live birth.

Unlike the ASRI data, data from a multicenter study involving 183 women who had had three or more spontaneous abortions showed a nonsignificant decrease in the live birth rate among patients randomly assigned to immunotherapy compared with the rate for a control group (36% versus 48%) (68). It has been argued, however, that more than 400 patients would have to be enrolled to obtain a reliable estimate of efficacy in a metaanalysis with the expectation of a 10% benefit and that results of trials enrolling fewer than 250 patients are more likely to be negative (69).

Although likely effective, the use of allogeneic leukocytes in the treatment of women with recurrent spontaneous abortions can be associated with risks similar to those associated with any other leukocyte transfusion. These include alloimmunization to leukocyte antigens and neonatal graft versus host disease. Such side effects appear to be rare, and the number of adversely affected infants in the immunized group (3%) was similar to the number in the control group who did not receive transfusions (12).

The mechanism of the beneficial action of allogeneic leukocyte immunotherapy in the care of patients with recurrent spontaneous abortion is unknown. It has been suggested that the observed beneficial clinical response may be associated with production of autoantiidiotypic antibodies (70), release of IL-1 (71), or a decrease in maternal IL-2 receptors (72).

Allogeneic Blood Transfusion and Inflammatory Bowel Disease

The recurrence rate after surgical treatment of intestinal obstruction or perforation in patients with Crohn's disease has been estimated to be approximately 50% 10 years after treatment (73). It has been suggested that immunologic mechanisms are involved in the pathogenesis of Crohn's disease. Tartter et al. (11) reported that patients with Crohn's disease have fewer circulating total lymphocytes and T lymphocytes than do healthy controls and that use of multiple allogeneic blood transfusions was associated with a significantly lower peripheral total lymphocyte and T-cell counts after surgery.

Several observational studies have been conducted to examine whether the postoperative recurrence rate among patients with Crohn's disease is affected by perioperative use of allogeneic blood transfusion. Pooled data suggested that the recurrence rate in the two groups is similar: 37.5% in the group who underwent transfusion versus 40.5% in the group who did not undergo transfusion (74–78). However, the available data are from retrospective studies and are difficult to compare because the studies had different follow-up periods and different surgical interventions were performed. In 1995, a metaanalysis of individual patient data on 622 patients with Crohn's disease showed no effect of perioperative allogeneic blood transfusions on subsequent need for surgical intervention, independent of age, sex, disease location, or extent of the resection (79).

Allogeneic blood transfusion has been reported to be a major risk factor in the development of infectious complications among patients with Crohn's disease who undergo a surgical procedure (49). Such an association did not reach statistical significance in another study (75). Because many factors can affect recurrence rates among patients with Crohn's disease as well as the rate of septic complications after resection, a large, well-designed, randomized clinical trial is needed to clarify the role of allogeneic blood transfusion in the disease activity of patients with this disorder.

ANIMAL STUDIES

Allogeneic Blood Transfusion and Tumor Growth

The relation between allogeneic blood transfusion and tumor growth has been examined extensively in various animal models. These are summarized in Table 60.4 (80). Data from both inbred and outbred animal models indicate that allogeneic blood transfusion accelerates tumor growth and enhances formation of metastatic nodules (81–85). The effect of allogeneic blood transfusion on growth of solid tumors has been investigated in murine models in our laboratory. In these experiments, mice that received allogeneic blood transfusions and were then inoculated intramuscularly with either syngeneic malignant melanoma (B16) cells or mastocytoma (P815) cells had larger tumors than did mice given syngeneic transfusions (81). Similar results were obtained when syngeneic B16 tumor cells were infused intravenously and the pulmonary nodules counted (81,82). Experiments performed to investigate the effect of tumor cell dose showed that the tumor growth–promoting effect associated with allogeneic blood transfusion was evident only when small numbers of tumor cells (1.25 to 2.5 $\times$ 10^5) were inoculated into the host animal. The tumor growth–promoting effect of allogeneic blood transfusion was not evident when large numbers of tumor cells were inoculated into the experimental animals. This finding suggests that the number of tumor cells inoculated, or tumor burden, has strong bearing on whether the tumor growth–promoting effect associated with allogeneic blood transfusion was manifest.

The influence of the timing of allogeneic blood transfusion in enhancing formation of pulmonary nodules in experimental animals has been examined. Studies with both inbred (mice) and outbred (rabbits) animals have shown that allogeneic blood transfusion has a tumor growth–promoting effect when administered before infusion of syngeneic tumor cells (83). In the murine model, male C57Bl/6J mice (MHC type H-2b) were the recipients, Balb/c mice (MHC type H-2d) were the allogeneic donors, and the tumor cells were syngeneic (H-2b) methylcholanthrene-induced fibrosarcoma cells. In the rabbit model, California Black rabbits were used as the allogeneic blood donors and New Zealand White rabbits were the allogeneic blood recipi-

TABLE 60.4. SUMMARY OF THE EFFECTS ON TUMOR GROWTH OF ALLOGENEIC BLOOD TRANSFUSIONS IN VARIOUS EXPERIMENTAL ANIMAL STUDIES

Effect	n
Stimulation of tumor growth	17
Inhibition of tumor growth	3
No effect	4
Total	24

n, number of studies showing the indicated effect.
Modified from Bordin JO, Blajchman MA. Blood transfusion and tumor growth in animal models. In: Vamvakas EC, Blajchman MA, eds. Immunodeficiency effects of allogeneic blood transfusion. Bethesda, MD: American Association of Blood Banks, 1999:29–42, with permission.

ents. The tumor cells were from a spontaneously occurring rabbit epithelial tumor known as VX-2 (83,84).

To better replicate the clinical situation, enhancement of tumor growth by allogeneic blood transfusion was investigated in experiments with mice and rabbits that received syngeneic and allogeneic transfusions after the inoculation with tumor cells. These data indicated that allogeneic blood transfusion enhances tumor growth in animals with established tumors (84). Another series of investigations with inbred mice only, provided similar evidence indicating that allogeneic blood transfusion after tumor cell engraftment enhances tumor growth (85).

Is has been shown that animals with either nonestablished or established tumors receiving unmodified allogeneic blood transfusions had significantly larger numbers of pulmonary nodules than did animals given leukoreduced allogeneic blood transfusions (83,84). The allogeneic blood transfusion-associated tumor growth–promoting effect was ameliorated by means of prestorage leukoreduction of the allogeneic blood but not by poststorage leukoreduction (83,84). In this context, it has been shown that animals given transfusions of allogeneic buffy-coat leukocytes had more pulmonary nodules than did animals that received either leukoreduced allogeneic blood or nonleukoreduced allogeneic plasma (84). Although results from experimental animals cannot necessarily be extrapolated to the clinical situation, results of these experimental studies with animals indicate that bedside (poststorage) leukoreduction of allogeneic blood components may not be very effective in preventing the tumor growth–promoting effect of allogeneic blood transfusion.

The issue whether stored syngeneic blood influences tumor growth in experimental animals has been explored (86). The data indicate that rabbits that received stored nonleukoreduced syngeneic blood transfusions had a median number of pulmonary nodules similar to that of control animals not given transfusions or animals given prestorage leukoreduced allogeneic blood. The results of these studies suggest that the transfusion of stored syngeneic blood (unmodified or prestorage leukoreduced) is not associated with a tumor growth–promoting effect, at least in this experimental animal model (86).

Allogeneic Blood Transfusion and Bacterial Infection

The data regarding the TRIM effect in animal models of infection are somewhat contradictory. Moreover, a variety of experimental conditions such as anesthesia, the presence of shock, trauma, type of surgery, blood volume, and timing and frequency of transfusion have been reported relevant (87–91).

In a series of experimental animal studies, Waymack et al. (87–90) found that animals that received allogeneic transfusions had immune impairment and a poorer response to a septic challenge than did animals that received syngeneic transfusions. In a burn model, these investigators observed that rats given allogeneic blood transfusions had a higher mortality than did rats given syngeneic blood or saline solution (91). In a model of bacterial peritonitis in rats, a significant adverse effect on survival was associated with allogeneic transfusion (88). In another study, allogeneic blood transfusion was associated with marked immune impairment to a bacterial challenge immediately after transfusion (92). Moreover, allogeneic blood transfusion, in particular with allogeneic leukocytes, was shown to adversely affect host resistance to a gut-derived infection with *Escherichia coli* in a murine model (93). It has been shown in a cecal ligation and puncture model with mice that transfusion of allogeneic blood greatly increases susceptibility to infection. The results of these studies also indicated that splenocytes of mice that received allogeneic transfusions produced increased quantities of the T_H2-type cytokines IL-4 and IL-10 and lesser amounts of IL-2, probably leading to increased antibody production and a decreased cell-mediated response (94). In contrast, in murine experiments with a bacterial peritonitis model in which syngeneic was compared with allogeneic blood transfusion, the latter was shown not to influence overall survival of animals challenged with *E. coli* (95). Although a clear negative effect of shock was detected, no adverse effect of transfusion, either syngeneic or allogeneic, was observed in a rat model (96).

MECHANISMS OF TRANSFUSION-ASSOCIATED IMMUNOMODULATION

Although the mechanisms causing the immunosuppressive effects of allogeneic blood transfusion have been debated extensively, the exact mechanism of this interesting biologic phenomenon has yet to be elucidated. A number of putative mechanisms have been postulated, and these are summarized in Table 60.5. The three major mechanisms accounting for much of the experimental data suggesting the occurrence of a TRIM effect include clonal deletion, induction of anergy, and immune suppression. Clonal deletion is inactivation and removal of alloreactive lymphocytes that would, for example, cause rejection of an allograft. Anergy implies immunologic unresponsiveness. Immune suppression suggests that the responding cell is being inhibited by another cell or by a cytokine (30,97). Antiidiotypic antibodies, which are predominantly of the V_H6 gene family, have been found in the serum of recipients of allogeneic blood transfusions and in patients with long-term functioning renal allografts (98). Allogeneic blood transfusion has been shown to alter various

TABLE 60.5. POSTULATED MECHANISMS OF THE TRANSFUSION-ASSOCIATED IMMUNOMODULATION EFFECT

Clonal deletion of specific lines of cells
Induction of suppressor cells
Production of antiidiotypic antibodies
Suppression of natural killer cell activity
Polarization of the immune system to type T_H2 cell responses
Altered T4/T8 ratio resulting in immunosuppression
Production of nonspecific biologic response modifiers
Mixed microchimerism
Selection of nonresponder type immune cells
Accumulation of soluble molecules (sFasL or sHLA-I) that inhibit the immune response
Induction of apoptosis, resulting in cell death of specific types of immune competent cells
Others

immunologic functions of recipients (Table 60.2). Results of investigations indicate that leukocytes lose their immunogenicity during storage; consequently transfusion of stored allogeneic blood may result in recipient T-cell anergy and thus transfusion-associated immunosuppression (19).

Results of in vitro studies have indicated that low-molecular-weight components in antihemophilic factor VIII preparations may inhibit the proliferative responses of peripheral blood mononuclear cells to phytohemagglutinin (29). In these studies, high-purity factor VIII concentrates have been shown to reduce induction of T-cell-activation molecules such as the IL-2 receptor (CD25), the transferrin receptor (CD71), CD38, the CD11a/CD18 ratio, and HLA-DR antigen expression (29). Evidence also has been provided to indicate that this inhibitory action of factor VIII concentrates was at least partly caused by contamination by transforming growth factor-β (99).

An extensive body of observational data has accumulated that indicates the allogeneic leukocytes present in cellular blood components likely cause many of the adverse effects observed in allogeneic transfusion recipients. These include transfusion reactions, HLA alloimmunization, graft versus host disease, transmission of infectious agents, and immunomodulation (1). All available clinical and experimental data suggest that transfused allogeneic leukocytes bearing class II HLA antigens appear to participate in the development of the immunomodulatory effects observed in recipients of allogeneic cellular blood products (1).

Allogeneic HLA antigens elicit an immune response by delivering at least two different signals to recipient T cells. It has been shown that HLA compatibility between an allogeneic blood donor and a recipient may result in persistence of circulating donor leukocytes in the recipient (100). The survival of small numbers of transfused allogeneic leukocytes in the circulation of the recipient, called *microchimerism,* may cause down-regulation of the immune response of the recipient and induce immune tolerance to donor alloantigens. It is possible that such microchimerism predisposes the recipient to development of a form of transfusion-associated graft versus host disease (100). Preliminary results of investigations of microchimerism performed with the polymerase chain reaction technique, indicate that leukocytes transfused from male donors can persist for 1 to 6 days in most women receiving multiple transfusions (101). The significance of microchimerism as the mechanism causing TRIM remains to be clarified (102,103).

Support for the hypothesis that TRIM is caused by transfused allogeneic leukocytes has come mainly from data from experimental studies with animals. These have shown that animals receiving allogeneic buffy-coat leukocytes have significantly more pulmonary tumor nodules than do animals given either plasma or prestorage-leukoreduced whole blood (84). It is possible that prestorage leukoreduction may prevent accumulation of soluble biologic mediators actively synthesized and released by the leukocytes present in the donor allogeneic blood during storage. It also is possible that such substances are involved in the immunomodulation observed after allogeneic blood transfusion. Transfused allogeneic leukocytes were identified as the blood component responsible for gut-derived infection in a murine infection model (93).

Further clues to the mechanism of the allogeneic TRIM have been provided by experimental studies with animals that show the tumor growth–promoting effect of allogeneic blood transfusions can be adoptively transferred to naive animals. These experiments have provided evidence that spleen cells harvested from animals that have received allogeneic transfusions can transfer the effect to naive animals (83). In these experiments, the number of pulmonary nodules found in animals that received spleen cells from animals that had received allogeneic transfusions was significantly higher than that found in animals that received spleen cells from animals that had received transfusions of syngeneic blood (83). This effect could not be adoptively transferred to naive animals given infusions of spleen cells derived from animals that had been given transfusions with prestorage-leukoreduced allogeneic blood. We have found that both B and T splenic lymphocytes must be transferred to produce the tumor growth–promoting effect associated with allogeneic blood transfusion in naive animals (unpublished observations, 1994).

Although the precise mechanism of TRIM has not been fully elucidated, the foregoing clinical and experimental animal data suggest that the TRIM effect is immunologically mediated and related to the presence of allogeneic donor leukocytes, or their products, in the transfused allogeneic cellular blood components. Although results from animal models cannot necessarily be extrapolated to the clinical situation, the data suggest that prestorage leukoreduction may be effective in ameliorating some of the immunosuppressive effects of allogeneic blood transfusion. Properly designed, prospective clinical studies are needed to ascertain whether patients with malignant disease undergoing curative surgery need leukoreduced blood products.

SUMMARY

A considerable body of literature has accumulated over the past three decades indicating that transfused allogeneic leukocytes can be associated with adverse effects on recipients. Appreciation that transfusion-associated immunosuppression may increase morbidity and mortality among recipients of allogeneic transfusions has become a major concern for practitioners of transfusion medicine. Whether this effect is clinically relevant for patients with malignant disease is still unproved (2). In contrast, much of the clinical data on the risk of postoperative infectious complications of allogeneic blood transfusion have been reasonably consistent and appear to indicate that recipients of nonleukoreduced allogeneic blood may well have increased susceptibility to bacterial infection (2,55,104).

Most of the considerable body of available information appears to indicate that the allogeneic leukocytes present in allogeneic blood components or their products have adverse biologic effects. These effects include nonhemolytic febrile transfusion reactions, alloimmunization to HLA antigens, graft versus host disease, and possibly the TRIM effects discussed earlier (1,2, 55). With regard to the latter, data from the animal models indicate that the TRIM effect is immunologically mediated and associated with allogeneic leukocytes. Moreover, the relevant experimental animal data suggest that prestorage leukoreduction, as opposed to poststorage leukoreduction, is effective in ameliorating growth enhancement of tumors associated with allogeneic blood transfusion (44,80,84). This ameliorative effect of prestorage leukoreduction, however, has not been fully evaluated in humans. The benefit of leukoreduction, either prestorage or poststorage, has not been fully established for the TRIM effect.

Vamvakas and Blajchman (2,104) provided two alternative interpretations for and against a policy to implement universal leukoreduction of all cellular blood products for the purpose of preventing TRIM and the other side effects of allogeneic leukocytes. Because of the high degree of suspicion of the available results of clinical studies, these authors believe an adverse TRIM effect probably does exist but that it may be small, possibly representing less than a 10% increase in the risk of postoperative infection (2). They postulate that this small magnitude of the adverse TRIM effect may have made its clinical existence difficult to document. They nonetheless indicate that a TRIM effect of 10% would still represent an important complication of allogeneic transfusion, probably one that ought to be prevented, if possible, in all patients by means of universal leukoreduction (2).

REFERENCES

1. Bordin JO, Heddle NM, Blajchman MA. Biologic effects of leukocytes present in transfused cellular blood. *Blood* 1994;84:1703–1721.
2. Vamvakas EC, Blajchman MA. Deletrious clinical effects of transfusion-associated immunomodulation: fact or fiction? *Blood* 2001;97: 1180–1195.
3. Brand A, Houbiers JGA. Clinical studies of blood transfusion and cancer. In: Vamvakas EC, Blajchman MA, eds. *Immunomodulatory effects of allogeneic blood transfusion.* Bethesda, MD: American Association of Blood Banks, 1999:145–190.
4. Chung M, Steinmetz OK, Gordon PH. Perioperative blood transfusion and outcome after resection for colorectal carcinoma. *Br J Surg* 1993;80:427–432.
5. Vamvakas E. Perioperative blood transfusion and cancer recurrence: meta-analysis for explanation. *Transfusion* 1995;35:760–768.
6. Blajchman MA. Allogeneic blood transfusions, immunomodulation and postoperative bacterial infection: do we have the answers yet? *Transfusion* 1997;37:121–125.
7. Jensen LS, Andersen AJ, Christiansen PM, et al. Postoperative infection and natural killer cell function following blood transfusion in patients undergoing elective colorectal surgery. *Br J Surg* 1992;79: 513–516.
8. Heiss MM, Mempel W, Jauch KW, et al. Beneficial effect of autologous blood transfusion on infectious complications after colorectal cancer surgery. *Lancet* 1993;342:1328–1333.
9. Vamvakas EC, Moore SB. Blood transfusion and postoperative septic complications. *Transfusion* 1994;34:714–727.
10. Opelz G. The role of HLA matching and blood transfusions in the cyclosporine era. *Transplant Proc* 1989;21:609–612.
11. Tartter PL, Heimann TM, Aufses AH Jr. Blood transfusion, skin test reactivity, and lymphocytes in inflammatory bowel disease. *Am J Surg* 1986;151:358–361.
12. Coulam CB, Clark DA, Collins J, et al. Worldwide collaborative observational study and meta-analysis on allogeneic leukocyte immunotherapy for recurrent spontaneous abortion. *Am J Reprod Immunol* 1994;32:55–72.
13. Austyn JM. Antigen uptake and presentation by dendritic leukocytes. *Semin Immunol* 1992;4:227–236.
14. Shoskes DA, Wood KJ. Indirect presentation of MHC antigens in transplantation. *Immunol Today* 1994;15:32–38.
15. Mincheff MS, Meryman HT. Costimulatory signals necessary for induction of T cell proliferation. *Transplantation* 1990;15:32–38.
16. Guinan EV, Gribben JG, Boussiotis VA, et al. Pivotal role of the B7: CD28 pathway in transplantation tolerance and tumor immunity. *Blood* 1994;84:3261–3282.
17. Rees RC. Cytokines as biological response modifiers. *J Clin Pathol* 1992;45:93–98.
18. Muylle L, Joos M, Wouters E, et al. Increased tumor necrosis factor α (TNF-α), interleukin 6 (IL-6) levels in the plasma of stored platelet concentrates: relationship between TNF-α and IL-6 levels and febrile transfusion reactions. *Transfusion* 1993;33:195–199.
19. Mincheff MS, Meryman HT, Kapoor V, et al. Blood transfusion and immunomodulation: a possible mechanism. *Vox Sang* 1993;65: 18–24.
20. Watson HG, Ludlam CA. Immunological abnormalities in haemophiliacs. *Blood* Rev 1992;6:26–33.
21. de Biasi R, Rocino A, Miraglia E, et al. The impact of a very high purity factor VIII concentrate on the immune system of human immunodeficiency virus–infected hemophiliacs: a randomized, prospective, two-year comparison with an intermediate purity concentrate. *Blood* 1991;78:1919–1922.
22. Seremetis SV, Aledort LM, Bergman GE, et al. Three-year randomised study of high-purity or intermediate-purity factor VIII concentrates in symptom free HIV-seropositive haemophiliacs: effects on immune status. *Lancet* 1993;342:700–703.
23. Hilgartner MW, Buckley JD, Operskalski EA, et al. Purity of factor VIII concentrates and serial CD4 counts. *Lancet* 1992;341: 1373–1374.
24. Mannucci PM, Brettler DB, Aledort LM, et al. Immune status of human immunodeficiency virus seropositive and seronegative hemophiliacs infused for 3.5 years with recombinant factor VIII. *Blood* 1994;83:1958–1962.
25. Goedert JJ, Cohen AR, Kessler CM, et al. Risks of immunodeficiency, AIDS, and death related to purity of factor VIII concentrate. *Lancet* 1994;344:791–792.
26. Lusher JM, Arkin S, Abildgaard CF, et al. Recombinant factor VIII for the treatment of previously untreated patients with hemophilia A. *N Engl J Med* 1993;328:453–457.
27. Bray GL, Gomperts ED, Courter S, et al. A multicenter study of recombinant factor VIII (recombinate): safety, efficacy and inhibitor risk in previously untreated patients with hemophilia A. *Blood* 1994; 83:2428–2437.
28. Madhok R, Gracie JA, Forbes CD, et al. B cell dysfunction in haemophilia in the presence of HIV-1 infection. *Thromb Haemost* 1991;65: 7–10.
29. Vermont-Desroches C, Rigal D, Blourde C, et al. Immunosuppressive property of a very high purity antihaemophilic preparation: a low molecular weight component inhibits an early step of PHA induced cell activation. *Br J Haematol* 1992;80:370–377.
30. Blajchman MA, Bordin JO. Mechanisms of transfusion-associated immunosuppression. *Curr Opin Hematol* 1994;1:457–461.
31. Kaplan J, Sarnaik S, Gitlin J, et al. Diminished helper/suppressor lymphocyte ratio and natural killer activity in recipients of repeated blood transfusions. *Blood* 1984;64:308–310.
32. Opelz G, Sengar DPS, Mickey MR, et al. Effect of blood transfusions on subsequent kidney transplants. *Transplant Proc* 1973;5:253–259.
33. Opelz G, Terasaki PI. Improvement of kidney-graft survival with increased numbers of blood transfusions. *N Engl J Med* 1978;299: 799–803.
34. Blajchman MA, Singal DP. The role of red blood cell antigens, histocompatibility antigens, and blood transfusions on renal allograft survival. *Transfus Med Rev* 1989;3:171–179.
35. van Twuyver E, Mooijaart RJD, tem Berge IJM, et al. Pretransplantation blood transfusion revisited. *N Engl J Med* 1991;325:1210–1213.
36. Norman DJ, Wetzsteon P, Barry JM, et al. Blood transfusion are beneficial in HLA-identical sibling kidney transplants. *Transplant Proc* 1985;17:23–26.
37. Ross WB, Yap PL. Blood transfusion and organ transplantation. *Blood Rev* 1990;4:252–258.
38. Sells RA, Scott MH, Prieto M, et al. Early rejection following donor-specific transfusion prior an HLA-mismatched living related renal transplantation. *Transplant Proc* 1989;21:1173–1174.
39. Opelz G, Vanrenterghem Y, Kirste G, et al. Prospective evaluation

of pretransplant blood transfusions in cadaver kidney recipients. *Transplantation* 1997;63:964–967.
40. Opelz G. Current relevance of the transfusion effect in renal transplantation. *Transplant Proc* 1985;17:1015–1021.
41. Horimi T, Terasaki PI, Chia D, et al. Factors influencing the paradoxical effect of transfusions on kidney transplants. *Transplantation* 1983; 35:320–323.
42. Bektas H, Jörns A, Klempnauer J. Differential effect of donor-specific blood transfusions after kidney, heart, pancreas, and skin transplantation in major histocompatibility complex–incompatible rats. *Transfusion* 1997;37:226–230.
43. Gantt CL. Red blood cells for cancer patients [Letter]. *Lancet* 1981; 2:363.
44. Bordin JO, Blajchman MA. Immunosuppressive effects of allogeneic blood transfusions implications for the patient with a malignancy. *Hematol Oncol Clin North Am* 1995;9:205–217.
45. Busch ORC, Hop HCJ, van Papendrecht MAWH, et al. Blood transfusions and prognosis in colorectal cancer. *N Engl J Med* 1998;328: 1372–1376.
46. Houbiers JGA, Bland A, van de Watering LMG, et al. Randomised controlled trial comparing transfusion of leucocyte-depleted or buffy-coat-depleted blood in surgery for colorectal cancer. *Lancet* 1994;344: 573–578.
47. Heiss MM, Jaucth KW, Delanoff C, et al. Blood transfusion modulated tumor recurrence a randomized study of autologous versus homologous blood transfusion in colorectal cancer. *J Clin Oncol* 1994,12:1859–1867.
48. Certhan JR, Wallace RB, Folsom AR, et al. Transfusion history and cancer risk in older women. *Ann Intern Med* 1993;119:8–15.
49. Tartter PI, Driefuss RM, Malon AM, et al. Relationship of postoperative septic complications and blood transfusions in patients with Crohn's disease. *Am J Surg* 1988;155:43–48.
50. Jensen LS, Andersen AJ, Tristrup SC, et al. Comparison of one dose versus three doses of prophylactic antibiotics, and the influence of blood transfusion, on infections complications in acute and elective colorectal surgery. *Br J Surg* 1990;77:513–516.
51. Murphy P, Heal JM, Blumberg N. Infection or suspected infection after hip replacement surgery with autologous or homologous blood transfusions. *Transfusion* 1991;31:212–217.
52. Mezrow CK, Bergstein I, Tartter PI. Postoperative infections following autologous and homologous blood transfusions. *Transfusion* 1992; 32:27–30.
53. Triulzi DJ, Vanek K, Ryan DH, et al. A clinical and immunological study of blood transfusion and postoperative bacterial infection in spinal surgery. *Transfusion* 1992;32:517–524.
54. Fernandez MC, Goulieb M, Menitove JE. Blood transfusion and postoperative infection in orthopedic patients. *Transfusion* 1992;32: 318–322.
55. Vamvakas EC, Blajchman MA, eds. *Immunomodulatory effects of allogeneic blood transfusion.* Bethesda, MD: American Association of Blood Banks, 1999.
56. Busch ORC, Hop WCJ, Marquet RL, et al. Autologous blood and infections after colorectal surgery. *Lancet* 1994;343:668–669.
57. Jensen LS, Kissmeyer-Nielsen P, Wolff B, et al. Randomized comparison of leucocyte-depleted versus buffy-coat-poor blood transfusion and complications after colorectal surgery. *Lancet* 1996;348:841–845.
58. Tartter PI, Mohandas K, Azar P, et al. Randomized trial comparing packed red cell blood transfusion with and without leukocyte depletion for gastrointestinal surgery. *Am J Surg* 1998;176:462–466.
59. Van de Watering LMG, Hermans J, Houbiers JGA, et al. Beneficial effect of leukocyte depletion of transfused blood on post-operative complications in patients undergoing cardiac surgery: a randomized clinical trial. *Circulation* 1998;97:562–568.
60. Dawes LG, Aprahamian C, Condon RE, et al. The risk of infection after colon injury. *Surgery* 1986;100:796–803.
61. Pinto V, Baldonedo R, Nicolas C, et al. Relationship of transfusion and infectious complications after gastric carcinoma operations. *Transfusion* 1991;31:114–118.
62. Vamvakas EC, Blajchman MA. Prestorage versus poststorage white cell reduction for the prevention of the deleterious immumodulatory effects of allogeneic blood transfusion. *Transfus Med Rev* 2000; 14: 23–33.
63. Smith JB, Cowchock FS, Lata JA, et al. The number of cells used for immunotherapy of repeated spontaneous abortion influences pregnancy outcome. *J Reprod Immunol* 1992;22:217–224.
64. Clark DA, Daya S, Coulam CB, et al. Recurrent Miscarriage Immunotherapy Trialists Group. Implications of human trophoblast karyotype for the evidence-based approach to the understanding, investigation, and treatment of recurrent spontaneous abortion. *Am J Reprod Immunol* 1996;35:495–498.
65. Mowbray JF, Gibbings C, Liddell H, et al. Controlled trial of treatment of recurrent spontaneous abortion by immunization with paternal cells. *Lancet* 1985;1:941–943.
66. Ho HN, Gill TJ, Hsieh HJ, et al. Immunotherapy for recurrent spontaneous abortions in a Chinese population. *Am J Reprod Immunol* 1991;25:10–15.
67. Gatenby PA, Cameron K, Simes RJ, et al. Treatment of recurrent spontaneous abortions by immunization with paternal lymphocytes: results of a controlled trial. *Am J Reprod Immunol* 1993;29:88–94.
68. Ober C, Karrisson T, Odem RR, et al. Mononuclear cell immunization in prevention of recurrent miscarriage: a randomised trial. *Lancet* 1999;354:365–369.
69. Clark DA. Other immunomodulatory effects of blood transfusion. In: Vamvakas EC, Blajchman MA, eds. Immunomodulatory effects of allogeneic blood transfusion. Bethesda, MD: American Association of Blood Banks, 1999:237–252.
70. Sugi Y, Makino T, Maruyama T, et al. A possible mechanism of immunotherapy for patients with recurrent spontaneous abortion. *Am J Reprod Immunol* 1991;25:185–189.
71. Faulk WP, Labarrere CA, Carson SD. Tissue factor: identification and characterization of cell types in human placentae. *Blood* 1990; 76:86–96.
72. Kilpatrick DC. Soluble interleukin-2 receptors in recurrent miscarriage and the effect of leukocyte immunotherapy. *Immunol Lett* 1992; 34:201–206.
73. Williams JG, Wong WD, Rothenberger DA, et al. Recurrence of Crohn's disease after resection. *Br J Surg* 1991;78:10–19.
74. Williams JG, Hughes LE. Effect of perioperative blood transfusion on recurrence of Crohn's disease. *Lancet* 1989;2:131–132.
75. Peters WR, Fry RD, Fleshman JW, et al. Multiple blood transfusions reduce the recurrence rate of Crohn's disease. *Dis Colon Rectum* 1989; 32:749–753.
76. Sutherland LR, Ramcharan S, Bryant H, et al. Effect of perioperative blood transfusion on recurrence of Crohn's disease [Letter]. *Lancet* 1989;2:1048.
77. Scott ADN, Ritchie JK, Phillips RKS. Blood transfusion and recurrent Crohn's disease. *Br J Surg* 1991;78:455–458.
78. Steup WH, Brand A, Weterman KH, et al. The effect of perioperative blood transfusion on recurrence after primary operation for Crohn's disease. *Scand J Gastroenterol* 1991;26:81–86.
79. Hollaar GL, Gooszen HG, Post S, et al. Perioperative blood transfusion does not prevent recurrence in Crohn's disease. *J Clin Gastroenterol* 1995;21:134–138.
80. Bordin JO, Blajchman MA. Blood transfusion and tumor growth in animal models. In: Vamvakas EC, Blajchman MA, eds. *Immunomodulatory effects of allogeneic blood transfusion.* Bethesda, MD: American Association of Blood Banks, 1999:29–42.
81. Shirwadkar S, Blajchman MA, Frame B, et al. Effect of allogeneic blood transfusion on solid tumor growth and pulmonary metastases in mice. *J Cancer Res Clin Oncol* 1992;118:76–180.
82. Shirwadkar S, Blajchman MA, Frame B, et al. Effect of blood transfusions on experimental pulmonary metastases in mice. *Transfusion* 1990;30:188–190.
83. Blajchman MA, Bardossy I, Carmen R, et al. Allogeneic blood transfusion-induced enhancement of tumor growth: two animal models showing amelioration by leukodepletion and passive transfer using spleen cells. *Blood* 1993;81:1880–1882.
84. Bordin JO, Bardossy L, Blajchman MA. Growth enhancement of established tumors by allogeneic blood transfusion in experimental

animals and its amelioration by leukodepletion: the importance of the timing of the leukodepletion. *Blood* 1994;84:344–348.
85. Francis DMA, Clunie GJA. Influence of the timing of blood transfusion on experimental tumor growth. *J Surg Res* 1993;54:237–241.
86. Blajchman MA. Immunomodulatory effects of allogeneic blood transfusions: clinical manifestations and mechanisms. *Vox Sang* 1998; 74[Suppl 2]:315–319.
87. Waymack JP, George CD, Pietsch JD, et al. Effect of varying number and volume of transfusions on mortality rate following septic challenge in an animal model. *World J Surg* 1987;11:387–391.
88. Waymack JP, Warden GD, Alexander JW, et al. Effect of blood transfusion and anesthesia on resistance to bacterial peritonitis. *J Surg Res* 1987;42:528–535.
89. Waymack JP, Robb E, Alexander JW. Effect of transfusion on immune function in a traumatized animal model, II: effect on mortality rate following septic challenge. *Arch Surg* 1987;122:935–939.
90. Waymack JP, Miskell P, Gonce S. Alterations in host defense associated with inhalation anesthesia and blood transfusion. *Anesth Analg* 1989;69:163–168.
91. Waymack JP, Gallon L, Barcelli U, et al. Effect of blood transfusions on macrophage function in a burned animal model. *Curr Surg* 1986; 43:305–307.
92. Galandiuk S, George CD, Pietsch JD, et al. An experimental assessment of the effect of blood transfusion on susceptibility to bacterial infection. *Surgery* 1990;108:567–571.
93. Gianotti L, Pyles T, Alexander JW, et al. Identification of the blood component responsible for increased susceptibility to gut-derived infection. *Transfusion* 1993;33:458–465.
94. Babcock GF, Alexander JW. The effects of blood transfusion on cytokine production by TH1 and TH2 lymphocytes in the mouse. *Transplantation* 1996;61:465–468.
95. Goldman M, Frame B, Singal DP, et al. Effect of blood transfusion on survival in a mouse bacterial peritonitis model. *Transfusion* 1991; 31:710–712.
96. Cue JI, Peyton JC, Malangoni MA. Does blood transfusions or hemorrhagic shock induce immunosuppression. *J Trauma* 1992;32: 613–617.
97. Dzik WH. Proposed mechanisms of the immunomodulatory effect of allogeneic blood transfusion. In: Vamvakas EC, Blajchman MA, eds. Immunomodulatory effects of allogeneic blood transfusion. Bethesda, MD: American Association of Blood Banks, 1999:73–93.
98. Singal DP, Leber B, Harnish DG, et al. Molecular genetic basis for the antiidiotypic antibody response associated with successful renal allograft survival in humans. *Transplant Proc* 1991;23:1059–1062.
99. Wadhwa M, Dilger P, Tubbs J, et al. Identification of transforming growth factor-β as a contaminant in factor VIII concentrates: a possible link with immunosuppressive effects in hemophiliacs. *Blood* 1994; 84:2021–2030.
100. Starzl T, Demetris A, Murase N, et al. Cell migration, chimerism and graft acceptance. *Lancet* 1992;339:1579–1582.
101. Adams PT, Davenport RD, Reardon DA, et al. Detection of circulating donor white blood cells in patients receiving multiple transfusions. *Blood* 1992;80:551–555.
102. Nusbacher J. Blood transfusion is mononuclear cell transplantation. *Transfusion* 1994;34:1002–1006.
103. Dzik WH. Mononuclear cell microchimerism and the immunomodulatory effect of transfusion. *Transfusion* 1994;34:1007–1012.
104. Vamvakas EC, Blajchman MA. Universal white-cell reduction: the case for and against. *Transfusion* 2001;41:691–712.

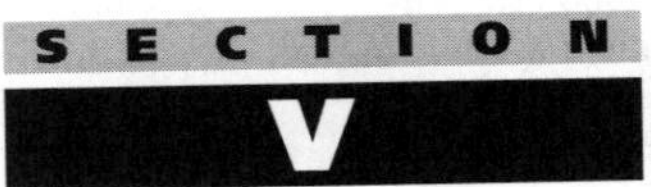

SPECIAL TOPICS

61

RED BLOOD CELL RADIOLABELING AND IN VIVO KINETICS

RICHARD J. DAVEY

Red blood cells can be labeled with selected radioactive nuclides. The subpopulation of these labeled cells can then be detected and measured in vivo. This technique has allowed specialists in transfusion medicine, hematology, and nuclear medicine to study normal red blood cell survival and kinetics. The use of red blood cells tagged with radionuclides confirmed the results of early red blood cell differential agglutination studies and established the normal red blood cell lifespan at 110 to 120 days (1). Radiolabeled red blood cells have proved useful in expanding our understanding of pathologic conditions such as immune red blood cell destruction and polycythemia vera. Labeled red blood cells also allow evaluation of new blood-processing technologies and new storage products.

RED BLOOD CELL RADIOLABELS USEFUL IN TRANSFUSION MEDICINE

The ideal red blood cell radiolabel should possess the characteristics in Table 61.1. A single radionuclide that possesses all of these characteristics does not exist. However, three radionuclides—chromium 51, technetium 99m, and indium 111—have proved very useful in the evaluation of red blood cell survival and kinetics in health and disease. Each has certain advantages and disadvantages that influence their applicability in selected situations. Each is relatively nontoxic to red blood cells and to recipients. The labels are not metabolized by red blood cells, nor are other cells relabeled in vivo.

An understanding of both radiation biophysics and fundamentals of nuclear medicine is essential if one is to use these tracers in clinical or laboratory settings (2). The γ-photon energy of the compound should fall in the optimal range of standard γ-counting instruments (100 to 300 keV). The yield of γ-photon emissions is the number of photons emitted per 100 radioactive decays. A high yield means that a lower radiation dose can be used to achieve adequate detection levels. The γ-photon energy, radioactive half-life, and elution characteristics of each label are shown in Table 61.2.

Chromium 51

The first clinically useful red blood cell radiolabel was described by Gray and Sterling in 1950 (3) and was quickly identified as a useful tool to determine red blood cell lifespan in vivo. The technical simplicity of labeling, excellent red blood cell uptake of the label, low toxicity, and low and stable rate of elution are the major advantages of ^{51}Cr. This radionuclide remains the standard against which all other red blood cell radiolabels have been compared.

Chromium 51 is produced by neutron activation and is usually supplied as sodium radiochromate ($Na[^{51}Cr]O_4$). The principal γ-photon emission occurs at an energy of 320 keV, slightly

TABLE 61.1. DESIRABLE CHARACTERISTICS OF A RED BLOOD CELL RADIOLABEL

Minimal radiation dose to the recipient
Nontoxic to the recipient
Specific for red blood cells
Nontoxic to red blood cells
No metabolism of the label by red blood cells
No elution of the label
No relabeling of other cells in vivo
Radioactive half-life appropriate for the study
Minimal manipulation of the cells during labeling

R.J. Davey: Department of Medicine, New York Blood Center, New York, New York.

TABLE 61.2. FEATURES OF RADIONUCLIDES USED FOR RED BLOOD CELL LABELING

Feature	Chromium 51	Technetium 99m	Indium 111
Radioactive half-life	27.7 d	6.0 h	2.8 d
Major γ-photon emissions (yield)	320 keV (9.8%)	140 keV (90%)	172/247 keV (90/94%)
Elution rate	1% a day	1% to 7% an hour	4% to 8% a day
Suitable for imaging	No	Yes	Yes

high for optimal detection in standard γ-counting instruments. Conversely, the yield of γ-photon emissions, 9.8%, is quite low, necessitating that a relatively high dose of the compound must be administered for optimal detection, especially in long-term survival studies. The high dose required for detection precludes the use of this compound for imaging studies, which require a high yield of γ-photon emissions. Hexavalent sodium radiochromate binds to red blood cells in two phases. First, the hexavalent chromate binds rapidly and reversibly to the red blood cell membrane and is reduced to the trivalent chromic form of the compound. The chromic ion binds more slowly and firmly to the β-globin chain of hemoglobin and probably to other intracellular ligands as well. Younger red blood cells take up slightly more label than do older cells. Not only is this bond quite firm, but also any unbound trivalent (reduced) chromium does not label other red blood cells. The overall labeling efficiency of ^{51}Cr is quite high, approximately 90%. Technical procedures have been published for labeling red blood cells with ^{51}Cr for transfusion compatibility (4) and for evaluation of blood storage and preservation systems (5).

The half-life of ^{51}Cr is 27.7 days, which is good for long-term red blood cell survival and kinetic studies. However, this is too long for short-term studies to determine red blood cell mass or for serial studies of red blood cells of differing phenotypes. Either the patient is exposed to radiation for an unnecessarily long time or the residual counts from early studies confound the determination of recoveries from a later study. Despite relatively firm binding characteristics, ^{51}Cr elutes from red blood cells over time. There is a loss of approximately 1.4% of the label within the first 24 hours, probably from a more loosely bound fraction of the compound. The elution rate subsequently remains relatively steady at between 0.56% and 2.04% per day (6). An elution correction of 1% per day is satisfactory for most clinical and investigational purposes. Nonradioactive isotopes of chromium have been investigated as red blood cell labels. Chromium 52–labeled red blood cells have in vivo survival times similar to those of red blood cells labeled with ^{51}Cr (7), but the isotope must be detected by means of atomic absorption spectroscopy.

Technetium 99m

Technetium 99m has characteristics different from those of ^{51}Cr that have made it quite useful as an adjunctive red blood cell radiolabel. This metastable compound is produced in the molybdenum generators present in many hospital nuclear medicine departments. Technetium 99m rapidly decays to technetium 99, which has a half-life of 6.02 hours. In doing so, it emits a γ-photon at 140 keV with a yield of 90%. This emission falls well within the range of γ-counting instruments. This radionuclide is used widely as an imaging agent because of the preparation, high yield, and ease of detection.

When incubated with red blood cells, ^{99m}Tc, as pertechnetate, labels hemoglobin and other intracellular ligands with a labeling efficiency of approximately 90%. The material, however, has a high and variable rate of elution. This characteristic, along with its short half-life, makes ^{99m}Tc unsuitable for red blood cell recovery and survival studies. However, it is useful for short-term procedures, such as determination of red blood cell mass (8), or for rapid, serial determination of the compatibility of red blood cells of differing phenotypes in highly immunized patients for whom transfusion is difficult (9).

Indium 111

Indium 111 has several favorable characteristics as a red blood cell label. It has two major γ-photon emissions, 173 keV and 247 keV, both with yields exceeding 90%. It is very useful as an imaging agent. Indium 111 must be chelated to traverse the red blood cell membrane and label intracellular proteins. Several chelating agents have proved useful, including 8-hydroxyquinoline, tropolone, oxine, and acetylacetone. The half-life of the compound is 2.83 days, which is suitable for determination of red blood cell mass, short -term red blood cell survival studies, and labeling of platelets and leukocytes (10).

There is a major technical difficulty with ^{111}In as a red blood cell label, namely its high and variable elution rate. There is 8% to 10% elution within 1 or 2 days, followed by approximately 4% per day. This restricts the use of this radionuclide to red blood cell mass, short-term survival, and red blood cell imaging studies.

Nonradioactive Red Blood Cell Labels

Radioactive red blood cell labels have proved useful and well tolerated. However, patients and study subjects are exposed to a low dose of radiation, and this is a concern, especially when studies are necessary in the care of infants and pregnant women. Therefore, investigators have explored methods to measure red blood cell kinetics and in vivo survival with nonradioactive methods. Biotin-labeled red blood cells have been studied to measure both circulating red blood cell volume (11) and red blood cell survival (12). Detection of the biotinylated red blood cells was determined with either iodine 125 streptavidin or flow cytometry and was compared with ^{51}Cr-labeled cells infused simultaneously. The red blood cell volume determined with biotinylated red blood cells agreed with that determined with ^{51}Cr-labeled cells. In the red blood cell survival study, approximately one half of the biotin was observed to leave the circulation in a few weeks. The remaining biotinylated red blood cells retained the biotin and had an approximately normal lifespan. Biotinylation of red blood cells, however, modifies selected red blood cell antigens (13), raising an important caution about using red blood cells labeled in this manner.

Flow cytometry, which is based on identification of differences between red blood cell antigens on donor and recipient red blood cells, has shown promise as a nonradioactive technique to assess red blood cell survival (14,15). Fluorescent cell linkers that can be detected with flow cytometry have been studied (16). These rather imprecise techniques may be limited, however, to general assessment of the survival of minor populations of transfused red blood cells to measure transfusion compatibility.

CLINICAL USES OF RADIOLABELED RED BLOOD CELLS

Alloimmune Red Blood Cell Destruction

Identification of alloimmune red blood cell antibodies usually is accomplished by skilled blood bank and reference laboratory technologists. Compatible red blood cells can then be provided, sometimes with the assistance of rare-donor registries. In vivo compatibility studies may be necessary, however, in the following circumstances: (a) multiple alloantibodies of unclear specificity, (b) an alloantibody of unclear clinical significance against a high-incidence antigen, (c) an unexplained hemolytic transfusion reaction, and (d) clinically significant alloantibodies masked by a strongly reactive autoantibody. In most cases, it is important to determine the suitability for transfusion of red blood cells of a specified phenotype. Short-term information regarding in vivo compatibility is preferred over precise determination of long-term red blood cell recovery. Small volumes of allogeneic red blood cells generally are used for these studies. If compatibility information is urgently needed from red blood cells of differing phenotypes, red blood cells labeled with ^{99m}Tc are preferred.

If there is time to study the immune destructive pattern in more detail, red blood cells labeled with ^{51}Cr usually are chosen. In this case, accurate determination of the patient's red blood cell mass is necessary to properly calculate the subsequent survival of the injected allogeneic cells. This can be performed by means of injecting a sample of autologous cells labeled with ^{99m}Tc (17). An alternative is to determine the 100% survival value (used to calculate red blood cell mass) from the ^{51}Cr counts obtained from a sample drawn 3 minutes after injection of the labeled cells. This allows complete mixing of the labeled cells but is not long enough for the initiation of most red blood cell immune destruction.

Red blood cells can be removed from the circulation by means of differing mechanisms of immune destruction, each defined by characteristic survival patterns. Representations of each of these four patterns are illustrated in Figure 61.1.

Normal Recovery

In a healthy subject, approximately 97% to 102% of fresh transfused red blood cells can be recovered at 60 minutes and 95% to 100% at 24 hours.

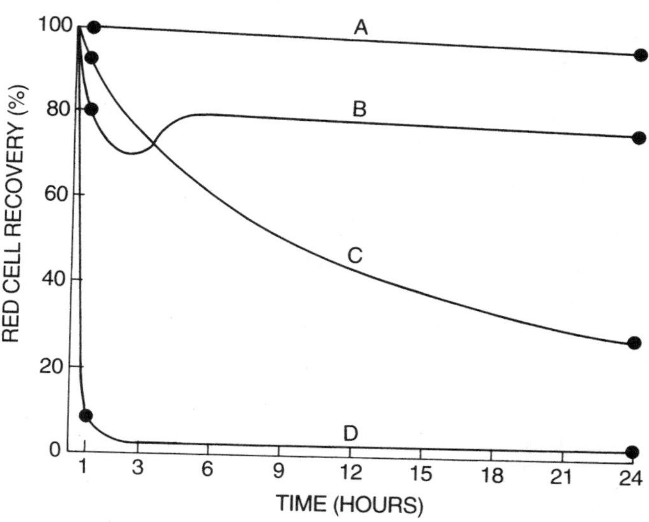

FIGURE 61.1. Red blood cell recovery curves 24 hours after transfusion show differing mechanisms of immune red blood cell destruction. **A:** Normal recovery. **B:** Partial complement activation with two-component extravascular destruction pattern (e.g., IgM anti-Le). **C:** No complement activation with single exponential extravascular destruction (e.g., IgG anti-D). **D:** Complete complement activation with intravascular destruction (e.g., anti-A). The 1-hour recovery percentage is not always predictive of transfusion safety.

Extravascular Destruction without Complement Activation (Single Exponential Recovery Curve)

Most immunoglobulin G (IgG) red blood cell alloantibodies do not activate complement. Destruction of incompatible cells is progressive, the recovery curve defined by a single exponential. The concentration and IgG subclass of the antibody and generation of inflammatory cytokines are important determinants of the rate of removal of the cells. The four IgG subclasses vary in efficiency in binding to Fc receptors on reticuloendothelial system (RES) macrophages. Immunoglobulin G3 often is associated with immune hemolysis, whereas IgG2 and IgG4 are inefficient in removing sensitized cells. Immunoglobulin G1, the most common subclass, varies in its capability to remove red blood cells. Immunoglobulin G1 often is present in higher titer than are the other subclasses, however, and is most often involved in IgG-mediated red blood cell destruction.

Antibodies of the Rh, Kell, Duffy, and Kidd blood systems usually are IgG and do not activate complement. These antibodies have a single exponential pattern of cell destruction. This pattern highlights the importance of extending red blood cell recovery studies to at least 24 hours. A 60-minute recovery may be above the 70% minimum required for transfusion safety, but the recovery may fall well below that standard at 24 hours. Transfusion based on the 60-minute recovery percentage alone may result in a severe hemolytic transfusion reaction.

Extravascular Destruction with Partial Complement Activation (Two-component Recovery Curve)

Antigen-antibody reactions following transfusion of incompatible red blood cells can activate complement. Most IgM and some IgG red blood cell alloantibodies initiate the complement activation sequence. Approximately 20 to 40 IgM molecules per red blood cell are required to activate complement. Immunoglobulin G molecules must be physically adjacent on the red blood cell membrane for complement activation to occur. Therefore, many more membrane-bound IgG molecules are required to initiate the complement cascade.

Often the kinetics of the antigen-antibody reaction result in partial complement activation with generation of the membrane-bound C3b complement fragment. The C3b fragment is subject to cleavage to C3bi by plasma factor I with plasma factor H as a cofactor. Red blood cells with membrane-bound C3b and C3bi adhere to complement receptors CR1 and CR3 on RES macrophages in the liver and spleen. These adherent red blood cells can be destroyed by means of phagocytosis or by antibody-dependent cell-mediated cytotoxicity. They may also undergo membrane damage and spherocytic change after partial phagocytosis.

Often only a small number of adherent red blood cells are damaged or destroyed by these mechanisms. Complement fragment C3bi on the remaining cells is degraded by plasma factors I and H to fragment C3c, which detaches from the cell, and fragment C3d,g, which remains attached to the cell surface.

Red blood cells coated with C3d,g do not effectively bind to the complement receptors of the RES. The cells detach from RES macrophages and circulate normally. These red blood cells may be protected from further complement-mediated damage as the inactive C3d,g fragments occupy complement-binding sites. A red blood cell recovery curve therefore shows early loss of C3b-coated red blood cells and normal survival of the remaining cells with C3d,g complement fragments on their membranes. The transfusion of a larger volume of these incompatible red blood cells is not likely to harm the patient and may result in a sustained transfusion benefit. An extensive review of the role of complement and complement receptors in transfusion medicine has been published (18). A simplified diagram of the classical complement pathway and its role in immune red blood cell destruction is shown in Figure 61.2.

Red blood cell antibodies that usually react optimally at temperatures below 37°C (e.g., Lewis, MNS, P1) often yield two-component recovery curves. If after the rapid early loss of cells, at least 70% of the infused cells are circulating at 24 hours, the patient can receive larger quantities of similar cells with little risk of rapid immune hemolysis.

Intravascular Destruction with Complete Complement Activation

Some red blood cell alloantibodies are efficient activators of complement, the most important by far being anti-A and anti-B. Complement is fully activated with clustering of C3b fragments on the red blood cell surface. The kinetics of the reaction result in formation of the C5b-C9 membrane attack complex. This complex is capable of damaging the red blood cell membrane to the extent that membrane integrity is lost and the cell is destroyed by means of osmotic lysis. Incompatible cells usually are hemolyzed within minutes. Transfusion of larger volumes of such red blood cells is contraindicated.

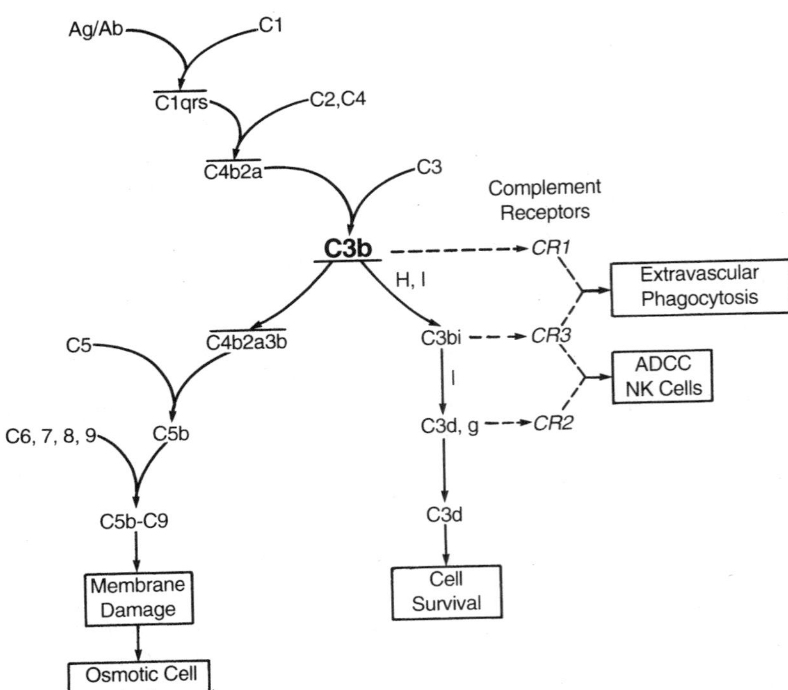

FIGURE 61.2. Simplified pattern of classical complement activation and its role in immune red blood cell destruction. Complete complement activation results in osmotic intravascular cell lysis. Partial complement activation results in the extravascular destruction of a percentage of the sensitized cells that adhere to reticuloendothelial system (RES) macrophages or to natural killer cells. Remaining, nonadherent, cells with membrane-bound component C3d,g have normal survival times. The kinetics of the reactions at the C3d phase determine the extent of intravascular and extravascular destruction. Most IgG antibodies do not activate complement, instead mediating red blood cell destruction by means of direct adherence of sensitized cells to RES macrophages.

Selected antibodies (e.g., Kidd) or groups of antibodies are of the IgG class activate complement. Complement and IgG appear to act synergistically in promoting red blood cell opsonization and destruction. The addition of complement to red blood cells sensitized with IgG enhances phagocytosis. Red blood cell recovery curves when both IgM and IgG antibodies are active show a rapid loss of a minor population of cells from IgM-mediated complement activation and a slower phase of red blood cell destruction mediated by the IgG antibody.

Autoimmune Red Blood Cell Destruction

The use of radiolabeled red blood cells to evaluate autoimmune red blood cell destruction is limited. In most cases of autoimmune hemolytic anemia, both allogeneic and autologous red blood cells are equally affected by the offending autoantibody. Red blood cell survival studies can add little to what can be determined by other clinical and laboratory studies. However, if an apparent specificity of the autoantibody can be determined (e.g., anti-e) and appropriately phenotyped (antigen-negative) allogeneic red blood cells can be obtained, in vivo study of these cells may be useful to determine their in vivo survival versus autologous cells. If the existence of a contributing but masked alloantibody is suspected, red blood cells that do not contain the respective antigen can be labeled and transfused to determine their survival versus autologous cells.

TABLE 61.3. DIFFERENTIAL FEATURES OF RECOVERY STUDIES TO EVALUATE IMMUNE RED BLOOD CELL DESTRUCTION AND RED BLOOD CELL STORAGE SYSTEMS

Immune red blood cell destruction (transfusion compatibility)
- Red blood cell age: Fresh cells (<5 d old). Avoids red blood cell loss due to storage factors.
- Red blood cell type: Allogeneic cells of a specific phenotype usually chosen.
- Volume infused: 1–3 ml. Small volume decreases risk of transfusion reaction.
- 100% recovery point: Determined from early samples obtained after mixing is complete.
- Interpretation: Shape and slope of the 24-hour recovery curve are predictive of clinical significance of red blood cell antibody.

Red blood cell storage and preservation
- Red blood cell age: Usually red blood cells stored for maximum time under experimental conditions.
- Red blood cell type: Autologous cells. Avoids risk of disease transmission or alloimmunization.
- Volume infused: Larger volume (15 ml) is easier to manipulate and requires a smaller radiation dose per cell.
- 100% recovery point: Determined by independent red blood cell mass study with different radioisotope (double-label method) or by back-extrapolation to zero-time (single-label method).
- Interpretation: Red blood cell recovery at 24 hours determines suitability (>75% mean recovery required).

Blood Storage Systems and Preservative Solutions

Studies of in vivo red blood cell recovery after storage in a new container, manipulation by a new process, or exposure to a new preservative solution are essential to evaluate the safety and efficacy of the new storage conditions or cell manipulation. The U.S. Food and Drug Administration requires that at least 75% of red blood cells exposed to a new process or solution be recovered 24 hours after they have been transfused. Although the technique for radiolabeling red blood cells for these purposes is similar to that used for determining transfusion compatibility, there are some important differences in the conduct of the test and interpretation of results. These differences are summarized in Table 61.3.

Autologous red blood cells that have been stored under the experimental conditions are chosen for these studies. Because autologous cells are used, a larger volume can be used for the study. Determination of the 100% recovery (zero-time) value is critical for storage studies. This value must be determined with accuracy so that 24-hour recovery can be properly calculated. This contrasts with the method in studies done to determine transfusion compatibility. Small volumes of allogeneic cells are used for compatibility studies. The shape of the recovery curve and the timing of cell destruction are of primary importance.

Chromium 51 is the radiolabel usually chosen for blood storage and preservation studies. The low and stable rate of elution and the relatively long half-life make it the label of choice. Correction ratios have been developed to compare ^{111}In and ^{99m}Tc with the chromium standard (19), but these radiolabels have not proved useful for labeling the stored red blood cells in these studies.

Technetium 99m is, however, helpful in determining the blood volume of the study subject, thus contributing to the accuracy of the 100% (zero-time) recovery value. The 3-minute survival value useful in studies of red blood cell immune destruction can lead to inaccuracy if used in a study of a blood storage system. Fresh red blood cells are used in an immune destruction study, whereas stored red blood cells are used in preservation and storage studies. Red blood cells are damaged during storage, the so-called storage lesion. These cells are immediately removed after transfusion. A 3-minute sample misses the cells that are immediately removed and therefore yields a falsely high 24-hour recovery value. Although back-extrapolation to zero-time from a series of early chromium-labeled samples yields acceptable results (5) and the results compare favorably with results obtained with two labels (20), many investigators use the double-label approach to these studies.

In a typical experiment, fresh autologous red blood cells are labeled with ^{99m}Tc, and stored or modified autologous red blood cells are labeled with ^{51}Cr. The samples are mixed before transfusion, thus canceling errors in making standards and counting samples. Because the fresh, unmodified technetium-labeled cells circulate normally, a 3-minute sample drawn after mixing is complete and counted for technetium can be used to determine red blood cell mass. This provides the volume of dilution for determination of the 100% recovery point of the experimental, chromium-labeled cells.

Red blood cells for transfusion are subjected to a variety of storage manipulations and conditions, all of which must be evaluated for safety and efficacy before they can be approved. Some of these manipulations are designed to improve red blood cell preservation and subsequent in vivo survival. Advances in plastic containers and plasticizing agents (21,22) and in anticoagulant-preservative solutions (23) have led to extended liquid storage of red blood cells with excellent posttransfusion survival characteristics. Most recent studies, however, are designed to evaluate the effect of other storage manipulations on red blood cells. γ-Irradiation of blood products, used to prevent posttransfusion graft versus host disease, negatively affects red blood cells. The dose of γ-irradiation has been studied to maximize the desired effect on donor lymphocytes while minimizing the damage to the stored (24,25) or frozen (26,27) red blood cells. The in vivo characteristics of red blood cells that have been enzymatically converted from group B to group O also have been studied with ^{51}Cr-labeled red blood cells (28). Prestorage leukocyte reduction and pathogen inactivation techniques are other examples in which poststorage red blood cell recovery studies have been used to evaluate advances in blood product manipulation and storage.

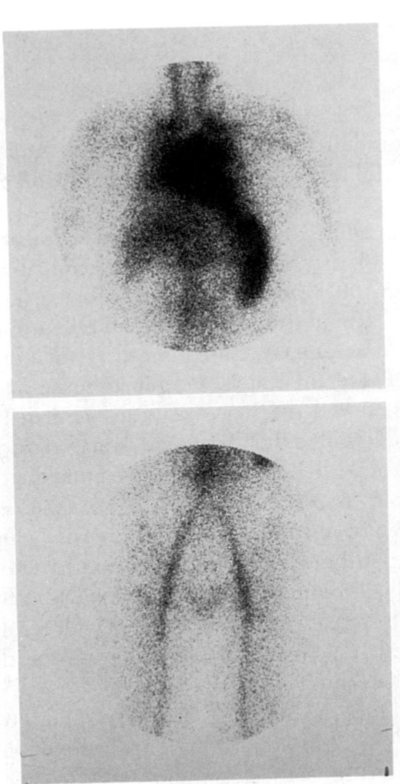

^{111}In Blood Pool Scan

FIGURE 61.3. Blood pool scan obtained with red blood cells labeled with indium 111. The characteristics of indium 111 as a radiolabel allow easy detection with standard imaging instruments. The heart, great vessels, and an enlarged spleen are evident. (From Anderson KC, Ness PM, eds. *Scientific basis of transfusion medicine.* Philadelphia: WB Saunders, 1994, with permission).

Diagnostic Imaging

Radiolabled red blood cells occasionally are used for blood pool scanning, localization and sizing of the spleen or accessory spleen, and visualization of vascular anomalies such as hemangioma. Red blood cells damaged by heat and labeled with ^{99m}Tc localize in the spleen and can be used to study that organ, although this technique is now rarely used. The blood pool can be imaged with red blood cells labeled with ^{111}In and differential organ uptake of the labeled red blood cells determined over time. Quantitative sequential counting and imaging can be performed and focused on a specific organ, such as the spleen or liver (Fig. 61.3). The extent of splenic red blood cell sequestration can thus be determined in cases of peripheral red blood cell destruction.

SUMMARY

Difficult clinical transfusion problems, although often solved with noninvasive clinical and laboratory studies, continue to occasionally necessitate in vivo evaluation of the survival of radiolabeled red blood cells of carefully selected phenotypes. The characteristics of the survival pattern of the radiolabeled cells can provide critical information about transfusion options for the patient. The effect of new developments in blood storage and preservation on red blood cells must be evaluated with radiolabeled recovery studies. In these situations, 24-hour red blood cell recovery must be determined with accuracy. The three radioisotopes discussed in this chapter can contribute to achieving these clinical and experimental goals. A clear understanding of the characteristics of each radionuclide is essential for appropriate use and interpretation of results. Close collaboration between the transfusion medicine specialist, the patient care physician, and the nuclear medicine department can ensure that these studies can be conducted with technical precision and minimal inconvenience or risk to the patient or to the study subject. Technical improvements in the availability, application, and interpretation of radiolabeled red blood cell studies will be welcome, especially in reducing the high and variable elution rates of ^{99m}Tc and ^{111}In. New lipophilic chelates for ^{111}In and modifications in the labeling procedures for ^{99m}Tc may enhance their usefulness.

Nonradioactive tracers and techniques, such as biotin and flow cytometry, would eliminate the low exposure of the patient to radioactivity. Nonradioactive isotopes such as chromium 52 may allow nonradioactive studies to be accurately performed. However, wide experience with the currently used radionuclides has shown that these agents are remarkably useful and safe. It is likely that they will continue to be used for the evaluation of immune red blood cell destruction and for the study of innovations in the manipulation, storage, and preservation of red blood cells.

REFERENCES

1. Ebaugh FG, Emerson CP, Ross JF. The use of radioactive chromium-51 as an erythrocyte-tagging agent for the determination of red cell survival in vivo. *J Clin Invest* 1953;32:1260–1276.

2. Heaton WAL. Fundamentals of blood element radiolabeling. In: Davey RJ, Wallace ME, eds. *Diagnostic and investigational uses of radiolabeled blood elements.* Bethesda, MD: American Association of Blood Banks, 1987:1–38.
3. Gray SJ, Sterling K. The tagging of red cells and plasma proteins with radioactive chromium. *J Clin Invest* 1950;29:1604–1613.
4. International Committee for Standardization in Hematology. Recommended method for radioisotope red-cell survival studies. *Br J Haematol* 1980;45:659–666.
5. Moroff G, Sohmer PR, Button LN. Proposed standardization of methods for determining the 24-hour survival of stored red cells. *Transfusion* 1984;24:109–114.
6. Garby L, Mollison PL. Deduction of mean red cell life-span from 51Cr survival curves. *Br J Haematol* 1971;20:527–536.
7. Al Sioufi H, Button L, Propper R, et al. A novel non-radioactive chromium method for red cell survival in humans. *Transfusion* 1985;24: 415a.
8. Jones J, Mollison PL. A simple and efficient method of labeling red cells with 99mTc for determination of red cell volume. *Br J Haematol* 1978;38:141–148.
9. Holt JT, Spitalnik SL, McMican AE, et al. A technetium-99m red cell survival technique for in vivo compatibility testing. *Transfusion* 1983; 23:148–151.
10. AuBuchon JP, Brightman A. Use of indium-111 as a red cell label. *Transfusion* 1989;29:143–147.
11. Mock DM, Lankford GL, Widness JA, et al. Measurement of circulating red cell volume using biotin-labeled red cells: validation against 51Cr-labeled red cells. *Transfusion* 1999;39:149–155.
12. Mock DM, Lankford GL, Widness JA, et al. Measurement of red cell survival using biotin–labeled red cells: validation against 51Cr-labeled red cells. *Transfusion* 1999;39:156–162.
13. Cowley H, Wojda U, Cipolone KM, et al. Biotinylation modifies red cells antigens. *Transfusion* 1999;39:163–168.
14. Read EJ, Crabill HE, Davey RJ. Flow cytometric determination of transfused red blood cell survival in a patient with autoimmune hemolytic anemia (AIHA). *Transfusion* 1985;25:451a.
15. Zeiler T, Muller JT, Hasse C, et al. Flow cytometric determination of RBC survival in autoimmune hemolytic anemia. *Transfusion* 2001;41: 493–498.
16. Read EJ, Cardine L, Yu M. Flow cytometric detection of human red cells labeled with a fluorescent membrane label: potential application to in vivo survival studies. *Transfusion* 1991;31:502–508.
17. Heaton WAL. Evaluation of posttransfusion recovery and survival of transfused red cells. *Transfus Med Rev* 1992;6:153–169.
18. Freedman J, Semple JW. Complement in transfusion medicine. In: Garratty G, ed. *Immunobiology of transfusion medicine.* New York: Marcel Dekker, 1994:403–434.
19. Marcus CS, Myhre BA, Angulo MC, et al. Radiolabled red cell viability, I: comparison of 51Cr, 99mTc, and 111In for measuring the viability of autologous stored red cells. *Transfusion* 1987;27:415–419.
20. Beutler E, West C. Measurement of the viability of stored red cells by the single isotope technique using 51Cr. *Transfusion* 1984:24: 100–104.
21. Davey RJ, Heaton WAL, Sweat LT, et al. Characteristics of leukocyte-reduced red cells stored in tri(2-ethylhexyl) trimellitate plastic. *Transfusion* 1994:34;895–898.
22. AuBuchon JP, Estep TN, Davey RJ. The effect of the plasticizer di-2-diethylhexylphthalate on the survival of stored red cells. *Blood* 1988; 71:448–452.
23. Hess JR, Rugg N, Knapp AD, et al. Successful storage of RBCs for 10 weeks in a new additive solution. *Transfusion* 2000;40:1012–1016.
24. Davey RJ, McCoy NC, Yu M, et al. The effect of pre-storage irradiation on posttransfusion red cell survival. *Transfusion* 1992;32:525–528.
25. Moroff G, Holme S, AuBuchon JP, et al. Viability and in vitro properties of AS-1 red cells after gamma irradiation. *Transfusion* 1999;39: 128–134.
26. Suda BA, Leitman SF, Davey RJ. Characteristics of red cells irradiated and subsequently frozen for long-term storage. *Transfusion* 1993;33: 389–392.
27. Valeri CR, Pivacek LE, Cassidy GP, et al. In vitro and in vivo measurements of gamma-radiated, frozen, glycerolyzed RBCs. *Transfusion* 2001;41:545–549.
28. Kruskall MS, AuBuchon JP, Anthony KY, et al. Transfusion to group A and O patients of group B RBCs that have been enzymatically converted to group O. *Transfusion* 2000;40;1290–1298.

62

HLA AND MOLECULAR TESTING

THOMAS M. WILLIAMS

The human major histocompatibility complex (MHC) resides on the short arm of chromosome 6. The complete genomic sequence of this region appears to contain 230 to 300 genes and to span 4 to 8 megabases, depending on where the telomeric boundary is drawn (1). Many of the genes in the MHC encode proteins involved in immune responses, including the class I and class II antigenic molecules of the HLA system; the class III molecules comprising complement components C2, C4, and tumor necrosis factor; and the peptide transporter proteins TAP1 and TAP2. This chapter focuses on the genetic structure of the MHC, current HLA nomenclature, tests for detecting HLA, and the biomedical significance of HLA antigens.

The existence of white blood cell antigens independent of red blood cell genetic systems was suggested as early as 1952. In 1958, Jan Dausset (2,3) detected, in a patient who had undergone multiple transfusions, the first leukocyte antibody (called Mac [HLA-A2]). This discovery was followed in 1958 by independent studies on similar antibodies in postpartum serum, reported by van Rood et al. (4) and Payne and Rolfs (5). These antibodies originally were thought to be autoimmune in nature or to be isoantibodies responsible for febrile (nonhemolytic) transfusion reactions. Early in 1960, Brunning et al. (6) found that these antibodies could be used to detect several diallelic genetic systems present on the cells of most tissues. Until 1964, advances in HLA typing were hampered by inconsistent and nonspecific leukoagglutination testing methods. This status changed with the development of the lymphomicrocytotoxicity assay by Terasaki and McClelland (7,8). In a slightly modified form, this test continued to be the standard for clinical HLA typing until the widespread adoption of nucleic acid–based methods in the 1990s.

In 1964, the first International Histocompatibility Workshop was held. Since then, 11 workshops have been held at 2- to 4-year intervals. These workshops are designed to confirm scientific findings and to develop unifying concepts regarding the MHC and to upgrade existing HLA nomenclature. Table 62.1 presents an overview of the workshops, listing the workshop number, year held, major theme, and number of HLA alleles known to exist at that time. In the third workshop (1967), it was established that the HLA antigens belonged to the same genetic system (9), and the term *HL-A,* coined from the Hu leukocyte system of Dausset et al. (10) and the LA system of Payne et al. (11), was assigned to identify this system. By 1970, it was established through skin grafting studies with human subjects, particularly families with HLA-identical siblings, that these antigens were important in organ transplantation (12). In 1973, it became clear from results of one-way mixed leukocyte cultures with homozygous testing cells that other genetic polymorphisms existed within the MHC (13). Also by 1973, the remarkable association of HLA and certain diseases became apparent (14, 15). In the late 1970s, HLA-D (mixed leukocyte culture defined) antigens were established (16), serologically detected antigens on B lymphocytes (HLA-DR [D-related]) were found to be closely related to the HLA-D antigenic products (17,18), and the existence of the HLA-C locus was confirmed (19).

From 1980 to 1987, advances in biochemistry, molecular biology, and the development of monoclonal antibodies to the MHC antigenic product markedly expanded knowledge about the MHC. Workshops during this time confirmed the existence of the DQ and DP loci (20,21) and focused on increasingly refined methods for identifying the burgeoning number of HLA

T.M. Williams: Department of Pathology, University of New Mexico, and Department of Genetics and Cytometry, TriCore Reference Laboratories, Albuquerque, New Mexico.

TABLE 62.1. HISTORICAL OVERVIEW

International Workshop	Year	Major Theme	Number of Known HLA Alleles
I	1964	Serologic techniques compared	—
II	1965	Standardize techniques and nomenclature	4
III	1967	One major genetic system named HL-A	12
IV	1970	International anti-sera analysis	20
V	1972	Population differences for HLA	32
VI	1975	Identification of D(DR) locus by cellular techniques; HLA-C locus confirmed	38
VII	1977	Serologic detection of DR antigens	60
VIII	1980	Compendium of HLA antigen frequencies	72
IX	1984	Introduction of RFLP molecular techniques; DQ/DP loci confirmed	90
X	1987	Standardization and application of RFLP; introduction of PCR/SSOPH typing	110
XI	1991	Standardization and application of PCR/SSOPH HLA class II typing to transplantation, disease association, and population genetics	300
XII	1996	Analysis of class I and class II alleles by means of DNA sequencing	600
—	2002	International Workshop XIII, May, 2002	1,350

RFLP, restriction fragment length polymorphism; PCR, polymerase chain reaction; SSOPH, sequence-specific oligonucleotide probe hybridization.

alleles and correlation of the serologic, biochemical, and molecular biologic findings related to the MHC. In the most recent international workshop, a primary focus was sequence-based typing and identification of class I and II alleles. It is interesting (Table 62.1) that the number of known HLA alleles gradually increased from 4 to 90 in two decades (1965 through 1985) but dramatically increased to 1,350 in the subsequent 15 years with the introduction of molecular genetic technology for allele identification.

MAJOR HISTOCOMPATIBILITY COMPLEX

The class I, II, and III genes of the MHC lie in a 4-megabase region of chromosome 6–8 megabases if one includes the more telomeric class I–related gene HFE and the butyrophilin family of genes (22).

The telomeric 2,000 kb of the MHC contains a number of genes, including those encoding the class I antigens (Fig. 62.1). The Class I HLA-A, B, and C genes reside in this region, as do the nonclassical MHC-Ib genes HLA-E, F, and G. HLA-E, F, and G are expressed at lower levels than are the classical genes, do not have the extensive polymorphism of the HLA-A, B, and C genes, and appear to have more limited functions in the immune system. Between the HLA-B locus and the tumor necrosis factor loci described later reside the MIC family of genes that encode variants of class I proteins. Loci within this family display extensive polymorphism and may encode proteins that interact with γδ T cells and participate in natural killer cell activation (23). Finally, the HFE gene responsible for genetic hemochromatosis lies approximately 4.3 megabases telomeric to HLA-A (24).

Centromeric of the HLA-B locus of the class I region is a 1-megabase segment traditionally called the class III region (Fig. 62.1) (22). This region has a dense and diverse array of genes, many with as yet unknown functions. Some of these class III genes encode proteins with functions in innate immunity and inflammation. This region includes the complement components C2, Bf (factor B protein of the alternate pathway of complement activation), and C4. In most persons, the C4 locus is duplicated as C4A and C4B, each encoding a functional, somewhat biochemically different, molecule. Members of the tumor necrosis family, also lie within the class III region. Other genes within the class III region, such as those encoding 21-hydroxylase enzymes involved in steroid metabolism, have no direct link to immunity. Although linkage to specific HLA alleles may be helpful in assessing 21-hydroxlase deficiency associated with congenital adrenal hyperplasia, direct genotyping is now possible.

The class II gene loci occupy approximately 1 megabase of DNA centromeric to the class III region (Fig. 62.1) (22). Within this region, are 18 closely linked loci that code for the α and β chains of the class II antigenic proteins. Proceeding from the telomeric to the centromeric boundaries of the region (Fig. 62.1), the first gene cluster is composed of several β-chain loci and one α chain locus that encode the HLA-DR antigens. The DRB1 and DRA loci (Fig. 62.1) are responsible for the DR1 to DR18 specificities, whereas the DRB3, DRB4, and DRB5 loci and DRA are responsible for the DR52, DR53, and DR51 specificities, respectively. Centromeric to the DRB genes are the DQ genes (Fig. 62.1D). The DQA1 and DQB1 loci encode the HLA-DQ specificities. Near the centromeric end of the MHC, the genes DPA1 and DPB1 encode the HLA-DPw1 to DPw6 specificities. The class II region also contains several pseudogenes related to the genes encoding the DR, DQ, and DP antigens with errors preventing successful transcription and translation. Other genes with important accessory functions to class I and II antigen presentation are present in the class II region. The LMP2 and LMP7 genes, the TAP1 and TAP2 genes, and the tapasin gene encode proteins that participate in protein degradation and peptide transport and loading in the class I system (25). The HLA-DM and HLA-DO encode proteins involved in peptide loading in the class II system.

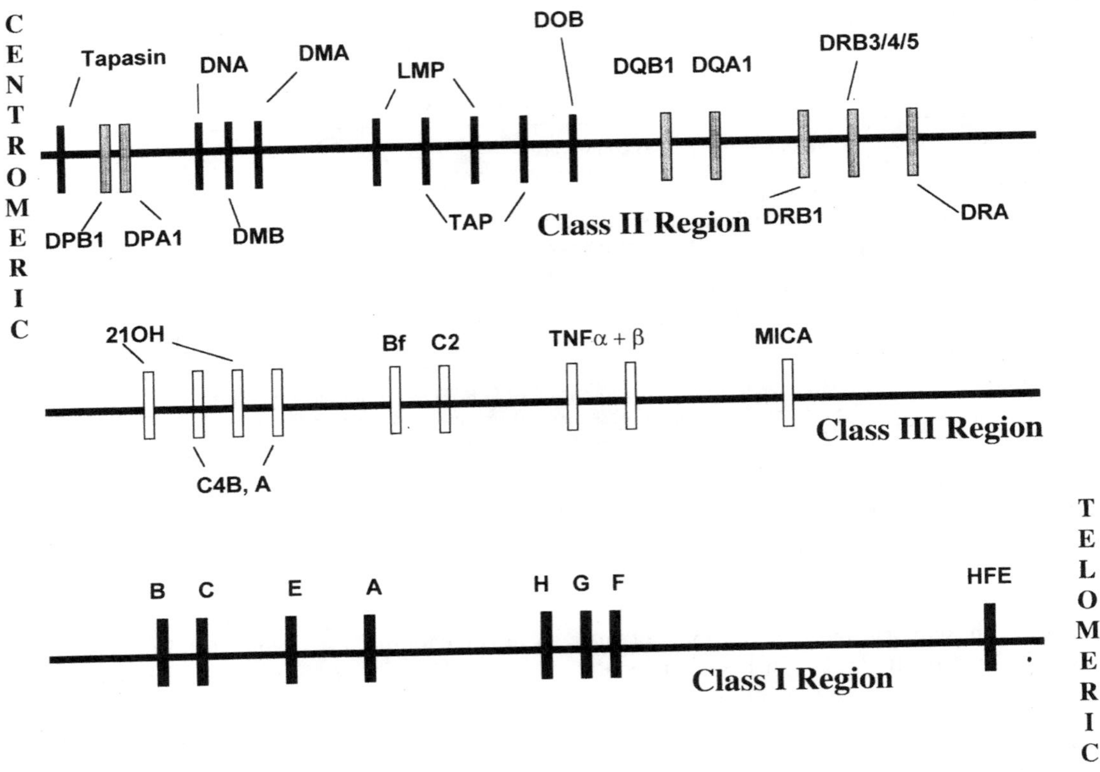

FIGURE 62.1. Selected genes in the major histocompatibility region on human chromosome 6 in the class I, II, and III regions. Distances between loci are not drawn to scale. For exact gene locations, see www.sanger.ac.uk/HGP/Chr6/MHC.shtml. (Modified from McCluskey J, Peh CA. The human leukocyte antigens and clinical medicine: an overview. *Rev Immunogenet* 1999;1:3, with permission.)

CLASS I AND II ANTIGENS AND THEIR FUNCTION

The structure, tissue distribution, and function of the glycoprotein antigenic products of the class I and class II genes of the MHC differ considerably. Both class I and class II antigens are heterodimeric, having three to four extracellular domains in addition to transmembrane and intracytoplasmic regions (26) (Fig. 62.2). Class I antigens are composed of a 45,000-d α heavy chain encoded by the HLA-A, B, and C gene loci noncovalently bound to a 12,000-d light chain, β_2-microglobulin, encoded by a gene locus on chromosome 12. The α chain is a transmembrane protein, whereas β_2-microglobulin is extracellular. Domains α_1 and α_2 contain variable amino acid sequences and thus represent the antigenic sites. The α_3 domain has constant sequences homologous to the constant regions of immunoglobulin proteins. The α_3 domain of the heavy chain and β_2 microglobulin are noncovalently associated with each other near the cell membrane. The α_1 and α_2 domains sit on top of them to form an peptide antigen-binding cleft with a floor of eight flat β sheets bound on the sides by two long α helixes, as illustrated in Figure 62.3. Most of the polymorphic amino acid changes of the class I histocompatibility antigen differences are associated with the floor or sides of this pocket, although some map to other domains (27,28).

Class II antigens are composed of a 33,000-d α chain noncovalently associated with a 28,000-d β chain (Fig. 62.2). The α chain is encoded by the A gene loci and the β chain by the B gene loci in the HLA-D region of the MHC. For example, the DQ antigen α and β chains are encoded by the DQA1 and DQB1 genes, respectively. The α_1 and β_1 domains are variable and form an antigen-binding groove similar to that described earlier (29). The α_2 and β_2 domains are relatively constant with immunoglobulin-like homology.

Class I antigens have a universal tissue distribution as plasma membrane proteins of all nucleated cells and platelets. Class II antigens have a limited tissue distribution primarily on antigen-processing cells such as B lymphocytes and macrophages, although they can be induced in several cell types, including endothelial cells.

Class I and II molecules acquire self and nonself peptides in their binding cleft and display them on the plasma membrane of cells for recognition by the T-cell antigen receptor (25). In the normal state, T cells that bind with high affinity to self peptides in the context of an individual's class I and II molecules are either deleted or suppressed by a variety of mechanisms to prevent autoimmune disorders. However, peptides derived from viruses, bacteria, and some parasites presented by the class I and class II molecules to T-cell antigen receptors evoke an immune response. Class I molecules primarily acquire 8- to 10-amino-

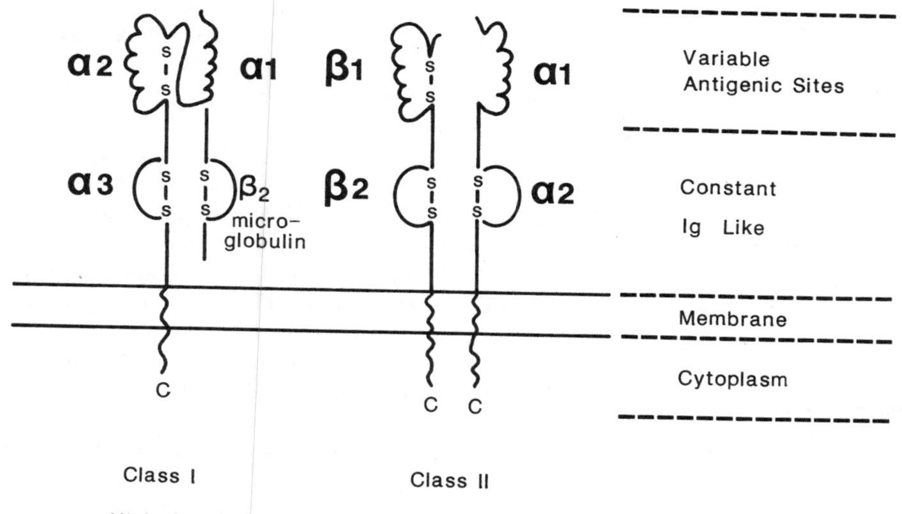

FIGURE 62.2. Simplified illustration shows the biochemical structure of class I and II antigens. (Modified from Strominger JL. Human histocompatibility antigens: genes and proteins. In: Pernis B, Vogel HJ, eds. *Cell biology of the major histocompatibility complex.* New York: Academic Press, 1985:19, with permission.)

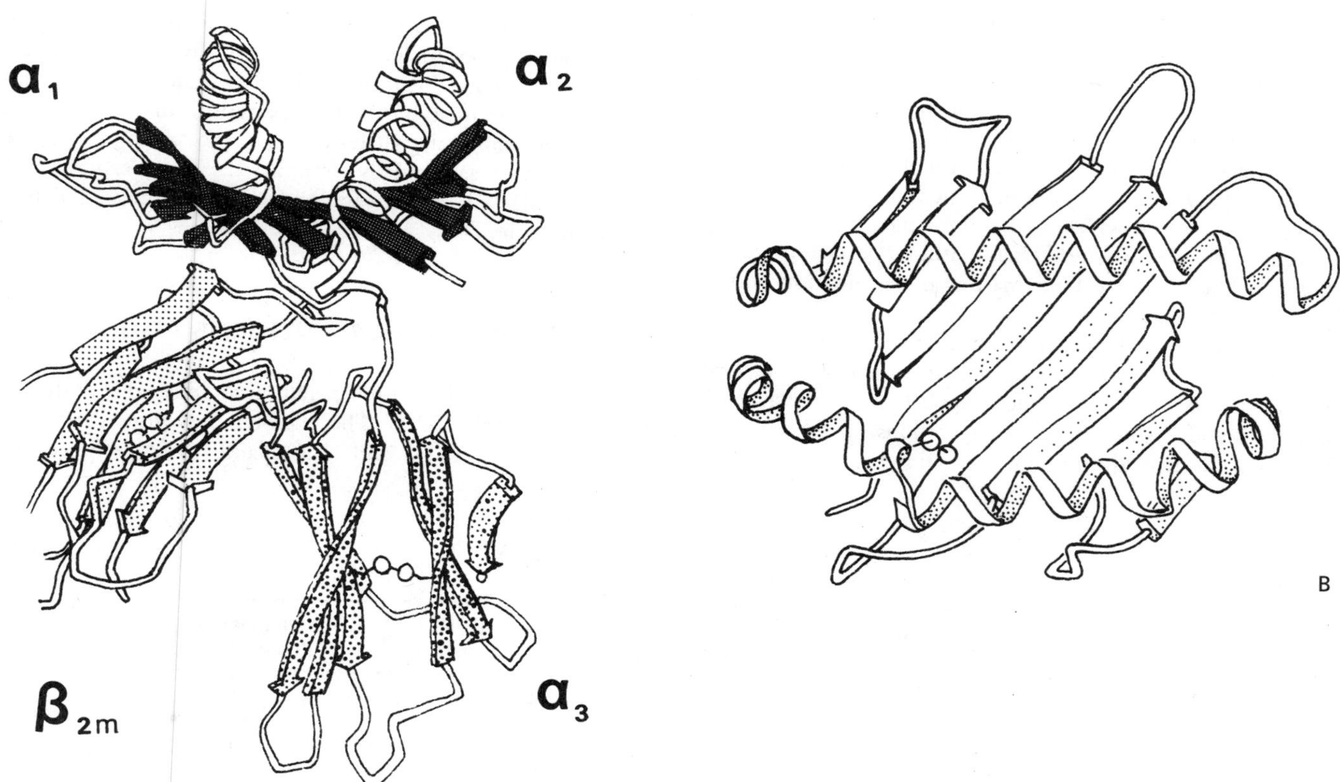

FIGURE 62.3. A: Side view of class I antigen molecule. **B:** View of the antigen-binding pocket looking down toward the cell membrane. (Modified from Bjorkman PJ, Saper MA, Samraoui B, et al. The foreign antigen binding site and T cell recognition regions of class I histocompatibility antigens. *Nature* 1987; 329:508,509, with permission.)

acid peptides generated by means of degradation of cytoplasmic proteins in the proteosome system. Class I antigens function as MHC restriction elements in the destruction of virus-infected target cells and present peptides to CD8 cytotoxic T cells. Class II molecules bind 13- to 25-amino-acid peptides of exogenous and endogenous origin degraded within the endosomal system. Class II antigens are MHC restriction elements that augment the sensitizing limb of the immune response and present peptides to CD4 helper T cells. Activation of CD8 and CD4 T cells then results in a program of cell division and differentiation resulting in cellular and humoral immune responses (25).

NOMENCLATURE AND POLYMORPHISM OF THE HLA SYSTEM

Table 62.2 illustrates the HLA gene loci, the variable polypeptide chains, the number of related serologic specificities, and the number of alleles within each specificity. In the class I region, the HLA-A, B, and C loci are all highly polymorphic with 100 to 412 known alleles (30). Multiple alleles are present within most of the known serotypes. For example, the A2 serotype has more than 51 alleles. In the class II region, the HLA-DRA locus is almost monomorphic, whereas the DRB genes are polymorphic, with hundreds of known alleles. The DQA1 and DQB1 genes and the DPA1 and DPB1 loci demonstrate similar but less extensive polymorphism. The DQA1, DPA1, and DPB1 allelic variation can be detected with DNA typing but not with serologic testing (31). The HLA system is the most polymorphous genetic system known to exist in humans. The number of possible different phenotypes possible from all combinations of these HLA alleles is greater than the global population. Fortunately, linkage disequilibrium in all human populations results in great overrepresentation of certain haplotypes, which makes finding HLA-identical individuals within a population for purposes such as unrelated bone marrow transplantation possible.

Exons in which most of the polymorphism in the class I (exons 2 and 3) and class II (exon 2) genes occurs encode the α_1 and α_2 and the α_1 and β_1 domains, which interact with bound peptides (30). New alleles appear to emerge at a fairly high rate and become fixed in populations, in theory, if they provide a selective advantage in presenting peptides from infectious organisms. New alleles are generated by means of point mutation, recombination, and gene conversion–like events (30, 31).

The nomenclature of the HLA system is established by an international committee sponsored by the World Health Organization and is updated frequently (32,33). Table 62.2 shows the general scheme for designating HLA antigens and alleles. Each serologic specificity is prefixed by the genetic system designation *HLA-*, followed by a letter denoting the encoded antigen (e.g., *A, B, C, DR*). This letter is followed by a digit indicating specificity (32). For example (Table 62.2), the A locus encodes the specificities HLA-A1 through A80; the B locus, HLA-B7 through B81; the C locus, HLA-Cw1 through Cw10; the DRA and DRB1 loci, HLA-DR1 through DR18; and the DQB1 and DQA1 loci, HLA-DQ1 through DQ9.

The nomenclature of the HLA system was first established with serologic data. Molecular data were introduced later according to the precise DNA sequences of each allele. The existing nomenclature had to be modified to accommodate this information. This modification is shown in Table 62.2. For class I alleles, because only the α chain is variable, the molecular designation is the system (HLA-), the locus (A, B, or C), an asterisk (*), and a four-digit number. The first two digits of this number correspond to the serologic specificity; for example, HLA-A*0301 is the first molecular allele of the HLA-A3 serologic specificity, and HLA-A*0302 is the second. In the class II region, because both the α and β chains can be variable, the locus designation must include the polypeptide chain responsible for the allele. For example, class II, HLA-DRB1*1501 is interpreted as HLA system, DR locus, β-1 polypeptide chain (*B1*), DR15 serologic specificity (*15* after the asterisk), first molecular allele (*01*). For molecular alleles that have no serologic equivalents, alleles are sequentially numbered; for example, HLA-DQA1*0101 is the first molecular allele of the α_1 polypeptide chain of the DQ.

DETECTION OF HLA ANTIGENS AND ALLELES

The detection of HLA is generally accomplished with three basic methods (Table 62.3). The microlymphocytotoxicity assay developed by Terasaki and McClelland (7) of peripheral blood

TABLE 62.2. HLA NOMENCLATURE

Genetic Locus	Encoded Polypeptide	Antigen or Associated Specificity	Allelic Equivalent	Number of Known Alleles
HLA-A	α	A1 to A80	A*0101 to *8001	207
HLA-B	α	B7 to B81	B*0702 to *8301	412
HLA-C	α	Cw1 to Cw10	Cw*0102 to *1802	100
DRA	α	DR1 to DR18	DRA*0101 to *0102	2
DRB1	β1		DRB1*0101 to *1608	271
DQA1	α	DQ1 to DQ9	DQA1*0101 to *0601	20
DQB1	β1		DQB1*0501 to *0402	45
DPA1	α1	DPw1 to DPw6	DPA1*0103 to *0401	19
DPB1	β1		DPB1*0101 to *8901	93

TABLE 62.3. DETECTION OF HLA ANTIGENS AND ALLELES

Serologic methods
HLA-A, B, and C: microlymphocytotoxicity test
HLA-DR and DO: modified microlymphocytotoxicity test, B-cell-enriched lymphocytes
Cellular methods
HLA-D(DR) and DQ: one-way mixed lymphocyte reaction (MLR) with
Homozygous testing cells
Primed lymphocytes (PLT)
Cloned T cells
HLA-DP: MLR in PLT or with T-cell clones
Nucleic acid–based methods for class I and II allele identification
Restriction fragment length polymorphism
Sequence-specific primer polymerase chain reaction
Sequence-specific oligonucleotide probe hybridization analysis
DNA sequencing with gel electrophoresis typing
Emerging DNA sequencing techniques

lymphocytes isolated from whole blood has been the standard test for the serologic detection of HLA-A, B, and C antigens. This is a complement-dependent test in which the addition of rabbit serum to HLA antibodies fixed to the lymphocyte membrane causes cell death. The end point is leakage or retention of fluorescent dyes from lymphocytes with damaged or intact cell membranes, respectively. Modifications of this test, primarily an increase in incubation time and isolation of B lymphocytes from peripheral blood, allow typing for the HLA-DR and DQ antigens (17).

Variations of the mixed leukocyte reaction (Table 62.3) with homozygous testing cells, primed lymphocytes, or T-cell clones are the primary methods for detecting HLA-D, DQ, and DP antigens (34–36). The mixed leukocyte reaction methods have been largely replaced by nucleic acid–based techniques for the detection of class II alleles.

The application of molecular genetic technology to the field of histocompatibility has led to an unprecedented expansion in our knowledge of the MHC at the molecular level. DNA sequences have been obtained for the HLA genes and alleles in a variety of populations worldwide (32). These sequence data have been useful for several reasons:

1. They have revealed the underlying DNA sequence variations among individuals (and therefore, amino acid variations) responsible for the antigenic differences in HLA molecules detectable with traditional serologic and cellular HLA testing.
2. They have made apparent the fact that results of serologic HLA tests define only broad groups of class I and class II alleles. Numerous subgroups of alleles distinguishable by sequence differences are present within these broad serologic groups. The result is a very large number of known alleles (37).
3. Sequence data have allowed detailed definition of the genetic basis of the HLA-mediated disease associations described later.
4. Knowledge of the DNA sequences of HLA alleles has facilitated the substitution of nucleic acid–based methods for serologic and cellular methods for clinical HLA typing.

A variety of methods have been developed to identify class I and II alleles. These range from restriction fragment length polymorphism assays to direct DNA sequencing (Table 62.3). Many laboratories have replaced or complemented serologic typing with DNA-based typing methods for several reasons. Precise identification of alleles not possible by serologic means may be clinically important in unrelated bone marrow transplantation, as discussed later. Second, nucleic acid–based typing can help resolve serologic typings compromised by cross-reactivity or complicated by clinical states resulting in pancytopenia or poor expression of HLA antigens on lymphocyte membranes. Third, even in the best circumstances, serologic typing may not be accurate, especially in ethnic groups with great diversity at loci such as HLA-B (38).

Sequence-specific Oligonucleotide Probe Hybridization

Relevant regions of the class I and class II genes are amplified from genomic DNA by means of the polymerase chain reaction (PCR) with two oligonucleotide primers that anneal to 5′ and 3′ flanking regions that are conserved (are identical) among individuals. Care must be taken in choosing primers to find ones that are locus specific (amplify HLA-A but not the related HLA-B locus, for example), that amplify all known alleles at a locus, and that result in roughly equal amplification of the two alleles in a heterozygous individual. After the PCR, the amplified DNA is blotted onto nylon membranes in a dot or slot blot format, denatured, and irreversibly fixed to the membrane by means of ultraviolet light exposure. Identification of the individual alleles is accomplished by means of hybridization of the blotted nylon membranes with a series of radiolabeled or nonradioactively labeled sequence-specific oligonucleotide probes (39). Probes are chosen to anneal to amplified regions of the class I and II genes that vary from allele to allele. Probes with nucleotide sequences perfectly complementary to the amplified DNA hybridize specifically to the PCR product target and can be visualized by means of autoradiography or colorimetry. With careful control of stringency conditions of hybridization and washing, these probes can detect single-base-pair differences, which result in single-amino-acid substitutions in the expressed proteins. Alleles are assigned on the basis of panels of positive and negative hybridization reactions with oligonucleotides specific for a particular allele or sequence. Sequence-specific oligonucleotide probe hybridization (SSOPH) typing is complex because it requires a substantial number of oligonucleotide probes to detect and differentiate among the large number of known class I and II alleles. However, it can be used for accurate mid- to high-resolution allele identification (40) and is most useful when large numbers of research or clinical cases must be typed.

Reverse dot blots and line blots take advantage of the fact that several oligonucleotide probes specific for alleles of interest can be immobilized on a single membrane (41). Products of the PCR from a single patient may then be hybridized to the membrane to allow relatively rapid HLA typing. However, reverse dot blots require that all probes on the membrane hybridize appropriately with their target sequences under identical hybridization and washing conditions. This is a challenging problem that requires considerable empirical experimentation with different probes for each target sequence.

Sequence-specific Primer Polymerase Chain Reaction

Polymerase chain reaction primers are designed so that their 3′-most 1–2 nucleotides are complementary to base positions within class I and II genes that differ for different alleles (42). Sequence-specific primers with 3′ ends that anneal perfectly to sequences present in a particular allele or allele subgroup result in productive DNA amplification. Other alleles or allele subgroups are not amplified. Gel electrophoresis can then be used to detect the presence or absence of PCR products of the appropriate size, and hybridization assays are avoided. Sequence-specific PCR is most useful for medium-resolution HLA typing and for initial quick identification of broad antigen groups, such as DR52. Then, SSOPH or DNA sequencing can be used to define microvariants of these specificities if necessary. Sequence-specific PCR requires 100 or more simultaneously performed PCR assays per patient to identify HLA-A, -B, and -DRB allele groups at serologically equivalent resolution. The method requires optimization to avoid failed amplification reactions in each run.

Sequence-based Typing

Sequence-based typing has the advantage of requiring only a limited number of primers for the PCR for each HLA locus. There is no need for a series of detecting oligonucleotide probes for each allele. Polymerase chain reaction products are prepared that will encompass the relevant polymorphic positions within the class I or II gene to be sequenced. Sequencing primers are annealed to the PCR products to generate sequencing ladders that are separated on a high-resolution gel. Any known or previously unknown allele in the population can be identified by means of inspection of the DNA sequence or electropherogram. Electropherograms must be of high quality for accurate detection of heterozygous positions in the sequenced PCR products. The development of high-throughput automated fluorescent DNA-sequencing machines, analysis software, and capillary electrophoresis systems has made this method less cumbersome. Direct sequencing for HLA typing is technically demanding but yields unparalleled precision in allele identification. As the number of known class I and II alleles continues to escalate, the SSOPH and sequence-specific PCR methods have become increasingly complex, making direct sequencing an increasingly attractive method for laboratories (43–45).

Choice of HLA Typing Method

Several factors influence a decision to use one HLA typing method over another (Table 62.4). Sequence-specific PCR and reverse SSOPH can be performed in a time (4 to 5 hours) appropriate for clinical situations such as cadaveric renal transplantation. DNA sequencing is a reasonable approach for situations such as unrelated bone marrow transplantation in which allele-level HLA matching of donors and recipients is desired and turnaround times of a few days to a week are acceptable.

GENOTYPES, PHENOTYPES, AND HAPLOTYPES

HLA antigens are expressed codominantly. The phenotype of expressed antigens for any given person is not equivalent to the genotype. Because HLA genes are closely linked on chromosome 6, they are inherited in units known as *haplotypes.* Each sibling of a family inherits one of two HLA haplotypes from each parent.

Figure 62.4 illustrates the segregation of haplotypes in a family of seven, focusing on the A, B, Cw, and DR serologic specific-

TABLE 62.4. CHARACTERISTICS AND APPLICATIONS OF HLA TYPING METHODS

Method	Resolution	Transplantation Application
Microlymphocytotoxicity	Serologic specificity	Solid-organ transplantation, investigation of presence of null alleles
Sequence-specific primer polymerase chain reaction	Serologic, higher resolution with large number of primers	Solid-organ and related stem-cell transplantation, well suited to low to moderate testing volume
Forward SSOPH	Serologic to allele level	Solid-organ and stem-cell transplantation, well suited to high-volume testing
Reverse SSOPH	Serologic, higher resolution with larger number of probes	Solid-organ and related stem-cell transplantation, suitable for low to moderate testing volume
DNA sequencing	Allele level	Unrelated stem-cell transplantation, resolution of typing problems with other methods, characterization of new alleles

SSOPH, sequence-specific oligonucleotide probe hybridization.

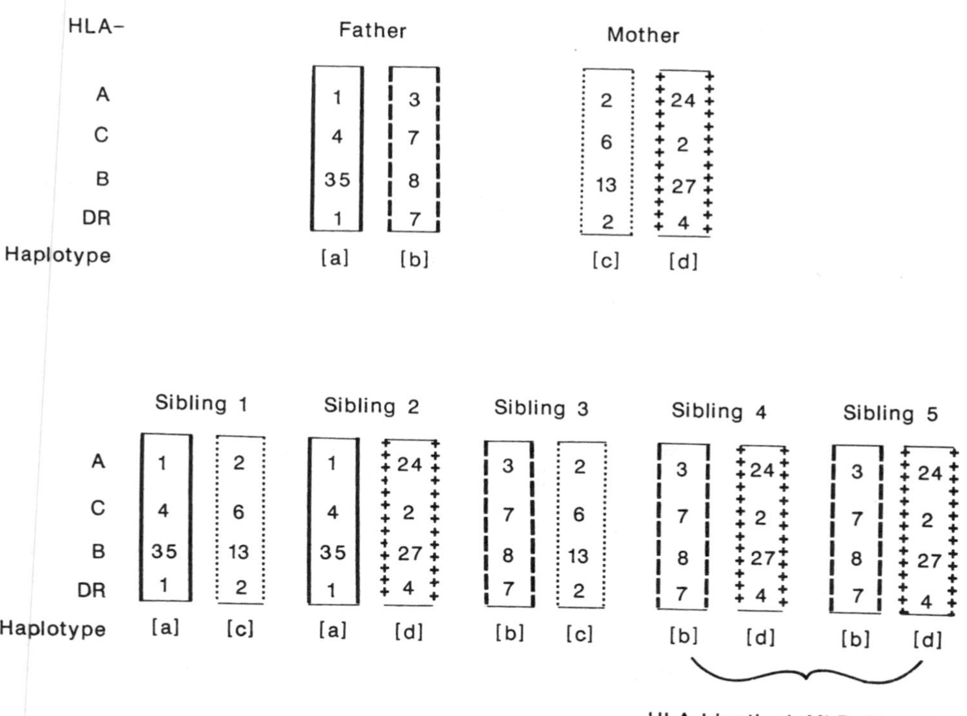

FIGURE 62.4. Typing of a family of seven persons for HLA-A, B, C, and DR antigens. The data reflect the genotypes of each family member as well as the parental haplotypes.

ities. Analysis of the data for a single individual does not allow assignment of the serologic types present to a specific paternally or maternally derived chromosome; that is, the typing data are unphased. Thus one cannot be certain whether the DR7 in sibling 3 is present on a chromosome carrying B8 or B13. However, analysis of the typing data for the entire family and the transmission of specificities to the children, makes it possible to phase each of the pairs of parental chromosomes and to determine haplotypes. For example, one of the paternal chromosome-6 pairs, haplotype *[a]*, contains HLA-A1, Cw4, B35, and DR1; the other paternal chromosome, haplotype *[b]*, includes HLA-A3, Cw7, B8, and DR7. Similarly, the maternal chromosome-6 pairs can be separated as haplotypes *[c]* and *[d]*. Each child in this family inherits *[a]* or *[b]* from the father and *[c]* or *[d]* from the mother. Each child differs from each parent by one HLA haplotype. Because there can be only four parental haplotypes, the chances are 1 in 4 that the siblings will have same paternal-maternal haplotypes (are HLA-identical), 1 in 2 that siblings will differ by one haplotype, and 1 in 4 that they will differ by two haplotypes. For example, siblings 4 and 5 are HLA-identical, and sibling 4 shares no haplotypes with sibling 1 and one haplotype with siblings 2 and 3. Because siblings 4 and 5 are genetically identical with regard to the MHC, their lymphocytes will not react in mixed leukocyte culture.

The difference between phenotypes and genotypes can be clarified even further with sibling 4 (Fig. 62.4) as an example. If family data were not available, this sibling's phenotype would be written as HLA-A3, A24; Cw2, Cw7; B8, B27; DR4, DR7. This implies lack of family data that would allow assignment of the A, C, B, and DR combinations to the appropriate haplotypes. With family data available, however, the genotype is written HLA-A3, Cw7, B8, DR7/A24, Cw2, B27, DR4. The slash in this statement clearly defines the two haplotypes inherited by this child.

Although HLA gene loci are closely linked, there is a low frequency of recombination during meiosis. The crossover rate is approximately 0.8% between the A and B loci and approximately 0.5% between the B and DR loci. For example, 1 of every 200 families exhibits recombination between the B and DR genes.

HLA allele and haplotype frequencies exhibit ethnic variation. Some alleles and hapotypes are widely distributed around the globe, and others are almost exclusively within a particular ethnic group. In population studies, the phenomenon of linkage disequilibrium is apparent in all groups. This term indicates that in randomly mating populations, the haplotype frequency for two or more linked gene loci is significantly higher than would be expected by chance alone. The expected frequency is obtained from the product of the gene frequencies of the involved genes. For example, among white persons, the observed A1, B8 haplotype frequency (7.0%) is approximately 4.4 times greater than the expected haplotype frequency (1.6%). These excess haplotype frequencies may exist for a variety of reasons, including high prevalence in the founders of a population and selective pressure from infectious organisms (46).

MEDICAL AND BIOLOGIC SIGNIFICANCE OF HLA

The HLA system plays a role in several areas of biomedical significance (Table 62.5). The ability to trace the appearance of novel HLA alleles in populations and to compare the frequencies of alleles among populations to gain information about human origins and migration in anthropologic and evolutionary studies is a fascinating field of inquiry but beyond the scope of this chapter (47). The extensive polymorphism of the HLA loci has been exploited for many years in identity testing; however, the use of microsatellite loci for this purpose has begun to supplant the use of HLA loci (see Chapter 63). The role of HLA class I typing to support platelet transfusion is described in Chapter 16.

Transplantation

Transplantation poses a special problem in medicine because the extreme polymorphism of the HLA loci make it unlikely that an unrelated donor of cells, tissues, or organs will be matched at an allele level or at a serologic level with a recipient without a concerted effort to identify matched donors and recipients. One solution is to identify an HLA-identical sibling, but many potential transplant recipients do not have access to these donors. For organ transplantation, powerful immunosuppressant drugs have made transplantation feasible with mismatched living and cadaveric donors and recipients. However, better HLA-A, B, and DR matching at a serologic level generally increases the half-life of the transplanted organ and decreases overall morbidity (48). Thus cadaveric donor kidneys are shared on a national basis with waiting recipients with end-stage renal failure who have no mismatches (49).

Finding well-matched donors of hematopoietic stem cells if there are no HLA-identical siblings is facilitated by resources such as the National Marrow Donor Program which has enrolled several million potential donors with known HLA types (50). The goal for unrelated stem cell donation is increasing allele-level matches for HLA-A, B, and DRB1, although the level of mismatching permissable and whether other loci such as HLA-C and DQB1 should be matched are controversial. Subtle allelic mismatches between stem cell donors and recipients appear to increase the risk of failure of engraftment of the transplanted cells and the risk of severe graft versus host disease (51,52). The use of umbilical cord blood stem cells and the depletion of T cells from transplanted cells may allow greater donor-recipient mismatches (53,54). Retrospective studies are underway to assess in a definitive manner the level of matching necessary for successful stem cell transplantation (55). Hematopoietic stem cell transplantation is discussed in Chapters 36 through 38.

There are two major mechanisms by which class I and II donor-recipient mismatches may adversely affect transplantation—production of anti-HLA antibodies and cell-mediated rejection. Transplant recipients become sensitized or produce antibodies directed against class I and class II specificities through several routes. Exposure to fetal HLA molecules encoded by paternal haplotypes during pregnancy, especially multiple pregnancies, can lead to the presence of long lasting, high-titer anti-HLA antibodies. Similarly, mismatched HLA antigens from previous organ donors and donors of transfused blood components can lead to sensitization. The presence of recipient preformed anti-HLA antibodies may lead to hyperacute rejection of a donor organ bearing the relevant HLA specificities (26). Therefore, laboratories maintain serum screening programs to detect and identify anti-HLA antibodies in waiting recipients so that inappropriate donors can be avoided. Immediately before transplantation, crossmatches to detect donor-directed anti-HLA antibodies are performed between donor lymphocytes and recipient serum by means of the microcytotoxicity assays described earlier or more sensitive flow cytometric technology (56).

Donor HLA antigens mismatched with recipient HLA antigens can elicit a strong cell-mediated immune response. As many as 10% of a recipient's T cells are able to recognize and respond to donor-mismatched HLA antigen (57). These responses contribute to acute rejection in organ transplantation and graft versus host disease in stem cell transplantation. HLA matching and immunosuppressive therapy help to mitigate this problem.

Disease Association

The association of certain HLA alleles and their encoded antigens with particular diseases, especially autoimmune disorders, has been known for some time. In more than 40 disorders, there is significant deviation in the frequency of HLA antigens from that of healthy controls (58) (Table 62.6). In general, HLA-associated diseases have certain common features. They are known or suspected to have an inherited component, usually have autoimmune features, and display a clinical course often featuring repeated acute relapses followed by remission. For most HLA-associated diseases, the etiologic factor is unknown and the pathophysiologic mechanism is incompletely understood. One hypothesis for the link between HLA antigens and disease suggests that a necessary but not sufficient requirement for disease development is the differential ability of a class I or II heterodimer encoded by a specific allele to present autoantigens to the T-cell receptor.

Two of the strongest HLA-associations are the DQB1*0602 allele with narcolepsy (59) and B*27 alleles with ankylosing spondylitis (58). Almost all patients with narcolepsy have the associated alleles; approximately 90% of patients with ankylosing spondylitis have the associated alelles. In white populations with-

TABLE 62.5. BIOMEDICAL SIGNIFICANCE OF THE HLA SYSTEM

Antigen presentation
Association with certain diseases
Organ and stem cell transplantation
Platelet transfusion
Population genetics and anthropology
Identity testing

TABLE 62.6. DISEASES ASSOCIATED WITH HLA ANTIGENS AND ALLELES

Disorder	Antigen or Allele Linkage	Comments
Class I or II Associations		
Ankylosing spondylitis	B*27 alleles	Useful in ruling out diagnosis of ankylosing spondylitis
Narcolepsy	DQB1*0602	Both the DQB1 locus or linked loci and alterations in hypocretin or orexin peptides; receptors appear to contribute to narcolepsy
Insulin-dependent diabetes mellitus	DRB1*03/*04, DQB1*02 and *03 alleles	Presence of DRB1*03/*04 confers a 25-fold relative risk
Rheumatoid arthritis	DRB1*04 alleles sharing epitope encoded by codons 67–74	May be most useful in predicting severity of disease
Cervical intrepithelial neoplasia and invasive cancer	B*07, DRB1*11, DQB1*0301, *0302, DRB1*1501, DQB1*0602	DRB1*13 alleles appear to be protective
Latency period before onset of AIDS	Homozygosity at HLA loci or A*29, B*35-Cw*04, B*54, *55 and *56, DRB1*11	Conversely, heterozygosity or B*14, Cw*08 appear protective
Mutation of Nonimmune Response Genes Within the Major Histocompatibility Complex		
21-Hydroxlase deficiency	Linked to cosegregating HLA haplotypes in families	Diagnosis by means of direct CYP21 genotyping
Hemochromatosis	A*03	Diagnosis by means of direct *HFE* genotyping
Complement component 2 (C2) deficiency	A*25, B*18, DR2	Diagnosis by means assessment of complement levels

out these disorders, the frequencies of DQB1*0602 (25% to 30%) and of the B*27 group (5% to 10%) are substantial but do not approach the frequencies among persons with these disorders. Thus the antigens involved are not unique to narcolepsy and ankylosing spondylitis but are overrepresented among affected persons. Approximately 3% of persons with a B*27 allele have ankylosing spondylitis, a risk approximately 100-fold greater than that among persons without B*27. Results of HLA testing that show the absence of DQB1*0602 or B*27 alleles is useful to help rule out a diagnosis of narcolepsy or ankylosing spondylitis for a patient. Results that show the presence of these alleles are less useful because of the prevalence of these alleles in the general population.

The association of HLA antigens with most other autoimmune disorders usually does not carry the high relative risk that narcolepsy and ankylosing spondylitis do. Although these HLA associations are generally less useful in diagnosis, they provide important insights into the pathophysiologic mechanism of these diseases and may help assess prognosis. For example, approximately 95% of patients with type 1 diabetes mellitus (formerly known as insulin-dependent diabetes mellitus) have either the DRB1*03 or the DRB1*04 allele or both (60). Patients heterozygous for DRB1*03/*04 have a relative risk for type 1 diabetes mellitus 3 to 6 times greater than that of patients with DRB1*03 or DRB1*04 alone or in combination with another DRB1 allele. Susceptibility to type 1 diabetes mellitus appears to be linked to haplotypes containing DRB1*03 or DRB1*04 with DQB1*02 and DQB1*03 alleles.

Many persons with rheumatoid arthritis have inherited DRB1*04 alleles encoding a common epitope. Heterozygosity and homozygosity for alleles encoding this epitope may be predictive of a more severe course of arthritis. Thus allele identification may be helpful in assessing prognosis (61).

A number of studies have been performed in an attempt to define specific HLA alleles that confer susceptibility or resistance to disorders such as cervical cancer (62,63) and acquired immunodeficiency syndrome (64,65) (Table 62.6). There appear to be HLA alleles that interact with other genetic and environmental factors to influence the outcome of these multifactorial diseases. However, results may vary somewhat among studies given the complexity of these disorders and differences in the ethnicity of the populations studied, the subtypes of the papillomaviruses and human immunodeficiency virus 1 involved, and the definition of cases and controls.

Because the MHC contains genes with no obvious role in immune system function, some diseases caused by point mutation or deletion of genes in this region cause disorders not directly related to immunity. However, because of linkage disequilibrium, overrepresentation of specific class I or class II antigens may occur in these disorders. Congenital adrenal hyperplasia is caused by mutations in the MHC class III region genes encoding 21-hydroxylase (66). Although linkage to specific HLA alleles is present in persons with congenital adrenal hyperplasia, direct genotyping is generally preferable for diagnostic purposes. Similarly, genetic hemochromatosis is caused by mutations in the HFE gene telomeric to the HLA-A locus (24). Although the presence of A*03 confers severalfold excess risk of hemochromatosis, the most direct route to genetic diagnosis is HFE genotyping.

SUMMARY

The HLA loci on chromosome 6 are composed of a series of class I and II genes that display a degree of naturally occurring polymorphism unmatched within the rest of the human genome.

This polymorphism appears to be maintained to ensure appropriate responses to the infectious organisms encountered by global human populations. The crucial role of the class I and II molecules is to bind to the degradation products of proteins and present them to T-cell antigen receptors for recognition as endogenous or foreign peptides. Major histocompatibility complex polymorphism has several consequences in medicine and biology beyond the normal immune response: (a) Major histocompatibility complex genetic variation can be exploited as a tool for anthropologic study of human migration and development. (b) Highly informative HLA loci have been useful for human identity testing. (c) Specific HLA alleles are associated with a propensity to development of particular disease entities, especially autoimmune disorders. (d) The challenge of finding HLA-matched donors and recipients presents special problems in stem cell and organ transplantation.

REFERENCES

1. Available at: www.sanger.ac.uk/HGP/Chr6/MHC.shtml.
2. Dausset J, Nema A. Presence d'une leuco-agglutinine dans le serum d'uncas d'agranulocytose chronique. *C R Soc Biol (Paris)* 1952;140: 534.
3. Dausset J. Iso-leuco anticorps. *Acta Haematol (Basel)* 1958;20:156.
4. van Rood JJ, Eernisse JG, van Leeuwen A. Leukocyte antibodies in sera from pregnant women. *Nature* 1958;181:735.
5. Payne R, Rolfs MR. Fetomaternal leukocyte incompatibility. *J Clin Invest* 1958;37:756.
6. Brunning JW, van Leeuwen A, van Rood JJ. Some studies concerning the localization and nature of leucocyte group substance in placental tissue. In: Proceedings of the Ninth Congress of the International Society of Blood Transfusion, Mexico, 1962. Basel: Karger, 1964:568.
7. Terasaki PI, McClelland JD. Microdroplet assay of human serum cytotoxins. *Nature* 1964;204:998.
8. Terasaki PI, McClelland JD, Park MS, et al. Microdroplet lymphocyte cytotoxicity test. In: Ray JG Jr, Hare DB, Peterson PW, et al., eds. *NIAID manual of tissue typing techniques, no. 76-545.* Washington, DC: US Department of Health, Education, and Welfare (NIH), 1977.
9. Ceppellini R, Curtoni ES, Mattuiz PL, et al. Genetics of leukocyte antigens: a family study of segregation and linkage. In: Curtoni ES, Mattiuz PL, Tosi RM, eds. *Histocompatibility testing 1967.* Copenhagen: Munksgaard, 1967:149.
10. Dausset J, Ivanyi P, Ivanyi D. Tissue alloantigens in humans: identification of a complex system (Hu-1)–histocompatibility testing 1965. *Ser Haematol* 1965;11:51.
11. Payne R, Tripp M, Weigle J, et al. A new leukocyte isoantigen system in man. *Cold Spring Harbor Symp Quant Biol* 1964;29:285.
12. Dausset J, Rapaport FT, Legrand L, et al. Skin allograft survival in 238 human subjects. In: Terasaki PI, ed. *Histocompatibility testing 1970.* Copenhagen: Munksgaard, 1970:381.
13. Jorgensen F, Lamm LU, Kissmeyer-Nielsen F. Mixed lymphocyte cultures with inbred individuals: an approach to MLC typing. *Tissue Antigens* 1973;3:232.
14. Brewerton C, Caffrey M, Hart F. Ankylosing spondylitis and HL-A27. *Lancet* 1973;1:904.
15. Schlosstein L, Terasaki PI, Bluestone R, et al. High association of an HL-A antigen, W27, with ankylosing spondylitis. *N Engl J Med* 1973; 288:704.
16. Thorsby E, Piazza A, eds. Joint report from the Sixth International Histocompatibility Workshop Conference, II: typing for HLA-D (LD-1 or MLC) determinants. In: Kissmeyer-Nielsen F, ed. *Histocompatibility testing 1975.* Copenhagen: Munksgaard, 1975:414.
17. Jones EA, Goodfellow PN, Bodmer JG, et al. Serological identification of HL-A-linked human "Ia-type" antigens. *Nature* 1975;256:650.
18. Bodmer JG. Summary and conclusions: Ia serology. In: Bodmer WF, et al., eds. *Histocompatibility testing 1977.* Copenhagen: Munksgaard, 1977:351.
19. Staub Nielsen L, Sandberg L, Mayr WR, et al. Report on an analysis of reagents defining antibodies against third locus HL-A antigens. In: Kissmeyer-Nielsen F, ed. *Histocompatibility testing 1975.* Copenhagen: Munksgaard, 1975:322.
20. Dausset J, Cohen D. HLA at the gene level. In: Albert ED, Baur MP, Mayr WR, eds. *Histocompatibility testing 1984.* Berlin: Springer-Verlag, 1984:22.
21. Bodmer WF. The HLA system, 1994. In: Albert ED, Baur MP, Mayr WR, eds. Histocompatibility testing 1984. Berlin: Springer-Verlag, 1984:11.
22. Rhodes DA, Trowsdale J. Genetics and molecular genetics of the MHC. *Rev Immunogenet* 1999;1:21–31.
23. Groh V, Steinle A, Bauer S, Spies T. Recognition of stress-induced MHC molecules by intestinal epithelial gamma delta T cells. *Science* 1998;279:1737.
24. Ehrlich R and Lemonnier FA. HFE: a novel nonclassical class I molecule that is involved in iron metabolism. *Immunity* 2000;13:585.
25. Watts C, Powls S. Pathways of antigen processing and presentation. *Rev Immunogenet* 1999;1:60.
26. McCluskey J, Peh CA. The human leukocyte antigens and clinical medicine: an overview. *Rev Immunogenet* 1999;1:3.
27. Bjorkman PJ, Saper MA, Samraoui B, et al. Structure of the human class I histocompatibility antigen, HLA-A2. *Nature* 1987;329:506.
28. Bjorkman PJ, Saper MA, Samraoui B, et al. The foreign antigen binding site and T cell recognition regions of class I histocompatibility antigens. *Nature* 1987;329:512.
29. Brown JH, Jardetzky TS, Gorga JC, et al. The three-dimensional structure of the human class II histocompatibility antigen HLA-DR1. *Nature* 1993;364:33.
30. Little AM, Parham P. Polymorphism and evolution of class I and II genes and molecules. *Rev Immunogenet* 1999;1:105.
31. Marsh SGE, Parham P, Barber LD. Evolution and anthropology of HLA. In: *The HLA facts book.* London: Academic Press, 2000:73.
32. Bodmer JG, Marsh SG, Albert ED, et al. Nomenclature for factors of the HLA system, 1998. *Tissue Antigens* 1999;53:407.
33. Available at: www. ebi. ac. uk/imgt/hla/.
34. Shaw S, Johnson AH, Shearer GM. Evidence for a new segregant series of B cell antigens that are encoded in the HLA-D region and that stimulate secondary allogeneic proliferative and cytotoxic responses. *J Exp Med* 1980;152:565.
35. Wank R, Schendel DJ. Genetic analysis of HLA-D region products defined by PLT. In: Albert ED, Baur MP, Mayr WR, eds. *Histocompatibility testing 1984.* Berlin: Springer-Verlag, 1984:289.
36. Flomenberg N. Functional polymorphisms of HLA class II gene products detected by T-lymphocyte clones: summary of the Tenth International Histocompatibility Workshop Cellular Study. In: Dupont B, ed. *Immunobiology of HLA: histocompatibility testing 1987.* Vol 1. New York: Springer-Verlag, 1989:532.
37. Schreuder GMTh, Hurley CK, Marsh SGE, et al. The HLA dictionary 1999: a summary of HLA-A, -B, -C, -DRB1/3/4/5, -DQB1 alleles and their association with serologically defined HLA-A, -B, -C, -DR, and -DQ antigens. *Tissue Antigens* 1999;54:409.
38. Mytilineos J, Lempert M, Middleton D, et al. HLA class I DNA typing of 215 "HLA-A, -B, -DR zero mismatched" kidney transplants. *Tissue Antigens* 1997;50:355.
39. Kimura A, Sasazuki T. Eleventh International Histocompatibility Workshop reference protocol for the HLA DNA-typing technique. In: Tsuji K, Aizawa M, Sasazuki T, eds. *HLA 1991: Proceedings of the Eleventh International Workshop and Conference.* Vol 1. Oxford, UK: Oxford University Press, 1992:397.
40. Ng J, Hurley CK, Baxter-Lowe LA, et al. Large-scale oligonucleotide typing for HLA-DRB1/3/4 and HLA-DQB1 is highly accurate, specific, and reliable. *Tissue Antigens* 1993;42:473.
41. Saiki RK, Walsh PS, Levenson CH, et al. Genetic analysis of amplified DNA with immobilized sequence-specific oligonucleotide probes. *Proc Natl Acad Sci U S A* 1989;86:6230.
42. Olerup O, Zetterquist H. HLA-DR typing by PCR amplification with sequence specific primers (PCR-SSP) in 2 hours: an alternative to sero-

logical DR typing in clinical practice including donor-recipient matching in cadaveric transplantation. *Tissue Antigens* 1992;39:225.
43. Wu J, Griffith BB, Bassinger S, et al. 1996. Strategies for unambiguous detection of allelic heterozygosity via direct DNA sequencing of PCR products: application to the HLA DRB1 locus. *Mol Diagn* 1996;1: 89–98.
44. Versluis LF, Rozumuller EH, Duran K, et al. Ambiguous DPB1 allele combinations resolved by direct sequencing of selectively amplified alleles. *Tissue Antigens* 1995;46:345.
45. Turner S, Ellexson ME, Hickman HD, et al. Sequence-based typing provides a new look at HLA-C diversity. *J Immunol* 1998;161:1406.
46. Alper CA, Awdeh Z, Yunis EJ. Conserved, extended MHC haplotypes. *Exp Clin Immunogenet* 1992;9:58.
47. Mack SJ, Erlich HA. HLA class II polymorphism in the Ticuna of Brazil: evolutionary implications of the DRB1*0807 allele. *Tissue Antigens* 1998;51:41.
48. Suthanthiran M, Strom TB. Renal transplantation. *N Engl J Med* 1994; 331:365–376.
49. Takemoto SK, Terasaki PI, Gjertson DW, et al. Twelve years' experience with national sharing of HLA-matched cadaveric kidneys for transplantation. *N Engl J Med* 2000;343:1078.
50. Kernan NA, Bartsch G, Ash RC, et al. Analysis of 462 transplantations from unrelated donors facilitated by the National Marrow Donor Program. *N Engl J Med* 1993;328:593.
51. Petersdorf EW, Longton GM, Anasetti C, et al. The significance of HLA-DRB1 matching on clinical outcome after HLA-A, B, DR identical unrelated donor marrow transplantation. *Blood* 1995; 86:1606.
52. Sasazuki T, Juji T, Morishima Y, et al. Effect of matching of class I alleles on clinical outcome after transplantation of hematopoietic stem cells from an unrelated donor. *N Engl J Med* 1998;339:1177.
53. Kurtzberg J, Laughlin M, Graham ML, et al. Placental blood as a source of hematopoietic stem cells for transplantation into unrelated recipients. *N Engl J Med* 1996;335:157.
54. Aversa F, Tabilio A, Velardi A. Treatment of high-risk acute leukemia with T-cell-depleted stem cells from related donors with one fully mismatched HLA haplotype. *N Engl J Med* 1998;339:1186.
55. Hurley CK, Baxter-Lowe LA, Begovich AB, et al. The extent of HLA class II allele level disparity in unrelated bone marrow transplantation: analysis of 1,259 national marrow donor program donor-recipient pairs. *Bone Marrow Transplant* 2000;25:385.
56. Gebel HM, Bray RA. Sensitization and sensitivity: defining the unsensitized patient. *Transplantation* 2000;69:1370.
57. Janeway CA, Travers P. Antigen recognition by T lymphocytes. In: Janeway CA, ed. *Immunobiology,* 3rd ed. New York: Garland Publishing, 1997:4:1.
58. Lechler R, ed. *HLA and disease.* London: Academic Press, 1994.
59. Pelin Z, Guilleminault C, Risch N, et al. HLA-DQB1*0602 homozygosity increases relative risk for narcolepsy but not disease severity in two ethnic groups. US Modafinil in Narcolepsy Multicenter Study Group. *Tissue Antigens* 1998;51:96.
60. Aitman TJ, Todd JA. Molecular genetics of diabetes mellitus. *Clin Endocrinol Metab* 1995;9:631.
61. Weyand CM, Hicok KC, Conn DL, et al. The influence of HLA-DRB1 genes on disease severity in rheumatoid arthritis. *Ann Intern Med* 1992;117:801.
62. Apple RJ, Becker TM, Wheeler CM, et al. Comparison of human leukocyte antigen DR-DQ disease associations found with cervical dysplasia and invasive cervical carcinoma. *J Natl Cancer Inst* 1995;87: 427–436.
63. Hildesheim A, Schiffman M, Scott DR, et al. Human leukocyte antigen class I/II alleles and development of human papillomavirus-related cervical neoplasia: results from a case-control study conducted in the United States. *Cancer Epidemiol Biomarkers Prev* 1998;7:1035–1041.
64. Carrington M, Nelson GW, Martin MP, et al. HLA and HIV-1: heterozygote advantage and B*35-Cw*04 disadvantage. *Science* 1999;283: 1748.
65. Hendel H, Caillat-Zucman S, Lebuanec H, et al. New class I and II HLA alleles strongly associated with opposite patterns of progression to AIDS. *J Immunol* 1999;162:6942.
66. White PC, Speiser PW. Congenital adrenal hyperplasia due to 21-hydroxylase deficiency. *Endocr Rev* 2000;21:245.

Rossi's Principles of Transfusion Medicine, Third Edition, edited by Toby L. Simon, Walter H. Dzik, Edward L. Snyder, Christopher P. Stowell, and Ronald G. Strauss. Lippincott Williams & Wilkins, Philadelphia © 2002.

63

PARENTAGE TESTING

DAVID W. GJERTSON

"Am I the father?" Although cases of disputed parentage may start with simple questions, laboratory tests often produce complex answers. "Inclusions" of parentage must always be qualified because shared genetic markers are not unique and merely corroborate assertions of parentage, and "exclusions" must be qualified because inconsistent genetic markers only suggest nonparentage because markers may be due to laboratory error or genetic anomaly. To fully resolve the question of parentage, one needs to quantify the errors and chance matches through inferential elements of genetic theory, statistical reasoning, and empiric knowledge. It is this inferential nature of parentage testing that distinguishes it from other clinical practices.

The purpose of this chapter is to clarify the genetic and statistical aspects of parentage testing and to briefly describe laboratory procedures. The chapter builds on a previous version written by Polesky (1) and begins with sections on historic background, basic principles, and selection of specific genetic markers routinely used in parentage testing. It continues with a discussion of the fundamental principles underlying the interpretation of standard parentage cases—situations where one putative father, an undisputed mother, and a child are tested. It ends with a discussion of nonstandard cases, including variations of paternity where a) the mother is not tested (motherless case), b) the putative father is deceased and his genetic markers are deduced from those of relatives (reconstruction case), and c) the putative father and child share an overwhelming number of genetic traits but mismatch at a single genetic marker (isolated single-locus inconsistency case). These are not necessarily mutually exclusive events, and the roles of tested individuals may interchange (i.e., disputed maternity). Often, several variations present themselves at once.

D.W. Gjertson: Departments of Biostatistics and Pathology and UCLA Immunogenetics Center, University of California, Los Angeles, California.

HISTORIC BACKGROUND

Any constant trait can be used to resolve questions of parentage. A constant trait has the following properties: a) is unaffected by age, disease, or other environmental conditions; b) is fully expressed at birth and remains constant throughout life; and c) is under strict genetic control so traits are inherited in a regular and reproducible manner. Before Mendel defined the gene, racial and other anthropologic measures had been used to exclude paternity. For example, Wiener (2) chronicled the practice of the ancient Carthaginians who relied on special committees for determining paternity. They examined all children at the age of 2 months and, if the resemblance to the father was not great enough, they condemned the children to death. In contradistinction, some native tribes of Central Australia did not put any faith in physical resemblance, because they did not believe in human fatherhood or that the nominal father had any share in procreation except that intercourse prepares a woman for conception (3). Pearson (4) summarized remarks made by Aristotle that skin color played a role when determining cases of doubtful paternity and, later, described the common practice by West Indies courts of deciding these matters based on skin mosaics and tints. In 1810, Archer (5) reported that a white woman, by intercourse with a white male and a black male, might conceive twins, one of whom is white, the other mulatto. Generally, however, physical characteristics (stature, skin and eye colors, earlobe shapes and other facial features, etc.) suffer two drawbacks that render them unacceptable for resolving parentage disputes. First, transmission of these traits is difficult to predict due to many genes interacting among themselves and with their environment (e.g., eye color may change with age and disease). Second and, perhaps more importantly, physical traits are readily apparent. A mother could identify a man who looks like her child and then make an accusation of paternity, but it would be circular for others to use the resemblance to corroborate her allegation.

The discovery by Landsteiner (6) of ABO markers and the establishment by von Dungern and Hirszfeld (7) that these factors were inherited started the modern incorporation of blood traits into the process of determining parenthood. Wiener summarizes early accounts of medicolegal applications of blood tests in several papers (8–10). Today, a laboratory's repertoire of tests includes markers on the red and white blood cells (e.g., human leukocyte antigen (HLA)-based evaluations), serum enzymes and proteins and, overwhelmingly, DNA-based markers. Reviews of the applications of these tests to paternity include those by numerous investigators (11–17).

In general, the methods for the detection of genetic markers and their inheritance patterns are firmly established and accepted by most courts throughout the world (18,19). European courts have relied on blood tests for excluding paternity since the 1920s (20) and for including paternity since the late 1950s (21). In the United States, blood tests have been accepted for the purpose of disproving paternity since the late 1930s (18), but the use of genetic evidence to prove paternity was of relatively recent onset (22). In 1976, the American Medical Association and the American Bar Association issued joint guidelines (18) suggesting that a statement on the likelihood of paternity be included in legal reports and, in 1983, the American Association of Blood Banks (AABB) issued guidelines for reporting estimates of inclusion probabilities in parentage test reports (23). Nowadays, the admissibility of genetic tests to prove or disprove claims of parentage is no longer in doubt (24)—some states have even deemed genetic testing conclusive. For example, in Tennessee, "an individual is conclusively presumed to be the father of a child if blood, genetic, or DNA tests show that the statistical probability of paternity is 99% or greater" (19).

Applications of laboratory tests to establish familial relationships include disputed fatherhood and motherhood, kidnapping, adoption, immigration, inheritance, interchange of infants at birth, and identification of human remains. Resolving disputed paternity is by far the most common application. As early as 1850, 5% of births in England and other parts of Europe were computed to be illegitimate (25). In 1968, 10% of live U.S. births were registered as illegitimate (26). By 1982, that number had increased to 17% (27), and present estimates exceed 30% of the 4,000,000 annual births (28). Over one-fourth of a million paternity cases are resolved by genetic testing each year (280, 510 cases documented by AABB for 1999; see www.aabb.org).

BASIC GENETIC PRINCIPLES UNDERLYING PARENTAGE TESTING

The classic ABO system (29–31) serves as a model to explain the basic principles involved when using blood tests for parentage cases. (Although DNA markers have largely supplanted traditional tests, the same genetic principles apply when analyzing DNA systems.) Agglutination of the two main antibody types, anti-A and anti-B, with antigens on the surface of red blood cells divides individuals into four elementary groups: a) AB, which reacts with both antibodies; b) A, which reacts only with anti-A; c) B, which reacts only with anti-B; and d) O, which reacts with neither antibody. These four groups are phenotypic expressions of an inherited genotype comprised of maternal and paternal genes or haplotypes. Bernstein (32) elucidated the exact mode of inheritance for these groups as simple or direct, meaning that groups are governed by single genes obeying Mendel's two laws.

Mendel's first law dictates that the alternate forms of the ABO genes (i.e., the two dominant alleles A and B, and the one recessive, silent allele O) have no permanent effect on one another when present in the same individual, but they segregate unchanged during meiotic division of the chromosomes by passing into different gametes. Mendel's second law asserts that genes on different chromosomes sort independently and can be predicted by rules of mathematic combination. Consider an individual who is phenotype A. Because the O allele is recessive to A, two genotypes (i.e., the homozygote, AA, and the heterozyote, AO) both give rise to the A phenotype. Even when using DNA-based tests, recessive genotypes must be considered, because single-fragment patterns may be due to silent or null alleles rather than due to true homozygosity or closely spaced fragments. If the individual is genotype AA, then the A allele will assort 100% of the time versus 50% if the AO genotype is present. The likelihood of a particular genotype is determined by the distribution of alleles in a defined population.

In general, estimating the distribution of alleles in the population is a complex process controlled by genetic as well as statistical sampling (33). Genetic sampling refers to variations that arise during the transmission of genetic material from generation to generation and that are influenced by forces of population size, mating structures, selection, and mutation. Statistical sampling refers to variations that arise when selecting individuals from within the same population and, for discrete genetic systems, that are governed by the multinomial theorem when every member of the population is equally likely to be chosen at any stage of sampling.

In 1908, G.H. Hardy and W. Weinberg derived simultaneously a rule that, when applicable, greatly simplifies estimating the distribution of alleles. A population is in Hardy-Weinberg equilibrium (HWE) whenever mating is random and mutation, selection, immigration, and emigration do not occur. Once in HWE, the processes of sexual reproduction alone do not alter the frequencies of genes, and frequencies will remain constant in every subsequent generation. In other words, estimates of frequencies of alleles are governed just by statistical sampling. A substantial body of evidence suggests that HWE can be practically assumed for genetic markers routinely used in parentage testing.

Strictly speaking, human populations cannot be in HWE because the forces of selection and mutation are ever present. Furthermore, multiple genetic systems may be physically linked when expressed on the same chromosome and may be dependent when expressed on different chromosomes due to population substructure (i.e., nonrandom assortment due to ethnic groups within racial designations marrying one another). The use of HWE and the *product rule* (another procedure of multiplying proportions of genes across independent loci to form a combined phenotype proportion) have been seriously questioned in forensic identification cases (34–36). Although methods exist for incorporating HW disequilibrium and population substructure into genetic calculations, empiric studies (37–42) assessing the use of the product rule and HWE have demonstrated that, for the major racial groups and for the routine markers used in parentage testing, corrections do not significantly alter the accuracy of calculations. For practical purposes, assuming HWE and independence across genetic systems yields valid results.

To conclude the ABO example, the assortment probability of the A gene from an A phenotype is derived assuming HWE. Let p, q and r be the frequencies for alleles A, B and O, respectively. (Note that we assume $p + q + r = 1$.) The distribution of possible ABO genotypes is derived from the multinomial theorem as: $(p + q + r)^2 = p^2 + 2pq + 2pr + q^2 + 2qr + r^2$, where p^2 is the frequency of genotype AA, 2pq is the frequency of genotype AB, and so on. The probability of genotype AA given phenotype A is $p^2 / (p^2 + 2pr)$ because the genotype is either AA or AO, and the probability of genotype AO given phenotype A is, therefore, $2pr / (p^2 + 2pr)$. The probability of transmitting the A gene equals the weighted average of each genotype's assortment probability with weights equal to the probabilities of the genotypes given the phenotype. Symbolically, the transmission probability equals $1 \times [p^2 / (p^2 + 2pr)] + 0.5 \times [2pr / (p^2 + 2pr)]$. For North American whites where $p = 0.26$ and $r = 0.67$, an A individual will transmit the A gene 58% of the time.

Complete coverage of all areas of genes and population genetics can be found in several reference works (33,43–45).

SELECTION OF GENETIC TESTS

Ideally, a test or test battery should efficiently exclude nonparents and include parents. In paternity testing, the statistic that measures the power of a test to eliminate nonfathers is the probability of exclusion (*A* for Ausschlußwahrscheinlichkeit, exclusion plausibility). *A* is the probability for a test to eliminate a falsely accused man given the constellation of mother-child genetic markers. Suppose that, in the ABO system, the mother is type O and the child is type B. Notwithstanding laboratory error or genetic anomaly (e.g. the Bombay phenotype for the mother) (30), B is the implied paternal marker. Let Q be the probability that B appears as an allele in the phenotype of a randomly selected individual of a given racial background. Then, $Q = 1 - (1 - q)^2$, where q is the frequency of B in that race, and $A = 1 - Q$. If $q = 0.07$ (a typical value for North American whites), then $Q = 0.14$, and $A = .86$, implying that 86% of wrongfully accused white men would be excluded as the father by the ABO blood test for this mother and child.

Prior to testing any member of a paternity trio, it is possible to estimate the average chance that testing will exclude parentage if the accused is not the parent. For each genetic system, an average power of exclusion ($\bar{A}$) can be calculated as the weighted average over all mother-child marker constellations based on the gene frequencies for alleles in the system. Wiener et al. (46) derived the general equation, $\bar{A} = pq(1 - pq)$, for a two-allele system, and Garber and Morris (47) derived the general equation for genetic systems of n codominant alleles. For more complex systems with recessive alleles and linked loci (e.g., HLA markers), Gjertson et al. (48) used empiric methods to estimate average powers of exclusion. Table 63.1 lists $\bar{A}$ for genetic systems commonly used in paternity testing. For example, the ABO system will exclude 14% of white nonfathers on average.

Many genetic systems (e.g., ABO) have limited power to exclude nonfathers; however, use of the product rule allows the results to be combined if test systems are independent, yielding a cumulative probability of exclusion:

$$\bar{A}_{CUM} = 1 - \prod_i (1 - \bar{A}_i),$$

where $\bar{A}_i$ is the average probability of paternity for system *i*. The power of combining independent tests is substantial. For example, combining ten tests, each with $\bar{A}$ of 0.14 (typical of the ABO antigens and many serum protein and enzyme systems) yields $\bar{A}_{CUM} = 1 - (1 - 0.14)^{10} = 78\%$. Combining four tests each with $\bar{A}$ of 0.9 (typical of HLA and some DNA systems) yields $\bar{A}_{CUM} = 99.99\%$. Such a battery would fail to exclude only 1 out of every 10,000 nonfathers.

Traditional Test Batteries

At present, there are approximately 75 to 100 genetic systems used to test cases of disputed parentage. Traditionally, laboratories chose a battery of serologic tests that provided an average power of exclusion above 95%. As seen in Table 63.1, there are several ways to achieve this goal by combining tests of HLA, red blood cell antigens, enzymes, and serum proteins (29–31; see Chapter 62).

The HLA system part of the major histocompatibility complex is one of the most powerful single genetic systems used in parentage testing ($\bar{A} = 95\%$ and 93% in blacks and whites, respectively). Although the HLA system consists of multiple loci (e.g., HLA-A, -B, -C, -D, -DR, -DP, and -DQ) located on chromosome 6, only serologic testing for antigens at the A and B loci are typically used in parentage testing. The usefulness of the HLA system in parentage testing relates to the great diversity and stability of antigens in all populations. Based on the close linkage of 20 A and 40 B specificities, it is possible to identify over 800 haplotypes and approximately 180,000 phenotypes.

Human leukocyte antigen typing depends on the observation of complement-dependent cytotoxicity whenever a viable lymphocyte suspension is incubated with the antibody (antiserum) having specificity for an antigen present on the surface of the test cells. To determine a person's HLA phenotype, it is necessary to type the cells with a large battery of antisera. Few antisera are monospecific, so two or more different sera are needed to define each antigen. All persons in a paternity case should be typed by the same laboratory at the same time in order to minimize the variability that can occur when cells are typed with reagents from different sources or lots.

ABO blood grouping has been the standard in cases of disputed parentage. When forward (cell) and reverse (serum) typ-

TABLE 63.1. AVERAGE PROBABILITIES OF EXCLUSION FOR U.S. BLACK AND WHITE NONFATHERS

System	Blacks	Whites	Ref
Classic Systems			
HLA	0.95	0.93	(48)
ABO	0.18	0.14	(48)
MNSs	0.34	0.30	(48)
Rh	0.18	0.26	(48)
Red Blood Cell Enzymes and Serum Proteins			
Phosphoglucomutase$_1$	0.31	0.32	(1)
Red blood cell acid phosphatase	0.17	0.24	(1)
Gamma marker (Gm)	0.19	0.21	(1)
Haptoglobin	0.19	0.18	(1)
Transferrin	0.11	0.18	(1)
Group Specific Component	0.22	0.31	(1)
DNA Systems			
VNTRs: probe/locus (enzyme)			
pAC256/D17S79 (PstI)	0.81	0.79	(16)
pa3'HVR/D16S85 (PvuII)	—	0.90	(77)
YNH24/D2S44 (HaeIII)	0.94	0.96	(78)
TBQ7/D10S28 (HaeIII)	0.98	0.96	(78)
EFD52/D17S26 (HaeIII)	0.95	0.91	(78)
SLI1335/D1S339 (HaeIII)	0.97	0.95	(78)
STRs			
HUMCSF1PO	0.63	0.56	(79)
HUMTHOX	0.51	0.35	(79)
HUMTH01	0.47	0.54	(79)
HUMvWA	0.65	0.64	(79)
D16S539	0.56	0.47	(79)
D7S820	0.52	0.59	(79)
D13S317	0.42	0.44	(79)
D5S818	0.56	0.45	(79)

HLA, human lymphocyte antigen; Rh, rhesus; VNTRs, variable number of tandem repeats; STRs, short tandem repeats.

ings are done, test results are usually unambiguous. If cells are typed as A or AB, subtyping is occasionally useful. In certain racial groups, ABO variants are more common than in others, and abnormal variants are possible. Examples of abnormal variants include the Bombay phenotype, in which persons fail to express an expected A or B antigen, and *cis* AB, in which persons inherit A and B as a single allele AB.

The Rh system is one of the most informative of the red blood cell antigen systems ($\bar{A}$ = 18% and 26% in blacks and whites, respectively). Serologic testing with anti-D, -C, -E, -c, -e (in E positives) and -Cw (in C positives) makes it possible to identify ten common phenotypes and numerous probable genotypes. In addition to the common types, several rare types have been described in which some of the expected antigens are missing or are suppressed. The specificity of the reagents used in routine Rh typing occasionally fails to detect the antigens present. This problem occurs because many of the antibodies recognize compound antigens. For example, anti-C often contains anti-Ce and does not react strongly with cells containing the haplotype CDE. When unusual findings occur in Rh typing, it is important to use different antisera and methods, to consider absorption and elution studies, and to study other family members.

The MNSs system is more likely to identify nonfathers than any other red blood cell antigen system ($\bar{A}$ = 34% and 30% in blacks and whites, respectively). In interpreting test results, it is important to be cautious about assigning genotype from the observed phenotype when a person types as positive for M, N, S, and s. In blacks, a frequently observed allele, S^u, can be misinterpreted as absence of an expected gene product. Persons appearing to be homozygous S or s can, in reality, be SS^u or sS^u. Other rare alleles include M^g and M^k. Typing reagents come from various sources (lectins, animal, human), and test results do not necessarily agree when the same sample is tested with different reagents. For this reason, independent duplicate tests and good quality control are essential for accurate results.

Other red blood cell groups include the Kell, Duffy, Kidd, Lewis, P, Lutheran, and Xg systems. The chance of obtaining useful information from these markers is limited because of their distribution in the population. Null alleles are present in all of these systems, and they are fairly common in Duffy. In blacks, the most common phenotype is Fy(a−b−). When expected antigens are not detected, absorption and elution studies are helpful to identify antigens that are nonreactive in agglutination tests.

There are dozens of red blood cell enzyme and serum protein systems for cases of disputed parentage used by various laboratories (1). Typing of their products is usually done by electrophoretic separation of protein bands, which are detected by staining, by immunofixation, or by a reaction with a specific substrate. Appropriate controls must be used with each electrophoretic run, and two trained technicians should read the patterns independently. When rare variants are found, they should be compared with specific controls or verified by an independent laboratory.

DNA Test Batteries

Traditional systems were limited to genetic variations expressed in the tested tissue (blood). Each tissue, however, contains a complete complement of DNA coding for all traits whether or not those traits are expressed in the tissue sampled. As a result, tests of DNA markers have largely supplanted the classic tests. The DNA tests generally have higher probabilities of exclusion, are less expensive, and are easier to perform. Currently, laboratories select a battery of DNA tests that provide an average power of exclusion well above 99%.

Compared to serologic tests, DNA batteries require fewer tests for the same level of exclusion so they reduce the quantity of tissue that needs to be drawn. This is a significant advantage of DNA testing over classic testing, because tissue other than blood can be used routinely to obtain results. More and more laboratories are collecting noninvasive biologic samples using buccal swabs.

The most widely used DNA tests detect restriction fragment length polymorphisms (RFLPs) by cleaving DNA with catalytic restriction enzymes recognizing specific nucleotide sequences. Markers are detected with radioactive, chemiluminescence, or colorimetric assays using the Southern method (49). Differences among individuals in the lengths of their fragments (usually measured in number of base pairs ranging from 500 to 10,000 pairs) are inherited characteristics that can be recognized by altered mobility of bands on agarose gel electrophoresis. The majority of RFLPs display genetic diversity by varying the number of tandem repeat (VNTR) units of core-sequence DNA (50). Typically, laboratories select a test battery of 3 to 4 VNTR loci (see Table 63.1) to provide an average power of exclusion above 99%.

Restriction fragment length polymorphism tests are not without difficulties. Although accuracy in DNA mobility measurements can be enhanced using densitometers, internal controls, and computer processing, inherent in electrophoresis systems is a resolution limitation that causes bands to have shape and width. Thus, a continuum of alleles, rather than discrete markers, is detected because measurement error is never zero. Typically, these measurement errors are 1% to 3% of band size. Closely spaced or overlapping RFLP bands will create ambiguous allelic assignments. Consequently, either statistically based matching criteria or modeling methods must be used in the analysis.

Incorporating DNA measurement variability into forensic and genetic analyses has been the subject of a number of recent reports (51,52). Most parentage laboratories doing RFLP testing use statistically based matching criteria—fixed or floating bins—to assign frequency values for RFLP alleles (53). Using split samples, laboratories evaluate their ability to reproduce results within and between runs and to routinely detect the minimum size difference between two bands. Two values, known as σ (within band measurement error) and δ (between band measurement error), are determined for each locus-probe-enzyme combination (54). In the fixed-bin method, the bin in which a band falls from a series of equal-sized bins over the range of observed alleles determines its frequency. In the floating-bin system, counting all database bands in a bin that is formed around the observed band plus or minus δ determines its frequency.

More recently, another class of VNTR loci that differ by two to six base-pair-repeat units has been used for parentage analysis. These loci are called short tandem repeats (STRs) and are detected using polymerase chain reaction (PCR) methodologies (55,56). The major advantages of STR-based markers compared to RFLP-based markers for parentage testing are a) the test methods are more amenable to automation (e.g., detection via capillary electrophoresis using the ABI Prism series of genetic analyzers), b) the DNA products are generally of discrete and separable lengths, and c) the conditions of sample storage are not usually critical. A major disadvantage of STR markers is that the number of alleles (usually 6 to 12) per system is fewer than those of the longer VNTRs (which have at least 20 discernable alleles) and, thus, individual STR systems have lower probabilities of exclusion (Table 63.1). Typically, laboratories need to select test batteries of 8 to 10 STR systems to provide an average power of exclusion above 99%. Because of the more limited polymorphism of STR loci, several marker systems may be amplified together or mixed prior to electrophoresis as long as the amplification conditions are compatible and the fragment sizes between loci do not overlap. Usually triplex or quadruplex systems of STRs can be assembled, and each multiplex provides an average power of exclusion similar to a single VNTR system.

EVALUATION OF A STANDARD PARENTAGE CASE

A standard parentage case begins with one witness, usually the mother (MO), accusing a man (herein called the tested man, TM) of fathering her child (CH), plus another witness, usually TM, denying paternity and implicating an alternative father, who is usually not tested. Blood or other tissue samples are taken under controlled conditions from the MO, CH, and TM, who can all be positively identified. These specimens, along with their recorded histories and witnessed consents, are sent to a parentage laboratory for genetic testing. Once specimens reach the laboratory, processing, testing, and interpretation are performed in a standard and verifiable manner, using proper written procedures and documenting strict compliance with these procedures in every case.

In the United States, several agencies accredit laboratories for parentage testing. Since 1990, the AABB has been the leading accrediting agency for parentage testing. The standards set forth by the AABB encompass all aspects of parentage testing, including specific qualifications, training and competence assessment of laboratory directors and other key personnel, equipment calibration and preventive maintenance, supplier qualifications, quality control and assurance, design control (including validation of test systems), reporting requirements, internal and external assessments, process improvement, facilities, and safety.

Exclusion Criteria

Upon completion of laboratory testing, examination of the genetic markers of MO and CH permits deduction of the paternal contribution by Mendel's laws. The paternal marker is commonly called the obligatory paternal gene (or genes in the case in which MO and CH share two markers—one by descent and the other by coincidence—leaving both markers undifferentiated). A failure to identify the obligatory gene(s) in TM constitutes a genetic inconsistency (an exclusion), and accumulated inconsistencies result in an opinion of nonpaternity. In the ABO example from the last section, in which the phenotypes of MO and CH were O and B, respectively, the obligatory paternal gene was B. If the phenotype of a TM were A, there would exist an ABO exclusion because he lacks the obligatory gene. Because of possible mutations and laboratory errors, most parentage laboratories require two or more independent genetic inconsistencies to consider issuing an opinion of nonpaternity.

A few parentage laboratories, relying solely on DNA-based evidence, are requiring three or more independent genetic inconsistencies (57). Because the chromosomal regions evaluated in parentage tests using practically all VNTR-RFLP and STR systems are in noncoding regions of DNA, their rates of mutations (ranging from 0.1% to 3%) are generally higher than those of classic systems (<0.1%) that code for proteins. Consequently, the plausibility of a false exclusion increases. Nevertheless, in parentage testing, samples typically are generous, permitting retesting and further DNA testing at will, by the original laboratory or referral to another laboratory if there is any doubt about mutation or laboratory error. (Also, alleged fathers have been known to have a friend substitute for them when specimens are collected.) If necessary, the entire procedure can be repeated because histories of participants are known.

Inclusion Criteria

Identifying the presence of the obligatory genes (or their possibilities) in the TM constitutes a genetic consistency (an inclusion of paternity). When TM matches CH, it is not sufficient to summarize the evidence by quoting A, $\bar{A}$, or $\bar{A}_{CUM}$ (or, equivalently, their complements of probabilities of matches by chance), because the values are based only on the markers of MO and CH and would not distinguish between tested men. In other words, these probabilities remain the same regardless of whether or not TM is excluded or included. The preferred approach for quantifying inclusions requires calculating the probability of paternity (*W* for Wahrscheinlichkeit der valterschaft, plausibility of paternity). The optimal properties of *W* for deciding paternity are well known and described in numerous papers (58–60). The logic of the calculation of *W* is presented next, followed by the principles and assumptions underlying its computational method.

Suppose two men (TM1 and TM2), unrelated to each other and to the MO, are named as possible fathers in a paternity case. All agree that the child's father is one of the two men, and no other evidence exists that distinguishes the men. The four individuals undergo genetic testing, and, for the sake of argument, assume that only one VNTR system (SLI1335/D1S339) is tested. (Normally, enough tests are conducted that one man would be excluded and, by the process of elimination, the other man would be the father.) The hypothetical results are shown in the left panel of Figure 63.1. The number, spacing, and position of bands corresponding to TM1 *(Lane 3),* TM2 *(Lane 4),* MO *(Lane 5),* and CH *(Lane 6)* are noted, and their sizes (in kilobase pairs, [kb]) are interpolated from the DNA molecular-size ladders placed in *Lane 1* and *Lane 11.* Because CH has a band at 2.13kb that is beyond 3% of band size for either of MO's bands (0.67kb and 2.67kb), this band is the obligatory paternal marker and, because both men possess a marker indistinguishable from this band, neither is excluded. Adding evidence that the two men and CH share a common band near 2.13kb are the results of coelectrophoresis experiments shown in *Lane 7* and *Lane 8.* MIX1 and MIX2 contain DNA aliquots from the CH mixed with each man's DNA, respectively. These "mixed lane" results demonstrate that possible band shifting during electrophoresis cannot explain the apparent matches among TM1, TM2, and CH. Summarized in the right panels of Figure 63.1 are the average sizes of the bands for the tested individuals under the two paternity hypotheses—TM1 fathered the child (top panel labeled *X*), and TM2 fathered the child (bottom panel labeled *Y*).

Suppose we have 1,000 such two-man cases, each resulting in the birth of one child. Without specifying the child's type and assuming that each man has equivalent fertility, 500 children would be fathered by men like TM1 and 500 by men like TM2. By Mendel's laws, the chance that a child, like CH, would result from a mating between TM1 and MO is 50%: a band near 2.13kb would assort from the man with probability 1 because he has been assigned a single band; a band near 2.67kb would assort from the mother with probability 0.5 because she has been assigned two bands; and a 2.13kb/2.67kb CH would be produced with probability $1 \times 0.5 = 50\%$. (For completeness, TM1 may truly have two coalesced bands, but this uncertainty does not affect *W*, because both bands are indistinguishable from one another as well as from the CH's band at 2.13kb. Further, he may have a null or silent allele but, to the extent that nulls are rare, this uncertainty does not alter *W* either.) Likewise, TM2 and MO would produce such an offspring 25% of the time because each adult has two bands. So, of the 500 children produced by TM1-type men, 250 (i.e., $500 \times 50\%$) children would appear to have the same genetic markers as CH; likewise, of the 500 children produced by TM2-type men, 125 (i.e., $500 \times 25\%$) would be expected to have the same genetic markers as CH. Thus, 375 (i.e., $250 + 125$) children would be produced who have the genetic markers like CH in our hypothetical case. But two-thirds of these 375 would be fathered by men of TM1's type and one-third by men of TM2's type. Men of TM1's type are twice as likely to produce such a child. Therefore, all else being equal (in accord with our hypothesis), the odds are 2 to 1 that TM1 is the father.

Even if TM2 does not show up for his blood test, we can still compute the odds. A randomly selected white would have a 6% chance of transmitting the 2.13kb marker to an offspring.

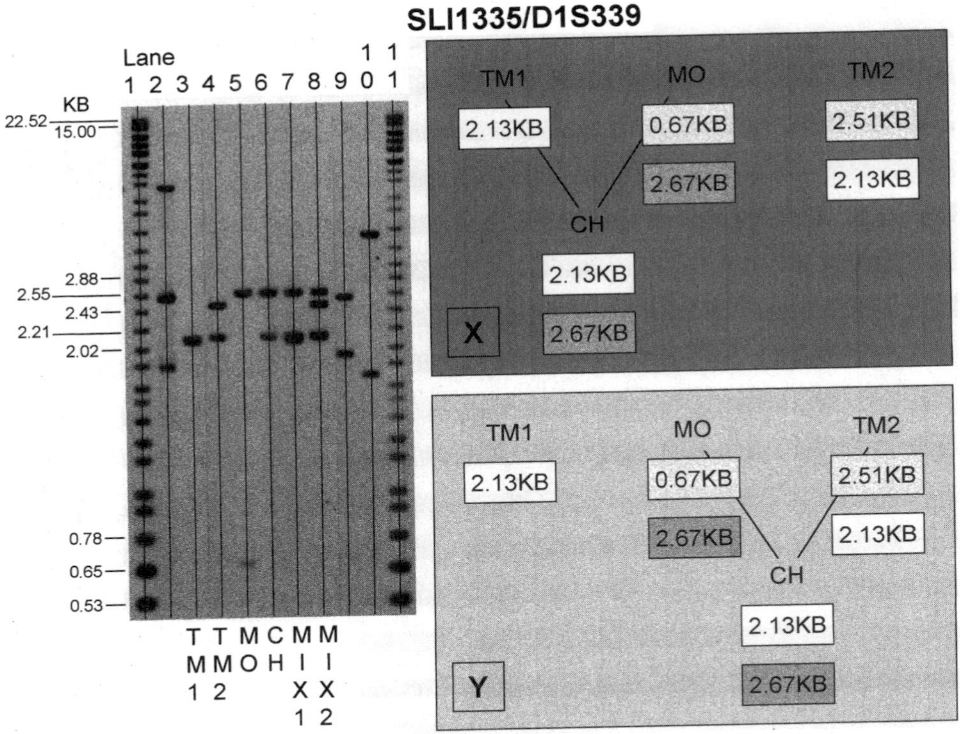

FIGURE 63.1. Example case showing a) the autoradiograph of genetic markers of TM1, TM2, MO, CH, MIX1 and MIX2 for one VNTR (SLI1335/D1S339) locus *(left panel),* and b) the average sizes of the detected bands for the tested individuals under the two paternity hypotheses: TM1 fathered the child *(top right panel labeled X),* and TM2 fathered the child *(bottom right panel labeled Y).*

It can be shown that the transmission probability for a marker from a randomly selected, but untested, individual is simply its frequency in the population (38). In floating-bin systems, it is determined by counting all database bands in a bin formed around the CH's band $\pm\delta = 2.13 \pm 2.13 \times (3\%) = 2.07 - 2.19$ kb. For whites, 203 of 3,238 bands (6%) fell into this interval. The untested TM2 and MO would produce an offspring like the CH 3% of the time (i.e., 0.5 × 6%). So, of the 500 children produced by untested TM2s, 15 (i.e., 500 × 3%) children would appear to have the same genetic markers as CH. Thus, 265 (i.e., 250 + 15) children would be produced who have the genetic markers like CH in our hypothetical case, but men of TM1's type would father 94% of those 265 children compared to 6% by untested TM2s. In other words, men of TM1's type are 15.67 times as likely to produce such a child compared to untested TM2 men. Therefore, all else being equal, the odds are 15.67 to 1 that TM1 is the father.

We may obtain the odds (or equivalently *W*) directly by computing and comparing the probabilities of producing a child under each of the two paternity hypotheses (X and Y). Under X (upper right panel of Figure 63.1), TM1's 2.13kb type mated with MO's 0.67kb/2.67kb type yields CH's 2.13kb/2.67kb type with probability 1 × 0.5 = 0.5. Under Y (lower right panel), an untested TM2 mated with MO yields CH's type with probability 0.06 × 0.5 = 0.03. Because each man was equally likely before paternity testing, we give equal weight of 0.5 to *X* and *Y*, and we conclude that the probability of paternity for TM1 is

$$W_{TM1} = (0.5) / [(0.5 + 0.03)] = 94\%$$

and the probability of paternity for the untested TM2 is

$$W_{TM2} = (0.03) / (0.5 + 0.03) = 6\%$$

In 1938, Essen-Möller (61) and his mathematic colleague, Quensel, devised a formula (generally known as the Essen-Möller formula) for the standard parentage case which enabled blood test findings to be expressed numerically as a probability of paternity. They arrived at the relationship shown above: $W = X / (X + Y)$ in which the sum of the probabilities of the hypotheses paternity (*X*) and nonpaternity (*Y*) equals 1. A somewhat different approach was suggested by Gurtler (21) to report the odds $PI = X / Y$ as the paternity index with large values suggesting fatherhood. The probability of paternity can be rewritten as

$$W = PI / (PI + 1)$$

In our hypothetical example, the VNTR system has significantly increased TM1's chances of being the true father compared to an untested man. $W = 94\%$ is higher than the prior chance of 50%. Most states require values exceeding 99%, so the results suggest examining other independent genetic systems such that, as a collection, the true father constellation becomes rare. If multiple, independent genetic markers are used in the diagnosis, the resulting probability of paternity W_{CUM} is given by a variation of the product rule

$$W_{CUM} = PI_{CUM} / (PI_{CUM} + 1)$$

where the cumulative PI for the series of independent tests is

$$PI_{CUM} = PI_1 \times PI_2 \times \ldots \times PI_N$$

Principles and Assumptions Underlying *W*

A rigorous formulation of *W* requires tedious computation and is described elsewhere (58). For DNA-based tests with unambiguous genotype assignment, tables of formulas exist for possible fragment-banding patterns, greatly simplifying the calculation (62). In complicated genetic systems (i.e., ones in which a single genotype cannot be deduced from a phenotype, like the ABO and HLA systems), the likelihood of a particular genotype among tested individuals needs to be determined from frequency tables for a defined population. The necessary steps are easily programmable and computer software exists that greatly expedites calculation. (For commercial software, see C. Brenner at www.dna-view.com.) Essen-Möller's equation assumes that the evidence other than the blood tests is equally balanced for and against paternity. Such an assumption, made by a laboratory, is sometimes justified on the basis that it has a neutral position. A better justification is that the assumption is made in order to illustrate the significance of the genetic evidence, which is summarized by the *PI*. Some laboratories present values of *W* under a variety of assumptions about the strength of the nongenetic evidence. A formula known as Bayes' theorem gives the probability of paternity *W* as a function of *PI* (that comes from the genetic evidence) and the prior probability of paternity π (that comes from the nongenetic evidence). Twenty-three years after Essen-Möller published his formula, Ihm (63) showed that the formula could be derived from a straightforward application of Bayes' theorem, a proposition introduced by the monk Thomas Bayes in 1763. The formula is

$$W\pi = (PI \times \pi) / [PI \times + (1 - \pi)]$$

Note that when $\pi = 0.5$, $W_{0.5} = PI / (PI + 1)$. Presentation of *W* at various prior probabilities facilitates the evaluation of evidence in cases in which there is more than one alternative father or the possible fathers differ in fertility or access. When the *PI* exceeds 1,000, even a prior probability as small as 1% results in a *W* value in excess of 90% (64–66).

Several other assumptions are necessary to properly interpret *W*. In parentage testing, the task of the laboratory is to perform the appropriate tests accurately and provide a biostatistical evaluation of the results. To use this information correctly, the judge needs to understand the basic principles and assess the assumptions underlying the evaluation. The assumptions can be categorized as fundamental, specific, empiric, and changeable.

Fundamental claims imply correctness in laws of genetics and mathematics. Specific assumptions include a) undisputed maternity, b) accurately identified subjects, and c) accurate lab results. Empiric assumptions involve a gene's frequency in a defined population. The need to estimate population frequencies on the basis of samples can introduce sampling error. Selvin has shown that large uncertainties in gene and haplotype frequencies may produce substantial variation in *PI* (67). Frequency tables are compiled from casework and can be sorted on the basis of race or ethnicity.

Changeable assumptions include randomness of mating (in which possible fathers are not related to the mother or to each other), race and, as mentioned above, the prior probability of paternity. For DNA-based tests, race is introduced to define a population of possible fathers in the formulation of *PI*. Gene frequencies are usually uncommon in each race or ethnic group but occasionally vary markedly from one racial group to the next. In practice, race is assigned by interview, and the alternative father's race is equated with that of the putative father. In casework, there exists a strong concordance in race among men who are tested when a mother identifies two or more men as possible fathers (38). In individual cases, a court or judge can consider the physical characteristics of the child and question any assumption about the race of the alternative father. In some cases, it is appropriate to test sensitivity in *W* based on various assumptions about the race of the father.

EVALUATION OF NONSTANDARD PARENTAGE CASES

What makes nonstandard parentage cases troublesome is the increased complexity when evaluating results. Cases include, but are not limited to, ones in which a) the mother is not tested (motherless case), b) the putative father is not tested and his genetic markers are deduced from those of relatives (reconstruction case), and c) the putative father and child share an overwhelming number of genetic traits but mismatch at a single genetic marker (isolated single-locus inconsistency case). The common themes among these cases are that more genetic information is missing, the missing information requires statistical imputation, and imputation generally increases the genetic uncertainty. For example, one needs to consider two obligatory paternal genes in most motherless cases, whereas usually one paternal gene is central to standard cases. Also, one must systematically evaluate four, as opposed to two, genetic markers for an untested putative father whose type is reconstructed after testing his heterozygous parents. Greater marker uncertainty decreases powers of exclusion and parentage indices alike, so that a greater number of genetic systems need to be investigated for the same accuracy as a standard case.

The types and frequencies of nonstandard parentage cases are rising. For example, at the University of California at Los Angeles (UCLA) in 1984, less than 0.1% of casework was motherless, whereas 10% of current casework is motherless (UCLA Tissue Typing Laboratory and Long Beach Genetics, Inc., raw data not shown). The variety of pedigrees requiring reconstruction has also grown as the number of reconstruction cases increases.

Much of the increase in nonstandard cases is due to the power of DNA-based tests, which allows laboratories to offer extended services. Some of the increase may be due to greater public awareness of the possibilities of parentage testing.

Valentin (68) and Asano et al. (69) formulated the general procedures whenever the mother was untested, and Ihm and Hummel (70) and Asano et al. (71) outlined the methods for calculating *W* using markers from relatives of deceased putative fathers. The most comprehensive report was prepared by Baur (72) and includes methods for calculating *W* for almost any type of dispute. For completeness, Brenner (73) discusses a computerized algorithm to settle arguments about the genetic relationship among any miscellaneous collection of people, and Wenk et al. (74) offer a method to summarize the genetic evidence that two persons are related when no other relatives are available for study (i.e., kinship studies).

Motherless Cases

The VNTR-D1S339 data in Figure 63.1 can be used to illustrate motherless cases by pretending MO's data in *Lane 5* does not exist. Without knowing MO's contribution, either of CH's two bands (at 2.13kb and 2.67kb) could have come from the father and, therefore, there are two possible obligatory paternity genes. To exclude a man, he must lack both bands. If Q is the probability that a 2.13kb or 2.67kb band appears as an allele in the phenotype of a randomly selected individual of a given racial background, then $Q = 1 - [1 - (q + r)]^2$ where q and r are the frequencies of the 2.13kb and 2.67kb bands, respectively. Let $A_{MO} = 1 - Q$, where the subscript MO denotes the motherless calculation. If $q = 0.06$ and $r = 0.05$ (values for North American whites compiled by Long Beach Genetics, Inc., who supplied the data), then $Q = 0.21$, and $A_{MO} = .79$, implying that 79% of wrongfully accused white men would be excluded as the father by the D1S339 test of CH only. Had MO been tested with the same results as before, $A = 88\%$. In other words, the power to exclude a falsely accused man has been reduced by 9 percentage points by not testing the MO. This reduction is typical for motherless cases. On average, $\bar{A}$ is reduced by ~10% whenever the MO is not tested (48).

Even though MO is not tested, the paternity of CH by either TM1 or TM2 is still consistent with the markers of these tested men and CH. Again, suppose TM2 is unavailable for testing. To calculate *W*, we must systematically impute the phenotype data of the missing MO.

One could list all the possible phenotypes for MO (without the knowledge of CH's phenotype), compute their probabilities as either 2xy or x^2 depending on zygosity and, finally, compute the conditional transmission probabilities for the 2.13kb and 2.67kb markers within each phenotype. However, because most phenotypes lack the 2.13kb or 2.67kb markers or both, most conditional transmission probabilities are zero. Alternatively, one can limit the calculation to just those phenotypes establishing a mother-child relationship knowing CH's phenotype.

The procedure is outlined as follows: Let M be the fictitious marker representing the collection of all other markers not near either 2.13kb or 2.67kb. M's frequency $m = 1 - (q + r)$ where q and r represent the band frequencies of the 2.13kb and 2.67kb markers, respectively. The relevant phenotypes for untested MO are a) 2.13, b) 2.13/2.67, c) 2.13/M, d) 2.67, and e) 2.67/M—otherwise, she would be excluded as the mother of CH.

For *X*, the case in which TM1 is assumed to be the father of CH, the relevant MO phenotypes further reduce to just types b, d, and e—otherwise TM1 would be excluded. TM1's 2.13kb type mated with each of MO's relevant types yields the CH's 2.13kb/2.67kb type with probability $(1 \times 0.5) \times 2qr + (1 \times 1) \times r^2 + (1 \times 0.5) \times 2rm$ where the values in parentheses represent transmission probabilities of TM1 and MO, respectively, according to Mendel's principles. The final element represents MO's relevant phenotype frequency under HWE. Simplifying with algebra, $X = r$.

Under *Y*, an untested TM2 mated with each of untested MO's five relevant types yields CH's type with probability $(r \times 1) \times q^2 + [(q + r) \times 0.5] \times 2qr + (r \times 0.5) \times 2qm + (q \times 1) \times r^2 + (q \times 0.5) \times 2rm$. (Note that the first element of each of *Y* term corresponds to the transmission probability for TM2's markers, which are known to us only in the statistical sense because he also was not tested.) With some algebra, $Y = 2qr$. (The result is intuitive, because the chance of observing CH's phenotype given two random, untyped parents is just its random frequency in the population.) If we give equal weight to *X* and *Y*, we conclude that the probability of paternity for TM1 is

$$W_{TM1} = (r) / [(r) + (2qr)] = 1 / (1 + 2q) = 89\%$$

To conclude, other than imputing MO's missing information, no other assumptions were necessary to evaluate a motherless case beyond those of a standard case. Once evaluated, the interpretation of exclusion or inclusion (i.e., *W*) remains the same.

Reconstruction Cases

Suppose TM1 is unavailable for testing, but tests could be made of some of his undisputed relatives. Analogous to the motherless case, it is possible to reconstruct his genetic markers and their frequencies and transmission probabilities from those of tested relatives. In Figure 63.1, let the bands in *Lane 3* and *Lane 4* now correspond to the father (F1) and mother (M1) of TM1 (i.e., the putative grandfather and putative grandmother), and let the bands in *Lane 5* and *Lane 6* remain those of the MO and CH. Again, the CH's band at 2.13kb is the obligatory paternal marker and, because at least one of the putative grandparents (in our specific scenario, both) possesses a marker indistinguishable from this band, they are not excluded as possible grandparents and, by descent, TM1 is not excluded either.

To obtain the probability of paternity, W_{REC}, we reconstruct TM1's transmission probability of the 2.13kb band from then phenotypes of F1 and M1. Tested man 1 has one of two possible D1S339 genotypes: 2.13kb/2.13kb (i.e., single-banded receiving a band near 2.13kb from each parent); or 2.13kb/2.51kb (i.e., double-banded receiving a band near 2.13kb from F1 and a band near 2.51kb from M1). The two genotypes are distinct and each occurs with 1:2 probability because M1 is double banded. Under *X*, TM1's possible types mated with MO's 0.67kb/2.67kb type yields CH's 2.13kb/2.67kb type with probability 0.5 × 1 × 0.5 + 0.5 × 0.5 × 0.5 = 0.375. Each term has three elements representing the probabilities of a) TM1 having a particular reconstructed genotype given the phenotypes of F1 and M1, b) the transmission probability of the 2.13kb marker from TM1, and c) the transmission probability for the 2.67kb marker from MO. Under *Y*, an untested TM2 mated with MO yields CH's type with probability 0.06 × 0.5 = 0.03. Because each man is equally likely to be the father before paternity testing, we give equal weight to *X* and *Y*, and we conclude that the probability of paternity for TM1 is

$$W_{REC} = (0.375) / (0.375 + 0.03) = 92\%$$

W_{REC} is only slightly smaller than W_{TM1} (94% from the standard case). Little information was lost regarding TM1's chances of transmitting a band near 2.13kb when both fictitious putative grandparents possessed copies of the obligatory gene. Previously, TM1 had a near-100% chance of transmitting at conception a band near 2.13kb when directly tested, and now he has a 75% chance of transmitting the band when indirectly tested through his parents.

The general principles of reconstruction cases can be extended to situations in which more information is unknown concerning the pedigree of the putative father. Let a subject in a pedigree be deemed external if neither parent is in the diagram, and extend the pedigree, if necessary, so that both parents are included for any member who is not external. Let a detailed pedigree (DP) be defined as the pedigree expanded to include the genetic markers of each member and the indication for each marker of a nonexternal member, whether it is maternal or paternal in origin. It is assumed that the DPs extend over the set of all DPs that are consistent with the tested individuals and that all of the DPs are distinct (i.e., the DPs are mutually exclusive and exhaustive). One can then compute a probability for each DP, starting with the externals whose probabilities are calculated as 2xy (double banded or heterozygotes) or x^2 (single banded or homozygotes). Probabilities for direct descendants of externals are then computed as products of the appropriate conditional probabilities (0.5 when a marker is received from a heterozygous external and 1 when a marker is received from a homozygous external) times the probabilities of the externals. One proceeds in like manner until all members have been accounted, and the result is the probability assigned initially to the DP, say, Q(DP). Next, the conditional probability for the DP given the observed phenotypes is given by

$$P(DP) = Q(DP) / \Sigma Q(DP),$$

where the sum (Σ) is over all distinct DPs. By summing over the appropriate DPs, one obtains the probabilities for the relevant genetic marker types for the putative father. From these, one can compute the probability that the putative father would transmit any given genetic marker.

The following situation illustrates the more general reconstruction case. Suppose that only the putative grandmother (M1 in *Lane 4*) was tested. Relative to TM1's pedigree, M1 is external and TM1 (albeit not tested) is a direct descendent. We extend the pedigree to include external F1 and list all sets of DPs that are consistent with the known markers of the pedigree. Just as in the motherless case, this means delineating the markers for F1 that are relevant and one additional fictitious marker corresponding to all the remaining markers. Under X, the relevant marker is the obligatory gene (band near 2.13kb). Let F represent the fictitious marker composed of all other markers not near either 2.13kb. Its frequency f = 1 − q where q is the frequency of the 2.13kb band. If q = 0.06, then f = 0.94.

From these markers come the relevant phenotypes for F1: a) 2.13, b) 2.13/F, and c) F. Next, combining M1's known type with F1's three possible types and an indication for each marker, whether it is maternal (m) or paternal (p) in origin, gives rise to 8 DPs. They are a) M1 = 2.13/2.51, F1 = 2.13, and TM1 = $2.13_m/2.13_p$; b) M1 = 2.13/2.51, F1 = 2.13, and TM1 = $2.51_m/2.13_p$; c) M1 = 2.13/2.51, F1 = 2.13/F, and TM1 = $2.13_m/2.13_p$; d) M1 = 2.13/2.51, F1 = 2.13/F, and TM1 = $2.51_m/2.13_p$; e) M1 = 2.13/2.51, F1 = 2.13/F, and TM1 = $2.13_m/F_p$; f) M1 = 2.13/2.51, F1 = 2.13/F, and TM1 = $2.51_m/F_p$; g) M1 = 2.13/2.51, F1 = F, and TM1 = $2.13_m/F_p$; and h) M1 = 2.13/2.51, F1 = F, and TM1 = $2.51_m/F_p$.

Using basic principles, we compute Q's and P's for each DP, then sum over the appropriate P(DP)s (the ones that contain the obligatory gene) to obtain the probabilities for the relevant genotypes for TM1. Without showing arithmetic details, there are three relevant genotypes for TM1: $2.13_m/2.13_p$, $2.13_m/F_p$, and $2.51_m/2.13_p$, with probabilities equal to 0.03, 0.03, and 0.47, respectively. Therefore, TM1's chance of transmitting the band near 2.13kb equals 0.28 (i.e., 0.03 × 1 + 0.03 × 0.5 + 0.47 × 0.5).

Mating of TM1's relevant type with MO's 0.67kb/2.67kb type yields CH's 2.13kb/2.67kb type with probability 0.28 × 0.5 = 0.14. As in the standard case, an untested TM2 mated with MO yields CH's type with probability 0.06 × 0.5 = 0.03. Because each man was equally likely to be the father before paternity testing, we give equal weight of 0.5 to *X* and *Y*, and we conclude that the probability of paternity for TM1 is

$$W_{REC} = 0.14 / (0.14 + 0.03) = 82\%$$

Now, W_{REC} is substantially smaller than W_{TM1} (94% from the standard case). The chances of TM1 having transmitted a band near 2.13kb have been reduced to 28% by not testing him and only testing one of his parents.

Isolated Single-locus Inconsistency Cases

A problematic outcome arises when there exists an isolated single-locus mismatch among many tested systems between the putative father and child. Mutation rates (μ) for VNTR and STR loci are on the order of 1:1,000 to 3:100, so absolute opinions of exclusion are unjustified based on just one of these systems, especially when all remaining systems yield a large combined *PI (residual PI)*. As pointed out by Fimmers et al. (75), modifying *PI* (or *W*) for a possible mutation pattern presents a practical, rather than theoretic, obstacle: the problem of identifi-

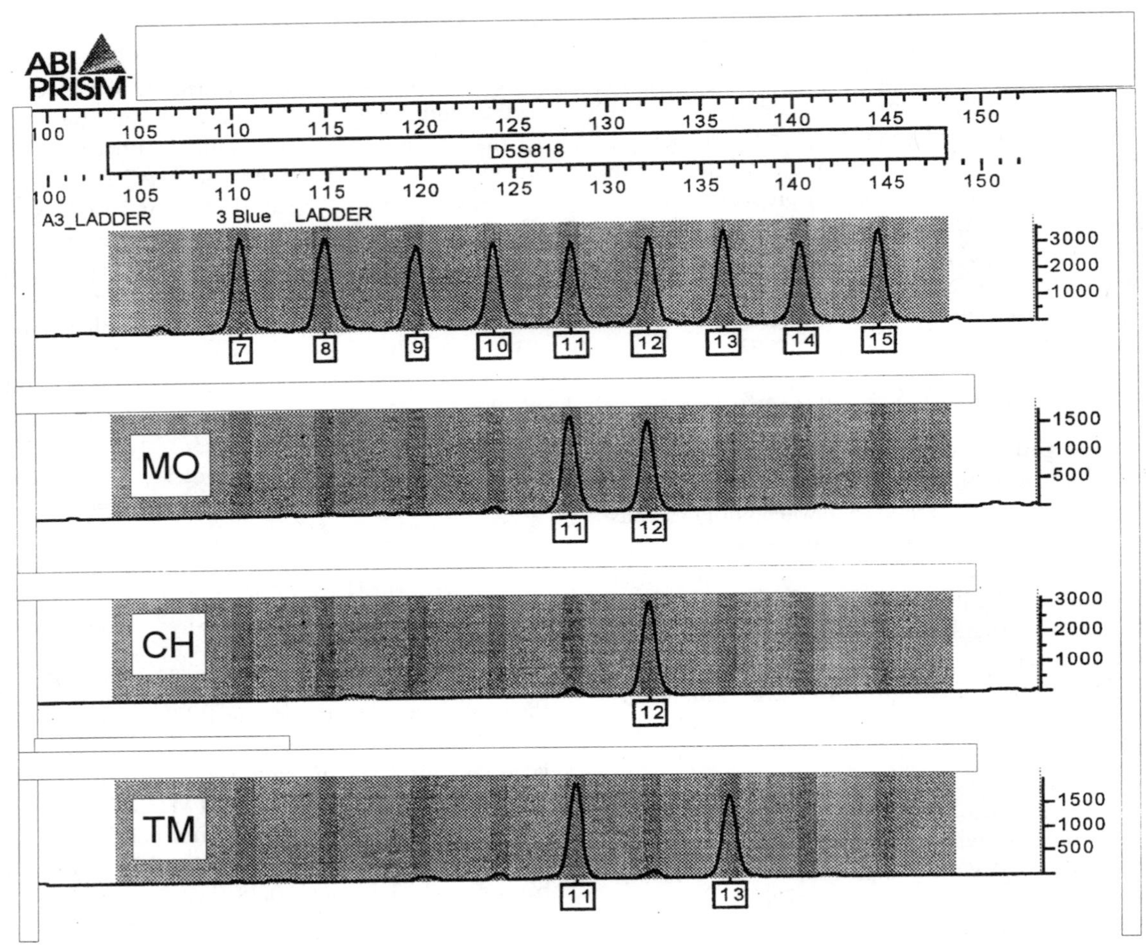

FIGURE 63.2. Example ABI Prism electropherograms showing a suspected DNA mutation between CH and TM for one STR (D5S818) locus.

ability when estimating parameters to describe specific mutational events.

Figure 63.2 illustrates a case whose subjects had an isolated mismatched STR system (D5S818) but otherwise had results from seven other STR loci (data not shown) consistent with paternity (*residual PI* = 1,774). (Note that duplicate testing of the MO and CH confirmed their genetic markers, implying that a simple sample exchange during the testing of the D5S818 system could not explain the isolated apparent exclusion.) In the D5S818 system, the TM possesses the 11 and 13 repeat-unit alleles, which do not appear in CH, so there exists a single-locus mismatch. Rarely, however, one of the TM's markers may mutate to produce a 12 repeat-unit allele. Alternatively, the TM may have produced an amorphous marker as the result of an unequal crossover or other anomaly during meiosis. Such a null or silent marker would be undetectable in both the TM and CH. Suppose $m_{I,J}$ equals the specific mutation fate for changing allele I to J where I and J come from the set of DNA fragments. Following Fimmers et al (75) instructions and ignoring null alleles, the *specific mutation PI* (PI_{SPC}) is roughly equal to

$$PI_{SPC} = (m_{11,12} + m_{13,12}) \;/\; 2f_{12},$$

where f_{12} represents the allele frequency of the 12-repeat-unit allele in a defined population. Unfortunately, this *PI* expression contains the specific mutation rates which usually lack precise estimation due to the degree of polymorphism in most DNA systems and the rarity of the phenomenon. Alternatively, an *average mutation PI* ($\overline{PI}$) can be derived on a per-system basis and substituted to compute an overall result as described next.

Initially, one tallies the frequency of cases displaying a single paternal discrepancy in the isolated system relative to a battery of DNA loci. The numerator equals this frequency, μ, because the banding pattern is either consistent with paternity or not. Under nonpaternity, the denominator depends on the chance of a correct exclusion. Hence, this probability equals the average probability of exclusion for nonfathers ($\bar{A}$). Then, the $\overline{PI}$ is given by

$$\overline{PI} = \mu \;/\; \bar{A}.$$

Returning to the example shown in Figure 63.2, $\mu = 0.0015$

(AABB Annual Report Summary for 1999) and $\bar{A}$ = 0.45 (Table 63.1) for the D5S818 system. Thus, $\overline{PI}$ = 0.0015 / 0.45 = 0.0033 and the overall PI = (0.0033) × (1,774) ≈6. If we give equal weight to TM's and an alternative man's prior probability of paternity, we conclude that W = 86% based on all the STR genetic information. Because PI greater than 100 is generally required for legal presumption, the overall results suggested that additional systems be tested for paternity after encountering the single isolated mismatch. Indeed, further laboratory testing was done using three VNTR systems, which did not demonstrate any additional exclusion. The final PI based on the 11 loci (including the isolated inconsistency) was 9,202 and W = 99.99%.

In practice, average mutation PI should be calculated by each laboratory using its empirically validated data, because values can vary depending on experimental conditions. Although the average mutation PI can be combined with remaining systems to obtain an overall result, one needs to be aware that, when using an average substitute, one is not making use of all of the information, and the actual mutation PI may be different for different banding patterns. To minimize the effects of possible extraneous PI values, one may use low estimates for the average mutation rate and routinely require that additional systems be tested for paternity after encountering a single isolated mismatch. The natural consequence is that, if the tested man is truly not the biologic father of the child, the probability of finding additional nonmatches leading to an opinion of exclusion is increased.

CONCLUSIONS

In the United States, about 45 laboratories are currently accredited by the AABB for parentage testing and, roughly, another 30 nonaccredited facilities offer to either perform or broker this service. (See www.aabb.org/About the AABB/Stds and Accred/aboutptlabs.pdf.) Among facilities, DNA-based technologies were used routinely on about 97% of all cases, whereas serology-based tests were used on only 3% of cases. The routine use of DNA-based genetic markers is the most significant development in the state-of-the-art of parentage testing in the last decade. Interestingly, the use of DNA tests in establishing paternity has been practically free of scientific controversy (as opposed to its use in criminal identification) due partly to its gradual introduction and partly because it was replacing already powerful conventional systems (e.g., HLA). The technical, genetic, and computational issues of parentage are the same regardless of whether DNA or serology-based tests are performed (80).

Technical issues are that specimens should be properly labeled, their chain of custody on transport to the laboratory should be documented and, once in the laboratory, they should be processed, tested, and interpreted in a standard and verifiable manner. The genetic issues are that systems used to resolve disputed parentage should be not only highly differentiated among individuals but also inherited in a regular and reliable pattern. Mutations do occur and, because they are expected to cause false mismatches rather than false matches, laboratories usually require two or more genetic inconsistencies to exclude a man from paternity. Computational issues include the validation of genetic marker frequencies and the product rule to combine results from two or more genetic systems. This chapter documented that these issues have been well resolved for both conventional and DNA tests.

Interestingly, the complexity of biostatistical evidence relied upon in parentage disputes has increased with the increased use of DNA-based tests. Variable number tandem repeat markers are detected chiefly by electrophoresis systems, with inherent resolution limitations leading to a continuum of alleles rather than discrete markers. To handle this uncertainty, the ideas of statistically-based matching criteria or Gaussian error models have been incorporated into the analysis. Further, electropherograms depicting STR results (Figure 63.2) needed statistical adjustment, too.

Beyond this, the sheer power of DNA systems has led clients to demand, and laboratories to accept, an increasing number of nonstandard parentage cases in which information is missing for one or more parties. Additional statistical methods were needed to impute this missing information. Because DNA mutation rates are larger than those of conventional markers, there is a higher incidence of problematic outcomes involving isolated mismatches among many tests between the putative father and child. Incorporating the possibility of mutation into parentage test results also complicates the evaluation. This chapter demonstrated that tools do exist to resolve a complex array of nonstandard parentage cases.

ACKNOWLEDGMENTS

The author wishes to acknowledge and thank Dr. John Taddie and Janice d'Autremont from Long Beach Genetics, Inc., for providing current data and casework for this chapter.

REFERENCES

1. Polesky HF: Applications of genetic marker typing in disputed parentage cases. In: Rossi EC, Simon T, Moss GS, et al., eds. *Principles of transfusion medicine,* 2nd ed. Baltimore: Williams & Wilkins, 1996: 849–861.
2. Wiener AS. Heredity and the lawyer. *Scientific Monthly* 1941;52: 139–146.
3. Read C. No paternity. *Journal of the Royal Anthropological Institute of Great Britain and Ireland* 1918;48:146–154.
4. Pearson K. Note on the skin-colour of the crosses between Negro and white. *Biometrika* 1909;6:348–353.
5. Archer F. Facts illustrating a disease peculiar to the female children of Negro slaves. *The Medical Repository* 1810;1:319–323.
6. Landsteiner K. Zur kenntnis der antifermentativen lytischen und agglutinierenden wirkungen des blutserums und der lymphe. *Zentralblatt für Bakteriologie* 1900;28:357–362.
7. von Dungern E, Hirszfeld L. Ueber vererbung gruppenspezifischer strukturen des blutes. *Zeitschrift für Immunitätsforschung und Experimentelle Therapie* 1910;6:284.
8. Wiener AS. *Blood groups and blood transfusions.* Springfield, IL: Charles C Thomas Publisher, 1935.
9. Wiener AS. *Rh-Hr blood types; applications in clinical and legal medicine and anthropology.* New York: Grune & Stratton, 1954.
10. Wiener AS. Forensic blood group genetics: critical historical review. *N Y State J Med* 1972;72:810–816.
11. Baird ML. DNA profiling: laboratory methods. In: Faigman DL, Kaye

DH, Saks MJ, et al., eds. Modern scientific evidence: the law and science of expert testimony. St. Paul: West Publishing, 1997:661–685.
12. Bryant NJ. *Disputed paternity: the value and application of blood tests.* New York: BC Decker, 1980.
13. Grumbaum BW, ed. Handbook for forensic individualization of human blood and bloodstains. Hayward, CA: Sartorius GmbH, 1981.
14. Lee CL. Current status of paternity testing. *Fam Law Q* 1975;9: 615–634.
15. Rolih SD, Judd WJ. *Serological methods in forensic science.* Arlington, VA: American Association of Blood Banks, 1985.
16. Smouse PE, Chakraborty R. The use of restriction fragment length polymorphisms in paternity analysis. *Am J Hum Genet* 1986;38: 918–939.
17. Terasaki PI. Resolution by HLA testing of 1,000 paternity cases not excluded by ABO testing. *J Fam Law* 1978;16:543–557.
18. Abbott JP, Miale JB, Jennings ER, et al. Joint AMA-ABA guidelines: present status of serologic testing. *Fam Law Q* 1976;10:247–285.
19. Faigman DL, Kaye DH, Saks MJ, et al., eds. Modern scientific evidence: the law and science of expert testimony, parentage testing, legal issues. St. Paul: West Publishing Co., 1997:748–760.
20. Schiff F. *Die Blutgruppen und ihre Anwendungsgebiete.* Berlin: Springer, 1933. (Translation in: *Selected contributions to the literature of blood groups and immunology.* Fort Knox, KY: US Army Medical Research Laboratory, 1971:329.)
21. Gurtler H. Principles of blood group statistical evaluation of paternity cases at the University Institute of Forensic Medicine Copenhagen. *Acta Med Leg Soc (Liege)* 1956;9:83–94.
22. Kaye DH, Kanwischer R. Admissibility of genetic testing in paternity litigation: a survey of state statutes. *Fam Law Q* 1988;22:109–116.
23. Walker RH, ed. *Inclusion probabilities in parentage testing.* Arlington, VA: American Association of Blood Banks, 1983.
24. Strong JW, ed. *McCormick on evidence,* 4th ed. St. Paul: West Publishing Co., 1992.
25. Goldsmid FH. Extracts from the tables and official information respecting the Prussian states for the year 1849, published by the Statistical Department at Berlin, and a few remarks by the translator. *Journal of the Statistical Society of London* 1860;23:201–221.
26. Stern C. *Principles of human genetics,* 3rd ed. San Francisco: Freeman, 1973.
27. Schutzman F. Interests of the Office of Child Support Enforcement, US Department of Health and Human Services. In: Walker RH, ed. *Inclusion probabilities in parentage testing.* Arlington, VA: American Association of Blood Banks, 1983:7–12.
28. Venture SJ, Martin JA, Curtin SC, et al. Births: final data for 1998. *Natl Vital Stat Rep* 2000;48:8.
29. Giblett ER. *Genetic markers in human blood.* Oxford: Blackwell Science, 1969.
30. Race RR, Sanger R. *Blood groups in man,* 6th ed. Oxford: Blackwell Science, 1975.
31. Salmon CJ, Cartron J, Rouger P. *The human blood groups.* Chicago: Year Book, 1984.
32. Bernstein F. Ergebnisse einer biostatischen zusammenfassenden betrachtung uber die erblichen blutstrukturen des menschen. *Klin Wochenschr*1924;3:1495.
33. Weir BS. *Genetic data analysis II.* Sunderland, MS: Sinauer Associates, 1996.
34. Lander ES. DNA fingerprinting on trial. *Nature* 1989;339:501–505.
35. Cohen JE, Lynch M, Taylor CE. Forensic DNA tests and Hardy-Weinberg equilibrium. *Science* 1991;253:1037–1038.
36. Lewontin RC, Hartl DL. Population genetics in forensic DNA typing. *Science* 1991;254:1745–1750.
37. Mickey MR, Gjertson DW, Terasaki PI. Empirical validation of the Essen-Möller probability of paternity. *Am J Hum Genet* 1986;39: 123–132.
38. Morris JW, Gjertson DW. The paternity index, population heterogeneity, and the product rule. In: Bar W, Fiori A, Rossi U, eds. *Advances in forensic haemogenetics 5.* Berlin: Springer-Verlag, 1993;435–437.
39. Morton NE. Genetic structure of forensic populations. *Proc Natl Acad Sci U S A* 1992;89:2556–2560.
40. Devlin B, Risch N, Roeder K. No excess of homozygosity at loci used for DNA fingerprinting. *Science* 1990;249:1416–1420.
41. Chakraborty R, Kidd K. The utility of DNA typing in forensic work. *Science* 1991;254:1735–1739.
42. Stivers DN, Chakraborty R. A test of allelic independence based on distributions of allele size differences at microsatellite loci. *Hum Hered* 1997;47:66–75.
43. Bodmer WF, Cavalli-Sforza LL. *Genetics, evolution and man.* San Francisco: Freeman, 1976.
44. Lewin B. *Genes,* 3rd ed. New York: John Wiley and Sons, 1987.
45. Li CC. *First course in population genetics.* Pacific Grove, CA: Boxwood Press, 1978.
46. Wiener AS, Lederer M, Polayes SH. Studies in isohemagglutination. IV: On the chance of providing non-paternity with special reference to blood groups. *J Immunol* 1930;19:259–282.
47. Garber RA, Morris JW. General equations for the average power of exclusion for genetic systems of n codominant alleles in one-parent and no-parent cases of disputed parentage. In: Walker RH, ed. *Inclusion probabilities in parentage testing.* Arlington, VA: American Association of Blood Banks, 1983:277–280.
48. Gjertson DW, Mickey MR, Terasaki PI. Empirical paternity exclusion rates. *Am J Forensic Med Pathol* 1987;8:123–126.
49. Southern EM. Detection of specific sequences among DNA fragments separated by gel electrophoresis. *J Mol Biol* 1975;98:503–517.
50. Nakamura Y, Leppert M, O'Connell P, et al. Variable number of tandem repeat (markers) for human gene mapping. *Science* 1987;235: 1616–1622.
51. Berry DA. Inferences using DNA profiling in forensic identification and paternity cases. *Statistical Science* 1991;6:175–205.
52. Roeder K. DNA fingerprinting: a review of the controversy. *Statistical Science* 1994;9:222–247.
53. Allen RW, Wallhermfechtel M, Miller MV. The application of restriction fragment length polymorphism mapping to parentage testing. *Transfusion* 1990;30:551–564.
54. Endean DJ. RFLP analysis for paternity testing: observations and caveats. Proceedings of the 1989 International Symposium on Human Identification. Madison, WI: Promega Corporation, 1989:55–76.
55. Mullis K, Faloona F, Scharf S, et al. Specific enzymatic amplification of DNA in vitro: the polymerase chain reaction. *Cold Spring Harbor Symposia on Quantitative Biology* 1986;51:263–272.
56. Edwards A, Civitello A, Hammond, et al. DNA typing and genetic mapping with trimeric and tetrameric tandem repeats. *Am J Hum Genet* 1991;49:746–756.
57. Gunn PR, Trueman K, Stapleton P, et al. DNA analysis in disputed parentage: the occurrence of two apparently false exclusions of paternity, both at short tandem repeat (STR) loci, in the one child. *Electrophoresis* 1997;18:1650–1652.
58. Baur MP, Elston RC, Gurtler H, et al. No fallacies in the formulation of the paternity index. *Am J Hum Genet* 1986;39:528–536.
59. Elston RC. Probability and paternity testing. *Am J Hum Genet* 1986; 39:112–122.
60. Mickey MR, Gjertson DW, Terasaki PI. Empirical validation of the Essen-Möller probability of paternity. *Am J Hum Genet* 1986;39: 123–132.
61. Essen-Möller E. Die Beweiskraft der Ahnlichkeit im vaterschaftsnachweis—theoretische grundlagen. *Mitteilungen der Anthropologischen Gesellschaft in Wien* 1938;68:9–53.
62. Traver M. Appendix 7: formulas for paternity index and RMNE values for simple codominant systems. In: *Guidance for standards for parentage testing laboratories.* Arlington, VA: American Association of Blood Banks, 2000:91.
63. Ihm P. Die mathematischen grundlagen, vor allem fur die statistische auswertung des serologischen und anthropologischen gutachtens. In: Hummel K, ed. *Die Medizinische Vaterschaftsbegutachtung mit Biostatistischem Beweis.* Stuttgart: Fischer, 1961;128–145.
64. Potthoff RF, Whittinghill M. Maximum-likelihood estimation of the proportion of nonpaternity. *Am J Hum Genet* 1965;17:480–494.
65. Hummel K, Kundinger O, Carl A. The realistic prior probability from blood group findings for cases involving one or more men. Part II. Determining the realistic prior probability in one-man cases (forensic

cases) in Freiburg, Munich, East Berlin, Austria, Switzerland, Denmark, and Sweden. In: Hummel K, Gerchow J, eds. *Biomathematical evidence of paternity.* Berlin: Springer-Verlag, 1981;81–87.

66. Baur MP, Rittner C, Wehner HD. The prior probability parameter in paternity testing. Its relevance and estimation by maximum likelihood. In: Lectures of the Ninth International Congress of the Society for Forensic Hemogenetics. Bern, 1981;389–392.
67. Selvin S. Some statistical properties of the paternity ratio. In: Walker RH, ed. *Inclusion probabilities in parentage testing.* Arlington, VA: American Association of Blood Banks, 1983;77–88.
68. Valentin J. Bayesian probability of paternity when mother or putative father are not tested: formulas for manual computation. *Hereditas* 1979; 149:405–416.
69. Asano M, Minakata K, Hattori H. Diagnosis of paternity for cases without the mother and without both mother and putative fathers based on blood group findings from the relatives. *Z Rechtsmed* 1980; 84:135–144.
70. Ihm P, Hummel K. A method to calculate the plausibly of paternity using blood group results of any relatives. *Z Immun-Forsch* 1975;149: 405–416.
71. Asano M, Minakata K, Hattori H. General formulas of the estimated likelihood ratio Y/X in the diagnosis of paternity of a deceased putative father. *Z Rechtsmed* 1980;84:125–133.
72. Baur MP. *Erweiterung des Essen-Möller-Modells und die praktische durchfuhrung der serologisch-biostatistischen abstammungsbegutachtung mit dem programmsystem P.A.P.I.* Bonn: Rheinische Friedrich-Wilhelms-Universitat, 1977.
73. Brenner CH. Symbolic kinship program. *Genetics* 1997;145:535–542. (Published erratum appears in *Genetics* 1997;147:following 398.)
74. Wenk RE, Traver M, Chiafari FA. Determination of sibship in any two persons. *Transfusion* 1996;36:259–262.
75. Fimmers R, Henke L, Henke J, et al. How to deal with mutations in DNA-testing. In: Rittner C, Schneider PM, eds. *Advances in forensic haemogenetics 4.* Berlin: Springer-Verlag, 1992:285–287.
76. Balazs I, Baird M, Clyne M, et al. Human population genetic studies of five hypervariable DNA loci. *Am J Hum Genet* 1989;44:182–190.
77. Allen RW, Bliss B, Pearson A. Characteristics of a DNA probe (pa3′HVR) when used for paternity testing. *Transfusion* 1989;29: 477–485.
78. Taddie J. Personnel communication, 2001.
79. Lins AM, Micka KA, Sprecher CJ, et al. Development and population study of an eight-locus short tandem repeat (STR) multiplex system. *J Forensic Sci* 1998;43:1–13.
80. Morris JW, Gjertson DW. Parentage testing; scientific status. In Faigman DL, Kaye D, Sates MJ, et al. *Modern scientific evidence: The law and science of expert testimony.* St. Paul: West Publishing, 1997; 760–778.

Rossi's Principles of Transfusion Medicine, Third Edition, edited by Toby L. Simon, Walter H. Dzik, Edward L. Snyder, Christopher P. Stowell, and Ronald G. Strauss. Lippincott Williams & Wilkins, Philadelphia © 2002.

64

TISSUE BANKING

JEANNE V. LINDEN

GROWTH OF TISSUE BANKING

Each year, tens of thousands of patients benefit from donated bone, cartilage, and tendons used to reconstruct and rehabilitate, corneas to avert or correct blindness, skin to treat burns, and reproductive tissue to redress infertility. Numerous other tissues are transplanted in medical practice for diverse clinical applications (Table 64.1). The most commonly transplanted allografts are bone, cornea, and skin (Table 64.2). The amount and variety of tissues collected, processed, and transplanted in the United States is difficult to determine because there is no national reporting system. In 1999, tissue banks distributed over 750,000 allografts for transplantation (1), including over 45,000 corneas (2). The number of musculoskeletal tissue allografts used annually is approximately 520,000 (2a). Skin is transplanted at the rate of about 7,740 square feet annually (2a). With improved preservation and processing techniques, transplantation of heart valves is now estimated at 4,900 annually (New York State Department of Health, unpublished data, 1999). These procedures require donation of cardiovascular tissue, musculoskeletal tissue and skin from over 20,000 cadaver donors (1) and eyes from 44,000 cadaver donors (2).

J.V. Linden: Department of Biomedical Sciences, New York State Department of Health and State University of New York, and Department of Pathology and Laboratory Medicine, Albany Medical College, Albany, New York.

In addition to tissues from cadaver donors, many tissues for clinical use are derived from living donors (Table 64.3), including semen and oocytes for use in artificial insemination and assisted reproductive technology procedures. In 1999, over 21,000 ejaculates were processed from 536 semen donors by New York State-licensed semen banks. These semen banks distributed over 60,000 vials of semen for artificial insemination. In addition, semen from 3,700 client depositors was collected and cryopreserved for later use (New York State Department of Health, unpublished data, 1999). Donor oocytes were used in approximately 10% of all assisted reproductive technology cycles carried out in the United States in 1998, or 7,756 cycles (3). Tissue from living donors also includes human milk to nourish low-birth-weight, premature infants. The Human Milk Banking Association of North America reports the existence of eight active member banks (4).

Because no comprehensive national usage figures are available, it is difficult to determine the rate of increase in the demand for tissues. However, novel uses for tissue in transplantation have emerged that were not envisioned just a few years ago. Amniotic membrane is transplanted to correct epithelial eye defects, bioengineered skin products are used for wound healing, and nerve tissue, from both cadaver and living donors, is transplanted to serve as a conduit for nerve regeneration in damaged limbs. In late 1998, the medical world was fascinated with the first hand transplant—there have been at least eight worldwide since. In the future, human pluripotent progenitor cells from embryos

TABLE 64.1. COMMON INDICATIONS FOR TISSUE TRANSPLANTATION

Tissue	Indications
Bone	Fill defects caused by malignancy or trauma
	Spinal fusion
	Revision for failed hip prosthesis
	Fill periodontal defects
Skin	Temporary covering for third-degree burns
Cornea	Corneal edema
	Herpetic scars
	Keratoconus
Heart valve	Replace damaged valves
Dura	Repair dura defect from trauma, malignancy
Fascia	Correct ptosis
Tendon	Replace injured knee ligament
Cartilage	Maxillofacial reconstruction
	Repaired damaged articular cartilage
Saphenous vein	Coronary artery bypass graft
	Leg revascularization
Reproductive tissue	Redress infertility
Amnion	Repair epithelial eye defects
Bioengineered tissue products	Diabetic ulcers
	Autologous skin or cartilage replacement

TABLE 64.2. ALLOGENEIC TISSUE DISTRIBUTED (ISSUED) FOR TRANSPLANT ANNUALLY IN THE UNITED STATES

Tissue	Units (Estimated)
Cadaver Tissue[a,b,c,d]	
Musculoskeletal tissue[a]	523,197
Cornea[b]	45,765
Pericardium[a]	9,577
Tendon[c]	8,624
Skin (sq ft)[a]	7,735
Fascia[c]	5,783
Heart valves[d]	4,900
Vessels[d]	4,100
Dura[c]	101
Living Donor Tissue[d,c]	
Semen (vials)[d]	>100,000
Oocyte/embryos[e]	30,963
Musculoskeletal tissue[d]	792
Amnion[d]	265

[a] American Association of Tissue Banks. Council of Accredited Member Tissue Meeting. March 2001.
[b] Eye Banks Association of America. Eye Banking Statistical Report. 1999.
[c] American Association of Tissue Banks. Survey of accredited tissue banks. 1996.
[d] New York State Department of Health (NYSDOH). Unpublished projected data based on 58,949 vials distributed by New York State-licensed tissue banks in 1999. (NYSDOH licenses semen banks located nationwide.)
[e] Centers for Disease Control. Society for Assisted Reproductive Technology (ART). Resolve. 1998 Assisted Reproductive Technology Success Rates. Based on 7,741 ART cycles using donor oocytes and four embryos transferred per cycle.

TABLE 64.3. KINDS OF DONORS PROVIDING TISSUE FOR TRANSPLANTATION

Cardiorespiratory and Neurologic Death	Living Donor
Cornea	Bone
Bone	Semen
Skin	Oocyte
Tendon	Amnion
Fascia	Fetal tissue
Heart valve	Nerve
Saphenous vein	Corneal limbus
Dura mater	
Cartilage	
Nerve	

may be used in the treatment of Parkinson disease, diabetes, and spinal cord injuries.

TISSUE DONATION

Tissue Donors

In contrast to organ donors, tissue donors do not need to have functioning circulation. Tissues such as bone, eyes, and skin can generally be collected up to 24 hours after cessation of the donor's cardiac and respiratory functions. Tissues such as bone and skin can be donated by organ donors with brain death, but more commonly, tissues are donated by other hospitalized patients who have experienced cardiorespiratory and neurologic death. Recently, tissue procurement practices have become more effective as a result of increased cooperation between tissue banks and organ procurement agencies through required referral statutes (5) (New York State PHL §4351). Several eye banks obtain a major portion of their donation referrals from medical examiners who have access to a large number of young, healthy individuals who experience sudden death and never reach a hospital (2).

Living Donors

The tissue most commonly donated by living donors is blood, the primary subject of this book, but living donors also provide other tissues (Table 64.3). Tissue donation by a living person generally is limited to renewable tissue, such as gametes, extraembryonic tissue, and human milk. Except for autografts, which are now sometimes cultured for expanded use in the burned patient, skin is almost always taken from cadavers and not from living donors. Cartilage can also be cultured for autologous transplant in knee repair. Bone can be obtained from living donors in the form of femoral heads and tibial plateaus that are removed and otherwise would be discarded during surgical procedures (total hip and knee replacements with prostheses). Recent attempts to transplant allogeneic nerve tissue have shown promise. The first such transplant from a living donor occurred in November, 2000 (CNN.com news report, November 17, 2000).

Required Referral for Tissue Donation

The availability of tissues for transplantation depends on strong public support, the presence of laws clearing legal barriers to donation, and the willingness of trained health professionals to approach the next-of-kin on the subject of donation. Key to this in the United States is a spirit of altruism and volunteerism coupled with the value of autonomous choice. In the United States, consent to donate is informed and voluntary with one exception. More than 60 eye banks are located in states with medical examiner laws that allow removal of corneas for transplantation under the following circumstances: a) the body is under the medical examiner's jurisdiction; b) autopsy is required by law; c) there is no known objection by the next-of-kin; and d) the removal will not disturb the body's appearance (6,7). These state laws presume consent and permit removal of eyes without an interview of the next-of-kin concerning the deceased's medical and social history and human immunodeficiency virus (HIV) or hepatitis risk behaviors. Two states, Maryland and California, expanded the law to cover non–medical examiner cases when a next-of-kin cannot be found (8). In 1992, 13,691 corneas were procured without consent under medical examiner laws. This represented 31% of all the corneas procured in the United States (6). In 1998, only 11 eye banks reported obtaining corneas through use of the states' medical examiner laws. Fifty-two other eye banks do not, for various reasons, take advantage of the medical examiner laws enacted in their respective states (9).

In the late 1980s, most states enacted required-request laws that sought to increase the supply of organs and tissues by requiring hospital personnel to request permission of the next-of-kin for organ and tissue donation at the time of a patient's death (if the prospective donor is medically eligible and there is a suitable need). In some states, such as New York, these laws were amended to require referral of all deaths to an organ procurement organization (OPO) or designated tissue bank so that specially trained persons will be available to request consent (New York State PHL §4351). Federal required-referral requirements were implemented through the Health Care Financing Administration's (HCFA) Hospital Conditions of Participation for Organ, Tissues and Eye Donation, effective August 21, 1998 (5). These rules mandate as a condition for Medicaid and Medicare reimbursement that all hospitals notify OPOs of all deaths and imminent deaths so that potential donors are identified and families are asked about donation. Hospitals must also work with at least one tissue bank and one eye bank to maximize donation opportunities. The effect of these required referral laws is not clear. In New York, where such a law went into effect on January 1, 1998, mixed results have been reported. Although a small increase in tissue donation has been realized statewide, certain metropolitan areas have reported a decline in eye donation. It is also not clear whether the increase in tissue donation in recent years is the result of required referral or of enhanced advertising campaigns and increased public awareness for organ and tissue donation (10). Under required referral, costs associated with around-the-clock reporting of deaths and imminent deaths are proving to be expensive in certain areas.

STRUCTURE AND FUNCTION OF A TISSUE BANK

System of Tissue Banking in the United States

Compared with the organ procurement and sharing system, the tissue bank complex in the United States is less organized. There are approximately 100 tissue banks in the United States that process musculoskeletal tissue, cardiovascular tissue, and skin. Although most are not for profit, a few for-profit companies process tissue for tissue banks. About 90% of the bone grafts used come from the 60 or more tissue banks accredited by the American Association of Tissue Banks (AATB). There are over 100 not-for-profit eye banks accredited by the Eye Bank Association of America (EBAA). Almost all cornea allografts used in the United States are provided by these eye banks. The safety and effectiveness of allografts is guided by national professional standards of AATB (11), EBAA (12), the American Society for Reproductive Medicine (ASRM) (13), and others. The U.S. Food and Drug Administration and several states, including New York, Florida, and California, have regulatory and licensure requirements (see section on regulation oversight of tissue banks below).

Public and Professional Education

Public altruism and the willingness of persons to be organ and tissue donors form the foundation of the transplant system. Effective public education is essential for successful organ and tissue donation programs (14). A major impediment to the procurement of more transplantable organs and tissues has been the failure of health care professionals to offer the next-of-kin the option of organ and tissue donation (15). Grieving relatives of a potential donor do not always spontaneously consider donation, but they should gently be offered the opportunity. This situation has been gradually improved by professional education and encouragement by federal and state legislation and initiatives (10). Media attention to organ and tissue transplantation has increased the recognition and credibility of OPOs and the public and professional support for donation. Some media inquiries, such as the *Orange County Register's* report entitled "The Body Brokers" (16), may serve to shake the public's confidence that donated tissues are handled with respect and do not result in excessive corporate profits.

Disease Transmission and Donor Suitability Criteria

When brain death is established, that patient is considered a cadaver, and the cadaver's suitability as a possible tissue donor can be determined. Despite a careful donor selection process, the risk of donor-to-recipient transmission of viral, bacterial, and fungal diseases remains (Table 64.4) (17). This risk is minimized by a careful review of the medical and social history, including HIV and hepatitis risk behaviors, physical examination, blood testing for infectious diseases, and autopsy results, if performed (Table 64.5). Evaluating the health history of the prospective donor is an important step in establishing the suitability of tissues for use and in preventing the transmission of infectious diseases to recipients. Certain criteria are used for selecting tissue donors (Table 64.5). General donor suitability criteria include the absence of systemic infection or any infectious or malignant disease transmissible by tissues. Cancer, with the exception of primary brain tumors without metastasis, generally disqualifies the tissue donor. The donor history review is specifically designed to exclude those at high risk for hepatitis or HIV (i.e., nonmedical injected drug users, men who have sex with other men, persons who exchange sex for money, persons with hemophilia or related clotting disorders, and other significant exposure to hepatitis or HIV) (11). Whenever possible, serologic tests should be performed on pretransfusion blood samples to avoid false-negative results in the event massive transfusions were given near the time of death (18). In the case of posttransfusion specimens, algorithms for determining hemodilution are available (11). Testing of postmortem blood specimens can be complicated by hemolysis, which can cause false-positive results in some hepatitis B surface antigen enzyme immunoassays (HBsAg EIAs) and false-negative results in some HIV nucleic acid tests. There are new tests on the market for HIV and hepatitis that have been validated for use with postmortem specimens. Infectious diseases can also be transmitted through transplant of tissue from living donors. Cases are well-documented in the semen banking arena (Table 64.6) (19).

In addition to the general selection criteria for donors, there are specific eligibility criteria for each tissue type to ensure that the donated materials will function adequately (Table 64.7). When practical, tissue from living donors is cryopreserved and quarantined prior to retesting the donor for HIV and hepatitis to rule out seroconversion during the time of storage. Specific regulatory requirements for quarantine generally apply to semen donors.

TABLE 64.4. INFECTIOUS DISEASES REPORTED TO HAVE BEEN TRANSMITTED BY TISSUE ALLOGRAFTS

Allografts	Infectious Disease
Bone	Hepatitis C
	Hepatitis, unspecified type
	HIV-1
	Bacteria
	Tuberculosis
Cornea	Hepatitis B
	Rabies
	Creutzfeldt-Jakob disease
	Cytomergalovirus (?)
	Bacteria
	Fungus
Dura	Creutzfeldt-Jakob disease
Heart valve	Hepatitis B
	Tuberculosis
Skin	Bacteria
	Cytomegalovirus (?)
	HIV-1 (?)
Pericardium	Creutzfeldt-Jakob disease
	Bacteria
Pancreatic islet	Bacteria

HIV, human immunodeficiency virus.
From Eastlund T. Infectious disease transmission through cell, tissue and organ transplantation. Reducing the risk through donor selection. *Cell Transplant* 1995;4:455–477, with permission.

TABLE 64.5. CADAVER TISSUE DONOR SELECTION STEPS TO PREVENT DISEASE TRANSMISSION

No Monetary Incentive to Donate
Health History Review
Interview with next of kin
Review of medical records
Interview with health care provider
Exclusion of those with infection, malignancy
No degenerative neurologic disease
No autoimmune disease
No human pituitary-derived hormone use
HIV, Hepatitis Risk-behavior Exclusions
Persons with clinical or laboratory evidence of HIV infection[a]
Men who have had sex with another man in past 5 years
Past or present nonmedical injections of drugs in past 5 years
Persons with hemophilia or related clotting disorders who have received clotting factor concentrates
Persons who engaged in sex for money or drugs in past 5 years
Persons who had sex with any of the above in past 12 months
Treatment for syphilis or gonorrhea in past 12 months
Prison inmate for at least 7 days in the past 12 months
Tattoo in past 12 months
Blood Tests
HBsAg
Anti-HIV-1/HIV-2
Anti-HCV
Anti-HTLV-1
Syphilis
Maternal HIV Testing and Risk Factor Exclusion if Donor <18 Months Old
Physical Examination
Unexplained jaundice
Evidence of intravenous drug use
Extend signs of infection
Autopsy Examination (If Performed)

HIV, human immunodeficiency virus; HBsAg, hepatitis B surface antigen; HTLV, human T-lymphotropic virus.
[a] Signs and symptoms are unexplained weight loss, night sweats, spots typical of Kaposi sarcoma on or under the skin or mucous membranes, swollen lymph nodes lasting more than 1 month, persistent white spots or unusual blemishes in the mouth, fevers above 99°F for more than 10 days, persistent cough and shortness of breath, persistent diarrhea.

Tissue Procurement

Tissues are collected aseptically in the operating room (with or without subsequent sterilization) or in the autopsy room (in which case the tissues are usually sterilized).

Informed Consent for Tissue Donation

In the spring of 2000, several highly publicized newspaper investigative series triggered a national debate on the ethics of procuring and processing tissue for profit (16). Questions were raised about the propriety of financial gain from tissue donation, diverting tissue needed for life-saving purposes to cosmetic uses, the inadequacies of informed consent, and the extent to which the tissue banking industry was monitored. An investigation

TABLE 64.6. TRANSMISSION OF INFECTIOUS DISEASES TO SEMEN RECIPIENTS

Authors	Agents and Diseases	No of Reported Cases/ No Women Exposed[a]	Transmissibility
Stewart *et al.* (9)	HIV-1	4/8	Yes
Chiasson *et al.* (10)	(donor)	1/134	—
Rekart (14)	—	2/24	—
Mascola (15)	—	1/89	—
		2/46	—
		1/10	—
CDC (12)	HIV-1 (husband-wife)	1/1	—
Berry *et al.* (17)	Hepatitis B virus	1/1	Yes
	Hepatitis C virus	0	Likely
Fiurmara (23)	Gonorrhea	1/1	Yes
Hansen *et al.* (25)	—	3/unknown	—
Barwin (30)	*Ureaplasma urealyticum*	1/1	Yes
Caspi *et al.* (31)	*Mycoplasma hominis*	1/1	Yes
Kleegman (32)	*Trichomonas vaginalis*	2/2	Yes
Moore *et al.* (33)	HSV-2	1/2	Yes
Nagel *et al.* (35)	*Chlamydia trachomatis*	1/1	Yes
Kleegman	Group B streptococcus	2/2	Yes
—	CMV	0	Possible
—	Human papilloma virus	0	Possible
—	HTLV-1	0	Likely
—	Syphilis	0	Possible

CDC, Centers for Disease Control; HIV, human immunodeficiency virus; HSV, herpes simples virus; CMV, cytomegalovirus; HTLV, human T-lymphotropic virus.
[a] Number tested, where applicable.
From Linden JV, Crister JK. Therapeutic insemination by donor II: a review of its known risks. *Repro Med Rev* 1995;4:19–29, with permission.

by the Department of Health and Human Services Office of Inspector General (OIG) followed. In its report, the OIG recommended that tissue banks make their finances public and enhance informed consent processes by describing potential uses of donated tissue and disclosing the bank's relationships with other companies (1). The OIG also recommended that the Food and Drug Administration expedite the publication of its proposed regulatory agenda for tissue banks. There is evidence that the industry is responding to concerns about diversion of tissue for cosmetic purposes. For example, one criticism has been that skin needed for medically necessary reconstruction is sometimes diverted for cosmetic surgical uses, thus creating shortages of skin for patients with burns (although the AATB's Council on Accredited Member Tissue Banks 2001 meeting cited a distribution problem rather than a shortage of transplantable skin). A large skin processor that extracts collagen for both medical reconstruction and cosmetic uses is offering skin procurers the option of using a dermatome designed to harvest skin in two layers (20). With the first pass, the dermatome peels away the top layer of skin suitable for burns. With the second pass, it removes the deeper dermal layer that may be processed for collagen extraction, which can be further processed to meet cosmetic surgical needs.

GENERAL PRINCIPLES OF TISSUE PRESERVATION AND TRANSPLANTATION

Preservation of tissues is much easier than preservation of vascularized solid organs. Effective tissue preservation methods include freezing, refrigeration, drying, and the use of chemicals. The maximal permissible length of storage depends on the tissue and the preservation method (Table 64.8). Storage conditions and dating periods have been set by national standard-setting organizations (11,12).

Excluding bone, which is usually freeze dried, the most common method of storing tissues is in cold temperatures, either refrigerated storage or cryopreservation and storage in the frozen state. For short-term storage, refrigeration at 4°C or freezing often suffices, whereas long-term storage usually requires a frozen state. Several tissues can be preserved by a variety of methods. Bone and dura mater can be effectively cryopreserved or lyophilized. Much of the lyophilized and cryopreserved human tissue used in transplantation serves a structural purpose and need not be preserved in a viable state (Table 64.9). These tissues are composed of an extracellular matrix (such as collagen) with few or no viable cells present to support the matrix after transplantation. In some tissue, such as the cornea, a single layer of viable donor cells is important. In other tissues, supportive host cells infiltrate and slowly replace the transplanted structure. For example, bone, connective tissue, and dura commonly are freeze dried and used largely as nonviable transplants of extracellular matrix permitting ingrowth of metabolically active host cells following transplantation. Other human tissues, such as blood, marrow, skin, cornea, and gametes, are stored by refrigeration or cryopreservation. For these tissues, posttransplantation viability is essential, and their usefulness after transplantation depends on maintaining not only metabolic activity but also the capacity

TABLE 64.7. TISSUE-SPECIFIC DONOR ELIGIBILITY CRITERIA

Bone and Connective Tissue
Age: 15–55 years if male and donated bone is for weight-bearing use; 15–45 years if female and donated bone is for weight-bearing use
No exposure to toxic substances that might accumulate in bone
No bone metabolic disease or significant connective tissue disorder
No radiation therapy to bone
No long-term, high-dose corticosteroid use
Skin
Age: 14–65 years
No skin infection or rash
Eye
Age: 1–80 years (5–50 years preferred)
No corneal defect or disease
Heart Valve
Age: 0–50 years
Weight: At least 5 pounds
No known heart disorder affecting valves
Semen
Age: 18–39 years
No inherited disease
Normal semen analysis
Negative semen culture for gonorrhea
Oocyte
Age: 21–34
No inherited disease
Saphenous Vein
Age: up to 55 years
No diabetes or significant hypertension
No varicose veins, significant atherosclerosis, or trauma to the vessels
Extraembryonic Tissue (Amnion, Umbilical Vein)
Age: full term at time of delivery
No meconium staining of amniotic fluid
No pelvic or vaginal infection
Consent of both parents

TABLE 64.9. POSTTRANSPLANT ROLE OF PRESERVED HUMAN TISSUE IN CLINICAL USE

Structural
Bone
Dura mater
Fascia lata
Tendon
Cartilage
Skin
Heart valve
Amnion
Cornea
Vein
Artery
Metabolic, Replicative
Red blood cell
Platelet
Bone marrow
Blood stem cells
Semen
Oocyte
Embryo
Fetal tissue
Parathyroid gland

TABLE 64.8. RECOMMENDED PRESERVATION CONDITIONS AND DATING PERIOD FOR HUMAN TISSUE

Tissue	Storage Condition	Dating Period
Bone	−40°C	5 years
—	−20°C	6 months
—	1–10°C	15 days
—	Liquid nitrogen	Not defined
—	Lyophilized, room temperature	5 years
Tendon	−40°C	5 years
Fascia lata	Lyophilized, room temperature	5 years
—	−40°C	5 years
Articular cartilage	−40°C	5 years
—	Liquid nitrogen, immersed	Not defined
Skin	1–10°C	14 days
—	−40°C	5 years
Cornea	2–6°C	14 days
Heart valve, vein, artery	−100°C	Not defined
Dura	Lyophilized, room temperature	Not defined
Semen	Liquid nitrogen, immersed	Not defined
—	Liquid nitrogen, vapor phase	Not defined

Adapted from Vengelen-Tyler V, ed. *Technical manual,* 13th ed. Bethesda, MD: American Association of Blood Banks, 1999:569, with permission.

to synthesize protein, to proliferate, or to differentiate. Therefore, effective cryopreservation is more difficult.

Bone Processing, Preservation, and Transplantation

Clinical Use of Bone Grafts

Bone allografts have many uses, including providing acetabular and proximal femur support for replacement of failed prosthetic hip joints, packing benign bone cysts, fusing the cervical or lumbar spine to correct disk disease or scoliosis, restoring alveolar bone in periodontal pockets, reconstructing maxillofacial deficits, or replacing resected bone involved with a slowly spreading bone malignancy (such as osteosarcoma). The latter procedure is accomplished with large osteochondral allografts that permit tumor resection and cure without limb amputation.

Usually, when bone grafting is needed, fresh autograft is taken from the patient's own iliac crest during surgery. Fresh bone autograft is the most effective material, but preserved allografts are practical alternatives that approximate the results obtained with fresh bone autograft (21). In some patients, an autograft is not an option because sufficient bone is not available. In addition, bone allografts reduce operating room time and the number of operative sites, leading to reduced morbidity and lower cost (Table 64.10). However, the use of bone allograft carries the risk of donor-to-recipient transmission of infectious disease (17), a risk that is minimized by careful donor selection and testing, and disinfection and sterilization during tissue processing. Bone for grafting usually is available in three forms: frozen, lyophilized, and (to a lesser extent) air dried.

Frozen Bone

Bone, collected under aseptic conditions in the operating room and subsequently frozen, is available in a wide variety of shapes and sizes from cadaveric donors, or as femoral heads or tibial plateaus obtained from living donors undergoing total joint replacement. This frozen bone is largely free of bacteria, but it does carry the risk of viral transmission. Diseases known to have been transmitted by unprocessed bone include HIV, tuberculosis, and hepatitis. Today, the risk of disease transmission by frozen bone is reduced greatly by careful review of donor health history, physical examination, autopsy results (if performed), and testing for HIV antibody, hepatitis C virus (HCV) antibody, HBsAg, human T-cell lymphotropic virus type I (HTLV-I), and syphilis. Some tissue banks also screen donors for hepatitis B core antibody. Transmission of bacterial or viral infection with bone allograft is a well-documented risk, but it is exceedingly low. For example, the risk of transmitting HIV through bone grafting has been calculated to be less than one per million grafts (22) and is even lower if grafts are subjected to sterilization using γ-irradiation or ethylene oxide. In one well-publicized case, whole frozen bone did transmit HIV, while bone from which the marrow had been removed did not (23). Frozen bone can cause alloimmunization from exposure to antigens on the attached connective tissues, marrow, and blood, although it apparently does not affect the outcome of the graft. Detailed reviews addressing the role of histocompatibility and the immune response in bone allograft transplantation have been published (24,25). Antibodies to histocompatibility antigens (24,25), blood group antigens (26), and bone matrix proteins have been induced by transplanted frozen bone. To avoid Rh alloimmunization, Rh-negative bone usually is selected if the bone has not been processed to remove red blood cells and the recipient is an Rh-negative female with child-bearing potential.

Aseptically collected cadaveric bone is cut into usable shapes and sizes under aseptic conditions. Each allograft is prepared further by removing extraneous tissue, culturing to detect bacteria, dipping in an antibiotic solution (optional), packaging, and storage at −40°C or lower. No further processing is required. Frozen cadaveric bone commonly is available as femoral head, proximal femur, distal femoral condyle, whole femur or tibia, iliac crest, and rib. Frozen bone can be stored up to 5 years at −40°C. This form of preservation does not maintain cellular viability; thus, frozen bone is used for structural support that depends on an intact calcified extracellular matrix or is used as filler to promote new bone formation. These storage periods have been chosen arbitrarily; there is no evidence that the biomechanical or osteoinductive properties of bone decline during frozen storage.

Bone that otherwise would be discarded can be collected from living donors during surgical procedures (total hip or knee replacements with prostheses). The suitability of a volunteer living donor is determined by a careful health history review and blood testing for HIV, HBsAg, HTLV-I, HCV, and syphilis (11). Many tissue banks also will test for hepatitis B core antibody. After bacteriologic culturing, these bone specimens usually do not undergo further processing and are stored frozen. Standards call for frozen bone from a living donor to be preserved at −40°C and not released for use until the donor has had a second negative HIV test on a new blood sample obtained 6 months after donation. This step is intended to eliminate donors who were in the early stage of HIV infection but were antibody negative at the time of donation (termed the *window period*).

TABLE 64.10. A COMPARISON OF BONE AUTOGRAFT AND ALLOGRAFT: ADVANTAGES AND DISADVANTAGES

Autograft Advantages
Unsurpassed incorporation
Histocompatible
Autograft Disadvantages
Limited supply
Donor site morbidity
Prolonged anesthesia
Increased blood loss
Allograft Advantages
Readily available, unlimited supply
Wide choice of size, shapes
Easy storage
Allograft Disadvantages
May transmit disease
Immunogenic

Lyophilized Bone

Bone can be obtained from cadavers in the hospital operating room or autopsy room. The bone is placed on ice for transport to a tissue laboratory, where it is frozen at −40°C or lower until further processing, which includes removal of surface tissues and internal fat, blood, and marrow by means of mechanical agitation, high-pressure water jets, and alcohol soaks. Then the bone is cut into clinically useful shapes and sizes (e.g., strips, blocks, dowels, struts, and cubes) or ground into powder. The bone allografts are then lyophilized to a residual moisture content of less than 5% and stoppered sterilely under vacuum. Samples of each batch are tested for sterility. Bone is often sterilized with ethylene oxide (27) or γ-irradiation. Some physicians prefer irradiation because of the possible carcinogenic risk associated with exposure to ethylene oxide residue (28).

Routine quality control testing of bone is designed to monitor safety rather than potency or efficacy. Potency can be studied by using assays for osteoinductive capacity and biomechanical properties, but these analyses usually are applied only when there is a change in the production process. Lyophilized bone is not viable and is brittle unless fully rehydrated prior to use. Lyophilized bone can be stored at room temperature for up to 5 years.

Bone collected aseptically in the operating room and processed aseptically can be lyophilized without use of a sterilant. Because the bone is bacteria free, final sterilization with ethylene oxide or γ-irradiation is not necessary. Although the bone is free of bacteria, it still has the potential to transmit viral diseases. Despite this risk, some physicians prefer aseptically processed, nonsterilized lyophilized bone because it, theoretically, has better osteoinductive capacity than sterilized bone and has no ethylene oxide residue.

Air-dried Bone

Air drying is an alternative to lyophilization that dehydrates bone and permits convenient storage at room temperature. Bone that has been prepared in small shapes and sizes can be air dried in a dehydrator or convection oven. The dried bone may be sterilized with ethylene oxide or irradiation. Some physicians prefer air-dried bone to lyophilized bone because lyophilization can reduce the biomechanical strength of grafts (29). There are conflicting data (30), and because there are no controlled clinical or in vitro studies demonstrating superiority of air-dried bone, the issue remains unresolved. It appears that air drying preserves the osteoinductive capacity of bone (31, 32). Lyophilizing bone at subzero temperatures is not necessary to preserve the bone morphogenic protein and other bone growth factors that reside in the extracellular matrix. Bone can be air dried slightly above room temperature without loss of osteoinductive capacity.

Sterilization of Bone Allografts

Sterilization of tissues has been accomplished by several methods, including heat, chemicals, ethylene oxide, and γ-irradiation. Some tissues are treated with antibiotics in vitro prior to storage, but this decontaminates only the surface and is effective against only bacteria. Both γ-irradiation and ethylene oxide are commonly used to sterilize bone, cartilage, dura, and tendon. Most bone grafts distributed in the United States are freeze dried and sterilized with chemicals, γ-irradiation or ethylene oxide gas.

γ-Irradiation of bone was introduced over 30 years ago and still is used widely (33). The minimal bacteriocidal level of γ-irradiation is 10,000–20,000 Gy. Uncontrolled human studies have shown that irradiated, calcified (33,34), and demineralized (31,35) bone grafts are clinically effective. Numerous studies have shown that mineralized bone allografts irradiated at 2.5 to 3 Mrad are also clinically effective. Clinical success rates of 85% to 91% have been reported (36,37). In controlled studies, the clinical effectiveness of bone allografts subjected to 25,000 Gy irradiation was comparable to that of nonirradiated bone grafts (38). Irradiated demineralized bone has active osteoinductive activity and has been effective in nonstructural clinical applications.

The introduction of bone sterilization by ethylene oxide gas simplified bone processing and facilitated the widespread use of sterilized, air-dried, and lyophilized bone products (27). The effects of ethylene oxide treatment on the biomechanical and osteoinductive capacity of bone allografts have been questioned, however. Controlled studies in animals demonstrate that repair of bone defects with lyophilized calcified bone grafts is not affected by sterilization with ethylene oxide (39). Ethylene oxide–treated, demineralized bone grafts have been effective in healing long bone segmental defects in rabbits (40) but have had reduced efficacy in rats (41). A controlled study in dogs demonstrated that the osteoinductive capacity of demineralized bone grafts sterilized with ethylene oxide is the same as that of nonsterilized bone (38), whereas a study in rats showed a reduction (42). Despite these discordant results, ethylene oxide–sterilized bone has been used widely.

Ear Ossicles

Ear ossicles are used for a special kind of bone graft to correct selected cases of deafness in which the patients' own ossicles have suffered congenital, traumatic, or postinfectious damage (43). Ear ossicles are procured by removing the temporal bone en bloc or as a core with a bone-plug cutter. The temporal bone can be stored temporarily, frozen for months, or preserved in formalin for up to 2 weeks, after which time the tympanic membrane and ossicular chain are dissected. The ossicles have been stored in Cialit (an organomercuric compound) at 1° to 2°C for up to 2 months (44), in buffered formaldehyde or 70% alcohol (45) for up to 1 year at room temperature. Alternatively, ossicles are dissected at the time of collection, lyophilized, and then sterilized with ethylene oxide gas or γ-irradiation (46). Lyophilized ossicles can be stored at room temperature for up to 5 years.

Connective Tissue Preservation and Transplantation

Cartilage and Meniscus

Human cartilage can be transplanted at weight-bearing or non-weight-bearing sites. For non-weight-bearing uses such as nasal reconstruction and mandibular or orbital rim augmentation (47), the graft provides structural support and need not be viable. To obtain the allograft, costal cartilage can be collected during surgery or in the autopsy room. The cartilage can be sterilized by γ-irradiation and stored in saline, or lyophilized, sterilized with ethylene oxide, and stored at room temperature.

Articular cartilage can be transplanted to weight-bearing articular surfaces to replace focal cartilage defects caused by trauma, particularly in the knee. Fresh cartilage is obtained as a femoral hemicondyle, tibial plateau osteochondral fragment, or as a measured segment removed with a template cutter that can be press fitted into a similarly cut area in the recipient. When cartilage is used for weight-bearing surfaces, it has been assumed that chondrocytes must survive collection and preservation and remain viable, producing normal cartilage matrix to maintain mechanical properties. It is assumed that chondrocytes deep within the cartilage matrix resist cell-mediated immune responses by the recipient and, if kept viable during storage, are able to survive after transplantation. Cartilage grafts from histoincompatible donors, stored less than 24 hours at 4°C, have survived for as long as 7 years after transplantation if the grafts developed a sound union and correct biomechanical conditions were met (48, 49). Articular cartilage collected in a sterile manner can be stored at 4°C in saline or electrolyte solutions with or without 10% fetal calf serum and antibiotics (50,51). Because optimal storage times have not been determined, articular cartilage often is transplanted within 24 hours of collection, but cartilage stored up to 72 hours at 4°C has been used. Cartilage slices stored in tissue culture media at 37°C in 5% carbon dioxide maintain in vitro cell viability for up to 60 days but have not been shown to be effective clinically (52). Cartilage cryopreserved with or without dimethyl sulfoxide (DMSO) maintains viability with variable degrees of success (53,54).

The use of a large osteochondral allograft, such as the femur with the articular cartilage attached, is thought to require preservation of cartilage viability to maintain biomechanical properties. To accomplish this, grafts have been stored at 4°C in electrolyte solutions for less than 24 hours (55), or have been frozen in 10% glycerol or 15% DMSO and stored at −70°C or lower (56–58). Following transplantation in humans and animals, the surface of the articular cartilage allografts undergoes degenerative changes in a few years.

Transplantation of menisci still is in the infant stage, and the indications for its use are undefined. The menisci are C-shaped disks of fibrocartilage interposed between the femoral condyles and tibia. The integrity and presence of the meniscus are essential for knee mechanics and biochemistry. Loss or disruption of the meniscus is associated with joint laxity and degenerative arthritis. Meniscal transplantation has been proposed as a method of providing a biologically and biomechanically acceptable structure to replace the damaged or removed meniscus. There have been unpublished reports of successful transplantation of menisci stored less than 24 hours at 4°C. However, fresh menisci usually are not available. Cryopreserved menisci have been used successfully in animals (59), but methods of preserving menisci are not well developed.

Tendon and Ligament

The knee is the joint most frequently involved in sports-related injury. Arthroscopic methods for replacing the anterior or posterior cruciate ligaments with autografts, allografts, or artificial tendons and ligaments have been developed. Despite the sacrifice or weakening of normal structures, the use of autografts appears to have the highest success rate and the lowest incidence of complications. Allografts used to replace the injured anterior cruciate ligament usually are derived from cadaveric patellar or Achilles tendons. Patellar and Achilles tendon allografts are usually stored frozen, but some are stored lyophilized (60). In vitro biomechanical properties of tendons do not seem to be affected greatly by freezing, lyophilizing, or ethylene oxide sterilization (61). There are, however, reports of synovitis and degeneration of transplanted lyophilized patellar tendon allografts that have been sterilized by ethylene oxide (62). Frozen tendon allografts are commonly sterilized by γ-irradiation, which can reduce their mechanical strength, particularly if the dose exceeds 2 Mrad (63). There is no evidence that maintenance of cellular viability during processing and storage is important to clinical effectiveness. The long-term efficacy of tendon allografts, as well as optimal processing and storage conditions prior to use, have not been determined.

Fascia Lata

The fascia lata is a broad fibrous membrane investing the thigh muscles. The thick lateral portion acts as a flattened tendon, with muscular insertions helping to maintain the trunk in an erect posture. It can be removed and transplanted as an autograft or allograft. As an allograft, fascia lata is used to suspend the upper eyelid to correct ptosis, to replace injured anterior cruciate ligaments (60), and to repair ankle, hip, and shoulder suspensions, (i.e., repair of the ruptured rotator cuff of the shoulder). Fascia lata usually is preserved by lyophilization, sterilized by ethylene oxide gas or γ-irradiation, and stored at room temperature for up to 5 years at a residual moisture of less than 5%. After rehydration, its biomechanical properties equal those of fresh frozen fascia lata (64).

Dura Mater

The dura mater is the outermost, toughest, and most fibrous of the three meningeal membranes covering the brain and spinal cord. The intracranial portion is collected, processed, stored, and distributed for several clinical uses, the most common being closure of dural defects caused by resection of tumor or repair of traumatic injury. Human dura allograft most commonly is preserved by lyophilization. Ethylene oxide and γ-irradiation are effective in preventing transmission of viruses and bacteria; however, Creutzfeldt-Jakob disease has been transmitted by dura mater sterilized by these two methods (65). Donors with a history of neurologic disorders are not accepted as dura mater donors. Lyophilization and ethylene oxide sterilization have not lessened the effectiveness of dura allografts (66). Reconstituted freeze-dried dura is thick and strong, holds suture well, and is incorporated into normal surrounding tissue without rejection.

Skin Preservation and Use

Human skin allograft is the dressing of choice for temporary grafting onto deep burn wounds whenever sufficient amounts of autografted skin are unavailable. Early excision of burn wounds and covering with cadaver skin allograft has shortened hospitalization and decreased mortality more than any other treatment (67). A skin allograft provides temporary coverage and acts as a barrier against loss of water, electrolytes, protein, and heat. It excludes bacterial infection and speeds reepithelialization. Skin allografts are replaced periodically until sufficient autograft skin can be obtained. A skin allograft also is used for unhealed skin defects (decubitus ulcers, autograft skin donor sites, pedicle flap donor sites, and traumatically denuded areas).

After collection, fresh skin can be stored at 2° to 8°C for up to 14 days (11). During storage, the medium is changed regularly (e.g., every 48 hours or as it acidifies as indicated by pH indicators). For refrigerated storage, standard tissue culture media, such as RPMI-1640, Eagle's minimum essential medium, or balanced salt solutions, commonly are used with or without added antibiotics. Viability is best maintained if the skin is free floating rather than rolled, and an optimal ratio of skin area-to-volume of medium has been established.

Skin also can be frozen to maintain viability and improve availability. Because of the decline of viability during refrigerated storage, it is best to initiate cryopreservation within 2 to 3 days of procurement. The cryoprotectant most commonly used is glycerol, which is used at concentrations of 10% or 15%, and skin is cryopreserved as strips (3- by 8-inch) on fine-mesh gauze in flat cryopreservation bags. Cryogenic damage is minimized by controlling the rate of freezing to about −1°C/min; however, the optimal rate has not been determined (68, 69). Many tissue banks use heat sinks rather than electronic controlled-rate freezers. Heat sinks involve aluminum plates or Styrofoam-insulated boxes, which are placed with skin directly into a −70°C mechanical freezer. This simple process provides a slow, controlled freezing rate and also maintains cellular viability (70). The AATB standards permit frozen storage in a mechanical freezer at about −70°C (−50° to −90°C), in the vapor phase of liquid nitrogen at −150°C (−100° to −196°C), or submerged in liquid nitrogen at −196°C (11). The maximal allowable storage period that maintains viability and structural integrity in the frozen state has not been determined. Cryopreserved skin allograft usually is transported from the tissue bank to the hospital on dry ice.

Skin generally is not preserved by lyophilization because there is decreased clinical efficacy when used in patients with burns. Lyophilized skin is sometimes used by oral surgeons to cover oral mucous membrane defects and speed reepithelialization.

Corneal Preservation and Transplantation

The cornea is one of the most frequently transplanted tissues, with over 45,000 transplanted annually in the United States. Corneal transplantation has increased and become highly effective because of improved suture material, better surgical instruments, and effective topical antiinflammatory medications to control rejection. The common conditions leading to transplantation are corneal edema, keratoconus, corneal regraft, and herpetic scars. Donor cells in the avascular full-thickness cornea graft enjoy long-term survival without the aid of histocompatibility matching because the recipient site is almost completely avascular. The failure rate of 5% to 10% might be improved, however, by human leukocyte antigen (HLA) matching (71). Systemic immunosuppressants are not used, but topical corticosteroids are routinely used.

Eyes are enucleated from the cadaver, preferably within 6 hours of death. The oldest method of storage for whole eyes is 4°C in a moist chamber. Most surgeons will not use corneas stored in this manner beyond 24 hours, even though the tissue appears to maintain enough endothelial cells for an efficacious graft for as long as 48 hours after collection. The most common form of storage is refrigeration at 4°C in a modified tissue culture medium. Prior to storage, the cornea and a rim of sclera are removed from the whole eye and placed in a tissue culture medium such as that introduced by McCarey and Kaufman in 1974 (M-K medium) containing 5% dextran (as an osmotic agent) plus an antibiotic (72). The antibiotic most commonly used is gentamicin. Routine testing of corneas after storage commonly shows gentamicin-resistant organisms, but these are usually of low pathogenic potential and do not cause posttransplant infection. The M-K medium maintains endothelium viability up to 4 days; however, most surgeons prefer to transplant corneas stored in M-K medium within 48 hours. The addition of chondroitin sulfate as an osmotic agent and membrane stabilizer in K-sol tissue culture media has extended 4°C storage for as long as 7 to 10 days (73). An alternative culture technique has been used at a few eye banks, and it has maintained sterile corneas in tissue culture medium at 34°C for as long as 5 weeks (74). Rarely, corneas are frozen with cryoprotectants.

Heart Valve Preservation and Transplantation

Since their introduction 3 decades ago, human heart valve allografts have been shown to be superior to mechanical or pig valves for aortic valve replacement. Human heart valve allografts do not require anticoagulation, have a lower incidence of thromboembolism, and appear relatively resistant to infection. After valve allograft transplantation, donor endothelium is not maintained, but donor fibroblasts have been seen as many as 9.5 years after transplantation (75). Because anticoagulation is unnecessary, human valvular allografts are the graft of choice for children and pregnant women, as well as for patients with infection in the aortic root. The use of valvular allografts has been slowed, because implantation is more difficult technically and valve allografts are not readily available.

To obtain valve allografts, hearts are collected aseptically in the operating or autopsy room, and the pulmonic and aortic valves are removed. Human heart valves initially were stored at 5°C in tissue culture medium containing antibiotics (76). However, cell viability was lost under these conditions after 48 hours. Subsequently, it was shown that cryopreserved heart valves are superior, based upon improved cell viability and a reduced incidence of valve degeneration, rupture, leaflet perforation, and valve-related death. For these reasons, human heart valves generally are cryopreserved (77), by exposure first to antibiotic solutions for 24 to 48 hours and then to a 10% DMSO solution in RPMI-1640 with 10% fetal calf serum added. Freezing is accomplished at a controlled rate of − 1°C per minute to − 40°C. Valves generally are stored in the vapor phase of liquid nitrogen. Heart valves can be stored indefinitely in liquid nitrogen, although the nature of any deterioration during storage is not well characterized. The viability of cryopreserved connective tissue matrix cells is maintained but at a lower level than in fresh valves (78), and endothelium viability is lost (79).

Peripheral Nerve Transplantation

Fresh autografts of peripheral sensory nerves are used in nerve repair. Although allografts ideally might repair peripheral nerve defects without sacrificing the patient's own nerve, frozen, irradiated, and lyophilized allografts have not functioned well enough to achieve clinical usefulness.

Parathyroid Preservation and Transplantation

Hypercalcemia, kidney stones, and other complications associated with hyperparathyroidism can be treated by surgical removal of the parathyroids. Hyperparathyroidism often is caused by a single parathyroid adenoma, but in 10% of cases, generalized parathyroid hyperplasia is found, requiring removal of all four parathyroids. Postoperatively, the lack of parathyroid hormone can result in permanent hypocalcemia in 5% of all patients. Because of this, autotransplantation of a small amount of parathyroid tissue is done during total parathyroidectomy to provide a controlled source of parathyroid hormone (80,81). The parathyroid tissue is placed in the sternocleidomastoid muscle, flexor muscle groups, or subcutaneous tissue of the forearm. The remaining parathyroid tissue can be divided, placed in vials of cold tissue culture medium, and cryopreserved using 10% autogeneic serum and 10% DMSO; the tissue then can be frozen under controlled conditions and stored in liquid nitrogen at − 196°C (81,82). Frozen parathyroid autograft can be used if the tissue immediately implanted proves to be insufficient, fails to function, or becomes infected. Cryopreservation with DMSO maintains cell viability as illustrated by postimplant amelioration of hypocalcemia and sustained elevation of parathyroid hormone in the venous effluent of the grafted (versus the nongrafted) forearm (81,83). Postthaw viability can also be demonstrated in vitro by the suppression of parathyroid hormone secretion by increasing calcium concentrations (81,84). The length of time that frozen parathyroid tissue can be stored is unknown.

Preservation and Use of Reproductive Tissue

Semen Cryobanking

Artificial insemination of a female with her partner's semen (client depositor program) or with anonymous-donor semen is established therapy for the clinical management of infertility (85). Cryopreserved semen is used for both forms of artificial insemination. In client depositor programs, cryopreserved semen is stored so that a male who might become sterile as a consequence of therapy for Hodgkin disease or testicular malignancy can provide semen for later use. Sperm can even be collected postmortem, but ethical issues regarding lack of consent have arisen. There are approximately 110 semen banks in the United States (86). In 1999, New York State–licensed semen banks processed 97,231 vials and distributed 62,722 vials of semen for use in artificial insemination (New York State Department of Health, unpublished data, 2000).

In anonymous-donor programs there is a library of donors from whom donated frozen semen specimens are available. This facilitates the matching of hair and eye color, race, or other genetically determined characteristics with those of the parents. Sexually transmitted diseases, including HIV, can be transmitted by semen from donors to women undergoing artificial insemination (19,87,88). Cryopreservation permits storage so that a donor can be retested 6 months after donation to prevent use of semen donated by a man recently infected and prior to developing detectable antibody (in the window period). The interval between HIV exposure and seroconversion to antibody averages about 22 days (89). National professional standard-setting organizations require and the federal government recommends that semen be stored frozen and the donor tested and found negative for HIV antibody at the time of semen donation and 6 months later (11,13,90). Other diseases and organisms transmissible by donor semen include hepatitis B, gonorrhea, *Ureaplasma urealyticum, Mycoplasma hominis, Trichomonas vaginalis,* and *Chlamydia trachomatis.* Transmission of HTLV-I, syphilis, HCV, and human papillomavirus (HPV) may also be possible (19).

The basic practices and techniques of semen cryopreservation have changed little because the cryopreservative glycerol was discovered accidentally by Polge et al. in 1949 (91). Glycerol remains the standard cryoprotectant, and liquid nitrogen the freezing and storage method. Freezing methods are designed to control the rate of temperature decline, and thermal shock is prevented initially by cooling the semen slowly in air or in a waterbath to 5°C before the actual freezing process in the vapor phase of liquid nitrogen, or in a programmable, controlled-rate freezing device. After freezing, semen can be stored in the liquid phase of liquid nitrogen indefinitely.

A defective pregnancy as the result of sperm injury during the freezing-thawing process is a theoretic concern that has not been demonstrated. Cryopreservation of semen does not influence the frequency of abortions, multiple births, sex of the offspring, infant body size, or intelligence (92). In fact, there is some evidence to indicate that cryopreserved semen actually might be safer than fresh semen. In one study (93), there were 0.7% birth defects and 7.7% spontaneous abortions with cryopreserved semen, whereas in the general population the rate of birth defects is 6% and the rate of spontaneous abortions is 10% to 18%.

Oocytes and Embryos

Since Louise Brown, the world's first "test tube baby," was delivered on July 25, 1978, there has been an explosion in the assisted reproductive technologies. There are at least 295 assisted reproductive technology programs in the United States (3). In 1999, over 50,000 embryos were created and stored in New York state; over 28,000 embryos were transferred into patients (New York State Department of Health, unpublished data, 1999).

Extraembryonic Tissue Preservation and Transplantation

Extraembryonic tissues that have been used occasionally for transplantation include the amnion and the umbilical vein. The fetal amnion has been used as a covering for nonhealing chronic leg ulcers, burns, raw surfaces following mastectomy, major oral cavity reconstruction, and vaginoplasties. It also has been used as a pelvic peritoneum substitute following pelvic exenteration and as a source of replacement enzymes for inborn errors of metabolism (94,95). The amnion is the smooth, slippery, glistening membrane lining the fluid-filled space surrounding the fetus. Most of the amnion is covered on the maternal side by the chorion, a slightly roughened membrane. The fetal amnion can be collected aseptically during cesarean section or during vaginal delivery. The amnion epithelium and its basement membrane can be separated by blunt dissection from the underlying chorion immediately after collection or after temporary storage. After sterile procurement during cesarean section, the amniotic membrane can be stored at 5°C in a combined antibiotic-electrolyte solution and used within hours. Amnions delivered vaginally and stored in antibiotic solutions at 4°C remain sterile for as long as 24 to 48 hours after collection (96), thus obviating the need for sterile procurement during cesarean section. Isolated instances of storage by lyophilization or cryopreservation have been reported.

Human umbilical vein allografts are used infrequently as vascular substitutes to provide venous access for hemodialysis or as an arterial bypass graft. Umbilical veins, however, have patency rates inferior to saphenous vein autografts and thus have been used only as a last resort. Because most umbilical veins are collected during vaginal delivery rather than aseptically during cesarean section, a sterilization step is usually added. The liquid storage medium and chemical fixative (glutaraldehyde and ethanol) sterilize the veins. However, these veins do not provide as suitable a substratum for endothelial cell adhesion and proliferation as do fresh saphenous veins. Umbilical veins also can be lyophilized and subsequently sterilized by γ-irradiation or ethylene oxide. γ-Irradiation leaves the umbilical vein hard and brittle, whereas ethylene oxide leaves it softer and more pliable.

Donor-recipient Matching

For most tissues, donor-recipient HLA matching rarely is done. Tissues such as bone, fascia, tendon, cartilage, and dura are not preserved or transplanted in a viable state, but rather serve as a support or matrix that the recipient's own cells enter and gradually replace. Immunologic rejection, therefore, is not a major problem, and blood group or HLA matching is unnecessary. There are exceptions, however. For repeated corneal grafts, immunologic rejection can occur; efforts then are made to use HLA-matched corneas in these patients (97).

The ABO antigens are of major importance in transplantation because they constitute very strong histocompatibility antigens. Because they are expressed on vascular endothelium, major ABO mismatching can cause rapid graft rejection due to endothelial damage by ABO antibodies, with subsequent widespread thrombosis within the graft. Therefore, ABO matching is important to the success of vascularized grafts (i.e., kidney, heart, liver, and pancreas). ABO matching is not important in tissue grafts (i.e., fascia, bone, heart valves, skin, and cornea).

Red blood cell Rh antigen mismatch has been reported to stimulate antibody formation following transplantation of frozen unprocessed bone obtained from living donors (26). Consequently, these bone allografts usually are matched with the donor for the Rh antigen if the recipient is a female with child-bearing potential.

BLOOD BANK SUPPORT OF TISSUE TRANSPLANTATION

Hospital blood banks and blood centers have been greatly affected by organ and tissue transplantation, as well as by new and increased demands for services. Blood banks are involved in transplantation in several ways, including a) providing traditional blood components; b) providing new or special blood components; c) assisting with organ procurement; d) taking responsibility for tissue procurement, processing, storage, and distribution; and e) providing specialized services.

The major demand on blood banks for organ transplants involves the use of traditional, and some special, blood components (see Chapter 43). Also, many hospital blood banks and regional blood centers have entered the field of tissue banking which, like blood banking, depends on carefully controlled and reliable donor recruitment, donor eligibility determination, collection, processing, storage, and distribution. Hospital blood banks and regional blood centers have the physical and administrative resources, as well as the processing and distribution capacities, to operate a tissue bank (98) (Table 64.11).

Currently, most human cadaver tissue (bone, skin, heart valves, veins, and tendons) is collected by an organ and tissue procurement agency or regional tissue bank and distributed directly to the operating room or to other hospital sections in which tissue transplantation occurs. Because of a lack of centralization, there could be inadequate records of storage conditions

TABLE 64.11. SPECIAL CAPABILITIES OF BLOOD BANKS TO BE TISSUE TRANSPLANTATION SERVICES

Network of volunteers and community support
Expertise in counseling
Reputation for dependable service
History of success in donor recruitment and selection
Commitment to community service and accountability
Skill in public education with a broad-based public information system
Commitment to research and development
Experience with federal and state regulations
24-hour-per-day, 7-day-per-week operation
Computerized inventory control
Skill in logistics management
Professional qualified medical and technical direction
Established fiscal relations with hospitals
Expertise in processing, storage, distribution
Expertise in the cryobiology of several cell types
Quality assurance expertise

and recipient identification. In one case involving an HIV-infected donor, the recipients of several of the tissues could not be identified from hospital records (23). The hospital blood bank has the capacity, experience, and skills to act as a central depot and distribution point for all human tissue and ensure that distribution records are maintained. Blood centers and blood banks with expertise in donor recruitment, donor eligibility determination, and cellular cryopreservation expertise are ideal for providing tissue transplantation services. Some blood banks or regional blood services already function as tissue banks in that they procure, process, store, and distribute tissues.

Follow-up and Reimbursement

Following donation, the donor body is reconstructed to permit normal funeral arrangements and viewing by the family. The organ donor coordinator's responsibilities continue after the transplant, in that a letter of appreciation is sent to the next-of-kin, giving information about the specific use of the donated organs and tissues. This communication serves as a liaison between the donor's family and the organ and tissue procurement agencies. Later contact is often reestablished to assist in the amelioration of grief and bereavement.

Reimbursement for tissue transplantation is similar to that for blood transfusion. The tissue bank recovers expenses through a service fee (per tissue) billed to the hospital which, in turn, charges the patient. Providers of health care insurance reimburse hospitals for most tissues.

REGULATORY OVERSIGHT OF TISSUE BANKS

With the rapid growth of all areas of the tissue banking industry, there has been an increasing need for accountability and measures that ensure safe, quality tissues are available for clinical use. Quality improvement can be effected through voluntary standards, and most tissue banks have incorporated the achievement of high standards into their goals. However, for tissue banks that are unable, or unwilling, to meet industry standards, regulatory intervention or enforcement may be necessary. Until recently, large segments of the tissue banking industry have been unregulated. A few states, specifically New York, Florida, and California, adopted licensure requirements in the early 1990s. The New York State Department of Health has the most comprehensive oversight program. Beginning in 1991, New York established administrative, licensure, and technical requirements for all entities that collect, process, store, or distribute tissue in New York. Currently, 623 tissue banks, including 31 cardiovascular tissue banks, 53 musculoskeletal tissue banks, 42 skin banks, 20 eye banks, 55 semen banks, 32 oocyte-embryo banks, 68 hematopoietic progenitor cell banks, and 72 nontransplant anatomic banks (banks providing bodies, body parts, and tissues for health professional education and medical research) are licensed to operate in New York. New York state regulations extend to the clinical use of tissue, such as physician's offices where semen is used in artificial insemination and hospitals and ambulatory surgery units that transplant tissue.

Federal regulation of tissue banks began with the publication, by the Food and Drug Administration, of Human Tissue Intended for Transplantation—Interim Rule in December 1993 (99). These regulations included infectious disease testing, donor screening, and record-keeping requirements for most tissues. Reproductive tissue, human milk, and bone marrow were specifically excluded. The Final Rule on Human Tissue Intended for Transplantation was published in July 1997 (100). These federal regulations are being supplanted by a series of regulations first announced in the Proposed Approach to the Regulation of Cellular and Tissue-based Products in March 1997 (101). The more comprehensive regulations and proposed rules now include reproductive tissues and hematopoietic progenitor cells and registration (86), suitability screening and testing (102), and good tissue practices (103, 104) requirements.

SUMMARY

In the United States, organ and tissue procurement has been organized to maximize availability in an equitable and efficient fashion that is fair to donor and recipient alike. Most of the organ procurement efforts have become systematic and organized under federal mandate; there is, however, a growing cooperation in the transplantation service industry to facilitate the demanding, yet necessary, tangential requirements of organ and tissue procurement and allocation. Successful tissue preservation has encouraged the use of bone grafts, cardiovascular tissue, and skin in the clinical setting. More recent adjuncts to transplantation include semen and embryo cryobanking. As technology in this area continues to expand, blood banks may play an increasingly important role in coordinating, supporting, and directing transplantation and transplant-related interventions.

REFERENCES

1. Department of Health and Human Services. Oversight in tissue banking. Informed consent in tissue donation; expectations and realities. Boston: Office of Inspector General; January 2001.
2. 1999 Eye banking statistical report. Washington, DC: Eye Bank Association of America; 2000.2a. American Association of Tissue Banks Mid Year Meeting. Council of Accredited Member Tissue Banks meeting, March 12, 2001.
3. 1998 Assisted reproductive technology success rates. Atlanta, GA: Centers for Disease Control and Prevention; American Society for Reproductive Medicine; Resolve; December 2000.
4. Guidelines for the establishment and operation of a donor human milk bank. Raleigh, NC: Human Milk Banking Association of North America; 2000.
5. Department of Health and Human Services. Hospital conditions of participation: identification of potential organ, tissue and eye donors and transplant hospitals provision of transplant related data. *Federal Register* 998 June 28:63:33856–33875.
6. Lee PP, Start W, Yand JC. Cornea donation laws in the United States. *Arch Ophthalmol* 1989;107:1585–1589.
7. Lee PP, Yang JC, McDonald PJ, et al. Worldwide legal requirements for obtaining corneas: 1990. *Cornea* 1992;11:102–107.
8. Mathews P. Whose body? People as property. *Curr Leg Probl* 1983; 36:192–239.
9. 1998 Eye Banking Statistical Report. Washington, DC: Eye Bank Association of America; 1999.
10. Department of Health and Human Services. Partners for the National Organ and Tissue Donation Initiative. *Federal Register* 1998 Sept 17:63:49702–49703.

11. Woll JE, Kasprisin D. Standards for tissue banking. McLean, VA: American Association of Tissue Banks, 2001.
12. Medical standards. Washington, DC: Eye Bank Association of America, 2000.
13. Guidelines for gamete and embryo donation. The American Society for Reproductive Medicine. *Fertil Steril* 1998;70[Suppl 3]:1S–13S.
14. Gallup Survey. The U.S. public's attitudes toward organ transplants/organ donation. Princeton, NJ: Gallup Organization, 1986.
15. Prottas, J, Batten HL. Health professionals and hospital administrators in organ procurement: attitudes, reservations and their resolutions. *Am J Public Health* 1988;78:642–645.
16. Katches M, Heisel W, Campbell R, et al. The body brokers. *Orange County Register* 2000 Apr 16–20.
17. Eastlund T. Infectious disease transmission through cell, tissue and organ transplantation. Reducing the risk through donor selection. *Cell Transplant* 1995;4:455–477.
18. Bowen PA II, Lobel SA, Caruana RJ, et al. Transmission of human immunodeficiency virus (HIV) by transplantation: clinical aspects and time course analysis of viral antigenemia and antibody production. *Ann Intern Med* 1988;108:46–48.
19. Linden JV, Critser, JK. Therapeutic insemination by donor II: a review of its known risks. *Reprod Med Rev* 1995;4:19–29.
20. Aoki N. Putting burn victims first, Beverley firm develops tissue bank network. *Boston Globe* 2001 Feb 28.
21. Eastlund T. Bone transplantation and bone banking. In: Lonstein JE, Bradford DS, Winter RB, et al., eds. *Textbook of scoliosis and other spinal deformities,* 3rd ed. Philadelphia: WB Saunders, 1995:581–595.
22. Buck BE, Malinin TI, Brown MD. Bone transplantation and human immunodeficiency virus: an estimate of risk of acquired immunodeficiency syndrome (AIDS). *Clin Orthop* 1989;240:129–136.
23. Simonds RJ, Holmberg SD, Hurwitz RL, et al. Transmission of human immunodeficiency virus type 1 from a seronegative organ and tissue donor. *N Engl J Med* 1992;326:726–732.
24. Stevenson S, Horowitz M. Current concepts review. The response to bone allografts. *J Bone Joint Surg* 1992;74A:939–950.
25. Friedlaender GE, Horowitz MC. Immune responses to osteochondral allografts: nature and significance. *Orthopedics* 1992;15:1171–1175.
26. Musclow CE, Dietz G, Bell RS, et al. Alloimmunization by blood group antigens from bone allografts. *Immunohematology* 1992;9:102–104.
27. Cloward RB. Gas-sterilized cadaver bone grafts for spinal fusion operations. A simplified bone bank. *Spine* 1980;5:4–10.
28. Hogstedt C, Aringer L, Gustavsson A. Epidemiologic support for ethylene oxide as a cancer-causing agent. *JAMA* 1986;255:1575–1578.
29. Pelker RR, Friedlander GE, Markham TC, et al. Effects of freezing and freeze-drying on the biomechanical properties of rat bone. *J Orthop Res* 1984;1:405–411.
30. Bright RW, Burchardt H. The biomechanical properties of preserved bone grafts. In: Friediander GE, Mankin HJ, Sell KW, eds. *Bone allografts: biology, banking and clinical applications.* Boston: Little, Brown and Company, 1983:241–247.
31. Glowacki J, Murray JE, Kaban LB, et al. Application of the biologic principle of induced osteogenesis for cranial facial defects. *Lancet* 1981;1:959–962.
32. Gepstein R, Weiss RE, Saba K, et al. Bridging large detects in bone by demineralized bone matrix in the form of a powder. *J Bone Joint Surg* 1987;69:984–992.
33. Bright RW, Smarsh JD, Gambill VM. Sterilization of human bone by irradiation. In: Friedlander GE, Mankin HJ, Sell KW, eds. *Bone allografts: biology, banking and clinical applications.* Boston: Little, Brown and Company, 1983:223–232.
34. DeVries PH, Badgley CE, Hartman JT. Radiation sterilization of homogenous bone transplants utilizing radioactive cobalt. *J Bone Joint Surg* 1985;40:187–203.
35. Sonis ST, Kaban LB, Glowacki J. Clinical trial of demineralized bone powder in treatment of periodontal defects. *J Oral Med* 1983;38:117–122.
36. Zasacki W. The efficacy of application of lyophilized, radiation-sterilized bonegraft in orthopedic surgery. *Clin Orthop* 1991;272:81–87.
37. Komender J, Malczewska H, Komender A, et al. Therapeutic effects of transplantation of lyophilized and radiation-sterilized allogeneic bone. *Clin Orthop* 1991;272:38–49.
38. Loty B, Courpied JP, Tomeno B, et al. Bone allografts sterilized by irradiation. Biological properties, procurement and results of 150 massive allografts. *Int Orthop* 1990;14:237–242.
39. Prolo DJ, Pedrotti PW, Burres K, et al. Superior osteogenesis in transplanted allogeneic canine skull following chemical sterilization. *Clin Orthop* 1982;168:230–242.
40. Janovec M, Dvorak K. Autolyzed antigen-extracted allogeneic bone for bridging segmented diaphyseal bone defects in rabbits. *Clin Orthop* 1988;229:249–255.
41. Cornell C, Lane JM, Nottebaert M, et al. Effect of ethylene oxide sterilization upon bone inductive properties of demineralized bone matrix. *Trans Orthop Res Soc* 1987;11:74.
42. Sherman P, Hollinger P. Bone implant sterilization-ethylene oxide versus cobalt 60 irradiation. Annual meeting abstracts. Boston: American Association Oral and Maxillofacial Surgery, 1988(abst).
43. Lang J, Kerr AG, Smyth GDL. Long-term viability of transplanted ossicles. *J Laryngol Otol* 1986;100:741–747.
44. Ars B, Decracmer W, Ars-Piret N. Tympano-ossicular allografts: morphology and physiology. *Am J Otolaryngol* 1987;8:148–154.
45. Sataloff RT, Roberts BR. Preservation of otologic homografts. *Am J Otolaryngol* 1986;7:214–217.
46. Smith MFW. Freeze-dried otologic implants. *J Otolaryngol* 1980;9:222–227.
47. Guerrerosantos J. Recontouring the middle third of the face with onlay cartilage plus free fascia graft. *Ann Plast Surg* 1987;18:409–420.
48. Kandel RA, Gross AE, Ganel A, et al. Histopathology of failed osteoarticular shell allografts. *Clin Orthop* 1985;197:103–112.
49. Oakeshott RO, Farine I, Pritzker KPH, et al. A clinical and histologic analysis of failed fresh osteochondral allografts. *Clin Orthop* 1988;233:283–294.
50. Garrett JC. Treatment of osteochondral defects of the distal femur with a fresh osteochondral allograft: a preliminary report. *Arthroscopy* 1986;2:222–226.
51. Schachar N, Cucheran DI, Frank CB. Viability of intact articular cartilage at various times after donor death. *Trans Orthop Res Soc* 1988;12:436.
52. Jiminez SA, Brighton CT. Storage and preservation of viable articular cartilage. In: Friedlander GE, Mankin HJ, Sell KW, eds. *Osteochondral allografts. biology, banking and clinical applications.* Boston: Little, Brown and Company, 1983:203–213.
53. Tomford WW, Mankin HJ. Investigational approaches to articular cartilage preservation. *Clin Orthop* 1983;174:22–27.
54. Tomford WW, Mankin HJ, Friedlander GE, et al. Methods of banking bone and cartilage for allograft transplantation. *Orthop Clin North Am* 1987;18:241–247.
55. Gross AE, McKee N, Linger F, et al. Surgical techniques and clinical experience with articular allografts at the knee. In: Friedlander GE, Mankin HJ, Sell KW, eds. *Osteochondral allografts. biology, banking and clinical applications.* Boston: Little, Brown and Company, 1983:289–298.
56. Friedlaender GE, Mankin HJ. Transplantation of osteochondral allografts. *Annu Rev Med* 1984;35:311–324.
57. Gitelis S, Heligman D, Quill G, et al. The use of large allografts for tumor reconstruction and salvage of the failed total hip arthroplasty. *Clin Orthop* 1988;241:61–70.
58. Malinin TI, Mnaymneh W, Lo HK, et al. Cryopreservation of articular cartilage. Ultrastructural observations and long-term results of experimental distal femoral transplantation. *Clin Orthop* 1994;303:18–32.
59. Arnocsky SP, McDevitt CA, Schmidt MB, et al. The effect of cryopreservation on canine menisci: a biochemical, morphologic, and biomechanical evaluation. *J Orthop Res* 1988;6:1–12.
60. Andrews M, Noyes FR, Barber-Westin SO. Anterior cruciate ligament allograft reconstruction in the skeletally immature athlete. *Am J Sports Med* 1994;22:48–54.
61. Bechtold JE, Eastlund DT, Butts MK, et al. The effects of freeze-

drying and ethylene oxide sterilization on the mechanical properties of human patellar tendon. *Am J Sports Med* 1994;22:562–566.
62. Jackson DW, Windler GE, Simon TM. Intra-articular reaction associated with the use of freeze-dried, ethylene oxide sterilized, bone-patella tendon-bone allografts in the reconstruction of the anterior cruciate ligament. *Am J Sports Med* 1990;18:1–10.
63. Gibbons MI, Butler DL, Grood ES, et al. Dose-dependent effects of γ-irradiation on the material properties of frozen bone-patellar tendon-bone allografts. *Trans Orthop Res Soc* 1989;14:513.
64. Thomas ED, Gresham RB. Comparative tensile strength study of fresh, frozen and freeze-dried human fascia lata. *Surg Forum* 1963; 14:442–443.
65. Yamada S, Aiba T, Endo Y, et al. Creutzfeldt-Jakob disease transmitted by a cadaveric dura mater graft. *Neurosurgery* 1994;34:740–744.
66. Rosomoff HL, Malinin TI. Freeze-dried allografts of dura mater: 20 years' experience. *Transplant Proc* 1976;8:133–138.
67. Muller MJ, Herndon DN. The challenge of burns. *Lancet* 1994;343: 216–220.
68. Ingham E, Matthews JB, Kearney JN, et al. The effects of variation of cryopreservation protocols on the immunogenicity of allogeneic skin grafts. *Cryobanking* 1993;30:443–458.
69. Kearney JN. Cryopreservation of cultured skin cells. *Burns* 1991;17: 380–383.
70. Konstantinow A, Muhlbauer W, Hartinger A, et al. Skin banking. A simple method for cryopreservation of split-thickness skin and cultured epidermal keratinocytes. *Ann Plast Surg* 1991;26:89–97.
71. Smolin G, Goodman D. Corneal graft rejection. *Int Ophthalmol Clin* 1988;28:30–36.
72. Bourne WM. Corneal preservation. In: Kaufman HE, McDonald MB, Barron BA, et al., eds. *The cornea.* New York: Churchill Livingstone, 1988:713–724.
73. Doughman DJ. Corneal tissue preservation. *Int Ophthalmol Clin* 1988;28:50–56.
74. Doughman DJ, Harris JE, Mindrup E, et al. Prolonged donor corneal preservation in organ culture: long-term clinical evaluation. *Cornea* 1992;1:7–20.
75. O'Brien MF, Stafford EG, Gardner MAH, et al. A comparison of aortic valve replacement with viable cryopreserved and fresh allograft valves, with a note on chromosomal studies. *J Thorac Cardiovasc Surg* 1987;94:812–823.
76. Khanna SK, Ross JK, Monro JL. Homograft aortic valve replacement: seven years' experience with antibiotic-treated valves. *Thorax* 1981; 36:330–337.
77. O'Brien MF, Stafford EG, Gardner MAH, et al. Cryopreserved viable allograft aortic valves. In: Yankoh AC, Hetzer R, Miller DC, et al., eds. *Cardiac valve allografts 1972–1987.* New York: Springer-Verlag, 1988:311–321.
78. Messier RH, Domkowski PW, Aly HM, et al. High energy phosphate depletion in leaflet matrix cells during processing of cryopreserved cardiac valves. *J Surg Res* 1992;52:483–488.
79. Loose R, Markant S, Sievers HH, et al. Fate of endothelial cells during transport, cryopreservation and thawing of heart valve allografts. *Transplant Proc* 1993;25:3247–3250.
80. Walker RP, Paloyan E, Kelley TF, et al. Parathyroid autotransplantation in patients undergoing a total thyroidectomy: a review of 261 patients. *Otolaryngol Head Neck Surg* 1994;111:258–264.
81. Rothmund M, Wagner PK. Assessment of parathyroid graft function after autotransplantation of fresh and cryopreserved tissue. *World J Surg* 1984;8:523–527.
82. Herrera MF, Grant CS, van Heerden JA, et al. The effect of cryopreservation on cell viability and hormone secretion in human parathyroid tissue. *Surgery* 1992;112:1096–1101.
83. Wells SA, Farndon JR, Dale JK, et al. Long-term evaluation of patients with primary parathyroid hyperplasia managed by total parathyroidectomy and heterotopic autotransplantation. *Ann Surg* 1980;192: 451–458.
84. Wagner PK, Rumpelt HJ, Krause U, et al. The effect of cryopreservation on hormone secretion in vitro and morphology of human parathyroid tissue. *Surgery* 1986;99:257–264.
85. Sherman JK. Current status of clinical cryobanking of human semen. In: Paulson ID, Negro-Vilar A, Lucena E, et al., eds. *Andrology. Male fertility and sterility.* New York: Academic Press, 1986:517–547.
86. Food and Drug Administration. 21 CFR Parts 207, 807 and 1271. Human cells, tissues, and cellular and tissue-based products; establishment registration and listing. *Federal Register* 2001 Jan 19:66: 5447–5469.
87. Mascola L, Guinan ME. Screening to reduce transmission of sexually transmitted disease in semen used for artificial insemination. *N Engl J Med* 1986;314:1354–1359.
88. Araneta MRG, Mascola L, Eller A, et al. HIV transmission through donor artificial insemination. *JAMA* 1995;273:854–858.
89. Busch MP. HIV and blood transfusion: focus on seroconversion. *Vox Sang* 1994;62[Suppl 3]:13–18.
90. Centers for Disease Control and Prevention. Guidelines for preventing transmission of human immunodeficiency virus through transplantation of human tissue and organs. *MMWR* 1994;43:1–17.
91. Polge C, Smith AU, Parkes AS. Revival of spermatozoa after vitrification and dehydration at low temperatures. *Nature* 1949;164: 666–669.
92. Karow AM. Human gametes. In: Karow AM, Pegg DE, eds. *Organ preservation for transplantation.* New York: Marcel Dekker, 1981: 377–409.
93. Sherman JK. History of artificial insemination and the development of human semen banking. In: LaSalle B, Rinfret AP, eds. *The integrity of frozen spermatozoa.* Washington, DC: National Academy of Sciences, 1978:201–207.
94. Matthew RN, Faulk WP, Bennett JP. A review of the role of amniotic membranes in surgical practice. *Obstet Gynecol Annu* 1982;11:31–58.
95. Scaggiante B, Pineschi A, Sustersich M, et al. Successful therapy of Neimann-Pick disease by implantation of human amniotic membrane. *Transplantation* 1987;44:59–61.
96. Trelford JD, Trelford-Saunder M. The amnion in surgery, past and present. *Am J Obstet Gynecol* 1979;134:833–845.
97. Forstot SL, Binder PS. Corneal transplantation. In: Chatterjee SN, ed. *Organ transplantation.* Boston: John Wright, 1982:557–588.
98. Meryman HT. The role of blood banks in the development of the regional tissue banking program. *Transplant Proc* 1976;8:241–244.
99. 21 CFR Parts 16, et al. Human tissue intended for transplantation; interim rule. *Federal Register* 1993 Dec 14:58:65514–65521.
100. 21 CFR Parts 16 and 1270. Human tissue intended for transplantation; final rule. *Federal Register* 1997 July 29:62:40429–40447.
101. Food and Drug Administration. Proposed approach to regulation of cellular and tissue-based products. *Federal Register* 1997 Mar 4:62: 9721–9722.
102. 21 CFR Parts 210, 211, 820, and 1271. Suitability determination of donors of human cellular and tissue-based products; proposed rule. *Federal Register* 1999 Sept 30:64:52696–52723.
103. 21 CFR Part 1271. Current good tissue practice for manufacturers of human cellular and tissue-based products; inspection and enforcement; proposed rule. *Federal Register* 2001 Jan 8:6:1508–1559.
104. Vengelen-Tyler V, ed. *Technical manual,* 13th ed. Bethesda, MD: American Association of Blood Banks, 1999:569.

Rossi's Principles of Transfusion Medicine, Third Edition, edited by Toby L. Simon, Walter H. Dzik, Edward L. Snyder, Christopher P. Stowell, and Ronald G. Strauss. Lippincott Williams & Wilkins, Philadelphia © 2002.

65

MEDICOLEGAL ASPECTS OF BLOOD TRANSFUSION

JAMES L. MACPHERSON
EDWARD M. MANSFIELD

Blood transfusions now save as many as 4 million lives each year. In its 1997 report, the U.S. Government Accounting Office (GAO) estimated that nearly one-half of all transfusions were provided to meet an urgent life-saving need (1). Although the GAO also reports that the blood supply has never been safer, some patients continue to be injured by transfusions. Nearly a score of deaths are reported each year to the Food and Drug Administration (FDA) because patients received the wrong blood (2). These deaths result from the same kind of misidentifications that the Institute of Medicine recently noted often occur in hospitals when patients get the wrong medicines (3). A study by British researchers concludes that official error reports are a mere tip of an iceberg of transfusion-related deaths (4). And despite all the new testing and screening of donors and the virtual elimination of human immunodeficiency virus (HIV) from the blood supply, dozens of infections, most non–life-threatening, are transmitted by transfusion each year.

Largely because of infections transmitted before the 1990s, litigation against blood providers (most often an independent or American Red Cross [ARC] blood center) has soared during the past 2 decades. The huge wave of transfusion-transmitted acquired immunodeficiency syndrome (AIDS) cases (estimated at well over 1,000), which began in the mid-1980s, has now been followed by a growing number of lawsuits alleging hepatitis C virus (HCV) infections resulting from transfusions. Estimates run as high as 300,000 for the number of Americans alive today who may have been infected with HCV as a result of blood transfusions during the last 50 years (5). While the risk of HCV infection today is less than 1 in 100,000 transfusion recipients, 30 years ago the risk was as high as one in five.

The hospital is a codefendant in nearly all lawsuits for transfusion injury against a blood provider (6). The usual claims against a hospital allege inadequate oversight of the blood provider or the physician ordering the blood transfusion or both. The patient's physician is a codefendant in nearly one-half of all transfusion injury cases, with claims ranging from inadequate informed consent and failure to offer alternatives (such as directed or autotransfusion) to the overuse of blood.

Transfusion-related litigation consumes significant time and resources for blood-banking professionals and physicians. Potential legal problems begin with donation (i.e., inadequate screening) and continue through transfusion (e.g., unnecessary transfusion and mix-ups).

Two competing trends have surfaced in this litigation re-

J.L. Macpherson: America's Blood Centers, Washington, D.C.
E.M. Mansfield: Belin, Lamson, McCormick, Zumbach and Flynn, Des Moines, Iowa.

cently. First, despite the prevalence of so-called state *blood shield* laws (which define blood providers as medical service providers and thus immunize them from claims of strict liability for product injuries) plaintiffs' attorneys have employed creative negligence theories to try to hold blood providers responsible for transfusion injuries. Claims by injured blood donors have also increased as many seek assurances that they are financially covered should the transient injury of a phlebotomy result in a long-term disability. Second, the U.S. Supreme Court's recent decisions requiring lower federal courts to act as "gatekeepers" of expert testimony have effectively raised, both in federal court and in many state courts, the level of medical proof required to present a valid case (7). In rejecting so-called junk or hypothetical science, courts have insisted that injury claims be supported by generally accepted scientific evidence. This latter trend has somewhat moderated the effects of the former trend, by restricting the ability of plaintiffs' lawyers to resort to novel theories against blood providers.

Another trend in transfusion-related litigation is the emergence of other dispute-resolution models. Importantly, the costs of litigation, the delays between the filing of a claim and trial, and the uncertainty of outcome have driven both plaintiffs and defendants to seek alternatives to the classic one-plaintiff–one-lawsuit model. In addition, the national blood organizations (i.e., America's Blood Centers, American Association of Blood Banks [AABB], and the ARC) have urged the adoption of alternative dispute resolution (ADR) mechanisms including mediation, arbitration, and no-fault compensation, to resolve disputes arising from blood injuries (8). Given that many recipients of HCV-tainted transfusions are asymptomatic for a prolonged period, but may require medical monitoring during that period, such lower-cost litigation alternatives are particularly well suited for this new set of transfusion-related claims. Additionally, class action lawsuits have come into greater use as a way to streamline the difficult process of managing multiple suits with similar claims.

Good risk and claims management approaches to all types of claims are often the key to resolving disputes early, cost effectively, and satisfactorily—from the perspective of both patient-donor and blood provider–hospital and physician. When a claim turns into a lawsuit, early neutral evaluation and mediation can still resolve the dispute. Although blood providers already take a largely no-fault approach to donor injury, interest continues in a similar approach to transfusion injury, as recommended by the Institute of Medicine in its report on lessons learned from HIV epidemic (9).

DONOR INJURY AND EMOTIONAL DISTRESS

Despite all the publicity surrounding disease transmission from blood transfusions, the most frequent claims today against blood providers come from donors injured during the phlebotomy, usually for transient nerve damage. Donating blood is very safe. Injuries to donors are rare and permanent injuries are virtually nonexistent. Each year and for no personal gain, millions of healthy individuals voluntarily subject themselves to the blood donation process. Nonetheless, five types of problems can occur during donations:

1. Hematoma (i.e., bleeding into tissue, which can result in temporary tenderness and discomfort);
2. Donor reactions (usually fainting, occasionally seizures, which may result in injuries from falls);
3. Arterial puncture (rare, but results in major and painful hematomas);
4. Nerve irritation (usually self-limiting but often requiring physician intervention); and
5. Introduction of infection (very rarely causing long-term disabilities) (10).

Donor injuries can occur despite the greatest care on the part of the phlebotomist.

In a medical negligence case, an injury or unwanted result does not necessarily mean fault or liability on the part of the provider. The injured person or plaintiff must prove that the health care practitioner fell below the "acceptable standard of practice" and that such conduct caused the particular outcome. This general concept also applies to injuries from a phlebotomy.

Nevertheless, in dealing with volunteer blood donors, many blood centers follow a policy of providing appropriate care and compensation for harm from a donation, regardless of whether the center was at fault. The reason is that blood centers rely on the good will of donors to ensure the adequacy of a local blood supply. Media reports of adversarial relationships from poor handling of infrequent donor injuries can easily dampen the altruistic motivations of a large number of individual donors and donor groups. Thus, providers often reimburse for reasonable medical expenses associated with the injury. Some donors may also seek reimbursement for consequential losses (such as lost wages).

The most difficult donor injury to manage is nerve irritation. Nerve injuries can take a long time to heal, thereby requiring patience and confidence in eventual recovery. To ensure that the nerve damage does not result in more than a temporary disability (and ultimately result in litigation), the blood center must often work closely and carefully with the injured donor and his or her physician. Blood centers that retain their own neurologic consultants can often preempt needless and often exacerbating treatments for donor injuries.

If the donor's claim goes to an attorney, the injured party (the plaintiff) may seek to invoke the evidentiary principle of *res ipsa loquitur* in a donor injury case. The Latin phrase means *the thing speaks for itself* and is applied when the circumstances of an injury are such that it almost had to be caused by the defendant's negligence. Two Louisiana courts come to opposite conclusions on the applicability of *res ipsa* in two donor nerve injury cases (11).

The actual number of donor injury cases is unknown, because there are at least a half dozen major insurers of blood providers (from blood center–owned captives to traditional commercial insurers) and they are reluctant to publish claims data. In a 1992 questionnaire, 53% of blood collectors from various regions of the United States reported that they were currently defending one or more donor injury claims (12). As noted above, most are resolved through good claims management procedures in which the blood center takes responsibility for helping the donor to resolve the injury while assuming no inherent liability.

A developing area of litigation involves erroneous notification of a test result or notice of false-positive or ambiguous test results. Blood providers perform over 150 million disease-marker tests on over 14 million donations each year. This includes well-established and highly sensitive and specific tests for HIV and HCV, as well as nucleic acid tests emerging from research use. It also includes tests that are poor markers for disease, such as the test for antibodies to the hepatitis B core (HBcAb) and the assay for elevated liver enzymes (alanine transaminase or ALT). Most tests are designed to be as sensitive as possible for detecting minute amounts of viral markers. However, the other side of the coin is that these tests yield high numbers of false-positive results (sometimes more false- than true-positive results). In addition, the high volume of testing and tracking provides more opportunities for donors to be advised erroneously that they have tested positive when their true status is negative.

A few donors have sought to recover for mental anguish and other damages for false reports of positive results (especially when the diagnosis is as devastating as HIV). In one case, a blood provider incorrectly told a donor that she had tested positive for HIV. She sued for emotional distress. The court rejected the claim, however, noting that she received the correct information within 24 hours (13). Whether a claim is allowed or not, damages for mental anguish are usually limited to the period of time the person is under a misimpression regarding his or her test result (14). Proper compliance with an organization's standard operating procedures (SOPs) and the test manufacturer's package inserts usually provides a strong defense.

Concerns about a donor's emotional reactions to a notification should not cause a blood bank to fail to give notice. Failure to notify a donor when additional harm is reasonably foreseeable has obvious public health consequences (such as secondary infections) and can lead to liability.

We anticipate increases in donor-initiated litigation (and indeed, all blood-related litigation) for several reasons. First, our society has become more litigious. Second, the public's focus on transfusion-related HIV and HCV has identified blood providers as a potential defendant for many types of injuries. Third, a high number of phlebotomies are performed on patients for autotransfusion purposes. These special-case donors are prone to difficulty with phlebotomies and to suffer complications. They may make legal claims because they view their treatment and injury as part of their relationship with the blood center. The typical volunteer donor, in contrast, views blood donation as a civic responsibility and often assumes the small risk from a blood collection. Fourth, and as noted above, the sheer number of transfusions and corresponding donations, as well as the complexity of maintaining and accurately transmitting information, combine to provide increasing opportunities for errors and misnotifications. This last factor, however, can be mitigated by the increasing adoption of information technology that can more accurately track donations from the donor to the patient, as well as the adoption of systems approaches (such as the ISO 9000 certification process) for training and error prevention and management.

A comprehensive risk management approach to donors, including preventive measures, is crucial. Informed consent forms and pre- and postdonation information forms for donors should undergo prior legal review to ensure they provide appropriate information about reasonably foreseeable adverse events and outcomes. Donation procedure SOPs have to be clear, comprehensive, and carefully followed by well-trained staff. Information should be given to donors about how to handle foreseeable post-donation problems, including how to report any difficulties to the blood center and information on emergency contacts. Further, the blood collector should have written procedures for handling any report of a donor injury. The persons responding to concerns from donors must be trained in the blood center's risk and claims management procedures. When the donor makes a claim for compensation, early consultation with the claims manager of a blood center's liability insurer can help ensure that a mismanaged claim does not frustrate a donor into seeking legal advice.

To safeguard against emotional injury claims, notification letters should follow a format approved by legal counsel and the blood center's medical director. Notification procedures should ensure that test results are reported accurately, confidentially, and to the correct person. The blood center should keep copies of all correspondence and a record of all follow-up discussions with the donor.

When a donor is deferred, it is important that statements to third parties about the reasons for deferral be accurate but no more detailed than necessary, to avoid potential liability for defamation or invasion of privacy. In one recent case, a plaintiff filed a defamation claim after his status as permanently deferred was communicated to another plasma center. The court rejected the claim, because the communication was truthful and was in accord with FDA-approved SOPs (15).

Consultation between the blood center's risk manager and the insurer's claims manager can identify prudent policies that help a donor through the injury while avoiding excess costs and further claims. Blood centers should not ask for liability releases from donors in exchange for any compensation without consultation with the insurer or legal counsel. Such action could prompt the donor to seek legal advice and exacerbate a claim that was being well managed. When the donor and blood center reach an impasse over what is reasonable compensation for an injury claim, mediation should be tried to avoid protracted and expensive litigation.

PRIVACY AND CONFIDENTIALITY OF BLOOD DONORS

In transfusion-transmitted AIDS and HCV cases, a recurring question has been the extent to which a plaintiff can obtain information about or from the implicated blood donor. A number of court decisions have addressed this issue. Often some form of limited but confidential discovery of the donor is permitted (16,17). The recent trend has been to allow the plaintiff not only to obtain the donor's personal and medical history, but also to conduct an "anonymous" donor deposition (16,18). However, a common thread running through nearly all of the cases, even those allowing discovery, has been to protect the identity of the donor from public disclosure. Because an implicated donor may have transmitted an infection, courts reason that he or she is entitled to the legal protections of privacy.

On the whole, court decisions seem to have attained a reasonable balance in this area. Courts reject the notion of "fishing expeditions" that seek to question or test one or more donors about possible risks they carried at the time of donation. But most courts allow the questioning of donors who were likely to be infected at the time of a patient's infectious transfusion because they subsequently were tested with positive results for an infectious agent. In such cases, the rationale for questioning a donor is to determine whether he or she was aware of a risk factor but donated anyway, or whether the donor did not defer because the blood provider conducted inadequate questioning on possible risk factors.

When the plaintiff seeks the identity of a donor for some reason other than his or her status as a possible source of infection, this may dictate a different outcome. For example, in a donor injury case, the blood center was ordered to disclose the names of other donors who had been present and might have been witnesses to the injury (19). Also, when the donor is no longer living, a court may decide that his or her privacy interest is lessened. Thus, in one case, the court ordered disclosure of the identity of a deceased donor to the plaintiffs, while taking elaborate precautions to ensure that the donor's identity did not become public (20).

In sorting through these questions, courts have had to weigh the plaintiff's need for information against the rights and interests of the blood donor and the blood provider. Courts have considered the donor's right to privacy, society's interest in a safe and adequate blood supply, the physician-patient privilege, and a plaintiff's ability to pursue his or her claims against a blood provider in deciding whether to allow discovery concerning a particular donor. These four factors are discussed below.

Constitutional Right to Privacy

Although our U.S. Constitution does not contain an express right to privacy, the U.S. Supreme Court has recognized an implied constitutional right to privacy in contexts not involving transfusion-transmitted diseases, such as contraception and abortion. These precedents are often cited in cases discussing the blood donor's right to privacy (21). Further, some state constitutions explicitly recognize a right to privacy.

Most courts addressing the constitutional privacy question have ruled that the donor has a right to privacy, including the right not to have his or her medical condition made public or to be harassed or embarrassed. However, recognition of a constitutional right to privacy has not necessarily precluded all discovery from or about the donor. Some courts have fashioned protective orders intended to balance between protecting the donor's constitutional right and allowing the plaintiff limited discovery (22,23). When a blood provider seeks to protect a donor's right to privacy, the constitutional argument should be vigorously pursued.

Protecting the Blood Supply

Another consideration against involving donors in the litigation process is that it creates a disincentive for members of the public to continue volunteering as blood donors, which could ultimately lessen the availability of blood to help patients in need. Introducing additional disincentives, such as more intrusive questioning and a longer donation process, puts even more pressure on the all-volunteer system (18). Hence, some courts have accepted the need to protect the volunteer donor system as a ground for precluding plaintiffs from obtaining information from donors (24,25). Other courts have classified the argument as speculative, stating that there is no hard evidence that the volunteer blood donor system has been or will be adversely affected (23). Still other courts have expressed the view that allowing plaintiffs to pursue the donor ensures "institutional accountability," thus protecting the quality of the blood supply (21).

Confidentiality by Statute

Many states have enacted statutes or regulations that protect the identity of those who have been diagnosed or, in some instances, tested for HIV. Other states by law require the identity of all blood donors to be maintained. Because these matters vary from state to state, each blood provider should be familiar with the laws of every state where it does business. Interpretations of these state laws also vary. One court has held that even a veiled deposition of a donor amounted to prohibited disclosure of identifying information under a strict construction of the California statute (26). The penalties for violation of state donor confidentiality laws can be steep, including criminal prosecution and civil sanctions.

Physician-patient Privilege

By legislation or court decision, most courts have recognized the confidentiality of physician-patient communications. This privilege generally protects information that a patient has provided to a health care provider in the course of medical treatment and precludes the health care provider from disclosing that information without the patient's permission. Yet courts have generally ruled that there is no physician-patient privilege between a blood center and donor (27). A New York case expresses a contrary but decidedly minority view (28). The chances of successfully resisting donor discovery on this ground are slim, and some defense counsel now choose not to raise this argument.

Actions Against Blood Donors

Rarely has personal liability of the volunteer blood donor been asserted. For one thing, blood banks aggressively protect the identities of their blood donors. Moreover, the individual blood donor will typically not be a source of significant financial recovery. Plaintiffs generally pursue institutional defendants, because those are the enterprises with insurance or assets if liability is found.

In a 1991 case in Washington, the possibility of suing the donor was supported by a single judge, who wrote that the rights of persons not infected with HIV are superior to those of HIV-infected persons. The majority of judges deciding the case disavowed this view (29). The decision does not provide details on the claim that the transfusion recipient wanted to file against the donor. Another case also discussed a potential claim against a donor but, again, without specifics (30). The future of litigation against blood donors is uncertain but, if the past is a guide, significant activity in this area is not likely.

Patient Informed Consent

Informed consent refers to advising patients of the risks and benefits of treatment so they can make informed choices. It is based on the long-standing principle that every human being of adult years and sound mind has a right to determine what shall be done with his or her own body.

In the context of a blood transfusion, a specific consent for transfusion that is documented (i.e., signed or written into the patient's chart) is preferable to a general consent for unspecified treatment. Although the risks from transfusions today are very low (often far lower than other treatments carrying more severe or frequent risks for which no specific consent is usually obtained), the legal legacy of the AIDS epidemic and unavoidable contamination of blood in rare cases compel physicians to continue to obtain a specific consent for transfusion. In very few states (e.g., California and New Jersey) do statutes determine what patients must be told about the risk of transfusion and the appropriateness and availability of alternatives to transfusion, such as autotransfusion or hemodilution during surgery.

Consent should be executed if possible by the patient, provided he or she is an adult and able to provide it, rather than by a representative such as a spouse. Many organizations have developed patient brochures (and at least one is available on line) for providing detailed information about transfusions, their risks, and alternatives (31). Institutions should have an SOP on what patients should be told about transfusions and whether that information is presented orally or as part of the written consent form. Quality assurance procedures should ensure compliance. Exceptions should be provided for true emergencies in which there is no opportunity to obtain consent (32).

A physician who treats without the patient's consent could be considered to have committed a *battery* and be held directly responsible for the consequences, including the transmission of an infectious disease (33). Some courts have drawn a distinction between a claim for treatment with no consent, which supports a battery claim, and treatment without informed consent, which leads to a professional negligence (malpractice) claim (34). Informed consent does not require the physician to provide the patient with all the information about a procedure that would be provided to, say, a medical student. Generally, a physician must disclose the information that a "reasonable" person would consider significant when deciding to accept or reject a certain treatment (33,35). The test of reasonableness is arguably subjective and subject to second guessing by a court or jury. However, what "most physicians" do (in transmitting information about the offsetting risks for receiving and not receiving blood and available alternatives) is often held to be the proper and therefore reasonable standard of care.

Before the AIDS era, physicians generally did not advise patients specifically of the possible consequences of a blood transfusion. In a case where a patient contracted HIV while undergoing back surgery, however, a court invoked the informed consent doctrine and stated, "A physician cannot inform a patient of all of the material risks of a surgical or operative procedure without also informing him of the risks involved with a blood transfusion where a transfusion is a potential part of the procedure" (33). In a recent case arising out of a 1991 transfusion, a court found that a plaintiff had presented sufficient evidence for trial when he showed that the blood transfusion consent form that he signed did not explain alternatives such as directed donations (36). Because the testing on this HIV-tainted transfusion conformed to then-current standards, the plaintiff likely would not have had a claim but for his assertion that the consent form was deficient.

Which health care provider bears responsibility for providing informed consent? In general, the physician who performs the medical procedure has the duty to inform the patient (37). However, a hospital that provides information to the patient may have "gratuitously undertaken" the obligation to obtain consent and thus may be liable if it does not properly and fully inform the patient of the risks and alternatives (33). Thus, an incomplete informed consent can be more problematic than none at all.

A competent adult may refuse a blood transfusion for religious reasons, as with a Jehovah's Witness (38), but a transfusion may be ordered for an adult *in extremis* even if his or her spouse has stated a religious basis for refusing blood (39). For children or pregnant women, the treating physician, usually in conjunction with the hospital, should request court intervention rather than risking the consequences of a personal decision.

TRANSFUSION LIABILITY ISSUES

Transfusion liability issues are the most vexing and serious legal hazards facing the blood banking professional. Thanks to blood shield statutes and the common law view that blood is a service rather than a product, transfusion-based liability is rarely strict. That is, the plaintiff must establish more than an injury resulting from a tainted transfusion. He or she must prove negligence. If the blood was screened using state-of-the-art techniques, this will often prove difficult. Nonetheless, in their search for negligent conduct, astute plaintiffs' lawyers have tried to probe every available decision point in the process, ranging from the decision to permit the donor to give blood, to the decision not to perform a surrogate test on the donor, to the decision not to perform a "look-back" after a donor's blood tested positive. Understanding these potential theories, and how negligence is defined, is critical to the blood banking profession.

Although liability for negligence is the dominant theory in transfusion-related litigation, it is helpful to have some grasp of the alternative theories of strict liability and breach of warranty. For reasons discussed below, these theories are unlikely to be successful against a transfusion medicine provider.

Strict Liability in Tort

A claim for strict liability focuses on the integrity of the product rather than the conduct of its maker or seller. Strict liability applies to "[o]ne who sells any product in a defective condition unreasonably dangerous to the user or consumer" (40). Strict liability does not mean absolute liability for any injury resulting from use of a product. There must be proof of a defect in the manufacture, design, labeling, or warning which makes the product unreasonably dangerous.

Strict liability was developed for three reasons: a) based on the concept that costs imposed by a defective and unreasonably dangerous product are best borne by the manufacturing or distributing enterprise, which can spread the economic loss, b) to promote accident prevention, and c) in some cases, as a surrogate for negligence, which may be difficult and expensive to prove. A fundamental purpose of strict liability is to force defective and unreasonably dangerous products off of the market. A contrary view holds, however, that strict liability has caused beneficial products to be removed from the market.

Yet, in transfusion-related litigation, the debate about the pros and cons of strict liability law has become largely an academic irrelevancy. That is because a legislative and judicial consensus has emerged that blood should not be treated as a product and, therefore, its sellers and suppliers should not be subject to strict liability. In 1998, when the American Law Institute adopted its Third Restatement of Torts (Products Liability), the authors expressly provided that strict liability rules would be inapplicable to blood. As the drafters of the Third Restatement explained:

> [L]egislation in almost all jurisdictions limits the liability of sellers of human blood and human tissue to the failure to exercise reasonable care, often by providing that human blood and human tissue are not products or that their provision is a service. Where legislation has not addressed the problem, courts have concluded that strict liability is inappropriate for harm caused by such product contamination (41).

Warranty Liability, Express or Implied

Warranty law is another source of potential claims against sellers of defective products. Warranties can be express (i.e., based on something that the seller said) or implied (i.e., based on the sale itself). Liability for an express warranty arises from a representation that a product will perform in a particular manner or with a stated level of safety. A physician's therapeutic reassurance such as "there will be no problem," usually is not deemed sufficient to generate liability (42).

As the name indicates, implied warranties are implied at law for reasons of public policy. The Uniform Commercial Code, which has been enacted in virtually all states, imposes warranties of merchantability and fitness on the seller of goods (43). Yet express and implied warranty theories generally are not available against blood providers for the same reasons that strict liability claims cannot be asserted. Either by common law, by statute, or by both, blood transfusions are uniformly regarded as a service rather than a sale of a good.

Providing Blood Is a Service, Not a Sale

Even without the benefit of a blood shield statute, courts at common law typically found that providing blood constituted a service rather than the sale of a product. *Common law* is the collection of rules developed by courts over time and announced in their opinions. American common law was inherited from the English judicial system before the American Revolution and has evolved through generations of court decisions since. Common law is distinct from statutes, which are enacted by the legislature (and generally can override the common law), and from regulations, which are adopted by administrative agencies.

The underpinning for the common law view that blood is a service can be seen in an early New York case (44). That court concluded that supplying blood at a hospital was subordinate to the paramount function of furnishing trained personnel and specialized facilities to restore the plaintiff's health. When the blood provider is not a hospital, some courts have taken a different view (45). Other courts have held that the service-versus-sale distinction does not depend on whether the blood provider was a hospital (46).

Blood Shield Statutes

After a 1966 Florida case overruled the prior common law rule in that state that classified blood as a service (47), legislatures in Florida and across the nation reacted by enacting statutes to ensure that blood services remained outside strict liability. Known as *blood shield statutes,* these laws are in place in virtually every state. Only New Jersey and the District of Columbia remain without blood shield statutes.

The statutes are not uniform. Some apply only to nonprofit enterprises or are limited to specific diseases. Most of the statutes do not expressly mention strict liability but have been interpreted to preclude recovery under that theory (48). Despite considerable variability, the purpose of these statutes—to place blood providers beyond the reach of strict liability and warranty law—has been achieved.

Courts have thus far turned away arguments that the statutes violate either the federal constitution or particular state constitution provisions (49).

Negligence Claims Arising out of Blood Transfusions

Although strict liability and implied warranty claims usually cannot be maintained in transfusion-transmitted disease cases, a claim for negligence is available to the injured party in every jurisdiction. Negligence focuses upon the conduct of the blood provider. A plaintiff suing for negligence carries the burden of proving three elements: a) a duty of due care was owed to the plaintiff (the standard of care) and that duty was breached, b) the breach of the standard of care caused or substantially contributed to plaintiff's injury, and c) the person was damaged by the causally related outcome. In a typical lawsuit, all three of these elements may be contested.

Standard of Care

Establishing the blood provider's standard of care continues to be significant in many transfusion cases. The prevailing view is that blood centers, like physicians, are entitled to a professional standard of care. As a practical matter, this means that the plaintiff must have an expert to support his or her lawsuit because a layperson cannot testify as to what a professional standard of care should be. Yet this broad area of agreement has not eliminated all areas of controversy.

Two questions continue to be hotly debated. First, will the courts apply a *hard* professional standard, which means that a blood center that meets industry standards is deemed to have met professional standards? Or, rather, is the applicable standard a *soft* one under which the plaintiff is permitted to argue that a reasonable professional would do something more than meet prevailing industry standards? A second current question is the extent to which courts should screen the qualifications and methodology of a proposed expert before letting that expert testify in front of a jury.

As noted, courts have generally viewed blood centers as medical professionals entitled to the professional standard of care. A Colorado appellate court decision, which had expressly discounted the professionalism of blood banking, was overruled by that state's supreme court (50). In a 1993 case, the Nevada Supreme Court echoed the views of many courts in saying that there is a clear and growing consensus of jurisdictions that view that the production and safeguarding of the nation's blood supply is a professional activity, entitled to a professional standard of care. "We are convinced that determinations concerning the testing of donated blood and the exclusion of categories of donors are better suited to professionally trained members of the industry rather than lay persons. Such determinations require professional expertise in adopting procedures necessary for securing healthy blood and blood products without dangerously impacting the availability of adequate blood supplies" (51).

In recent years, however, courts have diverged on whether the professional standard should be hard or soft. For example, in an important California case involving a patient with thrombotic thrombocytopenic purpura who contracted AIDS from plasma transfusions she received in 1984, the court dismissed the plaintiff's negligence claim based on the contention that the blood center should have offered directed donations. The court decided that the plaintiff was not entitled to a trial because the blood center's policy regarding directed donations conformed to AABB and FDA standards (52). In an Ohio case a similar view was adopted, noting that "under Ohio law, the duty of care in a professional negligence action is dictated solely by the profession's standard" (53).

On the other hand, in two other recent notable cases involving 1984 transfusions from which the patient contracted AIDS, both the Illinois Supreme Court and the District of Columbia Court of Appeals have ruled that complying with industry standards is not an absolute defense (54,55). A plaintiff, according to these courts, is entitled to show that the industry standard was itself unreasonable or deficient. By the same token, the very Colorado Supreme Court case that had found blood banking to be a professional endeavor also ruled that plaintiffs should be allowed to show that the screening and testing procedures followed by the national blood banking community, upon which the local blood bank relied, were deficient (50).

Screening Experts

In 1993, the U.S. Supreme Court decided the Daubert v. Merrell Dow Pharmaceuticals, Inc., case (7). This famous case, which involved a challenge to expert testimony on whether the morning sickness drug Bendectin caused birth defects, has ushered in an era of greater court skepticism about experts. In the Daubert case, the Supreme Court adopted a four-factor test for whether expert testimony should be admitted in federal trial courts: a) whether the theory or technique can be tested, b) whether it has been subjected to peer review and publication, c) the known or potential rate of error, and d) whether it has been generally accepted within the scientific community. Although these factors are not absolute prerequisites, the Daubert case on the whole has encouraged trial courts to look more closely at whether the scientific community would accept a particular expert's testimony before allowing a jury to hear it.

A recent Colorado case illustrates this trend. There a patient received a transfusion in 1993 that was contaminated with HIV because the donor had given blood during the so-called *window period.* The plaintiff's expert argued that the blood center should have followed a procedure of freezing and quarantining blood donations for at least 6 months and then retested its donors before releasing the blood. The court, however, found this approach was not sufficiently accepted within the scientific community and refused to allow the case to proceed to trial (56). Notably, this decision limits the practical effect of the Colorado Supreme Court's earlier ruling that industry standards are not conclusive. Under this precedent, a plaintiff may have trouble presenting the required expert testimony to support a standard other than the industry standard. In another recent application of the Daubert case, the Texas Supreme Court decided that a trial court acted properly in excluding the plaintiffs' expert and dismissing their transfusion-injury case when the expert had no medical degree and had obtained his doctoral degree by correspondence course from an unaccredited university (57).

Significant Chronologies

Needless to say, because the blood center's conduct is judged by a negligence standard, the dates of the donation and the transfusion are very important. Because the possibility that the then-unknown causative agent of AIDS could be transmitted by blood first arose in 1982, courts have been willing to resolve cases arising in the early 1980s in favor of the defendant without the necessity of a jury trial (58). Cases closer to 1985 may present issues of fact, which generally preclude summary disposition, and cases in 1983 and 1984 have sometimes been resolved by pretrial motion (59) and sometimes by jury trial (51).

On January 4, 1983, after AIDS was reported in hemophiliacs and one transfusion recipient (60,60a), a Public Health Service work group met to discuss "candidate sets of recommendation." This meeting has taken on an importance in transfusion-transmitted AIDS litigation. Unfortunately, no verbatim report of the meeting exists; there are a few secondhand and partially conflicting reports (61–64). By these accounts, participants stated conflicting positions regarding issues such as exclusion of all homosexuals and the use of one or the other of several surrogate tests, including one for the hepatitis B core antibody. Virtually all accounts of the meeting, including those "on the record" in litigation, agree that no consensus was reached. No written recommendations were issued by the Centers for Disease Control or this work group.

On January 13, 1983, the AABB, ARC, and Council of Community Blood Centers (now America's Blood Centers) issued a joint statement that was the first effort by any governmental or nongovernmental group to give guidance to blood banks. The joint statement called for physician education, increased use of autologous donations, consideration of cryoprecipitate as a safer alternative to pooled factor VIII, adding a description of signs and symptoms of AIDS to donor screening criteria, avoiding recruitment of donors from groups with high incidence of AIDS, and working with local gay groups to limit blood donations by those at high risk. Laboratory screening was mentioned but expressly not recommended (65).

A second joint statement by these organizations and the first recommendations on AIDS by the Food and Drug Administration (FDA) followed in March 1983. These recommendations were the same in general (and many specifics) as the January joint statement. Again, laboratory screening was not advocated. It was discussed but not recommended in March 1983 (66,67).

These documents have achieved notoriety in AIDS-transfusion litigation. Defense attorneys for blood banks generally cite compliance with these recommendations to support nonliability. Indeed, there is much objective evidence that the recommended steps were highly effective in reducing donations by individuals with known risk for HIV (68,69).

Litigation regarding plasma has centered on a somewhat different landscape of documents. On January 14, 1983, the National Hemophilia Foundation issued recommendations that included direct questioning of sexual preference and evaluation of laboratory tests to identify plasma donors at high risk for AIDS transmission (70). On January 28, 1983, the American Blood Resources Association issued recommendations (71). On March 24, 1983, the FDA issued its first recommendation for establishments collecting source plasma, which differed from the recommendation for volunteer blood banks in several respects, including that plasma donors were to be examined for lymphadenopathy and weighed for unexplained weight loss before each donation and that plasma collected from donors belonging to groups at increased risk be specially labeled (72).

As more became known about AIDS, additional refinements were made to recommended procedures, sometimes by nongovernmental entities and sometimes by the FDA. On January 3, 1984, a call back was suggested for areas of high incidence of AIDS (73). Within the same time frame, the Centers for Disease Control published details of the first 18 cases, which established that AIDS was transmissible by transfusion (74). This was the first confirmation of transfusion-transmitted AIDS to appear in a peer-reviewed publication. In December of 1984, the homosexual risk group was redefined by the FDA so that "multiple sexual partners" became "males who have had sex with more than one male since 1979" (75).

In April 1984, the discovery of the virus now known as HIV was reported, proving an infectious cause (76). A specific test first became available in March 1985 (77). In the interim, a very few number of blood centers, all but one in the San Francisco Bay Area with its high volume of AIDS cases, began using either the hepatitis B core antibody (anti-HBc) or T4:T8 cell ratio as surrogate tests for AIDS, although in July 1984 a study group under the auspices of the FDA recommended, by majority report, against the use of the anti-HBc test (78).

This factual backdrop surfaces in virtually every transfusion-associated AIDS case. As the number of hepatitis C transfusion cases has increased, a common chronology has emerged in those cases as well. The critical dates are: a) 1981 when papers were published finding a correlation between elevated liver enzyme alanine aminotransferase (ALT) levels and non-A non-B hepatitis, b) 1987 when ALT and hepatitis B core antibody testing were recommended by the AABB as surrogate tests for non-A, non-B hepatitis and became the standard, c) 1990 when the first generation hepatitis C test was introduced, and d) 1992 when the second-generation test was introduced.

Working from these fact patterns, plaintiffs have fashioned a number of negligence theories, such as failure to screen (as opposed to test) a donor properly, failure to perform surrogate testing, failure to advise on directed donations, and failure to conduct a proper look-back—which have been asserted in both HIV and HCV cases. Indeed, HCV cases are now reprising the same negligence theories that were first developed a decade or earlier in the HIV litigation. Generally speaking, these theories are cast in terms of duties that the defendant allegedly breached. The more important theories are discussed below.

Donor Screening

Experienced plaintiffs' expert witnesses and counsel can advance a variety of imaginative donor screening issues. Examples of donor screening issues include the phrasing of particular screening questions, the manner of communicating risk group information (oral or written), and the timing of when AIDS information was made available to prospective donors (before or at the time of attempted donation). When the blood bank's practice was consistent with professional and government recommendations, decisions for the blood provider have been entered on a number of occasions (79–81). However, donor screening issues have been discussed in some cases in which there was a judgment for the plaintiff (82).

Surrogate Testing

In AIDS litigation, plaintiffs regularly argue that prior to the spring of 1985, in the absence of a specific test for antibodies to HIV, blood providers should have performed a surrogate test on donated blood. For cases involving donations from mid-1984 to the licensing of the first specific test (March 1985), plaintiffs can point to the few San Francisco Bay Area blood banks that implemented the hepatitis B core antibody test, although at least one court has distinguished that practice by noting that these blood banks were in an area of high risk (51). Defendants can point out that blood banks performing surrogate tests were responsible for collecting less than 5% of the national blood draw.

They also can argue, with some anecdotal evidence, that premature implementation of a surrogate test led to publicity that could have attracted high-risk donors seeking an AIDS test. Some courts have rejected the surrogate testing theory as a basis for liability (58,79,80). However, there have been jury verdicts for plaintiffs in which one of the claims was based on surrogate testing (82).

In HCV cases, plaintiffs have argued that donated blood should have been tested for elevated ALT levels in the early 1980s as soon as reports had appeared of a correlation between elevated ALT levels and non-A non-B hepatitis. Recently, this argument was rejected in two separate cases, one that went to trial and the other that was decided on a motion for summary judgment (83,84). An earlier case, however, found that a blood center could have had a duty to perform ALT testing in 1986 (85).

Inventory Cases

With the implementation of HIV antibody testing, blood banks faced a dilemma: use the untested units of blood that were in inventory (sometimes already at the hospital) or attempt to replace those units with tested units. It would have been physically impossible to replace fully the nation's inventory of untested blood without using existing units. A few patients were infected with untested units that were in inventory. Plaintiffs have argued both successfully (86) and unsuccessfully (87) that the blood bank had a duty to recall and test all units. Since 1985, blood banks have usually attempted to test units in inventory when a new test is introduced (such as HCV testing in 1990).

Unnecessary Transfusions and the Failure to Use Autologous and Directed Transfusion

The treating physician is responsible for the decision to transfuse. The emergence of serious transmissible diseases has made it more important than ever that the decision be for sound medical reasons. If the indications for transfusion cannot be medically defended and the patient is injured, the physician may be held liable. The hospital laboratory cannot review every decision to transfuse but may help prevent the inappropriate use of blood by a regular audit of transfusions and by helping to educate the physician staff. These mandates come from the Joint Commission on Accreditation of Healthcare Organizations (88).

An Ohio jury awarded $12 million when a resident physician ordered a unit from the general blood supply even though autologous units already donated may have sufficed (89). An allegedly unnecessary plasma transfusion resulted in a large award against a neonatologist (90). Here and in other instances, the plaintiff's case was based on underlying malpractice in transfusion medicine that allegedly led to transmission of AIDS. In one recent decision, though, the court explicitly rejected a theory that the blood center had a "duty to educate" hospitals and physicians on use of directed donations (81).

Failure to suggest autologous or directed donations also has been argued to juries (79), although those arguments are unavailable in many cases because of the emergent nature of the procedure or the health of the patient. In the experience of the authors, lay jurors readily assume directed donations are risk free. Educating them to the contrary can be a difficult undertaking. At least one study involving hundreds of thousands of donations showed that directed donors can have far higher rates of disease markers than community volunteer donors (91).

Patient Notification

The purpose of a look-back program is to identify and notify earlier recipients of blood components from donors who are subsequently found to have certain infectious agents. Look-back was generally implemented for HIV in 1986 (92), for HTLV-I in 1989 (93), and for HCV in 1998 and 1999 (94). Typically, the potentially infectious component was donated before the availability of the blood test, or the donor was exposed too recently to the virus for the antibody to be detectable (during the window period). Look-back is triggered by a subsequent donation with a positive test result or by an outside report, such as from the hospital, of a suspected case of a transfusion-transmitted infectious agent.

Advising a possibly infected person of his or her condition to avert a public health risk is consistent with sound medical ethics. Information must be accurate and followed by counseling. The legal support for look-back rests on cases such as the well-known California decision holding that a psychotherapist who had reason to believe his patient was likely to harm another person had a duty to warn the person in danger (95). That decision has been followed by cases holding that a physician or hospital could be liable for failing to warn a patient that he or she had contracted HIV when he or she spread the disease to a partner (96,97). The most important factor underlying a duty to warn is the foreseeability of future harm.

A successful look-back program requires cooperation among the blood center, hospital or transfusion service, the recipient's physician, and local or state health agencies. Because the primary duty of patient care rests with the physician, the health care institution does not usually deal directly with the patient unless his or her physician is unavailable or unwilling to perform a look-back notification. In certain cases, public health authorities may take responsibility for notifying patients. Whatever mechanism is selected should ensure that all information is handled confidentially. As noted earlier, breaches in confidentiality in which information about infectious disease is involved can lead to serious legal sanctions. Written confirmation as part of look-back is usually preferable, but there may be circumstances, especially involving the patient, in which telephone or face-to-face communication by the physician should occur.

Following identification and notification, patients (and sometimes spouses, spouse equivalents, and children, as appropriate) should be tested and counseled. Because patients are unlikely to be aware of their possible exposure to disease, they should benefit from early diagnosis and possible prophylactic or therapeutic interventions and, through counseling and behavior modifications, limit the spread to third parties.

Ultimately, a physician must decide whether and how to inform the patient. The physician may decide that knowledge would be harmful or of little or no benefit. For example, if the physician is confident that the potentially infected person is elderly or in ill health and thus at very low risk for transmitting infection, there may be a considered decision made to spare the patient the emotional upset. However, if the balance between the benefits and detriments of notification is at all debatable, the physician's decision should be in favor of notice.

The AABB and FDA have issued detailed recommendations for look-back programs. Standards for blood banks and transfusion services, issued by the AABB, require the establishment of look-back procedures for HIV and HTLV-I and -II (98). In 1992, the FDA issued a guidance memorandum recommending that blood establishments conduct HIV look-back programs. In 1993, FDA and the Health Care Financing Administration published proposed HIV look-back rules in the Federal Register (99).

In the late 1990s, the FDA published important guidances relating to HCV look-back (94). Recently, a proposed class action was filed alleging that certain blood centers negligently failed to perform their look-back duties to notify recipients of HCV-contaminated transfusions (100). As successful early therapies (it is hoped) become increasingly available for HIV and HCV patients, and as FDA look-back requirements become more complex (and more ambiguous), one can expect to see additional look-back claims.

Standard-setting Claims

In recent years, some states have decided that national standard-setting organizations, in particular AABB, can be sued for alleged negligence in promulgating national standards. In a well-known 1996 case, the New Jersey Supreme Court held that AABB could be held liable to a recipient of an HIV-contaminated transfusion for not recommending surrogate testing before August 1984 (101). At least two courts in other states followed this analysis (102,103). Yet in a significant 1999 decision, the California Court of Appeal disagreed with the New Jersey court's reasoning. It found that AABB did not have a duty to make favorable recommendations regarding direct questioning of donors, directed donations, and surrogate testing (104).

Causation

As noted above, the plaintiff in a transfusion case also must prove causation, namely, that the violation of the standard of care was responsible for his or her injuries. Not surprisingly, the more cutting-edge theories, such as failure to perform surrogate testing, negligent look-back, or negligent standard setting, tend to pose more difficult causation questions (84,104,105). Hepatitis C cases also can present thorny causation problems, in large part because of the prevalence of nontransfusion sources for the infection.

The last 2 decades of transfusion litigation have resulted in controversies that will never be fully resolved. As often occurs in our noncentralized court system, judicial decisions have been inconsistent. Surrogate testing lacked scientific support at the time, and some experts believe it would have increased the number of transfusion-transmitted AIDS cases by, among other things, attracting high-risk donors anxious for a test result (the magnet theory). Three contemporaneous studies (two published and one unpublished) failed to find a benefit from surrogate testing (106,107). Direct questioning on sexual preference and conduct subsequently has been shown to be acceptable to donors (108) and better understood (109) but has never been shown actually to reduce the risk to recipients. However, donor attitudes in such recent studies may reflect changes in societal mores since 1983.

To defendants, litigation of the past decade represents a display of revisionist thinking and "Galileo's revenge" by experts who claim they were not heeded at the time. To the plaintiffs, however, these cases illustrate a failure of the blood establishment.

ALTERNATIVE DISPUTE RESOLUTION

The high cost and unwieldiness of the traditional tort system have led some parties to search for alternative dispute resolution mechanisms. The idea of alternative dispute resolution (or ADR) is hardly new, although its use in medical negligence cases developed in the 1980s. Alternative dispute resolution in the United States, primarily in the mercantile setting, predated the Declaration of Independence. It became officially institutionalized in this country in 1922 with the creation of a new educational organization known as the Arbitration Society of America (110).

Today litigants looking for a way to escape the court system face an almost bewildering array of ADR choices. These go by such names as arbitration, early neutral evaluation, mediation, med-arb (combining mediation and arbitration), minitrials, and more.

Some no-fault or fault-based claim settlement mechanisms also exist under the ADR umbrella. These include the fault-based patient compensation programs in Indiana, Florida, and Louisiana, the no-fault neonatal neurologic injury program in Virginia, and the federal no-fault vaccine injury program. Typically, a patient must submit his or her claim to an expert panel where liability is adjudged (on a fault or no-fault basis, depending how the system is set up) and an award offered. The patient usually can choose to accept the award as settlement of the claim or forever reject the award and pursue his or her claim in the courts. Colorado and Utah have designed pilot programs for extending no-fault compensation programs (similar to workers compensation) to medical malpractice claims.

In general, arbitration, which is supported by enforcement statutes in most states, is a method whereby a single person or panel makes a final and binding award after a process that is usually faster and less formal than a trial. Mediation is probably the fastest-growing ADR option. It is a form of assisted negotiation using an enlisted neutral third party, whose task is to aid the parties in a quest for voluntary settlement. Minitrials can take many forms but generally provide a format in which limited evidence is presented to a jury and either a recommendation is rendered (typically for use in a mediation) or a binding award is made (like an arbitration) (Dauer E, unpublished material).

Several years ago, the ARC completed a pilot program, working with the AABB, America's Blood Centers, and the Center for Public Resources (an ADR advocacy group). Typical of ADR programs, its objective was to achieve early resolution of the cases with lower defense and management costs, without adversely affecting the cost of indemnity or settlement value. The pilot program used a technique developed in the nonmedical setting called *early neutral evaluation* (ENE), in which a neutral evaluator (usually someone trained in mediation) hears the arguments on both sides (after limited discovery or an initial phase of an exchange of documents) and renders a judgment on the likely outcome and value of the outcome, if any. The parties can then try mediation to resolve the case or continue litigating. Key to the success of ENE is that all parties, not just the attorneys, participate in the process. This allows the principals to hear first hand what the other party has to say and to receive the opinion of the neutral evaluator. The ARC trial on about 15 cases resulted in settlements at or below values estimated by the defense, but at far lower costs for defense attorneys than had been anticipated. As expected, systems like ENE get to the "bottom line" sooner and more inexpensively than traditional litigation.

An unpublished study by AABB, America's Blood Centers, and ARC showed that 60% of all expenses in AIDS cases went to defense attorneys, with about 15% for plaintiffs' counsel and 25% in compensation. These numbers, in conjunction with the results of the ENE pilot, leave hope that more direct use of ADR may ensure that a higher proportion of indemnity payments go toward compensation of injured patients rather than being consumed by legal expenses.

A system model for a "neo-no-fault" compensation program for designated injuries relating to transfusion has been prepared (Dauer E, unpublished material). Following notice of an incident, the injured person is contacted, qualified, and offered an immediate settlement package. In exchange for a waiver of rights to litigate, future medical costs are guaranteed and mediation is followed, if necessary, by binding arbitration. A stipend to pay legal counsel is included. America's Blood Centers, AABB, and ARC designed a pilot study of the program that was to be tested in Arizona in the mid-1990s, but it was never was implemented because of defense concerns that, given the current low incidence of transfusion injuries, such a program might attract claims that otherwise might not be filed.

Many administrative and cost issues remain to be settled, but ADR appears to be an attractive alternative to the litigation arena, because it emphasizes the injured party's needs rather than demands driven by a hoped-for recovery.

CONCLUSION

It is essential to learn from the past. Alternative dispute resolution mechanisms for those inadvertently or unavoidably injured by blood donation are in place and work well. Similar programs need to be developed for transfusion injuries. These procedures can decrease litigation and, more importantly, ensure that a greater share of compensation actually goes to injured parties.

REFERENCES

1. US General Accounting Office. Blood Supply: FDA oversight and remaining issues of safety; and Blood supply: transfusion-associated risks. 1997 Feb 25; PEMD-97-1 and PEMD-97-1.
2. America's Blood Centers. Hemolytic transfusion reactions, part 1: biological product deviations (errors and accidents). *Blood Bulletin* 2000;3:1–2.
3. Institute of Medicine. *To err is human: building a safer health system.* National Academy Press, 1999.
4. Williamson LM et al. Serious hazards of transfusion (SHOT) initiative: analysis of the first two annual reports. *BMJ* 1999:319:16–19.
5. Reser RJ, Radnofsky BA. New wave of tainted blood litigation: hepatitis C liability issues. *Def Counsel J* 2000:67;306.
6. Dauer E. Alternatives for the management and resolution of claims arising from transfusion-associated injuries. Center for Public Resources, 1992.
7. *Daubert v Merrell Dow Pharmaceuticals, Inc,* 509 US 579 (1993).
8. Dauer, E. Alternative methods for managing transfusion-injury claims. Report of a pilot program: mediation and early neutral evaluation. American Red Cross, American Association of Blood Banks, and Council of Community Blood Centers, 1994.
9. Leveton, LB, Sox HC, Soto MA, eds. *HIV and the blood supply: an analysis of crisis decisionmaking.* National Academy Press, 1995.
10. Sataro PA. Blood collection. In: Kasprisin CA, Laird-Fryer B. *Blood donor collection practices.* Bethesda, MD: American Association of Blood Banks, 1993:83–104.
11. Compare *Congelton v Baton Rouge General Hospital,* 444 So 2d 175 (La App 1983) and *Montgomery v Opelous General Hospital,* 540 So 2d 312 (La 1989).
12. Responses to private questionnaire by Foster Robberson, 1992.
13. *Griffin v American Red Cross,* 1994 WL 675105 (ED Pa 1994).
14. *Carroll v Sisters of St Francis,* 868 SW2d 585 (Tenn 1993).
15. *Helmstadter v North American Biological, Inc,* 559 NW2d 794 (Neb App 1997).
16. *Marcella v Brandywine Hosp,* 47 F3d 618 (3rd Cir 1995).
17. Kevin Hopkins. Blood, sweat, and tears: toward a new paradigm for protecting donor privacy. *Va J Soc Policy L* 2000;7:141.
18. *DaBoutte v Blood Sys, Inc,* 127 FRD 122 (WD La 1989).
19. *Cook v American National Red Cross,* 1998 WL 46399 (D Kan 1998).
20. *Doe v American National Red Cross,* 151 FRD 71 (SD W Va 1993).
21. *Stenger v Lehigh Valley Hosp Ctr,* 530 Pa 426, 609 A2d 796 (1992).
22. *Snyder v Mekhjiarn,* 125 NJ 328, 593 A2d 318 (1991).
23. *Watson v Lowcountry Red Cross,* 974 F2d 482 (4th Cir 1992).
24. *Rasmussen v South Florida Blood Service,* 500 So 2d 533 (Fla 1987).
25. *LaBurre v East Jefferson General Hospital,* 555 So 2d 1381 (La 1990).
26. *Irwin Memorial Blood Bank v Superior Court,* 229 Cal App 3d 151, 279 Cal Rptr 911 (1991).
27. *Belle Bonfils Memorial Blood Center v District Court,* 763 P2d 1003 (Colo 1988).
28. *Krygier v Airweld, Inc,* 137 Misc 2d 306, 520 NYS2d 475 (1987).
29. *Doe v Puget Sound Blood Center,* 117 Wash 2d 772, 819 P2d 370 (1991).
30. *Coleman v American Red Cross,* 145 FRD 422 (ED Mich 1993).
31. Knowing Your Options, America's Blood Centers, 1999: www.americasblood.org.
32. Goldman EB. Signed consent: a legal perspective, part I. In: Widmann F, ed. *Informed consent for blood transfusion.* Arlington, VA: American Association of Blood Banks, 1989:33–39.
33. *Jones v Philadelphia College of Osteopathic Medicine,* 813 F Supp 1125 (ED Pa 1993).
34. *Shenefield v Greenwich Hospital Association,* 10 Conn App 239, 522 A2d 829 (Conn App 1987).
35. *Arato v Avedon,* 5 Cal 4th 1172, 23 Cal Rptr 2d 131, 858 P2d 598 (1993).
36. *Kotofsky v Albert Einstein Medical Center,* 2000 WL 1618475 (ED Pa 2000).
37. Ballengee BO, Fleetwood MJ. Legal issues in blood banking. In: Kasprisin CA, Laird-Fryer B. *Blood donor collection practices.* Bethesda, MD: American Association of Blood Banks, 1993:170.

38. *Public Health Trust of Dade County v Wons,* 541 So 2d 96 (Fla 1989).
39. *Application of President and Directors of Georgetown College,* 331 F2d 1000 (DC Cir), *cert denied,* 377 US 978 (1964).
40. Restatement (Second) of Torts § 402A.
41. Restatement (Third) of Torts (Products Liability) § 19.
42. *Van Zee v Witzke,* 445 NW2d 34 (SD 1989).
43. Uniform Commercial Code §§ 2-105, 2-314, 2-315.
44. *Perlmutter v Beth David Hospital,* 308 NY 100, 123 NE2d 792 (1954).
45. *Hansen v Mercy Hospital, Denver,* 40 Colo App 17, 570 P2d 1309 (1977), aff'd *sub nom Belle Bonfils Memorial Blood Bank v Hansen,* 195 Colo 529, 579 P2d 1158 (1978).
46. *Whitehurst v American National Red Cross,* 1 Ariz App 326, 402 P2d 584 (1965).
47. *Russell v Community Blood Bank,* 185 So 2d 749 (Fla Dist Ct App 1966), aff'd as modified, 196 So 2d 115 (Fla 1967).
48. *Royer v Miles Laboratory, Inc,* 107 Or App 112, 811 P2d 644 (1991).
49. *Smith v Paslode Corporation,* 799 F Supp 960 (ED Mo 1992), aff'd in part and rev'd in part, 7 F3d 116 (8th Cir 1993).
50. Compare *Quintana v United Blood Services,* 811 P2d 424 (Colo App 1991), with *United Blood Services v Quintana,* 827 P2d 509 (Colo 1992).
51. *Brown v United Blood Services,* 858 P2d 391 (Nev 1993).
52. *Spann v Irwin Memorial Blood Centers,* 40 Cal Rptr 2d 360 (App 1995).
53. *Zaccone v American Red Cross,* 872 FSupp 457 (ND Ohio 1994).
54. *Advincula v United Blood Services,* 678 NE2d 1009 (Ill 1996).
55. *Ray v American National Red Cross,* 696 A2d 399 (DC App 1997).
56. *Smith v Belle Bonfils Memorial Blood Center,* 976 P2d 344 (Colo App 1998).
57. *United Blood Services, Inc v Longoria,* 938 SW2d 29 (Tex 1997).
58. *Kozup v Georgetown University,* 663 F Supp 1048 (DDC 1987), aff'd in part, vacated in part, 851 F2d 437 (DC Cir 1988).
59. *Knight v Department of Navy,* 757 FSupp 790 (WD Tex 1991).
60. Centers for Disease Control. Possible transfusion-associated acquired immune deficiency syndrome (AIDS) California. *MMWR* 1982;31: 652–654.
60a. Centers for Disease Control. Update on acquired immune deficiency syndrome (AIDS) among patients with hemophilia A. *MMWR* 1982; 31:644–652.
61. Drake D. The disease detectives puzzle over methods of control. *Philadelphia Inquirer,* 1993 Jan 9:Vol 308, No 9.
62. Marx J. Health officials seek ways to halt AIDS. *Science* 1983;219: 271–272.
63. Check W. Preventing AIDS transmission: should blood donors be screened? *JAMA* 1983;249:567–570.
64. Perkins H. AIDS the controversy. *California Blood Bank Letter* 1983; 1:474–477.
65. Joint statement on acquired immune deficiency syndrome (AIDS) related to transfusion. American Association of Blood Banks, Council of Community Blood Centers, American Red Cross, 1983 Jan 13.
66. Joint statement on prevention of acquired immune deficiency syndrome. American Association of Blood Banks, Council of Community Blood Centers, American Red Cross, 1983 Mar 7.
67. Director, Office of Biologics, National Center for Drugs and Biologics. Memorandum to all establishments collecting human blood for transfusions. Recommendations to decrease the risk of transmitting acquired immune deficiency syndrome (AIDS) from blood donors. Food and Drug Administration. 1983 Mar 23.
68. Selik RM, Ward JW, Buehler JW. Trends in transfusion-associated acquired immune deficiency syndrome in the United States, 1982 through 1991. *Transfusion* 1993;33:890–893.
69. Busch MP, Young MJ, Samson SM, et al. Risk of human immunodeficiency virus (HIV) transmission by blood transfusions before implementation of HIV-1 antibody screening. *Transfusion* 1991;31:4–11.
70. Recommendations to prevent AIDS in patients with hemophilia. National Hemophilia Foundation, 1983 Jan 14.
71. ABRA recommendations on AIDS and plasma donor deferral. American Blood Resources Association, 1983 Jan 28.
72. Director, Office of Biologics, National Center for Drugs and Biologics. Memorandum to all establishments collecting source plasma (human). Recommendations to decrease the risk of transmitting acquired immune deficiency syndrome (AIDS) from plasma donors. Food and Drug Administration, 1983 Mar 24.
73. Joint statement on acquired immune deficiency syndrome (AIDS) and blood transfusion. American Association of Blood Banks, Council of Community Blood Centers, American Red Cross, 1984 Jan 3.
74. Curran JW, Lawrence DN, Jaffe H, et al. Acquired immunodeficiency syndrome (AIDS) associated with transfusion. *N Engl J Med* 1984; 310:67–75.
75. Acting Director, Office of Biologics Research and Review. Memorandum to all establishments collecting blood, blood components or source plasma and all licensed manufacturers of plasma derivatives. Revised recommendations to decrease the risk of transmitting acquired immunodeficiency syndrome (AIDS) from blood and plasma donors. Food and Drug Administration, 1984 Dec 14.
76. Department of Health and Human Services. Statement by Secretary Heckler. 1984 Apr 23.
77. Department of Health and Human Services. Statement by Secretary Heckler. 1985 Mar 2.
78. Rodell M, et al. Final report of the hepatitis B core antibody testing study group. 1984 July 16.
79. *Osborn v Irwin Memorial Blood Bank,* 7 Cal Rptr 2d 101 (App 1992).
80. *Doe v Greater New York Blood Program,* 700 A2d 377 (NJ Super App Div 1997).
81. *Giorno v Temple University Hosp,* 875 FSupp 267 (ED Pa 1995).
82. *JK and Susie L Wadley Research Institute and Blood Bank v Beeson,* 835 SW2d 689 (Tex App Dallas 1992).
83. *Sturm v University of Cincinnati Medical Center,* 739 NE2d 364 (Ohio App 2000).
84. *Grant v American National Red Cross,* 745 A2d 316 (DC App 2000).
85. *Hernandez v Nueces County Medical Soc Commun Blood Bank,* 779 SW2d 867 (Tex App 1989).
86. *Carroll, et al. v Blood Center of Southeastern Wisconsin, et al.,* No 753–411 (Wis Cir Ct 1988).
87. *Kirkendall v Harbor Insurance Company,* 698 F Supp 768 (WD Ark 1988), aff'd, 887 F2d 857 (8th Cir 1989).
88. Mintz PD. Hospital transfusion committee and quality assurance. In: Rossi E, Simon T, Moss G, eds. *Principles of transfusion medicine.* Baltimore: Williams & Wilkins, 1991:730.
89. *Jeanne v Hawkes Hospital of Mt Carmel,* No 90AP-599 (Ohio Ct App May 23, 1991).
90. *Edwards, et al. v Samaritan Health Service, et al.,* No CV 87–3569 (Ariz Super Ct 1990).
91. Starkey JM, MacPherson JL, Bolgiano DC, et al. Markers for transfusion-transmitted disease in different groups of blood donors, *JAMA* 1989;262:3452–3454.
92. Joint statement on look-back: notification of previous recipients of blood and components from donors who now have a confirmed positive test for anti-HTLV-III. American Association of Blood Banks, Community Council of Blood Centers, American Red Cross, 1986 June 16.
93. Memorandum to AABB institutional members: guidelines for notification & counseling of recipients of HTLV-I/II positive blood. American Association of Blood Banks, 1989 May 26.
94. 63 FR 13675 (March 20, 1998); 63 FR 56198 (Oct 21, 1998); 64 FR 33309 (June 22, 1999).
95. *Tarasoff v Board of Regents of University of California,* 17 Cal 3d 425, 131 Cal Rptr 14, 551 P2d 334 (1976).
96. *Reisner v Regents of the University of California,* 31 Cal App 4th 1195, 37 Cal Rptr 2d 518 (1995).
97. *Chamberry v Mt Sinai Hosp,* 615 NYS2d 830 (NY Sup 1994).
98. American Association of Blood Banks. *Standards for blood banks and transfusion services,* 15th ed. Arlington, VA: American Association of Blood Banks, 1993:34.
99. *Federal Register* 1993 June 30:58.
100. *Sturman v Rush-Presbyterian-St Lukes Medical Center,* No 00L 011069 (Cook County, Ill, 2000).
101. *Snyder v American Assn of Blood Banks,* 676 A2d 1036 (NJ 1996).
102. *Weigand v University Hosp of New York,* 659 NYS2d 395 (Sup 1997).

103. *Douglass v Alton Ochsner Medical Foundation,* 696 So2d 136 (La App 1997).
104. *NNV v American Assn of Blood Banks,* 89 Cal Rptr 2d 885 (App 1999).
105. *McKnight v American Red Cross,* 1994 WL 323861 (ED Pa 1994).
106. Simon TL, Bankhurst A. A pilot study of surrogate tests to prevent transmission of acquired immune deficiency syndrome by transfusions. *Transfusion* 1984;24:373–378.
107. Pindyck J, Waldman A, Zang E, et al. Measures to decrease the risk of acquired immunodeficiency syndrome transmission by blood transfusion. *Transfusion* 1985;25:3–9.
108. Silvergleid AJ, Leparc GF, Schmidt PJ. Impact of explicit questions and high risk activities on donor attitudes and donor deferral patterns. *Transfusion* 1989:29:362–364.
109. Mayo DJ, Rose Ann, Matchelt SE, et al. Screening potential blood donors at risk for human immunodeficiency virus. *Transfusion* 1991; 31:466–474.
110. Roth B, Wulff R, Cooper C. *The alternative dispute resolution practice guide.* 1993.

CASE 65A

ELECTIVE SURGERY IN A JEHOVAH'S WITNESS

HISTORY

A 42-year-old man was discovered to have microhematuria on a routine urinalysis done in the course of an annual physical examination. The rectal examination showed a small, firm prostate and the prostate-specific antigen (PSA) was elevated at 5.5 ng/ml (upper limit of reference range, 4.0 ng/ml). Needle biopsies of the prostate showed adenocarcinoma. The patient's medical history, review of systems, and physical examination were otherwise unremarkable. His hemoglobin level was 15.8 g/dl. The patient was raised in a Christian church of the Orthodox tradition but had become a Jehovah's Witness as a young adult. He was referred for prostatectomy to a hospital in which physicians had been performing surgery on Jehovah's Witness patients for several years.

The patient met initially with one of the staff urologists who reviewed the case and discussed the options. The decision was made to perform a radical retropubic prostatectomy. A meeting was then arranged which included the patient, his father, a representative from his church, the urologist, an anesthesiologist, and a transfusion medicine physician. The amount of blood typically lost in this procedure was discussed; the urologist cited a few examples from the literature as well as the experience in his own patients. Because the patient had a high hemoglobin level to begin with and no coronary artery disease, it was explained to him that he could probably tolerate the loss of one-half of his red blood cell mass with little risk.

The patient had done a lot of reading and had decided that he would not accept any blood component including red blood cells, platelets, plasma, cryoprecipitate, or albumin. He would, however, accept recombinant proteins such as factor VIII and erythropoietin. It was pointed out to him that recombinant erythropoietin contains human albumin, but he was willing to accept it because the albumin was being used as a stabilizer for the erythropoietin and was not actually being transfused. He also would not permit the infusion of his own blood once it had been removed from his body, hence preoperative autologous blood donation was not an option. Upon further discussion, he was willing to receive blood removed from him if it remained in a continuous circuit with his body. Diagrams were drawn to show him how acute normovolemic hemodilution and intraoperative red blood cell recovery and reinfusion (using a cell washer) could be performed while maintaining contact with his vascular space. Acute normovolemic hemodilution was a particularly attractive option, because it has been used effectively in prostatectomy to limit allogeneic blood use (1).

At the end of the discussion, a plan was agreed upon. Three or four units of blood would be withdrawn at the beginning of the procedure and replaced with crystalloid fluids. The blood would be maintained in the circuit with a return line and a three-way stopcock for use at the end of the procedure or in the event of intraoperative bleeding. If intraoperative bleeding became severe, a cell-washing device would be brought into the operating room and used, also in continuous circuit with the patient. The patient would also accept erythropoietin after the procedure if his physicians felt his hemoglobin level was dangerously low. The question of what to do in the face of life-threatening bleeding was discussed at this point. The patient was quite clear that he would not accept any other form of transfusion other than what he had just agreed to, even if it meant that he would die. He did not authorize any proxy to make that decision for him while he was under anesthesia.

Following the meeting, the urologist wrote up the plan and sent copies to everyone who had attended the meeting. He then met once again with the patient to review the plan and to have the patient sign the consent forms.

DISCUSSION

The Jehovah's Witnesses is a Christian sect which began as a Bible study group in the nineteenth century. By the end of the century, their beliefs had crystallized and they began to expound them through the publications of the Zion's Watchtower Tract Society. Central to their beliefs is the primacy of the Bible, which they consider to be the word of God and the source of all truth. In the early part of the twentieth century, the belief system and structure of the Jehovah's Witnesses were formalized and centralized under the leadership of a remarkable organizer, Joseph Franklin Russell. The organization now claims over one million members in the United States and more than five million worldwide.

One of the core beliefs is the injunction against blood transfusion, which is based on the interpretation of several passages of the Bible, principally Genesis 9:3–4 and Leviticus 17:14. Because these books of the Bible are historically attributed to Moses, they carry considerable authority. These passages were clearly not written with transfusion in mind and are subject to different interpretations, but the Jehovah's Witnesses are certainly entitled to their own interpretation, and arguing the point is neither productive nor appropriate. It is important to understand that the consequences an individual believer may suffer for transgression are severe, namely forfeiture of eternal life and a form of excommunication called *disfellowshipping.* In June of 2000, a statement appeared on the Watch Tower Society website (2) announcing that church members who received transfusions voluntarily need not be disfellowshipped. Several days later the statement disappeared and was replaced by a clarification that the Church would not automatically disfellowship a transfused member. However, in the act of accepting a transfusion, the member showed that he was turning his back on the Church and by that act was disassociating himself from the faithful. So although the Church would not excommunicate a transfused member, the member in effect excommunicated himself. The consequences were still loss of eternal life and shunning by members of the Church (3).

Therefore, when contemplating a course of medical intervention which might require transfusion, such as surgery or chemotherapy, a Jehovah's Witness faces a serious decision. It also demands a significant commitment on the part of the institution agreeing to care for such a patient, because the law has consistently supported the right of competent adults to refuse blood transfusion, even if it may result in death. The practitioners and institutions caring for these patients therefore have a legal as well as moral obligation to respect their wishes.

Before embarking on the care of Jehovah's Witnesses, an institution must decide first of all whether or not it has the resources, including experience with blood-sparing techniques and staff comfortable working under the restrictions imposed by the patients' beliefs. It may be that the most appropriate step is to refer the patients to a center which has had some experience caring for Jehovah's Witnesses. The process for planning for the care of Jehovah's Witnesses should enlist wide representation from the hospital including from the offices of the general counsel, risk management, pastoral care, and an ethicist. As part of this phase of planning, a review of informed consent policies should be undertaken, particularly with respect to incompetent adults, minors, emancipated minors, and fetuses. Although the courts support the rights of competent adults to refuse transfusion, they have generally regarded the preservation of the life of minors and fetuses to be in the interest of the state. The institution should be sure that its policies are explicit with respect to these special categories of patients.

Once this ground work has been laid, the next step is to arrange for a meeting with the patient, offering him the opportunity to include a spiritual advisor, who may be his own pastor or a representative from the Church with experience in health care issues. The principal care providers, usually the surgeon and the anesthesiologist, must be present, as well as others who might have a central role. Paradoxically, it is often extremely useful to have a transfusion medicine physician present because he or she is often well versed in strategies for minimizing blood use.

During this discussion, the therapeutic options (some of which might not entail blood loss) should be reviewed and the likelihood of their success compared. The usual amount of blood loss and the likelihood of life-threatening blood loss should be presented to the patient, using local data if possible. During this discussion, it should be determined which blood components (e.g., red blood cells, plasma, platelets) or products (e.g., albumin, factor VIII concentrate) the patient will accept. It may be necessary to describe how these components are prepared. All of the various options for minimizing blood transfusion should be explained, including hypotensive anesthesia, preoperative autologous blood donation, acute normovolemic hemodilution, intraoperative shed-blood recovery and reinfusion, and perioperative erythropoietin administration. It should be determined which of these the patient finds acceptable. Although there is some variability in terms of what different patients will accept, the amount and accessibility of information available from the Jehovah's Witness organization has somewhat standardized the options.

It is also important to discuss an endgame with the patient, what the caretakers will be permitted to do if death from blood loss is imminent. The patient should be offered the opportunity to appoint a proxy to make any such decisions for him while he is under general anesthesia or is otherwise incompetent to make decisions for himself. It is important for the patient to articulate clearly the preference to die rather than receive a transfusion.

Given the amount of information that must be covered and the number of decisions that need to be made, it is usually useful to write up a summary of the discussion and the plan which has been agreed to, and circulate it to those who attended the meeting. This step not only affords everyone an opportunity to clarify the plan, but it also gives the patient some time to reconsider his options. The patient may find it helpful to refer to various resources that the Jehovah's Witnesses can provide, which describe alternatives to transfusion. At least one follow-up meeting should be scheduled to answer the patient's questions or revise the plan. This document should be considered a part of the patient's informed consent for the procedure. Some institutions have a policy of requiring a written statement from the patient to document his desire to decline transfusion, even if it means that serious injury or death might ensue.

For a very thorough treatment of many aspects of transfusion and the Jehovah's Witnesses, the reader is referred to a series of articles in a single issue of *Transfusion Medicine Reviews* (4).

CODA

The patient underwent radical retropubic prostatectomy and pelvic lymph node dissection. Three units of blood were withdrawn at the beginning of the procedure and reinfused at the end; a cell washer was not needed. The tissue removed showed a moderately differentiated adenocarcinoma, Gleason score 6 out of 10. There was no extension beyond the capsule and two out of two lymph nodes were clear. His hemoglobin level was 15.6 g/dl before the procedure and 13.1 g/dl afterward. The estimated blood loss was 600 ml. The patient made an uneventful recovery and was discharged 3 days after surgery with a hemoglobin level of 13.7 g/dl. Ten months later, the PSA level was <0.2 ng/ml.

Case contributed by Christopher P. Stowell, M.D., Ph.D., Massachusetts General Hospital, Boston, MA.

REFERENCES

1. Monk, TG, Goodnough LT, Birkmeyer JD, et al. Acute normovolemic hemodilution is a cost-effective alternative to preoperative autologous blood donation in patients undergoing radical retropubic prostatectomy. *Transfusion* 1995;35:559–565.
2. Available at http://www.watchtower.org.
3. Muramoto O. Bioethical aspects of the recent changes in the policy of refusal of blood of Jehovah's Witnesses. *BMJ* 2001;322:37–39.
4. Multiple articles. *Transfus Med Rev* 1991;5:243–286.

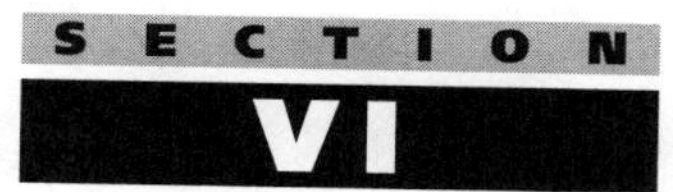

DELIVERY OF BLOOD SERVICES

66

ORGANIZATION OF BLOOD SERVICES IN THE UNITED STATES

JAY E. MENITOVE

During the early 1990s, compliance with the Food and Drug Administration's (FDA) current Good Manufacturing Practices (cGMPs) represented a paradigm change for blood collection agencies that previously followed good laboratory practices. In addition, cost containment pressures and declining or plateaued blood use led some blood organizations to adopt competitive business practices to increase market share in lieu of operating as quasiregulated monopolies serving static, regional areas. Mergers, acquisitions, and consolidations affected blood collection agencies in parallel with changes in the overall health care field. By the late 1990s, blood use increased after years of limited growth, competition was refocused to improve intraorganizational infrastructure, and blood centers raised charges to hospitals in an effort to align revenues with operating costs.

J.E. Menitove: Department of Internal Medicine, University of Missouri, and Community Blood Center of Greater Kansas City, Kansas City, Missouri, and School of Medicine, Kansas University, Kansas City, Kansas.

FACTORS AFFECTING BLOOD COLLECTION AGENCIES

During the 1980s and early 1990s blood collection agencies followed good laboratory practices. These agencies viewed themselves as service providers that operated regional laboratories in a relatively collegial environment. Cost increases were passed on to hospitals.

During the early to mid-1990s, dramatic changes occurred in the relationship between blood centers and the hospitals in their service regions. The previous paradigm in which hospitals received blood from their regional blood centers underwent challenge (1). The shift reflected a transition from a growth enterprise to a mature field. Although periodic blood shortages occurred, the overall decline in blood use rates that began in the mid-1980s in response to concerns about transfusion-transmitted human immunodeficiency virus (HIV), showed little change until the late 1990s. Throughout the 1990s, costs of collecting, processing, and testing voluntarily donated blood increased as a result of newly implemented HIV-2, HIV-antigen, and hepatitis C assays and more stringent regulation by the FDA.

Blood collection agencies found themselves struggling to conform to FDA-mandated current Good Manufacturing Practices and the transformation from service providers to product suppliers, (i.e., manufacturers of products). As manufacturers, blood centers sought to reduce errors, accidents, and nonconformities through standardization. Likewise, attempts to reduce costs of production led to creation of large, consolidated laboratories that performed infectious disease, ABO, Rh, and other testing. Competition among blood centers for hospital business replaced the earlier collegial relationship between the regional blood center and geographically contiguous hospitals. Price wars replaced pass-through cost adjustments in a foray to gain market share. Many blood centers dipped into reserves or encountered debt as price competition escalated and blood became a commodity rather than a service linking donors and recipients. Hospitals selected their blood suppliers on the basis of cost in addition to service.

By the late 1990s, the relationship between blood collection agencies and hospitals migrated from one focused on the cost of a commodity to a relationship valuing service, medical expertise, and patient outcomes. In some communities, blood centers and hospital systems established partnerships in which the blood center provided transfusion service activities in addition to blood and blood components. The change from price wars to value pricing occurred, because the quest for market share via low charges led to blood center debt without significant differences in overall market penetration, utilization increased, additional financial and personnel resources were needed, and costly new tests were added. For example, blood collection increased to 13.9 million units in 1999 from 12.6 million in 1997 (2–7). Nucleic acid testing (NAT) for hepatitis C and HIV was initiated in 1999 and 2000 (8–9).

BLOOD BANKING ORGANIZATIONS AND OVERSIGHT

The FDA is the ultimate governmental authority for ensuring the safety, purity, and potency of the blood supply in the United States. The agency exercises regulatory oversight through the Center for Biologics Evaluation and Research (CBER), which issues regulations and guidance about the collection of blood components used for transfusion or the manufacture of pharmaceuticals derived from blood, such as clotting factors, and establishes standards for the products. The CBER also regulates cell separation devices, blood collection containers, and viral screening tests. The CBER develops and enforces quality standards, inspects blood establishments, and monitors reports of biologic product deviation (previously error and accident reports) (10). The agency inspects all blood facilities at least every 2 years. Events affecting the safety, purity, or potency of a distributed biologic product that represent a deviation from cGMPs, applicable regulations or standards, specifications, or are unforeseen or unexpected must be reported to the FDA.

Several FDA advisory committees address contemporary issues. For example, the Blood Products Advisory Committee discusses license applications for infectious disease agents and scientific issues affecting blood safety and efficacy, including requirements for leukocyte reduction. The FDA's Transmissible Spongiform Encephalopathy Advisory Committee provides advice about transmission of variant Creutzfeldt-Jakob Disease (vCJD) through transfusion. The Department of Health and Human Services Blood Safety and Availability Committee provides additional input about scientific and technical issues but, unlike the FDA, is permitted to factor economic issues into its discussions.

Many blood collection agencies and transfusion services are affiliated with the national blood banking organizations, America's Blood Centers, the American Red Cross, and the American Association of Blood Banks.

America's Blood Centers (ABC), founded in 1962 as the Council of Community Blood Centers, is the trade organization for approximately 75 nonprofit, independently operated community blood centers located in 45 states. Each center is licensed by the FDA and maintains its own processes and procedures, quality assurance, and regulatory affairs. Individual centers decide whether to conduct blood testing or to contract for this service with other organizations. Member organizations collect 47% of the U.S. blood supply and subscribe to a community-based blood banking philosophy. Donated blood stays in the organization's community, and excess supplies are shared with other communities when available and needed.

The American Red Cross (ARC) provides approximately 46% of the U.S. blood supply through its national network of 36 regional blood services. Its management control is centralized and all regions operate under a single FDA license. Authority for the blood service operations is vested in the ARC's National Biomedical Services Board, rather than in local boards. American Red Cross Biomedical Headquarters in the Washington, D.C., area is responsible for training and quality assurance of its 36 regions. Blood testing has been consolidated into eight national testing laboratories. Research and development are conducted at regional centers and at the national Holland Laboratory in Virginia.

The American Association of Blood Banks (AABB), established in 1947, is the professional society for almost 8,000 individuals involved in blood banking and transfusion medicine and more than 2,200 institutions (community and ARC collection centers, hospital-based blood banks, and transfusion service laboratories). Individual members include physicians, scientists, administrators, medical technologists, blood donor recruiters, and public relations personnel. The AABB sets voluntary standards, a benchmark for judging performance, and accredits institutions that implement its standards (11).

COLLECTION AND TRANSFUSION OF BLOOD COMPONENTS

Collection

Calculations for quantifying U.S. blood collections and transfusions have been conducted periodically (1–6) (Table 66.1). Allogeneic whole blood collections peaked in 1986 and 1987, when approximately 13.6 million units were collected (including more than 240,000 units imported from Europe) or slightly more than 90 units per 1,000 U.S. residents aged 18 to 65 years. By 1997 this rate declined to approximately 72 units, raising significant concern that the supply might be insufficient to meet

TABLE 66.1. BLOOD COLLECTION AND TRANSFUSION DATA: 1980–1999

—	1980	1982	1984	1986	1987	1989	1992	1994	1997	1999
Collections × 10^{-6}										
Allogeneic										
Blood centers	9.7	11.1	11.5	12.1	12.1	11.9	11.5	11.3	11.0	12.3
Hospitals	1.2	1.3	1.3	1.3	1.3	1.4	1.4	.78	.78	.78
Imported	.27	.25	.29	.24	.27	.29	.21	.22	.20	.12
Total allogeneic	11.15	12.65	13.16	13.60	13.67	13.57	12.68	12.33	12.0	13.2
Autologous										
Blood centers	.014	.012	.023	.117	.184	.334	.702	.663	.386	.427
Hospitals	.014	.016	.035	.089	.213	.321	.415	.350	.257	.224
Total supply	11.17	12.68	13.22	13.81	14.07	14.23	13.79	13.34	12.60	13.9
Transfusions × 10^{-6}										
WBC and RBCs	9.9	11.47	11.98	12.16	11.61	12.06	11.31	11.11	11.52	12.4
Leukocyte-reduced[a]	—	—	—	—	—	—	7.7%	16.7%	21%	27%
Plasma	1.54	1.95	2.26	2.18	2.06	2.16	2.26	2.62	3.32	3.32
Platelets										
WBC-derived	2.9	3.60	4.57	5.06	4.86	5.15	4.69	3.58	3.40	3.04
Apheresis-derived	.056	.117	.168	.214	.262	.352	.607	.714	.940	1.003
% Apheresis	10.5	16.8	18.2	20.4	24.6	29.1	43.7	54.5	62.4	66.5

[a]WBC, white blood cell; RBC, red blood cell.
From references 2–7, with permission.

transfusion needs. Fortunately blood donations subsequently increased 3% to 4% per year (6).

Autologous collections increased following the onset of the AIDS pandemic, peaking in 1992 when 8% of blood collections were provided for self-use. By 1997 to 1999 only 4% to 5% of collected blood was donated for autologous use (5,6).

Hospitals collected 1.4 million (including 415,000 autologous units) of the 13.8 million units donated in 1992 (3). Subsequently, hospital-based whole blood collections declined in response to cost constraints and increased regulatory requirements, representing approximately 7% of current blood collections (5, 6).

Transfusion

Red blood cell transfusion rates were slightly in excess of 50 units per 1,000 residents in 1986 and 1987 (2). Concern about transfusion-transmitted infections, such as HIV and hepatitis, and educational efforts to maximize the appropriateness of transfusion therapy led to reductions in the number of transfusions. By 1997, the transfusion rate was 43 units per 1,000 residents (5). Leukocyte-reduced red blood cell transfusions increased from 7.7% to 40% to 50% of transfusions in the year 2000. Leukocyte reduction conducted at blood centers prior to storage superseded removal of white blood cells by filters attached to the infusion set at the time of transfusion (12).

Platelet transfusion growth slowed between 1992 and 1994, increased in 1997, and showed no change from 1997 to 1999. The source of platelet transfusions, however, evolved from whole blood to apheresis derived. Currently, apheresis platelets account for more than two-thirds of platelet transfusions. Fresh-frozen plasma transfusions showed unabated utilization pattern increases through 1997.

BLOOD DONOR RECRUITMENT

Blood donors give blood out of a sense of altruism, often in response to an organized blood drive. Other motivating factors include having family members or friends in need of a transfusion. Some donors provide blood after learning about shortages, and others donate to help a local child requiring transfusion. Occasionally, people donate solely to receive a token gift (13–16) (Fig. 66.1).

In general, the average blood donor donates 1.6 times per year. Two-thirds of donations are given at mobile blood drives, which may be held at the work place, in the community, or as religious-sponsored events. One-third of donations are provided at fixed site locations, predominately blood center facilities. Approximately 7% of donations are made at hospital-based permanent collection sites.

One-half of U.S. citizens have donated blood. Repeat donors, that is persons giving blood repeatedly, provide additional safety to the blood supply because of the low rate of seroconversion among those with previous negative test results. Retaining previous donors is also less costly than recruiting new donors. Persons returning within 6 months of their first donation are more likely to become long-term donors (13). College graduates return to donate more often than those with some college education. High school graduates or those with less education return even less frequently.

Reasons for not donating include being too busy, finding donation inconvenient, not being asked, or being physically unable to donate. Among prospective donors, 1% to 2% are deferred because of medical history information, 3% to 5% because of low hematocrit and hemoglobin levels, and 5 to 6% for other reasons.

Generational differences play a role in the likelihood that a person has been a blood donor. The proportion of Baby Boomers

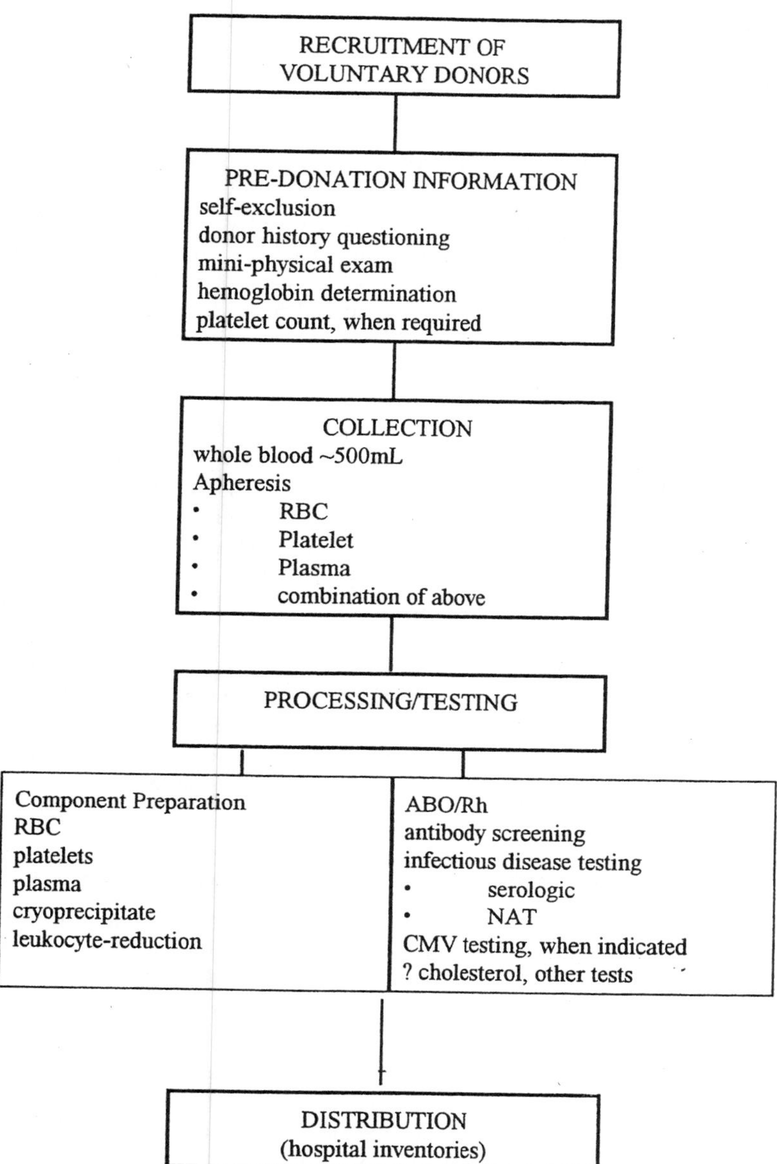

FIGURE 66.1. Blood recruitment, collection, processing, testing, and distribution.

(birth dates 1946 to 1962) who have donated blood is higher than that of Generation Xers (birth dates 1965 to 1977). Approximately 31% of blood donations collected at the Community Blood Center of Greater Kansas City in 1988 were given by those 26 to 35 years of age (Baby Boomers). In 1999, only 19% of the blood supply was provided by those in that age group (Generation Xers). This raises concern about meeting increasing demands for transfusions as the population ages. In 1980, 11.3% of the population was 65 or older, those with the highest frequency of transfusions. In 2000, this age group accounted for 13.0% of the population and is expected to increase by approximately 3 million persons by 2010.

DONOR MEDICAL EVALUATION

The tenets of blood donor screening include protecting the donor from mishaps associated with donation and obviating donations from those at risk of transmitting infectious agents or causing other adverse consequences to the recipient. The procedures for effecting these safeguards include prerecruitment information about behaviors that place people at risk for transmitting infectious agents and self-deferral if such behaviors occurred, donor history questioning in a private setting, lack of monetary inducements that might alter the veracity of answers to such questions, opportunities for donors to request removal of donated blood from the blood supply, and infectious disease testing.

As an example, concern about transmissible spongiform encephalopathy transmission by blood transfusion led to exclusion of persons residing in the United Kingdom for more than 3 months cumulatively between 1980 and 1996, the period of greatest risk of ingestion of tainted meat. Information about this subject and risk factors for contracting hepatitis and HIV are presented to persons before they donate, in an effort to deter donations from those with potentially hazardous exposures.

Donor history questions provide another opportunity to obtain information about potential risks to recipients. Donors are asked about a previous history of hepatitis or possible exposure to HIV to detect viral carriers. Other questions ask about use of potentially teratogenic medications such as etretinate, acitretin, isotretinoin, or finasteride (17).

Donors are asked, also, about their health status, including a history of vascular disease, medications prescribed by their physicians, and other questions to identify those at higher risk of complications following donation. The donor's pulse rate and rhythm and blood pressure must meet predetermined criteria. A blood sample is tested before donation to ensure the hemoglobin concentration is greater than 12.5 g/dl.

Donor history questions that indicate a reason for deferral or a previous positive infectious disease test result places donors in deferral registries. On occasion, previously deferred donors attempt to donate again. Reasons these donors reappear include a desire to obtain results of infectious disease testing, to receive community service credit, a misunderstanding about the reason for deferral, or as a result of erroneous recruitment by blood center staff (14). To offset undue incentives to donate in the volunteer system, FDA regulations limit the value of such items and prohibit those readily convertible to cash.

WHOLE BLOOD COLLECTION

Donors receive information about risk factors for transmitting infections through transfusion and are given an opportunity to self-defer if they have participated in such activities. Subsequently, donor history questioning, blood pressure, pulse rate, and temperature measurements are conducted, and a sample of blood is obtained for determining hemoglobin concentration. Donors receive information about the donation process and give their consent for blood collection.

Following an aseptic scrub procedure using povidone or tincture of iodine, donors provide approximately 500 ml of whole blood through venipuncture of an antecubital vein. An additional 25 ml of blood is obtained for ABO and Rh typing, red blood cell antibody screening, and infectious disease testing. Some blood collection agencies collect additional blood samples for cholesterol or other health screening as a public service and incentive to encourage donations. Following donation, donors partake in refreshments and leave the donation area after a brief interval. The total process takes 45 to 60 minutes.

REACTIONS AND INJURIES FOLLOWING WHOLE BLOOD DONATION

The symptom complex of dizziness, weakness, and pallor represents the most frequent adverse reaction associated with donation. These vasovagal reactions occur in 2% to 5% of blood donors and are characterized by increases in cardiac output and peripheral vascular sympathetic activity, and vasodilation (18). An associated increase in cardiac parasympathetic activity decreases the heart rate. The donor's skin is pale, cool, and moist. Thalamic activation occurs through emotional involvement and hyperventilation. Peripheral baroreceptor sensitivity plays an important role. The symptoms usually subside after the donor's legs are elevated, cold towels are placed on the forehead and back of the neck, and verbal reassurance is provided.

Syncope occurs in 0.08% to 0.34% of donors. Tetany or convulsive activity develops in 25% of those individuals with syncope. Syncope-related falls may cause injuries. The risk is highest among those less than 20 years of age and diminishes significantly in donors age 30 and older. Syncope occurs five-fold more often in first-time donors than in repeat donors. The risk is higher also in those weighing 110 to 120 pounds, the minimal weight for donors.

Severe reactions, those resulting in hospitalization, occur at a rate of approximately 1 per 200,000 allogeneic donations and 1 per 17,000 autologous donations (19). The latter may relate to underlying cardiac, vascular, and respiratory disease. First-time donors are at greater risk for severe reactions. In a nationwide study, older donors, especially those more than 60 years of age, had a higher frequency of hospitalization than younger donors. Of those requiring hospitalization, vasovagal attacks occurred in two-thirds of the studied cases and anginal episodes occurred in one-eighth. Additional events requiring hospitalization included blood leakage into muscle and fascial planes causing nerve and vascular compression, arteriovascular fistula formation, phlebitis, and pseudoaneurysms.

Hematoma, Arterial Puncture, Nerve Injury

Hematoma formation or bruising represents the most frequent donation-associated injury, occurring in 9% to 16% of donors. Although this event is self-limited, it causes concern because of associated soreness, discoloration, and the perception that bleeding persists. Other venipuncture-related injuries include the infrequent puncture of an artery instead of a vein. This leads rarely to a pseudoaneurysm, in which blood leakage becomes walled off by surrounding tissue. Acquired arteriovenous fistulae created by a channel between a lacerated vein and artery and development of a compartment syndrome from extravasating blood occluding capillaries and veins occur at very low incidence (20).

Local nerve injuries represent an infrequent but annoying problem for donors. Most sensory nerves lie deep to antecubital fossa veins. However, some nerves overlie or are intertwined with the veins. Venipuncture-induced nerve injuries cause donors to experience burning, shooting pain immediately or within hours after needle insertion, that tracks along the sensory nerve distribution. Such events occur once per 7,000 donations. Those causing donors to seek medical attention occur at a rate of 1 per 21,000 to 26,700 donations. Females are more likely than males to suffer this complication. These injuries occur despite properly performed venipunctures. Probing for venous cannulation and hematoma formation adversely affect the outcome. Most blood donors' symptoms resolve, but loss of sensation, hyperpathia, allodynia, and causalgia have been reported (20–22).

Iron Depletion

The donation of 450 to 500 ml of whole blood results in a loss of approximately 220 mg of iron. In general, men absorb 1 mg of iron per day from dietary sources, to replace 1 mg per day of iron losses through desquamation of gastrointestinal and genitourinary cells. Menstruating females require an additional 0.5 mg of iron per day to replace that lost through menses. The typical daily diet contains 24 mg of iron. Iron absorption increases from 1.0 to 1.5 mg/day to 4 to 5mg/day in those with iron deficiency. Iron absorption increases further in those taking iron supplements. The FDA-mandated minimal interval between donations is 56 days. As such, without increasing iron absorption from dietary sources as occur in the iron-deficient state or those taking supplemental iron, donors making multiple donations per year are at risk for depleting their iron stores and becoming iron deficient. As many as 24% of women donating once per year were considered iron deficient. Predonation hemoglobin concentration determinations serve as a crude measurement for detecting iron deficiency. Roughly 5% of donors are deferred because of low hemoglobin concentrations (23).

APHERESIS DONATIONS

An alternative to whole blood donation involves donations of red blood cells, platelets, plasma, or combinations of these components using cell separator devices (i.e., apheresis equipment) (24–26). Plateletpheresis collections have been conducted for more than 20 years but accounted for a minority of platelet transfusions through the mid-1990s. Apheresis platelets contain an equivalent platelet dose of 6 random-donor (i.e., whole blood–derived) platelet concentrates, limit the number of donors to whom patients are exposed, facilitate logistical issues for the transfusion service and nursing staff, and conform to the trend toward leukocyte reduction. Apheresis platelets routinely have fewer than 1×10^6 white blood cells/μL. Approximately one-half of platelet apheresis collections contain sufficient numbers of platelets to provide two routine doses.

In addition, apheresis technology permits the collection of two red blood cell units during one donation and combinations of red blood cell-plasma or red blood cell-platelet collections (27). These donations require approximately 45 to 90 minutes. At a time when collection needs are increasing and blood shortages occur, apheresis donations provide an opportunity to increase donated transfusion components without increasing the number of donors. The deferral period following a two-unit red blood cell donation is 16 weeks instead of 8 weeks. Up to 24 plateletpheresis donations are permitted per year. Predonation platelet counts are monitored, and all such counts must be greater 150,000/μL.

REACTIONS AND INJURIES FOLLOWING APHERESIS DONATION

Adverse reactions occur at a greater frequency following apheresis donation than after whole blood donation (28,29). During the cell separation procedure, the donor's blood is anticoagulated with citrate-containing solutions. Reinfusion of processed blood and accumulation of unmetabolized citrate leads to chills, discomfort, pallor, diaphoresis, nausea with or without emesis, chest tightness, extremity tingling or cramps, perioral paresthesias, a flushed sensation, blurred vision, throat numbness, and tachycardia. Such reactions occur in approximately 0.3% to 0.4% of donors undergoing apheresis procedures and are more common in first-time apheresis donors. Hypotension related to citrate, hypovolemia, or vasovagal reactions occurs in approximately 0.2% of donors. Venipuncture-related injuries such as hematoma formation, pain at the venipuncture site, and venous infiltration occur in up to 1.15% percent of donors. The red blood cells contained in the apheresis devices are not returned to the donor in 0.16% of procedures.

PROCESSING

Using centrifugation, red blood cell, platelet, and plasma components are separated from whole blood according to their density characteristics. Subsequently, the components are transferred from the whole blood container to satellite bags through integrally connected plastic tubing. Adding nutrients and saline to the red blood cells permits storage at 1° to 6°C for up to 42 days.

Platelets concentrated in approximately 50 ml of plasma maintain a 5-day shelf life at room temperature in monitored incubators when subjected to slow oscillation to keep the platelets suspended. Apheresis-derived platelets are stored under similar conditions.

Plasma intended for use as fresh-frozen plasma undergoes freezing within 8 hours of collection. It can be stored for up to 1 year at temperatures below −18°C.

Preparation of cryoprecipitate involves thawing frozen plasma at 4°C in a circulating water bath and then draining the supernatant plasma into an attached satellite bag. The remaining cold-precipitated material is then refrozen at −18°C and stored for up to 1 year.

Leukocyte reduction accomplished by passing whole blood through filters that remove white blood cells and platelets obviates the ability to produce whole blood–derived platelet concentrates. Alternatively, platelets may be separated by centrifugation prior to filtration, and the red blood cells and platelets passed through filters designed to remove white blood cells contained in each of these components. Filtration occurs no more than 72 hours after blood collection. Apheresis-derived platelets, in general, must contain fewer than 5×10^6 white blood cells per unit in order to qualify as leukocyte-reduced components.

TESTING

Each unit of blood undergoes testing for blood type and infectious disease agents.

ABO and Rh Testing

Donor centers test blood from each donation for ABO and Rh type using automated blood typing devices. Forward grouping occurs by addition of anti-A and anti-B reagents and reverse grouping by adding donor plasma to red blood cells demonstrated to display A or B antigens. Appropriate algorithms ensure concordance of forward and reverse grouping. That is, donor cells agglutinated by anti-A reagents must be accompanied by test results showing that the donor's serum agglutinated cells known to express B but not A antigens.

Red blood cells from first-time donors testing Rh negative undergo additional steps to determine if their cells express the weak-D antigen. The test results of all repeat donors are compared with those recorded previously. If discrepancies occur, the blood is not released until the variance is resolved.

Antibody Screening

Plasma from donor blood undergoes testing for unexpected clinically significant red blood cell antibodies. Alloantibodies against A or B antigens are expected in blood group B or A individuals, respectively, because these antibodies occur naturally. Unexpected alloantibodies refer to those against blood group antigens D, C, E, c, e, Kell, Kidd, and others. Because red blood cell components contain very little plasma, units with these alloantibodies are made available for transfusion with a label indicating the test results. Plasma from these donations is not distributed for transfusion, because recipients with red blood cell alloantigens corresponding to the alloantibodies may be opsonized by such antibodies and removed by the reticuloendothelial system.

Infectious Disease Testing

All donated blood undergoes serologic testing for antibodies against HIV-1 and -2, hepatitis C, hepatitis B core, and HTLV-I and -II, for hepatitis B surface antigen, for HIV p24 antigen (if not tested by approved NAT for HIV), and a serologic test for syphilis. Serologic testing for antibodies against cytomegalovirus (CMV) is performed on blood of selected donors.

Starting in 1999, NAT was instituted for the viral genomic sequences of hepatitis C virus (HCV) and HIV (8–9). These tests detect carriers of these viruses during the seronegative interval, or window period, between infection and seroconversion. For HIV, NAT detects infection approximately 10 days before seroconversion; for HCV detection occurs 57 days earlier. When introduced, NAT was conducted on pooled samples in fewer than 20 laboratories throughout the United States. Initial results corroborated the residual risk of HIV and HCV transmission estimated on the basis of serologic screening (30). Approximately 1 per 4.78 million donations was HIV seronegative and NAT positive, and 1 per 277,500 donations was HCV seronegative and NAT positive. Hepatitis B virus NAT will be introduced in late 2002. These tests increase costs for red blood cells by approximately 5% to 10%.

DISTRIBUTION

Blood and components become available for distribution to hospital inventories following completion of processing, testing, and record review.

Transfusion services routinely receive blood and components on prearranged schedules. The amount of blood stored at specific hospitals depends on the usage patterns and distance from the blood center. Availability and turnaround time are key components for determining allocations. Ad hoc shipments occur when patients require additional blood or nonroutinely stored blood components. Many donor centers maintain sophisticated red blood cell immunohematology laboratories for identifying compatible blood for patients with multiple red blood cell alloantibodies.

PLASMA PRODUCTS INDUSTRY

In contrast to recruitment, collection, processing, testing, and distribution of whole blood and blood components by nonprofit entities, the for-profit plasma industry produces intravenous immune globulin G (IVIG), albumin, and plasma-derived factor VIII and factor IX products, among others (Table 66.2). Approximately one dozen multinational companies fractionate plasma into preparations valued at more than $5.1 billion annually (31,32). More than 65% of the products are sold in the United States and Europe. In 1999, plasma product sales in the United States totaled $1.63 billion. If recombinant factors VIIa, VIII, and IX and monoclonal respiratory syncytial virus are included, the total market price reached $2.57 billion. Intravenous immune globulin represented 46% of the market. Other plasma derivatives include antithrombin III, fibrinogen, thrombin, and anti-D.

Twenty percent of plasma undergoing fractionation in the

TABLE 66.2. PRODUCTS DERIVED FROM PLASMA FRACTIONATION

Albumin
Polyvalent intravenous immune globulin (IVIG)
Coagulation factor concentrates
Factor VIII
Factor IX
Factor IX complex
Activated factor IX complex
Antithrombin III
Hyperimmune γ-globulin preparations
Rabies
Hepatitis B
Tetanus
Rh_oD (anti-Rh)
Respiratory syncytial virus
Polyvalent intramuscular immune globulin (IMIG)
Cytomegalovirus intravenous immune globulin (CMV-IMIG)
α_1-Antitrypsin
Fibrin glue (manufactured in Austria)

Rh, rhesus.

United States, or approximately 2 million liters, is recovered from volunteer whole blood donations. The source of the remaining 80% of plasma, or approximately 11 million liters, sent for fractionation comes from paid plasma donors who provide 500 ml or more of plasma (depending on size) during plasmapheresis procedures conducted as often as twice weekly.

The plasma industry undergoes intense regulation by the FDA and its trade organization, Plasma Protein Therapeutics Association Source (PPTA Source). The Quality Plasma Program devised by ABRA maintains requirements for plasma donors. Examples of regulations differing from volunteer whole blood donors include requirements that donors must present positive identification to show they live within a defined geographic area, undergo testing for opiates at periodic intervals, and take written tests to evaluate comprehension of donor history questions. Such donors, by FDA requirement, undergo an initial physical examination by physicians or specially trained allied health personnel, usually nurses. The examinations are repeated annually. Some centers use abbreviated screens on twice-per-week donors but must check hemoglobin and protein. Serum protein electrophoresis is done every 4 months to protect the donors against protein depletion, and syphilis testing is done at the same time. The industry also has a voluntary 60-day hold before pooling plasma to allow time to act on postdonation information. Donors must become qualified donors by a second acceptable donation within a 6-month period before their first donation is used for fractionation into injectable product.

Source plasma does not undergo anti-HTLV-I and -II testing because those viruses are intracellular. Anti-HBc testing would exclude many donors with antibodies against the hepatitis B surface antigen (anti-HBs) needed in IVIG. Units reactive for anti-HBc are included in shipments of recovered plasma. Some blood banks conduct process testing on plasma pools before fractionation, by means of NAT for hepatitis A or Parvovirus B19 genomes.

IMPACT OF NEW TRENDS

Forces driving changes in the 2000s include increases in blood use and reimbursement requirements for funding future transfusion medicine advances.

After a decade of little change in red blood cell utilization, 3% to 5% annual increases began in 1997. Innovative use of apheresis technology facilitates collecting more transfusion doses per donation, two units of red blood cells, two platelet transfusion doses, or red blood cell-platelet or red blood cell-plasma components. Apheresis collections offer additional advantages including components with $<5 \times 10^6$ white blood cells/μL, the requirement for leukocyte reduction.

This technology increases blood component availability but requires funding for implementation. Improved infectious disease testing technology by serologic and NAT enhances sensitivity and efficiency for current and emerging pathogens (e.g., vCJD). The costs associated with NAT may exceed $10 per donation, and those associated with universal leukocyte reduction add approximately $500 million annually to charges for blood components. Increased reimbursement from hospitals to blood centers rather than lower charges to gain market share marked a major paradigm shift in the early 2000s.

In parallel, transfusion medicine practitioners espoused blood utilization monitoring, best practice determinations, and outcomes investigations to promote efficient use of transfusion components. Blood centers, viewed as vendors of a product during the 1990s, reestablished value-added relationships in the early 2000s and provided blood management expertise to hospital partners. Improved information system technology for communicating and monitoring blood usage facilitated building this relationship.

Other technologic advances are reshaping blood center organizations. Methods for inactivating viruses and bacteria in single red blood cell, platelet, or plasma units (rather than application of these techniques in pooled units) are in clinical trials (33–36). Food and Drug Administration approval of these techniques would alter significantly the therapeutic ratio of transfusions and create a new approach to transfusion practice.

Oxygen-carrying substitutes are in clinical trials and platelet substitutes have been used in clinical situations (37,38). If proven effective and safe, these products will change transfusion practice. The brief intravascular dwell times of oxygen-carrying substitutes under development, however, may limit their use to emergency or resuscitation situations only.

Umbilical cord blood, as a source of hematopoietic progenitor cells, from related and nonrelated allogeneic donors provides effective treatment of malignant and nonmalignant hematologic disorders (39–42). Blood centers and hospitals have established programs to bank sufficient numbers of cord blood units for unrelated allogeneic stem cell transplants. Oversight of these programs, as proposed by the FDA, fosters development of cell expansion and gene insertion programs at facilities experienced with blood banking regulations, creating future opportunities for blood collection organizations.

SUMMARY

Blood services in the United States continue to evolve to meet the needs of hospitals in a managed care environment while delivering even safer products.

REFERENCES

1. Wood E. Providing blood components and services in the 20th century. Presented at the American Association of Blood Banks Annual Meeting, October 21, 1997, Denver, Colorado.
2. Surgenor DM, Wallace EL, Hao HS, et al. Collection and transfusion of blood in the United States, 1982–1988. *N Engl J Med* 1990;322: 1646–1651.
3. Wallace EL, Surgenor DM, Hao HS, et al. Collection and transfusion of blood and blood components in the United States, 1989. *Transfusion* 1993;33:139–144.
4. Wallace EL, Churchill DM, Surgenor DM, et al. Collection and transfusion of blood and blood components in the United States, 1992. *Transfusion* 1995;35:802–812.
5. Wallace EL, Churchill DM, Surgenor DM, et al. Collection and transfusion of blood and blood components in the United States, 1994. *Transfusion* 1998;38:625–636.

6. Blood collection and transfusion in the United States in 1997. Bethesda, MD: The National Blood Data Resource Center, 1999.
7. Comprehensive Report on Blood Collection and Transfusion in the United States in 1999. Bethesda, MD: The National Blood Data Resource Center,. 2001.
8. Dodd RY, Aberle-Grasse JM, Stramer SL. The yield of nucleic acid testing (NAT) for HIV and HCV RNA in a population of US voluntary donors: relationship to contemporary measures of incidence. *Transfusion* 2000;40[Suppl]:1S.
9. Pietrelli L, Strong DM, Holland PV, et al. Cobas ampliscreen HCV test, V2.0 minipool testing: clinical trial update for 13 US blood centers. *Transfusion* 2000;40[Suppl]:2S.
10. Food and Drug Administration, HHS. Reporting of biological product deviations in manufacturing. *Federal Register* 2000;65:66621–66622.
11. Gorlin JB. *Standards for blood banks and transfusion services,* 20th ed. Bethesda, MD: American Association of Blood Banks, 2000.
12. Vamvakas EC, Blajchman MA. Universal WBC reduction the case for and against. *Transfusion* 2001;41:691–712.
13. Ownby HE, Kong F, Watanabe K, et al. Analysis of donor return behavior. *Transfusion* 1999;39:1128–1135.
14. Munsterman KA, Grindon AJ, Sullivan MT, et al. Assessment of motivations for return donation among deferred blood donors. *Transfusion* 1998;38:45–50.
15. Strauss RG. Blood donations, safety, and incentives. *Transfusion* 2001; 41:165–167.
16. Sanchez AM, Ameti DI, Schreiber GB. The potential impact of incentives on future blood donation behavior. *Transfusion* 2001;41:78.
17. American Association of Blood Banks. Association Bulletin 99-10. New Uniform Donor History Questionnaire issued. December 2, 1999.
18. Trouern-Trend JJ, Cable RG, Badon SJ, et al. A case-controlled multicenter study of vasovagal reactions in blood donors: influence of sex, age, donation status, weight, blood pressure, and pulse. *Transfusion* 1999;39:316–320.
19. Popovsky MA, Whitaker B, Arnold NL. Severe outcomes of allogeneic and autologous blood donation: frequency and characterization. *Transfusion* 1995;35:734–737.
20. Newman BH. Donor reactions and injuries from whole blood donation. *Transfus Med Rev* 1997;11:64–75.
21. Horowitz SH. Venipuncture-induced causalgia: anatomic relations of upper extremity superficial veins and nerves, and clinical considerations. *Transfusion* 2000;40:1036–1040.
22. Newman BH. Venipuncture nerve injuries after whole-blood donation. *Transfusion* 2001;41:571.
23. Punnonen K, Rajamaki A. Evaluation of iron status of Finnish blood donors using serum transferrin receptor. *Transfus Med* 1999;9: 131–134.
24. Rugg N, Pitman C, Menitove JE, et al. A feasibility evaluation of an automated blood component collection system platelets and red cells. *Transfusion* 1999;39:460–464.
25. Elfath MD, Whitley P, Jacobson MS, et al. Evaluation of an automated system for the collection of packed RBCs, platelets, and plasma. *Transfusion* 2000;40:1214–1222.
26. Benjamin RJ, Rojas P, Christmas S, et al. Plateletpheresis efficiency: a comparison of the Spectra LRS and AMICUS separators. *Transfusion*1999;39:895–899.
27. Shi PA, Ness PM. Two-unit red cell apheresis and its potential advantages over traditional whole-blood donation. *Transfusion* 1999;39: 218–225.
28. Despotis GJ, Goodnough LT, Dynis M, et al. Adverse events in platelet apheresis donors: a multivariate analysis in a hospital-based program. *Vox Sang* 1999;77:24–32.
29. McLeod BC, Price TH, Owen H, et al. Frequency of immediate adverse effects associated with apheresis donation. *Transfusion* 1998;38: 938–943.
30. Kleinman SH, Stramer SL, Mimms L, et al. Comparison of preliminary observed yield of HCV and HIV minipool (MP) nucleic acid testing (NAT) with predictions from the incidence/window period (INC/WP) model. *Transfusion* 2000;40[Suppl]:4S.
31. The Marketing Research Bureau, Inc. The plasma fractions market in the United States—2000. Orange, CT.
32. The Marketing Research Bureau, Inc. The worldwide plasma fractions market—2000. Orange, CT.
33. Chapman J. Progress in improving the pathogen saftey of red cell concentrates. *Vox Sang* 2000;78[Suppl 2]:203–204.
34. Goodrich R. The use of riboflavin for the inactivation of pathogens in blood products. *Vox Sang* 2000;78[Suppl 2]:211–215.
35. Corash L. Inactivation of viruses, bacteria, protozoa and leukocytes in platelet and red cell concentrates. *Vox Sang* 2000;78[Suppl 2]: 205–210.
36. Pamphilon D. Review: viral inactivation of fresh frozen plasma. *Br J Haematol* 2000;109:680–693.
37. Mullon J, Giacoppe G, Clagett C, et al. Transfusion of polymerized bovine hemoglobin in a patient with severe autoimmune hemolytic anemia. *N Engl J Med* 2000;342:1638–1643.
38. Stowell CP, Levin J, Spiess BD, et al. Progress in the development of RBC substitutes. *Transfusion* 2001;41:287–299.
39. Stroncek DF, Confer DL, Leitman SF. Peripheral blood progenitor cells for HPC transplants involving unrelated donors. *Transfusion* 2000; 40:731–741.
40. Bensinger WI, Martin PJ, Storer B, et al. Transplantation of bone marrow as compared with peripheral-blood cells from HLA-identical relatives in patients with hematologic cancers. *N Engl J Med* 2001;344: 175–181.
41. Kaji EH, Leiden JM. Gene and stem cell therapies. *JAMA* 2001;285: 545–550.
42. Silberstein LE, Toy P. Research opportunities in transfusion medicine. *JAMA* 2000;285:577–580.

67

INTERNATIONAL ASPECTS OF BLOOD SERVICES

CELSO BIANCO

BLOOD SAFETY IN THE CONTEXT OF WORLD HEALTH

The tragedy of acquired immunodeficiency syndrome (AIDS) and concerns about transmission of disease by transfusion of blood and blood products have had global impact. Both developed and developing countries focused their public health systems on the epidemic and have worked toward improvement of their blood systems. The size and success of these efforts has been driven by public perception about risks, resources that could be diverted to the effort, and access to technology. Disparities are not necessarily related to the Gross Domestic Product (GDP). The United States spends a higher proportion of GDP than any other of the 191 member countries of the World Health Organization (WHO) on health care, but in the year 2000, according to the World Health Report (1), it ranked number 37 in general health care performance. However, public pressure encouraged the application of large resources and effort by both the private and the public sector, and the U.S. blood supply ranks among the safest in the world.

Most countries in the developing world confront a high disease burden and are struggling for resources and infrastructure in order to address their health care priorities. They are overwhelmed by infant mortality because of diarrhea, tuberculosis, malaria, AIDS, Chagas and other parasitic diseases, and hepatitis B. They are encouraged and supported by international organizations to develop basic public health measures such as mosquito control, vaccination, safe water, and safe waste disposal. Consequently, blood transfusion is a minor component of the budgets of these countries. There were, however, 36.1 million individuals with human immunodeficiency virus (HIV)/AIDS in the world at the end of 2000. The number of new infections reached 5.3 million and the number of deaths 3 million. About 21.8 million people have died of the disease since the beginning of the epidemic (1).

Blood transfusion issues, however, lag behind bigger problems, such as excessive use of injectable medications and the lack of affordable and disposable injection supplies. There is a belief in many countries that injected medications are more effective than those taken by other routes. In some countries like India, syringes are scavenged for resale. In Egypt, the proportion of new cases of hepatitis C attributable to unsafe injections exceeded 40% in 1996. The World Health Organization has produced a report on the safety of injections (http://www.who.int/inf-fs/en/fact231.html). Related to transfusion, few poor countries have implemented standards and quality systems that ensure that the right unit is available and transfused into the right patient. The frequency of hemolytic reactions is quite high in many countries, and there are no statistics to document the frequency. Often a patient will not receive a screened unit of blood, not because tests are unavailable but because the screened unit was not available when it was needed (J. Emmanuel, WHO, personal communication April 19, 2001).

BLOOD COLLECTIONS IN THE WORLD

Unfortunately, there is paucity of data about the status of the blood supply in the world. The World Health Organization estimates that there are 75 million donations a year, of which 45 million are made in developed countries and are tested for infectious diseases. Among the 30 million donations collected in developing countries, only 43% of the blood collected is screened for HIV, hepatitis B virus (HBV), hepatitis C virus (HCV), syphilis, and Chagas disease. Globally, WHO estimates that 5% to 10% of HIV infections are caused by transfusion of unsafe blood and blood products. Blood transfusion safety is covered by WHO on the following website: (http://

C. Bianco: Executive Vice President, America's Blood Center, Washington, D.C.

TABLE 67.1. TYPE OF WHOLE BLOOD DONATION ACCORDING TO THE WHO HEALTH DEVELOPMENT INDEX

—	Developing		Developed
—	Low HDI	Medium HDI	High HDI
Voluntary	31%	40%	98%
Replacement	61%	41%	2%
Paid	8%	19%	0%

WHO, World Health Organization; HDI, Health Development Index.
From World Health Organization. World Health Report. Geneva, 2000, with permission.

www.who.int/bct/main__areas__of__work/BTS/blood%20screening.htm).

Developed countries rely on volunteer, nonremunerated donors to maintain their blood supplies, but the vast majority of countries rely on replacement donors and paid donors. Table 67.1 shows a WHO estimate of distribution of blood donors according to the Health Development Index of the group of countries.

Replacement donor blood is demanded prior to admission to both public and private hospitals. Although some of the donors are family members, many are paid privately because patients need to reach the minimum number of donors. Difficulties collecting blood even from paid and replacement donors is the rule among developing and less-developed countries (2).

The Pan American Heath Organization (PAHO), a branch of WHO, has been somewhat successful in obtaining blood collection and screening data (3). Five of the 21 non-Latin Caribbean countries collect more than 50% of their blood from volunteer donors. However, the number of yearly collections is rather small, varying from a few hundred to a few thousand units a year. Eighty-seven percent of the 23,900 collections made in Jamaica, the largest of these countries, came from replacement donors. All the blood collected in this area is subjected to serologic screening for HIV and HBV. Only seven of these countries screen for HCV. Jamaica did not, at the time of the report. Among the 14 Latin American countries that provided data to PAHO, Argentina, Bolivia, Chile, Colombia, Costa Rica, Cuba, Ecuador, El Salvador, Honduras, Nicaragua, Panama, Paraguay, Uruguay, and Venezuela rely on replacement donors for their supply. Cuba collected 605,000 units in 1996, all from volunteer donors. These countries screen more than 97% of the collected blood for HIV, HBV, HCV, syphilis, and Chagas disease, with the exception of Bolivia, which collected 40,000 units and only 35% were screened. Great progress in the screening of blood donors was reported in Argentina between the years of 1995 and 1997, with extension of the screening to 97.97% of donors, leading to a ten-fold decrease in the risk of transmission of infection (4). Brazil was not included in the PAHO reports. However, data from the Brazilian Ministerio da Saude shows that the country, with a population of 163 million inhabitants, collected 1,664,000 units in 1999. In 1998, volunteer donors made 31% of the donations. All units were screened for the five mentioned infectious disease markers. See the following website: http://www.saude.gov.br/biblioteca/literatura/public__ti/Qualidade%20do%20Sangue.pdf.

The Pan American Heath Organization has also estimated the risk of transfusion-transmitted infectious diseases in Central and South America, based on 1993 and 1994 data and the known sensitivity of the screening assays and percentage of the units screened in the country (5). Table 67.2 summarizes some of the risks. The article does not estimate risk for Brazil, the largest country in South America. One estimate published in 1993 indicated that the risk of transmission of HIV in São Paulo was between 1:2,500 and 1:5,000 and was related to a high incidence rate. Improvements in donor selection and screening that occurred in recent years have probably lowered that rate (6).

The change from replacement to volunteer, nonremunerated,

TABLE 67.2. ESTIMATION OF THE PROBABILITY OF TRANSFUSION-TRANSMITTED INFECTION IN SOME COUNTRIES OF LATIN AMERICA

		Probability of Infection Per 10,000 Transfusions			
Country	Collections	HIV	HBV	HCV	Chagas
Bolivia	37,948	0.57	12.95	Not tested	219.28
Chile	217,312	0.00	0.20	41.82	5.87
Colombia	352,316	0.22	0.90	67.09	25.85
Costa Rica	50,692	0.00	0.34	Not tested	Not tested
Ecuador	98,473	0.95	3.39	9.38	2.06
El Salvador	48,048	0.00	2.42	16.97	17.75
Guatemala	45,426	0.00	10.71	49.74	7.35
Honduras	27,885	0.00	3.37	3.57	2.60
Nicaragua	46,001	0.00	14.21	20.43	2.1
Paraguay	32,893	0.00	6.99	Not tested	12.47
Peru	52,909	0.00	0.65	18.56	49.56
Venezuela	204,316	0.00	1.09	64.21	2.77

HIV, human immunodeficiency virus; HBV, hepatitis B virus; HCV, hepatitis C virus.
From Hamerschlak N, Pasternak J, Amato Neto V. Current risk of AIDS transmission by transfusion. *Rev Hosp Clin Fac Med Sao Paulo* 1993;48:183–185, with permission.

repeat donors has been very difficult for many countries. This has been attributed to cultural misunderstandings about blood donation, lack of expertise and resources for donor recruitment and retention, and inertia on the part of transfusion services and collecting agencies. The disadvantages of the one-time replacement donor are immense. These donors usually have a high prevalence of infectious disease markers. After screening there is a high rate of discard. For instance, in 1999 the rate of discard in Brazil reached 18% in certain regions, even with 27% volunteer donors. That rate was 26% in 1997. About one-half of the discards were caused by a positive test result for antibodies to the core antigen of hepatitis B, a federally required screening test for blood donors.

TRAGIC EXAMPLES OF PROBLEMS CONFRONTED BY DEVELOPING COUNTRIES

Romania reported 13 cases of AIDS to WHO in 1989. In 1990, 1,168 cases were reported, 97% of them in children. In many cases, this was associated with the practice of transfusion of infants and young children in public hospitals, to promote their development. Many cases were also attributed to the use of nonsterile needles in health care facilities. This event triggered the involvement of international organizations and some improvement in AIDS prevention and surveillance (7).

In Mexico City, following the introduction of HIV screening tests, the prevalence of antibodies in donors to a commercial plasmapheresis center increased from 6.3% to 9.2% in the subsequent 5 months. There was a direct relationship between the frequency of donation and seropositivity. A survey of employees disclosed the frequent reuse of disposable supplies (8). Subsequent investigation of the HIV epidemic in Mexico led some investigators to postulate that commercial plasmapheresis centers, located in 7 of the 24 Mexican states, played a major role in the dissemination of the infection (9).

In Pakistan, a survey of 141 transfusion recipients showed that 80% had never heard of viral hepatitis and 44% had never heard of AIDS. Forty-nine percent were not willing to pay an increased price for blood that was screened for blood-borne pathogens (10). In Zambia, the introduction of measures such as not collecting blood from prisoners and avoiding the use of expired test kits brought substantial improvement of the safety of blood transfusions (11). In Ethiopia, only blood destined for transfusion into children and foreigners is screened for HBV (12). A national survey of 1,147 patients on hemodialysis in Saudi Arabia showed that 68% were seropositive for HCV. Seropositivity correlated with longer-duration dialysis and blood transfusion. Nontransfused patients also had a prevalence of antibodies to HCV (13). In Thailand, the prevalence of antibodies to HIV among blood donors increased from 0.84% in 1988 to 4.04% in 1991. The use of paid donors was discontinued in 1993, leading to a decrease in prevalence to 3.34%. The prevalence of antibodies to HIV among replacement donors increased from 0.56% in 1988 to 5.82% in 1991. Screening of these donor populations with the HIV-1 p24 antigen assay greatly contributed to reduction of risk of infection by transfusion by removing seroconverting individuals from the donor pool (14).

ORGANIZATION OF BLOOD SERVICES IN DIFFERENT NATIONS

There is wide variability in the type of organization of blood services both in developed and developing countries. Many have reorganized in recent years in order to address criticisms related to mismanagement of the AIDS tragedy. In North America, the Canadian government carried out a long and detailed inquiry (15) that led to the substitution of the previous system, managed by the Canadian Red Cross, with an entirely new system. Hema-Quebec now covers the province of Quebec, and Canadian Blood Services covers the remainder of Canada. France reorganized its national system under a new centralized structure that eliminated the prominent role played by each major hospital in the 1980s and early 1990s. Holland centralized the management of their 23 blood centers into eight regional centers. The Swiss Red Cross reorganized its centers regionally and sold its plasma fractionation facility based in Bern to a private concern. The Australian Red Cross reorganized its blood system completely in order to modernize and prevent a government takeover. Brazil created a federally funded system of hemocentros that are based in each state and have assumed blood collection, testing, and distribution and have extended services to rural, underserved regions.

Many countries around the world, particularly developing countries, still have hospital-based systems that are federally or privately funded to run blood services. These systems still operate in many countries with medium-level resources. Examples are Mexico, with a small national system and a large number of hospital-based services, and Argentina, which had 551 hospital-based blood banks in 1996. Chile had 162 blood banks, Venezuela had 243, and Brazil over 2,000. India had 604 blood banks in 31 states. Interestingly, the World Health Report 2000 (1), published by WHO, points out that the main failings of many health systems are:

- Many health ministries focus on the public sector and often disregard the frequently much larger private sector health care.
- In many countries some, if not most, physicians work simultaneously for the public sector and in private practice. This means the public sector ends up subsidizing unofficial private practice.
- Many governments fail to prevent a "black market" in health, where widespread corruption, bribery, "moonlighting," and other illegal practices flourish. The black markets, which themselves are caused by malfunctioning health care systems and low income of health care workers, further undermine those systems.
- Many health ministries fail to enforce regulations that they, themselves, have created or are supposed to implement in the public interest.

There is immense variety in the structure of blood systems around the world. In developed countries most are either government run, like the French system, or are supported by direct government subsidies, like Canada and the United Kingdom. The local Red Cross manages some of these systems. Examples are Australia, Japan, Germany, Switzerland, and Finland. Italy, Portugal, and Argentina do not have national blood systems.

They have hospital-based blood banks, each providing for its own needs. Mexico has an incipient national system, but the majority of the collections takes place at state- and federally funded hospital blood banks. Brazil has created in the last 15 years at least one federally funded regional center (hemocentro) in each state. The hemocentros coexist with private blood centers, many of which are hospital based. Several of the private blood banks are American Association of Blood Banks (AABB) accredited and comply with ISO 9000.

Blood transfusion systems are changing rapidly in Europe as a result of the integration and desire for self-sufficiency promoted by the European Union (EU). The EU has promulgated standards for plasma derivatives that apply to all members. Standards for the collection and processing of whole blood are still the prerogative of each country. The ultimate goal of the organization is the establishment of a single standard for all blood and blood products for all member countries. There is an effort to establish common regulatory standards in the developed world through the International Conference on Harmonisation, of which the U.S. Food and Drug Administration is an active participant. Several documents generated by the conference are posted on the FDA website (http://www.fda.gov/cber).

Developing countries have a similar range of blood systems. The World Health Organization and PAHO have encouraged governmental involvement, the creation of national blood systems, and centralization of services like collections and testing, but often find substantial resistance from the private sector. However, international organizations have been successful in the promotion of quality standards that are gradually being implemented by these countries, within the limitations of their infrastructure and resources. The World Health Organization and PAHO have also generated training materials, both administrative and technical, for use by member countries. Organizations like International Society for Blood Transfusion (ISBT) have been quite successful in promoting quality standards in Eastern Europe and Asia. The AABB has devoted a substantial effort to the creation of international standards and accreditation and has collaborated with PAHO in the dissemination of these standards in Central and South America. The International Consortium for Blood Safety, an organization founded by Alfred Prince from the New York Blood Center, has focused on the development and dissemination of low-cost screening assays for developing countries. They have initiated programs in several areas of the world, including India and Paraguay.

In the United States, the Health and Human Services Committee on Blood Safety and Availability held a meeting dedicated to international issues in blood and blood transfusion in April 2001. Transcripts are posted on the Health and Human Services website (http://www.os.dhhs.gov/bloodsafety/). The meeting highlighted the role of U.S. agencies in the promotion of blood safety for less-developed countries. For instance, the National Institutes of Health have added a supplement dedicated to training in transfusion medicine to the Fogarty Program. The Centers for Disease Control and Prevention included in its global AIDS program the subject of transfusion. The meeting generated a number of suggestions for increased U.S. participation in the improvement of global blood safety.

SUMMARY

This chapter highlighted some of the global issues in transfusion medicine, the concern of developed countries about the wide gap in blood banking practices between developed and developing countries, and the desire to assist developing countries in their goal to achieve a safe and adequate blood supply. It also created an opportunity to express some of the observations derived from many years of involvement in international issues.

When asked about their goals, representatives of developing countries unanimously emphasize their desire to build blood systems that are as good as those in the United States and in the rest of the developed world. Many health care professionals in these countries have learned everything about the ideal models of blood transfusion safety through individuals trained abroad, scientific publications, and advertisements distributed by manufacturers of technology. These countries want the same technologies and approaches. They do not want to be considered second rate. An example is a recent decision made by the health authorities in India. Rapid tests are not acceptable for HCV or HIV screening. Enzyme-linked immunosorbent assay (ELISA)-type tests are now mandated. Essentially, most developing countries want to perform according to state-of-the-art standards. They want the same standards and the same tests. They reject less sophisticated tests. They struggle because of economic factors, not because of intellectual factors. Another important element impacting transfusion safety is national pride and the sanctity of blood. Brazil wrote into its constitution that blood could not be commercialized or exported, a reaction to abuses that took place over 30 years ago. China has forbidden payment of blood donors as recently as 2 years ago.

Unfortunately, current approaches used by organizations that assist developing countries contribute to the feelings of insufficiency and despair. Most programs focus on technology provided through the local governments. They provide short-term financial support, training in sophisticated institutions, equipment, and supplies. Trainees attend international meetings and are mesmerized by the impressive technology exhibits. They want it all. They return to their countries of origin and dream about setting up blood banks identical to those that they saw abroad. Some actually succeed in doing so. Then they realize that the system depends on the availability of qualified blood donors. This was not part of their training and was not mentioned by the local salesman pitching technologic wares. Trainees did not learn how to recruit volunteer blood donors. They did not learn how to create a sense of duty among the members of their community. They did not have resources to develop methods to deal with the frequent cultural barriers and myths about blood donation. In despair, they maintain their tradition of replacement donors.

The situation is aggravated by the uncritical adoption of testing standards of the developed world. For instance, Brazilian regulations require screening of all donors for hepatitis B core antibodies. Between 15% and 20% of donors in the Amazon area are positive for these antibodies. The proportion is 10% in other areas of the country. The units are collected and discarded. Furthermore, overzealous regulators require the performance of two different tests for HIV, Chagas disease, and syphilis. These wasted resources could be more appropriately applied to ongoing donor recruitment efforts leading to a stable base of loyal repeat donors.

To some degree, developed Western nations bear responsibility for the confusion about blood safety standards around the world. Despite the communication and interaction between regulatory agencies and blood banking organizations, countries cannot agree on procedures for the management of the safety of the blood supply. There is no better example than the plethora of irrational measures adopted to prevent the theoretic risk of transmission of variant Creutzfelt-Jakob disease (vCJD) by transfusion. England burns the plasma from every unit of blood that it collects and buys plasma from paid donors in the United States to fill its plasma fractionation plants. Portugal imports plasma for transfusion from Germany. Germany is considering discarding its plasma and obtaining it from other countries. And in the United States, a major blood banking organization decided that the recommendations of world experts on transmissible spongiform encephalopathies assembled by the Food and Drug Administration did not go far enough and wants to defer 6% to 9% of blood donors because of travel to Europe.

Global availability of safe blood transfusions can be achieved through the establishment of rational standards compatible with the infrastructure and resources of each country.

REFERENCES

1. World Health Organization. World Health Report. Geneva: World Health Organization, 2000.
2. Gibbs WN, Corcoran P. Blood safety in developing countries. *Vox Sang* 1994;67:377–381.
3. Blood Safety in the Americas. *Epidemiological Bulletin/PAHO* 1999; 20:8–9.
4. Schmunis GA, Zicker F, Segura EL, et al. *Transfusion* 2000;40: 1048–1053.
5. Schmunis GA, Zicker F, Pinheiro F, et al. Risk for transfusion-transmitted diseases in Central and South America. *Emerg Infect Dis* 1998;4: 5–11.
6. Hamerschlak N, Pasternak J, Amato Neto V. Current risk of AIDS transmission by transfusion. *Rev Hosp Clin Fac Med Sao Paulo* 1993; 48:183–185.
7. Hersh BS, Popovici F, Apetrei RC, et al. Acquired immunodeficiency syndrome in Romania. *Lancet* 1991;338:645–649.
8. Avila C, Stetler HC, Sepulveda J, et al. The epidemiology of HIV transmission among paid plasma donors, Mexico City, Mexico. *AIDS* 1989;3:631–633.
9. Volkow P, Perez-Padilla R, del-Rio C, et al. The role of commercial plasmapheresis banks on AIDS epidemic in Mexico. *Rev Invest Clin* 1998;50:221–226.
10. Luby SP, Niaz Q, Siddiqui S, et al. Patient's perceptions of transfusion risks in Karachi, Pakistan. *Int J Infect Dis* 2001;5:24–26.
11. Van Hoogstraten MJ, Consten EC, Henny CP, et al. Are there simple measurers to reduce the risk of HIV infection through blood transfusion in a Zambian district hospital? *Trop Med Int Health* 2000;5: 668–673.
12. Massenet D, Tesfaye G, Dandera B. Blood transfusion in Ethiopia. 1998;58:307–308.
13. Huraib S, al Rashed R, Aldrees A, et al. High prevalence and risk factors for hepatitis C in hemodialysis patients in Saudi Arabia. *Nephrol Dial Transplant* 1995;10:470–474.
14. Mundee Y, Kamtorn N, Chaiyaphruk S, et al. Infectious disease markers in blood donors in northern Thailand. *Transfusion* 1995;35: 264–267.
15. Krever, JH. Commission of inquiry on the blood system in Canada. Canadian Government Publishing, Ottawa, ON, 1997.

68

CURRENT GOOD MANUFACTURING PRACTICES

THOMAS F. ZUCK
P. ANN HOPPE

With the emergence of the acquired immunodeficiency syndrome (AIDS) during the early 1980s, the interest of the public as well as regulatory authorities in the safety of the blood supply increased dramatically. The vast majority of blood and blood components for transfusion are supplied in the United States by blood centers, which in this chapter refers to any establishment that draws blood from donors or processes blood and blood components for transfusion, whether the establishment is located in a free-standing facility or located in a hospital laboratory with a transfusion service. The concepts of current Good Manufacturing Practices (cGMP) apply equally to both. The scrutiny of these centers intensified concomitantly with the concerns about blood safety, and rigorous oversight continues today. This high level of oversight has been due, in part, to the reluctance of the public to accept involuntary risks, especially those associated with blood transfusions. It also has been difficult for the public to accept that unlimited resources are lacking and that reducing the risks of transfusions further will require trade-offs for risk reduction in other parts of the health care system (1). To illustrate with the example Keeney cited, decisions about buying an automobile with expensive safety equipment may preclude purchases to lower other health risks (1). Finally, because biologic systems are imperfect, reduction of transfusion risks to zero is not possible, regardless of the resources dedicated to achieve such a goal.

In order to optimize safety, compliance with the provisions of Title 21 of the Code of Federal Regulations (CFR) specifying cGMP that outline production process control requirements for the pharmaceutical industry continues to be the focus of inspections and guidelines by the Food and Drug Administration (FDA). Although guidelines do not exert the force of regulations because they have not met the requirements for federal rule making, they provide establishments with the FDA's expectations regarding the ability of blood centers to control production processes. Further, compliance minimizes the probability that unsuitable blood components will be made available, in contradistinction to released for transfusion. This is an even more restrictive definition than that used by the FDA to define reportable errors in which quality is defined as " . . . never releasing an unsuitable unit for transfusion or further manufacture" (2).

Current Good Manufacturing Practices embrace industrial rather than medical concepts. The subspecialty of transfusion medicine has been carved from other medical disciplines over the last 2 decades (3). Because blood center operations traditionally have been viewed as medical rather than industrial enterprises, the need to implement cGMP in blood centers was not immediately obvious. Further, implementation of cGMP has

T.F. Zuck: Hoxworth Blood Center, University of Cincinnati Medical Center, Cincinnati, Ohio.
P.A. Hoppe: Hoppe Regulatory Consultants, Decatur, Georgia.

been resisted by some blood banking professionals because they believed implementation would be detrimental to transfusion medicine as a medical discipline (4,5). Finally, it has been observed that health care organizations are not ideally suited for modern industrial management (6). Thus, blood centers have been required to separate operationally medical functions, such as providing consultations and patient care, from manufacturing activities, such as the production of red blood cells or platelets. The prevailing standards of medical care define the practice of the former, whereas cGMP govern the latter.

In this chapter a historic perspective and the elements of cGMP are presented and blood center supplementation of cGMP with statistical process controls and process innovation is introduced briefly.

HISTORIC PERSPECTIVE

Both the development of laws and regulations and the actual regulation of drugs and biologic products are exceedingly complex. Books and countless papers have been written on these subjects and only a most general overview can be presented here. In the simplest terms, Congress passes broad enabling legislation and operational regulations are then promulgated by regulatory agencies, primarily the FDA in the case of blood centers. Historically, many legislative and regulatory actions were taken through these pathways because of perceived disasters, most recently the emergence of AIDS and Creutzfeldt-Jakob disease.

Biologic products initially were regulated when Congress passed the Biologics Control Act in 1902 (7,8). The impetus for this act was provided by the deaths of several children following administration of an antitoxin contaminated with tetanus (8). Many provisions of this act established practices that remain part of current FDA law, 100 years later. Among these provisions is the requirement that a biologic product obtain premarket approval for the article to be shipped in interstate commerce. Historically, all food and drug manufacturers were required to register their firms and products with the FDA. In order to ship biologic products in interstate commerce, however, both establishment and product licenses were required. A product license would not be issued in the absence of an establishment license nor an establishment license granted unless the firm manufactured at least one licensed product. In that scheme, a *responsible head* (under current terminology, an authorized official, see below) served as the contact between the firm and the FDA.

Extensive changes to the regulations now require that a firm file only a biologics license application (BLA) to ship blood products in interstate commerce (9). These applications can be filed with paper copy, electronically, or a combination of both, and extensive guidance about filing has been published by the FDA (10). In addition, the term *responsible head* has been replaced by *authorized official,* and the responsibility for regulatory compliance rests with this person or persons designated to represent the firm. Firms that already hold approved establishment licenses and product licenses are issued a new biologics license when the FDA receives the first supplement to a firm's existing approved license. The approved product license along with the portion of the approved establishment license relevant to the requirements of the new regulation are deemed to constitute a biologics license under section 351 of the U.S. Public Health Service (PHS) act (11). The FDA has committed to work with sponsors to speed the process of biologics license regulatory review (12). Guidance for industry about submissions in the electronic format is available from the FDA, which also has established a docket in which it will publish those submission formats it can accept electronically (13,14).

The form used to apply to market a new drug or biologic (Form FDA 356[h]), or to supplement the old ELAs and PLAs, as well as to apply for a biologics license contains a certification section in which the applicant agrees, among other things, to comply with the cGMP provisions of the CFR. This certification clearly reinforces the emphasis by the FDA on cGMP.

The FDA has provided guidance to ensure compliance with the requirements for BLA submissions (15). This guidance partially echoes the scheme for interacting with the agency (FDA) about establishment license changes (section 601.12), which establishes reporting requirements and has been in effect for many years. The extent of FDA notification about a change is now categorized according to the significance of the change. Major changes, defined as presenting " . . . a substantial potential to have an adverse effect on the safety or effectiveness of the product . . . ", require a supplement submission and approval prior to distribution of a blood product in interstate commerce. Examples provided by the FDA requiring this most stringent level of regulation include implementation of a new production process for a blood component or a change in contractor to perform a portion of the manufacturing process, including infectious disease testing of blood donors.

Moderate changes that present a " . . . moderate potential to have an adverse effect on the safety or effectiveness of the product . . . " require notification of the agency at least 30 days prior to the distribution of a product affected by the changes. Included in this moderate category are changes in donor suitability, including donor deferral, or a change in manufacturer of automated donor apheresis equipment.

Moderate changes requiring supplemental submissions prior to distribution of a product affected by the change can also be made without waiting the 30 days. Labeling the application Supplemental Changes Being Effected at the time of submission is required for this regulatory treatment. Examples of these changes provided by the FDA include the use of an approved standard operating procedure (SOP) of another facility.

Minor changes are placed in the least stringent regulatory category. Such changes need only be included in the annual report. Examples of minor changes outlined by the FDA might include modification of quality control procedures that are consistent with the manufacturer's instructions, changes in radiation equipment used by the applicant or a contractor, or minor facility renovations.

From a practical standpoint, the changes brought by the single-license BLA have little impact on the day-to-day regulatory environment within which blood centers and transfusion services operate. The legal obligations with regard to cGMP remain unchanged, and the applicability of the cGMP elements described in greater detail below continues to expand. The FDA has encouraged licensees to communicate uncertainties about changes, including seeking guidance prior to implementing them (16). It also encourages cover letters with submissions to improve communications between the agency and a blood establishment. As noted, the authorized official has assumed the previous vital role of the responsible head in such interactions.

Recall authority of the FDA essentially remains unchanged by the recent licensing process modifications (21 CFR 7.40–7.59). All products manufactured in violation of FDA requirements are subject to recall. Following revocation or suspension of a license, the FDA may also order a recall of products already distributed by the firm. In 1902 and 1903, the PHS, then the enforcer of the act, focused on suspension and revocation of licenses as the basic enforcement mechanisms, with unannounced inspections occurring at least every 2 years. This compliance approach dominates current FDA enforcement philosophy in dealing with firms it views as noncompliant.

In 1905 Upton Sinclair published *The Jungle,* which described horribly unsafe and filthy practices in Chicago slaughterhouses—a public health disaster (17). Although Sinclair wrote the book as a social statement about abuse of the common working man, it is widely regarded as providing part of the impetus for the passage of the Pure Food and Drug Act of 1906. That law addressed the purity of food and drugs but neither their safety nor efficacy.

In 1909, at a time when inspections of biologic establishments were conducted by the Marine Hospital Service, then a component of the precursor to the current PHS, the concept of responsible head was developed. This person acted as a single point of interaction between the FDA and an establishment. As noted, the terminology for this person has been changed to authorized official.

Between 1909 and 1919 additional regulatory requirements were formulated to supplement the Biologics Control Act of 1902 (Table 68.1). Many of these provisions, such as training, production and control records, and lot release requirements, remain part of the regulations today. These provisions are framed as key elements of cGMP.

In 1938, a disaster again prompted congressional action. A pharmaceutical company marketed an elixir of sulfanilamide containing diethylene glycol, an alcohol closely related to a commonly used automobile radiator antifreeze. Unfortunately, this alcohol is extremely toxic and over 100 people, mostly children, died after ingesting the formulation. Simple toxicity tests would have demonstrated that the formulation was unsafe, but such tests were neither required nor performed. The Federal Food, Drug, and Cosmetic Act passed shortly thereafter required that the sponsor of a product subject to licensure prove its safety as well as its purity.

TABLE 68.1. EXAMPLES OF EARLY REGULATORY REQUIREMENTS

Immediate reporting of establishment changes
Demonstration of personnel training and competency
Maintenance of production records and controls
Lot release of articles
Labeling requirements

From Timm EA. 75 years compliance with biological regulations. *Food Drug Cosmet Law J* 1978;33:225–230, with permision.

In response to yet another disaster, the severe congenital defects caused by thalidomide in the late 1950s, the act was amended significantly in 1962 (Kefauver-Harris amendments). For the first time drugs were required to be proven effective, and this proof could be obtained only by clinical trials approved by the FDA prior to their undertaking. Unapproved drugs could not be distributed and given to patients until an exemption for the candidate drug was granted by the agency. These amendments completed the well-known approval or licensure triad: safety, purity, and efficacy.

An unusual provision of the CFR provides an additional pathway to ensure compliance with the regulations but at the same time relieves the FDA of many burdensome inspections. Section 601.22 permits unlicensed biologic products, such as recovered plasma, to be shipped for further manufacture while transferring the inspection responsibility from the FDA to the vendee of products declared to be in short supply. This provision applies particularly to unlicensed facilities, because it permits any registered establishment to ship unlicensed plasma in interstate commerce or internationally under Section 601.22, provided the vendee has documented that the product is in compliance with the provisions of the CFR.

In applying the requirements of cGMP to a firm, the distinction between licensure and registration is more technical than real. Licensure is required to ship licensed products in interstate commerce or internationally. Registration is required for all blood establishments, including those located in hospitals, that manufacture (collect, store, process, or distribute) blood components for transfusion or further manufacture. Registration requirements are outlined in 21 CFR, part 607; license requirements are in 21 CFR, part 601.

A major regulatory action was taken more recently when it was discovered that unsuitable units of blood were being released for transfusion or further manufacture by blood centers managed by the American Red Cross (ARC). In 1988, during an inspection of the National Headquarters of the ARC, the FDA found significant deficiencies. The agency entered into an agreement with the ARC that certain improvements would be made in their national systems (18). In the early 1990s, regulatory letters sent to some ARC centers cited failure to comply with provisions of section 211 of Title 21 of the CFR. Through these letters the FDA gave all the blood centers notice that they would be required to comply, not only with the cGMP portions of the 600 series (although technically parts, they are often referred to as series) mainly outlined in section 606, as they had been historically, but also with the provisions of the 200 series. This application of the more strict regulations by the agency was reinforced in many Form FDA-483s (the reports of observations by individual investigators left with blood centers following an FDA inspection). Frequently these observations suggested that the investigator(s) did not believe the establishment was in compliance with regulations, guidelines, or recommendations of the agency, including cGMP.

A pattern emerged in which blood centers gradually were being regulated as pharmaceutical manufacturers. Although there has been an outcry that this application of Title 21 was unwarranted, section 210.2(a) clearly states that the 600 and 200 series supplement one another. Only when there is a conflict does one take precedence, and in that case the more specific applies. This is not infrequent for blood centers, because sections 606 and 640 are more specific for blood centers than are many provisions of the 200 series.

In 1991, the FDA published a memorandum that outlined the more common deficiencies of blood establishments (19). Deficiencies were most frequently found in the areas of donor deferral, viral testing, following SOPs, and computer systems operations. Through this memorandum, the agency gave blood centers additional notice of its regulatory intent; this intent continues to be reinforced by recent actions of the agency.

In 1991, the FDA also published the first draft of proposed Quality Assurance Guidelines for Blood Establishments and held a workshop to receive input from the regulated establishments (20). It became very clear at this workshop that cGMP included quality systems and formed the cornerstone for FDA's intensified regulatory approach. It was reemphasized that blood centers producing blood and blood components are pharmaceutical manufactures and would be regulated as such.

CURRENT GOOD MANUFACTURING PRACTICES RATIONALE

As noted, cGMP is an industrial concept and, as such, its principles are rooted in industrial quality models (21). In the traditional detection model for quality (Fig. 68.1), testing of final product is used to discover production defects and weed out unsuitable products. Products are shipped with the knowledge that some percentage has undetected defects. It is left to the purchaser to discover a defective product and seek replacement. Detection has been the quality model generally used by health care facilities (22). But Deming, as well as others, emphasized that testing final products can not improve manufacturing quality—it can only describe it (23). The basis for this belief lies in the calculus of errors. Even a small variance in each process can

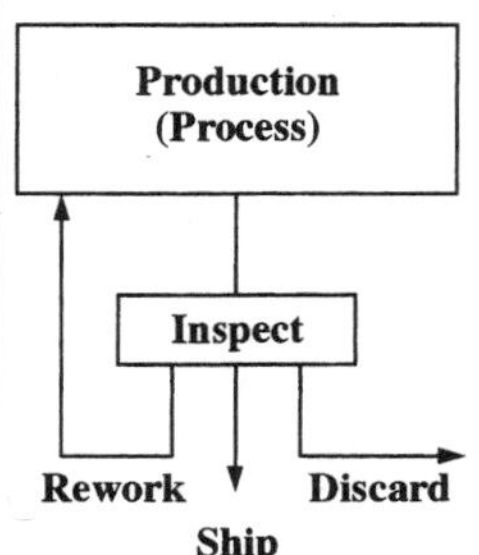

FIGURE 68.1. The detection model of quality control. Note the expensive consequences of failed inspections.

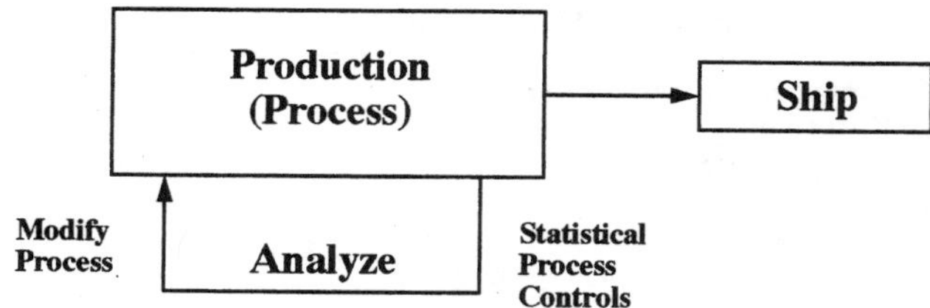

FIGURE 68.2. The prevention model of quality control. Note the similarity of this process with that of error management as diagrammed in Figure 68.4.

result in major product variation if numerous production steps are required. Thus, the detection model is no longer viewed as ideal for controlling biomedical manufacturing establishments. Product testing as the primary means of controlling quality in blood centers is particularly unsuitable because the quality of the raw materials—blood given by volunteer donors—cannot be completely controlled. Further, because each donation becomes a "lot" in the traditional pharmaceutical production sense, it is not feasible to perform additional tests on all products manufactured from each donation, that is, each lot. Finally, a blood product defect, such as contamination by an infectious agent that could have been intercepted by laboratory testing, may be discovered in a transfusion recipient only after disastrous consequences have ensued.

In contrast to the detection model, the prevention model (Fig. 68.2) seeks to obviate manufacturing variation by rigidly controlling manufacturing processes. In this model, it is assumed that employees will have lapses but that the design of the manufacturing systems will prevent such lapses from resulting in the release of components unsuitable for transfusion. This model is particularly apropos for blood centers because, as noted, neither the quality of the raw materials can be completely controlled nor each lot (a component) exhaustively tested. However, the manufacturing processes can be controlled with the objective of reducing lot-to-lot variation. The cGMP provide a roadmap for production controls and, as such, have been embraced by blood centers. The power of the elements of cGMP rests in their universality. As described below, each element can be applied to any manufacturing function, or skill box. In the context of this chapter, skill box refers to the smallest discrete step in a production process that can be described, characterized by the FDA, and controlled. The elements of cGMP are listed in Table 68.2. This division into elements is arbitrary but is based on an analysis of commonality of the requirements of Title 21 as they apply to all aspects of blood center operations. Thus, it is irrelevant whether they are applied to blood collection or to infectious disease testing; each element is applicable for each discrete blood center operation. The principle driving the elements rests in flow charts of operational production processes. In Figure 68.3 the general flow diagram of the production of platelets is shown. Optimally, cGMP elements are applied to each skill box in the manufacturing process. However, the cGMP elements should be viewed in the context of a blood center's entire production system. The safety of the blood supply is protected only by the application to the total system. The levels of protection (Table

TABLE 68.2. ELEMENTS OF CGMP

Standard operating procedures
Record keeping
Personnel management
Calibration
Validation
Labeling
Error management
Quality control and auditing
Facilities and equipment
Process and production change control

cGMP, current Good Manufacturing Practices.

TABLE 68.3. LEVELS OF PROTECTION OF THE BLOOD SUPPLY

Donor self-exclusion
Screening questions
Viral and surrogate testing
Deferral registries and duplicate search
Unit exclusion strategies
Confidential unit exclusion
Call-back programs

68.3) of the blood supply create a safety system with intentionally designed redundancies.

Standard Operating Procedures (§§ 211.100[a] and 211.22; §606.100[b])

Standard operating procedures management lies at the heart of quality manufacturing and cGMP compliance. In the context of blood center control for the purposes of this chapter, quality is narrowly defined as never releasing a product unsuitable for transfusion or further manufacture. Because blood and plasma centers are required to follow their own SOPs, each SOP creates unique regulatory requirements for that center. From a regulatory standpoint, this concept is significant in that compliance standards and regulatory requirements are created by individual center SOPs. Procedures are essential to ensure that all SOPs, including any changes, are reviewed and approved by the quality unit. Any deviation from established procedures should be documented and investigated. Such investigation should determine whether the deviation had an impact on quality. The results of such investigation should be reviewed and approved by the quality unit. A list of responsibilities of the quality unit are listed in Table 68.4.

Current Good Manufacturing Practices describe both the production methods used by blood centers to manufacture components and the manufacturing process controls in place. Section 211.22 requires approval of all SOPs by the quality control unit. As defined by the FDA, the quality control unit is an organizational entity with defined responsibilities and authority for controlling, through checking or testing, that specifications are met and quality systems are maintained. The FDA has explained that the quality control unit cited in 21 CFR 211 is equivalent to what is now called a quality program or quality assurance department. However, the principle of having a single "head" responsible for quality issues remains extant, without regard to what designations appear on an organizational chart. All matters that

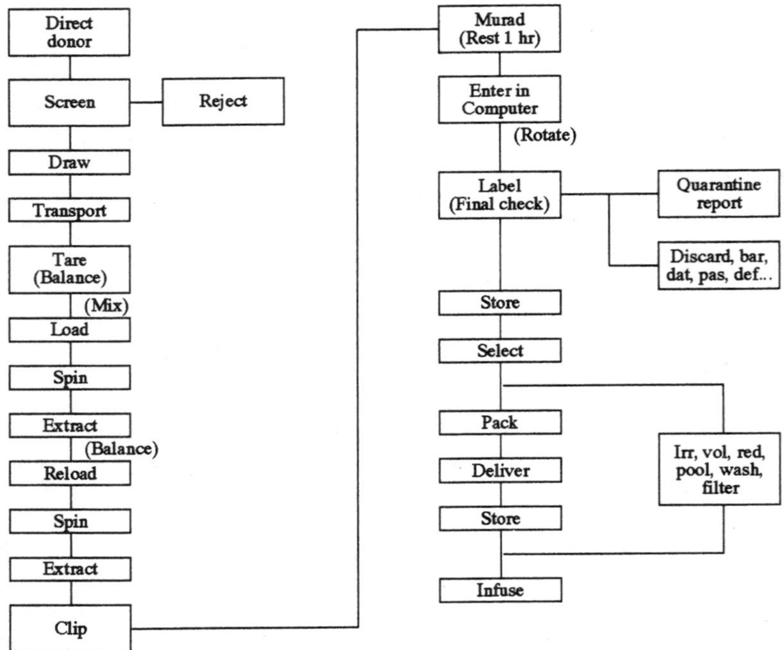

FIGURE 68.3. Simplified flow chart of platelet production. (From Zuck, TF. The good manufacturing concept. In: Sibinga CTS, Das PC, Heininger HJ, eds. *Good manufacturing practice in transfusion medicine.* Dordrecht, The Netherlands: Kluwer Academic Publishers, 1996, with permission.)

TABLE 68.4. QUALITY UNIT RESPONSIBILITIES

ATTRIBUTES OF THE REQUIRED UNIT
Responsibilities described in writing
Independent of production
Involved in all quality-related matters
Reviews and approves all quality-related issues
Adequate analytic control facilities at its disposal
UNIT RESPONSIBILITIES SHOULD INCLUDE, BUT NOT BE LIMITED TO THE FOLLOWING
Approve specifications
Approve test procedures, including process controls
Approve validation plans, protocols, or equipment
Review changes in product, process, or equipment and determine if revalidation is required
Approve specification changes, sampling plans, test procedures
Approve sampling procedures
Approve reference standards
Conduct analytic investigations and evaluate results
Approve testing materials
Provide analytical reports
Approve or reject intermediates and active pharmaceutical ingredients manufactured, processed, packed, or held under contract by another establishment
Gather data to support retest dates (stability testing)
Evaluate and approve contractors
Review batch records
Review complaints
Dispose of materials not meeting specifications
Dispose of materials returned to the establishment
Perform internal and external audits
Perform periodic assessments of procedures, policies, and responsibilities within the establishment's manufacturing and control operations

From FDA/CDER. Internationally harmonized guide for active pharmaceutical ingredients [Draft]. September 1, 1997, with permission.

relate to quality should funnel to a single person or group with broad knowledge of the entire blood center operation and access to the information necessary to assess the impact of proposed changes. These principles emphasize the importance with which the FDA views both the quality unit and SOPs.

Consensus has not developed about the level of detail that should be contained in blood center SOPs. It is generally agreed that they should be sufficiently explicit that a qualified technical person could, with minimal training, perform the described procedure and manufacture products that meet all requirements. Highly detailed SOPs require more frequent revision and are much more likely to be violated by center personnel, a failing that makes blood centers vulnerable during inspections, particularly if inspectors actually observe performance of procedures.

Every provision of a center's SOPs must reflect the manufacturers' instructions of licensed or approved systems used in the center. It is strongly recommended that planned deviations from a manufacturer's instructions occur only after submission to the FDA of the proposed alternative. Further, 21 CFR 211.100 requires that all deviations from SOPs, whether planned or inadvertent, must be documented. Change control of SOPs remains one of the more difficult issues for blood center management. Standard operating procedures to manage procedural changes are critical when implementing new and revised processes. Both meticulous change control and periodic review of SOPs during audits are essential to prevent "drift" in manufacturing processes.

A reference resource manual of SOPs of member centers maintained by the America's Blood Centers has proven to be a useful resource for supplying benchmarks for blood centers.

Record Keeping (§§606.160, 606.170, and 211.180 through 211.198)

Of the cGMP elements, record keeping is perhaps one of the most important, particularly from the perspective of preparing for inspections or defending a center's actions if legal issues arise. During inspection, it is assumed that an activity not documented was not performed. In general, the record-keeping requirements of the 200 series are more detailed and rigorous than those of the 600 series. However, the provisions of both series require concurrent, legible, indelible documentation of each production step (linked to the operator by dated signature or initials) and an audit trail for any changes subsequently made to records. Records of every lot must permit traceability and trackability of a product by both the manufacturer and the FDA during inspections and recalls. The latter may require reconstruction of manufacturing (including labeling) of a product that has been linked to an adverse reaction or other problem. Both the 200 and the 600 series require that records of adverse reactions and complaints be maintained. These records may be subject to scrutiny during inspections because they may indicate weaknesses in the manufacturing controls of an establishment. It is essential that the records of these events include an evaluation of the problem to determine if an investigation is warranted. If an investigation is performed, maintaining a detailed description of the process is critical. The records should document who made the decisions concerning whether the events also required a deviation report to FDA, whether look-back notifications or recalls are necessary and, if a device failure was involved, whether a Medical Device Report (MDR) was required in accordance with 21 CFR 803.

It is essential that the records extend to the training and competency of the personnel responsible for these decisions; that is, it is a cGMP requirement that only trained personnel be allowed to make these judgments. Important assignments such as these reporting functions should be identified in the position descriptions for the personnel. Meticulous records of compliance with cGMP elements are required to assure both upper management and the FDA that an establishment is in control. Control in this context can be defined as compliance in every respect with all of the establishment manufacturing SOPs and FDA requirements. During inspections of blood centers, whether by the private sector or regulatory bodies such as the FDA, the overriding investigational concern is whether an establishment is in control. Records should be designed to document control of manufacturing systems.

Record keeping is greatly facilitated by blood center computerization. Increasingly, information management and technology are being used to maintain batch records, document process control, and the like. Validation (see below) of computer systems used to maintain blood center records is the subject for extensive and detailed guidelines published by the FDA (24–30). Further, the FDA notified vendors of blood center software that these programs are medical devices subject to regulation (including 510k clearance processes), and blood centers must ensure that software used for control functions is a properly validated, 510k-cleared device, or equivalent (31–35). In the final section of this chapter, the application of information technology to improve process control though process innovation is briefly discussed further.

Personnel and Training (§§606.20, 211.22 through 211.34)

The requirements of the personnel regulations are designed to ensure that people engaged in the manufacture of biologics and drugs have sufficient education, training, and experience to perform their assigned functions. Section 211.22 also requires that employees be trained in cGMP by qualified individuals. Although these provisions present only the most general requirements, it has become recognized that several key components must be included as part of a personnel training program that complies with cGMP and that ensures SOPs are correctly implemented by all staff.

Training

Training should be performed formally by personnel with documented credentials attesting to their qualifications, and the records of training should include clearly defined objectives and course content. Training in general systems, such as computers, incident reporting, safety, and the like, are as important as technical training specific for an employee's tasks. Pre- and posttraining examinations are one acceptable way of documenting the attendance of the employee and that the training was effective. Refresher courses must be offered at predetermined appropriate frequencies and whenever a manufacturing or process control is changed. It is also critical that experience, education, and competency of staff and contractors be documented, without regard to whether they perform maintenance and repairs, training, auditing, or other staff functions, and particularly if they are expected to perform with little additional training after hire. In the absence of this training documentation and certification of credentials, it is critical that tasks performed be directly supervised; for example, records of laboratory equipment repair should be countersigned by the laboratory staff before the repairman leaves the premises.

Competency Testing

In addition to evaluations demonstrating effectiveness (pre- and posttraining testing) accompanying formal training, personnel should demonstrate continued competency by periodic examination, review of records they generate, and actual task performance. The results of these assessments should be retained by the quality unit as well as part of employees' training records. Personnel records should be subdivided to permit easy access to the training portions (and the corrective action relative to errors, if applicable) without divulging any confidential portion of the personnel record. If a weakness is detected, retraining and reevaluation become critical corrective actions. An employee who fails a competency evaluation (or makes a serious error in performance of duties) must not continue to perform that task without documented supervision until retraining and a satisfactory evaluation is recorded. The content of the assessment exercises is also a required record. It is not acceptable practice to discard the tests and maintain only the scores; however, maintaining a single master file copy of the test (versus every employee's copy) is acceptable as long as scores can be related to the appropriate test instrument.

Some employees may feel threatened by these activities; however, they can be approached constructively. Proper training improves the performances of all employees and they should be taught that they are better prepared to comply with cGMP through training. Employee acceptance can be improved by emphasizing that the performance of each employee is critical to the organization's success in complying with cGMP to ensure safe products, and that cGMP compliance is vital to the overall quality and regulatory compliance by blood center operations.

Retraining

Ad hoc training of employees who have experienced lapses and made errors forms a vital step in continuous improvement programs (see below). As with other forms of training, effectiveness must be documented. However, when there is a documented event that requires retraining, such as an error detected after a product has been released or an employee has failed a competency evaluation or proficiency testing, the retraining and its effectiveness must be documented as with other forms of training. However, citing retraining as the primary corrective action for an error is a double-edged sword; one must be prepared to answer the additional questions that derive from this conclusion, such as who else may need training. If this person's competency evaluation had inaccurately predicted the ability to perform, are there others failing to perform? Was the original training adequate or does the basic training need revision? What products may have been affected by inadequately trained staff? Is supervision of the employee adequate if the deficient performance was not detected until an error was made?

Calibration (§§606.60 and 211.68)

Calibration has been defined as the comparison of a firm's measurement systems with known standards. Because calibration requirements are not familiar concepts to some blood center personnel, an example may be helpful. A centrifuge used to manufacture platelets has multiple process points that can be calibrated. Among these are the centrifugation timer, its tachometer, and its brake timing. Subpart H (Laboratory Controls) of 21 CFR 606 outlines calibration requirements for several common devices used in blood collection, processing, and testing. Section 211.160(b)(4) outlines specific calibration provisions, requiring that all "instruments, apparatus, gauges, and recording devices must be calibrated under established protocols that specify periodicity." It is unclear how these provisions will ultimately be applied to blood centers, but there is increasing evidence that Team Biologics of the FDA, CBER, will apply all requirements stringently. Examples of deficiency citations that relate to cali-

TABLE 68.5. CALIBRATION DEFICIENCIES: SYNOPSIS OF WARNING LETTER CITATIONS

Written procedures for record keeping and equipment calibration are not followed.
Calibration logs, travel tickets, and donor files contained illegible corrections.
No documentation was available showing calibration of all equipment such as the donor scale, refrigerator alarm system, trip-scale temperature gauges, and thermometers used to monitor the incubator and freezer.
Records maintained for the incubator, freezer, and hematocrit analyzer revealed several instances of the equipment temperatures or calibration being outside acceptable ranges; no documentation was available to show that deviations were investigated or that corrective actions were implemented.
Equipment was not calibrated as prescribed in the standard operating procedures (SOPs) (21 CFR 606.60 @H1:) in that the RPM calibration and timer check of the centrifuge was not performed every 60 days as required in the written procedure and operator's manual; vital signs monitor was not calibrated every 6 months as required.
An employee failed to enter the reference pipette calibration constant as required by the firm's SOP.
The SOP for microliter pipette calibration does not require a time frame for review of the calibration records; as a result, review of records did not occur until 6 to 14 months later.
The apheresis department does not have an SOP requiring a time-frame for review of equipment maintenance and calibration.
No document is available to show calibration and maintenance of the recording thermometers.
Quality control checks on other laboratory equipment are not being performed in accordance with established written procedures.
Numerous records reviewed during the inspection contained illegible corrections, and there is no documentation that these records were reviewed by a supervisor.
Staff failed to calibrate the stopwatch used in the calibration of the Hematostat's timer, the tachometer used to calibrate the Hematostat's RPMs, and the sphygmomanometers.
Established written procedures for apheresis equipment calibration, monthly maintenance, and cleaning to avoid possible cross contamination, are not being followed.
There are no quality control and calibration records for the Diatek donor thermometer and the blood pressure cuff.
There are no quality control and calibration records, nor is there a written procedure for the quality control and calibration, for the scale used for collecting blood.
There were incomplete records of the quarterly performance testing of automatic cell washers and quarterly calibration checks of the Coulter counter instrument as required by the blood bank's written SOPs.
Records showed deficiencies related to the secondary review of analytic and calibration data.

CFR, Code of Federal Regulations; RPM, revolutions per minute.

bration issues are found in Table 68.5. Other areas that some centers fail to address are the qualification of the equipment that will be used to calibrate and the qualification of procedures and staff used by contractors performing calibration services. Blood centers retain full responsibility for ensuring that work will meet FDA requirements, whether it is done in-house or contracted.

In the 600 series, under Subpart D (Equipment), it is required that all production equipment be calibrated ". . . on a regularly scheduled basis as prescribed in the Standard Operating Procedures Manual." In section 606.60 the calibration requirements of common blood bank equipment are provided in tabular form. This table is incomplete, however, and many of the automated systems currently used in blood centers are not listed. Guidance then must be sought in section 211.68 and the manufacturer's instructions for the item (36).

As noted, blood centers must have a calibration SOP that specifies the center's policies regarding this requirement. Traditionally, blood centers have delegated responsibility for equipment calibration to the section in which the equipment is used. A more comprehensive approach is frequently used in the pharmaceutical industry in which a metrology unit is responsible for calibrating all equipment in the establishment. Scheduling can be computerized and can be integrated with process innovation system designs (see below). Centralized calibration of blood center measurement equipment provides several advantages, whether the metrology functions are provided by full- or part-time personnel, and is the preferred organizational approach. Management can easily review the calibration efforts of the establishment by consulting with one unit and one computer print-out, centralized file, or set of records.

Validation (§211.68)

Validation has been defined as documented evidence that provides a high degree of assurance that a specific process will consistently produce an outcome that meets its preestablished quality and performance specifications. Despite the lack of detailed validation requirements in either the 200 or 600 series, the FDA recently has focused on validation during center inspections, during workshops, and in guidelines and memoranda (20, 24–30). It has become clear that as blood bank systems continue to increase in complexity, validation of these systems will continue to be an important element of cGMP. During cGMP training, calibration frequently is confused with validation. The former deals with the assurance that critical measurement instruments for specific pieces of equipment used in the manufacture of blood components measure accurately.

Several aspects of validation recognized as critical: system description include validation plans and protocols (including established criteria for pass and fail), a defined process for review and acceptance of data including procedures for tracking and resolving all discrepancies, allocation of responsibility for the go ahead or no go decisions, and assessment of impact on operations and revalidation requirements.

System Description

Validation of a system cannot be achieved without an accurate description of the process that is to be validated. The description of the system should contain identification of all major pieces of equipment, software, hardware, and flow diagrams, as well as verbal characterizations of the systems or processes. This aspect of validation is of particular importance for computer systems for which, as noted, specific validation guidelines have been published by the FDA (24–30,37).

Validation

A key component of validation, whether retrospective or prospective, rests in developing and executing a validation protocol and planning its integration with operational systems. This protocol should prospectively specify the manner and documentation of system or process validation, the testing to be performed (including stress or boundary testing), and acceptable statistical outcomes. Test protocols should address all operational situations and all equipment or hardware that will be used, all sites, minimal and maximal load conditions, stress, interference, boundary conditions, and the like, that can reasonably be anticipated. The protocol should include the validation of the physical environment of the system (installation qualification, or IQ), the testing of the performance of the equipment as installed (performance qualification, or PQ), and the plan to follow up on the actual operation of the system by trained staff after integration in routine usage (operational qualification, or OQ) (28,37).

Revalidation Requirements

Protocols should specify when system and process revalidation should be undertaken. Revalidation is integrally linked to both process control (see below) and change control. The latter should be governed by change control SOPs.

Historically, validation requirements for blood centers developed bidirectionally. Blood centers explored what was doable for their legacy systems, and the FDA defined best methods for validation of blood center systems in general, enforcing validation requirements when failure to validate resulted in operational errors. The private sector offered language that would extensively revise the proposed language but not change its effectiveness (38), and the FDA finalized their draft guidance on validation of computer systems for all FDA related purposes (30). The understanding of regulatory expectations has increased to the point at which the industry no longer begs for additional guidance regarding systems and process validation (24). Further, much progress has been made in understanding the relationship of validation to process controls (see below).

Labeling (§§211.122–211.130; §606.120)

An important aspect of labeling of blood components lies in the definition of a lot or batch. In the 600 series, a lot is defined as " . . . having been thoroughly mixed in a single vessel." Clearly this definition relates only imprecisely to the production of blood components by blood centers and limits a *lot* to products from a single donor. Therefore, the term *batch* has more meaning in relation to release of products, and in the blood arena batch is usually defined as a group of products for which the laboratory tests were performed at the same time. Essentially, a batch release has the same meaning for blood centers as what the FDA has called a lot release. One of the difficulties created by these definitions rests in the inability to test each lot completely. This inability dictates that manufacturing controls must be in place to regulate product quality precisely, because only limited testing of final product is practical. In many blood centers, labeling is used as a control point to final check that a unit, or lot, is suitable for transfusion on further manufacture, and that other required work, such as testing for viral markers, has been performed on the batch. Each component is checked, usually by a computer, to ensure that all of the testing and record checking has been completed and that no disqualifying information appears in the past or current records of either the donor or the donated unit. If the product is stored for any period of time after the initial release, there must be procedures that ensure that any postdonation information received later or seroconversion of a donor results in appropriate interdiction of the products collected earlier, regardless of where they are stored.

Increasingly, blood centers are installing automated label printers that make on-demand custom labels for components only after an electronic record review has found each suitable for release. These systems also permit electronic label reconciliation to approach label accountability requirements of section 211.120. Product release systems permit automated checks as additional safeguards at the time the shipments are packed. Bidirectional bar coding permits encrypting a great deal of information about the unit on the label. The FDA has strongly encouraged transition to these systems through its support of the International Society of Blood Transfusion barcodes.

It is essential that labels be recognized as a critical control element requiring strict procedures for inventory, archives, and change control, as well as second-person checks of their acceptability for use (release to inventory) and approval of all changes. It is noteworthy that the recall provisions of 21 CFR 7.40–7.50 require a copy of reconstructed label of the product being recalled be provided to the FDA, regardless of the amount of time elapsed since the product was issued.

Error Management (21 CFR 211, §§606.160[b][7][iii] and 606.171[Final Rule] and 606.100[c]

Other than the obligation to report adverse reactions as provided in section 606.170 and the investigation of errors with documentation of corrective action as provided in section 606.100(c), an integrated error management system is not specifically required by the provisions of Title 21, although the rules in 21 CFR 606.171 mandate the reporting within 45 days of all biologic product deviations on released products. Table 68.6 has a summary of the reporting criteria and examples of reportable and nonreportable events. Traditionally, 21 CFR 600.14 has always required licensed facilities to report promptly any error that may affect the safety, purity, or potency of the product, and it was understood that a system was needed for capturing these events consistently. The FDA has recognized the importance of this cGMP element in a memorandum devoted to it (39), and after many years of debates and threats, the agency finally issued regulations that are more broadly applicable than any preceding policies, although they are narrowly directed.

The investigation and follow-up of deviations is critical to the successful improvement of blood center quality. Appropriate management of errors and accidents (or deviations in the current FDA terminology) forms the centerpiece of continuous improvement. Each blood center deviation should be treated as a "jewel" to be used as a case study for the staff to improve center processes. All facilities must develop SOPs for reporting, managing, and correcting errors and deviations. These SOPs should form the centerpiece of both blood center staff training and continuous improvement. Error management efforts and results

TABLE 68.6. SYNOPSIS OF FINAL RULE, EFFECTIVE MAY 7, 2001: REPORTING OF PRODUCT DEVIATIONS BY LICENSED MANUFACTURERS, UNLICENSED REGISTERED BLOOD ESTABLISHMENTS, AND TRANSFUSION SERVICES

Rule applies to all establishments: donor centers, blood banks, transfusion services
Reporting time not to exceed 45 days
Report by mail: Director, Office of Compliance and Biologics Quality, 1401 Rockville Pike, 200N (HFM-600), Rockville, MD 20853-1448; electronically: CBER's Web site: www.fda.gov/cber/biodev/biodev.htm
If the answers to the questions below are affirmative, the event is **reportable:**
Was the event associated with manufacturing?
Did the deviation affect safety, purity, or potency?
Did it occur in a licensee's or a contract facility?
Did the facility have control over the product when the deviation occurred?
Was the product distributed?
REPORTABLE BIOLOGIC PRODUCT DEVIATIONS
Event that may affect product purity, safety, or potency
Postdonation information potentially affecting safety
Compatibility sample collected from the wrong patient
Collection or processing materials did not meet specifications
FDA requirements not met on donor deferral and screening
Current or subsequent positive viral marker test
Donor screening (history, arm inspection, etc.) not recorded
Both confidential unit exclusion stickers not applied to unit
Donor deferral lists incorrectly checked
Outdated bag used for collection
Donor sample of unit clotted or hemolyzed
SOPs for collections inadequate or not followed
Collection time not documented or extended
Wrong time frame for collection or processing
Inappropriate use of special procedures
Testing not performed in accordance with instructions
Unsuitable samples used for testing
Mislabeling of ABO and the like
Storage or shipping temperatures incorrect
Failure to quarantine unsuitable units
Special orders not filled–CMV negative, for example
EXAMPLES OF NONREPORTABLE BIOLOGIC PRODUCT DEVIATIONS
Transfusion errors occurring outside the blood facility
Error corrected before distribution, safety not affected
Look-back procedures, retrieval, notification not followed
Donor protective measures not met (age, colds, flu, etc.)
Failure to check previous donation records
Labeling errors not affecting safety (short expiration, etc.)
Shipping paperwork errors
Units returned due to temperature deviations

FDA, Food and Drug Administration; SOPs, Standard Operating procedures; CMV, cytomegalovirus.
From Reporting of product deviations by licensed manufacturers, unlicensed registered blood establishments, and transfusion services: final rule. *Federal Register* 2001 May 7:21 CFR 606.171, with permission.

should be documented in the records of the quality control unit. Monitoring corrective action outcomes to ensure effectiveness is an essential part of the system for addressing corrections. Figure 68.4 illustrates a process diagram of error management. Note its similarity to the diagram of the prevention model of quality control (Fig. 68.2).

Because error management systems are not defined in Title 21, it has sometimes been considered difficult to outline a system that is certain to meet regulatory requirements; however, some

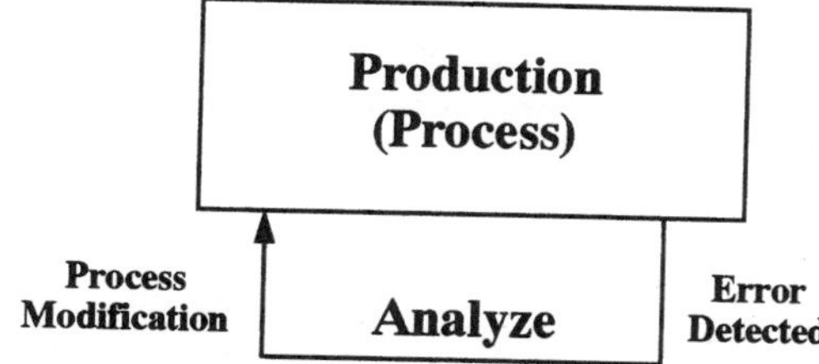

FIGURE 68.4. Error management process. Note similarity to the prevention model of quality control diagrammed in Figure 68.2.

attributes of good systems that have emerged both in blood centers and in industrial manufacturing concerns follow.

1. Employees at all levels in the organization are encouraged to report errors. Punitive policies to deal with lapses that result in errors will discourage reporting and hence opportunities for systems improvements may be lost.
2. Employees involved in the process in which an error was made should be involved with the resolution of the error and process change. The FDA also requires that staff be educated concerning the effect their errors have or potentially have on product quality; that is, it is required that they understand how their responsibilities have an impact on ensuring that only safe products are released.
3. Confirmation of the effectiveness of the corrective action is vital to ensure that the improved process continues to yield the expected results. Long-term evaluation should be undertaken at 6 or 12 months after a process improvement is completed.

Quality Control Unit and Internal Audits (§§600.10, 606.20, 211.22, 211.192, 211.180[e])

Meeting the quality system provisions of Title 21 facilitates compliance with cGMP. As noted, section 600.10 provides that an authorized official must be appointed to exercise control over all matters relating to compliance. Further, this designee must understand the scientific principles of manufacture. No similar provision is found in the 200 series. A licensed establishment must notify the FDA who has been designated as its authorized official(s) and must report any changes. Similarly, an unlicensed registered facility must identify a reporting official on FDA Form 2830 as part of its annual Blood Establishment Registration. The rationale for these provisions rests on the need for the agency to be able to deal with a responsible contact person in an establishment. Although the FDA permits the designation of alternative authorized officials, it takes no responsibility for the communication that must occur within a company; if a firm designates multiple authorized officials, the FDA may communicate with any one of them and the company must ensure that the information is disseminated appropriately. The authorized official can commit the establishment to certain courses of action, such as recalls, market withdrawals, and the like. Case law holds that upper management cannot avoid adverse consequences of noncompliance with regulatory requirements because a lower-ranking employee is designated the authorized official (40). Some experts believe that the chief executive officer should be the responsible head (authorized official) to indicate the commitment of senior management to the principles of cGMP (41). The Guideline for Quality Assurance in Blood Establishments states that, "A QC/QA Unit should report to management or its designee. In licensed firms, this unit should report to the Responsible Head who is the individual designated in the establishment license application to represent the firm in its regulatory activities with CBER [See 21 CFR 600.10(a) . . . ." (20). However, this is not wise unless regulatory compliance is a genuine part of the direct responsibilities and focus of this individual.

Section 211.22 states that an establishment must have a quality control unit (QC unit, quality program, or quality assurance [QA]) with several responsibilities designated in the code. Table 68.4 lists the responsibilities of the unit, including the authority to approve or reject all components and the approval of all written procedures used in the establishment. Although not required by the code, it is generally held that the QC unit should organizationally be distinct from manufacturing to ensure its independence, and this de facto requirement appears in FDA guidelines (20,42). In many blood centers the director of the QA unit reports to the chief executive officer. Such an organization table emphasizes to all blood center personnel the importance that senior management attaches to cGMP and quality in general.

Although internal audits are also not specifically required by the code, procedures to detect problems are required and internal audits are important to ensure that processes remain in control (see Production and Process Controls). Audits are included in the draft quality control guidelines and reference is made to section 211.180(e) which requires written procedures for evaluation of manufacturing records. Audits, whether performed by the facility staff, by customers, or by contracted third parties, can serve a more substantive role; they are active hunts for manufacturing problems. The key elements of an audit program are listed in Table 68.7. Integration of audits with error management offers an opportunity to augment continuous improvement efforts of blood centers proactively, the result of searching for errors and defects.

The quality control guidelines in effect since 1995 (and very similar to the 1991 and 1993 versions) suggest that audits focus on the adequacy of the critical control points outlined in the guidelines (20). One useful approach employs audits for the completeness of a cGMP element compliance throughout the center. For example, training and competency records could be reviewed in each unit throughout the center. In a second approach, a specific process can be audited and each skill box

TABLE 68.7. KEY ELEMENTS OF A BLOOD CENTER AUDIT PROGRAM

Written audit protocols
Audits of defined scope and purpose
Knowledgeable audit team members
Review of audit reports by authorized official
Referral of adverse finding for error management
Audit teams independent from production
Scheduled follow-up and reaudit

evaluated for compliance with all of the cGMP elements. Centers should develop audit procedures adaptable to their own operations.

Internal audits are considered confidential by the FDA and not available to blood center investigators unless fraud is suspected or there appears to be an imminent threat to public health. This policy is in place because if audit reports were reviewable by the FDA, audits might be discouraged. The FDA will also respect supplier audits as confidential internal audit information. However, it is critical that the center have readily available SOPs for audits, schedules demonstrating that all elements of operations are reviewed regularly (at least annually), processes for ensuring corrective and preventive action and follow-up, and formal closure notices to complete the records. It is also essential that any deviations discovered in the course of audits be properly documented in records that are available to FDA investigators.

Quality control units can be deployed to enhance the quality of blood center operations in a variety of ways. They can assume responsibility for personnel training, especially in cGMP, maintain calibration and validation records, design validation protocols, identify trends through statistical analysis, and the like. A well-directed QC unit can be of enormous value to both the authorized officials and the staff of the facilities in which it is established. It should be noted that QA staff are not the ideal staff to write SOPs, because they need to be the final approval authority and their objectivity cannot be ensured when reviewing their own work.

Facilities and Equipment (Multiple Sections of both the 600 and 200 series)

Most of the provisions in both series deal with sufficient space and flow design to prevent mix-ups and (in the case of interviewing blood donors, ensure privacy) and written procedures, schedules, and methods for maintenance and cleaning. To meet cGMP requirements, the contracts for cleaning, pest control, and maintenance must specify the materials to be used, the schedules and the procedures, and must show evidence of review and acceptance by the contracting facility. Such records must be reviewed by the firm periodically, and should meet cGMP documentation standards with dates and initials, no cross-outs, and the like. Signature logs should show dates of employment and training for the tasks performed, especially regarding avoidance of biohazards.

The segregation of unrelated activities and the preservation of clean and dirty pathways for both in-process materials and staff are basic cGMP principles. Section 606.40 emphasizes quarantine facilities, because it is critical to physically separate components unsuitable for release from those suitable for transfusion or further manufacture. Sterile supplies should be protected from inadvertent exposure to biohazard waste. Incoming goods must be physically separated from released-for-use inventory, and supplies with specific temperature requirements during storage (e.g., copper sulfate and plastic blood containers) must go promptly to monitored areas. All records must be protected against inadvertent loss or alteration, which translates to well-organized, locked storage or restricted-access areas. If off-site storage areas are used by licensed facilities, their licenses must include this supplement. The FDA has defined prompt retrieval of records to mean "availability within a few hours." Off-site storage of blood products by licensed facilities requires preapproval (license supplement) by the FDA and close oversight by the blood center to fulfill their responsibility to ensure that all FDA requirements will be met. Schedules of performance checks, as well as calibration, are provided in a table in section 606.60, but as with calibration requirements, much of the equipment used today is not specified in this table. Centers must develop their own schedules. In section 606.65 frequency of serologic reagent checks is specified.

Process and Production Controls (§§606.100, 606.140, 211.100, 211.101[c])

In a sense, all of the cGMP elements are embodied in production and process controls. The requirements for SOPs, calibration, and the like are outlined in these provisions as are a variety of quality control procedures. Significantly, the FDA explicitly accepts SOPs as provided by manuals of the American Association of Blood Banks and the American Red Cross (§606.100[d]). However, when these are referenced, it is important that the facility identify exactly which parts apply and determine that there is no conflict with manufacturer's directions or other FDA requirements. As previously emphasized, the determination that an establishment is in control is the most important attribute in the preservation of an establishment license.

CURRENT GOOD MANUFACTURING PRACTICES VIOLATIONS IN BLOOD ESTABLISHMENTS

In 1991, the FDA published common violations of cGMP in memorandum to establishments (19). The violations fell into four broad categories.

Donor Deferral

Deferral records were incomplete and multiple reasons for deferral were not recognized. Incomplete or inaccurate donor identification was noted as a recurring problem.

Viral Testing and Review of Testing Records

A variety of failures were outlined, including poor sample identification, failure to follow manufacturer's instructions, improperly qualified equipment, and samples tested numerous times without proper initial test invalidation (so-called, *testing to compliance*).

Computer Systems

Failure to validate computer systems and lack of documentation of computer training and validation of change procedures were cited frequently.

Standard Operating Procedures and Control of Operations

Standard operating procedures did not comply with FDA guidance and there was a lack of control of operations, especially in retesting of donor samples. Poor or absent change control procedures for SOPs were also frequently cited as deficiencies.

PROCESS CONTROL IMPERATIVE

Complying with cGMP and correcting deficiencies only begin to meet the public expectations for quality performance in manufacturing and distributing the nation's blood supply. Blood and plasma centers are developing quality improvement programs based on principles of continuous improvement, statistical process controls (SPC), and process innovation. The objective of these efforts is to reduce lot-to-lot variation in blood component manufacture and the risks of blood transfusion to as low as reasonably achievable, a concept that originated in the reduction of risks associated with exposure to ionizing radiation (43).

Continuous Improvement Initiatives

Continuous improvement initiatives are centered on error management by redesigning processes to prevent an error from recurring. They also embrace the prevention model of quality management that is rooted in SPC. As represented in Figure 68.2, this model monitors the various steps in manufacturing in an effort to determine which steps are and which are not in control. The many tools available to assist in these activities are too extensive and complex to be reviewed here. However, several of the more important ones relate directly to cGMP compliance. Statistical methods that are considered fundamental to SPC are frequency histograms (Pareto charts), Shewhart control charts (also called x, r charts), and process capability studies (44).

Histograms are useful in plotting the results of individual process outcomes and to prioritize corrective action. Figure 68.5 illustrates a histogram describing results of platelet concentrate manufacturing at one center. The Gaussian distribution of this histogram, provided it is similarly contoured and placed as on prior charts, suggests that the manufacturing processes are in control. A kurtotic or skewed distribution or a shift in the mean count to the right of left would suggest that processes may not be in control.

Shewhart or control charts are regarded as a singularly important tool of SPC to detect drift and variation in manufacturing processes (44). They permit identification of process weaknesses that result in lot-to-lot variation. When identified, process redesign can be undertaken to improve manufacturing and product quality.

Pareto charts offer another tool for blood center quality improvement (44). The frequency of cGMP problems discovered by audits or error management are charted on a histograph and give management the option of addressing first those problems that have both the most frequent occurrence and the highest likelihood of causing release of blood components unsuitable for transfusion. One of the difficulties of the current FDA inspection approach lies in its failure to differentiate a major from a very minor infraction. In a recent inspection documented on Form FDA-483, failure to perform specific gravity of a copper sulfate solution was cited as a cGMP violation of equal importance to performing faulty human immunodeficiency virus (HIV) donor screening (45). Unfortunately, neither the press

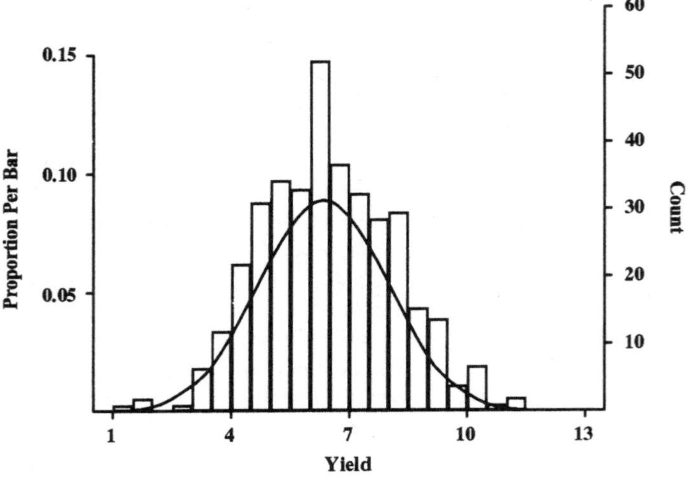

FIGURE 68.5. Platelet yield distribution. (From Zuck TF. Blood banking and transfusion medicine—past, present and future. *J Fla Med Assoc* 1993;80:20–24, with permission.)

and suppliers of electronic media nor the public understands the differences. In the United Kingdom, inspectional findings of blood centers are graded from critical (those that pose an imminent health hazard) to other (those of low probability of causing damage.) (Martin Bruce, personnel communication, 1994). This strategy permits both the inspected establishment and the public to assess the seriousness of the findings. Because the FDA has established grades of license change applications, perhaps a grading system based on the threat to public health posed by deficiencies could also be developed for those found in blood establishments. Such a grading system would help blood center staff to focus on those deficiencies most likely to affect the public health. Meanwhile, Pareto charting as a tool to determine priorities for error management within a blood center will partially compensate for current FDA blood center inspection and recall policies that do not grade the seriousness of deficiencies.

FUTURE INITIATIVES

Implementing cGMP represents only the initial effort to improve the safety of the blood supply by strengthening process controls in blood centers. Process innovation presents the next opportunity for centers to improve significantly the safety of the blood supply (46). To oversimplify, process innovation employs information technology (IT) to control manufacturing processes (47,48).

Initiated in industry to improve productivity, process innovation is being instituted in blood centers to improve quality and is defined in this chapter as the prevention of the release of units unsuitable for transfusion. Integrating computer control of manufacturing processes offers a significant advance to reduce further the risk of infectious disease transmission by blood transfusions. A few examples may illustrate the power of this strategy. Currently, blood center computer systems can be configured to prevent recruitment of deferred donors. Because deferred donors have been excluded from the rolls presented to telerecruitment departments, they can not be recruited. This principle can be extended. Figure 68.6 illustrates the capability of IT to control manufacturing processes. Personnel records can be linked with production records to prevent unsuitable employees from using their access codes to create batch records. Similarly, a centrifuge in need of calibration on a certain date could not be operated beyond that date to create a batch record for component manufacture. The power of linking IT with process controls lies in preventing the manufacture of components unsuitable for transfusion. Components not manufactured can not be released. Other examples of process innovation designed to increase the safety of the blood supply can be envisioned. More advanced systems will emerge as this technology is implemented in blood centers throughout the country. Definitive guidance on electronic signatures and electronic records has been issued (49).

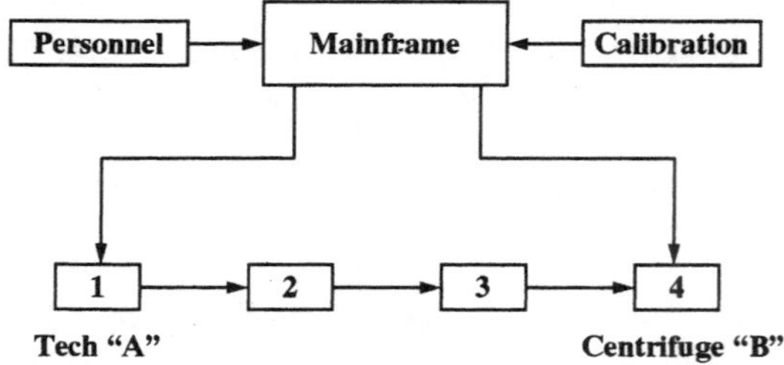

FIGURE 68.6. Theoretic process innovation in blood centers.

SUMMARY

In this chapter, the historic events that led to development of cGMP in the FDA regulation of the pharmaceutical industry and their recent more extensive application to blood establishments are reviewed. Many of the developments were driven by public health disasters or perceived disasters. The emergence of AIDS especially prompted increased regulatory rigor to be applied to blood centers. Vigorous application of cGMP principles to the production processes of blood and blood components has reduced, but not eliminated, risks associated with the transfusion of blood components. Fortunately, the availability of industrial models broadly applicable to blood centers has facilitated cGMP implementation.

Current Good Manufacturing Practices compliance now represents minimal performance standards for blood centers, and principles of continuous improvement and error rates as low as reasonably achievable have become the hallmarks of quality. Process innovation offers exciting mechanisms for extending the safety of an already exceedingly safe blood supply. Although in its infancy, IT will likely be featured prominently as a vital part of these innovations.

REFERENCES

1. Keeney RL. Decisions about life-threatening risks. *N Engl J Med* 1994; 311:193–196.
2. 21 CFR 606.171: Reporting of product deviations by licensed manufacturers, unlicensed registered blood establishments, and transfusion services: final rule. *Federal Register* 2001 May 7.
3. Klein HG. Transfusion medicine. The evolution of a new discipline. *JAMA* 1987;258:2108–2109.
4. Menitove JE. The recent emphasis on good manufacturing practices and the pharmaceutical approach damages blood banking and transfusion medicine as medical care activities. *Transfusion* 1993;33:439–442.
5. Polesky HF. *Should blood banks institute GMPs? Continuous flow.* Deerfield, IL: Baxter. 1993:10–11.
6. Laffel G, Blumenthal D. The case of using industrial quality management science in health care organizations. *JAMA* 1989;262: 2869–2873.
7. Timm EA. 75 years' compliance with biological regulations. *Food Drug Cosmet Law J* 1978;33:225–230.
8. Solomon JM. The evolution of the current blood banking regulatory climate. *Transfusion* 1994;34:272–277.
9. 69 FR 56441-56454: Biological products regulated under section 351 of the Public Health Service Act. Implementation of biologics license. Elimination of establishment license and product license: final rule. *Federal Register* 1999 Oct 20.
10. FDA/CBER guidance. Providing regulatory submissions to the Center for Biologics Evaluation and Research (CEBR) [on CD-ROM]. Biological Marketing Applications, November 1999.
11. CBER issues final rule implementing single biologics application. *ABC Newsletter* 1999 Oct 29:42:3–4.
12. Travis L. Quality consideration in electronic regulatory submissions. *Reg Affairs Focus* 2000 Sept:10–14.
13. Motise P. Part 11: electronic records, electronic signatures: answers to frequently asked questions. Available at: www.fda.gov.1999.
14. FDA guidance. Guidance for industry, providing regulatory submissions [on CD-ROM]. January 1999.
15. FDA Form 356(h). Instructions for completing biologic applications. Current edition, US Government Printing Office.
16. FDA/CBER guidance. Changes to an approved application. Biologic products: human blood and blood components intended for transfusion or for further manufacture. January 2000.
17. Sinclair U. *The Jungle.* Cambridge, MA: Robert Bently, 1905.
18. Letter of agreement between FDA and ARC, 1998.
19. FDA/CBER memorandum. Memorandum to all registered blood establishments; 1991 Mar 20.
20. FDA/CBER guideline. Guideline for quality assurance in blood establishments, 1995.
21. Smith G. *Statistical process control and quality improvement.* New York: Maswell MacMillan International Publishing Group, 1991.
22. Berwick DM. Continuous improvement as an ideal in health care. *N Eng J Med* 1989;320:53–55.
23. Deming WE. *Out of crisis.* Cambridge, MA: Massachusetts Institute of Technology Center for Advanced Engineering Study, 1986.
24. FDA/CBER guideline. Draft guidelines for the validation of blood establishment computer systems. *Federal Register* 1994 Sept 20: Docket No. 93 n-0394.
25. FDA/CBER memorandum. Requirements for computerization of blood establishments; 1989 Sept 8.
26. FDA/CBER memorandum. Recommendations for computerization of blood establishments; 1988 Apr 6.
27. Clark AS. Computer systems validation: an investigator's view. *Pharm Technol* 1988;Jan:61–66.
28. FDA/CDER guidance. Guide to inspection of computer systems in drug processing. Washington DC: US Government Printing Office; 1983 Feb.
29. Motise PJ. Validation of computerized systems in the control of drug processes: an FDA perspective. *Pharm Technol* 1984;8:40–45.
30. FDA. General principles of software validation; 1987 Jan 6.
31. Code of Federal Regulations, Title 21, Part 11 (21 CFR 11): Electronic records and signatures. Washington, DC: US Government Printing Office; 2000.
32. FDA/CBER guidance. Reviewer guidance for a premarket notification for blood establishment computer software; 1997 Jan 13.
33. FDA/CBER guidance. Letter to all licensed blood establishments: guidance for blood establishments concerning conversions to FDA-reviewed software products; 1995 Nov 13.
34. FDA/CBER memorandum, February 10, 1995. Letter to blood establishment computer software manufacturers; final published 1997 Jan 13.
35. GMP design controls review: special supplement to medical device approval letter. Washington Information Source Co; 1997 Apr.
36. FDA/CBER memorandum. Changes in equipment for processing blood donor samples; 1992 July 21.
37. FDA memorandum. Glossary of computerized system and software development technology; 1995 Aug.
38. Suggested revision of the computer validation guidelines submitted jointly by AABB, ARC, CCBC, 1994.
39. FDA/CBER memorandum. Responsibilities of blood establishments related to errors and accidents in the manufacture of blood and blood components; 1997 Mar 20.
40. *United States v. Park* 421 US 658 (1995).
41. Heaton A. Presentation to the Institute of Medicine Blood Forum; July 1994, Washington, DC.
42. FDA/CDER Draft. Internationally harmonized guide for active pharmaceutical ingredients; 1997 Sept 1.
43. Showby FD. Radiation and other risks. *Health Phys* 1965;11:879–887.
44. Pitt H. *SPC for the rest of us.* Reading, MA: Addison Wesley, 1993.
45. FDA. 483 inspectional findings, Toronto Center; 1994.
46. Davenport TH. *Process innovation.* Boston: Harvard Business School Press, 1993.
47. Zuck, TF. The good manufacturing concept. In: Sibinga CTS, Das PC, Heininger HJ, eds. *Good manufacturing practice in transfusion medicine.* Dordrecht, The Netherlands: Kluwer Academic Publishers, 1996.
48. Zuck TF. Blood banking and transfusion medicine—past, present and future. *J Fla Med Assoc* 1993;80:20–24.
49. FDA/CBER Draft. Guidance for Industry-21 CFR Part II, electronic records, electronic signatures glossary of terms August 29, 2001.

69

HOSPITAL TRANSFUSION SERVICES AND QUALITY ASSURANCE

PAUL D. MINTZ

A transfusion service is a complex enterprise characterized by high-volume, labor-intensive procedures performed under severe time pressure. Every aspect of its operation is scrutinized by an array of regulators, assessors, and inspectors. Staff and leadership performance are continually evaluated by clinicians, risk-managers, and administrators, and, not rarely, by attorneys, reporters, and patients. These constituencies are variably well informed but work under intense pressure as well. The many successes of the service are taken for granted, but one mistake can directly kill a person. A transfusion service never closes. The staff scrupulously follows detailed, frequently revised policies and procedures. They all must be trained and able to adapt these procedures to each unique situation and occasionally override them to respond to life-threatening crises. The director of a transfusion service must possess a broad range of clinical, technical, scientific, and administrative knowledge and judgment. The technologist requires a high level of intelligence, technical dexterity, and commitment to perform under intense pressures. Everyone who works in a transfusion service must be able to use a healthy dose of common sense. All of these activities occur in an environment of constant change. Technical and clinical innovations require immediate adaptation, and regulatory and accreditation requirements are revised frequently. There is a barrage of interruptions, yet everything must transpire in an environment of complete civility.

Transfusion service leaders are frequently asked to play a decisive role in difficult ethical decisions (e.g., autologous blood for patients who have positive serologic results for human immunodeficiency virus [HIV]), devise and implement rapidly large-scale initiatives (e.g., patient look-back programs for infectious diseases), and work successfully with vendors who are experiencing comparable pressure. The staff typically reports to administrators who do not have professional health care training and who exert relentless pressure for cost-containment and expense justification. The transfusion service environment poses challenges.

OVERVIEW

Blood bank, coined by Fantus (1), was the term originally applied to that area of a hospital in which blood was stored in containers for transfusion to patients. The dynamic role of the medical director and staff of this area in contemporary clinical practice make the term *transfusion service* more appropriate. This term better captures the responsibilities of ensuring safe transfusion practice and appropriate blood use. The transfusion service, in many instances, functions more as a trust fund than a bank. The U.S. Food and Drug Administration (FDA) and the American Association of Blood Banks (AABB) have their own nomenclature for the terms *blood bank* and *transfusion service* as described later. The generic term *transfusion service* is used throughout this

P.D. Mintz: Departments of Pathology and Internal Medicine and Clinical Laboratories and Blood Bank, University of Virginia Health System, Blood Bank and Transfusion Services, Charlottesville, Virginia.

chapter to describe all hospital facilities that engage in storing blood components and providing them for transfusion.

The *Standards for Blood Banks and Transfusion Services* of the AABB delineates the necessary elements for the organization of a transfusion service (2). The service must have a medical director with responsibility and authority for all medical and technical policies, processes, and procedures as well as for consultative services related to the care and safety of transfusion recipients. The medical director need not be responsible for the functions of the executive management of the service. These functions include overall responsibility and authority for the operations, quality system, compliance with standards and regulations, and review of the quality system. The FDA requires that a "blood establishment" be under the direction of a designated, qualified person who exercises control in all matters relating to compliance. The structure of each service may vary.

Many transfusion services now have a chief supervisor, who reports to a laboratory manager, who reports to the executive management of the hospital. In this arrangement, the medical director is not in a direct reporting relationship to those responsible for laboratory administration. This often excludes the medical director from authority in personnel, purchasing, budgeting, and other administrative matters. However, the Clinical Laboratory Improvement Act (CLIA) of 1988 mandates that the director of a laboratory have responsibility for its functions. The regulation states that the laboratory director must be a doctor of medicine or doctor of osteopathy (42 CFR 493.1443). This creates a situation in which the medical director has statutory responsibility without administrative authority. This dilemma must be solved with pragmatic cooperation between the administrators and the medical director.

The role of the transfusion service laboratory in performing pretransfusion compatibility testing has evolved dramatically from a matrix of elaborate protocols, including major and minor crossmatches and antibody detection tests performed at both room temperature and 37°C, to the present practice in many laboratories of performing a computer crossmatch when certain conditions are met for patients in whom no red blood cell alloantibody has been detected in current or previous testing (see Chapter 7) (3,4). At the same time, development of preoperative crossmatch guidelines and the introduction of performing only an ABO/Rh type and antibody detection test for patients unlikely to need transfusion in the perioperative period have been implemented to conserve transfusion service inventories (5–8).

The regulations established with the CLIA stipulate requirements for the qualifications of staff who perform or supervise the highly complex testing conducted within a transfusion service. The standards of the AABB and FDA Current Good Manufacturing Practices (CGMP) also require that the transfusion service have a process for personnel training and competency evaluation.

Written standard operating procedures are required by the FDA (21 CFR 606.160) and AABB standards (standard 6.1). A system must be in place to ensure process control for validation of processes and procedures, introduction and change of processes and procedures, proficiency testing, quality control, and the use of materials and other aspects of performance of procedures. This is required by the AABB standards and FDA CGMP. A defined system of documentation and record retention is also required by both (21 CFR 606.100, 606.140, and 606.160). Further aspects of AABB, FDA, and other accrediting requirements are as follows.

ROLE OF THE MEDICAL DIRECTOR

The medical director of the transfusion service should seize the opportunity to work with the clinical staff and hospital administration regarding all aspects of blood transfusion. The director should strive to be recognized and sought as the specialist in transfusion medicine within the institution. There are many ways to establish this role, but they typically require that the director develop and implement initiatives in a variety of areas. The medical director should develop a culture within the institution so that her or his advice is routinely sought. The role of the transfusion medicine specialist is to maintain a "central position in the flow of blood components and products" within the institution (9).

The heightened awareness of patients and physicians regarding the risks of blood transfusion therapy has made the role of the transfusion service director a more public one. This prominence has created receptiveness on the part of attending physicians to advice and education. With extensive knowledge of blood transfusion, the director should play an important role in the hemotherapeutic treatment of patients.

The transfusion service director serves as the principal educator of clinicians and house staff in blood transfusion practice. The director must be aware of the contemporary literature on the use of blood components, including consensus conference statements, practice guidelines, and emerging standards of practice. The director can educate the clinical staff on the availability of newly introduced blood components and pharmaceuticals (e.g., pathogen-inactivated blood components, fibrin sealant), and serve as an aggressive patient advocate for the introduction of these products for improved patient care (10). Interactions between the transfusion service director and the attending physician should be designed as educational and nonconfrontational and should be performed in the spirit of mutual patient advocacy.

The director should create a variety of opportunities for interaction with the clinical staff and should market his or her availability for consultation. In response to certain transfusion orders, the transfusion service director should contact the ordering physician. These informal queries serve the dual purpose of shaping improved patient care while informing physicians of the expertise available from the transfusion service. Each facility should develop its own list of situations in which a telephone call is initiated according to the scope of services of the facility. These can include requests for more than one platelet transfusion, more than 6 units of fresh-frozen plasma (FFP) per day for the same patient, a granulocyte concentrate, fresh blood, or a customized blood product (e.g., a cytomegalovirus-reduced-risk or irradiated product). If inventory issues dictate exceptions to practices (e.g., an Rh-negative patient will receive Rh-positive red blood cells), the medical director should call the patient's physician to explain the situation and suggest appropriate patient follow-up care.

Directors of transfusion services also should speak to a patient's physician when transfusion will be delayed owing to the presence of red blood cell alloantibodies or for any other reason. The director should review the laboratory and clinical data to assist in ordering of diagnostic tests and in blood transfusion management, particularly for patients who have received a large number of red blood cells without other components.

The review of laboratory information for patients receiving blood products provides the director with other opportunities to offer assistance. For example, the director may note refractoriness to platelet transfusions and offer prompt advice for diagnosis and management. Drug-induced platelet antibodies are not always detected by clinicians. A review by the transfusion service director of patients who do not respond to platelet transfusions is likely to uncover such occurrences. Each engagement between a transfusion service director and a clinician provides opportunities not only for improving an individual patient's care but also for forging relationships that will lead to future consultation.

Advice can be provided as the result of established testing algorithms within an institution. Approved by the medical staff, such reflexive systems can meet compliance requirements and lead to interpretive, billable reports that provide for efficient clinical care. Bleeding and thrombotic disorders are complex clinical situations that can be clarified more efficiently through directed laboratory testing algorithms. Red blood cell alloantibody identifications also lend themselves to interpretations by the transfusion service director regarding the likelihood of delays in blood availability and the potential clinical significance.

Requested consultations typically concern massive transfusion, therapeutic apheresis, refractoriness to platelet transfusion, unexpected perioperative bleeding, and invasive procedures possibly necessitating preprocedure platelet or plasma transfusion.

The director is responsible for evaluating all reported adverse events resulting from blood transfusions and making recommendations regarding future hemotherapy. The institution must have a procedure for assuring that adverse events are reported promptly to a physician caring for the patient and to the transfusion service. The FDA, AABB, and College of American Pathologists (CAP) all have regulations and standards regarding the evaluation and reporting of adverse effects of blood transfusion. The FDA requires that records be maintained of any reports of adverse reactions due to blood transfusion and that a thorough investigation of each reported reaction be conducted. All transfusion services must report deaths confirmed caused by a transfusion to the Office of Compliance, Center for Biologics Evaluation and Research, by telephone (301-827-6220) as soon as possible and by writing within 7 days, in accord with 21 CFR 606.170.

The AABB requires that a transfusion service have a process for the detection, reporting, and evaluation of suspected complications of transfusion (standard 7.3) and that all suspected transfusion complications are evaluated promptly and reviewed by the director (standard 7.3.2). The CAP requires that all transfusion reactions other than urticaria or circulatory overload be reported immediately to the laboratory (TRM.41750) and that documented procedures exist for actions to be taken in the event of a transfusion reaction (TRM.41700). In addition, the medical director must be involved in resolving a system failure in blood administration (TRM.41770). An interpretation by the director of all transfusion reaction investigations must be recorded in the patient's chart (TRM.42050).

A system must exist to inform patients of red blood cell alloantibodies. When communicated to physicians in the future, a delayed hemolytic transfusion reaction is avoided.

Cooperative efforts among physicians from different disciplines is important to improve the use and ongoing evaluation of blood products (11,12). For example, to ensure the appropriate use of FFP, the cooperative effort of hematologists knowledgeable in coagulation, treating physicians, and the transfusion service director often is useful. Similarly, the director may consult with hematologists to establish a threshold for prophylactic platelet transfusions that may be lower than current practice. Patients would be exposed to fewer blood products, resulting in institutional cost savings, conservation of the blood supply, and improved patient care.

The director should participate in the formulation of institutional policies to assure an adequate supply of blood to meet patient needs, review of procedures for blood administration, development and implementation of procedures for perioperative blood conservation and reinfusion, and consideration of alternatives to blood component transfusion (e.g., hematopoietic growth factors, blood substitutes when licensed). This provides leadership in shaping and standardizing transfusion practices in the institution.

The director must assure that appropriate processes for blood administration minimize the possibility of human error contributing to an adverse outcome. The standards of the AABB include accountability of the director for the care and safety of transfusion recipients (standard 1.1.1). A system of correct identification of patients is critical. Because most transfusions are performed by nurses, the transfusion service should work with the nursing services to assure that their procedures are appropriate and clear and to assure that appropriate education of the nursing staff occurs. Most hospitals require that two persons verify all of the appropriate information at the bedside before transfusion. The transfusion service director should take an active role in reviewing and assuring appropriate use of devices associated with transfusion, including filters and blood warmers. Policies regarding the addition of other fluids to blood components also should be reviewed by the director.

The director must participate actively in the quality assurance program related to blood transfusion. As described later, the director represents the transfusion service on the hospital transfusion committee.

The director can bring his or her clinical knowledge to bear on decisions regarding the extent of pretransfusion compatibility testing, the investigation of alloantibodies, the length of time specimens are held for subsequent testing, and the selection of components for inventory (e.g., type of fibrin sealant, timing of leukoreduction, type of platelet component, inventory of pathogen-inactivated components).

The foregoing activities provide for improved care, reduced costs, shorter hospital stays, and increased professional billing. The quiet accomplishment of a laboratory director in obtaining an adequate blood supply and making this available for transfusion are not services that typically serve as evidence of the director's contribution to patient care. Although the director may be held responsible for the failure to achieve these objectives, there may be a presumption that little effort or training was required to accomplish them. The transfusion service director, therefore, must strive not only to add value to medical care but also to be seen as adding value to medical care, ensuring his or her advice will be routinely sought and used (11).

QUALITY: AN OVERVIEW

Systems must be developed to prevent error and to anticipate and compensate for errors that will inevitably occur. Such a concept is also in the business interest of the institution. Systematic analyses of preventable complications in health care have typically shown that faulty systems are responsible for error more often than are individuals (13).

Quality may be defined as performance that meets or exceeds established expectations. Either outcomes or processes may be assessed to measure quality. A key component of improving quality is reducing variability in the outcome. For example, the instances of unacceptable turnaround time for release of a blood product can be reduced simply by reducing the variability, even if the mean time is not changed. When variance is reduced and consistency improved, control of a process is demonstrated, and benefits for interrelated systems are generated. For example, if there is minimal variability in turnaround times for release of blood products, transportation services and clinical services can coordinate their activities with this expectation. In addition to reducing variability, shifting the mean of a variable (e.g., reducing the time for product release) can also improve quality.

A data-driven approach to quality brings rigor to identifying defects, correcting them, and controlling processes to sustain improvement. The six sigma model of quality, in which organizations strive for error rates several standard deviations from the mean, is based on this model (14). Outcome data in transfusion medicine are typically related to the prevention of adverse events from various forms of cytopenia or factor deficiencies or to decreasing adverse effects of transfusion itself (15). Transfusions generally are supportive rather than primary therapy. Thus large-scale outcome analysis for blood transfusion is a formidable task. The primary goal of a quality assurance program for a transfusion service is to assure available and effective blood transfusion that is as safe as possible.

Quality assurance programs derived from industrial practices have been increasingly applied to clinical medicine (16,17). In these programs, the staff of an institution strives to create cycles of continuous improvement in the course of designing, measuring, assessing, and refining work processes. These improvement cycles are applicable to all levels of an organization (18) and have led to measurable improvements in health care (16).

A quality system (19,20) is a quality assurance program implemented to ensure that all parts of the processes of an enterprise work together to produce the expected output. In general, a quality system strives to identify process errors and defects and to eliminate them with sustainable changes through redesign of processes. Quality assurance is the totality of activities planned and performed to provide confidence that all procedures are functioning as expected. A quality assurance program must be designed and implemented to ensure that procedures are consistently performed. Elements of a quality assurance program include quality control procedures and standards for personnel, facilities, procedures, equipment, and record keeping. Audits are an integral component of a quality assurance program. As a matter of good practice, those responsible for quality assurance should report to senior management and not to operations personnel.

A data-driven problem-solving approach to quality assurance includes defining, measuring, analyzing, improving, and controlling processes. A quality program is a "spectrum of activities and processes that shape the characteristics of a product or service" (20). Any quality program must include a commitment from management to build quality into the system rather than just through inspection of a final product or service. There should be a spirit of cooperation between quality assurance and operations personnel. The goal is continuing improvement that will translate into improved patient care, regulatory and accreditation compliance, and good business practices.

Quality assurance efforts should focus on the aspects of the operation in which errors are known to be particularly troublesome or costly (21). The measurable outcome of the process monitored has to be defined at the outset. Knowing that certain specifications were met at a single time (quality control) suggests a likelihood that they will be met at other times, but it does not replace control of the processes. Process control is the collective set of actions taken to minimize variability in a process. Quality assurance of blood transfusion services involves each aspect of the process, from obtaining the blood supply and the patient specimen through monitoring of the patient once the transfusion is completed. Error management should be conducted by means of finding and solving system problems rather than placing blame and punishing individual workers for making a mistake. Such punitive management of error discourages reporting and decreases the potential for improvement.

Quality assurance plans must be manageable and clearly understood by the staff as well as by individual workers charged with compliance. A reasonable approach to documentation should be maintained. No purpose is served by collection of data without analysis and interpretation and without using the interpretation to improve a process. Once a process has been shown to result in minimal variation and to meet expectations, it is reasonable to consider whether requirements may then be raised. In this way, an effective quality assurance program can directly lead to increased operational efficiency.

Some believe that enthusiasm for the extension of industrial management theory into clinical laboratories should be tempered by the absence of cost benefit analysis (22). Clearly stating a program's expectations and measuring outcome can achieve the required cost benefit.

The development of a quality system in transfusion services allows certification by the International Organization for Standardization (ISO) 9000 quality management system that has been used by many businesses since 1986 (23). The ISO 9000 standards provide guidance in the development and implementation of an effective quality management system. It is not specific to any particular product or service but can be used generically by all enterprises. Complying with ISO 9000 standards does not mean that every product or service meets specific requirements. It means only that the quality system in use is capable of meeting them. The ISO standards basically require that an enterprise document its processes and then follow them as stated.

For any hospital quality assessment program to work successfully, physicians must give priority to the process, and hospital administration must make the necessary resources available to ensure its development, implementation, refinement, and ongoing support. Criteria used for evaluating clinical care should ideally be established from a scientific database. However, this information is not always available, and it may be necessary to use a consensus opinion (24). Implicit criteria are used when a designated expert reviews a particular case and judges the quality of care. Explicit criteria are specified in advance, before the assessment of individual cases is undertaken. Reviews based on implicit criteria can be individualized but are costly and inherently imprecise (25,26). Explicit criteria can be used to make reproducible assessments at a relatively low cost. They are, however, not responsive to the subtle variations in individual patients that can prompt different standards of therapeutic intervention. Implicit and explicit criteria frequently are combined in a particular quality assessment program of clinical practices. Explicit criteria often are used to separate cases that should not require further review (because they most likely have already met accepted standards of practice) from those that need to be reviewed individually (according to implicit criteria or a combination of implicit and explicit criteria). As institutions measure and assess various processes, criteria have to be modified as new clinical information becomes available and a different level of performance is required.

HISTORICAL PERSPECTIVE

Quality assessment of blood transfusion practice is not new. The first human transfusion was performed by Jean Denis in 1667 in Paris. Denis transfused animal blood into human beings and incurred the enmity of his colleagues, who preferred bloodletting as the therapy for most maladies. Eventually a decree was issued proscribing the performance of blood transfusion unless sanctioned by the Faculty of Medicine of Paris (27). This early prospective and retrospective auditing of blood transfusion certainly presented a more onerous burden of review and consequences than exists today.

Concern about abuse of blood has been noted as far back as 1936 (27). In 1951, the Ministry of Health in England called for the review of blood use at medical staff meetings. In the same year, an editorial in the *New England Journal of Medicine* noted the inappropriateness of some transfusions (28). A 1953 audit study concluded that only 241 of 290 transfusions were indicated (29). Additional publications between 1956 and 1960 (30–35) echoed this message, emphasized the physician's potential liability if an unnecessary transfusion were administered, and suggested the usefulness of audits. In 1961, the Joint Commission on the Accreditation of Hospitals and other experts emphasized the need to review transfusion practices (36,37).

By 1962, indications for blood transfusion were being included in the bylaws of hospitals (38). In the same year, the Joint Blood Council called for a review of transfusion practices by a medical staff committee (39). Several authorities recommended the establishment of a hospital transfusion board to review transfusion practices and called attention to the educational function such a committee would serve (40–43). A 1965 study showed that a large number of transfusions were inappropriate and could not be justified by the ordering physicians (44). In 1974, 14 of 46 Minnesota hospitals responding to a survey had procedures for reviewing indications for blood transfusion; among them, 25 had some form of transfusion committee (45).

REGULATORY AND ACCREDITATION REQUIREMENTS

A number of regulatory and accrediting agencies in the United States have developed standards regarding the quality assessment and improvement of blood transfusion practices. Since 1961, review of blood use has been an element of the accreditation process of the Joint Commission on Accreditation of Healthcare Organizations (JCAHO) (36). Between 1985 and 1991, the JCAHO required evaluation of all transfusions. After repeated blood utilization review consistently documented appropriate blood use, sampling became acceptable. Although a minority of hospitals complied with this extreme requirement, this standard was nevertheless the driving force behind blood utilization review in the United States. Since 1991, the JCAHO has made a series of modifications to this standard.

Food and Drug Administration

The FDA considers establishments that perform certain activities that it defines as manufacturing steps to be hospital blood banks, which are required to register annually using form FDA2830. A hospital blood bank is an entity that routinely collects or processes whole blood or blood components. These components may be collected by means of apheresis or prepared from whole blood. Processing includes freezing, deglycerolyzing, washing, irradiating, rejuvenating, or leukoreducing red blood cells. Hospital laboratories that solely prepare red blood cells or recovered plasma, pool platelets or cryoprecipitated AHF, or that issue bedside leukoreduction filters are considered hospital transfusion services, which are not required to register (21 CFR 607.65[f]).

Because blood and blood components are drugs under the Federal Food, Drug, and Cosmetic Act, the FDA CGMP regulations in 21 CFR 210 and 211, apply to the manufacture of these products. In addition, CGMP regulations for blood and blood components exist in 21 CFR 606. All of these regulations apply to FDA-defined hospital blood banks. The purpose of FDA registration is to allow the FDA to plan and perform routine CGMP inspections.

The Code of Federal Regulations requires a quality program. In 42 CFR 493.1701, it is mandated that "each laboratory establish and follow written policies and procedures for a comprehensive quality assurance program. . . . The laboratory's quality assurance program must evaluate the effectiveness of its policies and procedures; identify and correct problems . . . . All quality assurance activities must be documented." In 1995, the Center for Biologics Evaluation and Research produced a guideline to assist establishments in conducting quality programs in accord with applicable regulations. This guideline is available on the World Wide Web at http://www.fda.gov/cber/gdlns/gdeqa.txt.

Although the FDA does not routinely inspect hospital transfusion services, these services also engage in manufacturing in the view of the FDA, because compatibility testing, blood storage, labeling, and record keeping are considered steps in the manufacturing process. As such, transfusion services are also subject to CGMP regulations. Inspection of hospital transfusion services is overseen by the Centers for Medicare and Medicaid Services (formerly known as the Health Care Financing Administration) through a 1980 memorandum of understanding with the FDA that addresses inspection of these establishments. In an effort to reduce duplication of inspections, it was agreed that inspection of hospital transfusion services that are approved for Medicare reimbursement and that engage in compatibility testing but that neither routinely collect nor process blood components would be subject to inspection by the Centers for Medicare and Medicaid Services. This agreement pertains to responsibility for inspection only. No statutory authority transferred between the agencies. As part of the agreement, the Centers for Medicare and Medicaid Services adopted FDA regulations in 21 CFR 606 titled "Current Good Manufacturing Practice for Blood and Blood Components" and 21 CFR 640 titled "Additional Standards for Human Blood and Blood Components." These are the FDA requirements that have been incorporated into the CLIA regulations. Although the Centers for Medicare and Medicaid Services has financial authority, it does not have the direct regulatory authority of the FDA. Observations made by the Centers for Medicare and Medicaid Services may be communicated to the FDA, which can then directly inspect a hospital transfusion service.

All transfusion services, registered or unregistered and regardless of FDA nomenclature, must also comply with the regulations in 42 CFR 493 in accord with the Clinical Laboratory Improvement Amendments of 1988. For the purposes of CLIA certification, the Centers for Medicare and Medicaid Services retains responsibility for inspection of all transfusion services.

Many transfusion services may not be surveyed directly by the Centers for Medicare and Medicaid Services. Some are in an exempt state or have been accredited by an organization that has been granted deemed status by the Centers for Medicare and Medicaid Services (e.g., the CAP, the AABB, and the JCAHO). Inspections by an organization with deemed status satisfy certification requirements for the CLIA program (Table 69.1).

American Association of Blood Banks

The AABB has issued standards for blood banks and transfusion services accompanying an inspection and accreditation program since 1958. In 1990, the AABB recognized the need to develop a system of quality management applicable to the transfusion service environment. The purpose was to alter the approach to quality assessment and improvement from error detection to error prevention. This program has evolved since then to be consistent with FDA quality assurance guidelines and ISO 9000 standards. The AABB has formulated a list of quality system essentials (QSE) (Table 69.2). The intent of these essentials is to provide assurance that quality principles are applied consistently throughout the entire enterprise, not just within specific operational areas. Use of the QSE affords any transfusion service a guideline for organizing its activities and documentation. The use of audits for processes and systems provides an opportunity for considering each aspect of an activity and for influencing the quality of activities outside the immediate control of the transfusion service. Implementation of a quality management system provides for the routine capture of errors and accidents, some of which now are required to be reported to the FDA, as discussed later. The activities of a quality system involve data collection and analysis to select processes for internal audits. These internal audits provide information necessary to make process improvements to prevent errors.

Although not required by the AABB or others, a quality manual provides a convenient means of assuring that a transfusion service is meeting all the requirements of the QSE. One such manual has been published (46). This manual includes a matrix that links AABB QSE to source documents within the institution that demonstrate compliance. Existing procedure manuals can still be used.

The AABB assessment incorporates evaluation of the quality system at an institution and of each operational system. The quality system assessment is based on the same criteria for every facility. The operational systems, however, are identified by the activities performed within an individual facility. An example of implementation of the QSE has been published (46). The AABB standards (2) use the quality management system as a framework. Each of the ten chapters represents one of the AABB QSE.

The AABB inspection program has deemed status under the regulations of CLIA to perform on-site inspections of transfusion services to meet Center for Medicare and Medicaid Services requirements. This status means that the Center for Medicare and Medicaid Services has determined that the AABB accreditation process provides assurance that facilities meet or exceed conditions required by federal law and regulations. As such, a

TABLE 69.1. TRANSFUSION SERVICES SUBJECT TO INSPECTIONS BY OTHER AGENCIES

	Accreditation		
Inspecting Agency	AABB	CAP	JCAHO without AABB, CAP
AABB[a]	(Yes)	Yes	—
CAP[a]	Yes	(Yes)	—
JCAHO[a]	No	No	(Yes)
CMS	No	No	No

[a]Voluntary.
AABB, American Association of Blood Banks; CAP, College of American Pathologists; JCAHO, Joint Commission on the Accreditation of Healthcare Organizations CMS, Center for Medicine and Medicaid Services.

TABLE 69.2. QUALITY SYSTEM ESSENTIALS OF THE STANDARDS OF THE AMERICAN ASSOCIATION OF BLOOD BANKS

Organization
A structure that clearly defines and documents those responsible for the provision of blood components and services and the relationship of individuals responsible for key quality functions.
Resources
Policies, processes, and procedures to ensure the provision of adequate resources to perform, verify, and manage each of the activities of the transfusion service.
Equipment
Policies, processes, and procedures to ensure that calibration, maintenance, and monitoring of equipment conform to standards and applicable requirements.
Supplier and customer issues
Policies, processes, and procedures to evaluate the ability of providers to meet requirements consistently.
Process control
Policies and validated processes and procedures to ensure the quality of the blood components, tissue, and services provided and that procedures are conducted under controlled conditions.
Documents and records
Policies, processes, and procedures to ensure that documents are identified, reviewed, approved, and retained and that records are created, stored, and archived in accord with retention policies.
Incidents, errors, accidents; nonconformances; and complications
Policies, processes, and procedures to ensure the capture, assessment, investigation, and monitoring of deviations from, or of failures to meet, specified requirements. Definition of responsibility for review and authority for the disposition of nonconforming products and for appropriate reporting of deviations and failures.
Assessments: internal and external
Policies, processes, and procedures to ensure that external assessments are obtained at defined intervals and that internal assessments are conducted.
Process improvement through corrective and preventive action
Policies, processes, and procedures for data collection, analysis, and follow-up of issues that require corrective or preventive action.
Facilities and safety
Policies, processes, and procedures to the provision of a safe and adequate workplace.

laboratory accredited by the AABB does not need to be inspected routinely by the Center for Medicare and Medicaid Services. However, these facilities are subject to validation surveys and surveys performed in response to complaints by the Center for Medicare and Medicaid Services or state agencies on behalf of the Center for Medicare and Medicaid Services. The JCAHO also recognizes AABB accreditation status. Institutions that are AABB-accredited do not need to undergo transfusion service inspection by the JCAHO (Table 69.1).

Joint Commission on Accreditation of Healthcare Organizations

The JCAHO views transfusion services from a dual perspective. Standards are devoted both to the entire process of blood transfusion from blood ordering through infusion and to the laboratory procedures and practices. Two accreditation manuals have standards regarding blood transfusion. The *Comprehensive Accreditation Manual for Hospitals* (18) provides specific standards for hospitals that transfuse and monitor blood components. The *Comprehensive Accreditation Manual for Pathology and Clinical Laboratory Services* (47) contains technical standards that are patterned after the requirements of the Clinical Laboratory Improvement Amendments of 1988 and the standards of the AABB. This dual approach provides the JCAHO with the opportunity to assess the entire spectrum of clinical and laboratory blood transfusion practices. The JCAHO has deemed status with the Centers for Medicare and Medicaid Services (CMS) (Table 69.1).

Standards related to blood transfusion are included in the accreditation manual sections addressing the medical staff, care of patients, management of information, improvement of organization performance, environment of care, and sentinel event review. Among the salient standards, MS.8.1.3 states that the medical staff must have a leadership role in performance of activities related to blood transfusion. In addition, hemolytic transfusion reactions involving the administration of blood having major blood group incompatibilities are identified as reviewable sentinel events subject to specific review by the JCAHO. In the *Comprehensive Accreditation Manual* section of care of patients, standard TX.5 states that the medical staff must define the scope of assessment for procedures. Standard TX.5.1 states that "determining the appropriateness of a procedure for each patient is based, in part, on a review of the need to administer blood or blood components." Also in the section on care of patients, standard TX.5.2.2 mandates a process of informed consent for transfusion. In the section on management of information, the JCAHO stipulates that there must be adequate documentation of blood transfusion reactions. In the section on performance improvement, the commission mandates that confirmed transfusion reactions always elicit intense analysis (standard PI.4.3). This is reiterated in the *Laboratory Services Manual.* In this manual, standard LD.1.2 states that clinical laboratory services are regularly and conveniently available to meet the needs of individuals served. The JACHO cites, as an example of implementation for this standard, that in a small hospital where the director of the clinical laboratory is not a pathologist, arrangements should be made with a pathologist to provide expertise in clinical consultation for blood transfusion services and for review of all potential transfusion reactions. Standard QC.5.1 states that written policies and procedures for the blood bank service conform to the current edition of the AABB *Standards for Blood Banks and Transfusion Services.*

The *Laboratory Manual* has standards related to transfusion in the sections on official accreditation policies and procedures, quality control, leadership, improving organization performance, management of the laboratory environment, management of information, and sentinel events. Standard PI.3.1.1 in both manuals states that the organization must collect data to monitor the performance of processes that involve risks or may result in sentinel events and that these include the use of blood and blood components. As an example of evidence of performance for PI.3.1.1, the manual stipulates that surveyors should look at the use of blood and blood products. The 2000 *Comprehensive Manual* states that if the average number of transfusions per quarter is greater than 600, at least 5% of such transfusions be reviewed. If the average number of transfusions per quarter is less than 600, at least 30 transfusions must be reviewed. If there are fewer than 30 transfusions per quarter, all transfusions must be reviewed. The 2000–2001 *Laboratory Manual,* however, states that the organization can determine the detail and frequency of data collection for this activity and assure that its policy in this matter has been followed.

College of American Pathologists

The CAP laboratory accreditation program expects a participant laboratory to demonstrate that it is in compliance with the college's standards for laboratory accreditation. These standards relate to requirements for laboratory direction, physical facilities and safety, quality control and performance improvement, and inspection. Assessment of whether a laboratory meets the standards is accomplished through a series of checklists. The checklist questions are not standards but are considered tools for inspectors and directors to use in evaluating whether the laboratory is meeting standards. Most of the questions in the transfusion medicine checklist (section 5) are derived from the AABB *Standards for Blood Banks and Transfusion Services* and the relevant portions of the Clinical Laboratory Improvement Amendments of 1988. Any applicable question that cannot be answered "yes" is considered a deficiency and must be corrected within 30 days with the submission of supporting documentation for accreditation to be achieved. The inspector does not grant or deny accreditation, but may make a recommendation. The accreditation decision is made by the CAP Commission on Laboratory Accreditation. In addition to the on-site inspection program, the laboratory accreditation program of the college monitors proficiency testing performance of its participant laboratories. As does the AABB, the CAP has deemed status with the JCAHO and the Centers for Medicare and Medicaid Services (Table 69.1).

TRANSFUSION SERVICE ERROR REPORTING

On November 7, 2000, the FDA published a final rule amending the requirements for reporting errors and accidents (now termed *biological product deviations*) in the manufacturing of blood products. Manufacturing is defined as including "testing, processing, packing, labeling, storage, holding, or distribution" of both licensed and unlicensed blood components. Deviations and unexpected events in manufacturing that can affect the safety, purity, and potency of a product must be reported to the FDA under a new regulation (21 CFR 606.171) and an amended regulation (21 CFR 600.14). The new reporting requirement applies to licensed and unlicensed registered blood establishments and to unregistered transfusion services. Previously, only licensed blood establishments had to report errors and accidents. The FDA has devised a form, FDA-3486, for reporting these deviations. Information regarding this rule may be obtained at http://fda.gov/cber/biodev/biodev.htm.

Deviations must be reported only if the product was distributed. This is defined as having left the control of the establishment. If the product was not distributed, the incident still must be recorded in internal records per 21 CFR 606.160(b)(7)(iii). If the product was distributed, a report must be submitted to the Center for Biologics Evaluation and Research within 45 calendar days from the date information is acquired that reasonably suggests a reportable event occurred. The incident must also be recorded per 21 CFR 606.160(b)(7)(iii) and investigated per 21 CFR 606.100(c), 211.192 and 211.198. The FDA has stated that the purpose of this reporting system is to provide early warning of faulty processes as an indicator for potentially immediate problems that may be related to recalls and as surveillance for improving training and establishing guidance.

The deviation or unexpected event must occur in the facility or another facility under contract with the controlling facility. If a facility under contract to the hospital blood bank or transfusion service is responsible for a deviation, the hospital blood bank or transfusion service is responsible for reporting the problem if the product is distributed. The contract facility must perform an investigation but is not required to report. For example, if a test laboratory under contract to a hospital blood bank fails to provide viral marker testing and the unit is subsequently distributed, the blood bank must report this. If a transfusion service discovers that a unit is mislabeled with an extended outdate, the transfusion service must notify the blood center responsible for reporting to the FDA. The transfusion service would report this incident only if it further distributed the unit without correcting the label.

Deviations and unexpected events occurring within the facility or a facility under contract must be reported if they may affect the safety, purity, or potency of both licensed and unlicensed products that have been distributed. Examples of nonreportable events include a unit not being held at the appropriate temperature before transfusion after release from the blood bank, transfusion of a unit to the wrong patient, or failure by hospital staff to use a filter issued by the transfusion service. Reportable, unexpected events may occur even if all established procedures are followed within the transfusion service itself. An example of this would be a patient sample used for compatibility testing that was collected from the wrong patient.

Not reporting an event to the FDA within 45 days in and of itself constitutes a nonreportable deviation. A record-keeping deviation, such as failure to include the signature of the person preparing the unit in component preparation, would not be reportable because it would not affect the safety, purity, or potency of the product. A unit labeled with a shortened expiration date would also not be reportable, nor would a unit drawn too soon after the last donation. It would not be a reportable event if an allogeneic unit were issued when autologous blood was available. However, a unit labeled with an extended expiration date would be a reportable deviation. In summary, a deviation or unexpected event is reportable if all of the following criteria are met:

- It was associated with manufacturing.
- It occurred in the facility or at a contract facility.
- It may have affected the safety, purity, or potency of the product.
- The facility had control over the product.
- The product was distributed.

ERRORS IN TRANSFUSION PRACTICE

The extraordinary progress in microbiologic safety of blood transfusion in recent years (approximately a 10,000-fold reduction in the risk to patients from transfusion-transmitted HIV and hepatitis C virus infection) has not been matched by reducing the risk of nonviral serious hazards of transfusion. At present, hemovigilance programs established in the United Kingdom, Belgium, and Canada, all have documented that patients are still at considerable risk of adverse outcomes from noninfectious hazards of transfusion (48–50).

A recent review from the United Kingdom demonstrated that 54% of 618 reports received for major complications of transfusion documented transfusion of an incorrect unit of blood (48). Such voluntary reporting systems also indicate that there has been underreporting of noninfectious transfusion complications. Introduction of a notification system in Quebec resulted in a dramatic increase in the reporting of such incidents (50). Specimens obtained for compatibility testing whose ABO results do not match the results on record in the blood bank typically are not reported publicly as near-miss events. Similarly, samples drawn from the wrong patient that match by chance the historical record or that match the correct patient without a historical record also are not detected. Thus the true incidence of mistakes in the processes used to provide the correct unit to the patient is unknown. Errors in transfusion practices may actually be increasing. A recent report from one hospital documented a significant increase in problems with identification of patients, samples, and units from 1993 through 1999 (51).

Even without correcting for the underrecognition and underreporting of adverse events from noninfectious causes, the FDA has reported a transfusion-related death rate due to hemolytic reactions more than twice as high as that due to all infectious hazards combined. The reported incidence of fatal transfusion reactions owing to the infusion of ABO-incompatible blood has not improved significantly, as documented in reviews of data reported to the FDA or the New York State Department of Health between 1976 and the present (52–54). Such ABO-incompatible transfusions are the reported cause of death of as many as 24 patients each year in the United States (55). In the report by Linden (54), erroneous administration of a unit of blood was observed in 1 in 19,000 RBC units administered. One half of these events occurred outside the blood bank (administration to the wrong recipient 38%; phlebotomy errors 13%), and 15% of events involved multiple errors, the most common of which was failure to detect at the bedside that an incorrect unit had been issued. This study suggests that transfusion error continues to be a great risk, that most errors result from human mistakes and may be preventable, and that most of these events occur outside the blood bank, which is a strong argument for hospital-wide efforts at improving the process of transfusion safety. Numerous publications over the last 25 years consistent and widespread have documented the significance of errors in the process of transfusion without a significant commitment of financial resources directed toward improving safety in this area. At present, the risk that a patient will receive the wrong unit of blood in the United States is probably approximately 100 times the risk of acquiring hepatitis C virus or HIV by means of blood transfusion.

When an error occurs, corrective action must focus on an analysis of the processes in place that allowed the error to happen rather than simply disciplining employees. The questions that leadership should ask are, "Why was the procedure not followed correctly?" and "Why was it possible for the staff person to deviate from the policy in this way?" The answer to these questions should be documented and suitable actions taken to develop, implement, and evaluate improved processes to prevent error. It is insufficient to rely strictly on the vigilance of individuals to assure transfusion safety.

IMPROVING TRANSFUSION PRACTICE

A number of approaches have been used successfully to improve clinical transfusion practices. Toy (56) has summarized five processes for which there is published evidence of success.

One approach is to give lectures. Although many physicians may be reached simultaneously, it may be difficult to have a durable impact on transfusion practice. Publications on this approach have documented a decrease in inappropriate use of FFP from 53% to 22% through an educational conference program (57), a 75% decrease in the total number of red blood cells transfused in an obstetrics and gynecology service (58), and a 46% decrease in use of FFP over a 2-year period (59). The proportion of patients donating autologous blood decreased from 53% to 26%, the overall transfusion rate decreased from 10% to 7%, and the allogeneic transfusion rate did not change in a program that decreased unnecessary autologous collections without increasing the number of allogeneic transfusions (60).

A second approach is for a specialist in transfusion medicine to meet one-on-one with physicians. Although this is time-consuming, it can be particularly effective. Brief face-to-face conferences with surgeons reduced the proportion of transfusions not in compliance with criteria from 40% to 24%. Surgeons who participated in the study decreased their transfusion trigger significantly whereas control physicians did not (61). The use of autologous blood donation increased with visits to surgeons. No changes occurred in control hospitals where no visits were made. Interestingly, there was no increase in inappropriate use of autologous blood donations in study hospitals for procedures that required no preoperative blood order (62). Review of transfusions 1 day after administration with discussions with the ordering physician led to a reduction from 3.2% to 0.5% in the number of transfusions that failed to meet auditing criteria (63). In this study, the rate of unjustified transfusions decreased from 1.4% to 0% during a 1-year audit.

A third approach is to make patients rounds on a regular basis. This approach is time-consuming but directs physician attention to a particular patient who needs treatment and therefore may be particularly effective. A 77% reduction in the use of FFP over a 2-year period after implementation of a next-day review accompanied by an educational program has been demonstrated (64). The number of units transfused to patients with a hematocrit greater than 30% decreased from 30% to 10% when daily rounds were made (65).

A fourth approach is to review each transfusion order before the blood product is issued. This prospective review can be highly effective in improving transfusion practices. One mechanism for implementing this process is to have physicians select the indication for transfusion from a computerized order menu or by checking manually a transfusion order request form. Requests can also be reviewed by blood bank physicians and staff in conjunction with available laboratory data. Such a prospective review of blood utilization resulted in a significant reduction of allogeneic donor exposure in one study (66). Simpson (67) described how prospective audit of platelet transfusions, in which a substantial number of orders were initially denied or modified, resulted in significant improvement in platelet-ordering practices and a 56% reduction in platelet use over a 3-year period. An audit of platelet use followed by modified practice guidelines applied prospectively to requests for platelets led to a 14% decrease in the number of platelet units transfused during the following year (68). A mandatory pretransfusion approval program resulted in a 33% decrease in FFP transfusions (69). A decrease from 28.6% to 27.7% in the hematocrits of persons receiving transfused occurred, as did a reduction in the number of transfusion orders requiring review, after computerized screening of blood transfusion requests was implemented (70). A significant reduction in inappropriate platelet and FFP transfusions occurred after introduction of a new component request form that included transfusion guidelines (71). A significant decrease in inappropriate red blood cell, platelet, and FFP transfusions after the request form was modified to include indications for transfusion and relevant clinical and laboratory data was shown in another study (72).

A fifth approach to improving transfusion practices is to develop and implement algorithms. An intraoperative algorithm for transfusion in cardiac surgery has been reported successful (73).

Retrospective review of charts, while satisfying some accreditation requirements, has not been shown conclusively to influence transfusion practices when used as a single tool. Retrospective analyses can, however, augment utilization review when combined with other approaches. This activity, along with other approaches to reviewing the process of transfusion, and the development of review criteria are addressed later, in the section on the transfusion committee.

Combination of approaches has been successful in improvement of transfusion practice. Reviewing clinical and laboratory data for all transfusions with follow-up consultations substantially reduced the number of transfusions of red blood cells, platelets, FFP, and cryoprecipitate over a 4-year period (74). A 52% decrease in use of FFP occurred after implementation of a retrospective utilization audit, an educational program, a new FFP request form that required the ordering physician to indicate the reason for the request, and pathologist approval in cases lacking documentation of abnormal results of coagulation studies (75). The establishment of transfusion guidelines based on national standards accompanied by the implementation of a monitoring system that required physicians to record medical indications for all nonemergency transfusions and followed by selective retrospective auditing resulted in a 35.9% decrease in allogeneic donor exposures over a 3-year period (76). In a novel approach, a quality assessment program that permitted oversight of transfusionists' practices resulted in a decline from 50% to nearly zero in the percentage of transfusions at variance from institutional blood administration policy (77).

Educational strategies should be aimed at the attending physician who has the final responsibility for transfusion orders (78). One study showed that attending physicians had lower knowledge scores than did residents but exhibited more confidence in what they knew. Resident ordering practices were heavily influenced by the wishes of attending physicians. Most residents who answered the survey stated they had ordered transfusions they had judged unnecessary because a more senior physician had suggested that they do so. Multiinstitutional audits also serve as useful benchmarking tools (79).

TRANSFUSION MEDICINE COMMITTEE

A clinical staff committee concerned exclusively with practices and policies related to transfusion and the transfusion service has become routine in most hospitals. It may report to the health care evaluation office or committee, or the committee can report directly to the medical policy committee of the institution.

The membership of the transfusion committee should represent the departments that are the principal users of blood and blood components, such as hematology or oncology, surgery, and anesthesiology. Obstetrics and gynecology and pediatrics also should be represented if these departments are part of the hospital. In addition, staff from some of the surgical subspecialties (e.g., cardiovascular surgery) and from services with specialized needs (e.g., neonatal, emergency, intensive care) are appropriate representatives. The medical director of the transfusion service must be a committee member. The transfusion service supervisor can be a valuable resource concerning laboratory operations and the feasibility of proposed policies. Clinical staff members with special interests or expertise in transfusion medicine should be encouraged to accept appointment on the committee. Committee activities may prove educational for the participating physicians (80–82). Transfusion committee appointments should last several years so that expertise can be acquired and should be staggered to ensure continuity.

It is preferable for the blood bank director not to serve as chair of the transfusion committee. Changes in policy are more readily accepted if the transfusion committee is perceived as a distinct entity, independent of the transfusion service. As the expert, the director always has the opportunity to present views and shape policy. However, having a consumer of blood products serve as chair is likely to enhance the credibility, visibility, and effectiveness of the transfusion committee.

Other services in the hospital that often send representatives to the transfusion committee meetings include the hospital compliance office; the divisions of quality, risk, and utilization management of the health care evaluation office; the medical records department; medical and surgical nursing services; and the intravenous therapy team. If the hospital has a residency training program, it is helpful to have a resident physician present for committee meetings. The director of the blood center that supplies the hospital may be a valuable resource to provide comparisons of transfusion activities at different hospitals in the community (83). For example, if one hospital follows markedly different policies and does not encounter differences in outcome, this information can be the basis for adopting an alternative approach. When policies with medicolegal implications are under discussion (e.g., a policy for informed consent for blood transfusion, implementation of look-back procedures), it is useful to have the hospital attorney attend committee meetings.

A multidisciplinary transfusion committee can serve as an active and effective guiding force in the development of policies and procedures related to the transfusion of blood components. Physicians must give sufficient priority to this process, and the hospital administration must make the necessary resources available to ensure effective committee work. A prompt and thoughtful response to committee recommendations by hospital and clinical governing bodies is essential to creating the correct environment. In academic centers, department chairs should support the participation of faculty on clinical staff committees and appreciate that this is an important element of the faculty member's educational and service efforts. Data derived from the committee's work can serve as a source of clinical scholarship.

FUNCTIONS OF A TRANSFUSION COMMITTEE

Utilization Review

Although effective utilization review does not have to involve the transfusion committee, the participation of the committee can supplement other efforts. Functions addressed here can also be performed by transfusion service physicians prospectively or soon after transfusion.

Undertransfusion

A patient who needs a blood transfusion but does not receive one is more likely to be harmed than is a patient who receives a transfusion that is unnecessary. Most attention has been devoted to identifying unnecessary transfusions. However, hospital transfusion committees may want to determine whether patients who need transfusions are receiving them (84). For example, the members of the transfusion committee may want to review the medical records of patients with hemoglobin levels less than 5.5 or 5.0 g/dl who did not receive transfusions.

There is a great variability in transfusion practices among institutions. This variability illustrates the fact that clinical data indicative of the need for transfusion are so imprecise that indications for transfusion are not universally agreed upon. This prompts concern that undertransfusion may be a problem. In fact, higher transfusion thresholds than are conventionally recommended may be beneficial to some patients without cardiovascular disease. For example, a hematocrit less than 28% has been independently associated with risk of postoperative myocardial ischemia (85).

Undertransfusion can also occur if units of blood are not being released from the blood bank in a sufficiently timely manner (86). The publicity regarding the risks of transfusion and inappropriate transfusions and the strict policies, procedures, accreditation standards, and regulations governing blood banks may have combined to create undue concern about the release of blood components for transfusion. Results of CAP surveys have suggested that this may be the case. One survey (1991 Set J-D) concerned a 65-year-old man who arrived in the emergency department with symptoms of intestinal obstruction and a hematocrit of 22% was found to have an ABO blood grouping discrepancy. Fifty-three percent of 3,476 responding institutions indicated that they would not release red blood cells for transfusion until there was resolution of this discrepancy. This is an unfortunate response, because there would have been no harm in releasing group O red blood cells for this patient. In fact, there may have been considerable harm in not doing so. Another survey (1992 Set J-A) described a 29-year-old patient with Marfan syndrome who was group A Rh-negative who had undergone surgery for a dissecting aortic aneurysm that was complicated by considerable hemorrhage. More than 14% of 4,138 institutions who responded indicated that after the patient received 40 units of red blood cells, they "would not transfuse" a crossmatch-compatible group O Rh-positive unit into this patient, even though no group A red blood cells were available. Under these circumstances, it would be appropriate to transfuse even uncrossmatched group O Rh-positive blood. In a third survey (1985 Set J-B), 11.6% of institutions responded that they would have "refused to provide any component" to a patient to whom a "plasma-containing product must be given" who had red blood cell T activation.

Members of transfusion committees may want to ensure that blood bank technical staff are not delaying the release of urgently required components because of excessive concern about exceptions to routine practices.

Unnecessary Transfusion

Review of transfusion practices has the potential to improve the quality of clinical care, educate clinical staff, reduce costs, ensure regulatory and accreditation compliance, reduce the risk of litigation, provide information about the practices of individual physicians and specific clinical services, and establish consistent practices. Discussion of blood use in the care of specific patients prompted change in clinical practices in situations in which formal lectures had not (87). It is onerous and unnecessary to review intensively each transfusion in an institution. Rather, the transfusion service director and medical staff representatives of each hospital should determine the timing, scope, and intensity of the review. One approach used by many hospitals is to review only orders for transfusions for which certain predetermined screening criteria are not met. Intensive assessment of an individual case also may be initiated in response to concerns of a patient, provider, or third-party payer.

Timing of Utilization Review

Utilization review can be conducted prospectively or retrospectively. Prospective review requires verification by a reviewer that one or more criteria have been met before a blood component is made available for transfusion. Although this on-site validation is desirable and presumably the most beneficial, it is labor intensive and not always feasible in an emergency. Furthermore, in the care of an acutely ill patient, a discussion regarding transfusion practice may not always be conducive to effective education or may not be appropriate. Although prospective auditing may prove useful for customized blood products, such as irradiated components or unusually large orders, it is not likely to be feasible for all blood transfusions within an institution. Retrospective audits may be most effective if performed soon after the transfusion, for example, within 24 hours. Although common sense suggests that this prompt feedback would be useful to physicians, it requires a continuing effort and may not always be practical. Retrospective audits later are the least difficult to perform but also should be completed in as timely a manner as possible to be maximally effective. There are no data to substantiate the effectiveness of retrospective review alone in improving transfusion practices, although there are many reports of success with other approaches, some of which have been combined with retrospective review.

One method that has been used frequently requires prospective justification with either a computer-generated ordering menu or simply a requisition slip. In both cases, screening criteria are used as part of the ordering process. The ordering physician selects from a menu the transfusion criterion met by a particular patient or presents another clinical justification for transfusion. Table 69.3 contains examples of screening criteria that may be used. Screening criteria for adult (88,89) and pediatric (90,91) blood transfusion practices have been published. All or some of the orders in which another reason was provided as the indication for transfusion are reviewed more intensively, either before or after the transfusion. Transfusions thought to pose the greatest risk or be the most likely to be inappropriate can be reviewed. For hospitals that do not use screening criteria, these unusual transfusion episodes are a logical place to begin blood utilization review. Each type of component transfused in the institution should be reviewed, and each clinical service that uses blood should be evaluated.

If a retrospective review is conducted a long time after the transfusion, the reviewer must consider the information available to the clinician and the patient's clinical condition at the time the decision to perform transfusion was made.

Screening Criteria

Although screening criteria may be used to select transfusion episodes for intensive review, the criteria do not constitute a standard of practice. Not every patient who meets a screening criterion necessarily needs a blood transfusion, and there are patients who do not meet the screening criteria who may need a transfusion. It is necessary to differentiate between criteria used simply to select a medical record for further intensive review and what is appropriate clinical practice. Nevertheless, those who control the screening criteria exert great influence on clinical practice. Therefore the committee may want to review selectively some cases in which a transfusion has fallen within the criteria. Initially the criteria can be designed liberally to capture transfusion episodes in which inappropriate practices were most likely to have occurred. However, once these have been addressed, the criteria can be modified to become more restrictive. Differences in patient populations, professional judgment, and prevailing practices result in different screening criteria among hospitals. The clinical staff has overall responsibility for approving the screening criteria. The intriguing suggestion has been made that hospitals' clinical staffs should review each other to avoid the collegiality that arises within institutions (92).

The input and approval of practicing physicians are helpful to lessen the debate about the validity of screening criteria. The criteria should be limited to one or a few easily identified elements, and exceptions should be minimized. Policies regarding the administrative response to deficient transfusion practice should be publicized, so that there will be no surprises when blood utilization review is implemented. The screening criteria should be publicized regularly. If the criteria are not on an order menu, house staff and new members of the clinical staff should receive copies of the criteria, which should be disseminated throughout the institution.

Screening criteria should be evaluated on a regular basis. New clinical practices require reassessment of the criteria. Intensive assessment of a medical record or subsequent discussion about a specific clinical practice with a treating physician may prompt a revision of the criteria.

An alternative approach is a system in which the admission and discharge hematocrits of patients are used to determine the appropriateness of blood transfusions (93,94). The advantages of this system include possible elimination of extensive chart audits, individualization of reviews according to patient or procedure, and lack of dependence on a single hematocrit level at either admission or discharge, which can be misleading.

Consequences of Utilization Review

The JCAHO requires that credentialing of clinical staff include consideration of an individual's professional performance, judgment, and clinical skills (standards MS 5.12, MS 5.15). Peer review activities are specifically included in the JCAHO *Accreditation Manual* as sources of this information. Utilization review activities related to transfusion practice may be included in the credentialing process.

A retrospective utilization review must consider carefully the clinical situation at the time the transfusion was given. If, however, it is determined that a transfusion may have deviated from acceptable practice, the involved physician may be informed in writing and invited to provide an explanation for the transfusion in question. After the physician's response is received, the committee can make a final determination regarding the transfusion and inform the physician. Audit findings may be summarized for departments and divisions and should be made available to their chairs and directors. If blood transfusion practices are audited selectively, the review should be rotated so that at some point all of the divisions within the hospital are subject to review. Collected information should be sent regularly to the committee or individual to whom the transfusion committee reports. When particular problems with transfusion practices are identified, they should be subjected to repeated intense evaluation. The overall effect of the review program on clinical practices may be assessed as well.

It is important to communicate conclusions regarding appropriate transfusion practices to the clinical staff. These communi-

TABLE 69.3. CRITERIA THAT MAY BE USED TO PRECLUDE MORE INTENSIVE REVIEW OF ACCEPTABILITY OF BLOOD COMPONENT TRANSFUSION AND WHICH MAY BE INCORPORATED INTO BLOOD ORDERING FORMS OR COMPUTER PROGRAMS

Red Blood Cells
Hematocrit less than 25%
Acute blood loss greater than 20% of blood volume
Coronary or cerebral vascular disease and hematocrit less than 30%
More than 10% surface burns and hematocrit less than 30%
To improve oxygen delivery in patient with sepsis, septic shock, or acute respiratory distress syndrome, and hematocrit less than 36%
For neonates: hematocrit less than 40% with respiratory distress; otherwise, hematocrit less than 30% or blood loss more than 10% of blood volume

Platelet Concentrate
Bleeding or a planned invasive or surgical procedure and
Platelet count less than 80 × 10^9/L
or
Bleeding time longer than 7.5 min
or
Documented platelet function disorder
or
Administration of more than one blood volume of red blood cells and other volume-expanding fluids in previous 24 hours
Platelet count less than 100 × 10^9/L in a patient who
Has retinal or cerebral hemorrhage
or
Is recovering from a cardiopulmonary bypass procedure
Prophylactically for platelet count less than 20 × 10^9/L (<40 × 10^9/L in neonate)
Neonate with bleeding or a planned invasive or surgical procedure and platelet count less than 100 × 10^9/L

Fresh Frozen Plasma
Hemorrhage or a planned invasive or surgical procedure and
International normalized ratio 1.5 or higher (other than for central nervous system)
or
International normalized ration 1.3 or higher (for central nervous system)
Documented deficiency of factor II, V, VII, X, or XI
Administration of more than one blood volume of red blood cells and other volume-expanding fluids in previous 24 hours
Thrombotic thrombocytopenic purpura
Hemolytic uremic syndrome

Cryoprecipitate
Bleeding or a planned invasive or surgical procedure and
Documented deficiency of fibrinogen (<80 mg/dl)
or
Documented von Willebrand disease
or
Documented deficiency of factor XIII
or
Uremic platelet dysfunction (bleeding time longer than 7.5 min)

Cryoprecipitate-depleted Plasma
Bleeding or a planned invasive or surgical procedure and documented deficiency of factor II, V, VII, X, or XI
Thrombotic thrombocytopenic purpura
Hemolytic uremic syndrome

Granulocyte Concentrate
Neutropenia (<1 × 10^9/L) with documented infection unresponsive to antibiotics

Rh Immune Globulin
Postpartum Rh-negative mother with Rh-positive baby
Antepartum Rh-negative woman at 28 weeks of gestation or with risk of recent fetal-maternal hemorrhage or who received antepartum Rh immune globulin 12 weeks previously Rh-negative woman after abortion, ectopic pregnancy, miscarriage, or amniocentesis
Transfusion of Rh-positive cellular blood products to Rh-negative patient

These are not indications for transfusion.
Adapted from Mintz PD. Quality assessment and improvement of transfusion practices. *Hematol Oncol Clin North Am* 1995;9:219–232, with permission.

cations can reinforce good practices and can increase the openness of practitioners to future less supportive comments. Because an important element of any quality assessment program is the continuing education of the clinical staff, the auditing process should be designed more as a tutorial activity than as a punitive one. Improperly performed audits can antagonize those whom they are designed to instruct, thereby hindering acceptance of other well-designed programs. If the institutional leadership provides the necessary resources for the auditing process and physicians provide sufficient time and effort, utilization review can be an important element in documenting sustained excellence or continuing improvement in clinical practices.

Other Review Activities

In addition to auditing blood transfusion practices, the transfusion service or transfusion committee can pursue a number of other activities. Table 69.4 lists selected items regarding the ordering, dispensing, and administration of blood components that either the transfusion service or the committee may wish to monitor. The following are several broad reviews and activities that the committee may perform from year to year. Some of the elements listed in Table 69.4 are incorporated into these suggestions.

1. Review that transfusions are appropriately documented in the medical record. This activity should include a review of the documentation required by the institution's policies, including the process of obtaining informed consent. Such an audit can include a determination that consent has been obtained, that the patient's, witness's, and physician's signatures are included, and that the consent is appropriately dated and placed in the record in accord with institutional policy. The blood transfusion record can be audited to ensure that it includes the information the institution requires regarding the intended recipient's name, identification number, and ABO and Rh group; the component's unique identification number; the donor's ABO and Rh group; interpretation of compatibility tests; the volume administered, the expiration date or time of the component; time of transfusion; identification of the transfusionist; and information about patient monitoring during the transfusion. A systematic education program for transfusion nurses can improve documentation and monitoring procedures (95). The review can include verification that the medical record contains the documentation of the indications for transfusion, the prescription for the transfusion, and the outcome of the transfusion.
2. Review the institution's policies and procedures for proper patient, specimen, and blood component identification and other policies and procedures related to blood administration. Observe the administration of transfusions to ensure that proper patient and blood component identification has been completed. Boone et al. (96) found that careful monitoring can effectively identify correctable errors in blood administration. Review the adequacy of initial and continuing staff education.
3. Ensure that adequate policies and procedures exist for detecting, reporting, and evaluating transfusion reactions, and review the timeliness and adequacy of the investigations of these adverse events. Assess whether reasonable effort is made to ensure the reporting and evaluation of suspected instances of transfusion-transmitted infectious disease.
4. Evaluate the utilization of devices used in blood transfusion. The committee can ascertain that appropriate quality control has been performed on blood warmers and infusion pumps and that the devices used are appropriate for the purpose. Assure that personnel have been trained adequately in use of devices.
5. Review autologous blood collection and transfusion activities. A quality improvement team significantly improved the availability of autologous donor blood and had a far-reaching effect on quality improvement methods throughout one medical

TABLE 69.4. FACTORS TO CONSIDER IN MONITORING OF THE ORDERING, DISPENSING, AND ADMINISTRATION OF BLOOD COMPONENTS

1. Time request for blood component was received.
2. Was there a prescription for the transfusion?
3. Was the request submitted correctly?
4. Was the correct component selected for issue?
5. Was the component inspected?
6. Was the component outdated?
7. Was documentation before issue completed correctly?
8. Time transportation department was notified component was available.
9. Time component was issued.
10. Was the correct filter issued?
11. Was documentation regarding transportation completed correctly?
12. Time component was delivered by transportation.
13. Was the blood component unattended after release from the blood bank? Where was it?
14. Was informed consent obtained in accord with written procedure?
15. Were patient and blood component identification properly performed in accord with written procedure before transfusion was started?
16. Was documentation on the transfusion slip accurate and complete?
17. Were pretransfusion vital signs obtained and recorded?
18. Was filter attached properly?
19. Was arm and port preparation properly performed?
20. Time transfusion was started. Was this documented?
21. Were only approved solutions in contact with the component?
22. Were only approved solutions mixed with the component?
23. If used, was a blood warmer or infusion pump used in accord with written procedure?
24. Were vital signs obtained and recorded during the transfusion in accord with written procedure?
25. Was any transfusion reaction reported to a physician and the blood bank in accord with written procedure?
26. Time transfusion was completed. Was this documented?
27. Were vital signs taken and recorded, and was the patient observed after transfusion in accord with written procedures?
28. Were the component bag and other materials disposed of correctly?
29. Were written instructions about adverse reactions provided if the recipient was an outpatient or at home?
30. Was all documentation placed in the patient's permanent record in accord with written procedure?
31. Was the outcome of the transfusion documented in the medical record?

From Mintz PD, ed. *Transfusion therapy: clinical principles and practice.* Bethesda, MD: American Association of Blood Banks, 1999, with permission.

center (97). The committee can review how such services are being used, whether allogeneic blood was ever transfused when autologous blood was available, and whether autologous blood has been transfused more liberally than the committee deems appropriate. In view of the risks of bacterial contamination, clerical error, and hypervolemia that exist with autologous blood transfusion, the committee can reasonably require that the same standards used for allogeneic blood transfusion be used for autologous blood transfusion. An alternative, because autologous blood is safer, is for the transfusion committee to accept more liberal indications for transfusion of autologous blood. In either case, the same screening criteria can be used to determine which cases require more intensive review. This practice allows individual consideration of the use of autologous blood in situations in which allogeneic transfusion would be considered inappropriate. The collection, manipulation, and utilization of autologous blood collected intraoperatively, postoperatively, and after trauma also can be reviewed.

6. Review blood bank performance in such areas as timeliness of response to requests, productivity, and outdating of products.

7. Review the utilization of certain customized products such as irradiated blood.

8. Ensure that the last unit or units of several transfusions given sequentially are appropriate. A single low hemoglobin concentration or episode of bleeding can lead to the transfusion of several units of blood, of which the last or last few units may have been the least needed transfusions provided. These transfusions may not come routinely to the attention of the committee because the patient may have met a particular criterion initially. The committee may want to assure itself that when more than one unit of blood is transfused for a specific criterion, each of the units is truly indicated. In one study, two-unit transfusions were commonly given to patients undergoing total hip replacement when one unit would have sufficed (98). In another study, intertransfusion assessment was frequently not completed for postoperative patients (99). Results of another study suggested that determining the hematocrit immediately before administration of each unit of blood would have reduced by 25% the amount of blood transfused into patients undergoing colonic resection (100). Single-unit transfusion sometimes represents good practice. If one red blood cell transfusion increases oxygen delivery adequately, there is no need for additional transfusions.

9. Review whether the institution's guidelines for preoperative ordering of blood cross-matching (5) are followed. The effective use of preoperative cross-matching guidelines for elective surgery has been shown not to compromise patient care (101).

10. Review the veracity of the ordering physicians in choosing the criteria met to justify blood transfusion, if the institution has a system in which physicians indicate in advance the reason for the transfusion.

11. Review blood wastage due to failure to return unused units to the blood bank on a timely basis (102).

12. Review the hospital's look-back activities to ensure that they comply with federal regulations and guidelines and are being completed on a timely basis.

13. Review the timeliness and adequacy of delivery of blood components from the blood supplier. It may be helpful to invite blood center management to attend discussions regarding this issue.

14. Review blood bank proficiency testing, accreditation reports, and quality control results.

15. Determine, on occasion, the crossmatched to transfused ratio from selected services or within the entire institution. Although this calculation was emphasized in the past, its utility has frequently been overstated. There is no accreditation requirement to determine this statistic. However, institutions or selected departments or divisions may show a significantly elevated ratio, indicating that more blood is being crossmatched than is reasonably necessary. An appropriate ratio is less than 2.

16. Serve as an advocate for the blood bank to the hospital's clinical staff and administration for personnel, equipment, or space needs.

17. Assist in the development of hospital policies related to transfusion practices. In this regard, the members of the transfusion committee could help to shape policies regarding informed consent for blood transfusion, the availability of directed donations from friends or relatives of patients, and the development of look-back procedures for patients who may have received blood from donors subsequently known to have infection with an agent transmissible through blood transfusion.

Each transfusion committee should determine the topics it wants to consider. It should select areas that will help the institution achieve compliance with accreditation standards and regulatory requirements and focus on those most in need of systematic oversight or improvement.

The transfusion committee and others performing utilization review should be familiar with state laws and regulations governing the discoverability for legal proceedings of the committee's minutes, records, correspondence, and reports. The committee and others need to shape their practices accordingly. State statutes may prevent the routine release of these documents as a result of legal discovery proceedings but may permit courts to order the disclosure of such records if it is found that extraordinary circumstances make such an action desirable. Considerable caution must be taken regarding the content of all written records with respect to their discoverability.

SUMMARY

Although blood products typically represent only approximately 1% of a hospital's budget, transfusion is at once a life-saving and potentially life-threatening procedure. Remarkable progress has been made in reducing the transmission of viruses through blood transfusion, but this has not been matched in improved safety with respect to other important transfusion hazards. Although knowledge is still limited regarding indications for blood component transfusions, quality assessment programs for blood transfusion are needed to improve transfusion practice.

A successful quality program creates "an environment of watchful concern" (24) and is conducted in a professional, nonadversarial, and educational manner. Assessment of transfusion practices has the potential to enhance the knowledge and judgment of health care professionals, provide significant information about patient care, reduce the risk of litigation, decrease costs, ensure compliance with regulatory and accreditation requirements, conserve the blood supply, provide an opportunity to demonstrate quality and value to the public, and to help create, sustain, and document excellence in patient care.

REFERENCES

1. Fantus B. The therapy of Cook County Hospital. *JAMA* 1937;109: 128–131.
2. *Standards for Blood Banks and Transfusion Services,* 20th ed. Bethesda, MD: American Association of Blood Banks, 2000.
3. Barnes A, Wilson JK. The hospital transfusion service: management and administration. In: Rosse EC, Simon TL, Moss GS, et al, eds. *Principles of transfusion medicine,* 2nd ed. Baltimore: Williams & Wilkins, 1996:893–906.
4. Judd WJ. Modern approaches to pretransfusion testing. *Immunohematology* 1999;15:41–52.
5. Mintz PD, Nordine R, Henry JB, Webb W. Expected hemotherapy in elective surgery. *N Y State J Med* 1976;76:532–537.
6. Mintz PD, Lauenstein K, Hume J, et al. Expected hemotherapy in elective surgery: a followup. *JAMA* 1978;239:623–625.
7. Mintz PD, Haines AL, Sullivan MF. Incompatible crossmatch following nonreactive antibody detection test: frequency and cause. *Transfusion* 1982;22:107–110.
8. Mintz PD, Henry JB, Boral LI. Type and screen. *Clin Lab Med* 1982; 2:169–179.
9. Goodnough LT. What is a transfusion medicine specialist? *Transfusion* 1999;39:1031–1033.
10. Ness PM. Integrating the new generation of blood components into transfusion practice. *Transfusion* 1999;39:1027–1030.
11. AuBuchon JP. The role of transfusion medicine physicians. *Arch Pathol Lab Med* 1999;123:663–667.
12. Alving B, Alcorn K. How to improve transfusion medicine. *Arch Pathol Lab Med* 1999;123:492–495.
13. Leape LL, Bates DW, Cullen DJ, et al. Systems analysis of adverse drug events. *JAMA* 1995;274:35–43.
14. Pande PS, Neuman RP, Cavanagh RR. *The six sigma way: how GE, Motorola, and other top companies are honing their performance.* New York: McGraw-Hill, 2000.
15. Sherman LA. Outcomes in transfusion. *Arch Pathol Lab Med* 1999; 123:599–602.
16. Headrick LA, Neuhauser D. Quality healthcare. *JAMA* 1994;271: 1711–1712.
17. Kritchevsky SB, Simmons BP. Continuous quality improvement: concepts and applications for physician care. *JAMA* 1991;266: 1817–1823.
18. *Comprehensive accreditation manual for hospitals, 2000.* Oakbrook Terrace, IL: Joint Commission on Accreditation of Healthcare Organizations, 2000.
19. Hanson M. The "P's and Q's" of quality systems. *Arch Pathol Lab Med* 1999;576–569.
20. Nevalainen DE. The quality systems approach. *Arch Pathol Lab Med* 1999;123:566–568.
21. AuBuchon JP. Optimizing the cost-effectiveness of quality assurance in transfusion medicine. *Arch Pathol Lab Med* 1999;603–606.
22. Blumberg N. The costs and consequences of management fads and politically driven regulatory oversight. *Arch Pathol Lab Med* 1999; 123:580–584.
23. Peach RW, Ritter DS. *A pocket guide to implementing the ISO 9000 quality systems standard and QS-9000 requirements.* Methuen, MA: Goal QPC, 1996.
24. Donabedian A. The quality of care: how can it be assessed? *JAMA* 1988;260:1743–1748.
25. Goldman RL. The reliability of peer assessments of quality of care. *JAMA* 1992;267:958–960.
26. Caplan RA, Posner KL, Cheney FW. Effect of outcome on physician judgments of appropriateness of care. *JAMA* 1991;265:1957–1960.
27. Bock AV. Use and abuse of blood transfusions. *N Engl J Med* 1936; 215:421–425.
28. Garland J, Smith RM, Lanman TH, et al. Abuse of transfusion therapy [Editorial]. *N Engl J Med* 1951;245:745–746.
29. Straus B, Torres JM. Use and abuse of blood transfusion. *JAMA* 1953; 151:699–701.
30. Crisp WE. One pint of blood. *Obstet Gynecol* 1956;7:216–217.
31. Cantor D. A legal look at blood transfusions. *GP* 1957;16:82–84.
32. Crosby WH. Misuse of blood transfusions. *Blood* 1958;13: 1198–1200.
33. Crosby WH. Misuse of blood transfusions. *Med Bull US Army Eur* 1958;15:7.
34. Friesen R. The use and abuse of blood in abortions. *Can Med Assoc J* 1959;80:802–805.
35. Graham-Stewart CW. A clinical survey of blood-transfusion. *Lancet* 1960;2:421–424.
36. Bulletin of Joint Commission on Accreditation of Hospitals. Publication 26. March 1961.
37. MacDonald I. Editorial. *Bull LA County Med Assoc* 1961;91:57–58.
38. McCoy KL. The Providence Hospital blood conservation program. *Transfusion* 1962;2:3–6.
39. Joint Blood Council. Transfusion review program. *JAMA* 1962;180: 230–231.
40. Crosby WH. The hospital transfusion board. *Transfusion* 1962;2:1–2.
41. Powell NA, Johnston DG. Criteria for blood transfusion. *Calif Med* 1962;97:12–15.
42. Walz DV. An effective hospital transfusion committee. *JAMA* 1964; 189:660–662.
43. The transfusion of blood [Editorial]. *JAMA* 1964;189:116.
44. Dietrich EB. Evaluation of blood transfusion. *Transfusion* 1965;5: 82–88.
45. Swanson JO, Polesky HF. Transfusion review in Minnesota hospitals. *Minn Med* 1976;59:188–190.
46. Smith DM, Otter J. Performance improvement in a HTS: the American Association of Blood Banks quality systems approach. *Arch Pathol Lab Med* 1999;123:585–591.
47. *Comprehensive accreditation manual for pathology and clinical laboratory services.* Oakbrook Terrace, IL: Joint Commission on Accreditation of Healthcare Organizations, 2000–2001.
48. Williamson L, Cohen H, Love E, et al. The serious hazards of transfusion (SHOT) initiative: the UK approach to haemovigilance. *Vox Sang* 2000;78[Suppl 2]:291–295.
49. Baele PL, de Bruyere M, Deneys V, et al. Bedside transfusion errors: a prospective survey by the Belgium SAnGUIS Group. *Vox Sang* 1994; 66:117–121.
50. Robillard P, Blouin N, Hache D. Adverse transfusion reactions: experience of the Quebec Hemovigilance System. *Transfusion* 2000; 40[Suppl]:134S.
51. Butch SH. Comparison of seven years of occurrence reports. *Transfusion* 2000;40[Suppl]:159S.
52. Sazama K. Reports of 355 transfusion-associated deaths: 1976 through 1985. *Transfusion* 1990;30:583–590.
53. Honig CL, Bove JR. Transfusion-associated fatalities: review of Bureau of Biologics reports 1976–1978. *Transfusion* 1980;20:653–661.
54. Linden JV, Wagner K, Voytovich AE, et al. Transfusion errors in New York State: an analysis of 10 years' experience. *Transfusion* 2000; 40:1207–1213.
55. AuBuchon JP, Kruskall MS. Transfusion safety: realigning efforts with risks. *Transfusion* 1997;37:1211–1216.
56. Toy P. Guiding the decision to transfuse: interventions that do and do not work. *Arch Pathol Lab Med* 1999;123:592–594.
57. Barnette RE, Fish DJ, Eisenstaedt RS. Modification of fresh-frozen plasma transfusion practices through educational intervention. *Transfusion* 1990;30:253–257.
58. Morrison JC, Sumrall DD, Chevalier SP. The effect of provider education on blood utilization practices. *Am J Obstet Gynecol* 1993;169: 1240–1245.
59. Ayoub MM, Clark JA. Reduction of fresh frozen plasma use with a simple education program. *Am Surg* 1989;55:563–565.
60. Kanter MH, van Maanen D, Anders KH, et al. Study of an educa-

tional intervention to decrease inappropriate preoperative autologous blood donation: its effectiveness and the effect on subsequent transfusion rates in elective hysterectomy. *Transfusion* 1999;39:801–807.
61. Soumerai SB, Salem-Schatz S, Avorn J. A controlled trial of educational outreach to improve blood transfusion practice. *JAMA* 1993; 270:961–966.
62. Toy PT, McVay PA, Strauss RG, et al. Improvement in appropriate autologous donations with local education: 1987 to 1989. *Transfusion* 1992;32:562–564.
63. Renner SW, Howanitz JH, Fishkin BG. Toward meaningful blood usage review: comprehensive monitoring of physician practice. *Qual Rev Bull* 1987;13:76–80.
64. Shanberge JN. Reduction of fresh-frozen plasma use through a daily survey and education program. *Transfusion* 1987;27:226–227.
65. Giovanetti AM, Parravicini A, Baroni L et al. Quality assessment of transfusion practice in elective surgery. *Transfusion* 1988;28: 166–169.
66. Silver H, Tahhan HR, Anderson J, et al. A non-computer-dependent prospective review of blood and blood component utilization. *Transfusion* 1992;32:260–265.
67. Simpson MB. Prospective-concurrent audits and medical consultation for platelet transfusions. *Transfusion* 1987;27:192–195.
68. McCullough J, Steeper TA, Connelly DP et al. Platelet utilization in a university hospital. *JAMA* 1988;259:2414–2418.
69. Hawkins TE, Carter JM, Hunter PM. Can mandatory pretransfusion approval programmes be improved? *Transfus Med* 1994;4:45–50.
70. Lepage EF, Gardner RM, Laub RM, et al. Improving blood transfusion practice: role of a computerized hospital information system. *Transfusion* 1992;32:253–259.
71. Cheng G, Wong HF, Chan A, et al. The effects of a self-educating blood component request form and enforcements of transfusion guidelines on FFP and platelet usage. *Clin Lab Haematol* 1996;18: 83–87.
72. Tuckfield A, Haeusler MN, Grigg AP, et al. Reduction of inappropriate use of blood products by prospective monitoring of transfusion request forms. *Med J Aust* 1997;167:473–476.
73. Despotis RE, Grishaber JE, Goodnough LT. The effect of an intraoperative treatment algorithm on physician's transfusion practice in cardiac surgery. *Transfusion* 1994;34:290–296.
74. Lichtiger B, Fischer HE, Huh YO. Screening of transfusion service requests by the blood bank pathologist: impact on cost containment. *Lab Med* 1988;19:228–230.
75. Solomon RR, Clifford JS, Gutman SI. The use of laboratory intervention to stem the flow of fresh-frozen plasma. *Am J Clin Pathol* 1988; 89:518–521.
76. Rosen NR, Bates LH, Herod G. Transfusion therapy: improved patient care and resource utilization. *Transfusion* 1993;33:341–347.
77. Shulman IA, Lohr K, Derdiarian AK. Monitoring transfusionist practices: a strategy for improving transfusion safety. *Transfusion* 1994; 34:11–15.
78. Salem-Schatz SR, Avorn J, Soumerai SB. Influence of clinical knowledge, organizational context, and practice style on transfusion decision making: implications for practice change strategies. *JAMA* 1990;265: 476–483.
79. Toy PT. Effectiveness of transfusion audits and practice guidelines. *Arch Pathol Lab Med* 1994;118:435–437.
80. Maxwell JA, Sandlow LJ, Bashook PG. Effect of a medical care evaluation program on physician knowledge and performance. *J Med Educ* 1984;59:33–38.
81. Sandlow LJ, Bashook PG, Maxwell JA. Medical care evaluation: an experience in continuing education. *J Med Educ* 1981;56:580–586.
82. Bashook PG, Maxwell JA, Sandlow LJ. Increasing the educational value of medical care evaluation: a model program. *J Med Educ* 1982; 57:701–707.
83. Chapman RG. The role of the community blood center in improving transfusion practice. In: Wallas CH, Muller VH, eds. *The hospital transfusion committee.* Bethesda, MD:American Association of Blood Banks, 1982:87–94.
84. Mair B, Agosti SJ, Foulis PR, et al. Monitoring for undertransfusion. *Transfusion* 1996;36:533–535.
85. Hogue Jr CW, Goodnough LT, Monk TG. Perioperative myocardial ischemic episodes are related to hematocrit level in patients undergoing radical prostatectomy. *Transfusion* 1998;38:924–931.
86. Mintz PD. Undertransfusion [Editorial]. *Am J Clin Pathol* 1992;98: 150–151.
87. Bergin JJ. The composition and function of the hospital transfusion committee: historical perspective. In: Wallas CH, Muller VH, eds. *The hospital transfusion committee.* Bethesda, MD:American Association of Blood Banks, 1982:7–13.
88. Silberstein LE, Kruskall MS, Stehling LC, et al. Strategies for the review of transfusion practices. *JAMA* 1989;262:1993–1997.
89. Stehling L, Luban NLC, Anderson KC, et al. Guidelines for blood utilization and review. *Transfusion* 1994;34:438–448.
90. Blanchette VS, Hume HA, Levy GJ, et al. Guidelines for auditing pediatric blood transfusion practices. *Am J Dis Child* 1991;145: 787–796.
91. *Guidelines for conducting pediatric transfusion audits,* 3rd ed. Bethesda, MD: American Association of Blood Banks, 1992.
92. Epstein BH, Kaufman A. Hospital peer review: a new proposal. *JAMA* 1994;271:1485.
93. Goodnough LT, Verbrugge D, Vizmeg K, et al. Identifying elective orthopedic surgical patients transfused with amounts of blood in excess of need: the transfusion trigger revisited. *Transfusion* 1992;32: 648–653.
94. Goodnough LT, Vizmeg K, Riddell IV J, et al. Discharge haematocrit as clinical indicator for blood transfusion audit in surgery patients. *Transfus Med* 1994;4:35–44.
95. Devine P, McClure PL. Quality assurance of hospital transfusion practices: the role of nursing staff. *Qual Rev Bull* 1988;14:250–253.
96. Boone DJ, Steindel D, Herron R, et al. Transfusion medicine monitoring practices: a study of the College of American Pathologists/ Centers for Disease Control and Prevention Outcomes Working Group. *Arch Pathol Lab Med* 1995;119–1006.
97. Allison MJ, Toy P. A quality improvement team on autologous and directed-donor blood availability. *Jt Comm J Qual Improv* 1996;22: 801–810.
98. Gillham M, Mark A. A retrospective audit of blood loss in total hip joint replacement surgery at Middlemore Hospital. *N Z Med J* 1997; 110:294–297.
99. Andet AM, Goodnough LT. Determining transfusion appropriateness: limitations of the medical chart audit. *Clin Res* 1993;41:352A.
100. Tartter PI, Barron DM. Unnecessary blood transfusions in elective colorectal cancer surgery. *Transfusion* 1985;25:113–115.
101. Murphy WG, Phillips P, Gray A, et al. Blood use for surgical patients: a study of Scottish hospital transfusion practices. *J R Coll Surg Edinb* 1995;40:10–13.
102. Clark JA, Ayoub MM. Blood and component wastage report: a quality assurance function of the hospital transfusion committee. *Transfusion* 1989;29:139–142.

Rossi's Principles of Transfusion Medicine, Third Edition, edited by Toby L. Simon, Walter H. Dzik, Edward L. Snyder, Christopher P. Stowell, and Ronald G. Strauss. Lippincott Williams & Wilkins, Philadelphia © 2002.

INDEX

Page numbers followed by "f" indicate figures, and those followed by "t" indicate tables

B

C

D

E

H

I

J

K

M

P

S